Associate Editors

Merrill S. Kies, M.D.

Professor of Medicine
Department of Thoracic/Head and Neck Medical Oncology
University of Texas MD Anderson Cancer Center
Houston, Texas

Jesus E. Medina, M.D., F.A.C.S.

Paul and Ruth Jonas Professor and Chairman
Department of Otorhinolaryngology
The University of Oklahoma Health Sciences Center
Oklahoma City, Oklahoma

William M. Mendenhall, M.D.

Professor
Department of Radiation Oncology
University of Florida
Shands Hospital
Gainesville, Florida

Suresh K. Mukherji, M.D.

Chief of Neuroradiology and Head and Neck Radiology
Fellowship Program Director
Department of Radiology
Associate Professor of Radiology and Otolaryngology—Head and Neck Surgery
University of Michigan Health System
Ann Arbor, Michigan

Bernard B. O'Malley, M.D.

Attending Radiologist
Princeton Medical Center
Princeton, New Jersey

Bruce M. Wenig, M.D.

Professor of Pathology
Albert Einstein College of Medicine
Vice-Chairman for Anatomic Pathology
Department of Pathology and Laboratory Medicine
Beth Israel Medical Center and St. Luke's-Roosevelt Hospitals
New York, New York

Head and Neck Cancer

A Multidisciplinary Approach

Second Edition

Head and Neck Cancer

A Multidisciplinary Approach

Second Edition

Editors

Louis B. Harrison, M.D.
Clinical Director, Continuum Cancer Centers of New York
Chairman of Radiation Oncology, Beth Israel Medical Center and
St. Luke's Roosevelt Hospital Center
Co-Director, Institute for Head and Neck Cancer
Professor of Radiation Oncology, Albert Einstein College of Medicine
New York, New York

Roy B. Sessions, M.D., F.A.C.S.
Chairman, Department of Otolaryngology—Head and Neck Surgery
Co-Director, Institute for Head and Neck Cancer, Beth Israel Medical Center
Associate Director, Continuum Cancer Centers of New York
Professor of Otolaryngology—Head and Neck Surgery
Albert Einstein College of Medicine
New York, New York
Adjunct Professor, Department of Otolaryngology—Head and Neck Surgery
Georgetown University School of Medicine
Washington, DC

Waun Ki Hong, M.D.
American Cancer Society Professor
Samsung Distinguished University Chair in Cancer Medicine
Head, Division of Cancer Medicine
Professor and Chair, Department of Thoracic/Head and Neck Medical Oncology
University of Texas MD Anderson Cancer Center
Houston, Texas

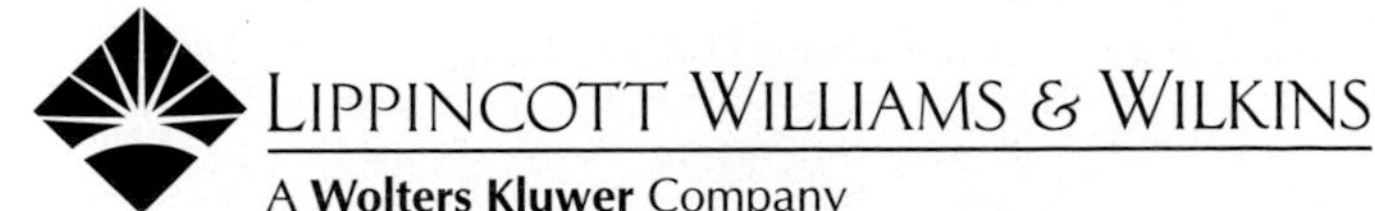

LIPPINCOTT WILLIAMS & WILKINS
A **Wolters Kluwer** Company
Philadelphia • Baltimore • New York • London
Buenos Aires • Hong Kong • Sydney • Tokyo

Acquisitions Editor: Jonathan Pine
Developmental Editor: Keith Donnellan
Project Editor: Sheila Higgins
Manufacturing Manager: Colin Warnock
Cover Designer: Christine Jenny
Compositor: Lippincott Williams & Wilkins Desktop Division
Printer: Maple Press

530 Walnut Street
Philadelphia, PA 19106 USA
LWW.com

Printed in the USA

First Edition published in 1998.

Library of Congress Cataloging-in-Publication Data

Head and neck cancer : a multidisciplinary approach / editors, Louis B. Harrison, Roy B. Sessions, Waun Ki Hong ; associate editors, William Mendenhall ... [et a.]. — 2nd ed.
p. ; cm.
Includes bibliographical references and index.
ISBN 0-7817-3369-3
1. Head—Cancer. 2. Neck—Cancer. I. Harrison, Louis B. II Sessions, Roy B. Hong, Waun Ki.
[DNLM: 1. Head and Neck Neoplasms—therapy. 2. Head and Neck Neoplasms—pathology. WE 707 H431724 2004]
RC280.H4H3845 2004
616.99'491—dc21 2003047507

---

10 9 8 7 6 5 4 3 2 1

To my mother and father, Lillian and Seymour Harrison, who have been outstanding parents, teachers, and friends. My respect and love for them, and my appreciation for all that they have done for me is unsurpassed.

L.B.H.

I dedicate this book to two groups: my cancer patients who have provided me with a bountiful harvest of gratification and the members of my family who have made innumerable sacrifices so that I might pursue my goals that, no matter how altruistic, have compromised their life-styles. My ever-supportive wife, Mary, and my children, Katharine, Elizabeth, Abigail, and Matthew, have provided a wonderful environment for my life beyond medicine. How fortunate I am for having shared all of this with courageous patients and with a wonderful family.

R.B.S.

I dedicate this book to my late brother, Dr. Suk Ki Hong, who was a Distinguished Professor at the State University of New York at Buffalo. He was my role model and the greatest inspiration for my entire academic career. In addition, I would like to express my deep appreciation to my wife, Mihwa, and our sons, Edward and Burton, for their unwavering support and encouragement.

W.K.H.

Contents

Part III. Basic Science and Pathology of Head and Neck Cancer

Contributing Authors

Nathalie Audet, M.D.
University of Toronto
Toronto, Ontario, Canada

Alejandro Berenstein, M.D.
Professor of Radiology, Neurology, and Neurosurgery
Albert Einstein College of Medicine
Director, Institute of Neurology and Neurosurgery
Director, Center for Endovascular Surgery
Beth Israel Medical Center
New York, New York

Luther W. Brady, M.D.
Distinguished University Professor
Hylda Cohn/American Cancer Society Professor of Clinical Oncology
Department of Radiation Oncology
Drexel University College of Medicine
Professor
Department of Radiation Oncology
MCP-Hahnemann University Hospital
Philadelphia, Pennsylvania

Randall L. Breau, M.D.
Associate Professor
Attending Surgeon
Department of Otolaryngology—Head and Neck Surgery
University of Arkansas for Medical Sciences
Little Rock, Arkansas

Ali W. Bseiso, M.D.
Department of Medical Oncology
The Marshfield Clinic
Marshfield, Wisconsin

Kenneth D. Burman, M.D.
Professor
Department of Medicine
The Uniformed Services University of the Health Sciences
Bethesda, Maryland
Clinical Professor
Departments of Medicine
Georgetown and George Washington Universities
Chief, Endocrine Section
Washington Hospital Center
Washington, DC

Robert M. Byers, M.D.
Professor
Department of Head and Neck Surgery
University of Texas MD Anderson Cancer Center
Houston, Texas

Joseph A. Califano III, M.D.
Assistant Professor
Department of Otolaryngology—Head and Neck Surgery
Johns Hopkins Medical Institutions
Baltimore, Maryland

John F. Carew, M.D.
Department of Otolaryngology
New York Presbyterian Hospital
New York, New York

Elise Carper, R.N., M.A., A.P.R.N., A.O.C.N.
Director of Nursing and Adult Nurse Practitioner
Department of Radiation Oncology
Beth Israel Medical Center
St. Luke's Roosevelt Hospital Center
New York, New York

Charles N. Catton, M.D.
Assistant Professor
Department of Radiation Oncology
University of Toronto
Staff Radiation Oncologist
Department of Radiation Oncology
Princess Margaret Hospital
Toronto, Ontario
Canada

Mark S. Chambers, D.M.D., M.S.
Associate Professor
Head and Neck Surgery
Department of Radiation Oncology
University of Texas MD Anderson Cancer Center
Houston, Texas

Gary L. Clayman, D.D.S., M.D., F.A.C.S.
Professor and Deputy Chairman
Department of Head and Neck Surgery
University of Texas MD Anderson Cancer Center
Houston, Texas

Jean-Marc Cohen, M.D.
Director of Cytopathology
Department of Pathology and Laboratory Medicine
Phillips Ambulatory Cancer Center
Beth Israel Medical Center PACC
New York, New York

June Corry, M.B.B.S., F.R.A.C.P., F.R.A.N.Z.C.R.
Senior Fellow
Department of Medicine
Melbourne University
Head, Head and Neck Unit
Department of Radiation Oncology
Peter MacCallum Cancer Institute
East Melbourne, Victoria
Australia

Peter D. Costantino, M.D.
Vice-Chairman and Co-Director
Center for Cranial Base Surgery
Department of Otolaryngology
St. Luke's-Roosevelt Hospital Center
Associate Professor
Department of Otolaryngology
Columbia University College of Physicians and Surgeons
New York, New York

Bruce Culliney, M.D.
Division of Hematology Oncology
Department of Medical Oncology
Beth Israel Medical Center
New York, New York

Bruce J. Davidson, M.D., F.A.C.S.
Professor and Chairman
Department of Otolaryngology—Head and Neck Surgery
Georgetown University Hospital
Washington, DC

Christopher M. DeBacker, M.D.
Volunteer Faculty
Department of Ophthalmology
California Pacific Medical Center
Staff Surgeon
Department of Ophthalmology and Plastic Surgery
St. Rose Hospital
San Francisco, California

Mark D. DeLacure, M.D.
Associate Professor
Department of Otolaryngology and Surgery (Plastic Surgery)
Chief, Division of Head and Neck Surgery and Oncology
New York University School of Medicine
New York, New York

Adam P. Dicker, M.D., Ph.D.
Associate Professor
Department of Radiation Oncology
Bodine Center for Cancer Treatment
Director, Clinical Research
Director, Division of Experimental Radiation Oncology
Thomas Jefferson University
Philadelphia, Pennsylvania

Jonathan J. Dutton, M.D., Ph.D.
Professor
Department of Ophthalmology
University of North Carolina at Chapel Hill
Chapel Hill, North Carolina

Avraham Eisbruch, M.D.
Associate Professor
Department of Radiation Oncology
University of Michigan
Associate Chairman
Department of Radiation Oncology
University of Michigan Hospital
Ann Arbor, Michigan

David W. Eisele, M.D., F.A.C.S.
Professor and Chairman
Department of Otolaryngology—Head and Neck Surgery
University of California, San Francisco
Attending Surgeon
Division of Head and Neck Surgery
U.C.S.F. Comprehensive Cancer Center
San Francisco, California

Stewart B. Fleishman, M.D.
Associate Clinical Professor
Department of Psychiatry
Albert Einstein College of Medicine
Bronx, New York
Director, Cancer Supportive Services
Beth Israel Medical Center/St. Luke's-Roosevelt Hospital Center
Continuum Cancer Centers of New York
New York, New York

Jorge E. Freire, M.D.
Assistant Professor
Department of Radiation Oncology
Hahnemann University Hospital
Philadelphia, Pennsylvania

Douglas K. Frank, M.D.
Assistant Professor of Otolaryngology—Head and Neck Surgery
Albert Einstein College of Medicine
Attending Surgeon
Department of Otolaryngology—Head and Neck Surgery
Institute for Head and Neck Cancer
Beth Israel Medical Center
New York, New York

Adam S. Garden, M.D.
Associate Professor
Department of Radiation Oncology
University of Texas MD Anderson Cancer Center
Houston, Texas

Gregg S. Gayre, M.D.
Assistant Professor
Department of Ophthalmology
University of North Carolina
Chapel Hill, North Carolina
Director of Aesthetic Services
Atlantic Eye and Face Center, PLLC
Cary, North Carolina

Ann M. Gillenwater, M.D.
Associate Professor and Associate Surgeon
Division of Surgery and Anesthesiology
Department of Head and Neck Surgery
University of Texas MD Anderson Cancer Center
Clinical Assistant Professor
Department of Otolaryngology
Baylor College of Medicine
Houston, Texas

Patrick J. Gullane, M.B., F.R.C.S., F.A.C.S.
Professor and Chair
Department of Otolaryngology
University of Toronto
Wharton Chair
Department of Head and Neck Surgery
Princess Margaret Hospital
Toronto, Ontario
Canada

Bruce G. Haffty, M.D.
Professor
Department of Therapeutic Radiology
Yale University School of Medicine
Vice Chair
Department of Therapeutic Radiology
Yale—New Haven Hospital
New Haven, Connecticut

Paul M. Harari, M.D.
Associate Professor
Department of Human Oncology
University of Wisconsin-Madison
Madison, Wisconsin

Louis B. Harrison, M.D.
Clinical Director
Continuum Cancer Centers of New York
Chairman of Radiation Oncology
Beth Israel Medical Center and St. Luke's Roosevelt Hospital Center
Co-Director, Institute for Head and Neck Cancer
Professor of Radiation Oncology
Albert Einstein College of Medicine
New York, New York

K. William Harter, M.D.
Professor and Vice-Chair
Department of Radiation Oncology
Georgetown University Medical Center/Lombardi Cancer Center
Washington, DC

Roy S. Herbst, M.D., Ph.D.
Associate Professor of Medicine
Associate Professor of Cancer Biology
Department of Thoracic/Head and Neck Medical Oncology
Chief, Section of Thoracic Oncology
University of Texas MD Anderson Cancer Center
Houston, Texas

F. Christopher Holsinger, M.D.
Assistant Professor
Department of Head and Neck Surgery
University of Texas MD Anderson Cancer Center
Houston, Texas

Waun Ki Hong, M.D.
American Cancer Society Professor
Samsung Distinguished University Chair in Cancer Medicine
Head, Division of Cancer Medicine
Professor and Chair
Department of Thoracic/Head and Neck Medical Oncology
University of Texas MD Anderson Cancer Center
Houston, Texas

John R. Houck, Jr., M.D.
Associate Professor
Department of Otorhinolaryngology
University of Oklahoma Health Sciences Center
Oklahoma City, Oklahoma

Kenneth S. Hu, M.D.
Assistant Professor
Department of Radiation Oncology
Albert Einstein College of Medicine
Attending Physician
Department of Radiation Oncology
Beth Israel Medical Center
New York, New York

Shyh-Min Huang, Ph.D.
Assistant Scientist
Department of Human Oncology
University of Wisconsin-Madison
Madison, Wisconsin

Ivo P. Janecka, M.D., M.B.A., F.A.C.S.
Professor of Surgery
Longwood Skull Base Program
Departments of Otolaryngology, Neurosurgery, and Plastic Surgery
Harvard Medical School
Boston, Massachusetts

Silloo B. Kapadia, M.D.
Professor
Department of Pathology
Penn State College of Medicine
Director, Surgical Pathology
Department of Anatomic Pathology
Penn State Milton S. Hershey Medical Center
Hershey, Pennsylvania

Merrill S. Kies, M.D.
Professor of Medicine
Department of Thoracic/Head and Neck Medical Oncology
University of Texas MD Anderson Cancer Center
Houston, Texas

Lawrence R. Kleinberg, M.D.
Assistant Professor of Oncology
Assistant Professor of Neurological Surgery
Johns Hopkins University School of Medicine
Baltimore, Maryland

Lydia T. Komarnicky, M.D.
Department of Radiation Oncology
MCP-Hahnemann University Hospital
Philadelphia, Pennsylvania

Janet I. Lee, M.D.
Resident
Department of Otolaryngology—Head and Neck Surgery
Baylor College of Medicine
Houston, Texas

Jean-Louis Lefebvre, M.D.
Professor, ENT and Head and Neck Surgery
Chief, Head and Neck Department
Centre Oscar Lambret
Lille, France

James C. Lemon, D.D.S.
Professor
Head and Neck Surgery
University of Texas MD Anderson Cancer Center
Houston, Texas

Eric J. Lentsch, M.D.
Assistant Professor
Department of Otolaryngology—Head and Neck Surgery
University of Louisville
Louisville, Kentucky

Charles Lu, M.D., S.M.
Assistant Professor of Medicine
Department of Thoracic/Head and Neck Medical Oncology
University of Texas MD Anderson Cancer Center
Houston, Texas

Anthony A. Mancuso, M.D.
Professor and Chairman
Department of Diagnostic Radiology
University of Florida College of Medicine
Gainesville, Florida

Jack W. Martin, D.D.S., M.S.
Professor
Chief, Section of Oncologic Dentistry
Department of Head and Neck Surgery
University of Texas MD Anderson Cancer Center
Houston, Texas

Marlene McGuire, R.N., M.A., N.P.C.
Department of Surgical Oncology
Cancer Institute of New Jersey
New Brunswick, New Jersey

Jesus E. Medina, M.D., F.A.C.S.
Paul and Ruth Jonas Professor and Chairman
Department of Otorhinolaryngology
The University of Oklahoma Health Sciences Center
Oklahoma City, Oklahoma

William M. Mendenhall, M.D.
Professor
Department of Radiation Oncology
University of Florida
Shands Hospital
Gainesville, Florida

Susan D. Miller, Ph.D.
Assistant Professor
Department of Otolaryngology—Head and Neck Surgery
Georgetown University Hospital
Washington, DC

Jason A. Moche, M.D.
Mt. Sinai Hospital
New York, New York

David A. Moffat, B.Sc., M.A., M.B.B.S., F.R.C.S.
Consultant in Otoneurological and Skull Base Surgery
Associate Lecturer
Department of Otolaryngology
University of Cambridge
Addenbrooke's-Cambridge University Hospital
Cambridge, United Kingdom

Suresh K. Mukherji, M.D.
Chief of Neuroradiology and Head and Neck Radiology
Fellowship Program Director
Department of Radiology
Associate Professor of Radiology and Otolaryngology—Head and Neck Surgery
University of Michigan Health System
Ann Arbor, Michigan

Mark R. Murphy, M.D.
Postdoctoral Residency Fellow
Department of Otolaryngology—Head and Neck Surgery
Columbia University
New York, New York

Jeffrey N. Myers, M.D., Ph.D., F.A.C.S.
Associate Professor
Surgeon
Department of Head and Neck Surgery
University of Texas MD Anderson Cancer Center
Houston, Texas

Bernard B. O'Malley, M.D.
Attending Radiologist
Princeton Medical Center
Princeton, New Jersey

Brian O'Sullivan
Professor
Department of Radiation Oncology
University of Toronto
Associate Director
Department of Radiation Oncology
Princess Margaret Hospital
Toronto, Ontario
Canada

Vassiliki A. Papadimitrakopoulou, M.D.
Associate Professor
Department of Thoracic/Head and Neck Medical Oncology
University of Texas MD Anderson Cancer Center
Houston, Texas

James T. Parsons, M.D.
Department of Radiation Oncology
Bethesda Memorial Hospital
Boynton Beach, Florida

Edmund D. Pellegrino, M.D.
Professor Emeritus of Medicine and Medical Ethics
Center for Clinical Bioethics
Department of Medicine
Georgetown University Medical Center
Washington, DC

Mark S. Persky, M.D.
Professor of Clinical Otolaryngology
Department of Otolaryngology
Albert Einstein College of Medicine
Bronx, New York
Vice-Chairman
Department of Otolaryngology—Head and Neck Surgery
Beth Israel Medical Center
New York, New York

Lester J. Peters, M.D.
Professor
Department of Pathology
University of Melbourne
Melbourne, Victoria
Australia
Director, Division of Radiation Oncology
Peter MacCallum Cancer Institute
East Melbourne, Victoria
Australia

David G. Pfister, M.D.
Associate Professor
Department of Medicine
Weill Medical College of Cornell University
Associate Member and Associate Attending Physician
Co-Leader, Head and Neck Cancer Disease Management Team
Department of Medicine
Memorial Sloan-Kettering Cancer Center
New York, New York

Russell K. Portenoy, M.D.
Professor
Department of Neurology
Albert Einstein College of Medicine
Bronx, New York
Chairman
Department of Pain Medicine and Palliative Care
Beth Israel Medical Center
New York, New York

Sanjay Prasad, M.D.
Department of Otolaryngology-Head and Neck Surgery
Georgetown University Medical Center
Washington, DC
Ear and Skull Base Associates
Rockville, Maryland

Julian J. Pribaz, M.D., M.B.B.S.
Professor of Surgery
Division of Plastic Surgery
Harvard University
Program Director
Harvard Plastic Surgery
Brigham & Women's Hospital
Boston, Massachusetts

Harry Quon, M.D., F.R.C.P.C.
Department of Radiation Oncology
Continuum Cancer Centers
Beth Israel Medical Center
St. Luke's-Roosevelt Hospital Center
New York, New York

John A. Ridge, M.D., Ph.D., F.A.C.S.
Associate Professor
Department of Otolaryngology and Bronchoesophagology
Temple University
Chief, Head and Neck Surgery
Fox Chase Cancer Center
Philadelphia, Pennsylvania

Danny Rischin, M.B.B.S., F.R.A.C.P.
Associate Professor
Department of Medicine
University of Melbourne
Head, Solid Tumor Developmental Therapeutics Program
Department of Medical Oncology
Peter MacCallum Cancer Institute
East Melbourne, Victoria
Australia

Geoffrey L. Robb, M.D., F.A.C.S.
Chairman and Professor
Department of Plastic Surgery
University of Texas MD Anderson Cancer Center
Houston, Texas

M. Alma Rodriguez, M.D., F.A.C.S.
Associate Professor
Ad-Interim Chair
Department of Lymphoma/Myeloma
University of Texas MD Anderson Cancer Center
Houston, Texas

Roy B. Sessions, M.D., F.A.C.S.
Chairman, Department of Otolaryngology—Head and Neck Surgery
Co-Director, Institute for Head and Neck Cancer
Beth Israel Medical Center
Associate Director
Continuum Cancer Centers of New York
Professor of Otolaryngology—Head and Neck Surgery
Albert Einstein College of Medicine
New York, New York
Adjunct Professor
Department of Otolaryngology—Head and Neck Surgery
Georgetown University School of Medicine
Washington, DC

Jatin P. Shah, M.D., F.A.C.S.
Professor of Surgery
Weill Medical College of Cornell University
Chief, Head and Neck Service
Elliot W. Strong Chair in Head and Neck Oncology
Department of Surgery
Memorial Sloan-Kettering Cancer Center
New York, New York

Ashok R. Shaha, M.D., F.A.C.S.
Professor of Surgery
Cornell University Medical Center
Attending Surgeon
Department of Surgery
Memorial Sloan-Kettering Cancer Center
New York, New York

Carol L. Shields, M.D.
Attending Surgeon
Ocular Oncology Service
Wills Eye Hospital
Philadelphia, Pennsylvania

Jerry A. Shields, M.D.
Professor
Department of Ophthalmology
Thomas Jefferson University
Director, Oncology Service
Wills Eye Hospital
Philadelphia, Pennsylvania

Dong M. Shin, M.D.
Professor of Medicine and Otolaryngology
Division of Hematology/Oncology
University of Pittsburgh Cancer Institute
Shadyside Hospital
Pittsburgh, Pennsylvania

David Sidransky, M.D.
Professor and Director
Head and Neck Cancer Research Division
Johns Hopkins University School of Medicine
Baltimore, Maryland

Benjamin D. Smith, M.D.
Resident
Department of Therapeutic Radiology
Yale University School of Medicine
Yale-New Haven Hospital
New Haven, Connecticut

Kevin T. Sperber, M.D.
Instructor
Department of Neurology
New York University School of Medicine
Director of Inpatient Services
Comprehensive Pain Treatment Center
Hospital for Joint Diseases
New York, New York

Margaret R. Spitz, M.D.
Professor and Chair
Department of Epidemiology
University of Texas MD Anderson Cancer Center
Houston, Texas

Bettie M. Steinberg, Ph.D.
Professor
Departments of Otolaryngology and Microbiology & Immunology
Albert Einstein College of Medicine
Bronx, New York
Chief, Division of Research
Department of Otolaryngology
Long Island Jewish Medical Center
New Hyde Park, New York

Erich M. Sturgis, M.D.
Assistant Professor
Department of Head and Neck Surgery
Department of Epidemiology
University of Texas MD Anderson Cancer Center
Houston, Texas

Lucian Sulica, M.D.
Assistant Professor
Department of Otolaryngology
New York Medical College
Valhalla, New York
Assistant Clinical Professor
Department of Otolaryngology
Albert Einstein College of Medicine
Bronx, New York
Director, Center for the Voice
Department of Otolaryngology
Beth Israel Medical Center
The New York Eye & Ear Infirmary
New York, New York

Michael H. Torosian, M.D.
Associate Professor
Department of Surgery
Temple University School of Medicine
Attending Surgeon
Department of Surgical Oncology
Fox Chase Cancer Center
Philadelphia, Pennsylvania

Randal S. Weber, M.D.
Department of Otorhinolaryngology—Head and Neck Surgery
University of Pennsylvania Health System
Philadelphia, Pennsylvania

Qingyi Wei, M.D., Ph.D.
Associate Professor
Department of Epidemiology
University of Texas MD Anderson Cancer Center
Houston, Texas

Bruce M. Wenig, M.D.
Professor of Pathology
Albert Einstein College of Medicine
Vice-Chairman for Anatomic Pathology
Department of Pathology and Laboratory Medicine
Beth Israel Medical Center and St. Luke's-Roosevelt Hospitals
New York, New York

Michael J. Zelefsky, M.D.
Associate Professor
Chief, Brachytherapy Service
Department of Radiation Oncology
Memorial Sloan-Kettering Cancer Center
New York, New York

Preface

The major goal in developing the first edition, *Head and Neck Cancer: A Multidisciplinary Approach,* was to create a standard of literary excellence based on a model of multidisciplinary collaboration. We believed this search would be built on the philosophy that cancer treatment in general, and especially head and neck cancer treatment, involves a sophisticated understanding of a very complex area: the anatomy, physiology, and pathophysiology associated with cancers and cancer treatment. The extraordinary functions of seeing, speaking, swallowing, hearing, and smelling depend on a symphony of parts working together, and the anatomic or physiologic alteration of that rhythm generally has a visible and immediate impact on life. The effectiveness in management of head and neck cancer, therefore, involves a seamless collaboration among surgical, radiation, and medical oncologists, as well as dentists, pathologists, radiologists, nurses, rehabilitation experts, and others. More than ever before, the editors and contributors of this textbook are committed to applying a multidisciplinary approach to these diseases. Currently, the standard of care in head and neck cancer is best achieved by adherence to the concept of professional inclusion, rather than isolation; pretreatment strategic planning coming out of tumor board discussions, data- and stage-based decision making, and in-depth support system capabilities are all essential to that philosophy.

Creating a standard that will span the generations is an ambitious endeavor, and should, it would seem, require a critical analysis of our initial effort, i.e., the first edition. We did just that, studying carefully from beginning to end the content of the first edition for clarity, readability, and appeal to the intended audience. Its substance and scientific endurance were scrutinized relative to these dynamic times. Data were changed when indicated, and we altered the first edition by eliminating or supplementing certain sections. We sought the critiques of many, listening and responding as objectively as possible. Therefore, we believe this second edition is a new book, rather than merely a revision of the first edition. Throughout the process of alteration, however, we have held true to the basic principles established for the first edition: the goal of head and neck oncologists should be to maximize the chance for cure while maintaining a strong emphasis on the individual's quality of life. Curing the cancer at any cost—i.e., returning the patient to society, cured but incapacitated—is no longer an accepted strategy and should be continually challenged. Strategies of organ preservation and function are, therefore, explored and emphasized throughout the text.

As a means of enhancing the standardization of treatment strategy development, we have added treatment algorithms to most site-specific chapters. In addition, much technical methodology in both radiation and surgery has been included in this edition, and discussion of diagnostic radiology has been increased substantially. Modern imaging is so integral to what is currently done that it is important for the oncologist to pay particular attention to this section.

Throughout this new edition, we have continued to emphasize scholarship, asking "why" as often as "how to." Finally, this edition reflects an added emphasis on translational research.

We have been delighted by the success of the first edition and that it won the prestigious Doody Award for Scientific Textbook in 2000. The development of this second edition has been done in an attempt to improve on the standard set by the first.

It has been especially gratifying to witness the coming together of this diverse group of authors. A majority of the contributors are preeminent in their particular area of expertise, and the editors appreciate their allowance of the intrusion into their already heavily committed schedules. In large measure, writing for a textbook reflects a commitment to education and the betterment of humankind. For us to express our gratitude for their efforts, while intangible, is heartfelt. Finally, we share the hope that the readers of this book will be aided in the care for their patients.

Louis B. Harrison, M.D.
Roy B. Sessions, M.D., F.A.C.S.
Waun Ki Hong, M.D.

PART I

General Principles of Management of Head and Neck Cancer

CHAPTER 1

Physical Examination of the Head and Neck

Douglas K. Frank and Roy B. Sessions

Compared with other anatomic regions of the body, the head and neck provides the diagnostician a unique advantage. Most of the upper aerodigestive tract, as well as facial and cervical soft tissue structures can be directly inspected, palpated, and even biopsied in the office setting. For the patient with head and neck cancer, a diagnosis is frequently made that correlates symptoms and complaints with physical findings.

Because the physical examination is not foolproof in detection and staging, the head and neck oncologist must frequently combine the information obtained from the physical examination with radiographic evaluation. Thus, the combination of traditional "laying on of the hands" and contemporary technology leads to accurate assessment and appropriate therapy.

In this chapter, following a brief discussion of history taking in the patient with head and neck cancer, the fundamentals of the physical examination will be presented by anatomic subsite. The typical physical signs and symptoms of neoplastic disease at these various subsites will also be highlighted, along with the ancillary diagnostic techniques of endoscopy and biopsy where applicable. Because radiographic techniques serve to enhance our clinical capacities, the types of imaging modalities available, as well as the circumstances for their use, will be highlighted in a separate section.

HISTORY TAKING IN PATIENTS WITH HEAD AND NECK CANCER

Most patients with a head and neck neoplasm present to the oncologist with signs or symptoms referable to their lesion. Occasionally a patient will be referred with (or found to have) an asymptomatic lesion which has been discovered on a routine head and neck examination. Symptomatic patients should be questioned about the duration and intensity of their signs and symptoms. Progression of any signs or symptoms should be noted, as well as the impact they make on daily functionality and quality of life.

A history of malignancy or premalignancy, particularly of the head and neck, should be noted. The patient's prior treatment(s) can significantly impact on methods available to manage the current disease. This is particularly problematic in patients with squamous cell carcinoma (SCC) of the upper aerodigestive tract because these patients can present with recurrent disease or second primary tumors despite having received high doses of external beam radiation therapy (EBRT) and or surgery. In such circumstances, further surgery or EBRT may not be feasible for the patient's current tumor.

All patients should be questioned regarding tobacco and alcohol usage, which are the agents typically associated with SCC (1). It should be noted, however, that an increasing percentage of younger patients with SCC present without this typical social history. In such patients there is some evidence to suggest that viruses, such as the human papilloma virus, may be linked to disease development (2).

Patients with suspected cutaneous neoplasms should be questioned about sun exposure. Because thyroid tumors (3) and certain lymphoproliferative disorders (4) can be associated with an antecedent exposure to nontherapeutic ionizing radiation, a careful history about such exposure should be taken.

A careful medical history should address comorbid conditions such as cardiovascular disease, pulmonary disease, diabetes, and immunodeficiency disorders. These diseases have a profound effect on prognosis of tumors such as SCC (5). Finally, one must consider the relevance of the age of the individual presenting with a suspected head and neck neoplasm. Both the histology and the presentation of head and neck neoplasia in the pediatric patient are different than in the adult, and the age of the patient as well as site of presentation can give clues as to the diagnosis prior to biopsy.

EXAMINATION OF THE SKIN OF THE HEAD AND NECK

Fair-skinned individuals with a long history of sun exposure harbor the greatest risk for developing a cutaneous malignancy (6,7). Nonmelanoma skin cancers may present as ulcerated, raised, or dry scaly lesions that bleed easily with manipulation. Melanomas are frequently pigmented and develop from preexisting lesions. Color variegation, irregular borders, and sudden growth are highly suggestive that malignant melanoma exists in a pigmented lesion (7). In many instances, the patient has not noted a skin lesion because of its location in the hair-bearing scalp or posterior neck. Disease is often discovered by a spouse, hairdresser, or physician. Less common cutaneous tumors such as sarcomas and those of the adnexal structures may appear as subcutaneous or highly expansive masses on examination.

After an overview of facial and neck skin, careful attention is paid to the ears and scalp. Disease can be obscured by the hair, thus it is important to examine the hair-bearing scalp in an organized fashion. The use of a magnifying glass can assist with the evaluation of smaller cutaneous lesions. Small nodular basal cell carcinomas may have a pearly appearance with fine surface blood vessels that are not easily seen without magnification.

Biopsy of the Skin of the Head and Neck

Suspected nonmelanoma skin cancers, such as basal and squamous cell carcinomas, can be biopsied by one of several techniques. These include shave, punch, incisional, as well as excisional biopsy. Anatomic location may best dictate which technique is used. Less invasive techniques such as shave biopsy are often performed proximal to vital structures or in cosmetically important areas.

Controversy exists as to the best technique to biopsy a suspected melanoma. Some evidence suggests that punch and incisional biopsy for melanoma may adversely affect patient outcome (8), possibly through displacing malignant cells into deeper tissues. For this reason, when possible, an excisional biopsy is preferred. The biopsy technique is probably less important in massive invasive melanomas.

EXAMINATION OF FACIAL STRUCTURES AND THE EARS

The careful evaluation of facial structures is an important, yet often overlooked aspect of the head and neck examination. Although some patients demonstrate an obvious mass or asymmetry of the face or related structures, careful evaluation may reveal subtle structural or neurologic abnormalities not previously noted by the patient. Such findings in turn may give clues about disease in inaccessible areas such as the orbits and paranasal sinuses.

General facial and orbital symmetry should be documented. Even subtle cheek swelling can be seen with soft tissue mesenchymal neoplasms, as well as paranasal sinus and oral cavity tumors that have ruptured through or distorted the facial bones. Pain and tenderness often accompany such swelling, but many patients are pain-free. Masses that present in this manner should be assessed for ulceration and skin fixation, as well as fixation to underlying structures. Attention should also be paid to decreased sensation (to light touch and pin prick) along the entire distribution of the trigeminal nerve. Both sensory and trigeminal motor abnormalities may suggest direct neural invasion at the site of known gross tumor (e.g., paranasal sinuses, orbit, oral cavity, skull base), or retrograde involvement of the nerve in the Meckel's cave. This latter scenario is occasionally encountered with neurotropic tumors such as adenoid cystic carcinoma (9), desmoplastic melanoma (10), and other lesions with an atypical neurotropic phenotype.

Facial asymmetries or masses may represent lymphatic or vascular malformations, and while they are not neoplasms, the manner in which they present must be understood so they can be distinguished from tumors. Lymphatic and vascular lesions frequently present in the perioral and periorbital regions. These types of lesions, particularly lymphatic malformations, can be quite extensive and extend to, or originate in, the neck. Obvious physical differences can be noted between lymphatic and vascular malformations. The former frequently do not present with overlying skin change and they are not usually compressible. The latter come in several varieties that can usually be distinguished based on physical examination characteristics. Low-flow vascular lesions can be distinguished from their high-flow counterparts by examination and by history (11,12).

Proptosis, often accompanied by diplopia or blurred vision, is a common finding with tumors that involve and distort intraorbital structures. There are a wide variety of such lesions that can involve the orbit and related structures. These can include lymphomas and pseudotumors, as well as epithelial lesions of intraorbital and surrounding cutaneous and adnexal structures. Paranasal sinus tumors, by direct extension, can also distort orbital structures. Limitation of extraocular movements and vision is frequently caused by the mass effect of tumors involving intraorbital structures. It should be kept in mind, however, that isolated abnormalities of either the third, fourth, or sixth cranial nerves (even without other orbital findings) can represent tumor infiltration into the cavernous sinus from an external skull base or intracranial site of primary disease. Such tumors can also create facial numbness by selectively affecting branches of the fifth cranial nerve.

Examination of the ear canal can be initially carried out with a handheld otoscope. Inspection of the canal skin and tympanic membrane is made. A discharge may conceal an underlying ear canal or middle ear tumor. An unresolving aural discharge, despite appropriate treatment, should be suctioned clear under binocular vision so that adequate assessment of the area can be made. This might even require general anesthesia. Cancer of the ear canal can be a deceiving problem. Pain accompanying a chronic aural discharge (especially bloody) is particularly worrisome for the presence of a neoplasm. A facial palsy, particularly one of gradual onset, may also be an indication of neoplastic disease in the middle ear and mastoid region (13). The nerve typically becomes involved by direct extension under these circumstances, either in its horizontal middle ear segment or vertical mastoid segment.

The first presenting sign of a nasopharyngeal cancer may be hearing loss and a sense of aural fullness secondary to eustachian tube obstruction and subsequent serous or acute otitis media (14). This disease should be ruled out in any adult patient with an unexplained middle ear inflammatory process detected on routine otoscopy (see "Examination of the Upper Aerodigestive Tract" later in the chapter). This is particularly the case in patients of Southeast Asian ancestry, where nasopharyngeal carcinoma is endemic (15). In adults in general, unilaterality of ear symptoms (infection, fullness, pain) should alert the physician to the possibility of malignancy.

Biopsy of Facial Structures and the Ears

Tumors of these areas can be sampled by transcutaneous fine-needle aspiration (FNA). This is a highly sensitive technique, particularly when interpreted by an experienced cytopathologist (16). When more tissue is required for diagnostic purposes, a more invasive biopsy technique of the underlying structures giving rise to the mass (e.g., paranasal sinuses) may be required using endoscopic instruments (see the following section, "Examination of the Upper Aerodigestive Tract"). Neoplasms presenting as intraorbital masses can also be biopsied with FNA. The FNA technique using ultrasound or computed tomography (CT) scan image guidance may be needed for deeper orbital neoplasms that cannot be directly visualized or palpated.

Neoplasms of the ear canal and middle ear structures are best biopsied with the small cup forceps biopsy technique. Although topical local anesthetic is often adequate for ear canal biopsy, general anesthesia may be required to adequately manipulate a tumor presenting in the middle ear.

EXAMINATION OF THE UPPER AERODIGESTIVE TRACT

The anatomic regions of the upper aerodigestive tract include the nasal cavity and paranasal sinuses, oral cavity, oropharynx, nasopharynx, hypopharynx, and larynx. Examination of the nasal cavity and pharyngeal axis has been greatly enhanced over previous years by the development of rigid and flexible fiberoptic equipment for use in the office setting (Fig. 1.1). Distal pharyngolaryngeal biopsy is even possible through some flexible fiberoptic instruments.

Examination of the entire upper aerodigestive tract is initially carried out with standard techniques of direct and indirect (mirror) visualization techniques, as well as by manual palpation. A fiberoptic evaluation for suspicious distal nasal and pharyngolaryngeal areas otherwise inaccessible is done after the aforementioned initial examination.

Examination of the Nasal Cavity

The initial examination of the upper aerodigestive tract commences with direct visualization of the nasal cavity with a nasal speculum and headlight/headmirror. The nasal speculum examination generally only affords inspection of the anterior nasal cavity, including the anterior nasal septum, inferior turbinate, and nasal vestibule. Topical decongestant and anesthesia are sprayed into the nose to assist in this examination, although this is generally reserved for fiberoptic evaluation. The most common nasal cavity neoplasms are SCC, minor salivary gland cancers, papillomas, and olfactory neuroblastomas, as well as neoplasms that have extended directly from the ethmoid and maxillary sinuses.

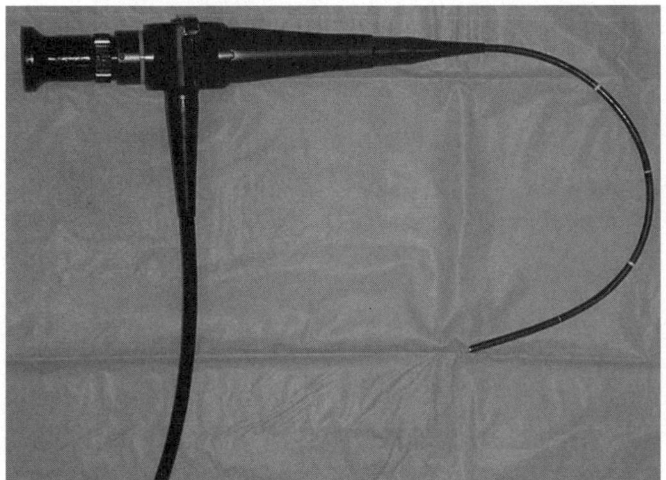

Figure 1.1 Standard flexible fiberoptic nasopharyngolaryngoscope used for upper aerodigestive tract evaluation in the office setting.

Tumor presence in the nasal cavity may be heralded by varying degrees of nasal obstruction, epistaxis, midfacial pain, midfacial mass, and even anosmia. Unexplained loss of smell, whether unilateral or bilateral, can be a presenting symptom of olfactory neuroblastomas (esthesioneuroblastomas) (17). Lesions eroding the anterior skull base can even present with the clear nasal discharge indicative of cerebrospinal fluid leak. Patients with any of these symptoms will need a fiberoptic examination (discussed later in the chapter) to assess disease extent and location, particularly when the tumor cannot be adequately seen through the anterior examination technique. Special mention should also be made of nasal obstruction and epistaxis as presenting signs in adolescent boys. Juvenile posterior nasal angiofibroma is unique to this category of patient and should be part of the differential diagnosis in this clinical situation (18).

Examination of the Oral Cavity

Examination of the anterior nasal cavity is followed by inspection of the oral cavity. This is best done with tongue blades, and a headlight/headmirror for illumination. The lips, buccal mucosa, and gingivobuccal sulci are inspected first. Any trismus is noted, and the patient's state of dentition evaluated. Next, the teeth and alveolar areas are examined, followed by the dorsal and ventral surfaces of the tongue, floor of mouth, and gingivolabial sulci. Again, tongue blades are invaluable in this examination for moving the soft tissues so that a complete inspection of areas of interest can be done. After the hard palate is visualized, the tongue is inspected for immobility and deviation. Deviation or atrophy usually represents hypoglossal nerve paralysis. The tongue deviates to the paralyzed side, and the loss of bulk is on that side as well. Oral cavity structures are tested for general sensation by touch with the tongue blades. Decreased sensation may suggest compromise of trigeminal nerve function, particularly the third division.

Most visible oral cavity cancers are SCCs, whereas the less common minor salivary gland tumors are submucosal (19). Ulcerative lesions on the mucosal surfaces typically bleed easily with manipulation. These cancers are often painful and tender. In fact, this sensitivity frequently motivates the patient with oral cancer to see a physician. An ill-fitting or painful denture may also herald the growth of neoplastic disease. White (leukoplakia) and red (erythroplakia) plaques on any of the mucosal oral cavity structures may be indicative of early or advanced premalignant disease (20–22). These lesions are frequently multiple and represent histologic change in a field of epithelium chronically exposed to carcinogens such as tobacco, both smoke-producing and smokeless. Premalignant oral cavity lesions frequently create a burning sensation.

Hematopoietic malignancies such as extranodal lymphomas can present in Waldeyer's ring tissues (palatine, lingual, and nasopharyngeal tonsils) (4,23). This diagnosis should be considered when a firm, nonulcerative, and nontender mass is noted in the tonsil or tongue base.

Palpation of oral cavity structures, particularly of gross tumor, is essential to the examination. Bimanual palpation is essential for proper evaluation of floor of the mouth and other structures in the area. This technique helps the clinician ascertain the size and thickness of the lesion (for staging purposes) as well as its mobility relative to other structures such as the jaw and underlying musculature.

Examination of the Oropharynx

The oropharynx should be inspected as a continuation of the oral cavity evaluation. Examination of the general area, however, is often hindered by an active gag reflex, and careful and gentle use of the tongue blade must be mastered. Any weakness or asymmetry of the gag reflex, suggesting glossopharyngeal nerve compromise, is noted. The tonsillar fossae with their anterior and posterior pillars are inspected first. Tonsil cancers, typically SCC, may not be obvious in deeply recessed tonsillar fossae. Upper neck pain, otalgia, and trismus may herald the presence of such tumors, which will typically present as firm, ulcerative, or endophytic masses in this area.

The tonsillar and soft palate examination is accomplished as one, and while it is unusual for neoplasms to originate on the latter, they may extend directly from the tonsil itself. Tumors of the deep parapharyngeal space can cause tonsil and palatal bulging as they expand medially (24) (Fig. 1.2), and as such can be misinterpreted as an oral/oropharyngeal problem by the inexperienced examiner. Some parapharyngeal space tumors can present with various degrees of dysphagia, dysarthria, and even partial obstruction of the upper aerodigestive tract. Tumors found in the parapharyngeal space include benign and malignant parotid and minor salivary gland tumors, schwannomas, paragangliomas, lymphomas, and metastatic SCCs (24).

Next, the glossopharyngeal sulci and tongue base are examined. The most anterior aspects of these structures can be visualized and palpated directly. The distal tongue base, however, cannot be directly visualized. Indirect mirror examination remains an invaluable technique for this part of the evaluation, and often creates a purer and wider angle view than fiberoptic techniques (discussed later in the chapter). Palpation of the tongue base for suspicious lesions or for patients in treatment follow-up is imperative, but this maneuver should be done at the end of the examination (once stimulated, the gag reflex can compromise any meaningful visualization of much of the area). While small tumors of the tongue base can be asymptomatic, larger tumors can be associated with varying degrees of local pain, blood-tinged sputum, and altered sound of breathing.

Examination of the Nasopharynx, Hypopharynx, and Larynx

Unlike the tongue base, the nasopharynx is best examined with a flexible fiberoptic scope. At the time that the base of tongue is examined with a mirror, the hypopharynx and larynx can often be seen. In many circumstances, the view afforded in this manner is excellent, and vocal fold movement as well as hypopharyngeal abnormalities can be seen. Sluggish true vocal fold mobility or paralysis may be from tumor mass effect in the region, tumor infiltration of the cricoarytenoid joint, or tumor compromise of the recurrent branch of the vagus nerve. The mirror is angled to afford inspection of the supraglottic larynx, pharyngoepiglottic folds, and pyriform fossae. Pooling of secretions is noted and may indicate an underlying mass or pharyngeal immobility secondary to vagus nerve compromise.

The most common malignancies of the hypopharynx and larynx are SCCs. Other tumors, such as minor salivary gland tumors, sarcomas, and neuroendocrine carcinomas can also occur in this anatomic region (25–29), but are very uncommon; generally these are distinguished from SCC by being submucosal, rather than surface lesions. Patients with cancers in the hypopharynx or larynx will present with varying degrees of hoarseness, dysphagia, odynophagia, otalgia (referred pain), and hemoptysis. The prevertebral tissue involvement of large hypopharyngeal tumors may distort the motion from side to side, which is elicited by grasping the larynx.

Certain areas of the upper aerodigestive tract, such as the superior and posterior nasal cavity and the nasopharynx, cannot be assessed by the routine physical examination. For visu-

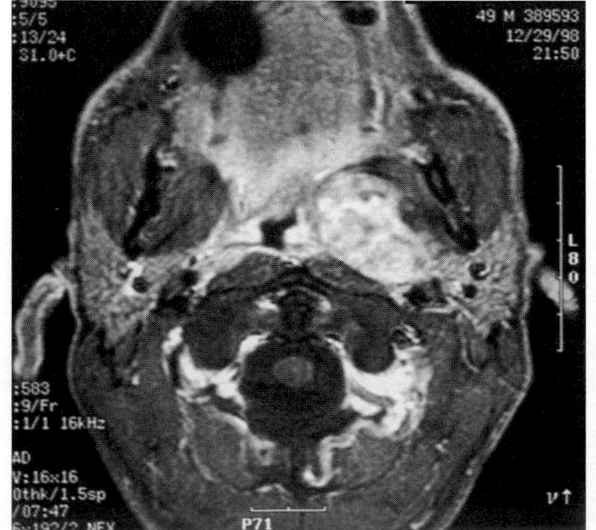

A

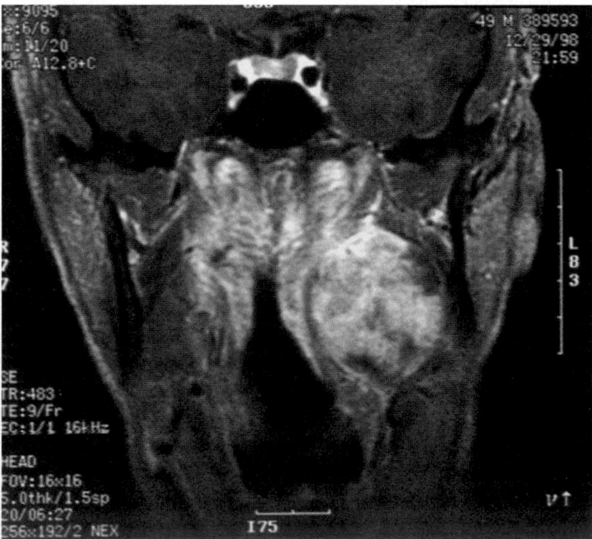

B

Figure 1.2 Axial (**A**) and coronal (**B**) magnetic resonance images of a left parapharyngeal space tumor compressing the left lateral oropharyngeal wall. On physical examination, this mass presented as a large bulge in the left oropharynx at the level of the lateral oropharyngeal wall and soft palate. It was not palpable as a neck mass. The patient presented with dysphagia. The tumor proved to be a carcinoma ex-pleomorphic adenoma.

alization of these areas, flexible or rigid fiberoptic endoscopy is very useful. Fiberoptic evaluation of the hypopharynx and larynx should always follow a suspicious mirror examination. This technology provides a more panoramic view of the area by which the examiner can evaluate subtle abnormalities and importantly, laryngeal sensation can be tested. A distinct advantage of the fiberoptic technique is that the tip of the scope can be used to test laryngopharyngeal sensation. Whereas decreased pharyngeal sensation indicates compromise of the glossopharyngeal nerve, decreased supraglottic sensation reflects the state of health of the internal branch of the superior laryngeal nerve, a branch of the vagus. Upper aerodigestive tract fiberoptic evaluation can almost always be accomplished in the office setting.

Biopsy of the Upper Aerodigestive Tract

Many areas of the upper aerodigestive tract, such as the nasal cavity and nasopharynx, the oral cavity, and the proximal oropharynx (tonsillar region), can be biopsied in the office setting using local infiltration or topical anesthesia. Patients with tumors that cannot be completely assessed in the office setting, and most patients with posterior oropharyngeal, hypopharyngeal, and laryngeal lesions should be biopsied in the operating room under general anesthesia.

Anterior nasal cavity lesions can usually be biopsied with a cup biopsy forceps. If, however, there is a possibility that a tumor may be arising from the superior nasal vault, this should not be done in the office setting. Imaging (see "Imaging of the Head and Neck" later in the chapter) should be obtained first to determine whether the tumor has intracranial communication. Posterior nasal cavity and nasopharyngeal lesions can often be biopsied in the office setting using rigid endoscopic guidance. In this anatomic region, the examiner should consider that certain tumors such as angiofibroma can be very vascular. When a potentially vascular lesion is identified based on its appearance (pulsatile, blue hue, etc.), appropriate imaging (as discussed later in the chapter) can often be diagnostic (18), obviating the need for a potentially dangerous biopsy.

Tumors of the oral cavity can be biopsied with either a punch or cup forceps. Tumors of the proximal oropharynx (tonsillar region) can be biopsied in a similar fashion. Adequate anesthesia as well as hemostasis can be obtained when a mixture of lidocaine and epinephrine is infiltrated into the tissues surrounding the site to be sampled. It is best not to infiltrate the tumor directly. The 4-mm punch has the advantage of delivering a specimen to the pathologist with little crush artifact. It also allows for precise orientation of tissue when there are concerns regarding tumor thickness—a prognostic factor for oral tumors such as tongue cancers (30,31).

Parapharyngeal space tumors presenting as oropharyngeal bulges can be biopsied transorally by the FNA technique. If there is suspicion that the mass may represent a vascular tumor such as a paraganglioma, imaging is usually diagnostic and allows the avoidance of a biopsy (see "Imaging of the Head and Neck" later in the chapter) (24).

Under some circumstances, tumors of the tongue base, hypopharynx, and larynx can be biopsied in the office setting using topical anesthesia and a fiberoptic scope that has an instrument port. The major disadvantages of this technique include relatively small and potentially nondiagnostic biopsies, as well as the inability to completely assess the extent of lesions in the awake and anxious patient. For these reasons, the hypopharynx and larynx should be evaluated under general anesthesia in the operating room. This also will ensure adequate biopsies and complete tumor assessment. Using a standard laryngoscope, the tongue base, posterior oropharyngeal wall, entire hypopharynx, esophageal inlet, and larynx can be inspected. Subglottic as well as ventricular extent of laryngeal cancers can be determined. True vocal fold fixation versus immobility from mass effect can be ascertained. The laryngoscope should be suspended when possible to assist in evaluating a laryngeal cancer.

Rigid and fiberoptic endoscopic techniques also allow the clinician to inspect and biopsy the esophagus. Patients with tumors in the proximal and distal esophagus usually present with varying degrees of dysphagia. Weight loss, hematemesis, and hemoptysis may also be prominent symptoms.

EXAMINATION OF THE NECK AND PAROTID REGION

The neck is an anatomically complex region that is examined by directed inspection and palpation. Multiple benign and malignant tumors can occur here. The neck itself can harbor malignant disease in its many lymph nodes metastatic from upper aerodigestive tract, thyroid gland, skin, lung, breast, and gastrointestinal and urologic tract sites. The neck can also be a site of primary cancers such as thyroid, salivary gland, lymphomas, and various types of sarcomas. The patient with any malignant tumor in the neck will frequently complain of a neck mass, and more often than not it is painless. Large cervical tumors such as those seen in the thyroid gland may compress upper aerodigestive tract structures, causing varying degrees of dysphagia or respiratory embarrassment. These latter symptoms may be especially troubling in more supine body positions.

The parotid region, while mostly overlying the posterior and lateral aspect of the face anterior to the pinna, also includes the upper lateral neck. This latter part of the gland overlies the superior third of the sternocleidomastoid muscle and is referred to as the tail of the parotid. The parotid gland, like other salivary glands, can be the primary site of various benign and malignant tumors of epithelial origin. The complex multicellular epithelial structure of salivary tissue serves as the origin of these multiple distinct tumor entities. The various distinct malignant parotid gland histologies can differ in their aggressiveness and prognosis (19). The parotid gland, with its associated lymph nodes, may also be the site of primary or disseminated lymphoma, or metastases of cancers from other head and neck locations. Cutaneous tumors such as melanoma and SCC can metastasize to the parotid region. The patient with a parotid tumor, like tumors at other neck sites, will most frequently complain of a mass with or without associated pain. Some patients with parotid tumors may present with a facial (cranial nerve VII) palsy even though the mass is not obvious. Facial nerve palsy along with associated pain, are ominous findings and usually imply that the tumor is malignant (19,32,33).

The lateral and central compartments of the neck are divided into levels for descriptive purposes (34). Table 1.1 describes the anatomic boundaries of these cervical lymph node levels. Lymph node metastases from tumors in certain upper aerodigestive tract subsites are more prone to spread to certain lymph node levels as opposed to others (35). There is a remarkable consistency to metastatic patterns.

The neck is palpated in a sequential fashion, encompassing all of the lymph node levels. One can begin in the submental and submandibular regions and progress along the anterior border of the sternocleidomastoid muscle to assess the jugular chain. The level I lymph nodes are best appreciated by bimanual examination (with a finger in the floor of the mouth and a hand on the neck). The posterior triangle and central compart-

TABLE 1.1 Cervical Lymph Node Levels

Neck level	Name of neck level	Description	Anatomic boundaries of neck level
I	Submental/submandibular group	Lymph nodes in the submental and submandibular triangles	Submental: anterior bellies of digastric muscles and hyoid bone Submandibular: anterior and posterior bellies of digastric muscle
II	Upper jugular group	Lymph nodes located around upper third of internal jugular vein and surrounding structures	Hyoid bone to skull base and posterior border of sternocleidomastoid muscle to lateral border of sternohyoid muscle
III	Middle jugular group	Lymph nodes located around the middle third of the internal jugular vein	Hyoid bone to the cricoid cartilage and the posterior border of the sternocleidomastoid muscle to the lateral border of the sternohyoid muscle
IV	Lower jugular group	Lymph nodes located around the lower third of the internal jugular vein	Cricoid cartilage to the clavicle and posterior border of the sternocleidomastoid muscle to the lateral border of the sternohyoid muscle
V	Posterior triangle group	Lymph nodes located around the lower half of the spinal accessory nerve and the transverse cervical artery	Anterior border of the trapezius muscle to the posterior border of the sternocleidomastoid muscle; clavicle is inferior border
VI	Anterior compartment group	Lymph nodes surrounding the midline visceral structures of the neck (includes perithyroidal and paratracheal lymph nodes)	Hyoid bone to suprasternal notch and medial border of carotid sheath to medial border of carotid sheath

Source: Adapted from Robbins KT, Medina JE, Levine PA, et al. Standardizing neck dissection terminology. *Arch Otolaryngol Head Neck Surg* 1991;117:601–605.

ments of the neck must also be palpated. Masses are noted for their size and whether or not they are mobile with respect to the overlying skin or underlying structures. Masses along the jugular chain (particularly those at levels II and III) may be fixed to the underlying carotid artery, a feature characterized by side-to-side mobility, but restricted motion up and down.

Neoplasms in the lower central compartment of the neck are typically of thyroid origin, although some laryngopharyngeal cancers can metastasize to lymph nodes in this area. Thyroid tumors typically move up and down during swallowing. Any patient with a thyroid neoplasm should also have their vocal fold mobility assessed. Paresis or paralysis of a true vocal fold in the presence of a thyroid mass suggests, but is not pathognomonic of malignancy.

It should be noted that solitary masses in the left supraclavicular fossa may represent a lymph node metastasis from a gastrointestinal, pelvic, breast, or thoracic primary malignancy. Such cervical metastatic lymph nodes are called sentinel nodes because they herald the presence of these anatomically distant cancers. It is a fact, however, that most malignant cervical adenopathy is metastatic, and most of these metastases come from primary sites in the head and neck.

Biopsy of the Neck and Parotid Masses

Most cervical and parotid region masses can be adequately sampled by the FNA technique. FNA is safe, highly sensitive and specific for the histologic diagnosis of benign and malignant lesions presenting in the head and neck (16). Excisional/incisional biopsy of cervical masses for initial diagnostic purposes is rarely recommended because it may interfere with future treatment strategies. An exception to this rule is the instance in which lymphoma is the suspected diagnosis because of the physical examination and initial FNA findings. In this instance a generous tissue sample is often desired for tumor characterization. In certain circumstances, FNA can yield this information through flow cytometry specimen processing (36).

IMAGING OF THE HEAD AND NECK

The most valuable diagnostic imaging techniques in head and neck oncology are CT scanning, magnetic resonance imaging (MRI), and ultrasound (37,38). Fluorine-18 fluorodeoxyglucose positron emission tomography (FDG-PET) is also being used in certain clinical situations. Its use continues to be analyzed (39–43), and early results of this technology suggest a valuable future. Imaging of the head and neck is typically performed for the following reasons:

- To evaluate the extent of primary tumor (and its potential regional metastases)
- To evaluate patients after treatment
- To evaluate patients with an unknown primary tumor who present only with cervical lymph node metastases.

Imaging of the Primary Tumor

The gold standard for imaging head and neck neoplasms, particularly as a first imaging study, is CT. Intravenous contrast material is frequently given during CT imaging to enhance diagnostic capabilities. CT can often delineate tumor soft tissue extent, beyond what is obvious by physical examination. CT can also help in the assessment of bony tumor involvement when the physical examination is unclear on this issue. In anatomic areas that are difficult to examine, but where tumor is suspected, CT can be very useful. The paranasal sinuses, the parapharyngeal space, the anterior and middle skull base, and the perilaryngeal spaces are examples of such locations.

CT imaging is very useful for the assessment of cervical lymph node metastases (44). It is not unusual for a patient to have a clinically negative neck despite radiographic evidence of lymph node disease. Patients with radiographic (or clinical) evidence of cervical metastases for an upper aerodigestive tract malignancy should also have CT imaging of the chest as these patients are at highest risk for the development of such tumor spread (45).

Although MRI is not useful for imaging bony involvement by primary head and neck tumors, it can give exquisite soft tissue and vascular detail. Although it is not recommended as the initial imaging study for delineating tumor extent, study characteristics along with geographic tumor location can often point to a particular histologic diagnosis. For example, parapharyngeal space tumors such as schwannomas and paragangliomas have characteristic MRI appearances (24). The superior soft tissue detail offered by MRI can also help to delineate tumor from entrapped secretions in paranasal sinus neoplasms (46).

Ultrasound is the most common modality used for thyroid imaging. Not only is it useful for delineating solid from cystic lesions, but it can also be used to localize smaller nodules for the purposes of FNA (sonographic-guided FNA) (47). At some centers, ultrasound is also used as a rapid clinical tool to assist in the detection of potential cervical metastases in patients with upper aerodigestive tract malignancies (48).

It is clear that imaging plays a fundamental role in the workup and evaluation of any patient with a head and neck neoplasm. The results of imaging may assist the clinician in the staging process by detecting local or regional extension of disease not obvious on the physical examination. Thus, the physical examination and selective imaging together optimize physical diagnosis and staging so that the most appropriate treatment can be rendered.

Imaging after Treatment

The patient who has completed treatment for a head and neck neoplasm often presents a clinical challenge to the diagnostician. Prolonging survival and quality of life depends on the early detection of locoregional recurrence of disease, as well as second primary head and neck tumors (specifically in the case of SCC). Patients treated for head and neck cancers often have undergone extensive resection with flap reconstruction, EBRT with or without chemotherapy, or interstitial radiation therapy. Any or all of these treatment techniques can significantly distort anatomy, making follow-up tumor surveillance difficult. Even in the absence of any obvious clinical abnormalities, periodic imaging of such difficult to examine patients is often useful. Because the area is altered by treatment, an imaging study (CT or MRI) is recommended 3 months after treatment to establish a new baseline.

Although CT and MRI studies are typically performed as initial and follow-up studies for the purposes of comparison, FDG-PET is gaining wider acceptance as a tool to assess the difficult to examine patient, especially in the posttreatment circumstance (39,42). Performed in the nuclear medicine department and relying on the greater uptake of glucose by more metabolically active malignant tissues, FDG-PET seems to be highly sensitive in this clinical situation, and perhaps even more so than traditional imaging modalities in detecting persistent or recurrent head and neck cancer. FDG-PET is also proving to be quite useful in detecting persistent or recurrent cancer in symptomatic patients with equivocal results on traditional imaging studies. FDG-PET seems to be able to predict with a relatively high degree of certainty which patients are most likely to have a positive biopsy result on endoscopic evaluation for persistent or recurrent disease (41).

Imaging of the Unknown Primary Tumor

Some SCCs may present as cervical lymph node metastases, without evidence of the primary upper aerodigestive tract malignancy, after a clinical and radiographic search. In many instances when SCC presents as cervical lymph node metastases (without other signs or symptoms), the primary tumor will either be found on office examination, in the operating room during diagnostic endoscopy, or on diagnostic imaging studies (49).

If the office examination of the upper aerodigestive tract is unrevealing in the patient with SCC in the cervical nodes, plans are usually made for a more detailed evaluation in the operating room under general anesthesia. Imaging prior to this operating room evaluation is important in that it can direct the clinician to suspicious sites of disease, thus minimizing the morbidity of potential multiple blind biopsies—the diagnostic yield of which is controversial.

CT with intravenous contrast, with its good soft tissue delineation, relatively low cost, and widespread availability, is a reasonable imaging study choice for the workup of the unknown primary SCC prior to evaluation under anesthesia. Positive or suspicious findings on CT can direct the surgeon to the site of the tumor and thus direct any biopsies. As more experience with FDG-PET accumulates, it is becoming clear that this modality can be highly sensitive in the detection of an unknown primary SCC (40). It should be ordered in centers where it is available when standard imaging modalities fail to detect the primary tumor.

In the patient with an unknown primary SCC and negative imaging studies, there remains controversy as to what should be done diagnostically at the time of the evaluation under anesthesia. The evaluation needs to include a thorough evaluation of the oral cavity and oropharynx (with attention to Waldeyer ring tissues), hypopharynx, nasopharynx, and larynx, as well as esophagus. The endoscopic, direct visualization, as well as palpation techniques outlined previously are used during this evaluation. When no tumor is encountered, some clinicians advocate random biopsies of the nasopharynx, tonsillar fossae, tongue base, and pyriform sinuses. There is no solid evidence supporting this multiple biopsy strategy, although there is some evidence that the yield for tonsillectomy alone may be quite high, thus justifying its use (49–51).

REFERENCES

1. Spitz MR. Epidemiology and risk factors for head and neck cancer. *Semin Oncol* 1994;21:281.
2. Gillison ML, Koch WM, Capone RB, et al. Evidence for a causal association between human papillomavirus and a subset of head and neck cancers. *J Natl Cancer Inst* 2000;92:709.
3. Goldman ND, Coniglio JU, Falk SA. Thyroid cancers. I: Papillary, follicular, and Hurthle cell. *Otolaryngol Clin North Am* 1996;29:593.
4. Finch S. Leukemia, lymphoma in atomic bomb survivors. In: Boice JD, Fraumeni J, eds. *Radiation carcinogenesis: epidemiology, and biological significance.* New York: Raven Press, 1984:37.
5. Singh B, Bhaya M, Stern J, et al. Validation of the Charleston comorbidity index in patients with head and neck cancer: a multi-institutional study. *Laryngoscope* 1997;107:1469.
6. Brash DE, Rudolph JA, Simon JA, et al. A role for sunlight in skin cancer: UV-induced p53 mutations in squamous cell carcinoma. *Proc Natl Acad Sci USA* 1991;88:10124–101248.
7. Lentsch EJ, Myers JN. Melanoma of the head and neck: current concepts in diagnosis and management. *Laryngoscope* 2001;111:1209.
8. Austin JR, Byers RM, Brown WD, et al. Influence of biopsy on the prognosis of cutaneous melanoma of the head and neck. *Head Neck* 1996;18:107.
9. Garden AS, Weber RS, Morrison WH, et al. The influence of positive margins and nerve invasion in adenoid cystic carcinoma of the head and neck treated with surgery and radiation. *Int J Radiat Oncol Biol Phys* 1995;32:619.
10. Beenken S, Byers R, Smith JL, et al. Desmoplastic melanoma: histologic correlation with behavior and treatment. *Arch Otolaryngol Head Neck Surg* 1989; 115:374.
11. Pappas DC, Persky MS, Berenstein A. Evaluation and treatment of head and neck venous vascular malformations. *Ear Nose Throat J* 1998;77:914.
12. Stal S, Hamilton S, Spira M. Hemangiomas, lymphangiomas, and vascular malformations of the head and neck. *Otolaryngol Clin North Am* 1986;19:769.

13. Testa JRG, Fukuda Y, Lowalski LP. Prognostic factors in carcinoma of the external auditory canal. *Arch Otolaryngol Head Neck Surg* 1997;123:720.
14. Sato H, Kurata K, Yen Y-H, et al. Extension of nasopharyngeal carcinoma and otitis media with effusion. *Arch Otolaryngol Head Neck Surg* 1988;114:866.
15. Wei WI. Nasopharyngeal cancer: Current status of management. *Arch Otolaryngol Head Neck Surg* 2001;127:766.
16. Karayianis SL, Francisco GJ, Schulmann GB. Clinical utility of head and neck aspiration cytology. *Diagn Cytopathol* 1988;4:187.
17. Levine PA, Gallagher R, Cantrell RW. Esthesioneuroblastoma: reflections of a 21-year experience. *Laryngoscope* 1999;109:1539.
18. Scholtz AW, Appenroth E, Kammen-Jolly K, et al. Juvenile nasopharyngeal angiofibroma: management and therapy. *Laryngoscope* 2001;111:681.
19. Spiro, RH. Salivary neoplasms: overview of a 35-year experience with 2,807 patients. *Head Neck Surg* 1986;8:177.
20. Armstrong WB, Meyskens FL. Chemoprevention of head and neck cancer. *Otolaryngol Head Neck Surg* 2000;122:728.
21. Khuri FR, Lippman SM, Spitz MR, et al. Molecular epidemiology and retinoid chemoprevention of head and neck cancer. *J Natl Inst Cancer* 1997;89:199–211.
22. Silverman S, Gorsky M, Lozada F. Oral leukoplakia and malignant transformation: a follow-up study of 257 patients. *Cancer* 1984;53:563.
23. Ezzat AA, Ibrahim EM, El Weshi AN, et al. Localized non-Hodgkin's lymphoma of Waldeyer's ring: clinical features, management, and prognosis of 130 adult patients. *Head Neck* 2000;23:547.
24. Olsen KD. Tumors and surgery of the parapharyngeal space. *Laryngoscope* 1994;104[Suppl 63]:1–28.
25. Alavi S, Calcaterra TC, Namazie A, et al. Glandular carcinoma of the larynx: the UCLA experience. *Ann Otol Rhinol Laryngol* 1999;108:485.
26. Berge JK, Kapadia SB, Myers EN. Osteosarcoma of the larynx. *Arch Otolaryngol Head Neck Surg* 1998;124:207.
27. Dei Tos AP, Dal Cin, P, Sciot R, et al. Synovial sarcoma of the larynx and hypopharynx. *Ann Otol Rhinol Laryngol* 1998;107:1080.
28. Klussmann JP, Eckel HE. Small cell neuroendocrine carcinoma of the larynx. *Ear Nose Throat J* 1999;78:22.
29. Lewis JE, Olsen KO, Inwards CY. Cartilaginous tumors of the larynx: clinicopathologic review of 47 cases. *Ann Otol Rhinol Laryngol* 1997;106:94.
30. Byers RM, El-Naggar AK, Lee Y-Y, et al. Can we detect or predict the presence of occult nodal metastases in patients with squamous carcinoma of the oral tongue? *Head Neck* 1998;20:138.
31. Onerci M, Yilmaz T, Gedikoglu G. Tumor thickness as a predictor of cervical lymph node metastasis in squamous cell carcinoma of the lower lip. *Otolaryngol Head Neck Surg* 2000;122:139.
32. Bron LP, O'Brien CJ. Facial nerve function after parotidectomy. *Arch Otolaryngol Head Neck Surg* 1997;123:1091.
33. Magnano M, Gervasio CF, Cravero L, et al. Treatment of malignant neoplasms of the parotid gland. *Otolaryngol Head Neck Surg* 1999;121:627.
34. Robbins KT, Medina JE, Levine PA, et al. Standardizing neck dissection terminology. *Arch Otolaryngol Head Neck Surg* 1991;117:601.
35. Lindberg R. Distribution of cervical lymph node metastases from squamous cell carcinoma of the upper respiratory and digestive tracts. *Cancer* 1972;29:1446.
36. Cannon CR, Richardson LD. Value of flow cytometry in the evaluation of head and neck fine-needle lymphoid aspirates: a 3-year retrospective review of a community-based practice. *Otolaryngol Head Neck Surg* 2001;124:544.
37. Foust RJ, Duong RT. Roles of computed tomography and magnetic resonance imaging diagnoses in the treatment of head and neck cancer. *Hematol Oncol Clin North Am* 1991;5:657.
38. Leuwer RM, Westhofen M, Schade G. Color duplex echography in head and neck cancer. *Am J Otolaryngol* 1997;18:254.
39. Farber LA, Benard F, Machtay M, et al. Detection of recurrent head and neck squamous cell carcinomas after radiation therapy with 2-^{18}F-fluoro-2-deoxy-D-glucose positron emission tomography. *Laryngoscope* 1999;109:970.
40. Jungehulsing M, Scheidhauer K, Damm M, et al. 2(^{18}F)-fluoro-2-deoxy-D-glucose positron emission tomography. *Otolaryngol Head Neck Surg* 2000;123:294.
41. Lonneux M, Lawson G, Ide C, et al. Positron emission tomography with fluorodeoxyglucose for suspected head and neck tumor recurrence in the symptomatic patient. *Laryngoscope* 2000;110:1493.
42. Lowe VJ, Boyd JH, Dunphy FR, et al. Surveillance for recurrent head and neck cancer using positron emission tomography. *J Clin Oncol* 2000;18:651.
43. Paulus P, Sambon A, Vivegnis D, et al. ^{18}FDG-PET for the assessment of primary head and neck tumors: clinical, computed tomography and histopathological correlation in 38 patients. *Laryngoscope* 1998;108:1578.
44. Merritt RM, Williams MF, James TH, et al. Detection of cervical metastasis: a meta-analysis comparing computed tomography with physical examination. *Arch Otolaryngol Head Neck Surg* 1997;123:149.
45. De Bree R, Deurloo EE, Snow GB, et al. Screening for distant metastases in patients with head and neck cancer. *Laryngoscope* 2000;110:397.
46. Som PM, Shapiro MD, Biller HF, et al. Sinonasal tumors and inflammatory tissues: differentiation with MR. *Radiology* 1988;167:803.
47. Boland GW, Lee MJ, Mueller PR, et al. Efficacy of sonographically guided biopsy of thyroid masses and cervical lymph nodes. *Am J Roentgenol* 1993;161:1053.
48. Van den Brekel MW, Castelijns JA, Stel HV, et al. Modern imaging techniques and ultrasound guided aspiration cytology for the assessment of neck node metastases: a prospective comparative study. *Eur Arch Otorhinolaryngol* 1993;250:11.
49. Mendenhall WM, Mancuso AA, Parsons JT, et al. Diagnostic evaluation of squamous cell carcinoma metastatic to cervical lymph nodes from an unknown head and neck primary site. *Head Neck* 1998;20:739.
50. McQuone SJ, Eisele DW, Lee D-J, et al. Occult tonsillar carcinoma in the unknown primary. *Laryngoscope* 1998;108:1605.
51. Randall DA, Johnstone PAS, Foss RD, et al. Tonsillectomy in diagnosis of the unknown primary tumor of the head and neck. *Otolaryngol Head Neck Surg* 2000;122:52.

CHAPTER 2

General Principles of Head and Neck Pathology

Bruce M. Wenig and Jean-Marc Cohen

The surgical pathologist is an integral member of the clinical team that administers to the head and neck cancer patient. The pathologist's role is multifactorial. In the simplest of terms, it is his or her job to render the correct diagnosis. However, that "final" goal is not an isolated achievement nor is the diagnosis the sole responsibility placed on the surgical pathologist. There are numerous factors that go into the diagnosis of cancer, not the least important of which are what type of cancer is it, how invasive is the tumor, are the surgical margins free of involvement, is there metastatic disease, and are there any pathologic features that may allow for predicting the biologic behavior for a given tumor.

This chapter is an overview of the pathologic issues relative to head and neck cancer. It begins with an overview of the general principles of the pathology of head and neck neoplasms, including the surgical pathology report, classification of tumors, histologic differentiation and grading of tumors, adjunct techniques to light microscopy in the diagnosis of head and neck cancers, histopathologic parameters in the assessment of head and neck tumors, and factors that may potentially impact prognosis. The second half of the chapter primarily focuses on head and neck squamous cell carcinoma (HNSCC) beginning with discussions on field carcinogenesis followed by the pathology of HNSCC. The latter subject includes discussion of precursor lesions of HNSCC (i.e., grading of epithelial dysplasia), invasive SCC, and variants of SCC. Because of space limitations, the pathology of salivary gland neoplasms, neuroendocrine neoplasms, thyroid and parathyroid lesions, mesenchymal and hematolymphoid neoplasms will not be included in this chapter. See Chapters 25–30 and 34 in this textbook for a discussion of these subjects.

SURGICAL PATHOLOGY REPORT AND TISSUE SPECIMEN

The pathology report is the document that contains the pathologist's diagnosis for a given surgical or cytologic specimen. The pathology report not only contains the diagnosis of the tumor but also may include the type, differentiation and histologic grade of the tumor, the extent of disease, including whether the tumor is invasive (*in situ* vs. submucosal invasion), whether the surgical margins are involved by tumor, whether there is neural or lymph–vascular space invasion, and whether nodal metastases and extranodal extension are present. In addition, the pathology report may contain the results of any adjunct studies that assist in establishing the diagnosis. Therefore, the pathology report includes information of prognostic and therapeutic importance. Further, the pathology report is a legal document that becomes a part of the patient's medical record.

The final histologic diagnosis is not an isolated achievement or the sole responsibility of the pathologist. In addition to the final diagnosis, the pathology report contains the gross and microscopic description of the specimen. For small specimens such as a biopsy, the gross description is relatively simple and straightforward. For larger surgical resections, like those often required for the head and neck cancer patient, the surgical specimen may be large and complex in its details. The complexity of the surgical specimen necessitates that the pathologist has a good functional understanding of the surgical anatomy of the region. It is the responsibility of the pathologist to properly evaluate the gross specimen, and to describe in detail the gross characteristics of the tumor to include its relationship to the surrounding structures. The proper sectioning of the specimen is equally important. Improper sectioning will result in erroneous evaluation of the specimen. To this end, the surgeon and pathologist must work in unison, especially in appropriately orientating a large resection specimen and determining the key aspects of the specimen (e.g., surgical margins) that require special attention. The sections that are taken by the pathologist will ultimately indicate whether the tumor involves the surgical margins or whether the surgical margins are free of tumor. The issue of surgical margin involvement will impact on the necessity for additional surgical intervention or the use of adjuvant therapy. Therefore, the proper gross evaluation of the specimen, including the sectioning for histologic evaluation, is a critical component in the overall management of the head and neck cancer patient.

It should be obvious that the pathologist's role as a member of the clinical team goes beyond the histologic evaluation of a tumor and the assigning of a name (i.e., a diagnosis). Certainly, the diagnosis of the tumor is important, but there are multiple additional factors that are equally important, perhaps even more important to the overall management and prognosis of the head and neck cancer patient. These issues will be discussed in detail later in this chapter.

The pathologist is entirely dependent on the tissue sampling that is received from the surgeon. Without the appropriate material, a diagnosis cannot be rendered. This is true for neoplastic, as well as nonneoplastic lesions. In general, necrotic or ulcerated tissue should be avoided as the diagnostic yield from this material is, at best, low. The viable tissue surrounding or deep to the ulcerated or necrotic tissue should be sampled. The most common types of neoplastic proliferations of the upper aerodigestive tract (UADT) originate from the surface epithelium. A critical parameter used by the pathologist in differentiating a reactive or benign surface epithelial lesion from a malignant neoplasm is the presence or absence of stromal invasion. Adequate sampling should therefore include the depth of the tissue so that the pathologist can evaluate the epithelial-to-stromal interface, and an assessment for the presence or absence of stromal invasion can be made. Without an adequate epithelial-to-stromal interface, a diagnosis cannot be made, resulting in frustration for the pathologist, surgeon and most importantly, the patient. The deficiency of proper sampling leads to diagnostic and therapeutic delays. Further, tissue sampling of any anatomic site results in secondary pathologic changes that may cause diagnostic dilemmas for the pathologist.

The sampling of lymph nodes should include the largest node available as the diagnostic yield will be greatest as compared with a more accessible but smaller lymph node. Another issue in tissue sampling is the proper fixation of a specimen. Once a surgical specimen is removed, the surgeon should not delay in placing the specimen in the appropriate fixative. Excessive delay in placing the surgical specimen in fixative will result in autolytic and other artifactual alterations in the tissue. In general, the fixative that is most commonly used by pathologists is formaldehyde. However, some specimens, especially lymph nodes removed for a possible diagnosis of lymphoma, may require special fixation. Some lymphoid-related antigens are lost by prior fixation so that in certain situations, the pathologist will want unfixed or fresh tissue to perform specific immunohistochemical, flow cytometric, or molecular biologic studies. The pathologist should be notified and consulted relative to the proper handling of the surgical material. Similarly, if it is anticipated that electron microscopy or cytogenetic evaluation will be required to assist in the diagnosis, then special fixatives, such as gluteraldehyde for electron microscopy and tissue culture medium (e.g., RPMI) will be required. When such circumstances are anticipated the pathologist should be notified prior to the procedure that the specimen may require special handling.

The surgeon or any member of the surgical team should not bisect or section a tumor once it is excised from the patient. This may cause problems for the pathologist in the gross evaluation of the specimen, in appropriate tissue sectioning, and in appropriate tissue fixation. Such improper handling of the excised tissues may compromise the excised specimen. The gross evaluation, sectioning, and histologic examination of the surgical specimen fall under the purview of the pathologist. The surgeon should sample or remove sufficient tissue for diagnosis and send it to the pathologist intact, properly labeled and with any specific requirements or requests that may be needed (e.g., specific surgical margins). The relationship of the surgeon and the pathologist is not adversarial but should be collegial, with both specialists working in unison. Only in this way will the primary goal be achieved, which is the well-being and proper care of the patient.

GENERAL PRINCIPLES OF HEAD AND NECK NEOPLASMS

Classification

See the site-specific chapters in this textbook for detailed classification of the tumors that arise in those sites. The general classification of malignant tumors of the head and neck are detailed in Tables 2.1 through 2.5.

Terminology

Cancer is defined as a malignant and invasive growth or tumor, tending to recur after excision and metastasize to other sites (1). The cell of origin for a given neoplasm (benign or malignant) is its *histogenesis.* In head and neck malignancies, the most common type of malignant tumor is one that arises from the surface squamous epithelium. Squamous epithelial malignant tumors are carcinomas. However, the head and neck are rich in nonsquamous epithelial-derived structures, so that epithelial malignancies (carcinomas) may originate from salivary glands (major and minor), cutaneous adnexae, thyroid

TABLE 2.1 Classification of Epithelial Malignancies of the Head and Neck

Cutaneous epithelial malignant tumors
- Squamous cell carcinoma
- Basal cell carcinoma
- Verrucous carcinoma
- Malignant cutaneous adnexal tumors

Mucosal epithelial malignant tumors
- Squamous cell carcinoma
  - Keratinizing type
  - Nonkeratinizing type
- Variants of squamous cell carcinoma
  - Verrucous carcinoma
  - Spindle cell squamous carcinoma
  - Basaloid squamous cell carcinoma
  - Adenosquamous carcinoma
  - "Lymphoepithelial" or undifferentiated carcinoma
- Adenocarcinoma of surface mucosal origin
- Adenocarcinoma of mucoserous gland origin

TABLE 2.2 Classification of Neuroectodermal Tumors of the Head and Neck

Tumors of the dispersed neuroendocrine cell system (DNES) (as it applies to the head and neck)

Central DNES
- Olfactory neuroblastoma

Peripheral DNES
- Malignant melanoma
- Neuroendocrine carcinomas
  - Carcinoid tumor
  - Malignant carcinoid tumor (atypical carcinoid)
  - Small cell carcinoma undifferentiated neuroendocrine carcinoma
- Peripheral nerve sheath tumors (schwannoma, neurilemoma, and malignant peripheral nerve sheath tumors)
- Paragangliomas
- Merkel cell carcinoma
- Others

follicular epithelium, as well as parathyroid glands. Gland-forming tumors are termed adenocarcinomas. It should be noted that surface squamous epithelium is capable of differentiating along glandular cell lines so that gland-forming malignancies (i.e., adenocarcinomas) may originate from a squamous epithelium (2).

In addition to being rich in epithelial structures, the head and neck also contain abundant nonepithelial structures. These nonepithelial components include bone, cartilage, muscle (skeletal and smooth), nerves, vascular channels, and lymphoid structures. Any one of these nonepithelial or mesenchymal structures may give rise to a malignant tumor. In general, malignant tumors of nonepithelial or mesenchymal structures are called sarcomas. The exception to this categorization would be lymphoproliferative tumors, which are called lymphomas. Finally, the head and neck contain neuroectodermal (peripheral and central) elements including melanocytes, neuroendocrine cells, Schwann cells, paraganglia, and olfactory neuroepithelial cells, any one of which may give rise to malignant tumors, such as malignant melanomas, neuroendocrine carcinomas, malignant peripheral nerve sheath tumors, malignant paragangliomas, and olfactory neuroblastomas.

The discussion on terminology would not be complete without detailing the alterations of the surface epithelium that may represent the precursor change(s) heralding the malignant transformation of that epithelial structure. Refer to the appropriate section under "Field Cancerization" later in the chapter for a discussion of this subject.

TABLE 2.3 Classification of Mesenchymal Malignancies of the Head and Neck

Soft tissue
- Lymphoproliferative
  - Malignant lymphomas (Non-Hodgkin and Hodgkin)
- Skeletal muscle
  - Rhabdomyosarcoma

Nerve
- Malignant peripheral nerve sheath tumors
- Vascular/Lymphatic
  - Angiosarcoma
  - Malignant hemangioendothelioma
  - Kaposi sarcoma
  - Hemangiopericytoma
- Smooth muscle
  - Leiomyosarcoma
- Fibrous tissue
  - Fibrosarcoma
  - Malignant fibrous histiocytoma
- Notochord cell remnant
  - Chordoma
- Undefined mesenchymal cell
  - Synovial sarcoma
  - Alveolar soft part sarcoma

Matrix-producing malignancies
- Bone
  - Osteosarcoma
- Cartilage
  - Chondrosarcoma
- Odontogenic

TABLE 2.4 Classification of Salivary Gland Malignancies

Epithelial
- Mucoepidermoid carcinoma
- Adenocarcinoma, not otherwise specified:
  - Low grade
  - High grade
- Acinic cell adenocarcinoma
- Adenoid cystic carcinoma
- Polymorphous low-grade adenocarcinoma
- Malignant mixed tumors
- Salivary duct carcinoma
- Basal cell adenocarcinoma
- Epithelial–myoepithelial carcinoma
- Clear cell adenocarcinoma
- Cystadenocarcinoma
- Undifferentiated carcinoma
- Oncocytic carcinoma
- Squamous cell carcinoma
- Sebaceous adenocarcinoma/lymphadenocarcinoma
- Myoepithelial carcinoma
- Adenosquamous carcinoma
- Mucinous adenocarcinoma

Mesenchymal

Malignant lymphomas
- Malignant lymphomas and Hodgkin disease

TABLE 2.5 Classification of Thyroid Gland and Parathyroid Gland Malignancies

Thyroid gland
- Epithelial (follicular cell origin)
  - Follicular carcinoma and variants
  - Papillary carcinoma and variants
  - Anaplastic carcinoma
  - Mucoepidermoid carcinoma
  - Squamous cell carcinoma
- Neuroectodermal (C cell origin)
  - Medullary carcinoma
- Lymphoproliferative
  - Malignant lymphomas (non-Hodgkin and Hodgkin disease)
- Mesenchymal
  - Angiosarcoma
  - Leiomyosarcoma
  - Malignant peripheral nerve sheath tumors
  - Others

Parathyroid gland
- Parathyroid carcinoma

Histologic Differentiation and Grade

The more a tumor recapitulates the appearance of the cell or tissue layer from which it arises, the better differentiated it is. This definition applies to virtually all malignant tumors, and perhaps it is most applicable to squamous epithelial tumors. A well-differentiated squamous carcinoma is one that has obvious keratinization and intercellular bridges. The keratinization appears as layered acellular eosinophilic material or appears within the cytoplasm of the cell as "glassy" eosinophilic deposits. Intercellular bridges are best viewed under oil immersion magnification but can be seen on high magnification as very thin lines lying in between (outside) the cells and connecting these cells to each other (Fig. 2.1). As a tumor becomes less differentiated, it "loses" its histologic similarities to its cell of origin. A poorly differentiated squamous carcinoma has little, if any, keratinization and the presence of intercellular bridges becomes less distinct or absent (Fig. 2.2). In this setting, direct derivation from the surface epithelium or the overall growth pattern assist in defining this tumor as a SCC. The same definitions of differentiation apply to gland-forming malignant tumors (adenocarcinomas) and to mesenchymal malignant tumors.

The phenotypic extreme on the poorly differentiated end of the spectrum may result in a "dedifferentiated" or "undifferentiated" tumor that loses its light microscopic similarities to its cell of origin. It is this type of neoplasm that often necessitates special pathologic studies (e.g., immunohistochemistry) to determine its histogenesis. A common example of this in head and neck sites is the spindle cell squamous carcinoma. This high-grade variant of squamous carcinoma is characterized by the presence of a malignant spindle cell neoplastic infiltrate. The malignant spindle cells are devoid of keratinization and intercellular bridges. The histologic appearance of the spindle-shaped cells, the growth pattern including interconnecting and ramifying fascicles, and the absence of squamous epithelial features, simulate the appearance of several malignant mesenchymal neoplasms, hence earlier terminology of these tumors as carcinosarcomas and sarcomatoid carcinomas. Immunohistochemistry plays an important role in defining this tumor and assisting in the final diagnosis. In the majority of cases, spindle cell squamous carcinomas will be cytokeratin-positive. However, in addition to losing its phenotypic characteristics, tumors that are poorly differentiated may also lose their genotypic markers (i.e., epitopes), resulting in false-negative immunohistochemical findings. In the situation of spindle cell squamous carcinomas, immunohistochemical markers of epithelial differentiation may not be present, yet this tumor is still epithelial in origin (see "Spindle Cell Squamous Carcinoma" later in the chapter).

The histologic grade of a tumor is dependent on its differentiation. The better differentiated a tumor is, the lower its histo-

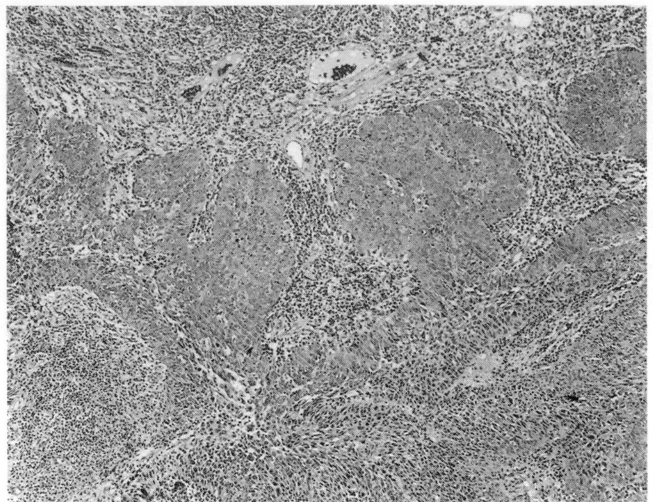

Figure 2.2 Poorly differentiated squamous cell carcinoma. In contrast to Figure 2.1, the invasive neoplasm seen here lacks evidence of squamous differentiation (e.g., keratinization or intercellular bridges). However, the overall growth pattern is one that is seen in association with squamous cell carcinomas. Although not shown in this illustration, this neoplasm was identified as arising from the surface epithelium establishing its diagnosis as a squamous cell carcinoma.

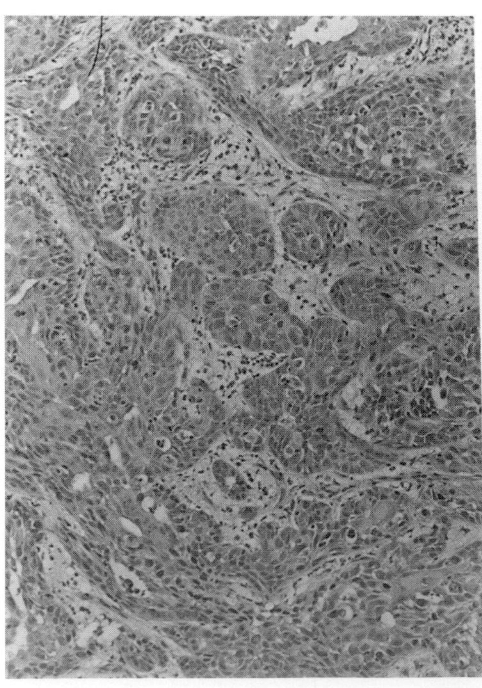

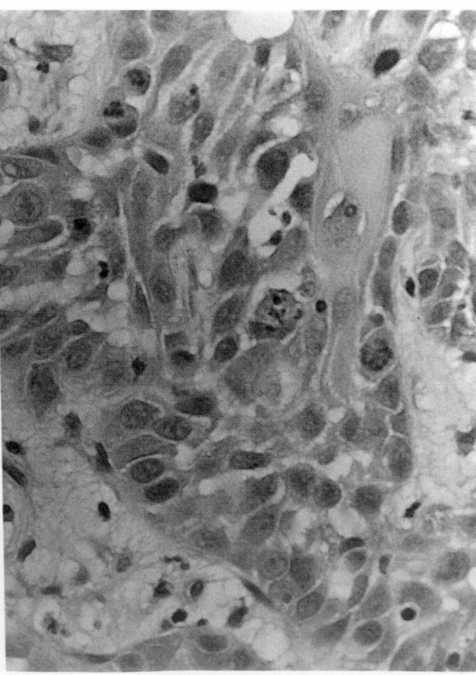

Figure 2.1 Well-differentiated squamous cell carcinoma. This tumor is invasive and is associated foci of individual cell keratinization (**left**) and intercellular bridges (**right**).

logic grade. A well-differentiated SCC is considered grade I, whereas a poorly differentiated SCC is a grade III. It stands to reason that better differentiated tumors tend to be DNA diploid or near DNA diploid with a lower cell proliferation rate (doubling time) and less likelihood of having aggressive behavior (locoregional recurrence or metastasis) in comparison to less differentiated or anaplastic tumors (3). This is not universally true. The extent and depth of invasion, and perhaps metastatic potential, may have no bearing on the histologic grade of a tumor, so that a histologic grade I SCC can be a high clinical grade cancer whereas a histologic grade III SCC may be a low clinical grade cancer. Nevertheless, prognostic correlation has been shown between histologic grade and clinical stage of SCCs of the UADT (3–8). In a multivariate analysis, Wiernik et al. (3) showed that tumor grading was an independent significant factor in the prediction of prognosis. These authors evaluated 1,315 patients with laryngeal SCC followed for a 10-year period and showed a highly significant difference between the survival and tumor-free rates for those with well-differentiated laryngeal SCC versus patients with anaplastic cancers, with the former having a better outcome than the latter (3).

Adjunct Tools in the Diagnosis of Head and Neck Tumors

As described earlier, the more a tumor recapitulates the appearance of its cell of origin, the better differentiated that tumor will be. Specific phenotypic characteristics for a given tumor, as seen by light microscopy, may immediately define that tumor type. For the pathologist, the light microscopic features of a malignant tumor that includes origin from the surface epithelium with the formation of keratin and intercellular bridges define a SCC. Given these features, the pathologist does not need to employ additional studies in determining the histogenesis of that tumor. Other examples may include a gland-forming tumor (adenocarcinoma), a melanin-rich malignant tumor (malignant melanoma), a tumor that is forming bone (osteosarcoma), and so on. However, not infrequently, the histogenesis of a malignant neoplasm is not readily apparent by light microscopy. The fact that the tumor is malignant may not be in dispute, but due to the absence of differentiation (undifferentiation), the histogenesis of the tumor becomes a guessing game. This is problematic to the surgical pathologist who wishes to categorize a tumor by its cell of origin. More important, the exact tumor type may require specific treatment protocols and have specific prognostic relevance. It is under these circumstances that the pathologist will use additional studies to determine the histogenesis of a given tumor, and therefore establish the correct diagnosis. Included among these studies are relatively simple tools such as histochemistry, immunohistochemistry, and electron microscopy, to more sophisticated modalities such as flow cytometry, cytogenetics, *in situ* hybridization, polymerase chain reaction, and other molecular biologic techniques.

HISTOCHEMISTRY

Through the understanding of biochemistry, histochemical techniques have been devised to clarify the chemical composition of a given pathologic lesion. Currently, there are numerous stains that the pathologist can use in the identification of various chemicals, as well as microorganisms. Examples include stains that will evaluate for the presence of carbohydrates or sugar residues such as the various mucins, stains for connective tissue components (cells, fibers, and ground substance), stains for pigments and minerals such as melanin, iron, lipofuscin, argentaffin and argyrophil granules, and stains for microorganisms. The results of these stains can be of critical importance in the diagnosis and differential diagnosis of a malignant tumor. An example of the application of histochemistry to the surgical pathology of malignant neoplasms could include an undifferentiated malignant neoplasm. The presence of positive staining with epithelial mucin stains may assist in the diagnosis of an adenocarcinoma. The absence of staining with epithelial mucin but positive staining with melanin stains (Fontana) may then indicate that the undifferentiated malignant neoplasm represents a (mucosal) malignant melanoma. Alternatively, an undifferentiated malignant neoplasm in the sinonasal tract that failed to stain with epithelial mucin or melanin stains but does stain with Bodian silver stain for neural fibers may then represent an olfactory neuroblastoma. As will be discussed in the following section, the presence of a specific immunohistochemical marker is not necessarily diagnostic for a specific tumor type as, to the consternation of surgical pathologists, there is much overlap in the staining characteristics of histogenetically different tumors. Refer to histotechnology manuals for a more in-depth discussion (9).

IMMUNOHISTOCHEMISTRY

Immunohistochemistry is the application of an immunologic procedure (antigen–antibody reaction) allowing for the recognition of intracellular molecular components (antigens) by light microscopic evaluation. The staining procedure involves the binding of a commercially prepared monoclonal antibody to an antigen located in the cell surface, within the cytoplasm or in the nucleus. The detection of the primary antibody is done by using a "secondary" antibody that is species-specific for the "primary" antibody. The visualization of the immunologic reaction involves the use of horseradish peroxidase or avidin–biotin complex (ABC method), and a chromogenic enzyme (usually diaminobenzidine) or a fluorescent label. Numerous antibodies are available that are developed against tumor antigens (thyroglobulin, leukocyte common antigen, prostate specific antigen, prostatic acid phosphatase, others), intracytoplasmic cellular components (intermediate filaments, neurosecretory granules, others), hormones (pituitary hormones, pancreatic polypeptide hormones, others), and microbiologic agents (herpes, cytomegalovirus, human immunodeficiency virus, others). The list of immunohistochemical markers and their diagnostic use is too numerous to be included. Table 2.6 lists a selection of immunohistochemical markers and their use in diagnostic surgical pathology. Fresh tissue is optimal for immunohistochemical studies. However, in most instances immunohistochemistry can be performed on formalin-fixed, paraffin-embedded tissue, including archival material. More recently, the development of the microwave technique has enhanced the ability to perform immunohistochemistry on archival material (10). In general, immunohistochemical staining takes from 2 to 3 days to complete and costs vary from approximately $50 to $100 per antibody to several hundred dollars for a fixed panel of antibodies. Immunohistochemistry has tremendous use and has largely supplanted electron microscopy as a diagnostic tool. The reasons for this are many, but two of the most significant are:

1. Less sampling problems as immunohistochemistry allows for the use of a more representative amount of tissue rather than the limited sampling constraints of ultrastructural analysis
2. Ultrastructural study requires special fixatives (e.g., gluteraldehyde) and the use of an electron microscope whereas immunohistochemistry only requires a light microscope.

TABLE 2.6 Immunohistochemical Stains

Cell type	Tumor	Stain
Epithelial	Papillomas, adenomas, carcinomas (squamous cell carcinoma, basal cell carcinoma, adenocarcinoma)	Cytokeratin, epithelial membrane protein (EMA); carcinoembryonic antigen (CEA) in adenocarcinomas and cutaneous adnexal tumors
Mucoserous cells of salivary gland	Benign mixed tumor, carcinomas	Cytokeratin, EMA
Myoepithelial cells	Benign mixed tumor, selected carcinoma with myoepithelial differentiation	Cytokeratin, EMA, CEA, S-100 protein, vimentin, calponin, muscle-specific actin, desmin, glial fibrillary acidic protein (GFAP), p63
Melanocytes	Malignant melanoma	S-100 protein, HMB-45, melan-A
Hematolymphoid cells:		
1. Lymphocytes, histiocytes	1. Non-Hodgkin malignant lymphomas	1. Leukocyte common antigen (LCA or CD45); lineage cell markers (B = L26 or CD20; T cell = UCHL-1 or CD45RO; CD3)
2. Plasma cells	2. Plasmacytomas	2. Monoclonal immunoglobulin light or heavy chains; plasma cell-associated antigens (PCA, PC, CD38); EMA
3. Langerhans histiocytes	3. Langerhans cell histiocytosis (e.g., eosinophilic granuloma)	3. S-100 protein; CD-1a
Neuroendocrine cells:	Neuroendocrine tumors:	
1. Paranglial cells	1. Paraganglioma	1a. Chief cells—chromogranin 1b. Sustentacular cells—S-100 protein
2. Neuroendocrine cells	2. Neuroendocrine carcinomas (carcinoid; malignant carcinoid; small cell carcinoma)	2. Chromogranin, synaptophysin, cytokeratin, neuron-specific enolase (NSE), S-100 protein, neurofibrillary protein; others
3. Merkel cells	3. Merkel cell carcinoma	3. Cytokeratin, including CK20; chromogranin; synaptophysin
Anterior pituitary	Pituitary adenoma, carcinoma	Cytokeratin, chromogranin, synaptophysin, NSE, S-100 protein, one or more pituitary peptide hormones (corticotropin, thyroid-stimulating hormone, growth hormone, luteinizing hormone, follicle-stimulating hormone, prolactin)
Thyroid follicular epithelium	Follicular adenoma, follicular carcinoma, papillary carcinoma	Thyroglobulin, thyroid transciption factor-1 (TTF-1), cytokeratin
Thyroid C-cell	Medullary carcinoma	Calcitonin, chromogranin, synaptophysin, CEA, TTF-1
Neural (Schwann cell)	Benign and malignant peripheral nerve sheath tumors, granular cell tumor	S-100 protein; GFAP; Leu-7 (CD57)
Skeletal muscle	Rhabdomyoma, rhabdomyosarcoma	Desmin, myoglobin, MyoD1, vimentin
Smooth muscle	Leiomyoma, leiomyosarcoma	Actins (muscle-specific and smooth muscle), desmin, caldesmon, vimentin
Adipose tissue	Lipomas, liposarcomas	Vimentin, S-100 protein
Endothelial cells	Vascular tumors (hemangioma, angiosarcoma)	Factor VIII-related protein, ulex europaeus, CD31, CD34
Chondrocytes	Chondromas; chondrosarcomas	S-100 protein; vimentin

This table is a partial listing of immunohistochemical stains.

Perhaps the greatest use of immunohistochemistry is its role in the differential diagnosis of an undifferentiated malignant neoplasm (Fig. 2.3), attempting to identify the origin of a metastatic malignant tumor or determining the histogenesis of a given malignant neoplasm. Included among the latter determinations would be separating B-cell lineage lymphomas from T-cell lineage lymphomas.

Based on the light microscopic appearance of a tumor, a panel of antibodies is used and algorithms followed in the differential diagnosis of a given neoplasm. It should be noted that there are only a very few tumor specific markers including thyroglobulin for thyroid follicular cell origin and prostate specific antigen or prostatic acid phosphatase for prostatic origin. As such, immunohistochemical reactivity alone is often not diagnostic but requires correlation with the clinical history, light microscopic features, and histochemical findings to arrive at the correct diagnosis. The use of controls in immunohistochemistry is critical to proper interpretation of the stains. A positive control indicates that the tissue being analyzed contains the antigen in question resulting in a positive immunohistochemical reaction. A negative control indicates that the tissue being analyzed does not contain the antigen in question, and there should be no immunoreactivity.

ELECTRON MICROSCOPY

The role of electron microscopy in diagnostic surgical pathology has waned since the advent of immunohistochemistry. Currently, ultrastructural evaluation plays a limited role in tumor diagnosis but is still used in those cases where light microscopy and immunohistochemistry may not provide the definitive answer as to the tumor type. More recently, the techniques of immunohistochemistry and electron microscopy have been wed to offer the best of both worlds.

FLOW CYTOMETRY, IMAGE ANALYSIS, AND CYTOGENETICS

Flow cytometry and image analysis attempt to quantitate relative DNA content distributions in tumors and, thereby, attempt to assess at the cellular level the potential biologic behavior of a given tumor (11,12). For flow cytometric measurement of DNA content (DNA ploidy), cell suspensions made by disaggregating solid tissue or paraffin-embedded tissue sections, fine-needle aspirates, or body fluids are used and passed ("flowed") in a linear stream through a laser beam for analysis. The light scatter emitted from the intrinsic cell qualities or fluorescent emissions from applied fluorochrome-labeled markers are detected by light sensors that convert the scatter or emissions into elec-

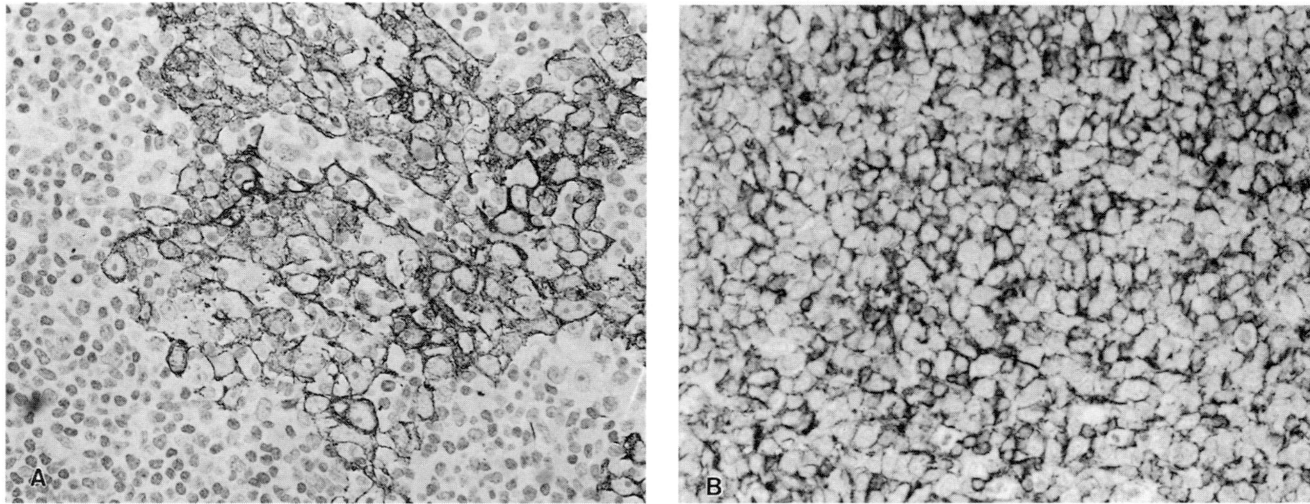

Figure 2.3 Immunohistochemical stains used in differentiating histomorphologically similar appearing undifferentiated nasopharyngeal neoplasms. **A:** The neoplastic cells react with cytokeratin confirming a diagnosis of nasopharyngeal undifferentiated carcinoma. Note the surrounding benign lymphocytes are nonreactive. **B:** The neoplastic cells react with leucocyte common antigen confirming a diagnosis of malignant lymphoma. This lymphoma was of B-cell origin as confirmed by immunoreactivity with B-cell specific antigens (not shown).

trical impulses. The latter are digitized and stored in a computer for data analysis using software programs. This analysis, resulting from the evaluation of thousands of cells per minute and consisting of up to 20,000 cell events, includes DNA histograms that relate to three phases of the cell cycle:

1. Resting G0 and cycling G1 phases that in a normal human cell population correspond to the amount of DNA in the 46 human chromosomes (designated 2C)
2. Synthetic (S) phase representing the doubling time of a given cell population
3. G2 and mitotic (M) phases that have twice the DNA content as the G0 and G1 cells (designated 4C for the double copy or tetraploid chromosome complement).

The S phase and G2 and M phases correspond to the proliferative fraction of cells in the population sampled. In this way, differences in DNA content from the normal diploid complement of chromosomes can be established in a given neoplasm and are expressed as the DNA index (13). A DNA index of 1 in a tumor would represent no detectable change in the DNA content from normal cells and would be a DNA diploid tumor. Abnormal changes in the DNA index of a tumor (DNA aneuploidy) include such changes as a DNA index of 2 (tetraploidy) or may also represent a loss of genetic material (DNA hypoploidy) resulting in a DNA index less than 1.

Flow cytometry has been extensively used for hematopoietic malignancies but has also been used for solid tumors, including head and neck malignancies (14–20). In general, these studies show that increased recurrence rates, shorter relapse times, distant metastasis, and shorter survival rates are present in those HNSCC with high DNA indices, high percent S-phase fraction, high proliferation rates, and DNA aneuploid tumors. The flow cytometric analysis of HNSCC needs to be viewed with caution. It might stand to reason that all DNA diploid tumors are benign or, at worst, are indolent neoplasms responding well to treatment while all DNA aneuploid tumors are malignant and aggressive neoplasms with poor response to treatment. In many instances these generalizations are true, but there are exceptions including DNA diploid tumors that had a bad clinical outcome (21), DNA aneuploid tumors that had a better prognosis than DNA diploid tumors (22), and tumors that are benign by light microscopic parameters with excellent long-term follow-up but proved to be DNA aneuploid (23). Therefore, the specificity and sensitivity of the DNA content of a given head and neck tumor as determined by flow cytometry is questionable, and it is apparent that the DNA content may not be an absolute criterion for benignancy or malignancy.

In image analysis or morphometry, light microscopic measurements are made on cells following cytologic preparation, touch imprints of tumors, or nuclear disaggregation from paraffin-embedded tissues. A microscopic image is captured by a video camera, digitized, and stored in a computer and, using computer software, is analyzed. Morphometric analysis is done on cell nuclei or on the cell itself examining quantitative measurements such as nuclear size, nuclear shape, cell volume, number of mitoses per unit area, and DNA content (24,25). Compared with flow cytometry, the histograms generated by image analysis are based on much fewer cell events and therefore are more unreliable. The advantage of image analysis is its ability to morphologic classification and to identify rare cell events. Morphometric analysis has been used to assess nuclear atypia and squamous intraepithelial neoplasias of the UADT (26–28). Using both flow cytometry and image analysis has distinct advantageous over using these studies independently. Further, both of these techniques have been used in conjunction with cell proliferation markers in the evaluation of proliferative capacity and biologic potential of various head and neck cancers (16,29).

Cytogenetic analysis allows for the detection of clonal chromosomal aberrations, many of which may be diagnostic for a particular tumor type. The value of cytogenetic evaluation in head and neck epithelial malignancies is of questionable use. However, evaluation of specific chromosomal abnormalities may be extremely valuable in the diagnosis of undifferentiated small round cell malignancies and in soft tissue tumors (30). In spite of the loss of differentiation in a neoplasm that may not be detectable by immunohistochemical or ultrastructural analysis, the characteristic chromosomal aberrations in these tumors appear to be retained and are critical in maintaining neoplastic transformation of that neoplasm (30). The characteristic cytogenetic aberrations of undifferentiated small round cell malignancies and soft tissue tumors (benign and malignant) are detailed elsewhere (30). For cytogenetic evaluation fresh, viable tumor should be taken and processed immediately in sterile tissue culture medium or in a physiologic buffer (e.g., RPMI or Hank's buffered salt solution). To prevent microbiologic contamination the tumor specimen should be taken using sterile equipment. It is imperative that viable tumor be sampled and that necrotic tumor or nonneoplastic tissue be excluded or only minimally sampled to increase the success of the cytogenetic analysis (30). The latter is less dependent on the amount of tumor sampled than on the quality of the tumor specimen such that cytogenetic evaluation can be performed from needle biopsies (30).

FINE-NEEDLE ASPIRATION BIOPSY

Fine-needle aspiration biopsy (FNAB) is a safe, inexpensive, rapid, and accurate procedure in the evaluation of almost any mass lesion. In the head and neck, FNAB is extensively used. The accessibility of the neck, salivary glands, thyroid gland, and orbit makes FNAB of lesions of these structures very practical. FNAB should be viewed as the initial procedure used in the assessment of a head and neck mass but it should not be the sole determinant by which a major operative resection is performed. FNAB is an invaluable diagnostic modality in the evaluation of a mass in the head and neck providing cytologic diagnosis that assists the clinician in the appropriate management of the patient. Touch-imprint cytology represents the pressing or "touching" of a microscopic slide against the cut surface of a tissue specimen followed by immediate fixation and staining. Imprint cytology may be especially helpful in the diagnosis of hematolymphoid lesions, in the evaluation of small biopsy specimens, or in biopsy material that is distorted or crushed. Several studies have found that touch-imprint cytology is as sensitive and perhaps more reliable than frozen section in the detection of micrometastases, especially in fatty lymph nodes that may be difficult to cut (31–33). Further, on-site assessment by a pathologist or in the frame of an FNAB clinic reduces the false-negative diagnosis and inadequacy rates, and increases the cost-effectiveness of FNAB (34,35).

For details on the technique of FNAB, refer to more comprehensive texts of cytopathology. The following sections provide a brief overview of FNAB of the specific anatomic sites of the head and neck.

Neck Mass

FNAB is a useful tool in the evaluation of a neck mass. The causes of neck masses or enlarged cervical lymph nodes are many, including reactive lymphadenopathies, infectious and granulomatous lymphadenitis, primary neoplasms (non-Hodgkin and Hodgkin lymphomas), and metastatic tumors (Fig. 2.4). In several reported studies that included a large number of cases, 25% to 60% of the aspirated enlarged lymph nodes showed reactive changes that were subsequently confirmed to be benign by either excisional biopsy or by close clinical follow-up of the patients who had benign clinical outcomes (36–40). In patients with known primary malignancies originating elsewhere or suspected of metastatic disease to cervical lymph nodes, FNAB is an extremely useful diagnostic tool, as the presence of nonlymphoid neoplastic cells are readily identifiable (41). In several series of FNAB of lymph nodes, metastatic cancer represented approximately 50% of the reported cases (36–40).

The diagnostic accuracy rate for FNAB diagnosis of non-Hodgkin malignant lymphoma ranges from 83% to 94% (40,42) whereas that for Hodgkin disease is from 83% to 98% (43,44).

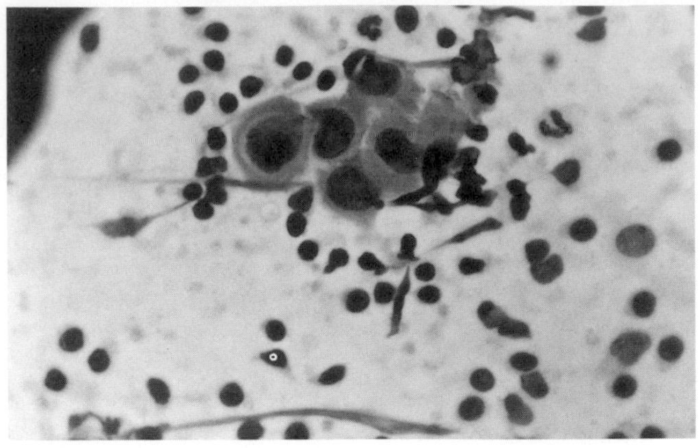

Figure 2.4 Fine-needle aspiration biopsy of a neck mass (lateral cervical lymph node) showing malignant cells with squamous features diagnostic for metastatic squamous cell carcinoma. Panendoscopic evaluation and biopsy identified the primary cancer to be of (ipsilateral) tonsillar origin.

Fine-needle aspiration biopsy findings in conjunction with flow cytometry or immunohistochemistry enables the subclassification of many non-Hodgkin lymphomas (45,46). Fine-needle aspiration biopsy can also be used in separating low-grade from high-grade non-Hodgkin malignant lymphoma. In a study by Russell and et al. (47), the authors had difficulty distinguishing among the low-grade malignant lymphomas but had no difficulty separating the low-grade from the high-grade malignant lymphomas by FNAB. Although the diagnostic accuracy for Hodgkin disease is high, the accuracy for subtyping the Hodgkin lymphoma is not, reported in one study to be 58% (46). A cytologic specimen cannot provide certain details relative to malignant lymphomas, including the architectural growth (i.e., follicular vs. diffuse), and it is very difficult to subtype Hodgkin disease by FNAB (46). Therefore, a presumptive diagnosis in an enlarged lymph node of malignant lymphoma made by FNAB should be followed by excisional biopsy with histopathologic evaluation. The excised lymph node should include the largest identifiable node to allow for histopathologic evaluation, as well as for immunohistochemical and molecular biologic studies. In general, the diagnostic accuracy for the presence of a tumor (sensitivity) and for the absence of a tumor (specificity) in lymph nodes is high ranging, from 87% to 100% and 88% to 98%, respectively (40,42,48).

Salivary Glands

Innumerable causes can contribute to enlargement of a salivary gland. These include many nonneoplastic and neoplastic (benign and malignant) proliferations. By far, the most common salivary gland tumor is a benign mixed tumor (pleomorphic adenoma). Therefore, the diagnostic accuracy of a salivary gland tumor is usually high. The diagnostic accuracy of FNAB of salivary gland tumors has been reported to include a sensitivity of 92%, specificity of 100%, and accuracy of 98% (49).

In general, the diagnosis of most salivary gland tumors by FNAB can be readily accomplished. However, a diagnosis by FNAB of certain specific salivary gland tumors, such as adenoid cystic carcinoma, low-grade polymorphous adenocarcinomas, and others, should be made with extreme caution. The cytologic features seen in these tumors can also be identified in benign mixed tumors. Further, it should be noted that when the differentiation of a benign from a malignant salivary gland tumor is based on the presence or absence of invasive growth, and not on the cytologic appearance, FNAB will not generate this information. It could be argued that any mass lesion of the salivary gland will ultimately require surgical intervention obviating the need for FNAB. Nevertheless, FNAB remains an excellent screening tool for salivary gland tumors more often than not, yielding enough information to guide the surgeon in his or her therapeutic approach. Despite the potential limitations of FNAB in the diagnosis of salivary gland tumors, it still remains an accurate diagnostic tool, quite comparable to frozen-section diagnosis (50,51).

Thyroid Gland

As with salivary gland tumors, the thyroid gland is readily accessible so FNAB has a very practical use with thyroid gland lesions. FNAB of the thyroid represents the first-line diagnostic procedure in the evaluation of a patient with a thyroid mass. The main purpose of thyroid gland FNAB is to distinguish between patients with benign nonneoplastic thyroid nodules that can be followed clinically from patients with a neoplasm (benign or malignant) that require surgical intervention (52). Not all solitary lesions of the thyroid require surgical intervention. FNAB may then offer the necessary diagnostic information for those thyroid lesions that can be nonsurgically monitored as compared with those that do require surgical removal (53). The diagnostic accuracy of thyroid FNAB is well established. The ability of thyroid FNAB to yield a positive aspirate in the presence of a neoplasm (sensitivity) (Fig. 2.5) and to be negative in the absence of a neoplasm (specificity) is high, reported in several large series to be more than 90% (53–56). Ultrasound-guided FNAB with on-site evaluation can increase the sensitivity and specificity of thyroid FNAB in lesions that are difficult to palpate (57). Of note, approximately 2% to 15% of smears are unsatisfactory for evaluation (58). In satisfactory smears, a thyroid tumor is diagnosed as benign in more than 60% of cases, malignant in approximately 5% of cases, and suspicious in the remainder of cases (52). Of the suspicious cases, approximately 20% followed by surgery will prove to be malignant (58). The accuracy of thyroid FNAB compares favorably to that of frozen-section diagnosis (59–61). In a study of 359 patients with thyroid nodules evaluated by FNAB and frozen section, Hamburger and Hamburger (62) report that in less than 1% of patients (3 cases) frozen section influenced the surgical procedure.

Similar to the challenges faced by the cytopathologist with FNAB of salivary glands, there are diagnostic limitations of thyroid gland FNAB, including those thyroid lesions in which the differentiation of a benign tumor from a malignant tumor is not predicated on the cytologic appearance but requires the identification of capsular or vascular invasion (i.e., follicular adenomas vs. follicular carcinomas). In this situation, cytology alone is not diagnostic and FNAB does not allow for this determination. It should be noted that oxyphilic changes (so-called Hürthle cells) represent a descriptive term and are not diagnostic for any specific thyroid lesion. Numerous thyroid lesions contain Hürthle cells including lymphocytic thyroiditis, adenomatoid nodules, follicular adenomas, follicular carcinomas, papillary carcinoma, and medullary carcinoma. Therefore, the presence of Hürthle cells on the FNAB of a thyroid lesion is not, in and of itself, diagnostic. Despite these potential limitations, FNAB is accurate in the diagnosis of thyroid tumors. Pathologic alterations seen in permanent sections of resected thyroid lesions following FNAB may result in worrisome histologic features that may be mistaken for malignant neoplasm (63,64). The post-FNA histologic changes occur in numerous lesions such as adenomatoid nodules, follicular adenoma and its variants, follicular carcinoma and its variants, papillary carcinoma and its variants, and hyperplastic lesions. Based on the type of reaction seen, post-FNA alterations may include acute or chronic type changes (65). Acute changes are usually identified within 3 weeks from the FNA to surgical removal and may include hemorrhage with hemosiderin-laden macrophages and granulation tissue (these represent the most common findings), localized follicular destruction, capsular alterations, atypical cytologic features with necrosis and mitoses, and nuclear atypia that typically occurs near the needle tract and includes nuclear enlargement with clearing of the nuclear chromatin. Chronic changes are usually identified more than 3 weeks from the FNAB to surgical removal and may include squamous or oxyphilic metaplasia, infarction, capsular alterations with foci of pseudoinvasive growth, vascular alterations, including artifactual implantation or "invasion" of tumor cells, dilated vascular spaces with thrombosis, organization, and papillary endothelial hyperplasia and endothelial cell atypia (65,66). Additional changes may include cyst formation with papillary growth, fibrosis, calcifications, and cholesterol granulomas. Oxyphilic cells occurring in all settings (metaplasia, follicular adenoma, follicular carcinoma, or papillary carcinoma) may be more sensitive to trauma due to the oxygen-sensitive mitochondria that predominate in these cells. Any compromise to the oxygen supply of the oxyphilic cells may result in degenerative changes, including hemorrhage, infarction, and papillary degeneration.

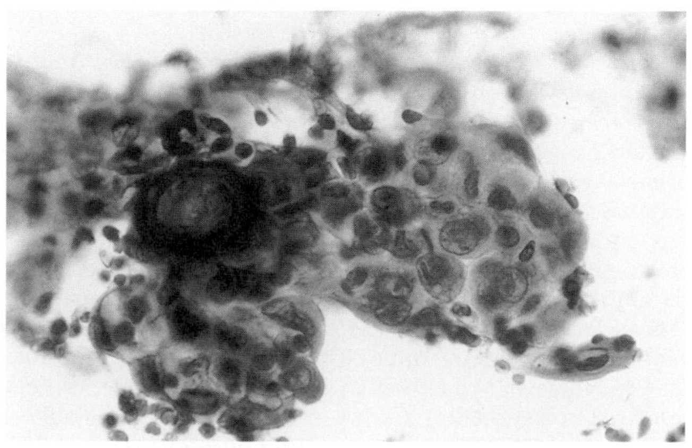

Figure 2.5 Fine-needle aspiration biopsy of a thyroid mass diagnostic for thyroid papillary carcinoma.

Orbital Lesions

Orbital FNAB is an accurate and beneficial procedure in the evaluation of orbital lesions, obviating the need for extensive surgery to arrive at a diagnosis. Orbital FNAB allows for the evaluation of deeply situated unresectable tumors that in the past required extensive surgery to generate material for diagnosis. Kennerdell et al. (67) evaluated 156 orbital lesions by FNAB and reported that 80% contained diagnostic material, 18% were insufficient for evaluation and 2% were either false-positive or false-negative. These authors indicate that insufficient aspirates were the result of a fibrous lesion, a lymphoproliferative process in which there were insufficient cells for diagnosis or an orbital apical location. According to Kennerdell et al. (67), the most common orbital lesions reported in their series were carcinomas (primary and metastatic), lymphoproliferative lesions, and inflammatory diseases. The accuracy of orbital FNAB is high. Char et al. (68), in a study of uveal melanomas, report an 89% positive identification rate. Shields et al., in a series of 159 cases of fine-needle aspiration of intraocular lesions, obtained an 88% adequacy rate, a sensitivity rate of 100%, and a specificity rate of 98% (69). Complications of orbital FNAB may include diffuse retrobulbar hemorrhage, blindness (transient or permanent), globe perforation, and brain-related complications (67). All serious complications occurred due to faulty techniques reaffirming the importance of experience in FNAB.

FROZEN SECTIONS

Frozen section analysis plays an important part in the treatment of the head and neck cancer patient. The appropriate use of intraoperative consultations (frozen sections) usually results in a definitive diagnosis with immediate therapeutic impact while the patient is in the operating room. The accuracy of frozen sections has been analyzed for general surgical cases (70–76), as well as specifically for head and neck surgery (77–83). The studies on general surgical cases and otolaryngologic cases show similar findings with a 95% to 98% diagnostic accuracy rate, a 2% to 4% error rate (including <2% false-negative and <1% false-positive), and less than 4% of cases being deferred for permanent section evaluation. Diagnostic errors may occur due to improper sampling, technical flaws, interpretive inaccuracies, and faulty communication (70,75,76,78,81,82).

Among the determinations made by frozen section analysis are:

- The evaluation of adequacy of surgical margins of resection
- The differentiation between nonneoplastic, benign, and malignant proliferations
- The evaluation of lymph nodes for the presence of metastatic disease
- The determination of specimen identification and specimen adequacy, including the verification of such organs as the parathyroid glands
- The determination of whether a given case requires special diagnostic testing best performed on frozen material, such as for lymphomas.

Arguably, the most common request of the pathologist by the head and neck surgeon at the time of intraoperative consultation is the assessment of the surgical margins. Successful local control of a malignant tumor depends on complete surgical excision of all the disease. There are many factors that impact on the assessment of the surgical margins, including the type of surgical specimen, proper orientation of the specimen, proper sectioning of the specimen, and obviously the correct interpretation of the histopathologic changes. Unfortunately, even in the best situations an intraoperative report of negative margins may be followed a few days later by a permanent section diagnosis of positive margins. Byers et al. (84) reported on the results of frozen section in 216 patients with neoplasms of the oral cavity, oropharynx, and hypopharynx. Three groups were identified, including 68% of the patients in whom the tumors were initially adequately resected on the basis of negative surgical margins, 23% of the patients who had positive surgical margins that necessitated additional surgical resection to assure the presence of negative surgical margins, and the remaining 9% of patients in whom negative-free margins by frozen section could not be obtained (84). The follow-up of these three groups included local recurrence rates of 14.4%, 20% and 80%, respectively, with the third group having the worst survival rates. Byers et al. concluded that the probability of local recurrence in head and neck cancer is reduced when the resection margins are determined by intraoperative frozen-section consultation (84). The use of intraoperative frozen sections will also allow the surgeon to extend the surgical resection without loss of orientation of the operative field, a potential problem when additional surgery is required in a second operation (84). Further, carcinoma remnants that have not been completely removed in the initial operation often are difficult to identify macroscopically, making their removal in a second operation more difficult (85). Spiro et al. (83) report an intraoperative frozen-section diagnostic accuracy of 89% for oral tongue cancer. These authors found that the diagnostic accuracy was the same whether the sample was taken from the patient or from the surgical specimen.

It must be noted that a diagnosis of margin(s) negative for carcinoma by frozen-section analysis does not guarantee complete tumor removal. Limitations include the choice of biopsy sampling sites and the fact that frozen-section results are not always confirmed by permanent sections (85). Ord and Aisner (86) evaluated the accuracy of frozen section in assessing margins in 49 patients with oral cancer resections. They found a frozen-section accuracy rate of 99%; however, 7 patients had final margins that were positive but had not been diagnosed as such at the time of the frozen section. Errors in interpretation and in sampling accounted for these discrepancies. Cooley et al. (87) found five discrepancies in 249 frozen sections of laryngeal SCC in which the frozen diagnosis was negative but the permanent sections revealed dysplasia or carcinoma *in situ*. These authors found that insufficient leveling of the frozen block resulted in these discrepancies. Their recommendation was that in examining margins for laryngeal SCC the frozen-section tissue should be completely sampled by examining several levels at the time of frozen section. Spiro et al. (83) reported that of the 131 samples taken intraoperatively whose margins were reported as negative, 13 were later reported to be positive following permanent sections. Although the frozen-section diagnosis of surgical margins is extremely accurate, they are not entirely reliable in eliminating positive margins in the final diagnostic report.

Another issue relative to the intraoperative histologic evaluation of tumor resection margins is the time factor. The identification of negative surgical margins by frozen section may require a large number of samples. The result of numerous frozen sections in conjunction with the possibility of neck dissection may be the prolongation of surgery. In a prospective study of 24 patients with oral SCC, Bähr and Stoll (85) advocate the removal of the regional lymphatic drainage while the frozen-section examination of the surgical margins is being performed to reduce the time of surgery.

Frozen-section consultations on mucosal surface lesions can be useful especially in differentiating inflammatory and neoplastic lesions. Histologic grading of a mucosal malignancy (i.e., SCC) may be problematic and is not advocated by frozen section. Artifactual distortion and sampling limitations may lead to erroneous conclusions relative to the histologic differentiation of the carcinoma. Postirradiation alterations may lead to false-positive diagnosis due to the presence of bizarre cytologic alterations in the epithelium, minor salivary glands, fibroblasts, skeletal muscle, and endothelial cells (88,89).

A mass lesion of virtually every head and neck anatomic site may initially be viewed by the surgical pathologist at the time of frozen-section consultation. Among the head and neck sites, salivary gland lesions, thyroid gland lesions, parathyroid gland lesions, cervical neck masses, and mucosal-based lesions are often assessed by frozen section. As discussed earlier in the section on FNAB, with the increased use of FNAB, the use of frozen sections, particularly for salivary gland and thyroid gland tumors, has diminished. For frozen-section consultation of head and neck lesions, the reliability in the diagnostic accuracy of salivary gland tumors has been the most questioned (90–94). However in a review of 301 salivary gland lesions evaluated by frozen section, Gnepp et al. (95) report a diagnostic accuracy rate of 98% with an adjusted accuracy rate of 95.7% when deferred diagnosis was included. These authors report that this overall accuracy was comparable to that for other regions of the body (95). Further, Luna indicates that the frozen-section diagnosis of salivary gland tumors "present no more serious problems than do frozen-section diagnoses elsewhere in the body" (96).

Frozen-section evaluation has also been extensively used for thyroid lesions. The lesions that are usually identifiable at frozen section include thyroid papillary carcinoma (conventional types), widely invasive follicular carcinoma, anaplastic carcinoma, and medullary carcinoma. Problems arise in the frozen-section diagnosis of a single encapsulated thyroid mass that has a follicular growth pattern. The differential diagnosis in this setting would include a follicular adenoma, follicular carcinoma, and the follicular variant of thyroid papillary carcinoma. The differentiation of a follicular adenoma from a follicular carcinoma is predicated on the presence or absence of capsular or vascular space invasion. This finding may only be present in a very limited aspect of the tumor. Sampling this area at frozen section would be purely fortuitous as, macroscopically, the invasive foci are not discernible. Thyroid papillary carcinomas in permanent sections often display characteristic ground-glass appearing nuclei, a feature that is usually not present in frozen sections of papillary carcinoma (97). Rosen et al. (98) point out that the relatively low-sensitivity of frozen-section diagnosis of thyroid carcinomas relate to these issues. Kingston et al. (99) report on the role of frozen section in distinguishing benign from malignant thyroid follicular neoplasms. Of 395 cases, 198 had frozen section at the time of surgery. Using the final histologic diagnosis as seen in permanent sections as the gold standard, these authors report that frozen section was accurate in 79% of the cases in differentiating follicular adenoma from follicular carcinoma with a sensitivity of 52% and a specificity of 100%; an incorrect diagnosis of a benign lesion was reported in 21% of the patients (99). Kingston et al. (99) compared the accuracy of frozen-section diagnosis to the accuracy of using clinical factors alone to predict malignancy, including age greater than 50 years, tumor size greater than 3 cm, and a history of previous neck irradiation. These three clinical features were shown by Davis et al. (100) to be strong predictors of malignancy in thyroid follicular neoplasms. Kingston et al. (99) found an equally low sensitivity between frozen section and clinical parameters, ranging from 38% to 53%, in predicting malignancy but that frozen section resulted in a much higher specificity and positive predictive value than any of the clinical parameters. These authors recommend the continued use of frozen section for thyroid follicular lesions as a guide to the required extent of surgery (99).

The frozen-section diagnosis of lymph nodes is considered to be extremely accurate. Gnepp, in a review of the literature, reports that an accuracy rate of 98.9%, excluding deferred diagnoses, with a 0.1% false-positive rate and a 1% false-negative rate (101). It should be noted that the lymph nodes represent the most frequently deferred specimen in frozen-section diagnosis, especially in the diagnosis of a lymphoma. In general, the diagnosis of a carcinoma in a lymph node is not problematic at frozen section. Lymph node frozen section has also been used for accurate staging of the head and neck patient. Rassekh et al. (102) compared intraoperative node examination (palpation and inspection) to frozen-section diagnosis in the identification of metastatic disease to cervical lymph nodes, thereby evaluating the surgeon's ability to predict nodal stage. These authors prospectively studied 108 necks in 79 patients and reported that the overall reliability for intraoperative staging (palpation and inspection) was 59.3% (64 of 108) as compared with 92.3% (24 of 26) for frozen-section biopsy, representing a highly significant difference ($p < 0.005$) (102). Although frozen-section biopsy was not performed on all cases, Rassekh et al. (102) concluded that upstaging the neck without frozen-section biopsy is much less reliable, and that frozen-section biopsy is needed prior to converting a selective node dissection to a radical or modified radical neck dissection. Manni and van den Hoogen (103) reached a similar conclusion.

As with any surgical procedure, there are contraindications for the use of frozen sections. Frozen section consultation should not be used:

- When the frozen-section diagnosis will not have any impact on surgery such as satisfying the curiosity of the surgical team
- If the tissue specimen is small and additional sampling is not planned (in which situation, frozen sections may be equivocal or the material is artifactually distorted by the frozen section technique hampering histologic evaluation following permanent sections)
- For heavily calcified or ossified tissue
- For certain lesions such as small cutaneous melanocytic lesions and lymphoproliferative lesions requiring special handling or extensive histologic evaluation for diagnosis.

Histopathologic Parameters in the Assessment of Head and Neck Tumors

SURGICAL RESECTION MARGINS

The evaluation of surgical margins of resection for the presence or absence of lesional tissue falls under the purview of the surgical pathologist. However, how the specimen is removed and the orientation of the specimen is the responsibility of the surgeon. This is particularly true for those cases in which the tumor is initially excised and the designated margins are separately removed, the tumor is removed in multiple parts, or the specimen is a complex *en bloc* excision requiring proper orientation by the surgeon for those margins that are of critical concern. Once removed and properly oriented, the specimen becomes the responsibility of the surgical pathologist.

In brief, the designated margins are painted with India ink or other similar colored pigments and then sections are submitted for histologic examination. Despite the stringent environment that goes into the processing of tissue, the dye is retained and the pathologist, by microscopic examination, can evaluate the relationship of the tumor to all surgical margins of the resection. Specimens in which no tumor or dysplasia is present at the surgical margins of resection are considered completely excised. "At the margin of resection" means that the neoplastic cells are seen in contact with or lie within millimeters of the pigment that was painted along the margin prior to sectioning (Fig. 2.6). In this situation, the specimen is considered incompletely excised, requiring a wider excision to be assured that all viable tumor cells have been adequately removed.

Some discrepancy can be found in the literature as to what constitutes a positive or negative resection margin. Although some authors only include invasive carcinoma at the margin as positive, excluding carcinoma *in situ*, dysplasia, and gross residual disease (104), most pathologists would agree with the classification of positive margins set forth by Loree and Strong (105). In their review of 398 patients with primary oral cavity carcinoma, Loree and Strong (105) classified positive margins into four categories, including lesional tissue within 0.5 mm of the surgical margin (so-called close margins), dysplastic epithelium at the margin, carcinoma *in situ* at the margin, and invasive carcinoma at the margin. Suffice to say that the evaluation of dysplasia under optimal circumstances can be subjective (see "Field Cancerization" later in the chapter) let alone at the time of frozen-section where tissue distortion and artifact create additional diagnostic difficulties potentially result-

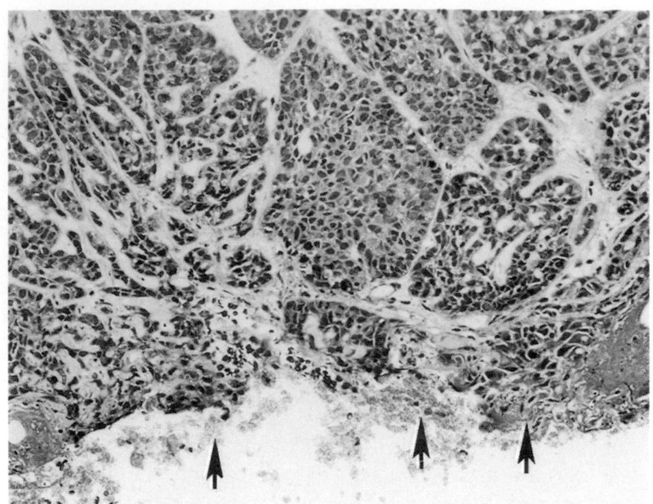

Figure 2.6 This malignant neoplasm is identified in continuity with the edge of the resection margin. The latter, seen at the bottom of the illustration, is delineated by the presence of pigment (*arrowheads*). As such, this tumor is "at the margin of resection" and is incompletely excised.

ing in misdiagnoses, including over diagnosis and under diagnosis.

The presence of lesional tissue within 5 mm of the inked surgical margin, regardless of whether it is invasive carcinoma or carcinoma *in situ*/severe dysplasia, places a patient at a nearly equal risk for local recurrence (106). The question of how wide a tumor should be excised is the responsibility of the surgeon. However, for some specimens such as the laryngeal SCC, free margins up to 2 mm may be sufficient (Fig. 2.7) while for a similar tumor at another site, such as the hypopharynx where submucosal spread may be more of a problem and the oral cavity, wider margins (5–10 mm) are optimal. The incidence of positive surgical margins is quite variable, ranging from as low as 3% (107) in some studies to as high as 60% in other studies (108). Certainly, this variability in "positive surgical margins" is dependent on multiple factors, not the least important of which may be the definition of what constitutes a positive margin.

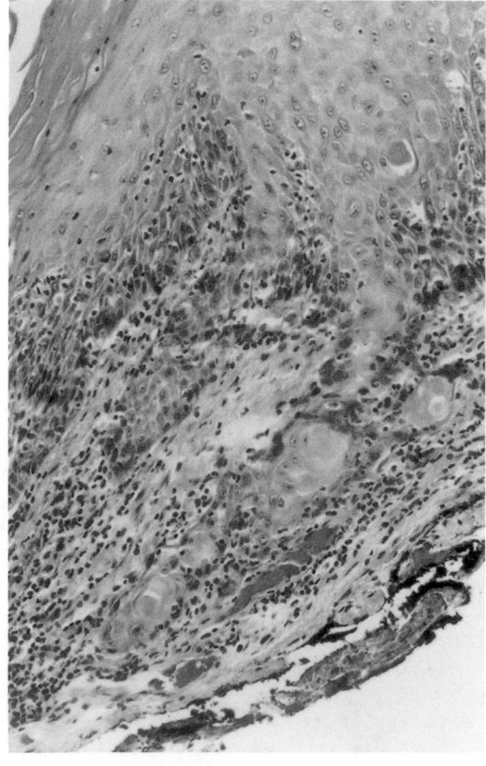

Figure 2.7 Laryngeal squamous cell carcinoma measuring approximately 2 mm from the inked surgical resection margin (bottom).

Jacobs et al. (109) found that of the entry population of 696 patients in their study, 112 patients (16%) with stage III and IV operable tumors had positive surgical margins. These authors indicate that the 16% represented a national average rather than an institutional incidence (109). In comparison to patients with negative margins, patients with positive margins had a significantly higher rate of local failure (21% vs. 9%, $p = 0.0003$) and distant failure (20% vs. 12%, $p = 0.42$) but a similar incidence of regional (nodal) failure (109). Patients with positive surgical margins were most often seen in nonglottic primary cancers and with increasing incidence as the node stage increased. The patients with positive margins had a higher rate of distant metastasis and died more rapidly than patients with positive margins with lower nodal status (109). The survival of the patients with positive margins was approximately one half of that of patients with negative margins. The addition of chemotherapy did not significantly alter the survival of patients with positive margins (109). These authors report a median survival of 19 months in patients with positive margins essentially equating to the expected outcome for patients with inoperable cancer.

Scholl et al. (110) report that in 54 of 268 patients (20.1%) with lingual SCC, the carcinoma was not initially completely removed (i.e., positive margins at frozen section). When additional surgery resulted in negative margins, the local recurrence rate was worse than if the initial margin was negative. These authors also found that positive mucosal margins were more often present in T1 and T2 tumors and positive soft tissue margins were more common in T3 and T4 lesions (110). Looser et al. (107) report that 71% of patients with positive margins had recurrent disease at the primary site compared with 32% of patients with negative margins. Spiro et al. (83) report an intraoperative frozen-section diagnostic accuracy of 89% for oral tongue cancer. These authors report that the diagnostic accuracy was the same whether the sample was taken from the patient or from the surgical specimen. Positive or close margins (within one high power field) were associated with significant increase in local recurrence ($p < 0.003$) (83).

Other studies have shown that implications of a positive surgical margin for SCC of the head and neck are associated with increased local failure and decreased survival rates. Loree and Strong (105) report that the overall local recurrence rate in the group of tumor-positive margins was 36% as compared with 18% for the tumor-negative margin group. Further, these authors showed a statistically significant difference in the 5-year survival rate between the tumor-positive margin patients (52% 5-year survival) as compared with the tumor-negative margin patients (52% 5-year survival). Although postoperative radiotherapy was found to reduce the local recurrence rate in the positive-margin patients, the overall 5-year survival rates between margin-positive and margin-negative patients was not affected by postoperative radiotherapy (105).

An additional factor that impacts on local recurrence is tumor size. The lower the clinical stage or pathologic class the better the ability to achieve local control and the overall better survival rates (84,107). Loree and Strong found the incidence of positive margins was directly proportional to the increasing tumor size (105). Scholl et al., in their evaluation of oral tongue

SCC, indicate in the presence of complete surgical removal of all disease to include macroscopic disease and histologically negative margins without neural invasion that adjunctive therapy does not improve local control as compared with surgery alone (110). In another study, van Es et al. (111) report that for T1 and T2 carcinomas of the mobile tongue and floor of mouth the single most important parameter in determining local recurrence is the histopathologic evaluation of margin status and that other histopathologic parameters are essentially irrelevant in predicting recurrence.

The presence of positive margins does not always translate into failure of local control; however, the overwhelming majority of patients with recurrent disease at the primary site have positive margins. The ability to completely resect a squamous carcinoma of the head and neck weighs heavily in the surgeon's decision to use surgery in the attempt to eradicate the cancer, and the presence of disease (gross or microscopic) at the surgical margins represents a key prognostic feature for patient survival. Batsakis notes that from 5% to 10% of carcinomas resist the surgical goal of clear margins regardless of tumor stage (112). He further notes that the survival of patients with free margins is related to the tumor stage of their carcinoma (112). The identification of negative margins is not a guarantee for the absence of local recurrence. The larynx perhaps is an outlier in regard to positive margins and local recurrence. Compared with extralaryngeal mucosal sites, patients with primary laryngeal SCC with positive surgical margins have a significantly lower incidence of local recurrence. Bauer et al. (113) report that of a total population of 111 patients with laryngeal SCC, 39 (35%) had positive surgical margins. Of these 39 patients, 7 (18%) developed local recurrence while 4 of the remaining 72 patients (6%) with negative margins developed local recurrence (113). These findings suggest that margin status and local recurrence are site-dependent and assists in explaining why surgeons are more apt to accept nearer margins for laryngeal carcinoma (free margins up to 2 mm) but require wider margins (5–10 mm) for carcinomas of extralaryngeal mucosal sites. Among the extralaryngeal sites with significant recurrence rates following negative surgical margin determination are the oral cavity and pharynx, including the hypopharynx (84,107). Intraoral sites with negative margins but significant recurrence rates include the palate, tonsil, buccal mucosa, tongue, gingiva, floor of mouth, and lip (107).

Mucosal margins are not the only tissue margins. Surgical margins of resection may include all soft tissue components including adipose tissue, skeletal muscle, bone, and neural structures. The latter are of particular concern in those tumors that have a propensity for neurotropism, such as adenoid cystic carcinoma of salivary glands. Bone, in particular the osseous margins of resection of the mandibular region, pose an especially significant issue in regard to carcinomas of the alveolar ridge, floor of mouth, lower buccal sulcus, and lower retromolar region. Carcinomas of these sites are among those with the highest rate of recurrence. As such, the evaluation of the mandibular bone for the presence and extent of involvement is a key determinant in patient management (114). The clinical determination of mandibular involvement is not reliable because one third of histologically proven carcinomatous invasion of the mandible show no clinical indication of (preoperative) bone involvement (115). Spread of oral carcinoma to the mandible typically occurs by direct invasion rather than by metastasis, lymph–vascular space spread, or through the nerves. The frozen-section assessment is difficult given the inherent difficulties in performing frozen section on bone. Touch preparations or imprints of the osseous stump can be performed. Evaluation of the nonosseous soft tissue is not a reliable indicator vis-à-vis osseous involvement. In their evaluation of local control of oral and oropharyngeal carcinomas with clinically determined mandibular bone involvement, Dubner and Heller (116) found a 19% recurrence rate following marginal mandibulectomy and 6% following segmental mandibulectomy. In this study local recurrence was not dependent on tumor size, node stage, invasion of the mandible, or radiotherapy. In those patients who recurred following segmental mandibulectomy, the recurrent disease was present within extraosseous soft tissues.

TISSUE SHRINKAGE AND SURGICAL MARGINS

The reliability of measuring the resection margins is impacted by postremoval changes, especially those related to tissue shrinkage. It is obvious that obtaining adequate tumor-free surgical margins is critical for the successful management of the patient with cancer. Any discussion on surgical resection margins would not be complete without a discussion on tissue shrinkage in the pathologic processing of resected tissues. Disparate surgical margin lengths of resected specimens between the *in vivo* measurements by the surgeon and the *in vitro* measurements by the pathologist have been reported for head and neck resection specimens (117,118) and non-head and neck resection specimens (119–122). Johnson et al. (117) found a mean tissue shrinkage of 31% ($p < 0.0001$) from the initial *in situ* measurement by the surgeon to the final microscopic assessment of oral cavity and lingual surface mucosal margins by the pathologist. These authors report that to obtain 5 mm of histopathologically clear margin an *in situ* margin of resection of at least 8 to 10 mm needs to be taken. In their evaluation of oral SCCs, Beaumont and Hains (118) found a reduction of 46% from the planned surgical margin before resection to the microscopically measured margin following pathologic preparation (minimum of 10 mm measured *in situ* surgical margin and average of 5.8 mm following fixation). These authors report significant differences in the longitudinal diameter of the whole specimen from *in situ* to fresh states ($p < 0.0004$) and in the diameter of the tumor from the fresh state to fixed states ($p < 0.0000$) with the most significant shrinkage reported from the fresh state to the fixed state with a mean shrinkage of 4.82 mm. Goldstein et al. (120), in their evaluation of colorectal resection specimens, found that bowel segments shrank to a median length of 3 cm or 40% of their original *in vivo* length after being removed from the patient and left in an unfixed state for 10 to 20 minutes. After formalin fixation the free-floating ends shrank an additional 0.85 cm. Overall, after fixation colon segments shrank 57% of their original *in vivo* length. However, the majority of the tissue shrinkage occurred within the first few minutes after removal of the specimen and only 30% of the tissue shrinkage was attributed to formalin fixation. Similarly, Johnson et al. (117) found that the greatest proportion of shrinkage occurred immediately on resection. Although there are very few studies assessing the shrinkage of tissue margins it is apparent that a significant amount of tissue shrinkage occurs from the moment the tissue is excised to the time the pathologist reviews the histologic preparation of the excised tissues. Such tissue shrinkage should be taken into account and accommodated for by the surgeon at the time of the operation.

MOLECULAR BIOLOGY IN THE ASSESSMENT OF SURGICAL MARGINS ("MOLECULAR MARGINS")

Brennan et al. (123) used molecular biologic markers in assessing histopathologic-negative surgical margins and negative lymph nodes for patients with SCC of the head and neck. In 52% of the patients studied, *p53* mutations were found in the tumor margins that were identified as free of tumor by conventional histologic examination. Mutations of *p53* were found in 21% of the lymph nodes that were negative for tumor by conventional histologic examination. In 38% of the patients with *p53*-positive margins, the tumor recurred locally. The authors concluded that the presence of *p53* mutations in surgical margins and in lymph nodes that were negative for tumor by light microscopic examination portended a substantially higher risk for local recurrent disease than those patients without *p53* mutations in their surgical specimens (123). In their opinion, molecular biologic studies augmented conventional light microscopy in identifying cancer at surgical margins and in lymph nodes, and also may improve the prediction of local tumor recurrence (123). Subsequent to the study by Brennan et al., Ball et al. (124) evaluated *p53* immunostaining of surgical margins in predicting local recurrence of oral and oropharyngeal SCC. These authors found that there was a sample odds ratio test predicting a 5.333 times higher chance of local recurrence in patients with at least one *p53*-positive surgical margin.

When overexpressed in model cell lines, eIF4E is a translation initiation factor and powerful oncogene (125). It has been reported to be elevated in HNSCC but not in benign lesions and its overexpression may represent an early step in malignant transformation (125). Immunohistochemical analysis for eIF4E expression has shown it to be consistently elevated in patients with SCC. In a study by Franklin et al. (125) of laryngeal and hypopharyngeal carcinoma, 92% (12 of 13 cases) of patients with negative eIF4E in histologically negative surgical margins were free of locoregional recurrences whereas 67% (12 of 18 patients) with overexpressed eIF4E in the surgical margins developed recurrences (disease-free interval of 31.95 months). These authors report significant differences in the Kaplan-Meier survival curves for eIF4E-positive and eIF4E-negative margins ($p = 0.0002$).

Batsakis, in a comprehensive review from the pathologist's perspective in the assessment of surgical excision margins in HNSCC, made a number of cogent recommendations (106). He indicated that sole reliance of margins as assessed on the resected specimen should be discouraged and he suggested that, when feasible, the intraoperative evaluation of tissue surrounding the specimen should be made and that should be regarded as the "true margin." The histologic definition of what constitutes a "positive" should be uniformly accepted and applied. Molecular margins as presently constituted have not yet supplanted conventional methods of evaluating surgical resection margins.

Pathologic Tumor, Node, Metastasis System for the Classification of Malignant Tumors

The World Health Organization uses a staging system to describe the anatomic extent of a malignant tumor (126). This assessment of tumor includes three components: T for the extent of the primary tumor; N for the presence or absence of regional lymph node metastasis; and M for the presence or absence of distant metastasis. This classification system includes both clinical and pathologic parameters, and often these parameters will coincide. The following sections will include the pathologic parameters used in the TNM staging system for malignant tumors supplemented by pathologic features not necessarily part of the TNM system but which may impact on prognosis and treatment.

TUMOR SIZE, THICKNESS, AND LOCATION

The TNM system used tumor size (T) to indicate the extent of disease. Lower T staged tumors measure less than 2 cm; intermediate staged tumors measure between 2 and 4 cm; higher staged tumors measure more than 4 cm (126). It is generally considered that the size of a tumor represents an independent variable in its prognosis. Larger tumors (T3 and T4) have been reported to correlate with increased local recurrence as well as with decreased 2- and 5-year survival rates (84). However, larger tumors are not necessarily indicative of a worse prognosis and smaller tumors do not necessarily confer an indolent biologic behavior. Some head and neck tumors, such as in the oral cavity, may have a large surface component (high T stage), but these tumors are only superficially invasive and have a favorable prognosis. Similarly, large tumors of the thyroid gland measuring more than 5 cm may be entirely encapsulated with an associated favorable outcome. Conversely, small head and neck tumors may be deeply invasive and have a poor prognosis despite their small size. Some examples of this phenomenon occur with small cell (oat cell) neuroendocrine carcinomas of the head and neck, extranodal angiocentric T-cell malignant lymphomas of the sinonasal tract, and mucosal malignant melanomas. Therefore, although there is some validity to a larger malignant tumor conveying a worse prognosis, this is not universally true and should not unequivocally be used as an independent variable of prognosis.

The predictive value of tumor thickness or quantitative measurement of depth of invasion has been used for cutaneous malignant melanomas (127,128). A similar quantitation does not apply for mucosal malignant melanomas (129). Studies of SCCs of the UADT have attempted to correlate the extent of invasive cancer with the likelihood of cervical lymph node metastasis or prognosis (130–134). The findings in these studies vary in predicting at what depth of infiltration a SCC is more apt to metastasize. Spiro et al. (130) retrospectively evaluated the predictive value of tumor thickness in T1, T2, and T3 N0 SCCs of the oral tongue and floor of mouth. Tumor thickness greater than 2 mm correlated best with treatment failure, manifested as the presence of regional node metastases in 38% of the patients with tumors greater than 2 mm as compared with 7.5% for tumors ≤2 mm (minimal follow-up of 2 years). These authors concluded that in the N0 patient, tumor thickness greater than 2 mm, regardless of tumor size, merited elective neck dissection. Mohit-Tabatabai et al. (131) found a strong statistical correlation between tumor thickness and regional metastasis. In their study, patients with floor of mouth squamous cancers staged as T1 or T2 and N0 measuring ≤1.5 mm, 1.6 to 3.5 mm, and greater than 3.5 mm had corresponding regional metastases in 2%, 33%, and 60%, respectively (mean follow-up of 69 months) (131). These authors concluded that floor of mouth cancers measuring more than 1.6 mm should have elective neck dissections (131). Other studies of oral cancers have also shown a statistical correlation between the depth of invasion and presence of regional metastasis although the depth of tumor varied in each study. Fakih et al. (135) found that the tumor size cut-off at which nodal recurrence did or did not occur was 4 mm, for Rasgon et al. (136) and Platz et al. (137) the tumor size cut-off was 5 mm. However, there are a number of studies in which a statistical correlation could not be found between tumor thickness and nodal metastasis or prognosis (133,138,139). Karas et al. (134) examined the relationship of tumor thickness as determined in biopsy specimens with the tumor thickness in the final resected specimens in patients with floor of mouth cancers. They found that in biopsy specimens with tumor thickness of ≤1 mm that the tumor thickness in the final specimens would be less than 2 mm ($p = 0.055$), and that tumor thickness greater than 2 mm in the biopsy material measured greater than 3.5 mm in the final specimen ($p = 0.0001$) (134). These authors suggested that the information from the biopsy samples could be extrapolated and correlated to the findings of other investigators who correlated tumor thickness in oral cavity cancers with likelihood of regional metastasis, to suggest the possible needs for prophylactic neck dissection. In the study by Karas et al. (134), tumor thickness measuring between 1 and 2 mm was too variable to be of predictive value.

In regard to other sites, Baredes et al. (140) found that in 44 patients with variably staged soft palate SCCs (7 as T1, 14 as T2, 16 as T3, and 7 as T4), none of the patients with a tumor thickness of less than 2.86 mm had nodal metastasis, 60% of patients with tumor thickness greater than 2.86 mm but less than 3.12 mm had metastatic disease, and all patients with tumors greater than 3.12 mm had nodal metastasis. They concluded that there was a significant correlation between tumor thickness and the presence of nodal disease and that this association was more direct than that between T stage and nodal disease (140). Baredes et al. also report that thicker lesions had poorer survival (140). Frierson and Cooper (132) evaluated 187 SCCs of the lower lip and found that the tumor thickness strongly correlated with nodal metastasis. For these authors, nodal metastasis occurred in 74% of patients with cancers measuring ≥6 mm suggesting that lip squamous cancers of that thickness need elective neck dissections. Moore et al. (141) and Urist et al. (142) also identified depth of invasion and tumor thickness as important prognostic parameters in UADT cancers. In 1995, Zitsch et al. (8) reviewed a series of 1,252 patients with lip cancer over a 47-year period. These authors did not measure tumor thickness, but among multiple parameters available in 1,036 patients they found tumor size impacted on prognosis with those lip cancers measuring greater than 3 cm (T2 or greater) having a higher rate of nodal metastases (16% of patients) than those that measured less than 3 cm (6% of patients) (8). Further, the range of 5-year survival rate for patients whose tumors measured greater than 3 cm was 30% to 50% in contrast to 90% 5-year survival rates for patients whose tumors measured less than 3 cm (8). Based on their findings, Zitsch et al. suggested aggressive management for lip cancer ≥3 cm (8).

The location of a tumor in the UADT may have an impact on the depth of invasion and potential for metastatic disease. As an example, the glottic area of the larynx quantitatively has less vascular spaces than other anatomic sites of the larynx. Therefore, for histologically similar carcinomas of equal invasive growth, those arising in the glottic area may be less likely to metastasize as compared with supraglottic or subglottic cancers due to less availability of vascular spaces in this anatomic site. This may also apply to other mucosal sites of the head and neck. However, tumor location does play an extremely important factor in tumor identification and in prognosis. Cancers that present earlier in the course of disease will have a better prognosis than those cancers that remain undetectable until they present at a more advanced stage of disease. Some examples of the former include tumors that present in areas that are visible to the patient (e.g., cutaneous sites of the head and neck) or result in symptomatology in the earlier stages of disease (e.g., true vocal cord). Patients with cancers of these sites may be diagnosed and treated while their tumors are still of a lower clinical stage or in areas which are readily accessible to complete surgical resection without functional compromise or involvement of vital structures. In contrast, patients who have cancers that arise in areas in which symptoms may not develop early or whose symptomatology simulates nonspecific pathologic processes, such as cancers of the hypopharynx, paranasal sinuses, and middle ear, may only be detected in the advanced stages of disease with large tumors, extensive invasive growth, involvement of vital structures, difficult localization for complete removal, portending a poor outcome. Cerezo et al. found strong statistic correlation between the site of the primary tumor and prognosis (143). In a multivariate analysis of 492 patients with squamous carcinoma of the head and neck, these authors found that patients with primary tumors of the larynx and nasopharynx had higher survival rates than patients with carcinoma of the oropharynx, mobile tongue, floor of mouth, retromolar trigone, and hypopharynx (143). They correctly attributed this discrepancy to the ability to control locoregional disease or better tumor response to adjuvant therapy (i.e., radiation or chemotherapy). Doweck et al. (144) evaluated 250 patients with advanced head and neck cancer and found that patients with hypopharyngeal carcinoma were at greater risk for developing distant metastasis than patients with carcinoma of the oral cavity, oropharynx, and larynx.

PATTERN OF INVASION, NODAL AND DISTANT METASTASIS, AND MULTIPLE MALIGNANCIES IN HEAD AND NECK CANCER

The pattern and extent of invasion, nodal and distant metastasis, and multiple primary malignant tumors have prognostic significance in the head and neck cancer patient.

Pattern of Invasion

Invasive cancers composed of dyscohesive cells, loose bands, small nests or solitary dispersed tumor cells ("diffuse spread") (Fig. 2.8) are regarded as prognostically unfavorable with a greater tendency to metastasize as compared with cancers invading in cohesive nests or having pushing borders (134,145–148). The reasons for this may relate to the basal lamina distribution in these invasive patterns. In single cell or small irregular aggregate invasion, there is less likely to be expression of collagen type IV or laminin that normally is seen in the basal lamina (146). This suggests that single cell or small irregular aggregate invasion may represent active invasion into the stromal tissue. In contrast, large cords or cohesive aggregates of invasive carcinoma into the submucosa (Fig. 2.9) do retain expression of continuous or focal regions of collagen IV or laminin with separation of the invasive tumor from the host stroma by intact basal lamina (146). This suggests that invasive nests have ceased active invasion, and that there is an attempt to recapitulate the normal epithelium by epithelial organization and maturation (146). Tumors with a "diffuse spread" invasive pattern decreased survival to 30% to 40% as compared with 80% to 90% survival in patients with a more cohesive or "pushing" pattern of invasion (146,147).

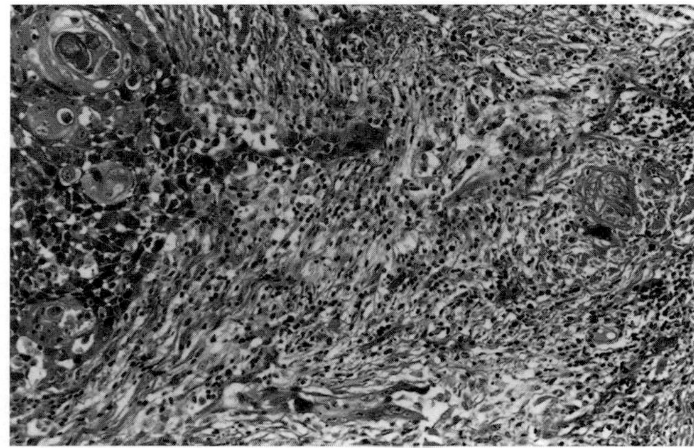

Figure 2.8 Poorly differentiated squamous cell carcinoma invading as dyscohesive or dispersed tumor cells. This pattern of invasion is considered as "diffuse spread" and is regarded as prognostically unfavorable with a greater tendency to metastasize.

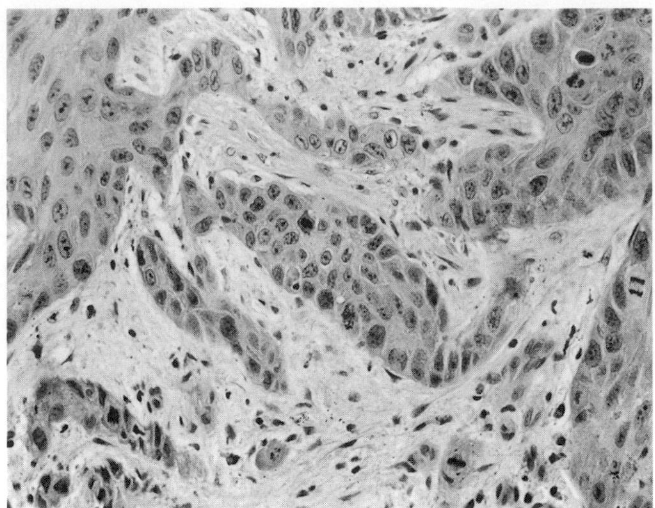

Figure 2.9 In contrast to the tumor shown in Figure 2.8, the invasive cancer seen here shows cohesive nests. This pattern of invasion is prognostically more favorable as compared with tumors with "diffuse spread" invasive patterns.

The pattern of invasion for oral SCC relative to local recurrence and survival was analyzed by Spiro et al. for 150 previously untreated patients (83). These authors assigned grades to the pattern of invasion with grade 1 representing well-defined "pushing" border to grade 4 representing diffuse infiltration and cellular dissociation, including single cell infiltration. The grade to the pattern of invasion was determined based on the appearance of tumor at the deepest point of invasion, and was modified from prior studies by Anneroth et al. (149) and Byrne et al. (150). Grade 2 included invasive tumors in which the advancing edge infiltrated in solid cords, bands, or strands; grade 3 had margins containing small groups or cords of infiltrating cells (83) Spiro et al. found that there was increased incidence of nodal and distant metastases ($p < 0.0003$ and $p < 0.01$, respectively), as well as a significant decrease in survival ($p < 0.01$) with higher grades of infiltration (i.e., grades 3 and 4) as compared with lower grades of infiltration (i.e., grades 1 and 2) (83). However, the grade of infiltration had no impact on local recurrence. These authors noted that the carcinomas with higher grades of infiltration tended to be larger and occurred in younger patients.

Floor of mouth carcinomas may grow in a radial or superficial manner spreading along the surface epithelium only (intraepithelial) but not invading through the basement membrane (151). This is akin to cutaneous melanomas in which the tumor may have a radial (superficial) growth phase as compared with a vertical growth phase characterized by invasive growth into the submucosal compartment. Like cutaneous melanomas, floor of mouth cancers require the occurrence of a critical depth of invasion for there to be a significant increase risk for developing nodal metastasis. Carbone et al. (152) describe the so-called superficial extending carcinoma of the hypopharynx in which there is extensive invasion of the lamina propria by SCC that was predominantly limited to the lamina propria by lateral spread of the tumor. These authors indicate that invasion into underlying muscle could be present but is restricted to few microscopic foci, and deeply infiltrating carcinoma may coexist with a "superficial extending carcinoma." Carbone et al. suggest that the "superficial extending carcinomas" may represent the pharyngeal counterpart to early gastric and esophageal cancer, and that like those gastrointestinal tumors, the pharyngeal tumors were potentially curable and a favorable prognosis was suggested (152). Subsequently, the so-called superficial extending carcinoma involving the laryngeal region was reported (153,154). Ferlito et al. (155) indicate that the "superficial extending carcinoma" should be considered as an early stage carcinoma (stage 2) with minimal invasion into the lamina propria and capable of metastatic disease.

LYMPH–VASCULAR SPACE INVASION, NEUROTROPISM, AND SOFT TISSUE INVASION

The presence of tumor within lymphatic spaces or blood vessels (Fig. 2.10) does not necessarily indicate that metastatic disease is present or will develop. However, several studies have demonstrated a statistical correlation between the identification of vascular space invasion and nodal metastasis (133,156–158). Sarbia et al. (159) evaluated the incidence and prognostic significance of blood vessel invasion (BVI), lymph vessel invasion (LVI), and neural invasion (NI) in SCC of the esophagus. These authors found a higher incidence of all three variables in higher pathologic and clinical stage tumors than in patients with lower pathologic and clinical stage tumors. Further, 5-year survival rates were significantly lower in patients with BVI and LVI than in patients without these findings (159). These authors report no prognostic significance with the presence of neural invasion (Fig. 2.11). Nevertheless, the presence of neurotropism in SCC of various UADT sites should be considered an adverse finding in head and neck malignancies indicative of a tumor's biologic aggressiveness as determined by an increased incidence of local recurrence, nodal metastasis, or decreased patient survival (132,139,158,160–162). Similarly, extension into soft tissue structures such as fat and muscle, or cartilaginous and osseous invasion by SCC of the head and neck general indicates a higher clinical stage tumor associated with a higher incidence of nodal metastasis (158,163). It has been thought that hyaline cartilage is resistant to invasive cancer (164) and that in the larynx, there is preferential invasion of squamous carcinoma into ossified cartilage as compared with nonossified cartilage. However, Michaels (165) has not found this to be true. Michaels identified extensive invasion of laryngeal squamous carcinoma into nonossified cricoid and thyroid cartilage (165). The invasion and destruction of bone by cancer is thought to be performed

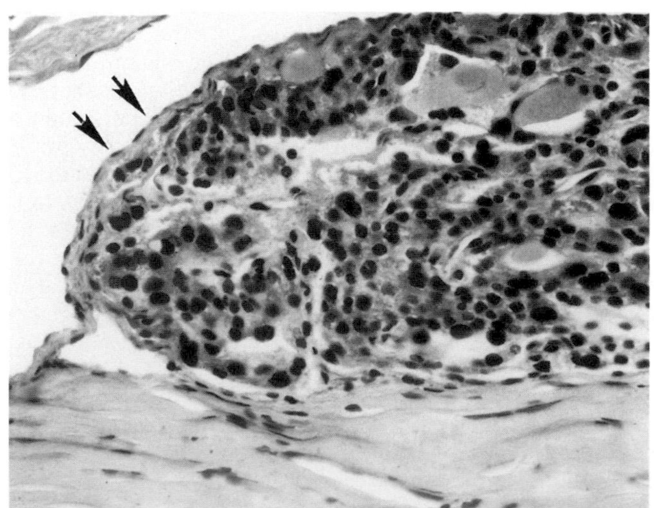

Figure 2.10 Parathyroid carcinoma showing vascular space invasion. Toward the left side of the illustration the endothelial cells lining this vascular space are seen (*arrowheads*) but become attenuated or lost due to the intravascular invasion of this tumor.

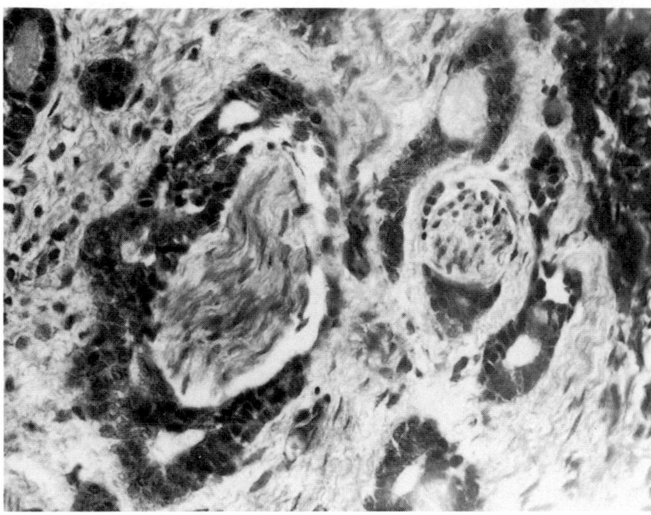

Figure 2.11 Adenoid cystic carcinoma of the parotid gland showing perineural invasion.

by osteoclasts mediated by prostaglandins (166) rather than by the direct action of the invasive cancer.

LYMPH NODES

The presence of lymph node or distant metastasis is correlated with increased morbidity and mortality in association with most malignancies. A notable exception would be thyroid papillary carcinoma, which generally is an indolent tumor even in the presence of nodal metastasis. For head and neck metastatic carcinoma to lymph nodes, several factors may have prognostic significance, including the presence of extracapsular extension by the tumor, site of nodal metastasis, number of lymph nodes with metastatic disease, node fixation, and tissue response to metastatic tumor. The presence of nodal metastasis with extension of the tumor outside the capsular confines of the lymph node and into perinodal soft tissues (extracapsular spread, or ECS) (Fig. 2.12) is generally considered an adverse

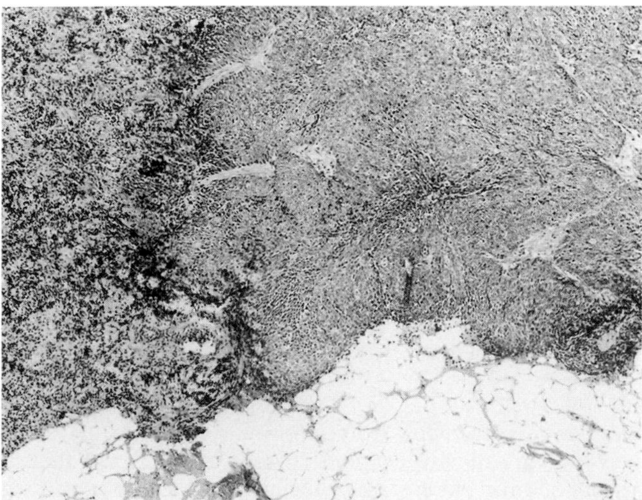

Figure 2.12 Metastatic carcinoma to a cervical neck lymph node with extracapsular extension. The remnant of the lymph node is seen at the left. The majority of the lymph node has been replaced by metastatic carcinoma, which shows extension into perinodal adipose tissue (lower portion of illustration). Extracapsular spread is considered an adverse prognostic finding.

finding associated with increased risk for recurrent disease, increased risk for distant metastasis, and a reduction in long-term survival by up to 50% (143,158,167–177). Extracapsular spread is further subdivided based on whether it was found microscopically or whether this feature was evident by gross examination. Macroscopic ECS is associated with an even greater risk for recurrent disease than by microscopic determination alone (158,178). Further, lymph nodes measuring more than 3 cm demonstrate a greater than 75% incidence of ECS (167,171,173,174). Johnson et al. (179) advocate the use of postoperative adjuvant therapy (radiation or chemotherapy) in the presence of transcapsular extension. Similarly, Leemans et al. (175,176), in two separate studies, advocate the use of adjuvant systemic therapy in patients with ECS. More recently, Myers et al. (177) reaffirmed that ECS is the most significant predictor of both regional recurrence and the development of distant metastasis accounting for decreased survival of patients with SCC of the oral tongue. Of the 260 patients in their study, 146 patients (56%) were pathologically node-negative (pN0), 75 patients (28%) were pathologically node-positive without ECS (pN+/ECS–), and 45 patients (17%) were node-positive with ECS (pN+/ECS+). Following the order of pN0, pN+/ECS– and pN+/ECS+, the 5-year disease specific and overall survival rates for these patients were 88% and 75%; pN+/ECS– were 65% and 50%; pN+/ECS+ were 48% and 30%; the overall recurrence rates were 19.8%, 34.2%, and 51.1%, respectively; the regional failure rates were 11.5%, 19.2%, and 28.9%, respectively; and the distant metastases rates were 3.3%, 8.2%, and 24.4%, respectively. Based on their findings the authors advocate the use of intensive regional and systemic adjuvant therapy for patients with ECS.

The site of metastatic disease may impact on overall prognosis. Patients with a nodal metastasis to the lower neck area have a worse prognosis than patients in whom the metastatic deposits are limited to the upper neck (168,180,181). McLaughlin et al. (182) found that abnormal retropharyngeal adenopathy, as determined by radiographic assessment (computed tomography scan, magnetic resonance imaging), was a predictor of outcome in SCC of the head and neck. Patients with squamous carcinoma of the head and neck of varying T stages (I–IV) and varying N stages (N0–N3), followed for a minimum of 2 years, had rates of neck relapse and distant metastasis that were significantly higher with retropharyngeal adenopathy (182); the rates of 5-year relapse-free survival and absolute survival were significantly lower (182).

The prognostic implication of whether metastatic tumor is found in a single lymph node or whether multiple nodes harbor disease has been debated. A number of studies have found that there is no prognostic significance in the absolute number of positive lymph nodes (183,184). However, other studies have found prognostic significance in the number of lymph nodes containing metastatic cancer, showing an inverse relationship between the absolute number of lymph nodes containing metastatic cancer and survival (143,144,167,171,172,175,176, 185). Doweck et al. (144) in their study on 250 patients with advanced head and neck cancer reported that the most accurate predictor of distant metastasis was the number of neck levels with clinical evidence of disease. Patients with more than one level of nodal metastases had an odds ratio of 3.17 for having distant metastasis. Of these patients 36% had distant metastasis compared with 17.9% if only one level of the neck was involved and 10.2% if the neck was negative. There is no specific cut-off in the number of positive lymph nodes associated with decreased survival. In a number of studies, the involvement by metastatic tumor in 3 or more lymph nodes appeared to be a predictor of distant metastasis and decreased survival

(143,175,176). Olsen et al. (158) found no significance when the number of lymph nodes involved was between 1 and 3, but when 4 or more lymph nodes were positive for metastatic tumor, there was a significant statistical correlation with 2-year recurrence-free survival (51% with at least 4 lymph nodes compared with 79% with 1–3 positive lymph nodes). Spiro et al. (185) report that the presence of bilateral nodal metastases is an adverse prognostic finding associated with a worse prognosis in comparison to patients with unilateral metastatic disease. Mamelle et al. (186) retrospectively evaluated 914 patients with SCC of various head and neck sites who underwent lymph node dissection in an attempt to determine prognostic factors relative to nodal disease. These authors report that in a multivariate analysis the most significant prognostic factors were the site of the positive node in or out of the sentinel node area ($p < 0.001$) and the number of positive nodes ($p < 0.001$), and that a more accurate approach was obtained by combining both factors (186). The presence of nodal metastasis in four or more lymph nodes located out of the sentinel node area was associated with decreased 5-year survival rates and increased likelihood of metastatic disease (186). Mamelle et al. (186) report that in the multivariate analysis, ECS was a nonsignificant risk factor in survival or distant metastatic spread ($p = 0.09$) but was significant in their univariate analysis ($p < 0.001$).

The presence of clinically palpable cervical lymph nodes has also been reported to be associated with increased risk for distant metastases. Vikram et al. (187) found the incidence of distant metastasis to be higher (25%) in patients who presented with palpable cervical lymph nodes than in those patients who did not. Similarly, Alvi and Johnson (188) found that 93% of their patients who developed distant metastasis as the first site of failure had palpable neck disease compared with 42% without distant metastasis.

Several studies have evaluated the presence of node fixation and stromal desmoplasia with prognosis. Cerezo et al. (143) and Leemans et al. (175) found that the presence of lymph node fixation was an adverse finding showing statistical significance influencing the inability to control regional disease or in adversely affecting the survival rates. Similarly, Olsen et al. (158) found that the presence of stromal desmoplasia (defined as fibroblastic proliferation in response to metastatic tumor), reduced the 2-year recurrence-free period from 86% in patients without stromal desmoplasia to 32% in patients with stromal desmoplasia. Olsen et al. (158) indicate that the desmoplastic stromal response was usually found with extracapsular tumor spread and suggested that this probably represented an unexplained host–tumor interaction. A desmoplastic tissue response in other infiltrating cancers such as the breast and gastric cancers, have also been associated with a poor prognosis. An interesting phenomenon relates to the desmoplastic response in nasopharyngeal cancers. Not infrequently, nasopharyngeal carcinomas of the undifferentiated and nonkeratinizing types do not elicit a stromal response to invasive growth whereas nasopharyngeal carcinomas of the keratinizing type do cause a desmoplastic response. Both the undifferentiated and nonkeratinizing carcinomas are radioresponsive cancers having a better 5-year survival rate as compared with the radioresistant keratinizing type of carcinoma. Perhaps, in these specific tumor types, the presence or absence of a host-generated desmoplastic response affects the radiosensitivity of the tumor, ultimately affecting the prognosis.

DISTANT METASTASIS

Distant metastasis by hematogenous spread to visceral sites from a head and neck squamous carcinoma most commonly includes spread to the lungs, liver, and bone (189). Distant metastatic tumor from a head and neck squamous carcinoma carries ominous clinical importance generally heralding the demise of the patient over relatively short periods of time despite all attempts at controlling disease (190). Among the factors that may be associated with distant metastatic tumor are the histologic type of cancer, tumor size, and the status of cervical lymph node involvement. Several of the more recently described high-grade variants of squamous carcinoma, including the basaloid SCC and adenosquamous carcinoma, often present as large tumors that are deeply invasive associated with nodal and distant metastasis. The reason for this aggressive behavior at presentation is not completely understood.

Both the tumor size (T stage) and the cervical node involvement (N stage) have been shown to have a high incidence of distant metastases (143,176,191–193). In addition to N stage, the number of lymph nodes involved, the number of lymphatic chains involved, and the presence of ECS, have all been shown to be associated with an increased incidence of distant metastasis (143,144,172,175,176). Cerezo et al. (143), in a multivariate analysis of 492 patients with metastatic neck disease from SCC of the head and neck, found that when three or more lymph nodes had metastatic disease the distant recurrence-free survival was reduced to 41% as compared with 84% when one lymph node was involved and 57% when two lymph nodes were involved. These same authors also found that when two or more lymphatic chains contained metastatic tumor, the distant recurrence-free survival was reduced to 40% as compared with 74% when one lymphatic chain was involved (143). In an autopsy study of 112 patients who had SCC of the head and neck, Nishijima et al. (189) found that nodal status was a significant prognostic factor in the presence of distant metastases. Of the 41 patients (37%) in their study who were found to have distant metastases at the time of death, 53 patients had tumor in cervical lymph nodes (189). Of these 53 patients, 26 patients had evidence of distant metastases, which represents a positive correlation between nodal status and development of distant metastasis ($p < 0.01$). Nishijima et al. (189) further combined their patients into those who had tumor at the primary site with those who had tumor in cervical lymph nodes (classified as cancerous lesions above the clavicle), and found of these 82 patients, 43% had distant metastases ($p < 0.05$). These authors concluded that distant metastasis occurred most frequently in patients with residual or recurrent disease in the neck. They reported no correlation between the T and N stage, anatomic site of the primary tumor, or presence or absence at controlling disease at the primary site with the frequency of developing distant metastases. The authors indicate that in their patients, the T and N stages were determined at the time of the initial examination (when the patients were alive). Irrespective of the T or N stage, these patients ultimately died of their tumors and so it was thought that the initial T and N stages may not have played a significant role in the analysis of patients who died of advanced disease (189).

Skin involvement by mucosal SCC of the head and neck is uncommon, and usually is an indication of advanced or recurrent disease (194). Cole and McGuirt (195) have shown that cutaneous involvement from a primary mucosal SCC has adverse prognostic implications. These authors found that the presence of direct cutaneous extension from a mucosal SCC was associated with a mean survival of 7 months whereas intradermal lymphatic spread carried a mean survival of 3 months; involvement of facial skin had an overall better prognosis than when there was involvement of neck skin with 12-month and 3-month median survival, respectively (195).

SECOND MALIGNANCY

In spite of the recent advances in the therapeutic management of the head and neck cancer patient, the overall survival of these patients has not substantially improved. A prime reason for the absence of improved overall survival of the head and neck cancer patient is their increased risk for developing a second primary malignancy. Compared with the standard population, the head and neck cancer patient is at greater risk (10–30 times) of developing a second primary malignancy (196) with the frequency varying from less than 5% (197) to as high as 36% (198), with many studies in the 15% to 25% range (199–201). Criteria used in defining multiple primary carcinomas include that the tumors be separate and distinct (at least 2 cm apart) without any dysplasia in the intervening mucosa and that the second primary tumor does not represent a metastasis or recurrent tumor (197). The diagnosis of a second primary tumor such as in the lung includes the presence of a solitary lesion that is histologically distinct from the primary tumor (201). Second primary malignancies occurring within a 6-month period from the discovery of the primary cancer are termed *synchronous tumors,* whereas second primary malignancy that occurs after the 6-month period from the discovery of the first tumor are referred to as *metachronous tumors.* Most of the second malignancies develop in other UADT mucosal sites (199,200,202). Non-head and non-neck sites in which second malignancies develop include the lungs (200–202), esophagus (200,201,203), and bowel (200,202). Most often, the histology of the second primary malignant neoplasm is a squamous carcinoma (201,203) but other histologic types such as adenocarcinomas may occur (202). Some of the more recently defined high-grade variants of SCC, including the basaloid cell squamous carcinoma and adenosquamous carcinoma, are notorious for the presence of multiple concurrent primary tumors in mucosal sites of the head and neck at the time of initial presentation.

Factors that may play a significant role in the development of a second malignancy include the site of the original primary cancer, the age of the patient, the size of the primary tumor, the status of regional lymph nodes, and the use of tobacco and alcohol. Head and neck second malignancies are more likely to develop when the primary cancer is in the oral cavity, hypopharynx, or oropharynx than if the index tumor is of laryngeal origin (200–202). Patients who developed their tumors prior to 60 years of age may be at greater risk for developing a second primary malignancy (201,202). Jones et al. (202) showed that patients with lower stage index tumors (T1 and T2) and patients who had no nodal metastasis (N0) at the presentation of their index tumor, were more likely to develop a second malignancy than patients with higher stage index tumors and patients who did have nodal metastasis at the presentation of their index tumor ($p < 0.0001$ and 0.0003, respectively). Lippman and Hong (204) also identify the threat of a second malignancy in early-stage head and neck index cancer patients. Patients with index tumors of the head and neck who smoke tobacco (>20 pack-years) and consume alcohol are at significant increased risk for developing a second malignancy than those who do not smoke or drink (201). Survival rates after the second cancer are influenced by the site of the second malignancy and persistent use and abuse of tobacco and alcohol (201). Second malignancies of the lung and esophagus portend a significantly worse prognosis than second malignancies of other head and neck sites with 5-year survival rates from the diagnosis of the second malignancy of 2% (for lung) and 3% (for esophagus) versus 20% for second head and neck malignancies (201). Continued use of tobacco and alcohol also adversely affected survival rates, with 5-year survival rates of 5% for smokers versus 20% for nonsmokers, and 6% for drinkers versus 27% for nondrinkers (201). Despite a modicum of increased overall survival in some groups, the development of a second malignancy is almost always fatal (201).

The site of the second malignancy differs for different index tumors. Head and neck and esophageal second primary malignancies are more prevalent after oral cavity and pharyngeal index tumors, whereas the development of a second primary tumor of the lung was most common after a laryngeal index tumor (200,202). Haughey et al. (200) suggest a shared mucosal susceptibility between the index tumor and the second malignancy to account for this phenomenon. A common "digestive tract axis" is shared between oral cavity, pharynx and the esophagus, while the larynx and lung share a common "respiratory tract axis." This shared mucosal susceptibility is a variation on the "field cancerization" concept, which highlights the importance of carcinogen activation of an entire exposed mucosa. The concepts of "field cancerization" and mutagen sensitivity, a possible marker for the development of secondary malignancy, will be discussed in the next section in relationship to carcinogenesis.

Increased glutathione S-transferase (GST) expression, a carcinogen detoxifying enzyme, may represent a possible "marker" for the development of secondary malignancies in the head and neck cancer patient. In patients with primary oral SCC who developed a second primary head and neck malignancy, Bongers et al. (205) identified increased expression of GST in the normal tissues in direct vicinity of the index tumor in comparison to matched controls. These authors believed that increased GST had predictive value for the development of a second primary tumor (205).

The critical issue for the otolaryngologist in the evaluation and planned treatment of the patient with head and neck cancer is to be acutely aware of the possibility that the patient has or will develop a second primary malignancy. The diagnosis of a primary head and neck cancer should initiate panendoscopic evaluation of the entire UADT, as well as the lower aerodigestive tract and esophagus to exclude the possibility of a synchronous second primary cancer, with vigilant follow-up care given the possibility of developing a metachronous cancer. The results of these findings may ultimately impact on the diagnostic approach, treatment protocol, and prognostic impact for that patient. The development of a second primary malignancy is in all likelihood a multifactorial process combining genetic and environmental risks. The development of a second primary cancer may potentially be predictive on the basis of sophisticated molecular biologic assessment.

FIELD CANCERIZATION

In 1953, Slaughter et al. (206) introduced the concept of "field cancerization," suggesting the importance of carcinogen activation of an entire exposed mucosa. These authors postulated that multiple, independent, carcinogenic events occurred in separate cells due to exposure of the "preconditioned epithelium" or "condemned mucosa" to a carcinogenic agent. The field of preconditioned epithelium or "condemned mucosa" became activated or broke down into cancer producing multiple, separate carcinomas rather than a tumor from a single cell that becomes malignant (206). Subsequent studies confirmed the "field cancerization" phenomenon in which significant dysplastic changes affect a wide epithelial mucosal field in patients at high risk for developing cancer (e.g., heavy smokers and drinkers) (207–209). The concepts of "field cancerization" and "condemned mucosa" explain the greater risk to the head and neck cancer patient for the development of a second primary malignancy which in turn plays a significant factor in tendency for these tumors to recur or persist despite therapeutic intervention, with adverse impact on survival.

Using the same observation made by Slaughter et al. (206), Carey (210) and Worsham et al. (211) proposed an alternative hypothesis suggesting that a single focus of tumor develops and spreads laterally by arborization without disrupting the adjacent normal mucosa. Worsham et al. (211) evaluated synchronous but separate carcinomas (primary floor of mouth and pyriform sinus lying 6 to 7 cm apart) and metachronous carcinomas (recurrences of these tumors after radiotherapy) in a single patient to determine whether the tumors were of common or independent clonal origin. Histologically, the two tumors shared a similar morphology, including invasive moderate to poorly differentiated keratinizing SCCs. The authors found that all four tumors were of monoclonal origin and suggested that in some patients second primary cancers may arise at distant sites because of the lateral spread of malignant clones. This lateral spread presupposes the multiple factors required for active neoplastic cell motility with penetration of extracellular matrices (212). Studies by Bedi et al. (213) and Califano et al. (214) support these observations. Bedi et al. (213) using X chromosome inactivation and loss of heterozygosity analysis in multiple HNSCC from eight female patients showed high probability that second primary tumors were progeny of the same clone, supporting the idea that many second primary tumors represent extensions of the initial tumor clone. Califano et al. (214) demonstrated that apparently normal mucosa surrounding preinvasive and microinvasive HNSCCs shared common genetic aberrations with the tumor supporting the concept proposed by Worsham et al. (211).

Squamous Cell Carcinoma

In the head and neck region, the most common lesion encountered by the otolaryngologist and the pathologist relates to alterations of the surface squamous epithelium. The following sections focus on the squamous epithelial alterations of the UADT, including precursor lesions, SCC, and variants of SCC.

Terminology

In the head and neck, the most common clinical and pathologic problems confronted by the surgeon and pathologist relate to the alterations of the mucosal epithelium. A brief overview of the clinical and pathologic terminology used in the diagnosis of these lesions is in order.

Leukoplakia is a clinical term that describes any white lesion on a mucous membrane. A leukoplakic lesion is usually associated with a mucosal thickening and is not indicative of underlying malignant tumor.

Erythroplakia is a clinical term that describes any red lesion on a mucous membrane. An erythroplakic lesion is often indicative of an underlying malignant tumor.

Hyperplasia is the thickening of an epithelial surface as a result of an absolute increase in the number of cells.

Acanthosis is the hyperplasia and thickening of the stratum malpighian (the nucleated, viable portion of the epidermis or epithelium consisting of the basal, squamous, and granular layers).

Pseudoepitheliomatous hyperplasia is the exuberant reactive or reparative overgrowth of squamous epithelium (hyperplasia) displaying no cytologic evidence of malignancy but may be mistaken for an invasive SCC.

Keratosis can be described as an increase in the amount of surface keratin (hyperkeratosis). For the larynx, which normally is a nonkeratinizing epithelium, the use of the term *hyperkeratosis* is redundant; the term "keratosis" therefore is preferable.

Parakeratosis is the presence of nuclei in the keratin layer.

Dyskeratosis is the abnormal keratinization of epithelial cells.

Ulceration is the erosion or loss of the surface epithelium.

Metaplasia is a benign alteration that results in a change from one histologic tissue type to another. It generally occurs as a result of tissue insult or injury.

Koilocytosis is a descriptive term for the cytoplasmic vacuolization of squamous cells. This morphologic change is suggestive of viral (human papillomavirus) infection.

DYSPLASIA AND INTRAEPITHELIAL NEOPLASIA

Dysplasia and **intraepithelial neoplasia** is the spectrum of abnormal epithelial maturation and cellular aberrations that may or may not precede an invasive carcinoma. Dysplasia is synonymous with atypia. The ovarian cervix is the prototypic epithelium defining dysplastic changes. Dysplasia is graded into mild, moderate, and severe depending on the extent of involvement of the surface epithelium. In general, the lesser the degree of dysplasia, the less likely there will be transformation to an invasive carcinoma. Conversely, the higher the grade of dysplasia, the more likely there will be progression to an invasive carcinoma. In the UADT, particularly in the larynx, severe dysplasia (i.e., carcinoma *in situ*) is not a prerequisite for the development of an invasive SCC. In other words, invasive carcinoma may develop in an epithelium with only mild dysplastic changes.

CARCINOMA *IN SITU*

As classically defined, carcinoma *in situ* (CIS) represents full thickness mucosal epithelial dysplastic change without violation of the basement membrane For all intents and purposes, severe dysplasia is synonymous with CIS. As previously noted, in the upper airways, CIS (as classically defined) is not a requirement prior to the development of an invasive SCC. The latter may arise from the basal epithelial layer in the absence of overlying dysplastic changes. Therefore, in this setting, the definition of CIS can be expanded to include those lesions in which the mucosal alterations are so severe that there would be a high probability for the progression to an invasive carcinoma if left untreated. Extension of the dysplastic process to involve the mucoserous glands is still considered as CIS and not invasive carcinoma.

EARLY, SUPERFICIALLY, OR MICROSCOPIC INVASIVE SQUAMOUS CELL CARCINOMA

These terms describe SCC in which there is penetration of the basement membrane with invasion of the carcinoma into the underlying submucosal compartment. The identification of *superficial* or *microinvasive* carcinoma is significant given the presence of vascular spaces high in the lamina propria and the potential, even in the presence of "early" invasive cancer, for metastatic disease.

Clinical Alterations of the Surface Epithelium

The clinical appearance of premalignant or "incipient" lesions of the mucosal surfaces of the UADT include leukoplakic, erythroplakic, or speckled leukoplakia reflecting the presence of a white, red, or mixed white/red lesion, respectively. Among these clinical changes, erythroplakic lesions are commonly associated with ominous histopathologic alterations, including severe dysplasia, CIS, or invasive carcinoma. In contrast, leukoplakic lesions are not necessarily a premalignant lesion and may demonstrate a spectrum of histopathologic changes ranging from an increased surface keratinization without dysplasia to invasive keratinizing squamous carcinoma. Leukoplakic lesions, in contrast with erythroplakic lesions, tend to be well defined with demarcated margins. Although the risk for developing a malignancy in a leukoplakic lesion is low, there is still a risk (approximately 10%–12%) of malignant transformation (215,216). The clinical appearance of a mixed white and red lesion, called *speckled leukoplakia,* carries an intermediate risk between "pure" leukoplakic and "pure" erythroplakic lesions for the development of a malignancy (217), but speckled leukoplakia should be viewed as a variant of erythroplakia (215,217,218). In a study of 236 patients with asymptomatic intraoral carcinoma, Mashberg and Feldman (218) report that 64% of the lesions were red or predominantly red (erythroplakic), 23% were equally red and white (speckled leukoplakia), and 12% were white or predominantly white (leukoplakic).

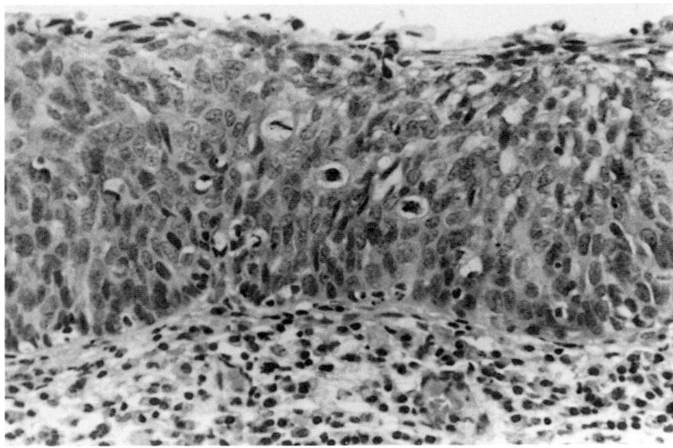

Figure 2.13 Laryngeal (glottic) carcinoma *in situ* "classic" or nonkeratinizing type. There is full-thickness dysplasia with replacement of the squamous epithelium by atypical, small, immature basaloid cells, including numerous mitotic figures in the absence of surface keratinization. The dysplastic cells are confined to within the surface epithelium and do not penetrate the basement membrane into the submucosa.

Histopathology of Squamous Epithelial Neoplasia

PRECURSOR LESIONS

Precursor lesions to squamous epithelial lesions of the UADT present diagnostic challenges in that the majority of dysplastic epithelial changes are of the keratinizing type to which the continuum of mild to moderate to severe dysplasia to invasive carcinoma that characterizes the nonkeratinizing dysplasias does not consistently apply. This results in problems in the histologic grading of these changes and raises questions about what constitutes a diagnosis of severe dysplasia. In this context the justification of using the designation CIS, relative to keratinizing dysplasia, becomes questionable.

Leukoplakia, erythroplakia, and speckled leukoplakia are not histopathologic terms. The qualitative intraepithelial alteration in a malignant direction is referred to as dysplasia. Dysplasia is, for all intents and purposes synonymous, with atypia although dysplasia has been used in relation to architectural abnormalities while atypia has been used for cytomorphologic changes.

Histologic criteria for the diagnosis of intraepithelial neoplasia of the UADT include both cytomorphologic and maturation abnormalities. These alterations include the proliferation of immature or "uncommitted" cells characterized by a loss of cellular organization or polarity, nuclear pleomorphism (variations in the size and shape of the nuclei), increase in nuclear size relative to the cytoplasm, increase in the nuclear chromatin (hyperchromasia) with irregularity of distribution, and increased mitoses, including atypical forms in all epithelial layers. The dysplastic changes may or may not be associated with keratosis or dyskeratosis. The location of the architectural and cytomorphologic changes within the epithelium represents key diagnostic parameters in the assessment of UADT epithelial dysplasia.

The paradigm for grading epithelial dysplasia is the one used for the uterine cervix. In the uterine cervix the "classic" or nonkeratinizing form of dysplasia commonly occurs. The increasing gradations of cervical intraepithelial neoplasia (CIN) include mild (CIN I), moderate (CIN II), and severe (CIN III) with the latter representing full-thickness replacement of the squamous epithelium by atypical, small, immature basaloid cells and is referred to as carcinoma *in situ* (CIS) (Fig. 2.13). This grading scheme is reproducible and is clinically useful. However, the "classic" or nonkeratinizing dysplasia of the uterine cervix is uncommon in the UADT, especially in the laryngeal glottis (219). In contrast, most of the intraepithelial neoplasias of the UADT are keratinizing dysplasias. Using the definition of CIS of the uterine cervix that requires loss of maturation of squamous epithelium, a keratotic lesion cannot be CIS because keratosis requires maturation of the squamous epithelium. Therefore, the use of the specific term CIS in keratinizing dysplasias has been questioned (220) and is likely inappropriate in this setting. A more appropriate designation is of severe keratinizing intraepithelial dysplasia.

The criteria for evaluating keratinizing dysplasias are less defined and the diagnosis of severe keratinizing intraepithelial dysplasia remains controversial. The definition of severe dysplasia in the UADT, especially in the laryngeal glottis is broader than the highly reproducible pattern seen in the uterine cervix and includes a microscopically heterogenous group of lesions (220). In the setting of keratinizing dysplasia where surface maturation is retained with only partial replacement of the epithelium by atypical cells, severe dysplasia includes those lesions in which the epithelial alterations are so severe that there would be a high probability for the progression to an invasive carcinoma if left untreated (Fig. 2.14). Severe dysplasia shows the presence of aberrant cell maturation with dyskeratotic cells and mitotic figures with or without atypical forms above the basal zone (221). These alterations often occur in the presence of surface keratinization (Fig. 2.15). In the evaluation of UADT dysplasia the presence of surface keratinization is not significant (222), however, finding dyskeratotic cells represents an important clue to the presence of significant dysplasia (223).

Grading Epithelial Dysplasia of the Upper Aerodigestive Tract

The histopathologic interpretation and grading of epithelial dysplastic changes in the UADT are imprecise and subjective. Given the complexities in the issues relative to UADT intraep-

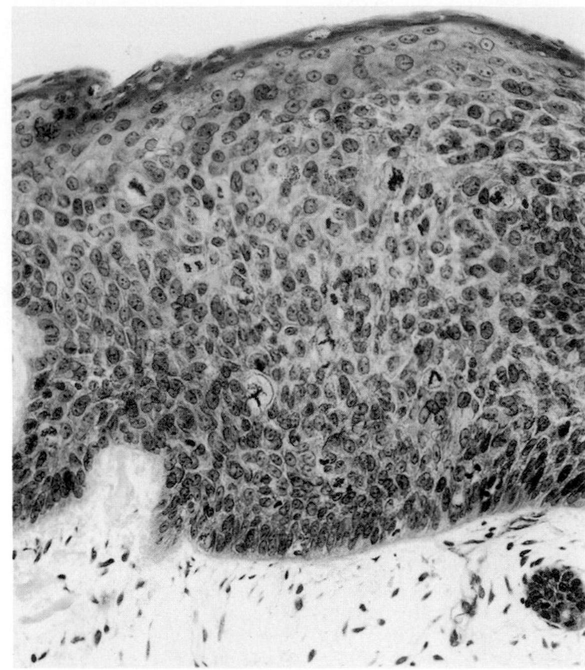

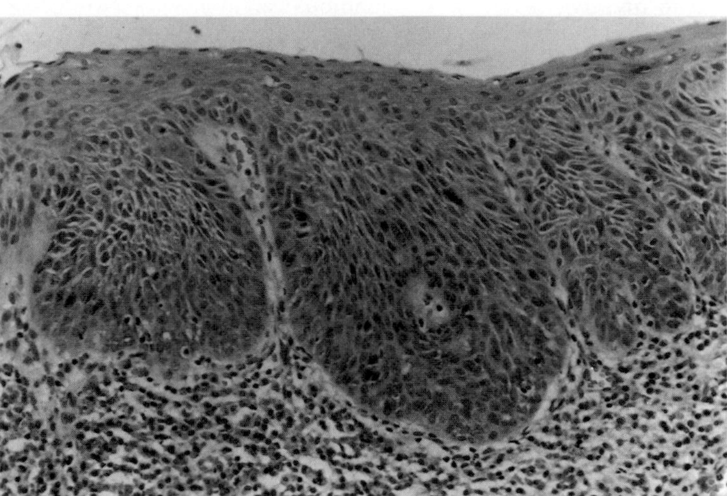

Figure 2.14 **A:** Laryngeal (glottic) keratinizing dysplasia. Surface maturation is retained with replacement of the squamous epithelium by atypical cells, including numerous suprabasal mitotic figures. Although there is not full thickness dysplasia, the lesion is considered as severe dysplasia given that the epithelial alterations are so severe that there is a high probability for the progression to an invasive carcinoma if left untreated. **B:** Similar alterations as those seen in **A**, but the bulbous downward growth adds concern for the evolution to invasive carcinoma.

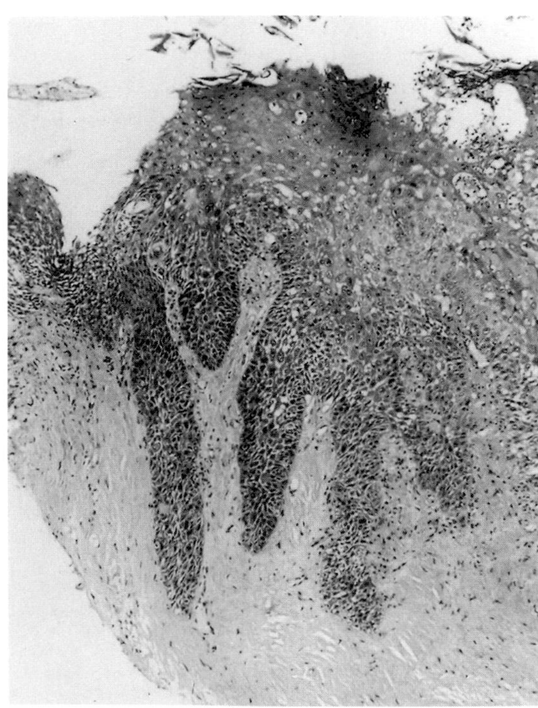

Figure 2.15 Laryngeal biopsy showing keratosis and severe dysplasia with superficial invasion. This epithelium does not show full thickness dysplasia (i.e., carcinoma *in situ*). The dysplastic alterations are limited to the lower portion of the epithelium but are still considered severe, and the angulated downward extension of this severely dysplastic epithelium is sufficient to consider this superficially invasive.

ithelial lesions, confusion and misunderstandings may occur between the clinician and the pathologist that may result in inappropriate management of the patient. Uniformity in terminology is desirable so that there is a correlation between the pathologic diagnosis and the clinical importance of that diagnosis. In an attempt to standardize the terminology of UADT intraepithelial lesions using a grading system akin to that of the cervical mucosa, Crissman and Zarbo (224) used the terminology of squamous intraepithelial neoplasia (SIN) with SIN I equivalent to mild dysplasia, SIN II to moderate dysplasia, and SIN III to severe dysplasia. Similar gradations using the terminology of laryngeal intraepithelial neoplasia (LIN) have been proposed (225). More recently, the Ljubljana classification of laryngeal precancerous lesions was proposed (226). In this system the terms used include simple hyperplasia (i.e., keratosis without atypia), abnormal hyperplasia (i.e., keratosis with atypia), atypical hyperplasia (i.e., severe dysplasia), and CIS. These systems have conceptual validity but may not be entirely applicable from a practical standpoint in the UADT. Currently, the preferred grading for dysplastic epithelial alterations of the UADT include mild, moderate, and severe dysplasia depending on the degree and extent of cellular and maturation alterations that are present.

Regardless of the terminology employed, close interaction between the pathologist and the clinician is required so that each individual understands the impact of their respective findings and the importance to the patient in therapy and prognosis.

Risk of Progression

The end point for the grading of dysplasia is to convey to the clinician what is the potential biologic behavior of a given epithelial lesion. Keratotic epithelium without dysplasia carries a very low risk for developing subsequent carcinoma with reported incidences from 1% to 5% (224,226–232). In contrast, keratotic epithelium with dysplasia is associated with an increased risk for the subsequent progression or development of premalignant or overtly carcinomatous changes varying from 11% to 18% of cases (224,226–232). This risk for malignant transformation represents an increase from three to five times as compared with carcinoma arising in keratotic lesions without atypia. Bouquot and Gnepp (233) found greater variability relative to risk progression of keratosis with and without atypia in their review of the literature. Nevertheless, the potential value in grading keratotic dysplasias is apparent from the review by Barnes of the literature (232) in which the risk for developing invasive carcinoma in mild, moderate, and severe dysplasia was 5.7%, 22.5%, and 28.4%, respectively. Other studies have shown that severe dysplasia is associated with increased incidences of persistent disease or progression to invasive carcinoma (234–237). Bauer and McGavran (238) indicated that if enough sections are taken, microinvasive carcinoma will be found in laryngeal lesions that have keratosis with cytologically atypical cells.

Another important point to recognize is the clinical concern attached to a diagnosis of severe keratinizing intraepithelial neoplasia. This clinical concern is due to the fact that severe dysplasia is often multifocal and frequently occurs adjacent to or near synchronous foci of invasive carcinoma. Further, this form of dysplasia has a rate of progression to invasive carcinoma that is greater than that of "classic" CIS (234,237,239). A diagnosis of severe dysplasia requires therapeutic intervention, as well as clinical evaluation of the entire UADT to exclude the possible presence of additional foci of dysplasia or carcinoma.

In general, mild and moderate dysplasias are thought to be reversible alterations. Circumstantial evidence supports the idea that preinvasive dysplasias are potentially reversible following cessation or removal of an instigating factor such as tobacco use (240). The problem of predicting the malignant potential of a dysplastic lesion is greatest in cases of moderate dysplasia. It is virtually impossible to differentiate the moderately dysplastic lesions that are reversible from those that represent the earliest forms of neoplastic transformation (235). Therefore, a diagnosis of moderate dysplasia should engender enough concern to the clinician to warrant close patient follow-up. Recurrence or persistence of this dysplasia may be indicative of malignant transformation. The determination of whether a mild to moderate dysplasia is reactive or neoplastic, although a desirable goal, is not always achievable. The clinically abnormal lesions that show limited cytologic and maturation abnormalities falling under the designation of reactive atypias or hyperplastic lesions represent reversible changes that rarely, if ever, progress to carcinoma. These lesions are responsive to conservative management. Epithelial hyperplasia (acanthosis) is a common finding and can be seen without atypia or in association with atypia. In hyperplasia there usually is an irregular contour to the basal zone and there may be protrusion of the epithelium below adjacent epithelium, possibly suggesting a microinvasive carcinoma. A diagnosis of microinvasive carcinoma should be reserved for those examples in which there is definitive evidence of dissociated squamous cells at the epithelial-to-stromal interface. Epithelial hyperplasias may be caused by an infectious agent (e.g., fungi) and fungal stains may be useful to identify the causative microorganism.

Immunohistochemical evaluation for type IV collagen and laminin has been used in the evaluation of intraepithelial lesions. Sakr et al. (241) found that basal lamina was prominent and continuous in normal and reactive hyperplasias, was usually prominent and continuous in mild to moderate dysplasia, and was thinned and occasionally discontinuous in severe dysplasia or CIS.

Microinvasive, Superficial, or "Early" Invasive Squamous Cell Carcinoma

Microinvasive SCC is a cancer that infiltrates into the superficial compartment of the lamina propria. As simple as this may appear, the diagnosis of superficially invasive SCC can be subjective with no unanimous definition among pathologists. For laryngeal lesions, some authors consider microinvasive cancer to include the presence of scattered malignant cells within the submucosa just below the basement membrane (242) or within 1 to 2 mm of the basement membrane (224,243,244), whereas other authors believe that microinvasive carcinoma is present when tongues or discrete foci of malignant epithelium invade through the basement membrane (245). Barnes defines microinvasive carcinoma as invasive SCC that extends into the stroma no more than 0.5 mm as measured from the adjacent (nonneoplastic) epithelial basement membrane (232). Irrespective of its specific definition, a diagnosis of microinvasive carcinoma excludes those lesions that are restricted to the surface epithelium or CIS (Tis) and those carcinomas that are deeply invasive into muscle and cartilage and extralaryngeal structures (T2 or greater tumors). Also, the presence of lymph–vascular space invasion would exclude a diagnosis of microinvasive carcinoma. Of note, extension of the dysplastic process to involve the seromucinous glands is still considered as CIS and not invasive carcinoma (Fig. 2.16). The clinical manifestations and appearance of microinvasive SCC are similar to those of CIS. In the larynx, full cord mobility is present. Any dysfunction in vocal cord mobility (fixation) by definition indicates muscle invasion, which excludes a diagnosis of microinvasive cancer.

Histologically, microinvasive carcinoma can occur in two unrelated phases. The first is the development from and as a

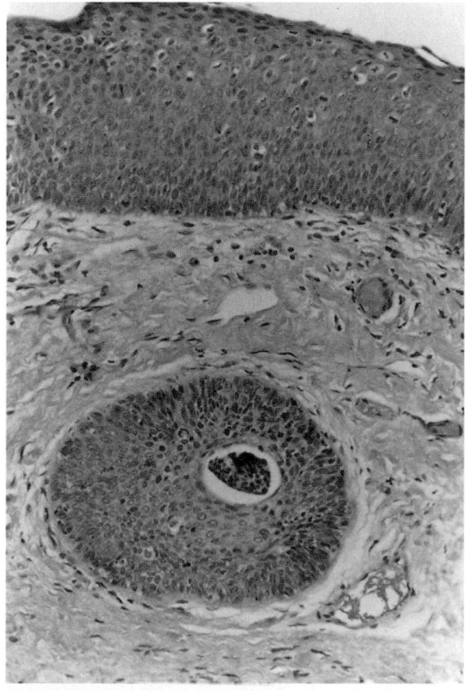

Figure 2.16 Laryngeal (glottic) carcinoma *in situ* (CIS) of the surface epithelium with extension of the dysplastic process to involve the seromucinous glands. The extension to seromucinous glands is still considered as CIS and not invasive carcinoma.

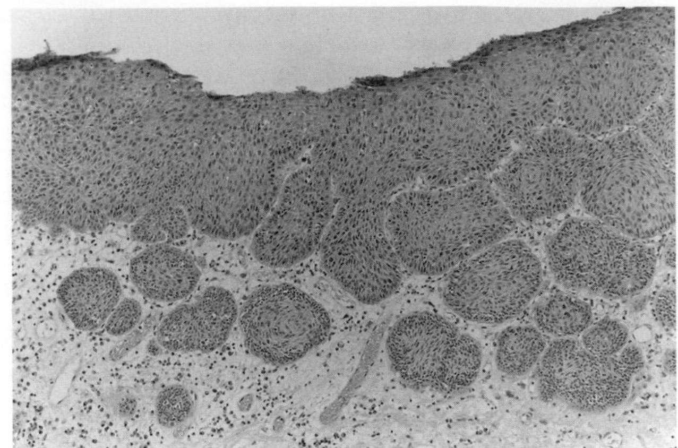

Figure 2.17 Laryngeal (glottic) microinvasive squamous cell carcinoma developing as a continuum from carcinoma *in situ*.

continuum of CIS (Fig. 2.17). The second is invasion from an epithelium demonstrating no evidence of CIS. In the UADT, particularly in the larynx, severe dysplasia (i.e., CIS) is not a prerequisite for the development of an invasive SCC. Such invasive carcinomas "drop off" or "drop down" from the basal cell layer with the overlying mucosa showing no evidence of dysplasia (Fig. 2.18). In all examples of invasive carcinoma the invasive nests must be cytologically malignant with dysplastic changes, dyskeratosis and mitotic figures, including atypical forms. The tumor nests have an irregular outline with infiltrative borders. The presence of invasive cancer generally results in stromal induction or a desmoplastic host response that includes edematous change immediately around the tumor nests with granulation tissue and fibrosis.

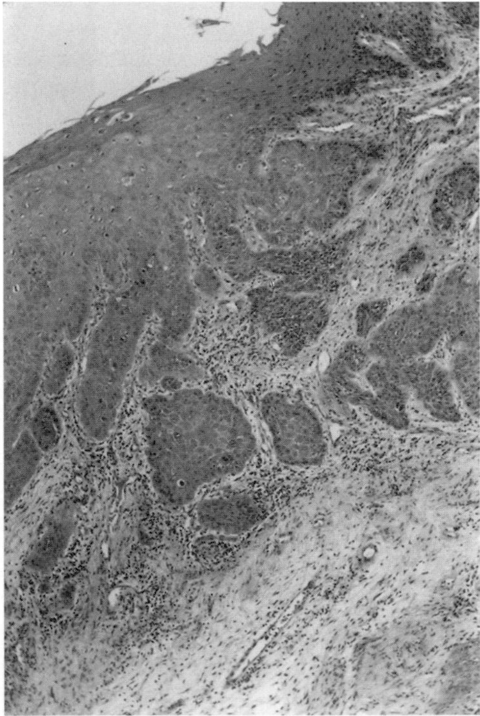

Figure 2.18 Laryngeal (glottic) invasive squamous cell carcinoma developing from the basal zone of the surface epithelium in which most of the epithelium is free of dysplastic changes (so-called drop-off carcinoma).

Microinvasive cancer is a biologically malignant lesion potentially capable of gaining access to lymphatic or vascular channels in the lamina propria that may result in metastatic disease. For microinvasive carcinoma of the laryngeal glottis, several studies have shown that the clinical significance is similar to CIS/severe dysplasia that with appropriate therapy (excision or radiotherapy) progression of disease from a microinvasive to a more invasive carcinoma does not occur (236,237,242–245). This may be due to the earlier clinical manifestations produced by glottic cancers leading to an earlier diagnosis of cancer before it has invaded into deeper aspects of the larynx. Glottic microinvasive cancers are generally not associated with metastatic disease due to the fact that the glottic portion of the larynx has quantitatively less lymph–vascular spaces as compared with the supra- and subglottis. In contrast to the laryngeal glottis, supraglottic microinvasive carcinomas are associated with metastatic disease in approximately 20% of patients (246).

The concept of so-called superficially extending carcinoma of the larynx and hypopharynx was introduced as the morphologic equivalent to early carcinoma of the upper gastrointestinal tract (232,247,248). As it is defined, superficially extending carcinoma includes those SCCs that invade beyond what is considered as microinvasion or superficial invasion (i.e., not beyond the lamina propria) without invasion into adjacent muscle or cartilage.

Invasive Squamous Cell Carcinoma

The clinical (gross) appearance of invasive SCC is quite variable and includes ulcerated, flat, exophytic, verrucoid, or papillary growths. The histologic appearance of invasive SCC may be as variable as the gross appearance without specific correlation between the gross appearance and the histopathologic findings. Invasive SCC of the UADT includes keratinizing and nonkeratinizing carcinomas varying from well differentiated to poorly differentiated. Severe dysplasia/CIS of the surface epithelium may be a common component found in association with invasive SCC; this component need not be present. For all types of SCC the presence of invasion is diagnostic of a malignancy. Invasion can be as single (dyscohesive) cells or small irregular aggregates or can appear as large cords or cohesive aggregates. In addition, a desmoplastic stromal response and foreign body reaction to keratin in the stroma may assist in identifying invasion. Invasive cancer will efface the normal architecture and may be associated with lymph–vascular space invasion, neurotropism, and invasion into muscle, bone, and cartilage. Once the cancer invades beyond a few millimeters or extends into muscle, cartilage, or other soft tissue components outside the anatomic structure from which it originates, then the tumor becomes a higher clinical stage neoplasm with the potential for a more aggressive behavior. Immunohistochemical studies have shown that that the presence or absence of basement membrane components around invasive cancer correlated with the pattern of tumor invasion (241). The pattern of tumor invasion (single cell vs. large cords) represents an inherent biologic parameter of tumor aggressiveness (224,241).

Pitfalls in the Diagnosis of Invasive Squamous Cell Carcinoma

Sampling is a major issue in the evaluation of SCC of the UADT. In the absence of adequate representative tissue including epithelial-to-stroma interface, one should be circumspect relative to a diagnosis of SCC. Diagnostic pitfalls in the diagnosis of SCC include pseudoepitheliomatous hyperplasia (249), necrotizing sialometaplasia (250), juxtaoral organ of Chievitz (250), and radiation atypia.

Pseudoepitheliomatous hyperplasia (PEH) is an exuberant reactive epithelial response to a variety of stimuli, including chronic inflammatory conditions, infections, trauma, and neoplasms. Pseudoepitheliomatous hyperplasia is classically associated with granular cell tumor (GCT), which is a benign neoplasm of probable peripheral nerve sheath origin often occurring in the oral cavity (tongue, lips) and larynx. In the setting of GCT the epithelial response may be so extensive as to be indistinguishable from SCC. Close attention to the presence of the GCT intimately associated with the PEH will assist identifying this epithelial proliferation as reactive rather than neoplastic. To this end, S100 protein may be of assistance in identifying the presence of the GCT. Further, a helpful diagnostic clue in not diagnosing the PEH associated with GCT as malignant is the fact that the epithelial proliferation does not extend below the depth of the GCT. Infections such as fungi and mycobacteria may induce PEH simulating SCC. Fungi within the depth of the surface epithelium or even within the submucosa may result in PEH of the surface epithelium; special stains may be of assistance in the identification of fungal forms.

Necrotizing sialometaplasia (NS) represents a benign, self-healing (reactive) inflammatory process of salivary gland tissue that clinically and histologically may be mistaken for a malignant neoplasm. Necrotizing sialometaplasia most commonly involves the intraoral minor salivary glands, in particular the palate, but major salivary glands as well as the minor salivary glands of virtually every site in the UADT can be affected. The most common presenting problem is that of a painless ulcerated lesion or a nodular swelling. The lesions are usually asymptomatic but may be associated with pain, numbness or a burning sensation, and dysphagia. The pathogenesis for NS is believed to be secondary to an ischemic event with compromise of the vascular supply to salivary glands leading to ischemic necrosis. The ischemia may be iatrogenically induced following an operative procedure, trauma (post-intubation), or radiotherapy. Necrotizing sialometaplasia may occur *de novo*, unassociated with a traumatic event, or it may occur in association with other nonneoplastic lesions or in association with a neoplasm (benign or malignant).

Necrotizing sialometaplasia typically appears as a deep, craterlike ulcerative lesion measuring from 1 to 3 cm. However, the lesion may appear as a submucosal nodular swelling that may slough leaving a craterlike ulcer. The histologic appearance is that of lobular necrosis of the salivary glands with preservation of the lobular architecture of the minor salivary glands. The histologic hallmark is squamous metaplasia of residual acinar and ductal elements. The necrotic lobules consist of acinus-sized pools of mucin, which may extend into adjacent tissue eliciting a granulation tissue reaction with associated acute and chronic inflammation. The lobular architecture is maintained and the metaplastic lobules vary slightly to moderately in size and shape, and have smooth edges surrounded by granulation tissue and an intense mixed acute and chronic inflammatory reaction. The squamous cells are bland in appearance with uniform nuclei and abundant eosinophilic cytoplasm with occasional preservation of ductal lumina or scattered mucocytes. Mucicarminophilic material is seen within lumina and within the cytoplasm of residual mucocytes. With regeneration, mitoses, individual cell necrosis, enlarged nuclei, and prominent nucleoli can be seen. Associated findings include ulcerated mucosa and PEH. Pseudoepitheliomatous hyperplasia results when the metaplastic lobules present in excretory ducts and merge with surface epithelium. This reaction may be so striking that it makes differentiation from an infiltrating SCC very difficult.

The juxtaoral organ of Chievitz (JOC) is a normal microscopic structure of unknown function located at the angle of the mandible, bilaterally, in close association with the buccal nerve near the buccotemporalis fascia. Given the proximity to nerves, these nonneoplastic epithelial structures may be confused with carcinomatous invasion of nerves. This is especially true during intraoperative consultation in a patient with known oral SCC. The JOC is typically not grossly visualized but may be sampled and sent for frozen section. Histologically, the JOC is composed of well-defined clusters of epithelial cells that may show the presence of intercellular bridges and palisading nuclei. The cells are cytologically bland and lack pleomorphism or mitotic activity. Keratinization is typically absent despite the presence of intercellular bridges.

Radiation-related changes and the differentiation of radiation-induced epithelial changes from recurrent/persistent SCC present one of the more challenging diagnostic dilemmas, even for the most experienced surgical pathologist. This differentiation cannot always be achieved by conventional light microscopy and unfortunately there are no adjunct modalities that may assist in remedying this diagnostic conundrum. Helpful features that may suggest radiation alterations of benign epithelium include the retention of a rounded appearance to the epithelial nests, absence of dysplastic epithelial changes, absence of atypical mitoses, and presence of secondary epithelial and stromal alterations associated with radiation injury, including smudged appearing nuclei, stromal fibrosis with atypical stromal cells, and endothelial cell atypia.

Histologic Prognostic Indicators

Among the histologic findings that may impact on the prognosis in HNSCC include:

- status of the surgical resection margins
- tumor size, thickness, and location of the lesion
- pattern of invasion
- involvement of lymph–vascular spaces
- invasion of soft tissue structures including nerves, bone, and cartilage
- nodal metastasis with or without extranodal extension of tumor
- distant metastasis
- host response
- neovascularization
- presence of multiple malignancies (224,251,252).

DNA analysis and oncogene expression (e.g., *p53*, cyclin D1 protein) have been reported to have prognostic importance in HNSCC (253–255).

Morphologic Subtypes of Squamous Cell Carcinoma

Numerous variants of HNSCC are known (Table 2.7). The diagnostic criteria and diagnostic problems associated with some of these specific subtypes of HNSCC are discussed in the following sections.

TABLE 2.7 Head and Neck Squamous Cell Carcinoma (SCC) and Variants

Conventional SCC
Papillary SCC
Verrucous carcinoma
Spindle-cell squamous carcinoma
Basaloid SCC
Nasopharyngeal carcinoma
Adenoid SCC
Adenosquamous carcinoma

PAPILLARY (EXOPHYTIC) SQUAMOUS CELL CARCINOMA

Papillary (exophytic) SCC represents an uncommon but distinct subtype of head and neck SCC (256–258). The demographics for this subtype of SCC are similar to those of conventional SCC with the tendency to affect men more than women, and occurring in adults with a mean age in the seventh decade of life. Papillary SCCs have a predilection to the larynx, oral cavity, oro- and hypopharynx, and sinonasal tract (256–258). The larynx is the most common site of occurrence. Symptoms vary according to the site of involvement. Papillary SCC usually arise *de novo* without identification of a coexisting benign lesion such as a papilloma, although association with precursor papilloma or occurrence in patients with previous history of a papilloma at the site of the papillary SCC has been reported (258). Human papillomavirus (HPV) by *in situ* hybridization and polymerase chain reaction have been detected in papillary SCC (258).

Papillary SCC is most often seen as a solitary lesion with an exophytic or papillary growth. Tumor size may range from 2 mm up to 4 cm. Histologically, papillary SCC has filiform growth with fingerlike projections and identifiable fibrovascular cores or a broad-based bulbous to exophytic growth with rounded projections resembling a cauliflower-like growth pattern in which fibrovascular cores can be seen but tend to be limited to absent (Fig. 2.19). The squamous epithelium is cytologically malignant and this malignant epithelium identifies these tumors as carcinomas separating them from papillomas. Surface keratinization is generally limited and often absent. Definitive invasion may be difficult to demonstrate in biopsy specimens, with the carcinomatous epithelium suggesting an *in situ* process rather than invasive carcinoma. However, the extent of growth with the formation of a clinically appreciable exophytic mass goes beyond the general concept of an *in situ* carcinoma. These tumors should be considered as being invasive even in the absence of definitive stromal invasion.

Surgery is the treatment of choice; adjunctive therapy may be used. The majority of papillary SCCs are low clinical stage (T2) and their behavior overall is similar to conventional SCC of similar stage (258), although some authors report a better overall prognosis for papillary SCC than for conventional SCC when matched for T stage (257).

The differential diagnosis of papillary SCC includes laryngeal papillomatosis (LP), conventional SCC, and verrucous carcinoma (VC). Laryngeal papillomatosis is distinguished by its bland epithelial proliferation. Cytologic abnormalities may be seen in LP and they tend to be focal when present, but do not approach the level of dysplasia seen in papillary SCC. Verrucous carcinoma is characterized by a verrucous growth pattern with marked keratosis in layers or tiers, absent nuclear atypia, absent mitotic activity beyond the basal layer, and a pushing rather than infiltrative pattern of invasion. These features contrast with those seen in papillary and exophytic SCC.

VERRUCOUS CARCINOMA

Verrucous carcinoma is a highly differentiated variant of SCC, with locally destructive but not metastatic capabilities. Verrucous carcinoma affects men more than women and generally occurs in the sixth and seventh decades of life. Verrucous carcinoma can occur anywhere in the UADT. The most common sites of occurrence, in descending order, include oral cavity, larynx, nasal fossa, sinonasal tract, and nasopharynx (259–262). Symptoms vary according to site. In the larynx hoarseness is the most common complaint; less frequent symptoms include airway obstruction, hemoptysis, and dysphagia. In the oral cavity, mass with or without pain is often noted. In the sinonasal tract airway obstruction is most common. In the nasopharynx dysphagia is typically encountered. The most common site of occurrence of VC in the larynx is the glottic area. Oral cavity VCs most commonly arise on the buccal mucosa and gingiva.

The etiology of VC remains speculative and includes tobacco smoking or chewing. Viral-induction appears to be a legitimate etiologic factor in the development of VC but a causal relationship has not been clearly identified. The active role of HPV is more likely as a promoter in the multistep process of carcinogenesis in squamous cells of the UADT (263–265).

Verrucous carcinomas appear as tan or white, warty, fungating or exophytic, firm to hard masses of varying size measuring up to 9 to 10 cm in diameter. In general, the tumors are attached by a broad base. The histologic appearance of VC is that of a benign-appearing squamous cell proliferation requiring the following characteristics for diagnosis:

- Uniform cells without dysplastic features or mitoses
- Marked surface (ortho)keratinization ("church-spire" keratosis)
- Broad or bulbous rete pegs with a pushing but not infiltrative margin (Fig. 2.20).

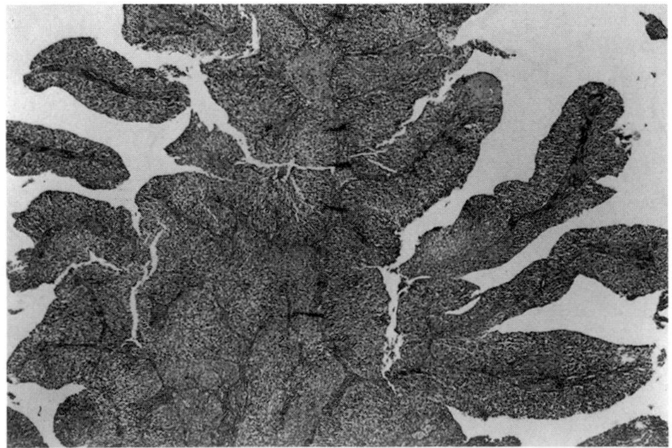

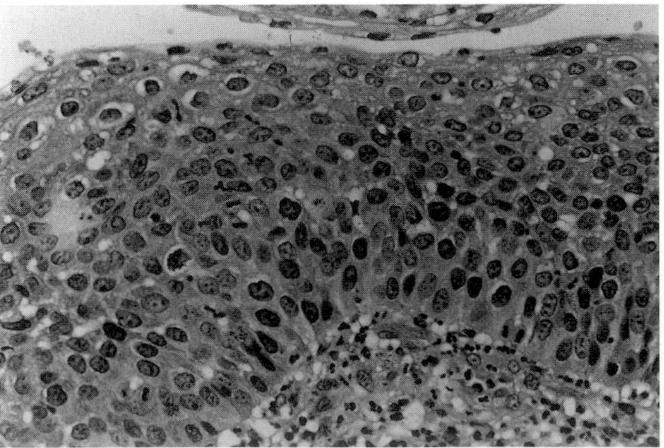

Figure 2.19 Papillary squamous cell carcinoma. **Left:** Papillary epithelial neoplasm with fibrovascular cores devoid of surface keratinization. **Right:** Higher magnification shows the presence of cytologically malignant epithelial cells.

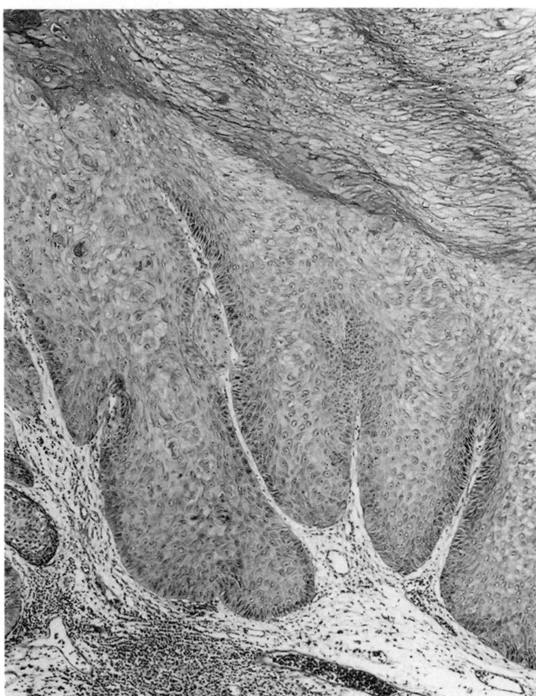

Figure 2.20 Verrucous carcinoma of the larynx characterized by an epithelial proliferation of uniform cells without dysplastic features or mitoses, marked surface keratinization, and broad or bulbous rete pegs pushing downward into the submucosa.

A mixed chronic inflammatory cell infiltrate composed of lymphocytes, plasma cells, and histiocytes may be prominent along the adjacent stroma. The pathologic diagnosis of VC may be extremely difficult and require multiple biopsies over several years prior to identification of diagnostic features supporting appropriate interpretation. Both clinicians and pathologists should be aware of this fact. To this end, adequate biopsy material is critical to interpretation and should include a good epithelial–stromal interface. The pathologist should not over interpret a verrucoid lesion as a carcinoma without seeing the relationship of the more superficial aspects of the lesion to the underlying stroma.

Surgery (conservation or total laryngectomy) is the definitive diagnostic modality. The literature supports the dogma that radiotherapy is contraindicated in the treatment of VC. The reason for this is the purported induction of anaplastic transformation of VC following radiotherapy. However, similar transformations can occur following surgery, cryosurgery, and even without any treatment. Therefore, radiotherapy is not contraindicated in the treatment of VC and can be used in selected clinical settings, including those patients with advanced disease or patients who are not good surgical candidates. Metastatic tumor spread to regional lymph nodes is rare and distant metastases do not occur. The prognosis is excellent following complete surgical removal. Local recurrence may occur if incompletely excised. Cervical adenopathy may be associated with VC representing reactive changes and not metastatic disease.

The differential diagnosis of VC includes a variety of lesions, including reactive keratosis, epithelial hyperplasia, or pseudoepitheliomatous hyperplasia; verruca vulgaris; (keratotic) squamous papilloma or papillomatosis; and Schneiderian papillomas and keratoacanthoma (when VC affects cutaneous sites). However, VC must be differentiated from the "conventional" type of SCC. The differentiation of VC from a "conventional" type of carcinoma is based on the presence or absence of cytologic abnormalities. Dysplastic features limited in scope and confined to the basal zone areas can be seen in VC. Any dysplastic features greater than this should exclude a diagnosis of VC. Hybrid neoplasms composed of VC and coexisting conventional SCC occur (261,262) and have been reported in up to 20% of cases (261). Careful evaluation of the depth of the lesion is important to exclude this possibility.

Proliferative verrucous leukoplakia (PVL) and verrucous hyperplasia represent interrelated and irreversible mucosal lesions of the oral cavity and UADT with a propensity to progress to either VC or conventional types of SCC (266–268). Proliferative verrucous leukoplakia is a rare aggressive form of oral leukoplakia with a tendency to recur, often with multifocal oral involvement, and to undergo malignant transformation. Proliferative verrucous leukoplakia is most common in elderly women (mean age in the eighth decade of life) with a long history (decades) of oral leukoplakia. Proliferative verrucous leukoplakia most commonly begins on the buccal mucosa followed by the hard and soft palate, alveolar mucosa, tongue, floor of mouth, gingiva, and lip. Although a history of tobacco use is present in a high percentage of patients (>50%), a significant minority of patients has no history of tobacco use. The diagnosis of PVL in its early stages is virtually impossible due to the innocuous appearance of the lesions. The clinical and pathologic appearance in the early stages of PVL is no different than any other type of leukoplakic lesion. Clinically, the lesion is a flat, thickened keratosis with the histologic appearance of a nondysplastic keratosis. With progression of disease, the lesions become multiple, multifocal, and confluent, with an exophytic or warty (verrucoid) appearance. It is in the latter clinical form that squamous cancer (VC or conventional SCC) is seen. Any given lesion may show a combination of verrucous hyperplasia, VC, and conventional well-differentiated SCC. Given the fact that PVL is associated with VC in a high percentage of cases, some authors believe that PVL should be considered as a premalignant condition or an early biologic form of VC (267,269). This would then obviate the confusion, both clinically and pathologically, that surrounds the use of the term *verrucous hyperplasia* in describing these oral cavity lesions. Proliferative verrucous leukoplakia is composed of hyperplastic squamous epithelium with regularly spaced, verrucous epithelial projections and associated hyperkeratosis. Proliferative verrucous leukoplakia is a sharply defined lesion and in contrast to the downward growth into the underlying submucosal compartment by the bulbous rete pegs in VC, the hyperplastic epithelium in PVL remains superficial (without submucosal invasion) and does not extend deeper than that of the adjacent epithelium. This raises the issue of adequate sampling and the difficulties in differential diagnosis on incisional biopsy material. To exclude the presence of submucosal invasion, complete excision of the lesion allowing for histologic examination of the entire lesion is most appropriate. The treatment of PVL is by surgical excision. However, disease-free survival rates following surgery are low due to recurrence and multifocal involvement. Radiotherapy has not been shown to be effective in controlling disease.

Rarely, verruca vulgaris (VV) may occur in the larynx and presents difficulties in differentiation from VC. In VV there is a prominent keratohyaline granular layer, parakeratosis, and sharp acanthotic pegs, all features that are not present in VC (270).

SPINDLE CELL SQUAMOUS CARCINOMA

Spindle cell squamous carcinoma (SCSC) is defined as a tumor composed of conventional SCC (*in situ* or invasive carcinoma) associated with a malignant spindle cell stromal component. Synonyms include "sarcomatoid" carcinoma, carcinosarcoma, pleomorphic carcinoma, metaplastic carcinoma, collision tumor, pseudosarcoma, and Lane tumor.

The overwhelming majority of SCSC occur in men (85%) most frequently in the sixth to eighth decades of life. Spindle cell squamous carcinoma can occur anywhere in the UADT. The most common sites in descending order of occurrence include the larynx (true vocal cords more than false vocal cords and supraglottis), oral cavity (lips, tongue, gingiva, floor of mouth, buccal mucosa), skin, tonsils, and pharynx. Symptoms vary according to site. In the larynx hoarseness, voice changes, airway obstruction, and dysphagia are all common. In the oral cavity or skin a mass or nonhealing sore with or without pain may be noted. In the sinonasal tract and nasopharynx airway obstruction, pain, epistaxis, discharge, facial deformity, unilateral otitis media, and orbital symptoms are often encountered. There is no specific correlation with known risk factors (alcohol, tobacco, or environment/occupation). Spindle cell squamous carcinoma has been reported in areas of prior irradiation.

Spindle cell squamous carcinoma is often a grossly polypoid or fungating mass commonly found in the larynx, hypopharynx, oral cavity, and sinonasal tract (271). Variations in the gross appearance may correlate with the primary site of occurrence. In the larynx the appearance may be polypoid or exophytic; in the sinonasal tract and nasopharynx the appearance may be fungating or ulcerative. Spindle cell squamous carcinomas are firm, tan-white, gray, or pink masses varying in size from 1 to 6 cm.

The histologic features that define SCSC include the identification of a malignant, undifferentiated spindle cell proliferation and the presence of a conventional squamous cell component (Fig. 2.21). The latter includes either *in situ* squamous carcinoma or frankly invasive differentiated squamous carcinoma. The spindle cell component generally is the dominant cell type. The spindle cell proliferation is usually hypercellular and pleomorphic with large, hyperchromatic nuclei, prominent nucleoli, and many mitoses (typical and atypical). Necrosis is not uncommon. The spindle cell proliferation may be sparsely cellular (hypocellular) with marked stromal collagenization (so-called collagenized SCSC), but nuclear pleomorphism and mitotic figures are still present. The growth pattern varies and includes fascicular, storiform, or palisading; an associated myxomatous stroma may be present. Heterologous elements, including bone and cartilage may be present and may even be malignant (chondrosarcomatous or osteosarcomatous foci).

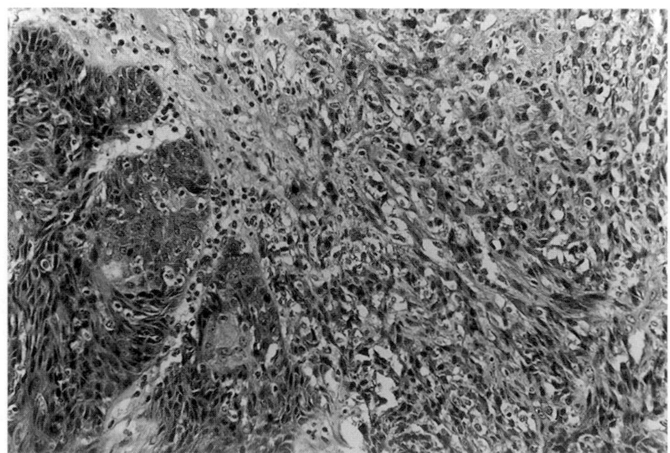

Figure 2.21 Laryngeal (glottic) spindle cell squamous cell carcinoma. The neoplastic infiltrate includes differentiated squamous cell carcinoma (left) intimately associated with a malignant spindle-shaped and pleomorphic cellular component.

The spindle cells are cytokeratin immunoreactive in the majority of cases (272–276) but in up to 40% of cases may be cytokeratin-negative (273). Cytokeratin staining may vary from focal to diffuse. Expression of vimentin and various myogenic markers (desmin, actins) have been reported (274–277). S-100 protein and HMB-45 are negative. Ultrastructurally, in the majority of cases, SCSCs show evidence of epithelial derivation, including desmosomes, tonofilaments, and macula adherens (272,278). The histogenesis of the spindle cells is controversial as evidenced by the array of names given to this tumor.

Epithelial derivation is supported by the intimate association with conventional SCC and the presence of cytokeratin immunoreactivity in the majority of cases and lack of immunoreactivity with other antibodies. Despite the presence of heterologous elements, including malignant bone or cartilage, neither of these components has been reported to metastasize and in all probability they represent a metaplastic phenomenon. Identical immunohistochemical *p53* expression patterns in the epithelial and spindle cell components of SCSC support the concept that these phenotypically divergent cell populations share similar developmental pathways and divest the concept that SCSC represents a reactive process or a collision tumor between epithelial and mesenchymal components (279).

Surgery is the preferred therapy. Radiotherapy may be used as an adjunct to surgery but neither radiotherapy nor chemotherapy has merit as the sole therapeutic modality. The prognosis is dependent on the clinical stage but, in general, is considered poor. Polypoid lesions may behave less aggressively than flat, ulcerative tumors, perhaps correlating with limited (superficial) invasion. Vocal cord lesions which manifest symptoms early in the disease course may have a better prognosis than SCSC arising in other sites (supraglottis, hypo- and nasopharynx) where symptoms occur only after the tumor has become large and extensively infiltrative. Metastatic disease primarily occurs to cervical lymph nodes and lung, and may include conventional SCC alone, SCSC alone, or both conventional and SCSC.

The squamous cell component of SCSC may be limited and require multiple sectioning for identification, or it may be absent. The differential diagnosis includes myofibroblastic or fibroblastic proliferations, mucosal malignant melanoma, and sarcomas including malignant fibrous histiocytoma, fibrosarcoma, malignant peripheral nerve sheath neoplasm, osteosarcoma, and chondrosarcoma. These sarcomas, while uncommon in relation to a mucosal surface of the head and neck region, do occur. In general, these tumors are deeply seated in any given location and do not usually result in a polypoid mass protruding from a mucosal surface. As a rule, in the absence of any other confirmatory studies (i.e., immunohistochemistry, electron microscopy), a malignant spindle cell neoplasm of a mucosal surface of the UADT presenting as a polypoid lesion or identified in more superficial locations of the submucosa, should be considered as an SCSC. This is true even in the absence of a squamous carcinomatous component, the presence of heterologous matrix-producing elements, or in the absence of cytokeratin immunoreactivity.

Reactive and neoplastic lesions composed of myofibroblastic cells include nodular fasciitis-like lesions and inflammatory myofibroblastic tumors (IMT), and have been reported as occurring in the larynx (280). These lesions are moderately cellular with a proliferation of spindle-shaped cells, but do not display a striking degree of nuclear pleomorphism. Mitotic figures may be encountered but atypical mitoses are not seen. The findings of atypical mitoses should prompt consideration of a true malignancy. Although the lesions are not encapsulated, they do not exhibit the insidious pattern of infiltration of adjacent tissues that is characteristic of more aggressive lesions. The lesions may fill the submucosal region, abutting the basement membrane on which the mucosal epithelial cells are resting; however, the spindle cell proliferation does not infiltrate into the mucosal epithelial cells. Nevertheless, the overlying mucosa may appear atrophic in areas. These lesions are cytokeratin-negative. In addition, the myofibroblastic cell component may be muscle-specific actin (HHF35), smooth muscle actin, and vimentin-positive. Recent evidence has shown the presence of anaplastic lymphoma kinase (*ALK*) gene rearrangements and expression in IMT indicating oncogenic *ALK* expression as an important mechanism in the pathogenesis of IMT and supports the concept that IMTs are neoplastic (281–283).

BASALOID SQUAMOUS CELL CARCINOMA

Basaloid squamous cell carcinoma (BSCC) is a high-grade variant of SCC with a predilection to the base of the tongue, supraglottic larynx, hypopharynx, and palatine tonsil (284,285). Basaloid squamous cell carcinoma is histologically characterized by an invasive neoplasm composed of basaloid cells intimately associated with either a dysplastic squamous epithelium, *in situ* SCC, or invasive SCC.

Basaloid squamous cell carcinoma occurs more commonly in men than in women and predominantly occurs in the sixth to seventh decades of life. These tumors have a predilection for the hypopharynx (pyriform sinus), larynx (supraglottis), and tongue. Symptoms depend on the site of occurrence and include hoarseness, dysphagia, pain, or a neck mass. Etiologic factors include excessive alcohol or tobacco use. The cell of origin has not definitively been identified but in all probability is a single totipotential cell capable of divergent differentiation and located either in the basal cell layer of the surface epithelium or within seromucous glands.

Grossly, these tumors are described as firm to hard, tan-white masses often with associated central necrosis measuring up to 6 cm in greatest dimension. Infrequently, they may be exophytic in appearance. Histologically, BSCC is an invasive neoplasm composed of basaloid cells with an associated squamous component and demonstrating a variety of growth patterns, including solid, lobular, cribriform, cords, trabeculae, and glandlike or cystic growth (Fig. 2.22). The basaloid cell component is the predominant cell type and consists of cells with pleomorphic, hyperchromatic nuclei, scanty cytoplasm, and increased mitotic activity (Fig. 2.22). Peripheral nuclear palisading may be present. Comedonecrosis is seen in the center of the neoplastic lobules. Intercellular deposition of a hyalin or mucohyalin material can be seen and is similar in appearance to the reduplicated basement membrane material seen in some salivary gland tumors. Infrequently, a spindle cell component may be identified and true neural-type

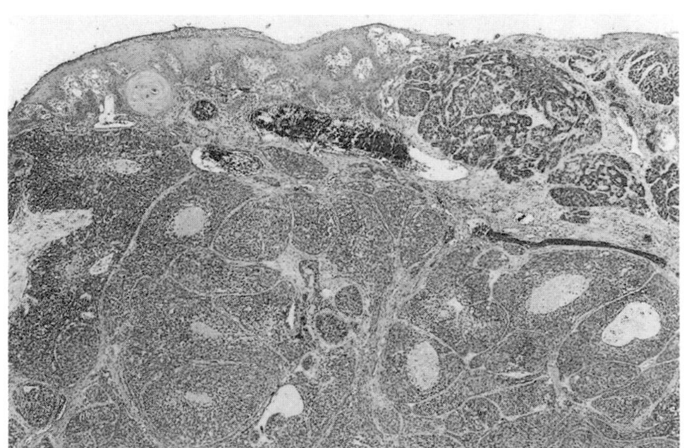

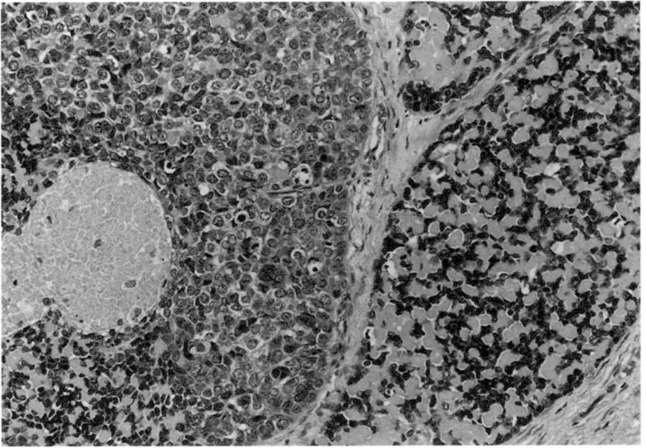

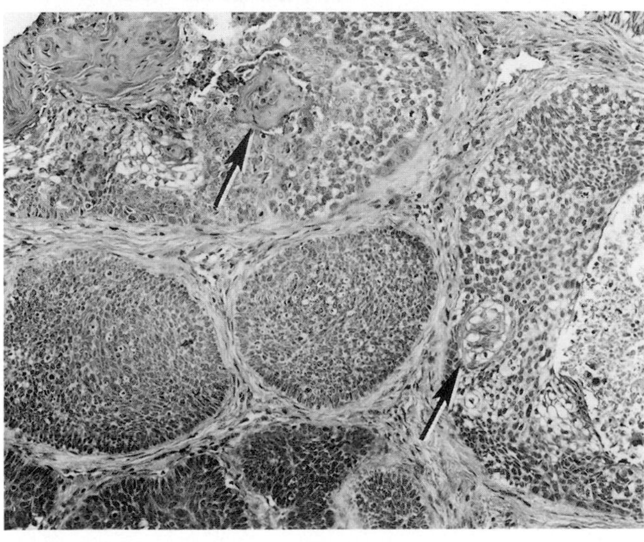

Figure 2.22 Basaloid squamous cell carcinoma of the hypopharynx. **Top left:** The tumor originated from the surface epithelium. The infiltrative component shows a predominant lobular growth with foci of central necrosis. **Top right:** Toward the left there is a neoplastic lobule with central necrosis composed of malignant, pleomorphic, basaloid-appearing cells; toward the right the presence of basement membrane like extracellular material is reminiscent of salivary gland tumors. **Bottom:** Typically the squamous component of this tumor is focally seen in a neoplasm that is predominantly composed of pleomorphic, basaloid-appearing cells. Areas of squamous differentiation (*arrows*) are present.

rosettes may rarely be present (286). The squamous component includes dysplastic squamous epithelium, foci of abrupt keratinization, *in situ* SCC, or invasive SCC. The squamous foci typically are a minor component (Fig. 2.22) and may be focally present yet absent in biopsies. Continuity with the surface epithelium may be seen.

Histochemical stains may show periodic acid-Schiff and Alcian blue-positive material within the cystic spaces. Immunoreactivity is consistently present with epithelial markers, including cytokeratins (AE1/3, 34E12,CAM5.2), epithelial membrane antigen (EMA), and carcinoembryonic antigen (CEA) (285–287). Neuroendocrine markers (i.e., chromogranin and synaptophysin), and HMB-45 are negative. Basaloid squamous cell carcinoma may express neuron specific endase (NSE) but is considered as nonspecific. Variable expression can be seen with vimentin, S-100 protein, and actin. Electron microscopy (EM) shows the features of SCC, including cell groups with numerous and prominent tonofilament bundles, increased desmosomes, and epithelial pearls and loose stellate granules or replicated basal lamina within the cystic spaces (284,288) and absence of glandular differentiation (288). Flow cytometry studies have shown that patients with BSCC whose tumors were DNA aneuploid had better mean survival periods than those with diploid DNA tumors.

The treatment of choice for BSCC includes radical surgical excision and as a result of both early regional lymph node as well as distant visceral metastases, radical neck dissection and supplemental radio- and chemotherapy may be included in the initial management protocol. Basaloid squamous cell carcinoma is an aggressive, high-grade tumor with increased tendency to be multifocal, deeply invasive, and metastatic. Metastases occur via lymphatics and blood vessels with sites of predilection including regional and distant lymph nodes, lung, bone, skin, and brain. Metastases include both basaloid and squamous cell components. Basaloid squamous cell carcinoma is a rapidly fatal neoplasm associated with high mortality rates within the first year following diagnosis.

Shallow biopsies may belie the depth and extent of invasion and may not be representative of the lesion leading to erroneous classification. The differential diagnosis of BSCC primarily includes adenoid cystic carcinoma and small cell (undifferentiated) neuroendocrine carcinoma. Adenoid cystic carcinoma is characterized by the presence of a proliferation of basaloid cells with homogenous-appearing hyperchromatic nuclei lacking significant pleomorphism and generally devoid of mitotic activity. Further, squamous differentiation is not a component of adenoid cystic carcinoma. Small cell neuroendocrine carcinoma may be difficult to differentiate from BSCC by light microscopy. This is an important differentiation as small cell neuroendocrine carcinomas are treated nonsurgically with radiation and systemic chemotherapy. Morice and Ferreiro (287) compared the immunoreactive profile of BSCC from small cell neuroendocrine carcinoma and adenoid cystic carcinoma. These authors found that while rare examples of BSCC may be reactive with neuroendocrine markers, including chromogranin and synaptophysin, these markers are typically positive in small cell neuroendocrine carcinoma but absent in BSCC.

UNDIFFERENTIATED CARCINOMA (LYMPHOEPITHELIOMA-LIKE OR NASOPHARYNGEAL-TYPE)

Undifferentiated carcinoma is a variant of SCC, commonly of nasopharyngeal origin or Waldeyer ring origin (i.e., base of tongue, palatine tonsils, and adenoids) that arises from the surface epithelium. According to the World Health Organization (WHO) nasopharyngeal carcinomas are divided into two histologic subtypes: keratinizing, and nonkeratinizing (289). The nonkeratinizing type is further subdivided into nonkeratinizing differentiated and nonkeratinizing undifferentiated (Table 2.8). Synonyms for undifferentiated carcinoma include lymphoepithelioma, Regaud and Schmincke types of lymphoepithelioma, and transitional carcinoma.

TABLE 2.8 World Health Organization (WHO) Classification of Nasopharyngeal Carcinoma

WHO type I
Keratinzing squamous cell carcinoma
WHO type II
Nonkeratinizing differentiated
Nonkeratinizing undifferentiated

Overall, nasopharyngeal carcinoma is an uncommon neoplasm in the United States, accounting for approximately 0.25% of all cancers (290,291). In China, it accounts for 18% of all cancers. Nasopharyngeal carcinoma affects men more than women and occurs over a wide age range but is most common in the sixth decade of life. Irrespective of the histologic type the clinical presentation is similar and includes neck mass, hearing loss, nasal obstruction, nasal discharge, epistaxis, pain, otalgia, and headache. The signs and symptoms are often subtle and nonspecific leading to delay in diagnosis and eventual presentation with advanced disease. The lateral wall of the nasopharynx (fossa of Rosenmüller) is the most common site of occurrence. Lymphoepithelioma-like carcinomas can be found in nonnasopharyngeal head and neck sites, including the larynx and hypopharynx (292,293).

The suggested etiologic factors include:

- Genetic and geographic: increased incidence in China especially in southern (Kwantung province) and northern provinces and Taiwan; although the incidence among Chinese people decreases after emigration to low-incidence areas, it still remains higher than in non-Chinese populations; HLA-A2 histocompatibility locus has been suggested as the marker for genetic susceptibility to nasopharyngeal carcinoma.
- Epstein-Barr virus (EBV): elevated titers of anti-EBV antibodies are associated with nasopharyngeal carcinoma (undifferentiated and nonkeratinizing types) (294); however, no clear cause and effect has been established between the presence of EBV and the development of nasopharyngeal carcinoma.
- Other suggested implicating factors are diet, poor hygiene, and environmental conditions (295).

Radiologic findings on plain film radiographs are variable and nonspecific and include a soft tissue mass, bone destruction, and sinus opacity. Computed tomography may demonstrate bone invasion, including invasion of the base of skull and expansion of sinuses with progression of disease.

The gross appearance of nasopharyngeal carcinoma varies from a mucosal bulge with an overlying intact epithelium to a clearly demonstrable mass with extensive involvement of the surface epithelium to a totally unidentifiable lesion fortuitously sampled and identified by microscopic evaluation. Three histologic types are identified based on the predominant appearance and include:

1. Keratinizing
2. Nonkeratinizing (Fig. 2.23)
3. Undifferentiated (Figs. 2.24 and 2.25).

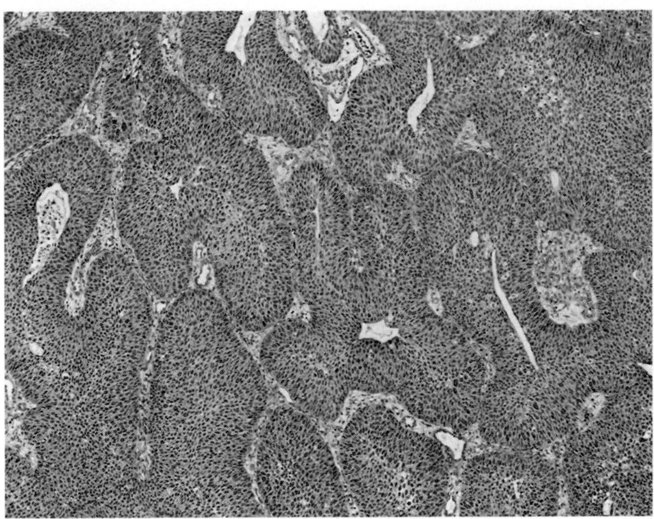

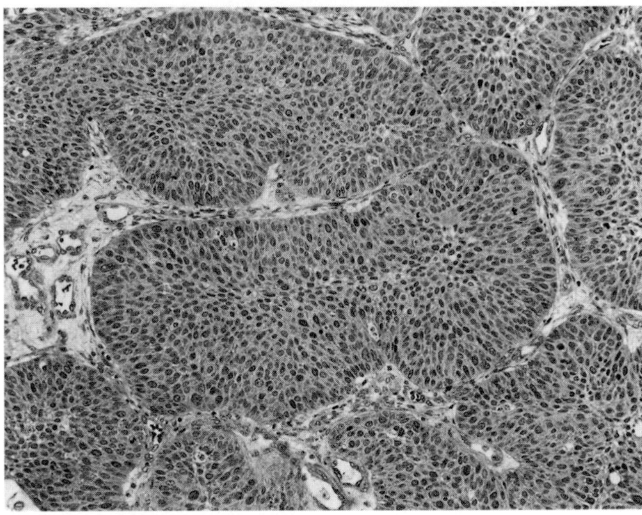

Figure 2.23 Nasopharyngeal nonkeratinizing carcinoma, differentiated type. **Left:** This carcinoma is characterized by the presence of wide interconnecting cords of neoplastic cells. **Right:** At higher magnification, the cellular infiltrate of the nasopharyngeal nonkeratinizing carcinoma, differentiated type shows the absence of keratinization.

For a description of the histologic features see Table 2.9.

As a result of the anatomic constraints imposed by the nasopharynx and the tendency of these neoplasms to present in an advanced stage, supervoltage radiotherapy (6,500–>7,000 rads) is considered the treatment of choice. Responsiveness to radiation varies per histologic type and thereby impacts on prognosis. The keratinizing subtype is not radioresponsive. These tumors have a tendency to remain localized without (nodal) dissemination. However, based on the radioresistance, the 5-year survival rate is in the range of 20% to 40% (295). The nonkeratinizing subtype is variably radioresponsive. These tumors have a tendency to metastasize to regional lymph nodes. Based on their relative radioresponsiveness, the 5-year survival rate is in the range of 60% (295). The undifferentiated subtype is radiosensitive. These tumors have a tendency to metastasize to regional lymph nodes. Nevertheless, despite the tendency to disseminate and to be the least differentiated of all the subtypes based on their radiosensitivity, the 5-year survival rate is approximately 60% (295). Factors that may affect prognosis include:

- Clinical stage
- Patient age. The younger the age the better the prognosis, which probably correlates to the fact that nasopharyngeal carcinoma occurring in younger patients is predominantly of the undifferentiated type
- Lymph node metastasis (positive nodes decrease survival by approximately 10%–20%).

The sole use for chemotherapy is for widespread disease. The Regaud and Schmincke types of nasopharyngeal carcinoma refer

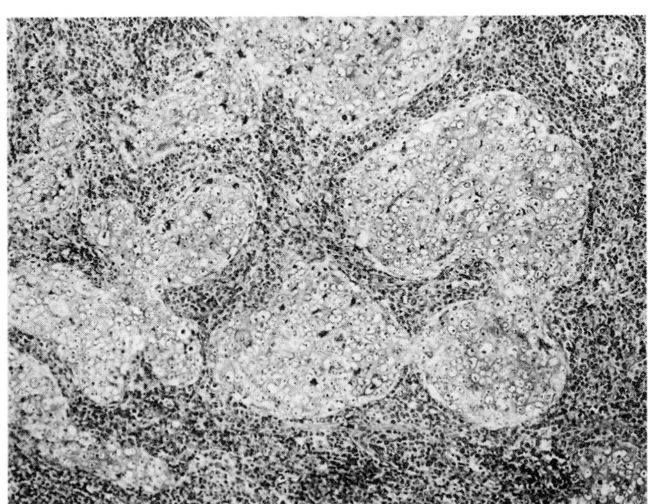

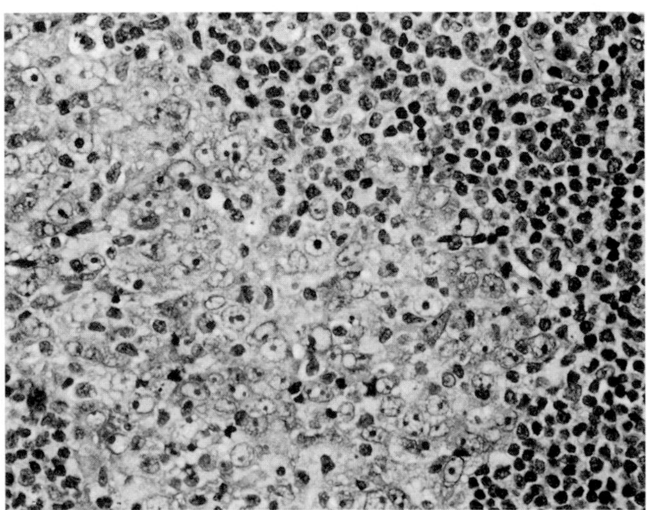

Figure 2.24 Nasopharyngeal nonkeratinizing carcinoma, undifferentiated type, cohesive growth. **Left:** The neoplastic nests are readily identified, standing out as distinct nests or syncytium from the surrounding benign lymphocytic cell population. **Right:** At higher magnification, the neoplastic cells include enlarged nuclei with vesicular chromatin, indistinct cell borders, and prominent eosinophilic nucleoli.

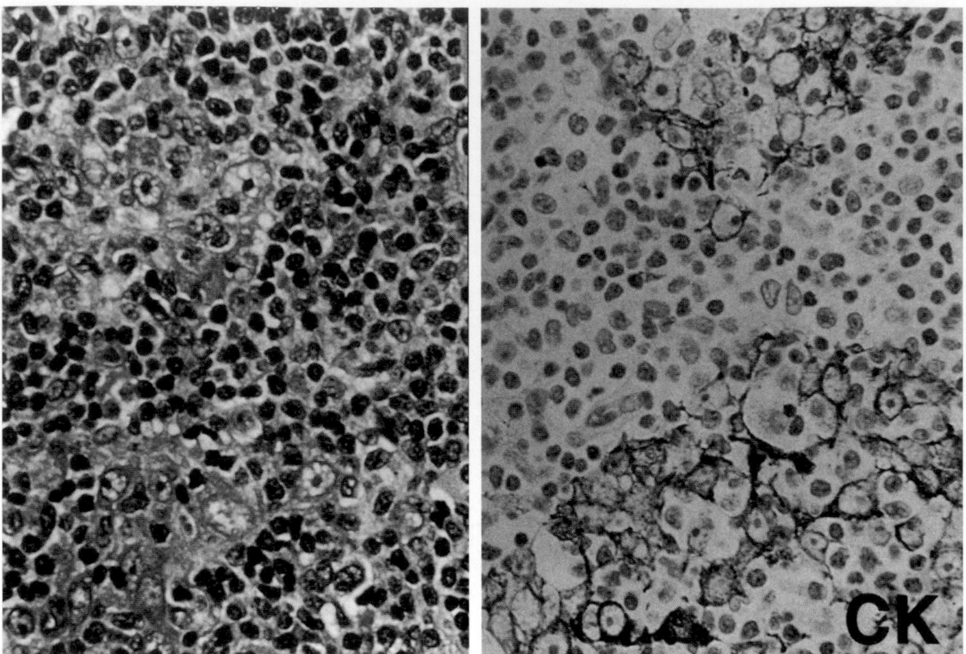

Figure 2.25 Nasopharyngeal nonkeratinizing carcinoma, undifferentiated type. **Left:** Often there is an absence of desmoplasia in association with this invasive carcinoma making identification of the malignant cells difficult, as seen in this high magnification. **Right:** Cytokeratin (CK) immunoreactivity is needed to confirm the epithelial nature of the cells.

to those neoplasms with syncytial versus individual cell invasive growth patterns, respectively; these designations and their correlated growth have no bearing on the biology of the disease.

The differential diagnosis of nasopharyngeal carcinoma includes non-Hodgkin malignant lymphoma (large cell or immunoblastic), mucosal malignant melanoma, and rhabdomyosarcoma. Differentiation is readily achieved by appropriate immunohistochemical staining.

Metastatic Neoplasms to the Neck Region from an Occult Primary Neoplasm

By definition, an occult metastasis includes the presence of an overt neck mass harboring a histologically proven metastatic neoplasm in the absence of a clinically detectable primary neoplasm. The most common clinical manifestation of a metastatic tumor to the neck from an occult primary neoplasm is that of a unilateral, fixed mass. The demographics of this entity include a more common occurrence in men than women, and it most frequently occurs in the fifth to seventh decades of life (296). The majority of metastatic tumors to the cervical lymph nodes take origin from a head and neck primary tumor and, therefore, the most common histologic appearance is that of an SCC. By far, the nasopharynx, tonsils, and base of tongue, collectively referred to as the Waldeyer tonsillar ring, are the areas harboring the occult primary tumor in the majority of squamous carcinomas metastatic to the neck (296). Other common but less frequent sites of the occult tumor include the thyroid gland (papillary carcinoma), hypopharynx, and larynx (supraglottic region). Metastatic tumors to the neck are not limited to origin

TABLE 2.9 Nasopharyngeal Carcinoma

Features	Keratinizing	Nonkeratinizing	Undifferentiated
Percent of cases	Approximately 25%	Least common (<15%)	Most common (>60%)
Sex/age	M>F; 6th decade	M>F; 6th decade	M>F; bimodal 2nd and 6th decades
Histology	Keratinization, intercellular bridges; conventional squamous cell carcinoma graded as well, moderately or poorly differentiated; desmoplastic response to invasion	Little to absent keratinization, growth pattern similar to transitional carcinoma of the bladder; typically, absence of desmoplastic response to invasion	Absent keratinization; syncytial growth, cohesive or noncohesive cells with round nuclei, prominent eosinophilic nucleoli, scant cytoplasm and mitoses; prominent nonneoplastic lymphoid component; typically, absence of desmoplastic response to invasion
IHC	CK-positive	CK-positive	CK-positive; LCA- and DES-negative
EBV	Weak association	Strong association	Strong association
Treatment	Radioresponsiveness is not good	Variably radioresponsive	Radiosensitive
Prognosis	10%–20% 5-year survival	35%–50% 5-year survival	60% 5-year survival

CK, cytokeratin; DES, desmin; EBV, Epstein-Barr virus; IHC, immunohistochemistry; LCA, leukocyte common antigen.

from a head and neck neoplasm but may represent primary occult neoplasms from organ systems in the thorax, abdomen, and pelvis (296). The most common primary site for a metastatic tumor originating from below the clavicle is the lungs. Virtually every organ may be the primary focus of a metastasis to the head and neck. A malignant neoplasm of the head and neck that has an unusual histologic appearance or that presents difficulty in its histologic classifying should alert the pathologist to the possibility that the neoplasm may represent a metastasis from a distant site.

Except for the metastatic thyroid papillary carcinoma, the histologic appearance of metastatic cystic (squamous cell) carcinoma to cervical lymph nodes does not allow confirmation of a specific site of origin. This is especially true for keratinizing SCCs, the origin of which could be from any head and neck mucosal site. However, metastatic tumors with the morphologic appearance which includes nonkeratinizing or undifferentiated carcinoma are strongly suggestive of origin from the Waldeyer tonsillar ring. Pacchioni et al. (294) evaluated 25 cases of occult metastasis to cervical lymph nodes for the presence of EBV by *in situ* hybridization following fine-needle aspiration biopsies of the neck mass and correlated with the histology of the surgical specimens (after locating the primary site of origin). These authors report that EBV was expressed in all seven metastases that ultimately proved to have originated from the nasopharynx, whereas the remaining 18 cases (not of Waldeyer ring origin) were EBV-negative. Paccioni et al. (294) indicate that detection of EBV in cervical metastatic foci may assist in localization of the occult primary to the Waldeyer ring.

Controversy exists between the diagnoses of metastatic cystic SCC versus a carcinoma arising in a branchial cleft cyst (branchiogenic carcinoma). Martin et al. (297) established the criteria for the diagnosis of a branchiogenic carcinoma, including:

1. The metastatic tumor occurs along the line extending from a point anterior to the tragus along the anterior border of the sternocleidomastoid muscle to the clavicle.
2. The histology supports origin from a branchial cleft-derived structure.
3. The histology supports carcinoma arising in the wall of an epithelial-lined cyst.
4. A minimum of 5-year follow-up demonstrates no evidence of a primary source for this neoplasm.

Despite the fulfillment of these criteria it is highly unlikely that carcinoma arises in a branchial cleft cyst (298–300). Rather, all these cystic nodal lesions represent metastatic cystic SCC most often originating from a primary tumor in the Waldeyer tonsillar ring (300). The primary Waldeyer ring neoplasm may be so small as to defy clinical detection but nevertheless is capable of metastasizing.

Treatment for the occult metastatic tumor is not fixed and is dependent on the clinical stage, location of the lymph node(s) involved, and histologic appearance of the tumor. A combination of surgery (neck dissection) and radiotherapy is the preferred therapeutic approach (296,301–303). The single most important factor in prognosis is the clinical stage (296,302). Other factors that correlate with prognosis include the location of the lymph node (e.g., supraclavicular nodal involvement has a poor prognosis) and the histologic appearance (e.g., metastatic adenocarcinomas have worse survival rates).

The lymphatic drainage to the cervical lymph nodes is predictable and the anatomic location of the metastatic focus assists in the search for the primary focus. The diagnostic workup for a patient with a metastatic tumor in the neck of occult primary origin includes:

1. Panendoscopic evaluation of the upper respiratory tract including direct laryngoscopy, bronchoscopy, and esophagoscopy.
2. The biopsy of any mucosal abnormality and if no abnormalities are grossly seen, random biopsies, especially of the Waldeyer tonsillar ring (nasopharynx, tonsil, and base of tongue), are indicated.
3. Radiographs.

REFERENCES

1. *Webster's encyclopedic unabridged dictionary of the English language.* New York: Random House, 1989:216.
2. Gnepp DR, Heffner DK. Mucosal origin of sinonasal tract adenomatous neoplasms. *Mod Pathol* 1989;2:365.
3. Wiernik G, Millard PR, Haybittle JL. The predictive value of histological classification into degrees of differentiation of squamous cell carcinoma of the larynx and hypopharynx compared with the survival of patients. *Histopathology* 1991;19:411.
4. McGavran JR, Hellquist HB, Michaels L. The incidence of cervical lymph node metastases from epidermoid carcinoma of the larynx and their relationship to certain characteristics of the primary tumor. *Cancer* 1961;14:655.
5. Arthur K, Farr HW. Prognostic significance of histologic grade in epidermoid carcinoma of the mouth and pharynx. *Am J Surg* 1972;124:489.
6. Crissman JD, Liu WY, Gluckman JL, et al. Prognostic value of histopathologic parameters in squamous cell carcinoma of the oropharynx. *Cancer* 1984; 54:2995.
7. Crissman JD. Tumor-host interactions as prognostic factors in histologic assessment of carcinomas. *Pathol Annu* 1986;21:29.
8. Zitsch RP III, Park CW, Renner GJ, et al. Outcome analysis of lip carcinoma. *Otolaryngol Head Neck Surg* 1995;113:589.
9. Prophet EB, Mills B, Arrington JB, et al. *Laboratory methods in histochemistry.* Washington, DC: Armed Forces Institute of Pathology, 1992:1.
10. Shi SR, Key ME, Kalra KL. Antigen retrieval in formalin-fixed, paraffin-embedded tissues: an enhancement method for immunohistochemical staining based on microwave oven heating of tissue sections. *J Histochem Cytochem* 2001;39:741.
11. Lovett EJ III, Schnitzer B, Keren DF, et al. Application of flow cytometry to diagnostic pathology. *Lab Invest* 1984;50:115.
12. Pesce CM. Defining and interpreting diseases through morphometry. *Lab Invest* 1987;56:568.
13. Hiddemann W, Schumann J, Andreeff M, et al. Convention on nomenclature for DNA cytometry: committee on nomenclature, society for analytical cytology. *Cancer Genet Cytogenet* 1984;3:181.
14. Johnson TS, Williamson KD, Cramer MM, et al. Flow cytometric analysis of head and neck carcinoma DNA index and s-fraction from paraffin-embedded sections: comparison with malignancy grading. *Cytometry* 1985;6:461.
15. Chauvel P, Courdi A, Gioanni J, et al. The labelling index: a prognostic factor in head and neck carcinoma. *Radiother Oncol* 1989;14:231.
16. Lampe HB. DNA analysis of head and neck squamous cell carcinoma by flow cytometry. *Laryngoscope* 1993;103:637.
17. Sakr W, Hussan M, Zarbo RL, et al. DNA quantification and histologic characteristics of squamous cell carcinoma of the upper aerodigestive tract. *Arch Pathol Lab Med* 1989;113:1009.
18. Kokel WA, Gardine RL, Sheibani K, et al. Tumour DNA content as a prognostic indicator in squamous cell carcinoma of the head and neck region. *Am J Surg* 1988;156:276.
19. Guo YC, DeSanto L, Osetinsky GV. Prognostic implication of nuclear DNA content in head and neck cancer. *Otolaryngol Head Neck Surg* 1989;100:95.
20. Kearsely JH, Bryson G, Battistutta D, et al. Prognostic importance of cellular DNA content in head and neck squamous cell cancers. A comparison of retrospective and prospective series. *Int J Cancer* 1991;47:31.
21. Luna MA, El Naggar A, Parichatikanond P, et al. Basaloid squamous cell carcinoma of the upper aerodigestive tract: clinicopathologic and DNA flow cytometric analysis. *Cancer* 1990;66:537.
22. Goldsmith MM, Cresson DH, Arnold LH, et al. DNA flow cytometry as a prognostic indicator in head and neck cancer. *Otolaryngol Head Neck Surg* 1987;96:307.
23. Joensuu H, Klemi PJ, Eerola E. DNA aneuploidy in follicular adenomas of the thyroid gland. *Am J Pathol* 1986;124:373.
24. Hall TL, Fu YS. Applications of quantitative microscopy in tumor pathology. *Lab Invest* 1985;53:5.
25. Pesce CM. Defining and interpreting diseases through morphometry. *Lab Invest* 1987;56:568.
26. Hellquist H, Olofsson J, Gröntoft O. Carcinoma in situ and severe dysplasia of the vocal cords. A clinicopathological and photometric investigation. *Acta Otolaryngol (Stockh)* 1081;92:543.
27. Böcking A, Auffermann W, Vogel H, et al. Diagnosis and grading of malignancy in squamous epithelial lesions of the larynx with DNA cytomorphometry. *Cancer* 1985;56:1600.
28. Munck-Wikland E, Kuylenstierna R, Lindholm J, et al. Image cytometry

DNA analysis of dysplastic squamous epithelial lesions in the larynx. *Anticancer Res* 1991;11:597.
29. Landberg G, Tan EM, Roos G. Flow cytometric multiparameter analysis of proliferating cell nuclear antigen/cyclin and Ki-67 antigen: a new view of the cell cycle. *Exp Cell Res* 1990;187:111.
30. Fletcher JA. Cytogenetic analysis of soft tissue tumors. In: Weiss SW, Goldblum JR, eds. *Enzinger and Weiss's soft tissue tumors.* St. Louis: Mosby, 2001; 125.
31. Aust R, Stahle J, Stenkvist B. The imprint method for cytodiagnosis of lymphadenopathies and of tumors of the head and neck. *Acta Cytol* 1971;15:123.
32. Gentry JF. Pelvic lymph node metastases in prostatic carcinoma. The value of touch imprint cytology. *Am J Surg Pathol* 1986;10:718.
33. Suen KC, Wood WS, Syed AA, et al. Role of imprint cytology in intraoperative diagnosis: value and limitations. *J Clin Pathol* 1978;31:328.
34. Mayall F, Denford A, Chang B, et al. Improved FNA cytology results with a near patient diagnosis service for non-breast lesion. *J Clin Pathol* 1998; 51:541.
35. Brown LA, Coghill SB. Cost effectiveness of a fine needle aspiration clinic. *Cytopathology* 1992;3:275.
36. Frable WJ. Thin-needle aspiration biopsy. A personal experience with 469 cases. *Am J Clin Pathol* 1976;65:168.
37. Frable MAS, Frable WJ. Fine needle aspiration biopsy revisited. *Laryngoscope* 1982;92:1414.
38. Kline TS, Kannan V, Kline IK. Lymphadenopathy and aspiration biopsy cytology: review of 376 superficial nodes. *Cancer* 1984;54:1076.
39. Gertner R, Podoshin L, Fradis M. Accuracy of fine needle aspiration biopsy in neck masses. *Laryngoscope* 1984;94:1370.
40. Ramzy I, Rone R, Schultenover SJ, et al. Lymph node aspiration biopsy-diagnostic reliability and limitations: an analysis of 350 cases. *Diagn Cytopathol* 1985;1:39.
41. Schultenover SJ, Ramzy I, Page CP, et al. Needle aspiration biopsy: role and limitations in surgical decision making. *Am J Clin Pathol* 1984;82:405.
42. Qizilbash AH, Elavathil LJ, Chen WC, et al. Aspiration biopsy of lymph nodes in malignant lymphoma. *Diagn Cytopathol* 1985;1:18.
43. Kardos TF, Vinson JH, Behm FQ, et al. Hodgkin's disease: diagnosis by fine-needle aspiration biopsy-analysis of cytologic criteria from a selected series. *Am J Clin Pathol* 1986;86:286.
44. Das DK, Gupta SK, Datta BN, et al. Fine needle aspiration cytodiagnosis of Hodgkin's disease and its subtypes. I. Scope and limitations. *Acta Cytol* 1990; 34:329.
45. Young NA, Al-Saleem T. Diagnosis of lymphoma by fine-needle aspiration cytology using the revised European-American classification of lymphoid neoplasms. *Cancer (Cancer Cytopathol)* 1999;87:325.
46. Chhieng DC, Cohen J-M, Cangiarella JF. Cytology and immunophenotyping of low- and intermediate-grade non-Hodgkin's lymphomas with a predominant small-cell component. *Diagn Cytopathol* 2001;24:90.
47. Russell J, Skinner J, Orell S, et al. Fine needle aspiration cytology in the management of lymphoma. *Aust NZ J Med* 1983;13:365.
48. Shaha A, Webber C, Marti J. Fine needle aspiration in the diagnosis of cervical lymphadenopathy. *Am J Surg* 1986;152:420.
49. Stewart CJR, Mackenzie K, McGarry GW, et al. Fine-needle aspiration cytology of salivary gland: a review of 341 cases. *Diagn Cytopathol* 2000;22:139.
50. Cohen MB, Ljung BME, Boles R. Salivary gland tumors: fine-needle aspiration vs frozen section diagnosis. *Arch Otolaryngol Head Neck Surg* 1986;112: 867.
51. Layfield LJ, Tan P, Galsgow BJ. Fine-needle aspiration of salivary gland lesions. Comparison with frozen section and histologic findings. *Arch Pathol Lab Med* 1987;111:346.
52. Davidson HG, Campora RG. Thyroid. In: Bibbo M, ed. *Comprehensive cytopathology.* Philadelphia: WB Saunders, 1991:649.
53. Suen KC, Quenville NF. Fine needle aspiration biopsy of the thyroid gland: a study of 304 cases. *J Clin Pathol* 1983;36:1036.
54. Frable MA, Frable WJ. Thin needle aspiration biopsy of the thyroid gland. *Laryngoscope* 1980;90:1619.
55. Åkerman M, Tennvall J, Biörklund A, et al. Sensitivity and specificity of fine needle aspiration cytology in the diagnosis of tumors of the thyroid gland. *Acta Cytol* 1985;29:850.
56. Ramacciotti CE, Pretorius HT, Chu EW, et al. Diagnostic accuracy and use of aspiration biopsy in the management of thyroid nodules. *Arch Intern Med* 1984;144:1169.
57. Baloch ZW, Tam D, Langer J, et al. Ultrasound-guided fine-needle aspiration biopsy of the thyroid: role of on-site assessment and multiple cytologic preparations. *Diagn Cytopathol* 2000;23:425.
58. Boey J, Hsu C, Collins RJ. False-negative errors in fine-needle aspiration biopsy of dominant thyroid nodules. A prospective follow-up study. *World J Surg* 1986;10:623.
59. Bugis SP, Young JEM, Archibald SD, et al. Diagnostic accuracy of fine-needle aspiration biopsy versus frozen section in solitary thyroid nodules. *Am J Surg* 1986;152:411.
60. Hamburger JI, Husain M. Contribution of intraoperative pathology evaluation to surgical management of thyroid nodules. *Endocrinol Metab Clin North Am* 1990;19:509.
61. Kopald LH, Layfield LJ, Mohrmann R, et al. Clarifying the role of fine-needle aspiration, cytologic evaluation and frozen section examination in the operative management of thyroid cancer. *Arch Surg* 1989;124:1201.
62. Hamburger JI, Hamburger SW. Declining role of frozen section in surgical planning for thyroid nodules. *Surgery* 1985;98:307.
63. LiVolsi VA, Merino MJ. Worrisome histologic alterations following fine-needle aspiration of the thyroid (WHAAFT). *Pathol Annu* 1994;29(Pt 2):99.
64. Gordon DL, Gattuso P, Castelli M, et al. Effect of fine needle aspiration on the histology of thyroid neoplasms. *Acta Cytol* 1993;37:651.
65. Chan JKC, Tang SK, Tsang WYW, et al. Histologic changes induced by fine needle aspiration. *Adv Anat Pathol* 1996;3:71.
66. Tsang K, Duggan MA. Vascular proliferation of the thyroid: a complication of fine needle aspiration. *Arch Pathol Lab Med* 1992;116:1040.
67. Kennerdell JS, Slamovits TL, Dekker A, et al. Orbital fine-needle aspiration biopsy. *Am J Ophthamol* 1985;99:547.
68. Char DH, Miller TR, Ljung B-M, et al. Fine needle aspiration biopsy in uveal melanomas. *Acta Cytol* 1989;33:599.
69. Shields JA, Ehya H, Eagle RC, et al. Fine needle aspiration of biopsy of suspected intraocular tumors. *Ophthalmology* 1993;11:1677.
70. Holaday WJ, Assor D. Ten thousand consecutive frozen sections. A retrospective study focusing on accuracy and quality control. *Am J Clin Pathol* 1974;61:769.
71. Dehner LP, Rosai J. Frozen section examination in surgical pathology. *Minn Med* 1977;60:769.
72. Kaufman Z, Lew S, Giffel B, et al. Frozen-section diagnosis in surgical pathology. A prospective analysis of 526 frozen sections. *Cancer* 1986;57:377.
73. Rogers C, Klatt EC, Chandrasoma P. Accuracy of frozen-section diagnosis in a teaching hospital. *Arch Pathol Lab Med* 1987;111:514.
74. Sawady J, Berner JJ, Siegler EE. Accuracy of and reason for frozen sections: a correlative, retrospective study. *Hum Pathol* 1988;19:1019.
75. Howanitz PJ, Hoffman GG, Zarbo RJ. The accuracy of frozen-section diagnosis in 34 hospitals. *Arch Pathol Lab Med* 1990;114:355.
76. Zarbo RJ, Hoffman GG, Howanitz PJ. Interinstitutional comparison of frozen-section consultation: a College of American Pathologists q-probe study of 79,647 consultations in 297 North American institutions. *Arch Pathol Lab Med* 1991;115:1187.
77. Ferreiro JA, Myers JL, Bostwick DG. Accuracy of frozen section diagnosis in surgical pathology: review of 1-year experience with 24,880 cases at Mayo Clinic Rochester. *Mayo Clin Proc* 1995;70:1222.
78. Saltzstein SL, Nahum AM. Frozen section diagnosis: accuracy and errors; uses and abuses. *Laryngoscope* 1973;83:1128.
79. Remsen KA, Lucente FE, Biller HF. Reliability of frozen section diagnosis in head and neck neoplasms. *Laryngoscope* 1984;94:519.
80. Ikemua K, Ohya R. The accuracy and usefulness of frozen-section diagnosis. *Head Neck* 1990;12:298.
81. Gandour-Edwards R, Donald PJ, Wiese D. The accuracy and clinical utility of frozen section in head and neck surgery. Evidence at a university medical center. *Head Neck* 1993;15:33.
82. Gandour-Edwards RF, Donald PJ, Lie JT. Clinical utility of intraoperative frozen section diagnosis in head and neck surgery. A quality assurance perspective. *Head Neck* 1993;15:373.
83. Spiro RH, Guillamondegui O, Paulino AF, et al. Pattern of invasion and margin assessment in patients with oral tongue cancer. *Head Neck* 1999;21:408.
84. Byers RM, Bland KL, Borlase B, et al. Prognostic and therapeutic value of frozen section determination in the surgical treatment of squamous carcinoma of the head and neck. *Am J Surg* 1978;136:525.
85. Bähr W, Stoll P. Intraoperative histological evaluation of tumor resection borders without prolonging surgery. *Int J Oral Maxillofac Surg* 1992;21:90.
86. Ord RA, Aisner S. Accuracy of frozen sections in assessing margins in oral cancer resection. *J Oral Maxillofac Surg* 1997;55:663.
87. Cooley ML, Hoffman HT, Robinson RA. Discrepancies in frozen section mucosal margin tissue in laryngeal squamous cell carcinoma. *Head Neck* 2002;24:262.
88. Barney PL. Histopathologic problems and frozen section diagnosis in diseases of the larynx. *Otolaryngol Clin North Am* 1970;3:493.
89. Berthrong M, Fijardo LF. Radiation changes in surgical pathology. II. Alimentary tract. *Am J Surg Pathol* 1981;5:153.
90. Miller RH, Calcaterra TC, Paglia DE. Accuracy of frozen section diagnosis of parotid lesions. *Ann Otol Rhinol Laryngol* 1979;88:573.
91. Hillel AD, Fee WE Jr. Evaluation of frozen section in parotid gland. *Surgery* 1983;109:230.
92. Wheelis RF, Yarrington CT Jr. Tumors of the salivary glands: comparison of frozen-section diagnosis with final pathologic diagnosis. *Arch Otolaryngol* 1984;110:76.
93. Granick MS, Erickson ER, Hanna DC. Accuracy of frozen-section diagnosis in salivary gland lesions. *Head Neck Surg* 1985;7:465.
94. Rigaul NR, Miller P, Lore JM Jr, et al. Accuracy of frozen section diagnosis in salivary gland neoplasms. *Head Neck Surg* 1986;8:442.
95. Gnepp DR, Rader WR, Cramer SF, et al. Accuracy of frozen section diagnosis in salivary gland. *Otolaryngol Head Neck Surg* 1987;96:325.
96. Luna MA. Uses, abuses and pitfalls of frozen section diagnoses in diseases of the head and neck. In: Barnes L, ed. *Surgical pathology of the head and neck.* New York. Marcel Dekker Inc, 2001:1.
97. Hapke MR, Dehner LP. The optically clear nucleus. A reliable sign of papillary carcinoma of the thyroid? *Am J Surg Pathol* 1979;3:31.
98. Rosen Y, Rosenblatt P, Salzman E. Intraoperative pathologic diagnosis of thyroid neoplasms. Report on experience with 504 specimens. *Cancer* 1990;66: 2001.
99. Kingston GW, Bugis SP, Davis N. Role of frozen section and clinical parameters in distinguishing benign from malignant follicular neoplasms of the thyroid. *Am J Surg* 1992;164:603.

100. Davis NL, Grodon M, Germann E, et al. Clinical parameters predictive of malignancy of thyroid follicular neoplasms. *Am J Surg* 1991;161:567.
101. Gnepp DR. Frozen sections. In: Gnepp DR, ed. *Pathology of the head and neck.* New York: Churchill Livingstone, 1988:1.
102. Rassekh CH, Johnson JT, Myers EN. Accuracy of intraoperative staging of the N0 neck in squamous cell carcinoma. *Laryngoscope* 1995;105:1334.
103. Manni JJ, van den Hoogen FJ. Supraomohyoid neck dissection with frozen section biopsy as a staging procedure in the clinically node-negative neck in carcinoma of the oral cavity. *Am J Surg* 1991;162:373.
104. Zieske LA, Johnson JT, Myers EN, et al. Squamous cell carcinoma with positive margins. Surgery and post operative irradiation. *Arch Otolaryngol Head Neck Surg* 1986;112:863.
105. Loree TR, Strong EW. Significance of "positive" margins in oral squamous cell carcinoma. *Am J Surg* 1990;160:410.
106. Batsakis JG. Surgical excision margins: a pathologist's perspective. *Adv Anat Pathol* 1999;6:140.
107. Looser KG, Shah JP, Strong EW. The significance of "positive" margins in surgically resected epidermoid carcinomas. *Head Neck Surg* 1978;1:107.
108. Mantravadi RVP, Haas RE, Leibner EJ, et al. Postoperative radiotherapy for persistent tumor at the surgical margin in head and neck cancers. *Laryngoscope* 1983;93:1337.
109. Jacobs JR, Ahmad K, Casiano R, et al. Implications of positive surgical margins. *Laryngoscope* 1993;103:64.
110. Scholl P, Byers RM, Batsakis JG, et al. Microscopic cut-through of cancer in the surgical treatment of squamous carcinoma of the tongue. Prognostic and therapeutic implications. *Am J Surg* 1986;152:354.
111. van Es RJJ, Amerongen N, Slootweg PJ, et al. Resection margin as a predictor of recurrence at the primary site for T1 and T2 oral cancers. Evaluation of histopathologic variables. *Arch Otolaryngol Head Neck Surg* 1996;122:521.
112. Batsakis JG. Surgical margins in squamous cell carcinoma. *Ann Otol Rhinol Laryngol* 1988;97:213.
113. Bauer WC, Lseinski SG, Ogura JH. The significance of positive margins in hemilaryngectomy specimens. *Laryngoscope* 1975;85:1.
114. Cleary KR, Batsakis JG. Oral squamous cell carcinoma and the mandible. *Ann Otol Rhinol Laryngol* 1995;104:977.
115. Weisman RA, Kimmelman CP. Bone scanning in the assessment of mandibular invasion by oral cavity carcinoma. *Laryngoscope* 1982;92:1.
116. Dubner S, Heller KS. Local control of squamous cell carcinoma following marginal segmented mandibulectomy. *Head Neck* 1993;15:29.
117. Johnson RE, Sigman JD, Funk GF, et al. Quantification of surgical margin shrinkage in the oral cavity. *Head Neck* 1997;19:281.
118. Beaumont DG, Hains JD. Changes in surgical margins in vivo following resection and after fixation. *Aust J Otolaryngol* 1992;1:51.
119. Gardner ES, Sumner WT, Cook JL. Predictable tissue shrinkage during frozen section histopathologic processing for Mohs micrographic surgery. *Dermatologic Surg* 2001;27:813.
120. Goldstein NS, Soman A, Sacksner J. Disparate surgical margin lengths of colorectal resection specimens between in vivo and in vitro measurements. The effects of surgical resection and formalin fixation on organ shrinkage. *Am J Clin Pathol* 1999;111:349.
121. Silverman MK. Golomb FM, Kopf AW, et al. Verification of a formula for determination of preexcision surgical margins from fixed-tissue melanoma specimens. *J Am Acad Dermatol* 1002;27:214.
122. Sondenaa K, Kjellvold KH. A prospective study of the length of the distal margin after low anterior resection for rectal cancer. *Int J Colorectal Dis* 1990; 5:103.
123. Brennan JA, Mao L, Hruban RH, et al. Molecular assessment of histopathological staging in squamous-cell carcinoma of the head and neck. *N Engl J Med* 1995;332:429.
124. Ball VA, Righi PD, Tejada E, et al. P53 immunostaining of surgical margins as a predictor of local recurrence in squamous cell carcinoma of the oral cavity and oropharynx. *Ear Nose Throat J* 1997;76:818.
125. Franklin S, Pho T, Abreo FW, et al. Detection of the protooncogene eIF4E in larynx and hypopharynx cancers. *Arch Otolaryngol Head Neck Surg* 1999;125:177.
126. American Joint Committee on Cancer. *Manual for staging of cancer,* 3rd ed. Philadelphia: JB Lippincott Co, 1988.
127. Clarke WH, From L, Bernardino EA, et al. The histogenesis and biologic behavior of primary human malignant melanoma of the skin. *Cancer Res* 1969;29:705.
128. Breslow A. Thickness, cross-sectional area and depth of invasion in the prognosis of cutaneous melanoma. *Ann Surg* 1970;172:902.
129. Wenig BM. Laryngeal mucosal malignant melanoma: a clinicopathologic, immunohistochemical and ultrastructural study of four cases and a review of the literature. *Cancer* 1995;75:1568.
130. Spiro RH, Huvos AG, Wong GY, et al. Predictive value of tumor thickness in squamous carcinoma confined to the tongue and floor of the mouth. *Am J Surg* 1986;152:345.
131. Mohit-Tabatabai MA, Sobel HJ, Rush BF, et al. Relation of thickness of floor of mouth stage I and stage II cancers to regional metastasis. *Am J Surg* 1986; 152:351.
132. Frierson HF Jr, Cooper PH. Prognostic factors in squamous cell carcinoma of the lower lip. *Hum Pathol* 1986;17:346.
133. Ravasz LA, Hordijk GJ, Slootweg PJ, et al. Uni- and multivariate analysis of eight indications for post-operative radiotherapy and their significance for local-regional cure in advanced head and neck cancer. *J Laryngol Otol* 1993; 107:437.
134. Karas DE, Baredes S, Chen TS, et al. Relationship of biopsy and final specimens in evaluation of tumor thickness in floor of mouth carcinoma. *Laryngoscope* 1995;105:491.
135. Fakih AR, Rao RS, Borges AM, et al. Elective versus therapeutic neck dissection in early carcinoma of the tongue. *Am J Surg* 1989;158:309.
136. Rasgon BM, Cruz RM, Hilsinger RL, et al. Relation of lymph-node metastasis to histopathologic appearance in oral cavity and oropharyngeal carcinoma: a case series and literature review. *Laryngoscope* 1989;99:1103.
137. Platz H, Fries R, Hudec M, et al. The prognostic relevance of various factors at the time of first admission of the patient. *J Max-Fac Surg* 1983;11:3.
138. Close LG, Brown PM, Vuitch MF, et al. Microscopic invasion and survival in cancer of the oral cavity and oropharynx. *Arch Otolaryngol Head Neck Surg* 1989;115:1304.
139. Morton RP, Ferguson CM, Lambie NK, et al. Tumor thickness in early tongue cancer. *Arch Otolaryngol Head Neck Surg* 1994;120:717.
140. Baredes S, Leeman DJ, Chen TS, et al. Significance of tumor thickness in soft palate carcinoma. *Laryngoscope* 1993;103:389.
141. Moore C, Kuhns JG, Greenberg RA. Thickness as a prognostic aid in upper aerodigestive tract cancers. *Arch Surg* 1986;121:1410.
142. Urist MM, O'Brien CJ, Soong SJ, et al. Squamous carcinoma of the buccal mucosa: prognostic factors analysis. *Am J Surg* 1987;154:411.
143. Cerezo L, Millan I, Torre A, et al. Prognostic factors for survival and tumor control in cervical lymph node metastases from head and neck cancers. A multivariate analysis. *Cancer* 1992;69:1224.
144. Doweck I, Robbins T, Vieira F. Analysis of risk factors predictive of distant failure after targeted chemoradiation for advanced head and neck cancer. *Arch Otolaryngol Head Neck Surg* 2001;127:1315.
145. McGavran MH, Bauer WC, Ogura JH. The incidence of cervical lymph node metastases from epidermoid carcinoma of the larynx and their relationship to certain characteristics of the primary tumor. A study based on the clinical and pathological findings for 96 patients treated by en bloc laryngectomy and radical neck dissection. *Cancer* 1961;14:55.
146. Crissman JD, Liu WY, Gluckman JL, et al. Prognostic value of histopathological parameters in squamous cell carcinoma of the oropharynx. *Cancer* 1984; 54:2995.
147. Yamamoto E, Mikayawa A, Kohama G. Mode of invasion and lymph node metastasis in squamous cell carcinoma of the oral cavity. *Head Neck Surg* 1984;6:938.
148. Jakobsson PA, Eneroth GM, Kollander D, et al. A histological classification and grading of malignancy in carcinoma of the larynx. *Acta Radiol* 1973;12:1.
149. Anneroth G, Batsakis J, Luna M. Review of the literature and a recommended system of malignancy grading in oral squamous carcinomas. *Scand J Dent Res* 1987;95:229.
150. Byrne M, Koppang HS, Lilleng R, et al. New malignancy grading is a better prognostic indicator than Broder's grading in oral squamous carcinoma. *J Oral Pathol Med* 1989;18:432.
151. Crissman JD, Gluckman J, Whiteley J, et al. Squamous cell carcinoma of the floor of the mouth. *Head Neck Surg* 1980;3:2.
152. Carbone A, Micheau C, Bosq J, et al. Superficial extending carcinoma of the hypopharynx: report of 26 cases of an underestimated carcinoma. *Laryngoscope* 1983;93:1600.
153. Sulfaro S, Volpe R, Barzan L, et al. Superficial extending carcinoma of the larynx. *Laryngoscope* 1988;98:1127.
154. Carbone A, Volpe R, Barzan L. Superficial extending carcinoma (SEC) of the larynx and hypopharynx. *Pathol Res Pract* 1992;188:729.
155. Ferlito A, Carbone A, DeSanto LW, et al. "Early" cancer of the larynx: the concept as defined by clinicians, pathologists, and biologists. *Ann Otol Rhinol Laryngol* 1996;105:245.
156. Poleksic S, Kalwaic HJ. Prognostic value of vascular invasion in squamous cell carcinoma of the head and neck. *Plast Reconstr Surg* 1978;61:234.
157. Close LG, Burns DK, Reisch J, et al. Microvascular invasion of cancer of the oral cavity and oropharynx. *Arch Otolaryngol Head Neck Surg* 1987;113:1191.
158. Olsen KD, Caruso M, Foote RL, et al. Primary head and neck cancer. Histopathologic predictors of recurrence after neck dissection in patients with lymph node involvement. *Arch Otolaryngol Head Neck Surg* 1994;120: 1370.
159. Sarbia M, Porschen R, Borchard F, et al. Incidence and prognostic significance of vascular and neural invasion in squamous cell carcinoma of the esophagus. *Int J Cancer* 1995;61:333.
160. Byers RM, O'Brien J, Waxler J. The therapeutic and prognostic implications of nerve invasion in cancer of the lower lip. *Int J Radiat Oncol Biol Phys* 1978;4:215.
161. Goepfert H, Dichtel WJ, Medina JE, et al. Perineural invasion in squamous skin cancer of the head and neck. *Am J Surg* 1984;148:542.
162. Soo K, Carter RL, O'Brien CJ, et al. Prognostic implications of perineural spread in squamous carcinoma of the head and neck. *Laryngoscope* 1986; 96:1145.
163. Pittam MR, Carter RL. Framework invasion by laryngeal carcinomas. *Head Neck Surg* 1982;4:200.
164. Kuettner KE, Pauli BU, Soble L. Morphological studies on the resistance of cartilage to invasion by osteosarcoma cells in vitro and in vivo. *Cancer Res* 1878;38:277.
165. Michaels L. *Pathology of the larynx.* Berlin: Springer-Verlag, 1978:1.
166. Carter RL, Tanner NSB. Local invasion by laryngeal carcinoma: the importance of focal (metaplastic) ossification within laryngeal cartilage. *Clin Otolaryngol* 1979;4:283.

167. Snow GB, Annyas AA, Van Slooten EA, et al. Prognostic factors of neck node metastasis. *Clin Otolaryngol* 1982;7:185.
168. Kalnins IK, Leonard AG, Sako K, et al. Correlation between prognosis and degree of lymph node involvement in carcinoma of the oral cavity. *Am J Surg* 1977;134:450.
169. Johnson JT, Myers EN, Bedetti CD, et al. Cervical lymph node metastasis: incidence and implications of extracapsular carcinoma. *Arch Otolaryngol* 1985;111:534.
170. Snyderman NL, Johnson JT, Schramm VL, et al. Extracapsular spread of carcinomas in cervical lymph nodes: impact upon survival in patients with carcinomas of the supraglottic larynx. *Cancer* 1985;56:1597.
171. Richard JM, Sancho-Garnier H, Michaeu C, et al. Prognostic factors in cervical lymph node metastasis in upper respiratory and digestive tract carcinomas: study of 1713 cases during a 15-year period. *Laryngoscope* 1987;97:97.
172. Leemans CR, Tiwari R, van der Waal I, et al. The efficacy of comprehensive neck dissection with or without postoperative radiotherapy in nodal metastases of squamous cell carcinoma of the upper respiratory and digestive tracts. *Laryngoscope* 1990;100:1194.
173. Hirabayashi H, Koshii K, Kohei U, et al. Extracapsular spread of squamous cell carcinoma in neck lymph nodes: prognostic factor of laryngeal cancer. *Laryngoscope* 1991;101:502.
174. Esclamado RM, Carroll WR. Extracapsular spread and the perineural extension of squamous cell cancer in the cervical plexus. *Arch Otolaryngol Head Neck Surg* 1992;118:1157.
175. Leemans CR, Tiwari R, Nauta JJP, et al. Regional lymph node involvement and its significance in the development of distant metastases in head and neck carcinoma. *Cancer* 1993;71:452.
176. Leemans CR, Tiwari R, Nauta JJP, et al. Recurrence at the primary site in head and neck cancer and the significance of neck lymph node metastases as a prognostic factor. *Cancer* 1994;73:187.
177. Myers JN, Greenberg JS, Mo V, et al. Extracapsular spread. A significant predictor of treatment failure in patients with squamous cell carcinoma of the tongue. *Cancer* 2001;92:3030.
178. Carter RL, Bliss JM, Soo KC, et al. Radical neck dissections for squamous carcinomas: pathological findings and their clinical implications with particular reference to transcapsular spread. *Int J Radiat Oncol Biol Phys* 1987;13:825.
179. Johnson JT, Myers N, Srodes CH, et al. Maintenance chemotherapy for high-risk patients. A preliminary report. *Arch Otolaryngol* 1985;111:727.
180. Stell PM, Morton RP, Singh SD. Cervical lymph node metastases: the significance of the level of the lymph node. *Clin Oncol* 1983;9:101.
181. Grandi C, Alloisio M, Moglia D, et al. Prognostic significance of lymphatic spread in head and neck carcinomas: therapeutic implications. *Head Neck Surg* 1985;8:67.
182. McLaughlin MP, Mendenhall WM, Mancuso AA, et al. Retropharyngeal adenopathy as a predictor of outcome in squamous cell carcinoma of the head and neck. *Head Neck* 1995;17:190.
183. Schuller DE, McGuirt WF, McCabe BF, et al. The prognostic significance of metastatic cervical lymph nodes. *Laryngoscope* 1980;90:557.
184. Johnson JT, Barnes EL, Myers EN, et al. The extracapsular spread of tumors in cervical node metastasis. *Arch Otolaryngol* 1981;107;725.
185. Spiro RH, Alfonso AE, Farr HW, et al. Cervical lymph node metastasis from epidermoid carcinoma of the oral cavity and oropharynx. A critical review assessment of current staging. *Am J Surg* 1974;128:562.
186. Mamelle G, Pampurik J, Luboinski B, et al. Lymph node prognostic factors in head and neck squamous cell carcinoma. *Am J Surg* 1994;168:494.
187. Vikram B, Strong E, Shah J, et al. Failure at distant sites following multimodality treatment for advanced head and neck cancer. *Head Neck* 1984; 6:730.
188. Alvi A, Johnson JT. Development of distant metastasis after treatment of advanced-stage head and neck cancer. *Head Neck* 1997;19:500.
189. Nishijima W, Takooda S, Tokita N, et al. Analyses of distant metastases in squamous cell carcinoma of the head and neck and lesions above the clavicle. *Arch Otolaryngol Head Neck Surg* 1993;119:65.
190. Probert JC, Thompson RW, Bagshaw MA. Patterns of spread of distant metastases in head and neck cancer. *Cancer* 1974;53:342.
191. Merino OR, Lindberg RD, Fletcher GH. An analysis of distant metastasis from squamous cell carcinoma of the upper respiratory and digestive tracts. *Cancer* 1977;40:145.
192. Dennington ML, Carter DR, Meyers AD. Distant metastases in head and neck carcinoma. *Laryngoscope* 1980;90:196.
193. Pack RJ. Distant metastases from head and neck cancer. *Cancer* 1984;53:342.
194. Brownstein MH, Helwig EB. Spread of tumors to the skin. *Arch Dermatol* 1973;107:80.
195. Cole RD, McGuirt WF. Prognostic significance of skin involvement from mucosal tumors of the head and neck. *Arch Otolaryngol Head Neck Surg* 1995; 121:1246.
196. Fijuth J, Mazeron JJ, Le Péchoux, et al. Second head and neck cancers following radiation therapy of T1 and T2 cancers of the oral cavity and oropharynx. *Int J Radiat Oncol Biol Phys* 1992;24:59.
197. Warren S, Gates DC. Multiple primary malignant tumors: a survey of the literature. *Am J Cancer* 1932;16:1358.
198. Hong WK, Lippman SC, Itri L, et al. Prevention of second primary tumors with isotretinoin in squamous cell carcinoma of the head and neck. *N Engl J Med* 1990;323:795.
199. Gluckman JL, Crissman JD, Donegan DO. Multicentric squamous-cell carcinoma of the upper aerodigestive tract. *Head Neck Surg* 1980;3:90.
200. Haughey BH, Gates GA, Arfken CL, et al. Meta-analysis of second malignant tumors in head and head cancer: the case for an endoscopic screening protocol. *Ann Otol Rhinol Laryngol* 1992;101:105.
201. Schwartz LH, Ozsahin M, Zhang GN, et al. Synchronous and metachronous head and neck carcinomas. *Cancer* 1994;74:1933.
202. Jones AS, Morar P, Phillips DE, et al. Second primary tumors in patients with head and neck squamous cell carcinoma. *Cancer* 1995;75:1343.
203. Shapshay SM, Hong WK, Fried MP, et al. Simultaneous carcinomas of the esophagus and upper aerodigestive tract. *Otolaryngol Head Neck Surg* 1980; 88:373.
204. Lippman SM, Hong WK. Second malignant tumors in head and neck squamous cell carcinoma: the overshadow threat for patients with early-stage disease. *Int J Radiat Oncol Biol Phys* 1989;17:691.
205. Bongers V, Snow GB, De Vries N, et al. Second primary head and neck squamous cell carcinoma predicted by the glutathione S-transferase expression in healthy tissue in direct vicinity of the first tumor. *Lab Invest* 1995;73:503.
206. Slaughter DP, Southwick HW, Smejkal W. "Field cancerization" in oral stratified squamous epithelium. Clinical implications of multicentric origin. *Cancer* 1953;6:963.
207. Berg JW, Schottenfeld D, Ritter F. Incidence of multiple primary cancers. III. Cancers of the respiratory and upper digestive system as multiple primary cancers. *J Natl Cancer Inst* 1970;44:263.
208. Cohn AM, Peppard SB. Multiple primary malignant tumors of the head and neck. *Am J Otolaryngol* 1980;1:411.
209. Licciardello JTW, Spitz MR, Hong WK. Multiple primary cancer in patients with cancer of the head and neck: second cancer of the head and neck, esophagus and lung. *Int J Radiat Oncol Biol Phys* 1989;17:467.
210. Carey TE. Field cancerization: are multiple primary cancers monoclonal or polyclonal? *Ann Med* 1996;28:183.
211. Worsham MJ, Wolman SR, Carey TE, et al. Common clonal origin of synchronous primary head and neck squamous cell carcinomas: analysis by tumor karyotypes and fluorescence in situ hybridization. *Hum Pathol* 1995;26:251.
212. Stetler-Stevenson WG, Aznavoorian S, Liotta LA. Tumor cell interactions with the extracellular matrix during invasion and metastasis. *Ann Rev Cell Biol* 1993;9:541.
213. Bedi GC, Westra WH, Gabrielson E, et al. Multiple head and neck tumors: evidence for common clonal origin. *Cancer Res* 1995;26:251.
214. Califano J, van der Riet P, Westra W, et al. Genetic progression model for head and neck cancer: implications for field cancerization. *Cancer Res* 1996; 56:2484.
215. Mashberg A, Samit A. Early diagnosis of asymptomatic oral and oropharyngeal squamous cancers. *CA Cancer J Clin* 1995;45:328.
216. Silverman S, Gorsky M, Lozada F. Oral leukoplakia and malignant transformation. *Cancer* 1984;53:563.
217. Mashberg A. Erythroplasia: the earliest sign of asymptomatic oral cancer. *J Am Dent Assoc* 1978;96:615.
218. Mashberg A, Feldman LJ. Clinical criteria for identifying early oral and oropharyngeal carcinoma: erythroplasia revisited. *Am J Surg* 1988;156:273.
219. Crissman JD, Zarbo RJ. Quantitation of DNA ploidy in squamous intraepithelial neoplasia of the laryngeal glottis. *Arch Otolaryngol Head Neck Surg* 1991;117:182.
220. Fechner RE, Mills SE. Premalignant lesions of the larynx. In: Silver C, ed. *The larynx.* Philadelphia: WB Saunders, 1991:2.
221. Crissman JD, Gnepp DR, Goodman ML, Hellquist H, Johns ME. Pre-invasive lesions of the upper aerodigestive tract. Histologic definitions and clinical implications (a symposium). *Pathol Annu* 1987;22:311.
222. Blackwell KE, Fu YS, Calcaterra TC. Laryngeal dysplasia. A clinicopathologic study. *Cancer* 1995;75:457.
223. Mills SE, Gaffey MJ, Frierson HF Jr. Conventional squamous cell carcinoma. In: *Tumors of the upper aerodigestive tract and ear. Atlas of tumor pathology.* Fascicle 26. Third series. Washington, DC: Armed Forces Institute of Pathology, 2000:45.
224. Crissman JD, Zarbo RJ. Dysplasia, in situ carcinoma, and progression to invasive squamous cell carcinoma of the upper aerodigestive tract. *Am J Surg Pathol* 1989;13[Suppl 1]:5.
225. Friedmann I, Ferlito A. Precursors of squamous cell carcinoma. In Ferlito A, ed. *Neoplasms of the larynx*. Edinburgh: Churchill Livingstone, 1993:97.
226. Gale N, Kambic V, Michaels L, et al. The Ljubljana classification: a practical strategy for the diagnosis of laryngeal precancerous lesions. *Adv Anat Pathol* 2000;4:240.
227. Crissman JD. Laryngeal keratosis and subsequent carcinoma. *Head Neck Surg* 1979;1:386.
228. McGavran MH, Bauer WC, Ogura JH. Isolated laryngeal keratosis: its relation to carcinoma of the larynx based on clinicopathologic study of 87 consecutive cases with long-term follow-up. *Laryngoscope* 1960;70:932.
229. Norris CM, Peale AR. Keratosis of the larynx. *J Laryngol Otol* 1963;77:635.
230. Gabriel CE, Jones DG. Hyperkeratosis of the larynx. *J Laryngol Otol* 1973; 87:129.
231. Henry RC. The transformation of laryngeal leukoplakia to cancer. *J Laryngol Otol* 1979;93:447.
232. Barnes L. Diseases of the larynx, hypopharynx and esophagus. In: Barnes L, ed. *Surgical pathology of the head and neck.* New York: Marcel Dekker, 2001:127.

233. Bouquot JE, Gnepp DR. Laryngeal precancer: a review of the literature, commentary, and comparison with oral leukoplakia. *Head Neck* 1991;13:488.
234. Hellquist H. Lundgren J, Oloffsson J. Hyperplasia, keratosis, dysplasia and carcinoma in situ of the vocal cords—a follow-up study. *Clin Otolaryngol* 1982;7:11.
235. Crissman JD, Zarbo RJ. Quantitation of DNA ploidy in squamous intraepithelial neoplasia of the laryngeal glottis. *Arch Otolaryngol Head Neck Surg* 1991;117:182.
236. Miller AH, Fisher HR. Clues to the life history of carcinoma in-situ of the larynx. *Laryngoscope* 1971;81:1475.
237. Crissman JD, Zarbo RJ, Drozdowicz S, et al. Carcinoma in-situ and microinvasive squamous carcinoma of the laryngeal glottis. *Arch Otolaryngol Head Neck Surg* 1988;114:299.
238. Bauer WC, McGavran MH. Carcinoma in situ and evaluation of epithelial changes in laryngopharyngeal biopsies. *JAMA* 1972;221:72.
239. Böcking A, Auffermann W, Vogel H, et al. Diagnosis and grading of malignancy in 23 squamous epithelial lesions of the larynx with DNA cytomorphometry. *Cancer* 1985;56:1600.
240. Auerbach O, Hammond EC, Garfinkel L. Histologic changes in the larynx in relation to smoking habits. *Cancer* 1970;25:92.
241. Sakr WA, Zarbo RJ, Jacobs JR, et al. Distribution of basement membrane in squamous cell carcinoma of the head and neck. *Hum Pathol* 1987;18:1043.
242. Miller AH. Carcinoma in situ of the larynx—clinical appearance and treatment. In: Alberti PW, Bryce DP, eds. *Centennial conference on laryngeal carcinoma*. New York: Appleton-Century-Crofts, 1976.
243. Gillis TM, Incze MS, Vaughan CW, et al. Natural history and management of keratosis, atypia, carcinoma in situ and microinvasive cancer of the larynx. *Am J Surg* 1983;146:512.
244. Padovan IF. Premalignant laryngeal lesions-a laryngologist's viewpoint. In: Alberti PW, Bryce DP, eds. *Centennial conference on laryngeal carcinoma*. New York: Appleton-Century-Crofts, 1976.
245. Friedmann I. Precancerous lesions of the larynx. In: Alberti PW, Bryce DP, eds. *Centennial conference on laryngeal carcinoma*. New York: Appleton-Century-Crofts, 1976.
246. DeSanto LW. Cancer of the supraglottic larynx: a review of 260 patients. *Otolaryngol Head Neck Surg* 1985;93:705.
247. Carbone A, Micheau C, Bosq J, et al. Superficial extending carcinoma of the hypopharynx: report of 26 cases of an underestimated carcinoma. *Laryngoscope* 1983;93:1600.
248. Ferlito A, Carbone A, DeSanto LW, et al. "Early" cancer of the larynx: the concept as defined by clinicians, pathologists, and biologists. *Ann Otol Rhinol Laryngol* 1996;105:245.
249. Mills SE, Gaffey MJ, Frierson HF Jr. Benign squamous proliferations. In: *Tumors of the upper aerodigestive tract and ear. Atlas of tumor pathology*. Fascicle 26. Third series. Washington, DC: Armed Forces Institute of Pathology, 2000:21.
250. Mills SE, Gaffey MJ, Frierson HF Jr. Miscellaneous tumor-like lesions. In: *Tumors of the upper aerodigestive tract and ear. Atlas of tumor pathology*. Fascicle 26. Third series. Washington, DC: Armed Forces Institute of Pathology, 2000:355.
251. Crissman JD, Liu WY, Gluckman JL, et al. Prognostic value of histopathologic parameters in squamous cell carcinoma of the oropharynx. *Cancer* 1984; 54:2995.
252. Lampe HB. DNA analysis of head and neck squamous cell carcinoma by flow cytometry. *Laryngoscope* 1993;103:637.
253. Sakr W, Hussan M, Zarbo RL, et al. DNA quantification and histologic characteristics of squamous cell carcinoma of the upper aerodigestive tract. *Arch Pathol Lab Med* 1989;113:1009.
254. Watling DL, Gown AM, Coltrera MD. Overexpression of p53 in head and neck cancer. *Head Neck* 1992;14:437.
255. El-Naggar AK, Steck K, Batsakis JG. Heterogeneity of the proliferative fraction and cyclin D1/CCND1 gene amplification in head and neck squamous cell carcinoma. *Cytometry* 1995;21:47.
256. Crissman JD, Kessis T, Shah KV, et al. Squamous papillary neoplasia of the upper aerodigestive tract. *Hum Pathol* 1988;19:1387.
257. Thompson LDR, Wenig BM, Heffner DK, et al. Exophytic and papillary squamous cell carcinoma of the larynx: a clinicopathologic series of 104 cases. *Otolaryngol Head Neck Surg* 1999;120:718.
258. Suarez PA, Adler-Storthz K, Luna MA, et al. Papillary squamous cell carcinomas of the upper aerodigestive tract: a clinicopathologic and molecular study. *Head Neck* 2000;22:360.
259. Batsakis JG, Hybels R, Crissman JD, et al. The pathology of head and neck tumors: verrucous carcinoma, part 15. *Head Neck Surg* 1982;5:29.
260. Ferlito A, Recher G. Ackerman's tumor (verrucous carcinoma) of the larynx. A clinicopathologic study of 77 cases. *Cancer* 1980;46:1617.
261. Medina JE, Dichtel W, Luna MA. Verrucous-squamous carcinomas of the oral cavity. A clinicopathologic study of 104 cases. *Arch Otolaryngol* 1984; 110:437.
262. Luna MA, Tortoledo ME. Verrucous carcinoma. In: Gnepp DR, ed. *Pathology of the head and neck*. New York: Churchill Livingstone, 1988:497.
263. McKaig RG, Baric RS, Olshan AF. Human papillomavirus and head and neck cancer: epidemiology and molecular biology. *Head Neck* 1998;20:250.
264. Dyson N, Howley PM, Münger K, et al. The human papillomavirus-16 E7 oncoprotein is able to bind the retinoblastoma gene product. *Science* 1989; 243:934.
265. Gillison ML, Koch WM, Capone RB, et al. Evidence for a causal association between human papillomavirus and a subset of head and neck cancers. *J Natl Cancer Inst* 2000;92:709.
266. Shear M, Pindborg JJ. Verrucous hyperplasia of the oral mucosa. *Cancer* 1980; 46:1855.
267. Hansen LS, Olson JA, Silverman S. Proliferative verrucous leukoplakia. A long-term study of thirty patients. *Oral Surg Oral Med Oral Pathol* 1985;60: 285.
268. Murrah VA, Batsakis JG. Proliferative verrucous leukoplakia and verrucous hyperplasia. *Ann Otol Rhinol Laryngol* 1994;103:660.
269. Batsakis JG, Suarez P, el-Naggar AK. Proliferative verrucous leukoplakia and its related lesions. *Oral Oncol* 1999;35:354.
270. Fechner RE, Mills SE. Verruca vulgaris of the larynx. A distinctive lesion of probable viral origin confused with verrucous carcinoma. *Am J Surg Pathol* 1982;6:357.
271. Berthelet E, Shenouda G, Black MJ, et al. Sarcomatoid carcinoma of the head and neck. *Am J Surg* 1994;168:455.
272. Zarbo RJ, Crissman JD, Venkat H, et al. Spindle-cell carcinoma of the aerodigestive tract mucosa: an immunohistologic and ultrastructural study of 18 biphasic tumors and comparison with seven monophasic spindle-cell tumors. *Am J Surg Pathol* 1986;10:741.
273. Ellis GL, Langloss JM, Heffner DK, et al. Spindle-cell carcinoma of the aerodigestive tract: an immunohistochemical analysis of 21 cases. *Am J Surg Pathol* 1987;11:335.
274. Lewis JE, Olsen KD, Sebo TJ. Spindle cell carcinoma of the larynx: review of 26 cases including DNA content and immunohistochemistry. *Hum Pathol* 1997:28:664.
275. Nakleh RE, Zarbo RJ, Ewing S, et al. Myogenic differentiation in spindle cell (sarcomatoid) carcinoma of the upper aerodigestive tract. *Appl Immunohistochem* 1993;1:58.
276. Ophir D, Marshak G, Czernobilsky B. Distinctive immunohistochemical labeling of epithelial and mesenchymal elements in laryngeal pseudosarcoma. *Laryngoscope* 1987;97:490.
277. Ellis G, Langloss JM, Enzinger FM. Coexpression of keratin and desmin in a carcinosarcoma involving the maxillary alveolar ridge. *Oral Surg Oral Med Oral Pathol* 1985;60:410.
278. Balercia G, Bhan AK, Dickersin GR. Sarcomatoid carcinoma: an ultrastructural study with light microscopic and immunohistochemical correlation of 10 cases from various anatomic sites. *Ultrastruc Pathol* 1995;19:249.
279. Ansari-Lari MA, Westra WH. Immunohistochemical p53 expression patterns in sarcomatoid carcinomas of the upper respiratory tract. *Mod Pathol* 2001;14: 148A.
280. Wenig BM, Devaney K. Bisceglia M. Inflammatory myofibroblastic pseudotumors of the larynx: a clinicopathologic report of eight cases including immunohistochemical and ultrastructural analysis. *Cancer* 1995;76:2217.
281. Coffin CM, Patel A, Perkins S, et al. ALK1 and p80 expression and chromosomal rearrangements involving 2p23 in inflammatory myofibroblastic tumor. *Mod Pathol* 2001;14:569.
282. Cook JR, Dehner LP, Collins MH, et al. Anaplastic lymphoma kinase (ALK) expression in the inflammatory myofibroblastic tumor: a comparative immunohistochemical study. *Am J Surg Pathol* 2001;25:1364.
283. Rubin BP, Lawrence BD, Perez-Atayde A, et al. TPM-ALK fusion genes and ALK expression in inflammatory myofibroblastic tumor. *Mod Pathol* 2000;13: 15A.
284. Wain SL, Kier R, Vollmer RT, et al. Basaloid-squamous carcinoma of the tongue, hypopharynx and larynx. *Hum Pathol* 1986;17:1158.
285. Banks ER, Frierson HF Jr, Mills SE, et al. Basaloid squamous cell carcinoma of the head and neck: a clinicopathologic and immunohistochemical study of 40 cases. *Am J Surg Pathol* 1992;16:939.
286. Weineke J, Thompson LDR, Wenig BM. Basaloid squamous cell carcinoma of the nasal cavity and paranasal sinuses. *Cancer* 1999;85:841.
287. Morice WG, Ferreiro JA. Distinction of basaloid squamous cell carcinoma from adenoid cystic and small cell undifferentiated carcinoma by immunohistochemistry. *Hum Pathol* 1998;29:609.
288. Hewan-Lowe K, Dardick I. Ultrastructural distinction of basaloid-squamous carcinoma and adenoid cystic carcinoma. *Ultrastr Pathol* 1995;19:371.
289. Shanmugaratnam K, Sobin LH, Barnes L, et al. *World Health Organization histological classification of tumours. Histological typing of tumours of the upper respiratory tract and ear,* 2nd ed. Berlin: Springer-Verlag, 1991.
290. Easton JM, Levine PH, Hyams VJ. Nasopharyngeal carcinoma in the United States. A pathologic study of 177 US and 30 foreign cases. *Arch Otolaryngol* 1981;106:88.
291. Dickson RI, Flores AD. Nasopharyngeal carcinoma: an evaluation of 134 patients treated between 1971–1980. *Laryngoscope* 1985;95:276.
292. Ferlito A, Weiss LM, Rinaldo A, et al. Lymphoepithelial carcinoma of the larynx, hypopharynx, and trachea. *Ann Otol Rhinol Laryngol* 1997;106:437.
293. MacMillan C, Kapadia SB, Finkelstein SD, et al. Lymphoepithelial carcinoma of the larynx and hypopharynx: study of eight cases with relationship to Epstein-Barr virus (EBV) and p53 gene alterations, and review of the literature. *Hum Pathol* 1996;27:1172.
294. Pacchioni D, Negro F, Valente G, et al. Epstein-Barr virus by in situ hybridization in fine-needle aspiration biopsies. *Diagn Mol Pathol* 1994; 3:100.
295. Barnes L. Nasopharyngeal carcinoma. In: Barnes L, ed. *Surgical pathology of the head and neck.* New York: Marcel Dekker Inc, 2001:527.

296. Luna MA. The occult primary and metastatic tumors to and from the head and neck. In: Barnes L, ed. *Surgical pathology of the head and neck.* New York: Marcel Dekker Inc, 2001;1421.
297. Martin H, Morfit MH, Ehrilich G. The case for branchiogenic cancer (malignant branchioma). *Ann Surg* 1950;132:867.
298. Batsakis JG, McBurney TA. Metastatic neoplasms to the head and neck. *Surg Gynecol Obstet* 1971;133:673.
299. Compagno J, Hyams VJ, Safavian M. Does branchiogenic carcinoma really exist? *Arch Pathol Lab Med* 1976;100:311.
300. Thompson LD, Heffner DK. The clinical importance of cystic squamous cell carcinomas in the neck: a study of 136 cases. *Cancer* 1998;82:944.
301. Schwarz D, Hamberger AD, Jesse RH. The management of squamous cell carcinoma in cervical lymph nodes in the clinical absence of a primary lesion by combined surgery and radiotherapy. *Cancer* 1981;48:1746.
302. Shenoy AM, Hasan S, Nayak U, et al. Neck metastasis from an occult primary—the Kiwai experience. *Indian J Cancer* 1992;29:203.
303. Shah JP, Lydiatt W. Treatment of cancer of the head and neck. *CA Cancer J Clin* 1995;45:352.

CHAPTER 3

Prognostic Factors in Patients with Head and Neck Cancer

Benjamin D. Smith and Bruce G. Haffty

Treatment of head and neck cancer requires accurate risk stratification to determine the type and extent of therapy needed and the expected clinical outcome. Physical examination, diagnostic imaging studies, and pathologic review enable the clinician to determine the size and extent of the primary tumor, the status of cervical lymph nodes, and the likelihood of distant metastatic disease, thus generating an accurate tumor, node, metastasis (TNM) stage for each patient. In addition to TNM staging, other clinical and pathologic factors not routinely incorporated into the staging system have been shown to influence response to therapy and eventual outcome. These factors may be categorized as follows:

1. Prognostic factors related to the primary tumor
2. Prognostic factors related to the cervical lymph nodes
3. Prognostic factors related to patient demographics
4. Prognostic factors related to the patient's general medical condition.

In addition to clinical and pathologic factors, recent interest has focused on identifying molecular factors that may influence clinical outcome. These molecular markers not only provide useful prognostic information, they also serve as targets for novel pharmacotherapies that would antagonize cellular proliferation by interfering with specific cellular processes. Molecular factors that influence tumor behavior fall into several broad categories including protooncogenes, tumor suppressor genes, growth factors, immune-related factors, loss of heterozygosity at various genetic loci, total cellular DNA content, and parameters related to the kinetics of *in vivo* tumor growth.

When considering prognostic factors in head and neck cancer, several specific outcomes merit attention. In addition to disease-free and overall survival, the relationship between a specific prognostic factor and local recurrence, regional recurrence, and distant metastatic disease must be considered. Factors specifically related to local recurrence may necessitate wider surgical resection, increased dose or altered fractionation of external beam radiotherapy, or the use of brachytherapy boost to the primary tumor bed. Factors specifically related to regional recurrence may prompt prophylactic neck dissection or radiotherapy in the clinically N0 neck or determine the type of neck dissection selected in patients with clinically positive cervical lymph nodes. Finally, factors predictive of distant metastases may prompt more aggressive screening for concomitant disease below the clavicles before attempting radical locoregional treatment (1).

FACTORS RELATED TO THE PRIMARY TUMOR

Tumor Dimensions

Tumor size and extent of invasion determines clinical and pathologic T stage for head and neck squamous cell carcinoma

(HNSCC). Although the evolution and use of the staging system for head and neck cancer is more completely discussed elsewhere in this textbook, this section will specifically focus on the relationship between tumor dimensions and outcome as addressed in clinical studies. T stage is determined clinically by measuring the maximal surface diameter of a mucosal neoplasm or pathologically by measuring the maximal cross-sectional diameter of a resected tumor. Because tumors arising from mucosal surfaces do not conform to spherical geometry, the maximal tumor diameter does not perfectly correlate with either tumor depth or tumor volume.

As the primary determinant of T stage, maximum tumor diameter has traditionally been considered an important risk factor for the presence of concomitant nodal metastases, local recurrence, and poor survival. For example, in two studies conducted on a total of 603 patients with HNSCC, Magnano et al. found that T stage was a consistent, independent predictor of pathologically positive cervical lymph nodes (2,3). In addition, pathologic maximal tumor diameter has been shown to predict local recurrence in tumors arising from the lower lip (4), oral cavity and oropharynx (5), and larynx (6). Finally, most studies (5,7–10), though not all (11), have shown a univariate association between either clinical or pathologic tumor diameter and survival.

One limitation of using tumor size as a prognostic determinant was highlighted by Moore et al. who stratified 155 patients with oral squamous cell carcinoma (SCC) based on surface diameter of the primary tumor (7). Eighty-four percent of patients with tumors ≤2 cm survived disease-free for 3 years, compared with 52% of patients with tumors larger than 2 cm. However, no significant differences in survival existed between tumors with surface diameters in the following three groups: 2.1 to 3 cm, 3.1 to 4 cm, and greater than 4 cm. Thus, although a gross trend exists between surface diameter and survival, this trend does not follow a simple dose-response relationship. In a follow-up study conducted on 151 patients with oral and oropharyngeal SCC, Moore et al. compared the prognostic ability of tumor surface diameter and tumor thickness in predicting concomitant nodal metastases and 3-year disease-free survival (12). As shown in Figure 3.1, tumor thickness is a more consistent predictor of nodal metastasis and survival than surface diameter.

The correlation between invasion depth and risk for concomitant cervical node metastases has been confirmed in multiple studies. For example, as shown in Table 3.1, Yuen et al. found that tumor thickness was significantly associated with nodal metastasis, local recurrence, and disease-free survival in a cohort of 85 patients with oral tongue carcinoma (13). In multivariate analysis, tumor thickness was the only significant predictor of nodal metastasis, but failed to predict local recurrence or disease-free survival. Furthermore, in a series of 76 patients with carcinoma of the tongue who all received neck dissection, Woolgar demonstrated that the mean reconstructed thickness of tumors with pathologically positive cervical lymph nodes was 19 mm, compared with 10 mm in patients without metastases (14). Tumors with a large mucosal surface area but minimal invasion were not at increased risk for nodal metastases. In such cases, clinical and pathologic T stage may overestimate the likelihood of concomitant nodal disease. The relationship between tumor thickness and risk for cervical lymph node metastases has been confirmed for several sites of the head and neck including lower lip (4,15), oral cavity, and oropharynx (16–25). Finally, multivariate analysis has shown that increased tumor thickness predicts locoregional recurrence (26,27) and poor survival (26) in oral cavity tumors. Hence, tumor thickness allows for more accurate prognostication than tumor diameter and should be incorporated into decisions regarding treatment of the clinically N0 neck.

In addition to consideration of maximal tumor diameter and thickness, use of computed tomography (CT) enables the calculation of total tumor volume. In a series of 63 patients with supraglottic primaries treated with primary irradiation, Mancuso et al. found that tumor volume calculated from pretreatment CT scans was an independent predictor of local control, with local control rates of 89% in tumors less than 6 cm^3 and 52% in tumors ≥6 cm^3 (28). Furthermore, in a study of 103 patients with supraglottic SCC, tumor volume as calculated from pretreatment CT was a stronger predictor of locoregional failure than clinical T stage in multivariate analysis (29). Hence, calculation of tumor volume using diagnostic imaging provides important prognostic information that can supplement traditional clinical staging.

Margin Status

The presence of residual carcinoma at the margins of surgical resection is an important risk factor for local recurrence in HNSCC. Although the presence of positive margins may indicate an error in surgical judgment at the time of resection, it may also imply a more biologically aggressive tumor that extends microscopically through the muscle bundles, submucosal lymphatics, and perineural spaces (30). The precise definition of "positive margins" varies depending on the study and may include invasive tumor within 5 mm of the final surgical margins, carcinoma *in situ* involving the final surgical margin, and dysplasia involving the final surgical margin. In a review of resections for head and neck cancer performed at Memorial-Sloan Kettering Cancer Center, Looser et al. classified 1,775 cases according to final margin status (31). After excluding patients with gross residual disease, they identified 62 patients with microscopically positive margins, defined as either cancer within 0.5 cm of the margin, marked atypia or premalignant changes in the margin, carcinoma *in situ* in the margin, or invasive carcinoma in the margin. Interestingly, patients in all four of these groups experienced increased local recurrence rates, ranging from 64% in patients with invasive cancer at the margin to 85% for patients with carcinoma *in situ* at the margin, compared with a local recurrence rate of 32% in patients with negative margins. Despite a clear relationship between positive margins and local recurrence, this study failed to show any clear trends between margin status and survival.

Many other studies have confirmed the prognostic importance of margin status in head and neck cancer. The presence of positive margins has been shown to predict local or locoregional recurrence for the following sites: lower lip (4), oral cavity (27,32,33), buccal mucosa (34), oral tongue (35,36), oral and oropharyngeal tongue (37,38), base of tongue (39), oral cavity and oropharynx (40), larynx (41,42), and all sites combined (43–47). Furthermore, the presence of positive margins predicts poor overall survival in univariate analysis for the following sites: oral cavity (33), oral tongue (48), oral and oropharyngeal tongue (38), oral cavity and oropharynx (17), base of tongue (39), supraglottic larynx (49), larynx (8,42,50), and all sites combined (43,44,51,52). Whether or not margin status is an independent predictor of survival remains somewhat controversial, with two studies confirming an independent association (42,52) but six others failing to find an association (5,8,9,43,49,53). Margin status has not been shown to predict regional or distant recurrent disease.

Given the negative prognostic implications of positive margins, Byers et al. demonstrated that use of intraoperative frozen sections can identify those patients with initially positive margins and thus allow resection of additional tissue to remove residual carcinoma and reduce the risk for local recurrence (51). In this cohort of 216 patients with SCC arising from the oral cav-

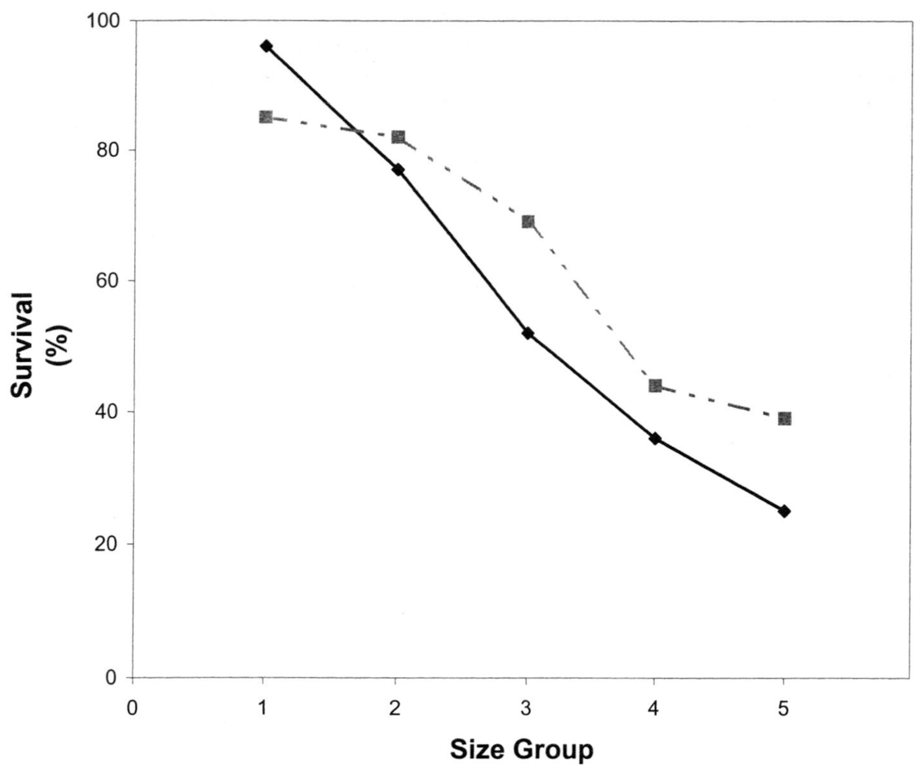

A

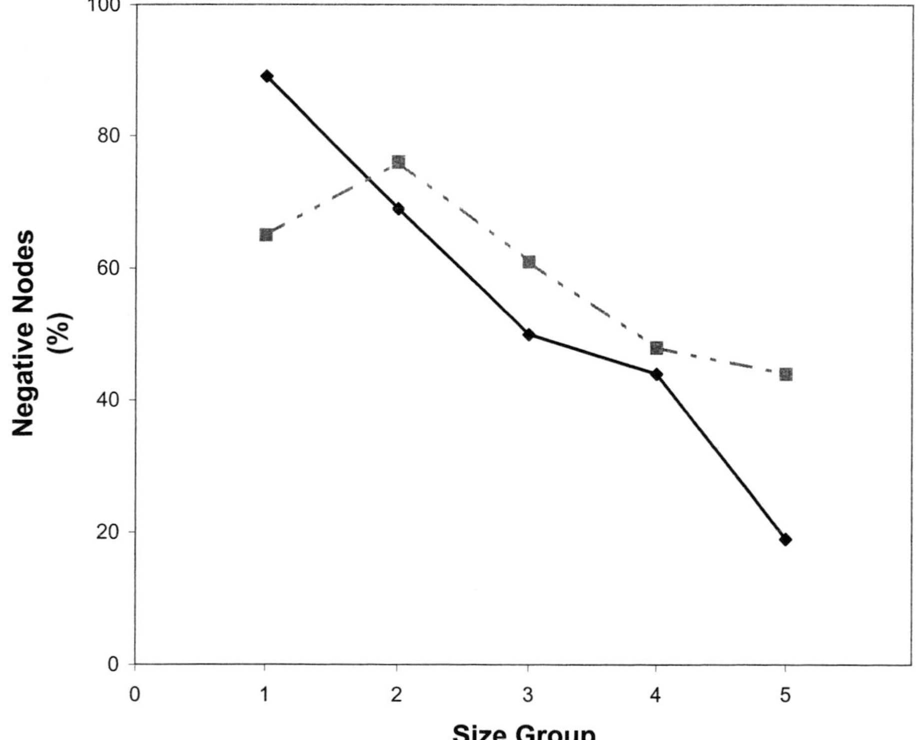

B

Size Group	Thickness (mm)	Surface Diameter (mm)
1	1-3	1-10
2	4-6	11-20
3	7-12	21-30
4	13-18	31-40
5	>18	>40

C

Figure 3.1 The relationship between tumor thickness (*solid line*) and surface diameter (*gray broken line*) with respect to survival **(A)** and nodal positivity **(B)** in 151 oral cavity and oropharyngeal cancers. Cut-offs for the size groups are presented in **C**. (Adapted from Moore C, Kuhns JG, Greenberg RA. Thickness as prognostic aid in upper aerodigestive trace cancer. *Arch Surg* 1986;121:1410–1414.)

TABLE 3.1 Tumor Thickness and Prognosis in Oral Tongue Squamous Cell Carcinoma

Thickness	No. of patients	Nodal metastasis (%)	Local recurrence (%)	5-year disease-free survival (%)
<3 mm	10	10	0	100
3–9 mm	44	50	11	77
>9 mm	31	65	26	60

See Yuen et al. (13).

ity, oropharynx, and hypopharynx, patients with initially positive margins on frozen section received additional resection to achieve final negative margins. Local recurrence in this group was 13%, compared with a local recurrence rate of 12% in patients with negative margins on initial frozen section. Patients with positive final margins had an 80% local recurrence rate. Hence, use of intraoperative frozen-section analysis of surgical margins may result in a clinically significant reduction in local recurrence.

However, in a follow-up study of 268 patients with SCC of the tongue, those patients with initially positive margins who were ultimately rendered negative had an increased risk for local recurrence and death compared with patients with negative frozen-section margins (30). Thus, the authors recommend use of postoperative radiotherapy in all patients with initially positive frozen-section margins. One additional concern regarding the use of intraoperative frozen sections to determine margin status is potential inaccuracy, with one study reporting a 14% (7/49) false-negative rate for oral cancer (54).

For those patients with persistently positive margins, postoperative external beam radiotherapy remains an important component of therapy. However, even with combined modality therapy, most investigators (34,43,46,55), although not all (56), report an increased incidence of local recurrence in those patients with positive margins. One important factor influencing local control in patients with positive margins is dose of postoperative radiotherapy. This has been noted by Zelefsky et al. who reported a 7-year actuarial local control rate of 92% in patients who received greater than 60 Gy, compared with 44% in patients who received less than 60 Gy (56). In addition, interest has grown in using postoperative brachytherapy, either alone or following postoperative external beam radiotherapy, to improve local control in patients with positive margins (57–60). Beitler et al. report a study of 29 patients with microscopically close or positive margins after curative surgery treated with postoperative external beam radiotherapy to a median dose of 60 Gy followed by iodine-125 permanent implant designed to deliver a cumulative lifetime dose of 120 to 160 Gy to the high-risk target volume (60). This treatment strategy resulted in a 92% 2-year actuarial local control rate and clearly merits further study in a phase III randomized trial.

Malignancy Grading

Pathologists have long recognized the potential prognostic significance of cellular morphology in SCC. In 1920, Broders proposed a four-tiered grading system for carcinoma of the lip that was based on the proportion of the neoplasm resembling normal squamous epithelium (61). This grading system provides an easily assessed scheme for assessing tumor differentiation and roughly correlates with prognosis, as poorly differentiated tumors are more likely to recur and reduce survival (49,62–69). Broders grading system has been criticized, however, for its subjectivity and failure to consistently predict survival in multivariate modeling (9,33,49,70–72). The lack of independent significance of Broders grading system may be due to the association between higher grade (more poorly differentiated) and advanced stage apparent in data from the National Cancer Data Base (73).

In 1973, Jakobsson proposed a semiquantitative grading system that considered not only histologic parameters of the tumor cell population but also the host–tumor interface (74). Parameters describing the tumor cell population included structure and growth of the neoplasm, degree of keratinization, nuclear pleomorphism, and the frequency of mitoses. The tumor–host interface was assessed for mode of invasion, degree or stage of invasion, vascular invasion, and lymphoplasmacytic cellular response. When this classification system was applied to a series of 42 patients with laryngeal SCCs treated with radiotherapy, tumors with high malignancy grade were more likely to recur and result in death with disease. However, in a subsequent multivariate analysis conducted on 77 patients with oropharyngeal cancer, Crissman et al. found that invasion pattern was the only histologic parameter that independently predicted survival (75). None of the other histologic parameters, either independently or as a composite score, were significant predictors of outcome.

In 1987, Anneroth et al. reviewed efforts to devise a malignancy grading system and proposed that grading consist of six morphologic features: degree of keratinization, nuclear polymorphism, number of mitoses, pattern of invasion, stage of invasion, and lymphoplasmacytic infiltration (76). In 1989, Bryne et al. applied Anneroth's grading system to only the most anaplastic fields in the most invasive areas of the tumor (Table 3.2) (77). In two cohorts of 68 and 61 patients with oral SCC, invasive cell grading (ICG) was a highly significant, independent, and reproducible predictor of survival (77–79). Those patients with a total malignancy score between 5 and 10 experienced a 57% 5-year survival, compared with 19% 5-year survival in patients with malignancy scores greater than 10. Furthermore, Broders grading system failed to correlate with

TABLE 3.2 Invasive Cell Grading System

	Score			
Morphologic feature	**1**	**2**	**3**	**4**
Degree of keratinization	Highly keratinized (>50% of the cells)	Moderately keratinized (20%–50% of the cells)	Minimal keratinization (5%–20% of the cells)	No keratinization (0%–5% of the cells)
Nuclear polymorphism	Little nuclear polymorphism (>75% mature cells)	Moderately abundant nuclear polymorphism (50%–75% mature cells)	Abundant nuclear polymorphism (25%–50% mature cells)	Extreme nuclear polymorphism (0%–25% mature cells)
Number of mitoses (high power field)	0–1	2–3	4–5	>5
Pattern of invasion	Pushing, well-delineated infiltrating borders	Infiltrating, solid cords, bands, or strands	Small groups or cords of infiltrating cells	Marked and widespread cellular dissociation in small groups or in single cells (n < 15)
Lymphoplasmacytic infiltration	Marked	Moderate	Slight	None

See Bryne et al. (77).

survival in both cohorts. The authors concluded that histologically invasive regions might be responsible for the clinical behavior of HNSCC. Further study of ICG conducted by other groups has shown that a high ICG score strongly predicts the presence of occult cervical metastases and extracapsular extension (14,16,19). Due to the strong correlation between ICG and concomitant nodal metastases, this factor should be considered in decisions regarding elective treatment of the clinically negative neck.

In addition to assessment of malignancy grade, many studies have attempted to determine which individual histologic parameters contribute most strongly to prognosis. Several studies suggest that pattern of invasion may predict outcome independent of other histologic parameters. Tumors that infiltrate in small groups or cords of cells, or infiltrate with marked cellular dissociation, may behave more aggressively. For example, Spiro et al. found that oral tongue SCCs with high-grade pattern of invasion were more likely to present with concomitant nodal metastases, develop distant metastases, and result in death (80). In addition, for oral carcinoma that invades the mandible, high-grade invasion pattern increases the rate of mandibular margin positivity and local recurrence and results in a fourfold increased risk for death with disease in multivariate analysis (81). The correlation between aggressive pattern of invasion and poor locoregional control (4,24,28,37,82–84) and survival (10,17) has been noted in several other studies.

In addition to pattern of invasion, lymphoplasmacytic infiltration of the tumor bed has been considered as a potential independent marker of prognosis. In a study of 396 patients with HNSCC, multivariate analysis revealed that the presence of lymphocytic intratumoral and peritumoral infiltrates decreased the risk for concomitant cervical lymph node metastases, whereas a plasmocytic infiltrate increased the risk (2). In addition, at least two studies have reported a correlation between leukocyte infiltration and improved locoregional control in univariate modeling (22,24).

Perineural Invasion

Infiltration of perineural spaces occurs in up to 52% (85) of HNSCCs and was first noted to influence surgical and adjuvant treatment strategies by Ballantyne et al. in 1963 (86). Perineural invasion (PNI) may result in dysphagia secondary to involvement of the vagal trunk (87) or pain and hypesthesia along the territories of the glossopharyngeal or trigeminal nerves (87,88). Computed tomographic findings suggestive of PNI include obliteration of the fat within the pterygopalatine fossa, enlargement of neural foramina, and increased enhancement in the region of the Meckel cave (89). In addition, a study of 48 patients with oral tongue, base of tongue, or floor of mouth SCC, used CT to identify the presence of vascular or perineural invasion with a sensitivity of 88% and a specificity of 83% using criteria including "aggressive" tumor margins, invasion of the sublingual space, and direct adjacency to the lingual vasculature (90).

Perineural invasion may be mediated by the presence of nerve cell adhesion molecule (NCAM) on the surface of SCCs, which engages in homophilic binding with NCAM expressed in neural and perineural tissues. In two studies of 76 and 66 patients with HNSCC, expression of NCAM on the surface of neoplastic cells was significantly associated with PNI detected on review of pathologic sections (91,92).

Numerous clinical studies have identified PNI as an important predictor of poor prognosis. In tumors arising from the lower lip (4,15,51), oral tongue (25), oral cavity (18,19,85), larynx (93), and all sites combined (2,3) the presence of PNI in or surrounding the primary tumor increased the risk for concomitant cervical metastases. Furthermore, following definitive treatment of HNSCC, the presence of PNI in the primary tumor increased the risk for local recurrence (4,85,94,95), regional recurrence (64), locoregional recurrence (22,24,96,97), poor cause-specific survival (85,96), and poor overall survival (48,96). However, primary tumors positive for PNI do not result in a higher rate of distant metastases (98).

The association between PNI and local recurrence may result from either centrifugal or centripetal propagation of malignant cells along the perineural space and away from the primary tumor. Most primary tumors will only disseminate up to 2 cm along the perineural space (99), although PNI 12 cm from the primary tumor has been reported (86). As a result, PNI may allow malignant cells to evade surgical excision or radiotherapy and result in local recurrence. In addition, the association between PNI and regional recurrence implies that these tumors may be more biologically aggressive. The association between PNI and tumor aneuploidy, a known marker of poor prognosis, supports this hypothesis (100).

Despite the clear importance of PNI, the percent of mucosal HNSCCs positive for PNI varies widely in the literature, from 5% (95) to 52% (85). This discrepancy may result from a tendency to identify PNI only when large, named nerves are involved. However, although PNI of small, unnamed nerves may not result in clinical symptoms, the relationship between PNI and prognosis is independent of nerve diameter (85). Hence, all HNSCC pathologic specimens should be closely examined for PNI, even in nerves less than 1 mm in diameter.

Vascular Invasion

One additional histologic parameter not considered in traditional malignancy grading schemes for HNSCC is vascular invasion, the presence of neoplastic epithelium within an endothelial-lined channel. Vascular invasion is a frequent finding in head and neck tumors, occurring in more than 50% of pathologic specimens (5,14,101). As with tumor depth and pattern of invasion, vascular invasion may identify tumors with an aggressive biologic nature due to their ability to invade normal anatomic structures. Indeed, vascular invasion has been shown to correlate with the presence of concomitant cervical metastases in both univariate (14,17,94,101) and multivariate models (2,3,25,102). In addition, the presence of vascular invasion in the primary tumor specimen has been noted to increase the risk for subsequent locoregional recurrence in oral cavity, oropharyngeal, and laryngeal SCC treated surgically (5,64,94). However, in a cohort of 135 patients with oral cavity SCC treated with surgery followed by postoperative radiotherapy, vascular invasion did not independently predict poor locoregional control, suggesting that postoperative radiotherapy may mitigate the poor prognosis associated with vascular invasion (32,80). Vascular invasion has also been associated with increased risk for distant metastatic disease (5,71). To date, little data exist regarding the significance of vascular invasion as an independent predictor of mortality in head and neck cancer patients.

FACTORS RELATED TO THE CERVICAL LYMPH NODES

Number of Positive Lymph Nodes

The number of cervical lymph nodes histologically positive for SCC provides one of the simplest, and perhaps most important, prognostic markers in head and neck cancer. Mamelle et al. retrospectively reviewed 914 patients who received cervical lymph node dissection as a component of initial therapy for oral cavity, oropharyngeal, hypopharyngeal, and laryngeal SCC (103). Patients with palpable lymph nodes greater than 3 cm underwent radical lymph node dissection, and all other patients underwent selective neck dissection on sentinel nodes with immediate pathologic evaluation. Those patients with positive sentinel nodes then received ipsilateral modified radical neck dissection and contralateral selective neck dissection. Thus, all patients, regardless of their clinical N stage, received pathologic evaluation of their cervical lymph nodes. Those patients with positive cervical lymph nodes received 50 Gy to the neck with a 15 Gy boost in areas of extracapsular spread. Lymph node number exhibited a strong dose-response correlation with distant metastasis and survival (Fig. 3.2). In multivariate analysis stratified by tumor site and patient age, number of positive nodes was a significant, independent predictor of survival. Furthermore, although extracapsular spread and node location (upper vs. middle vs. lower neck) were significant predictors of survival in univariate analysis, after controlling for number of lymph nodes, they lost their prognostic significance. Thus, with this particular treatment algorithm, the number of positive nodes emerged as an important independent predictor of prognosis.

The importance of positive cervical nodes has been noted in many other studies and appears to correlate with risk for regional recurrence and distant metastasis. Studies have demonstrated a correlation between increasing number of positive nodes and regional recurrence in patients with advanced SCC who receive postoperative radiotherapy (104), patients who do not receive radiotherapy (64), patients with oral cavity (65) and hypopharyngeal or lateral epilaryngeal primary tumors (105), and patients who receive neck dissection for mucosal HNSCC from any site (106,107). Furthermore, number of positive nodes clearly predicts risk for distant metastatic disease for all sites of HNSCC (11,98,103,108–112). Number of positive nodes predicts both regional recurrence (64) and distant recurrence (111) even after controlling for other prognostic variables in multivariate analysis.

Finally, the number of positive cervical lymph nodes consistently correlates with survival in univariate analysis for all major sites of HNSCC (9,62,65,104,105,108,113–117). The relative importance of extracapsular extension versus number of positive nodes remains somewhat controversial. In addition to the Mamelle et al. study (103), Moe et al. found node number to predict poor survival independent of extracapsular extension in 159 patients with advanced laryngeal cancer (11). However, cohorts of 136 patients with clinically node positive oral cavity cancer (63) and 281 patients with supraglottic cancer (49) found that extracapsular extension, not number of positive nodes, was an independent predictor of poor survival. Differences in treatment modalities and stratification of pathologic variables may explain some of the differences noted in these studies. Regardless, patients with either multiple positive lymph nodes or extracapsular extension are at risk for recurrence and should be considered for aggressive therapy.

Extracapsular Extension

Extracapsular extension (ECE) occurs in roughly 60% of patients with positive cervical nodes and is associated with N stage (118,119). A study of 337 patients undergoing neck dissection as a component of therapy for HNSCC found that ECE was present in 10.5% (18/171), 35% (26/75), 55% (35/64), and 74% (20/27) of clinically N0, N1, N2 and N3 patients, respectively (117). The extent of ECE can be stratified into the following three levels based on the morphology of the involved cervical lymph nodes:

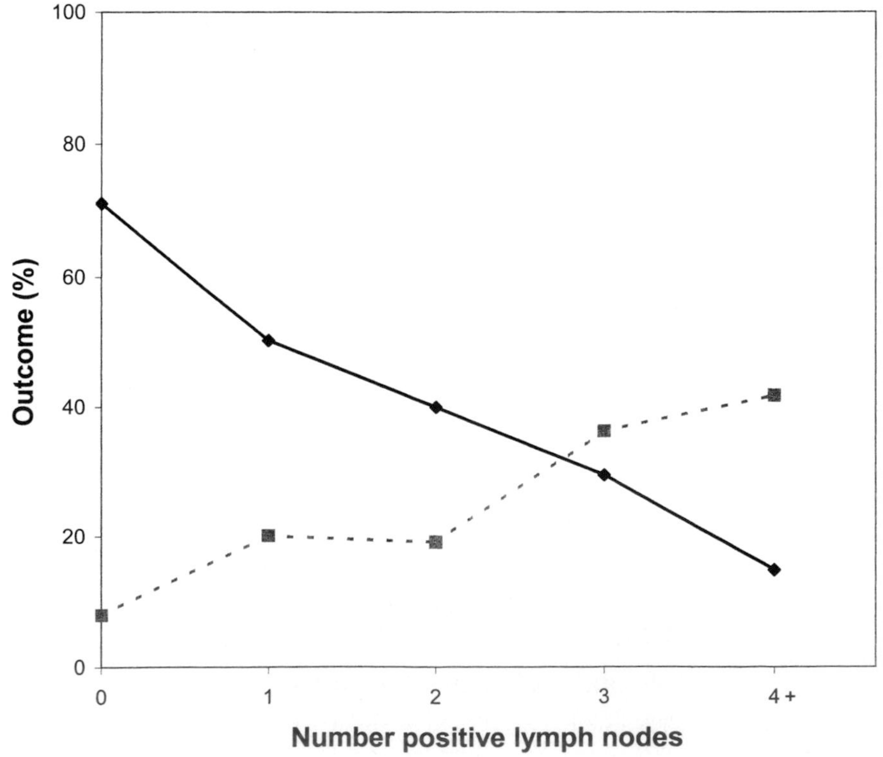

Figure 3.2 Number of positive cervical lymph nodes as a predictor of distant metastasis (*gray broken line*) and 5-year overall survival (*solid line*) in a cohort of 914 patients undergoing lymph node dissection for a primary head and neck squamous cell carcinoma. (Data from Mamelle G, Pampurik J, Luboinski B, et al. Lymph node prognostic factors in head and neck squamous cell carcinomas. *Am J Surg* 1994;168:494–498.)

1. Macroscopic extracapsular spread with involvement of adjacent anatomic structures such as the internal jugular vein or skeletal muscle
2. Macroscopic extracapsular spread confined to the perinodal fibro-adipose tissue
3. Microscopic extracapsular spread (14).

As a general marker of tumor invasiveness and biologic aggressiveness, some authors have proposed that the presence of ECE in cervical lymph nodes may predict recurrence at the primary site. This hypothesis remains unresolved, as two studies conducted on a total of 207 patients with laryngeal cancer noted a significant association (120,121), but two other studies conducted on a total of 392 patients with HNSCC have not confirmed this association (105, 118).

Regardless of its relationship with local recurrence, ECE is a significant determinant of prognosis due to its association with increased risk for recurrence in the neck and distant metastatic disease. For example, in a review of 284 patients with HNSCC who received neck dissection as a component of initial therapy, the presence of gross or microscopic ECE tripled the risk for neck recurrence in multivariate modeling (64). In addition, patients with gross ECE were 1.5 times as likely to develop regional recurrence as compared with patients with microscopic ECE, although this trend did not reach statistical significance. Many other series have confirmed this relationship for the following sites: oral tongue (14), oral cavity and oropharynx (5,32,97), hypopharynx and lateral epilarynx (105), pyriform sinus (9), supraglottic larynx (120,122,123), larynx (121,124,125), and all sites combined (72,104,106,107,126). The association between ECE and regional recurrence is independent of other prognostic variables in HNSCC (64,107,124).

The presence of ECE also increases the risk for distant metastatic disease. In a review of 281 patients who received a neck dissection as a component of initial therapy for HNSCC, the presence of ECE tripled the risk for distant metastasis as the first site of failure (19.1% in ECE-positive patients vs. 6.7% in ECE-negative patients) (109). These findings have been reproduced in several large studies (98,108,110,117). Currently, no study has examined whether the relationship between ECE and distant metastatic disease is independent of the number, size, and location of positive cervical lymph nodes.

In addition, ECE is a significant predictor of poor disease-free, cause-specific, and overall survival. In a retrospective study of 281 patients with supraglottic SCC treated with surgery with or without postoperative radiotherapy, pathologic node-negative patients experienced a 5-year overall survival of 65%, compared with 49% in node-positive patients without ECE and 20% in node-positive patients with ECE (49). In a multivariate model constructed from relevant clinicopathologic covariables, the presence of ECE conferred the highest risk of death, resulting in a sixfold increased risk of death due to primary tumor compared with node-negative patients. In contrast, patients with positive nodes but no ECE experienced a threefold increased risk of death due to disease. This independent association between ECE and poor cause-specific or overall survival has been confirmed for the following sites: oral cavity (63), oral cavity and oropharynx (5), supraglottic larynx (62), larynx and hypopharynx (125), and all sites combined (52,107,124).

The importance of ECE as compared with other pathologic factors was underscored in a prospective randomized clinical trial conducted by Peters et al. that evaluated radiation dose in the postoperative setting (127). In this trial, patients with ECE experienced significantly higher locoregional recurrence rates than patients without ECE. In addition, in the subset of patients without ECE, only those patients with four or more adverse risk factors experienced a locoregional recurrence rate comparable to those patients with ECE. Adverse factors examined included oral cavity primary, close or positive margins, PNI, two or more positive nodes, largest node greater than 3 cm, Zubrod score ≥2, and delay in starting radiotherapy. As a result, the study authors concluded that ECE is the dominant pathologic risk factor in HNSCC. Furthermore, this study showed that, in patients with ECE, locoregional control increased from 52% to 74% as dose increased from 57.6 Gy to 63 Gy. No such dose-response was evident in patients without ECE, suggesting that tumors with ECE require higher postoperative doses to achieve adequate locoregional control.

Due to the poor prognosis associated with ECE, several investigators have explored the potential benefit of adjuvant chemotherapy in this patient population. Johnson et al. report a nonrandomized study of patients with HNSCC with histologically documented ECE (128,129). Fifty patients received 6 months of methotrexate, 5-fluorouracil, and leucovorin following surgery and postoperative radiation and 47 patients were treated with surgery and radiation alone. Although the study was not randomized, the two treatment groups did not differ significantly with respect to age, tumor site, Karnofsky performance status, number of positive nodes, and percent of nodes with ECE. Five-year adjusted survival was 54% in the group treated with adjuvant chemotherapy compared with 17% in the historical controls. The potential benefit of adjuvant chemotherapy was confirmed in a prospective randomized trial that evaluated the use of concurrent weekly cisplatin and postoperative radiation in a cohort of patients with stage III and IV HNSCC and histologically documented ECE (130). Forty-eight percent (19/39) of the patients who received concurrent chemoradiation experienced disease recurrence, compared with 68% (30/44) of the patients who received postoperative radiotherapy alone. Concurrent chemoradiotherapy significantly improved overall survival, disease-free survival, and locoregional recurrence-free survival but did not decrease the incidence of distant metastatic disease.

Node Location

The anatomic location of positive cervical lymph nodes has classically been described by dividing the neck into five anatomic levels (131). Level I refers to nodes within the submandibular and submental triangles. Levels II, III, and IV refer to the chain of nodes along the upper, middle, and lower third of the jugular vein, respectively. Level V refers to nodes along the spinal accessory nerve and within the posterior cervical triangle. Using these categories, Mamelle et al. defined sentinel nodes as those nodal groups that provide the primary lymphatic drainage for a particular site within the head and neck (103). Thus, the sentinel nodes for oral cavity tumors were defined as levels I, II, and III; the sentinel nodes for oropharyngeal, hypopharyngeal, and laryngeal tumors were defined as levels II and III. Applying this classification to cervical node pathologic specimens from 914 patients with HNSCC, Mamelle et al. found that the presence of nodal metastases outside the sentinel node region independently decreased 5-year survival by more than 50% and nearly doubled the rate of distant metastasis. Furthermore, node location (in or out of the sentinel area) predicted survival independent of number of positive nodes and extracapsular spread. The increased risk for regional recurrence, distant recurrence, and death associated with positive low cervical lymph nodes has been noted in several other studies of patients with HNSCC (11,40,105,111,113,114,116,132,133). Finally, de Bree et al. found that 33% of patients with HNSCC with low jugular lymph node metastases showed evidence of concomitant distant metastatic disease on preoperative CT of the thorax (1). Clearly, patients with positive lymph nodes outside of the sentinel node regions merit aggressive preoperative screening for distant disease and are at increased risk for treatment failure and death following aggressive locoregional therapy.

Node Size

The diameter of the largest metastatic cervical lymph node contributes to the assessment of N stage in HNSCC and may correspond with total tumor burden. In a review of 250 radical neck dissection specimens, Carter et al. found that pathologic nodal size greater than 2 cm correlated with increased risk for regional recurrence (107). However, several other studies have failed to determine a relationship between node size assessed clinically or pathologically and either regional recurrence or locoregional recurrence (40,42,106). In contrast, Mamelle et al. found that nodal size increased the risk for distant metastases, with patients having nodal diameter less than 3 cm experiencing a distant metastasis rate of 22%, compared with 35% for patients with nodal diameter between 3 and 6 cm and 49% for patients with nodal diameter greater than 6 cm (103). Furthermore, in a multivariate analysis of clinical parameters only, node size was a significant predictor of poor overall survival. In contrast, other studies have not found an independent relationship between pathologically assessed nodal size and survival when other relevant pathologic variables are considered (9,42,107, 125). Thus, the diameter of the largest positive cervical lymph node may serve as a helpful clinical predictor of outcome but does not appear to exert an independent prognostic when pathologic factors are considered.

DEMOGRAPHIC PARAMETERS

Age

Age is a commonly considered covariable and is known to influence outcome in certain types of cancer. For example, patient age and attendant comorbidities may influence the vigor of the immune response directed against the tumor and the patient's ability to tolerate maximal therapy. In addition, head and neck cancers arising in patients at either extreme of the age continuum may result from different etiologic agents and thus manifest different clinical outcomes. For example, Schantz et al. found that cultured lymphocytes from nonsmoking young adults with HNSCC were more susceptible to bleomycin-induced chromosome damage than lymphocytes from older smokers with HNSCC and healthy control subjects, suggesting that genetic susceptibility to environmental carcinogens may influence the risk for HNSCC in young adults (134). Investigators have noted an increase in the incidence of oral tongue cancer in adults younger than 40 years, thus prompting additional interest in the risk factors, natural history, and optimal treatment of HNSCC in the young (48).

Risk factor profiles indicate that young adults with HNSCC are less likely to have prior exposure to tobacco or alcohol and are more likely to be female (135,136). With respect to clinical outcome, Siegelmann-Danieli et al. examined a retrospective cohort of 87 oral tongue SCC patients, 30 of whom were 45 years of age or younger at time of diagnosis (136). In this study, age did not influence relapse rates, cancer-free survival, and overall survival in both univariate and multivariate analysis. Similarly, Verschuur et al. conducted a retrospective case-control study on 185 previously untreated patients with HNSCC younger than 40 years and control subjects matched for site, sex, and date of presentation (135). Age did not influence cause-specific survival in univariate or multivariate analysis. However, older patients were twice as likely to develop second primary SCCs of the upper aerodigestive tract (14% vs. 7%), possibly due to their increased use of tobacco products. The effect of young age remains controversial, as one report on 1,030 HNSCC cancer patients found that patients older than 40 years were twice as likely to develop recurrent disease as patients younger than 40, even after controlling for TNM stage, primary tumor site, and comorbidity (137). Hence, the importance of young age as a prognostic factor in patients with head and neck cancer is unclear and treatment decisions should not be based solely on patient age.

Head and neck cancers in older adult populations also present a different epidemiologic profile. In a study of 161 older adult patients with HNSCC, Leon et al. found that patients older than 70 years are less likely to use tobacco and alcohol and more likely to be female (138). The decreased consumption of tobacco and alcohol in older adult patients with HNSCC correlates with a lower incidence of *p53* mutations in this population (139). With respect to survival, although Leon et al. demonstrated that older adult laryngeal cancer patients experienced worse overall survival, cause-specific survival was not influenced by patient age. Furthermore, in a prospective study of 203 head and neck cancer patients, advanced age correlated with worsening 2-year overall survival in univariate analysis, but this association was not significant when adjusted for TNM stage and the presence of comorbidities (140). Thus, although older adult patients with HNSCC may present with different risk factor profiles, the overall tumor behavior and cause-specific survival does not differ substantially from those patients between the ages of 40 and 70.

Sex

Sex is not generally considered a significant determinant of survival in patients with head and neck cancer. Indeed, most large series have failed to find a significant difference in outcome with respect to sex (67,69,141–146). Only one relatively large study conducted on 278 patients with stage I to IV laryngeal cancer found an independent association between sex and survival (42). In this study, female patients experienced a 75.6% 3-year overall survival, compared with 62.9% in male patients. However, the disease-free interval was nearly identical, 60.4 months in women and 59.7 months in men. Thus, it is likely that the survival benefit experienced by women was more likely due to differences in comorbidity between the sexes rather than difference in intrinsic tumor behavior. Clearly, the literature strongly suggests that no clinically meaningful differences in outcome exist for men and women with HNSCC.

Race

Data from the National Cancer Data Base indicate that African-American, non-Hispanic patients are almost twice as likely to present with stage IV disease as compared with their white counterparts (73). In a total of 295,022 cases of cancer from the head and neck reported from 1985 to 1994 in the United States, 40% of African Americans presented with stage IV disease, compared with 24% of whites and 26.4% of Hispanics. However, in one large retrospective study conducted on 1,632 patients with laryngeal cancer (144), and in a prospective study conducted on 649 patients with HNSCC (67), race was not a significant predictor of overall survival in univariate analysis. Furthermore, in a prospective study conducted on 203 patients with head and neck cancer, black race was associated with poor

2-year overall survival in univariate analysis, but this association was no longer significant after controlling for stage and comorbidity (140). These studies suggest that the biologic aggressiveness of HNSCC does not differ between white and black patients. However, more thorough screening of black populations is clearly necessary to enable early detection and successful treatment.

Alcohol and Tobacco Exposure

Exposure to alcohol and tobacco has long been recognized as an important risk factor for the development of HNSCC. Exposure to these carcinogens results in specific molecular insults that promote neoplasia. For example, cigarette smoking has been associated with overexpression of the protooncogene bcl-2, a protein known to inhibit apoptosis (147). In addition, concurrent use of alcohol and tobacco has been associated with a high rate of nonspecific mutations in the tumor suppressor gene *p53* (148). Perhaps as a result of these deleterious mutations, prior or continued use of alcohol and tobacco in patients with head and neck cancer is a risk factor for poor outcome. Furthermore, use of these substances has been associated with immunosuppression, malnutrition, and impaired tissue oxygenation resulting in hypoxic radioresistance.

The most rigorous exploration of the relationship between alcohol consumption and outcome in head and neck cancer patients resulted from a prospective study of 649 patients who received in-depth questioning near the time of diagnosis regarding alcohol consumption, treatment for alcoholism, abstinence from alcohol prior to the diagnosis of cancer, and alcohol-related health problems (67). The authors used the Michigan Alcoholism Screening Test (MAST) to devise a three-tier alcohol severity staging system to allow rapid risk stratification of head and neck cancer patients. Stage A included nonalcoholics and abstinent (less than one drink per week) alcoholics without a history of alcohol-related systemic health problems. Stage B included abstinent alcoholics with a history of alcohol-related systemic health problems and alcoholics currently drinking without a history of alcohol-related systemic health problems. Stage C included alcoholics who were currently drinking and had a history of alcohol-related systemic health problems. Patients in stages B and C were more likely to die from any cause following treatment for HNSCC. In addition, after adjusting for other potential predictors of survival, stage C patients were two times more likely to die from head and neck cancer as stage A patients. The authors speculate that alcohol intake may influence outcomes by contributing to immunosuppression and malnutrition.

Of note, this study provided indirect evidence that interventions to eliminate alcohol intake may help to improve outcomes. After controlling for relevant covariables, alcoholics abstinent at the time of diagnosis were half as likely to die as alcoholics who were currently drinking. Eighty percent of abstinent alcoholics had received formal treatment for their alcoholism, either through inpatient programs or Alcoholics Anonymous.

The interaction between cigarette smoking and response to radiotherapy was demonstrated in a prospective study of stage III and IV HNSCC patients treated with primary irradiation with or without concomitant 5-fluorouracil (149). Any smoking during the 6½-week course of radiotherapy decreased the complete response rate from 74% to 45%, the 2-year survival rate from 66% to 39%, and the median survival from 30 months to 16 months. In addition, mortality was influenced by the length of time between smoking cessation and initiation of treatment, with a risk reduction of 40% for those patients who quit less than 12 weeks prior to diagnosis and of 70% for patients who quit more than 1 year prior to diagnosis. In multivariate analysis, smoking was the only significant predictor of survival, with those who abstained 2.5 times more likely to survive. The authors speculated that the deleterious impact of smoking may be related to lower levels of activity of natural killer cells, reduced cell-mediated immunity, and increased blood carboxyhemoglobin concentrations resulting in tissue hypoxia and increased radioresistance (150). The adverse effect of continued smoking during radiotherapy has also been noted in two studies conducted on patients with T1 and T2 glottic carcinomas treated with primary radiation (151,152). In addition to mortality, continued smoking roughly doubles the risk for long-term complications in patients with T1 glottic cancer treated with primary radiation (153).

To evaluate the effect of alcohol and tobacco consumption on the risk for second primary malignancies, Day et al. conducted a nested case-control study composed of 80 case patients with second cancers and 189 sex- and survival-matched oral cancer patients free of second cancers (154). The risk for a second primary tumor of the aerodigestive tract (oral cavity, pharynx, larynx, esophagus, and lung) increased with both number of cigarettes smoked per day and years of cigarette smoking, peaking at 4.7 for those patients who smoked 40 or more cigarettes per day for 20 or more years. Similarly, consumers of 15 or more drinks per week of beer experienced 3.8 times the risk for aerodigestive tract second primary tumors when compared with nondrinkers or light drinkers (0–4 drinks per week). There was little or no excess risk for hard liquor and wine drinking.

Day et al. also investigated the relationship between cessation of smoking or drinking at time of diagnosis and risk for second primary tumor. Cessation of smoking at the time of diagnosis did not decrease the risk for second primary tumors within the first 5 years after diagnosis. However, risk was significantly reduced 5 years after smoking cessation. Thus, smoking cessation at time of diagnosis may reduce the long-term risk for second primary tumors. No clear trend existed between cessation of alcohol consumption and risk.

Due to the well-documented deleterious effects of tobacco and alcohol use, in addition to data suggesting that abstinence from these substances may improve outcomes, substance abuse counseling and cessation programs should be integrated into the care of head and neck cancer patients.

FACTORS RELATED TO THE PATIENT'S GENERAL MEDICAL CONDITION

Comorbid Illness

Comorbidity refers to the presence of other diseases, illnesses, or conditions in addition to the index cancer. Although not included in TNM staging, comorbidity directly influences the care of cancer patients, selection of initial treatment modalities, and evaluation of treatment effectiveness. Using a four-tiered classification (none, mild, moderate, and severe), Piccirillo found that 21% of head and neck cancer patients have moderate or severe comorbidity (140). Examples of moderate comorbidity included poorly controlled hypertension, past stroke with residua, and history of an alcoholic seizure. Severe comorbidity included congestive heart failure or myocardial infarction within the last 6 months, recent stroke, and severely decompensated alcoholism (155). In a prospective study of 203 patients with primary head and neck cancer, the presence of comorbidity was a significant, independent predictor of 2-year survival, even after controlling for type of initial treatment, age, and TNM stage (140). Patients with moderate comorbidity were nearly three times as likely to die within 2 years when compared with patients with no or mild comorbidity. Additionally, a retrospective multi-institutional study of 70 head and neck cancer patients 45 years of age and younger revealed that comorbidity is an independent predictor of tumor-specific and disease-free survival (156,157).

Given the importance of comorbidity as a predictor of survival, efforts have been made to develop new systems for staging head and neck cancer that combine TNM staging with symptom-severity and comorbidity indices. The general scheme for such a staging system of oral cavity cancer is presented in Figure 3.3. Of note, the most advanced stage, stage D, is determined solely by the presence of severe comorbidity or moderate or severe symptom severity. Hence, advanced TNM stage alone is not sufficient to merit placement in the worst prognostic category. Using multivariate modeling, the investigators convincingly demonstrated that this model was more strongly predictive of disease-free and overall survival than TNM staging alone in a retrospective cohort of 277 patients with oral cavity SCC (155). Similar results were obtained in other retrospective studies conducted on oral cavity (158), oropharyngeal (159), and laryngeal (160) cancers. Clearly, the combination of comorbidity, symptom severity, and TNM stage holds promise for more accurate prognostication in head and neck cancer and merits prospective validation (140).

Nutritional Status

Malnutrition is common in patients with head and neck cancer and attributable to a number of causes including poor dietary habits, excessive alcohol consumption, local tumor effects, tumor-induced cachexia, and the effects of various therapies (161). In 1984, Goodwin and Torres applied a prognostic nutritional index to a retrospective cohort of 50 consecutive patients with advanced head and neck cancer to determine if nutritional

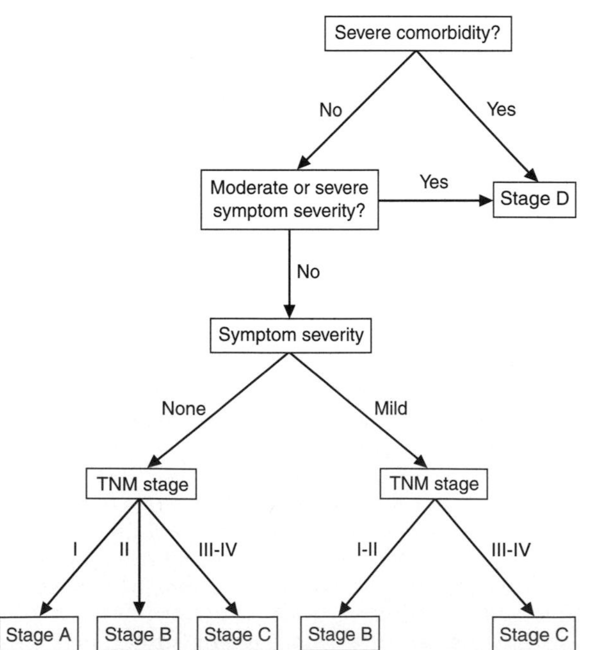

Figure 3.3 Decision tree for clinical-severity staging of oral cavity cancer. (From Pugliano FA, Piccirillo JF, Zequeira MR, et al. Clinical-severity staging system for oral cavity cancer: five-year survival rates. *Otolaryngol Head Neck Surg* 1999;120:38–45.)

status influenced postoperative complications and survival (162). The prognostic nutrition index considers serum albumin, serum transferrin, triceps skin-fold thickness, and cutaneous delayed hypersensitivity to mumps, streptokinase-streptodornase, or candida. This index was generated from retrospective review of 161 patients undergoing gastrointestinal surgery and then prospectively validated in 100 patients as an indicator of risk for postoperative complications (163). Goodwin and Torres found that 89% (8/9) of patients with a prognostic nutrition index greater than 39% had major postoperative complications, compared with 14% (4/29) of patients with prognostic nutrition index ≤39%. In addition, 64% (9/14) of the patients with prognostic nutrition index greater than 39% died of their disease within 1 year, compared with 28% (10/36) of patients with prognostic nutrition index ≤39%.

Prognostic nutrition index is calculated as follows:

$$158\% - 16.6\,(\mathrm{ALB}) - 0.78\,(\mathrm{TSF}) - 0.2\,(\mathrm{TFN}) - 5.8\,(\mathrm{DH})$$

where ALB is serum albumin (g/dL); TSF is triceps skin-fold thickness in mm; TFN is serum transferrin level (g/dL); and DH is cutaneous delayed hypersensitivity reaction to mumps, streptokinase-streptodornase, or candida graded as 0 (nonreactive), 1 (<5 mm induration), or 2 (≥5 mm induration).

The relationship between nutritional status, postoperative complications, and survival has been further explored in several prospective studies. In an analysis of six different nutritional parameters, 10% weight loss in the 6 months preceding surgery was the only significant, independent predictor of major postoperative complications in a cohort of 64 patients with T2 to T4 carcinomas of the oral cavity, oropharynx, hypopharynx, and larynx (164). In a subsequent study, 5% weight loss in the 6 months preceding initial treatment for advanced HSNCC was identified as an independent predictor of poor disease-specific survival in men but not women (165). Unfortunately, a randomized trial of preoperative tube feeding in 49 severely malnourished (weight loss >10% of body weight) head and neck cancer patients failed to show a decrease in complications or a survival benefit (166). As noted in a review on cancer cachexia and glucose metabolism, the multiple metabolic derangements present in malnourished patients with cancer create a catabolic state that cannot be overcome simply by the provision of excessive calories (167).

Clearly, malnutrition increases the risk for postoperative complications and may even affect disease-specific survival. Future research may focus on identifying novel nutritional prognostic factors such as serum amino acid profiles (161) and zinc levels (168) and on optimizing preoperative nutritional status.

Anemia

Anemia may influence tissue oxygenation and thus worsen local control and survival in patients who receive radiotherapy as a component of their treatment. This hypothesis has been consistently supported in numerous retrospective studies as presented in Table 3.3 (169). For example, in a study of 109 patients with T1 and T2 SCC of the glottic larynx treated with primary radiation, 2-year local control was 95% in patients with pretreatment hemoglobin concentration of 13 g/dL, compared with 66% local control in patients with hemoglobin less than 13 g/dL (170). Multivariate analysis revealed that hemoglobin was the only significant predictor of local control and survival in this cohort. Another study of 735 patients with early stage glottic cancer noted that pretreatment hemoglobin was an independent predictor of local recurrence (171). In more heterogeneous studies encompassing most primary sites for head and neck cancer, higher hemoglobin level (14.5 in men and 13.0 in

TABLE 3.3 Studies Correlating Anemia and Outcome

Author	Description of patients	Treatment given	MVT	Local/regional recurrence	Survival	Measure of anemia
Overgaard et al. 1986 (172)	950 larynx or pharynx SCC	RT	No	Yes ($p < 0.01$)	OS ($p < 0.01$)	Hemoglobin <14.5 g/dL for men and <13.0 g/dL for women pretreatment
van Acht et al. 1992 (180)	357 T1–4 N0–2 glottic or supraglottic SCC	RT	Yes	NR	DFS ($p < 0.05$)	Hemoglobin <11.0 mmol/L for men and <10.0 mmol/L for women at day 35 of RT
					OS ($p > 0.05$)	Decrease in hemoglobin ≥1.0 from before treatment to day 35 of RT
Fein et al. 1995 (170)	109 T1–2 N0 glottic larynx SCC	RT and surgical salvage	Yes	Yes ($p < 0.01$)	NR	Hemoglobin ≤13 g/dL pretreatment
Dubray et al. 1996 (169)	217 T1–4 N0–3 oral cavity and oropharynx SCC	RT and surgical salvage	Yes	Trend ($p = 0.06$)	OS ($p = 0.04$)	Hemoglobin <13.5 g/dL for men and <12.0 g/dL for women pretreatment
Tarnawski et al. 1997 (179)	847 T1–4 N0–2 laryngeal supraglottic SCC	RT	Yes	Yes ($p < 0.0001$)	NR	Hemoglobin as continuous variable and change in hemoglobin during treatment period
Lee et al. 1998 (175)	451 stage III or IV HNSCC	RT	Yes	Yes ($p = 0.003$)	OS ($p = 0.0007$)	Hemoglobin <14.5 g/dL for men and <13.0 g/dL for women pretreatment
Overgaard et al. 1998 (176)	422 (414 eligible) T1–4 N0–3 pharynx and supraglottic larynx SCC	RT and surgical salvage	Yes	Yes ($p = 0.001$)	Trend DFS and recurrence ($p = 0.09$)	Hemoglobin <9.0 mmol/L for men and <8.0 mmol/L for women pretreatment
Warde et al. 1998 (171)	735 T1–2 glottic SCC	RT	Yes	Yes ($p < 0.05$)	NR	Hemoglobin <10.0 g/dL to <14.0 g/dL
Lutterbach et al. 2000 (177)	258 T1–4 glottic SCC	Surgery	Yes	Yes ($p < 0.05$)	NR	Hemoglobin <13.0 g/dL for men and <12.0 g/dL for women pretreatment
Glaser et al. 2001 (178)	191 T2–4 N0–3 M0 oral cavity or oropharynx SCC	RT, CTX, surgery	No	Yes ($p < 0.05$)	OS ($p < 0.05$)	Hemoglobin <14.5 g/dL with or without exogenous erythropoetin treatment

CTX, chemotherapy; DFS, disease-free survival; HNSCC, head and neck squamous cell carcinoma; MVT, multivariate; NR, not reported; OS, overall survival; RT, radiotherapy; SCC, squamous cell carcinoma.

women) was associated with improved locoregional control and survival in patients treated with radiotherapy (172–176). An analysis of 258 patients with surgically treated glottic cancer demonstrated that low hemoglobin levels (<13.0 in men and <12.0 in women) before radiotherapy correlated with poor locoregional control (177). This suggests that anemia may influence outcome in head and neck cancer patients independent of its influence on hypoxic radioresistance.

Although no clinical trials have yet been published in the literature, results of a recent retrospective nonrandomized cohort study of 191 patients with T2 to T4, N0 to N3, M0 SCC of the oral cavity or oropharynx treated with chemoradiotherapy and surgery suggest therapeutic benefit from exogenous administration of erythropoietin (178). Similar to results of other studies, low hemoglobin was a significant prognostic indicator of incomplete pathologic response to neoadjuvant therapy, reduced locoregional control, and poor overall survival. However, addition of exogenous recombinant human erythropoietin (r-HuEPO) in patients with hemoglobin less than 14.5 significantly improved their response compared with those patients with low hemoglobin who did not receive r-HuEPO. Moreover, patients with low hemoglobin receiving r-HuEPO did not differ in tumor control and survival compared with patients with normal hemoglobin. Use of r-HuEPO was successful in producing significant increases in hemoglobin level during the treatment period. In multivariate analysis, hemoglobin level after neoadjuvant therapy appeared to be a stronger prognostic indicator of outcomes compared with pretreatment hemoglobin level. Interestingly, this finding is supported by results of a retrospective analysis of patients who did not receive any exogenous erythropoietin, which suggested that hemoglobin level after radiotherapy could be equally or more important than pretreatment hemoglobin level for predicting local control (179). Another retrospective study on patients with glottic or supraglottic SCC indicated that decreases in hemoglobin during radiotherapy, even with relatively normal baseline hemoglobin, showed a trend toward poorer disease-free survival (180). As a whole, these results suggest that, for a variety of SCC sites, exogenous administration of erythropoietin in patients with anemia before or during radiotherapy may become a promising adjunct therapy for improving tumor response and survival. Clearly, future randomized trials should assess whether correction of malignancy-induced anemia with exogenous erythropoietin will result in improved local control and survival in head and neck cancer patients (181).

MOLECULAR PROGNOSTIC FACTORS

The vast array of molecular factors studied in head and neck cancer can be divided into several broad categories. Protooncogenes code for proteins that promote cellular proliferation. A protooncogene is transformed into an oncogene when its protein product becomes unresponsive to the normal regulatory processes that control cell division. Activation of protooncogenes occurs by point mutations, chromosomal translocations, or gene amplification. At the cellular level, an oncogene exerts a dominant phenotype over its protooncogene counterpart because only one copy of an oncogene is necessary to promote neoplasia. In contrast, tumor suppressor genes (anti-oncogenes) inhibit cellular proliferation. At the cellular level, both copies of a tumor suppressor gene must be mutated to promote neoplasia. Another class of markers includes proteins and growth factors that mediate the interaction between neoplastic cells and their local microenvironment. In addition to these specific molecular markers expressed in neoplastic cells, other factors such as tumor ploidy and the rate of tumor cell proliferation may yield important prognostic information.

p53

p53 is a transcription factor with tumor suppressor function that negatively regulates the cell cycle and serves to protect the integrity of the genome. Its gene resides on chromosome 17p13 and is composed of 11 exons spanning 20 kb in length (182). In response to certain types of DNA damage, *p53* protein levels increase resulting in G1 arrest or apoptosis (183–186). *p53* mediates G1 arrest through transactivation of at least two genes: *p21WAF1CIP1*, an inhibitor of the G1 cyclin-dependent kinases essential for the G1/S transition, and *GADD* (45), a gene implicated in growth arrest and DNA excision repair (185,187,188). *p53* induction also results in apoptosis, presumably when the extent of DNA damage exceeds the capacity of cellular repair mechanisms (189). Thus, *p53* protects the cell from propagating mutations to subsequent generations and is considered the "guardian of the genome" (183).

Loss of *p53* function may contribute to tumor aggressiveness by promoting resistance to radiation and chemotherapy, accelerated growth in hypoxic conditions, and tumor neovascularization. When compared with cells with wild-type *p53*, *p53* mutant cell lines exhibit more resistance to ionizing radiation and certain chemotherapeutic agents (190–192). This evidence leads to the hypothesis that tumors lacking a functional *p53* gene will exhibit a radioresistant and chemotherapy-resistant phenotype due to a deficiency in DNA damage-induced apoptosis (188). This hypothesis has been strengthened by experiments conducted with *p53* mutant cell lines derived from HNSCCs. Transfection with an adenoviral vector or a liposomal system containing a functional *p53* gene resulted in a dose-dependent increase in radiation sensitivity, restoration of the G1 checkpoint, and induction of apoptosis (193–196). *p53* may also mediate hypoxia-induced apoptosis. Graeber et al. demonstrated that mutations in *p53* reduce hypoxic cell death and confer a competitive advantage to cells growing in a hypoxic environment (197). Thus, mutations in *p53* may increase the number of hypoxic cells, conferring hypoxia-mediated radioresistance. Finally, loss of *p53* function results in the down-regulation of thrombospondin-1, an inhibitor of angiogenesis (198). Indeed, a strong correlation between *p53* overexpression, a surrogate marker for *p53* gene mutation, and both elevated tumor microvessel density and vascular endothelial growth factor (VEGF) expression has been reported in HNSCC (199,200). As a whole, the data from basic science studies support the hypothesis that *p53* mutations contribute to biologically aggressive tumor behavior by conferring resistance to radiotherapy and chemotherapy and by promoting angiogenesis.

Inactivation of *p53* is a common event in HNSCC and may result from spontaneous or tobacco-induced mutations (148) or from sequestration by cellular proteins such as mdm2 (201) or the E6 viral oncoprotein of human papillomavirus (HPV) (202). Detection of *p53* mutations has been attempted through both protein-based and DNA-based techniques. Many studies have used immunohistochemistry (IHC), capitalizing on the differential expression of wild-type and mutant *p53*. Wild-type *p53* has a half-life of 20 minutes, whereas many *p53* mutations confer stability to the protein and thus result in higher intracellular levels detectable via IHC (182). Unfortunately, this technique often fails to detect nonsense or frameshift mutations that result in *p53* protein truncation (203). Furthermore, induction of wild-type *p53* in response to DNA damage can result in sufficient quantities for IHC detection. Saunders et al. sequenced all coding exons of the *p53* gene from 39 laryngeal SCCs and found that *p53* IHC resulted in a 64% concordance, 42% false-positive rate, and 23% false-negative rate (204). Larger studies that examined only the conserved regions of the *p53* gene reported 59% to 71% concordance with IHC (203,205). Thus, although relatively simple and inexpensive, IHC is not an accurate method for detecting *p53* mutations.

DNA-based techniques for detection of *p53* mutations have focused on exons 5 through 8, a highly conserved region that codes for a DNA-binding domain (182). However, studies have found that 20% to 25% of *p53* gene mutations lie outside the conserved region (206,207), although these mutations may not influence *in vivo p53* function. Finally, loss of heterozygosity at the *p53* gene locus has been examined using polymorphic markers and fluorescent *in situ* hybridization (FISH) (208–210).

Studies correlating *p53* mutation with outcome in HNSCC are compiled in Table 3.4. Results of these studies remain mixed; however, several excellent studies have demonstrated an association between directly sequenced *p53* mutations and resistance to radiotherapy. In the largest study to employ direct sequencing, Koch et al. evaluated the prognostic significance of *p53* mutations in exons 5 through 9 in 110 HNSCCs treated with either primary or adjuvant radiotherapy (139). These tumors spanned all major sites for HNSCC and included all clinical stages. In multivariate analysis, patients with *p53* mutations were 2.4 times more likely to develop locoregional recurrence, equal to the risk for locoregional recurrence conferred by the presence of positive cervical lymph nodes. In contrast, *p53* expression as assessed via IHC failed to correlate with any outcome variable (203). Similarly, two other studies showed that *p53* mutation, but not protein overexpression, predicted poor locoregional control and survival in cohorts composed of 58 and 68 patients with HNSCC, most of whom received radiotherapy (211,212). Furthermore, a study conducted on 22 incidences of recurrent HNSCC previously treated with radiation found that 21 of the 22 recurrences had evidence for *p53* inactivation by either gene mutation, mdm2 overexpression, or HPV infection (213). In contrast to these three studies, Gallo et al. examined 85 patients with mainly early stage HNSCC treated with primary irradiation and found that *p53* mutation resulted in trends toward poor locoregional control and disease-free survival in univariate analysis, but was not predictive of disease-free or cause-specific survival in multivariate modeling (214). Furthermore, the only study to sequence all expressed exons in the *p53* gene failed to show a relationship between *p53* mutation and local recurrence in laryngeal SCCs treated with radiotherapy. However, this study had limited power due to the inclusion of only 35 patients (206). Although results remain mixed, evidence suggests that *p53* mutation may be an important predictor of radioresistance and poor locoregional control.

In addition to the relationship between *p53* mutation and response to radiotherapy, several groups have considered the relationship between directly sequenced *p53* mutations and response to chemotherapy. In a cohort of 105 patients with HNSCC treated with platinum- and fluorouracil-based induction chemotherapy, Temam et al. directly sequenced all coding regions of the *p53* gene from biopsy specimens taken prior to the initiation of chemotherapy. Multivariate modeling revealed that tumors with a mutant *p53* gene were 70% less likely to experience major response to chemotherapy and, independently, tumors with high levels of *p53* protein expression were

TABLE 3.4 Studies Correlating p53 Mutation and Outcome

Author	Description of patients	Treatment given	MVT	Detection of p53 abnormality	% positive	Local/ regional recurrence	Survival	Notes
p53 sequencing in primary radiotherapy series:								
Overgaard et al. 1998 (212)	68 HNSCC (stage not specified)	RT + nimorazole	Yes	IHC DGGE + sequencing exons 5–9	67% 47%	No Yes (HR = 4.1)	No CSS (HR = 4.8)	*p53* mutants at risk for LR recurrence
Saunders et al. 1999 (204)	35 laryngeal SCC (mainly T1–2)	Primary RT	No	IHC sequenced exons 2–11	67% 48%	No No	NR NR	*p53* status not correlated with local failure
Gallo et al. 1999 (214)	85 HNSCC (mostly T1–2 N0)	Primary RT	Yes	SSCP + sequencing exons 5–8	45%	No	No	*p53* mutants trended to LR failure in univariate analysis only (*p* = 0.10)
p53 sequencing in heterogeneous series:								
Koch et al. 1996 (139)	110 stage I–IV HNSCC	68 surgery + RT 42 primary RT	Yes	Sequenced exons 5–9	44%	Yes (RR = 2.4)	No	*p53* mutants more likely to develop LR recurrence
Erber et al. 1998 (219)	86 stage I–IV HNSCC	surgery (68 received post-operative RT)	No	Sequenced exons 5–8	15% (DNA contact mutations)	NR	DFS (*p* = 0.05) OS (*p* = 0.01)	Only DNA contact mutations conferred poor prognosis
Mineta et al. 1998 (211)	58 stage I–IV oral and oropharyngeal SCC	Mostly primary or preoperative RT	Yes	IHC SSCP + sequencing exons 5–8	74% 18%	NR NR	No CSS (RR = 9.9)	

Author	Description of patients	Treatment given	MVT	Detection of p53 abnormality	% positive	Response to CTX	Survival	Notes
p53 assessment in chemotherapy series:								
Temam et al. 2000 (207)	105 stage III–IV HNSCC	Induction of cisplatin and 5-FU	Yes	IHC sequenced exons 2–11	61% 37%	Yes (*p* = 0.05) Yes (*p* = 0.01)	NR NR	Both *p53* IHC and mutation were independent predictors of response
Cabelguenne et al. 2000 (215)	106 stage I–IV HNSCC	Induction of cisplatin and 5-FU	Yes	*p53* LOH DGGE + sequencing exons 4–9	54% 68%	Trend Yes (RR = 2.7)	NR NR	Presence of *p53* mutation or anti-*p53* serum antibodies conferred highest risk of not responding (RR = 4.9)
Etienne et al. 1999 (218)	82 stage II–IV HNSCC	61 induction cisplatin/5-FU, 21 concurrent chemoRT	Yes	Immunolumino-metric assay	NR	Trend for chemoRT group only	No	*p53* status correlated with poor CSS in univariate but not MVT analysis
Shiga et al. 1999 (217)	68 stage II–IV HNSCC	Induction cisplatin and 5-FU or paclitaxel	Yes	IHC	37%	No	DFS (*p* = NS) OS (*p* = 0.001)	
Warnakulasuriya et al. 2000 (216)	111 stage III–IV HNSCC	Multiple different CTX regimens (8 received RT alone)	Yes	IHC	32%	NR	DFS (*p* = 0.04) OS (*p* = 0.02)	

5-FU, 5-fluorouracil; CSS, cause-specific survival; CTX, chemotherapy; DFS, disease-free survival; DGGE, denaturing gradient gel electrophoresis; HNSCC, head and neck squamous cell carcinoma; HR, hazard ratio; IHC, immunohistochemistry; LOH, loss of heterozygosity; LR, local-regional; MVT, multivariate analysis; NR, not reported; NS, not significant; OS, overall survival; RT, radiotherapy; RR, relative risk; SCC, squamous cell carcinoma; SSCP, single-strand conformation polymorphism.

60% less likely to experience a major response (207). The correlation between *p53* overexpression and resistance to chemotherapy persisted in the subset of patients with wild-type *p53*, suggesting that *p53* IHC conveys independent prognostic information in patients treated with chemotherapy. An additional study conducted on 106 patients with HNSCC treated with cisplatin and 5-fluorouracil neoadjuvant chemotherapy screened for *p53* mutations using denaturing gradient gel electrophoresis (DGGE) on polymerase chain reaction (PCR) products from exons 4 through 9 of the *p53* gene followed by direct sequencing of those exons that demonstrated a variant DGGE pattern (215). In agreement with Temam et al., this study found that *p53* mutation was the only significant predictor of response to chemotherapy in multivariate analysis, with *p53* mutant tumors 63% less likely to respond to chemotherapy. At least three other studies have reported a correlation between *p53* overexpression and poor survival in patients with HNSCC who receive chemotherapy (216–218). Thus, strong evidence supports a role for *p53* alterations in predicting poor initial response and long-term survival following treatment with chemotherapy.

At least one group has considered whether the location of *p53* mutations influences the clinical phenotype of HNSCC. Erber et al. sequenced exons 5 through 8 and assessed for loss of heterozygosity at the *p53* allele in 86 oral cavity, oropharyngeal, hypopharyngeal, and laryngeal SCCs, stage I to IV (219). All patients received surgical resection, and 79% (68/86) received postoperative radiotherapy. Twenty-eight percent (24/86) of tumors exhibited a mutation within structural components of the *p53* gene, and 15% (13/86) of tumors exhibited mutations within regions critical for DNA binding of the *p53* protein. DNA contact mutations were associated with nodal positivity, advanced stage, and poor recurrence-free and overall survival in univariate analysis. Furthermore, in the subset of stage IV patients, the presence of contact mutations correlated with poor overall survival. No such correlation between structural mutations and stage at presentation or outcome was observed. These results imply that *p53* mutations resulting in the specific loss of DNA binding and thus transcriptional regulation result in radioresistance and particularly poor survival. The clinical significance of specific *p53* mutations clearly merits further study.

In contrast to the compelling relationship between *p53* gene mutations and resistance to radiotherapy and chemotherapy, the prognostic value of *p53* expression as assessed by IHC remains controversial. Overexpression of *p53* has been associated with poor outcome in the following cohorts: 69 patients with HNSCC, T1 to T4 N0 to N3, treated with surgery or radiotherapy (220); 106 patients with oropharyngeal SCC, stages II to IV, treated with surgery (88 received adjuvant radiotherapy) (221); 88 patients with stage I to IV laryngeal cancer treated surgically (12 received adjuvant radiotherapy) (222); 98 patients with HNSCC treated with primary radiotherapy (223); and 102 patients with T1 N0 M0 glottic SCC treated with primary radiotherapy (224). Despite these promising results, *p53* expression has not correlated with outcome in the following large studies: 51 patients with T1 SCC of the ventral tongue or floor of mouth treated with surgery alone (225); 69 patients with T2 to T4 oral and oropharyngeal SCC treated with surgery alone (226); 115 patients with HNSCC stage I to IV treated with surgery (73 received postoperative radiotherapy) (227); 85 patients with T1 to T4 oral tongue SCC treated with surgery or radiotherapy (228); 86 patients with T1 to T2 glottic SCC treated with primary radiotherapy (229); and 68 patients with stage I to IV nasopharyngeal carcinoma treated with radiotherapy (230). Finally, at least two studies have reported an association between *p53* overexpression and favorable outcome in 99 stage I to IV laryngeal cancers treated with surgery or radiotherapy (231) and in 103 patients with T1 to T4 N0 to N3 oropharyngeal SCC treated with surgery and postoperative radiation (200). The variation in these studies may in part be attributable to differences in antibodies used, antigen retrieval methods, scoring of *p53* positivity, primary tumor site, and treatment modalities. Given these contradictory results, the value of *p53* IHC as a determinant of prognosis in patients with HNSCC remains unclear.

Angiogenesis-Related Markers

Angiogenesis, the sprouting of new blood vessels from a preexisting endothelium, enables the growth of tumors beyond microscopic size (232,233). Many growth factors and cytokines, including the VEGF family, basic and acidic fibroblast growth factor (bFGF, aFGF), interleukin-8 (IL-8), and platelet-derived endothelial cell growth factor (PD-ECGF) have been shown to promote angiogenesis (234). The VEGF family consists of five members including VEGF, P1GF, VEGF-B, VEGF-C, VEGF-D, and the Orf virus VEGFs (VEGF-E) (235). Of these factors, VEGF plays a pivotal role in vasculogenesis and angiogenesis; VEGF-C is a potent inducer of lymphangiogenesis (236). Receptors for the VEGF family include VEGFR-1, VEGFR-2, and VEGFR-3, also known as *flt*, KDR/*flk-1*, and *flt4*, respectively (235). VEGFR-1 and VEGFR-2 are expressed on vascular endothelium, whereas VEGFR-3 is expressed in the lymphatic endothelium.

Vascular endothelial growth factor, a 34 to 50 kDa dimer composed of two identical disulfide-linked subunits that arise from differential splicing of a single gene (237), is frequently expressed in HNSCC (238) and has received the most study as a potential mediator of angiogenesis. Overexpression of VEGF may result from hypoxia-induced up-regulation of transcription and eIF4E-mediated up-regulation of translation (239–241). Because hypoxic tumors display increased radioresistance, VEGF protein levels may serve as a surrogate marker for hypoxic radioresistance. Furthermore, angiogenic activity may influence a tumor's metastatic potential by exposing it to a greater endothelial surface area, thus increasing the likelihood of hematogenous dissemination (242). In addition, once a tumor has formed a distant micrometastasis, it must recruit a vascular supply to proliferate to a clinically relevant size.

Angiogenic activity can be assessed in archival tumor tissue directly by staining with antibodies targeted against proteins that reside on endothelial cells, such as factor VIII, CD-31, and CD-34. In addition, expression of angiogenesis-promoting factors has been assessed via IHC and enzyme-linked immunosorbent assay. Expression of both VEGF and PD-ECGF has been reported to correlate with microvessel density (MVD) in HNSCC (199,200,243).

Studies that assessed tumor angiogenesis using immunohistochemical staining of microvessels are presented in Table 3.5 (244). Elevated tumor MVD has been shown to correlate with risk for concomitant cervical lymph node metastasis in oral cavity (245–247) and nasopharyngeal carcinomas (248,249). Furthermore, elevated MVD has been shown to correlate with risk for regional relapse in clinically N0 oral cavity carcinomas treated with surgery (250,251). The prognostic value of MVD in more heterogeneous series has been mixed, with one study of 97 stage I to IV laryngeal cancers reporting a significant association between elevated MVD and poor disease-free survival (252), but at least three other studies failing to uncover a relationship between MVD and prognosis (253–255).

Several groups have also examined the relationship between tumor MVD and response to radiotherapy. High MVD predicted local recurrence in 139 stage I to IV oropharyngeal tumors treated with primary irradiation, thus suggesting that tumors with intense neovascularization are more resistant to radiotherapy (256). However, a study of 31 T1 and T2 laryngeal cancers found the opposite and suggests that poorly vascularized tumors are more likely to manifest hypoxic radioresistance (257). Finally, intermediate MVD predicted favorable local control and survival in 76 stage III and IV HNSCCs treated with either induction chemotherapy followed by radiation or concurrent chemoradiation (258). These authors suggested that tumors with poor neovascularization may recur due to inadequate drug delivery coupled with hypoxic radioresistance whereas tumors with intense neovascularization recur due to their ability to undergo rapid repopulation in optimally oxygenated conditions. Clearly, although tumor MVD may correlate with nodal disease and regional recurrence, the relationship between MVD and radiosensitivity, chemosensitivity, and prognosis remains unclear and merits further study in large, homogeneous cohorts.

Directly assessing expression of angiogenic factors offers another approach to the study of tumor angiogenesis. High levels of VEGF and PD-ECGF have been shown to correlate with the presence of concomitant nodal metastases in both nasopharyngeal and oral cavity carcinomas (247–249,259). Furthermore, expression of VEGFR-3 on lymphatic endothelium within the region of the primary tumor significantly correlates with concomitant nodal metastasis, suggesting that lymphangiogenesis may increase the likelihood of spread to the cervical lymph nodes (259). In addition, VEGF overexpression appears to be a relatively consistent predictor of poor prognosis in clinical series. In a retrospective study of 56 stage II to IV oral and oropharyngeal SCCs treated with surgical excision and postoperative radiotherapy, VEGF expression predicted poor local control and increased risk for distant metastatic disease (260). In multivariate modeling, VEGF emerged as an independent predictor of poor disease-free and overall survival. Mineta et al.

TABLE 3.5 Studies Correlating Tumor Microvessel Density and Outcome

Author	Patients	Treatment	MVT	Marker	Local recurrence	Regional recurrence	Survival	Notes
Radiotherapy series:								
Rowchowdhury et al. 1996 (244)	30 stage I–IV nasopharyngeal cancers	RT (3 received concurrent bleomycin)	No	Factor VIII	No	No	DFS ($p = 0.05$) OS ($p = 0.02$)	*High* MVD predicts distant metastasis and poor survival
Giatromanolaki et al. 1999 (258)	76 stage III–IV HNSCC	Induction CTX or concurrent CRT	Yes	CD-31	Yes ($p < 0.0001$)	NR	OS ($p = 0.007$)	*Intermediate* MVD associated with best local control and survival
Kamijo et al. 2000 (257)	31 T1-2 laryngeal SCC	RT	Yes	CD-31	Yes ($p = 0.01$)	NR	NR	*Low* MVD tumors 16 times more likely to recur locally
Aebersold et al. 2000 (256)	139 stage I–IV oropharyngeal SCC	RT (27 received concurrent CTX)	Yes	CD-31	Yes ($p = 0.03$)	NR	OS ($p < 0.0001$)	*High* MVD tumors 9 times more likely to recur locally

CRT, chemoradiotherapy; CTX, chemotherapy; DES, disease-free survival; HNSCC, head and neck squamous cell carcinoma; MVD, microvessel density; MVT, multivariate analysis; NR, not reported; OS, overall survival; RT, radiotherapy; SCC, squamous cell carcinoma.

also demonstrated that VEGF expression as measured with Western blotting independently predicted poor disease-free survival in a cohort of 60 patients with stage I to IV HNSCC (261). The univariate correlation between VEGF expression and poor outcomes has been reported in at least three smaller cohorts as well (35,262,263). In contrast, VEGF levels did not correlate with overall survival in a cohort of 156 patients with stage I to IV HNSCC (255). Nevertheless, most studies support the hypothesis that VEGF overexpression predicts poor outcome and larger, confirmatory studies are needed.

The relationship between VEGF expression and response to primary radiotherapy remains uncertain. In a cohort of 41 patients with oral SCC treated with preoperative radiotherapy, Shintani et al. found that VEGF overexpression correlated with failure to undergo major pathologic response to radiotherapy (264). In contrast, Aebersold et al. found no correlation between VEGF levels and local failure in 139 stage I to IV oropharyngeal SCCs treated with primary irradiation (256). Clearly, additional studies are needed to assess the relationship between VEGF expression and radioresistance.

Cyclin D1

Cyclin D1, also known as PRAD1, is a protooncogene located on chromosome 11q13 (265) that serves as the rate-limiting controller of G1-phase progression through the cell cycle (266). In response to extracellular mitogens, cyclin D1 levels increase and complex with the cyclin-dependent kinases cdk4 or cdk6 to mediate progression through G1 by phosphorylation of the retinoblastoma protein. In HNSCC, alterations in cyclin D1 protein levels may result from up-regulation of translation (240,241) or from genomic inversions, translocations, or gene amplification (173, 267). Overexpression of cyclin D1 shortens the G1 interval and reduces the dependence of the cell on mitogens for proliferation. For example, Zwijsen et al. found that overexpression of cyclin D1 in a human epithelial breast cancer cell line reduced the fraction of cells entering quiescence under conditions where growth factors were limited, resulting in accelerated growth (268). Such observations suggest that deregulation of cyclin D1 may increase the overall aggressiveness of certain cancers by desensitizing cellular proliferation to inhibitory signals.

In HNSCC, deregulation of cyclin D1 has been measured using a variety of methods. At the protein level, several studies have assessed cyclin D1 expression using IHC. At the DNA level, a number of techniques including cytogenetics, Southern blot analysis, PCR gene amplification, and FISH have been used to measure cyclin D1 gene amplification (269).

Although the exact prognostic significance of cyclin D1 deregulation has not been completely determined, current evidence suggests a relationship between cyclin D1 amplification and poor prognosis (Table 3.6). In patients with clinically negative cervical lymph nodes, expression of cyclin D1 in the primary tumor independently confers a fourfold increased risk of finding histologically positive cervical lymph nodes on neck dissection (270). Bova et al. found cyclin D1 overexpression to predict increased risk for poor disease-free and overall survival in 148 patients with stage I to IV oral tongue SCC treated with surgery (52 patients received postoperative radiotherapy) (271). Similarly, Michalides et al. found that cyclin D1 overexpression was an independent predictor of shortened disease-free interval in 115 stage I to IV HNSCCs treated with surgery (73 received postoperative radiotherapy) (272). In addition, Pignataro et al. demonstrated that cyclin D1 overexpression independently doubled the risk for tumor relapse in 149 stage I to IV laryngeal SCCs treated with surgery (63 received postoperative radiation) (273). At least five other studies conducted on smaller cohorts of 45 to 94 patients have shown a relationship between cyclin D1 deregulation and poor prognosis in HNSCC (227,261,274–278). In contrast, Muller et al. failed to find a relationship between *11q13* amplification and disease-free or overall survival in 280 HNSCCs, T1 to T4 N0 to N3, treated with either surgery alone (79 patients) or surgery and postoperative radiotherapy (201 patients) (279). Only one other study conducted on 50 patients failed to correlate cyclin D1 amplification with outcome (280). Finally, Yoo et al. found high cyclin D1 protein expression to be protective against local recurrence in a case-control study of 60 T1 and T2 N0 laryngeal SCCs treated with primary radiation (281). Thus, the cumulative weight of evidence implicates cyclin D1 deregulation, particularly as assessed through IHC, as an important determinant of poor disease-free and overall survival in HNSCC treated with surgery with or without adjuvant radiation. More data are clearly needed with regard to the prognostic significance of cyclin D1 in patients treated with primary irradiation.

In addition to the relationship between cyclin D1 amplification and poor prognosis, a specific A/G polymorphism that modulates splicing of cyclin D1 mRNA may also influence prognosis (282). Matthias et al. examined 384 patients with HNSCC, stage I to IV, treated with surgery and other appropriate modalities (283). Cyclin D1 genotype did not influence susceptibility to HNSCC and did not correlate with T stage, N

TABLE 3.6 Studies Correlating Cyclin D1 Status and Outcome

Author	Description of patients	Treatment given	Marker	% positive	MVT	Local control	Survival	Notes
Meredith et al. 1995 (275)	56 stage I–IV HNSCC	Surgery and/or RT and/or CTX	11q13 amplification	39%	No	NR	CSS ($p = 0.001$) OS ($p = 0.002$)	
Bellacosa et al. 1996 (276)	51 stage I–IV laryngeal SCC	Surgery, 5 received postoperative RT	Cyclin D1 amplification	18%	Yes	NR	OS ($p = 0.04$)	
Akervall et al. 1997 (227)	75 stage I–IV HNSCC	Surgery and/or RT and/or CTX	11q13 cytogenetics	12%	Yes	NR	CSS ($p = 0.005$)	Correlation between cyclin D1 expression and survival observed only for tumors with strong staining
			IHC	41%		NR	CSS ($p = 0.05$)	
Fortin et al. 1997 (280)	50 SCC (38 OC, 12 OP), stage I–IV	Surgery and/or RT and/or CTX	11q13 amplification	20%	No	NR	No	
Kyomoto et al. 1997 (277)	45 HNSCC, T1–4, N0–2	Surgery alone	Cyclin D1 amplification	25%	Yes	NR	OS ($p = 0.002$)	IHC predicted OS in univariate but not MVT
			IHC	53%		NR	No	
Michalides et al. 1997 (272)	115 stage I–IV HNSCC	Primary surgery (72 received postoperative RT)	IHC	50%	Yes	No	DFS ($p = 0.05$)	Overexpression correlates with recurrence when all sites considered
Muller et al. 1997 (279)	280 stage I–IV HNSCC	201 surgery + postoperative RT	11q13 amplification	57%	Yes	NR	No	
		79 surgery alone		35%		NR	No	
Nogueira et al. 1998 (278)	56 stage I–IV HNSCC	"Curative intent"	Cyclin D1 amplification	33%	No	NR	No	Amplification correlates with recurrence when all sites considered ($p = 0.007$)
Pignataro et al. 1998 (273)	149 stage I–IV laryngeal SCC	Surgery (63 received postoperative RT)	IHC	32%	Yes	NR	DFS ($p = 0.02$) OS ($p = 0.06$)	Cyclin D1 expression associated with alcohol and tobacco consumption
Bova et al. 1999 (271)	148 stage I–IV oral tongue SCC	Surgery (53 received postoperative RT)	IHC	68%	Yes	NR	DFS ($p = 0.05$) OS ($p = 0.02$)	Cyclin D1 expression plus loss of *p16* expression associated with worst prognosis
Mineta et al. 2000 (261)	94 stage I–IV tongue SCC	Surgery (not otherwise specified)	IHC	19%	No	NR	OS ($p = 0.04$)	
Yoo et al. 2000 (281)	30 T1–2, N0 laryngeal SCC, non-recurrent	RT	IHC	67%	No	Yes ($p = 0.02$)	NR	Low cyclin D1 levels predicted local recurrence
	30 T1–2, N0 laryngeal SCC, recurrent			37%				

CSS, cause-specific survival; CTX, chemotherapy; DFS, disease-free survival; HNSCC, head and neck squamous cell carcinoma; IHC, immunohistochemistry; MVT, multivariate analysis; NR, not reported; OC, oral cavity; OP, oropharynx; OS, overall survival; RT, radiotherapy; SCC, squamous cell carcinoma.

stage, patient age, or sex. Homozygosity for the G allele, the GG genotype, was associated with poorly differentiated tumors. When controlling for the relationship between genotype and differentiation, the GG genotype correlated with poor disease-free survival in laryngeal and pharyngeal tumors. Future investigations along this avenue of research should be conducted to determine the relationship between this genotype and cyclin D1 function within malignant cells.

Epidermal Growth Factor Receptor and Transforming Growth Factor-α

The receptor tyrosine kinase epidermal growth factor receptor (EGFR) and its ligand transforming growth factor-α (TGF-α) are frequently overexpressed in HNSCC (284,285). Activation of EGFR induces autophosphorylation, resulting in activation of several signaling pathways including Ras-MAP kinase, phospholipase C, phosphatidylinositol 3-kinase, and signal transducers and activators of transcription (286,287). In HNSCC, autocrine activation of EGFR by TGF-α functions to promote cellular proliferation and inhibit apoptosis. For example, *in vitro* experiments conducted on HNSCC-derived cell lines demonstrated that inhibition of TGF-α with antisense oligonucleotides and inhibition of EGFR with antisense oligonucleotides, monoclonal antibodies, or specific inhibitors of EGFR kinase activity resulted in reduced cellular proliferation (288,289). Furthermore, *in vivo* transfection of a vector expressing EGFR antisense oligonucleotides resulted in growth inhibition and induction of apoptosis in nude mice tumor xenografts (290).

EGFR expression may also modulate tumor radioresistance. In murine tumors, Akimoto et al. found that the magnitude of EGFR expression positively correlated with increased radioresistance and inversely correlated with radiation-induced apoptosis (291). In addition, blockade of EGFR with the monoclonal antibody C225 enhances radiosensitivity of SCCs both *in vitro* and *in vivo.* In cell lines derived from patients with HNSCC, concomitant C225 administration and radiotherapy results in enhancement of radiosensitivity, in part because inhibition of EGFR results in down-regulation of anti-apoptotic proteins such as Stat3 and thus promotes radiation-induced apoptosis (292,293). Furthermore, *in vivo* experiments suggest that concomitant C225 infusion and radiotherapy inhibit DNA damage repair and tumor angiogenesis while promoting central tumor necrosis and granulocyte infiltration (294,295). Clearly, inhibition of EGFR activity holds promise as a novel mechanism for enhancing tumor radiosensitivity.

Elevation of EGFR protein expression in HNSCC occurs most frequently through activation of EGFR gene transcription (284, 285), although gene amplification may also occur (296, 297). The mechanism of EGFR transcriptional control remains largely unknown, although evidence suggests that wild-type *p53* may suppress EGFR transcription in HNSCC cell lines (298). Overexpression of EGFR in HNSCC has been assessed primarily via quantitative radioligand receptor assay (RRA) or via quantitative IHC using computerized image analysis. Of note, Grandis et al. found that computerized image analysis correlated strongly with EGFR and TGF-α mRNA levels, whereas scoring by individuals did not correlate with mRNA levels (285).

In agreement with laboratory data, clinical studies have established a relationship between EGFR expression and poor prognosis (Table 3.7) (299). Initial evidence for the prognostic use of EGFR levels derived from Dassonville et al., who found that EGFR expression independently predicted poor relapse-free survival in 109 stage I to IV HNSCC patients treated primarily with either chemotherapy or surgery (300). A follow-up study revealed that for patients treated with induction chemotherapy or concurrent chemoradiation, EGFR positivity failed to predict initial response to chemotherapy but was a significant predictor of poor cause-specific survival (218). Maurizi et al. used RRA to establish an independent relationship between EGFR expression and poor disease-free and overall survival in 140 stage I to IV laryngeal SCCs treated primarily with surgery (301). Subsequent multivariate analysis revealed that EGFR levels were an important determinant of regional recurrence, with a 5-year metastasis-free survival of 66% for EGFR-negative tumors and 15% for EGFR-positive tumors (302). Similarly, Grandis et al. used quantitative IHC to show that increasing levels of both TGF-α and EGFR predicted poor disease-free and cause-specific survival in a cohort of 91 stage I to IV HNSCCs (303) treated with surgery (56 received postoperative radiotherapy). Finally, Wen et al. report that TGF-α, but not EGFR, predicted recurrent disease in 68 early stage laryngeal SCCs treated with primary radiation (304). Thus, the cumulative weight of clinical studies supports a role for EGFR and TGF-α protein levels in determining poor prognosis for patients treated with surgery or chemotherapy. Clearly, further clinical studies are required to establish EGFR expression as a risk factor for patients treated with primary irradiation.

Molecular Determinants of Margin Status

Local recurrence remains a significant cause of treatment failure despite optimal surgical resection with negative final surgical margins. As a result, interest has developed in identifying molecular aberrations detectable in surgical margins that would allow for identification of histologically occult residual disease. Brennan et al. explored this hypothesis in a group of 25 primary HNSCCs resected with negative surgical margins (305). Only primary tumors with a characterized *p53* mutation were included in the series. DNA was extracted from the resected surgical margins followed by PCR amplification of exons 5 through 9 on the *p53* gene, cloning into a bacteriophage vector, and subsequent amplification in *Escherichia coli*. From 500 to 1,000 clones from each margin were probed with an oligonucleotide sequence specific for the *p53* mutation found in the original primary tumor. Using this technique, 13 of 25 patients

TABLE 3.7 Studies Correlating EGFR Expression and Outcome

Author	Description of patients	Treatment given	MVT	Marker	Method (% positive)	Local/regional recurrence	Survival	Notes
Dassonville et al. 1993 (300)	109 stage I–IV HNSCC	73 CTX, 29 surgery, 6 RT, 1 none	Yes	EGFR	RRA	NR	DFS ($p = 0.03$)	EGFR status correlated with OS in univariate but not MVT
Wen et al. 1996 (304)	68 stage I–II laryngeal SCC	RT alone	No	TGF-α EGFR	IHC: 56% IHC: 43%	Yes ($p < 0.01$) No	No No	Qualitative IHC only
Maurizi et al. 1996 (301)	140 stage I–IV laryngeal SCC	Surgery (postoperative RT not mentioned)	Yes	EGFR	RRA: 20%	NR	OS ($p = 0.0001$) DFS ($p = 0.01$)	
Almadori et al. 1999 (302)	140 stage I–IV laryngeal SCC	Surgery (postoperative RT not mentioned)	Yes	EGFR	RRA: 20%	Yes ($p = 0.001$)	NR	EGFR status independently predicts regional recurrence
Grandis et al. 1998 (303)	91 stage I–IV HNSCC	Surgery (56 received postoperative RT)	Yes	TGF-α EGFR	IHC	NR NR	CSS ($p = 0.0001$) CSS ($p = 0.0001$)	EGFR status divided into tertiles using computerized image analysis
Etienne et al. 1999 (218)	82 stage II–IV HNSCC	61 induction cisplatin/5-FU, 21 concurrent chemoRT	Yes	EGFR	RRA	NR	CSS ($p = 0.009$)	
Xia et al. 1999 (299)	47 stage I–IV oral SCC	Surgery	No	EGFR	IHC	NR	OS ($p < 0.0001$)	Qualitative IHC used to divide sample into three levels of EGFR expression

5-FU, 5-fluorouracil; CSS, cause-specific survival; CTX, chemotherapy; DFS, disease-free survival; EGFR, epidermal growth factor receptor; HNSCC, head and neck squamous cell carcinoma; IHC, immunohistochemistry; MVT, multivariate model; NR, not reported; OS, overall survival; RT, radiotherapy; RRA, radioligand receptor assay; SCC, squamous cell carcinoma; TGF-α, transforming growth factor-alpha.

were found to have *p53* mutations within histologically negative margins. Of these 13 patients, 5 developed local recurrence at the site of the positive margin whereas none of the patients with *p53*-negative margins developed local recurrence (p = 0.02). This technique clearly offers promise for identifying those patients at risk for local recurrence who may benefit from aggressive adjuvant therapy. However, widespread clinical application remains difficult to its technical demands, expense, and time-consuming nature.

Eukaryotic initiation factor 4E (eIF4E), an mRNA cap-binding protein that up-regulates translation, offers several advantages over *p53* in the assessment of molecular margin status (240,241). First, eIF4E is overexpressed in 100% of HNSCCs (306). In contrast, *p53* mutations are present in roughly 45% of primary tumors and thus *p53* margin status is only assessable in these cases. Furthermore, eIF4E expression in surgical margins is readily assessable via IHC, which is less technically difficult and more commonly available than the method employed by Brennan et al. (305). In a study of 54 patients with stage I to IV laryngeal SCC treated with surgery (16 received postoperative radiotherapy), eIF4E-positive margins were noted in 59% (32/54) of the cases (306). Of these, 67% (21/32) had recurrent disease (9 local, 9 regional, and 3 distant). In contrast, of the 22 patients with eIF4E-negative margins, 18% (4/22) experienced a recurrence (2 local, 1 regional, 1 distant) (p = 0.0007 by log-rank test). This study also used IHC to assess *p53* expression in surgical margins. *p53*-positive margins were noted in only 6 cases and appeared to be a less sensitive predictor of recurrence than eIF4E status. One additional study conducted on 65 patients with stage I to IV HNSCC treated with surgery (40 received postoperative radiotherapy) showed in multivariate analysis that eIF4E-positive margins resulted in a sevenfold increased risk for locoregional failure (307). Thus, eIF4E expression as assessed via IHC is a strong predictor of risk for recurrence and may prove useful in clinical decision making.

Loss of Heterozygosity at Other DNA Loci

A common pathway toward malignancy is the loss of function of both alleles of a tumor suppressor gene. This often occurs through an inactivating mutation of one allele followed by loss of heterozygosity (LOH), the genetic deletion of the remaining functional allele. Hence, regions of the genome consistently deleted in a given tumor type suggest the presence of a tumor suppressor gene at that locus. Loss of heterozygosity is assayed by comparing the PCR product of a polymorphic microsatellite marker amplified from normal tissue with the same marker amplified from neoplastic tissue. The presence of two distinct marker alleles in the normal tissue and only one marker allele in the neoplastic tissue represents a positive test for LOH. Common regions of LOH in HNSCC are given in Table 3.8 (123,209,274,308–322).

Loss of heterozygosity at multiple alleles may correlate with prognosis in HNSCC. Partridge et al. found that LOH at either *3p24-26, 3p13, 9p21,* or *18q21.1* was associated with poor survival in a cohort of 48 HNSCCs (312). Furthermore, the fraction of alleles displaying LOH was a significant independent predictor of poor locoregional control and survival. Similarly, Li et al. assessed for LOH at *3p21, 3p25-26, 8pter-21.1, 13q14,* and *17p12* in a group of 27 HNSCCs treated with surgery (309). In this group, LOH at two or more loci was correlated with death with disease (4 out of 13 patients with LOH at two or more loci dead with disease vs. 0 out of 14 patients with LOH at less than two loci). These studies demonstrate that LOH at multiple loci is likely a marker of aggressive disease and poor prognosis in HNSCC.

Additional studies have assessed individual genetic loci as potential predictors of outcome. Partridge et al. examined LOH at chromosome 3p in a group of 48 oral SCC treated surgically (313). Loss of heterozygosity at 3p in early stage oral SCC significantly correlated with reduced disease-free and overall survival (mean survival 42 months in LOH-positive tumors vs. 102 months in LOH-negative tumors). Scholnick et al. reported LOH at 8p21-23 in a cohort of 59 supraglottic laryngeal SCCs treated with surgical excision (311). Allelic loss at 8p23 was found to be a statistically significant, independent predictor of tumor recurrence and death caused by the primary tumor. Finally, Lazar et al. report that LOH at 11q23 was associated with risk for recurrent disease in 52 stage II to IV HNSCCs (274). This evidence suggests that assessment for LOH at certain loci may prove valuable in establishing prognosis for patients with HNSCC.

TABLE 3.8 Common Regions of LOH in HNSCC

Chromosomal region	Reference	Date
3p, 5q, 9q, 11q, 17p	Ah-see et al. (308)	1994
3p, 8p, 13q, 17p	Li et al. (309)	1994
3p, 8p, 9p, 9q, 11q	el-Naggar et al. (310)	1995
3p, 13q, 17p	Bockmuhl et al. (317)	1996
3p, 9p	Ishwad et al. (123)	1996
13q	Maestro et al. (314)	1996
3p24–26, 3p21.3–22.1, 3p12.1–14.2	Partridge et al. (313)	1996
3p25.1	Rowley et al. (315)	1996
8p23	Scholnick et al. (311)	1996
11q23, 11q25	Uzawa et al. (316)	1996
7q, 10q, 11p, 11q, 15q, 20p	Bockmuhl et al. (319)	1997
18q11.1–q12.3 and 18q21.1–q23	Jones et al. (318)	1997
11q23	Lazar et al. (274)	1998
7q21.3-qter	Wang et al. (320)	1998
16q24 and the p53 and pRB loci	Gleich et al. (208,209)	1996, 1999
13q34, 13q14.3, 13q12.1	Gupta et al. (321)	1999
22q11.2–q12.3	Poli-Frederico et al. (322)	2000

HNSCC, head and neck squamous cell carcinoma; LOH, loss of heterozygosity.

DNA Ploidy

DNA aneuploidy, the presence of an abnormal amount of nuclear DNA, is associated with poor prognosis in most human solid tumors. The amount of cellular DNA can be quantitated using flow cytometry, a technique for measuring nuclear DNA content in solution, or image analysis, a method of quantitating nuclear DNA in tissue sections. A meta-analysis published in 1991 reviewed 26 studies on ploidy in HNSCC (323). In a total of 1,984 tumors, 37% were diploid, 54% were aneuploid, and 10% were polydiploid. Meta-analysis of survival in the 10 relevant studies showed a strong increase in deaths in nondiploid tumors. Analysis by site revealed a significant increase in mortality in nondiploid oral cavity tumors (5 studies) but no significant difference in mortality with respect to ploidy in laryngeal tumors (5 studies). Ploidy failed to predict recurrence (2 studies) and response to radiation (2 studies).

Studies conducted subsequent to this meta-analysis are presented in Table 3.9. In general, these studies support the conclusion that nondiploid tumors are associated with poor prognosis. The presence of aneuploidy in oral cavity, oropharyngeal, and hypopharyngeal SCCs has been shown to correlate with risk for concomitant nodal metastasis (324,325). Furthermore, a prospective study conducted on 429 stage I to IV oral cavity SCCs treated with surgery found that aneuploidy independently predicted increased risk for locoregional failure and poor disease-free survival (325). When restricted to 116 patients with T1 to T4 N0 oral cavity SCCs treated with excision of the primary tumor only, aneuploidy independently predicted risk for

TABLE 3.9 Studies Correlating Ploidy and Outcome

Author	Description of patients	Treatment given	MVT	Local/regional recurrence	Survival	Notes
Heterogeneous series:						
Tytor et al. 1990 (329)	176 stage I-IV oral SCC	Surgery and/or RT	Yes	NR	OS ($p < 0.01$)	Aneuploid tumors responded better to preoperative RT, nondiploidy predicted worse OS in multivariate analysis
Kearsley et al. 1991 (330)	172 stage I-IV HNSCC	Not specified	Yes	NR	DFS ($p < 0.0001$) OS ($p < 0.001$)	Aneuploidy predicted poor recurrence-free and OS in multivariate analysis
Rua et al. 1991 (332)	53 T1-3 N0 laryngeal SCC	Surgery and/or RT and/or CTX	No	NR	Trend for OS ($p = 0.10$)	
Zatterstrom et al. 1991 (328)	72 stage I-IV HNSCC	Surgery and/or RT and/or chemotherapy	Yes	NR	No	Nondiploidy correlated with poor OS in univariate but not multivariate analysis
Welkoborsky et al. 1995 (331)	40 stage I-IV glottic SCC	Surgery (5 received postoperative RT)	Yes	Yes ($p = 0.006$)	OS ($p = 0.0003$)	Nondiploidy predicted local/ regional recurrence and OS in multivariate analysis
Syms et al. 1995 (333)	94 T1-4 pN+ oral cavity and oropharynx SCC	Surgery (90 received postoperative RT)	No	NR	No	
Hemmer et al. 1998 (326)	116 T1-4 clinically N0 oral SCC	Surgery without neck dissection	Yes	Yes ($p < 0.05$)	OS ($p < 0.05$)	Aneuploidy independent predictor of regional metastatis and poor OS
Danic et al. 1999 (327)	36 laryngeal SCC (stage not specified)	Surgery	Yes	NR	No	Aneuploidy associated with poor OS in univariate analysis but not after controlling for proliferative activity
Sampedro et al. 1999 (334)	91 stage I-IV larynx and pharynx SCC	Surgery (48 received postoperative RT)	No	No	No	
Hemmer et al. 1999 (325)	429 stage I-IV oral SCC	Surgery (adjuvant therapies not mentioned)	Yes	Yes ($p < 0.01$)	DFS ($p < 0.001$)	Aneuploidy independent predictor of local-regional failure and poor relapse-free survival
Radiotherapy series:						
Walter et al. 1991 (336)	29 T1 N0 M0 glottic SCC	RT	No	Yes ($p = 0.02$)	NR	*Aneuploidy* predictor of local recurrence in case-control study
Westerbeek et al. 1993 (335)	44 T1 glottic SCC	RT	Yes	Yes ($p = 0.02$)	NR	*Aneuploidy* independent predictor of local failure
Fu et al. 1994 (340)	143 stage III–IV HNSCC	RT (RTOG protocols 79–13, 79–15, 83–13)	Yes	No	No	*Aneuploidy* predicted poor local-regional control and OS in univariate analysis but lost significance after controlling for stage, site, and p105
Toffoli et al. 1995 (337)	72 T1–2 N0 laryngeal SCC	RT	Yes	Yes ($p < 0.01$)	NR	*Diploidy* independent predictor of local failure
Zackrisson et al. 1997 (339)	89 stage I–IV HNSCC	Primary RT (33 patients received post-RT surgery)	Yes	No	No	*Aneuploidy* predicted poor local control in univariate analysis but lost significance after controlling for N stage and Tpot
Yip et al. 1998 (338)	51 stage I–IV nasopharyngeal cancers	RT	No	Yes (p not given)	OS ($p < 0.01$)	*Aneuploidy* correlated with local-regional recurrence, distant metastasis, and poor OS
Begg et al. 1999 (206)	476 stage I–IV HNSCC	RT	Yes	No	No	Pooled data from 11 centers in Europe

HNSCC, head and neck squamous cell carcinoma; MVT, multivariate analysis; NR, not reported; OS, overall survival; RT, radiotherapy; RTOG, Radiation Therapy Oncology Group; SCC, squamous cell carcinoma.

developing regional recurrence following initial therapy (326). Most other studies conducted on cohorts treated with various combinations of surgery, radiotherapy, and chemotherapy have confirmed an association between aneuploidy and poor survival in univariate (327,328) or multivariate analysis (329–331). Despite three studies that found no correlation between ploidy and outcome (332–334), most of the literature including large prospective studies and a meta-analysis concurs that aneuploid tumors are more likely to recur and result in death following standard treatment.

Several studies have also specifically examined the relationship between ploidy and radioresistance in cohorts treated with primary irradiation. In the largest study, pooled data from 11 centers in Europe found that aneuploidy did not correlate with locoregional control in 476 stage I to IV HNSCC patients treated with primary radiotherapy (206). However, when limited to early stage glottic SCC treated with primary radiation, two studies have found aneuploidy to predict local failure (335,336) whereas one study found diploidy to predict local failure (337). In a cohort of patients with nasopharyngeal cancer, aneuploidy correlated with locoregional recurrence in 51 patients treated with primary irradiation (338). Two additional studies conducted on more heterogeneous cohorts reported a correlation between aneuploidy and poor locoregional control in univariate analysis (339,340). However, after controlling for relevant clinicopathologic covariables, aneuploidy failed to predict response to radiation in these cohorts. Thus, the literature remains controversial regarding aneuploidy and radioresistance; ploidy currently does not influence selection of patients for primary radiotherapy.

Cellular Proliferation and Kinetics Markers

The kinetics of tumor growth have been hypothesized to modulate clinical outcomes in patients treated with protracted radiotherapy. Fast-growing tumors are more likely than slow-growing tumors to repopulate an irradiated tumor bed during the course of conventional radiotherapy and thus result in local failure (341). However, accelerated fractionation shortens the total treatment time and thus may serve to decrease the risk for local recurrence. Indeed, numerous clinical studies have now demonstrated that local control worsens as overall treatment time is increased, whereas accelerated fractionation schedules result in improved local control (342). Theoretically, if fast-growing tumors could be identified prior to the start of radiotherapy, an appropriate fractionation schedule could be selected to maximize local control. The rate of tumor growth can be estimated through *in vivo* labeling of tumor tissue with bromo- or iodo-deoxyuridine (BrdUrd and IdUrd, respectively) several hours before biopsy. Using either flow cytometry or IHC, the amount of incorporated BrdUrd or IdUrd is measured. This measurement allows for calculation of the labeling index (LI, the fraction of cells in S-phase), the time spent in S-phase (Ts), and the potential doubling time of the tumor population (Tpot) (206,343).

The most comprehensive study of cell kinetics parameters included prospective data from 11 European centers that treated a total of 476 stage I to IV HNSCC patients with primary, conventionally fractionated radiotherapy (206). Treatment was given in an overall time of at least 6 weeks to a minimum dose of 60 Gy and median follow-up was 30 months for surviving patients. Fifty-one percent of patients had local recurrence and 53% died. In univariate analysis, the only kinetics parameter associated with local control was LI ($p = 0.03$), with tumors that had a low LI (<5%) doing significantly better than tumors with a high LI (>15%). However, in multivariate analysis, no kinetics parameters predicted locoregional control. Similarly, a short Ts was associated with improved overall survival in univariate analysis ($p = 0.01$), but this association disappeared in multivariate analysis. This study therefore suggested that cell kinetics parameters as assessed via flow cytometry are not independent predictors of local failure in patients with HNSCC treated with primary radiotherapy. As a result, novel approaches to the determination of tumor cell proliferation during the course of treatment may be needed to accurately predict the likelihood of local control and select appropriate fractionation schedules.

REFERENCES

1. de Bree R, Deurloo EE, Snow GB, et al. Screening for distant metastases in patients with head and neck cancer. *Laryngoscope* 2000;110:397–401.
2. Magnano M, De Stefani A, Lerda W, et al. Prognostic factors of cervical lymph node metastasis in head and neck squamous cell carcinoma. *Tumori* 1997;83:922–926.
3. Magnano M, Bongioannini G, Lerda W, et al. Lymph node metastasis in head and neck squamous cells carcinoma: multivariate analysis of prognostic variables. *J Exp Clin Cancer Res* 1999;18:79–83.
4. de Visscher JG, van den Elsaker K, Grond AJ, et al. Surgical treatment of squamous cell carcinoma of the lower lip: evaluation of long-term results and prognostic factors—a retrospective analysis of 184 patients. *J Oral Maxillofac Surg* 1998;56:814–820.
5. Close LG, Brown PM, Vuitch MF, et al. Microvascular invasion and survival in cancer of the oral cavity and oropharynx. *Arch Otolaryngol Head Neck Surg* 1989;115:1304–1309.
6. Foote RL, Buskirk SJ, Stanley RJ, et al. Patterns of failure after total laryngectomy for glottic carcinoma. *Cancer* 1989;64:143–149.
7. Moore C, Flynn MB, Greenberg RA. Evaluation of size in prognosis of oral cancer. *Cancer* 1986;58:158–162.
8. Pera E, Moreno A, Galindo L. Prognostic factors in laryngeal carcinoma. A multifactorial study of 416 cases. *Cancer* 1986;58:928–934.
9. Del Valle-Zapico A, Fernandez FF, Suarez AR, et al. Prognostic value of histopathologic parameters and DNA flow cytometry in squamous cell carcinoma of the pyriform sinus. *Laryngoscope* 1998;108:269–272.
10. Bundgaard T, Bentzen SM, Wildt J, et al. Histopathologic, serologic, epidemiologic, and clinical parameters in the prognostic evaluation of squamous cell carcinoma of the oral cavity. *Head Neck* 1996;18:142–152.
11. Moe K, Wolf GT, Fisher SG, et al. Regional metastases in patients with advanced laryngeal cancer. Department of Veterans Affairs Laryngeal Cancer Study Group. *Arch Otolaryngol Head Neck Surg* 1996;122:644–648.
12. Moore C, Kuhns JG, Greenberg RA. Thickness as prognostic aid in upper aerodigestive tract cancer. *Arch Surg* 1986;121:1410–1414.
13. Yuen AP, Lam KY, Wei WI, et al. A comparison of the prognostic significance of tumor diameter, length, width, thickness, area, volume, and clinicopathological features of oral tongue carcinoma. *Am J Surg* 2000;180:139–143.
14. Woolgar JA. Carcinoma of the tongue: pathological considerations in management of the neck. *J R Soc Med* 1996;89:611–615.
15. Frierson HF, Cooper PH. Prognostic factors in squamous cell carcinoma of the lower lip. *Hum Pathol* 1986;17:346–354.
16. Giacomarra V, Tirelli G, Papanikolla L, et al. Predictive factors of nodal metastases in oral cavity and oropharynx carcinomas. *Laryngoscope* 1999;109:795–799.
17. Woolgar JA. T2 carcinoma of the tongue: the histopathologist's perspective. *Br J Oral Maxillofac Surg* 1999;37:187–193.
18. Martinez-Gimeno C, Rodriguez EM, Vila CN, et al. Squamous cell carcinoma of the oral cavity: a clinicopathologic scoring system for evaluating risk of cervical lymph node metastasis. *Laryngoscope* 1995;105:728–733.
19. Woolgar JA, Scott J. Prediction of cervical lymph node metastasis in squamous cell carcinoma of the tongue/floor of mouth. *Head Neck* 1995;17:463–472.
20. Fukano H, Matsuura H, Hasegawa Y, et al. Depth of invasion as a predictive factor for cervical lymph node metastasis in tongue carcinoma. *Head Neck* 1997;19:205–210.
21. Asakage T, Yokose T, Mukai K, et al. Tumor thickness predicts cervical metastasis in patients with stage I/II carcinoma of the tongue. *Cancer* 1998;82:1443–1448.
22. Unal OF, Ayhan A, Hosal AS. Prognostic value of p53 expression and histopathological parameters in squamous cell carcinoma of oral tongue. *J Laryngol Otol* 1999;113:446–450.
23. Mohit-Tabatabai MA, Sobel HJ, Rush BF, et al. Relation of thickness of floor of mouth stage I and II cancers to regional metastasis. *Am J Surg* 1986;152:351–353.
24. Hosal AS, Unal OF, Ayhan A. Possible prognostic value of histopathologic parameters in patients with carcinoma of the oral tongue. *Eur Arch Otorhinolaryngol* 1998;255:216–219.
25. Maddox WA, Urist MM. Histopathological prognostic factors of certain primary oral cavity cancers. *Oncology (Huntingt)* 1990;4:39–42.
26. Spiro RH, Huvos AG, Wong GY, et al. Predictive value of tumor thickness in squamous carcinoma confined to the tongue and floor of the mouth. *Am J Surg* 1986;152:345–350.
27. Jones KR, Lodge-Rigal RD, Reddick RL, et al. Prognostic factors in the recurrence of stage I and II squamous cell cancer of the oral cavity. *Arch Otolaryngol Head Neck Surg* 1992;118:483–485.
28. Mancuso AA, Mukherji SK, Schmalfuss I, et al. Preradiotherapy computed tomography as a predictor of local control in supraglottic carcinoma. *J Clin Oncol* 1999;17:631–637.
29. Hermans R, Van den Bogaert W, Rijnders A, et al. Value of computed tomography as outcome predictor of supraglottic squamous cell carcinoma treated by definitive radiation therapy. *Int J Radiat Oncol Biol Phys* 1999;44:755–765.
30. Scholl P, Byers RM, Batsakis JG, et al. Microscopic cut-through of cancer in the surgical treatment of squamous carcinoma of the tongue. Prognostic and therapeutic implications. *Am J Surg* 1986;152:354–360.
31. Looser KG, Shah JP, Strong EW. The significance of "positive" margins in surgically resected epidermoid carcinomas. *Head Neck Surg* 1978;1:107–111.
32. Parsons JT, Mendenhall WM, Stringer SP, et al. An analysis of factors influencing the outcome of postoperative irradiation for squamous cell carcinoma of the oral cavity. *Int J Radiat Oncol Biol Phys* 1997;39:137–148.
33. Jones AS. Prognosis in mouth cancer: tumour factors. *Eur J Cancer B Oral Oncol* 1994;30B:8–15.
34. Fang FM, Leung SW, Huang CC, et al. Combined-modality therapy for squamous carcinoma of the buccal mucosa: treatment results and prognostic factors. *Head Neck* 1997;19:506–512.
35. Eisma RJ, Spiro JD, Kreutzer DL. Role of angiogenic factors: coexpression of interleukin-8 and vascular endothelial growth factor in patients with head and neck squamous carcinoma. *Laryngoscope* 1999;109:687–693.
36. Lam KY, Ng IO, Yuen AP, et al. Cyclin D1 expression in oral squamous cell carcinomas: clinicopathological relevance and correlation with p53 expression. *J Oral Pathol Med* 2000;29:167–172.
37. Kirita T, Okabe S, Izumo T, et al. Risk factors for the postoperative local recurrence of tongue carcinoma. *J Oral Maxillofac Surg* 1994;52:149–154.
38. El-Husseiny G, Kandil A, Jamshed A, et al. Squamous cell carcinoma of the oral tongue: an analysis of prognostic factors. *Br J Oral Maxillofac Surg* 2000;38:193–199.
39. Machtay M, Perch S, Markiewicz D, et al. Combined surgery and postoperative radiotherapy for carcinoma of the base of radiotherapy for carcinoma of the base of tongue: analysis of treatment outcome and prognostic value of margin status. *Head Neck* 1997;19:494–499.
40. Shah JP, Cendon RA, Farr HW, et al. Carcinoma of the oral cavity. Factors affecting treatment failure at the primary site and neck. *Am J Surg* 1976;132:504–507.
41. Naude J, Dobrowsky W. Postoperative irradiation of laryngeal carcinoma—the prognostic value of tumour-free surgical margins. *Acta Oncol* 1997;36:273–277.

42. Kowalski LP, Franco EL, de Andrade Sobrinho J, et al. Prognostic factors in laryngeal cancer patients submitted to surgical treatment. *J Surg Oncol* 1991; 48:87–95.
43. Amdur RJ, Parsons JT, Mendenhall WM, et al. Postoperative irradiation for squamous cell carcinoma of the head and neck: an analysis of treatment results and complications. *Int J Radiat Oncol Biol Phys* 1989;16:25–36.
44. Zieske LA, Johnson JT, Myers EN, et al. Squamous cell carcinoma with positive margins. Surgery and postoperative irradiation. *Arch Otolaryngol Head Neck Surg* 1986;112:863–866.
45. Wang ZH, Million RR, Mendenhall WM, et al. Treatment with preoperative irradiation and surgery of squamous cell carcinoma of the head and neck. *Cancer* 1989;64:32–38.
46. Vikram B, Strong EW, Shah JP, et al. Failure at distant sites following multimodality treatment for advanced head and neck cancer. *Head Neck Surg* 1984; 6:730–733.
47. Chen TY, Emrich LJ, Driscoll DL. The clinical significance of pathological findings in surgically resected margins of the primary tumor in head and neck carcinoma. *Int J Radiat Oncol Biol Phys* 1987;13:833–837.
48. Myers JN, Elkins T, Roberts D, et al. Squamous cell carcinoma of the tongue in young adults: increasing incidence and factors that predict treatment outcomes. *Otolaryngol Head Neck Surg* 2000;122:44–51.
49. Nicolai P, Redaelli de Zinis LO, Tomenzoli D, et al. Prognostic determinants in supraglottic carcinoma: univariate and Cox regression analysis. *Head Neck* 1997;19:323–334.
50. Bradford CR, Wolf GT, Fisher SG, et al. Prognostic importance of surgical margins in advanced laryngeal squamous carcinoma. *Head Neck* 1996;18:11–16.
51. Byers RM, Bland KI, Borlase B, et al. The prognostic and therapeutic value of frozen section determinations in the surgical treatment of squamous carcinoma of the head and neck. *Am J Surg* 1978;136:525–528.
52. Barra S, Barzan L, Maione A, et al. Blood transfusion and other prognostic variables in the survival of patients with cancer of the head and neck. *Laryngoscope* 1994;104:95–98.
53. Huang D, Johnson CR, Schmidt-Ullrich RK, et al. Incompletely resected advanced squamous cell carcinoma of the head and neck: the effectiveness of adjuvant vs. salvage radiotherapy. *Radiother Oncol* 1992;24:87–93.
54. Ord RA, Aisner S. Accuracy of frozen sections in assessing margins in oral cancer resection. *J Oral Maxillofac Surg* 1997;55:663–669;discussion 669–671.
55. Jacobs JR, Ahmad K, Casiano R, et al. Implications of positive surgical margins. *Laryngoscope* 1993;103:64–68.
56. Zelefsky MJ, Harrison LB, Fass DE, et al. Postoperative radiation therapy for squamous cell carcinomas of the oral cavity and oropharynx: impact of therapy on patients with positive surgical margins [Erratum appears in *Int J Radiat Oncol Biol Phys* 1993;25:935]. *Int J Radiat Oncol Biol Phys* 1993;25:17–21.
57. Vikram B, Mishra S. Permanent iodine-125 implants in postoperative radiotherapy for head and neck cancer with positive surgical margins. *Head Neck* 1994;16:155–157.
58. Pernot M, Aletti P, Carolus JM, et al. Indications, techniques and results of postoperative brachytherapy in cancer of the oral cavity. *Radiother Oncol* 1995;35:186–192.
59. Chao KS, Emami B, Akhileswaran R, et al. The impact of surgical margin status and use of an interstitial implant on T1, T2 oral tongue cancers after surgery [See comments]. *Int J Radiat Oncol Biol Phys* 1996;36:1039–1043.
60. Beitler JJ, Smith RV, Silver CE, et al. Close or positive margins after surgical resection for the head and neck cancer patient: the addition of brachytherapy improves local control. *Int J Radiat Oncol Biol Phys* 1998;40:313–317.
61. Broders AC. Squamous-cell epithelioma of the lip. *JAMA* 1920;74:656–664.
62. Morales-Angulo C, Val-Bernal F, Buelta L, et al. Prognostic factors in supraglottic laryngeal carcinoma. *Otolaryngol Head Neck Surg* 1998;119:548–553.
63. Noguchi M, Kido Y, Kubota H, et al. Prognostic factors and relative risk for survival in N1-3 oral squamous cell carcinoma: a multivariate analysis using Cox's hazard model. *Br J Oral Maxillofac Surg* 1999;37:433–437.
64. Olsen KD, Caruso M, Foote RL, et al. Primary head and neck cancer. Histopathologic predictors of recurrence after neck dissection in patients with lymph node involvement. *Arch Otolaryngol Head Neck Surg* 1994;120: 1370–1374.
65. Cooke LD, Cooke TG, Forster G, et al. Prospective evaluation of cell kinetics in head and neck squamous carcinoma: the relationship to tumour factors and survival. *Br J Cancer* 1994;69:717–720.
66. Hirabayashi H, Koshii K, Uno K, et al. Extracapsular spread of squamous cell carcinoma in neck lymph nodes: prognostic factor of laryngeal cancer. *Laryngoscope* 1991;101:502–506.
67. Deleyiannis FW, Thomas DB, Vaughan TL, et al. Alcoholism: independent predictor of survival in patients with head and neck cancer. *J Natl Cancer Inst* 1996;88:542–549.
68. Beenken SW, Krontiras H, Maddox WA, et al. T1 and T2 squamous cell carcinoma of the oral tongue: prognostic factors and the role of elective lymph node dissection. *Head Neck* 1999;21:124–130.
69. Roland NJ, Caslin AW, Nash J, et al. Value of grading squamous cell carcinoma of the head and neck. *Head Neck* 1992;14:224–229.
70. Bourhis J, Dendale R, Hill C, et al. Potential doubling time and clinical outcome in head and neck squamous cell carcinoma treated with 70 Gy in 7 weeks. *Int J Radiat Oncol Biol Phys* 1996;35:471–476.
71. Janot F, Klijanienko J, Russo A, et al. Prognostic value of clinicopathological parameters in head and neck squamous cell carcinoma: a prospective analysis. *Br J Cancer* 1996;73:531–538.
72. Shingaki S, Suzuki I, Kobayashi T, et al. Predicting factors for distant metastases in head and neck carcinomas: an analysis of 103 patients with locoregional control. *J Oral Maxillofac Surg* 1996;54:853–857.
73. Hoffman HT, Karnell LH, Funk GF, et al. The National Cancer Data Base report on cancer of the head and neck. *Arch Otolaryngol Head Neck Surg* 1998; 124:951–962.
74. Jakobsson PA, Eneroth CM, Killander D, et al. Histologic classification and grading of malignancy in carcinoma of the larynx. *Acta Radiol Ther Phys Biol* 1973;12:1–8.
75. Crissman JD, Liu WY, Gluckman JL, et al. Prognostic value of histopathologic parameters in squamous cell carcinoma of the oropharynx. *Cancer* 1984; 54:2995–3001.
76. Anneroth G, Batsakis J, Luna M. Review of the literature and a recommended system of malignancy grading in oral squamous cell carcinomas. *Scand J Dent Res* 1987;95:229–249.
77. Bryne M, Koppang HS, Lilleng R, et al. New malignancy grading is a better prognostic indicator than Broders' grading in oral squamous cell carcinomas. *J Oral Pathol Med* 1989;18:432–437.
78. Bryne M, Koppang HS, Lilleng R, et al. Malignancy grading of the deep invasive margins of oral squamous cell carcinomas has high prognostic value. *J Pathol* 1992;166:375–381.
79. Bryne M. Prognostic value of various molecular and cellular features in oral squamous cell carcinomas: a review. *J Oral Pathol Med* 1991;20:413–420.
80. Spiro RH, Guillamondegui O, Paulino AF, et al. Pattern of invasion and margin assessment in patients with oral tongue cancer. *Head Neck* 1999;21: 408–413.
81. Wong RJ, Keel SB, Glynn RJ, et al. Histological pattern of mandibular invasion by oral squamous cell carcinoma. *Laryngoscope* 2000;110:65–72.
82. Yamamoto E, Kohama G, Sunakawa H, et al. Mode of invasion, bleomycin sensitivity, and clinical course in squamous cell carcinoma of the oral cavity. *Cancer* 1983;51:2175–2180.
83. Odell EW, Jani P, Sherriff M, et al. The prognostic value of individual histologic grading parameters in small lingual squamous cell carcinomas. The importance of the pattern of invasion. *Cancer* 1994;74:789–794.
84. Pameijer FA, Hermans R, Mancuso AA, et al. Pre- and post-radiotherapy computed tomography in laryngeal cancer: imaging-based prediction of local failure. *Int J Radiat Oncol Biol Phys* 1999;45:359–366.
85. Fagan JJ, Collins B, Barnes L, et al. Perineural invasion in squamous cell carcinoma of the head and neck. *Arch Otolaryngol Head Neck Surg* 1998;124: 637–640.
86. Ballantyne AJ, McCarten AB, Ibanez ML. The extension of cancer of the head and neck through peripheral nerves. *Am J Surg* 1963;106:651–667.
87. Carter RL, Pittam MR, Tanner NS. Pain and dysphagia in patients with squamous carcinomas of the head and neck: the role of perineural spread. *J R Soc Med* 1982;75:598–606.
88. Boerman RH, Maassen EM, Joosten J, et al. Trigeminal neuropathy secondary to perineural invasion of head and neck carcinomas. *Neurology* 1999;53: 213–216.
89. Curtin HD, Williams R, Johnson J. CT of perineural tumor extension: pterygopalatine fossa. *AJR Am J Roentgenol* 1985;144:163–169.
90. Mukherji SK, Weeks SM, Castillo M, et al. Squamous cell carcinomas that arise in the oral cavity and tongue base: can CT help predict perineural or vascular invasion? *Radiology* 1996;198:157–162.
91. McLaughlin RB, Montone KT, Wall SJ, et al. Nerve cell adhesion molecule expression in squamous cell carcinoma of the head and neck: a predictor of propensity toward perineural spread. *Laryngoscope* 1999;109:821–826.
92. Vural E, Hutcheson J, Korourian S, et al. Correlation of neural cell adhesion molecules with perineural spread of squamous cell carcinoma of the head and neck. *Otolaryngol Head Neck Surg* 2000;122:717–720.
93. McGavran MH, Bauer WC, Ogura JH. The incidence of cervical lymph node metastases from epidermoid carcinoma of the larynx and their relationship to certain characteristics of the primary tumor. *Cancer* 1961;14:55–66.
94. Yilmaz T, Hosal AS, Gedikoglu G, et al. Prognostic significance of vascular and perineural invasion in cancer of the larynx. *Am J Otolaryngol* 1998;19: 83–88.
95. Lydiatt DD, Robbins KT, Byers RM, et al. Treatment of stage I and II oral tongue cancer. *Head Neck*1993;15:308–312.
96. Soo KC, Carter RL, O'Brien CJ, et al. Prognostic implications of perineural spread in squamous carcinomas of the head and neck. *Laryngoscope* 1986;96: 1145–1148.
97. Mendenhall WM, Parsons JT, Mancuso AA, et al. Definitive radiotherapy for T3 squamous cell carcinoma of the glottic larynx. *J Clin Oncol* 1997;15: 2394–2402.
98. Alvi A, Johnson JT. Development of distant metastasis after treatment of advanced-stage head and neck cancer. *Head Neck* 1997;19:500–505.
99. Carter RL, Foster CS, Dinsdale EA, et al. Perineural spread by squamous carcinomas of the head and neck: a morphological study using antiaxonal and antimyelin monoclonal antibodies. *J Clin Pathol* 1983;36:269–275.
100. Rubio Bueno P, Naval Gias L, Garcia Delgado R, et al. Tumor DNA content as a prognostic indicator in squamous cell carcinoma of the oral cavity and tongue base. *Head Neck* 1998;20:232–239.
101. Close LG, Burns DK, Reisch J, et al. Microvascular invasion in cancer of the oral cavity and oropharynx. *Arch Otolaryngol Head Neck Surg* 1987;113: 1191–1195.
102. Resnick JM, Uhlman D, Niehans GA, et al. Cervical lymph node status and survival in laryngeal carcinoma: prognostic factors. *Ann Otol Rhinol Laryngol* 1995;104:685–694.
103. Mamelle G, Pampurik J, Luboinski B, et al. Lymph node prognostic factors in head and neck squamous cell carcinomas. *Am J Surg* 1994;168:494–498.
104. Mantravadi RV, Skolnik EM, Haas RE, et al. Patterns of cancer recurrence in the postoperatively irradiated neck. *Arch Otolaryngol* 1983;109:753–756.

105. Lefebvre JL, Castelain B, De la Torre JC, et al. Lymph node invasion in hypopharynx and lateral epilarynx carcinoma: a prognostic factor. *Head Neck Surg* 1987;10:14–18.
106. Snow GB, Annyas AA, van Slooten EA, et al. Prognostic factors of neck node metastasis. *Clin Otolaryngol* 1982;7:185–192.
107. Carter RL, Bliss JM, Soo KC, et al. Radical neck dissections for squamous carcinomas: pathological findings and their clinical implications with particular reference to transcapsular spread. *Int J Radiat Oncol Biol Phys* 1987;13: 825–832.
108. Grandi C, Alloisio M, Moglia D, et al. Prognostic significance of lymphatic spread in head and neck carcinomas: therapeutic implications. *Head Neck Surg* 1985;8:67–73.
109. Leemans CR, Tiwari R, Nauta JJ, et al. Regional lymph node involvement and its significance in the development of distant metastases in head and neck carcinoma. *Cancer* 1993;71:452–456.
110. Hart AK, Karakla DW, Pitman KT, et al. Oral and oropharyngeal squamous cell carcinoma in young adults: a report on 13 cases and review of the literature. *Otolaryngol Head Neck Surg* 1999;120:828–833.
111. Cerezo L, Millan I, Torre A, et al. Prognostic factors for survival and tumor control in cervical lymph node metastases from head and neck cancer. A multivariate study of 492 cases. *Cancer* 1992;69:1224–1234.
112. Pitman KT, Johnson JT. Skin metastases from head and neck squamous cell carcinoma: incidence and impact. *Head Neck* 1999;21:560–565.
113. O'Brien CJ, Smith JW, Soong SJ, et al. Neck dissection with and without radiotherapy: prognostic factors, patterns of recurrence, and survival. *Am J Surg* 1986;152:456–463.
114. Trible WM, Dias A. Cervical lymph node metastases. Prognosis related to level and distribution. *Arch Otolaryngol* 1964;79:247–249.
115. Hibbert J, Marks NJ, Winter PJ, et al. Prognostic factors in oral squamous carcinoma and their relation to clinical staging. *Clin Otolaryngol* 1983;8:197–203.
116. Kalnins IK, Leonard AG, Sako K, et al. Correlation between prognosis and degree of lymph node involvement in carcinoma of the oral cavity. *Am J Surg* 1977;134:450–454.
117. Pinsolle J, Pinsolle V, Majoufre C, et al. Prognostic value of histologic findings in neck dissections for squamous cell carcinoma. *Arch Otolaryngol Head Neck Surg* 1997;123:145–148.
118. Johnson JT, Barnes EL, Myers EN, et al. The extracapsular spread of tumors in cervical node metastasis. *Arch Otolaryngol* 1981;107:725–729.
119. Johnson JT, Myers EN, Bedetti CD, et al. Cervical lymph node metastases. Incidence and implications of extracapsular carcinoma. *Arch Otolaryngol* 1985;111:534–537.
120. Devineni VR, Simpson JR, Sessions D, et al. Supraglottic carcinoma: impact of radiation therapy on outcome of patients with positive margins and extracapsular nodal disease. *Laryngoscope* 1991;101:767–770.
121. Prim MP, De Diego JI, Hardisson D, et al. Extracapsular spread and desmoplastic pattern in neck lymph nodes: two prognostic factors of laryngeal cancer. *Ann Otol Rhinol Laryngol* 1999;108:672–676.
122. Myers EN, Alvi A. Management of carcinoma of the supraglottic larynx: evolution, current concepts, and future trends. *Laryngoscope* 1996;106: 559–567.
123. Ishwad CS, Ferrell RE, Rossie KN, et al. Loss of heterozygosity of the short arm of chromosomes 3 and 9 in oral cancer. *Int J Cancer* 1996;69:1–4.
124. Gavilan J, Prim MP, De Diego JI, et al. Postoperative radiotherapy in patients with positive nodes after functional neck dissection. *Ann Otol Rhinol Laryngol* 2000;109:844–848.
125. Brasilino de Carvalho M. Quantitative analysis of the extent of extracapsular invasion and its prognostic significance: a prospective study of 170 cases of carcinoma of the larynx and hypopharynx. *Head Neck* 1998;20:16–21.
126. Carter RL, Barr LC, O'Brien CJ, et al. Transcapsular spread of metastatic squamous cell carcinoma from cervical lymph nodes. *Am J Surg* 1985;150: 495–499.
127. Peters LJ, Goepfert H, Ang KK, et al. Evaluation of the dose for postoperative radiation therapy of head and neck cancer: first report of a prospective randomized trial. *Int J Radiat Oncol Biol Phys* 1993;26:3–11.
128. Johnson JT, Myers EN, Schramm VL, et al. Adjuvant chemotherapy for high-risk squamous-cell carcinoma of the head and neck. *J Clin Oncol* 1987;5: 456–458.
129. Johnson JT, Myers EN, Mayernik DG, et al. Adjuvant methotrexate-5-fluorouracil for extracapsular squamous cell carcinoma in cervical metastasis. *Laryngoscope* 1990;100:590–592.
130. Bachaud JM, Cohen-Jonathan E, Alzieu C, et al. Combined postoperative radiotherapy and weekly cisplatin infusion for locally advanced head and neck carcinoma: final report of a randomized trial. *Int J Radiat Oncol Biol Phys* 1996;36:999–1004.
131. Spiro RH, Alfonso AE, Farr HW, et al. Cervical node metastasis from epidermoid carcinoma of the oral cavity and oropharynx. A critical assessment of current staging. *Am J Surg* 1974;128:562–567.
132. Ellis ER, Mendenhall WM, Rao PV, et al. Does node location affect the incidence of distant metastases in head and neck squamous cell carcinoma? *Int J Radiat Oncol Biol Phys* 1989;17:293–297.
133. Kowalski LP, Bagietto R, Lara JR, et al. Prognostic significance of the distribution of neck node metastasis from oral carcinoma. *Head Neck* 2000;22: 207–214.
134. Schantz SP, Hsu TC, Ainslie N, et al. Young adults with head and neck cancer express increased susceptibility to mutagen-induced chromosome damage. *JAMA* 1989;262:3313–3315.
135. Verschuur HP, Irish JC, O'Sullivan B, et al. A matched control study of treatment outcome in young patients with squamous cell carcinoma of the head and neck. *Laryngoscope* 1999;109:249–258.
136. Siegelmann-Danieli N, Hanlon A, Ridge JA, et al. Oral tongue cancer in patients less than 45 years old: institutional experience and comparison with older patients. *J Clin Oncol* 1998;16:745–753.
137. Lacy PD, Piccirillo JF, Merritt MG, et al. Head and neck squamous cell carcinoma: better to be young. *Otolaryngol Head Neck Surg* 2000;122:253–258.
138. Leon X, Quer M, Agudelo D, et al. Influence of age on laryngeal carcinoma. *Ann Otol Rhinol Laryngol* 1998;107:164–169.
139. Koch WM, Brennan JA, Zahurak M, et al. p53 mutation and locoregional treatment failure in head and neck squamous cell carcinoma. *J Natl Cancer Inst* 1996;88:1580–1586.
140. Piccirillo JF. Impact of comorbidity and symptoms on the prognosis of patients with oral carcinoma [Letter; Comment]. *Arch Otolaryngol Head Neck Surg* 2000;126:1086–1088.
141. Bataini JP, Asselain B, Jaulerry C, et al. A multivariate primary tumour control analysis in 465 patients treated by radical radiotherapy for cancer of the tonsillar region: clinical and treatment parameters as prognostic factors. *Radiother Oncol* 1989;14:265–277.
142. Callery CD, Spiro RH, Strong EW. Changing trends in the management of squamous carcinoma of the tongue. *Am J Surg* 1984;148:449–454.
143. Griffin TW, Pajak TF, Gillespie BW, et al. Predicting the response of head and neck cancers to radiation therapy with a multivariate modelling system: an analysis of the RTOG head and neck registry. *Int J Radiat Oncol Biol Phys* 1984; 10:481–487.
144. Smith RR, Caulk R, Frazell E, et al. Revision of the clinical staging system for cancer of the larynx. *Cancer* 1973;31:72–80.
145. Easson EC, Palmer MK. Prognostic factors in oral cancer. *Clin Oncol* 1976;2: 191–202.
146. Stell PM. Prognosis in mouth cancer: host factors. *J Laryngol Otol* 1992;106: 399–402.
147. Gallo O, Bianchi S, Porfirio B. Bcl-2 overexpression and smoking history in head and neck cancer. *J Natl Cancer Inst* 1995;87:1024–1025.
148. Brennan JA, Boyle JO, Koch WM, et al. Association between cigarette smoking and mutation of the p53 gene in squamous-cell carcinoma of the head and neck. *N Engl J Med* 1995;332:712–717.
149. Browman GP, Wong G, Hodson I, et al. Influence of cigarette smoking on the efficacy of radiation therapy in head and neck cancer. *N Engl J Med* 1993;328:159–163.
150. Overgaard J, Nielsen JE, Grau C. Effect of carboxyhemoglobin on tumor oxygen unloading capacity in patients with squamous cell carcinoma of the head and neck. *Int J Radiat Oncol Biol Phys* 1992;22:407–410.
151. Terhaard CH, Snippe K, Ravasz LA, et al. Radiotherapy in T1 laryngeal cancer: prognostic factors for locoregional control and survival, uni- and multivariate analysis. *Int J Radiat Oncol Biol Phys* 1991;21:1179–1186.
152. Benninger MS, Gillen J, Thieme P, et al. Factors associated with recurrence and voice quality following radiation therapy for T1 and T2 glottic carcinomas. *Laryngoscope* 1994;104:294–298.
153. van der Voet JC, Keus RB, Hart AA, et al. The impact of treatment time and smoking on local control and complications in T1 glottic cancer. *Int J Radiat Oncol Biol Phys* 1998;42:247–255.
154. Day GL, Blot WJ, Shore RE, et al. Second cancers following oral and pharyngeal cancers: role of tobacco and alcohol. *J Natl Cancer Inst* 1994;86:131–137.
155. Pugliano FA, Piccirillo JF, Zequeira MR, et al. Clinical-severity staging system for oral cavity cancer: five-year survival rates. *Otolaryngol Head Neck Surg* 1999;120:38–45.
156. Singh B, Bhaya M, Stern J, et al. Validation of the Charlson comorbidity index in patients with head and neck cancer: a multi-institutional study. *Laryngoscope* 1997;107:1469–1475.
157. Singh B, Bhaya M, Zimbler M, et al. Impact of comorbidity on outcome of young patients with head and neck squamous cell carcinoma. *Head Neck* 1998;20:1–7.
158. Ribeiro KC, Kowalski LP, Latorre MR. Impact of comorbidity, symptoms, and patients' characteristics on the prognosis of oral carcinomas. *Arch Otolaryngol Head Neck Surg* 2000;126:1079–1085.
159. Pugliano FA, Piccirillo JF, Zequeira MR, et al. Clinical-severity staging system for oropharyngeal cancer: five-year survival rates. *Arch Otolaryngol Head Neck Surg* 1997;123:1118–1124.
160. Piccirillo JF. Importance of comorbidity in head and neck cancer. *Laryngoscope* 2000;110:593–602.
161. Scioscia KA, Snyderman CH, Wagner R. Altered serum amino acid profiles in head and neck cancer. *Nutr Cancer* 1998;30:144–147.
162. Goodwin WJ Jr, Torres J. The value of the prognostic nutritional index in the management of patients with advanced carcinoma of the head and neck. *Head Neck Surg* 1984;6:932–937.
163. Buzby GP, Mullen JL, Matthews DC, et al. Prognostic nutritional index in gastrointestinal surgery. *Am J Surg* 1980;139:160–167.
164. van Bokhorst-de van der Schueren MA, van Leeuwen PA, Sauerwein HP, et al. Assessment of malnutrition parameters in head and neck cancer and their relation to postoperative complications. *Head Neck* 1997;19:419–425.
165. van Bokhorst-de van der S, van Leeuwen PA, Kuik DJ, et al. The impact of nutritional status on the prognoses of patients with advanced head and neck cancer. *Cancer* 1999;86:519–527.
166. van Bokhorst-De Van Der Schueren MA, Quak JJ, von Blomberg-van der Flier BM, et al. Effect of perioperative nutrition, with and without arginine supplementation, on nutritional status, immune function, postoperative morbidity, and survival in severely malnourished head and neck cancer patients. *Am J Clin Nutr* 2001;73:323–332.

167. Tayek JA. A review of cancer cachexia and abnormal glucose metabolism in humans with cancer [Review; 111 refs]. *J Am Coll Nutr* 1992;11:445–456.
168. Doerr TD, Marks SC, Shamsa FH, et al. Effects of zinc and nutritional status on clinical outcomes in head and neck cancer. *Nutrition* 1998;14:489–495.
169. Dubray B, Mosseri V, Brunin F, et al. Anemia is associated with lower local-regional control and survival after radiation therapy for head and neck cancer: a prospective study. *Radiology* 1996;201:553–558.
170. Fein DA, Lee WR, Hanlon AL, et al. Pretreatment hemoglobin level influences local control and survival of T1-T2 squamous cell carcinomas of the glottic larynx. *J Clin Oncol* 1995;13:2077–2083.
171. Warde P, O'Sullivan B, Bristow RG, et al. T1/T2 glottic cancer managed by external beam radiotherapy: the influence of pretreatment hemoglobin on local control. *Int J Radiat Oncol Biol Phys* 1998;41:347–353.
172. Overgaard J, Hansen HS, Jorgensen K, et al. Primary radiotherapy of larynx and pharynx carcinoma—an analysis of some factors influencing local control and survival. *Int J Radiat Oncol Biol Phys* 1986;12:515–521.
173. Izzo JG, Papadimitrakopoulou VA, Li XQ, et al. Dysregulated cyclin D1 expression early in head and neck tumorigenesis: in vivo evidence for an association with subsequent gene amplification. *Oncogene* 1998;17:2313–2322.
174. Hoyer M, Jorgensen K, Bundgaard T, et al. Lack of predictive value of potential doubling time and iododeoxyuridine labelling index in radiotherapy of squamous cell carcinoma of the head and neck. *Radiother Oncol* 1998;46: 147–155.
175. Lee WR, Berkey B, Marcial V, et al. Anemia is associated with decreased survival and increased locoregional failure in patients with locally advanced head and neck carcinoma: a secondary analysis of RTOG 85-27. *Int J Radiat Oncol Biol Phys* 1998;42:1069–1075.
176. Overgaard J, Hansen HS, Overgaard M, et al. A randomized double-blind phase III study of nimorazole as a hypoxic radiosensitizer of primary radiotherapy in supraglottic larynx and pharynx carcinoma. Results of the Danish Head and Neck Cancer Study (DAHANCA) Protocol 5-85. *Radiother Oncol* 1998;46:135–146.
177. Lutterbach J, Guttenberger R. Anemia is associated with decreased local control of surgically treated squamous cell carcinomas of the glottic larynx. *Int J Radiat Oncol Biol Phys* 2000;48:1345–1350.
178. Glaser CM, Millesi W, Kornek GV, et al. Impact of hemoglobin level and use of recombinant erythropoietin on efficacy of preoperative chemoradiation therapy for squamous cell carcinoma of the oral cavity and oropharynx. *Int J Radiat Oncol Biol Phys* 2001;50:705–715.
179. Tarnawski R, Skladowski K, Maciejewski B. Prognostic value of hemoglobin concentration in radiotherapy for cancer of supraglottic larynx. *Int J Radiat Oncol Biol Phys* 1997;38:1007–1011.
180. van Acht MJ, Hermans J, Boks DE, et al. The prognostic value of hemoglobin and a decrease in hemoglobin during radiotherapy in laryngeal carcinoma. *Radiother Oncol* 1992;23:229–235.
181. Sturgis EM, Gianoli GJ, Miller RH, et al. Avoiding transfusion in head and neck surgery: feasibility study of erythropoietin. *Laryngoscope* 2000;110: 51–57.
182. Levine AJ. p53, the cellular gatekeeper for growth and division. *Cell* 1997;88: 323–331.
183. Lane DP. Cancer. p53, guardian of the genome. *Nature* 1992;358:15–16.
184. Lane DP. The regulation of p53 function: Steiner Award Lecture. *Int J Cancer* 1994;57:623–627.
185. Hunter T. Braking the cycle. *Cell* 1993;75:839–841.
186. Yonish-Rouach E, Resnitzky D, Lotem J, et al. Wild-type p53 induces apoptosis of myeloid leukaemic cells that is inhibited by interleukin-6. *Nature* 1991;352:345–347.
187. el-Deiry WS, Harper JW, O'Connor PM, et al. WAF1/CIP1 is induced in p53-mediated G1 arrest and apoptosis. *Cancer Res* 1994;54:1169–1174.
188. Blank KR, Rudoltz MS, Kao GD, et al. The molecular regulation of apoptosis and implications for radiation oncology. *Int J Radiat Biol* 1997;71:455–466.
189. Sionov RV, Haupt Y. The cellular response to p53: the decision between life and death. *Oncogene* 1999;18:6145–6157.
190. Lowe SW, Ruley HE, Jacks T, et al. p53-dependent apoptosis modulates the cytotoxicity of anticancer agents. *Cell* 1993;74:957–967.
191. Lowe SW, Schmitt EM, Smith SW, et al. p53 is required for radiation-induced apoptosis in mouse thymocytes. *Nature* 1993;362:847–849.
192. Clarke AR, Purdie CA, Harrison DJ, et al. Thymocyte apoptosis induced by p53-dependent and independent pathways. *Nature* 1993;362:849–852.
193. Chang EH, Jang YJ, Hao Z, et al. Restoration of the G1 checkpoint and the apoptotic pathway mediated by wild-type p53 sensitizes squamous cell carcinoma of the head and neck to radiotherapy. *Arch Otolaryngol Head Neck Surg* 1997;123:507–512.
194. Liu TJ, el-Naggar AK, McDonnell TJ, et al. Apoptosis induction mediated by wild-type p53 adenoviral gene transfer in squamous cell carcinoma of the head and neck. *Cancer Res* 1995;55:3117–3122.
195. Pirollo KF, Hao Z, Rait A, et al. p53 mediated sensitization of squamous cell carcinoma of the head and neck to radiotherapy. *Oncogene* 1997;14: 1735–1746.
196. Xu L, Pirollo KF, Chang EH. Transferrin-liposome-mediated p53 sensitization of squamous cell carcinoma of the head and neck to radiation in vitro. *Hum Gene Ther* 1997;8:467–475.
197. Graeber TG, Osmanian C, Jacks T, et al. Hypoxia-mediated selection of cells with diminished apoptotic potential in solid tumours. *Nature* 1996;379:88–91.
198. Dameron KM, Volpert OV, Tainsky MA, et al. Control of angiogenesis in fibroblasts by p53 regulation of thrombospondin-1. *Science* 1994;265: 1582–1584.
199. Giatromanolaki A, Fountzilas G, Koukourakis MI, et al. Neo-angiogenesis in locally advanced squamous cell head and neck cancer correlates with thymidine phosphorylase expression and p53 nuclear oncoprotein accumulation. *Clin Exp Metastasis* 1998;16:665–672.
200. Grabenbauer GG, Muhlfriedel C, Rodel F, et al. Squamous cell carcinoma of the oropharynx: Ki-67 and p53 can identify patients at high risk for local recurrence after surgery and postoperative radiotherapy. *Int J Radiat Oncol Biol Phys* 2000;48:1041–1050.
201. Chen CY, Oliner JD, Zhan Q, et al. Interactions between p53 and MDM2 in a mammalian cell cycle checkpoint pathway. *Proc Natl Acad Sci U S A* 1994;91: 2684–2688.
202. Levinson W, Jawetz E. *Medical microbiology and immunology.* Stamford, CT: Appleton & Lange, 1998:547.
203. Taylor D, Koch WM, Zahurak M, et al. Immunohistochemical detection of p53 protein accumulation in head and neck cancer: correlation with p53 gene alterations. *Hum Pathol* 1999;30:1221–1225.
204. Saunders ME, MacKenzie R, Shipman R, et al. Patterns of p53 gene mutations in head and neck cancer: full-length gene sequencing and results of primary radiotherapy. *Clin Cancer Res* 1999;5:2455–2463.
205. Calzolari A, Chiarelli I, Bianchi S, et al. Immunohistochemical vs molecular biology methods. Complementary techniques for effective screening of p53 alterations in head and neck cancer. *Am J Clin Pathol* 1997;107:7–11.
206. Begg AC, Haustermans K, Hart AA, et al. The value of pretreatment cell kinetic parameters as predictors for radiotherapy outcome in head and neck cancer: a multicenter analysis. *Radiother Oncol* 1999;50:13–23.
207. Temam S, Flahault A, Perie S, et al. p53 gene status as a predictor of tumor response to induction chemotherapy of patients with locoregionally advanced squamous cell carcinomas of the head and neck. *J Clin Oncol* 2000; 18:385–394.
208. Gleich LL, Li YQ, Biddinger PW, et al. The loss of heterozygosity in retinoblastoma and p53 suppressor genes as a prognostic indicator for head and neck cancer. *Laryngoscope* 1996;106:1378–1381.
209. Gleich LL, Li YQ, Wang X, et al. Variable genetic alterations and survival in head and neck cancer. *Arch Otolaryngol Head Neck Surg* 1999;125:949–952.
210. Hartig G, Zhang J, Voytovich GM, et al. Fluorescent in situ hybridization evaluation of p53 gene deletions at a tumor interface of lingual carcinoma. *Laryngoscope* 2000;110:1474–1478.
211. Mineta H, Borg A, Dictor M, et al. p53 mutation, but not p53 overexpression, correlates with survival in head and neck squamous cell carcinoma. *Br J Cancer* 1998;78:1084–1090.
212. Overgaard J, Sorensen SB, Stausbol-Gron B, et al. TP53 mutation is an independent prognostic marker for poor outcome of radiotherapy in squamous cell carcinoma of the head and neck. *Int J Radiat Oncol Biol Phys* 1998;42 [Suppl]:146.
213. Ganly I, Eckhardt SG, Rodriguez GI, et al. A phase I study of Onyx-015, an E1B attenuated adenovirus, administered intratumorally to patients with recurrent head and neck cancer [Erratum appears in *Clin Cancer Res* 2000;6: 2120]. *Clin Cancer Res* 2000;6:798–806.
214. Gallo O, Chiarelli I, Boddi V, et al. Cumulative prognostic value of p53 mutations and bcl-2 protein expression in head-and-neck cancer treated by radiotherapy. *Int J Cancer* 1999;84:573–579.
215. Cabelguenne A, Blons H, de Waziers I, et al. p53 alterations predict tumor response to neoadjuvant chemotherapy in head and neck squamous cell carcinoma: a prospective series. *J Clin Oncol* 2000;18:1465–1473.
216. Warnakulasuriya S, Jia C, Johnson N, et al. p53 and P-glycoprotein expression are significant prognostic markers in advanced head and neck cancer treated with chemo/radiotherapy. *J Pathol* 2000;191:33–38.
217. Shiga H, Heath EI, Rasmussen AA, et al. Prognostic value of p53, glutathione S-transferase pi, and thymidylate synthase for neoadjuvant cisplatin-based chemotherapy in head and neck cancer. *Clin Cancer Res* 1999;5:4097–4104.
218. Etienne MC, Pivot X, Formento JL, et al. A multifactorial approach including tumoural epidermal growth factor receptor, p53, thymidylate synthase and dihydropyrimidine dehydrogenase to predict treatment outcome in head and neck cancer patients receiving 5-fluorouracil. *Br J Cancer* 1999;79: 1864–1869.
219. Erber R, Conradt C, Homann N, et al. TP53 DNA contact mutations are selectively associated with allelic loss and have a strong clinical impact in head and neck cancer. *Oncogene* 1998;16:1671–1679.
220. Shin DM, Lee JS, Lippman SM, et al. p53 expressions: predicting recurrence and second primary tumors in head and neck squamous cell carcinoma. *J Natl Cancer Inst* 1996;88:519–529.
221. Caminero MJ, Nunez F, Suarez C, et al. Detection of p53 protein in oropharyngeal carcinoma. Prognostic implications. *Arch Otolaryngol Head Neck Surg* 1996;122:769–772.
222. Jackel MC, Sellmann L, Dorudian MA, et al. Prognostic significance of p53/bcl-2 co-expression in patients with laryngeal squamous cell carcinoma. *Laryngoscope* 2000;110:1339–1345.
223. Raybaud-Diogene H, Fortin A, Morency R, et al. Markers of radioresistance in squamous cell carcinomas of the head and neck: a clinicopathologic and immunohistochemical study. *J Clin Oncol* 1997;15:1030–1038.
224. Narayana A, Vaughan AT, Kathuria S, et al. p53 overexpression is associated with bulky tumor and poor local control in T1 glottic cancer. *Int J Radiat Oncol Biol Phys* 2000;46:21–26.
225. Gluckman JL, Pavelic ZP, Welkoborsky HJ, et al. Prognostic indicators for squamous cell carcinoma of the oral cavity: a clinicopathologic correlation. *Laryngoscope* 1997;107:1239–1244.
226. Veneroni S, Silvestrini R, Costa A, et al. Biological indicators of survival in

patients treated by surgery for squamous cell carcinoma of the oral cavity and oropharynx. *Oral Oncol* 1997;33:408–413.
227. Akervall JA, Michalides RJ, Mineta H, et al. Amplification of cyclin D1 in squamous cell carcinoma of the head and neck and the prognostic value of chromosomal abnormalities and cyclin D1 overexpression. *Cancer* 1997;79: 380–389.
228. Xie X, Boysen M, Clausen OP, et al. Prognostic value of Le(y) and H antigens in oral tongue carcinomas. *Laryngoscope* 1999;109:1474–1480.
229. Pai HH, Rochon L, Clark B, et al. Overexpression of p53 protein does not predict local-regional control or survival in patients with early-stage squamous cell carcinoma of the glottic larynx treated with radiotherapy. *Int J Radiat Oncol Biol Phys* 1998;41:37–42.
230. dos Santos CR, Goncalves Filho J, Magrin J, et al. Involvement of level I neck lymph nodes in advanced squamous carcinoma of the larynx. *Ann Otol Rhinol Laryngol* 2001;110:982–984.
231. Hirvikoski P, Kumpulainen E, Virtaniemi J, et al. p53 expression and cell proliferation as prognostic factors in laryngeal squamous cell carcinoma. *J Clin Oncol* 1997;15:3111–3120.
232. Folkman J. Tumor angiogenesis: therapeutic implications. *N Engl J Med* 1971; 285:1182–1186.
233. Folkman J. Tumor angiogenesis. *Adv Cancer Res* 1985;43:175–203.
234. Klagsbrun M, D'Amore PA. Regulators of angiogenesis. *Annu Rev Physiol* 1991;53:217–239.
235. Veikkola T, Karkkainen M, Claesson-Welsh L, et al. Regulation of angiogenesis via vascular endothelial growth factor receptors. *Cancer Res* 2000;60:203–212.
236. Heimdal JH, Aarstad HJ, Klementsen B, et al. Peripheral blood mononuclear cell (PBMC) responsiveness in patients with head and neck cancer in relation to tumour stage and prognosis. *Acta Otolaryngol* 1999;119:281–284.
237. Klagsbrun M, Soker S. VEGF/VPF: the angiogenesis factor found? *Curr Biol* 1993;3:699–702.
238. Denhart BC, Guidi AJ, Tognazzi K, et al. Vascular permeability factor/vascular endothelial growth factor and its receptors in oral and laryngeal squamous cell carcinoma and dysplasia. *Lab Invest* 1997;77:659–664.
239. Dvorak HF, Brown LF, Detmar M, et al. Vascular permeability factor/vascular endothelial growth factor, microvascular hyperpermeability, and angiogenesis. *Am J Pathol* 1995;146:1029–1039.
240. Zimmer SG, DeBenedetti A, Graff JR. Translational control of malignancy: the mRNA cap-binding protein, eIF- 4E, as a central regulator of tumor formation, growth, invasion and metastasis. *Anticancer Res* 2000;20:1343–1351.
241. De Benedetti A, Harris AL. eIF4E expression in tumors: its possible role in progression of malignancies. *Int J Biochem Cell Biol* 1999;31:59–72.
242. Hlatky L, Tsionou C, Hahnfeldt P, et al. Mammary fibroblasts may influence breast tumor angiogenesis via hypoxia-induced vascular endothelial growth factor up-regulation and protein expression. *Cancer Res* 1994;54:6083–6086.
243. Fukuiwa T, Takebayashi Y, Akiba S, et al. Expression of thymidine phosphorylase and vascular endothelial cell growth factor in human head and neck squamous cell carcinoma and their different characteristics. *Cancer* 1999;85: 960–969.
244. Roychowdhury DF, Tseng A Jr, Fu KK, et al. New prognostic factors in nasopharyngeal carcinoma. Tumor angiogenesis and C-erbB2 expression. *Cancer* 1996;77:1419–1426.
245. Artese L, Rubini C, Ferrero G, et al. Microvessel density (MVD) and vascular endothelial growth factor expression (VEGF) in human oral squamous cell carcinoma. *Anticancer Res* 2001;21:689–695.
246. Alcalde RE, Shintani S, Yoshihama Y, et al. Cell proliferation and tumor angiogenesis in oral squamous cell carcinoma. *Anticancer Res* 1995;15: 1417–1422.
247. Alcalde RE, Terakado N, Otsuki K, et al. Angiogenesis and expression of platelet-derived endothelial cell growth factor in oral squamous cell carcinoma. *Oncology* 1997;54:324–328.
248. Guang-Wu H, Sunagawa M, Jie-En L, et al. The relationship between microvessel density, the expression of vascular endothelial growth factor (VEGF), and the extension of nasopharyngeal carcinoma. *Laryngoscope* 2000; 110:2066–2069.
249. Wakisaka N, Wen QH, Yoshizaki T, et al. Association of vascular endothelial growth factor expression with angiogenesis and lymph node metastasis in nasopharyngeal carcinoma. *Laryngoscope* 1999;109:810–814.
250. Williams JK, Carlson GW, Cohen C, et al. Tumor angiogenesis as a prognostic factor in oral cavity tumors. *Am J Surg* 1994;168:373–380.
251. Shpitzer T, Chaimoff M, Gal R, et al. Tumor angiogenesis as a prognostic factor in early oral tongue cancer. *Arch Otolaryngol Head Neck Surg* 1996;122: 865–868.
252. Beatrice F, Cammarota R, Giordano C, et al. Angiogenesis: prognostic significance in laryngeal cancer. *Anticancer Res* 1998;18:4737–4740.
253. Hegde PU, Brenski AC, Caldarelli DD, et al. Tumor angiogenesis and p53 mutations: prognosis in head and neck cancer. *Arch Otolaryngol Head Neck Surg* 1998;124:80–85.
254. Dray TG, Hardin NJ, Sofferman RA. Angiogenesis as a prognostic marker in early head and neck cancer. *Ann Otol Rhinol Laryngol* 1995;104:724–729.
255. Salven P, Heikkila P, Anttonen A, et al. Vascular endothelial growth factor in squamous cell head and neck carcinoma: expression and prognostic significance. *Mod Pathol* 1997;10:1128–1133.
256. Aebersold DM, Beer KT, Laissue J, et al. Intratumoral microvessel density predicts local treatment failure of radically irradiated squamous cell cancer of the oropharynx. *Int J Radiat Oncol Biol Phys* 2000;48:17–25.
257. Kamijo T, Yokose T, Hasebe T, et al. Potential role of microvessel density in predicting radiosensitivity of T1 and T2 stage laryngeal squamous cell carcinoma treated with radiotherapy. *Clin Cancer Res* 2000;6:3159–3165.
258. Giatromanolaki A, Koukourakis MI, Georgoulias V, et al. Angiogenesis vs. response after combined chemoradiotherapy of squamous cell head and neck cancer. *Int J Cancer* 1999;80:810–817.
259. Moriyama M, Kumagai S, Kawashiri S, et al. Immunohistochemical study of tumour angiogenesis in oral squamous cell carcinoma. *Oral Oncol* 1997;33: 369–374.
260. Smith BD, Smith GL, Carter D, et al. Prognostic significance of vascular endothelial growth factor protein levels in oral and oropharyngeal squamous cell carcinoma. *J Clin Oncol* 2000;18:2046–2052.
261. Mineta H, Miura K, Ogino T, et al. Prognostic value of vascular endothelial growth factor (VEGF) in head and neck squamous cell carcinomas. *Br J Cancer* 2000;83:775–781.
262. Eisma RJ, Spiro JD, Kreutzer DL. Vascular endothelial growth factor expression in head and neck squamous cell carcinoma. *Am J Surg* 1997;174:513–517.
263. Maeda T, Matsumura S, Hiranuma H, et al. Expression of vascular endothelial growth factor in human oral squamous cell carcinoma: its association with tumour progression and p53 gene status. *J Clin Pathol* 1998;51:771–775.
264. Shintani S, Kiyota A, Mihara M, et al. Association of preoperative radiation effect with tumor angiogenesis and vascular endothelial growth factor in oral squamous cell carcinoma. *Jpn J Cancer Res* 2000;91:1051–1057.
265. Motokura T, Bloom T, Kim HG, et al. A novel cyclin encoded by a bcl1-linked candidate oncogene. *Nature* 1991;350:512–515.
266. Sherr CJ. D-type cyclins. *Trends Biochem Sci* 1995;20:187–190.
267. Jares P, Fernandez PL, Campo E, et al. PRAD-1/cyclin D1 gene amplification correlates with messenger RNA overexpression and tumor progression in human laryngeal carcinomas. *Cancer Res* 1994;54:4813–4817.
268. Zwijsen RM, Klompmaker R, Wientjens EB, et al. Cyclin D1 triggers autonomous growth of breast cancer cells by governing cell cycle exit. *Mol Cell Biol* 1996;16:2554–2560.
269. Alavi S, Namazie A, Calcaterra TC, et al. Clinical application of fluorescence in situ hybridization for chromosome 11q13 analysis in head and neck cancer. *Laryngoscope* 1999;109:874–879.
270. Capaccio P, Pruneri G, Carboni N, et al. Cyclin D1 expression is predictive of occult metastases in head and neck cancer patients with clinically negative cervical lymph nodes. *Head Neck* 2000;22:234–240.
271. Bova RJ, Quinn DI, Nankervis JS, et al. Cyclin D1 and p16INK4A expression predict reduced survival in carcinoma of the anterior tongue. *Clin Cancer Res* 1999;5:2810–2819.
272. Michalides RJ, van Veelen NM, Kristel PM, et al. Overexpression of cyclin D1 indicates a poor prognosis in squamous cell carcinoma of the head and neck. *Arch Otolaryngol Head Neck Surg* 1997;123:497–502.
273. Pignataro L, Pruneri G, Carboni N, et al. Clinical relevance of cyclin D1 protein overexpression in laryngeal squamous cell carcinoma. *J Clin Oncol* 1998; 16:3069–3077.
274. Lazar AD, Winter MR, Nogueira CP, et al. Loss of heterozygosity at 11q23 in squamous cell carcinoma of the head and neck is associated with recurrent disease. *Clin Cancer Res* 1998;4:2787–2793.
275. Meredith SD, Levine PA, Burns JA, et al. Chromosome 11q13 amplification in head and neck squamous cell carcinoma. Association with poor prognosis. *Arch Otolaryngol Head Neck Surg* 1995;121:790–794.
276. Bellacosa A, Almadori G, Cavallo S, et al. Cyclin D1 gene amplification in human laryngeal squamous cell carcinomas: prognostic significance and clinical implications. *Clin Cancer Res* 1996;2:175–180.
277. Kyomoto R, Kumazawa H, Toda Y, et al. Cyclin-D1-gene amplification is a more potent prognostic factor than its protein over-expression in human head-and-neck squamous-cell carcinoma. *Int J Cancer* 1997;74:576–581.
278. Nogueira CP, Dolan RW, Gooey J, et al. Inactivation of p53 and amplification of cyclin D1 correlate with clinical outcome in head and neck cancer. *Laryngoscope* 1998;108:345–350.
279. Muller D, Millon R, Velten M, et al. Amplification of 11q13 DNA markers in head and neck squamous cell carcinomas: correlation with clinical outcome. *Eur J Cancer* 1997;33:2203–2210.
280. Fortin A, Guerry M, Guerry R, et al. Chromosome 11q13 gene amplifications in oral and oropharyngeal carcinomas: no correlation with subclinical lymph node invasion and disease recurrence. *Clin Cancer Res* 1997;3:1609–1614.
281. Yoo SS, Carter D, Turner BC, et al. Prognostic significance of cyclin D1 protein levels in early-stage larynx cancer treated with primary radiation. *Int J Cancer* 2000;90:22–28.
282. Betticher DC, Thatcher N, Altermatt HJ, et al. Alternate splicing produces a novel cyclin D1 transcript. *Oncogene* 1995;11:1005–1011.
283. Matthias C, Branigan K, Jahnke V, et al. Polymorphism within the cyclin D1 gene is associated with prognosis in patients with squamous cell carcinoma of the head and neck. *Clin Cancer Res* 1998;4:2411–2418.
284. Grandis JR, Tweardy DJ. Elevated levels of transforming growth factor alpha and epidermal growth factor receptor messenger RNA are early markers of carcinogenesis in head and neck cancer. *Cancer Res* 1993;53:3579–3584.
285. Grandis JR, Melhem MF, Barnes EL, et al. Quantitative immunohistochemical analysis of transforming growth factor-alpha and epidermal growth factor receptor in patients with squamous cell carcinoma of the head and neck. *Cancer* 1996;78:1284–1292.
286. Hackel PO, Zwick E, Prenzel N, et al. Epidermal growth factor receptors: critical mediators of multiple receptor pathways. *Curr Opin Cell Biol* 1999;11: 184–189.
287. Grandis JR, Zeng Q, Drenning SD. Epidermal growth factor receptor—medi-

ated stat3 signaling blocks apoptosis in head and neck cancer. *Laryngoscope* 2000;110:868–874.

288. Grandis JR, Chakraborty A, Zeng Q, et al. Downmodulation of TGF-alpha protein expression with antisense oligonucleotides inhibits proliferation of head and neck squamous carcinoma but not normal mucosal epithelial cells. *J Cell Biochem* 1998;69:55–62.
289. Rubin Grandis J, Chakraborty A, Melhem MF, et al. Inhibition of epidermal growth factor receptor gene expression and function decreases proliferation of head and neck squamous carcinoma but not normal mucosal epithelial cells. *Oncogene* 1997;15:409–416.
290. He Y, Zeng Q, Drenning SD, et al. Inhibition of human squamous cell carcinoma growth in vivo by epidermal growth factor receptor antisense RNA transcribed from the U6 promoter. *J Natl Cancer Inst* 1998;90:1080–1087.
291. Akimoto T, Hunter NR, Buchmiller L, et al. Inverse relationship between epidermal growth factor receptor expression and radiocurability of murine carcinomas. *Clin Cancer Res* 1999;5:2884–2890.
292. Huang SM, Bock JM, Harari PM. Epidermal growth factor receptor blockade with C225 modulates proliferation, apoptosis, and radiosensitivity in squamous cell carcinomas of the head and neck. *Cancer Res* 1999;59: 1935–1940.
293. Bonner JA, Raisch KP, Trummell HQ, et al. Enhanced apoptosis with combination C225/radiation treatment serves as the impetus for clinical investigation in head and neck cancers. *J Clin Oncol* 2000;18:47S–53S.
294. Huang SM, Harari PM. Modulation of radiation response after epidermal growth factor receptor blockade in squamous cell carcinomas: inhibition of damage repair, cell cycle kinetics, and tumor angiogenesis. *Clin Cancer Res* 2000;6:2166–2174.
295. Milas L, Mason K, Hunter N, et al. In vivo enhancement of tumor radioresponse by C225 antiepidermal growth factor receptor antibody. *Clin Cancer Res* 2000;6:701–708.
296. Eisbruch A, Blick M, Lee JS, et al. Analysis of the epidermal growth factor receptor gene in fresh human head and neck tumors. *Cancer Res* 1987;47:3603–3605.
297. Yamamoto T, Kamata N, Kawano H, et al. High incidence of amplification of the epidermal growth factor receptor gene in human squamous carcinoma cell lines. *Cancer Res* 1986;46:414–416.
298. Grandis JR, Zeng Q, Drenning SD, et al. Normalization of EGFR mRNA levels following restoration of wild-type p53 in a head and neck squamous cell carcinoma cell line. *Int J Oncol* 1998;13:375–378.
299. Xia W, Lau YK, Zhang HZ, et al. Combination of EGFR, HER-2/neu, and HER-3 is a stronger predictor for the outcome of oral squamous cell carcinoma than any individual family members. *Clin Cancer Res* 1999;5:4164–4174.
300. Dassonville O, Formento JL, Francoual M, et al. Expression of epidermal growth factor receptor and survival in upper aerodigestive tract cancer. *J Clin Oncol* 1993;11:1873–1878.
301. Maurizi M, Almadori G, Ferrandina G, et al. Prognostic significance of epidermal growth factor receptor in laryngeal squamous cell carcinoma. *Br J Cancer* 1996;74:1253–1257.
302. Almadori G, Cadoni G, Galli J, et al. Epidermal growth factor receptor expression in primary laryngeal cancer: an independent prognostic factor of neck node relapse. *Int J Cancer* 1999;84:188–191.
303. Grandis JR, Melhem MF, Gooding WE, et al. Levels of TGF-alpha and EGFR protein in head and neck squamous cell carcinoma and patient survival. *J Natl Cancer Inst* 1998;90:824–832.
304. Wen QH, Miwa T, Yoshizaki T, et al. Prognostic value of EGFR and TGF-alpha in early laryngeal cancer treated with radiotherapy. *Laryngoscope* 1996; 106:884–888.
305. Brennan JA, Mao L, Hruban RH, et al. Molecular assessment of histopathological staging in squamous-cell carcinoma of the head and neck [See comments]. *N Engl J Med* 1995;332:429–435.
306. DeFatta RJ, Nathan CA, De Benedetti A. Antisense RNA to eIF4E suppresses oncogenic properties of a head and neck squamous cell carcinoma cell line. *Laryngoscope* 2000;110:928–933.
307. Nathan CA, Franklin S, Abreo FW, et al. Analysis of surgical margins with the molecular marker eIF4E: a prognostic factor in patients with head and neck cancer. *J Clin Oncol* 1999;17:2909–2914.
308. Ah-See KW, Cooke TG, Pickford IR, et al. An allelotype of squamous carcinoma of the head and neck using microsatellite markers. *Cancer Res* 1994;54: 1617–1621.
309. Li X, Lee NK, Ye YW, et al. Allelic loss at chromosomes 3p, 8p, 13q, and 17p associated with poor prognosis in head and neck cancer. *J Natl Cancer Inst* 1994;86:1524–1529.
310. el-Naggar AK, Hurr K, Batsakis JG, et al. Sequential loss of heterozygosity at microsatellite motifs in preinvasive and invasive head and neck squamous carcinoma. *Cancer Res* 1995;55:2656–2659.
311. Scholnick SB, Haughey BH, Sunwoo JB, et al. Chromosome 8 allelic loss and the outcome of patients with squamous cell carcinoma of the supraglottic larynx. *J Natl Cancer Inst* 1996;88:1676–1682.
312. Partridge M, Emilion G, Pateromichelakis S, et al. The prognostic significance of allelic imbalance at key chromosomal loci in oral cancer. *Br J Cancer* 1999;79:1821–1827.
313. Partridge M, Emilion G, Langdon JD. LOH at 3p correlates with a poor survival in oral squamous cell carcinoma. *Br J Cancer* 1996;73:366–371.
314. Maestro R, Piccinin S, Doglioni C, et al. Chromosome 13q deletion mapping in head and neck squamous cell carcinomas: identification of two distinct regions of preferential loss. *Cancer Res* 1996;56:1146–1150.
315. Rowley H, Jones A, Spandidos D, et al. Definition of a tumor suppressor gene locus on the short arm of chromosome 3 in squamous cell carcinoma of the head and neck by means of microsatellite markers. *Arch Otolaryngol Head Neck Surg* 1996;122:497–501.
316. Uzawa K, Suzuki H, Komiya A, et al. Evidence for two distinct tumor-suppressor gene loci on the long arm of chromosome 11 in human oral cancer. *Int J Cancer* 1996;67:510–514.
317. Bockmuhl U, Schwendel A, Dietel M, et al. Distinct patterns of chromosomal alterations in high- and low-grade head and neck squamous cell carcinomas. *Cancer Res* 1996;56:5325–5329.
318. Jones JW, Raval JR, Beals TF, et al. Frequent loss of heterozygosity on chromosome arm 18q in squamous cell carcinomas. Identification of 2 regions of loss—18q11.1-q12.3 and 18q21.1-q23. *Arch Otolaryngol Head Neck Surg* 1997; 123:610–614.
319. Bockmuhl U, Petersen S, Schmidt S, et al. Patterns of chromosomal alterations in metastasizing and nonmetastasizing primary head and neck carcinomas. *Cancer Res* 1997;57:5213–5216.
320. Wang XL, Uzawa K, Miyakawa A, et al. Localization of a tumour-suppressor gene associated with human oral cancer on 7q31.1. *Int J Cancer* 1998;75:671–674.
321. Gupta VK, Schmidt AP, Pashia ME, et al. Multiple regions of deletion on chromosome arm 13q in head-and-neck squamous-cell carcinoma. *Int J Cancer* 1999;84:453–457.
322. Poli-Frederico RC, Bergamo NA, Reis PP, et al. Chromosome 22q a frequent site of allele loss in head and neck carcinoma. *Head Neck* 2000;22:585–590.
323. Stell PM. Ploidy in head and neck cancer: a review and meta-analysis. *Clin Otolaryngol* 1991;16:510–516.
324. Welkoborsky HJ, Bernauer HS, Riazimand HS, et al. Patterns of chromosomal aberrations in metastasizing and nonmetastasizing squamous cell carcinomas of the oropharynx and hypopharynx. *Ann Otol Rhinol Laryngol* 2000; 109:401–410.
325. Hemmer J, Nagel E, Kraft K. DNA aneuploidy by flow cytometry is an independent prognostic factor in squamous cell carcinoma of the oral cavity. *Anticancer Res* 1999;19:1419–1422.
326. Hemmer J, Kraft K, Kreidler J. The significance of DNA flow cytometry in predicting survival and delayed clinical manifestation of occult lymph node metastasis to the untreated neck in patients with oral squamous cell carcinoma. *J Craniomaxillofac Surg* 1998;26:405–410.
327. Danic D, Milicic D, Prgomet D, et al. Prognostic factors in carcinoma of the larynx: relevance of DNA ploidy, S-fractions and localization of the tumour. *J Laryngol Otol* 1999;113:538–541.
328. Zatterstrom UK, Wennerberg J, Ewers SB, et al. Prognostic factors in head and neck cancer: histologic grading, DNA ploidy, and nodal status. *Head Neck* 1991;13:477–87.
329. Tytor M, Olofsson J, Ledin T, et al. Squamous cell carcinoma of the oral cavity. A review of 176 cases with application of malignancy grading and DNA measurements. *Clin Otolaryngol* 1990;15:235–252.
330. Kearsley JH, Bryson G, Battistutta D, et al. Prognostic importance of cellular DNA content in head-and-neck squamous-cell cancers. A comparison of retrospective and prospective series. *Int J Cancer* 1991;47:31–37.
331. Welkoborsky HJ, Hinni M, Dienes HP, et al. Predicting recurrence and survival in patients with laryngeal cancer by means of DNA cytometry, tumor front grading, and proliferation markers. *Ann Otol Rhinol Laryngol* 1995;104: 503–510.
332. Rua S, Comino A, Fruttero A, et al. Relationship between histologic features, DNA flow cytometry, and clinical behavior of squamous cell carcinomas of the larynx. *Cancer* 1991;67:141–149.
333. Syms CA 3rd, Eibling DE, McCoy JP Jr, et al. Flow cytometric analysis of primary and metastatic squamous cell carcinoma of the oral cavity and oropharynx. *Laryngoscope* 1995;105:149–155.
334. Sampedro A, Alvarez C, Martinez J, et al. Cell proliferation activity and kinetic profile in the prognosis and therapeutic management of carcinoma of the pharynx and larynx. *Otolaryngol Head Neck Surg*1999;121:476–481.
335. Westerbeek HA, Mooi WJ, Hilgers FJ, et al. Ploidy status and the response of T1 glottic carcinoma to radiotherapy. *Clin Otolaryngol* 1993;18:98–101.
336. Walter MA, Peters GE, Peiper SC. Predicting radioresistance in early glottic squamous cell carcinoma by DNA content. *Ann Otol Rhinol Laryngol* 1991; 100:523–526.
337. Toffoli G, Franchin G, Barzan L, et al. Brief report: prognostic importance of cellular DNA content in T1-2 N0 laryngeal squamous cell carcinomas treated with radiotherapy. *Laryngoscope* 1995;105:649–652.
338. Yip TT, Lau WH, Chan JK, et al. Prognostic significance of DNA flow cytometric analysis in patients with nasopharyngeal carcinoma. *Cancer* 1998;83: 2284–2292.
339. Zackrisson B, Gustafsson H, Stenling R, et al. Predictive value of potential doubling time in head and neck cancer patients treated by conventional radiotherapy. *Int J Radiat Oncol Biol Phys* 1997;38:677–683.
340. Fu KK, Hammond E, Pajak TF, et al. Flow cytometric quantification of the proliferation-associated nuclear antigen p105 and DNA content in advanced head & neck cancers: results of RTOG 91-08. *Int J Radiat Oncol Biol Phys* 1994; 29:661–671.
341. Begg AC. The clinical status of Tpot as a predictor? Or why no tempest in the Tpot! *Int J Radiat Oncol Biol Phys* 1995;32:1539–1541.
342. Haustermans K, Fowler JF. Is there a future for cell kinetic measurements using IdUrd or BdUrd? *Int J Radiat Oncol Biol Phys* 2001;49:505–511.
343. Begg AC, McNally NJ, Shrieve DC, et al. A method to measure the duration of DNA synthesis and the potential doubling time from a single sample. *Cytometry* 1985;6:620–626.

CHAPTER 4

General Principles of Head and Neck Radiology

Bernard B. O'Malley and Suresh K. Mukherji

Cross-sectional imaging usually provides staging information that supplements or complements the clinical examination of the head and neck. This is particularly true in patients with limitations to the examination such as those in pain or with trismus, a stocky build, or posttreatment changes. There is no "routine" scan of the head and neck whether at a primary or tertiary care center. The design of any scan should be made in light of the pertinent clinical history. Incumbent on the imaging subspecialist is helping to narrow down the clinical pre-scan differential diagnosis. Although some sites are not routinely scanned prior to intervention sometimes imaging reveals benign causes of clinically suspicious masses. (Fig. 4.1). For the purpose of consistency, an imaging division must establish a menu of imaging protocols (Fig. 4.2) and must maintain strict quality control of the end product. The protocols are designed both to stage the primary site carefully and to stage the neck accurately (Fig. 4.3) (1). In design of all scans, some consideration should be given to the eventual need to correlate between modalities, typically computed tomography (CT) and magnetic resonance imaging (MRI) (Fig. 4.4). The choice of modality used for any stage of a given disorder should reflect an agreement between the clinical and radiologic members of the interdisciplinary team. This latter consideration often is driven both by standard of care and by the relative availability of scanners and skills of the interpreter.

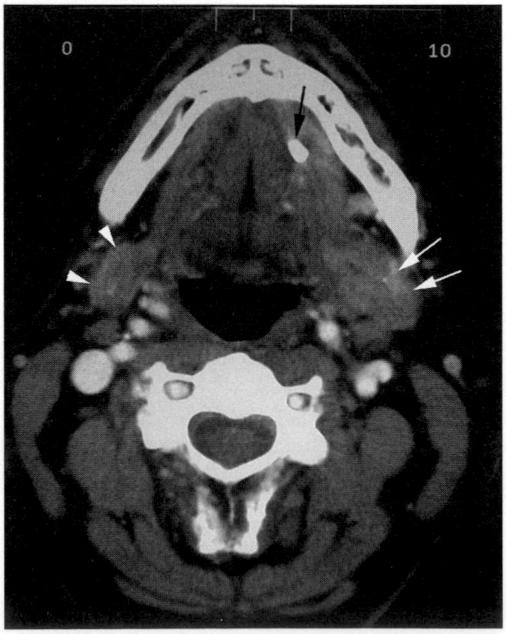

Figure 4.1 Pseudomass of the neck. The left submandibular gland (*white arrows*) is swollen compared with the right (*white arrowheads*) due to an obstructing calculus (*black arrow*) within the left Wharton duct.

The interpretation of any scan must be performed by an interdisciplinary team member who knows staging criteria and the impact of suspected findings on the management options for the patient. Awareness of common relapse rates and patterns will reduce the possibility of misinterpreting a second primary as local progression (2). We find it productive to survey a scan blinded to the clinical history (Fig. 4.5) before a more directed analysis of the scan in light of the given clinical history. This approach minimizes "tunnel vision" and prevents a bias toward the significance of the findings. The reader should not be fooled by imaging artifacts (Fig. 4.6) (3), secondary phenomena (Fig. 4.7), or anatomic variants (Figs. 4.8–4.10) that might cause overstaging or prompt an unnecessary, possibly disastrous intervention. Careful analysis and description also prompts timely preoperative consultation with additional subspecialists when lesions, or their treatment, will compromise cosmetically or functionally sensitive structures.

The interpretation should address all the relevant issues at the primary site—tumor volume, local invasion, lymph node staging (4), comorbid signs, and unanticipated findings (Fig. 4.5)—in reference to the clinical course of disease. Often a conclusion cannot (and should not) be rendered without direct consultation or clinical correlation with the ordering physician(s). Occasionally, one must review the office chart directly. The final impression of the report should be succinct and unambiguous. Serious or unexpected abnormalities should prompt a phone

Patient Name ____________

MSK# ____________

NEURORAD/HEAD AND NECKRAD
CT PROTOCOLS

c- / c+
Ionic
Non Ionic

HEAD- Head holder, standard, occiput-palate, 22cm FOV (small FOV peds)

□ #1- Brain Routine

□ #2- Brain- PostOp, Trauma, Correlate

□ #3- Head/Orbits, Head/Sinuses (cover down to teeth for sinus)

□ #4- Head/IACs

□ #5- Stereotactic (Surgeons' Copy)

SINUS- Head Holder, Detail, 15cm FOV to include petrous apex, Cover down to Teeth

□ #1- Sinus- Axial Only 5x4 (3x2 if much dental amalgam)
□ #2- Sinus- Axial +/- Coronal (3x2 if much dental amalgam)

□ #3- Sinus -

Multiplanar -	Coronal	then	Axial
much amalgam	5x5	then	3x3
minml amalgam	3x3	then	5x5

ORBITS- Head Holder, Detail, 15cm FOV (12 Peds)

□ #1 Orbits- Axial only 3 x 2 or 1.5 x 1.5 (1.0 x 1.0)

□ #2 Orbits-

Multiplanar -	Coronal	then	Axial
much amalgam	5x5	then	3x2 (or 1.5 x 1.5)
minml amalgam	3x3	then	3x2 (or 1.5 x 1.5)

Petrous Temporal Bone- Head Holder (axials), EDGE Algorithm, 15cm FOV
retro to Detail Algorithm, 18cm FOV

Coronal 1.5 mm, 3x2mm, 5x4mm
Axial 3x2mm, 1.5x1.5mm

NECK PROTOCOLS- Table Top, Detail, 22cm FOV, Inject LEFT ARM.

□ #1- Routine Survey: PTB ← 5x5 → Hyoid ← 10x10 → Arch

□ #2- Nasophx (angle): Mid-Orbit Plane ← 5x5 → Hyoid ← 10x10 → Arch
Parotid (NO angle): Mid-Orbit Plane ← 5x5 → Hyoid ← 10x10 → Arch

□ #3- Oral/Tongue/FOM: EAC ← 5x5 → larynx ← 10x10 → Arch (REANGLE PRN)

FOR #4 AND #5 NECK - ORAL CONTRAST - ESOPHACAT (or standard as tolerated)

□ #4- Larynx/Pyriform: EAC ← 5x5 → Carina PLUS SFOV Laynx @ 3x2mm (or 1.5mm)

□ #5- (para)Thyroid: PreContrast - Hyoid ← 10x10 → Carina
PostContrast - EAC ← 5x5 → Carina (or bottom of mass)

□ #6- Brachial Plexus: Overlapping small (5x5) and large (10x10) FOV from C-¾ to T-4

□ **MANDIBLE** 1:1 PROTOCOL 25cm FOV, BONE Algorithm, Parallel to Lower Edge
5x5mm or 3x3mm PRINT "OR COPY" of body only @ 1.33 mag on 2/1 print format

□ **DENTA SCAN** - Helical 1mm x 1mm 15 FOV - no angle; chin vertical
Bone - retro std

____
RADIOLOGIST

A

Figure 4.2 Imaging protocols. **A:** Memorial Sloan-Kettering Cancer Center (MSKCC) computed tomography protocol worksheet. *(continued)*

MSKCC Division of Neuroradiology
MR Imaging Protocols

HEAD:

MODIFIED #1 BRAIN #1 HEAD

#2 BRAIN Frontal Parietal POST MOD #2 F P
Temporal Occipital FOSSA T O

#3 BRAIN (midline) 3/1peds 4/1adults HiRes T-2

SELLA/PITUITARY

HEAD/NECK:

HEAD/ORBITS IAC PARANASAL

NASOPHARYNX PTB TONGUE/ORAL CAVITY

MODIFIED B. PLEX/THYROID

MRA: NECK COIL -- 2D TOF BIFURCATION TO SKULL BASE
3D PC @ BIFURCATION
HEAD COIL -- 3DTOF CIRCLE OF WILLIS
3DPC CIRCLE OF WILLIS - VENC = _____
3DPC POST FOSSA - VENC = _____
2DPC SAGITTAL SINUS

SPINE:
CERVICAL // EXT'd CERV -- _____ // THORACIC // _____--EXT'd LSS // LSS

TOTAL SPINE- START UPPER LOWER

GAD TOTAL SPINE - BASELINE Upper s -- Lower s/c -- Upper c
FOLLOW UP Lower s -- Upper s/c -- Lower c
GAD LSS lepto style

PLEXUS
BRACHIAL PLEX - ATT'N R/L LUMBAR PLEXUS -- ATT'N R/L

GAD BRACH PLX -- R/L GAD LUMB PLEX -- R/L

HYBRID B PLEX / C-SPINE R/L GAD HYB L PLX/L-SPINE R/L

B

Figure 4.2 (continued) **B:** MSKCC magnetic resonance imaging protocol worksheet. *EAC,* external auditory canal; *FOV,* field of view; *IAC,* internal auditory canal; *LSS,* lumbosacral spine; *PTB,* petrous temporal bone; *SFOV,* small field of view.

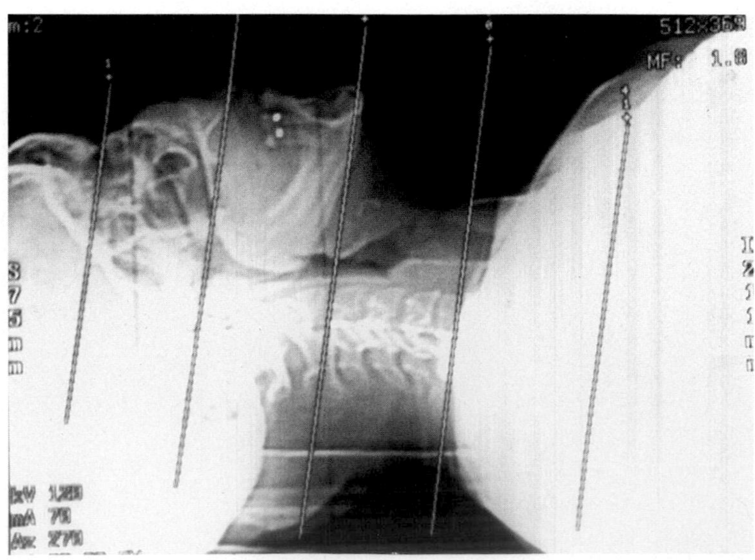

Figure 4.3 Standard axial prescription of computed tomography scan that covers the skull base to the superior mediastinum. Head is neutral. Not all sections are shown. Images usually are 5-mm thick through the neck.

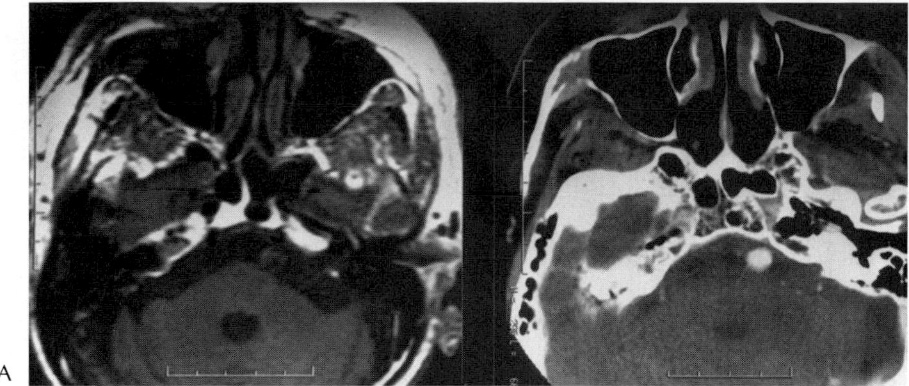

Figure 4.4 Correlation of different imaging modalities. Axial magnetic resonance imaging **(A)** and computed tomography **(B)** of the same patient before and after treatment interval, showing the value of being able to correlate between different modalities at different times if there are parallels in design of imaging protocols.

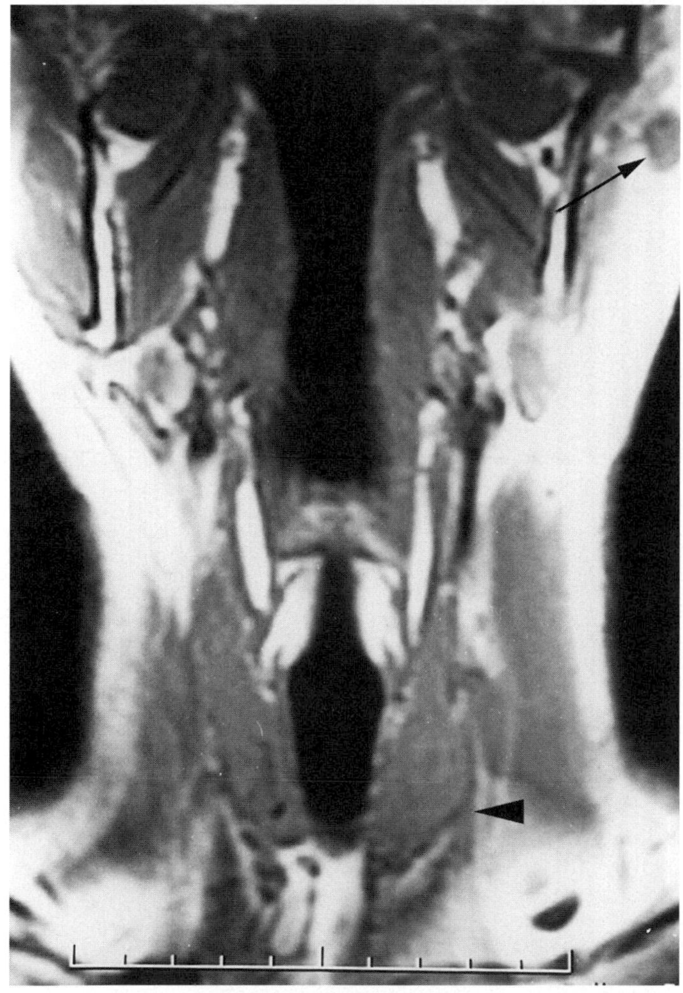

Figure 4.5 Survey coronal (T1-weighted) view of the neck for adenopathy before scan of lesion in left parotid gland (*arrow*), revealing an additional lesion in the left lobe of the thyroid gland (*arrowhead*). The index parotid gland lesion proved to be benign hyperplasia, whereas the thyroid contained papillary cancer.

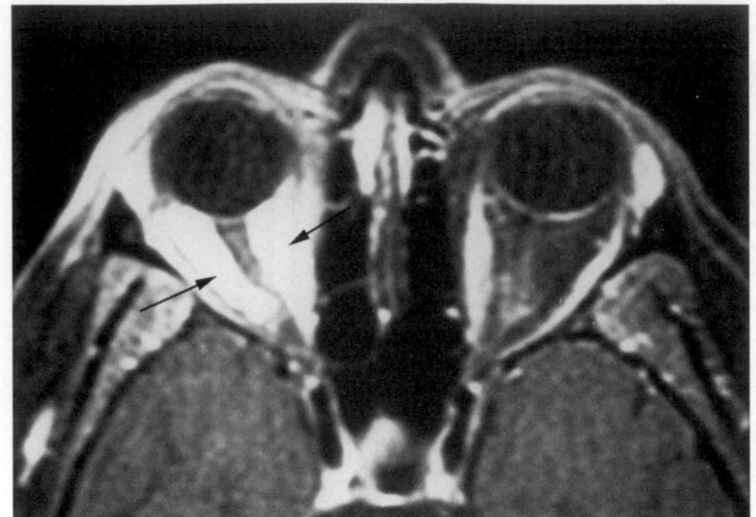

A

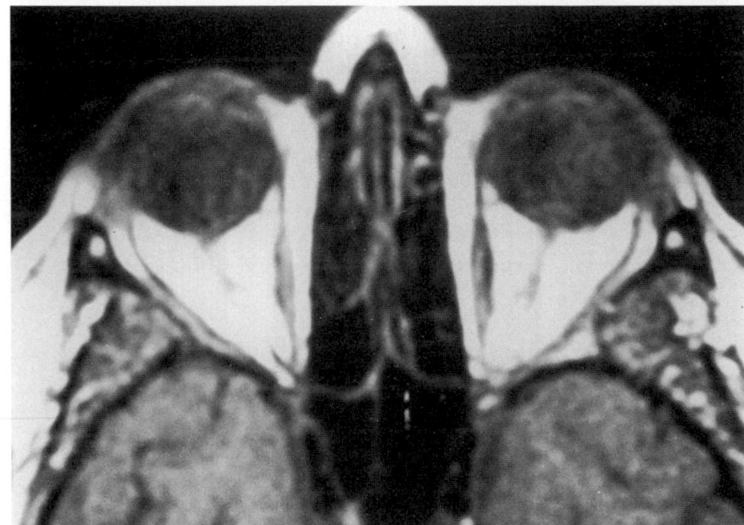

B

Figure 4.6 Imaging artifacts. **A:** Artifactual hyperintensity of right retrobulbar compartment (*arrows*) on fat-suppressed version of axial contrast-enhanced, T1-weighted magnetic resonance imaging. **B:** Normal appearance confirmed by precontrast axial T1-weighted view without fat suppression.

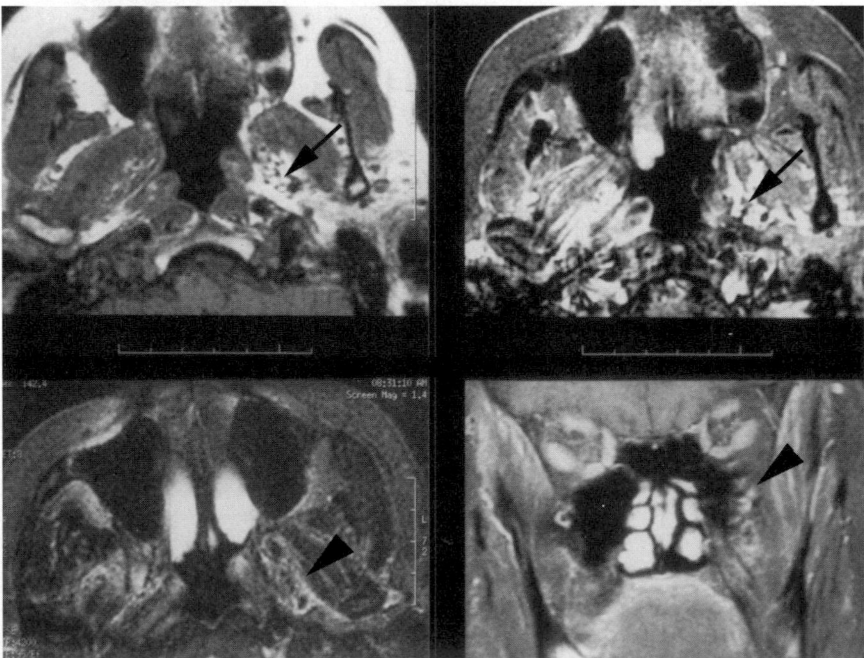

Figure 4.7 Variant anatomy of parapharyngeal space. **Clockwise from top left:** Magnetic resonance imaging (MRI) in axial T1-weighted; fat-suppressed axial contrast enhanced; T1-weighted and coronal T1-weighted and axial T2-weighted MRI views; showing pseudomass of fatty atrophy (*arrows*) of left lateral pterygoid muscle, which suppresses on T2- and T1-weighted series (*arrowheads*).

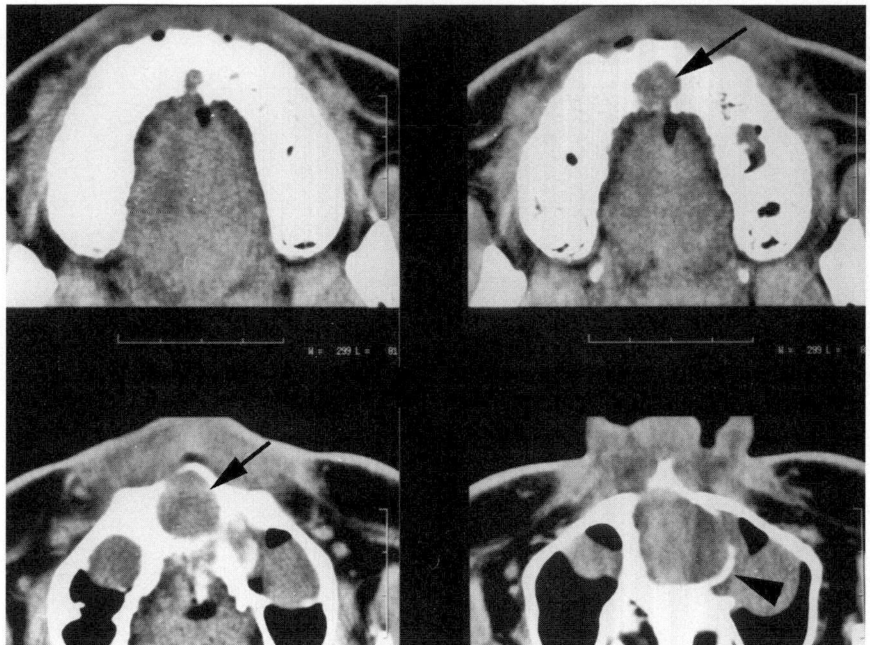

Figure 4.8 Developmental anomaly presenting as a nasal cavity mass. Contrast-enhanced axial views of a fissural cyst (*arrows*) bulging across the left nasal cavity, deforming the party wall of the antrum (*arrowhead*).

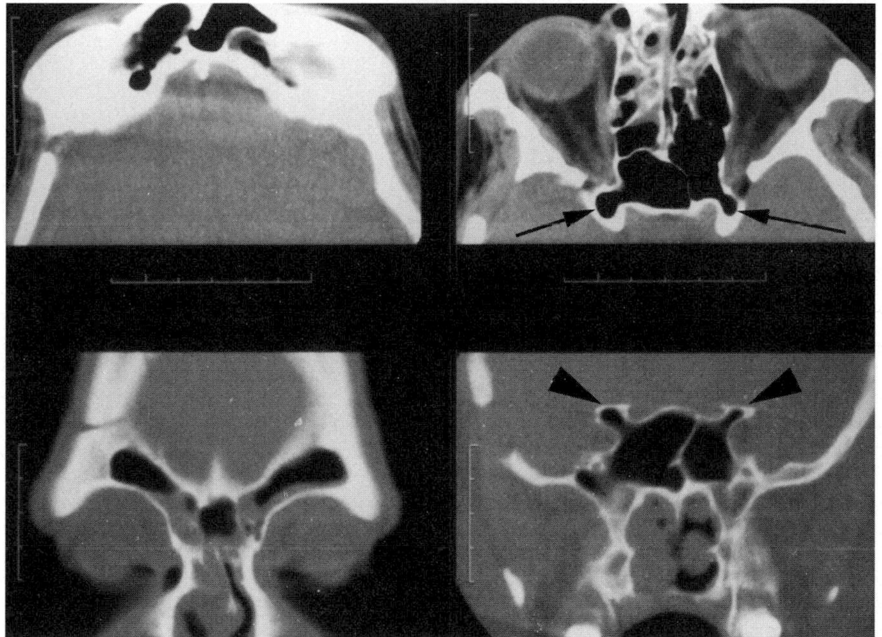

Figure 4.9 Developmental variant aeration of both anterior clinoid processes in the axial (*arrows*) and direct coronal (*arrowheads*) plane in a patient after prior frontotemporal craniotomy.

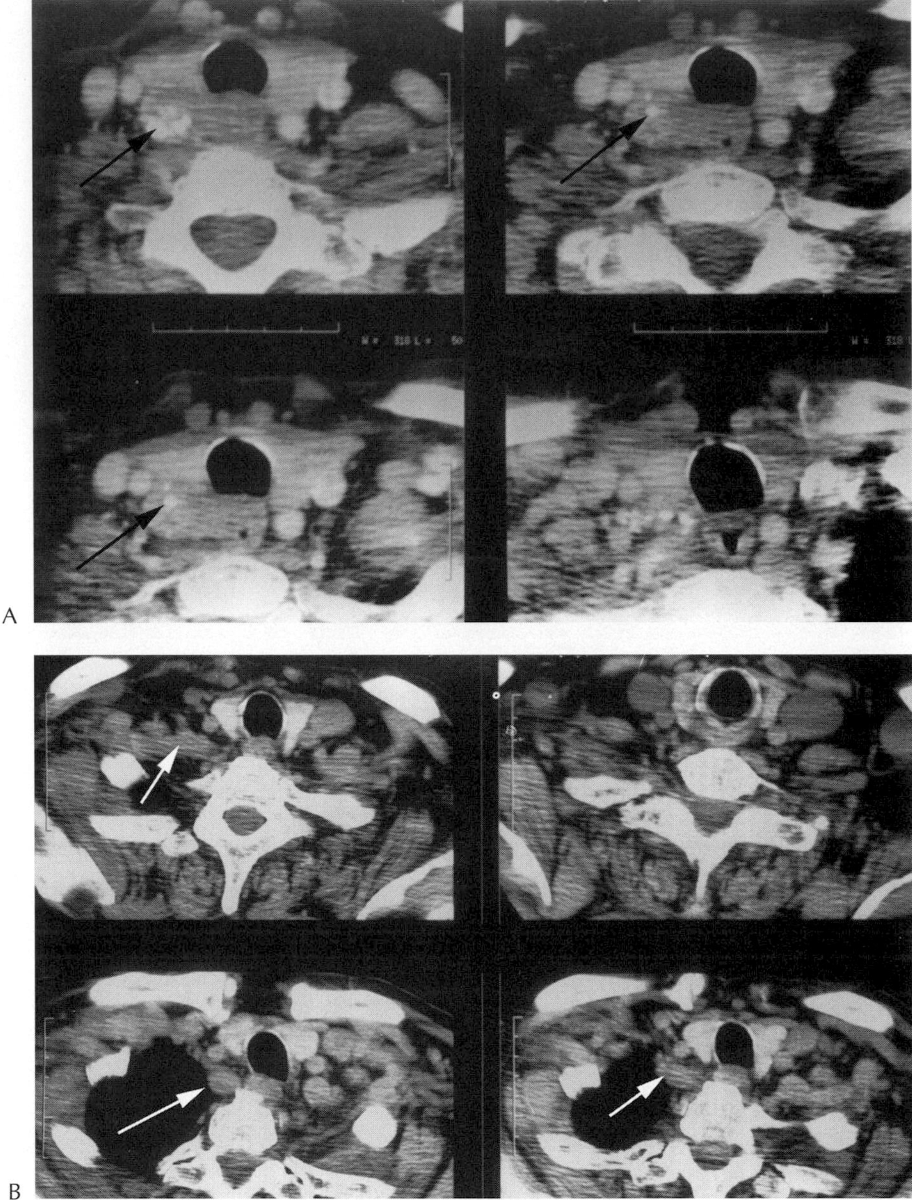

Figure 4.10 Imaging of variant pseudomass. **A:** Developmental variant pseudomass. Contrast-enhanced axial computed tomography (CT) images through neck base show value of intravenous contrast confirming aberrant right subclavian artery (*arrows*) masquerading as a calcified mass of the right lobe of thyroid gland. **B:** Developmental variant producing pseudomass. Serial contrast-enhanced axial CT through inlet showing pseudomasses of right tracheoesophageal groove due to aberrant right subclavian artery (*arrows*).

call to the appropriate party. Graphic notations in the chart from the radiologist can promote simple and accurate information within the interdisciplinary team (Fig. 4.11). One must be keenly aware of the standard appearances of operative reconstructions to maximize the potential for detecting subclinical recurrences (5). Comparison to prior scans or correlation with other concurrent imaging modalities is essential and should be performed by the imaging subspecialist. Correlating the reports from prior and current scans can give a false impression of the significance of reported findings. The language used in the report is pivotal when a potential abnormality has been identified. The comment "further evaluation" has a connotation very different from "follow-up evaluation." *Follow-up evaluation* implies that in the absence of an adequate comparison examination, the significance of a finding cannot be known until the next interval scan. *Further evaluation* implies that a finding is suspicious enough to warrant additional imaging to better characterize its significance. When further evaluation by a certain modality is suggested, anticipated possibilities must be specified so that the correct technique is applied to answer a specific question.

Follow-up surveillance-type scanning requires consistency of scan techniques between appointments to determine early changes. Quality control is a constant process, and new technical staff members require careful in-service training. We use our report not only to convey results but also to indicate the scan protocol that was used or whether a different protocol may be necessary at the next imaging interval.

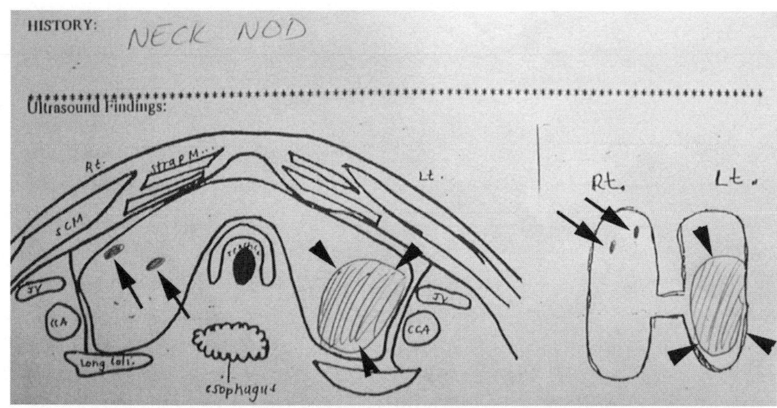

A

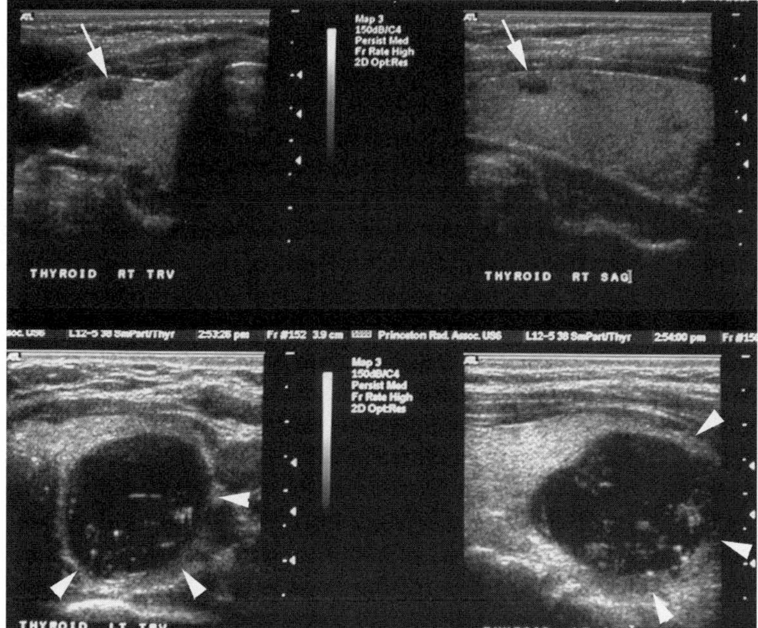

B

Figure 4.11 Thyroid worksheet. **A:** Worksheet shows position of lesions in the axial (left) and coronal (right) portrayal. **B:** High-resolution sonogram of the thyroid gland. Top panel shows right lobe with small nodule at upper pole (*white arrows*) in axial (left) and sagittal (right) planes. Bottom panel shows left lobe with complex cyst expanding the lower pole in axial (left) and sagittal (right) planes.

CHOICE OF MODALITY

Several considerations are available in selecting the modality with which to investigate a head and neck disorder. The primary consideration is the condition of the patient. Most patients are ambulatory and free of debilitating pain and present with stable respiratory status. However, these latter situations are atypical in patients with advanced lesions or in the immediate postoperative condition. Patients should be prepared properly before transfer to radiology and should be capable of providing consent for their scans and procedures. It is not uncommon to encounter a patient from a clinic who is too uncomfortable for scanning because of a preceding biopsy.

Simple radiographic examinations are associated with few, if any, contraindications. These roentgenograms can be obtained at the bedside and in the operating room and require minimal patient cooperation. The exposures are brief (split-second) and therefore less susceptible to patient motion. The information they provide is simple but vital and reassuring (e.g., tube placement, abnormal sponge count, and pneumothorax). To obtain more detailed information, the patient has to be stabilized and cooperative for transfer to an imaging suite and positioning on an imaging table.

Fluoroscopic examinations are supervised by a physician, and the safety of the patient is balanced against the need for obtaining results from the test. Fluoroscopically guided therapeutic procedures require a cooperative patient to allow safe completion of the procedure; angiographic examinations should not be attempted on uncooperative patients. The most common problem contributing to motion is the patient's inability to manage secretions, particularly in the standard supine imaging position (Fig. 4.12). This results in swallowing motion artifact, which degrades evaluation of structures related to the oral cavity and pharynx and larynx.

Cross-sectional examinations require cooperative patients for a number of reasons. Each individual CT section requires 1 to 2 seconds' exposure for adequate image formation. Detailed examinations require several thin sections, which increase the scan time and therefore the risk that the patient will move or swallow during the examination. This activity results in a less-than-diagnostic examination but also results in image misregistration, compromising the completeness of the study and producing serious distortion of any attempted reformatted projection.

Patient and structural motion are an even greater problem with MRI. Conventional imaging sequences require 2 to 3 minutes of scan time for adequate spatial resolution. Fast imaging techniques vary, depending on the type of scanner,

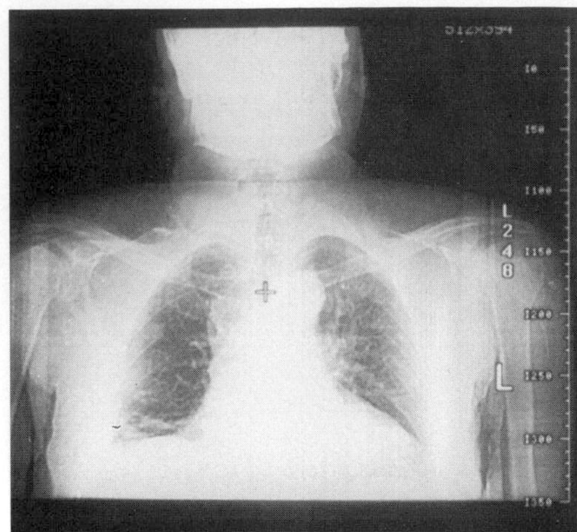

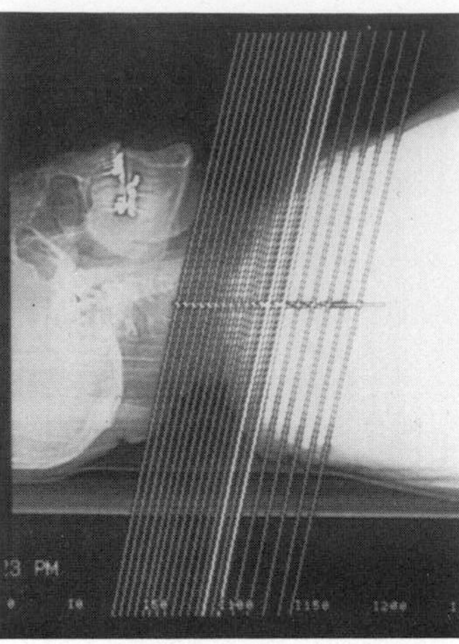

Figure 4.12 Frontal and lateral "scout" images from which scans are prescribed. **Right:** A computed tomography protocol for disorders involving the thoracic inlet or brachial plexus, where thin, small field-of-view sections of the central compartment are overlapped by thicker large field-of-view sections that cover the supraclavicular and axillary spaces with less beam-hardening artifact.

but can be performed in less than a minute, with a corresponding loss of spatial resolution and increase in imaging artifacts. Unlike the CT process, wherein an individual section can be repeated in a few seconds, the entire MRI sequence is degraded by intermittent motion, and the success of a repeat sequence will not be known until it is repeated entirely. Regardless of the modality used, any baseline examination obtained should be comprehensive so as to properly diagnose and stage a lesion or lesions, particularly when the consultation is generated by a symptom rather than by a palpable abnormality (Fig. 4.13).

COMPUTED TOMOGRAPHY

Aside from the foregoing considerations, the most common choice for imaging of head and neck disorders is CT or MRI. The main advantage of CT is the speed at which patients can be scanned and rescanned. Additional advantages are the widespread availability of CT scanners, the relative comparability of CTs from different institutions, and the clinical acceptance of CT images, the appearance of which has not changed substantially over the years. Given the wide variety of sequences available with MRI, CT might be characterized more accurately as more

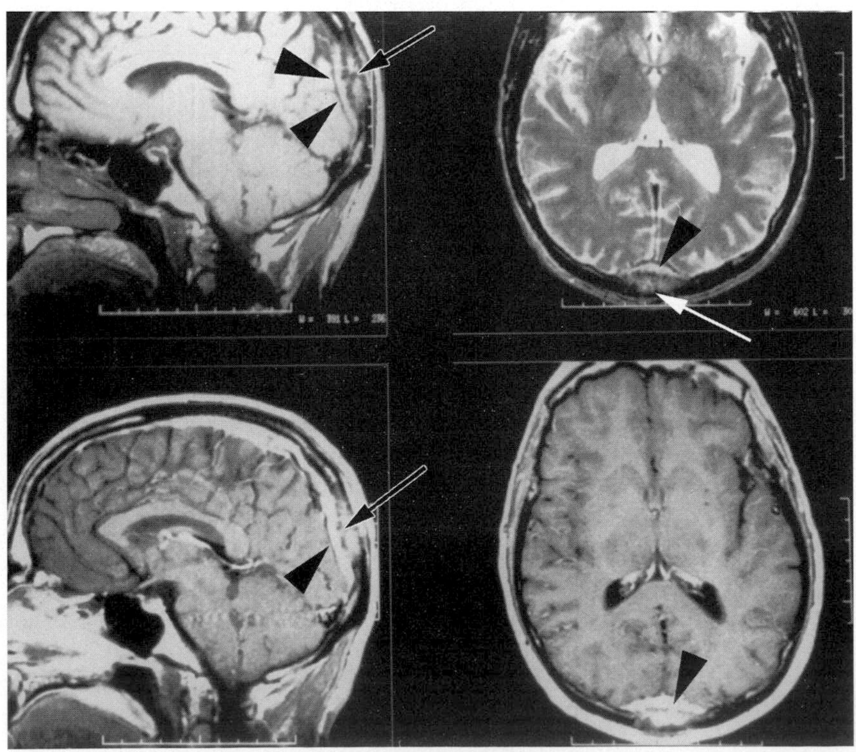

Figure 4.13 Baseline examinations should be comprehensive. Papilledema and visual decline prompted request for orbital magnetic resonance imaging (MRI). Sagittal and axial MRI reveal occipital bone metastasis (*arrows*) with epidural component (*arrowheads*) compromising the distal superior sagittal sinus, a remote cause of papilledema.

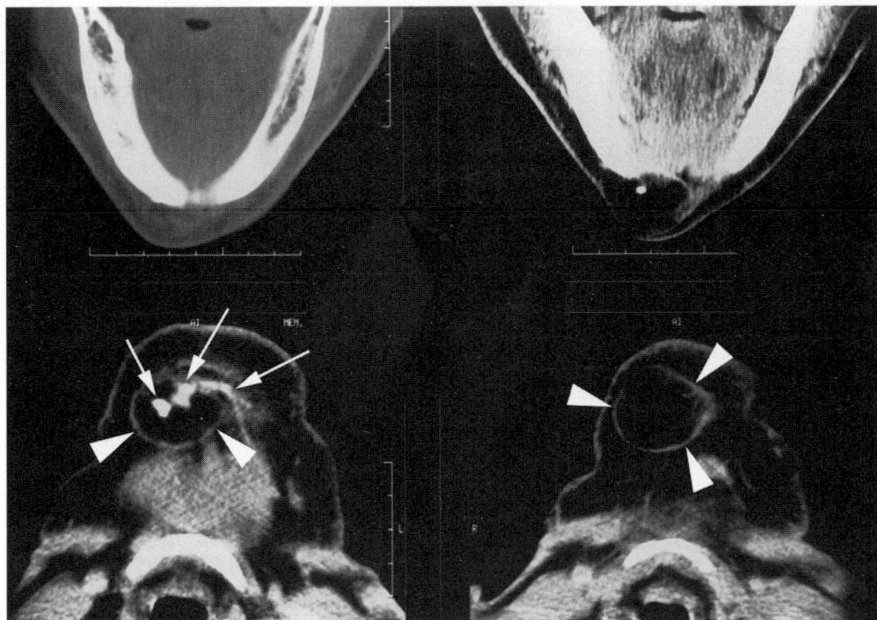

Figure 4.14 Limited but capable tissue resolution of computed tomography (CT). Semicoronal contrast-enhanced CT excludes mandibular or floor-of-mouth origin of submental mass. Axial CT shows capacity of CT to resolve the calcium (*short arrow*), soft-tissue (*long arrow*), and fat components surrounded by a capsule (*arrowheads*) of a dermoid lesion.

efficient, consisting only of precontrast or postcontrast series, usually limited to the axial plane. Few lesions can be diagnosed as to histology or grade by cross-sectional imaging before resection (Fig. 4.14). Tissue discrimination with CT, although less sensitive than MRI, is based on the attenuation by a spectrum of several different tissue densities. They simply are divided into air, fat, soft tissue, and bone (calcium). The advent of intensity modulated radiation therapy (IMRT) has increased the significance of CT for treatment planning (6), therefore requiring continued recognition of anatomic and pathologic variations revealed by CT. Proper processing of CT data through computer algorithms, followed by appropriate photographic "window-level" settings, is necessary to reveal minor abnormalities and the true extent of disease. CT staff must be trained to perform these functions routinely.

Most CT scans are accomplished with axial scans of the neck at 3- to 5-mm section thickness and axial (with or without coronal) images of the primary site at 2- to 3-mm section thickness. Few sites require 1.0- to 1.5-mm section thickness.

Generally, the procedure starts with CT as the primary modality in patients who can tolerate iodinated intravenous contrast. The CT examination addresses the most common issues for staging of the primary site and is an adjunct for evaluation of the neck (Fig. 4.15). In addition to lymph node staging CT has a strong negative predictive value for invasion of the prevertebral muscle plane (7). Any question not addressed fully by the initial comprehensive CT scan can be answered by MRI (8). Furthermore, the MRI can be a more focused examination (9) in the face of the preceding CT results.

If a patient cannot tolerate MRI, a more detailed CT examination may be appropriate. MRI has less of the previously touted advantage of multiplanarity over CT now that later-generation CT scanners have the ability to scan larger areas with thin, often overlapping or helical (spiral) sections that provide robust data sets. Reformatted coronal and sagittal projections, or projections in every imaginable plane, are possible with on-board computer-based CT consoles or off-board workstations (Figs. 4.16 and 4.17). Although CT can resolve the basic tissue densities within the body (Fig. 4.14), generally it requires intravenous contrast to maximize tissue contrast. Intravenous contrast enhances blood vessels intensely but also improves discrimination among the soft tissues and fascial planes in the neck. Additional postbolus delayed images are useful in revealing intrinsic masses of solid organs such as salivary neoplasms (10). Careful application of intravenous contrast is recommended for CT scans of certain regions prone to artifacts such as the thoracic inlet (Fig. 4.18). Healthy renal status is the

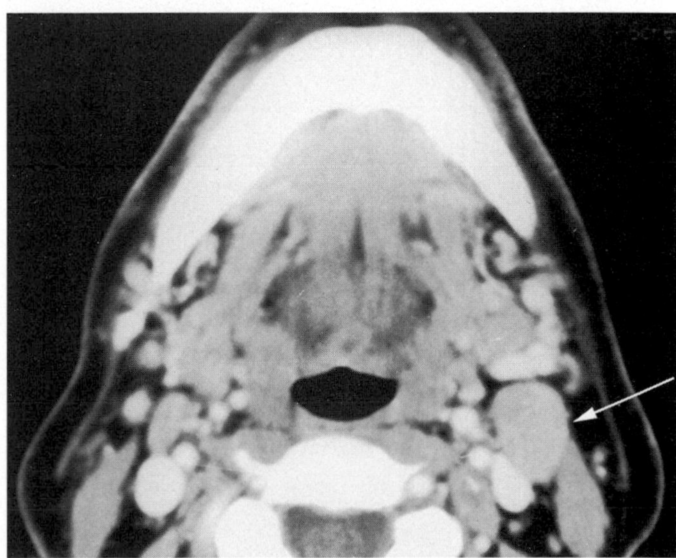

Figure 4.15 Contrast-enhanced axial computed tomography scan showing an enlarged left level II lymph node (*arrow*) that is nearly isodense to muscle.

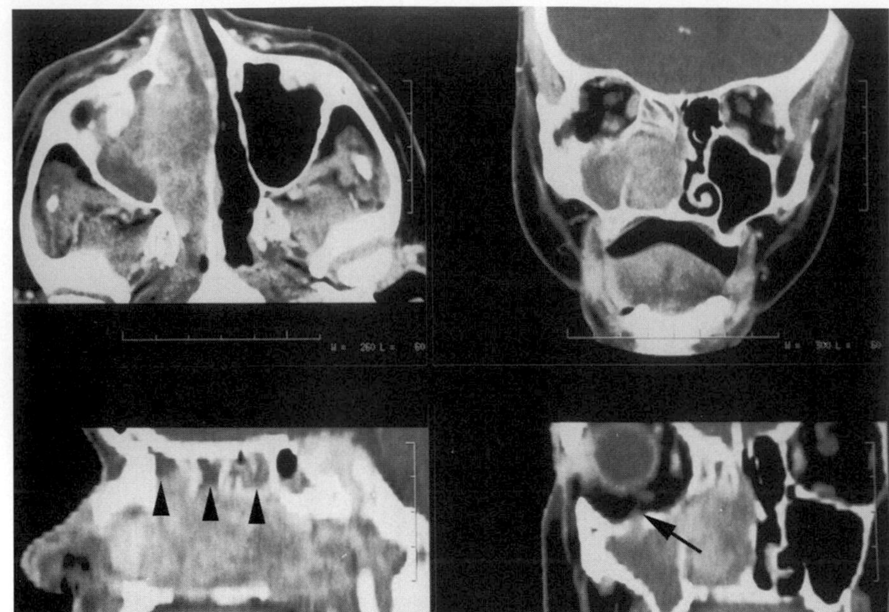

Figure 4.16 Value of reformatted views. Direct coronal and axial contrast-enhanced computed tomography of sinuses in a cooperative patient. Reformatted coronal view (**bottom**) demonstrates involvement of infraorbital groove (*arrow*) as well as the direct coronal view (**top**). The reformatted parasagittal view shows tumor infiltration limited to the lower segment of the ethmoid complex (*arrowheads*).

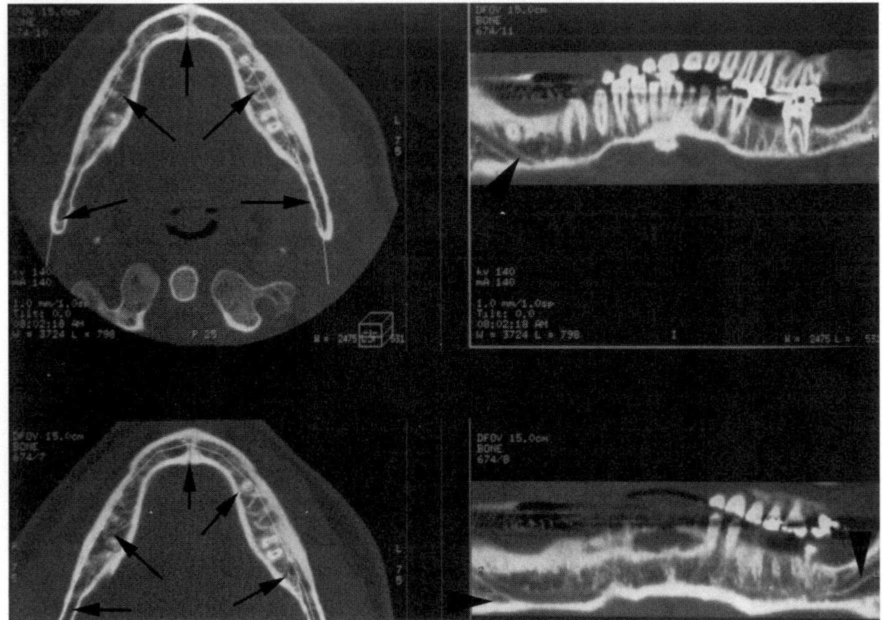

Figure 4.17 Bone window of panoramic views of the mandible (**right**) at two different positions, as shown from corresponding manual tracing (*arrows*) on the axial view (**left**). These views show the relationship of the tooth roots to the cancellous bone and alveolar canal (*arrowheads*). (DentaScan, GE Medical Systems, Milwaukee, Wis.)

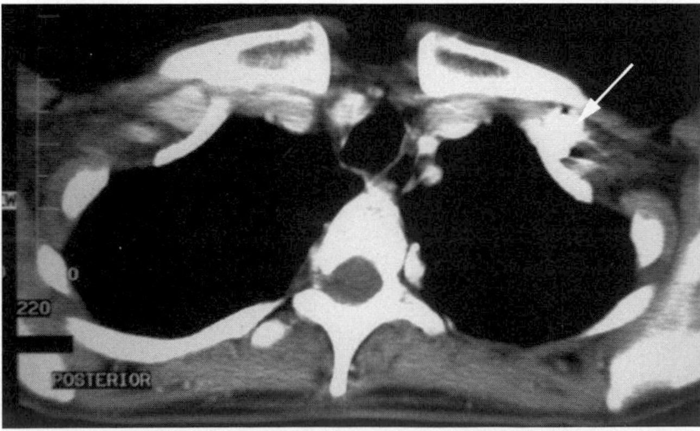

Figure 4.18 Contrast technique. Enhanced axial image through the thoracic inlet with detailed evaluation of anatomy. Saline push at end of injection prevents streak artifact from densely opacified left subclavian vein (*arrow*).

requirement for contrast excretion. Coordination with dialysis is necessary for end-stage patients who can manage the fluid load. Contrast should not be administered to patients with partly compromised or declining renal function.

For evaluation of the skull base, the alternate recommendation of modalities must be determined for each case. This issue requires consideration of two factors. The most important is determining the component of the bone that is at risk. Although CT is the better modality for evaluation of cortical bone and can demonstrate permeative destruction of cancellous bone, MRI is more sensitive to disturbance in signal related to early disease within the marrow space of cancellous bone. The second factor to consider is the mechanism of osseous involvement. Squamous cancer usually causes cortical destruction or erosion along a front of growth, a condition readily identified with appropriate CT technique. Imaging of the lingual plate of the mandible, the orbital floor, and the anterior and central skull base requires high-resolution CT. In most sites CT is more specific but MRI has a strong negative predictive value (11) that perhaps replaces CT when negative.

Other histopathologic processes have a different, more permeative mechanism involving both sides of an osseous barrier, with little (if any) cortical bone change. Lymphoma, adenocarcinoma, and esthesioneuroblastoma therefore require MRI for complete evaluation.

Bone detail is translated readily from CT data set to accurate three-dimensional models. Simple two-dimensional renderings of tumor outlines can be projected onto the frontal and lateral scout images (Figs. 4.19 and 4.20) to assist in radiation treatment planning around vital radiosensitive structures. Finally, CT provides an excellent environment for imaging-guided percutaneous biopsy and aspiration or pain management procedures. CT also has applications for assisting in the more precise placement of brachytherapy catheters at the nasopharynx (12).

MAGNETIC RESONANCE IMAGING

The advantages of MRI are several, and the capabilities of MRI scanners will continue to increase well beyond the potential for improvement of CT. The immediate but less obvious feature is that many head and neck lesions can be staged with MRI without the requirement for intravenous contrast (as with CT) (13). Of course, contrast-enhanced images lend additional confidence to the interpretation of the MRI scan (14). MRI has become more integral in pretreatment baseline staging of some head and neck cancers with the model being nasopharyngeal cancer (15).

An example of the role of noncontrast-enhanced MRI is correlation with radionuclide scans of the neck and upper mediastinum in patients being followed for thyroid cancer (16). The capacity of the computers in the MRI scanner to modify the outgoing or incoming signal from the patient provides a nearly infinite variety of possible sequences for evaluating the soft tissues of the aerodigestive tract and related organ systems. This variety may be the reason why nonradiologists are less comfortable looking at the scans in their offices, especially when the techniques and equipment vary from office to office. Imaging departments must strike a balance between implementing evolving improvements and maintaining, over time, a consistency between scans that the entire interdisciplinary team must understand. Even without intravenous contrast, MRI provides superior contrast resolution between different tissue types in the body (13), neoplastic and otherwise. This capability is especially true at the time of initial staging, before any intervention or treatment.

Once surgery and radiation therapy have occurred, the signal abnormalities on MRI become more confluent, and distinguishing what might be residue or recurrent disease as a group from changes related to treatment becomes more challenging (17). Contrast-enhanced series, usually with background or fat

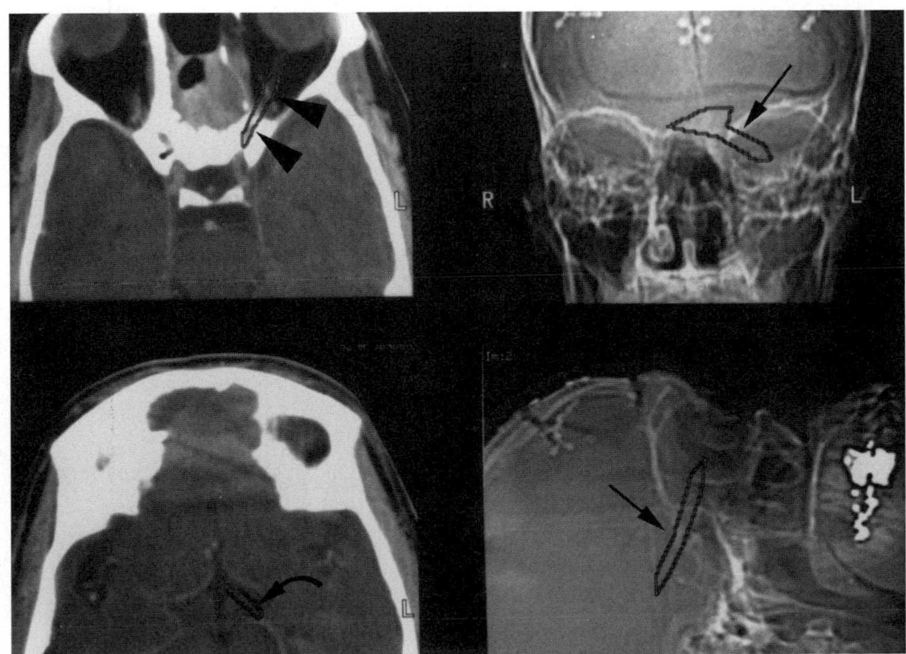

Figure 4.19 Computed tomography (CT) for treatment planning. Enhanced axial CT images locate segments of the optic nerves (*arrowheads*), chiasm, and tracts (*curved arrow*), which are transposed to scout frontal and lateral views (*arrows*) with "correlate" function to help to plan treatment portals.

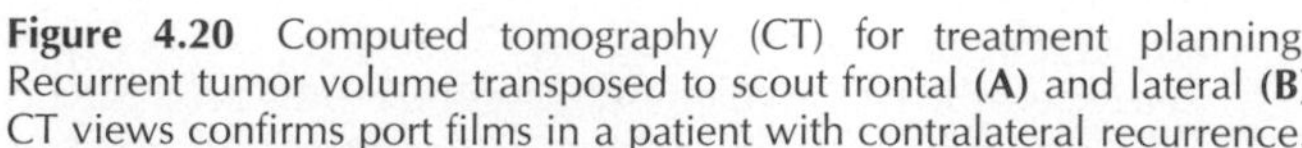

Figure 4.20 Computed tomography (CT) for treatment planning. Recurrent tumor volume transposed to scout frontal **(A)** and lateral **(B)** CT views confirms port films in a patient with contralateral recurrence.

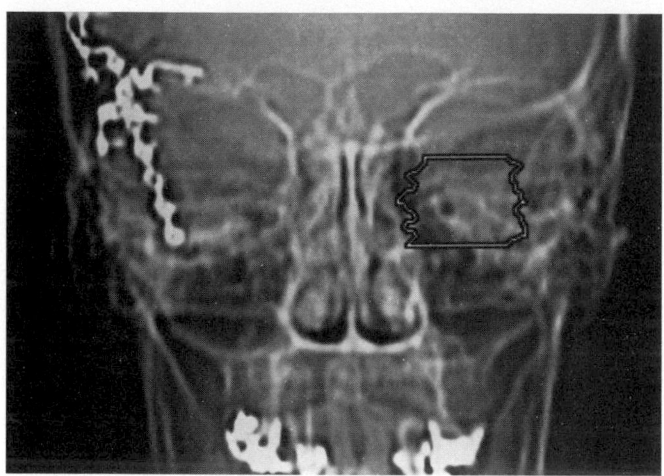

A

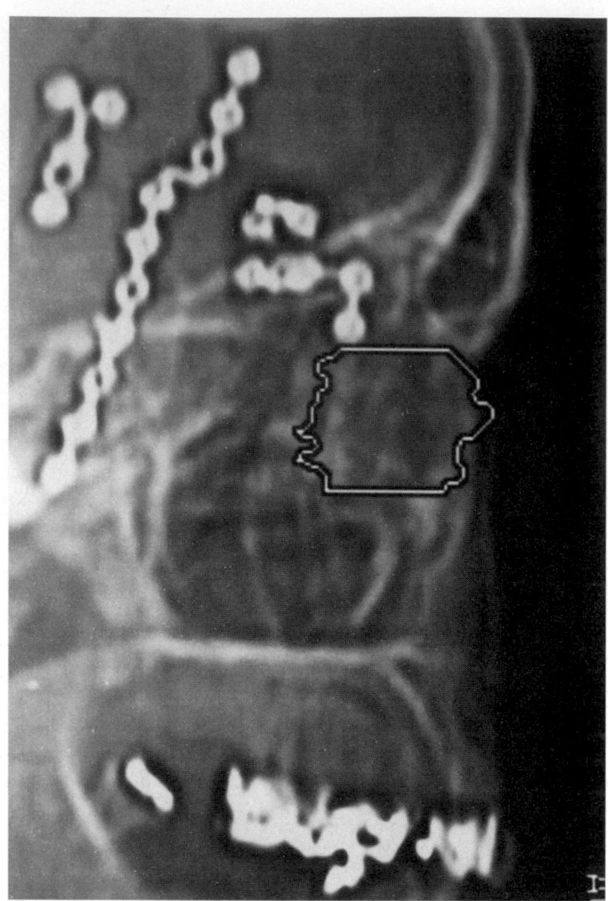

B

suppression, lengthen the MRI scan time to this end. Comparison with prior scans becomes crucial during follow-up, but a familiarity with the postoperative appearance of various primary sites (5,18) is necessary if one is to make useful comments about the first baseline conducted after surgery (Fig. 4.21). Imaging where a recurrence in any given patient will occur becomes more difficult over time, and revisiting the original images is recommended even if no apparent change occurs in a patient's more recent scans.

The freedom to select any imaging plane with MRI allows the imaging subspecialist to choose the projection along which disease extension is demonstrated best. This capability is especially useful at the fissures and foramina of the skull base. Even greater spatial resolution can be achieved with the use of devices called *surface coils*. Rather than receiving and resolving signal from a large region of the head or neck, the scanner can bring all the resolution to bear on the complexity of a smaller structure by the application of a small receiver coil to the surface of the body over the region of interest (Fig. 4.22). This technique is particularly helpful for superficial lesions with infiltrating deep components.

Magnetic resonance scanners also have the capacity to evaluate some physiologic parameters. The most widely known is magnetic resonance angiography. Modification of spin-echo and (more commonly) gradient-echo sequences allows one to noninvasively survey arterial or venous blood flow without

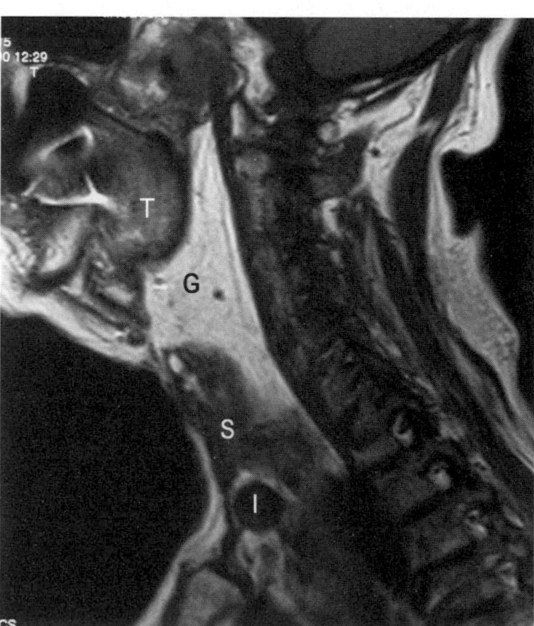

Figure 4.21 Postoperative imaging. Sagittal T1 magnetic resonance imaging of neck after laryngectomy and pharyngeal reconstruction. Note fat of myocutaneous free flap (*G*) situated below base-of-tongue anastomosis (*T*) above stoma (*S*) and innominate artery (*I*).

A

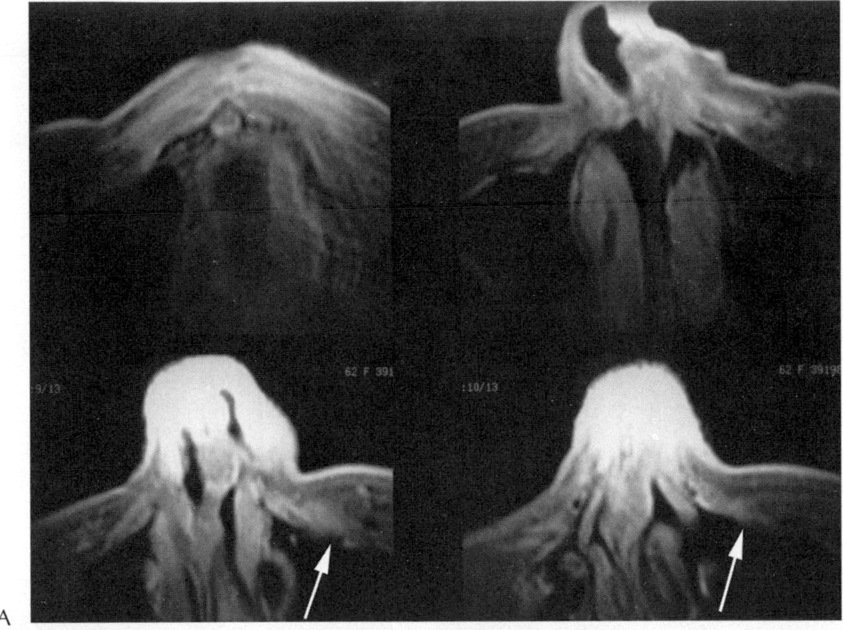

B

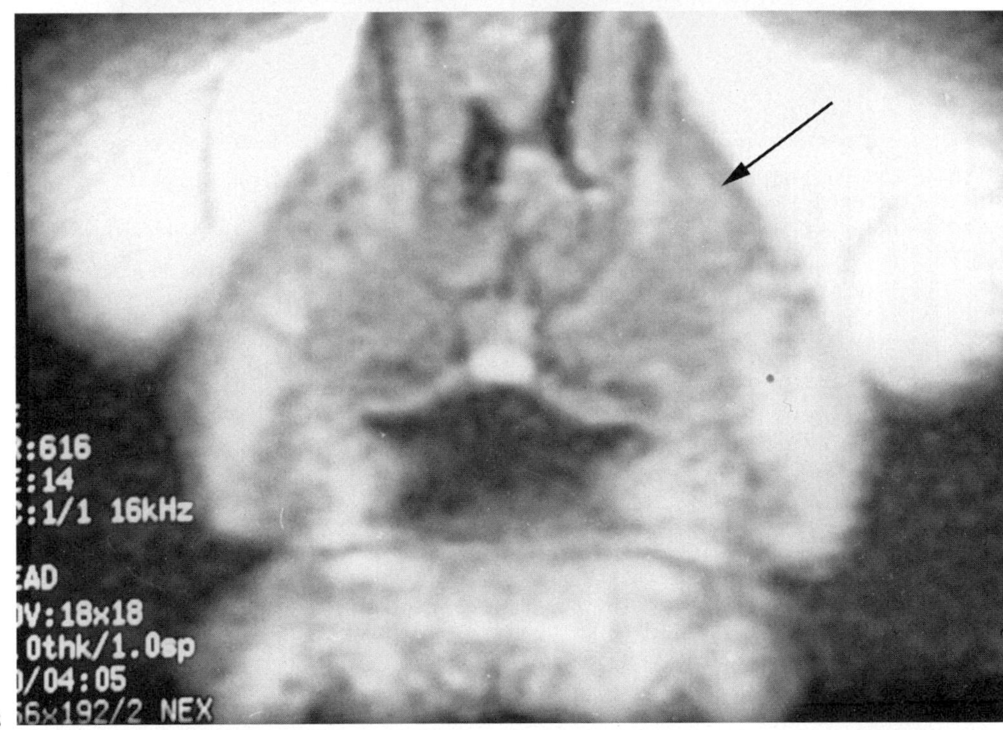

Figure 4.22 Value of surface coil scan. Serial contrast-enhanced, axial, T1-weighted views **(A)** show greater resolution of left premaxillary infiltration (*arrows*) from nasal skin cancer than does magnified coronal T1-weighted view from **(B)** head coil segment of scan (*arrow*).

(see Fig. 28.27B) or with (Fig. 4.23) intravenous contrast. The more familiar conventional spin-echo technique demonstrates the tissue structures surrounding vessels better than the intraluminal contents, which are a signal void (Fig. 4.24). Gradient-echo sequences highlight blood flow as a bright signal presence and allow an adjustable degree of adjacent tissue discrimination or suppression. This simple noninvasive evaluation, however, does not provide all the information that catheter angiography reveals. Such features as vascularity, arteriovenous shunting, relative contribution of multiple feeding vessels, and intraluminal (back) pressure are not obtained. Though these elements may require catheter angiography, the duration of the angiogram can be abbreviated by information gained from the preceding magnetic resonance angiography (19).

Another capability of the MRI scanner is magnetic resonance spectroscopy. The original thrust of clinical MRI development was the hope of determining the presence or absence of disease by the signal characteristics of the tissue. Recent *in vitro* investi-

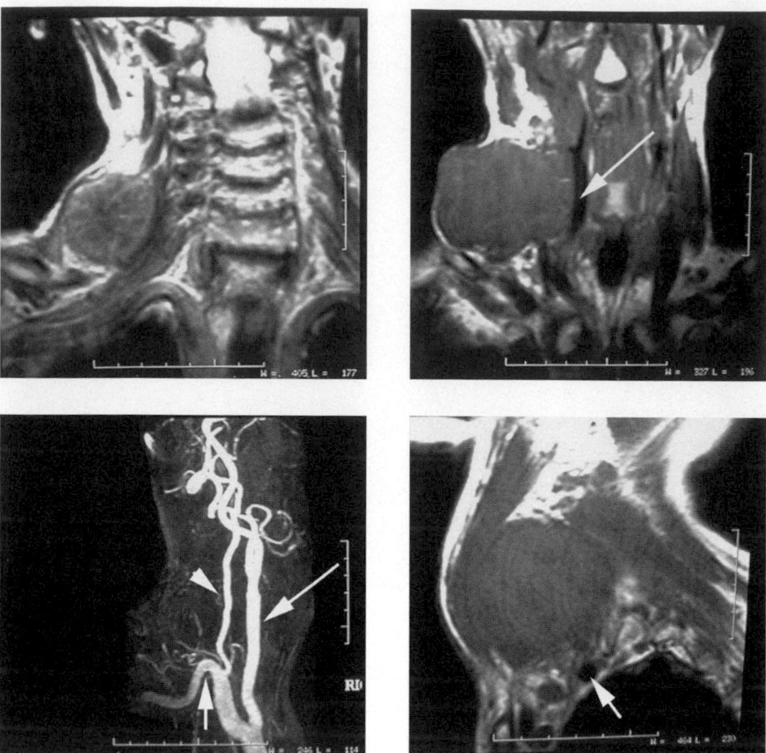

Figure 4.23 Magnetic resonance angiography (MRA). **Clockwise from top left:** T2 coronal, T1 coronal, T1 sagittal, and projected image from MRA show large mass at base of right neck displacing the common carotid artery (CCA) (*long arrow*), but not compromising the CCA or subclavian artery (*short arrow*) or the vertebral artery (*arrowhead*).

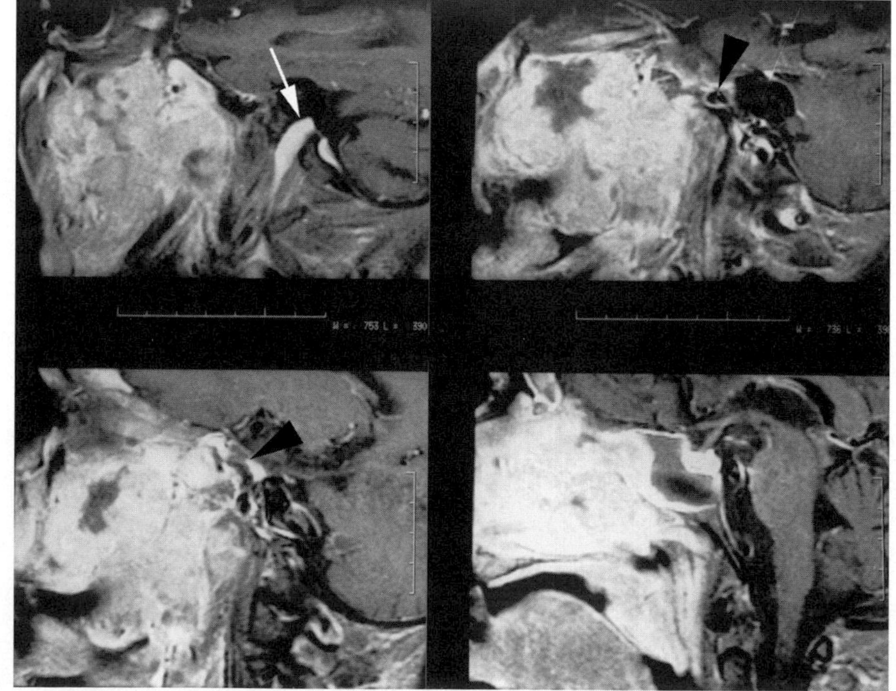

A

Figure 4.24 **A:** Vascular visualization on conventional magnetic resonance imaging.

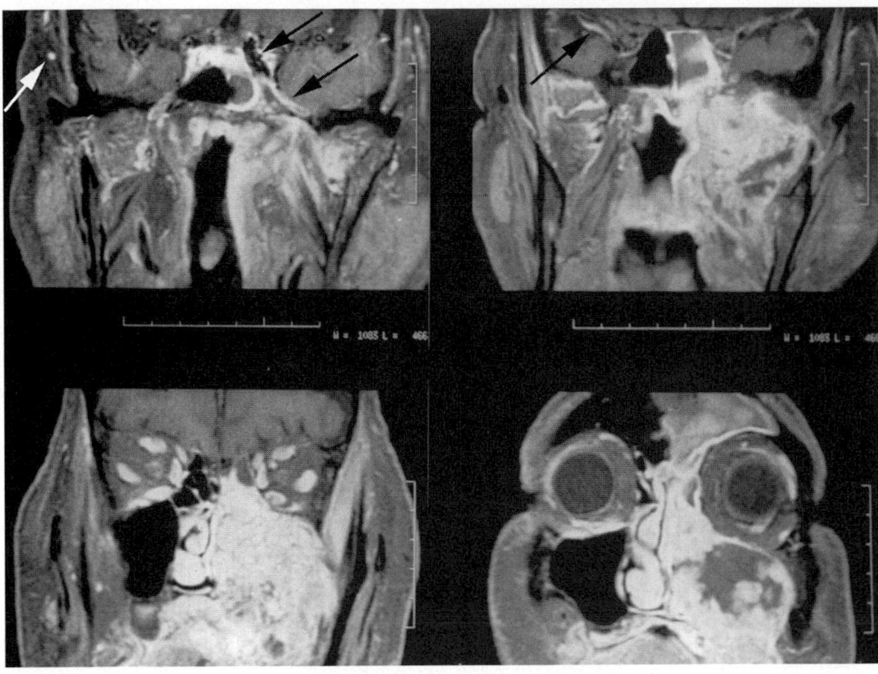

B

Figure 4.24 (continued) B: Serial sagittal, contrast-enhanced, T1-weighted views of advanced sinonasal tumor shown in coronal contrast series. Venous blood is bright (*arrows*) owing to slow velocity. Internal carotid signal is void owing to high velocity (*arrowheads*).

gations have suggested that the most reliable proton magnetic resonance spectroscopy (^{1}H-MRS) markers, which can distinguish squamous cell carcinoma (SCC) from normal muscle of the extracranial head and neck, are the relative levels of choline (Cho) and creatine (Cr) (20,21). Elevation of the Cho/Cr ratio appears to be a consistent finding for SCC and has also been identified in analysis of various SCC cell cultures and SCC containing cervical metastatic lymph nodes (20). These *in vitro* findings have been demonstrated in *in vivo* studies performed in patients with SCC of the extracranial head and neck. Analysis with ^{1}H-MRS of SCC performed at 1.5 T has demonstrated significant elevation of the Cho/Cr ratio in patients with tumors compared with normal tongue muscle. The spectra for normal tongue muscle are dominated by a broad lipid peak centered between 1.3 and 0.9 ppm (20). The Cho and Cr peaks are typically not detected in *in vivo* normal muscle using single voxel technique (20,22). It should be emphasized that the Cho/Cr ratio is nonspecific and cannot distinguish between tumors nor can it differentiate between grades of squamous cell carcinoma or metastatic potential. However, this ratio may be used as a spectral tumor marker if one is attempting to identify a malignancy or attempting to differentiate recurrent tumor from nonmalignant posttreatment changes in the extracranial head and neck using ^{1}H-MRS.

The upper aerodigestive tract is an inherently difficult area to perform MRS. To obtain highly resolved spectra, a very homogeneous magnetic field is required in the area to be examined (i.e., $\leq$0.1 ppm deviation in the magnetic field). Numerous structural interfaces exist in this region that result in large magnetic field inhomogeneities. In many cases, these large field inhomogeneities cannot be corrected by the use of magnetic field shim. Susceptibility artifact from the paranasal sinuses, mandible, and pharyngeal airway often prohibits analysis of low-volume tumors located adjacent to these structures. Pulsations from the carotid artery result in rhythmic field inhomogeneities and may prevent spectral analysis of lesions that involve the poststyloid parapharyngeal space (22). Magnetic resonance spectroscopy is also limited due to motion artifact. This is a common problem in older patients with obstructing airway lesions that are required to lie flat during image acquisition.

Another advantage of MRI is its earlier detection of central nervous system abnormalities regardless of whether they are related to the head and neck lesion or to its treatment. The lower brain and basal cisterns are easily seen and should be examined carefully for abnormalities. The future challenge of MRI will be to accomplish all the foregoing functions with scanners that have a less confining architecture without giving up imaging speed or efficiency. Open-architecture scanners usually are limited to low field strength, narrowing their applicability.

SONOGRAPHY

Sonography has a varied role in head and neck oncology, depending on institutional patterns. Imaging departments are most familiar with thyroid and vascular sonography in the neck. Sonographic lymph node staging can be learned and applied readily but remains limited for evaluation of the high lateral retropharyngeal and retrosternal sites. However, sonography can facilitate fine-needle aspiration of indeterminate lymph nodes found by any modality (23). Doppler interrogation has been helpful in characterizing internal lymph node architecture lymph nodes that are normal in size as well as enlarged. Distortion of the normal hilar vascular pattern correlates with metastatic tumor involvement. The subjective nature of that feature is reduced with Doppler assessment of the volume of lymph node blood flow, noted to increase with "power

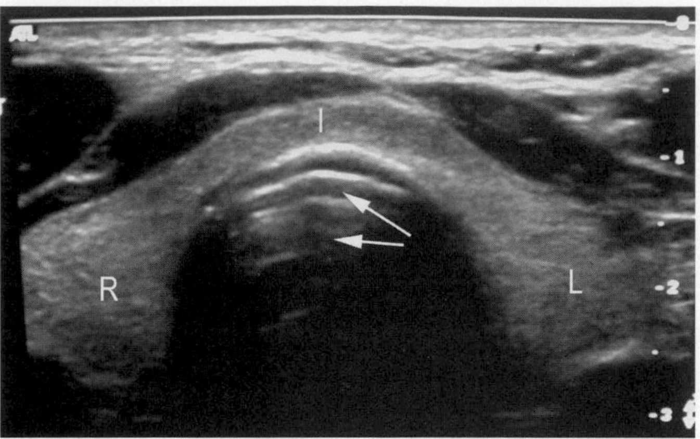

Figure 4.25 Extended field-of-view sonography. New transducers allow broader whole organ coverage for better anatomic depiction of right (*R*) and left (*L*) lobes and isthmus (*I*). Artifact from tracheal ring (*arrows*).

Doppler" analysis. Occasional sonographically guided biopsies are performed on thyroid or other superficial lesions. Sonography for local tumor staging has been advocated but probably is best considered by experienced operators an adjunct to the in-clinic examination, perhaps eliminating the need for examination under anesthesia in selected cases. Some would advocate sonography for evaluation of the tongue (24) but it is markedly limited for follow-up evaluation. Sonography of the major salivary glands can be helpful in confirming whether a lesion has breached the capsule of the gland. A technical innovation wherein an "extended field of view" captures a more panoramic layout of the organ may make sonography more widely acceptable in the neck and thyroid bed (Fig. 4.25). Evaluation of the reconstructed pharynx has been reported to be reliable using standard (25) and endoscopic methods (26).

NUCLEAR MEDICINE

Nuclear medicine imaging is based on the ability to detect minute change in metabolism, which frequently predates visible change in anatomy. It depends on, and is limited by, the availability of radiopharmaceuticals capable of showing the metabolic pathway of interest. Its shortcoming is its limited spatial resolution as compared with the exquisite detail achieved by CT or MRI. However, the iodine-131 scan, one of the earliest nuclear medicine procedures developed, is still the mainstay of imaging of well-differentiated thyroid cancer both for its ability to detect minute quantities of functional thyroid tumor and for evaluation of known or occult metastases for the possibility of radioiodine treatment.

Gallium scan for lymphoma also is a well-established and widely available technique. It is based on the propensity of most lymphomas to concentrate gallium. It is used mainly in the primary staging of lymphoma and, in those cases in which the lymphoma is gallium-avid, in the follow-up monitoring of chemotherapy (Fig. 4.26).

Parathyroid imaging is another area in which nuclear medicine frequently is used for location of parathyroid adenoma or hyperplasia. It is especially useful in cases of recurrence after surgery, in which the anatomy may be distorted, or when the parathyroid gland may be in ectopic locations. The agent used most commonly is sestamibi scan with early and delayed images (Fig. 4.27; see also Color Plate 1 following page 524). Some investigators combine sestamibi scan with technetium 99m-pertechnetate or iodine-123 thyroid scan for better delineation of the parathyroid neoplasm. Thallium-201 with ^{99m}Tc-pertechnetate thyroid scan and image subtraction also has been used with very good results.

Positron emission tomography (PET) is a functional imaging technique that depicts tissue metabolic activity (Fig. 4.28). As most tumors show increased glycolytic activity compared with non-neoplastic tissues, fluorine-18–labeled fluorodeoxyglucose (FDG), a glucose analog, has proven to be a very useful marker of tumor activity in many parts of the body. The radiopharmaceutical, ^{18}F-FDG, has been shown to be highly accurate in detecting tumor activity based on the usually increased glycolysis in tumor tissues. Tumor tissue also has less well-developed mechanisms for exporting glucose compared with normal cells. Anatomic imaging relies on change in size of the primary tumor and extent of adenopathy for assessment of tumor progression or treatment response. Following surgery or radiation therapy it can be difficult to detect residual or recurrent tumor clinically, though findings such as the presence of a mass, increasing pain, or soft tissue necrosis may suggest it. Recurrent disease may also be difficult to detect on post-therapeutic CT and MRI studies due to edema, scarring, and flap reconstruction (27,28). Early identification of persistent or recurrent tumor may increase the effectiveness of early salvage therapy. Accurate identification of granulation tissue may prevent unnecessary biopsy. Biopsy of an irradiated area may precipitate tissue necrosis (29). This is a particular problem in the larynx, where chondronecrosis may result in laryngectomy. FDG-PET can be very effective in this setting as it is not limited by anatomic distortion as are CT and MRI, and the PET result may increase the yield and diagnostic accuracy of biopsy.

The sensitivity for detection of disease generally ranges from 80% to 100%, whereas specificity ranges from 43% to 100%. False positives are a significant issue necessitating close clinical and imaging correlation. A negative result is generally highly reassuring, as the negative predictive value of FDG-PET has been shown to be high (30). Most FDG-PET scans are performed in patients at risk for recurrent disease because of clinical suspicion. The role of FDG-PET in routine surveillance of the post-therapy head and neck cancer patient has not yet been determined, though it has been suggested (31). Stokkel et al. (30) suggest that in patients suspected of having recurrent laryngeal or hypopharyngeal cancer in whom FDG-PET is negative, endoscopy may be omitted for at least 6 months and possibly up to a year, resulting in considerable cost saving.

Imaging usually starts approximately 45 minutes to 1 hour after intravenous injection of FDG. The field of view should include at least the entire neck, the base of skull, and the superior mediastinum. Both the emission images and the transmission images (for attenuation correction) are acquired. For a modern PET scanner, the typical section thickness and spatial resolution are between 4 and 5 mm. Both the emission (uncorrected) and the attenuation-corrected images are reconstructed in the transaxial plane and reformatted into coronal and sagittal planes. For adequate analysis, all three orthogonal planes can be reviewed. Because of the limited *anatomic* resolution of the PET scanning as compared with CT or MRI and owing to the small size of structures in the head and neck, it is imperative that these views be interpreted by an expert reader and correlated with the corresponding MRI or CT images (Fig. 4.29). When available, image co-registration allows precise matching of the functional activity to the anatomic structure. Hybrid combined CT/PET scanners allow near-perfect registration of anatomic and metabolic abnormalities. Nuclear scans acquired on modified conventional gamma cameras provide important

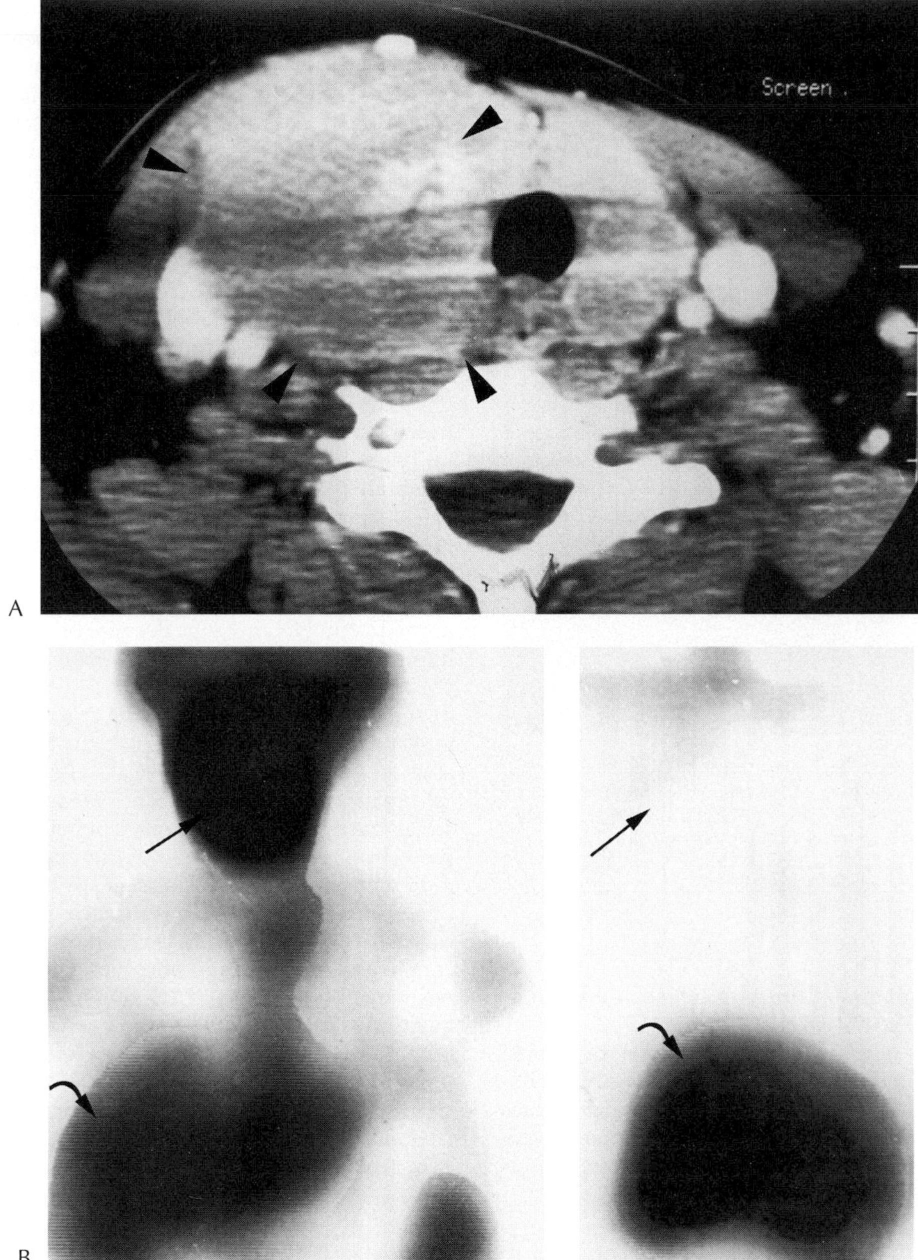

Figure 4.26 Correlation between modalities. **A:** Enhanced axial computed tomography view of heterogeneous enlargement of thyroid gland with large right lobe mass (*arrowheads*) diagnosed, by fine-needle aspiration, as lymphoma. **B:** Gallium scan at diagnosis (**left**) and follow-up (**right**) showing value of local and systemic staging and follow-up to resolution of nuclear activity with resolution of neck uptake (*arrows*). Normal liver uptake (*curved arrows*).

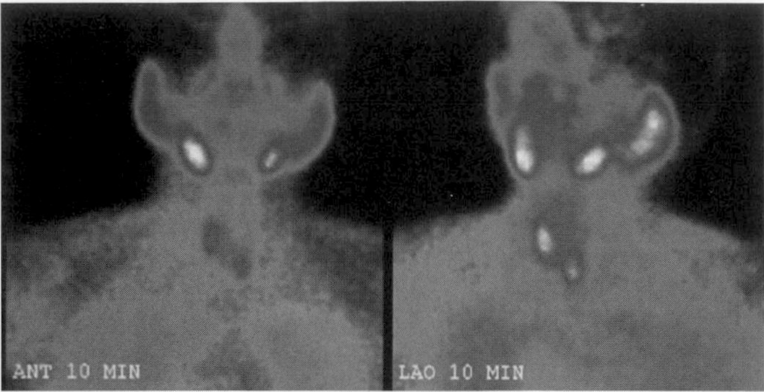

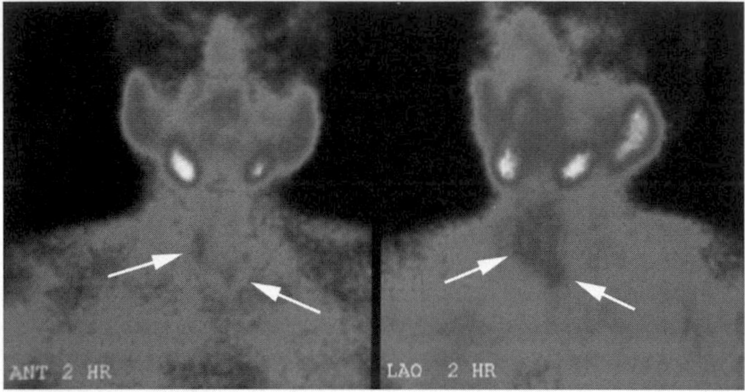

Figure 4.27 Parathyroid imaging. Technetium sestamibi nuclear scans in the early phase (**top**) and delayed phase (**bottom**) show multiple bilateral sites of retained activity in a patient with multifocal parathyroid hyperplasia. *Ant,* anterior; *LAO,* left anterior oblique. (See Color Plate 1 following page 524.)

adjunctive staging information at the mandible and nasopharynx (32) in patients who cannot have PET scans.

Another metabolic imaging technique that has been shown to be useful for evaluating head and neck SCC is ^{201}Tl single photon emission computed tomography (SPECT). Several studies have demonstrated that SCC is thallium-avid. Previous investigators have suggested that ^{201}Tl may be able to detect lesions larger than 1 cc (33). Initial results have shown that ^{201}Tl SPECT may be helpful in attempting to differentiate recurrent tumor from posttreatment changes and may be more accurate than CT or MR imaging for making this important distinction. Valdes-Olmes reported a higher diagnostic accuracy for ^{201}Tl SPECT (sensitivity = 93%, specificity = 78%) than compared with CT/MRI (sensitivity = 76%, specificity = 30%) (34). Mukherji et al. report a higher specificity ^{201}Tl SPECT (sensitivity = 88%, specificity = 94%) compared with CT (sensitivity = 100%, specificity = 24%) when attempting to identify recurrent tumor (35). These results of ^{201}Tl SPECT compare favorably with those previously reported for FDG-PET, which has previously been discussed, and ^{99m}Tc-sestamibi. Leitha at al. reported a sensitivity and specificity of 95.3% and 78.4%, respectively, for the ability of ^{99m}Tc-sestamibi to differentiate recurrent head and neck SCC from posttreatment changes (36).

There are potential advantages of ^{201}Tl SPECT over FDG. Thallium-201 SPECT may be superior to PET-FDG for imaging nasopharyngeal carcinoma and other skull base tumors. Unlike FDG, background uptake of ^{201}Tl by normal brain is low. Conspicuity of nasopharyngeal and skull base tumors may be reduced with PET-FDG, as these tumors are directly adjacent to normal brain FDG activity. Because of the low background activity of the normal brain, these tumors are well-delineated with ^{201}Tl imaging (35).

Initial reports have suggested that ^{201}Tl SPECT may be used for both predicting response to definitive radiotherapy and for assessing response within 6 weeks after completion of nonsurgical organ preservation therapy. Nagamachi et al. (36a) demonstrate that quantitative measures of ^{201}Tl uptake may be useful in predicting response of SCC of the upper aerodigestive tract to radiotherapy alone. Mukherji et al. have suggested that ^{201}Tl SPECT may be a reliable technique for assessing response to treatment when performed within 6 weeks after completion of combined chemotherapy and radiation therapy (33). As previously mentioned, FDG-PET is unreliable due to a high false-negative rate for predicting treatment response when performed within 1 to 2 months after completion of radiotherapy (37). These initial results suggest that ^{201}Tl may be able to predict radioresponsiveness and assess the success of treatment earlier than can be done with FDG-PET or cross-sectional imaging. However, further studies are needed to confirm these initial results.

A,B

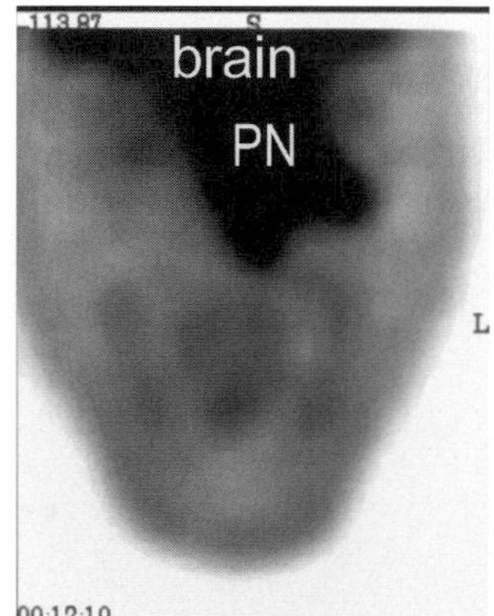

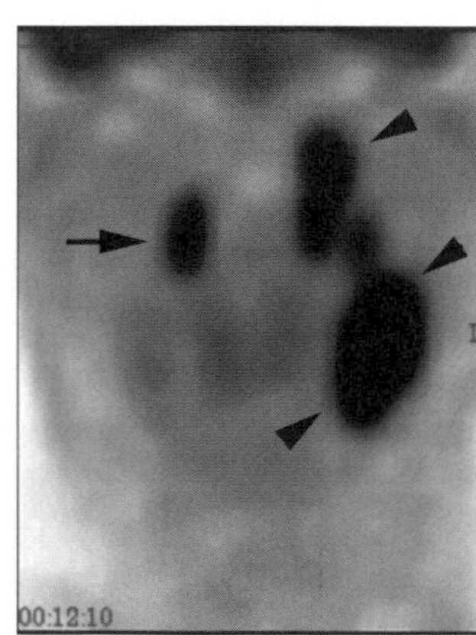

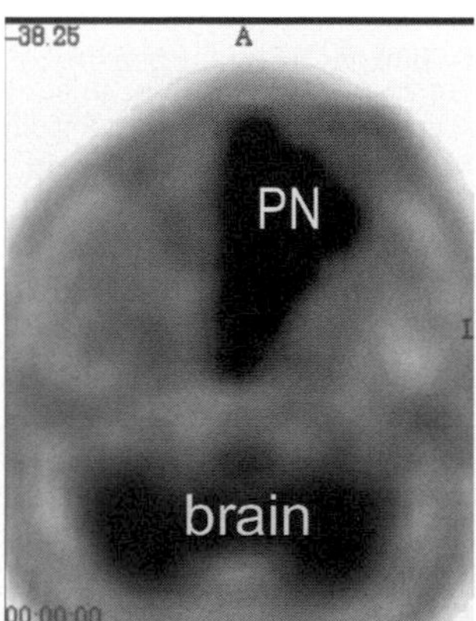

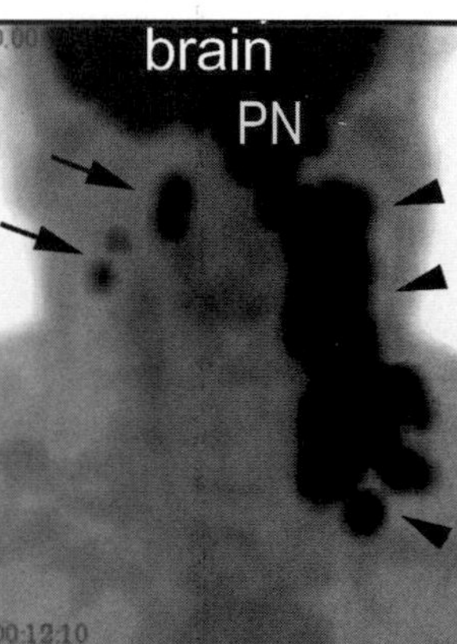

C,D

Figure 4.28 Fluorodeoxyglucose–positron emission tomography nuclear imaging of lymphoma of paranasal cavity. **(A)** Coronal paranasal, **(B)** coronal cervical, **(C)** axial paranasal, and **(D)** composite coronal views show the left paranasal (*PN*) primary lymphoma, right (*arrows*) and extensive left (*arrowheads*) cervical adenopathy. Background shows brain activity.

A

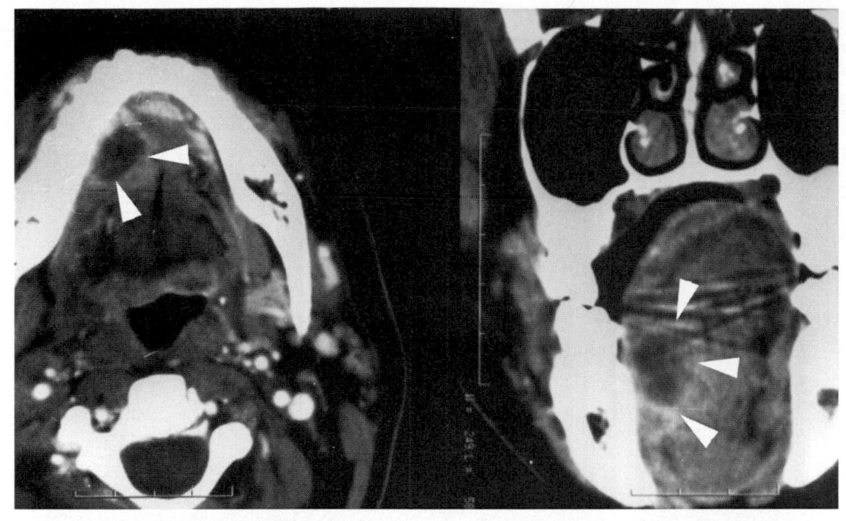

B

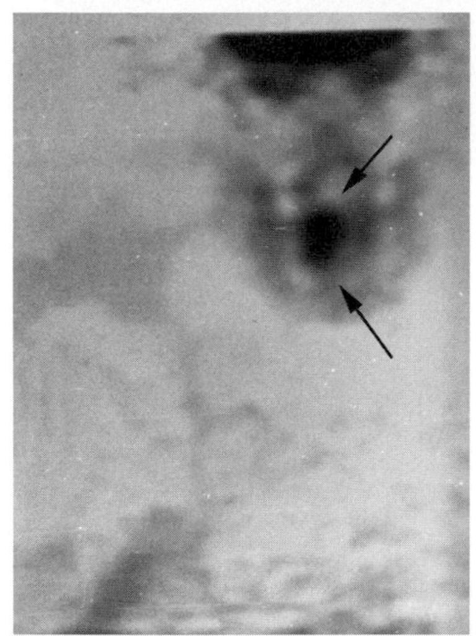

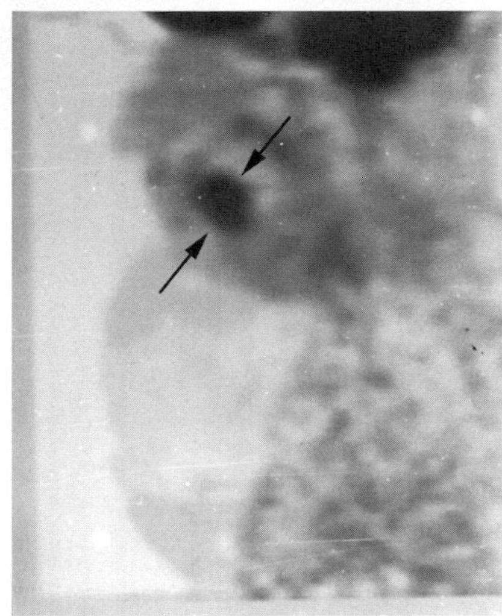

Figure 4.29 Correlation between modalities. **A:** Contrast-enhanced computed tomography in axial (left) and coronal (right) planes show necrotic process (*arrowheads*) thought clinically to be treatment-related induration. **B:** A fluorodeoxyglucose–positron emission tomography scan in coronal (**left**) and sagittal (**right**) plane excludes necrosis and confirms tumor recurrence (*arrows*).

ANGIOGRAPHY

Angiography can provide diagnostic information and a therapeutic option in the head and neck region. Diagnostic angiography is particularly useful in predicting the vascularity of a mass and the number and extent of feeding and draining vessels (see Fig. 28.28). Angiographic features also help characterize lesions in such critical locations as the skull base, where differentiation between meningioma, glomus tumor, and metastasis is useful pretreatment information. Preoperative particle embolization can help to decrease operative time through improved control of hemorrhage.

These procedures should be performed by a subspecialty angiographer and should be coordinated carefully with the timing of the definitive surgical resection. Test carotid balloon occlusion can be performed safely through the transfemoral approach. The procedure is requested when carotid bypass, sacrifice, or operative difficulty is anticipated. The head and neck circulation should be studied in an efficient manner to minimize catheter time. Cross-circulation should be confirmed before temporary occlusion (Fig. 4.30). Repeated checks to confirm the completeness of the test occlusion are necessary for absolute exclusion of

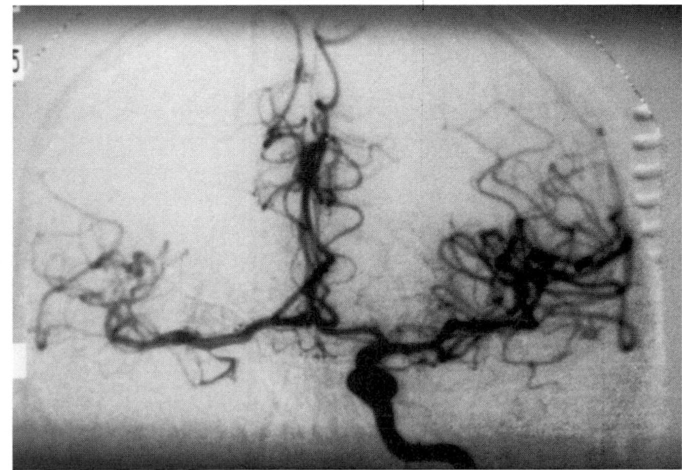

Figure 4.30 Catheter angiography. Left internal carotid injection showing cross-circulation to right anterior and middle cerebral arteries before testing carotid balloon occlusion of right internal carotid artery.

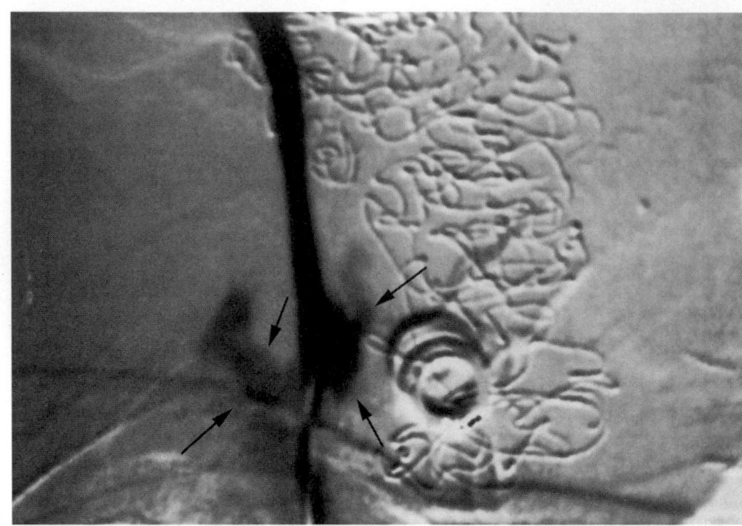

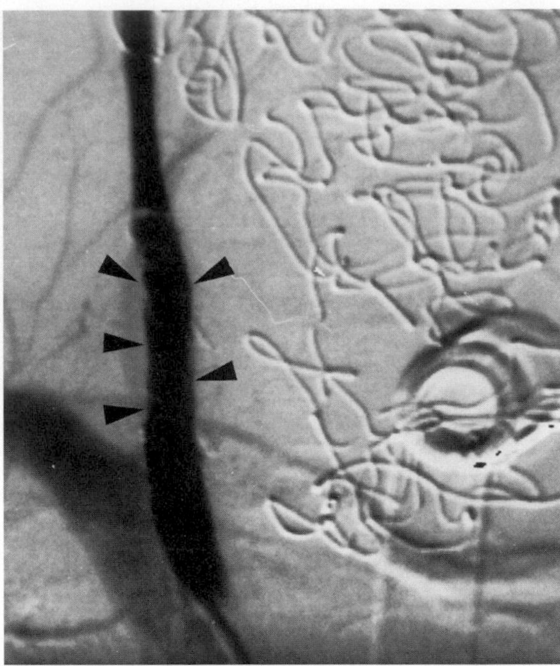

Figure 4.31 Therapeutic angiography. **A:** Selective right common carotid artery injection shows brisk contrast extravasation (*arrows*) into parastomal region at carotid rupture. Postembolization shows resolved leak after endovascular coil placement (*arrowheads*). **B:** Persistent antegrade distal carotid flow due to disseminated intravascular coagulation.

a false-tolerance result. The carotid "stump pressure" (back pressure) should be monitored and referenced to the patient's systemic blood pressure. Hypotensive challenge or nuclear brain–blood flow studies are helpful for additional predictability of perioperative brain schemia or infarction. Selective intraarterial chemotherapy through a transfemoral or transtemporal artery approach allows for decreased systemic toxicity at the cost of slightly greater local toxicity (38–40).

Emergency carotid angiography is requested much less frequently with the widespread use of vascularized flaps. Temporary or permanent occlusion of the carotid artery or its branches can be performed with appropriate consent and planning (Fig. 4.31).

INTERVENTIONAL PROCEDURES

Occasionally, imaging-guided percutaneous biopsy procedures are necessary (Figs. 4.32–4.35) (41,42). The most common situation is the presence of a radiographically apparent

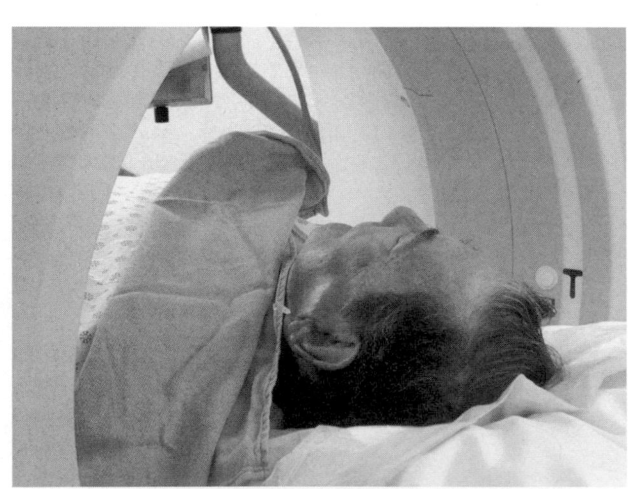

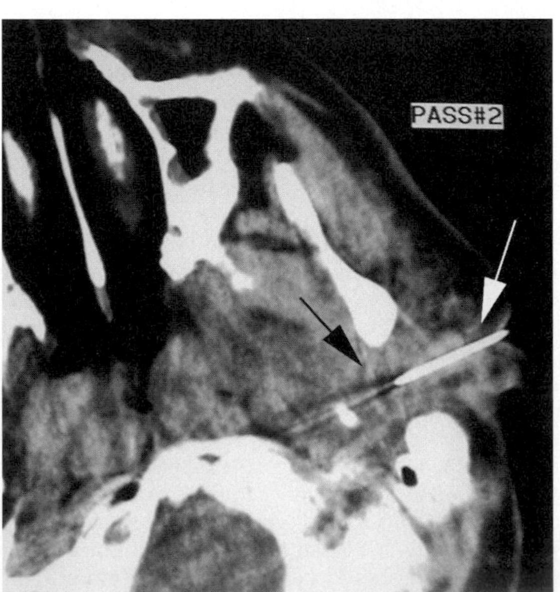

Figure 4.32. Interventional computed tomography (CT). **A:** Patient positioned and draped in supine scanning within wide CT gantry with needle anterior to the tragus. **B:** Control axial image shows needle penetrating the skin (*white arrow*) and needle tip within parotid mass (*black arrow*).

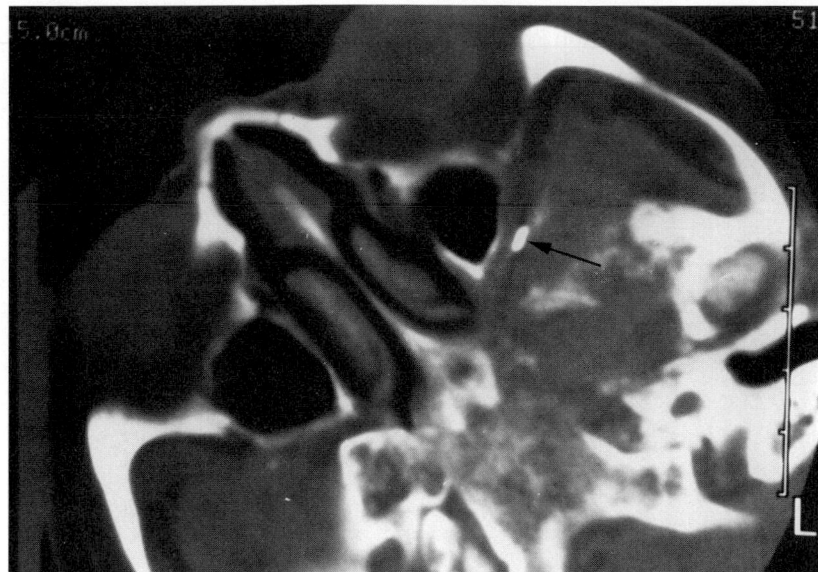

Figure 4.33 Interventional computed tomography (CT). CT shows needle placement (*arrow*) for percutaneous CT-guided biopsy of inaccessible lesion deep within the pterygomaxillary space with recurrent skin cancer.

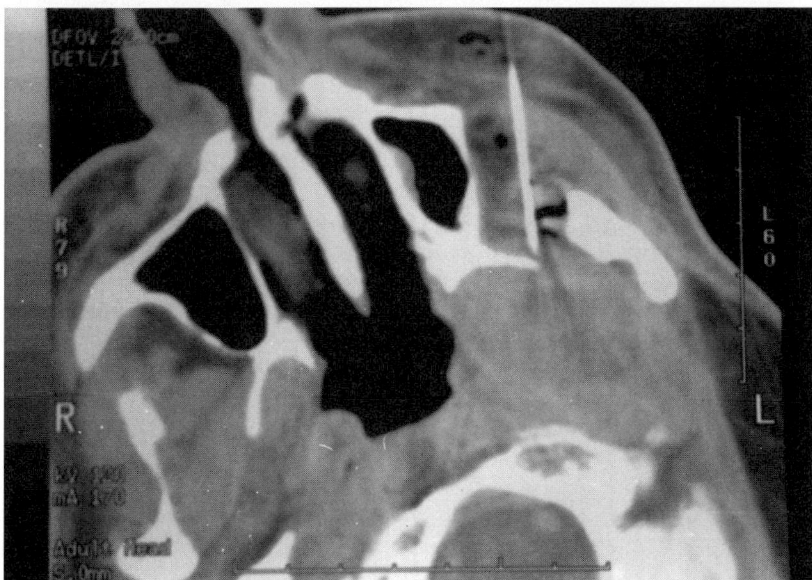

Figure 4.34 Interventional computed tomography (CT). Axial CT shows needle placement in the masticator space in a patient with deep recurrence of squamous cell carcinoma of the retromolar trigone.

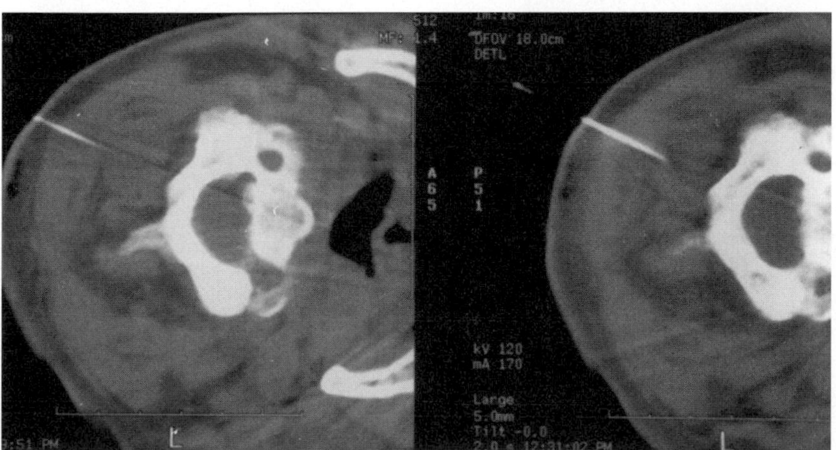

Figure 4.35 Interventional computed tomography (CT). Axial CT with patient in the decubitus position shows needle placement in nonpalpable paraspinal lymph node, confirming progression.

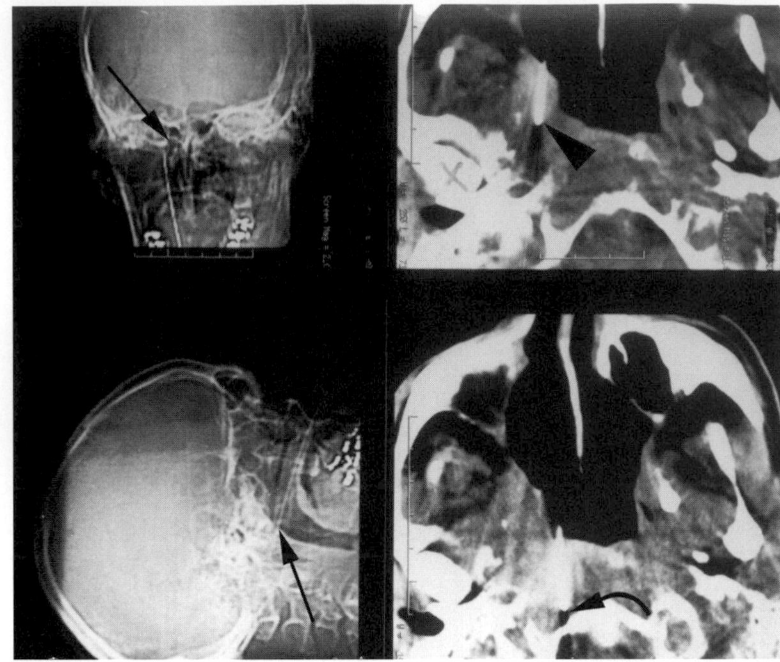

Figure 4.36 Interventional computed tomography (CT). Novel transnasal CT-guided approach to nasopharyngeal disease under intravenous sedation. Undiagnosed disease status after two endoscopic biopsies accessed with 20-gauge needle tip (*arrows*) in mucosal space (*arrowhead*) and within the basiocciput (*curved arrow*) of the skull base via indwelling sterile nasal trumpet. The diagnosis is granulomatous disease.

abnormality that is not palpable clinically. Other indications are the presence of a lesion too close to vital structures to allow a safe office biopsy, confirmation of recurrence deep to a well-healed flap, preoperative determination of the histologic type or grade of a deep-seated lesion, and pretreatment differentiation of suspected progression in a patient with two different primary tumors. Though some of these might be attempted with fluoroscopic guidance, CT control provides a more accurate demonstration of safe needle trajectories. An equally important consideration is the confirmation of needle-tip position in the appropriate part of the lesion (Figs. 4.36 and 4.37). This certainty helps in determining the relative need for an operative procedure or continued attempts at the percutaneous approach when the specimen is deemed inadequate by the on-site cytotechnologist or is believed to be nondiagnostic on the final pathology report. The opening of the CT gantry is relatively accommodating for needle manipulation minimizing claustrophobia (Fig. 4.32). Image reconstruction occurs

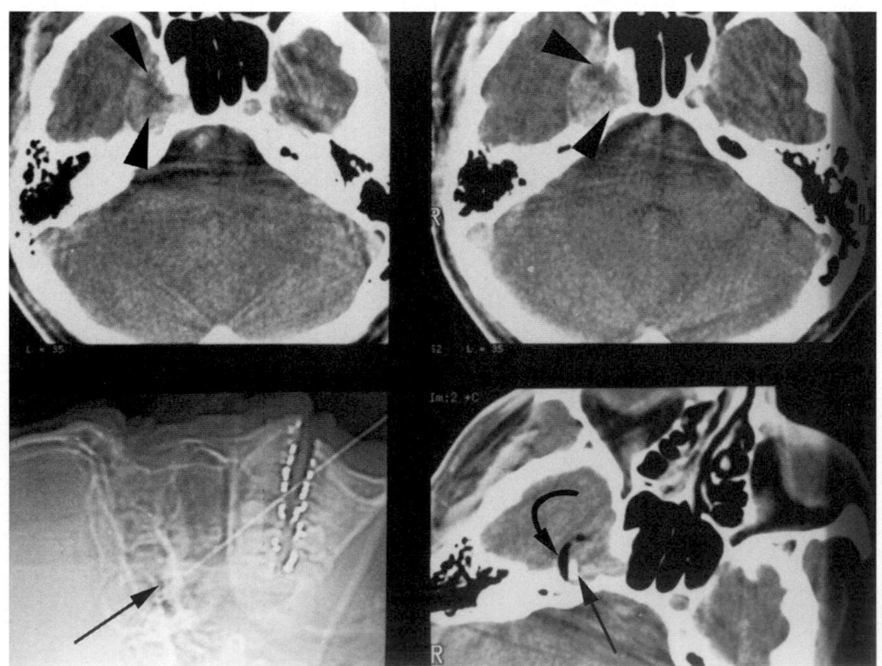

Figure 4.37 Interventional computed tomography (CT). Percutaneous CT-guided biopsy of right cavernous sinus mass (*arrowheads*) under anesthesia. A 20-gauge needle advanced transfacially into cavernous mass (*arrows*) via foramen ovale with air, confirming extradural location (*curved arrow*).

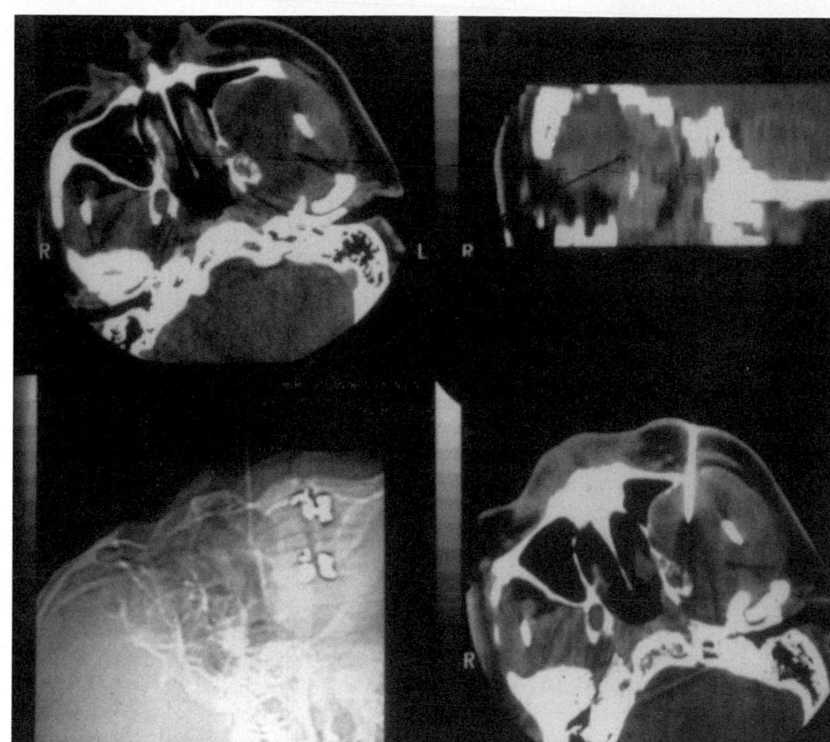

Figure 4.38 Transfacial biopsy. **Clockwise from top left:** Axial computed tomography (CT), reformatted oblique parasagittal CT, postplacement CT axial and scout views. Large, well-marginated left retromaxillary mass with confirmation of 18-gauge needle tip. The diagnosis is neuroma.

within seconds, revealing important soft-tissue or bony landmarks.

The procedures are performed using 20- to 25-gauge needles, with appropriate consent for bleeding, infection, and nerve injury. Larger-gauge needles can be used with caution in the appropriate setting (Fig. 4.38) (43). Biopsies of vascular lesions are obtained, first ensuring that informed consent has been obtained because bleeding might ensue.

THREE-DIMENSIONAL IMAGING

Occasionally, three-dimensional renderings are necessary to better appreciate the orientation of a mass. These models can be constructed from CT (44) or MRI data sets. Simple models consisting of a few tissue-type components can be created in a relatively semiautomated fashion by a technologist and can be crosschecked by the physician (Fig. 4.39). More complex models

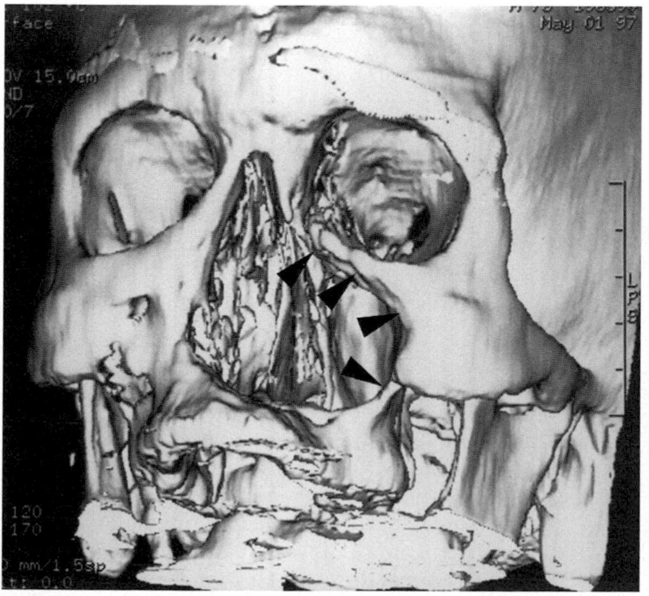

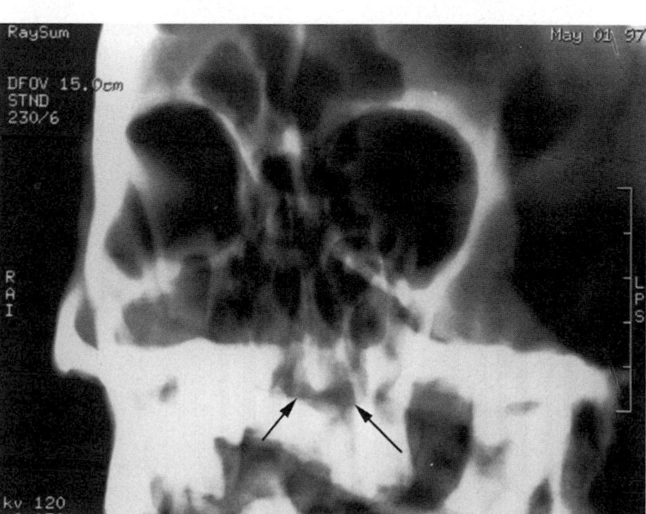

Figure 4.39 Three-dimensional imaging. **A:** Surface rendering of facial bones showing erosive change due to a squamous cancer of the nasal vestibule (*arrowheads*). **B:** Radiographic-appearing "ray sum" projection of same view from axial computed tomography data. The defect shown in the maxillary bone on the ray sum projection (*arrows*) is not apparent on the surface rendering.

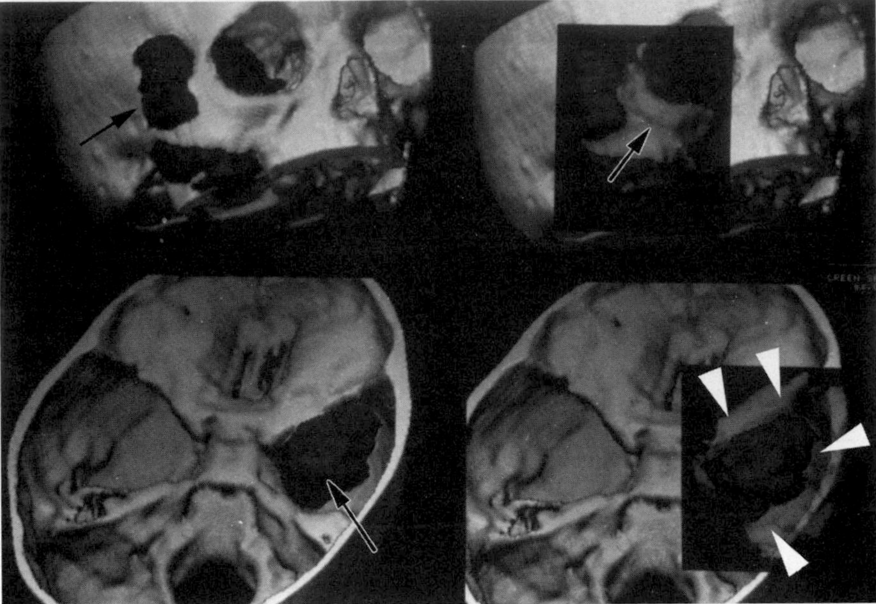

Figure 4.40 Three-dimensional imaging. Surface rendering of skull showing mass arising within the sphenoid bone (*arrows*). The "see-through" view renders the regional bone translucent to allow visualization of the extraosseous component (*arrowheads*) of the mass, which otherwise would be out of the operating surgeon's sight.

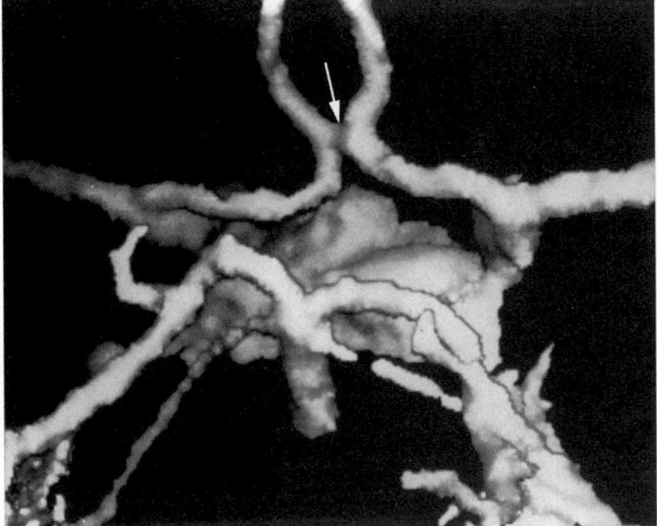

Figure 4.41 Computed tomographic (CT) angiography. Three-dimensional computer rendering of the circle of Willis created from a contrast-enhanced, thin, axial CT examination. The image confirmed the presence of a well-developed anterior communicating artery (*arrow*) in a patient in whom an attempted test carotid occlusion could not be performed.

demonstrating the lesion and its relationship to surrounding structures require greater "up-front" physician input and are created from a significantly greater number of thinner sections (see Fig. 28.31B). Therefore, an accurate model can rarely be performed retrospectively from a routine scan, but the scan must be planned carefully and processed before importing it to the three-dimensional workstation.

Various components of the model can be shown separately or in combination. Layers of overlying soft tissue or bone can be rendered translucent, facilitating the choice of operative approach (Fig. 4.40). Views showing the anticipated operation at various stages of completion help in planning brachytherapy and reconstructive efforts. These models contribute to operative planning and coordination of multiple surgical teams and also can help trainees to understand what otherwise may take years to appreciate from cross-sectional images alone. An added benefit is using the model to help patients to understand the gravity of their lesion and the corresponding informed consent.

One type of three-dimensional rendering that can be produced from CT data is CT angiography. After appropriate contrast bolus technique, the axial images through the skull base can be processed to extract the high attenuation of the intraarterial contrast (Fig. 4.41).

Various clinical syndromes present to the head and neck subspecialist; most are pain- related, for which a structural cause is sought. Carefully planned scans can be designed to outline the various developmental (Fig. 4.42), neoplastic (Figs. 4.43 and 4.44), and malignant (Fig. 4.45) causes of these complaints. Imaging-guided procedures can be performed percutaneously to alleviate pain in this population with complex disease- and treatment-related problems (45).

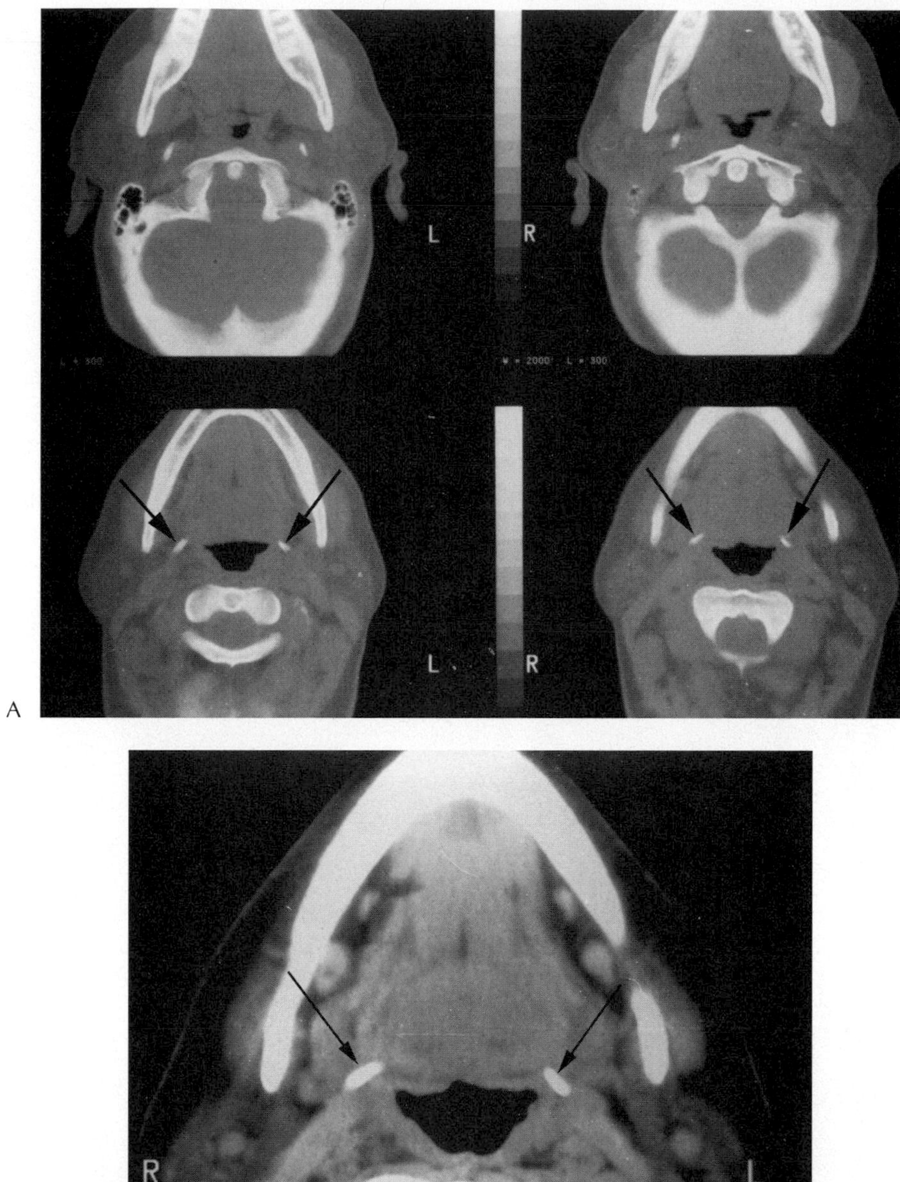

Figure 4.42 Pain syndrome. Serial axial computed tomography (CT) bone windows **(A)** and single-axial CT tissue window **(B)** show bilateral calcification of the stylohyoid ligaments (*arrows*) in a patient with painful swallowing (Eagle syndrome).

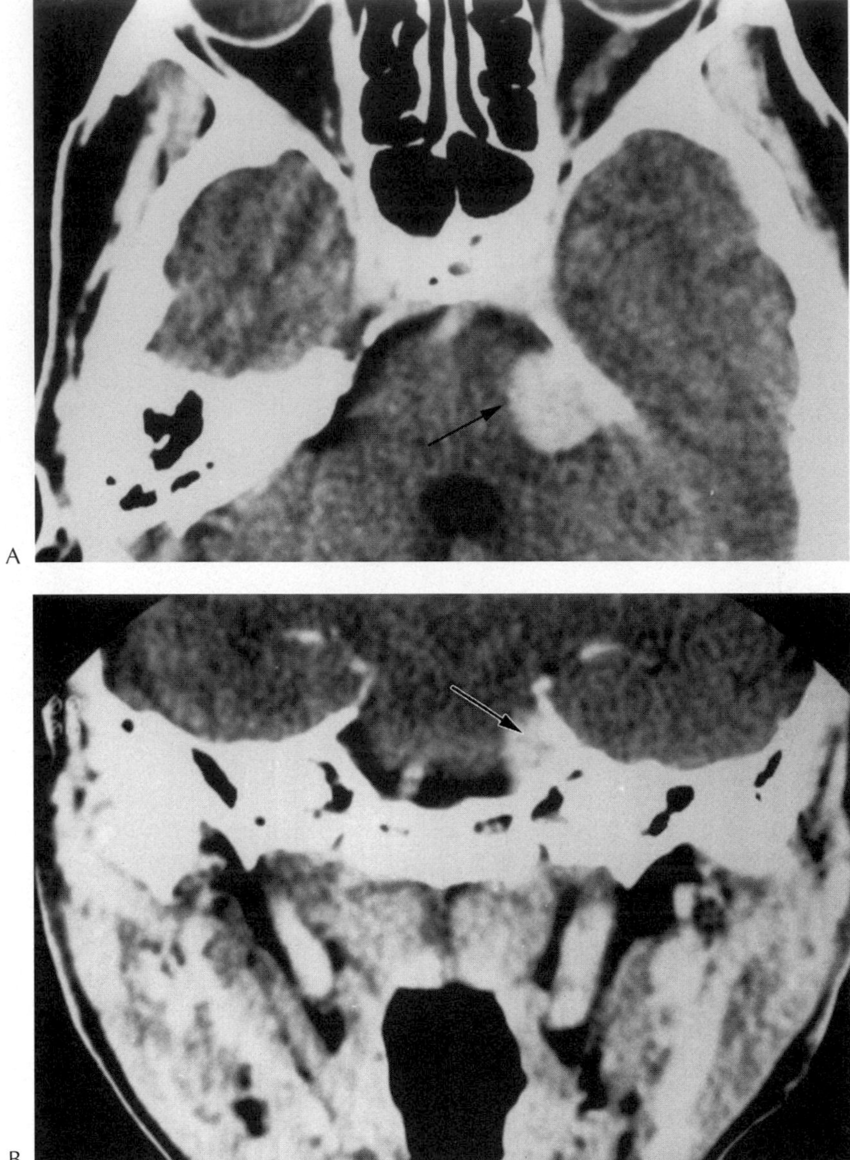

Figure 4.43 Pain syndrome. Enhanced axial **(A)** and direct coronal **(B)** computed tomography images of small meningioma impinging on fifth nerve root entry zone (*arrows*) in a patient with hemifacial pain.

FOLLOW-UP IMAGING

At some subsites follow-up imaging has been shown to provide no positive influence on survival (46). Follow-up imaging commonly is used to lend confidence to the clinical examination. Decisions about follow-up must strike a balance between the availability of resources and the need for diagnostic certainty. Algorithms are a popular way of managing individual patients. This method is helpful but might be better considered in global-practice terms. Certainly, many patients would be more reassured if they knew their posttreatment PET scan showed no suspicious activity. However, a busy clinician might serve the patient cohort better by asking which two or three of the 50 patients seen in a clinic day would benefit from a PET scan.

Timing of follow-up imaging includes various stages: during treatment, immediately after operation or completion of therapy, and early and late scanning. Immediate postoperative scanning rarely is necessary to establish completeness of resection, except for piecemeal-type removal or when gross residual disease is left *in situ*. Outside of investigational protocol requirements, this practice may not be necessary. Early and late follow-up scanning is occasionally requested. The need for imaging support of the status of "no evidence of disease" depends on the ability to examine the primary site. With the widespread application of complex grafts and higher therapeutic radiation dosing, follow-up imaging is becoming more necessary as the clinical examination becomes less reliable.

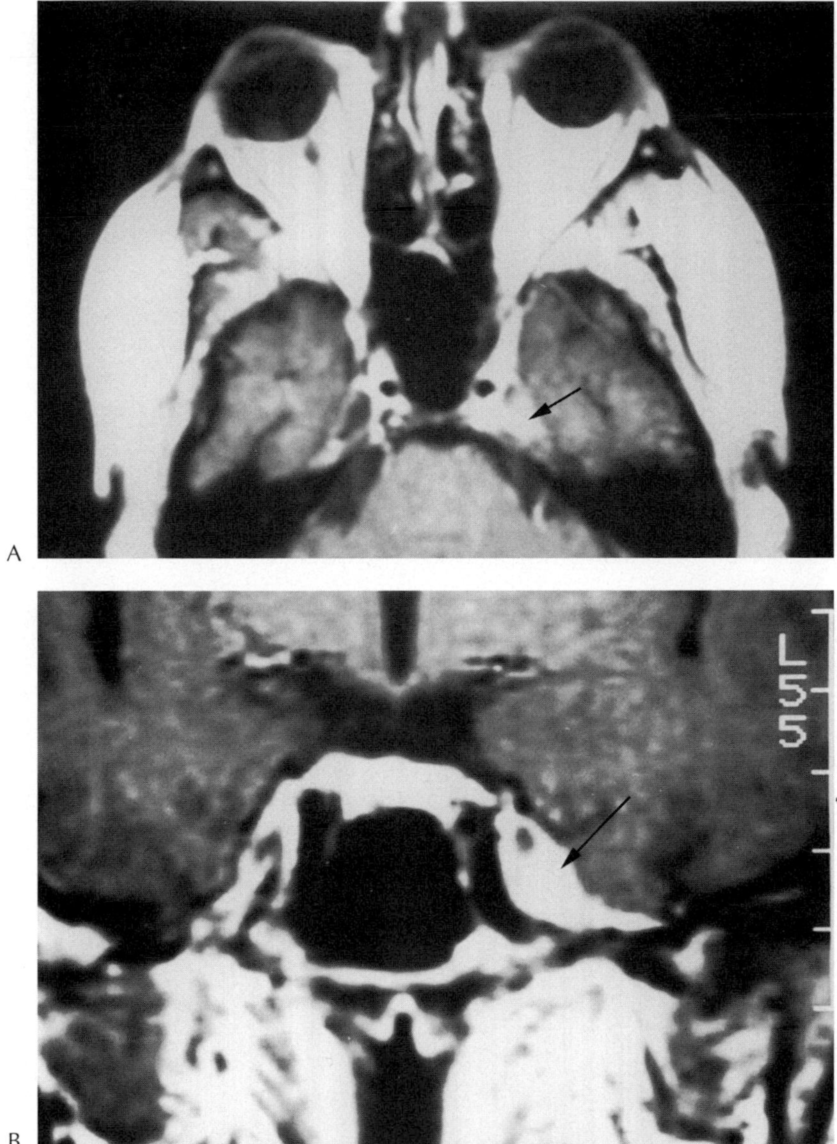

Figure 4.44 Pain syndrome. Enhanced axial **(A)** and coronal **(B)** T1-weighted magnetic resonance imaging views showing a small cavernous lesion (*arrows*) within the left Meckel cave in a patient with painful hemifacial spasm.

The discussion of the choice of modality cannot take place in the absence of the issue of frequency of follow-up scanning. In the immediate perioperative or postirradiation time frame, the gross loss of tissue planes markedly compromises CT and (to a greater extent) MRI interpretation (Fig. 4.46). Given this limitation, using the simpler, less costly modality (CT) makes sense. Furthermore, if the region of interest is well outlined by CT, this may be the modality of choice for treatment protocols that require frequent imaging. The only limiting factor would be contraindication to intravenous CT contrast, which is typical in the setting of renal dysfunction of platinum-based regimens. MRI could be held in reserve for periodic intervals or when CT does not confirm a new suspicious clinical finding.

An important question that is often asked concerns the best time to perform posttreatment imaging when attempting to determine primary site response following nonsurgical organ preservation therapy. Accurate assessment helps identify patients who have successfully responded from those who failed treatment and may benefit from early salvage surgery. Previous studies have suggested that changes in tumor size can predict treatment response. Posttreatment imaging appears to be most reliable for predicting primary site response when performed approximately 3 to 4 months following the completion of definitive radiotherapy (20,27). Complete radiologic resolution of the lesion on the posttreatment study compared with a pretreatment study

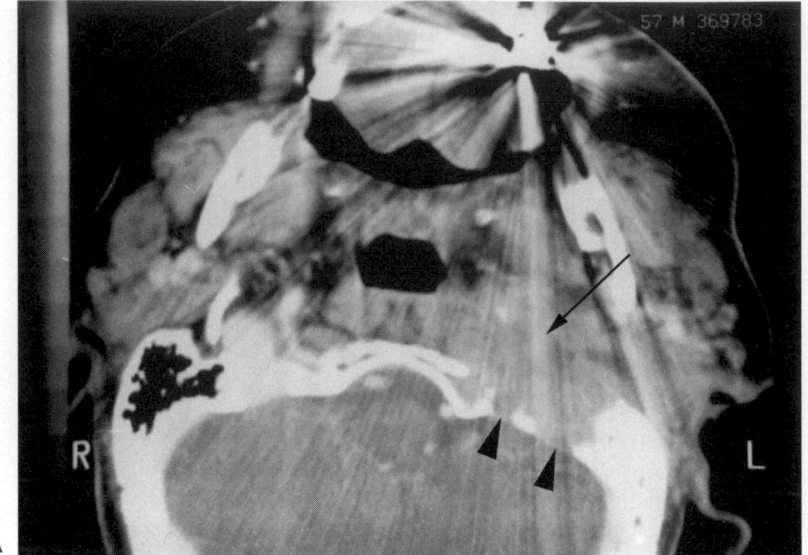

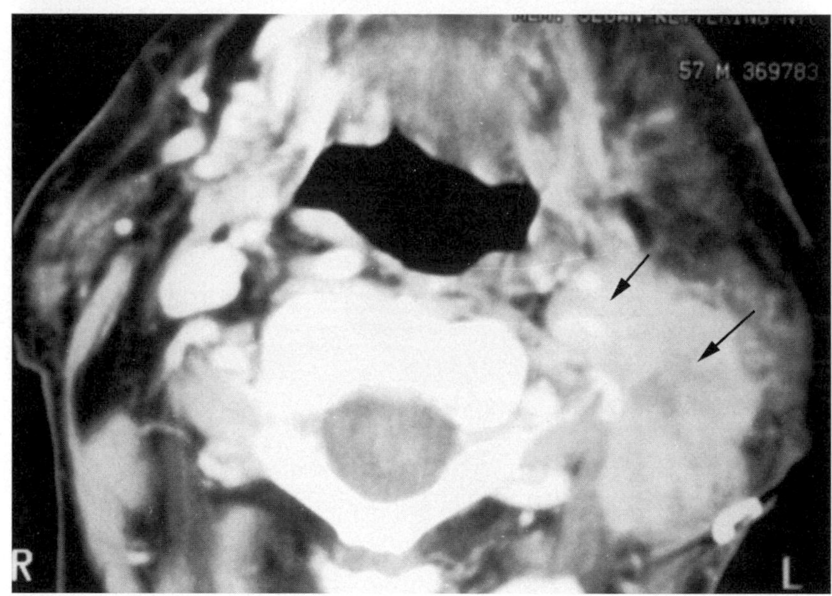

Figure 4.45 Syncope syndrome. Enhanced axial computed tomography at skull base **(A)** and upper neck **(B)**, showing metastatic disease to carotid space (*arrows*) and skull-base destruction (*arrowheads*) in a patient with carotid syncope.

strongly suggests a successfully controlled primary site. Patients with a persistent mass at the primary site that has undergone less than 50% reduction in size are indicative of treatment failure. Partial resolution of a mass, defined as 50% to 75% reduction in size, is an indeterminate finding (20,27). These patients require further imaging and close clinical observation. On follow-up studies, interval enlargement of a persistent mass is suggestive of recurrent disease or laryngeal necrosis. However, stability of the mass over a 2-year period is suggestive of fibrosis and scarring. Imaging modalities aimed at measuring metabolic activity such as ^{18}F-FDG PET or ^{201}Tl-SPECT may prove beneficial in differentiating between recurrent disease and radiation change (35,47,48).

The increasing role of concomitant chemotherapy and radiotherapy (chemoradiation) for organ preservation and treatment of unresectable head and neck SCC have resulted in investigations aimed at determining if CT can be used to noninvasively predict the response of lymph nodes following therapy. It is possible that accurate prediction of the presence of tumor within lymph nodes following chemoradiation with CT may preclude the need for planned neck dissection in

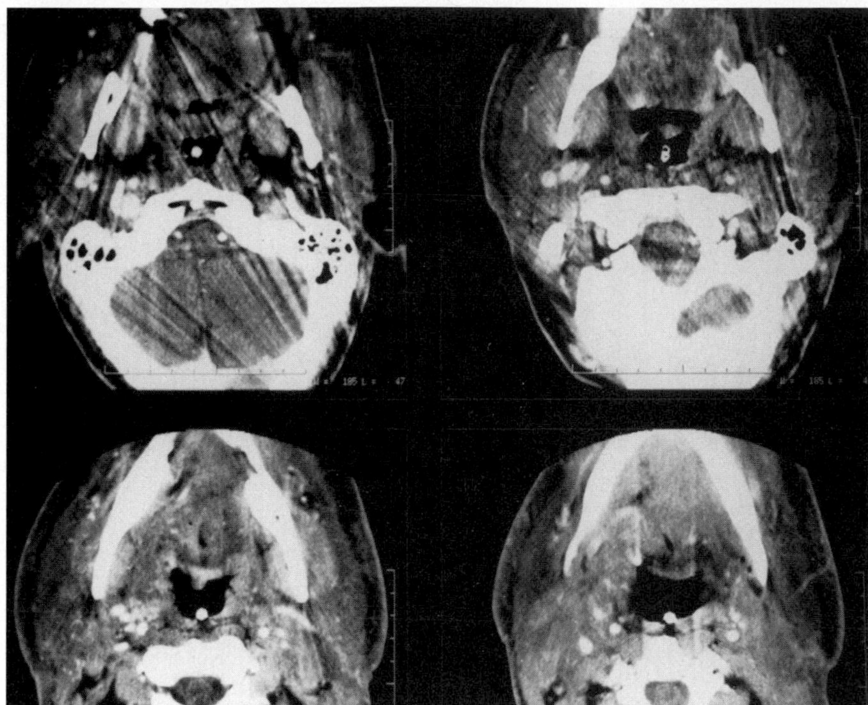

Figure 4.46 Serial contrast-enhanced axial sections, showing limited diagnostic capacity of postoperative scans in the perioperative time frame due to poorly defined tissue planes.

patients with pretreatment nodal metastases. Labadie et al. report that a reduction in posttreatment of nodal tumor volume (NTV) of an individual lymph node by 90% compared with pretreatment NTV correlates with a high degree of negative pathologic findings for tumor in that node following planned neck dissection performed 6 weeks after completion of chemoradiation (49). These initial studies suggest that changes in NTV can predict nodal response. Thus, an argument can me made that a favorable imaging response can preclude planned neck dissection in a recently treated neck thereby reducing patient morbidity. However, the effect of such an alteration in standard treatment on overall survival needs to be investigated.

REFERENCES

1. Madison MT, Remley KB, Latchaw RE, et al. Radiologic diagnosis and staging of head and neck squamous cell carcinoma. *Radiologic Clin N Am* 1994;32: 163–181.
2. Talmi YP, Horowitz Z, Wolf M, et al. Delayed metastases in skin cancer of the head and neck: the case of the "known primary." *Ann Plast Surg* 1999;42: 289–292.
3. Anzai Y, Lufkin RB, Jabour BA, et al. Fat-suppression failure artifacts simulating pathology on frequency-selective fat-suppression MR images of the head and neck. *AJNR Am J Neuroradiol* 1992;13:879–884.
4. Som PM. Detection of metastasis in cervical lymph nodes: CT and MR criteria and differential diagnosis [Review]. *AJR Am J Roentgenol* 1992;158:961–969.
5. Bely-Toueg N, Halimi P, Laccourreye O, et al. Normal laryngeal CT findings after supracricoid partial laryngectomy. *AJNR Am J Neuroradiol* 2001;22: 1872–1880.
6. Hunt MA, Zelefsky MJ, Wolden S, et al. Treatment planning and delivery of intensity-modulated radiation therapy for primary nasopharynx cancer. *Int J Radiat Oncol Biol Phys* 2001;49:623–632.
7. Righi PD, Kelley DJ, Ernst R, et al. Evaluation of prevertebral muscle invasion by squamous cell carcinoma. Can computed tomography replace open neck exploration? *Arch Otolaryngol Head Neck Surg* 1996;122:660–663.
8. Lemort M. Computed tomography (CT) in head and neck tumors: technique and indications [Review]. *J Belge de Radiologie* 1994;77:60–66.
9. Barakos JA. Advances in magnetic resonance imaging of the head and neck [Review]. *Topics Magn Reson Imaging* 1994;6:155–165.
10. Groell R, Doerfler O, Schaffler GJ, et al. Contrast-enhanced helical CT of the head and neck: improved conspicuity of squamous cell carcinoma on delayed scans. *AJR Am J Roentgenol* 2001;176:1571–1575.
11. Chung TS, Yousem DM, Seigerman HM, et al. MR of mandibular invasion in patients with oral and oropharyngeal malignant neoplasms. *AJNR Am J Neuroradiol* 1994;15:1949–1955.
12. Kremer B, Klimek L, Andreopoulos D, et al. A new method for the placement of brachytherapy probes in paranasal sinus and nasopharynx neoplasms. *Int J Radiat Oncol Biol Phys* 1999;43:995–1000.
13. Ross MR, Schomer DF, Chappell P, et al. MR imaging of head and neck tumors: comparison of T1-weighted contrast-enhanced fat-suppressed images with conventional T2-weighted and fast spin-echo T2-weighted images. *AJR Am J Roentgenol* 1994;163:173–178.
14. Hudgins PA. Contrast enhancement in head and neck imaging [Review]. *Neuroimaging Clin N Am* 1994;4:101–115.
15. Chong VF, Mukherji SK, Ng SH, et al. Nasopharyngeal carcinoma: review of how imaging affects staging. *J Comput Assist Tomogr* 1999;23:984–993.
16. Scott AM, Macapinlac H, Zhang J, et al. Image registration of SPECT and CT images using an external fiduciary band and three-dimensional surface fitting in metastatic thyroid cancer. *J Nuclear Med* 1995;36:100–103.
17. Leslie A, Fyfe E, Guest P, et al. Staging of squamous cell carcinoma of the oral cavity and oropharynx: a comparison of MRI and CT in T- and N-staging. *J Comput Assist Tomogr* 1999;23:43–49.
18. Som PM, Urken ML, Biller H, et al. Imaging the postoperative neck [Review]. *Radiology* 1993;187:593–603.
19. Gomori JM. Vascular evaluation of head and neck masses by magnetic resonance imaging. *Israel J Med Sci* 1992;28:262–267.
20. Mukherji SK, Schiro S, Castillo M, et al. Proton MR spectroscopy of squamous cell carcinoma of the extracranial head and neck: in vitro and in vivo studies. *AJNR Am J Neuroradiol* 1997;18:1057–1072.
21. Mukherji SK, Schiro S, Castillo M, et al. Proton MR spectroscopy of squamous cell carcinoma of the upper aerodigestive tract: in vitro characteristics. *AJNR Am J Neuroradiol* 1996;17:1485–1490.
22. Mukherji SK. *Clinical applications of magnetic resonance spectroscopy.* New York: John Wiley and Sons, 1998.
23. Baatenburg de Jong RJ, Knegt P, Verwoerd CD. Reduction of the number of neck treatments in patients with head and neck cancer [Review]. *Cancer* 1993;71:2312–2318.

24. Narayana HM, Panda NK, Mann SB, et al. Ultrasound versus physical examination in staging carcinoma of the mobile tongue. *J Laryngol Otol* 1996;110:43–47.
25. Lee JH, Sohn JE, Choe DH, et al. Sonographic findings of the neopharynx after total laryngectomy: comparison with CT. *AJNR Am J Neuroradiol* 2000;21: 823–827.
26. Chak A, Canto MI, Cooper GS, et al. Endosonographic assessment of multimodality therapy predicts survival of esophageal carcinoma patients. *Cancer* 2000;88:1788–1795.
27. Mukherji SK, Mancuso AA, Kotzur IM, et al. Radiologic appearance of the irradiated larynx. Part I. Expected changes. *Radiology* 1994;193:141–148.
28. Hudgins PA, Burson JG, Gussack GS, et al. CT and MR appearance of recurrent malignant head and neck neoplasms after resection and flap reconstruction. *AJNR Am J Neuroradiol* 1994;15:1689–1694.
29. Fu KK, Woodhouse RJ, Quivey JM, et al. The significance of laryngeal edema following radiotherapy of carcinoma of the vocal cord. *Cancer* 1982;49:655–658.
30. Stokkel MP, Terhaard CH, Hordijk GJ, et al. The detection of local recurrent head and neck cancer with fluorine-18 fluorodeoxyglucose dual-head positron emission tomography. *Eur J Nucl Med* 1999;26:767–773.
31. Anzai Y, Carroll WR, Quint DJ, et al. Recurrence of head and neck cancer after surgery or irradiation: prospective comparison of 2-deoxy-2-[F-18]fluoro-D-glucose PET and MR imaging diagnoses. *Radiology* 1996;200:135–141.
32. Kao CH, Tsai SC, Wang JJ, et al. Comparing 18-fluoro-2-deoxyglucose positron emission tomography with a combination of technetium 99m tetrofosmin single photon emission computed tomography and computed tomography to detect recurrent or persistent nasopharyngeal carcinomas after radiotherapy. *Cancer* 2001;92:434–439.
33. Mukherji SK, Gapany M, Neelon B, et al. Evaluation of 201T1 SPECT for predicting early treatment response in patients with squamous cell carcinoma of the extracranial head and neck treated with nonsurgical organ preservation therapy: initial results. *J Comput Assist Tomogr* 2000;24:146–151.
34. Valdes Olmos RA, Balm AJ, Hilgers FJ, et al. Thallium-201 SPECT in the diagnosis of head and neck cancer. *J Nuclear Med* 1997;38:873–879.
35. Mukherji SK, Gapany M, Phillips D, et al. Thallium-201 single-photon emission CT versus CT for the detection of recurrent squamous cell carcinoma of the head and neck. *AJNR Am J Neuroradiol* 1999;20:1215–1220.
36. Leitha T, Glaser C, Pruckmayer M, et al. Technetium-99m-MIBI in primary and recurrent head and neck tumors: contribution of bone SPECT image fusion. *J Nucl Med* 1998;39:1166–1171.
36a. Nagamachi S, Moshi M, Jinnouchi S. The use of ^{201}T1-SPECT to predict the response to radiotherapy in patients with head and neck cancer. *Nucl Med Commun* 1996;17:935–942.
37. Greven KM, Williams DW 3rd, Keyes JW Jr, et al. Positron emission tomography of patients with head and neck carcinoma before and after high dose irradiation [See comments]. *Cancer* 1994;74:1355–1359.
38. Claudio F, Cacace F, Comella G, et al. Intraarterial chemotherapy through carotid transposition in advanced head and neck cancer. *Cancer* 1990;65:1465–1471.
39. Imai S, Kajihara Y, Munemori O, et al. Superselective cisplatin (CDDP)-carboplatin (CBDCA) combined infusion for head and neck cancers. *Eur J Radiol* 1995;21:94–99.
40. Shimizu T, Sakakura Y, Hattori T, et al. Superselective intraarterial chemotherapy in combination with irradiation: preliminary report. *Am J Otolaryngol* 1990;11:131–136.
41. Zanella FE, Valavanis A. Interventional neuroradiology of lesions of the skull base [Review]. *Neuroimaging Clin N Am* 1994;4:619–637.
42. Robbins KT, vanSonnenberg E, Casola G, et al. Image-guided needle biopsy of inaccessible head and neck lesions. *Arch Otolaryngol Head Neck Surg* 1990;116: 957–961.
43. Mukherji SK, Turetsky D, Tart RP, et al. A technique for core biopsies of head and neck masses. *AJNR Am J Neuroradiol* 1994;15:518–520.
44. Silverman PM, Zeiberg AS, Sessions RB, et al. Helical CT of the upper airway: normal and abnormal findings on three-dimensional reconstructed images. *AJR Am J Roentgenol* 1995;165:541–546.
45. Erickson SJ, Hogan QH. CT-guided injection of the stellate ganglion: description of technique and efficacy of sympathetic blockade. *Radiology* 1993;188:707–709.
46. Cooney TR, Poulsen MG. Is routine follow-up useful after combined-modality therapy for advanced head and neck cancer? *Arch Otolaryngol Head Neck Surg* 1999;125:379–382.
47. Mukherji SK, Drane WE, Tart RP, et al. Comparison of thallium-201 and F-18 FDG SPECT uptake in squamous cell carcinoma of the head and neck. *AJNR Am J Neuroradiol* 1994;15:1837–1842.
48. Fischbein N, Anzai Y, Mukherji SK. Application of new imaging techniques for the evaluation of squamous cell carcinoma of the head and neck. *Semin Ultrasound CT MR* 1999;20:187–212.
49. Labadie RF, Yarbrough WG, Weissler MC, et al. Nodal volume reduction after concurrent chemo- and radiotherapy: correlation between initial CT and histopathologic findings. *AJNR Am J Neuroradiol* 2000;21:310–314.

CHAPTER 5

Intensity Modulated Radiotherapy of Head and Neck Cancer

Avraham Eisbruch

In traditional irradiation of head and neck cancer, the placement of the radiation fields and their shapes are based on the bony anatomy acquired by the simulator diagnostic-quality films. During the late 1980s, advancements in computer technology and imaging introduced methods to identify the targets on computed tomography (CT) scans and display the radiation beams in three dimensions relative to the anatomy. In addition, calculation of and display of the radiation dose distributions and methods to evaluate and compare rival plans using dose-volume histograms (DVHs) became available. The introduction of multileaf collimators facilitated an increase in the number of beams that could be delivered without a large extension of treatment time. Treatment could now be delivered from multiple angles, including non-coplanar directions, when required. The result was the emergence of three-dimensional conformal radiotherapy (3DCRT), which allowed better precision of irradiation delivery to image-based targets and some improvements in sparing noninvolved critical tissue. Early studies of the use of 3DCRT in head and neck cancer examined cancer of the larynx (1), nasopharynx (2), hypopharynx (3), and paranasal sinuses (4). These studies demonstrated a significant benefit from 3DCRT in better coverage of the tumors and reduced doses to critical tissue compared with standard techniques. In the community, 3DCRT became widely used, essentially relying on the traditional arrangement of three fields while using beam's eye views to ensure adequate coverage of the targets ("standard 3D"). This use of 3D technology has mostly been applied to the boost phase of treatment. An analysis of the results of 3DCRT of nasopharyngeal cancer at Memorial Sloan Kettering Hospital showed no difference in the outcome of patients treated with standard techniques compared with patients whose boost phase was delivered with 3DCRT (5). These authors concluded that further benefit would be gained if highly conformal doses were delivered throughout therapy, not just during the boost phase, although more advanced techniques will be required for this end. Intensity modulated radiotherapy (IMRT) is an emerging technology that facilitates an even higher degree of dose conformality, and offers opportunities for additional clinical gains.

INTENSITY MODULATED RADIOTHERAPY: GENERAL ASPECTS

Intensity modulated radiotherapy (IMRT) implies the use of radiation fields whose intensity varies across the field, depending on the thickness of the target and the existence of critical organs or critical noninvolved tissue in their path. Treating the targets with multiple beams of varying intensity allows a relatively uniform dose in an irregularly shaped target while avoiding a high dose to the surrounding structures. Two technological developments made IMRT possible: the introduction of computer-controlled multileaf collimators, and the development of computerized optimization, or "inverse planning", that determines the intensity of the beams which is required to satisfy a specified set of dose distributions.

Most IMRT delivery systems use either tomotherapy or conventional multileaf collimators. In tomotherapy, the patient is treated using a narrow slit beam, similar to the tomography techniques used in diagnostic CT. The commercial MIMiC® system, developed by NOMOS® Corporation (Cranberry Township, Pa.), is mounted on a conventional accelerator and delivers treatment to a narrow slice of the patient while the accelerator rotates around the patient. Beamlets of varying intensities are created by moving the MIMiC leaves in and out of the beam during the gantry rotation around the patient.

Because the beam "slice" is narrow, it is necessary to move the couch with great precision to obtain sequentially treated "slices" without gaps or overlaps. A helical tomotherapy design, currently being developed at the University of Wisconsin, is similar in its operation to the helical CT. Unlike the serial tomotherapy described previously, this design will avoid the requirements to abut subsequent slices, thus improving the safety and reliability of the system. Delivering IMRT using a conventional multileaf collimator can be made in a "dynamic" or "static" form. In the "dynamic" form, the leaves at each gantry position are swept across the target while the beam is on and their speed determines the radiation fluence. In "static" or "segmental" multileaf IMRT, each field consists of multiple segments with different intensities. This form of IMRT is offered by most manufacturers of linear accelerators.

The complexity of IMRT plans cannot usually be achieved by forward, iterative process alone used in 3DCRT plans. Computer-based optimization process, called inverse planning, is instead being used. Inverse planning demands the planner to state the treatment goals, usually in terms of the dose or dose/volume goals for the targets and the constraints for the critical normal tissue (the objective, or cost function). The computer attempts to achieve the desired outcome by iteration through numerous possible beam intensities. The desired solution is the dose distribution that minimizes the variance of the delivered dose relative to the objective function. For each target and noninvolved organ or tissue, an importance factor or weight is assigned, and the objective function is the sum of the variance terms representing each structure of interest, multiplied by the importance factor. Because the variance is the sum of the squares of the differences between the prescribed and the delivered doses, this approach is called a *quadratic objective function,* and is the one used in most optimization systems. A publication by the Intensity Modulated Radiation Therapy Collaborative Working Group summarizes the consensus regarding IMRT planning, delivery, commissioning, radiation safety and quality assurance, and details recommendations about target volume and dose specification (6). This publication is recommended for readers who are interested in more detailed discussions about the general aspects of IMRT.

INTENSITY MODULATED RADIOTHERAPY FOR HEAD AND NECK CANCER

The anatomy of the neck is complex, with many critical and radiation-sensitive organs in close proximity to the targets. Tight dose gradients around the targets that limit the doses to the noninvolved tissue, features characteristic of IMRT, are desirable and offer the potential for therapeutic gains. Noninvolved tissue, the sparing of which may offer tangible gains, includes the major salivary glands, minor salivary glands dispersed within the oral cavity, the mandible, and the pharyngeal musculature. In the cases of nasopharyngeal and paranasal sinus cancer, critical normal tissue that may be partly spared using IMRT includes the inner and middle ears, the temporomandibular joints, temporal brain lobes, and the optic pathways.

In addition to noninvolved tissue sparing, IMRT offers a potential for improved tumor control by reducing the constraints on the tumor dose due to critical organs (e.g., the spinal cord, brainstem, and the optic pathways) that occasionally limit the tumor boost doses in conventional radiotherapy (RT). This is achieved by specifying a maximal dose to the critical organs, and a high penalty in the optimization process if that dose is exceeded. In addition, IMRT eliminates the need for posterior neck electron fields, commonly used in conventional RT, and their associated dose deficiencies. IMRT in the head and neck is more feasible than in other sites, since organ motion is practically absent. The only factor that has to be taken into account is patient setup uncertainties. This can be addressed by using adequate immobilization and by assessing the resulting setup variations.

Patient Selection

Head and neck IMRT is work-intensive and lengthens treatment time. Not every patient is expected to benefit; those who would benefit most are patients with paranasal sinus cancer where the targets are near the optic pathways, patients with oropharyngeal or nasopharyngeal cancer in whom standard RT fields would encompass most of the salivary glands, and patients in whom standard techniques would require a compromise in the tumor dose, due to proximity of the tumor to the spinal cord or brainstem. Patients with laryngeal cancer and clinically noninvolved neck, receiving treatment to the larynx alone or requiring irradiation of the neck encompassing the jugulodigastric nodes but not extending to the base of skull, may not benefit from IMRT compared with simpler techniques. The same applies to patients requiring irradiation to the ipsilateral neck alone.

Immobilization

Head and neck immobilization is typically performed using a thermoplastic mask with several attachment points to the treatment table, and a head support. Several commercial systems are available. Typically, immobilization with these systems results in daily setup errors of few millimeters, on average (7). These errors require an extension of the targets by 3 to 5 mm to ensure adequate irradiation (see "The Planning Tumor Volumes" later in the chapter). It is important to extend the mask to include the lower neck and shoulders, if targets in the lower neck and the supraclavicular nodes are included in the IMRT plans. An alternative used in some institutions is to treat the lower neck with an anterior field, and match this field with the IMRT fields using a split-beam technique. In these cases, the head and upper neck alone need to be immobilized.

Imaging

The simulation contrast-enhanced CT is in most cases the only imaging modality required for the delineation of the targets. Magnetic resonance imaging (MRI) is limited by its sensitivity to artifacts, difficulty in interpretation, long examination time, and cost. Magnetic resonance imaging is a necessary adjunct to CT for tumors close to the base of skull (i.e., nasopharyngeal and paranasal sinus cancer), where it provides better details of tumor extension and better details of the parapharyngeal and retropharyngeal spaces compared with CT (8). Fluorodeoxyglucose-positron emission tomography (FDG-PET) has been found to add significantly to the information gained from CT regarding the tumor extent in lung cancer (9). In contrast, series of head and neck cancer where CT, MRI and FDG-PET were obtained, and surgery was then performed to validate the primary tumor extent and involvement of the lymph nodes, reported a rather limited benefit of FDG-PET compared with CT/MRI (10). This modality remains, for the time being, a research tool for defining the extent of the target (an exception is defining the target in recurrent cancer, where FDG-PET has demonstrated a higher sensitivity than CT or MRI). In all cases, the findings of a careful clinical examination, including direct endoscopy under anesthesia, form the basis for assessing the extent of the primary tumor.

Selection and Outlining of the Targets

A major potential pitfall of IMRT is the failure to select and delineate the targets accurately. This is especially relevant in head and neck cancer, where a high risk for subclinical local and nodal disease exists, and where adequate irradiation of the lymph nodes at risk is crucial for locoregional control and survival. For example, in standard three-field head and neck RT, the first echelon and the retropharyngeal nodes are treated routinely when the primary tumor is targeted. In contrast, these nodes will not be adequately irradiated by IMRT if they are not specified on the planning CT.

Target Definitions in the Head and Neck

The gross target volumes (GTVs) consist of the primary tumor and of lymph nodes with apparent or suspected metastasis. The primary tumor GTV is defined using radiologic and clinical assessment. Lymph node GTVs include nodes with radiologic criteria of involvement (diameter >1 cm; in the case of the jugulodigastric nodes, >1.1–1.5 cm), smaller nodes with spherical rather than ellipsoid shape, nodes containing inhomogeneities suggestive of necrotic centers, or a cluster of three or more borderline nodes (11). The clinical target volume (CTV) surrounding the primary tumor consists of tissue perceived to contain microscopic, subclinical tumor extension. In addition to the primary tumor CTV, the lymphatic CTVs consist of nodal areas that are at risk for metastatic disease but do not match the radiologic criteria of involved nodes.

Delineation of the Primary Tumor Clinical Target Volume

Factors used for assessing the extent of the CTV margins in each case include tumor site, size, stage, differentiation, and morphology (exophytic vs. ulcerative, infiltrative vs. pushing front). Rather than expand the GTV uniformly, we recommend outlining the CTV on the planning CT on slice-by-slice basis. Knowledge of the anatomic and clinical patterns of tumor extension, and clinical judgment, as well as a familiarity with head and neck imaging, are necessary for accurate estimation of the CTV margins around the tumor. Specific recommendations for each tumor site have been detailed elsewhere (12).

Selection and Delineation of the Lymphatic Clinical Target Volumes

Our knowledge of the pattern and risk for lymphatic drainage from different head and neck sites is based on the classic anatomic work of Rouviere (13), reviewed recently (14), the assessment of the location and prevalence of clinical neck metastasis by Lindberg (15), and the large experience with elective neck dissections providing information about microscopic metastases, reported by Byers and Shah (16,17). A division of the neck to six levels has been developed by surgeons from Memorial Hospital and revised by Robbins et al. (18,19), allowing standardized and improved reporting of the nodal involvement and the surgical therapy of the neck. Adoption of this system for identification and outlining of the nodal CTVs for IMRT is highly recommended. It should be emphasized that the retropharyngeal nodes, which are not routinely dissected surgically, are not considered in the surgical neck levels classification, but are important targets in the irradiation of nasopharyngeal and other advanced head and neck cancer. Reviews of the risk for metastases to each neck level (20), and of the neck levels at risk for each tumor site and stage (12) have recently been published. Several publications are recommended for identifying the neck levels on the planning CT scans. An imaging-based nodal classification, using CT or MRI-based criteria that correspond to the surgical anatomic landmarks, has been developed by head and neck radiologists (21). In addition, several excellent articles have been published by radiation oncologists demonstrating how to outline the lymph node neck levels as CTVs on the planning CT scans (20,22,23) or axial MRI (20).

In the postoperative cases, the surgical specimens provide information that helps in determining the neck levels at risk. Neck dissection disrupts some anatomic landmarks used to define the borders between the levels. On the other hand, the surgical bed is apparent on the CT scan and should be encompassed entirely within the CTV. It is often impossible to distinguish between the primary tumor resection and the adjacent neck dissection bed, and they are encompassed within a unified CTV. Neck levels in which microscopic extracapsular lymph node extension has been found are considered high-risk volumes and are assigned a higher dose (see later).

The Planning Tumor Volumes

Once the GTVs and CTVs are outlined on the axial CT images, a uniform expansion of these targets is performed to obtain the planning tumor volumes (PTVs) that accommodate setup uncertainties, typically by 3 to 5 mm. Doses are prescribed to the PTVs or to comparable "growth" areas in some commercial planning systems. When the targets are close to the skin, as may occur in postoperative cases, the PTV may extend beyond the surface. In such cases, the PTV should be "edited" back to the surface. If the PTV extends to the skin but the skin is not at a high risk, the external body contour may be defined as a noninvolved organ for the optimization system. This facilitates avoiding excessive dose to the skin.

Similar to the expansion of the targets to yield the PTVs, there is a need to accommodate uncertainties regarding the critical normal organs, especially the spinal cord, brainstem, and the optic pathways that may lie in regions of steep dose fall-off near the targets. This can be accomplished by expanding these organs uniformly, yielding the planning risk volumes (PRVs). At the University of Michigan, the spinal cord is expanded by 0.5 cm to yield the spinal cord PRV. The maximal accepted doses are 45 Gy to the spinal cord and 50 Gy to the PRV. Similarly, the optic nerves and chiasma are expanded by 3 to 5 mm for treatment plans of nasopharynx or paranasal sinus tumors.

An example of the delineation of the targets and noninvolved structures in a case of oropharyngeal cancer is provided in Figure 5.1 (see Color Plate 2 following page 524).

Dose Prescription and Specification and Normal Tissue Dose Constraints

The delivery of a single plan throughout the course of treatment provides better dose conformality compared with several consecutive plans, commonly practiced in standard RT for head and neck cancer (24). When a single plan is prescribed, the gross tumor PTV receives both a higher total dose and a higher dose per fraction compared with the PTVs of the subclinical disease. Because of the differences in the daily fraction doses, a correction of the total dose to yield the normalized total dose (NTD) for a 2 Gy fraction regimen is required when the fraction dose is different from standard fractionation. An

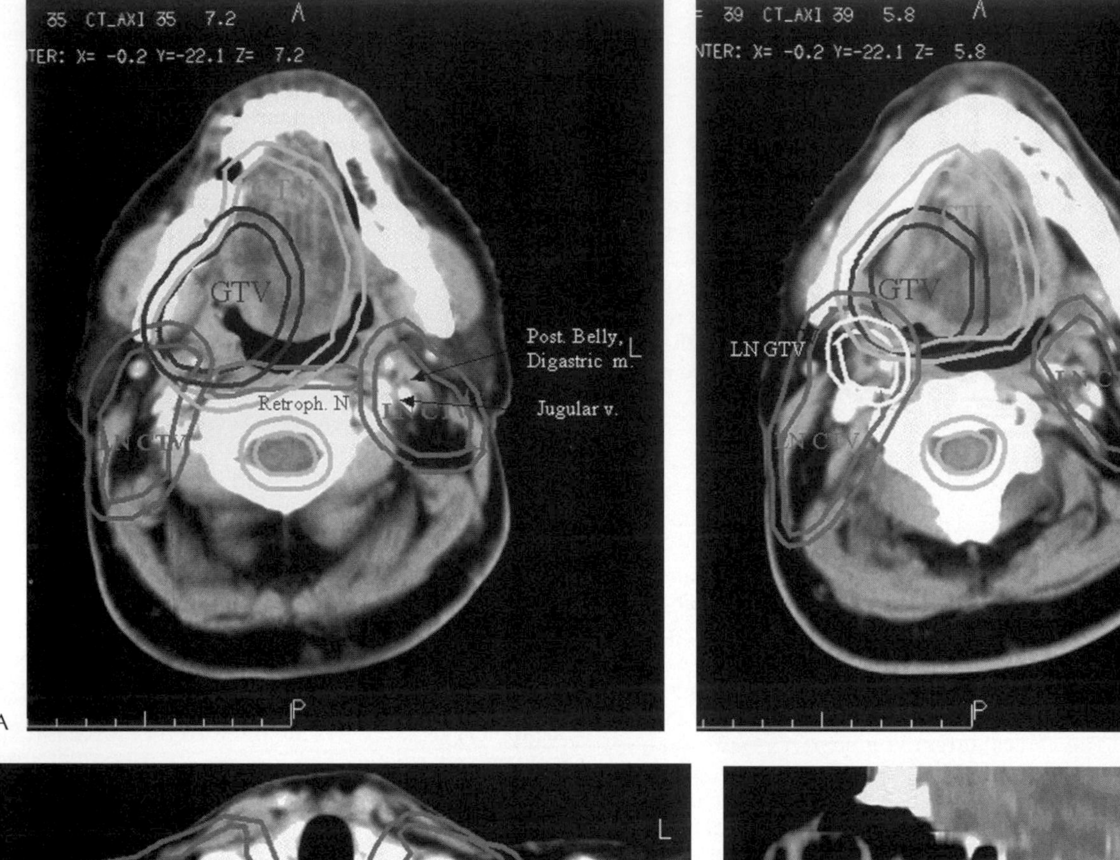

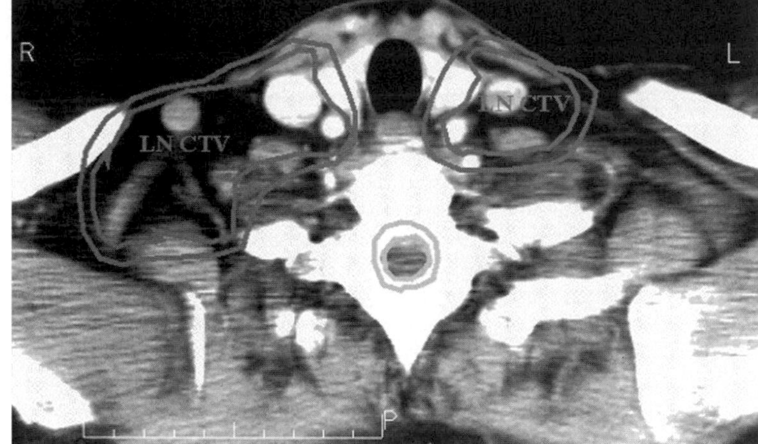

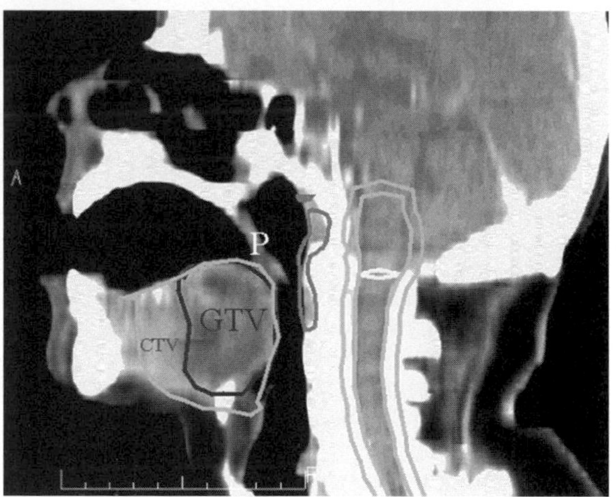

Figure 5.1 The targets outlined on planning computed tomography (CT) in a case of stage T2, N1 carcinoma of the right tonsil, involving the lateral base of tongue. The gross target volume (*GTV*), primary tumor clinical target volume (*CTV*), and lymphatic GTV and CTVs are each expanded uniformly by 0.5 cm to yield the corresponding planning tumor volume (*PTV*). **A:** Level II nodal targets in the ipsilateral neck, and the retropharyngeal nodes bilaterally, are outlined through the base of skull. Level II nodes in the contralateral neck are outlined up to the level in which the posterior belly of the digastric muscle crosses the jugular vein. Cephalad to this level, only the ipsilateral level II nodal CTVs and the retropharyngeal nodes are outlined. In cases where the contralateral neck contains clinical or radiologic evidence of metastasis, or in the case of nasopharyngeal cancer, level II is outlined through the base of skull bilaterally. **B:** Nodal metastasis in the LN neck is outlined as a nodal GTV, expanded to yield its PTV. **C:** In the LN lower neck, nodal levels IV and V are included in the CTV. Only level IV is outlined in the contralateral lower neck (the contralateral neck did not have clinical evidence of metastasis). **D:** A sagittal reconstruction of the CT may help in the assessment of the extent of disease. On axial images, it is difficult to distinguish the soft palate from the base of the tongue that contains the targets. The sagittal view facilitates the exclusion of the soft palate (*P*) from the targets. (See Color Plate 2 following page 524.)

extensive discussion of this issue is provided by Mohan et al. (24). There are two general approaches to dose prescription. The first would be prescribing a total dose delivering standard fraction dose to the gross disease PTV (e.g., 70 Gy over 35 fractions), and low fraction doses to the subclinical disease PTVs: 63 Gy to the high-risk and 58.1 Gy to lesser-risk elective targets that over 35 fractions would deliver fraction doses of 1.8 Gy and 1.66 Gy, yielding NTD of 60 Gy and 50 Gy, respectively (the NTDs are calculated for late-reacting tissue, assuming an α/β of 3 Gy). When used for advanced disease, this schedule is expected to be delivered concurrent with chemotherapy. The second strategy is to deliver a higher-than-standard fraction dose to the gross disease PTV, adjusting the total dose to yield NTD near 70 Gy, and standard fraction doses to the elective PTVs. Such a strategy was adopted by the Radiation Therapy Oncology Group (RTOG) study of IMRT for oropharyngeal cancer (RTOG study H-0022). In this study, the gross disease PTV receives a total of 66 Gy in 30 fractions, 2.2 Gy per fraction. PTVs of high-risk subclinical disease receive 60 Gy, and low-risk PTVs receive 54 Gy, at 2.0 and 1.8 Gy per fraction, respectively. This results in the gross disease PTV receiving NTD of 70 Gy over 6 weeks, similar to the total time and dose delivered by an accelerated RT regimen (25). A more aggressive reported regimen delivers a total of 60 Gy in 25 fractions (2.4 Gy per fraction) to the gross disease and 50 Gy (2.0 Gy per fraction) to electively treated volumes, yielding an NTD of 66 Gy delivered over 5 weeks (26). If we take into account the relatively target large dose inhomogeneity produced by IMRT, it would be apparent that large tissue volumes within the targets receive even higher fraction doses, and higher NTDs, than those calculated for the prescribed doses. A phase I dose escalation study in which the fraction size and the total dose to the gross disease PTVs are escalated is currently being conducted at the Medical College of Virginia (27). It is postulated that limiting the high-dose treated volume to the target alone by IMRT may reduce the risk for late complications arising from large fraction doses (26,27). However, critical normal tissues at risk in the head and neck (i.e., nerves, noninvolved mucosa, blood vessels, bone, etc.) are embedded within the targets and are at risk for late toxicity. These schemes, therefore, should only be practiced within well-defined clinical trials. As yet, the follow-up periods of published head and neck cancer IMRT series are not sufficient to assess the risk for late complications arising from higher-than-standard fraction doses and total NTDs delivered to the targets (26,28).

Dose and dose/volume specifications are made to impose constraints on the DVHs of the targets, noninvolved tissue of interest, and nonspecified tissue outside the targets. RTOG protocol H-0022 specifies the prescription dose as the dose that encompasses at least 95% of the PTV. No more than 20% of the PTV can receive more than 110% and no more than 1% of the PTV can receive less than 93% of the prescribed dose. To limit hot spots outside the targets, the protocol specifies that no more than 1% of the tissue outside the PTVs can receive more than 110% of the prescribed dose. This is done by adding a dose constraint for all nonspecified tissue (all tissue outside the targets and the specified organs), to prevent volumes of high dose outside the targets.

Dose constraints regarding critical organs are usually stated in terms of the maximal dose. Commonly applied constraints in the head and neck are maximal doses of 45 Gy to the spinal cord, 54 Gy to the brainstem, 70 Gy to the mandible, and 50 to 55 Gy to the optic pathway. These constraints were derived from standard irradiation, where the organ at risk receives irradiation at a standard daily fraction dose for part of the therapy course and is then fully shielded. In contrast, IMRT typically delivers lower daily fraction doses to these organs throughout therapy. In addition, the maximal dose derived from the DVH represents only a small organ volume, whereas standard RT delivers any specified dose homogeneously to relatively large volumes. In most instances, therefore, the same dose constraints are more conservative when applied to IMRT compared with standard RT. Conversely, steep fall-off of doses near the critical organs may increase the risk for inadvertent overdosage to these organs due to motion and setup uncertainties. This issue can be addressed by a uniform expansion of the critical organs to yield the PRVs, as discussed previously. Organs with parallel functional architecture require specification of the mean dose or partial organ volume dose, rather than the maximal dose. Examples are the specification in RTOG protocol H-0022 of the maximal mean dose to the parotid salivary glands at 26 Gy, or limiting the dose to at least 50% of the gland volume to less than 30 Gy, and constraining the dose to two thirds of the larynx at less than 50 Gy.

Optimization Process

The PTVs and noninvolved organs lie in close vicinity, or overlap with each other. It is necessary to assign weighting factors (or penalty/importance factors) to each target and organ that determine the relative importance of fulfilling their dose specifications or constraints. These weighting factors are derived following an iterative, trial and error process that requires refinement for each patient to produce an optimal plan. These factors differ among the various optimization systems. Examples of penalty factors for head and neck cancer plans were provided by several authors (29,30). It was noted that because normal structure doses are penalized during optimization only if they exceed the limits set by the user, the constraints need to be more stringent than the clinical criteria (30). At the University of Michigan, the optimization system uses a cost function that strives to minimize the dose to some noninvolved structures in addition to setting a maximal dose constraint that facilitates a reduction of the doses to these organs (31). Also, using a combination of linear and high-power objective functions (in addition to the quadratic objective function used in most commercial systems), strict head and neck target dose homogeneity could be achieved (31).

In addition to the physical dose and dose/volume optimization criteria, several investigators examined the use of biologic/clinical criteria as a basis for optimization in the head and neck. These investigations include optimization using the probability of uncomplicated tumor control (32), tumor control probability (TCP) and normal tissue complication probability (NTCP) (33), and the equivalent uniform dose concept (EUD), which is defined as the biologically equivalent dose that, if given uniformly, will lead to the same cell kill in the tumor volume as the actual nonuniform dose distribution (34). The latter investigators found that optimizing using EUD as the cost function is superior to optimization using dose or dose/volume. Work at the University of Michigan comparing various biologic factors and dose or dose/volume as the bases for optimization found that the balancing of power and weights, rather than the specific cost function, is the determining factor for the optimization results (35). Biologic cost functions are expected to be superior to dose-based functions when the parameters of the biologic models, derived from clinical dose-response and dose-complication data, are known with greater confidence. An example is the optimization of advanced paranasal sinus cancer plans, where optic pathway NTCPs derived from patient complication data were used for the critical organ cost function (36).

Number and Directions of the Beams

While tomotherapy uses arcs around the patient, IMRT using multileaf collimator (MLCs) requires decisions regarding the number and orientation of the beams. It has been suggested that if the number of segments (or beamlets) is large enough, the direction of the beams is not important, and coplanar beams arranged equidistant around the patient's head and neck would achieve satisfactory results. Most investigations of IMRT of head and neck with MLCs use this approach. The beam number should be odd, to prevent opposed beams that would increase hot spots near their entrance to the neck. Nine beams arranged equidistant (40 degrees apart) were found to be optimal: they provided better dose distributions than five or seven beams, whereas fifteen beams did not seem to improve the plans (27). An optimization of the angles of the beams was found to be unnecessary by some authors (27) whereas others reported an improvement in head and neck plans when optimized, non-coplanar beam angles were used (37). This issue continues to be a subject to research, while current recommended field arrangement for IMRT of head and neck cancer with MLCs is nine equidistant, coplanar fields (Fig. 5.2; see also Color Plate 3 following page 524).

Specific Sites

NASOPHARYNX

Intensity modulated radiotherapy of the nasopharynx represents opportunities in sparing many critical noninvolved structures and improved tumor coverage, as detailed previously. These improvements have been demonstrated in several treatment planning exercises in nasopharyngeal and oropharyngeal tumors, where IMRT plans were compared with "standard 3D" plans in the same patients (26,27,29,30,38–41). However, to translate the advantage apparent in planning to a clinical benefit, it is crucial to outline the targets adequately. This may be more difficult in the case of nasopharyngeal cancer compared with other tumor sites. The GTV should be derived from an MRI that has been registered with the planning CT, as discussed previously. The CTV should adequately encompass potential subclinical tumor extension at the base of skull, detailed elsewhere (12). Lymph node CTVs should include level II nodes through the base of skull, as well as levels IB and III through V bilaterally, and the retropharyngeal nodes (see references 20, 22, and 23 for details regarding the outlining of the neck lymph node levels on the planning CT). Specified critical tissues include the major salivary glands, optic nerves and chiasm, brainstem, spinal cord, inner ears, temporomandibular joints, and mandible. Options for the prescribed doses and constraints for noninvolved organs are detailed previously under "Dose Prescription and Specification and Normal Tissue Dose Constraints. " An example of the targets and IMRT dose distributions in a case of nasopharyngeal cancer is provided in Figure 5.3 (see Color Plate 4 following page 524).

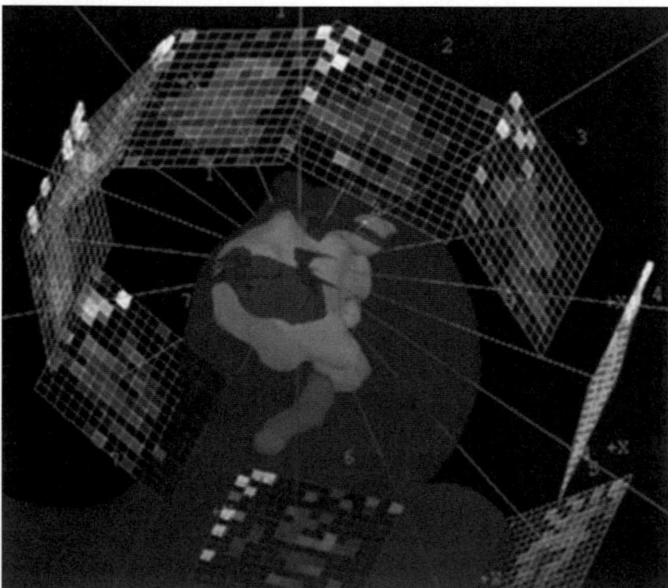

Figure 5.2 Beam arrangement for intensity modulated radiotherapy using a multileaf collimator. Nine coplanar, equidistant beams are used, each containing 1 × 1 cm or 0.5 × 0.5 cm pencil "beamlets." (See Color Plate 3 following page 524.)

The largest clinical series of IMRT of nasopharyngeal cancer has been reported by investigators at the University of California in San Francisco (42). In a recent update of this series (28) they reported 67 patients treated between 1995 and 2000. The GTV dose was 2.12 to 2.25 Gy per fraction to a total of 65 to 70 Gy and the CTV dose was 1.8 to 2.0 Gy per fraction to a total of 50 to 60 Gy. To prevent underdosing of the targets, the prescribed doses were typically the minimal doses encompassing the targets.

The resulting delivered mean GTV dose was 74.5 Gy, at mean GTV fraction doses of 2.24 to 2.4 Gy. The resulting NTD (calculated for late-responding tissue) was 80 Gy. This regimen yielded excellent locoregional tumor control: 97% at median follow-up of 31 months, with reasonable acute toxicity. The authors stated that no excessive late effects were observed. However, longer follow-up is still required for adequate assessment of the late toxicity.

PARANASAL SINUSES

Similar to the nasopharynx, MRI is required for accurate delineation of the GTV when the tumor is near the base of skull. Defining the extent of the CTV depends on the sinuses involved and tumor extent, discussed in detail elsewhere (12). The main obstacle for adequate tumor irradiation is the proximity of the optic pathways to the target in advanced cases. In these cases, IMRT can provide adequate target coverage while sparing the optic pathways (Fig. 5.4; see also Color Plate 5 following page 524). The group from Royal Marsden Hospital used MLC-based IMRT employing standard arrangement of beams: an anterior and two half-blocked lateral fields (43). They found that compared with 3DCRT, using the same beam arrangement, IMRT significantly reduced the dose to the optic nerves and improved PTV coverage. The group from Ghent University in Belgium used a combination of five to seven equally spaced MLC beams and additional non-coplanar beams that improved, in their experience, dose distributions (44). They reported early results in 11 patients, in whom the maximal dose to the optic pathways and brainstem was limited to 60 Gy while the PTV received 70 Gy. No vision toxicity was noticed over a short follow-up period in these patients. MLC-based IMRT planning of patients with non-resectable maxillary sinus cancer at the University of Michigan found no substantial difference between plans using an anterior and two lateral fields, compared with nine equidistant beams arranged around the patient. Thus, the use of a field arrangement considered optimal in standard radiotherapy benefits IMRT by reducing beam numbers and reducing the complexity of treatment delivery. Significant improvement in the doses to the optic pathways, compared with 3D conformal RT plans, was noted. IMRT plans of 13 patients with non-resectable paranasal sinus tumors demonstrated doses to the contralateral optic nerve and to the chiasma that were within known tolerance (<60 Gy), while

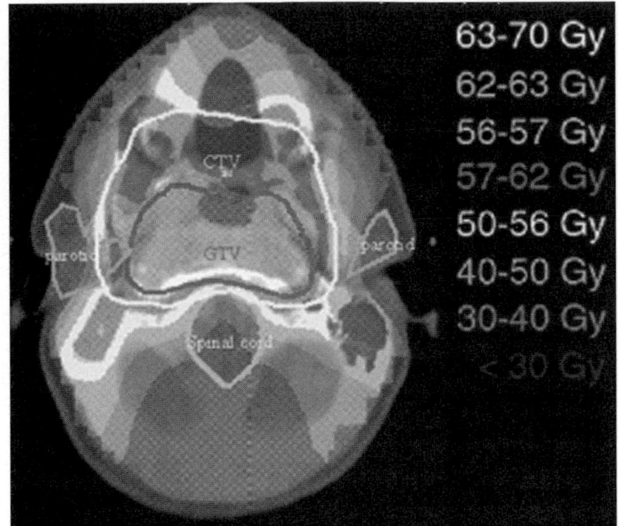

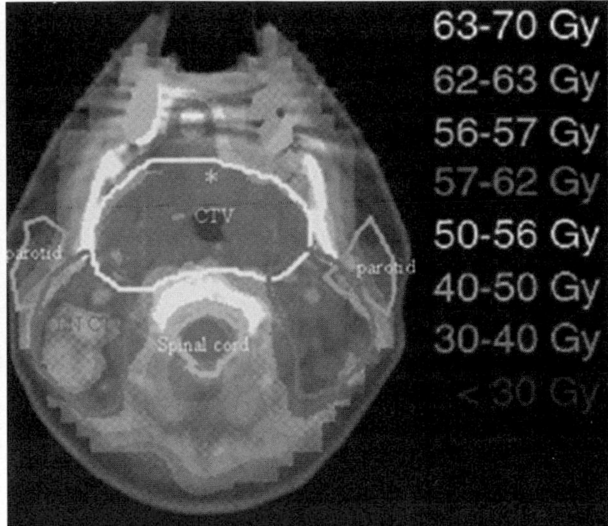

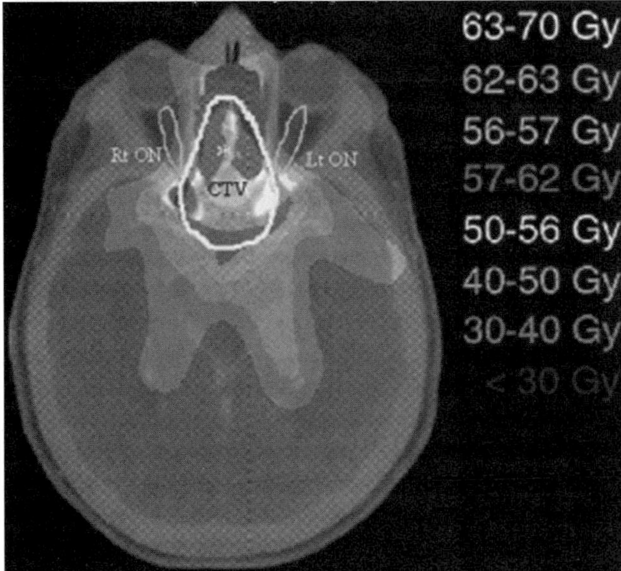

Figure 5.3 Targets and doses in intensity modulated radiotherapy of nasopharyngeal cancer. **A:** The gross target volume (*GTV*) was outlined following registration of the planning computed tomography with diagnostic magnetic resonance imaging. The clinical target volume (*CTV*) includes the base of skull, the posterior paranasal sinuses, the clivus, and the parapharyngeal space. **B:** Caudal to the GTV, the CTV contains the parapharyngeal and posterior pharyngeal space through midtonsils. Level II nodal CTVs are outlined through the base of skull bilaterally. **C:** The CTV encompasses the sphenoid and cavernous sinuses in locally advanced cases. Limiting the dose to the optic pathways is an important objective of planning. **D:** Dose-volume histograms of the case described in **A–C**. Both parotid glands are spared while the targets are adequately irradiated. (See Color Plate 4 following page 524.)

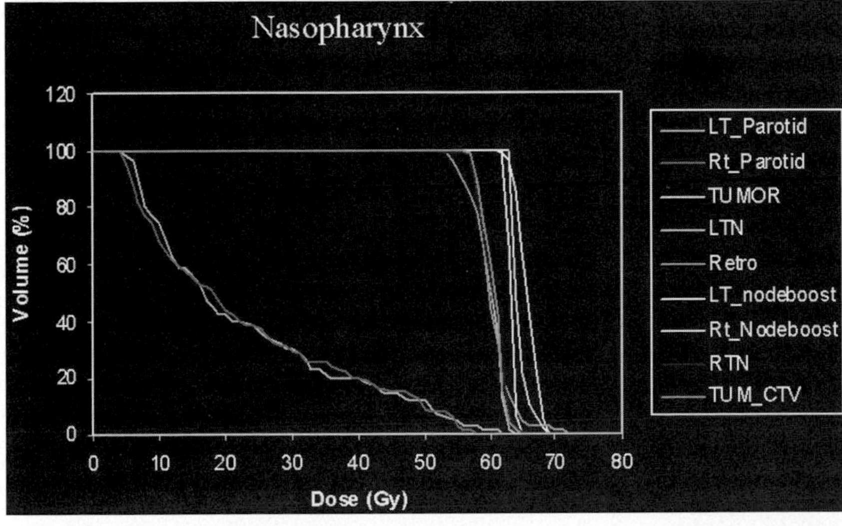

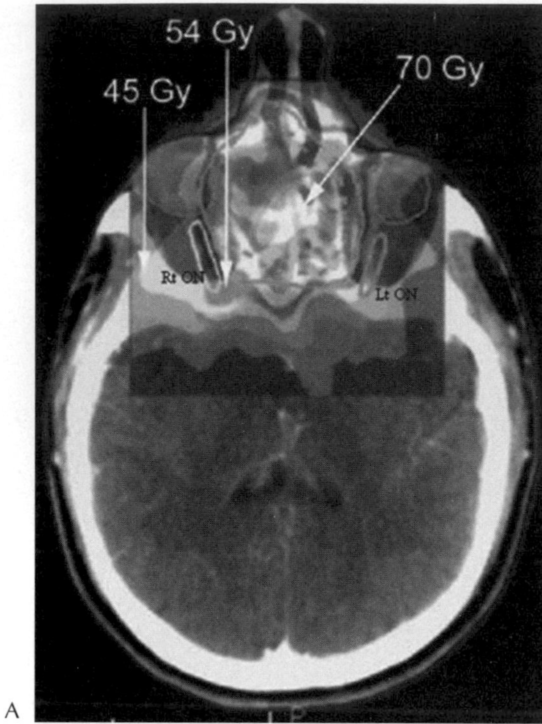

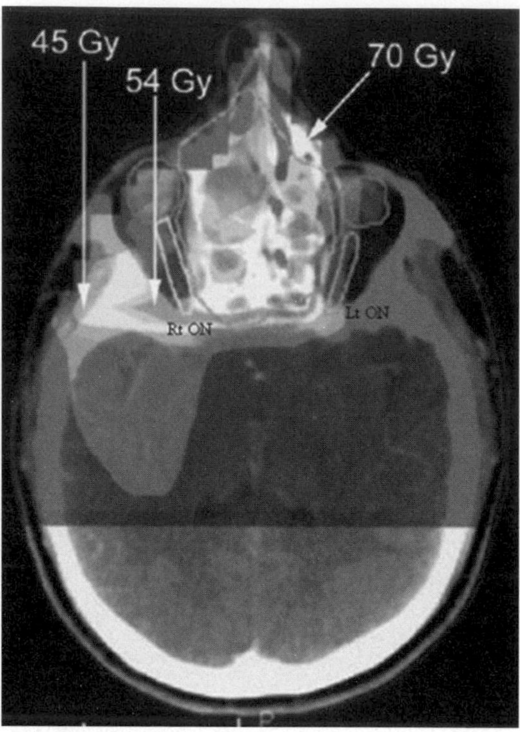

Figure 5.4 A,B: Isodoses of intensity modulated radiotherapy for advanced paranasal sinus cancer. Sparing the optic pathways was a major planning objective. (See Color Plate 5 following page 524.)

the ability to spare the ipsilateral optic nerve depended on the anatomic relationships between the PTV and the nerve. Optimization using NTCP of the optic nerves as an objective function was found to facilitate planning and provide a basis for the assessment of the clinical trade-off between PTV coverage and ipsilateral optic nerve sparing (36).

OROPHARYNX

Outlining of the primary tumor and lymph node CTVs and GTVs depends on tumor location and extent. In general, for lateralized tumors, the ipsilateral level II nodal CTV is outlined through the base of skull. The contralateral nodes at highest risk are the jugulodigastric nodes in level II. On CT axial images, these nodes lie below the level in which the posterior belly of the digastric muscle crosses the jugular vein. This is also the uppermost extent of radical neck dissection. At the University of Michigan, the most cephalad contralateral level II nodal CTV is outlined in these images. However, the contralateral nodal level II CTVs in patients with clinical evidence of nodal involvement in the contralateral neck or in those with midline tumors are outlined through the base of skull. In all patients, if the retropharyngeal nodes are at risk, they are outlined bilaterally through the base of skull. An example of the dose distributions obtained by IMRT in a case of oropharyngeal cancer is shown in Figure 5.5 (see Color Plate 6 following page 524). Details of dose prescriptions, critical organ dose constraints, and quality assurance procedures for the treatment of early oropharyngeal cancer are provided in RTOG protocol H-0022, available at the Website of RTOG (www.RTOG.org).

The pattern of locoregional tumor recurrence after IMRT of head and neck cancer at the University of Michigan, where the majority of patients had oropharyngeal cancer, was reported by Dawson et al. (45). Almost all recurrences appeared in-field, in high-risk volumes that had received the full prescribed dose. An update of this study includes 98 patients, mostly with oropharyngeal cancer, treated with primary (41 patients) or postoperative (57 patients) multisegmental IMRT. At a median follow-up of 40 months (range, 6–84 months), 15 locoregional failures (15%) occurred. Of these, 12 recurred in-field, and 3 were marginal recurrences, where less than 95% of the tissue volume harboring the recurrent tumor had received the prescribed dose. The cases with marginal recurrences included a patient with a history of neck surgery for oral cancer, treated with RT for tumor recurrence. Tumor subsequently recurred in unpredicted lymph nodes and in subcutaneous tissue. This case highlights the unpredictability of the lymphatic drainage in patients with a history of surgery, who therefore may not be suitable candidates for IMRT. Another patient had oral cancer with multiple level II-IV microscopic nodal metastasis. This patient had a marginal recurrence in paratracheal nodes (level VI), which highlights the risk at any neck level when adjoining levels are involved. A third patient with oropharyngeal cancer recurred marginally in ipsilateral retropharyngeal nodes. No patient recurred in the contralateral level II near the base of skull, an area that had been spared in many patients, and no patient recurred in the spared parotid glands. Careful examination and reporting of the pattern of locoregional recurrence by radiation oncologists treating head and neck cancer with IMRT is essential to further understand and improve it.

NONINVOLVED ORGAN SPARING WITH INTENSITY MODULATED RADIOTHERAPY: CLINICAL RESULTS

Several clinical studies assessed the use of IMRT in parotid salivary gland sparing and in reducing xerostomia. When the doses and treated parotid gland volumes were correlated with the parotid salivary output after multisegmental IMRT, it was

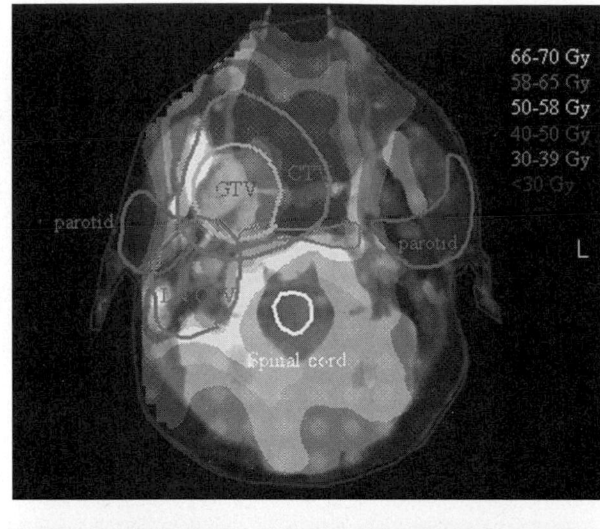

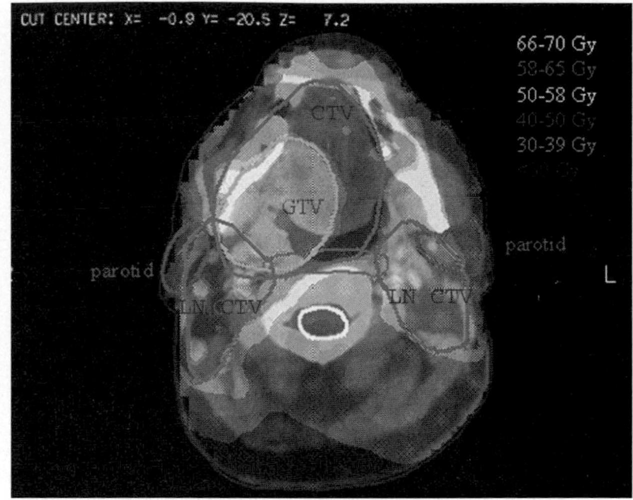

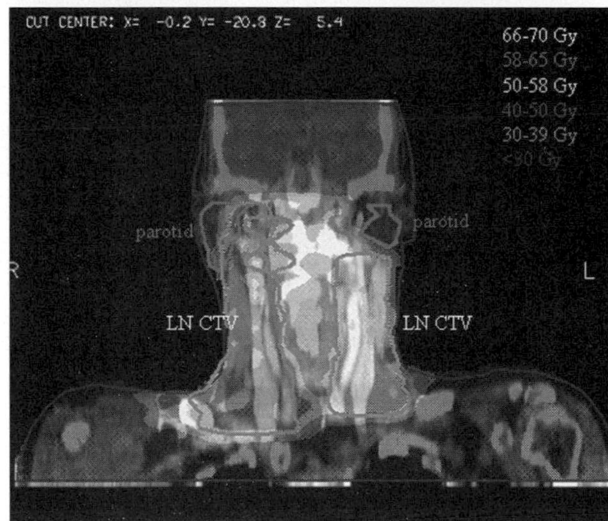

Figure 5.5 **A–C:** Isodoses of intensity modulated radiotherapy for the patient described in Figure 5.1. The contralateral parotid gland received a low dose (mean, 17 Gy) and the ipsilateral gland a moderate dose (mean, 32 Gy). CTV, clinical target volume; GTV, gross target volume. (See Color Plate 6 following page 524.)

found that the large majority of the glands receiving a mean dose of more than 26 Gy did not produce measurable saliva and did not recover, whereas glands receiving lower mean doses produced variable salivary output that increased over time (46). One year after RT, parotid glands receiving a moderate dose (mean dose of 17–26 Gy) recovered, on average, to the pre-RT salivary production levels. Analysis of a validated patient-reported xerostomia questionnaire showed that xerostomia improved significantly over time, in tandem with the increase in saliva production (47). Two years after radiation, xerostomia reported by patients receiving parotid-sparing bilateral neck radiation was only slightly worse than in patients receiving unilateral neck RT. Factors found to be statistically significant predictors of patient-reported xerostomia included the mean dose to the major salivary glands and the mean dose to the oral cavity, representing radiation received by the minor salivary glands. An improvement to mild or no xerostomia during the second year was also reported using the RTOG toxicity scale, following IMRT for nasopharyngeal cancer (28,42). It is apparent from these and other studies (48) that the sparing of the salivary glands, made possible by IMRT, achieves tangible gains in the retention of the salivary production and in xerostomia symptoms.

Additional potential functional gains from IMRT compared with conventional radiotherapy include swallowing and speech measures following aggressive chemo-irradiation, reported to be superior using IMRT compared with standard RT (49). Further quantitative assessment of the potential gains in organ sparing using IMRT will enhance our understanding of the role of this technology in the treatment of head and neck cancer.

REFERENCES

1. Coia L, Galvin J, Sontag M, et al. Three dimensional photon treatment planning in carcinoma of the larynx. *Int J Radiat Oncol Biol Phys* 1991;21:183–192.
2. Leibel S, Kutcher G, Harrison L, et al. Improved dose distributions for 3D conformal boost treatment in carcinoma of the nasopharynx. *Int J Radiat Oncol Biol Phys* 1991;20:823–833.
3. Esik O, Schlegel W, Boesecke R, et al. Three dimensional radiotherapy planning for laryngeal and hypopharyngeal cancer. *Radiother Oncol* 1991;20:238–244.
4. Roa WH, Hazuka MB, Sandler HM, et al. Results of primary and adjuvant CT-based 3-dimensional radiotherapy for malignant tumors of the paranasal sinuses. *Int J Radiat Oncol Biol Phys* 1994;28:857–865.
5. Wolden SL, Zelefsky MJ, Hunt MA, et al. Failure of a 3D conformal boost to improve radiotherapy for nasopharyngeal carcinoma. *Int J Radiat Oncol Biol Phys* 2001;49:1229–1234.
6. Intensity Modulated Radiation Therapy Collaborative Working Group. Intensity modulated radiotherapy: current status and issues of interest. *Int J Radiat Oncol Biol Phys* 2001;51:880–914.
7. Gilbeau L, Octave-Prignot M, Renard L, et al. Comparison of setup accuracy of three different thermoplastic masks for the treatment of brain and head and neck tumors. *Radiother Oncol* 2001;58:155–166.
8. Som PM. The present controversy over the imaging method of choice for evaluating the soft tissues of the neck. *AJNR Am J Neuroradiol* 1997;18:1869–1872.
9. Pieterman RM, van Putten JW, Meuzelaar JJ, et al. Preoperative staging of non-small cell lung cancer with positron-emission tomography. *N Engl J Med* 2000; 343:254–261.

10. Schechter NR, Gillenwater AM, Byers RM, et al. Can positron emission tomography improve the quality of care for head and neck cancer patients? *Int J Radiat Oncol Biol Phys* 2001;51:4–9.
11. Brekel van den NWM, Stel HV, Castelijns JA, et al. Cervical lymph node metastasis: assessment of radiologic criteria. *Radiology* 1990;177:379–384.
12. Eisbruch A, Foote RL, O'Sullivan B, et al. Intensity-modulated radiation therapy of head and neck cancer: emphasis on the selection and delineation of the targets. *Semin Radiat Oncol* 2002;12:238–249.
13. Rouviere H. Lymphatic systems of the head and neck. Ann Arbor, MI: Edwards Brothers, 1938. Tobias MJ, translator.
14. Mukherji SK, Armao D, Joshi VM. Cervical nodal metastases in squamous cell carcinoma of the head and neck: what to expect. *Head Neck* 2001;23:995–1005.
15. Lindberg RD. Distribution of cervical lymph node metastases from squamous cell carcinoma of the upper respiratory and digestive tracts. *Cancer* 1972;29: 1446–1449.
16. Byers RM, Wolf PF, Ballantyne AJ. Rationale for elective modified neck dissection. *Head Neck Surg* 1988;10:160–167.
17. Shah JP. Patterns of cervical lymph node metastasis from squamous carcinomas of the upper aerodigestive tract. *Am J Surg* 1990;160:405–409.
18. Robbins KT, Medina JE, Wolfe GT, et al. Standardizing neck dissection terminology. Official report of the Academy's committee for head and neck surgery and oncology. *Arch Otolaryngol Head Neck Surg* 1991;117:601–605.
19. Robbins KT. Integrating radiological criteria into the classification of cervical lymph node disease. *Arch Otolaryngol Head Neck Surg* 1999;125:385–387.
20. Gregoire V, Coche E, Cosnard G, et al. Selection and delineation of lymph node target volumes in head and neck conformal radiotherapy. Proposal for standardizing terminology and procedure based on the surgical experience. *Radiother Oncol* 2000;56:135–150.
21. Som PM, Curtin HD, Mancuso AA. An image-based classification for the cervical nodes designed as an adjunct to recent clinically based nodal classification. *Arch Otolaryngol Head Neck Surg* 1999;125:388–396.
22. Nowak PJCM, Wijers OB, Lagerwaard FJ, et al. A three-dimensional CT-based target definition for elective irradiation of the neck. *Int J Radiat Oncol Biol Phys* 1999;45:33–39.
23. Wijers OB, Levendag PC, Tan T, et al. A simplified CT-based definition of the lymph node levels in the node negative neck. *Radiother Oncol* 1999;52:35–42.
24. Mohan R, Wu Q, Manning M, et al. Radiobiological considerations in the design of fractionation strategies for intensity modulated radiation therapy of the head and neck. *Int J Radiat Oncol Biol Phys* 2000;46:619–630.
25. Fu KK, Pajak TF, Trotti A, et al. RTOG phase III randomized study to compare hyperfractionation and two variants of accelerated fractionation to standard fractionation radiotherapy for head and neck squamous cell carcinomas: first report of RTOG 9003. *Int J Radiat Oncol Biol Phys* 2000;48:7–16.
26. Butler EB, The BS, Grant WS, et al. SMART (simultaneous modulated accelerated radiation therapy) boost: a new accelerated fractionation schedule for the treatment of head and neck cancer with intensity modulated radiotherapy. *Int J Radiat Oncol Biol Phys* 1999;45:21–32.
27. Wu Q, Manning M, Schmidt-Ullrich R, et al. The potential for sparing of parotids and escalation of biologically equivalent dose with intensity modulated radiation treatments of head and neck cancers: a treatment design study. *Int J Radiat Oncol Biol Phys* 2000;46:195–205.
28. Lee N, Xia P, Akazawa P, et al. Intensity modulated radiotherapy in the treatment of nasopharyngeal carcinoma: an update of the UCSF experience. *Int J Radiat Oncol Biol Phys*2002;53:12–22.
29. Chao KSC, Low D, Perez CA, et al. Intensity-modulated radiation therapy in head and neck cancer: the Mallincrodt experience. *Int J Cancer* 2000;90:92–103.
30. Hunt MA, Zelefsky MJ, Wolden S, et al. Treatment planning and delivery of intensity-modulated radiation therapy for primary nasopharyngeal cancer. *Int J Radiat Oncol Biol Phys* 2001;49:623–632.
31. Vineberg KA, Eisbruch A, Kessler ML, et al. Is uniform target dose possible in IMRT plans for head and neck cancer? *Int J Radiat Oncol Biol Phys* 2002;52: 1159–1172.
32. Agren AK, Brahme A, Turesson I. Optimization of uncomplicated control for head and neck tumors. *Int J Radiat Oncol Biol Phys* 1990;19:1077–1085.
33. De Neve W, De Gersem W, Derycke S. Clinical delivery of IMRT for relapsed or second-primary head and neck cancer using a multileaf collimator with dynamic control. *Radiother Oncol* 1999;50:301–314.
34. Wu Q, Mohan R, Niemierko A. IMRT optimization based on the generalized equivalent uniform dose (EUD). *Int J Radiat Oncol Biol Phys* 2002;52:224–235.
35. Vineberg KA, McShan DL, Kessler ML, et al. Comparison of dose, dose-volume, and biologically-based cost functions for IMRT plan optimization. *Int J Radiat Oncol Biol Phys* 2001;51[Suppl 1]:71(abst).
36. Tsien C, Eisbruch A, McShan R, et al. IMRT for locally advanced paranasal sinus cancer: application of clinical decisions in the planning process. *Int J Radiat Oncol Biol Phys* 2003;55:776–784.
37. Pugachev A, Li JG, Boyer AL, et al. Role of beam orientation optimization in intensity modulated radiation therapy. *Int J Radiat Oncol Biol Phys* 2001;50: 551–560.
38. Eisbruch A., Marsh LH, Martel MK, et al. Comprehensive irradiation of head and neck cancer using conformal multisegmental fields: assessment of target coverage and noninvolved tissue sparing. *Int J Radiat Oncol Biol Phys* 1998;41: 559–568.
39. Van Dieren EB, Nowak PJCM, Wijers OB, et al. Beam intensity modulation using tissue compensators or dynamic multileaf collimation in three-dimensional conformal radiotherapy in cancer of the oropharynx and larynx, including the elective neck. *Int J Radiat Oncol Biol Phys* 2000;47:1299–1309.
40. Boyer AL, Geis P, Grant W, et al. Modulated beam conformal therapy for head and neck tumors. *Int J Radiat Oncol Biol Phys* 1997;39:227–236.
41. Xia P, Fu K, Wong GW, et al. Comparison of treatment plans involving intensity-modulated radiotherapy for nasopharyngeal carcinoma. *Int J Radiat Oncol Biol Phys* 2000;48:329–337.
42. Sultanem K, Shu HK, Xia P, et al. Three-dimensional intensity-modulated radiotherapy in the treatment of nasopharyngeal carcinoma: the University of California-San Francisco experience. *Int J Radiat Oncol Biol Phys* 2000;48: 711–722.
43. Adams E, Nutting CM, Convey DJ, et al. Potential role of intensity modulated radiotherapy in the treatment of tumors of the maxillary sinus. *Int J Radiat Oncol Biol Phys* 2001;51:579–588.
44. Claus F, De Gershem W, De Wagter C. An implementation strategy for IMRT of ethmoid sinus cancer with bilateral sparing of the optic pathways. *Int J Radiat Oncol Biol Phys* 2001;51:318–331.
45. Dawson LA, Anzai Y, Marsh L, et al. Local-regional recurrence pattern following conformal and intensity modulated RT for head and neck cancer. *Int J Radiat Oncol Biol Phys* 2000;46:1117–1126.
46. Eisbruch A, Ten Haken R, Kim HM, et al. Dose, volume and function relationships in parotid glands following conformal and intensity modulated irradiation of head and neck cancer. *Int J Radiat Oncol Biol Phys* 1999;45: 577–587.
47. Eisbruch A, Kim HM, Terrell JE, et al. Xerostomia and its predictors following parotid-sparing irradiation of head and neck cancer. *Int J Radiat Oncol Biol Phys* 2001;50:695–704.
48. Chao KSC, Deasy JO, Markman J, et al. A prospective study of salivary function sparing in patients with head and neck cancers receiving intensity-modulated or three-dimensional radiation therapy: initial results. *Int J Radiat Oncol Biol Phys* 2001;49:907–916.
49. Mittal B, Kepka A, Mahadevan A, et al. Use of IMRT to reduce toxicity from concomitant radiation and chemotherapy for advanced head and neck cancer. *Int J Radiat Oncol Biol Phys* 2001;51[Suppl 1]:82(abst).

CHAPTER 6

Dental Oncology and Maxillofacial Prosthetics

Jack W. Martin, Mark S. Chambers, and James C. Lemon

Rehabilitation of function, aesthetics, and prevention of infection, should be the major concerns of the treatment team prior to treatment and following the elimination of disease in the head and neck cancer patient. In caring for patients, most cancer treatment centers use a team approach, wherein members from each involved discipline (e.g., surgery, radiotherapy, dental therapy, chemotherapy, and speech therapy) determine their roles in the overall treatment. Patients with head and neck cancer should be referred to an oncologic dentist or maxillofacial prosthodontist during their initial medical workup to evaluate their oral and dental health. The results of this evaluation can then be integrated into the primary treatment plan. Early dental intervention can decrease the risk factors for radiation-induced osteoradionecrosis in the head and neck and chemotherapy-induced systemic infection. Early intervention can also allow surgically removed anatomic structures, such as the maxilla, to be immediately replaced with a prosthesis during the primary ablative procedure (1,2).

ORAL AND DENTAL ANATOMY

Surgeons, radiotherapists, and medical oncologists who treat patients with head and neck cancer should be familiar with oral and dental anatomy so that they can accurately communicate with their dental colleagues. Adult teeth are routinely used as landmarks to document the location of tumors of the jaws and to plan intraoral resections and prosthetic procedures before and after surgery. The most commonly used scheme for this purpose is the universal numbering system, which is used worldwide to identify the position and type of adult teeth. In this system, adult teeth are numbered sequentially from 1 to 32, starting with the right maxillary third molar and proceeding around the arch to the left third molar, down to the left mandibular third molar, and then around the mandibular arch to the right third molar. Missing or impacted teeth are counted in this system (3). Anatomic structures of the maxilla and mandible are important in retention and support of prostheses used in rehabilitation of patients with head and neck cancer. In the maxilla, the tissues important for the support and retention of prostheses are the tuberosity, alveolar ridge, and hard palate. In the mandible, the major supporting structures are the alveolar ridge, retromolar pad, and buccal shelf. Of course, sound and periodontally healthy teeth in both arches are very important in retention and support of prostheses. Conservation of the supporting tissue, consistent with oncologic principles used in the eradication of disease, should be a goal of the surgeon and medical oncologist (4,5).

ORAL AND DENTAL EVALUATION

Throughout treatment and follow-up care, the surgeon, radiation oncologist, and medical oncologist should be able to recognize oral pathology secondary to poor dental status; such pathology may include advanced periodontal disease, gross dental caries, tissue irritation secondary to poorly fitting prostheses, and poor oral hygiene. Plaque and calculus formation on teeth is an indication of poor oral hygiene. Preliminary findings of the initial medical examination should be noted. The patient should then be referred to an oncologic dentist, who should do a thorough radiographic and oral/dental examina-

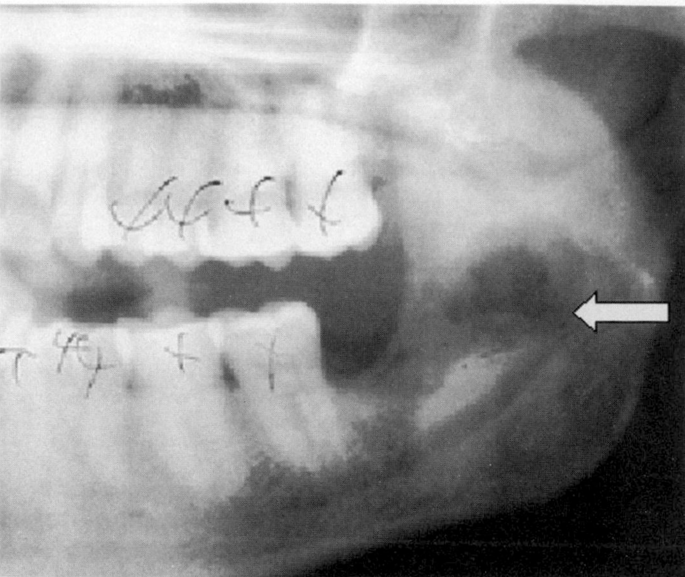

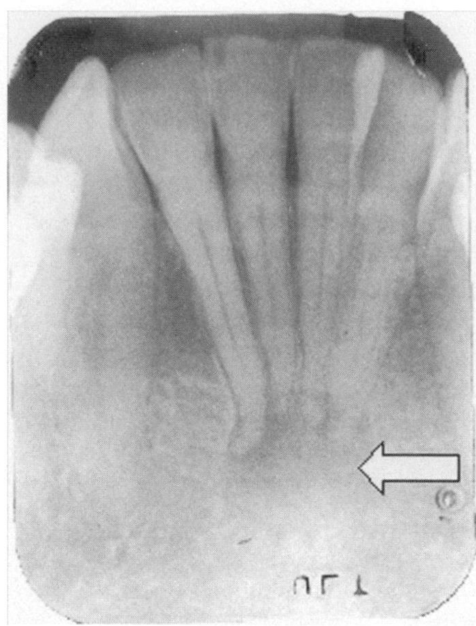

Figure 6.1 X-rays obtained in the dental office are relatively inexpensive, easily obtained, and can be diagnostic. The panoramic x-ray (**left**) shows a cancer in the ramus of the mandible. A periapical x-ray (**right**) shows an abscess associated with the anterior mandibular teeth in a patient with lymphoma.

tion and make impressions of dental and facial structures as appropriate. Panoramic, periapical, bitewing, and occlusal x-rays can be diagnostic and are inexpensive and easily obtained in the dental office (Fig. 6.1) (6). Casts obtained from impressions of the maxilla, mandible, and face can be useful in treatment planning, surgical prosthesis fabrication, and posttreatment rehabilitation. Teeth with a poor prognosis should be extracted before irradiation or chemotherapy (Fig. 6.2). This may require general anesthesia, intravenous sedation, or local anesthesia, depending on the difficulty of dental surgery and the patient's mental and physical status. Performing dental surgical procedures at the time of the primary ablative procedure may decrease the time the patient must wait before starting adjunctive treatments such as irradiation or chemotherapy. Reducing sites of infection decreases the chances of osteoradionecrosis in patients who undergo irradiation and infectious episodes in patients who receive chemotherapy (7).

Initially, posttreatment for at least one year after therapy for cancer follow-up of patients by the oncologic dentist is mandatory. Patients who undergo irradiation of the head and neck may experience dry mouth (xerostomia) and an increase in oral or dental problems such as infection and caries. All members of the treatment team should understand the importance of fluoride and at each follow-up appointment should encourage the patient to use a fluoride rinse (8–10). In many instances patients can be referred back to their general dentist for routine dental care after the initial posttreatment period.

In summary, thorough oral and dental evaluation by an oncologic dentist documents the oral and dental pathology before cancer treatment is begun. The results of the oral/dental evaluation enable the treatment team to inform the patient about rehabilitation, reduce or eliminate the sites of potential infection, and reveal important information that will be useful during treatment and rehabilitation. To ensure appropriate medical and legal responsibility, a dentist should be included as a member of the treatment team (11).

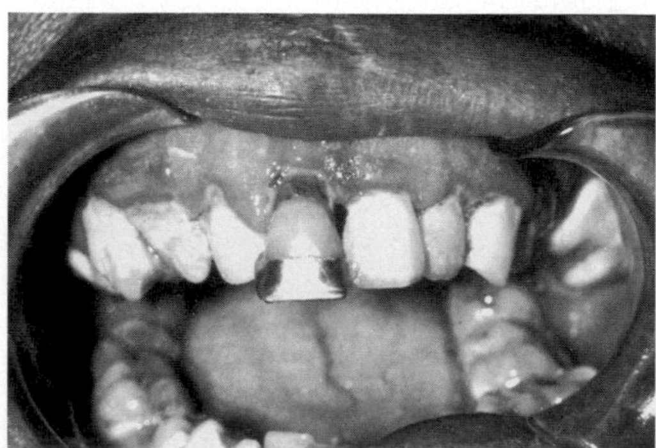

Figure 6.2 Patient with poor oral hygiene and periodontal disease will need multiple dental extractions prior to chemotherapy or radiation therapy. This can be done at the primary ablative procedure or at a separate procedure under local, intravenous, or general anesthesia.

INTRAORAL PROSTHETIC REHABILITATION

Usually there are three phases of prosthetic rehabilitation: surgical, interim, and definitive. Each phase may span several months to one year, depending on size and the location of the tumor and on the type of treatment required. Initially, surgical and interim prostheses may require frequent follow-up appointments and adjustments. Patients who undergo surgery that involves the maxilla and sinus may experience leakage from the mouth through the nose. Meticulous oral and dental hygiene are important, and physical therapy may be necessary to increase or maintain oral opening.

Maxilla

Cancer involving the maxillary sinus, hard palate, and alveolus may cause substantial postoperative speech and swallowing problems. Surgical considerations that may improve prosthetic rehabilitation of patients who receive a maxillectomy are as follows:

1. When operating on a dentate patient, surgeons should make the alveolar cuts through the socket of an extracted tooth. (When cuts are made between teeth both teeth may be lost.)
2. When making the palatal cut, as much of the supporting tissue (e.g., premaxilla, tuberosity, and alveolar ridge) as possible should be conserved, consistent with oncologic principles.
3. As a general rule, a split-thickness skin graft (STSG) should be placed in the maxillary defect. A well-placed STSG reduces secretions, facilitates oral hygiene, and provides a sound tissue base for a prosthesis.
4. The palatal mucosa, if it is not affected by disease, can be retained and used to line the midline portion of the palatal cut. This tissue is extremely resistant to the abrasive forces of the prosthesis.
5. The inferior and middle turbinates should be removed to allow extension of the prosthesis into the defect area and to ensure that a good seal is obtained.
6. Mandibular molar teeth on the side of the maxillectomy should be extracted if the opposing maxilla and teeth are resected. These teeth can pose a hygiene problem and are essentially nonfunctional after a posterior maxillectomy. This problem is particularly significant when the resection extends inferiorly in the cheek mucosa.
7. When possible, the maxillectomy should be performed intraorally, thus eliminating the facial incision and resulting disfigurement (Fig. 6.3) (12).

A surgical obturator prosthesis placed at the time of the ablative procedure restores the palatal contour, which is important in speech and swallowing. This prosthesis can be ligated to the remaining teeth with wire or retained with a bone screw in the edentulous patient. The surgical obturator prosthesis may allow the patient to speak and swallow almost immediately after surgery and, in turn, may obviate the need for a nasogastric tube (Fig. 6.4). The prosthesis maintains proper lip and cheek support during initial healing and thus, increases resistance to the contracture and subsequent facial deformity or scar tissue Patients scheduled for maxillectomy should be referred to the oncologic dentist during their initial evaluation so that there is adequate time for fabrication of this prosthesis (13).

An interim obturator prosthesis is placed at the time the surgical obturator and packing are removed. The interim obturator prosthesis is modified as necessary to accommodate healing during the initial healing phase (Fig. 6.5). A minimum of 5 to 10 appointments may be needed to adjust and modify the prosthesis (14).

A definitive obturator prosthesis is made after the surgical defect has stabilized. This prosthesis maximizes aesthetics and function. The average life span of the definitive obturator prosthesis is 3 to 5 years, and close follow-up is important to ensure an accurate fit (Fig. 6.6) (15).

Reconstruction of the maxilla in patients who have received a maxillectomy with free flaps is becoming increasingly popular. In some cases the use of free flaps may be an excellent alternative to the obturator prosthesis, whereas in others this option may not offer acceptable aesthetic or functional results. Older adults, mentally challenged individuals, and those who have lost the dexterity to place and remove a prosthesis should be considered for free-flap reconstruction. Patients who demand a functional and aesthetic restoration after reconstruction with a free flap should be referred to a maxillofacial prosthodontist prior to the procedure so that information concerning rehabilitation can be considered before the procedure (16).

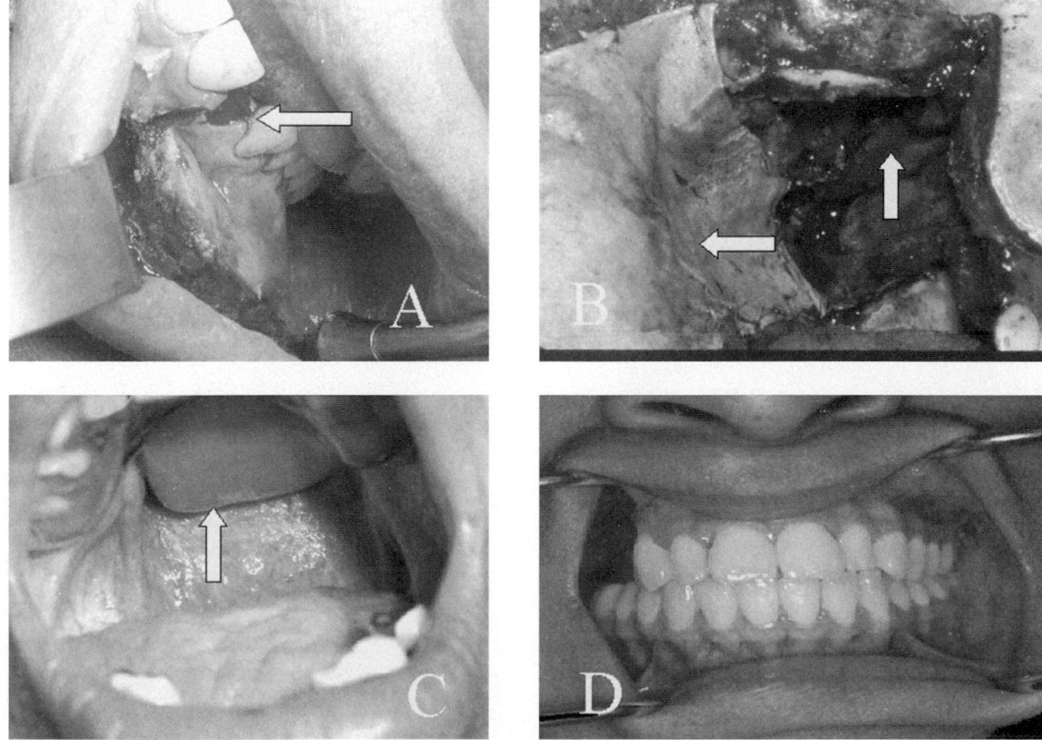

Figure 6.3 Important surgical considerations in maxillectomy. **A:** Make alveolar cuts through extraction socket in dentate patients. **B:** Remove inferior and middle turbinates and place split-thickness skin graft. **C:** Remove total soft palate to improve prosthesis function. **D:** Perform intraoral resection and spare premaxilla when possible.

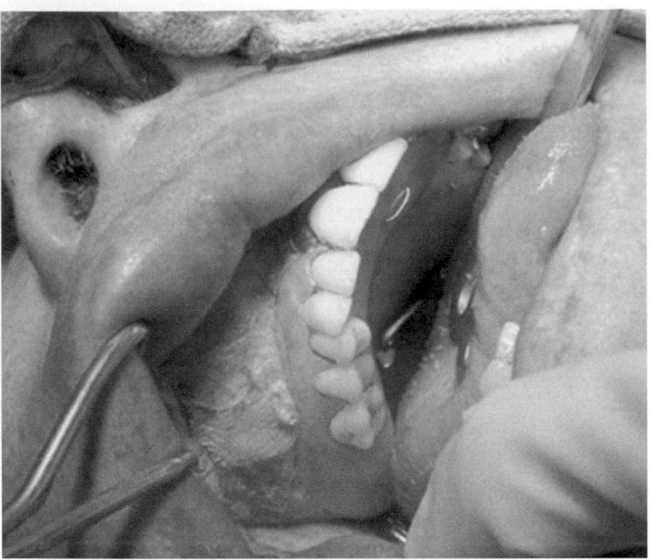

Figure 6.4 Surgical obturator prosthesis retained by interdental wiring negates the use of a nasogastric tube and fixates the split-thickness skin graft reconstruction during initial healing. It also provides postoperative aesthetics and supports the cheek and lips, which resist facial contracture. This prosthesis is removed along with the packing in 5 to 7 days.

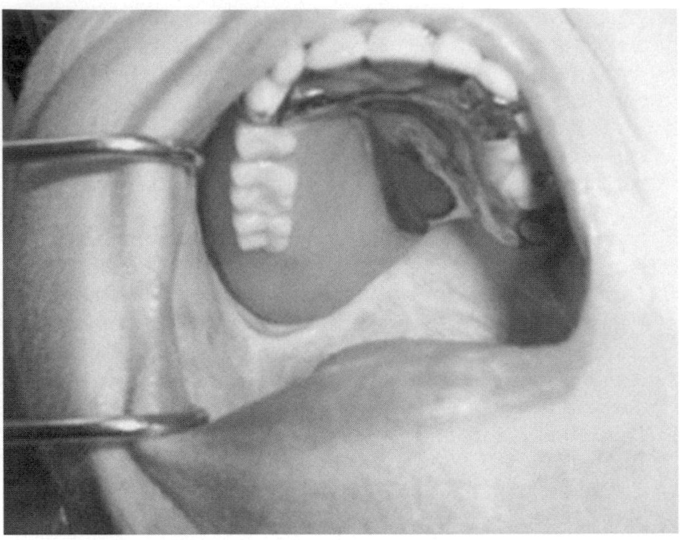

Figure 6.6 Definitive obturator prosthesis in place. This prosthesis maximizes function and aesthetics.

Soft Palate

When the soft palate is involved in the surgical procedure, the surgeon must consider whether the remaining soft palate will be useful in prosthetic rehabilitation. In most cases, when the remaining soft palate is nonfunctional it should be completely removed. Removal of the soft palate allows easy access to the pharynx for fabrication of the prosthesis. Sometimes, a thin strip of soft palate can be vitally important for prosthesis retention in patients with limited supporting tissue, such as when a bilateral total maxillectomy has been done (Fig. 6.7) (17). When resection of the soft palate is anticipated, an intraoperative dental consultation may be indicated. Primary radiation treatment of the soft palate may cause incompetency of the soft palate owing to fibrosis. In this situation, prosthetic rehabilitation may be impossible because of poor access to the oral pharynx. In some cases, surgical removal of the soft palate may be required before prosthetic rehabilitation. Prosthetic rehabilitation may not restore the pretreatment function because of radiation-induced fibrosis in the muscles of the pharyngeal walls. These muscles are important in compensating for the missing soft palate (18).

Mandible

Patients requiring a mandibulectomy may need surgical stents to assist the surgeon in realignment of the mandibular frag-

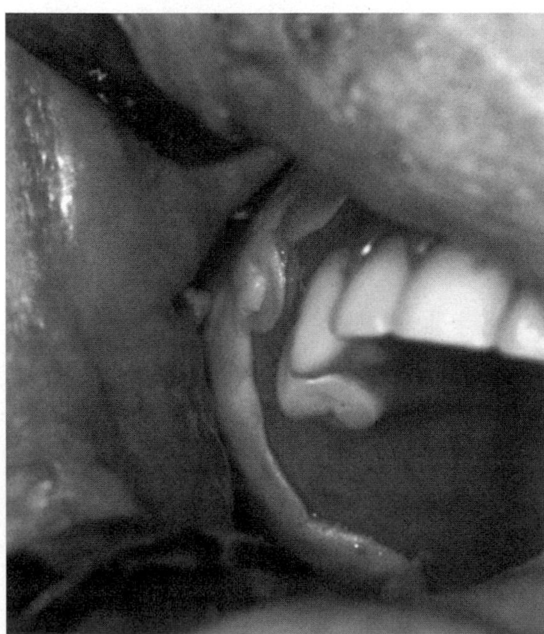

Figure 6.5 Interim obturator prosthesis is placed after removal of the surgical obturator prosthesis. This prosthesis must be followed closely and modified to accommodate healing. It is usually worn for 3 to 6 months until the surgical defect stabilizes.

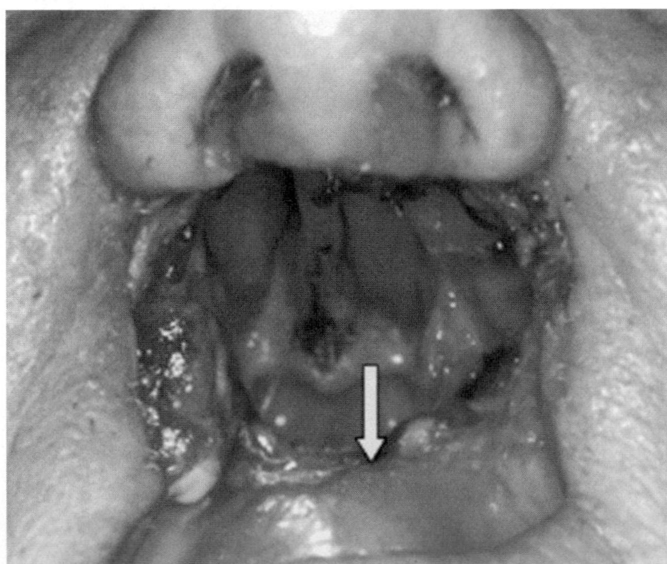

Figure 6.7 Midface resection with total bilateral maxillectomy. Soft palate (*arrow*) is retained for retention and support of obturator prosthesis.

ments before reconstruction. These stents are custom made and require preoperative fabrication. Reconstruction plates are devices used for restoration, construction, reconstruction, or improvement in the shape and appearance of missing, defective, damaged, or misshapen body features. These plates must be bent with precision to ensure a proper relationship between the mandible and the maxilla. Arch bars may also aid in realignment and stabilizing the mandible during reconstruction (19). The maxillary teeth opposing mandibular reconstruction may need to be extracted to prevent trauma to bone and soft tissue flaps. When reconstruction is not being considered for a patient who has received a mandibulectomy, removal of the condyle and ramus on the affected side prevents migration of these structures medially toward the maxilla. Such migration can make prosthetic rehabilitation more difficult (20).

In general, soft tissue coverage of the mandible when free flaps are used does not provide adequate supporting tissue for prosthetic rehabilitation (Fig. 6.8). Vestibuloplasty is a surgical procedure designed to restore alveolar ridge support by reducing the attachment of muscles to the buccal, labial, and lingual aspects of the jaw and thinning the existing tissue, such as flaps used in the initial reconstruction. Split-thickness skin grafts are important because they provide a sound tissue base for a prosthesis and also can be used to separate the floor of the mouth from the buccal mucosa (Fig. 6.9) (21). When the tongue is sutured to the buccal or labial mucosa, prosthetic rehabilitation is limited if not impossible. As with the maxilla, conservation of the supporting tissue in the mandible, consistent with removal of disease, is important. Dental implants can be placed in the non-irradiated native or reconstructed mandible and may be critical to the stability and retention of the mandible prosthesis. Maxillary and mandibular resection dentures can be fabricated for patients who do not receive reconstructive surgery after mandibulectomy.

Tongue

Speech and swallowing dysfunction are common problems in postglossectomy patients. Tumors of the oral cavity often involve contiguous structures and resections within the floor of the mouth are likely to involve the tongue's bulk, tissue and muscle attachments, or innervation.

Palatal augmentation prostheses are removable palatal prostheses that reshape the hard palate to improve contact between the tongue and palate during speech and swallowing (Fig. 6.10). These prostheses may be needed to correct impaired tongue mobility as a result of surgery, trauma, or neurologic/motor deficits. Resection sites that are most likely to affect oral components of speech and swallowing are the oral tongue, anterior or posterior mandible, floor of mouth, and base of tongue (22).

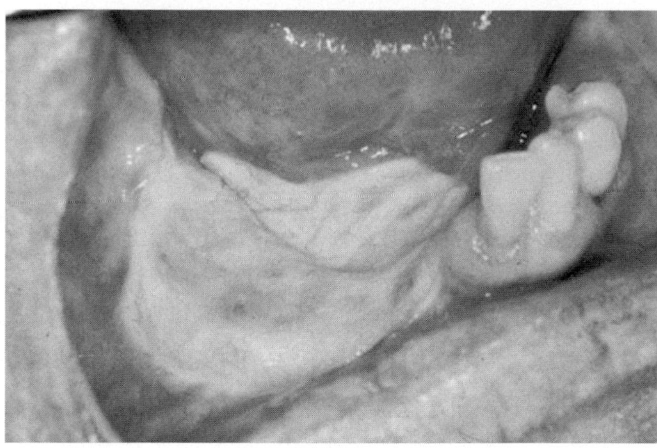

Figure 6.9 Fibula reconstruction of mandible with split-thickness skin graft vestibuloplasty and dental implant placement. Patient is now ready for prosthetic rehabilitation.

The greatest improvement in function results when movement of the residual tongue tissue is retained. Replacing lost tissue bulk with soft tissue may obliterate some of the space that cannot be controlled by the limited range of motion of the tongue. Patients with the greatest movement of the residual tongue benefit the most from the augmentation prosthesis, and patients with a mobile tongue tip have the best function. The use of thinner microvascular flaps for closure of the surgical site allows the residual innervated portion of the tongue to function with minimal impairment of movement. The palatal augmentation prosthesis offers rehabilitation advantages for patients with impaired function of the tongue. The ultimate treatment goal is maximum restoration of speech and swallowing, which may require the combination of soft tissue and prosthetic reconstruction.

Oral Hygiene Procedures

Oral hygiene is one of the most important aspects of postoperative care. Initially, the surgical defect should be irrigated with

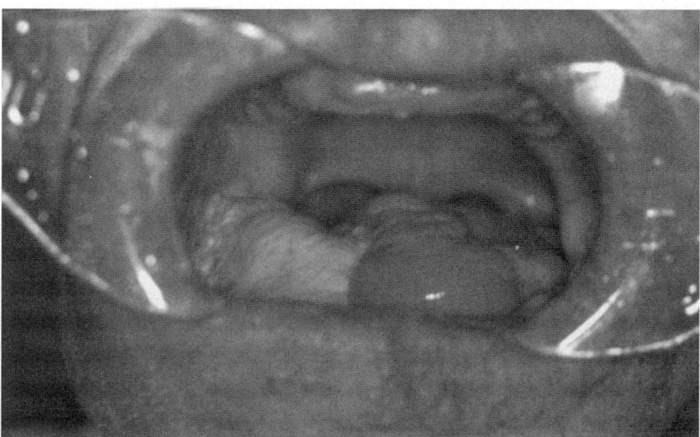

Figure 6.8 Fibula reconstruction of mandible with skin paddle reconstructing floor of mouth and covering mandible. This skin paddle is movable, thick, and not satisfactory for prosthesis support.

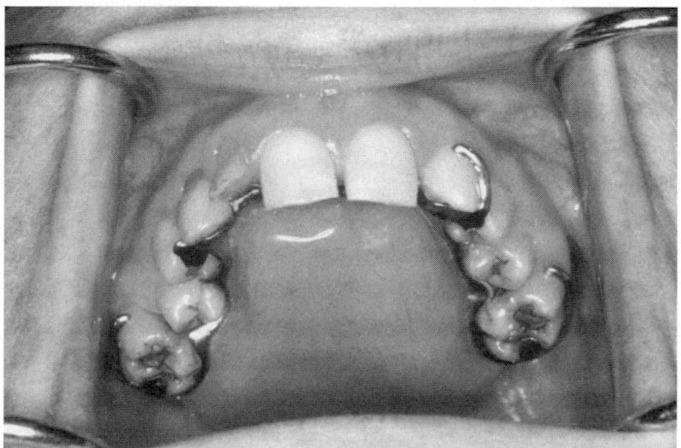

Figure 6.10 Patient with total glossectomy reconstructed with free flap and palatal augmentation prosthesis. Prosthesis functions against free flap and improves speech and swallowing.

a gravity irrigation system. After initial healing, a power-spray unit such as Water Pik (Teledyne Dental, Buffalo, N.Y.) can be used by the patient. The patient should be instructed in the proper use of the lavage system. Initially after surgery, the patient should rinse three times a day with a saline solution made by adding 1 teaspoon of salt and 1 teaspoon of sodium bicarbonate to 16 oz of water. The irrigation system must provide enough pressure to ensure that the rinse reaches all parts of the surgical defect. Routine dental hygiene (i.e., tooth brushing and flossing) should be started as soon as possible. Patients are usually apprehensive about resuming the brushing and flossing of teeth because of concerns that doing so may harm the surgical site. However, if healing proceeds normally, using a power-spray system beginning 4 weeks after surgery should not pose a problem. During the fourth week of healing, a 1:1 dilution of 3% hydrogen peroxide in water can be added to the oral hygiene routine. A sponge-tipped applicator (e.g., Oral-Swab, Crystal Lake, Ill.) may be used to clean the skin graft portion of the defect. After the surgical site has been cleaned, the entire oral cavity—including the teeth, tongue, cheek, and remaining hard palate—is cleaned (13,23).

Physical Therapy

Conventional oral physiotherapy (i.e., oral opening exercises) should be performed during and after radiation treatment, especially if the pterygoid regions are included in the radiation treatment fields (24). If oral opening is reduced following surgery, a series of tongue blades can be inserted between the posterior teeth until maximum opening is obtained. The blades are held in place for several minutes to allow the forming scar tissue to stretch, and then another tongue blade is added until a pain threshold is reached.

Various commercial devices to aid in mouth opening are available. One such device, the Therabite mouth opener (Atos Medical, Milwaukee, Wis.) opens the mouth in a manner that is similar to a car jack lifting a car (Fig. 6.11). Each of these devices, however, has advantages and disadvantages. Users of these devices must take care to ensure that teeth do not incur orthodontic movement or damage. The edentulous patient can use his or her fingers, placing them between the maxillary and mandibular ridges, to pry open the mouth. The exercises can be combined with extraoral palpation and stretching of the cheek and upper lip to keep the tissue as pliable as possible. During the first 4 weeks, the patient should be instructed to do these stretching exercises 3 or 4 times a day (15 minutes each session). In addition a trained physical therapist can institute more advanced means of physical therapy, such as electrotherapy, ultrasound therapy, and isometric exercises. Oral-opening measurements should be recorded to help both the clinician and the patient measure progress resulting from these exercises. In many cases, these physiotherapy techniques should be continued for at least 1 year. If a patient has a sudden loss of oral opening, the dentist should immediately suspect and rule out recurrence of disease (25).

OSSEOINTEGRATED DENTAL IMPLANTS

Dental implants have become very popular over the past 15 to 20 years, but indiscriminate placement of these implants can decrease their effectiveness and increase the cost of rehabilitation dramatically. In patients with a normal mandible and maxilla, the success rate is between 90% and 95% (26). However, in patients with a reconstructed mandible, the success rate may be lower, depending on the quantity and quality of the recipient bone. Careful planning is required before an implant is placed in any patient. Implants may be the only means by which prostheses can be retained.

Patients who have undergone a free fibula tissue transfer placed using microvascular techniques make excellent recipients of implants. However, the number, positioning, and spacing between implants is critical in prosthesis fabrication. These details are best dealt with after reconstruction, in a separate procedure, when a surgical stent made by the dentist responsible for rehabilitation can help guide the surgeon in the exact alignment and positioning of the implants. The information needed to obtain proper fit and positioning of prostheses can be determined only by postoperative evaluations. Some implant systems require two-staged surgical procedures whereas others require only one stage. The type of implant used should be the choice and responsibility of the dentist responsible for the prosthetic rehabilitation of the patient (Fig. 6.12) (27). Patients requiring postoperative radiation may not be candidates for implants. This subject is dis-

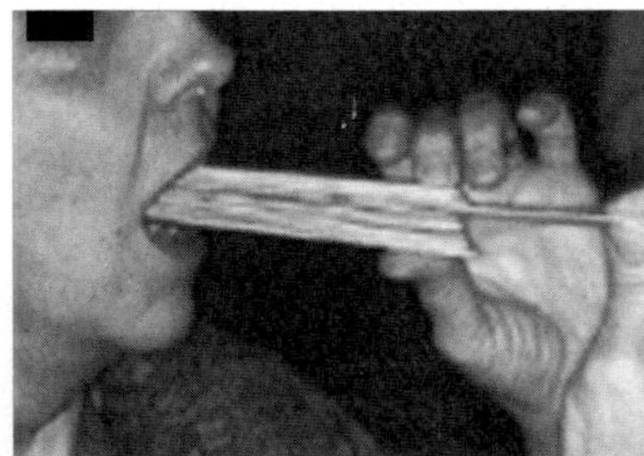

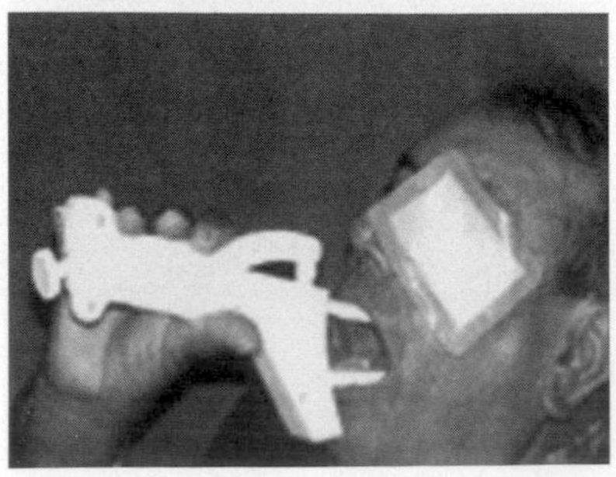

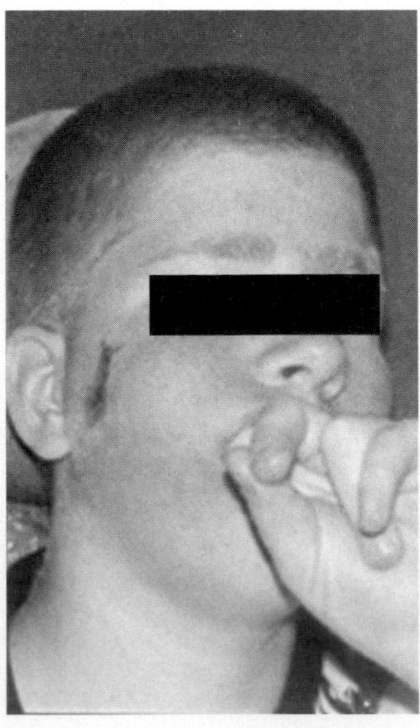

Figure 6.11 Physical therapy is a very important aspect in the care of the head and neck surgery patient. This figure illustrates tongue blades and the Therabite mouth opener (Atos Medical, Milwaukee, Wis.), that help maintain oral opening during initial healing along with facial massage and stretching.

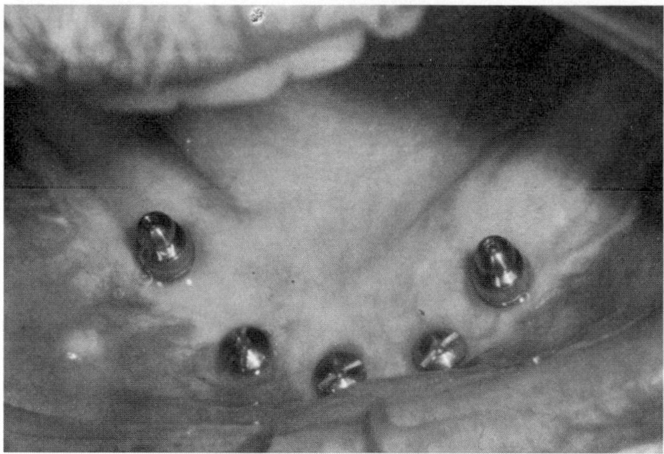

Figure 6.12 Patient reconstructed with fibula graft and dental implants. Number and position of implants are determined by dentist responsible for rehabilitation.

cussed later in the chapter in the section "Care of Patients with Head and Neck Cancer Treated with Radiation."

EXTRAORAL IMPLANTS

At the beginning of 1993, only one extraoral implant system had been approved by the U.S. Food and Drug Administration; however, more have been approved since then and are currently available. Like their intraoral counterparts, extraoral implants are placed in two stages; however, with extraoral implants 4 to 6 months are usually allowed to pass for them to become integrated before they are uncovered. Extraoral implants can be of great benefit for retention and stability of facial prostheses when correctly placed but do not always guarantee a successful prosthesis (28). Other retentive systems available for facial prostheses are adhesives. Undercuts in the defect, if properly prepared, also can be used to retain prostheses. When contact between intraoral and extraoral defects results from surgery, the facial portion of the prosthesis can be retained via its attachment to an intraoral component.

FACIAL PROSTHETICS

In general, a successful prosthesis is aesthetic, retentive, and tissue compatible. In addition, a prosthesis should be simple in design so that the patient can place and remove it easily. Materials used in constructing facial prostheses should be easy to clean, color stable, resistant to bacteria and fungal growth, durable, and well tolerated by tissues. The two materials that meet these criteria most fully are methylmethacrylate (plastic) and medical-grade silicones. Extraoral prostheses may be combined with intraoral prostheses to enhance retention and aesthetics.

General Rehabilitative Principles for Ablative and Reconstructive Surgery Involving Facial Structures

GENERAL PRINCIPLES

Numerous general surgical principles can be applied to placement of prostheses at all facial sites. Although basic, these principles are extremely important in ensuring the success of facial prostheses:

1. Smooth and round off all bony margins at the conclusion of the ablative procedure.
2. Place a STSG on any exposed bone or periosteum that is not covered with free tissue or a pedicle flap.
3. Remove unsupported tissue tags.
4. Take replacement tissues from areas that best match the tissues surrounding the recipient bed.
5. When using free tissue transfer flaps or pedicle flaps to repair the surgical defect, take care not to over bulk the surgical site in a patient for whom a prosthesis is planned.

ORBIT

When the orbital contents are removed in conjunction with a maxillary resection, reconstruction of the infraorbital rim improves the facial contour and enhances the prosthetic rehabilitation. This reconstruction can be accomplished by using a free-tissue transfer with bone. If the bony structures of the orbit are left intact, an STSG can be placed in the defect, thus allowing a prosthesis contact with the tissue at the depth of the defect (Fig. 6.13). Care must be exercised in placing the

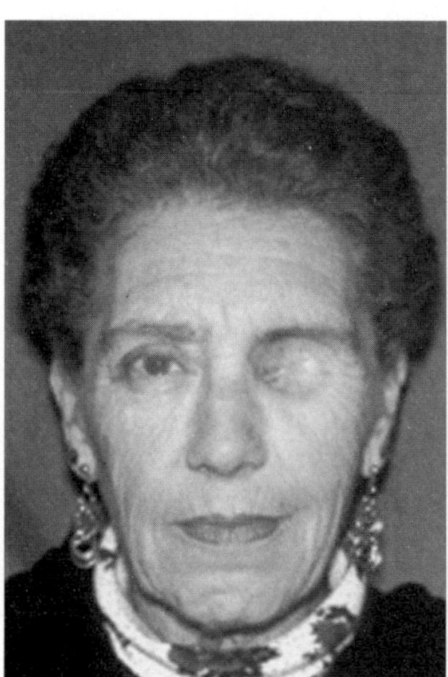

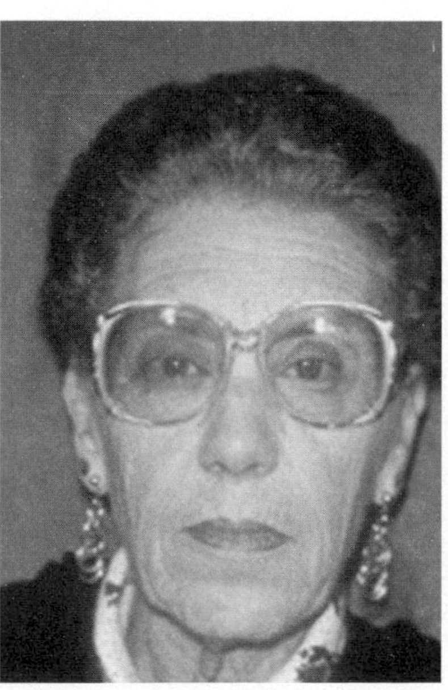

Figure 6.13 This figure illustrates an excellent split-thickness skin graft (STSG) reconstruction of an orbital defect and rehabilitation with an orbital prosthesis. If the bony structures of the orbit are left intact, an STSG should be placed in the defect. This allows placement of an orbital prosthesis that contacts the tissue at the depth of the defect.

STSG so that the normal position of the eyebrow is maintained. Alternatively, free-tissue transfer can be used to obliterate the defect entirely.

NOSE

Patients who undergo partial or total rhinectomy can be adequately rehabilitated using a removable prosthesis. An STSG should be placed in the defect to stabilize the borders of the defect and to maintain a normal lip position. For patients undergoing total rhinectomy, it is especially important that the inferior border of the nasal defect be fixated and that a dam at the inferior border of the defect be created. If the defect cannot be skin-grafted, the surgeon should consider positioning the mucocutaneous junction as far posteriorly into the defect as possible. This measure will fixate the border and help form a dam. If possible, the nasal spine should be spared and the mucosa of the septum skin-grafted.

EAR

The superior rim and tragus should be spared if possible (Fig. 6.14). If supported by cartilage, the superior rim can be used to support eyewear. The tragus can be used to hide anterior margins to improve aesthetics. The STSG can tolerate tissue adhesives used to retain facial prostheses and will also improve hygiene (29).

MIDFACE

To enhance prosthetic rehabilitation at midface sites, several special considerations must be made before and during the reconstructive procedure (28). During the ablative procedure, the surgical team should conserve as much of the maxilla and associated structures as possible. Respiratory mucosa should be removed from the remaining vomer, nasal floor, and sinuses and an STSG should be placed (21). The STSG will allow extension of the removable facial prosthesis into these areas if this extension later becomes necessary and will stop secretions from the replaced respiratory mucosa (crusting), thus improving overall hygiene (30).

A free flap with bone can be placed to improve the retention and support of the facial prosthesis. Sufficient space for this purpose is critical because if the graft is placed too far anteriorly, the aesthetics of the facial prosthesis can be diminished. If the reconstruction infringes on this space, placement of the prosthesis may be impossible. In this case another surgical procedure to reposition the graft would be needed before prosthesis fabrication. The free-graft reconstruction should be done after irradiation if implants are indicated. Once irradiated, the capacity of the bone for implant placement is severely diminished or lost because its osteogenic potential and microvascularity are decreased (31).

CARE OF PATIENTS WITH HEAD AND NECK CANCER TREATED WITH RADIATION

The clinical use of radiation is a complex process involving many professionals and a variety of interrelated functions. The aim of radiation therapy is to deliver a precisely measured dose of radiation to a defined target volume, thus eradicating the tumor while causing minimal damage to surrounding healthy tissue (32). More than 80% of patients diagnosed with head and neck cancer receive a course of radiation therapy as a component of their treatment.

Complications

A healthy oral status before radiation therapy reduces the risk for complications from therapeutic administration of ionizing radiation to the head and neck. These complications can be categorized as either acute (e.g., mucositis, infectious stomatitis, alteration of taste or smell acuity, dermatitis, pain, inflammation, and difficulty swallowing) or chronic (e.g., xerostomia, caries, abnormal development, fibrosis, trismus, photosensitivity, osteoradionecrosis, and pain) (33–35). The severity of treatment-induced morbidity depends on multiple factors such as the radiation dose, energy source, volume of tissue treated, pretreatment performance status, and pretreatment periodontal condition (36). The volume of tissue irradiated is susceptible to dermatitis and mucositis, which are often accompanied by salivary gland hypofunction, dysgeusia, dysphagia, odynophagia, hypovascularity of soft and hard tissues, fibrosis, or trismus (33,36,37). Widespread oral melanotic hyperpigmentation and hypopigmentation have been reported. Developmental abnormalities of the dentition and jaws may occur in children undergoing head and neck radiation therapy (38–41). In patients of all ages, altered tissues within the volume of tissue irradiated are highly susceptible to infectious processes, especially with fungal organisms, such as

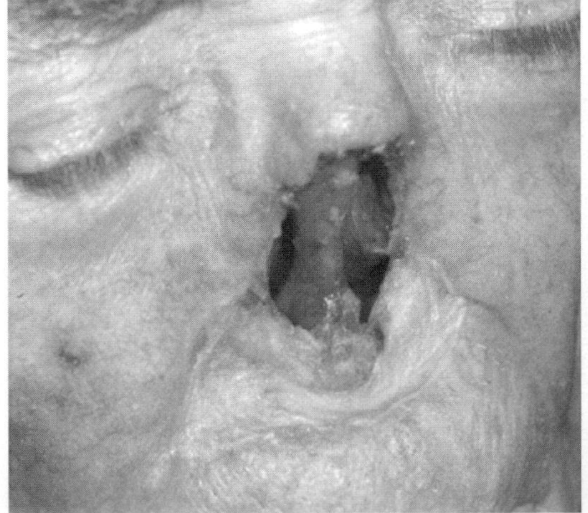

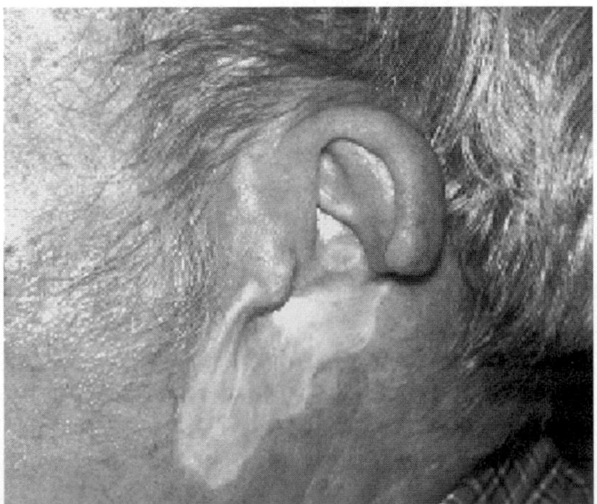

Figure 6.14 Nasal defect that represents basic principles for surgical preparation of facial defects. A split-thickness skin graft reconstruction that stabilizes the borders of the defect and no tissue tags is shown. The superior rim and tragus should be spared if possible when dealing with ear defects.

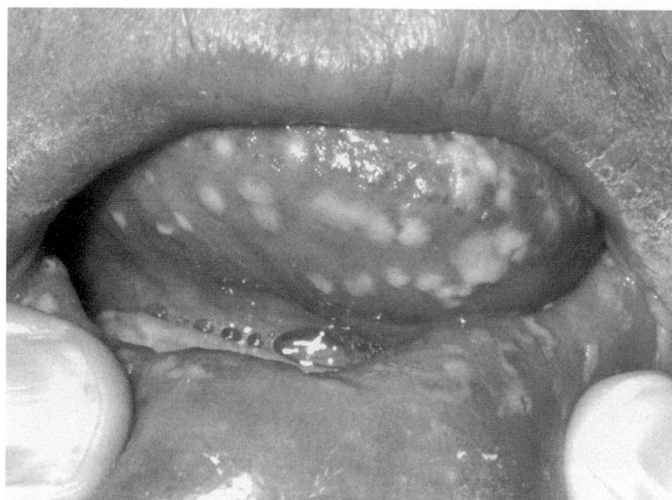

Figure 6.15 Oral candidiasis in a patient undergoing external beam radiation therapy for a base of tongue primary carcinoma.

Candida albicans or other *Candida* species; bacterial infections, especially with streptococci and staphylococci; and viral infections, especially with herpes simplex virus (Fig. 6.15) (42,43).

Mucositis

Oral mucositis generally occurs 5 to 7 days after initiation of external beam radiation therapy (Fig. 6.16). Oral mucosal changes depend on the fractionation, energy source, total dose of radiation, and oral and dental status (36). When an electron beam is used with high-energy photon beams in the treatment of deep lesions, the mucosal reactions on the side of the entering beam may consist of patchy or confluent exudate, whereas the contralateral side may show only erythema. During the course of radiation therapy, the mucosa becomes thin as a result of direct cell death and the sloughing off of rapidly replicating epithelial cells (44).

Eliminating all secondary sources of irritation such as alcohol, smoking, and coarse products that can further dehydrate oral tissues can decrease the severity of oral mucositis. Hot foods, alcohol- or phenol-containing mouth rinses, and sodium (45) should be avoided. Treatment of mucositis typically consists of palliative pain reduction therapy. Physicians have advocated several agents for topical use, including benzydamine hydrochloride, allopurinol, sucralfate suspension, kamillosan, povidone-iodine, antacids, sodium bicarbonate, local anesthetic agents (such as lidocaine hydrochloride), chlorhexidine gluconate, oral suspension of prostaglandin E_2, and aloe vera with the active ingredient acemannan (45–49). Unfortunately, very few clinical trials have examined these substances, and the results have shown only moderate clinical efficacy (50,51). Good oral hygiene is essential to improving oral comfort and reducing the risk for oral contamination. Bacterial, fungal, and viral infections can occur as superinfections with mucositis but are less likely to induce septicemia in patients undergoing radiation therapy than in patients receiving chemotherapy (33). Patients receiving a concurrent regimen of radiation therapy and chemotherapy may be at a greater risk for infectious mucositis than patients treated with either therapy alone. With fungal infections, such as oral candidiasis, the pathogenesis can be invasive, refractory to treatment, and potentially septic (42). Candidiasis can manifest as pseudomembranous, hyperplastic, or atrophic (erythematous) oral lesions (42). The sites most frequently affected are the tongue, buccal mucosa, hard or soft palate, or the commissurae labiorum oris (i.e., angular cheilitis) (Fig. 6.17). Treatment consists of such topical antifungal agents as nystatin oral suspension or clotrimazole troches, depending on the degree of xerostomia (42,52,53).

To avoid oral infections and to reduce the mucositis that may arise from radiation therapy, patients must frequently rinse the oral cavity to reduce oral microorganisms and to maintain mucosal hydration. Such oral lavage can be performed by rinsing with a solution of 1 teaspoon of sodium bicarbonate dissolved in 12 oz. water several times each day to alkalinize the oral cavity and to keep the oral and oropharyngeal tissues moist. Mouth rinses, saliva substitutes, and gustatory stimulants are frequently abandoned by patients treated with head and neck radiation therapy because the effect is short-lived or not effective (33). Such patients should be encouraged to increase water intake, decrease acidic and carbonated beverage intake, and decrease sodium intake.

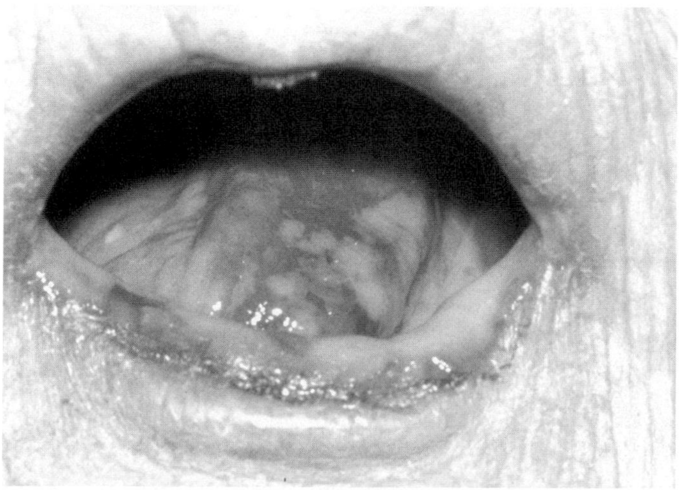

Figure 6.16 Radiation-induced mucositis in a patient receiving treatment for a squamous cell carcinoma of the oral tongue with metastatic disease in the cervical region.

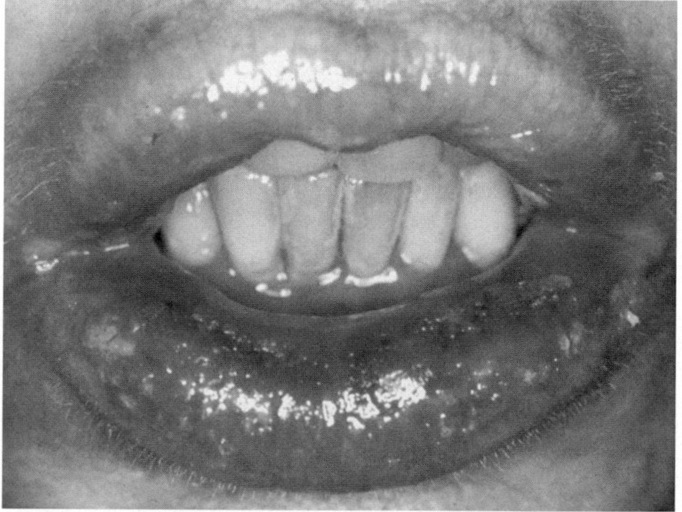

Figure 6.17 Patient undergoing radiation therapy to the oral cavity with angular cheilitis in the bilateral commissures and a candidal infection on the lower labial tissues.

Osteoradionecrosis

Radiation can permanently destroy cellular elements of bone and thus limit the potential for wound maintenance and the ability to heal after infection or trauma (e.g., dental extraction and alveoloplasty) (54,55). The risk for complications following trauma or oral surgical procedures in an irradiated field can be highly significant, depending on a predetermined threshold of irradiation, and result in osteoradionecrosis (Fig. 6.18) (36). For these reasons, elective oral surgical procedures, such as extractions or soft tissue surgery, are contraindicated within an irradiated field owing to hypovascularity, hypocellularity, and hypoxia (Fig. 6.19) (33). Nonsurgical dental procedures that can safely be performed include routine restorative procedures, oral prophylaxis, radiography, and endodontic and prosthodontic procedures.

If oral surgical intervention is required after radiation therapy, the clinician should discuss the volume of tissue irradiated and specific treatment parameters with the treating radiation therapist and should request a copy of the simulation or port films and treatment summary. Preoperative hyperbaric oxygen therapy may increase the potential of wound healing while minimizing the risk for osteoradionecrosis by promoting angiogenesis and osteogenesis (Fig. 6.20). Hyperbaric oxygen therapy must be used as an adjunct to débridement (sequestrectomy), wound care, parenteral antibiotics (as dictated by bone culture results), and composite bone and muscle grafts by free tissue transfer (subject to the availability of the requisite microvascular skills) (56,57). Antibiotics are chosen on the basis of macro- or microdilution sensitivity testing.

Hyperbaric oxygen therapy is time-consuming and expensive and must be performed in an accredited wound care center. However, compared with a postradiation surgical treatment consisting of radical débridement and reconstruction, hyperbaric oxygen treatment can be cost-effective. Hyperbaric oxygen also may preclude the need for jaw amputation, large resection, or microvascular surgery. The Marx protocol, consisting of 20 preoperative hyperbaric oxygen treatments followed by 10 postoperative treatments, is the standard treatment regimen (56,58). Optimal oral health must be maintained during and after radiation therapy. However, to avoid soft tissue injury during the postradiation healing period, patients must curtail all but the most basic oral hygiene procedures (i.e., brushing, flossing, and fluoride therapy). Following initial recovery from radiation effects, nonsurgical periodontal therapy, usually with prophylactic antibiotic coverage, is appropriate for treatment of the periodontium within the radiation field. It is important to detect and treat dental caries or traumatic dental injury that could lead to disease. If postradiation extractions are necessary, hyperbaric oxygen therapy, along with a specific oral care regimen, is indicated to augment wound healing (56). In such cases, tissues should be managed gently, and antibiotic coverage is required. Local anesthetics containing epinephrine should be avoided, when possible, to prevent further vascular constriction (59). Workers have reported successful placement of endosseous implants in irradiated fields, with a pretreatment regimen of hyperbaric oxygen (Fig. 6.21) (60,61). In contrast, osteoradionecrosis has been initiated by such elective surgical intervention (61,62).

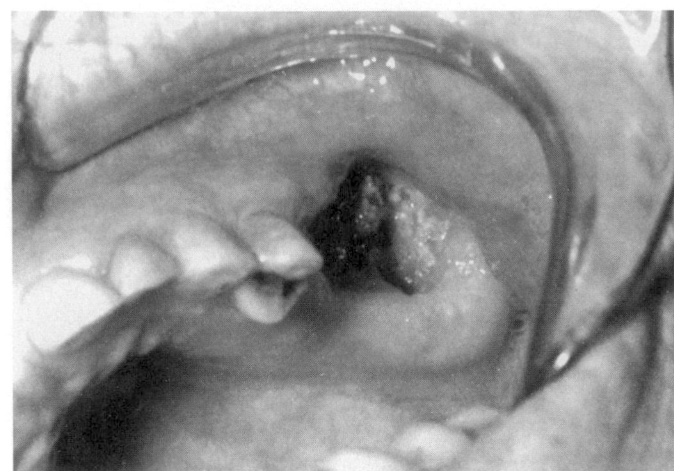

Figure 6.19 Osteoradionecrosis in the posterior maxilla secondary to a tooth extraction. This patient has radiation-induced hypovascularity in the bilateral maxillae secondary to irradiation of the soft palate and tonsil.

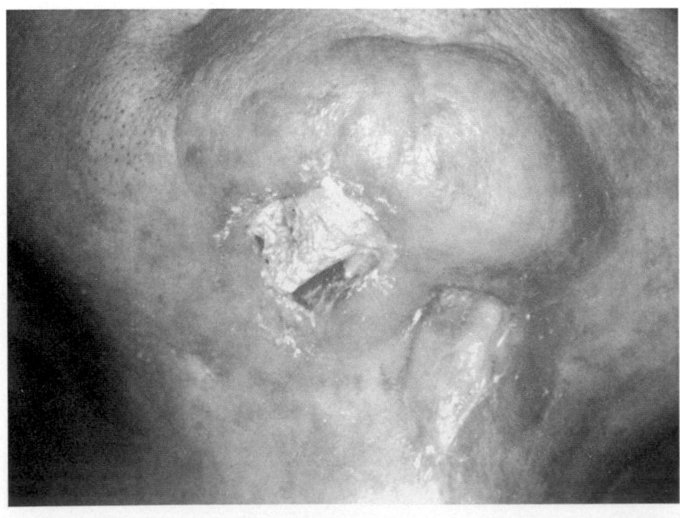

Figure 6.18 Osteoradionecrosis in the anterior mandible secondary to trauma from a motor vehicle accident. The mandible and upper cervical region were in the radiated field.

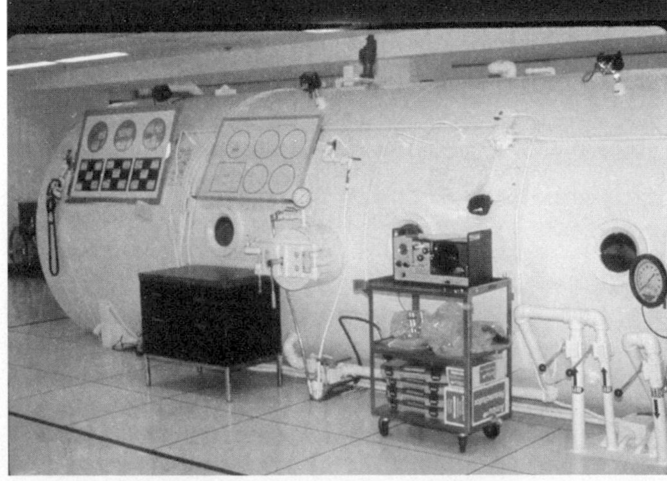

Figure 6.20 A multiplace hyperbaric chamber. Patients will undergo hyperbaric oxygen treatment using the Marx protocol (90 minutes of treatment, breathing 100% oxygen at 2.2–2.5 atmosphere absolute); 20–30 preoperative treatments are followed by 10–20 postoperative treatments.

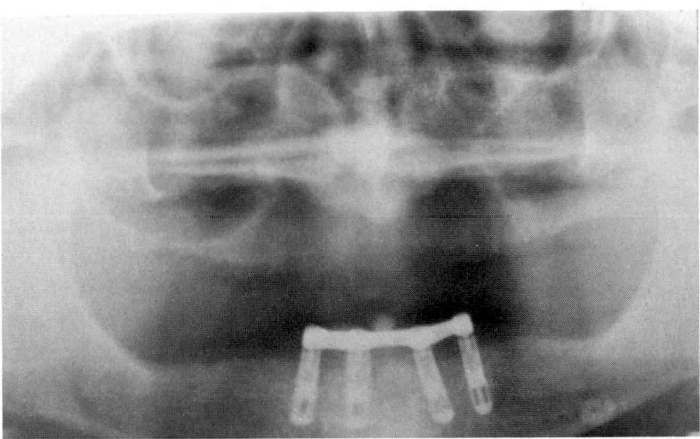

Figure 6.21 A panoramic radiograph revealing endosseous implants (2 years posttreatment) placed in an irradiated mandible following pre- and postoperative hyperbaric oxygen therapy. By torque evaluation and clinical/radiographic assessment, the implants are considered osseointegrated without evidence of necrosis.

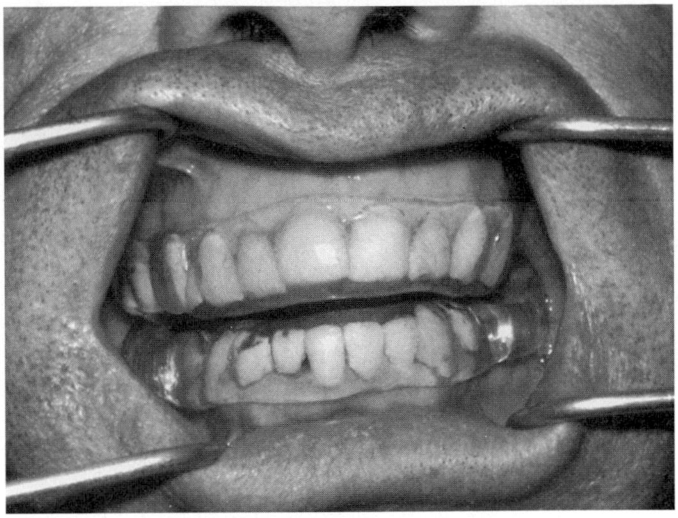

Figure 6.23 Fluoride carrier filled with 0.4% stannous fluoride and in position over maxillary and mandibular dentition.

Dental Caries and Xerostomia

CARIES

Dental caries is a common postradiation morbid sequela in patients with head and neck cancer treated with radiation therapy (63). Irradiation of major salivary glands leads to qualitative and quantitative changes in salivary secretions, reducing the buffering capacity of saliva (64). The result is a cariogenic environment, particularly in patients who ingest a diet high in carbohydrates or sucrose (Fig. 6.22). Susceptibility to caries is not limited to the dentition within the volume of tissue irradiated. Patients who have undergone irradiation should be treated with a specific prophylactic regimen consisting of flossing, brushing, and fluoride therapy. Fluoride treatment consists of a daily application of 0.4% stannous fluoride or 1.1% sodium fluoride (33,36,64). In adults with xerostomia, fluoride leaches out of the enamel within 24 hours; thus, the fluoride regimen must be performed daily to ensure optimal protection. The most efficient method of fluoride application is to use a custom-made polyprophylene fluoride carrier that completely covers, and extends slightly beyond, the tooth surface (Fig. 6.23) (36). Patients load the carriers with fluoride gel and place them onto the dentition daily for 10 minutes. Patients who receive low doses of radiation and are expected to have a slight degree of xerostomia can use a toothbrush to apply the fluoride gel (65). A daily fluoride program can decrease postradiation dentinal hypersensitivity; remineralize cavitated enamel matrices; and, more importantly, inhibit caries-forming organisms (33,36).

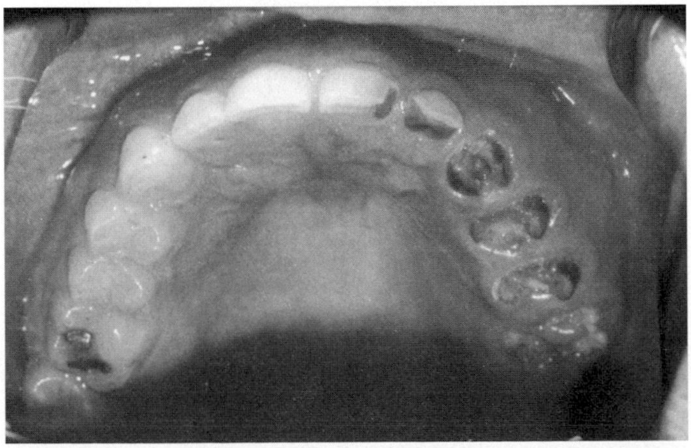

Figure 6.22 Radiation-induced caries in a patient who has received unilateral external beam radiation treatment for a parotid gland tumor with cervical nodal involvement.

XEROSTOMIA

Sialagogue therapy, such as with cholinergic agonists (e.g., pilocarpine hydrochloride), has been shown to provide clinically significant relief of symptoms of postradiation xerostomia (66,67). Other rinses reported to decrease oral discomfort related to xerostomia or mucositis contain cytokines, aloe vera derivatives, or antibiotics. When administered intravenously, during radiation therapy, amifostine, a free radical scavenger, has been shown to diminish toxic effects of irradiation on salivary glands.

If these guidelines are followed, healthy oral tissues can be maintained following radiation therapy. Achievement of this goal depends on the patient's cooperation and compliance, which should be verified by clinicians at follow-up appointments.

CARE OF PATIENTS WITH HEAD AND NECK CANCER TREATED WITH CHEMOTHERAPY

Most patients with cancer receive chemotherapy as a single- or multiple-drug regimen, either alone or in combination with other therapies (68,69). The duration of treatment ranges from several months to years, depending on how long the therapy remains effective or how long the patient can tolerate it. Because chemotherapeutic agents damage mitotically active normal tissue cells or multiplying tumor cells, chemotherapy often induces toxicity in the hematopoietic cells, skin, and aerodigestive tract (34,68). Such toxicity may cause treatment-induced complications in the oral cavity, especially if myelosuppression has occurred. Many of the sequelae of chemotherapy are similar to those induced by radiation therapy but are sometimes more episodic depending on the dosing schedule or chemotherapeutic agents administered.

Oral Complications

Acute oral conditions detected during the evaluation of the oral and dental status of patients with cancer must be treated before chemotherapy if the patient's health or hematologic values permit or, if not, when the opportunity arises between treatment cycles and when an appropriate performance status has been established. Chronic problems should not go unattended but should be treated strategically as the patient continues with chemotherapy (34). Through appropriate coordination, acute problems can be treated promptly. If left untreated, chronic conditions may become acute at a time when the patient's physical well-being or hematologic parameters will not allow oral treatment intervention.

Oral/Dental Treatment

During oncologic chemotherapy, the treatment plan for patients with cancer should be simple, practical, and functional in relation to the oral or dental health and should not be in the realm of cosmetic dentistry, fixed prosthodontics, or advanced periodontal therapy (34). Dental specialists face an almost overwhelming temptation to give aesthetic possibilities undue consideration while not recognizing the difficulty patients face in coping with their cancer diagnosis and undergoing drug therapies that have serious side effects (33–35).

The dentoalveolar complex should be thoroughly evaluated for microbial reservoirs or sanctuaries (e.g., plaque, calculus, or periodontal pockets), and these infectious foci should be eliminated before the start of chemotherapy (Fig. 6.24) (70). A diminished periodontal status presents a risk for infection. Clinically, however, the risk for infection depends on multiple interacting factors such as oral hygiene, immuno-myelosuppressive status, chemotherapeutic agents used, prophylactic or therapeutic antimicrobial agents used, and the degree of periodontal pathology.

To minimize the risks for periodontal infection, it is important to develop simple and practical guidelines for maintaining periodontal health and for diagnosing, preventing, and treating periodontal infections during therapy (33,70). Patients with cancer should make regular dental visits for overall dental assessment. Patients receiving chemotherapy can undergo a dental cleaning provided that they meet the following hematologic conditions: first, an absolute neutrophil count of approximately 1,000 per mm^3 a level at which the risk for developing an infection is minimal; and second, a platelet count greater than 50,000 per mm^3 with a normal coagulation profile (71). The administration of prophylactic antibiotics is essential in combating induced bacteremia, immunocompromised status, and potential hypofunction of the white blood cells introduced by chemotherapy. The American Heart Association recommends a viable antibiotic regimen for subacute bacterial endocarditis prophylaxis before periodontal procedures. The second dose should be given 6 to 8 hours after the loading dose (72).

Patients with an uninfected dentition and good periodontal health do not pose a diagnostic treatment challenge, nor do patients with advanced periodontal disease that mandates immediate surgical intervention. However, patients with increased loss of attachment with furcation involvement or periodontal pocket formation with furcation involvement pose a treatment dilemma (34). Patients in whom the soft tissue parallels the bone loss and in whom pocket depth is normal can be treated with regular periodontal care and maintenance. Extraction should be considered only for patients with pathologic mobility of dentition or with a fulminant periapical abscess (33). Patients with moderate to advanced periodontal disease present a greater challenge and would, under usual circumstances, receive instructions for infection prophylaxis and dental hygiene, as well as surgical correction. However, the feasibility of such comprehensive therapy during chemotherapy can be limited by several factors, including performance status, type of malignant disease, cycling of chemotherapy, and hematologic competence. The clinician should strive to provide a thorough scaling and to encourage maintenance through exceptional plaque control (i.e., brushing, flossing, and use of chlorhexidine gluconate) (33–35,73). To reduce the risk for sepsis, extractions should be considered for patients with any exacerbated acute periodontal infection. This oral surgical correction should be performed at the appropriate time in the treatment cycle or when the patient's cancer is in complete remission (Fig. 6.25). If chemotherapy is on hold, periodontal surgery could be considered, provided that the hematologic status is appropriate. The oncologic dentist must discuss with the treating medical oncologist the patient's oral status, treatment plan, and contraindica-

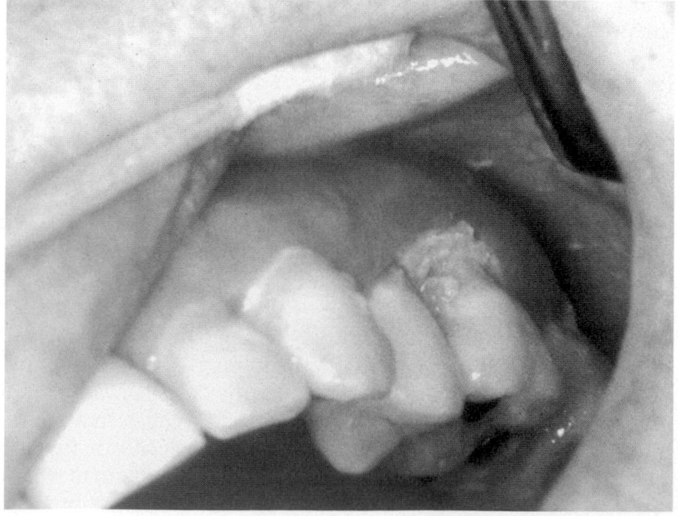

Figure 6.24 Heavy calculus and plaque on dentition providing a sanctuary for microbial and fungal activity.

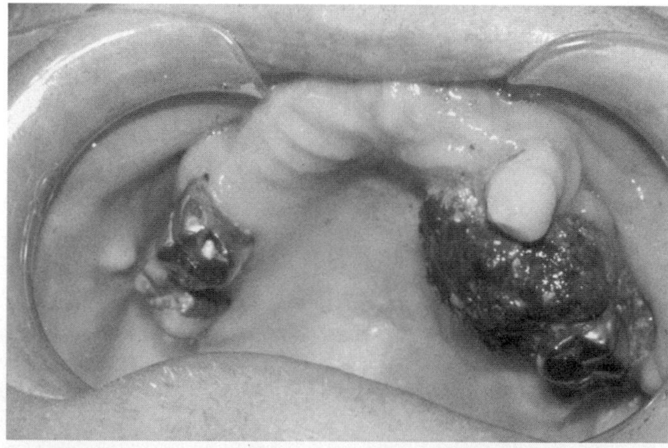

Figure 6.25 Postextraction site with an organized clot in a pancytopenic patient undergoing myelosuppressive chemotherapy. This patient is at their nadir and should have had no oral surgical intervention until the recovery phase of therapy with hematologic stability. Patient required random donor platelets with antibiotic therapy and a surgical débridement.

tions to surgical intervention, as well as the appropriate timing of oral treatment intervention (33–35,68).

Brushing and flossing of the teeth should continue to be the standard of dental care for patients who routinely brush and floss. However, as in the general population, many patients with cancer either do not floss or floss only infrequently. Thus, clinicians either may instruct patients to floss or may stress brushing techniques only. In most cases, patient factors and limited time parameters do not permit the patient to become proficient in flossing techniques (33). Patients who floss regularly are instructed to modify the flossing technique in certain clinical situations. First, patients are instructed to floss gently when the lining of the oral cavity starts to become sensitive to thermal changes or food substances, as sensitivity indicates mucosal thinning due to suppressive effects of chemotherapy on the normally proliferative epithelium (45). Second, patients are instructed to floss only to the gingiva when the platelet count decreases to less than 50,000 per mm^3. This technique removes most of the debris from this area (34).

In controlling plaque accumulation, it is important to minimize the risk for gingival inflammation, the oral bacterial load, and the potential for infection. Along with routine brushing and flossing, rinsing with chlorhexidine gluconate should be initiated when patients begin chemotherapy. Such rinsing is an adjunct to ideal oral–periodontal care and can also be used when indications arise, such as oral mucosal changes secondary to chemotherapy and subsequent increased soft tissue sensitivity (33,34,73). Patients undergoing chemotherapy should be encouraged to rinse with a dilute saline and sodium bicarbonate solution (5%) to reduce adherent mucoid debris on oral soft tissues, lubricate oral mucosal and oropharyngeal tissues, and elevate the pH of oral fluids (35). Patients experiencing nausea and anorexia should be encouraged to rinse with the sodium bicarbonate and saline solution several times throughout the day to reduce oral acidity and minimize the mucosal insult.

Another challenge that patients with cancer face in oral care is the risk for local infection or septicemia associated with dental implants. If an implant with its restorative component poses a risk for infection for patients under normal circumstances, this risk will be intensified during chemotherapy. Interventional antibiotics and aggressive hygiene have limited ability to control infection caused by a poorly integrated endosseous implant, whereas a well-integrated implant should not pose problems if its integrity is maintained with effective dental hygiene practices (74,75).

Appropriate evaluation of the oral cavity and correction of existing oral and dental pathology can minimize, and in some cases eliminate, treatment-limiting toxicities, such as mucositis, oral infections, and bleeding, that necessitate chemotherapy dose reduction or termination (68).

Mucositis

A diagnosis of oral mucositis should be reserved for oral tissue changes that are the direct cytotoxic effects of chemotherapy. The most common acute complication of chemotherapy, mucositis, has a specific, defined mechanism of progression: mucosal erythema progresses to oral sensitivity and then to mucosal denudation (Fig. 6.26) (45,50). All other factors must be ruled out before a condition is diagnosed as mucositis, as an incorrect diagnosis of mucositis could cause unnecessary delay, reduction in the dose, or complete discontinuance of effective chemotherapy (34). Incorrect mucosal assessment can also lead to improper care and treatment and thus to the persistence of this mucosal pathology. This problem can be further compounded by superinfection, pain, decreased nutritional intake, bleeding, or a focus for sepsis, effects that increase the treatment morbidity, costs, length of hospital stay, need for additional antibiotic therapy, and need for parenteral nutritional support.

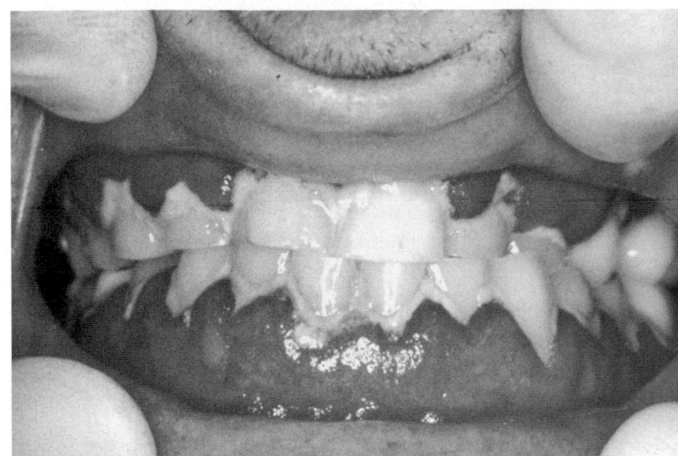
Figure 6.26 Chemotherapy-induced oral mucositis (World Health Organization grade III).

Chemotherapy agents known to produce mucositis are antimetabolites, antibiotics, and alkalating and vinca alkaloids (45,76). In cases of appropriately diagnosed mucositis, the emergence of mucosal toxicity would be expected to coincide with the administration of the chemotherapy. However, mucosal herpes simplex virus infections occurring early in the chemotherapy cycle can mimic mucositis. Failure to collect diagnostic cultures with each mucosal reaction can lead to a misdiagnosis of mucositis, in which case the infection would go untreated (77). Culturing at this early stage of therapy is essential for differentiating mucositis from infectious stomatitis that can be caused by a bacterial, fungal, or viral agent and that is usually associated with low hematologic values (Fig. 6.27) (33–35). Oral mucosal infectious agents must be correctly identified and treated, because the loss of mucosal integrity creates a portal of entry for systemic infection in immunocompromised patients (78).

Chemotherapy-induced pancytopenia, combined with mucositis, can lead to oral infection and bleeding events.

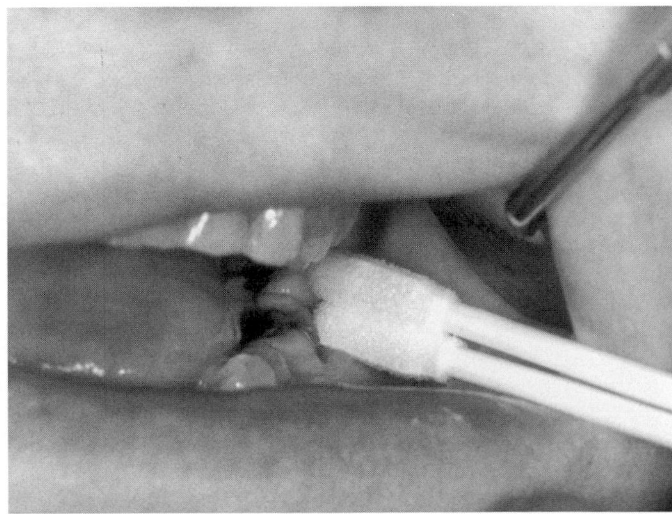
Figure 6.27 Culturing of an oral bacterial infection.

Patients may also have severe thrombocytopenia (platelets <20,000/mm^3) and neutropenia (neutrophils <500/mm^3) despite having normal-appearing oral mucosa. Serious complications, such as hemorrhagic diathesis or sepsis, can occur if hematologic parameters are not considered in the treatment of the oral cavity. Thus, clinicians should conduct a benefit-versus-risk analysis of the intended therapy and should thoroughly assess the hematologic values before each treatment intervention. Treatment guidelines based on such assessments have been established.

Diet

Although generally unrecognized, diet profoundly influences the stability of the oral tissues and can cause mucosal problems when a patient is undergoing cancer therapy (33). During the myelosuppressive phase of therapy or when the mucosa is thinned owing to chemotherapy, the diet should consist of nontraumatizing, soft foods that cannot puncture, abrade, or otherwise damage the vulnerable mucosal epithelium. Hard or abrasive food items can lead to increased pain, infection, or bleeding episodes.

All patients receiving chemotherapy are at risk for oral complications, and some patients are at a greater risk than others, depending primarily on the type of malignancy and the aggressiveness of the cancer treatment. Patents with hematologic malignancies (e.g., leukemia and lymphoma) have a greater risk than patients with solid tumors (e.g., breast cancer, lung cancer, and sarcomas), because the protective elements that maintain bodily homeostasis are part of the malignant process of hematologic malignancies (68). Additional aggressive therapy that is given cyclically or that allows hematologic recovery before the start of the next cycle further increases the risk for oral complications in these patient populations.

Viral and Bacterial Infection

Viral reactivity may lead to severe oral or disseminated infections during periods of myelo-immunosuppression. In particular, herpes simplex virus infections are often associated with severe, painful, and prolonged ulcerations atypical of those found in immunocompetent hosts (Fig. 6.28) (33–35,77). Suspected herpes simplex virus lesions should be treated with antiviral agents, such as acyclovir, administered orally or intravenously and managed as described previously for patients who receive radiation therapy. The diagnosis should be established using viral cultures, direct immunofluorescence or other rapid diagnostic tests, and histologic examination (77,79). Bacterial infections following chemotherapy can cause localized mucosal lesions, sialoadenitis, periodontal abscesses, pericoronitis, or acute necrotizing ulcerative gingivitis (34). Because systemic infection is a serious complication in neutropenic patients, constant vigilance must be maintained to prevent or manage oral infections of any type. Because antileukemic therapy is designed to achieve myelosuppression, this risk may be higher among patients with leukemia than among those with solid tumors (33). Oral infections should be treated with selected antibiotic combinations (broad-spectrum antibiotics), including an agent effective against anaerobic Gram-negative bacilli such as *Pseudomonas, Klebsiella*, or enterobacteria, which are often found in the oral cavity of immunocompromised individuals (33–35). Oral microbial culture testing should be done to ensure antibiotic sensitivity and resistance selection and to assist in identification of the causative organisms.

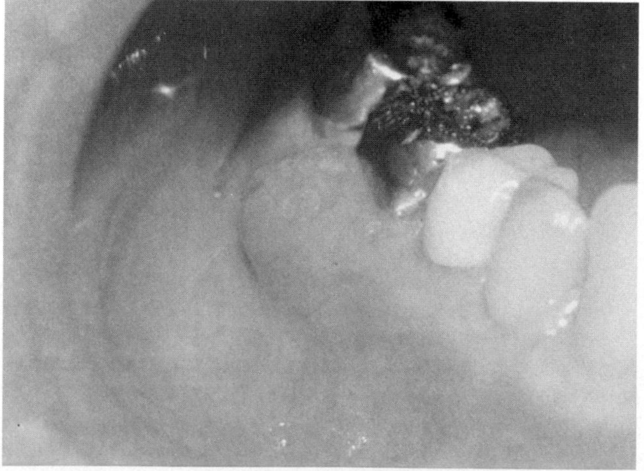

Figure 6.28 Culture-positive herpes simplex virus on the buccal mucosal tissue. Patient placed on an antiviral regimen. Herpes simplex virus is an often overlooked and under diagnosed oral condition.

REFERENCES

1. Martin JW, Lemon JC, King GE. Maxillofacial restoration after tumor ablation. In: Schusterman MA, ed. *Clinics in plastic surgery*. Philadelphia: WB Saunders, 1994;87–96.
2. Lemon JC, Martin JW, Jacob RF. Prosthetic rehabilitation. In: Weber RS, Miller MJ, Goepfert H, eds. *Basal and squamous cell skin cancers of the head and neck*. Philadelphia: Williams & Wilkins, 1996:305–312.
3. Fuller JL, Deneky GE. *Concise dental anatomy and morphology*, 2nd ed. Chicago: Year Book Medical Publishers, 1984:9.
4. Beumer JP, Curtis TA. Restoration of acquired hard palate defects. In: *Maxillofacial rehabilitation: prosthodontic and surgical considerations*. St. Louis: Mosby, 1979:188.
5. King GE, Jacob RFK, Martin JW. Oral and dental rehabilitation. In: Johns ME, ed. *Complications in otolaryngology: head and neck surgery*. Philadelphia: BC Decker, 1986:131.
6. Langland OE, Langlois RP, Morris CR. *Principle and practice of panoramic radiology*. Philadelphia: WB Saunders, 1982.
7. Lingeman RE, Singer MJ. Evaluation of the patient with head and neck cancer. In: Sven JY, Myers EN, eds. *Cancer of the head and neck*. New York: Churchill Livingstone, 1981;15.
8. Toth BB, Martin JW, Fleming TJ. Oral and dental care associated with cancer therapy. *Cancer Bull* 1991;43:397–402.
9. King GE, Toth BB, Fleming TJ. Oral dental care of the cancer patient. *Texas Dent J* 1988;105:10–11.
10. Toljanic JA, Saunders VW Jr. Radiation therapy and management of the irradiated patient. *J Prosthet Dent* 1984;52:852–858.
11. King GE, Lemon JC, Martin JW. Multidisciplinary teamwork in the treatment and rehabilitation of the head and neck cancer patient. *Texas Dent J* 1992;June: 9–12.
12. Martin JW, Jacob RF, Larson DL, et al. Surgical stents for the head and neck cancer patient. *Head Neck Surg* 1984;7:44.
13. Martin JW, Austin JR, Chambers MS, et al. Postoperative care of the maxillectomy patient. *ORL—Head and Neck Nurs* 1994;12:15–20.
14. King GE, Chambers MS, Martin JW. Patient appointments during interim obturation: is it cost-effective? *J Prosthod* 1995;4:168–172.
15. Martin JW, Lemon JC, King GE. Oral and facial restoration after reconstruction. In: Kroll S, ed. *Reconstructive plastic surgery for cancer*. St. Louis: Mosby, 1996:130–138.
16. Schusterman MA, Reece GP, Miller MJ, et al. The osteocutaneous free fibula flap: is the skin paddle reliable? *Plast Reconstr Surg* 1992;90:787.
17. Beumer JP, Kurrasch M, Kagawa T. Prosthetic restoration of oral defects secondary to surgical removal of oral defects secondary to surgical removal of oral neoplasms. *Calif Dent Assn J* 1982;10:47–54.
18. Conley S, Gosain A, Marks S, et al. Identification and assessment of velopharyngeal inadequacy. *Am J Otolaryngol* 1997;18:38–46.
19. King GE, Martin JW, Lemon JC, et al. Maxillofacial prosthetic rehabilitation combined with plastic and reconstructive surgery. *MD Anderson Oncol Case Rep Rev* 1993;8:1–11.
20. DeSanto LW, Thawley SE, Genden EM. Treatment of tumors of the oropharynx: surgical therapy. In: Thawley, Panje, Batsakis, et al., eds. *Comprehensive management of head and neck tumors*, Vol 1, 2nd ed. Philadelphia: WB Saunders, 1999:806–859.
21. Teichgraeber J, Larson DL, Castaneda O, et al. Skin grafts in intraoral reconstruction: a new stenting method. *Arch Otolaryngol Head Neck Surg* 1984;101:463.

22. Godoy AJ, Perez DG, Lemon JC, et al. Rehabilitation of a patient with limited oral opening following glossectomy. *Intl J Prosthod* 1991;4:70–74.
23. Krugmen M, Beumer J. Maxillectomy cavity care with a pulsating stream irrigator. *Eye Ear Nose Throat Mon* 1975;54:104.
24. Kottke FJ, Stillwell GK, Lehmann JF. *Krusen's handbook of physical medicine and rehabilitation*, 3d ed. Philadelphia: WB Saunders, 1982:102–123.
25. Barrett NV, Martin JW, Jacob RF, et al. Physical therapy techniques in the treatment of the head and neck patient. *J Prosthet Dent* 1988;59:343.
26. Adell R, Lekholm U, Rockler B, et al. A 15-year study of osseointegrated implants in the treatment of the edentulous jaw. *Int J Oral Surg* 1981;10: 387–416.
27. Granstöm G, Tjellström A, Branemark PI, et al. Bone anchored reconstruction of the irradiated head and neck cancer patient. *Otolaryngol Head Neck Surg* 1993;108:334–343.
28. Lemon JC, Chambers MS, Wesley PJ, et al. Rehabilitation of a midface defect with reconstructive surgery and facial prosthetics: a case report. *Int J Oral Maxillofac Implants* 1996;11:101–105.
29. Parr GR, Goldman BM, Rahn AO. Maxillofacial prosthetic principles in the surgical planning for facial defects. *J Prosthet Dent* 1981;46:323.
30. Marunick MT, Harrison R, Beumer J. Prosthodontic rehabilitation of midfacial defects. *J Prosthet Dent* 1985;54: 553–560.
31. Parel SM, Holt R, Branemark P-I, et al. Osseointegration and facial prosthetics. *Int J Oral Maxillofac Implants* 1986;1:27–29.
32. Lowe O. Pretreatment dental assessment and management of patients undergoing head and neck irradiation. *Clin Prevent Dent* 1986;8:24–30.
33. Chambers MS, Toth BB, Martin JW, et al. Oral and dental management of the cancer patient: prevention and treatment of complications. *Support Care Cancer* 1995;3:168–175.
34. Toth BB, Chambers MS, Fleming TJ, et al. Minimizing oral complications of cancer treatment. *Oncology* 1995;9:851–858.
35. Toth BB, Chambers MS, Fleming TJ. Prevention and management of oral complications associated with cancer therapies: radiotherapy/chemotherapy. *Texas Dent J* 1996;113:23–29.
36. Fleming TJ. Oral tissue changes of radiation-oncology and their management. *Dent Clin North Am* 1990;34:223–237.
37. Shrout MK. Managing patients undergoing radiation. *J Am Dent Assoc* 1991; 122:69–70,72.
38. Barrett AW, Porter SR, Scully C, et al. Oral melanotic macules that develop after radiation therapy. *Oral Surg Oral Med Oral Pathol* 1994;77:431–434.
39. Dahllöf G, Krekmanova L, Kopp S, et al. Craniomandibular dysfunction in children treated with total-body irradiation and bone marrow transplantation. *Acta Odontol Scand* 1994;52:99–105.
40. Dahllöf G, Rozell B, Forsberg CM, et al. Histologic changes in dental morphology induced by high dose chemotherapy and total body irradiation. *Oral Surg Oral Med Oral Pathol* 1994;77:56–60.
41. Brown AT, Sims RE, Raybould TP, et al. Oral gram-negative bacilli in bone marrow transplant patients given chlorhexidine rinses. *J Dent Res* 1989;68: 1199–1204.
42. Toth BB, Martin JW, Chambers MS, et al. Oral candidiasis: a morbid sequelae of anticancer therapy. *Texas Dent J* 1998;115:24–29.
43. Bergman OJ. Oral infections and septicemia in immunocompromised patients with hematologic malignancies. *J Clin Microbiol* 1988;26:2105–2109.
44. Sonis S, Clark J. Prevention and management of oral mucositis induced by antineoplastic therapy. *Oncology* 1991;5:11–18.
45. Borowski B, Benhamou E, Pico JL, et al. Prevention of oral mucositis in patients treated with high-dose chemotherapy and bone marrow transplantation: a randomized controlled trial comparing two protocols of dental care. *Eur J Cancer B Oral Oncol* 1994;30B:93–97.
46. Pfeiffer P, Madsen EL, Hansen O. Effect of prophylactic sucralfate suspension on stomatitis-induced by cancer chemotherapy. A randomized, double-blind cross-over study. *Acta Oncologica* 1990;29:171–173.
47. Loprinzi CL, Cianflone SG, Dose AM. A controlled evaluation of an allopurinol mouthwash as prophylaxis against 5-fluorouracil-induced stomatitis. *Cancer* 1990;65:1879–1882.
48. Wadleigh RZG, Redman RS, Graham ML. Vitamin E in the treatment of chemotherapy-induced mucositis. *Am J Med* 1992;92:481–484.
49. Gordon B, Spadinger A, Hodges E. Effect of granulocyte-macrophage colony-stimulating factor on oral mucositis after hematopoietic stem-cell transplantation. *J Clin Oncol* 1994;12:1917–1922.
50. National Institutes of Health Consensus Development Conference statement. Oral complications of cancer therapies: diagnosis, prevention, and treatment. *J Am Dent Assoc* 1989;119:179–183.
51. Hurst PS. Dental considerations in management of head and neck cancer. *Otolaryngol Clin North Am* 1985;18:573–603.
52. Peterson DE. Dental care for the cancer patient. *Compendium Cont Educ Dent* 1983;4:115–120.
53. Muzyka BC, Glick M. A review of oral fungal infections and appropriate therapy. *J Am Dent Assoc* 1995;126:63–72.
54. Beumer J, Silverman S Jr, Benak SB Jr. Hard and soft tissue necrosis following radiation therapy for oral cancer. *J Prosthet Dent* 1972;27:640–644.
55. Epstein JB, Giuseppe R, Wong FL. Osteoradionecrosis: study of the relationship of dental extractions in patients receiving radiotherapy. *Head Neck Surg* 1987;10:48–54.
56. Marx RE, Johnson RP. Studies in the radiobiology of osteoradionecrosis and their clinical significance. *Oral Surg Oral Med Oral Pathol Oral Radiol Endod* 1987;64:379–390.
57. Mansfield MJ, Sanders DW, Heimbach RD. Hyperbaric oxygen as an adjunct in the treatment of osteoradionecrosis of the mandible. *J Oral Surg* 1981;39: 585–589.
58. Marx RE, Johnson RP, Kline SN. Prevention of osteoradionecrosis: a randomized prospective clinical trial of hyperbaric oxygen versus penicillin. *J Am Dent Assoc* 1985;111:49–54.
59. Wescott WB. Dental management of patients being treated for oral cancer. *CDA J* 1985;13:42–47.
60. Bundgaard T, Tandrup O, Elbrond O. A functional evaluation of patients treated for oral cancer. A prospective study. *Int J Oral Maxillofac Surg* 1993;22: 28–34.
61. Granström G, Jacobsson M, Tjellström A. Titanium implants in irradiated tissues: benefits from hyperbaric oxygen. *Int J Oral Maxillofac Implants* 1992;7: 15–25.
62. Epstein JB, Wong FLW, Stevenson-Moore P. Osteoradionecrosis: clinical experience and a proposal for classification. *J Oral Maxillofac Surg* 1987;45:104–110.
63. Schubert MM, Izutsu KT. Iatrogenic causes of salivary gland dysfunction. *J Dent Res* 1987;66(S):680–688.
64. Keene HJ, Fleming TJ. Prevalence of caries-associated microflora after radiotherapy in patients with cancer of the head and neck. *Oral Surg Oral Med Oral Pathol Oral Radiol Endod* 1987;64:421–426.
65. Keene HJ, Fleming TJ, Toth BB. Cariogenic microflora in patients with Hodgkin's disease before and after mantle field radiotherapy. *Oral Surg Oral Med Oral Pathol* 1994;78:577–581.
66. Johnson JT, Feretti GA, Nethery WJ, et al. Oral pilocarpine for post-irradiation xerostomia in patients with head and neck cancer. *N Engl J Med* 1993;329: 390–395.
67. LeVeque FG, Montgomery M, Potter D, et al. A multicenter, randomized, double-blind, placebo-controlled, dose-titration study of oral pilocarpine for treatment of radiation-induced xerostomia in head and neck cancer patients. *J Clin Oncol* 1993;11:1124–1131.
68. Fleming ID, Brady LW, Mieszkalski GB, et al. Basis for major current therapies for cancer. In: Murphy GP, Lawrence W, Lenhard RE, eds. *American Cancer Society Textbook of Clinical Oncology*, 2nd ed, Atlanta: American Cancer Society, 1995:96–134.
69. Bakemeier RF, Oazi R. Basic concepts of cancer chemotherapy and principles of medical oncology. In: Rubin P, ed. *Clinical oncology: a multidisciplinary approach for physicians and students*, 7th ed. Philadelphia: WB Saunders, 1993: 105–116.
70. Toth BB, Martin JW, Fleming TJ. Oral complications associated with cancer therapy: An M. D. Anderson Cancer Center experience. *J Clin Periodontol* 1990;17:508–515.
71. Bodey GP. Quantitative relationship between circulating leukocytes and infection in patients with acute leukemia. *Ann Intern Med* 1966;64:328–340.
72. Dajani AS, Taubert KA, Wilson W, et al. Prevention of bacterial endocarditis: recommendations by the American Heart Association [review]. *Circulation* 1997;96:358–366.
73. Epstein JB, Vickars L, Spinelli J, et al. Efficacy of chlorhexidine and nystatin rinses in prevention of oral complications in leukemia and bone marrow transplantation. *Oral Surg Oral Med Oral Pathol* 1992;73:682–689.
74. Karr RA, Kramer DC, Toth BB. Dental implants and chemotherapy complications. *J Prosthet Dent* 1992;67:683–687.
75. Sager RD, Theis RM. Dental implants placed in a patient with multiple myeloma: report of a case. *J Am Dent Assoc* 1990;121:699–701.
76. Toth BB, Fleming TJ. Oral care for the patient with cancer. *Highlights on Antineoplastic Drugs* 1990;8:27–35.
77. Tang ITL, Shepp DH. Herpes simplex virus infection in cancer patients: prevention and treatment. *Oncology* 1992;6:101–109.
78. Meurman JH, Pyrhönen S, Teerenhovi L, et al. Oral sources of septicaemia in patients with malignancies. *Oral Oncology* 1997;33:389–397.
79. Poland J. Prevention and treatment of oral complications in the cancer patient. *Oncology* 1991;5:45–62.

CHAPTER 7

Nutritional Management of Patients with Head and Neck Cancer

Michael H. Torosian and John A. Ridge

Patients with head and neck cancer are often malnourished. Besides cancer, other factors causing malnutrition in this patient population are poor dietary habits, smoking, and alcohol intake. Protein-calorie malnutrition is characterized by weight loss, hypoalbuminemia, decreased skeletal muscle mass, reduced fat stores, anemia, and immune system suppression. Side effects of all forms of antineoplastic therapy, including surgery, radiation therapy, and chemotherapy, contribute to the development of malnutrition. Clinical studies have demonstrated that malnutrition is associated with increased morbidity and mortality after major oncologic surgery (1–4), and, furthermore, it decreases patient tolerance to both radiation therapy and chemotherapy.

Because head and neck cancer patients are susceptible to the adverse consequences of malnutrition, appropriate nutrition intervention can reduce morbidity and improve tolerance to antineoplastic therapy. This chapter summarizes the mechanisms of development of cancer cachexia, the clinical implications of malnutrition, and the routes and clinical efficacy of nutrition support in head and neck cancer patients.

DEVELOPMENT OF CACHEXIA

The etiology of cachexia in head and neck cancer patients is complex and multifactorial. Cancer cachexia is a clinical syndrome consisting of anorexia, weight loss, severe tissue wasting, asthenia, and organ system dysfunction. There are three major physiologic mechanisms—metabolic, obstructive, and treatment-related—responsible for the development of cachexia in head and neck cancer patients. The extent to which each of these factors contributes to the development of cachexia in an individual patient varies depending on tumor type, tumor stage, medical comorbidities, dietary habits, and other clinical factors. Throughout the course of one's illness, the relative importance of each of these factors on nutritional status can change. An accurate assessment of the causative factors of cachexia in patients with head and neck cancer is essential for determining and implementing an effective strategy to address their malnutrition.

Anorexia is common in patients with advanced head and neck cancer. Although the cause of cancer-related anorexia is unknown, dysfunction of the normal mechanisms that stimulate appetite can play a major role in its development. For example, tumors of the oral cavity and nasopharynx can significantly alter taste and olfactory sensation. Such alterations can cause markedly reduced food intake, a sensory dysfunction that is often exacerbated by cancer surgery, chemotherapy, and radiation therapy. Severe mucositis, decreased salivation, and pain related to the cancer and its therapy can produce anorexia and further development of malnutrition.

It has been suggested that leptin, a hormone secreted by adipose tissue, may play a role in the development and persistence of anorexia in cancer patients (5). Under normal conditions, weight loss causes leptin levels to decrease, which stimulates the hypothalamus to trigger a feeding response (6). Despite persistent and progressive weight loss in the cancer patient, anorexia persists suggesting dysfunction of the leptin-mediated hypothalamic feeding response (5,7).

Widespread abnormalities in energy, carbohydrate, lipid, and protein metabolism are known to occur in cancer patients (8–10). Aberrations in energy expenditure exist in the majority of patients with cancer. Although it was initially hypothesized that increased energy expenditure accounted for weight loss in these patients, clinical studies of energy metabolism have found that energy expenditure can be normal, increased, or decreased in these patients. In a study of 200 malnourished cancer patients with gastrointestinal malignancy, 59% of cancer patients exhibited abnormal energy expenditure (33% decreased and 26% increased resting energy expenditure). Other significant metabolic alterations found in cancer patients include increased rates of protein turnover (with protein breakdown typically exceeding protein synthesis); lipid catabolism, including depletion of total body fat and changes in body composition; and alterations in carbohydrate metabolism, including increased Cori cycle activity, glucose intolerance, impaired insulin sensitivity, decreased glucose oxidation, and increased rates of gluconeogenesis (8,10,12–14). These metabolic alterations cause significant dysfunction of the adaptive mechanisms that maintain homeostasis under normal conditions and contribute to cachexia in the cancer patient.

Although the etiology of cancer cachexia remains unknown, systemic factors that significantly alter host metabolism certainly contribute to the cachectic state. Two metabolic classes of cachexia mediators believed to be important in its pathogenesis are cytokines and regulatory hormones. These circulating factors cause a cascade of catabolic effects leading to the syndrome of cachexia. Cytokines are soluble proteins secreted by host tissues in response to malignancy, sepsis, and other pathologic events. Cytokines function by multiple mechanisms including autocrine (i.e., same cell), paracrine (i.e., adjacent cells), and systemic (i.e., distant cells) effects. Specific cytokines that have been implicated in the development of cancer cachexia include tumor necrosis factor (TNF), interferon-α, interleukin-1, and interleukin-6 (15,16).

Tumor necrosis factor, or cachectin, is secreted by macrophages, and studies *in vivo* have demonstrated that TNF can produce anorexia, weight loss, skeletal muscle loss, depletion of fat stores, hypoproteinemia and increased total body water (17). However, the entire syndrome of cancer cachexia cannot be reproduced by the action of TNF alone. Furthermore, it is difficult to detect circulating levels of TNF, even in patients with advanced malignancy. Another potential cachexia mediator is interleukin-1, which causes anorexia, pyrexia, hypotension, decreased systemic vascular resistance, increased cardiac output, and alterations in hepatic protein synthesis (18). Interleukin-6 causes many of the same effects as TNF or interleukin-1, and is secreted by macrophages stimulated by TNF or interleukin-1 (19). Although cytokines certainly play a role in its development, the relative importance of these circulating proteins in the etiology of cancer cachexia remains to be determined.

Regulatory hormones are important metabolic mediators and also play a critical role in the syndrome of cancer cachexia. The catabolic changes associated with cancer, sepsis, and other pathophysiologic stresses are typically characterized by decreased insulin and increased glucagon levels. The insulin/glucagon ratio is an index of host anabolism. A significant reduction of this ratio establishes a catabolic hormonal environment. This catabolic state cannot be reversed by insulin administration alone because of the associated compensatory increase in glucagon secretion (20). In fact, in animal models in which insulin has been given in an attempt to reverse the cachectic state, an excessive glucagon response can occur, resulting in a further reduction in the insulin/glucagon ratio (21). In our laboratory, insulin combined with the somatostatin analog octreotide was found to significantly increase the insulin/glucagon ratio; octreotide was provided to prevent the compensatory release of glucagon associated with exogenous insulin administration. By using the triple combination of insulin, octreotide, and growth hormone, increased carcass weight and improved nutritional status could be achieved in tumor-bearing animals. No stimulation of mammary cancer growth was found with this anabolic hormone therapy.

In addition to the metabolic theories proposed to explain cachexia, head and neck cancer patients are vulnerable to local effects of their tumors. Physical obstruction caused by head and neck cancers can prevent adequate intake of nutrients, resulting in significant weight loss and cachexia. These tumors can also impair mastication, cause swallowing dysfunction, and promote aspiration. The end result of these local effects of head and neck cancers is a significant reduction in protein-calorie intake.

In distinct contrast to the metabolic, circulating factors causing cancer cachexia, the local effects of head and neck cancers can be easily reversed by providing adequate nutrient intake. Depending on primary tumor site and extent of disease, treatment or bypass of the primary tumor (for example, by inserting a percutaneous gastrostomy tube for feeding) can completely reverse the catabolism caused by local effects of head and neck cancers. Accurate clinical assessment and appropriate nutrition intervention can create an anabolic environment when malnutrition results predominantly from the local effects of head and neck cancers or their treatment.

Finally, all forms of antineoplastic therapy contribute to the development of cachexia. Fasting for preoperative testing and postoperative recovery, postsurgical ileus, anorexia, and comorbid conditions commonly cause extended periods of inadequate nutrient intake. Chemotherapy and its associated adverse effects such as nausea, vomiting, anorexia, diarrhea, and mucositis may limit oral intake or impair nutrient absorption to further compromise an already malnourished patient. Radiation therapy to the head and neck can adversely alter taste sensation, decrease salivation, impair olfactory sense, and cause severe mucositis, greatly reducing spontaneous nutrient intake. During periods of antineoplastic therapy, it is critically important to avoid prolonged periods of reduced nutrient intake to prevent clinical morbidity and improve tolerance to surgery, chemotherapy, and radiation therapy.

CLINICAL IMPLICATIONS OF MALNUTRITION

The clinical relevance of malnutrition has been demonstrated by many studies that report increased morbidity and mortality in malnourished patients. Although numerous nutritional and metabolic parameters have been studied with regard to clinical outcome, weight loss and serum albumin levels are the simplest and most important tests of prognostic significance. As early as 1977, Costa (22) demonstrated that weight loss was a better predictor of death in lung cancer patients than performance status, tumor histology, or type of chemotherapy. DeWys (23) found a positive correlation between weight loss and both decreased survival and lowered performance status in most cancer patients. Mullen (3) developed a multifactorial prognostic nutritional index that stratified patients according to risk of developing complications after major cancer surgery. The most important factor of this predictive model was the circulating serum album level; other factors in this predictive equation included serum transferrin level, triceps skinfold measurement, and delayed cutaneous hypersensitivity reaction (3,24). Thus, it was recognized early on that malnutrition was associated with increased morbidity and mortality of cancer patients. However, reversing malnutrition in the cancer patient and demonstrating that nutrition support reduces cancer-related morbidity and mortality have been difficult.

CLINICAL EFFICACY OF NUTRITION SUPPORT

Numerous clinical trials have been conducted over the past three decades to investigate the effect of nutrition support on the outcome of cancer patients. Initial retrospective studies suggested that morbidity and mortality of cancer patients could be reduced with the provision of adequate nutrition support. However, subsequent prospective randomized study results have been in conflict with these early, retrospective reports (8,25). Prolonged nutrition support has limited efficacy except in select clinical situations.

The Perioperative Veterans' Affairs Total Parenteral Nutrition Cooperative Study most conclusively demonstrated the utility of preoperative total parenteral nutrition (TPN) in patients undergoing major cancer surgery (26). A significant reduction of postoperative complications was observed in severely malnourished patients undergoing laparotomy or thoracotomy in patients receiving TPN compared with the control group. The severely malnourished group represented less than 5% of the surgical patients in this study. Patients receiving TPN who were not malnourished or had borderline malnutrition showed an increased rate of infectious complications. An important exception to these results involves the use of nutrition support in bone marrow transplant patients (27). In patients receiving bone marrow transplantation, TPN has been found to improve overall survival, improve disease-free survival, and decrease the rate of relapse compared with control patients. As chemotherapy regimens become more aggressive and toxic, additional select groups of patients may be identified who will benefit from the use of nutrition support.

Nutritional Support for Patients with Head and Neck Cancer

Nutrition support for patients with head and neck cancer may be considered in terms of their relationship to treatment. Patients (a) may be awaiting treatment, (b) may have undergone resection, (c) may be undergoing radiation therapy or chemotherapy, or (d) may have completed treatment. Efforts to address problems with nutrition are strongly influenced by these factors. As a result, no single approach to providing adequate calorie and protein intake is appropriate for all patients. Randomized trials of nutritional support specifically for head and neck cancer patients have not been performed. Clinically, there are substantial variations in practice. However, some guiding principles should be observed.

Parenteral Nutrition

The overwhelming majority of patients with head and neck cancer have intact gut function. The chief sources of their difficulty in maintaining adequate nutritional status are mechanical factors. Dysphagia, odynophagia, and aspiration all have the potential to interfere with oral intake. However, once food has entered the esophagus, most patients are able to digest it. Hence, patients who present with head and neck neoplasms seldom require parenteral nutritional support. Patients who will not eat, cannot eat, or cannot eat enough will generally respond promptly to enteral nutritional maneuvers.

Untreated Patients

Most patients with cancer of the *oral cavity*, who often have difficulty maintaining adequate intake of normal (or even of soft) foods, are able to handle liquid nutritional preparations easily. Difficulty swallowing liquids is seldom a problem for patients whose tumor arises anterior to the faucial arch. Many patients with cancers of the oropharynx, larynx, and hypopharynx are also able to take liquids despite profound dysphagia with solid foods. For such patients, liquid nutrient supplements to their usual diet can be recommended before resection or the inception of radiation treatment. Unfortunately, most patients who are encouraged to supplement their diet fail to take liquid supplements in adequate amounts to compensate for the shortfall. As a result, they remain in a catabolic state despite attempts to improve their nutritional status through supplementation of their ordinary diet.

Such patients are probably best served by instructing them to view a liquid nutrient preparation as the mainstay of their diet, allowing "supplementation" with their food of choice. Few patients who take 2,000 kcal/day of a liquid nutrient preparation desire substantial additional intake, but (if compliant) they should be able to maintain or to improve their nutritional status through such an approach.

Untreated patients with many cancers of the *oropharynx, hypopharynx,* and *larynx* have such difficulty swallowing liquids that efforts to maintain (or improve) their nutritional status through oral agents fail. Many such individuals are unable to drink the necessary 2,000 to 2,400 cc/day required to maintain hydration and to meet nutritional goals. For these patients, and for those who are already receiving treatment, feeding tubes represent the best method for providing an adequate diet.

Nasogastric and gastrostomy tubes are those most commonly employed. Nasogastric tubes are placed with low morbidity. They are unsightly, uncomfortable, and all too often become dislodged. Hence, patient acceptance of even short-term nasogastric feeding at home is limited. Gastrostomy tubes are not generally visible to others, and, when properly placed, are not readily dislodged. However, their placement requires a surprisingly painful procedure, and neither leakage nor irritation about the site can be ignored as sources of discomfort and concern to patients and their caregivers.

Pretreatment counseling, the nature of the proposed cancer treatment, the time until therapy is initiated, and the quality of home nursing support may all influence the approach taken toward feeding tubes. If treatment commences within days and entails an operation, then logistical difficulties are likely to compromise meaningful nutrition support through a feeding tube before treatment. However, patients who are undergoing nonsurgical management of their head and neck cancers may require feeding tubes for weeks.

Postoperative Nutrition Support

Most patients who undergo resection of T1-T2 cancers of the *oral vestibule, oral tongue, floor of mouth,* and *mandibular alveolus* are able to maintain adequate hydration by oral intake within 3 days (if there are no intraoral suture lines). Patients who undergo a *maxillectomy* can usually begin full oral intake even sooner. Current length of stay after surgery for many such cancers is less than 3 days, so patients may be unable to take enough fluids by mouth alone when they are discharged from the hospital (28). Nonetheless, most are able to maintain hydration and nutrition within days of discharge. Despite the distaste most patients harbor toward nasogastric feeding tubes, these tubes serve the overwhelming majority of patients well in the interval between their operation and the time when they are able to maintain themselves with an oral diet.

Resection of T3-T4 cancers of the *oral cavity* and *oropharynx* is likely to be accompanied by longer hospitalization and more profound functional problems than those that follow surgical treatment of T1-T2 cancers. Even when healing is uncomplicated (and oral intake may resume in fairly short order), it is common for such patients to require nutritional supplementation until they can maintain sufficient oral intake. Though prospective evaluation of costs and quality of life has not been undertaken, creation of a gastrostomy tube is clinically justified when the anticipated duration of nutrition support exceeds 2 weeks. Patients who undergo pharyngectomy, resection of the tongue base, composite resection of the mandible, and flap reconstruction are at substantial risk for long-term dependence on tube feedings (29).

After total *laryngectomy* very few patients have difficulty resuming oral intake. Though there are substantial variations in practice surrounding the reintroduction of oral feeding, it is usually uneventful and well tolerated. Catheters for tracheoesophageal puncture may serve as feeding tubes. Gastrostomy tubes are seldom needed. The situation after partial laryngectomy is different. Some procedures engender considerable aspiration and difficulty swallowing, whereas others do not. Individual patient participation plays an important role in recovery. It may be difficult to predict the duration of feeding tube support for patients who have undergone a partial laryngectomy, but all too many patients require some sort of feeding tube support for months. Hence, gastrostomy tubes are often necessary even after uncomplicated partial laryngectomies (30).

Although some authors have recommended creation of gastrostomy tubes for all patients who undergo major resections of head and neck cancer, the morbidity of gastrostomy should not be ignored (31). Many gastrostomies undertaken in pursuit of such a policy may not prove necessary during the postoperative recovery period. Patients who are eating normally have a low tolerance for their gastrostomy tubes, and usually desire their prompt removal. It is often difficult to persuade patients to allow a gastrostomy tube to remain in place to be available for support during a planned course of postoperative radiation.

However, when complications (such as flap loss, development of a large fistula, or life-threatening aspiration) prevent the inception of oral feeding, gastrostomy tubes represent important adjuncts to supportive care. In the face of increased wound care requirements, repeated trips to the operating room, and other sources of stress, gastrostomy tubes are more comfortable for patients and easier for the nursing staff to maintain than are nasogastric feeding tubes.

Nutritional Support During Treatment

Treatment of head and neck cancers with *radiation* results in mucosal injury, odynophagia, xerostomia, and dysgeusia. Weight loss is the rule (32–34). Treatment schedules that involve acceleration of dosage (with shorter treatment time), increased radiation dose (often with hyperfractionation), or concomitant administration of chemotherapy with radiation are associated with profound and prolonged mucositis. A substantial minority of patients treated with concurrent chemoradiation remains dependent on tube feeding for months. Some never are able to resume a normal diet. Hence, when patients are receiving modern radiation treatment with curative intent, attention should be directed to nutrition support and swallowing from the inception of treatment planning.

Loss of weight and decline in the ability to eat are insidious. Patients seldom have problems during the initial 2 weeks of therapy. Problems with nutrition are typically recognized during the fourth week of treatment. Efforts to increase oral intake usually fail in this setting, and the placement of a feeding tube is only delayed. Severe decline in nutritional status is accompanied by increased need for hospitalization and all too often by treatment breaks. Hence, patients are probably best served if the clinicians address an impending problem with oral nutrition before radiation therapy begins. This represents an opportunity to create a gastrostomy and to instruct the patient (and caregivers) in its use before difficulty swallowing precipitates a significant problem with nutrition (or even hydration).

Treatment of head and neck cancer with *chemotherapy*, whether in a palliative setting or as part of a potentially curative regimen, is typically associated with stomatitis or mucositis. Patients with recurrent tumor are often nutritionally compromised (either by recurrent tumor or by sequelae of their initial treatment). Gastrostomy tubes are often beneficial for such individuals, and their use may prevent hospitalization for dehydration, which otherwise often complicates palliative treatment of patients with head and neck tumors.

Nutritional Support After Treatment

Most patients who are treated for head and neck cancer develop problems with nutrition that persist for years, even if they have been cured of their tumors. Some problems are relatively subtle and many are subject to compensatory mechanisms (such as change in diet). However, some patients are plagued with mechanical problems such as stricture and decline in excursion of the tongue base and larynx that create tremendous problems with resumption of an oral diet. The mechanisms through which these problems develop are not fully understood, and preventive maneuvers have not been widely adopted. Even seemingly simple questions—such as, Should esophageal dilation be regularly performed after head and neck radiation?—have not been addressed in a systematic fashion. There are wide variations in management approaches to such problems, and current clinical research is only now beginning to address them.

Placing Feeding Tubes

Although prolonged nasogastric tube placement has advocates, most patients with head and neck cancer who require long-term tube placement are best served by a gastrostomy (35). Gastric feedings with most liquid commercial supplements are well tolerated after a period of accommodation. Jejunostomy tubes may also be employed, but they impose logistical problems because delivering large volumes of tube feeding to the small intestine may precipitate diarrhea and dumping symptoms. As a result, jejunostomy feedings typically entail inconvenient infusions, rather than bolus feeding "meals." Their use should probably be restricted to the relatively unusual cases where the integrity of the stomach must be preserved or where prior stomach operations prevent gastrostomy placement.

Gastrostomies may be created in several ways. Percutaneous endoscopic gastrostomy (PEG) is currently the most common. Kits from many manufacturers are available in operating rooms and endoscopy suites. Transoral placement of a feeding tube may require pulling it past a head and neck cancer—a likely source of tumor implantation in the gastrostomy site (36). Tubes may be introduced directly through the abdominal wall, which may diminish the risk for tumor developing at the gastrostomy exit site (Fig. 7.1).

Tubes placed into the stomach through the abdominal wall by radiologists under image guidance are often of small diameter. They are more subject to occlusion and their fittings may be more difficult for elderly or infirm patients and caregivers to manage than larger tubes typically placed through other techniques.

An open "surgical" gastrostomy may be performed under general or local anesthesia if tumor or stricture precludes access to the stomach through the esophagus. Gastrostomy tubes may also be placed with excellent demonstration of anatomy using laparoscopy (37). If maintenance of the gastroepiploic arcade along the greater curve of the stomach is imperative, then techniques that permit placement of the feeding tube under direct vision are superior to the "blind" percutaneous approaches, which may (rarely) result in injury to structures surrounding the stomach.

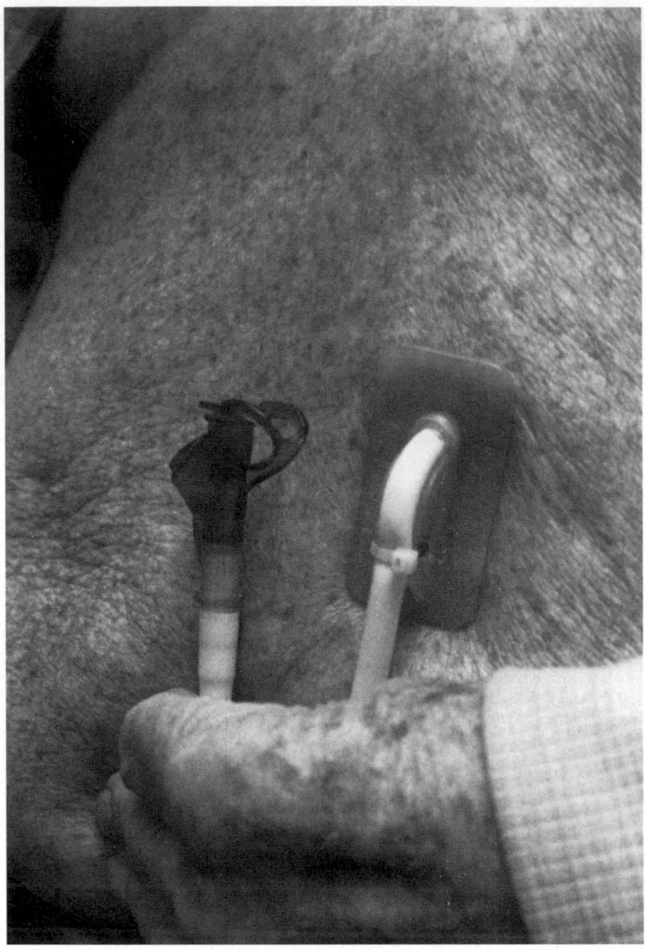

Figure 7.1 Gastrostomy tube in a patient.

Prior placement of a gastrostomy tube (the site of which has closed) does not constitute a contraindication to PEG placement. It may be difficult to reestablish access to the stomach through the prior track, so patients and physicians should be prepared for a procedure similar in scope to the initial gastrostomy placement. Furthermore, although most gastrostomy sites close within hours of tube removal, a few percent actually have become mature gastrocutaneous fistulae. These persist and fail to heal even after the tube has been removed. Surgical closure is needed for these persistent fistulae.

Jejunostomy tubes may also be used to provide enteral nutrition. Need to preserve or transpose an undamaged stomach, prior gastrectomy, and antecedent gastric restrictive procedures represent the most common indications for jejunostomy tube placement for patients with head and neck cancers. Percutaneous endoscopic jejunostomy (PEJ), laparoscopic jejunostomy, and open jejunostomy have all been employed. Though a PEJ is often feasible, open or minimally invasive surgical techniques should be part of the therapeutic approach if a jejunostomy is anticipated.

CONCLUSION

Patients with head and neck cancers present some unique challenges and opportunities for providing nutrition support. The local effects of head and neck cancers, postsurgical anatomic and functional deficits, and local treatment-related effects from radiation therapy can be counteracted by providing enteral nutrition distal to the head and neck region. As previously discussed, current technology provides convenient access for enteral nutrient provision. Although enteral feeding can reverse those aspects of malnutrition related to the local effects of head and neck cancers and their treatment, the component of cachexia due to systemic factors remains much more difficult to treat.

Nutrition support has been shown to increase tolerance and reduce toxicity associated with both chemotherapy and radiation therapy. Nutrition support can effectively replete or maintain nutritional status of head and neck cancer patients during courses of chemotherapy or radiation treatments. Support of host nutritional status is imperative during these treatments to reduce adverse effects, to minimize interruption of treatment schedules, and to maximize antineoplastic activity in head and neck cancer patients.

REFERENCES

1. Copeland EM, Daly JM, Dudrick SJ. Nutrition as an adjunct to cancer treatment in the adult. *Cancer Res* 1977;37:2451–2456.
2. Smale BF, Mullen JL, Buzby GP, et al. The efficacy of nutritional assessment and support in cancer surgery. *Cancer* 1981;47:2375–2381.
3. Mullen JL. Consequences of malnutrition in the surgical patient. *Surg Clin North Am* 1981;61:465–473.
4. Rhoads JE, Alexander CE. Nutritional problems of surgical patients. *Ann NY Acad Sci* 1955;63:268–272.
5. Inui A. Cancer anorexia-cachexia syndrome: current issues in research and management. *CA Cancer J Clin* 2002;52:72–91.
6. Schwartz MW, Seeley RJ. Neuroendocrine responses to starvation and weight loss. *N Engl J Med* 1997;336:1802–1811.
7. Schwartz MW, Dallman MF, Woods SC. Hypothalamic response to starvation: implications for the study of wasting disorders. *Am J Physiol* 1995;269:949–957.
8. Torosian MH, Daly JM. Nutritional support in the cancer-bearing host. *Cancer* 1986;58:1915.
9. Lindholm K, et al. Metabolism in peripheral tissues in cancer patients. *Cancer Treat Rep* 1981;65[Suppl]:79.
10. Brennan MF. Uncomplicated starvation versus cancer cachexia. *Cancer Res* 1977;37:2359.
11. Knox LS, et al. Energy expenditure in malnourished cancer patients. *Ann Surg* 1983;197:152.
12. Holroyde CP, Reichard GA. Carbohydrate metabolism in cancer cachexia. *Cancer Treat Rep* 1981;65[Suppl]:55.
13. Shaw JH, Wolfe R. Glucose and urea kinetics in patients with early and advanced gastrointestinal cancer. The response to glucose infusion, parenteral feeding, and surgical resection. *Surgery* 1987;101:181.
14. Edmonston JH. Fatty acid mobilization and glucose metabolism in patients with cancer. *Cancer* 1966;19:277.
15. Nakahara W. A chemical basis for tumor host relations. *J Natl Cancer Inst* 1960; 24:77.
16. Langstein H, et al. Reversal of cancer cachexia by antibodies to interferon-gamma but not cachectin-tumor necrosis factor. *Surg Forum* 1989;40:408.
17. Beutler B, Cerami A. Cachectin and tumor necrosis factor as two sides of the same biological coin. *Nature* 1986;320:584.
18. Woloski BMRNJ, Fuller GM. Identification and partial characterization of hepatocyte stimulating factor from leukemia cell lines: comparison with interleukin I. *Proc Natl Acad Sci USA* 1985;82:1443.
19. Powanda MC, Beisel WR. Hypothesis: leukocyte endogenous mediator/endogenous cryogen/lymphocyte activating factor modulates the development of nonspecific and specific immunity and affects nutritional status. *Am J Clin Nutr* 1982;35:752.
20. Unger RH. Glucagon and the insulin: glucagon ratio in diabetes and other catabolic illness. *Diabetes* 1981;20:834.
21. Bartlett DL, et al. Growth hormone, insulin and somatostatin therapy of cancer cachexia. *Cancer* 1994;73:1499.
22. Costa G. Cachexia, the metabolic component of neoplastic diseases. *Cancer Res* 1977;37:2327–2335.
23. Dewys WD. Anorexia in cancer patients. *Cancer Res* 1977;37:2354–2358.
24. Mullen JL, Gertner MH, Buzby GP, et al. Implications of malnutrition in the surgical patient. *Arch Surg* 1979;114:121–125.
25. Koretz RL. Parenteral nutrition: Is it oncologically logical? *J Clin Oncol* 1934;2:534.
26. The VA Total Parenteral Nutrition Co-operative Study Group. Perioperative total parenteral nutrition in surgical patients. *N Engl J Med* 1991;325:525.
27. Weisdorf SA, et al. Positive effect of prophylactic total parenteral nutrition on long-term outcome of bone marrow transplantation. *Transplantation* 1987;43:833.

28. Heller KS, Dubner S. Achievable hospital lengths of stay for head and neck cancer surgery. Society of Head and Neck Surgeons Scientific Program, 1997.
29. Schweinfurth JM, Boger GN, Feustel PJ. Preoperative risk assessment for gastrostomy tube placement in head and neck cancer patients. *Head Neck* 2001;23: 376–382.
30. Rademaker AW, Logemann JA, Pauloski BR, et al. Recovery of postoperative swallowing in patients undergoing partial laryngectomy. *Head Neck* 1993;15: 325–334.
31. Lillemoe KD. Complications of percutaneous gastrostomy. In: Eisele D, ed. *Complications in head and neck surgery.* St. Louis: Mosby, 1993:292–300.
32. Adelstein DJ, Saxton JP, Lavertu P, et al. Maximizing local control and organ preservation in Stage IV squamous cell head and neck cancer with hyperfractionated radiation and concurrent chemotherapy. *J Clin Oncol* 2002;20:1405–1410.
33. Beaver ME, Methane KE, Roberts DB, et al. Predictors of weight loss during radiation therapy. *Otolaryngol Head Neck Surg* 2001;125:645–648.
34. Lee JH, Machtay M, Unger LD, et al. Prophylactic gastrostomy tubes in patients undergoing intensive irradiation for cancer of the head and neck. *Arch Otolaryngol Head Neck Surg* 1998;124:871–875.
35. Mcklhail TM, Adelstein DJ, Rybicki LA, et al. Enteral nutrition during the treatment of head and neck carcinoma: is a percutaneous endoscopic gastrostomy tube preferable to a nasogastric tube? *Cancer* 2001;91:1785–1790.
36. Sinclair JJ, Scolapio JS, Stark ME, et al. Metastasis of head and neck carcinoma to the site of percutaneous endoscopic gastrostomy: case report and literature review. *JPEN J Parenter Enteral Nutr* 2001;25:282–285.
37. Edelman DS. Laparoendoscopic approaches to enteral access. *Semin Laparosc Surg* 2001;8:195–201.

CHAPTER 8

Symptom Management and Supportive Care for Head and Neck Cancer Patients

Elise Carper, Stewart B. Fleishman, and Marlene McGuire

In head and neck cancer patients, complex care issues are best addressed by a multidisciplinary approach. Preservation of form and function are key elements in the overall management of head and neck patients. However, eating, swallowing, and speech often are altered significantly in ways that severely affect a patient's overall quality of life. Physical, social, and psychological well-being are greatly affected by the potential disfigurement and dysfunction resulting from disease and its treatment (1).

Several methods of treatment of head and neck cancer are well established. Radiation therapy, surgery, and chemotherapy, and various combinations of these three therapeutic modalities, comprise today's optimal treatment modalities (2,3). Investigative treatment methods include biologic therapy, immunotherapy, and gene therapy. The treatment regimen for a specific patient depends on tumor site, stage, histology, and other factors. Treatment is composed of a single modality or combined methods. Each treatment method entails both general symptom management and specific care related to each treatment modality's distinctive side effects.

This chapter presents symptom management strategies for patients receiving treatment for cancers of the head and neck. We begin with a discussion of general symptoms common to all modalities, and then discuss treatment-specific symptoms and their management. A discussion of long-term symptom management follows, and we conclude with a discussion of end of life care.

Comprehensive symptom management that anticipates patient needs helps patients participate in care, complete all treatments without interruption as recommended by their health care team, and adjust to changes in function and appearance brought about by cancer and its treatment (4). Providing comprehensive symptom management to head and neck cancer patients is uniquely challenging, but it is critical to successful treatment outcomes.

At the time of initial contact with patients, actual and potential patient problems need to be identified. These may include physical, psychological, spiritual, practical, social, and cultural issues. A general principle of symptom management includes education of patients and significant others with respect to cancer diagnosis, plan of care, treatment-related side effects and their management, and various tests and procedures comprising workup and treatment. To provide the most comprehensive and effective care, factors affecting patient learning (e.g., education level, language barrier, and unfamiliarity with the medical system) are identified and addressed proactively.

TREATMENT DECISION MAKING

From the moment of diagnosis, throughout treatment and into the follow-up phase, patients enter the world of cancer and its treatment, a world filled with jargon and procedures that are unknown or unfamiliar to them. Fear of this unknown creates much anxiety and confusion and can lead to delays in decision making, inability or unwillingness to follow treatment plans, and inability to participate actively in one's own care.

With varied options for treatment of head and neck cancers, patients and families face often complicated decisions *before* treatment begins. Similar to breast cancer, patients with head and neck cancers are often directed to the modality of the physician consulted (surgery, radiation therapy, neoadjuvant chemotherapy) as the initial treatment approach. Discovering alternatives may entail second or even third consultations, perhaps at treatment centers far from home. Having absorbed the message that cancer should be treated with the lowest tumor burden, a time pressure to decide on a treatment course quickly heightens anxiety while processing new, copious, and sometimes frightening information.

Despite rather complete discussions of the relative benefits and risks of treatment, most patients are extremely vulnerable, making such decisions with full cure their immediate goal. With increasing efficacy, more patients survive longer, with morbidities that seem remote at the time of first consultation, but alter their lives in the months and years to come. With the increasing emphasis on organ preservation, multimodal treatment may prolong the initial course of time away from work or other daily activities. With disfigurements minimized, xerostomia, hearing loss, or other seemingly "minor" adjustments become ever so more bothersome when survival has been achieved. Open discussion of these potential long-term effects *early* in the treatment planning promotes longer-term satisfaction with care, and prepares patients and families for the rigors of treatment and the subsequent months or years.

MANAGEMENT OF COMMON TOXICITIES

Pain Management

Pain is a significant problem that affects 50% to 80% of patients with cancer and disturbs overall quality of life (5). Pain in the head and neck patient can be disease-related or treatment-related or a combination of both (2,5,6).

Nearly all patients who receive radiation therapy to the head and neck experience pain at some point during treatment (2,6). It is important to stress to patients, from the beginning of therapy, that some discomfort is expected and that comfort measures, including pain medications should be used early to minimize the dosages. Timely communication between patients and families and the oncology treatment team is critical to ensure prompt pain medication titration and management.

Pain management for patients with head and neck cancer should follow established guidelines, based on the original principles elucidated by the World Health Organization (WHO) and the Agency for Health Care Policy and Research (AHCPR) (7,8), which are briefly reviewed here. Pain should be evaluated regularly, classified as mild, moderate, or severe, and then treated via an algorithm. Pain assessment should be part of the initial consultation and each follow-up visit. Patients are asked to rate their pain level on a scale of 0 to 10, where 0 describes no pain, 5 describes moderate pain, and 8 to 10 describe severe pain or "the worst you can imagine." The location, intensity, and duration of pain and any aggravating or associated activities or sensations are assessed. Patients' current medication regimen is evaluated for appropriateness and efficacy. Often, patients present in acute pain that is inadequately controlled because of patients' lack of knowledge, fear of narcotic dependency, fear of acknowledging disease progression, or poor clinical management (5). Patients may have comorbid conditions that exacerbate cancer pain.

Postoperative pain is controlled with parenteral narcotics initially, administered by continuous intravenous route, patient-controlled analgesia (PCA), or subcutaneous injection, converted to an oral analgesic via the nasogastric tube or by mouth. Mild pain should be treated by acetaminophen-based products, rather than aspirin or nonsteroidal antiinflammatories, which can reduce platelet aggregation and impede healing or optimal cosmesis. Moderate levels of pain should be managed with codeine-based analgesics (9,10). Severe pain should be treated with morphine or fentanyl-based regimen. With any class of opiates, analgesics with a short half-life should be prescribed based on their period of effectiveness, usually every 3 hours to establish needs, then converted to longer acting preparations orally or parenterally. Oral codeine or morphines can be dosed twice a day. Another option is the transdermal fentanyl patches. Typical doses range from 25 to 200 μg per hour. The patch is especially suited to patients who have difficulty in taking medications orally, and its use is very simple. A new patch is applied to clean, dry skin every 3 days; patients are instructed to rotate sites, to remove the old patch before applying a new patch, and to clean completely any residual drug from the skin of the old site. The patches are not to be cut to deliver a partial dose as the contents leaks out. Transdermal patches should *not* be used without a lead-in of short-acting opiates.

Fentanyl is also available in a transmucosal delivery system (Actiq; Cephalon, West Chester, Pa.), placed in the mouth, which may be advantageous for patients with mouth or neck pain. Though Food and Drug Administration (FDA) approved, it is currently under study for this group in particular. The short-acting version of the same drug, or a close congener, should be used for "breakthrough" pain so that the underlying long-acting dose can be optimized (2,11). Regular breakthrough doses signal a need for higher doses of the long-acting preparation, unless the cause is expected to resolve quickly.

Severe pain may require continuous narcotic intravenous infusion delivered through a subcutaneous peripheral site or centrally through an indwelling central venous catheter. A PCA pump commonly is used because it delivers both maintenance and "basal" dose of analgesia plus a patient-controlled "rescue" dose for breakthrough pain. Morphine, hydromorphone (Dilaudid; Abbott Laboratories, Abbott Park, Ill.), fentanyl, and methadone are common drugs used for PCA infusion. This method is used frequently for patients with bony metastases and end-stage disease.

With any opiate, care must be given to monitor constipation and sedation, as well as mouth dryness or urinary retention, which may elicit change in dose, preparation, or delivery route. When initiating any narcotic analgesic, patients are instructed to increase fluid intake by at least 1 L per day, and to use a docusate based stool softener (Colace) liberally and daily to prevent constipation. A laxative such as Senokot may be added, perhaps on alternate days to avoid dependence and ensure regular evacuation. Patients who can take medications by mouth should be instructed to take the medication with food or a supplement to minimize potential nausea. Head and neck patients usually prefer liquid preparations. Additionally, patients are advised to use the anesthetic solution containing 2% viscous Xylocaine before taking elixirs (prepared with alcohol), because the latter often burn inflamed mucosa.

For patients who lack reimbursement for prescription drugs, significant out-of-pocket expenses may mount using most long-acting preparations. If these expenses are a barrier to proper care, a less expensive alternative is methadone, which in many states can be dispensed by local pharmacies in tablet form. It is a long-acting opiate that can treat both the incident and neuropathic components of cancer pain. Patient and family education is essential to reinforce the idea that methadone is not only for maintenance and withdrawal from illicit drugs. Review of the plan with the local pharmacist will ensure that it is kept on hand as well as reinforce the treatment goals.

A routine barrier to adequate analgesic treatment is the fear that opiates of any class when used for cancer pain from illness or treatment will become addictive. Patients with a preexisting dependence or substance abuse themselves are the most vulnerable patients, and their management should respect both this predisposition and their need for adequate analgesia (12). Ironically, patients who have been dependent on opiates, barbiturates, or benzodiazepines in the past likely will need higher than expected doses for pain relief. Such a contradictory pattern mandates good communication and very clear dosage parameters. This involves a minority of patients who are overrepresented among those with head and neck cancers who have a higher incidence of substance abuse. For the majority of patients without substance abuse histories, using adequate amounts of analgesics is an obstacle because they also fear addiction, although it is this group that is least likely to overuse.

Education of patients and family regarding pain management is important (5). As health care has changed and patient care has shifted more to the outpatient area and to patients' homes, knowledge of how to manage pain must be provided to caregivers. Mode of action, expected side effects of pain medications, and implementation of a bowel regimen are important aspects of patient and caregiver teaching. Written and verbal instructions and information should be given.

LOCAL ANALGESIA

Topical anesthetics for relief of mouth and throat pain may be indicated. This is especially true for patients receiving radiotherapy. Patients need careful instruction on how, where, and when to apply topical medications. A solution composed of equal parts 2% viscous lidocaine (Xylocaine), diphenhydramine (Benadryl), and aluminum hydroxide-magnesium hydroxide-simethicone (such as Mylanta or Maalox) often is helpful in relieving generalized mouth and throat pain. Patients are instructed to swish 10 to 15 mL of this solution in their mouths for 30 to 60 seconds, to gargle, then to spit out the solution (oral fields) or swallow (hypopharynx, tongue, and larynx fields). This short-acting anesthetic should be taken before meals, at bedtime, and as needed up to eight times in a 24-hour period. Overuse could cause cardiac arrhythmia.

Ulcerations and discrete areas of inflammation, such as scatter-related (from dental fillings) lateral tongue lesions, are often very painful. An ointment containing benzocaine, which may be obtained without prescription, may be helpful in providing a protective film over the area to promote healing and provide near-immediate acute relief of pain. Patients are instructed to apply the ointment directly to the inflamed area by using a cotton-tipped applicator or their fingers. Again, patients must be cautioned not to overuse this cardiac stimulant.

RESIDUAL PAIN

Neuropathic pain throughout the face, especially throughout the ear and mandible, serves as a constant reminder of their cancer to a minority of patients who have undergone multimodal treatment. Often mechanical in origin with resulting nerve compression or irritation, these symptoms are treated with custom-designed oral appliances, exercises, or anticonvulsants. Tricyclic antidepressants and anticonvulsants with their track record in neuropathic pain syndromes are a reasonable alternative depending on comorbidities (13). To maintain multidisciplinary collaboration, an evaluation by a dentist or oral surgeon would be beneficial, which should include evaluation for rehabilitative dental obturators as clinically indicated. Of course, persistent or recurrent cancer should be carefully ruled out in these circumstances.

Fatigue

Cancer and its treatments are a leading cause of fatigue. Though the mechanisms of fatigue are not well understood, research has shown fatigue to be an extremely common symptom for patients with cancer, and to negatively affect overall quality of life (14,15). All head and neck cancer treatment modalities—surgery, chemotherapy, and radiation—contribute to the development of fatigue. Depression and stress can also be very important contributors to fatigue and to sleeplessness. Surgery that adversely affects a patient's ability to eat can cause nutritional deficit and metabolic abnormalities. Chemotherapy often results in weakness, dehydration, and myelosuppression. Daily head and neck radiation treatments, though only minimally affecting bone marrow, are known to cause fatigue, the cause of which is probably a combination of nutritional factors, anemia, self-care demands, trouble sleeping, and so on. All modalities demand an increase in the body's self-repair mechanisms, which of itself may cause fatigue because of heightened physiologic demands.

Patients with cancer of the head and neck are often anemic at presentation, which undoubtedly contributes to fatigue and decreased quality of life. Prevalence of anemia is under current investigation. Harrison et al. (16) reported a retrospective study of 574 randomly selected patients undergoing radiation therapy. The study, not limited to head and neck, demonstrated that anemia is a common problem in the radiation setting. For the purposes of the study, anemia was defined as hemoglobin (Hg) <12 g/dL. Of the 574 randomly selected patients, 12% were receiving radiation therapy for cancers of the head and neck. Sixteen percent of head and neck patients were mildly to moderately anemic (Hg <12 and >10 g/dL) before beginning radiation therapy, and 32% became anemic during treatment (16% mild-moderate anemia, 16% severe, Hg <9.9 g/dL). Interestingly, the degree of negative change in Hg level during treatment from baseline was increased in the head and neck population compared with other cancer sites. This study remains ongoing.

The efficacy of radiation therapy, as defined by survival and increased locoregional control, is negatively affected by anemia. Lee et al. (17) reported an analysis of the Radiation Therapy Oncology Group (RTOG) protocol 85-27, in which low Hg levels were found to be strongly associated with decreased efficacy of treatment. In this prospective study of persons with advanced-stage cancers of the head and neck, a statistically significant reduction in survival and locoregional control was associated with Hg less than 14.5 g/dL in men and 13.0 g/dL in women. For patients with oral and oropharyngeal squamous cell carcinoma (SCC) receiving preoperative chemoradiation therapy, low pretreatment Hg levels have been found in a recent study (18) to be an independent poor prognostic factor, but one that could be reversed by the use of recombinant human erythropoietin (r-HuEPO). In this study, 10,000 units r-HuEPO was given three to six times a week to attain and maintain Hg >12.5 g/dL. The administration of erythropoietin is being intensely studied to see whether it can improve outcomes in patients receiving radiation therapy. It is already approved for patients receiving chemotherapy, with or without radiation therapy.

Quality of life is improved by administration of epoetin alfa in patients receiving chemotherapy (19). Several administration schedules are used, including 10,000 units three times per week or a subcutaneous injection of 40,000 units given weekly. A weekly complete blood count is drawn, with continued administration of erythropoietin based on Hg findings. Typically, mild anemia (Hg <12.0 g/dL but >10.0 g/dL) responds after four weekly injections. A more severe anemia requires a more protracted treatment course. Patients tolerate these injections well, with only occasional skin rashes noted (18,19).

Nausea and Vomiting

Nausea and vomiting are common side effects of chemotherapy and can result in weight loss, severe dehydration, and electrolyte imbalances (20,21). The most common fear of patients concerning chemotherapy is of uncontrolled nausea and vomiting (21). Fortunately, recent advances in antiemetics provide improved control of chemotherapy-related nausea and vomiting and improved quality of life for most patients.

A pretreatment assessment of patients' dietary habits, history of nausea and vomiting, anxiety level, and personality traits, along with the knowledge of which chemotherapeutic agents will be used, can help to identify those patients most at risk for severe nausea and vomiting. Typically, nausea and vomiting occur within the first 2 hours after administration of chemotherapy, and this acute phase can last for 24 hours. Delayed nausea and vomiting occur 24 hours after chemotherapy and can last 3 to 5 days or longer. In this case, urgent admission to the hospital may become necessary to provide intravenous hydration and antiemetics.

Anticipatory nausea occurs on sight of or entry to the hospital before treatment. It can also be initiated by the sight and smell of certain foods (21). Such measures as relaxation techniques, guided imagery, and especially premedication with benzodiazepine antiemetics the night before and the morning of treatment can be very helpful.

Antiemetic protocols using medications both before and after chemotherapy administration are common and can be very detailed (21). Written information describing each medication's actions and side effects is reviewed with patients, and time is spent with patients to ensure their comprehension. One regimen consists of granisetron, 2 mg, and dexamethasone (Decadron), 20 mg, given orally before administration of the chemotherapy, then Decadron in tapering doses from 8 to 4 mg orally, plus metoclopramide (Reglan), 10 mg three times daily after the chemotherapy for 2 days. Lorazepam (Ativan) can be added to this regimen, given either orally or intravenously as needed for unrelieved nausea and emesis. Choosing an agent from each pharmacologic class (dopamine blockers, 5-HT_3 blockers, benzodiazepines, antihistamines, corticosteroids, or cannabinoids) is preferred to capitalize on synergistic effects. Adequate antiemetic prescriptions are provided for patients on discharge, along with written instructions to call the health care team with any questions or concerns.

Bowel Disturbances

Both diarrhea and constipation are common expected side effects of therapy (21,22). Normal bowel and bladder function of patients is determined before treatment during the consultation. Patients are advised to report to the health care team any diarrhea, defined as three or more loose or watery stools in a 24-hour period. Patient management is focused on identifying and treating the cause of the diarrhea while replacing lost fluids, electrolytes, and nutrition. Patients are questioned regarding their diets and possible overuse of stool softeners or laxatives. Treatment with hydration and antidiarrheals usually is sufficient, along with adjustments in foods and medications. Nutritional supplements taken by mouth or used in tube feedings may cause diarrhea; switching to another formula may be helpful (10). Stool cultures and gastrointestinal evaluations are indicated for persistent diarrhea. Excessive diarrhea may require hospitalization.

Ideally, bowel movements should be soft and formed and occur once daily or every other day. Vinca alkaloids often cause constipation, which in turn causes anorexia, bloating, abdominal cramps, and nausea (23). Pain medications can also increase constipation by reducing peristalsis. Nursing assessment of patients' typical dietary habits, fluid intake, activity, and medications is undertaken to identify potential problems. Teaching is directed to increasing fiber in the diet, increasing fluid intake, and increasing activity as possible. A preventive bowel regimen such as docusate (Colace), 100 mg three times per day, plus Senokot, two tablets twice daily, is recommended and adjusted according to a patient's bowel pattern. Ongoing assessment and titration of medications is an important nursing function.

Nutritional Management

Head and neck cancer patients who receive optimal nutrition throughout the treatment management period have improved outcomes and less morbidity. Larger centers have access to the experience of trained dietitians or nutritionists. In smaller treatment settings, nutritional counseling is often implemented by nurses or physicians' assistants. Simply reminding patients to eat, with the encouragement of their families, is inadequate. A series of common obstacles—sensory, mechanical, and physiologic—prevent this advice from producing the desired effect. When the cancer involves the nose, mouth, and throat, taste buds can be affected. Without the proper moisture from salivary glands to aid their function, food becomes unappealing. Mechanical obstruction from the tumor prevents effective chewing and swallowing. Surgical interruption of involved muscles worsens function further prior to healing. Chemotherapy and radiation therapy can intensify dysfunction, with dry mouth and taste perturbation. Fatigue and inadequate intake forms the matrix of a downward spiral, in which patients become too tired to eat, then more fatigued as their intake decreases, amplifying the fatigue. Mucositis, stomatitis, and esophagitis discourage eating even more. Constipating analgesics making elimination harder and discourage intake even further. Progressive disease can greatly increase caloric need, putting the system into huge deficit, resulting in cachexia. Outwardly, it seems as if the patient just "isn't trying" or is depressed, without evaluating the full clinical picture described (24).

Nearly all patients who receive radiation therapy to the head and neck have difficulty in maintaining nutritional intake (2,21,25). Care goals are to assist patients to maintain weight and proper nutrition to promote wound healing, and to avoid breaks in treatment that can have an adverse impact on the overall effectiveness of cancer therapy (10). For most patients receiving radiation therapy, constipation is a problem related to decreased activity, fluid intake, and narcotic use. Patient education focuses on teaching how to increase protein and calorie intake, how to effectively use oral or enteral nutritional supplements, and how to maintain normal bowel functioning during treatment.

A thorough baseline nutritional assessment is critical to planning effective interventions to attain these goals (20) (see Chapter 7). Interventions center on educating patients and significant others about the importance of good nutrition during radiation therapy. This involves explaining the reasons for potential weight loss and nutritional deficit during and immediately after treatment (related to anorexia, taste changes, xerostomia, mucositis, and fatigue). Written materials such as "Eating Hints" (available free from the National Institutes of Health) are helpful for teaching patients and include sections on high-calorie, high-protein, soft-textured foods and liquid diets that are especially appropriate for head and neck cancer patients.

Perioperative Nutritional Management

Before surgery, a comprehensive nutritional assessment should be performed on all surgical patients. This is especially true for head and neck patients, whose tumors may affect physiologic function and alter the patients' already poor nutritional status due to their lifestyles of tobacco and alcohol abuse. More severe cases of malnutrition can be seen with patients who have large intraoral lesions, oropharyngeal cancers, and hypopharyngeal cancers (26). Dietary consultations are arranged at this juncture for patients who are malnourished. Nutritional support is initiated including oral supplementation, or if necessary, a nasogastric tube is placed before surgery for enteral feeding support. Often by providing oral analgesics prior to meals, nutrition can be greatly improved as pain and symptoms are lessened.

Maintaining adequate nutrition for patients after head and neck surgery is challenging (2,20). Some extensive operations require that patients receive nothing by mouth for several days. Nasogastric tubes generally are placed during these operations to provide access for nutritional support. Percutaneous endoscopic gastrostomy (PEG) tube placement is performed if long-term nutritional support is anticipated. If a nasogastric tube or PEG is in place, feedings usually commence within 24 hours after the presence of gastrointestinal motility is established.

Patients' feedings begin with water and gradually increase to full-strength supplement (e.g., Osmolite or Glucerna [Ross Pharmaceuticals, Columbus, Oh.] for diabetics). Feedings can be given either by gravity or by pump. Consultation with a dietitian is advised to calculate patients' caloric needs. Patients are monitored for side effects such as diarrhea or regurgitation related to the enteral feedings (2,20). Maintaining a patient's body weight at the presurgical level is ideal.

Surgical procedures involving large portions of oral tongue, the base of the tongue, the floor of the mouth, the retromolar trigone, or the supraglottic larynx may result in postoperative dysphagia. It is important to closely monitor patients' caloric intake by mouth and order appropriate food consistencies (soft or pureed). These individuals often need postoperative swallowing rehabilitation to adequately maintain their nutrition. Swallowing therapy focuses on promoting optimal oral intake with prevention of aspiration (27). Therapy entails determining positional changes during eating that will assist in compensating for structural changes in anatomy and of selecting the proper food consistencies.

Patients who have undergone a pharyngolaryngectomy with a gastric pull-up or removal of the entire pharynx, larynx, and esophagus with mobilization of the stomach into the neck/chest will have no problems with dysphagia, but are at risk for postprandial dumping syndrome (26). Nutritional interventions include instructing patients to limit liquid intake during meals, to eat five to six small meals a day, and to sit upright while eating and for 1 hour after meals. This decreases the risk for regurgitation due to the loss of the lower esophageal sphincter muscle.

Some individuals, even with intense swallowing rehabilitation, are unable to maintain their nutrition without the lifelong use of a gastrostomy tube. Accepting this device can be extremely difficult for patients because of the role food plays in our society. Significant help to integrate this device into everyday life is needed to assist patients in adjusting to this functional change.

Nutritional Needs During Radiation Therapy/Chemotherapy

Ongoing assessment of patients' nutritional status is very important. Patients may experience a rapid weight loss while on treatment as the degree of mucositis and anorexia increases. Daily weights, taken during the same period as the daily mouth spray, are an excellent way of trending weight loss and provide a mechanism for quick intervention. Weekly assessment for potential or present nutritional deficit should always include an examination of the mouth for degree of mucositis, xerostomia, ulcerations, fungal infections, or other factors that influence patients' ability to nourish themselves.

Symptom management may include arranging a dental consultation to adjust an appliance, a dietary consultation for those patients with special dietary needs (diabetics, vegetarians), and a consultation for placement of a PEG feeding tube. Symptoms related to the cancer or side effects of radiation that negatively affect patients' ability to nourish themselves are noted, and proper interventions are employed (25). Prescribing antiemetics and mucolytics may be necessary to optimize dietary intake/absorption.

Patients are encouraged to begin dietary changes (to high-calorie, high-protein foods) immediately, to offset future dietary deficit. All patients should begin nutritional supplementation (e.g., regular or sugar-free Carnation Instant Breakfast, Ensure Plus), in anticipation of potential weight loss related to radiation therapy (28). The goal of supplementation is to maximize calorie and protein intake for optimal tissue repair. The type and amount of supplements needed vary according to individual patient needs (e.g., sugar-free diet, inadequate diet) and attributes (e.g., age, body mass, activity level, previous weight loss) (20).

Problems of supplement intolerance may be helped by a consultation with a nutritionist. Patients (especially those treated with hyperfractionated or accelerated radiation, or treated on two machines) should be encouraged to take supplements throughout the day because timing of treatments often causes them to miss meals. A consultation for PEG placement is made if patients demonstrate persistent weight loss or inadequate oral intake.

Asking patients to keep a food diary, listing what they were able to eat over a 24-hour period, is a helpful way of assessing specific food preferences and taste aversions (10,20). This knowledge also helps to demonstrate to patients how little they actually were able to eat and how important supplementation is in maintaining weight. Weekly assessment of supplement use (e.g., name, amount taken, and frequency of feedings) and of any side effects from the supplements (e.g., nausea, diarrhea, eructation, flatulence, bloating) is an important way of supporting a patient's ability to maintain normal weight.

Assessment of patients' social support needs is essential. Are patients able to prepare food? If not, is there someone in the home who can perform this task? Are patients physically able to obtain supplements? Are supplements accessible? Will insurance cover the cost of supplements? Can patients afford to buy them? What other stresses in the home affect patients' ability to care for themselves? Referral to social services for assistance with these issues, which exert a strong impact on patients' abilities to cope with treatment, often is necessary. Social services consultations (social workers and financial counselors) should be initiated as soon as possible to ensure that essential support is available to patients to obtain food/supplements as needed.

A common problem for patients taking pain medications or using supplements is changes in bowel function (10). Patients are assessed for constipation and are encouraged to drink plenty of fluids, to exercise as possible, and to use a stool softener. If diarrhea is a problem, patients are encouraged to increase their intake of fluids to prevent dehydration and to use an antidiarrheal agent. Dehydration is especially dangerous when patients are receiving concomitant chemotherapy; these patients must be carefully assessed daily.

Follow-up Nutritional Needs

After completion of radiation, continued assessment for nutritional deficit is important (25). Patients should be weighed at each visit, and this weight compared with the end-of-treatment weight. If patients continue to lose weight 4 weeks after radiation therapy has been completed, a consultation with a nutritionist is indicated. Dental follow-up may be indicated for ill-fitting dentures and appliances (caused by changes in weight during treatment). Patients are reminded of their high risk for dental caries after radiation therapy and of the need for good oral hygiene, lifelong fluoride treatments (if applicable), and regular, close follow-up with a dentist. They are encouraged to avoid sweets, alcohol, tobacco, and other irritants.

Continued mucositis, persistent dysphagia, severe xerostomia, and continued anorexia all contribute to patients' inability to maintain or gain weight and are addressed in follow-up with prescribed medications and referral to a dentist or nutritionist or both (20). Patients who exhibit persistent dysphagia are referred to a speech pathologist for swallowing rehabilitation. Patients should be assessed for PEG dependence. Most patients who receive a PEG during radiation therapy should be taking a full, regular diet 3 to 6 months after treatment. They are assisted with a schedule for the tapering of feedings and the resumption of a normal diet and are encouraged to follow up with the gastroenterologist regarding the PEG. After completion of radiation therapy, all patients should be encouraged to continue taking in a well-balanced, healthy diet, avoiding irritants, tobacco, and alcohol to decrease the risk for second malignancies.

Ideally, after surgery, chemotherapy, or radiation therapy, patients are given a plan to advance their diet by an experienced nurse, nutritionist, or physician. Patients should begin to advance their diet as tolerated, starting with thick liquids if they have been NPO or fed parenterally. Thin liquids (e.g., water) are more difficult to swallow. Commercial preparations (e.g., Thick-it, Precision Foods, St. Louis, Mo.) can be added to most liquid foods. Prepackaged supplements should be used as intended, not replacing foods but rather in addition to them. The choice of foods is personal and cultural, with virtually every group having a milk-, rice-, or soy-based drink. Lactose may thicken mucosal secretions in those sensitive to it. If tolerated, foods inherently soft or pureed add variety to further encourage eating. Spices may stimulate appetite or burn locally. Of the four basic tastes—bitter, acid, sweet, and salty—the latter two are best tolerated by most. Methodically adding one new food each day, as in switching an infant from formula to solids, helps sort out the tolerable foods from those that irritate. Patients will advance steadily with this approach, which also provides many tasks for family members who have been sidelined by professional and hospital staff during the acute treatment phases and are eager to "do something."

SURGICAL CONSIDERATIONS

Surgical Evaluation

Surgical intervention is contingent on the general medical condition of a patient, tumor histology, and presence of distant metastases. Choice of treatment modality and its associated cure rates must also be considered. The type of surgical procedure performed varies based on site and size of the tumor, the presence of metastatic disease in the cervical lymph nodes, and the need for immediate reconstruction. Operative sites can be closed primarily or secondarily. More extensive resections involving large defects require immediate reconstruction to improve functional capacity and cosmesis. Reconstruction can be performed with local flaps, split-thickness skin grafts, pedicle flaps, or microvascular free flaps, which are used when vascularized soft tissue or bone is harvested from a donor site to a recipient site. Ultimately, the primary goal of oncologic surgery is the eradication of primary and metastatic disease with preservation of optimal patient function and quality of life.

Perioperative Period

A proactive approach is used to arrange various consultative services before surgery for patients who are expected to have significant postoperative rehabilitation needs. This serves to facilitate smooth recovery and enhance patients' relationships with the rehabilitation team. Speech consultations and counseling are arranged perioperatively for all patients who are undergoing glossectomy or total laryngectomy. The dental service is consulted if a patient requires a prosthetic device to improve oral function and cosmesis. Referrals to social services are initiated for patients with anticipated discharge needs. Smoking and alcohol cessation should also be initiated during this preoperative period.

Postoperative Period

Postoperative care is based on patient care needs specific to the performed procedure; however, some general principles of symptom management apply. Interventions focus on maintaining fluid and electrolyte balance, ensuring patency of surgical drains, assessing flaps and grafts, airway management, and providing nutritional support, oral care, pain control, wound care, psychological support, and postoperative rehabilitation. During the postoperative period, fluid and electrolyte balance is assessed carefully by strict calculation of intake and output during each shift. Clinical assessment, including auscultation of lung fields for fluid overload and daily weights, is performed every 8 hours.

Care of Surgical Drains and Flaps

Surgical interventions involving a neck dissection and reconstruction with a pedicle flap or microvascular flap require intraoperative placement of at least one drain to prevent hematoma or seroma formation. Management of surgical drains and flaps requires special care. Maintaining the patency of surgical drains is crucial and is accomplished by stripping the drainage tubing periodically, noting the amount, color, and consistency of the drainage, and documenting this information. Systematic assessment of suture lines and flap sites should be performed to assess for vascular integrity, noting complications such as dehiscence, hematoma formation, infection, and breakdown.

Flaps and grafts are assessed for warmth, color, capillary refill, and drainage. Blood supply to microvascular free flaps is evaluated at frequent intervals by Doppler auscultation over the flap site. Any change in free-flap pulse might indicate vessel occlusion. Vasoconstriction to the flap areas must be avoided. If a tracheostomy is in place, ties are not used with a myocutaneous flap or a microvascular free flap, as ties may constrict blood flow to the graft. Instead, tracheostomy tubes are sutured in place.

Care of Neck Dissection

Following a neck dissection a surgical drain is placed. Drainage of 100 to 150 mL is not uncommon in the initial postoperative period (29). Any rapid increase in the amount of drainage fluid or change in color from serosanguineous to bloody may indicate hematoma formation and necessitates prompt attention.

Profuse, milky white drainage after neck dissection is indicative of a chyle fistula. This occurs more frequently during left radical neck dissection, when the thoracic duct of the lymphatic system is injured. Chyle fistulae are managed conservatively by pressure dressings and low-fat diets. Surgical ligation may be required if conservative measures fail.

After radical neck dissection, patient teaching includes instruction in range-of-motion exercises, which are necessary to help prevent "shoulder syndrome," a condition that occurs as a result of denervation of the trapezius muscle and associated shoulder asymmetry. Studies have shown that even with preservation of the spinal accessory nerve there may be a temporary phase of dysfunction (30). Therefore, range-of-motion exercises should be initiated in these patients. Additionally, some patients may require more intensive physical therapy to improve their shoulder mobility. Debilitated patients may be referred to licensed physical therapists for exercises to improve range of motion and muscle strength (31). Often, these sessions are held three times per week and may continue for up to a year. Appropriate medications, especially to manage any neuropathic pain related to soft issue and nerve injury, are important.

Airway Management

Tracheostomy is performed during more extensive surgical procedures to prevent airway compromise secondary to edema (32). Initially, patients return from the recovery room with a cuffed tracheostomy tube in place, which usually is changed to an uncuffed tube after 5 to 7 days. Suctioning is conducted every 2 hours and otherwise as needed. The inner cannula is cleaned every 4 hours and as needed with water and a tracheostomy brush. Humidity through a tracheostomy collar prevents drying of the tracheal mucosa and facilitates removal of secretions. Normal saline, 3 to 5 mL, can be instilled into the tracheostomy tube and then suctioned out to remove more tenacious secretions (32). An aerosol bronchodilator such as albuterol (Proventil) can also be of use. Providing tracheostomy patients with a means by which to communicate is essential and is readily accomplished with a "magic slate" or writing tablet.

Patient education is key for patients who have had a laryngectomy or who are being discharged with a temporary tracheostomy. Patients must be independent in self-care tasks before discharge. Necessary supplies are provided at the time of discharge, and home health care is arranged as needed.

Oral Care and Wound Care

Many patients are not allowed oral intake following surgical procedures or have intraoral incisions, making meticulous oral hygiene essential. Oral care involves oral irrigation using tap water and a combination of baking soda and salt. Many institutions also provide low-power sprays with a solution of saline and sodium bicarbonate to cleanse the mouth of debris and provide comfort to patients. Intraoral obturators and dental prosthesis should be removed prior to providing any mouth care. After discharge, patients should perform oral care rinses and irrigations at home.

Surgical incisions are evaluated closely for signs of infection and are cleansed with half-strength peroxide and normal saline every 8 hours and otherwise as needed. Complications such as wound breakdown and fistula formation initially are treated conservatively, with débridement and packing. However, larger fistulae or fistulae that occur in a previously irradiated area may require surgical management with reexcision, drain placement, or subsequent flap closure.

RADIATION THERAPY CONSIDERATIONS

Symptom management of patients undergoing radiotherapy begins with a thorough physical assessment of those areas of the patient directly within the treatment portals. The skin, mouth, neck, and throat of most head and neck patients are within the treatment field and, in some cases, the nose, ears, eyes, scalp, upper chest, and back also are within the radiation field. Any anatomic changes related to cancer or its treatment (e.g., intraoral defect after a maxillectomy, orbital exenteration) and any resulting functional deficits (e.g., reliance on an obturator to eat and speak, dysphagia, decreased visual acuity and depth perception) are also noted in this initial assessment.

A baseline evaluation of patients' general oral hygiene and status of oral mucous membranes is obtained through examination. It is important to inspect all surfaces of the oral cavity and observe for redness, swelling, and tenderness of mucous membranes; yellow or white plaques, ulcers, or vesicles; a foul odor; incomplete healing of surgical incisions; and evidence of ill-fitting dental appliances or dentures (9,33). Assess current oral hygiene by determining the patient's use of toothpaste, mouthwash, and dental floss.

After surgery, patients often perform oral irrigations, which cleanse the surgical area of debris, minimize risk for infection, and moisten tissues to provide comfort. Most patients require a dental evaluation before they begin radiation therapy. This involves x-rays to determine any pretreatment dental care needs, and instruction in appropriate dental prophylaxis. In certain patients, dental appliances might require frequent adjustments by the dentist during the treatment period, to ensure proper fit (9).

Location, type, and severity of symptoms experienced by patients receiving radiation therapy to the head and neck are related to a number of factors. Radiation factors include the total dose of radiation delivered, the treatment field and pathway of radiation beams, the dose per fraction and number of fractions per day, the volume of tissue treated, and the duration of the treatment course. Patient and cancer treatment–related factors include the patient's baseline medical condition, the patient's age, and the use of chemotherapy or surgery before, after, or concurrent with the radiation (2,3).

Mucositis

The structures of the head and neck are lined with mucous membranes made up of rapidly cycling cells that are very sensitive to radiation. Acute symptoms experienced by patients receiving radiation therapy are the result of mucosal damage (34). Mucositis is an expected side effect of radiation therapy to the head and neck. Severity varies from mild discomfort to severe pain. Assessment of each patient's risk for severe mucositis begins at consultation, when both patient-related and treatment-related factors are evaluated (2,34). A list of risk factors is provided in Table 8.1.

At consultation, patients are informed of expected mucous membrane reactions from radiation therapy. Reaction of the mouth and throat to radiation generally begins 2 weeks after starting therapy and continues up to 4 weeks after completion

TABLE 8.1 Risk Factors for Mucositis

Patient factors
- Poor nutritional status, poor dental hygiene, and dental caries all have negative effect
- Immunosuppression (long-term steroid use) increases wound healing
- Poorly fitting dentures or oral appliances
- Cultural habits (use of spicy foods or chewing betal nuts), drinking alcohol, smoking or chewing tobacco

Treatment factors
- Dose, duration of treatment, and site of treatment
  - More sensitive—pharyngeal wall, soft palate, tonsillar pillars, buccal mucosa, lateral tongue, and floor of mouth
  - Less sensitive—hard palate, gingival ridge, and vocal cords
- Concomitant chemotherapy
- Surgical procedures resulting in altered anatomy (transplanted tissue responds to radiation as it would in original body site)
- Metallic dental work or surgical plates will increase "scatter" radiation to proximal mucosa

Developed by Carper E. Department of Radiation Oncology, Continuum Cancer Centers of New York, 2002.

TABLE 8.2 Patient Self-Care Regimen for Oral Hygiene

Rinse your mouth and gargle four to six times per day, before and after meals is suggested. Use the following solution:
1 qt water
1 tsp salt
1 tsp baking soda

Use a soft toothbrush or toothette and mild toothpaste (e.g., Biotene, or Arm and Hammer Baking Soda Toothpaste) after every meal and at bedtime. Be sure to clean your dental appliance or dentures at this time. vContinue flossing gently if this is your habit. If you don't normally floss, do not begin flossing during radiation therapy.

Avoid any mouthwashes containing alcohol.

Use a lip moisturizer frequently. Be sure to remove prior to your treatment!

Wear your fluoride trays (without fluoride) during your treatments if ordered.

Use a humidifier or vaporizer in the bedroom. Warm and cool mist are equally effective; the water becomes room temperature by the time it reaches you. Whichever "steamer" you choose, it should be cleaned *daily* and filled with *fresh water.* Position it to direct the spray toward your head. This humidifies secretions that thicken during radiation.

Avoid any oral irritants: spicy foods, scratchy-textured foods (pretzels), *any* type of smoke, and *all* alcohol.

Try to minimize talking by creating a "phone call tree" (updating one to two people per day and asking them to pass on this information to others you designate). Talking can be painful and exhausting.

Developed by Carper E. Department of Radiation Oncology, Continuum Cancer Centers of New York, 2002.

of treatment (33,35). Expected, normal reactions may include redness, swelling, tenderness, pain, difficulty in swallowing, and hoarseness. Patients are reassured that these effects are temporary, that measures are available to minimize their discomfort, and that they will be supported to ensure their completion of treatment.

Minimal research has been done to determine the most effective oral care regimen. Studies have demonstrated, however, that a systematic, consistent mouth care regimen is needed throughout radiation (9,11). Care focuses on promoting patients' oral hygiene to minimize risk for infection, providing measures to treat infection should it occur, and increasing patients' comfort. Patients are taught a self-care regimen that includes the key elements listed in Table 8.2, which is individualized as needed.

Patients are instructed to reduce irritation of mucous membranes during treatment by avoiding chemical irritants such as tobacco, alcohol, commercial mouthwash, spices (e.g., pepper, chili powder, horseradish, curry powder), and citrus fruits and juices (e.g., orange, lemon, lime, grapefruit, pineapple, and tomatoes). Physical irritants to be avoided include very hot or very cold foods and hard or coarse foods (e.g., toast, crackers, raw vegetables, potato chips, pretzels) and loose or ill-fitting dentures. Dietary changes to cool foods and fluids (e.g., ice pops, ice cubes, ice cream, sherbet, yogurt), a pureed or liquid diet, and increased use of nutritional supplements are helpful during the course of radiation.

A daily spray of normal saline, delivered under low pressure, cleanses the mouth, liquefies mucus, and provides comfort to patients. During this spray, a gentle flow of saline is directed to all surfaces of the oral cavity and oropharynx. This continues until the patient's mouth is clean and moist. Patients with oral cavity, oropharynx, and nasopharynx cancers may benefit most from this regimen, as the extent of irradiated mucous membranes can be quite extensive. An additional benefit of the daily oral spray is that it provides an opportunity for an assessment of the patient's physical, nutritional, psychosocial status, and a determination of any pain management or dental needs. Dental appliances should be adjusted by the dentist as needed and, in most cases, worn only when necessary during therapy (10).

Throughout the course of radiation, patients are assessed for signs of mucositis: redness, swelling, or tenderness of mucous membranes, yellow-white coating over mucous membranes, or ulceration or bleeding of mucous membranes. The oral cavity is also inspected for early signs of infection. *Candida albicans*, evidenced by white patches, is the most common cause of infection in patients receiving head and neck radiation (33,34). If patients develop *Candida* infection, an appropriate antifungal medication (such as Diflucan) should be prescribed. It's important to instruct patients on a proper medication schedule and to monitor them closely to assess response.

PREVENTION OF MUCOSITIS-RELATED TREATMENT BREAK

Patients with moderate to severe mucositis need intensive symptomatic support. They are at high risk for malnutrition, weakness, or pain to a degree that may necessitate a treatment break, with a resultant possible decrease in treatment effectiveness. Early identification and management of mucositis is critical. Intensive nutritional support, early placement of a PEG, and heavy reliance on supplements are often necessary and common, especially for patients receiving concomitant therapies. Often a combination of both systemic pain medications and local anesthetics is used throughout the treatment course, with timely titration of medication and an appropriate bowel regimen employed. A thorough discussion of pain and its management can be found earlier in this chapter. See Table 8.3 for an example of a pain medication regimen used for patients receiving radiation therapy.

When radiation therapy is complete, reinforcement of self-care measures that promote oral comfort and adequate nutrition is essential. Often, mucositis escalates for 1 to 2 weeks after completion of radiation. Typically, resolution of mucositis is complete within 6 to 8 weeks, and patients begin to resume normal activities of speaking and eating. Patients are informed that prolonged use or stress of the voice may lead to hoarseness even months after treatment, and they are encouraged to avoid smoke and fumes. A slow and gradual increase in texture of

TABLE 8.3 Managing Acute Pain During Radiation Therapy: A Sample Medication Regimen

Weeks 1 to 2 of treatment	Weeks 3 to 7 of treatment and for 4 to 8 weeks following completion of radiation therapy
Ibuprofen, Tylenol, or Cox-2 inhibitors (Vioxx, Celebrex) Orobase with benzocaine—apply topically to discrete areas of irritation Magic Mouthwash (equal parts Mylanta, viscous Xylocaine, and Benadryl), 10 cc before meals, bedtime, and prn; up to 8 times/day total	Oxyfast elixir, 20 mg/mL, 0.25–0.5 cc q2–3h prn, up to 6 cc/24 hours Duragesic patch, 25–100 μg, q72h Colace, two capsules/liquid equivalent, t.i.d. Senakot, two tablets/liquid equivalent, qhs–b.i.d. as needed Fleet oil retention followed by regular Fleet enema q 3 days as needed

Developed by Carper E. Department of Radiation Oncology, Continuum Cancer Centers of New York, 2002.

foods (from liquid to soft to regular) and the cautious addition of seasoned foods is advised. Pain medications and stool softeners are tapered and discontinued as soon as possible.

MUCOSITIS—PHARMACOLOGIC INTERVENTIONS

Despite only limited studies on efficacy, commonly used oral regimens to minimize mucositis do exist. Daily rinses of a mixture of water and salt (plus or minus sodium bicarbonate) are commonly used due to their cleansing and soothing abilities. Treatments other than local anesthetics and narcotics are used to diminish the severity of mucositis. Some of the more commonly reported nonanalgesic pharmacologic agents under study are described below.

Sucralfate oral suspension has been shown to significantly diminish gastric ulceration and has been studied for efficacy in minimizing radiation mucositis. Early studies showed a trend toward decreased mucositis in patients who used sucralfate. A prospective double-blind study comparing sucralfate and placebo demonstrated no statistically significant difference in mucositis, but patients in the sucralfate group reports less oral pain and used less narcotic analgesics (36).

Benzydamine HCl, a nonsteroidal agent with analgesic, antimicrobial, antiinflammatory, and anesthetic properties, was used in a recent safety and efficacy trial (37). Patients receiving radiation therapy were randomized to receive a 0.15% benzydamine oral rinse or placebo, to be used four to eight times daily during radiation therapy, and for 2 weeks following completion of treatment. Patients being treated daily up to 5,000 cGy who used the medication had significantly ($p = 0.006$) reduced erythema and ulceration by almost 30% compared with patients on placebo. Interestingly, benzydamine was not effective when patients received accelerated radiation therapy doses (defined here as ≥220 cGy/day). The medication was well tolerated, without significant adverse effects.

Use of granulocyte-macrophage colony-stimulating factor (GM-CSF) systemically in cancer is common. A potential new treatment of mucositis involving topical GM-CSF was studied in a prospective, randomized, open, parallel-grouped fashion. Stage II and IV head and neck patients used the solution and were compared as to degree of oral mucositis, perception of pain, incidence of secondary infection, and change in blood counts. No statistical differences were noted, and the study was discontinued early because of the extremely high cost of GM-CSF mouthwash (38).

Other agents under investigation include antimicrobials, and pharmacologic modulators such as glutamine, silver nitrate, and corticosteroids. Studies using less traditional agents are underway such as capsaicin in the form of a pepper candy, vitamins, and other antioxidants. Cryotherapy in the form of ice chips and popsicles is being looked at for radiation-induced mucositis, and even honey as an oral bacterial modulator is under review (39).

Xerostomia

Xerostomia is a common and often irreversible effect of head and neck irradiation. It is related to treatment of the major salivary glands and ubiquitous minor salivary glands throughout the oral cavity (35). Patients may describe decreased amounts of saliva; thicker saliva; difficulty in talking, eating, and swallowing; and changes in taste. Tenacious secretions, tongue-surface changes, cracked lips, and difficulty retaining dental appliances are common. The degree of xerostomia is highly variable and unpredictable from patient to patient. Xerostomia can begin during radiation therapy and often is permanent. Some patients claim that they have experienced late improvement that became noticeable several years after radiation therapy, but this, too, is highly variable.

Symptom management for patients with xerostomia involves teaching ways to increase oral moisture, making needed dietary changes, and minimizing the risk for caries. To increase moisture, patients are encouraged to take frequent sips of water or other liquids throughout the day (a thermos or aerosol pump spray bottle is helpful), to rinse their mouths before eating to provide immediate mouth moisture, and to use a humidifier whenever possible and especially at night. Sour, sugarless hard candy or gum can stimulate saliva flow. Patients should avoid mouth-drying substances such as caffeine, tobacco, and alcohol. Some patients try artificial salivas and mouth-moisturizing products and report relief.

Patient diets must be modified to increase intake of fluids and juices, unless otherwise contraindicated, and to decrease intake of dry or sticky foods (10). Crackers, toast, and peanut butter are examples of such foods that should be avoided. Gravies, sauces, and condiments to moisten foods are encouraged. Prevention of caries associated with xerostomia involves a lifelong adherence to the use of fluoride, as prescribed by patients' dentists. Patients also are encouraged to rinse frequently with a mixture of bicarbonate and water (9,11), as previously described.

XEROSTOMIA—PHARMACOLOGIC INTERVENTIONS

Amifostine (WR-1065) is a drug that has a protective effect on salivary gland functioning. The protective effect is selective, due to a greater uptake of drug in salivary glands as compared with neoplastic tissues. In a randomized trial (40), patients with previously untreated head and neck SCC were given daily radiotherapy (1.8–2.0 Gy) to doses of 50–70 Gy. Patients were randomized to receive amifostine, 200 mg/m^2, IV, 15 to 30 minutes before each radiation treatment. Results of this study showed a reduction of both acute and chronic xerostomia in the patients given amifostine ($p < 0.0001$) and no statistical change in locoregional (LRC), disease-free survival (DFS), or overall survival (OS). Fifty-three percent of the patients receiving amifostine had at least one episode of nausea/vomiting, which is a common side effect of the drug. Other side effects include transient hypotension and skin rashes/allergic reactions. More studies are ongoing to determine if amifostine delivered subcutaneously will have comparable efficacy.

Pilocarpine (Salagen) has been evaluated for its efficacy in relieving symptoms of postradiation xerostomia (41). At varying dosages of 2.5, 5.0, and 10.0 mg taken three times a day, salivary flow was improved to a statistically significant level. Patients reported mild to moderate sweating as the most common side effect. Zimmerman et al. (42) performed a retrospective review of xerostomia, defined as oral dryness, oral discomfort, and difficulty with sleep, speech, and eating. Patients who received concomitant pilocarpine during radiation therapy were compared with those who did not receive the drug. The group receiving pilocarpine reported significantly less xerostomia, as measured by patients' subjective reports.

One report describes one patient's use of butter, margarine, and vegetable oil in small amounts to relieve xerostomia after treatment with radiation therapy (43). The authors describe three case studies in which this practice appears to have eased xerostomia. Many other anecdotal reports exist, but no definitive study has as yet demonstrated that a specific product is most effective in relieving xerostomia; this remains an area of much-needed research.

Skin Reaction

A thorough skin assessment of patients before the start of radiation is essential and includes evaluating patients' risk for impaired skin integrity (see Table 8.4 for risk factors to be evaluated). Inspection of skin within the planned treatment field (both the entrance and exit sites) and allows one to note any obvious risk factors. Care of the patient at this time focuses on explaining what effect radiation will have on the skin and what patients can and should do to minimize the reaction and maximize their comfort. Giving patients a simple description of the expected skin reaction decreases their anxiety and enlists them in necessary self-care measures.

TABLE 8.4 Risk Factors for Impaired Skin Integrity

Treatment-related factors
- Large treatment field
- Specific susceptible treatment fields
  - Thin epidermis (face, neck)
  - Bony prominences (clavicle)
  - Body folds (ear lobe, pinna, nose)
  - Incision line or wound
  - Peristomal skin
- Treatment with electron-beam therapy
- Treatment with tangential fields
- Radiation given postoperatively
- Radiation given after or concurrently with chemotherapy

Patient-related factors
- Poor nutritional status
- Fair complexion
- History of severe skin reactions to sun exposure
- Diabetes
- Other conditions that affect skin healing ability (lupus, scleroderma, human immunodeficiency virus, burned skin, skin donor sites, etc.)

Source: Adapted from Kelvin JF, Absolon P, Bodansky B, et al. *Radiation oncology standards of patient care.* New York: Department of Radiation Oncology, Memorial Hospital for Cancer and Allied Diseases, 1996.

A radiation skin reaction is an expected, normal, and temporary side effect of radiation therapy (44–47). The acute reaction begins 2 to 3 weeks after starting radiation and continues 3 to 4 weeks after completion of therapy (44,46). The radiation effects are cumulative and may progress from mild to severe—from erythema, through hyperpigmentation, to dry desquamation (dryness, pruritus), and possible moist desquamation. In general, most skin reactions subside gradually over the 2 to 6 weeks after cessation of radiation therapy. It is important to warn chemotherapy patients of recall reactions within the treatment field, which may occur with particular agents [doxorubicin (Adriamycin), dacarbazine (DTIC), bleomycin] (44,46).

Moist desquamation, in which loss of the epidermis leads to open, weeping skin, can occur in skinfold areas (ear lobes) and at the point where two treatment fields match. Moist desquamation places skin at risk for infection and fluid losses (46), and can cause significant anxiety and discomfort (47). Severe moist desquamation can lead to a treatment break, which may affect the overall effectiveness of radiation treatment (48).

Describing to patients the purpose of skin care measures to minimize pain, decrease incidence of skin breakdown, and decrease infection is vital (45). As most of the measures used to care for skin are done by patients, it is important to obtain their active involvement. Although many anecdotal interventions for treatment of radiation skin reaction are described in the literature, little research has been conducted to determine the optimal regimen. Skin care measures, generally agreed on, are described in Table 8.5.

Detailed instructions for skin care during treatment should be provided to patients both in written form and orally. These instructions include how to cleanse and moisturize skin within the treatment field. Cleansing skin within treatment portals involves washing the skin gently with warm water, using only very mild soaps (e.g., Dove, unscented, or Basis soaps) (45,49,50), and rinsing well before gently patting the skin dry.

Moisturizing treated skin using a hydrophilic moisturizer (e.g., Aquaphor, Eucerin Creme, aloe vera gels) is recommended (46,47). Patients should apply moisturizer two to three times per day (depending on risk for breakdown of specific tissue), being careful to wash any residual moisturizer off the skin before treatment. On any day on which treatment is not given (weekends, holidays), moisturizer should be applied after washing in the morning and again at bedtime. Patients should be instructed to prevent irritation of radiated skin by avoiding physical irritants (e.g., tight-fitting clothing and shaving), chemical irritants (e.g., perfumes, cosmetics, deodorants, and moisturizers other than those recommended), extreme heat or cold, and prolonged, direct sun exposure (49).

During radiation therapy, patients' skin is assessed at least weekly and more often as needed for the degree of skin discomfort experienced, presence of scaling or pruritus, tissue breakdown, or moist desquamation. Patients receiving concomitant chemotherapy, cranial radiation, or nasopharynx radiation may note peeling of the scalp, pruritus, and alopecia (44). Such patients are instructed to use a mild shampoo and to apply the recommended moisturizer frequently to the scalp (45). Any signs and symptoms of skin infection (fever, increased pain, purulent or foul-smelling discharge) should be evaluated promptly, drainage should be cultured if present, and antibiotics prescribed.

Skin care continues after radiation therapy has been completed. This includes assessment of skin reaction resolution, reinforcement of the need for lifelong prevention of further skin injury by use of a sunblock (sun protection factor 45), and the avoidance of extreme heat or cold to skin in the treated area.

TABLE 8.5 Skin Care Guidelines for Patients

Skin that receives radiation therapy needs special care. Though a skin reaction is expected and temporary, it can sometimes be uncomfortable. The following tips address how you can help yourself (and your skin) during your course of therapy. These are only guidelines, and if you have any questions or concerns, you should speak with your nurse or physician.

General skin care instructions:

Wash skin in the treatment field with a mild soap; Dove unscented or Basis is preferred.

Apply Aquaphor ointment to the skin immediately after each treatment and at bedtime. On weekends, holidays, or any day in which you do not receive radiation therapy, apply the ointment in the morning and at night.

Your skin should be free of any ointment during the treatment. If necessary, wash your skin immediately prior to each treatment.

Do not apply any other skin cream, makeup, after-shave, or cologne to the area being treated. If you are uncertain about this, please speak with a nurse.

Avoid constrictive clothing, starched collars, tight ties, and other irritants to the skin during your course of radiation therapy.

Always use a sunscreen, SPF-45, when in the sun for greater than 10 minutes, and where a face shading hat when possible.

Dry desquamation (flaky, itchy skin):

Increase frequency of moisturizer, and decrease use of soap.

Cornstarch may be used on shoulders and back. Do not use in moist skin folds.

Topical 0.5% hydrocortisone cream applied with Aquaphor twice daily may reduce itching.

Benadryl 25 to 50 mg may help at bedtime but will increase oral dryness.

Moist desquamation (moist, blistered skin):

Goals are to prevent infection, reduce pain, and prevent treatment breaks.

Keep skin clean but minimize use of soap and water when possible. Air-dry after washing. Fanning may feel cooling.

Continue with use of moisturizer unless directed to stop use. May add frequent soothing and cooling applications of refrigerated, alcohol-free aloe vera gel.

Sivadene ointment may be prescribed. Use as directed by your team.

You may be given nonstick dressings to cover the affected area to prevent clothing from sticking.

If you are uncomfortable, ask your team for medication to reduce discomfort.

Remember, a skin reaction is expected, temporary, and reversible. It commonly takes 2 to 3 weeks to fully recover.

If you have a fever, or notice foul-smelling discharge or increased discomfort, speak with your medical team immediately.

Developed by Carper E. Department of Radiation Oncology, Continuum Cancer Centers of New York, 2002.

Long-term effects of radiation therapy on skin are noted months or years after completion of radiation therapy and may include thinning of epithelium (with increased risk for skin injury), telangiectasia, loss of sweat and sebaceous glandular function, and hyperpigmentation or hypopigmentation.

CHEMOTHERAPY CONSIDERATIONS

Concomitant Chemotherapy and Radiotherapy

Combined-modality organ- and function-preserving programs average 4 to 5 months in duration and are intensive, requiring maximum patient compliance. Organ and function preservation is applicable to patients with advanced carcinomas of the larynx, oropharynx, and hypopharynx in whom surgical management would require total laryngectomy or major oropharyngeal resection. Treatment involves the use of both radiation therapy and chemotherapy; therefore, patients experience an increased severity of side effects as compared with those who undergo only one form of therapy (2,3,51). Neck surgery often follows the chemoradiation treatment program.

A combined-modality program used for laryngeal preservation may consist of an induction phase of chemotherapy followed by intermittent chemotherapy given throughout an aggressive course of radiation (3). More commonly, a concomitant chemoradiation therapy regimen is used. The chemotherapy agents most commonly used neoadjuvantly are cisplatin and 5-fluorouracil administered on an every-3-week cycle. Each of three cycles requires that the patient be hospitalized for 5 days for the chemotherapy administration, which is followed by a 2-week recovery period. Cisplatin (100 mg per m^2) is given intravenously on Day 1 only. A continuous infusion of 5-fluorouracil (1,000 mg per m^2) is given intravenously over 5 days through an infusion pump to prevent acute toxicity and cardiac impairment. Three to four weeks after completion of the three cycles, radiation is initiated and single-agent cisplatin is given twice during the radiation phase (51). In concomitant regimens, single-agent cisplatin is given twice during the radiation phase, on treatment Days 1 and 22, and several cycles of chemotherapy are given adjuvantly, after radiation is completed.

A thorough history and physical examination and endoscopic evaluation are performed prior to initiation of chemotherapy. Routine studies ordered include a baseline electrocardiogram, chest roentgenogram, hematologic studies, and kidney and auditory function studies. A computed tomographic scan of the head and neck area is also obtained. Nutrition and dental consultations are necessary for patients with significant weight loss, chronic dysphagia, and poor dentition.

Common side effects associated with cisplatin are nausea, vomiting, diarrhea, constipation, renal toxicity, hearing loss, peripheral neuropathies, alopecia, and myelosuppression. Common adverse effects associated with 5-fluorouracil include diarrhea, nausea, vomiting, stomatitis, mucositis, rash, and neurologic dysfunction (23). Patients should be given written educational materials, in the form of booklets, pamphlets, or fact cards that succinctly describe the chemotherapeutic drugs' early and late side effects and ways to manage them.

Care during chemotherapy involves providing adequate patient education on the drugs and their side effects, prescribing/administering the drugs, and providing follow up on drug-related side effects (23,52). In general, all patients who undergo chemotherapy experience increased fatigue, anorexia, and heightened anxiety. Adequate teaching about the treatment planned and adjusting both patients' diets and activities can contribute to decreasing anxiety and maximizing appetite and energy.

Cisplatin administration places kidneys in danger of cytotoxic injury unless the drug is diluted adequately and excreted effectively (2,23). Early detection of dehydration during patients' chemotherapy treatments (21) is critical. On initial consultation, patients are encouraged to increase oral fluid intake by at least 2 quarts per day. This increased intake is a requirement for the 12-hour urine collection to measure urinary creatinine clearance before and after each chemotherapy cycle and is an essential part of preparing for cisplatin administration.

Patients receive aggressive hydration and mannitol-based diuretics during cisplatin administration to prevent acute renal toxicity. Increased micturition is the normal, expected result, for which patients must be prepared. Patients are asked to assist in accurately assessing urinary output by using urinals or bedpans (4). Accurate recording of fluid intake, whether intravenous, oral, or enteral, is essential. Electrolytes, serum creatinine, and urea nitrogen are drawn periodically to assess kidney function. Elevated levels can indicate dehydration and renal toxicity. After chemotherapy administration and the return home, patients must maintain an increased fluid intake and monitor their frequency of urination. Despite thorough teaching, abrupt onset of emergent dehydration can occur, and patients may require admission to the hospital for treatment of this condition with intravenous fluids.

Unresectable disease can be treated with single-agent chemotherapy, multidrug chemotherapy, radiation therapy, or multimodal therapy (22,23). The most commonly used combination chemotherapy regimen is cisplatin, 100 mg/m^2 intravenous bolus, on day 1, and 5-fluorouracil, 1,000 mg/m^2 intravenous continuous infusion, on days 1 to 4. Typically, patients are cycled every 3 to 4 weeks with a clinic appointment between cycles to assess response and toxicities. Disease presentation and response of disease to the drugs determine whether patients will receive the full three cycles. Patients' clinical performance and toxicity profile also are considered.

Single-agent therapy does not require that patients be hospitalized except for those who receive paclitaxel (Taxol) as a 24-hour infusion. Treatments are given in the outpatient department and usually are tolerated well. Patients' white blood cell levels are checked before each chemotherapy treatment and must exceed 3.0. The chemotherapy dose is escalated gradually on the basis of patient presentation and white blood cell levels. A paclitaxel infusion can be administered over a 3-, 6-, or 24-hour infusion period. Patients are advised that paclitaxel may cause allergic reactions.

Premedication of dexamethasone (Decadron), 20 mg orally the night before and the morning of treatment, intravenous Benadryl, and intravenous cimetidine or ranitidine immediately before paclitaxel administration minimize risk for severe reaction. Patients are observed for a reaction, and the infusion is discontinued immediately if one is observed.

Myelosuppression

Myelosuppression is a near-universal effect of chemotherapy (21,33). Therefore, patient teaching always includes a simple explanation of chemotherapy's myelosuppressive activity. Depletion of white blood cells predisposes patients to infection, and patients are instructed to avoid any known sources of infection, to pay scrupulous attention to hygiene, and to avoid large crowds. Patients are strongly urged to use a thermometer to check their temperature each day at home. Fevers of 100.5°F and higher must be reported to the health care team. A white blood cell level then is checked and, if neutropenic (an absolute neutrophil count <500/mm^3), hospital admission for antibiotics becomes an immediate priority.

Chemotherapy may also suppress red blood cell and platelet cell production, leading to anemia and thrombocytopenia. Thrombocytopenia increases risk for bleeding, and so patients are instructed about the importance of safety. They also are told to immediately report to the health care team any signs of active bleeding (e.g., delayed clotting, excessive bruising, gingival bleeding, or headaches).

Anemia may be very debilitating, with patients reporting severe fatigue and shortness of breath. A recent study suggests anemia may be associated with hypoxic tumor cell resistance to the cytotoxic agents commonly used in head and neck chemotherapy regimens (53). Historically, blood transfusions were used in cases of profound anemia or when patients developed persistent unrelieved fatigue. Because of potential risks with transfusion, the hemoglobin level became very low before transfusion was used. Today, epoetin alfa is often given to patients receiving chemotherapy or concomitant chemotherapy and radiation therapy, before profound anemia occurs, to attain and maintain Hg levels near 12.0 g/dL. This has not only decreased the number of transfusions required by patients, but also has led to improved quality of life (18,19,53).

Mild fatigue is a common and cumulative effect of chemotherapy. Such correctable causes as anemia and fluid or electrolyte imbalances should be ruled out. Stressors such as commuting to the hospital for treatment and dealing with the discomfort of toxicities, pain, and emotional strain all contribute to general malaise. The importance of balancing rest and activity is stressed. Some patients need to take a nap during the day, to which they may be unaccustomed.

Some chemotherapeutic agents (5-fluorouracil, methotrexate) can cause severe mucositis and diarrhea (54). Mucositis and stomatitis also can occur during radiation, and, for patients receiving both radiation therapy and chemotherapy, mucositis is both severe and prolonged (3,20,23,33,35). Chronic mucositis and stomatitis can be so debilitating that patients are unable to eat or drink. Weight loss and dehydration result in unscheduled hospitalizations and higher cost of care. Scheduled treatments may be postponed, and the chemotherapy dose will be reduced with the next treatment. Pain medication, intravenous hydration, and antifungal agents plus oral saline sprays often are used to manage severe cases of mucositis. Placement of a feeding tube is mandated to provide adequate nutrition in the presence of acute dysphagia and rapid weight loss.

Alopecia

Alopecia is one of the most obvious and public side effects of chemotherapy. Loss of hair is a vivid and ever-present reminder to patients of their diagnosis and of the treatment that they are receiving. A change in their body image occurs, and patients become self-conscious (1,55). Women often wear wigs or turbans, whereas men usually choose baseball caps, hats, or bandannas (55). Patients are reassured that the alopecia usually is temporary and that hair will likely grow back within a few months of treatment completion. All patients are encouraged to attend a "Look Good, Feel Better" program, sponsored by the American Cancer Society and available in most areas of the country. Maintaining a normal hygiene and makeup routine is encouraged to promote self-confidence during intensive treatment schedules (1).

LONG-TERM EFFECTS

Disfigurement and Dysfunction

The head and neck region is highly significant to body image because of its visibility and prominence. Body image incorporates the individual's perception of self as a social, psychological, and physiologic entity (1). Emphasis on the physical attractiveness of a person is reflective of modern society; as a result, many head and neck cancer patients experience great difficulty with socialization, reintegration with society, and self-esteem. Disfigurement and dysfunction occur as an aftermath of surgery and with visible, protruding, progressive disease. Those patients who undergo orbital exenteration or major reconstructive surgery (e.g., nasal surgery) face many psychological and physical hurdles in their recovery (1,56,57).

The combined efforts of a dedicated health care team can be instrumental in this recovery. Each member should ascertain the degree of disfigurement and dysfunction and provide practical tips on coping strategies. Patients who feel in control of their care and who make decisions regarding care feel more self-assured. Patients' sense of self and personal motivation, as well as support from caregivers, are keys to recovery (4,6).

Sensitivity and patience are necessary, and treating patients respectfully is essential. Staff must be aware that disfigured patients sitting in a crowded waiting room for lengthy periods of time may feel self-conscious and markedly uncomfortable. For some patients, communication may be clumsy (e.g., via a writing pad or a mechanical apparatus for laryngectomy patients) and time-consuming. Direct eye contact with the patient, without grimacing, is imperative. Asking about aspects of a patient's life (e.g., family routines, work, or news items) beyond the cancer reinforces the concept that cancer occurs in the context of a work and home life.

Fear of Recurrence

Often, patients hesitate to contact the health care team for fear of learning the possible meaning behind toxicities and changes in their physical strength or appearance and denial of cancer itself (4,6,21). It is incumbent on providers to establish good rapport with patients and to provide reassurance and encouragement within the uncertainty that the cancer brings to both patients and their caregivers. Patients must feel safe if they are to verbalize their fears to ensure that important information regarding their health is communicated to the health care team. It is very important that the health care team triages patients who require earlier, more intensive intervention and closer follow-up as early as possible in treatment so support is given in a timely way.

Many patients experience emotional relief just by discussing their fears and feelings. However, in some cases, referral to behavioral health specialists trained in or familiar with cancer may be indicated, such as for patients with a personal or family history of substance abuse disorders, clinical depression, or long-standing mental illness. Social services may be helpful with transportation, financial, or home care issues, and it may be appropriate to offer spiritual support through pastoral counselors at health care or religious institutions.

DISEASE PROGRESSION/END OF LIFE CARE

Some patients may present initially with advanced disease, in a debilitated state, and often with intractable pain. Single-agent therapy, investigational drug studies, and best supportive care are treatment options available for advanced disease, whether primary, recurrent, or metastatic. This is a difficult time for patients, families, and the health care team. Decision making is complex. Patients coming to the hospital on a frequent and regular basis become weary and discouraged, and may quietly be giving up hope. Caregivers may feel guilty relief when the patient or loved one is admitted to the hospital; it is then that they finally receive a respite from the overwhelming physical and emotional demands of caregiving.

In cases of advanced disease, the health care team must communicate openly and clearly with patients and their families, predicting when possible a poor prognosis and limited life expectancy. Any further treatment is described in terms of palliation, not cure. Often, an advance directive (living wills, health care power of attorney, health care proxies) must be obtained at a time of great emotional strain for patients and families. Whenever possible, the subject of advance directives should be initiated before terminal illness occurs (5).

Collaboration with social services is required and provides information and assistance on transportation, financial aid, home care, and hospice availability. Consistent social services, introduced earlier in the trajectory of illness provide additional support for patients, their caregivers, and the health care team. Long-distance commuters, foreign nationals, and those for whom English is a second language have specific barriers to treatment and a significant need of social services. Language barriers not only impede patients' understanding but also affect their ability to comply with treatment directives. Providers are asked to ensure that the translations are accurate, which is often difficult for untrained family members who are likewise emotionally distraught.

Home care may be helpful in many situations. Patients who are elderly or who live alone or with working relatives need to rely on professional caregivers or community-based volunteers. Patients become debilitated as their cancer progresses or if they experience treatment toxicities. Tracheostomy care, tube feedings, wound care, and general home care assistance by an home care aide and supervised by a professional nurse can be provided by home care agencies until such time as patients and caregivers are unable to manage care independently.

As patients' conditions deteriorate and chemotherapy or other treatment options are no longer available, hospice care should be considered. Hospice is most commonly provided in the home, and in certain locales at a freestanding center. The goal of care is to focus on comfort care and provide a much-needed respite for primary caregivers (58). Pain management, assistance with activities of daily living, and intravenous hydration can be provided. Death and death-related issues are approached gently, depending on the willingness of patients and caregivers to discuss such issues (5,58). This may be an opportune time for both patients and families to resolve personal concerns and accept death. Spiritual counseling is offered as appropriate to each patient (59).

Caregivers must be reassured that members of the health care team still are available should unmanageable complications occur in the home (e.g., airway distress and intractable pain). Most fears of patients and caregivers relate to the manner in which patients will die, and these can be discussed sensitively and openly. The fear of severe pain or of choking to death is realistic, and so end of life care concentrates on symptom management: providing relief of pain and suffering, and maintaining a viable airway. Practical and spiritual support for family members and caregivers during the dying process and afterward in bereavement are cornerstones that the care hospice provides.

CONCLUSION

Prevention and detection of head and neck cancer are best achieved through continued education of the public. Head and neck screening programs are offered at some institutions. Avoidance of alcohol and tobacco is stressed, and referral to supportive programs is provided (60). Education continues to be important once an individual receives a diagnosis of head or neck cancer and requires treatment. For many, lifestyle is altered once they are affected by cancer, and their lives can be fraught with personal and practical problems. Relieving the burden of cancer and its treatment plays a significant role in the overall treatment.

Caring for patients with head and neck cancers requires the use of both the science and the art of symptom management. Interventions to maintain the airway, to provide nutritional support, to care for the skin, to help relearn swallowing and communicating, and to ensure adequate pain relief all are essential aspects to the successful management of this complex group of patients. Superimposed are the accompanying emotional and psychological needs attached to the multidisciplinary treatment programs. Many patients are eager to learn new ways of eating and communicating and adapt readily. Even new ways of breathing can be learned successfully. Patients rely on the team to teach them what they must learn and to encourage them and their families through the difficult weeks and months of treatment. Patients and families need the team to teach and organize home care, whether the outcome is cure, disease control, progression, or death.

REFERENCES

1. Dropkin M. Coping with disfigurement and dysfunction after head and neck surgery: a conceptual framework. *Semin Oncol Nurs* 1989;5:213.
2. Bildstein CY. Head and neck malignancies. In: Groenwald SL, Frogge MH, Goodman M, et al., eds. *Cancer nursing principles and practice.* Boston: Jones and Bartlett, 1993:1114.
3. Hirshfield-Bartek J. Combined-modality therapy. In: Dow KH, Hilderley LJ, eds. *Nursing care in radiation oncology.* Philadelphia: WB Saunders, 1992:251.
4. Dodd MJ. Patterns of self care in cancer patients receiving radiation therapy. *Oncol Nurs Forum* 1984;11:23.
5. Haisfield ME, McGuire DB, Krumm S, et al. Patients' and healthcare providers' opinions regarding advance directives. *Oncol Nurs Forum* 1994;21:1179.
6. Hilderley LJ. Pain and fatigue. In: Dow KH, Hilderley LJ, eds. *Nursing care in radiation oncology.* Philadelphia: WB Saunders, 1992:57.
7. World Health Organization. *Cancer pain relief.* Geneva: WHO, 1986.
8. Jacox A, Carr D, Payne R, et al. *Clinical practice guideline number 9: management of cancer pain.* AHCPR publication 94-0592:139-41. Washington, DC: U.S. Department of Health and Human Services, Public Health Service, Agency for Health Care Policy and Research, 1994.
9. Madeya ML. Oral complications from cancer therapy: part 2: nursing implications for assessment and treatment. *Oncol Nurs Forum* 1996;23:808.
10. Iwamoto RR. Altered nutrition. In: Dow KH, Hilderley LJ, eds. *Nursing care in radiation oncology.* Philadelphia: WB Saunders, 1992:69.
11. Dudjak LA. Mouth care for mucositis due to radiation therapy. *Oncol Nurs Forum* 1987;10:131.
12. Passik S, Portenoy R. Substance abuse disorders. In: Holland J, et al., eds. *Psycho-oncology,* 2nd ed. New York: Oxford University Press, 1998:516–586.
13. Levy M. Pharmacologic treatment of cancer pain. *N Engl J Med* 1996;335: 1124–1132.
14. Cella D. Factors influencing quality of life in cancer patients: anemia and fatigue. *Semin Oncol* 1998;25[Suppl 7]:43–46.
15. Portenoy RK, Miaskowski C. Assessment and management of cancer-related fatigue. In: Berger AM, Portenoy RK, Weissman DE, eds. *Principles and practice of supportive oncology.* Philadelphia: JB Lippincott, 1998:109–117.
16. Harrison, L, Shasha D, Shiaova L, et al. Prevalence of anemia in cancer patients undergoing radiation therapy. *Semin Oncol* 2001;28:54–59.
17. Lee WR, Berkey B, Marcial V, et al. Anemia is associated with decreased survival and increased locoregional failure in patients with locally advanced head and neck carcinoma: a secondary analysis of RTOG 85-27. *Int J Radiat Oncol Biol Phys* 1998;42:1069–1075.
18. Glaser C, Millesi W, Kornek G, et al. Impact of hemoglobin level and use of recombinant erythropoietin on efficacy of preoperative chemoradiation therapy for squamous cell carcinoma of the oral cavity and oropharynx. *Int J Radiat Oncol Biol Phys* 2001;50:705–715.
19. Demetrie G, Kris M, Wade J, et al. Quality-of-life benefit in chemotherapy patients treated with epoetin alfa is independent of disease response or tumor type: results from a prospective community oncology study. *J Clin Oncol* 1998; 16:3412–3425.
20. Skipper A, Szeluga DJ, Groenwald SL. Nutritional disturbances. In: Groenwald SL, Frogge MH, Goodman M, et al., eds. *Cancer nursing principles and practice.* Boston: Jones and Bartlett, 1993:620.
21. Camp-Sorrell D. Chemotherapy: toxicity management. In: Groenwald SL, Frogge MH, Goodman M, et al., eds. *Cancer nursing principles and practice.* Boston: Jones and Bartlett, 1993:331.
22. Harris LL, Smith S. Chemotherapy in head and neck cancer. *Semin Oncol Nurs* 1989;5:174.
23. Knobf MT, Durivage HJ. Chemotherapy: principles of therapy. In: Groenwald SL, Frogge MH, Goodman M, et al., eds. *Cancer nursing principles and practice.* Boston: Jones and Bartlett, 1993:270.
24. Fleishman S. Cancer cachexia. In: Holland J, et al. *Psycho-oncology,* 2nd ed. New York: Oxford University Press, 1998:468–475.
25. Wilson PR, Herman J, Chubon SJ. Eating strategies used by persons with head and neck cancer during and after radiotherapy. *Cancer Nurs* 1991;14:98.
26. McGuire M. Nutritional care of surgical oncology patients. *Semin Oncol Nurs* 2000;16:128–134.
27. Logemann J. Swallowing and communication rehabilitation. *Semin Oncol Nurs* 1989;5:205.
28. Arnold C, Richter M. The effect of oral nutritional supplements on head and neck cancer. *Int J Radiat Oncol Biol Phys* 1989;16:1595.
29. Sigler B, Schuring L. *Ear, nose, and throat disorders.* St. Louis: Mosby, 1993:1.
30. McGuire M. Current trends in management of head and neck cancer. *Dev Supp Cancer Care* 1990;3:30–39.
31. Tunkel RS, Lachmann EA. Rehabilitative medicine. In: Berger AM, Portenoy RK, Weissman DE, eds. *Principles and practice of supportive oncology.* Philadelphia: JB Lippincott, 1998:681–690.
32. Martin L. Management of the altered airway in the head and neck cancer patient. *Semin Oncol Nurs* 1989;5:182.
33. Goodman M, Ladd LA, Purl S. Integumentary and mucous membrane alterations. In: Groenwald SL, Frogge MH, Goodman M, et al., eds. *Cancer nursing principles and practice.* Boston: Jones and Bartlett, 1993:734.
34. Beck S. Prevention and management of oral complications in the cancer patient. In: Hubbard SM, Greene PE, Knobf T, eds. *Current issues in cancer nursing practice.* Philadelphia: JB Lippincott, 1991:1.
35. Madeya ML. Oral complications from cancer therapy: I. pathophysiology and secondary complications. *Oncol Nurs Forum* 1996;23:801.
36. Epstein JB, Wong FLW. The efficacy of sucralfate suspension in the prevention of oral mucositis due to radiation therapy. *Int J Radiat Oncol Biol Phys* 1994;28: 693–698.
37. Epstein JB, Silverman S Jr, Paggiarino DA, et al. Benzydamine HCL for prophylaxis of radiation-induced oral mucositis: results from a multicenter, randomized, double-blind, placebo-controlled clinical trial. *Cancer* 2001;15: 875–885.
38. Sprinzl GM, Galvan O, de Vries A, et al. Local application of granulocyte-macrophage colony-stimulating-factor (GM CSF) for the treatment of oral mucositis. *Eur J Cancer* 2001;37:1971–1975.
39. Sela M, Maroz D, Gedalia I. Streptococcus mutans in saliva of normal subjects and neck and head irradiated cancer subjects after consumption of honey. *J Oral Rehabil* 2000;27:269–270.
40. Brizel, David M. Phase III randomized trial of amifostine as a radioprotector in head and neck cancer. *J Clin Oncol* 2000;18:3339–3345.
41. Rieke JW, Haferman MD, Johnson JT, et al. Oral pilocarpine for radiation-induced xerostomia: integrated efficacy and safety results from two prospective randomized clinical trials. *Int J Radial Oncol Biol Phys* 1995;31:661.
42. Zimmerman RP, Mark RJ, Tran LM, et al. Concomitant pilocarpine during head and neck irradiation is associated with decreased posttreatment xerostomia. *Int J Radiat Oncol Biol Phys* 1997;37:571.
43. Kusler DL, Rambur BA. Treatment for radiation-induced xerostomia: an innovative remedy. *Cancer Nurs* 1992;15:191.
44. Sitton E. Early and late radiation-induced skin alterations. Part I: mechanisms of skin changes. *Oncol Nurs Forum* 1996;19:801.
45. Sitton E. Early and late radiation-induced skin alterations. Part II: nursing care of irradiated skin. *Oncol Nurs Forum* 1996;19:907.
46. McDonald A. Altered protective mechanisms. In: Dow KH, Hilderley LJ, eds. *Nursing care in radiation oncology.* Philadelphia: WB Saunders, 1992:96.
47. Hilderly L. Skin care in radiation therapy: a review of the literature. *Oncol Nurs Forum* 1983;10:51.
48. Cox JD, Pajak TF, Marcial VA, et al. Interruptions adversely affect local control and survival with hyperfractionated radiation therapy of carcinomas of the upper respiratory and digestive tracts. New evidence for accelerated proliferation from RTOG Protocol 8313. *Cancer* 1992;69:2744.
49. Dim D, Macchia R, Gozza A, et al. Management of acute radiodermatitis. *Cancer Nurs* 1993;16:366.
50. Frosch P, Kligman A. The soap chamber: a new method for assessing the irritancy of soaps. *J Am Acad Dermatol* 1979;1:35.
51. Pfister D, Strong E, Harrison LB, et al. Larynx preservation with combined chemotherapy and radiation therapy in advanced but resectable head and neck cancer. *J Clin Oncol* 1991;9:850.
52. Reymann PE. Chemotherapy: principles of administration. In: Groenwald SL, Frogge MH, Goodman M, et al., eds. *Cancer nursing principles and practice.* Boston: Jones and Bartlett, 1993:293.
53. Littlewood TJ. The impact of hemoglobin levels on treatment outcomes in patients with cancer. *Semin Oncol* 2001;28:49–53.
54. Dodd MJ, Larson PJ, Dibble SL, et al. Randomized clinical trial of chlorhexidine versus placebo for prevention of oral mucositis in patients receiving chemotherapy. *Oncol Nurs Forum* 1996;23:921.
55. Foltz AT, Gaines G, Gullatte M. Recalled side effects and self-care actions of patient receiving inpatient chemotherapy. *Oncol Nurs Forum* 1996;23:679.
56. Schleper J. Prevention, detection, and diagnosis of head and neck cancers. *Semin Oncol Nurs* 1989;5:139.
57. Hong W, Doos W. Chemoprevention of head and neck cancer. *Otolaryngol Clin North Am* 1985;18:543.
58. McMillan SC, Mahon M. The impact of hospice services on the quality of life of primary caregivers. *Oncol Nurs Forum* 1994;21:1189.
59. Cooley ME. Bereavement care. *Cancer Nurs* 1992;15:125.
60. Hecht JP, Emmons KM, Brown RA, et al. Smoking interventions for patients with cancer: guidelines for nursing practice. *Oncol Nurs Forum* 1994;21:1657.

CHAPTER 9

General Principles of Reconstructive Surgery for Head and Neck Cancer Patients

Mark D. DeLacure

INTRODUCTION AND HISTORICAL PERSPECTIVE

Reconstructive surgery of the head and neck patient has undergone tremendous advancement over the past three decades, fueled largely by the increased application of microneurovascular free tissue transfer techniques to postablative defects. This modern era has been preceded by the fundamental contributions of many surgeons from the fields of plastic and reconstructive surgery, otolaryngology–head and neck surgery, neurosurgery, oral and maxillofacial surgery, and general surgery. The concepts of immediate reconstruction (1) and the contribution of the deltopectoral fasciocutaneous flap (2) were followed by the application of the then newly defined myocutaneous flaps of the mid-1970s, in particular, the pectoralis major myocutaneous flap (3).

Despite the report of the successful microvascular transfer of a jejunal interposition flap in 1959 (4), the modern era of clinical reconstructive microsurgery began in the early 1970s with increased refinement in instrumentation and technique, the description of new transfers, and the search for new applications of previously described flaps. This characterized the next decade with the reports of large series of the free jejunum interposition (5), the radial forearm fasciocutaneous flap for oral reconstruction (6), and, in particular, the fibula free flap for oromandibular reconstruction (7). The recognition of the superiority of these techniques and the development of multidisciplinary teams and simultaneous interdependent operative procedures have resulted in aesthetic and functional restoration of the head and neck patient to a heretofore unprecedented level.

The availability of an increased armamentarium of reliable reconstructive options has given the head and neck surgeon increased confidence in the application of radical ablative or intensive therapeutic approaches to advanced and recurrent disease. It has also given surgeons increased responsibility in anticipating and planning the reconstructive requirements for a particular procedure and for choosing appropriate support teams to achieve the highest possible level of form and function in returning patients to their premorbid existence. General principles of defect analysis and of flap design, anatomy, and physiology apply across all techniques and must be emphasized.

The traditional concept of the *reconstructive ladder* begins defect analysis with a hierarchical approach to the suitability of techniques to a particular defect, emphasizing simplicity, and ascending from simple to complex. It begins at the bottom rung with primary closure reconstruction, ascending from skin grafting to local flaps, through regional flaps, distant flaps, and on to the microneurovascular free tissue transfer of composite blocks of tissue at the top of the ladder. Surgeons must realize, however, that they are not obligated to push their patients though all or most of these steps and that many times the concept of the reconstructive *elevator,* advancing directly to microsurgical technique from the initial preoperative planning phase is most appropriate (e.g., anterior oromandibular reconstruction after composite resection). Conversely, the surgeon must not be extravagant in the application of advanced technique and must always have multiple contingency plans in place in the event of flap failure or recurrence of disease. Defect considerations include volume, composition (soft tissue, bone), location (proximity to vital structures, need for external/internal surfaces), and general status (i.e., previously operated, irradiated, infected, need for oronasocranial or oropharyngocervical separation, and the like). Functional considerations include the provision of sensibility, bone stock for skeletal framework and osseointegration, secretory mucosal surface, pliability, and so forth. Flap donor sites have been largely well defined and chosen for acceptability of residual functional or aesthetic deficit.

PRIMARY CLOSURE

Excisions oriented to allow closure within or parallel to relaxed skin tension lines result in aesthetic incisional scar placement. Despite its inherent simplicity, primary closure should avoid undue tension to avoid broadening of surgical scars. Undermining of adjacent normal skin margins may facilitate these efforts. Otherwise, graft and local flap techniques should be incorporated into the closure.

Most partial glossectomy defects can be closed per primam without significant impact on long-term speech and swallowing function. With the exception of primary closure of access incisions for neck dissection, mandibulotomy, and parotidectomy, flap techniques are commonly required in head and neck procedures.

SKIN GRAFTS

Skin grafts have primary application in small defects of the oral cavity and ear, maxillectomy cheek flap, temporalis fascia flap, coverage of muscle or omental free flaps in scalp reconstruction, and coverage of the radial forearm and fibula free flap donor sites. In the oral cavity, they allow the surgeon to overcome tethering and restriction of mobility, which can result from primary closure and critically affect orolingual function. Skin grafts generally heal well over fat, muscle, perichondrium, and fascia. They heal over meninges or periosteum but afford neither adequate protection nor stable coverage in these contexts. Inasmuch as such grafts are completely dependent on the recipient bed for survival via neovascularization, they are unsatisfactory for many previously operated, irradiated, or frankly infected sites, which are variably characterized by ischemic scar tissue, relative soft tissue hypovascularity, and inflammatory response. Such grafts are harvested with a dermatome in split-thickness skin graft (STSG) fashion, usually from the lateral thigh or buttock. Thickness should vary according to need from about 0.0012 to 0.0015 inch; thinner grafts exhibit easier take, but more contracture, than thicker grafts. Meshing allows expansion of a sheet graft to larger dimensions and is generally restricted to scalp resurfacing contexts in the head and neck region.

Donor sites in smaller harvests are best managed with an occlusive semipermeable dressing left in place for about a week, and larger donor sites covered by Xeroform gauze until separation. Vacuum-assisted closure (VAC) devices have also been used. Topical anesthetic creams (EMLA®;AstraZeneca, Wilmington, DE) may ease donor-site discomfort, which may well overshadow the larger cephalic procedure. Successful graft take is characterized by effective immobilization (to allow vascular ingrowth) utilizing a nonadherent antibiotic-impregnated bolster, intraoral prosthodontic device, and/or quilting sutures or staples. Additional requirements for success include meticulous hemostasis (avoidance of hematoma) and infection control (enzymatic dissolution), which includes timely removal of bolster dressings prior to significant bacterial colonization.

Full-thickness skin grafts (FTSGs) are appropriate for many small, externally visible facial defects. They are characterized by generally superior color match, contour, and texture, less contracture (secondary) potential, and poorer take than STSGs. Common donor sites include postauricular and upper eyelid (thin), and preauricular, nasolabial, and supraclavicular skin for thicker grafts. Templates should be slightly oversized due to primary contracture when FTSGs are harvested. Such grafts are usually taken with scalpel and subsequently thinned of subcutaneous fat (parasitic to new dermal blood supply) with scissors. Composite grafts of acellular dermal allograft plus patient STSG offers yet another approach to soft tissue resurfacing.

LOCAL SKIN FLAPS

Local skin flaps are primarily applied in the reconstruction of external facial defects and are characterized by superior color match (in comparison to grafts), contour, and texture, and ease of application/availability. Commonly used designs include advancement, rotation, bilobe, island transposition, and rhomboid transposition (Fig. 9.1). *In situ* tubing of such flaps can be

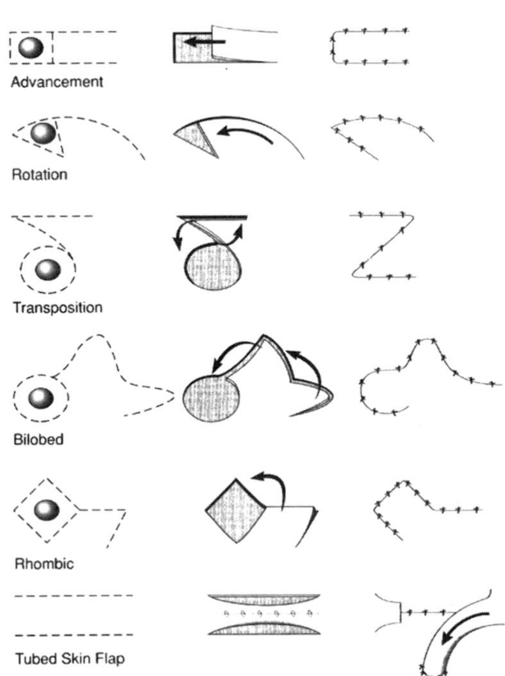

Figure 9.1 Six common designs for local skin flap reconstruction of head and neck defects, usually resulting from the resection of early staged cutaneous carcinomas.

useful in re-creating specialized structures (helical rim, alar rim, columella).

These flaps are perfused based on subdermal plexuses, and generally observe traditional length-to-width ratios of 3:1 or less. Improved understanding of the microvascular blood supply of the face has refined our understanding and application of these designs (8). Viscoelastic properties of skin and soft tissues such as creep, stretch, and stress relaxation are important concepts in local skin flap applications and often require a balanced contribution from flap, donor site, and recipient site to achieve the desired result. Tension, infection, and cigarette smoking all impact wound healing in this type of flap and mandate attention to detail in operative planning, execution, and counseling. The reader is referred to two excellent atlases in planning the design of such flaps (9,10).

One of the most common applications of this type of flap is the nasolabial flap (11). Rhomboid flap designs can transfer hair-bearing scalp to frontotemporal defects and are also good general designs inasmuch as six different rhomboid flap designs can be devised for any single defect. The Mustardé rotation-advancement flap for cheek and lower eyelid reconstruction also relies on these principles.

REGIONAL FLAPS

As the distance of required flap transposition increases, the incorporation of a defined axial blood supply becomes critical. This is further discussed in the section on myocutaneous flaps later in this chapter, and it becomes a critical consideration in the paramedian forehead (supratrochlear), Abbé, Abbé-Estlander (superior labial), and facial artery myomucosal (FAMM) flaps (12). The paramedian forehead flap remains a fundamental tool for major nasal reconstruction as refined by Burget and Menick (13), as well as for medial cheek reconstruction. Abbe designs transfer not only skin but also labial mucosa to compensate for soft tissue deficiency in lip reconstruction. The Washio postauricular flap and Mutter or epaulet flap are of historical interest and have largely been supplanted by free tissue transfer techniques. The temporal fascias (superficial or temporoparietal and deep) may be transferred as a bilobate flap pedicled on the superficial temporal system and may be thought of as a transferable bed for STSG placement in auricular reconstruction. The layers are highly vascular and pliable. This flap also has potential intraoral application (cheek, palate) independently and as part of temporalis muscle transfers, and may be transposed either pre- or retrozygomatically. Accurate knowledge of facial nerve anatomy and of the nuances of the anatomy of this region is critical to confident surgery without complication. This anatomy has been described in detail by Stuzin (14,15).

The deltopectoral and forehead flaps are of historical interest, and the recognition of defined territories of overlying skin, perfused by perpendicularly oriented myocutaneous perforating vessels, fueled many of the advancements in head and neck reconstructive work through the 1970s (16). This vascular orientation allowed circumferential suture around skin islands transferred with such flaps without compromising viability. Although the description of the pectoralis major myocutaneous flap in 1978 was the most significant of this genre of flaps, the latissimus dorsi and trapezius flaps have also been explored in various head and neck applications. Myocutaneous flaps allowed the predictable transfer of significant volumes of soft tissue (skin island, subcutaneous fat, and muscle) into major ablative head and neck defects. Such flaps demonstrated reliability and consequent versatility of application far in excess of their regional cutaneous and fasciocutaneous counterparts and allowed extension of the scope of ablative surgery and of functional reconstruction of the era. Sinocranial, orocervical, and pharyngocutaneous separation could now be reliably achieved. Single-stage major reconstructions became the norm. Primary closure reduced donor-site morbidity significantly in contrast to previous fasciocutaneous designs. The application of these flaps as vehicles for the transfer of vascularized segments of bone (trapezius-scapular, pectoralis-rib, latissimus-rib, sternocleidomastoid-clavicle) was an important historical step toward the microvascular transfer of bone.

The concept of angiosomes (17) has challenged and extended the dogma that such flaps could reliably transfer only skin directly overlying the muscle component of a myocutaneous flap. The angiosome is a volume of tissue supplied by a single-source artery and vein. Adjacent angiosomes are connected by a system of "choke" arteries (oscillating). Adjacent angiosomes may be captured in tissue transfer after interruption of the adjacent source artery through the reversal of physiologic blood flow. Once harvested tissue is extended *beyond* adjacent angiosomes (once removed), the incidence of necrosis is significantly elevated.

Pectoralis Major

The pectoralis major myocutaneous flap remains the major myocutaneous pedicled tissue transfer in head and neck reconstruction and continues to be a workhorse in selected applications. Its ease of development and application remain fundamental parts of the armamentarium of the contemporary head and neck surgeon. The flap is based on the pectoral branch of the thoracoacromial artery off the second portion of the axillary artery. The architecture of the axial supply follows that generally observed throughout the body, namely that the axial pedicle enters the muscle from its undersurface, running in a fat plane up to its intramuscular course. While traditional incisional designs have avoided crossing the horizontally disposed deltopectoral flap and required flap dissection beneath a bridge of uninterrupted skin, the increased difficulty of flap dissection is obviated by a continuous serpiginous incision (burning an historical bridge) joining the vertical limb of a neck dissection incision. (It is highly unlikely that a deltopectoral fasciocutaneous flap would be called on anymore to salvage a failed pectoralis major flap, thus invalidating this carryover of dogma from the early and unproven days of the pectoralis flap.) The contribution of the lateral thoracic artery to this flap is insignificant in the final analysis of most transfers.

Refinements in technique include developing the entire flap as an island design, allowing the transposition of a minimal amount of tissue over the clavicle, thus reducing external deformity. Section of the pectoral nerve branches to the muscle ensures that the pedicle is not compressed against it when rotated into a defect and also that the flap muscle component will atrophy and contour to external defects more rapidly and more acceptably.

Transfer of the flap through the neck most easily follows radical lymphadenectomy procedures in which the sternocleidomastoid muscle is sacrificed, the transposed pectoralis muscle affording reliable coverage to exposed critical neurovascular structures. The arc of rotation of the flap allows it to reliably reach the levels of the hard palate and superior helix. The flap may be applied to defects of nearly any configuration in structures inferior to these levels. Simultaneous harvest without patient repositioning is a significant advantage. The flap may be tubed on itself to form an interposition conduit for pharyngoesophageal reconstruction in salvage situations.

A medially based generic curvilinear lunar skin paddle design facilitates primary closure of the donor site and minimizes the transfer of breast parenchyma and deformity in female patients. Preoperative marking should include the horizontal level of the contralateral nipple to minimize vertical deformity on closure. Flap dissection is based on the direct visualization of the pedicle, which is directed inferolaterally.

Disadvantages include the potential transfer of hair-bearing skin into the oral cavity and the sheer bulkiness of this flap. This sometimes mandates the transfer of the flap as a muscle-only design, which can be used for the coverage of external defects in combination with other techniques and then skin grafted. Transposition of the flap, as with all pedicled designs, is limited by the arc of rotation of the flap pedicle—here, over the clavicle.

Common contemporary applications include major vascular coverage, radionecrotic wounds, large oral cavity defects, large parotid and neck defects, superior mediastinal and peristomal defects, and the salvage of free flap complications (Fig. 9.2A,B).

Such inferiorly pedicled flaps all exhibit an often relentless tendency toward dehiscence and/or fistulization the more superior the insetting requirement. In addition to the geometric contribution to this phenomenon is that the most distal aspect of the skin paddle (and most poorly perfused and vulnerable) is necessarily inset into the superiormost and often most critical coverage requirement areas. Partial flap loss, dehiscence, stricture (through the requirement for secondary wound healing and ischemic scar contracture), fistulization, and the like, are not uncommon phenomena despite the significant possibilities of myocutaneous flaps.

Latissimus Dorsi

This muscle is based on the thoracodorsal pedicle from the versatile subscapular system of flaps. It is a broad, thin muscle that can be transposed into the head and neck region either subcutaneously or via a transaxillary approach (18). Although its range of application as a pedicled flap and its transferred soft tissue volume are similar to that of the pectoralis, decubitus positioning, decreased reliability, and a high incidence of donor-site morbidity make this a tertiary choice for free tissue transfer techniques and the pectoralis.

The latissimus dorsi flap is a first-line choice, however, as a muscle flap for the microsurgical reconstruction of massive scalp defects. As a free tissue transfer, it is characterized by a huge available surface area; thin, pliable consistency; a long, large caliber; and an anatomically consistent vascular pedicle, facilitating ease of anastomosis in the neck. A meshed STSG completes the reconstruction.

Trapezius

Both vertically and transversely oriented skin paddle designs may be taken with this flap, which is based on the occipital and descending cervical branches of the external carotid and transverse cervical vessels, respectively (19). Applications of this flap and its variations were explored throughout the 1970s and 1980s. Although capable of reaching the midline neck, posteriorly situated defects were best suited to reconstruction with this method. Elegant anatomic studies have accurately documented variations in the vascular anatomy of these vessels (20). Previous neck dissection status is an important consideration inas-

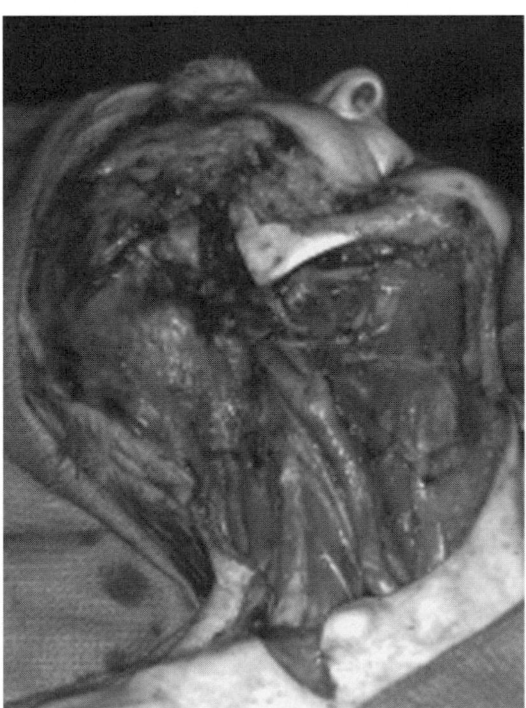

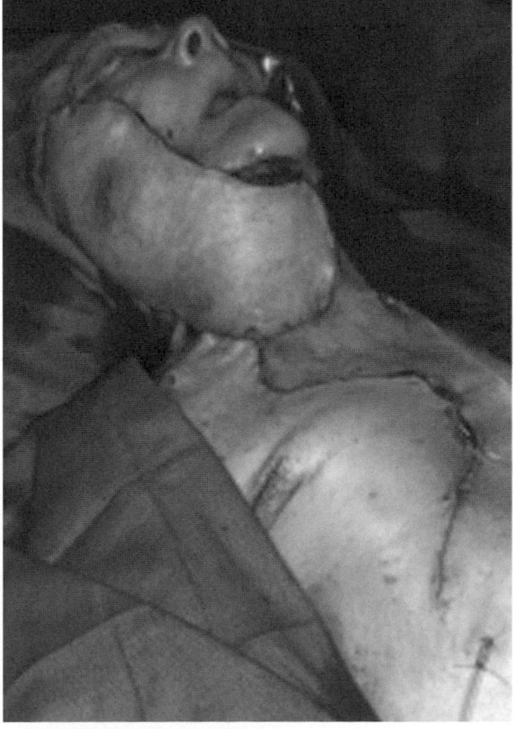

Figure 9.2 **A:** Defect status postradical resection of advanced stage metastatic malignant parotid tumor in octogenarian patient. High volume and high surface area requirement includes lateral canthus, infratemporal fossa, mandibulectomy, hemi neck, and great neurovascular structures. **B:** Pedicled pectoralis major myocutaneous flap reliably reconstructed the entire defect while allowing primary donor site closure. This was the most appropriate and efficient reconstructive option for this elderly patient with significant comorbidity considerations, despite expertise in microsurgical free tissue transfer techniques.

much as the exact status of the transverse cervical vessels is often unmentioned in the operative notes of previously treated patients. Significant disadvantages are those of the pedicled latissimus transfer above in addition to the occasional requirement for donor-site skin grafting, making this flap a tertiary option.

OTHER FLAPS

Myocutaneous flaps based on the platysma and sternocleidomastoid muscles have been described but offer little advantage in contemporary reconstruction. A more common potential application is that of the sternocleidomastoid muscle as a superiorly pedicled muscle flap to bolster posterior oral and laryngopharyngeal suture lines. Rotation is limited by the spinal accessory nerve's entry into the anterior border of the muscle. In the context of staging supraomohyoid neck dissection or modified radical techniques, this is particularly facilitated. High-stage neck disease as well as extracapsular extension of metastatic disease would be contraindications to this application.

Similarly, the levator scapula and posterior scalene muscles may be detached from their insertions as superiorly based muscle flaps for similar applications. Bipedicled and inferiorly unipedicled strap muscle flaps (e.g., omohyoid) survive via microvascular supply transmitted through their origins and insertions and from neovascularization by surrounding tissues more centrally. These muscles are occasionally useful for reconstruction of partial laryngeal and tracheal defects after conservation and extended conservation procedures.

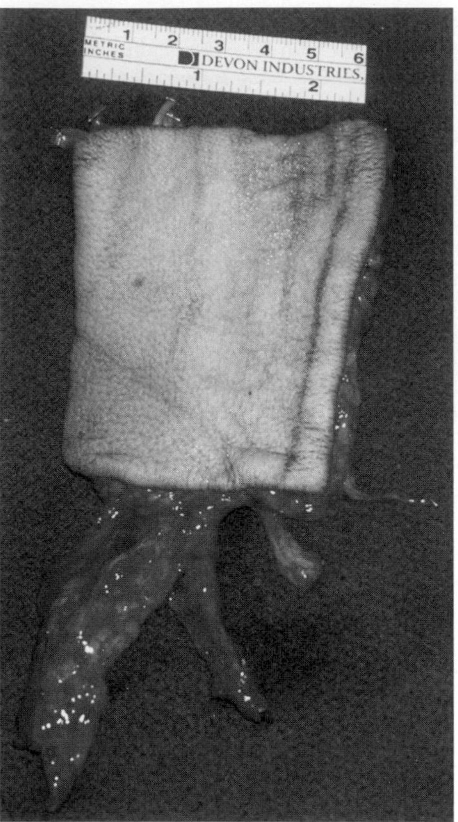

Figure 9.3 Fasciocutaneous microneurovascular forearm free flap ready for transfer. Left to Right foreground: vascular pedicle, palmaris longus tendon, antebrachial cutaneous nerves (see Ref. 2). A free flap is a composite block of tissue based on a defined vascular pedicle and territory. The block is "free" of the geometric restrictions imposed on pedicled flaps, which must remain attached through their vascular pedicles. This technique has revolutionized head and neck reconstruction since clinical application in the 1970s. These techniques are particularly applicable to large defects of the skull base, midface, oral cavity, pharynx, and mandible.

FREE MICRONEUROVASCULAR TISSUE TRANSFER

Clinical microsurgery has provided the single most important contribution to reconstruction of the head and neck patient in the last three decades, restoring patients to a heretofore unprecedented degree of form and function. It is now possible to replace resected or missing tissues with nearly identical tissue types (e.g., mucosa, bone, sensate skin, composites), volumes, and character. Many of the most significant drawbacks inherent to pedicled myocutaneous transfers can be more than adequately addressed through the thoughtful selection of microsurgical techniques.

The "free flap" is a composite block of tissue (fascia, muscle, fat, bone, skin, visceral conduit) perfused by a defined anatomic vascular pedicle and its subsequent myocutaneous or fasciocutaneous perforating vessels (Fig. 9.3). It is geometrically "free" of limitations imposed by the requirements of an attached pedicle. In another sense, such transfers are "free" of limitations imposed by restricted tissue types, which could be reasonably transferred to the head and neck region via available locoregional pedicles. Properly executed flap design and development usually produce a reconstruction with a vascularity that is superior to its historical counterparts or alternatives. This, in addition to the advantages above, has decreased the incidence of dehiscence, fistulization, partial flap loss, stricture, and the like. Microsurgical technique has allowed ablative surgeons to extend their resective techniques in more radical directions in both curative- and palliative-intent procedures through providing unprecedented reliability and versatility of design. Despite numerous studies on multiple simultaneous free flap reconstructions, such microsurgical tours de force rarely offer significant advantage over a well-planned single flap design in excess of a very real increase in risk and morbidity. Similar planning considerations facilitate the avoidance of vein grafts in the overwhelming majority of cases.

The discipline of reconstructive microsurgery demands a degree of discipline and experience as well as applied technical expertise that mandate significant additional training and commitment. It is a responsibility of the head and neck surgeon to foster the development of the multidisciplinary simultaneous two-team approach.

As important as the actual microsurgical anastomosis are the preoperative planning, flap selection, flap development, and perioperative care of the microsurgical patient. Characteristics of the ideal donor site include:

- Long, large caliber, anatomically consistent vascular pedicle
- Minimal donor-site morbidity—functional, aesthetic
- Simultaneous two-team approach
- Where applicable:
  - Provision for functional motor capability
  - Sensibility
  - Secretory mucosa
- Bone stock capable of accepting osseointegrated implants

Patient Selection

The most significant application of microsurgical technique to reconstructive head and neck surgery is in posttumor ablation.

In general, most patients who are candidates for curative-intent resective procedures producing defects that would benefit from free flap reconstruction are candidates for this technique. Numerous publications have documented the safety and efficacy of such procedures in the elderly. The general principle of "keep it simple" must prevail, for example, over the desire to reconstruct a posterolateral composite mandible defect with a fibula in a edentulous septuagenarian diabetic with severe coronary artery disease, just for the sake of reestablishing radiographic bony continuity. Prohibitive or prognostic comorbid factors must be considered and respected in the planning phase. Age, chronic obstructive pulmonary disease (COPD), hypertensive vasculopathy and arteriosclerotic vascular disease, malnutrition, alcoholism, and active smoking all undoubtedly contribute to a potentially compromised outcome—regardless of technique—and are common denominators in the head and neck cancer patient population. None of these factors, however, is absolutely prohibitive to the application of these techniques. Similarly, many of these entities have systemic impact and donor-site considerations in terms of donor vessels and wound healing, particularly the lower extremity fibula donor site.

Microsurgical techniques are also safe in the pediatric population but demand a very high level of expertise and capability.

Previous treatment history is of critical importance in preoperative planning, with particular reference to recipient vessels. This is amplified if the patient has been treated elsewhere, given the ambient lack of detail pertinent to microsurgical issues present in most operative notes. Vein grafts are usually avoidable through careful planning with regard to flap choice, recipient vessels, and contingency planning in such cases. Irradiation affects not only the microcirculation but also major vessels in terms of accelerating atherosclerotic degeneration, intimal and media thickening, and increasing endothelial friability and dehiscence. Attention to technical detail is of the utmost importance in such cases, which provide a significant challenge to even the most experienced team. Previous surgery either independent of or in addition to radiation history adds an additional degree of difficulty in terms of recipient vessel dissection, quality, and choice.

Points of Technique

Many aspects of resective surgery should be modified when a microsurgical transfer is anticipated. Routine sacrifice of the external jugular vein destroys a potential recipient vein or vein graft conduit and can usually be thoughtfully avoided. Major arterial and venous vessels that are to be transected should be handled with the utmost technical care and sacrificed somewhat away from their takeoff to provide a satisfactory stump for end-to-end anastomosis. This includes the internal jugular vein stump in radical dissections where end-to-side techniques can be applied to a stump of satisfactory length in creating a functional end-to-end flow configuration (21).

Flap ischemia times are generally to be minimized but are rarely defining issues in flap survival. Most times are less than 1 hour, with the exception of osseous transfers, which usually require osteosynthesis insetting of skeletal components prior to revascularization. Enteric (jejunum), muscle, and osteocyte components of flaps are most sensitive to ischemia. Complete dissection of the flap *in situ* and microscopic positioning and recipient vessel preparation *prior* to pedicle transection maximize success and minimize overall ischemic time. Flap cooling with iced saline throughout the ischemic period significantly reduces the tissues' metabolic demand and extends available time (warm versus cold schemia time) prior to the onset of critical and irreversible changes.

Complications

In the most expert of hands, flap failure occurs in about 5% of cases or less, including the most complex of reconstructions. Free flap loss is usually, but not always, an all-or-none phenomenon. Most failures occur within the first 72 hours of revascularization. The majority of anastomotic failures should be successfully salvaged through timely recognition and revision (22). A myriad of philosophies of perioperative management and monitoring techniques exists, and these techniques are largely an individual, idiosyncratic, and theoretical art. It may be that specialized instrumentation for free flap monitoring serves to improve survival only through increasing the vigilance of the nursing staff caring for the patient rather than through some intrinsic superiority to clinical observation alone (23).

Vessel wall dissection, disruption, and suture puncture result in endothelial discontinuity and exposure of thrombogenic subendothelial collagen. Platelet aggregation is enhanced through the production of the prostaglandin thromboxane-A_2 by activated platelets. Acute thrombosis is largely based on this physiologic phenomenon in addition to unfavorable mechanical factors (endothelial flaps, valves, adventitial inclusion, leaks, pleating, size mismatch, etc.) that may be present. This forms the basis for postoperative aspirin administration and for acute infusions of low molecular weight dextran-40 after revascularization. Bolus doses of 1,000 to 3,000 units of heparin are typically given just before pedicle transection and again just before flap reperfusion. Systemic heparinization does not occur and is not continued. Minidose heparin infusions are sometimes continued in cases requiring vein grafts or in revision cases. Restoration of endothelial continuity occurs over the ensuing 2 weeks.

Maintenance of perfusion through normal blood pressures is ensured by euvolemic status and by not attempting to overly modulate blood pressure in hypertensives. Similarly, the maintenance of normothermia minimizes peripheral vasoconstriction and sympathetic outflow, which are generally deleterious to microvascular blood flow. Attention to detail in flap design and insetting (pedicle geometry, tension, kinking) should minimize the need for special head positioning. A reverse Trendelenburg position to about 15 to 30 degrees is preferred and relatively favorable with regard to general edema, intracranial pressure, and venous outflow, and relatively unfavorable with regard to arterial inflow, cerebrospinal fluid (CSF) leak, and maintenance of slight neck extension.

The irreversible failure of reperfusion through a microvascular anastomosis is termed the "no reflow phenomenon" and has as its basis ischemia and endothelial cell swelling, luminal occlusion, and the release of toxic free radicals with ongoing distal soft tissue damage and necrosis.

Subsequent sections in this chapter address commonly used flap transfers and issues of selection and design.

Radial Forearm Flap

This flap is a fasciocutaneous design with sensate capabilities based on the *radial* vessels. It was one of the first flaps commonly applied to head and neck reconstruction (intraoral) and represents one of the most common transfers in contemporary reconstruction. Fasciocutaneous vessels are transmitted to the skin paddle via the lateral intermuscular (brachioradialis-flexor carpi radialis) septum. The flap may incorporate a monocortical segment of the radius bone (up to 10 cm) by including a cuff of flexor pollicis longus muscle. Sensate capabilities are provided by the *lateral and medial antebrachial cutaneous nerves*. The phe-

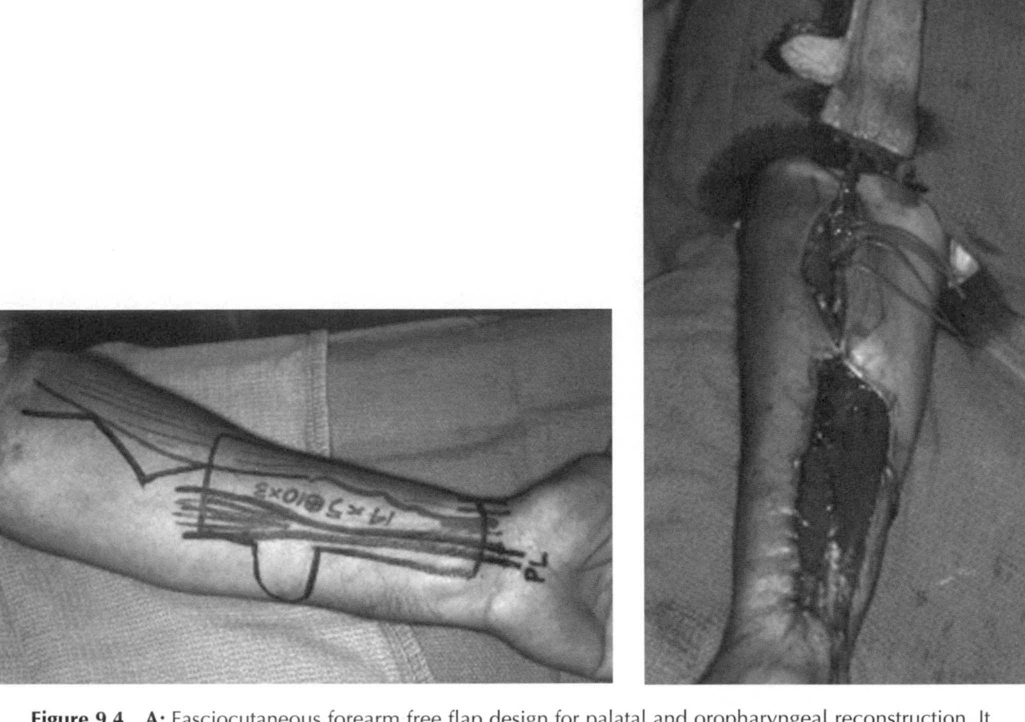

A B

Figure 9.4 **A:** Fasciocutaneous forearm free flap design for palatal and oropharyngeal reconstruction. It will include the palmaris longus tendon that will be sewn into residual pharyngeal constrictor muscles laterally. **B:** Completed dissection of radial forearm microvascular fasciocutaneous free flap. The flap (background) remains attached and perfused by the radial artery and concomitant vein(s) until the recipient site is ready for microsurgical anastomosis.

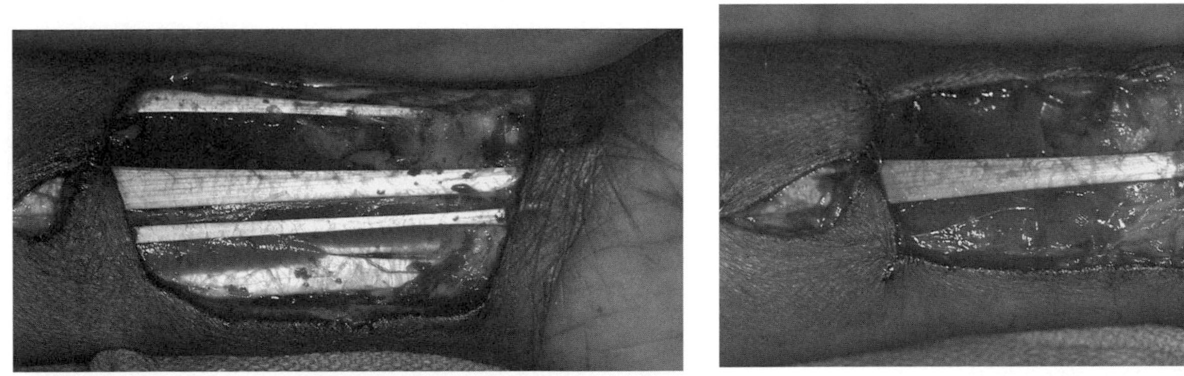

A B

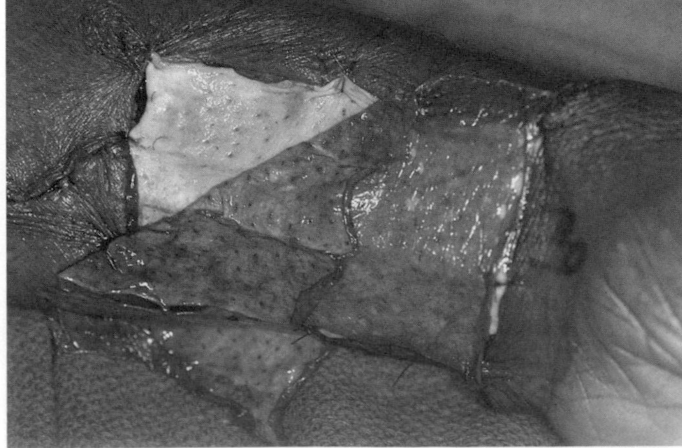

C

Figure 9.5 **A:** Typical defect after dissection of the radial forearm fasciocutaneous free flap. **B:** Perimeter skin is advanced centrally and tacked down to minimize overall dimensions of defect. Musculature is imbricated over exposed tendons where possible. Flexor carpi radialis tendon remains exposed, covered by a veil of paratenon. **C:** Acellular dermal allograft (Alloderm®)—autologous split thickness skin graft composite reconstruction of forearm defect. A tie-over bolster dressing and immobilization splint are then placed and maintained for about 1 week.

nomenon of "sensory upgrading" has been observed in sensate reconstruction of the oral cavity where the transferred forearm flap, anastomosed to the recipient lingual nerve, demonstrates greater fidelity in two-point discriminatory capability *after transfer* into the mouth than when *in situ* in the forearm *prior to* transfer (24). This is believed to be due to a greater cortical representation devoted to orolingual structures subserved by the lingual nerve.

In addition to the capabilities above, the flap's most intrinsic advantage is its thin, pliable soft tissue component, which has made it outstanding for intraoral reconstruction. This has facilitated tongue mobility in particular, and allowed reconstitution of contours, sulci, vestibules, and the like, with relative ease. Inclusion of the palmaris longus tendon with the flap offers some theoretical advantage in suspending the flap laterally in palatal and total lower lip reconstruction (25). The flap is also well suited to pharyngeal, laryngeal, and esophageal defects as a patched or tubed flap, and to complex external defects such as cheek, forehead, and nose (Fig. 9.4A,B). Drawbacks to this flap center around its distal and outwardly obvious donor-site deformity with mandatory skin grafting in most applications (Fig. 9.5A–C). In long-term follow-up, the impact is greatly diminished and well accepted by most. The bone stock provided by this transfer is usually inadequate and far inferior to alternatives where osseointegrated implantation is anticipated for oromandibular rehabilitation (26). The combination of reconstruction plate plus fasciocutaneous flap, while apparently an attractive alternative to composite bone containing free flaps, is usually an inferior choice in anterior reconstruction, and in application it is often neither time- nor resource-conserving.

Lateral Arm Flap

This flap is a fasciocutaneous design with sensate capabilities based on the posterior branches of the *radial collateral* vessels. Fasciocutaneous perforators are transferred to the overlying skin through the lateral intermuscular (brachialis, brachioradialis-triceps) septum. It may incorporate the *posterior cutaneous nerve of the arm* for sensate capability or the *posterior cutaneous nerve of the forearm* for vascularized interpositional grafting. Transfer of a portion of the humerus and fascia-only designs have been described. The skin and subcutaneous tissues of this region of the arm are somewhat thicker and less pliable than the forearm counterpart. Pedicle caliber is similar to the radial forearm vessels. Flap geometry involving pedicle entry in the midportion of the cutaneous paddle complicates application to certain defects. Flap pedicle dissection is more difficult and it is of shorter length than that of the radial forearm flap. This flap has advantages in that the donor site may be closed primarily with a single linear scar positioned in a location easily camouflaged by clothing, including short sleeves. This may be more appropriate to female and younger patients. In the male patient, this area of the arm may bear less hair than the forearm, making this flap a better choice for intraoral reconstructions in such patients.

Latissimus Dorsi

The latissimus dorsi is most commonly transferred as a muscle-only flap for the reconstruction of massive scalp defects. It is skin grafted with a meshed STSG for final resurfacing. The flap is based on the *thoracodorsal* pedicle, which is part of the subscapular system of flaps. The branch to the serratus anterior may be sacrificed, producing a very long pedicle of large caliber, facilitating anastomosis in the neck. The muscle is broad and thin, facilitating insetting over the calvarial contour. This flap does offer sensate capability, although motor reconstruction has been described. A lateral decubitus harvesting requirement usually mandates intraoperative position change and is a relative disadvantage.

Rectus Abdominus

This flap is based on the deep inferior epigastric vascular pedicle and is generally transferred as a myocutaneous flap or as a muscle-only flap. It does not support sensate needs and is usually not applied as a functional motor reconstruction. The flap may be designed in a multitude of orientations but is usually oriented vertically or horizontally [transverse rectus abdominus muscle (TRAM)]. This transfer has found particular application in the reconstruction of skull base defects where the muscle component may be used to reliably seal off the subarachnoid space and the overlying soft tissue to pad and resurface massive scalp and forehead soft tissue and skeletal defects. The flap is capable of supporting a large volume of overlying soft tissue and finds additional application in massive combined head and neck defects (Figs. 9.6 and 9.7). Vertical designs are commonly used in the reconstruction of total glossectomy defects.

Simultaneous flap harvest and resection are conducted with ease. Unilateral transfers may result in measurable abdominal wall weakness, which is well compensated by retained obliques, contralateral rectus, and muscle-sparing harvest techniques. This weakness is not noticed in most individuals. Herniation potential should be minimal with attention to detail in closure and with muscle-sparing harvest.

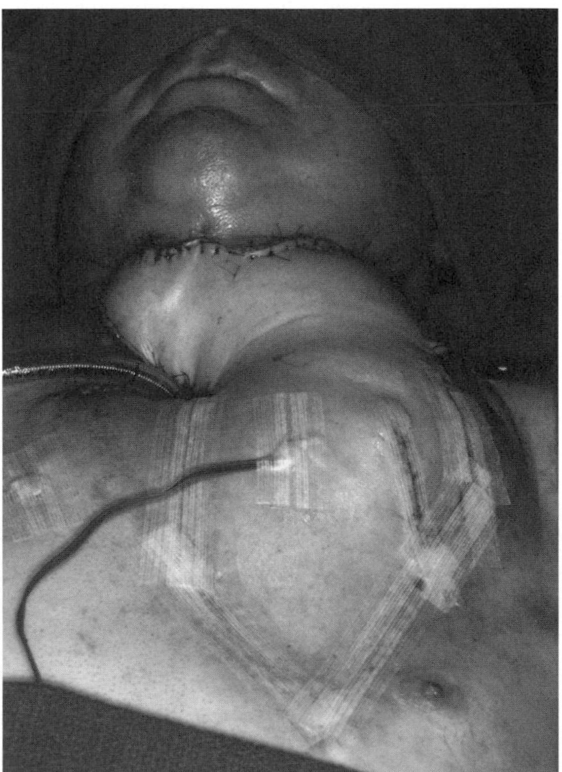

Figure 9.6 Quadripod modification of transverse rectus abdominus myocutaneous free flap for reconstruction of defect secondary to resection of peristomal recurrence. Considerations include full-thickness chest wall, exposed lung, great vessels, and brachial plexus. Microvascular free tissue transfer techniques have revolutionized the reconstruction of massive high volume, high surface area defects in previously operated and radiated fields.

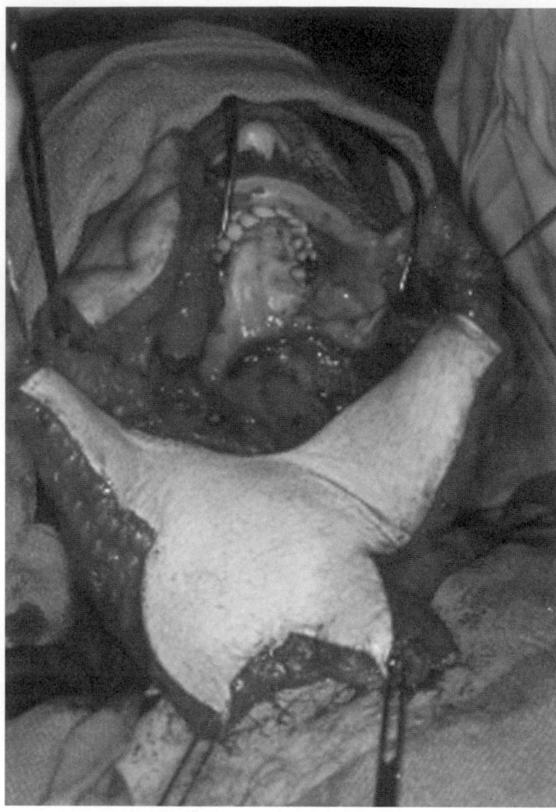

A

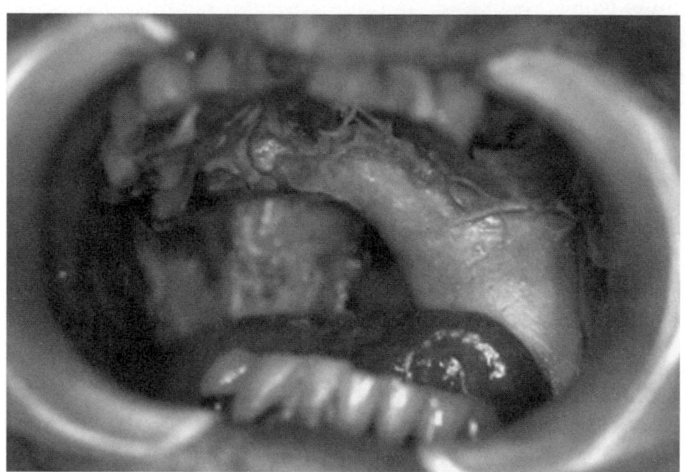

B

Figure 9.7 **A:** Quadripod modification of transverse rectus abdominus myocutaneous (TRAM) microvascular free flap for reconstruction of multiplanar oropharyngeal defect. Microsurgical free tissue transfer techniques have revolutionized the reconstruction of massive high volume, high surface area defects in previously operated and radiated fields. **B:** Multiplanar oropharyngeal reconstruction through quadripod modification of the TRAM microvascular free flap at 1 month after surgery.

Fibula

This transfer has revolutionized functional and aesthetic oromandibular reconstruction and rehabilitation since its application to the mandible. Subsequent refinements in technique have extended its application and usefulness. The flap is based on the *peroneal* vessels of the tibial-peroneal trunk, and the cutaneous component is perfused primarily by septocutaneous vessels transmitted via the posterior crural septum (Fig. 9.8A,B). Skin and muscle (flexor hallucis longus) may be reliably transferred with the bone and may be critical components in intraoral and external resurfacing (skin) and in submandibular contouring (flexor). These soft tissue components may be differentially inset, adding flexibility in the application of this flap.

The osseous component may be used to reconstruct the entire mandible (Fig. 9.9). Its dimensions are aesthetically ideal

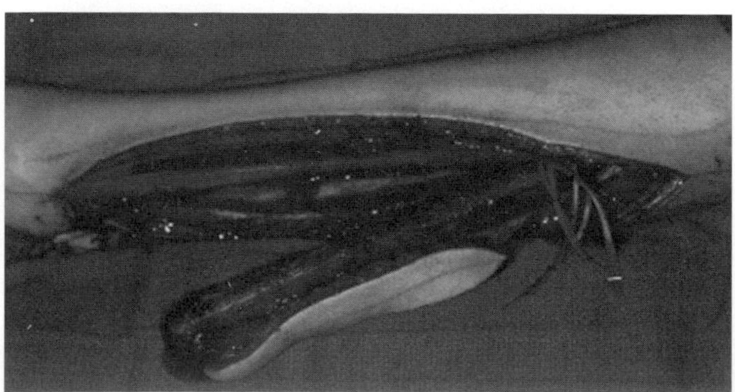

A

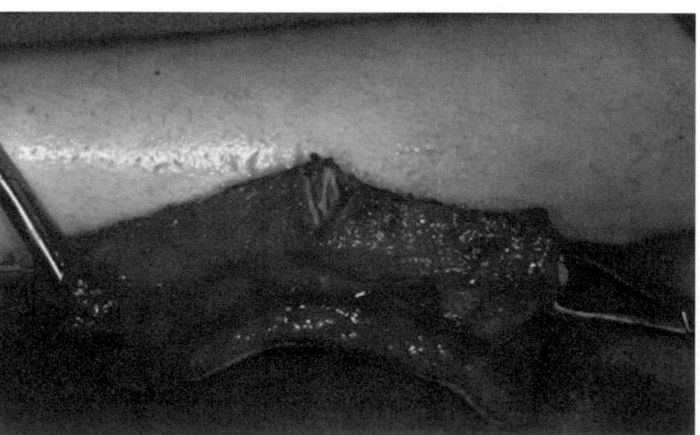

B

Figure 9.8 **A:** Osteomyocutaneous fibula free flap in situ. Cutaneous paddle may be positioned intraorally or extraorally, or both, depending on associated soft tissue requirements. Bone only designs are also common. **B:** Double closing wedge osteotomies retain medial periosteal attachments that allow anatomic skeletal reconstruction and centripetal perfusion of the bone after rigid internal fixation.

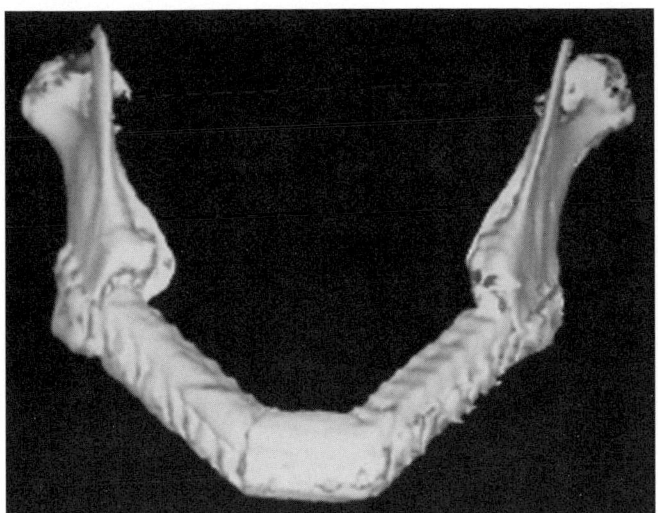

Figure 9.9 Angle-to-angle fibular free flap (skeletal component) reconstruction of mandible in three-dimensional computed tomographic reformatting. Note anatomic contouring and dimension of neomandible through two double-closing wedge osteotomies and titanium miniplate fixation.

for mandibular reconstruction and functionally ideal for osseointegrated implant placement. Simultaneous and independent maxillary reconstruction has also been accomplished with this flap (27) (Fig. 9.10A,B). More recent refinements of this transfer have included the *lateral sural cutaneous nerve*, adding sensate capability to the skin paddle.

Disadvantages of this flap are occasional difficulties in soft tissue wound healing characteristic of the lower extremity and the potential involvement of pedicle vessels with atherosclerotic vascular disease. Studies of postoperative function have demonstrated no significant long-term donor-site morbidity and only short-term ankle stiffness (28). An STSG is occasionally required to resurface the donor site in larger reconstructions.

The potential for osseointegrated implantation of dental prostheses represents a significant technical advancement over tissue-borne prosthodontics with the direct transfer of masticatory force to the underlying bone (Fig. 9.11A,B). It is important to realize, however, that this is an expensive and multistaged series of procedures, out of reach financially for most head and neck patients. This is despite the potential for primary implant placement at the time of flap transfer. In most series, fewer than one quarter of patients complete this rehabilitative sequence.

Iliac Crest

This flap is based on the *deep circumflex iliac artery system* (DCIA) and is capable of transferring large amounts of soft tissue and bone into massive defects. The composite flap may include skin, subcutaneous tissue, iliac crest, and the internal oblique muscle. Disadvantages have centered around the sheer volume of tissue and potential donor-site morbidity. The capability of differential insetting of flap components is an attractive feature of this transfer (29). Excepting the most demanding situations, this flap has been relegated to a secondary role behind the fibula flap for most oromandibular defects. Simultaneous flap harvest and resection are conducted with ease. This flap does not support motored or sensate reconstructions.

Jejunum

Interposition reconstruction of segmental pharyngoesophageal or high cervical esophageal defects is well suited to this flap, which is based on the accompanying *mesenteric* arcade vessels. The transverse cervical vessels are particularly good for recipient anastomosis if preserved in neck dissection procedures. A "sentinel loop" may be developed and brought out through the neck incision for monitoring of this otherwise buried flap (30). The advantage of transferring a secretory mucosal surface to the oral and pharyngeal axis is real, particularly in the context of radiation therapy. In such instances, the flap may be divided along its antimesenteric border and inset as a patch graft.

Potential disadvantages are those of laparotomy and enteric anastomosis. Endoscopic flap harvest may minimize donor-site morbidity. A feeding jejunostomy is required. An advantage of this flap over the gastric transposition is the ability to superiorly inset the flap to *any* level defect, whereas the transposed, pedicled stomach often has difficulty reaching above the tongue base (31,32). The superior vascularity of the transferred jejunum

A

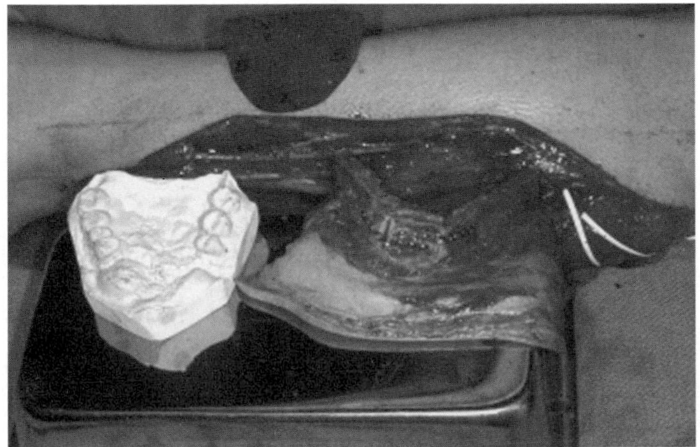

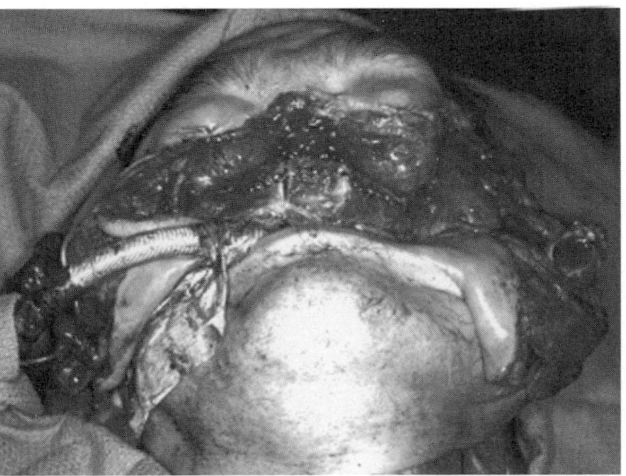

B

Figure 9.10 **A:** Using templates and dental models, the formerly straight bone is osteotomized and miniplate fixated while perfused in the leg. This minimizes schemia time and maximizes viable osteocyte transfer. **B:** Total bilateral maxillectomy reconstruction through fibula osteomyocutaneous free flap.

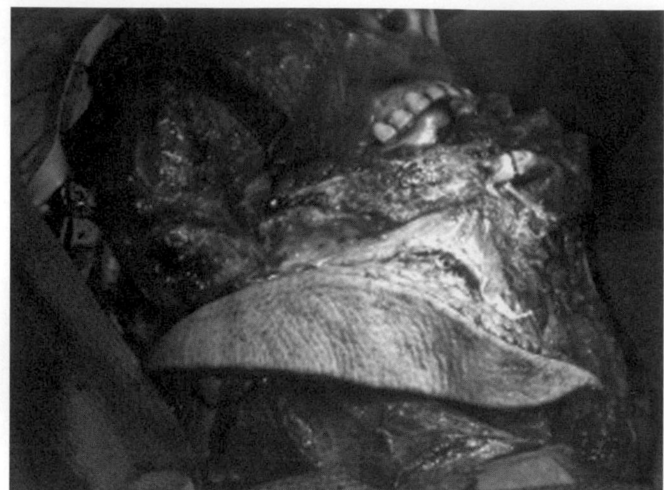

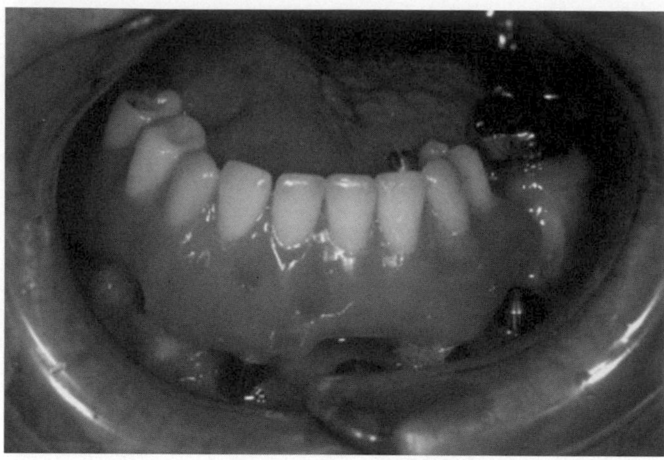

A B

Figure 9.11 **A:** Fibula osteomyocutaneous free flap internally fixated to residual mandible in anatomic relationship. The soft tissue component may be rotated intraorally or extraorally to reconstruct associated defects and to facilitate monitoring of the skeletal component. **B:** The implant bone mandibular prosthesis transmits masticatory force directly to the fibula bone through its osteointegrated implant abutments. This construct is biomechanically much more favorable than conventional tissue borne prosthodontics.

may reflect a lower dehiscence and fistulization rate than the relatively distal and ischemic stomach at this level of insetting. The jejunal transfer is limited by the level at which it is easy and safe to perform anastomosis to the remaining esophagus (thoracic inlet) without the need for thoracotomy and/or additional risk for intrathoracic anastomotic leak or fistula (the inferior level is *not* an issue for gastric transposition). Additional disadvantages include two circumferential enteric anastomoses in the neck (stomach—one anastomosis only), the propensity to anastomotic stricture requiring dilation therapy, and the lack of total esophagectomy recognizing the increased risk profile for synchronous and metachronous carcinomas, submucosal direct extension, and skip metastasis from more inferiorly positioned primaries. The mesenteric vessels must be respected for their friability and tendency toward rosetting and intimal separation.

SITE/FUNCTION-SPECIFIC CONSIDERATIONS

Reconstruction of the Scalp

The specialized hair-bearing tissues of the scalp are generally unyielding and require careful planning in reconstruction of mid-sized defects. Small defects may be closed with a variety of local rotation-advancement flap designs incorporating galeatomy and skin-grafted donor-site defects that are small and easily camouflaged by neighboring hair. Mid-sized defects may be handled by skin grafting pericranium and later tissue expansion of adjacent scalp, with its attendant morbidity in terms of cranial deformity and discomfort while under expansion. The Orticochea 3 and 4 flap designs are of great use in these defects and have been applied to defects as large as 20 square centimeters. Microsurgical technique has also aided this area of reconstruction in cases of scalp loss or ablation through skin-grafted latissimus dorsi transfer to reliably cover exposed calvarium with durable, easily contoured soft tissue. Aesthetic reconstruction of the frontal hairline is optimally performed with microsurgical transfer of a contralateral superficial temporal vessel-based Juri flap providing a normodirectional hair stream.

Skull Base Reconstruction

Separation of the intracranial contents and CSF compartment from oral and nasal cavity bacteria contamination, air entry, and from CSF leak are axiomatic. Physical protection of the brain where craniectomy is of significant size or critically located is a secondary but occasionally critical consideration. Dural closure is critical in the anterior cranial fossa and a variety of biomaterials are available for patch closure of such defects. This is often augmented with fibrin glues and fat grafts. The galea-pericranial flap is most commonly used to achieve oronasocranial separation in craniofacial procedures. The temporalis muscle is also available for this purpose. Large-scalp flaps may be mobilized to achieve surface closure with posterior donor-site STSG placement to complete the reconstruction. Larger orbitocranial and lateral defects are most commonly addressed with the TRAM flap, placing the muscle component against the brain and basal skull defect. Calvarial reconstruction in this context is generally unnecessary.

Craniofacial defects not requiring flap reconstruction and with sizable craniectomy and usable overlying soft tissue are usually appropriate for cranioplasty, which may be achieved with a variety of materials. In contrast to pediatric cranial vault reconstruction, the creation of an extended donor site for autologous bone is generally unnecessary and often inappropriate to the oncologic population. This statement is possible due to eminently biocompatible implant materials such as hydroxyapatite (HA) cements and bioresorbable and titanium mesh (Fig. 12A–C). Polymethylmethacrylate implants should be relegated to the archives of skull base reconstruction and were poor alternatives to bone grafts in their time. Mesh implants are easily contoured to the depths of such three-dimensional defects to dampen the pulsations of the underlying brain and to provide a scaffolding on which to place and mold the HA cement inlay. Surface contouring is then easily achieved to absolute anatomic precision. Bioresorbable mesh may be considered in cases requiring surveillance imaging or adjuvant radiotherapy, as it is radiotransparent and does not obfuscate such imaging studies.

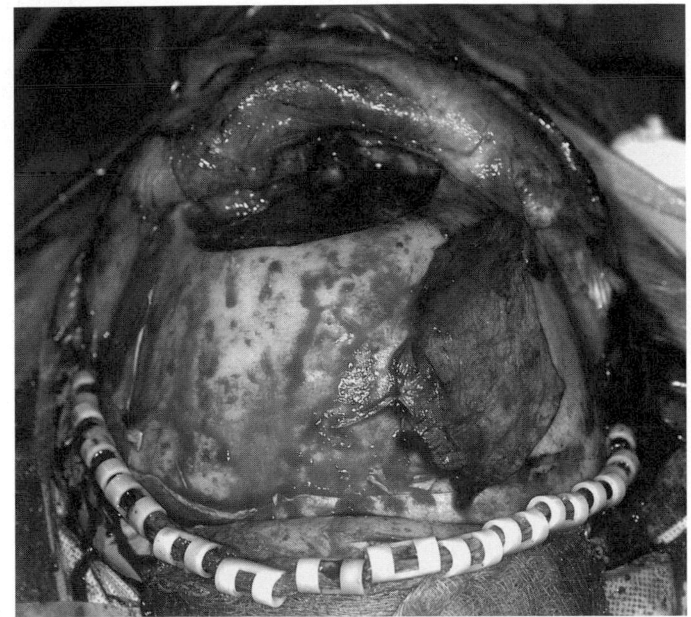

A

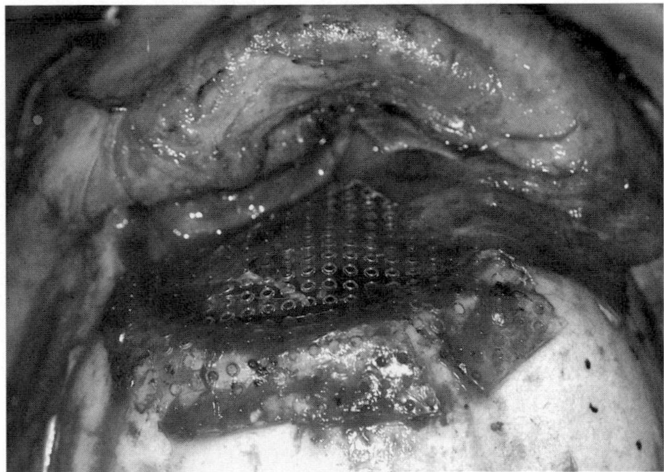

B

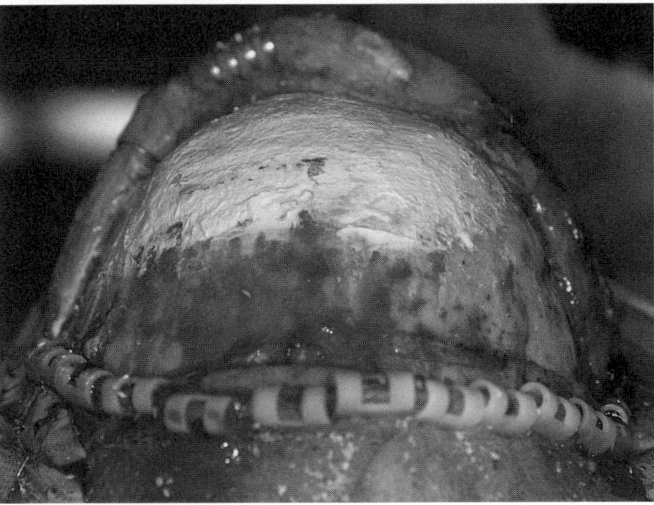

C

Figure 9.12 **A:** Full-thickness fronto-orbital defect viewed from vertex through bicoronal flap exposure. Galea-pericranial flap in right temporal field. This will be transposed beneath cranioplasty materials to ensure sinonasocranial separation and to minimize risk for descending infection, cerebrospinal fluid leak, and pneumocephalus. **B:** Resorbable mesh (polylactic acid-polygyglycolic acid copolymer) is inset into deep aspect of defect to dampen effects of brain pulsation on the orbit and on overlying cranioplasty cement during setting phase. It will degrade in about 18 months through hydrolysis. The galeal-pericranial flap is transposed beneath it. Screw fixation (resorbable or titanium) provides internal fixation at the perimeter. This biomaterial is radiotransparent and facilitates both the delivery of therapeutic radiation and postoperative surveillance diagnostic imaging studies. **C:** Hydroxyapatite cement completes the cranioplasty reconstruction. It is able to fill complex three-dimensional defects and can be sculpted to recreate any anatomic contour requirement. This biomaterial is eminently biocompatible and is capable of osteointegration where its perimeter is on contact with native bone.

Oral Cavity/Oropharynx

The mandible is of fundamental importance to the functions of mastication, deglutition, and articulation, and to the aesthetics of the lower third of the face. Interruption of the continuity of the mandibular arch, therefore, has the potential to profoundly affect these vital processes and to compromise critical protective, communicative, and sustentative functions. It is through the provision of a stable gnathic base via its alveolar process and teeth, and in providing muscular attachments to support the larynx (suprahyoid musculature), tongue (floor of mouth muscular sling, e.g., mylohyoid muscles), anteroposterior axial attachments for extrinsic tongue musculature (e.g., genioglossus muscles), and muscles of mastication (elevator) and mandibular depressor group muscles that it expresses its functional importance. Ablative disruption of these aspects of functional anatomy may contribute to airway compromise and aspiration (collapse of anteroposterior projection affecting oropharyngeal level patency) and malnutrition (decrease in masticatory efficiency through loss of teeth, muscular attachments), and profoundly disturb communicative function. Lower facial aesthetics are influenced by the inferior mandibular contour, transverse width, anteroposterior projection of the mentum, and vertical height. Disturbances of these aspects of mandibular function are manifest in the "Andy Gump" deformity, orthognathic dentofacial syndromes of chin deficiency or prominence, with or without malocclusion and abnormal lip posture, and cherubic facies.

Unrestricted movement of the tongue is critical to both articulation and the oral motor phase of swallowing function. The maintenance of this range of motion is of paramount importance in considerations of oral cavity reconstruction. Partial glossectomy defects of both oral and base tongue can usually be closed primarily with little if any long-term loss of function. Even small tongue defects extending onto the floor of mouth or sulcus regions will be severely and disproportionately compromised by the tethering effect of primary closure here. In this defect, a bolstered STSG applied to exposed floor of mouth and tongue musculature maintains both mobility and sulcular anatomy and provides a far superior functional result. Glossectomies approximating hemitongue resection should be addressed with free tissue transfer technique using either forearm (most applications) or lateral arm (selected applications). Sensate reconstructions should generally be attempted here to augment residual tongue function. Major glossectomies over one half should be reconstructed with the vertical design of the rectus free flap. The retention of a sliver of contralateral tongue usually offers no considerable function and may be discarded. The caudal aspect of the flap is inset into the vallecula region. The muscle portion of the flap is inset into the mandible via holes drilled into its lower border, re-creating the sling configuration of the native structure. This usually leaves the bulk of the flap filling the residual volume of the oral cavity. No attempt is made to close the skin island down to the muscle surface or any other structure. Exposed fat will granulate, mucosalize, and contract into a construct remarkably similar in appearance to the native structure. As flap size reduction occurs, functional and understandable articulation is achieved by some as is oral alimentation, even with retention of the residual larynx.

Sensibility in the oral cavity is primarily subserved by the lingual and inferior alveolar nerves, with disruption resulting in uncontrollable drooling and ineffective oral preparation of a food bolus. Despite proof of the phenomenon of sensory upgrading and the technical elegance of neural anastomosis and theoretical sophistication of sensate flap reconstructions, functional outcome in most patients falls far short of normality. Nonetheless, the rational application of these techniques clearly benefits a few and should be appropriately applied.

Major palatectomy may be well addressed through the forearm free flap (Fig. 9.13). Retention of the palmaris tendon facilitates anatomic and possibly functional reconstruction. Skin grafting the deep (nasopharyngeal) side of the flap may minimize contracture and resultant velopharyngeal insufficiency. This technique may allow patients to wear either no prosthodontic device or a smaller, more manageable one.

Orbitomaxillary defects represented an early application of free flap transfers in the midface. The increasing application of microsurgical techniques to maxillectomy defects offers the promise of obviating cumbersome prosthodontic devices, which may be difficult to maintain and manipulate. As with the mandible, the ability to reconstruct a bony alveolar arch is not often followed by meaningful dental implant reconstruction. This reality has made the TRAM flap (non–bone-containing) the commonest transfer to the maxilla region. Nonetheless, osteotomized fibular flaps are intriguing, and may be the only practical solution for the total bilateral defect. Continued exploration of such composite maxillary reconstructions should be pursued, as this represents one of the few remaining underexplored areas in microsurgical head and neck reconstruction. A goal here may be to augment and provide a base for more refined and smaller prosthodontic devices.

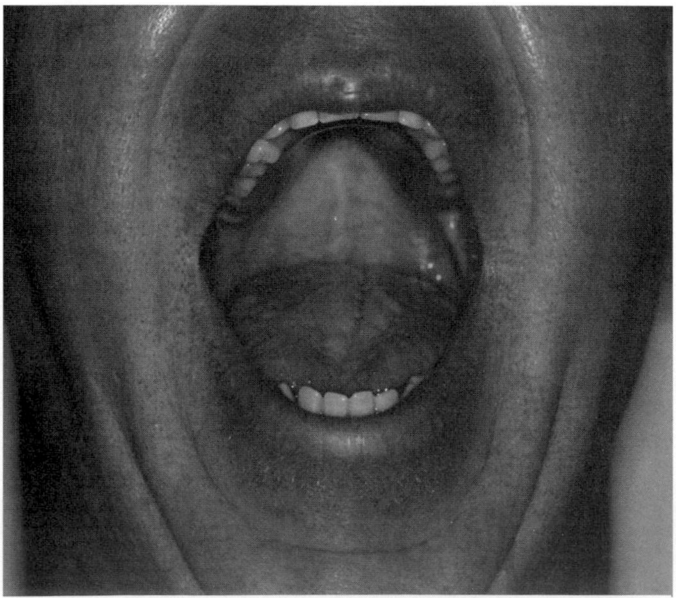

Figure 9.13 Total soft palatal reconstruction through fasciocutaneous forearm free flap (see design, Fig. 9.4A).

Pharyngolaryngeal Axis

Advanced hypopharyngeal and laryngeal tumors in both primary and organ-sparing protocol failure contexts require laryngopharyngectomy, leaving major, nearly or completely circumferential defects that must be reconstructed to restore continuity of the alimentary tract. Although primary closure is occasionally possible, patch reconstructions of either radial forearm or pectoralis to residual posterior remnant mucosa are more often required. The forearm is preferable due to its pliability characteristics, as are exploited in oral cavity reconstruction. Circumferential defects may be reconstructed with tubed radial forearm, pectoralis, jejunum, or gastric transposition. Tubed pectoralis should increasingly be of historical interest, given the superiority of the alternative flaps. Determinants of jejunum versus stomach include superior extent of defect (jejunum—unrestricted; stomach—base of tongue) as well as inferior extent of resection (jejunum—thoracic inlet; stomach—includes total esophagectomy). Inferior extent of resection considerations also apply to tubed flaps (pectoralis, forearm).

Microsurgical Reconstruction of Facial Paralysis

Long-standing cases of facial paralysis are characterized by end-organ (mimetic musculature) atrophy and fibrosis. Similar loss of function follows radical ablative cases, in which these muscles of facial expression are resected. Dynamic rehabilitation of such patients may be achieved through free tissue transfer techniques, centering on the reconstruction of lower third movements, specifically smiling. The sequence begins with the identification of contralateral buccal branches of the facial nerve and cross-face nerve grafting using a reversed sural nerve graft. After clinical evidence of the arrival of fibers to the affected side (about 1 year), the microsurgical transfer of gracilis *(medial femoral circumflex-obturator)*, serratus *(subscapular-long thoracic)*, or pectoralis minor *(subclavian branches)* muscle may be performed with microvascular and microneural anastomosis. Muscle insetting is from zygoma to commissure, emphasizing smile reconstruction. Advantages of this dynamic functional reconstruction include volitional and symmetric emotive firing of the reconstructed hemiface. Disadvantages include the requirement for multistaged procedures and additional procedures for periocular and upper facial rehabilitation.

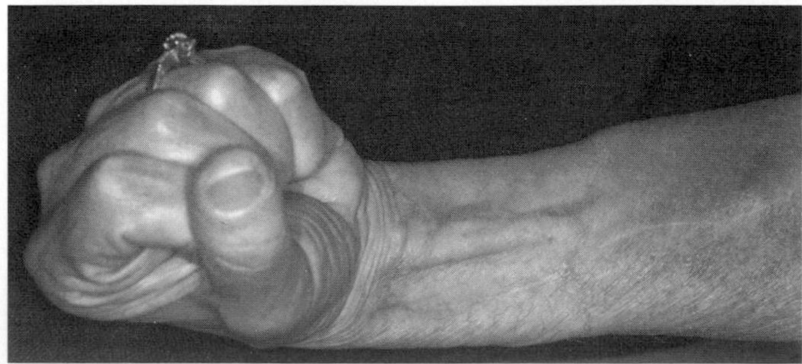

Figure 9.14 Composite grafting techniques (acellular dermal allografts + autologous STSG) have significantly impacted form and function for this visible and active donor site.

ALLOPLASTIC IMPLANTATION AND THE MODULATION OF WOUND HEALING

The science of alloplastic implantology continues to evolve, and application to aesthetic surgery should be sought in other texts. Major reconstruction of the head and neck involves primarily implant systems for osteosynthesis and reconstruction of bony discontinuity and biomaterials aimed at decreasing donor-site morbidity (e.g., bone extenders—hydroxyapatite cement; soft tissue replacement and regeneration—acellular dermal allograft) (Figs. 9.14 and 9.15A–C). Titanium is the basic rigid internal fixation material and is eminently biocompatible as a permanent implant. Absolute attention to detail in the proper application of these systems is essential and must resist an oft prevalent "hardware store" mentality (33). Autogenous bone grafts remain the material of choice for craniomaxillofacial reconstruction, and in these cases calvarial bone, rigidly fixated to adjacent skeletal components, has essentially replaced rib and iliac crest. A clear understanding of issues surrounding the surgery and healing of bone is essential to success (34). Continuity defects of the mandible spanning 4 to 6 cm in relatively favorable recipient beds (e.g., nonunion, comminution) may be grafted with tricortical grafts from the iliac crest. Longer defects or hostile recipient beds mandate revascularized free tissue transfer techniques if they are to be predictably reconstructed.

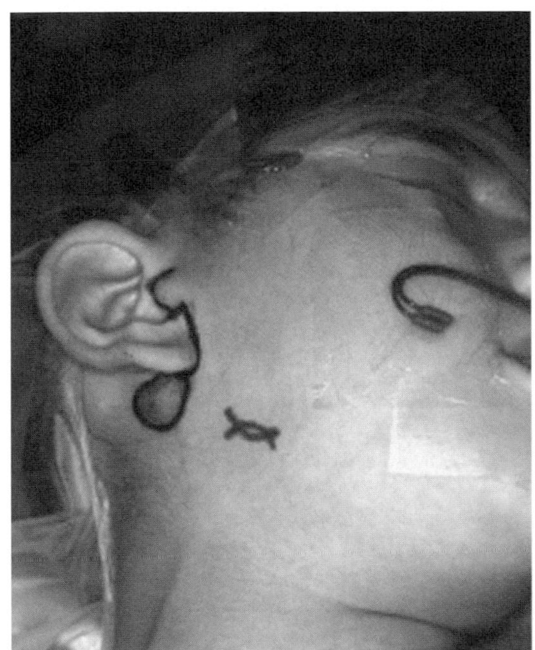

A

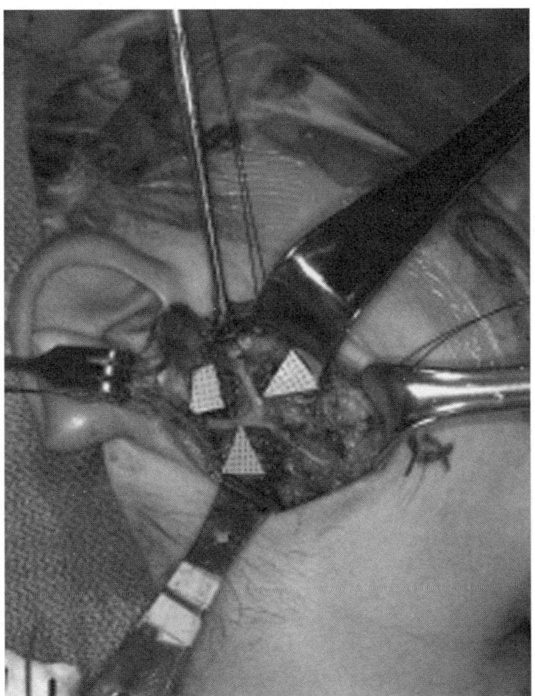

B

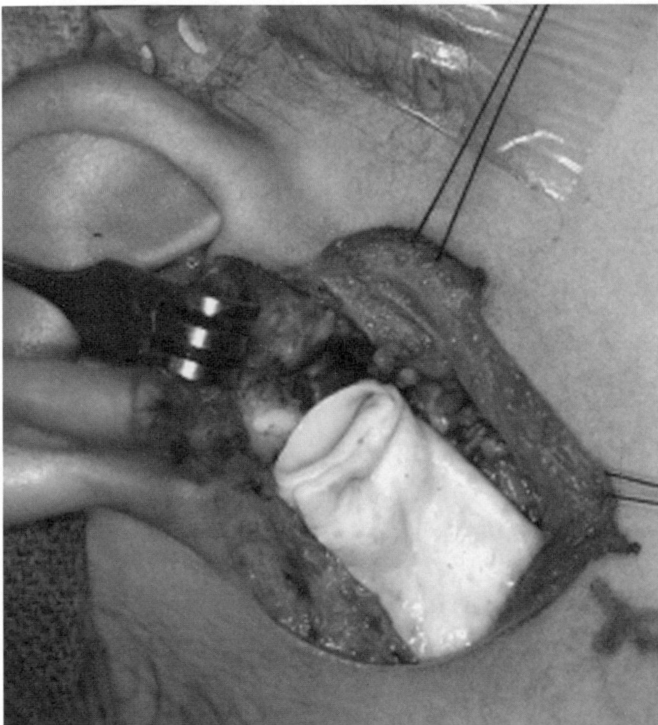

C

Figure 9.15 **A:** Recurrent congenital first branchial cleft cyst in 8-year-old girl. **B:** Defect after resection of recurrent first branchial cleft cyst including deep lobe parotid resection. **C:** Rolled acellular dermal allograft implant (Alloderm®) to ameliorate contour abnormality subsequent to radical parotid region surgery. There is evidence that the development of Frey syndrome may be diminished through the application of this technique.

THE FUTURE

Prefabrication through tissue engineering promises to extend our current spectrum of flaps with the potential to customize flap tissue types (composite mucosal and/or bone containing flaps) and composition and is a logical outgrowth of microsurgical technique. Similarly, the potential for organ transplantation has been realized with laboratory and clinical investigation in progress.

Functional outcomes assessment studies comparing various reconstructive techniques must be completed to allow rational reimbursement schedules that match the complexity and intensity of such efforts.

CONCLUSION

Contemporary reconstructive techniques, largely relying on microsurgical free tissue transfer, have restored head and neck cancer patients to a heretofore-unprecedented level of form and function. Indeed, the perhaps greatest contributions to this field in the past three decades have come from reconstructive plastic surgery. The contrast to similar patients of even a few decades ago is truly a remarkable testament to surgical creativity and technical advancement. By way of comparison, ablative procedures performed over this same time frame have undergone little change since their original descriptions at the turn of the 20th century (neck dissection, laryngectomy) and in the first half of the 20th century. Despite our current ability to restore multiple tissue types to radiographic normality, facsimiles of normal form, and semblances of sensibility, this population of unfortunate patients remains far from normal in functional outcomes assessment because of the complex integrated requirements of this region. It may well be that we have maximized our refinement of currently available reconstructive techniques over the past decade and must now look to advances from molecular oncology to reach the next set of functional and aesthetic goals for these patients through the performance of less radical and disruptive ablative procedures as allowed by therapeutic advancements from that field.

REFERENCES

1. Edgerton MT. Replacement of lining to oral cavity following surgery. *Cancer* 1951;4:110.
2. Bakamjian VY. Total reconstruction of pharynx with medially based deltopectoral skin flap. *NY State J Med* 1968;1:2771.
3. Ariyan S. The pectoralis major myocutaneous flap. A versatile flap for reconstruction in the head and neck. *Plast Reconstr Surg* 1979;63:73.
4. Seidenberg B, Rosznak SS, Hurwittes, et al. Immediate reconstruction of the cervical esophagus by a revascularized isolated jejunal segment. *Ann Surg* 1959;149:162.
5. Coleman JJ, Searles JM, Hester TR, et al. Ten years experience with free jejunal autograft. *Am J Surg* 1987;154:394–398.
6. Soutar DS, McGregor IA. The radial forearm flap in intraoral reconstruction: the experience of 60 consecutive cases. *Plast Reconstr Surg* 1986;78:1.
7. Hidalgo D. Fibula free flap: a new method of mandible reconstruction. *Plast Reconstr Surg* 1989;84:71.
8. Whetzel TP. Arterial anatomy of the face: an analysis of vascular territories and perforating cutaneous vessels. *Plast Reconstr Surg* 1992;89:591–603.
9. Baker SR, Swanson NA. *Local flaps in facial reconstruction.* St. Louis: Mosby, 1995.
10. Jackson LT. *Local flaps in head and neck reconstruction.* St. Louis: Mosby, 1985.
11. Shumrick KA. The anatomic basis for the design of forehead flaps in nasal reconstruction. *Arch Otolaryngol Head Neck Surg* 1992;118:373–379.
12. Pribaz J. A new intraoral flap: facial artery musculomucosal (FAMM) flap. *Plast Reconstr Surg* 1992;90:421–429.
13. Burget GC, Menick FJ. *Aesthetic reconstruction of the nose.* St. Louis: Mosby, 1994.
14. Stuzin JM. The anatomy and clinical applications of the buccal fat pad. *Plast Reconstr Surg* 1990;85:29–37.
15. Stuzin JM. Anatomy of the frontal branch of the facial nerve: the significance of the temporal fat pad. *Plast Reconstr Surg* 1989;83:265–271.
16. Schuller DE, Mountain RE. Head and neck reconstructive surgery. In: Lee KJ, ed. *Essential otolaryngology,* 6th ed. Norwalk, CT: Appleton & Lange, 1995: 941–967.
17. Taylor G, Palmer J. The vascular territories (angiosomes) of the body: experimental study and clinical applications. *Br J Plast Surg* 1987;AO:1–l3.
18. Sabatier RE, Bakamjian VY. Transaxillary latissimus dorsi flap reconstruction in head and neck cancer. *Am J Surg* 1985;50:427–434.
19. Urken ML, Naidu R, Lawson W, et al. The lower trapezius island musculocutaneous flap revisited. Report of 45 cases and a unifying concept of the vascular anatomy. *Arch Otolaryngol Head Neck Surg* 1991;117:502.
20. Netterville JL, Wood D. The lower trapezius flap: vascular anatomy and surgical technique. *Arch Otolaryngol Head Neck Surg* 1991;117:73.
21. DeLacure MD, Kuriakose MA, Spies AL. Clinical experience in end-to-side anastomosis with a microvascular anastomotic device. *Arch Otolaryngol Head Neck Surg* 1999;125:869–872.
22. Hidalgo DA, Jones CS. The role of emergent exploration in free-tissue transfer: a review of 150 consecutive cases. *Plast Reconstr Surg* 1990;86:492–498.
23. Jones NF. Discussion of monitoring of free flaps with surface-temperature recordings: Is it reliable? *Plast Reconstr Surg* 1992;89:500–502.
24. Boyd B, Mulholland S, Gullane P, et al. Reinnervated lateral antebrachial cutaneous neurosome flaps in oral reconstruction: Are we making sense? *Plast Reconstr Surg* 1994;93:1350–1362.
25. Sadove R, Luce E, McGrath P. Reconstruction of the lower lip and chin with the composite radial forearm-palmaris longus free flap. *Plast Reconstr Surg* 1991;88:209.
26. Frodel JL, Funk GF, Capper DW, et al. Osseointegrated implants: a comparative study of bone thickness in four vascularized bone flaps. *Plast Reconstr Surg* 1993;92:449–458.
27. Sadove R, Powell L. Simultaneous maxillary and mandibular reconstruction with one free osteocutaneous flap. *Plast Reconstr Surg* 1993;92:141–146.
28. Anthony JP, Rawnsley JD, Benhaim P, et al. Donor leg morbidity and function after fibula free flap mandible reconstruction. *Plast Reconstr Surg* 1995; 96:146–152.
29. Urken ML, Vickery C, Weinberg H, et al. The internal oblique-iliac crest osseomyocutaneous free flap in oromandibular reconstruction: report of 20 cases. *Arch Otolaryngol Head Neck Surg* 1989;115:339–349.
30. Bradford CR, Esclamado RM, Canoll WR. Monitoring of revascularized jejunal auto-grafts. *Arch Otolaryngol Head Neck Surg* 1992;18:1042–1044.
31. Spiro RH. Gastric transposition for head and neck cancer: a critical update. *Am J Surg* 1991;162:348–352.
32. Inoue Y. A retrospective study of 66 esophageal reconstructions using microvascular anastomoses: problems and our methods for atypical cases. *Plast Reconstr Surg* 1994;94:277–284.
33. DeLacure MD, Friedman CD. Metal plate and screw technology. *Otolaryngol Clin North Am* 1994;27:983–1000.
34. DeLacure MD. The physiology of bone healing and bone grafts. *Otolaryngol Clin North Am* 1994;27:859–874.

CHAPTER 10

Quality-of-Life Issues in Patients with Head and Neck Cancer

Russell K. Portenoy and Kevin T. Sperber

Historically, the overarching mission of the oncologist has been the eradication or control of neoplasms. This focus clearly is justified in the management of head and neck cancers, many of which are potentially curable, or controllable for long periods, if current antineoplastic therapies are employed.

Tumor control cannot suffice as the only goal of care, however. Management strategies may be needed to address a broad range of disturbances that result from the tumor or from the interventions used to control it. These disturbances, any one or a combination of which can profoundly undermine quality of life (QOL), often include refractory symptoms such as xerostomia or pain, functional impairments in speech and eating, and psychological problems such as depression (1–16). A decline in QOL may complicate the long-term outlook for any patient with head and neck cancer, including patients who are cured.

The acknowledgment by clinicians that QOL concerns are a fundamental aspect of care for patients with head and neck cancer is reflected by a growing interest in the investigation of QOL concerns in this population. During the last decade, an increasing number of studies have assessed the epidemiology of symptoms or psychosocial functioning, or have directly measured QOL end points during clinical trials of antineoplastic therapies (17). The measurement of QOL as a secondary outcome in clinical trials is particularly noteworthy and mirrors a trend apparent in studies of other tumor types (18–24). In the population with head and neck cancer, the diversity of treatment approaches and the evidence that very divergent therapies can yield similar survivals for some tumors (25) highlight the importance of these QOL end points as a means by which to distinguish the risks and benefits associated with different antineoplastic treatments.

In the population with head and neck cancer, therefore, the focus on primary antineoplastic treatment approaches should not minimize the importance of QOL measurement or interventions to improve QOL. Clinicians who treat patients with head and neck cancer should understand the QOL construct, address QOL concerns in the clinical setting, and continue to support the measurement of QOL end points in clinical trials to evaluate the short- and long-term costs and benefits of various treatments (26–32).

DEFINITION OF QUALITY OF LIFE

Although there is no single accepted definition, quality of life is most appropriately considered to be a construct that reflects the individual's perception of overall well-being. Some authors have emphasized that QOL may be understood as the perceived difference between the present condition and a condition that is desired (33). The term *health-related QOL* (34) is used to refer to those issues that apply specifically to the experience of illness.

The construct of health-related QOL has two main characteristics: subjectivity and multidimensionality (24). These characteristics are relevant to both the clinical assessment of QOL concerns and the measurement of QOL in therapeutic trials.

Subjectivity

Although an observer can make useful inferences about a patient's QOL based on behavioral observations (35), QOL is fundamentally a subjective appraisal of well-being by the individual. The reliability and validity of observer ratings are inherently suspect, particularly as the information about the perceptions and experiences that influence QOL becomes more detailed. Indeed, several surveys have confirmed that clinician and patient evaluation of QOL parameters are not highly correlated (6,36–38), and a survey that compared pain ratings of cancer patients and their physicians noted that clinician accuracy was especially poor when assessing patients who had the most severe pain (39). The latter finding suggests that inferences about subjective states may be most uncertain at a level of patient distress that is most clinically relevant.

The inherent subjectivity of health-related QOL implies that changes over time in QOL outcomes can occur as a result of shifting perceptions related to the disease, independent of the disease, or both. Although a problem may be overtly unchanged, such as aphonia after laryngectomy, the QOL implications of the problem cannot be assumed to be static. Over time, the problem's impact on QOL may shift with the patient's perception of the disease, availability of treatment or support services, physical or psychosocial functioning, family status, or other factors. Similarly, problems that evolve, such as gradual loss of the ability to eat, are likely to worsen QOL progressively, but the extent and course of the decline cannot be assumed in the context of the same unpredictable constellation of perceptions.

The variability of subjective QOL assessments implies that the most accurate understanding of QOL (or the impact of a specific intervention on QOL) is best achieved through a systematic, longitudinal evaluation of selected subjective outcomes. This applies equally to the evaluation of QOL in the clinical setting and in therapeutic trials.

Multidimensionality

The concept of multidimensionality reflects the observation that the very diverse perceptions or experiences that influence QOL can be usefully clustered into categories, which are usually termed *domains* or *dimensions.* It is assumed that a global measure of QOL actually derives from the patient's integration of perceptions and experiences in these varying domains (33,40). On the basis of extensive clinical experience and empiric investigations, some of which have been performed in the head and neck cancer population (see later), a large number of potential domains can be proposed for assessment of QOL. Most investigators emphasize the value of an assessment that acquires information about the physical, psychological, and social domains. Other domains, such as the spiritual, may be equally important, but, to date, have not been the focus of QOL research in the head and neck cancer population.

Each of the broad dimensions that contribute to an understanding of QOL actually subsumes many distinct elements, any one or group of which could be assessed as part of a comprehensive QOL evaluation (Table 10.1). The psychological dimension, for example, may refer to mood, psychological symptomatology, psychiatric diagnoses, positive skills or traits (e.g., coping), or any of numerous discrete concepts such as body image or sexuality. Similarly, the physical dimension could emphasize the experience of symptoms, overall physical functioning, specific capabilities (e.g., speaking, eating), or other features.

The multidimensionality of the QOL construct implies that global health-related QOL, the individual's overall perception of well-being in relation to the disease, cannot be defined by an assessment that is limited to a particular set of specific symptoms or functional concerns, such as impaired swallowing, or to one single dimension, such as physical well-being. The most accurate and clinically useful information about QOL can be acquired by evaluating a range of problems in different domains. Although a limited assessment can be informative, it should not be equated with a global evaluation of QOL.

CLINICAL IMPLICATIONS OF THE QUALITY-OF-LIFE CONSTRUCT

Clinicians who manage patients with head and neck cancer routinely assess and manage a range of disturbances that influence

TABLE 10.1 Multiple Dimensions of Quality of Life and Examples of the Types of Concerns That Could Be Addressed Within Each Dimension

Major dimensions	Generic concerns	Disease-specific concerns
Physical well-being	Common symptoms	Xerostomia, dysphagia, and other symptoms related to the disease or therapy
	Performance status	Impaired speech, swallowing, and other impairments related to the disease or therapy
Psychological well-being	Psychological symptoms (e.g., depression, anxiety)	
	Adaptation	
	Body image	Effect of disfigurement
	Intimacy, sexuality	
Social well-being	Interpersonal contacts	
	Social support	
	Family integrity	
	Marital relationship	
Other dimensions		
Role functioning	Ability to work	
	Maintaining social and familial roles	
Spiritual and religious	Religious beliefs	
	Involvement with organized religion	
	Regrets versus contentment	
	Emptiness versus sense of meaning	
Relationship with health care providers		
Financial		

overall QOL. A multidimensional evaluation of QOL concerns usually includes information about symptom distress, psychological state, physical and psychosocial functioning, status of the family, need for practical assistance at home, and other matters suggested in the interaction with the patient. Although all clinicians address these concerns at various points during the course of a patient's illness, assessment of the most salient QOL concerns on a routine, ongoing basis is less common. With few exceptions, therapies to manage a decline in QOL are not proactive but rather are driven by an obvious deterioration in the patient's status or a crisis in one area or another.

Clinicians who are equipped with a more detailed, ongoing understanding of QOL concerns might be better able to improve routine assessment and management of such concerns. This understanding may help identify problems that could be managed at an earlier and more treatable stage, locate patients at increased risk (41), and target medical resources.

Common Quality-of-Life Concerns in the Clinical Setting

Patients with head and neck cancer may experience a decline in QOL as a result of a broad range of adverse perceptions and experiences. Information about these outcomes continues to be limited, despite a growing number of reports. The descriptive data available are valuable but only begin to illuminate the nature of QOL disturbances associated with head and neck cancer and how these patients differ from the general population (26–32,34).

PHYSICAL SYMPTOMS AND FUNCTIONAL IMPAIRMENTS

Studies that have used validated instruments to assess symptoms and functional impairments in the head and neck cancer population are limited. Sample sizes have been small, and the heterogeneity in tumor location, presence or absence of active disease, and primary treatment approaches has impeded collection of sufficient data about any one subgroup. Cross-sectional assessment, variation in the evaluation of comorbid conditions, and lack of adequate comparison groups further confound the interpretation and generalization of results. Given these limitations, all conclusions about the prevalence, characteristics, and impact of persistent symptoms and functional impairments remain tentative.

This notwithstanding, there is evidence that both persistent symptoms and functional impairment in speech and eating are highly prevalent in all populations with head and neck cancer, including long-term survivors. For example, a cross-sectional survey of 50 patients 1 to 6 years after curative therapy (surgery alone, 28%; radiation alone, 18%; or both, 54%) observed that 24% to 38% reported high levels of the following symptoms: dry mouth, trouble swallowing, mucus production, pain in mouth or tongue, trouble with taste, appetite disturbance, trouble speaking on the telephone, sleep disturbance, and constipation (6). Another cross-sectional survey of 204 patients 7 to 11 years after curative radiation therapy identified similarly high prevalence rates of dry mouth, mucus production, and swallowing difficulties (8). Problems with speech were the major disturbance identified in a cross-sectional study of 48 patients 4 to 26 months after surgery (9). A survey of 117 patients that focused on pain noted that 83.8% of previously untreated patients with stage III or IV disease complained of this symptom; the mean duration (plus or minus standard deviation) was 6.2 ± 5.9 months, and the mean intensity (plus or minus standard deviation) on a 10-point numeric scale was 5.0 ± 2.7 (42). An earlier longitudinal survey demonstrated that pain on presentation is a significant predictor of pain 3 months after treatment (43).

Although the adverse impact of unrelieved symptoms and persistent functional disturbances on overall QOL is likely to be severe, this relationship has received very little empiric evaluation. One survey demonstrated that pain and dysphagia are associated with weight loss after radiation therapy (44), and another study determined that QOL 12 months after treatment was largely determined by pain, dysphagia, and disturbances in speech (45).

Fatigue is among the most common symptoms experienced by patients with cancer. Although there are no data that clarify the prevalence and impact of this symptom among populations with active or cured head and neck cancer, studies in other cancer populations have underscored the need to address this problem as a major factor in cancer-related QOL (46–48).

The causes of cancer-related fatigue are multifactorial, and an algorithmic approach to the assessment and management of fatigue emphasizes the need to evaluate potential treatable causes and comorbidities (48). Among the important treatable causes are anemia, major depressive disorder, sleep disturbance, and side effects of centrally acting medications.

The known association between anemia and fatigue combined with anecdotal observations suggesting treatment-related benefits on energy level and QOL led to a number of studies designed to explore the effects of epoetin alfa on fatigue and QOL in cancer patients undergoing treatment for anemia. In two community-based studies, more than 4,300 anemic cancer patients with various tumor types who were receiving chemotherapy were treated with a starting dose of 10,000 units of epoetin alfa three times weekly (49,50). The dose was increased to a maximum of 60,000 units weekly after 1 to 2 months if the hematologic response was inadequate. Three quarters of the patients in these studies had solid tumors, and 2% had head and neck malignancies.

In both studies, epoetin alfa significantly increased hemoglobin levels and reduced transfusion requirement. In addition, energy level, activity level, and overall QOL improved significantly over baseline levels, and these changes correlated directly with hemoglobin change from baseline. A further analysis demonstrated that improvement in fatigue occurred in all categories of tumor response. Patients who achieved a complete response, partial response, or stable disease rating, but who had no increase in hemoglobin, did not have a meaningful or significant increase in QOL.

The data from these two large studies were subjected to an incremental analysis designed to evaluate the relationship between marginal changes in hemoglobin level and changes in reported fatigue. This analysis demonstrated that fatigue improved at each level of hemoglobin change, and that the maximal change in fatigue occurred between hemoglobin levels of 11 and 12 g/dL.

Another community-based, open-label study of 302 patients evaluated epoetin alfa 40,000 units s.c. weekly (51). Treatment was well tolerated and again produced increased hemoglobin level, reduced transfusion requirement, and improved QOL independent of tumor response to chemotherapy.

Two more recent trials, one placebo controlled (52) and one open label (53), provided yet additional data in support of the link between hemoglobin and fatigue, and the improvement in QOL that could follow treatment for anemia. In the controlled trial, 375 patients with solid or nonmyeloid hematologic malignancies receiving varied chemotherapy regimens were randomly assigned to receive epoetin alfa or placebo; significant improvements in hemoglobin and QOL outcomes occurred only in the group that received active therapy. The open-label trial demonstrated benefits among those who were not receiving chemotherapy at the time of treatment.

These studies strongly suggest that epoetin alfa–induced improvement in hemoglobin correlates significantly with clinically significant improvements in fatigue, functional status, and overall QOL in anemic cancer patients receiving chemotherapy. The studies exemplify the value of QOL measurement in developing interventions that could have an important favorable influence on the long-term outcomes of cancer therapy.

Systematic prospective surveys and controlled trials are needed to characterize these QOL concerns further. The data available do not clarify important differences among tumors that arise at different sites or the differences that result from the various therapies used for these tumors (26,27,29,30). The time courses of these problems, which could best be elucidated through longitudinal studies, also are unknown.

PSYCHOLOGICAL SYMPTOMS AND PSYCHOSOCIAL DISTURBANCES

A high potential for psychosocial distress in patients with head and neck cancer has been hypothesized on the basis of prevalent comorbidity, specifically alcohol abuse, and the relatively low educational status and social support that characterize many in this population (2). Although sufficient survey data have been collected to confirm a high prevalence of distress, little is known yet about the specific types of psychological disturbance or their effect on overall QOL. The data in this area, like the information about symptoms and functional disturbances, are compromised by the limited number of studies, the diverse methodologies of assessment, and the marked heterogeneity among patients with head and neck cancer. Additionally, the extant studies have not clarified adequately the type of problems that might undermine psychological or social wellbeing, which may include mood disorders and other psychiatric states, family conflict, or lack of social resources or support.

Nonetheless, numerous surveys have suggested a high rate of psychological problems and impaired psychosocial functioning among patients with head and neck cancer (1,5,7,54–60). A cross-sectional survey of 48 long-term survivors, for example, used a validated questionnaire and observed scores consistent with depression in 40% (57). In a cross-sectional survey of 204 patients 7 to 11 years after curative radiation therapy, a validated psychiatric screening tool was used to identify a high level of psychological distress in 30%; multivariate analysis demonstrated that psychological distress was significantly associated with impaired cognitive function, reduced social well-being, and pain (7). A study of 172 patients who underwent partial or complete laryngectomy recorded sexual dysfunction in more than 20% and a poor adjustment to work in more than 25%; a comparison of partial and complete laryngectomy patients found that QOL was most influenced by the presence of a stoma (10).

A cross-sectional survey of 55 patients highlighted the effect of access to information about the disease on the psychosocial well-being of patients with head and neck cancer (61). The extent of available information about disease severity and prognosis had a greater influence on adjustment than did the severity of the disease. The more informed patients were better adjusted in interpersonal relationships, including family relationships, but also had more anxiety and expressed more fears about health and symptoms.

GLOBAL QUALITY OF LIFE

Although a growing number of surveys have used validated QOL instruments to collect information about overall QOL (3,6–9,62–71), the interpretation of these data is difficult because of the lack of comparison groups and the methodologic concerns described previously. For example, a longitudinal study of a heterogeneous sample of 75 head and neck cancer patients [mixed diagnoses and stages; treated with surgery alone (60%), radiation alone (8%), or both (32%)] suggested that global QOL declines in the immediate posttreatment period and then returns to baseline in most patients 3 months later (62). This study was designed to validate a new instrument rather than to explore clinical issues, however, and only mean data are provided; there is no evaluation of patient subgroups, including the group with relatively poor QOL scores at 3 months.

Although considerable work has been performed to characterize the population with head and neck cancer in terms of the varied quality-of-life domains, few definitive data are available. In part, this can be explained by the rapid changes that have occurred in the area of QOL assessment during the last decade. The advent of reliable and valid instruments (see later), which has greatly expanded the options for survey methodologies, is recent, and only now are these instruments being included in studies of QOL concerns. Additionally, the lack of adequate data reflects the challenges inherent in the disease. To acquire clinically relevant information, survey methods must be developed to address the heterogeneity in tumor site, stage, treatment, and outcomes.

Barriers to the Management of Quality-of-Life Concerns

As more information accumulates about the prevalent QOL concerns experienced by patients with head and neck cancer, clinicians can apply this information to facilitate more efficient treatment programs, pursue more informed therapeutic decision making about primary therapy, and help explain the disease and its management to the patient and family. Progress in clinical application is likely to be slow, however, owing to numerous barriers. Awareness of these barriers, which can be ascribed to the patient, to the clinician, and to the health care system, is the first step in diminishing their impact.

As a fundamentally subjective phenomenon, QOL cannot be addressed unless patients report their concerns accurately. Unfortunately, the ability of the patient to communicate cannot be assumed. Patient-related problems in communication have been empirically demonstrated in the assessment of cancer pain (72) and can be presumed to affect other issues as well. Communication may be limited because the patient perceives the problem to be socially unacceptable (e.g., the report of emotional disturbances by men) or because of stoicism or a desire to be a "good" patient. Some patients fear that complaints about QOL concerns will distract the physician from the task of cancer therapy. Others are inhibited by fear of worsening the situation merely by discussing it or by concern about the type of intervention that may be suggested by the physician (e.g., opioid analgesics for pain). Finally, communication may be impaired in special populations, such as the elderly, the demented, those with severe psychiatric disorders (including active chemical dependency), and those whose first language is different from that of the clinician.

Clinicians must be aware of these impediments to patient communication. The lack of a spontaneous complaint should not be taken simply as an indication that no problem exists. Assessment should be viewed as an active process, through which patients are reassured of the importance of QOL and their major concerns are elicited.

Many clinician-related barriers to the effective management of QOL concerns also exist. Most clinicians spend very limited time with each patient, and the need to treat acute problems or to explain the risks and benefits of antitumor therapies may take precedence. Clinicians who perceive their roles primarily in terms of disease-related therapy may not address other concerns, even if time permits. Knowledge of symptom control measures, psycho-oncology, and other aspects of palliative care also may be limited. Deficiencies have been well demonstrated in oncologists' knowledge of basic pain management approaches (73), and it is very likely that similar deficiencies impede clinicians' progress in addressing other QOL concerns.

Some aspects of the health care system itself may be barriers to improvement in QOL-directed therapies. Reimbursement for interventions that may be valuable for QOL, such as physical therapy, drugs for symptom control, and home care nursing, varies with the type of insurance; many patients lack coverage for some or all of these measures. Within each hospital or outpatient medical system, expertise in the variety of areas related to QOL, such as pain management, rehabilitation, palliative care, and psycho-oncology, may not exist. Professionals may have no options for referral to specialists when refractory problems are identified. The lack of specialists also limits the opportunities for education and role modeling that may be essential to improve management by primary caregivers. Like the patient-related and clinician-related barriers to improvement in QOL-directed therapies, these problems in the health care system must be recognized and, to the extent possible, redressed.

Palliative Care: A Model for Addressing Quality-of-Life Concerns

The available data suggest that a substantial proportion of patients who undergo curative therapy for head and neck cancer experiences persistent problems that undermine QOL. Although detailed information is lacking, these problems may relate to symptom distress, functional losses, psychosocial disturbances, or some combination of these problems. For these patients, the disease is no longer a therapeutic issue. Management strategies need address only those factors that prevent a satisfactory QOL.

Management of QOL concerns may be more complicated for those patients who are not cured. Although prolonged periods of stability might ensue, the disease is anticipated to progress and, in all likelihood, to result ultimately in death. The complex symptomatology and functional disturbances experienced by patients with progressive head and neck cancer demand a comprehensive approach to palliative care, particularly as the need for interventions intensifies toward the end of life.

Although the concept of palliative care now is firmly established within the broad field of oncology, its parameters are not well defined. However, an evolving consensus exists, which is exemplified in the definition of palliative care promulgated by the World Health Organization (74):

> Palliative care is the active total care of patients whose disease is not responsive to curative treatment. Control of pain, of other symptoms, and of psychological, social and spiritual problems is paramount. The goal of palliative care is the achievement of the best possible QOL for patients and their families.

Palliative care is best conceptualized as the therapeutic model applied to address those factors that undermine the QOL or the opportunity to die with comfort and dignity. As such, it is a fundamental part of medical practice, the "parallel universe" to therapies directed at cure or prolongation of life.

All physicians who treat patients with incurable diseases are engaged in palliative care. Recognition of the range of factors that may undermine QOL facilitates a detailed assessment, which, in turn, allows the development of a therapeutic strategy designed to ameliorate the most important of these factors. The primary clinician can coordinate a treatment team that can address unrelieved symptoms, psychological distress, functional deterioration, or other concerns. At the end of a patient's life, the primary clinician may continue in this role or assist a hospice program in providing comprehensive care. At any point during the course, referral to a specialist in palliative care, if available, may be helpful. Physicians who specialize in palliative medicine have specialist-level skills in assessment and symptom control (75), and maintain access to an interdisciplinary team. These specialists in palliative care perceive their role as similar to that of specialists in any other discipline of medicine: resource persons to other primary caregivers, primary caregivers when the challenges of the case warrant this involvement, and educators and researchers in the field of palliative care.

The goals expressed in this definition of palliative care initially found expression in the hospice movement, which has been concerned primarily with improved care for the dying. In the United States, hospice has evolved as a system for the delivery of end-of-life care to patients who are no longer receiving primary therapies. The broader concept of palliative care described in the definition of the World Health Organization encompasses a level of care well beyond this version of hospice. Palliative care aims to address the physical, psychosocial, and spiritual concerns that contribute to the quality of both life and death throughout the course of incurable, life-threatening diseases. Although the need for palliative care interventions intensifies at the end of life, the core concerns are salient for the patient and family throughout the course of the disease. The palliative care model accepts the need for strong physician input on an ongoing basis, expresses a willingness to use aggressive tertiary interventions for appropriate patients, and endorses the need for research to improve quality of care and advance the scientific foundation of treatment.

All physicians who treat patients with persistent or recurrent head and neck cancer must become comfortable with palliative care as an active therapeutic endeavor that is applied throughout the course of the illness. Clinicians must reject the unfortunate and untrue position that the lack of a curative or life-prolonging treatment means that "nothing can be done." Both the patient and caregivers are served better if the clinician has communicated successfully from the start that palliative care is as central to medical care as is primary treatment for the disease or its complications. Patients who have learned that help is available to them so that they can live with the disease are more likely to accept the transition to a phase without primary treatment. Although the intensity with which palliative care is provided may increase after life-prolonging therapies are exhausted, patients who have been exposed to this model of care are able to perceive a continuity characterized by the ongoing desire of the clinician to manage symptoms and address other QOL concerns. In such a context, the referral to a palliative care specialist, if needed, is not viewed as a defeat but merely as a way to obtain expert care.

RESEARCH IMPLICATIONS OF THE QUALITY-OF-LIFE CONSTRUCT

The ability to measure QOL concerns has many implications for research. As described previously, QOL assessment instruments and methods can be applied to epidemiologic studies of selected problems, such as uncontrolled symptoms or psychological distress. These surveys can elucidate the prevalence, characteristics, and impact of symptoms and functional disturbances, and have clear implications for the targeting of therapeutic resources after successful therapy.

In clinical investigations of antineoplastic therapies, measurement of QOL concerns can yield data that are complementary to such traditional outcomes as survival and tumor response. Although the effort required to measure QOL over time can be substantial, intensive psychometric research during the last two decades has provided a strong scientific foundation for this effort.

Measurement of QOL outcomes during clinical trials can yield many potential benefits. After a therapeutic approach has been introduced in the clinical setting, knowledge of the range of associated QOL outcomes may help the clinician to position the therapy among other approaches that produce similar rates of response. The availability of these data encourages evidence-based decision making as a complement to the usual reliance on intuition and experience. The importance of this evidence-based reasoning has been underscored by research findings that suggest the imprecision inherent in clinical guesswork. For example, a comparative trial of continuous versus intermittent chemotherapy for breast cancer yielded the counterintuitive finding that the treatment associated with lesser patient burden, that is, intermittent therapy, actually yielded a greater negative impact on QOL (76). Another study of patients with sarcoma demonstrated that limb sparing, intuitively a preferred approach, did not actually improve QOL (77).

The availability of valid information about QOL outcomes in clinical decision making is particularly important when comparative trials demonstrate no clear survival advantage among various treatment approaches. For example, the clinical importance of the demonstration that a larynx preservation protocol yields survival similar to laryngectomy and radiation therapy (25) could be potentially illuminated by careful QOL assessment.

This use of QOL data to clarify the "price" that must be paid for an effective antineoplastic therapy can be formalized into cost-utility analyses (78). These analyses represent an effort to incorporate patient preferences and QOL outcomes into the more traditional evaluation of cost benefit. They are clearly relevant in assessing therapies for head and neck cancer, which may produce morbidities (e.g., persistent symptoms or functional loss) that produce long-term impairments in QOL. These QOL impairments can be quantitated and combined with the direct medical costs incurred by patients as they seek help for adverse outcomes. With sufficient information about QOL, these analyses can clarify the advantages and disadvantages of various treatment options.

To date, these potential benefits of QOL assessment have only started to be explored in populations with head and neck cancer. Although the number of scientific reports is growing, there are yet relatively few carefully performed epidemiologic studies of QOL concerns and almost no clinical trials that incorporated systematic QOL evaluation. This situation will not improve until investigators acquire a working knowledge of QOL assessment methodologies.

QUALITY-OF-LIFE ASSESSMENT: PRACTICAL CONSIDERATIONS

Given the complexity of the QOL construct, the diverse characteristics of patients with head and neck cancer, and the varying needs of investigators and clinicians, no one method of QOL measurement can be applied to every situation. The lack of a single optimal method complicates the matter for most investigators, who may have difficulty selecting appropriate QOL assessment instruments and methodologies. A practical understanding of the instruments available and the options for QOL measurement is needed to encourage a more informed judgment.

Generic, Multidimensional Quality-of-life Instruments

Detailed information about a specific domain related to QOL can be elicited using a questionnaire designed and validated for the purpose of this assessment. Each of these specific instruments may be useful to assess a phenomenon that contributes to QOL in the cancer population, but none should be used alone to characterize fully the QOL construct. For example, each of the many instruments that evaluate varying types of psychosocial dysfunction (79), symptom distress (80,81), or performance status (82–84) may illuminate an aspect of QOL, but none can be viewed as a measure of global QOL. As discussed later, these instruments can be used in a QOL assessment paradigm based on the employment of multiple instruments.

Generic, multidimensional questionnaires have been developed and validated to assess QOL in varying cancer populations or populations with diverse types of medical illness (Table 10.2). All evaluate, at minimum, physical, psychological, and social well-being. Most have valid total scores that depict overall QOL and subscale scores that reflect well-being in each of the major dimensions. As generic measures, they capture information common to many populations. The cancer-specific instruments may yield results that are generalizable across tumor types; when administered to different cancer populations, they offer the opportunity for direct comparisons of the outcomes evaluated.

The earliest attempt at multidimensional assessment consisted of a series of visual analog scales, each of which evaluated a specific (e.g., pain) or general (e.g., global well-being) influence on QOL (85). These so-called linear analog self-assessment (LASA) scales have been used in trials and appear to be effective. The psychometrics are not as well established as are other multidimensional instruments, however, and the validity of subscale scores is unclear. These limitations favor the use of one of the newer multidimensional instruments, if feasible.

The QL-Index was an early, cancer-specific, multidimensional QOL measure that originally was validated as an observer-rated scale and then was adapted as a patient-rated scale (35). It uses only five items to screen various domains and usually is coadministered with a single-item, patient-rated, global measure of well-being, which is known as the Uniscale. Although it has yielded meaningful data in numerous studies (86), the QL-Index has been largely supplanted by longer and more detailed self-assessment instruments. The QL-Index can be recommended in the setting of very limited resources or extreme patient burden.

The Functional Living Index–Cancer (FLIC) was the first cancer-specific, multidimensional QOL instrument to undergo extensive psychometric evaluation (87). It has been used in numerous surveys and some clinical trials, one of which raised concerns about patient burden in a debilitated population (88). More recent trials, however, have established the potential for very high compliance rates with instruments as long and detailed as the FLIC (89), suggesting that compliance may be influenced more by the method of administration than by the number or type of items. Although it assesses multiple domains, the FLIC was designed to yield only a single global score indicative of QOL. The lack of valid subscale scores is a major limitation. One study used factor analysis to proffer subscales (90), but this approach requires replication and has not been applied.

Newer cancer-specific QOL instruments provide both subscale scores and a global QOL score. The availability of valid subscale scores, which may identify variation in the domains

TABLE 10.2 Examples of Generic Multidimensional Quality-of-Life (QOL) Instruments

Instrument	Comment
Functional Living Index–Cancer (FLIC)	Multidimensional; good psychometrics; subscales recently proffered but little experience in their use; lack of subscales to date has encouraged the use of newer QOL scales
European Organization for Research and Treatment of Cancer (EORTC) QLQ-C30	Newest revision of well-validated, multidimensional instrument that has both global QOL and subscale scores (EORTC QLQ-C30) (61), can be combined with validated head and neck cancer module; experience in clinical trials limited, but basic instrument plus module likely to be useful for QOL assessment in head and neck cancer trials
Functional Assessment of Cancer Therapy (FACT)	Well-validated, multidimensional QOL scale; includes global and subscale scores; has a specific version for head and neck cancer with "additional concerns" section developed for this population; limited experience in clinical trials setting, but likely to be useful for QOL assessment in head and neck cancer trials
Cancer Rehabilitation Evaluation System (CARES)	Well-validated, multidimensional QOL scale that provides global and subscale scores; not specific for head and neck cancer; limited experience in clinical trials setting, but likely to be useful for QOL assessment in head and neck cancer trials; short form possibly particularly useful for clinical trials
Linear Analogue Self-Assessment (LASA)	Consists of multiple visual analog scales, each of which screens a particular domain; multidimensional, but psychometrics of global and subscale scores not elaborated; not specific for head and neck cancer; limited experience in clinical trials setting, but likely to be useful for QOL assessment in head and neck cancer trials
Medical Outcomes Study Scale (MOS SF-36)	Well-validated, multidimensional scale that provides global and subscale scores; assesses general health status; not cancer-specific; limited experience in clinical trials setting, but could be useful for QOL assessment in head and neck cancer trials; nonetheless, a cancer-specific instrument is usually preferred
Sickness Impact Profile (SIP)	Well-validated, multidimensional scale for general health status; not cancer-specific; provides extensive information about function; limited experience in clinical trials setting, but not likely to be useful in head and neck clinical trials because of its length
McMaster Health Index Questionnaire (MHIQ)	Well-validated multidimensional scale for general health status; not cancer-specific; limited experience in clinical trials setting, but could be useful for QOL assessment in head and neck cancer trials; nonetheless, a cancer-specific instrument is usually preferred
Nottingham Health Profile	Well-validated, multidimensional scale for general health status; not cancer-specific; limited experience in clinical trials setting, but could be useful for QOL assessment in head and neck cancer trials, despite an emphasis on severe impairment; nonetheless, a cancer-specific instrument is usually preferred

affected most by an intervention, is a distinct advantage. These measures include the Functional Assessment of Cancer Therapy (FACT) (91), the QLQ-C30 of the European Organization for Research and Treatment of Cancer (EORTC QLQ-C30) (92), and the Cancer Rehabilitation Evaluation System (93). Although these scales all evaluate physical and psychosocial well-being, they vary in the specific questions they ask to assess these domains and in the range of other perceptions queried. No comparative studies have been conducted, and the relative advantages and disadvantages of these instruments in selected populations are unknown. For this reason, the best approach is an empiric one: an investigator should review the items and assess the degree to which the scale appears to capture the important issues for the study population in question. Both the EORTC QLQ-C30 and the FACT scale have supplemental modules for the assessment of concerns specific to head and neck cancer, which may offer a substantial advantage for studies in these populations (see later).

Other multidimensional scales have been developed for use in general populations of the medically ill (Table 10.2). These include the SF-36 form of the Medical Outcomes Study (MOS SF-36) (94), the Sickness Impact Profile (SIP) (95), the McMaster Health Index Questionnaire (96), and the Nottingham Health Profile (97). Although none has been used much in a clinical trials setting, an investigator may find advantages in one or another depending on the objectives and design of the study and the characteristics of the population. In general, however, a cancer-specific instrument is more likely to be a sensitive measure of QOL issues in a cancer population.

Instruments for Head and Neck Cancer

Some instruments, including a few that are multidimensional, have been developed to assess specific QOL concerns in populations with head and neck cancer (Table 10.3). As discussed later, an assessment methodology that includes one or more of these scales can provide useful information that would not be acquired through the use of a generic, multidimensional instrument alone.

The University of Washington Quality of Life Head and Neck Questionnaire (UW QOL) is a nine-item, patient-rated, multidimensional instrument that includes questions about pain, disfigurement, speech, swallowing, and performance status (62). Longitudinal evaluation in a cohort of patients with head and neck cancer demonstrated high test-retest reliability and concurrent validity using the Sickness Impact Profile as the standard. Given its brevity and the lack of items that assess psychological or social status, the UW QOL questionnaire should be viewed as a limited screen of relevant outcomes, rather than a comprehensive multidimensional instrument. It may be an informative addition to a broader evaluation.

The University of Michigan Head and Neck Quality of Life (HNQOL) (64,70) is an interviewer-administered questionnaire composed of 21 items assessing four domains: pain, emotion, communication, and eating. Each item is rated on a 5-point Likert scale. Preliminary testing for reliability and validity has been done with good results. Further validation is needed to fully determine this instrument's usefulness.

The Functional Status in Head and Neck Cancer–Self Report (FSH&N-SR) is another multidimensional, self-reporting meas-

TABLE 10.3 Examples of Quality-of-Life (QOL) Instruments Designed for Use in Populations with Head and Neck Cancer

Instrument	Comment
University of Washington Quality of Life Head and Neck (UW QOL)	Nine-item scale that assesses symptoms and several functional outcomes; given limited coverage, may be most useful if combined with other measures; has reliability and validity in initial study
University of Michigan Head and Neck Quality of Life (HNQOL)	Interviewer-administered, 21-item questionnaire assessing four domains—pain, emotion, communication, and eating; has reliability and validity in initial study
Functional Status in Head and Neck Cancer Self-Report (FSH&N-SR)	Fifteen-item scale that assesses symptoms and several functional outcomes; given limited coverage, may be most useful if combined with other measures; has reliability and validity in initial study
Head and Neck Quality of Life Questionnaire	Comprehensive, multidimensional measure that comprises two previously validated measures and additional items; assesses symptoms, cognitive and psychosocial status, life satisfaction, and other concerns, and is designed to be head and neck cancer–specific; has reliability and validity in initial study
Head and Neck Cancer Module of the EORTC QLQ-C30	Designed to be coadministered with the generic, multidimensional QOL measure developed by the European Organization for Research and Treatment of Cancer (EORTC); well-validated scale that assesses symptoms prevalent in head and neck cancer and some functional concerns
Head and Neck Cancer Module of the FACT scale	Coadministered with the generic, multidimensional QOL measure, the Functional Assessment of Cancer Therapy (FACT) scale; assesses symptoms prevalent in head and neck cancer and some functional concerns; not independently validated
Head and Neck Cancer Performance Status Scale	Validated, observer-rated scale that yields scores for understandability of speech, normalcy of diet, and ability to eat in public; may be very useful if combined with other measures
Head and Neck Radiotherapy Questionnaire	Well-validated, interviewer-administered, 22-item questionnaire that assesses the status of the oral cavity, throat, digestive function, energy level, and psychosocial functioning; may be a very useful measure of acute morbidity due to radiation in populations with head and neck cancer
Quality of Life—Radiation Therapy Instrument Head and Neck Module (QOL-RTI/H&N)	A 39-item, self-assessed questionnaire using a 10-item Likert response scale consisting of five domains—functional, emotional, family, socioeconomic, and general; it gives broader coverage than the HNRQ but has not been extensively tested
Quality of Life Questionnaire for Advanced Head and Neck Cancer (QLQ)	A 19-item, self-assessed questionnaire consisting of 15 questions rated on a four-point Likert-type scale and four questions rated on a five-point scale
Mayo Clinic Postlaryngectomy Questionnaire	Forty-eight-item scale that evaluate symptoms and psychosocial functioning after laryngectomy; has not been independently validated but appeared to function well in a large, cross-sectional study of postlaryngectomy patients (10)
Linear Analogue Self-Assessment (LASA) Scale for Voice Quality	Sixteen linear analog scales that assess voice quality after therapy for laryngeal cancer; has not been independently validated but may be useful if voice quality is a primary end point

ure that focuses on symptoms and functional outcomes (71). Issues for assessment were identified from interviews with 114 head and neck cancer patients. The 15 items evaluate xerostomia, pain, fatigue, breathing, and disturbances in speech, swallowing, eating, and movement of the upper body. Psychometric evaluation provided evidence of construct validity, discriminative and convergent validity, and good internal consistency. Like the UW QOL questionnaire, this instrument evaluates a limited range of domains and should not be viewed as a comprehensive multidimensional questionnaire. It, too, may be most useful if combined with other instruments.

Another approach to the development of head and neck cancer–specific multidimensional QOL assessment involved the creation of a questionnaire that combines two previously validated measures, one evaluating cognitive and psychosocial status, and the other evaluating life satisfaction, with newly devised questions that assess demographics, symptoms, and global well-being (98). A pilot study in 84 patients suggested that the measures used to construct the questionnaire could be used to generate valid subscale scores and that the questionnaire overall has adequate reliability and validity. Although further study is needed to confirm the utility of this scale, it represents a strong effort to derive a comprehensive multidimensional QOL assessment tool that is truly specific to head and neck cancer.

The head and neck cancer modules designed to be coadministered with the EORTC QLQ-C30 and the FACT scale, respectively, also assess a selected group of symptoms (e.g., xerostomia and dysphagia) and some functional concerns that are relatively unique to this population. The EORTC instrument has been independently validated (99). The ability to acquire specific, clinically relevant information through the use of these modules addresses the major disadvantages of the generic, multidimensional questionnaires.

Other instruments evaluate more specific concerns. A validated, observer-rated head and neck cancer performance status scale yields separate scores for intelligibility of speech, normalcy of diet, and ability to eat in public (84). Although this instrument provides information about a limited area of function related to QOL, its simplicity and clinical relevance recommend its use.

The Head and Neck Radiotherapy Questionnaire (HNRQ) evaluates the acute morbidity after radiation therapy for head and neck cancer and has been well validated in a clinical trial context (100). This instrument has been advocated as an appropriate outcome measure in studies that incorporate a radiation treatment arm.

Another tool for evaluating patients being treated with radiotherapy is the Quality of Life Radiation Therapy Instrument Head and Neck Module (QOL–RTI/H&N) (64,69). It is a 39-item self-assessed questionnaire using a 10-item Likert response scale. Although both internal consistency and reliability have been favorable, it has been used on only a small group of patients, and further validation and testing on larger population would be beneficial. It can be used in the same population as the HNRQ, but it includes more nonphysical symptoms and a wider range of QOL issues.

The impact of advanced disease in head and neck cancer patients can be evaluated by the Quality of Life Questionnaire for Advanced Head and Neck Cancer (QLQ) (68). This questionnaire is focused on four major domains: physical, functional/mood, psychological, and attitude toward treatment. No data on reliability and only minimal data on validity are available.

Functioning after laryngectomy has been assessed with the Mayo Clinic Postlaryngectomy Questionnaire, a 48-item scale that evaluates symptoms and psychosocial functioning after laryngectomy (10). This instrument has not been formally validated but appeared to function well in a large cross-sectional study of postlaryngectomy patients. Another scale used a simple 16-item LASA approach to assess patients' ability to speak after treatment for laryngeal cancer (101). This measure could be used if voice quality is perceived to be a primary end point in studies of this disorder.

Issues in the Selection of a Methodology for Clinical Trials

Numerous issues must be resolved in selecting and implementing a methodology for QOL assessment in clinical investigations. A thoughtful approach to this process is likely to yield a method that optimally balances feasibility with the accumulation of valid and comprehensive data.

GENERAL APPROACH

To clarify the major issues in the selection of a methodology for QOL assessment, Osoba et al. (102) have developed an algorithm for the selection of QOL measures that describes a series of decision points, each of which depends on the objectives, preferences, and resources of the investigator or clinician (Fig. 10.1). The first decision point clarifies the purpose of the QOL assessment: (a) screening for problems, (b) profiling patient characteristics, or (c) identifying patient preferences. The type (or types) of assessment instruments appropriate for the study is guided by this overall objective. A brief, multidimensional QOL questionnaire may be an appropriate single measure if the goal is to screen a population for problems that could compromise QOL. A combination of several measures may be needed to provide more detailed information if the goal is a population profile of selected QOL outcomes.

The second decision point elaborates the method for data collection: interview or questionnaire. Typically, questionnaires have usually been used in clinical investigations because methodology is simplified and there are no concerns about interrater reliability. If necessary, a questionnaire can be read to a patient who is unable to complete it without assistance. Interviews may be most useful when obtaining exploratory information about previously unstudied experiences. The process of creating quantitative data from interview material can be challenging, however, and may require coding of transcripts by independent observers. Nonetheless, interviews can yield very illuminating data if carefully performed. The development of a new questionnaire, for example, often begins with an interview, which can be very helpful in defining appropriate content.

The third decision point relates to the target of the assessment: generic or specific to a disease or treatment. Generic instruments (labeled "universal, or core" in Fig. 10.1) may be sufficient in many settings, and, with the advent of valid multidimensional instruments, allow the acquisition of screening information about a broad range of QOL concerns that may be useful across tumor types. These instruments do not acquire information about the specific problems that characterize a disease or a treatment and, for this reason, may obscure clinically relevant distinctions or fail to identify a particular concern that is prominent in relatively small numbers of patients. In the head and neck cancer population, for example, detailed information about the prevalence and impact of dysphagia and speech disturbances may be essential to an understanding of QOL but will not be assessed by use of a generic questionnaire. The use of a generic questionnaire alone would not be appropriate in a clinical investigation of a head and neck cancer therapy if what one desires is a detailed evaluation of the effect of this therapy on these outcomes. To achieve such a goal, a more disease-specific approach should be implemented.

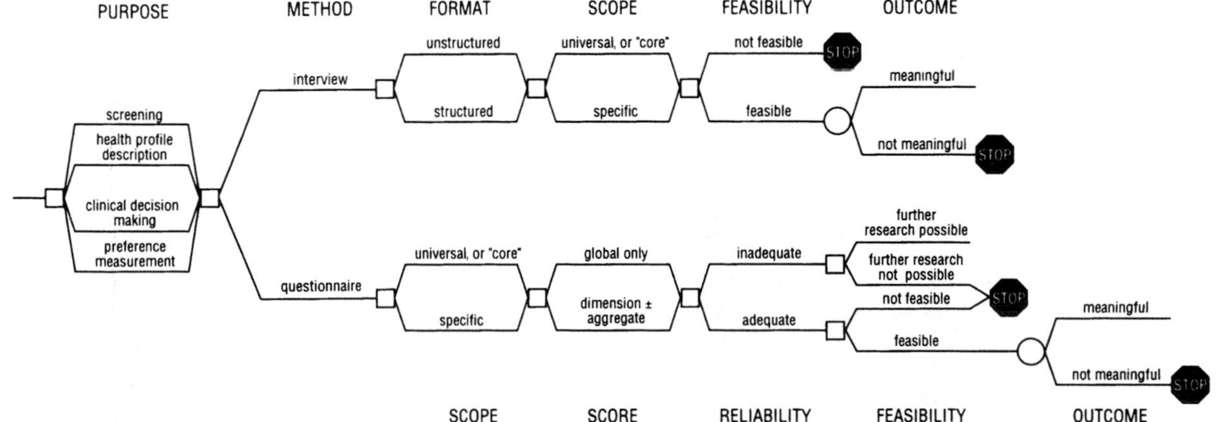

Figure 10.1 Algorithm for the selection of quality-of-life measures. Each decision point must be resolved through consideration of the objectives, preferences, and resources maintained by the investigator or clinician. This approach illustrates the broad range of options available for quality-of-life assessment and encourages the use of a methodology targeted to the needs of the study. (Adapted from Osoba D, Aaronson N-K, Till JE. A practical guide for selecting quality of life measures in clinical trials and practice. In: Osoba D, ed. *Effect of cancer on quality of life*. Boca Raton, FL: CRC Press, 1991:89, with permission.)

The fourth decision point relates to the scope of the QOL assessment. The resources for QOL data collection—time, personnel, and economic resources—usually are limited, and the burden of data gathering that can be placed on patients must be carefully considered. In planning most studies, an accommodation must be made between the breadth of information that would be desirable and the constraints imposed by resource limitations and respondent burden. If resources are sufficient to allow only the administration of a brief instrument at relatively long intervals, generic instruments that screen the various QOL dimensions may be the only feasible approach. If, however, resources are adequate to allow the administration of a questionnaire packet followed by a telephone contact to ensure completion, it may be possible to obtain detailed information that profiles a range of QOL outcomes. Similarly, the general condition of the patient population must be considered. The detailed assessment that may be possible in relatively healthy patients with early disease may be excessive for more debilitated patients with advanced cancer.

SINGLE VERSUS MULTIPLE INSTRUMENTS

As discussed previously, the benefits of the generic, multidimensional QOL instruments—simplicity, breadth, generalizability, and potential for both subscales and aggregate scores—are balanced by several disadvantages. None of these scales offers much detail about any single domain, and all may miss entirely the important influences on QOL that are specific to a particular population, disease, treatment, or clinical setting. These disadvantages may be a major concern when such a scale is administered as the only QOL assessment tool. The recent development of head and neck cancer–specific, comprehensive, multidimensional QOL questionnaires may represent important progress, but further experience with these measures is required before their value can be judged.

The administration of a group of specific scales, each of which is selected to evaluate a separate QOL concern in the population under study, can obviate the limitations of the multidimensional instrument. Using the purpose of the study for a basis, the investigator may choose to combine one or more head and neck cancer–specific instruments with other validated measures that assess particular concerns, such as coping or social functioning. This approach might enhance the accuracy of the assessment, better target the evaluation to the aims of the study, and provide the investigator with more flexibility than would be possible with multidimensional scales. However, this approach assumes a great deal of knowledge on the part of the investigator and may increase the practical burdens on both the investigator and patients. It also reduces the opportunity for comparisons across populations.

An alternative method that potentially eliminates these disadvantages combines a small number of selected measures targeted to specific concerns with a generic, multidimensional instrument. This approach, involving a core plus supplemental measures, has been applied in two ways. In the first, coordinated modules specific to a disease site or treatment setting are developed in association with a core instrument (91,103,104). As described previously, modules for the assessment of patients with head and neck cancer have been coordinated with the QOL instrument of the EORTC (99) and the FACT scale.

In the second approach, supplemental measures unrelated to the core instrument are coadministered to obtain detailed information about relevant issues. Performance status is routinely assessed separately, typically using a brief, observer-rated scale. The Karnofsky Performance Status scale, for example, provides information about physical functioning (82) that may complement the physical well-being subscale of a multidimensional measure. In a similar manner, a scale that evaluates psychological distress, social functioning, or symptoms can be added to provide useful detail about these specific concerns.

Physical and psychological symptoms are highly prevalent in all cancer populations (80,81,105–114), including patients with head and neck cancer (1,4,6–8,10,11,42,62,71,84,100,115), and the addition of a detailed symptom assessment to a generic, multidimensional scale may be a particularly valuable approach. Although all generic QOL instruments include symptom-related information, none provides much detail about a broad range of symptoms or global symptom distress. None includes measurement of some of the most common symptoms (e.g., xerostomia) in head and neck cancer patients. Extensive information about symptoms can be acquired with a nonvalidated symptom checklist, which is the most common approach used in clinical trials, or, preferably, with a validated comprehensive symptom measure, specifically the Rotterdam Symptom Checklist (81) or the Memorial Symptom Assessment Scale (80). Another validated instrument, the Symptom Distress Scale, includes a small number of symptoms and is best considered a measure of global symptom distress (116,117). Information about pain, an important symptom in head and neck cancer (42,105,115), can be acquired using a simple pain intensity scale (e.g., verbal categorical, numeric, or analog) or a more comprehensive instrument, the Brief Pain Inventory, which evaluates pain intensity and pain-related interference in various spheres of function (118–120).

These symptom scales are not specific for head and neck cancer, of course. In some circumstances, the use of a scale that focuses on the prevalent symptoms in this particular population may provide more detail. As described previously, several brief questionnaires developed in populations with head and neck cancer include such relevant symptom information (Table 10.3). Given the brevity of these scales, it would be possible to coadminister a comprehensive symptom measure and a brief head and neck cancer–specific measure if a detailed assessment of symptoms was a major goal of the study. The use of the head and neck cancer–specific modules associated with the EORTC QLQ-C30 or the FACT scale may be another means of acquiring information about the symptoms that are prevalent in this population.

The foregoing considerations suggest a particularly useful approach to a comprehensive QOL assessment in the head and neck cancer population. One of the generic, multidimensional instruments with a supplemental head and neck module—specifically the EORTC QLQ-C30 or the FACT scale—could be used as the core instrument, to which a small number of carefully selected other measures might be added to capture information about those concerns that are not adequately screened or that require more detail. As noted earlier, a general performance status scale usually is routinely included. A comprehensive symptom measure, specifically the Memorial Symptom Assessment Scale (80) or Rotterdam Symptom Checklist (81), might be considered if symptom prevalence, characteristics, and impact are salient outcomes. If additional data pertaining to symptoms or functional outcomes are not covered sufficiently by the modules, information about these outcomes can be obtained with no patient burden by the addition of the observer-rated head and neck performance status scale (84), or with minimal burden by the addition of one of the brief patient-rated head and neck cancer–specific instruments, such as the UW QOL (62) or the FSH&N-SR (71). Other supplemental instruments might be considered in the postradiation (100) or postlaryngectomy (10) setting. Although separate measures of psychological or social functioning are added less commonly, one or more of these instruments should be considered if the impact on these dimensions is highly salient.

Occasionally, no validated instrument exists for the assessment of a critically important issue. For example, the effect of a specific treatment-related morbidity on selected occupations may be highly relevant depending on the objectives of the study. In these situations, a small number of additional questions must be devised.

TYPE OF STUDY

In epidemiologic studies that profile a patient population, the selection of instruments must be determined by the specific questions under investigation. For example, a study designed to clarify the prevalence, characteristics, and impact of pain in a cancer population might be most informative if specific pain measures are combined with a generic, multidimensional QOL instrument (121).

The potential value of QOL end points in randomized clinical trials now is widely acknowledged. The use of QOL assessment methods in nonrandomized trials is more controversial. Quality of life data collected in single-arm trials may be inaccurate or prone to misinterpretation due to bias or placebo effect. This possibility must be weighed against the potential advantages, specifically the valuable information that might be obtained by comparing changes in QOL outcomes with changes in the tumor or other medical outcomes after an intervention. For example, the evaluation of QOL end points could help to determine the degree to which a new therapy might have important palliative effects on symptoms or functional disturbances, even in the absence of significant tumor shrinkage. Quality of life assessment during nonrandomized trials may also be useful when precisely measuring tumor reduction is difficult, such as occurs in prostate or pancreas cancer (122). Finally, formal evaluation of QOL in early trials could clarify the type of evaluation that would be most informative in later comparative studies.

The distinction between so-called explanatory and pragmatic clinical trials (123) may be informative when evaluating the potential advantages and disadvantages of a comprehensive QOL assessment in nonrandomized studies. The major goal of an explanatory trial is to elucidate a biologic principle, whereas a pragmatic trial is designed primarily to clarify the clinical role of a treatment. Quality of life assessment is most likely to be advantageous in nonrandomized trials that have a pragmatic intent; it is more likely to be superfluous in those that are primarily explanatory.

TIMING OF ASSESSMENT

The timing of QOL assessments during a clinical trial is influenced by a variety of factors. These include the type of treatment and its mode of administration, the course of the biologic effects produced by the treatment, the expected course of the treatment's impact on QOL concerns, the objectives of the assessment, the capacity of the patients to comply, and the resources available to the investigator. A minimum of three assessments has been advocated for chemotherapy trials: baseline, time of maximum adverse effects, and end of therapy (20). Although this minimal assessment probably will capture the important persistent changes induced by the treatment, it offers no information about the time course of these changes. These time course data can be very useful in planning treatment strategies to manage the adverse effects associated with a new therapy or in developing hypotheses about causal relationships.

In chemotherapy trials, an assessment immediately before each treatment cycle, or every other cycle, is likely to be more informative than are assessments at longer intervals. This type of monitoring often is incorporated easily into the treatment schedule of the study drug. In contrast, QOL monitoring after other types of primary therapy, such as radiation or a surgical procedure, is not well defined and must be decided on a case-by-case basis. Considerations affecting this decision making include both the time course of treatment effects and the specific aims. For example, the QOL outcomes after radiation therapy may be viewed in terms of acute and subacute effects or long-term effects. In a study that compares radiation therapy with another treatment, a comprehensive evaluation of QOL outcomes could include frequent assessments during the period immediately after treatment and less frequent assessments for a period sufficient to assess long-term effects. Depending on the goals of the study, the latter period could extend for years (7,8).

METHODOLOGIC CONTROLS

The feasibility of repeated QOL assessments depends on developing methods to ensure the accuracy of the data and to reduce the likelihood of missing data. Although inevitably some patients will be lost prematurely from the study owing to illness or death, relocation, or mere preference, and others will fail to complete all questionnaires, these problems can be minimized. If possible, questionnaires should be read to patients who are unable to manage them without assistance, and provisions should be made for completion of questionnaires at home. If the latter approach is feasible, it requires an option for mail return and is best implemented using a reminder telephone call from an investigator. If a patient is unable to complete an assessment, a follow-up call should determine the cause of this attrition.

CONCLUSION

The QOL construct has profound implications in populations with head and neck cancer. After treatment, many patients experience long-term morbidity, including refractory symptoms, psychosocial disturbances, and impairments in such basic functions as speech and eating. All patients, including those who ultimately are cured, may experience a decline in QOL sufficient to compromise the benefits gained from antitumor therapy. In the clinical setting, careful assessment is necessary for developing therapeutic strategies designed to ameliorate the factors that undermine QOL. Palliative care is the appropriate medical model for addressing QOL concerns in those with persistent disease. For patients who cannot be cured, the goal of palliative care is to improve QOL at all disease stages.

The QOL construct also has important research implications. Systematic QOL assessment can yield clinically relevant data in epidemiologic studies and clinical trials of antineoplastic therapies. A decade of intensive research has yielded numerous validated instruments, including many that are specific to the head and neck cancer population. Although the methodologies that may be used to acquire accurate data are evolving, an investigator usually can develop a feasible assessment protocol that addresses the major purposes of the study. Intensive efforts now are needed to encourage QOL measurement in all clinical trials. The impact of this information on therapeutic decision making is likely to be very positive.

REFERENCES

1. Rapoport Y, Kreitler, Chaitchik S, et al. Psychosocial problems in head and neck cancer patients and their change with time since diagnosis. *Ann Oncol* 1993;4:69.
2. Breitbart W, Holland J. Psychosocial aspects of head and neck cancer. *Semin Oncol* 1988;15:61.
3. Rathmell AJ, Ash DV, Howes M, et al. Assessing quality of life in patients treated for advanced head and neck cancer. *Clin Oncol* 1991;3:10.

4. Mohide EA, Archibald SD, Tew M, et al. Postlaryngectomy quality of life dimensions identified by patients and health care professionals. *Am J Surg* 1992;164:619.
5. Pruyn J, Jong P, Bosman L, et al. Psychosocial aspects of head and neck cancer—a review of the literature. *Clin Otolaryngol* 1986;11:469.
6. Bjordal K, Freng A, Thorvik J, et al. Patient self-reported and clinician-rated quality of life in head and neck cancer patients: a cross-sectional study. *Eur J Cancer* 1995;3:235.
7. Bjordal K, Kaasa S. Psychological distress in head and neck cancer patients 7–11 years after curative therapy. *Br J Cancer* 1995;71:592.
8. Bjordal K, Kaasa S, Mastekaasa A. Quality of life in patients treated for head and neck cancer: a follow-up study 7–11 years after radiotherapy. *Int J Radiat Oncol Biol Phys* 1994;28:847.
9. Jones E, Lund VJ, Howard DJ, et al. Quality of life of patients treated surgically for head and neck cancer. *J Laryngol Otol* 1992;106:238.
10. DeSanto LW, Olsen KD, Rohe DE, et al. Quality of life after surgical treatment of cancer of the larynx. *Ann Otol Rhinol Laryngol* 1995;104:763.
11. Watt-Watson J, Graydon J. Impact of surgery on head and neck cancer patients and their caregivers. *Nurs Clin North Am* 1995;30:659.
12. Schwartz S, Patrick L, Yueh B. Quality of life outcomes in the evaluation of head and neck cancer treatments. *Arch Otolaryngol Head Neck Surg* 2001;127:617.
13. Gritz E, Carmack C, de Moor Carl, et al. First year after head and neck cancer: quality of life. *J Clin Oncol* 1999;17:352.
14. Hammerlid E, Silander E, Hornestam L, et al. Health-related quality of life three years after diagnosis of head and neck cancer: a longitudinal study. *Head Neck* 2001;23:113.
15. Rogers S, Hannah L, et al. Quality of life 5–10 years after primary surgery for oral and oropharyngeal pharyngeal cancer. *J Craniomaxillofacial Surg* 1999;27:187.
16. Epstien J, Robertson, Emertson S, et al. Quality of life and oral function in patients treated with radiation therapy for head and neck cancer. *Head Neck* 2001;23:389.
17. Morton RP. Evolution of quality of life assessment in head and neck cancer. *J Laryngol Otol* 1995;109:1029.
18. Cella DR. Quality of life: concepts and definition. *J Pain Symptom Manage*1994;9:186.
19. Gotay CC, Kom EL, McCabe MS, et al. Quality of life assessment in cancer treatment protocols: research issues in protocol development. *J Natl Cancer Inst* 1992;84:575.
20. Moinpour CM, Peig P, Metch B, et al. Quality of life end points in cancer clinical trials: review and recommendations. *J Natl Cancer Inst* 1989;81:485.
21. Osoba D. Lessons learned from measuring health-related quality of life in oncology. *J Clin Oncol* 1994;12:608.
22. Nayfield SG, Ganz PA, Moinpour CM, et al. Report from a National Cancer Institute (USA) Workshop on Quality of Life Assessment in Cancer Clinical Trials. *Qual Life Res* 1992;1:203.
23. Donovan K, Sanson-Fisher RW, Redman S. Measuring quality of life in cancer patients. *J Clin Oncol* 1989;7:959.
24. Cella DR, Tulsky DS. Measuring quality of life today—methodological aspects. *Oncology* 1990;4:29.
25. Department of Veterans Affairs Laryngeal Cancer Study Group. Induction chemotherapy plus radiation compared with surgery plus radiation in patients with advanced laryngeal cancer. *N Engl J Med* 1991;324:1685.
26. Rogers SN, Lowe D, Humphris P. Distinct patient groups in oral cancer: a prospective study of perceived health status following primary surgery. *Oral Oncol* 2000;36:529.
27. de Graeff A, de Leeuw R, Ros W, et al. A prospective study on quality of life of laryngeal cancer patients treated with radiotherapy. *Head Neck* 1999;21:291.
28. Epstein J, Robertson M, Emerton S, et al. Quality of life and oral function in patients treated with radiation therapy for head and neck cancer. *Head Neck* 2001;23:38.
29. de Graeff A, de Leeuw R, Ros W, et al. A prospective study on quality of life of patients with cancer of the oral cavity or oropharynx treated with surgery with or without radiotherapy. *Oral Oncol* 1999;35:27.
30. List M, Siston A, Haraf D, et al. Quality of life and performance in advanced head and neck cancer patients on concomitant chemoradiotherapy: a prospective examination. *J Clin Oncol* 1999;17:1020.
31. Campbell B, Marbella A, Layde P. Quality of life and recurrence concern in survivors of head and neck cancer. *Laryngoscope* 2000;110:895.
32. de Graeff A, de Leeuw R, Ros W, et al. Long-term quality of life of patients with head and neck cancer. *Laryngoscope* 2000;110:98.
33. Calman KC. Definitions and dimensions of quality of life. In: Aaronson NK, Beckmann JH, eds. *The quality of life of cancer patients.* New York: Raven Press, 1987:1.
34. Hammerlid E, Taft C. Health-related quality of life in long-term head and neck cancer survivors: a comparison with general population norms. *Br J Cancer* 2001;84:149.
35. Spitzer WO, Dobson AJ, Hall J, et al. Measuring the quality of life of cancer patients. A concise QL-Index for use by physicians. *J Chronic Dis* 1981;34:585.
36. Presant CA. Quality of life in cancer patients: who measures what? *Am J Clin Oncol* 1984;7:571.
37. Slevin, Plant H, Lynch D, et al. Who should measure quality of life, the doctor or the patient? *Br J Cancer* 1988;57:109.
38. Kahn SB, Hums PS, Harding SP. Quality of life and patients with cancer: a comparative study of patient versus physician perceptions and its implications for cancer education. *J Cancer Educ* 1992;7:241.
39. Grossman SA, Sheidler VR, Swedeen K, et al. Correlation of patient and caregiver ratings of cancer pain. *J Pain Symptom Manage* 1991;6:53.
40. Ware JE. Measuring functioning, well-being, and other generic health concepts. In: Osoba D, ed. *Effect of cancer on quality of life.* Boca Raton, FL: CRC Press, 1991:7.
41. de Graeff A, de Leeuw R, Ros W, et al. Pretreatment factors predicting quality of life after treatment for head and neck cancer. *Head Neck* 2000;22:389.
42. Saxena A, Gnanasekaran N, Andley M. An epidemiological study of prevalence of pain in head and neck cancers. *Indian J Med Res* 1995;102:28.
43. Keefe FJ, Brantley A, Manuel G, et al. Behavioral assessments of head and neck cancer pain. *Pain* 1985;23:327.
44. Johnston CA, Keane TJ, Prudo SM. Weight loss in patients receiving radical radiation therapy for head and neck cancer: a prospective study. *J Enteric Parenter Nutr* 1982;6:399.
45. Morton RP. Life satisfaction in head and neck cancer patients. *Clin Otolaryngol* 1995;20:499.
46. Vogelzang NJ, Breitbart W, Cella D, et al. Patient, caregiver, and oncologist perceptions of cancer-related fatigue: results of a tripart assessment survey. The Fatigue Coalition. *Semin Hematol* 1997;suppl 2:4–12.
47. Curt GA, Breitbart W, Cella D, et al. Impact of cancer-related fatigue on the lives of patients: new findings from the fatigue coalition. *Oncologist* 2000;5:353–360.
48. Portenoy RK, Itri LM. Cancer-related fatigue: guidelines for evaluation and management. *Oncologist* 1999;4:1–10.
49. Demetri GD, Kris J, Wade J, et al. Quality-of-life benefit in chemotherapy patients treated with epoetin alfa is independent of disease response of tumor type: results from a prospective community oncology study. *J Clin Oncol* 1998;16:3412.
50. Glaspy J, Bukowski R, Steinberg D, et al. Impact of therapy with epoetin alfa on clinical outcomes in patients with non-myeloid malignancies during cancer chemotherapy in community oncology practice. *J Clin Oncol* 1997;15:1218.
51. Gabrilove JL, Cleeland CS, Livingston RB, et al. Clinical evaluation of once-weekly dosing of epoetin alfa in chemotherapy patients: improvements in hemoglobin and quality of life are similar to three-times-weekly dosing. *J Clin Oncol* 2001;19:2875.
52. Littlewood TJ, Bajetta E, Nortier JW, et al. Effects of Epoetin alfa on hematologic parameters and quality of life in cancer patients receiving nonplatinum chemotherapy: results of a randomized, double-blind, placebo-controlled trial. *J Clin Oncol* 2001;19:2865.
53. Quirt I, Robeson C, Lau CY, et al. Epoetin alfa therapy increases hemoglobin levels and improves quality of life in patients with cancer-related anemia who are not receiving chemotherapy and patients with anemia who are receiving chemotherapy. *J Clin Oncol* 2001;19:4126.
54. David DJ, Barritt JA. Psychosocial aspects of head and neck cancer surgery. *Aust N Z J Surg* 1977;47:584.
55. Olson M, Shedd DP. Disability and rehabilitation in head and neck cancer patients after treatment. *Head Neck Surg* 1978;1:52.
56. Dretmer B, Ahlbom A. Quality of life and state of health for patients with cancer in the head and neck. *Acta Otolaryngol* 1983;96:307.
57. Morton RP, Davies ADM, Baker J, et al. Quality of life in treated head and neck cancer patients: a preliminary report. *Clin Otolaryngol* 1984;9:181.
58. Dropkin MJ. Coping with disfigurement and dysfunction after head and neck cancer surgery: a conceptual framework. *Semin Oncol Nurs* 1989;5:213.
59. Langius A, Bjorvell H, Lind MG. Functional status and coping in patients with oral and pharyngeal cancer before and after surgery. *Head Neck* 1994;16:559.
60. Bunston T, Mings D. Developing an instrument to determine the symptom management and nonmedical needs of patients with head and neck cancer. *Curr Opin Oncol* 1994;1:26.
61. Kreitier S, Chaitchik S, Rapoport Y, et al. Psychosocial effects of level of information and severity of disease on head and neck cancer patients. *J Cancer Educ* 1995;10:144.
62. Hassan SJ, Weymuller EA. Assessment of quality of life in head and neck cancer patients. *Head Neck* 1993;15:485.
63. Rogers S, Lowe D, Brown J, et al. A comparison between the University of Washington Head and Neck Disease-Specific Measure and the Medical Short Form 36. EORTC QOQ-C33 and EORTC Head and Neck 35. *Oral Oncol* 1998;34:361.
64. Ringash J, Bezjak A. A structured review of quality of life instrument for head and neck cancer patients. *Head Neck* 2001;23:201.
65. Cella D. *F.A.C.I.T manual,* version 4. Evanston, NY: Center on Outcomes, Research and Education, Evanston Northwestern Health Care and Northwestern University, 1997.
66. Morton R, Witterick I. Rationale and development of a quality of life instrument for head and neck cancer patients. *Am J Otolaryngol* 1995;16:284.
67. Morton R. Quality of life and cost-effectiveness. *Head Neck* 1997;19:243.
68. Rathmell A, Ash D, Howes M, et al. Assessing quality of life in patients treated for advanced head and neck cancer. *Clin Oncol* 1991;3:10.
69. Johnson D, Casey L, Noriega D. A pilot study of patient quality of life during radiation therapy treatment *Qual Life Res* 1994;3:267.
70. Terrell J, Navanti K, Esclamado R, et al. Head and neck cancer specific quality of life. *Arch Otolaryngol Head Neck Surg* 1997;123:1125.
71. Baker C. A functional status scale for measuring quality of life outcomes in head and neck cancer patients. *Cancer Nurs* 1995;18:452.

72. Ward SE, Goldberg N, Miller-McCauley V, et al. Patient-related barriers to management of cancer pain. *Pain* 1993;52:319.
73. Von Roenn JH, Cleeland CS, Gonin R, et al. Physician's attitudes and practice in cancer pain management: a survey from the Eastern Cooperative Oncology Group. *Ann Intern Med* 1993;119:121.
74. World Health Organization. *Technical report series 804, cancer pain and palliative care.* Geneva: World Health Organization, 1990:11.
75. Doyle D, Hanks GW, MacDonald RN, eds. *Oxford textbook of palliative medicine,* 2nd ed. Oxford: Oxford University Press, 1998.
76. Coates A, Gebski V, Bishop JF, et al. Improving the quality of life during chemotherapy for advanced breast cancer. A comparison of intermittent and continuous treatment strategies. *N Engl J Med* 1987;317:1490.
77. Sugarbaker PH, Barofsky IK, Rosenberg SA, et al. Quality of life assessment in patients in extremity sarcoma clinical trials. *Surgery* 1982;91:17.
78. Drummond W, Stoddart GL, Torrance GW. *Methods for the economic evaluation of health care programmes.* Oxford: Oxford Medical Publishers, 1987.
79. Cella DF, Jacobsen PB, Lesko LM. Research methods in psycho-oncology. In: Holland JC, Rowland JH, eds. *Handbook of psychooncology.* New York: Oxford University Press, 1989:737.
80. Portenoy RK, Thaler HT, Kornblith AB, et al. The Memorial Symptom Assessment Scale: an instrument for the evaluation of symptom prevalence, characteristics and distress. *Eur J Cancer* 1994;30A:1326.
81. de Haes JCJM, van Knippenberg FCE, Neijt JP. Measuring psychological and physical distress in cancer patients: structure and application of the Rotterdam Symptom Checklist. *Br J Cancer* 1990;62:1034.
82. Yates JW, Chalmer B, McKegney FP. Evaluation of patients with advanced cancer using the Karnofsky Performance Status. *Cancer* 1980;40:2220.
83. Schag CC, Heinrich RL, Ganz PA. Karnofsky Performance Status revisited: reliability, validity and guidelines. *J Clin Oncol* 1984;2:187.
84. List MA, Pitter-Sterr C, Lansky SB. A performance status scale for head and neck cancer patients. *Cancer* 1990;66:564.
85. Priestman TJ, Baum M. Evaluation of quality of life in patients receiving treatment for advanced breast cancer. *Lancet* 1976;24:899.
86. Wood-Dauphinee, Williams JI. The Spitzer Quality of Life Index: its performance as a measure. In: Osoba D, ed. *Effect of cancer on quality of life.* Boca Raton, FL: CRC Press, 1991:170.
87. Schipper H, Clinch J, McMurray A, et al. Measuring the quality of life of cancer patients: the Functional Living Index–Cancer. Development and validation. *J Clin Oncol* 1984;2:472.
88. Ganz PA, Haskell CA, Figlin RA, et al. Estimating the quality of life in a clinical trial of patients with metastatic lung cancer using the Karnofsky Performance Status and the Functional Living Index–Cancer. *Cancer* 1988;61:849.
89. Sadura A, Pater J, Osoba D, et al. Quality of life assessment: patient compliance with questionnaire completion. *J Natl Cancer Inst* 1992;84:1023.
90. Morrow GR, Lindke J, Black P. Measurement of the quality of life in patients: psychometric analyses of the Functional Living Index–Cancer. *Qual Life Res* 1992;1:287.
91. Cella DF, Tulsky DS, Gray G, et al. The Functional Assessment of Cancer Therapy scale: development and validation of the general measure. *J Clin Oncol* 1993;11:570.
92. Aaronson NK, Ahmedzai S, Bergman B, et al. The European Organization for Research and Treatment of Cancer QLQ-C30: a quality of life instrument for use in international clinical trials in oncology. *J Natl Cancer Inst* 1993;85: 365.
93. Ganz PA, Schag CAC, Lee JJ, et al. The CARES: a generic measure of health-related quality of life for patients with cancer. *Qual Life Res* 1992;1:19.
94. Stewart AL, Hays RD, Ware JE. The MOS short-form general health survey: reliability and validity in a patient population. *Med Care* 1988;26:724.
95. Bergner M, Bobbitt RA, Carter WB, et al. The Sickness Impact Profile: development and final revision of a health status measure. *Med Care* 1981;19:787.
96. Chambers LW, MacDonald LA, Tugwell P, et al. The McMaster Health Index Questionnaire as a measure of quality of life for patients with rheumatoid disease. *J Rheumatol* 1982;9:780.
97. Hunt S, McKenna SP, McEwen J, et al. The Nottingham Health Profile: subjective health status and medical consultations. *Soc Sci Med* 1981;15A:221.
98. Morton RP, Witterick IJ. Rationale and development of a quality of life instrument for head and neck cancer patients. *Am J Otolaryngol* 1995;16:284.
99. Bjordal K, Kaasa S. Psychometric validation of the EORTC core quality of life questionnaire, 30-item version and a diagnosis-specific module for head and neck cancer patients. *Acta Oncol* 1992;31:311.
100. Brownian GP, Levine MN, Hodson DI, et al. The head and neck radiotherapy questionnaire: a morbidity/quality of life instrument for clinical trials of radiation therapy in locally advanced head and neck cancer. *J Clin Oncol* 1993;11:863.
101. Llewellyn-Thomas HA, Sutherland I-U, Hogg SA, et al. Linear analogue self-assessment of voice quality in laryngeal cancer. *J Chron Dis* 1984;37:917.
102. Osoba D, Aaronson N-K, Till JE. A practical guide for selecting quality of life measures in clinical trials and practice. In: Osoba D, ed. *Effect of cancer on quality of life.* Boca Raton, FL: CRC Press, 1991:89.
103. Aaronson NK, Bakker W, Stewart A, et al. Multidimensional approach to the measurement of quality of life in lung cancer clinical trials. In: Aaronson NK, Beckmann JH, eds. *The quality of life of cancer patients.* New York: Raven Press, 1987:63.
104. Aaronson NK, Bullinger M, Ahmedzai S. A modular approach to quality of life assessment in cancer clinical trials. *Recent Results Cancer Res* 1988;111:238.
105. Grond S, Zech D, Lynch J, et al. Validation of World Health Organization guidelines for pain relief in head and neck cancer. *Ann Otol Rhinol Laryngol* 1993;102:342.
106. Portenoy RK, Thaler HT, Kornblith AB, et al. Symptom prevalence, characteristics and distress in a cancer population. *Qual Life Res* 1994;3:183.
107. Curtis EB, Kretch R, Walsh TD. Common symptoms in patients with advanced cancer. *J Palliat Care* 1991;7:25.
108. Dunphy YP, Amesbury BDW. A comparison of hospice and homecare patients: patterns of referral, patient characteristics and predictors of place of death. *Palliat Med* 1990;4:105.
109. Dunlop GM. A study of the relative frequency and importance of gastrointestinal symptoms and weakness in patients with far-advanced cancer [student paper]. *Palliat Med* 1989;4:37.
110. Reuben DB, Mor V, Hiris J. Clinical symptoms and length of survival in patients with terminal cancer. *Arch Intern Med* 1988;148:1586.
111. Derogatis LR, Morrow GR, Fetting J, et al. The prevalence of psychiatric disorders among cancer patients. *JAMA* 1983;249:751.
112. Craig TJ, Abeloff NM. Psychiatric symptomatology among hospitalized cancer patients. *Am J Psychiatry* 1974;131:1323.
113. Levine PM, Silberfarb PM, Lipowski ZJ. Mental disorders in cancer patients: a study of 100 psychiatric referrals. *Cancer* 1978;42:1386.
114. Massie MJ, Holland JC. Overview of normal reactions and prevalence of psychiatric disorders. In: Holland JC, Rowland JH, eds. *Handbook of psychooncology.* New York: Oxford University Press, 1989:273.
115. Vecht CJ, Hoff AM, Kansen PJ, et al. Types and causes of pain in cancer of the head and neck. *Cancer* 1992;70:178.
116. McCorkle R, Young K. Development of a symptom distress scale. *Cancer Nurs* 1978;1:373.
117. Kukull WA, McCorkle R, Driever M. Symptom distress, psychosocial variables and survival from lung cancer. *J Psychosoc Oncol* 1986;4:91.
118. Daut RL, Cleeland CS, Flannery RC. The development of the Wisconsin Brief Pain Questionnaire to assess pain in cancer and other diseases. *Pain* 1983;17: 197.
119. Portenoy RK, Kornblith AB, Wong G, et al. Pain in ovarian cancer: prevalence, characteristics, and associated symptoms. *Cancer* 1994;74:907.
120. Portenoy RK, Miransky J, Thaler HT, et al. Pain in ambulatory patients with lung or colon cancer: prevalence, characteristics and impact. *Cancer* 1992;70: 1616.
121. Ferrell BR, Wisdom C, Wenzl C. Quality of life as an outcome variable in the management of cancer pain. *Cancer* 1989;63(suppl):2321.
122. Moore MJ, Osoba D, Murphy K, et al. Use of palliative endpoints to evaluate the effect of mitoxantrone and low-dose prednisone in patients with hormonally resistant prostate cancer. *J Clin Oncol* 1994;12:689.
123. Schwartz D, Lellouch J. Explanatory and pragmatic attitudes in therapeutic trials. *J Chron Dis* 1967;20:637.

CHAPTER 11

General Principles of Rehabilitation of Speech, Voice, and Swallowing Function After Treatment of Head and Neck Cancer

Susan D. Miller and Lucian Sulica

Over the past three decades, concern for restoration of function has become a primary goal in the treatment of persons with head and neck cancer. Conservation surgery, radiation therapy, sensate flap reconstruction, and larynx-sparing protocols have all received attention in the effort to maintain or reestablish functional speech, voice, and swallowing in these patients. More important than any single technique, multidisciplinary collaborative management, with contributions from the head and neck surgeon, radiation oncologist, medical oncologist, reconstructive surgeon, speech pathologist, prosthodontist, dental oncologist, nutritionist, nurse oncologist, psychologist, audiologist, and social worker, has proved instrumental in achieving these aims. Although the value of such an approach is widely recognized, it is occasionally difficult to form a truly integrated treatment plan from the varied backgrounds and foci of the members of the therapeutic team. This chapter synthesizes the points of view of an otolaryngologist and a speech pathologist in pursuit of the same goal: optimal functional outcome for the patient. The collaboration needed to produce it has mirrored in many ways the professional cooperation necessary to clinical care. Differences in terminology, emphasis, and theoretic approach must be recognized, discussed candidly, and resolved jointly. In doing so, a member of the team learns from another, allowing subtle modifications in approach to benefit the patient. The disagreements that remain often reflect real gaps in scientific knowledge, not necessarily evident when approaching a problem from a more narrow perspective, and serve to direct future inquiry.

PRETREATMENT ASSESSMENT

Where quality-of-life issues, such as speech, voice, and swallowing, are concerned, the informed patient may be the person best suited to assessing needs, and as a result provides invaluable input to the team. To do this effectively, patients must first learn a great deal about subjects of which they likely know little or nothing. Thus, the inclusion of the patient begins with pretreatment counseling.

Preoperative consultation with the speech pathologist should be scheduled soon after the physician has made a definitive diagnosis and initial recommendations for treatment. During this visit, the speech pathologist reviews what the patient already knows and explains normal anatomy and physiology and anticipated functional changes. Patients with glottic carcinoma treated with radiation should be counseled regarding vocal changes, such as hoarseness, and swallowing difficulties that may occur during or following radiotherapy. Patients undergoing oral, pharyngeal, or conservation laryngeal surgery should be counseled regarding their immediate postsurgical course, and the likely need for temporary nasogastric and tracheostomy tubes. Short- and long-term rehabilitation strategies for speech, voice, and swallowing should be discussed. If oral communication will not be a possibility after extensive oral cavity surgery, patients need information about augmentative or alternative communication devices. Patients scheduled for total laryngectomy learn of voicing alternatives available to them. Frequently, patients consent to trial use of an electrolarynx on their neck or intraorally, and order the recommended device prior to surgery. We have found that patients who are willing to experiment with speech devices before surgery feel more "in control" and comfortable that they will be able to express their needs. Patients and their families may want to meet a patient volunteer who has undergone similar surgery. An important goal of pretreatment counseling is for the speech pathologist to establish rapport with the patient, so that the patient has a speech professional, in addition to the physician, with whom to address concerns.

DIAGNOSTIC EVALUATION

Speech

Reading samples, including standardized articulation sentences, nonnasal and nasal paragraphs, and conversational speech samples, should be recorded from persons whose tongue, velum, or jaw will be affected by surgery. These samples establish baseline articulation, fluency, rate, dialect, intonation, and nasality patterns. A spectrogram that portrays frequency, intensity, and format information regarding resonant frequencies of the vocal tract provides additional data regarding tongue placement and resonance. Standardized articulation testing typically is not performed for patients undergoing treatment for early or later stage laryngeal carcinoma unless modification of the articulating structures is planned. However, the speech pathologist should listen for and document any perceived articulation, fluency, rate, or dialect patterns during conversation with the patient. The speech pathologist examines orofacial structures, sensation, and function. Plans for pretreatment dental care or postoperative radiation are discussed as they may impact articulation, voice, and deglutition. Preoperative hearing status should be assessed for patients with reduced hearing acuity, as these individuals may have difficulty monitoring intelligibility and precision of their articulation.

Swallowing

If swallowing problems are present prior to treatment, a modified barium swallow (MBS) (1) or fiberoptic endoscopic evaluation of swallowing (FEES) (2) should be performed. Sensory testing, an addition to the FEES examination (FEEST) (3), is an evolving modality, the importance of which has yet to be established in the context of treatment of head and neck cancer. These studies will be performed after surgery, if dysphagia exists, and a baseline examination is useful in the development of a management strategy. The MBS is a videofluoroscopic study of the motor aspects of the oral, pharyngeal, and esophageal stages of the swallow with varying food consistencies. It permits measured amounts of barium bolus to be followed from the lips to the stomach and can assess the effects of compensatory strategies such as head position, chin tuck, and so forth (4). For patients with oral-stage dysphagia, the MBS is the procedure of choice. If pharyngeal or laryngeal problems exist, the FEES or FEEST can be performed at bedside. The FEES employs a fiberoptic nasopharyngoscope to directly observe the pharyngeal and laryngeal structures during the pharyngeal phase of the swallow. A bolus of contrasting color is utilized to note premature spillage into the hypopharynx or laryngeal vestibule before swallowing, vocal fold closure, and the presence of residue in the hypopharynx and laryngopharynx after a swallow. Penetration or aspiration may be identified after a swallow, although they cannot be directly observed (5). The MBS and FEES primarily analyze the motor components of swallowing. Laryngeal sensory testing involves the delivery of air pulses of measured intensity to the mucosa of the larynx via a nasopharyngoscope. By observing patient response, or, in the case of a patient with altered consciousness, activation of the laryngeal adductor reflex, sensation can be quantified. Most of the work to establish morbid thresholds has been performed in the context of stroke, but sensory testing holds promise for more accurate assessment of postoperative swallowing deficits (3).

Voice

Baseline acoustic and aerodynamic analysis should be performed on all patients with voice change, and with special care in early glottic cancer patients whether undergoing radiation or microsurgical excision. Measures of fundamental frequency, frequency perturbation (jitter), amplitude, amplitude perturbation (shimmer), and noise to harmonic ratio are obtained from a sustained vowel /a/. Instruments such as the Computerized Speech Laboratory (Kay Elemetrics Corp., Lincoln Park, Nj.), Speech Viewer III (IBM, Austin, Tx. Dr. Speech (Tiger Electronics, Seattle, Wa.) and Speech Master III (Speech-Master, Vero Beach, Fl.) can be used to obtain these measures quickly. Baseline airflow rates, subglottal pressure, and laryngeal resistance measures can be calculated using the Aerophone II (Kay Elemetrics Corp.), Glottal Enterprise (Syracuse, Ny.), or Nagashima Phonatory Function Analyzer (Kelleher Medical, Richmond, Va.). Like all automated instruments, these offer convenience and efficiency, but they are not a substitute for a well-informed operator. The accuracy of data depends entirely on a conscientious, intelligent professional collecting it. Documentation of these measures prior to treatment and at specific intervals during and after treatment is essential for objective comparison of vocal changes following microsurgery or radiation therapy for early glottic carcinoma.

POSTTREATMENT INTERVENTION

Speech and Swallowing After Oral Cavity Surgery

Restoration of speech and swallow function after glossectomy appears to be highly dependent on (a) the quantity and mobility of residual tongue after surgery; (b) the reconstructive technique; (c) the integrity of motor and sensory nerve supply to the specific tissue; (d) the functional recovery following reconstruction; (e) the degree of scarring and fibrosis to the residual tongue musculature after surgery and radiation; (f) the early intervention of speech therapy; and (g) patient psychosocial factors such as age, medical condition, motivation, and family support (6–8). Patients undergoing resections of the anterior portion or less than 50% of the mobile tongue may present with a delayed swallowing reflex and reduced ability to manipulate the bolus in the oral cavity (5). The return of normal speech intelligibility and deglutition for small, anterior tongue lesions less than 12 cm has been reported (9,10). Articulation deficits are mild and often characterized by a lateral lisp. Speech therapy should focus on oral motor exercises to achieve adequate linguoalveolar and linguopalatal contact for accurate phoneme productions.

Patients with larger tongue lesions present with poor bolus formation, poor bolus manipulation, delayed elicitation of the swallow reflex, and increased oral transit time due to decreased tongue bulk and mobility (1) and reduced glossopalatal closure (11). Compensatory speech patterns, such as contacting the tongue behind the lower teeth, are used to obtain intelligible linguoalveolar (t,d,n,l,s,z) and linguopalatal (sh,ch) sound production if the tongue cannot contact the alveolar ridge or palate. If contact remains difficult, a palatal prosthesis can lower the palate and aid linguopalatal contact (5,12).

When more than 50% of the tongue is sacrificed, when the base of tongue, floor of mouth, or lateral pharyngeal walls are altered, or when an extensive oral lesion requires a composite resection, including total glossectomy, radical neck dissection, or mandibulectomy, speech and swallowing difficulties are profound (13–15). Salibian et al. (16) found that the successful outcome of swallowing and speech correlated with the shape and position of the tongue root and the surface area of the floor of the mouth. Reconstruction for large tumors of the tongue and floor of mouth using split-thickness skin grafts, reinnervated rectus abdominis (10,17), and pectoralis major (18) myocutaneous tissue flaps and microvascular free flaps result in more functional speech and swallowing than does primary closure (19,20). The bilobed, sensate radial forearm flap allows optimal functional speech and swallowing return after extensive oral cavity surgery (21–23). The bilobed design allows for one portion of the muscle flap to provide bulk for restoring the floor of the mouth, whereas the other portion provides volume to the "mobile" tongue (22). Excellent speech and swallowing has been reported using the infrahyoid muscle flap for medium-sized defects in the floor of the mouth, tongue, buccal mucosa, and lateral pharyngeal wall (24). Excellent to good functional speech and swallowing outcome was reported in 18 of 20 base of tongue carcinoma patients (11/12 T1 and T2 patients; 8/9 T3 and T4 patients) treated with external beam irradiation followed by an interstitial implant boost with iodine 125 several weeks later (25). However, sensory testing reveals that radiation significantly diminishes intraoral two-point discrimination in patients so treated, probably permanently (26).

As reconstructive techniques and organ preservation protocols multiply, additional diagnostic studies such as videosonography (27), high-speed cineradiography (28), and perfusion manometry (29) may become useful to measure and compare functional aspects of swallowing recovery. The short- and long-term effects of radiotherapy, chemotherapy, and/or surgery on the sensory aspects of swallowing also will become more apparent as sensory testing becomes an integral part of cancer management.

Voice and Swallowing Changes After Treatment of Laryngeal Cancer

The issue of voice quality is especially important for patients with early glottic carcinoma, because both radiation and endoscopic resection can achieve adequate oncologic results. Both modalities can also improve voice for most patients, but available data on their relative merit can be difficult to interpret for two principal reasons. First, there are no universally accepted measures of voice outcome comparable to 5-year survival in head and neck oncology. Study results vary, depending on the combination of acoustic, aerodynamic, stroboscopic, or perceptual data reported. Thus some studies report that voice returns to normal with treatment (30–32), whereas others, generally those relying more heavily on quantitative information, report persistent abnormal values (33–37). Second, recovery of vocal function can be a long process. For example, some studies show significant abnormalities 6 months after radiation treatment that improve slowly over months to years (34,38). Mucosal wave may take as long as 1 year to return (38). Just as there is no consensus on voice measures, there is no agreement as to when a voice result can be considered "final." Posttreatment intervals in the literature vary from 3 months (12) to 10 years (34). Furthermore, improvement probably occurs at a slower rate after radiation than after surgery, so a comparison of patients at the same point following treatment may not be useful.

Of the two therapeutic modalities, radiation is the better studied. Patterns of rapid improvement, marked deterioration and recovery, and general fluctuation have all been observed following treatment (31,32). Although there is widespread agreement that voice quality ultimately improves, there is less consensus regarding whether the radiated voice ever becomes normal. Studied as a whole, early glottic carcinoma patients at least 1 year after completion of radiation therapy were found to have poorer voice than age- and sex-matched controls in a number of studies (33,36,37,39). By 9 months, all 25 patients in one study regained 90% to 100% of normal voice, when evaluated by a calculated voice analysis (32). Of 60 patients with T1 disease studied before and at various intervals up to 10 years after radiotherapy, 55% to 85% achieved normal voice quality, both by perceptual and quantitative assessment, compared with age- and sex-matched controls (34). A similar study, which included some T2 lesions, found normal return of voice in 67% of patients, as assessed by their physicians (40). Various factors tended to compromise the voice result: increased patient age (34), complications during the course of treatment (40), continued smoking (34,40), and mucosal stripping for initial diagnosis (34,40). Behrman et al. (41) have highlighted the difficulties in separating postradiation voice changes from age-related dysphonia.

Despite observed differences from normal, postradiation voice has been the benchmark against which surgical results are measured. Studies in which patients undergoing radiation therapy are compared with stage-matched patients undergoing endoscopic resection have generally found that voice tends to be superior following radiation (42,43). An analysis of results of endoscopic resection by Hirano et al. (35) noted postoperative hoarseness to occur more often than after radiation, to be characterized by breathiness rather than by strain, and to be proportional to the amount of vocalis muscle resected. Subsequent studies have expanded on these observations. McGuirt et al. (44) found that voice quality after surgery can be equivalent to that of irradiated patients in patients with unilateral T1 disease sparing the anterior commissure, subglottis, and arytenoid. Conversely, transglottic resection, partial or complete resection of the arytenoid, and resection of the anterior commissure all resulted in significant compromise of voice in a study of patients 6 months or more after endoscopic resection (45). Endoscopic laser resection with surgical margins of 2 mm or less has been proposed to spare as much vocal fold thickness as possible (46). The oncologic efficacy of this approach remains to be established conclusively, but narrow-margin excision results in better voice than the more extensive traditional cordectomy, comparable with voice after radiation (46).

In general, poor voice quality after surgery is the result of incomplete glottic closure (35,44,45,47), in contrast to postradiation dysphonia, which results mainly from fibrosis and stiffness of the vocal folds (36,37,39,41). Therefore, surgery is best suited to lesions amenable to excision with minimal tissue loss. These can be difficult to identify in the office, even with stroboscopy (48), and the surgeon must stand ready to alter treatment plans if a lesion is unexpectedly extensive at microlaryngoscopy.

Little data regarding voice outcome has accumulated in advanced laryngeal carcinoma, both because organ preservation protocols are relatively new, and because the benefits of retaining the larynx seem self-evident. Evaluation of a small number of patients after chemoradiation for stage III and IV disease, aimed primarily at identifying reliable indicators of vocal function, revealed functional voice in the majority of subjects (42). When voice and speech quality of laryngectomees is compared with that of radiated patients and of normal control subjects, there are surprisingly few acoustic differences between the treated groups (49). Perceptual ratings, however, clearly identify decreased intelligibility, voice quality, and speech acceptability in the laryngectomized patients. In one study, however, self-rating of quality of life by patients after laryngectomy did not differ from that of patients treated with radiation only, although verbal handicap was worse (43).

Available research on voice outcomes, while yielding an abundance of data, has left significant ambiguities. As in analyses of benign voice disorders, the correlation between perceptual and quantitative data can be poor. In most study designs, objective data are collected and translated into a conclusion about functional status by a health care professional. Yet voice is exclusively a quality-of-life issue; logic suggests that patients may be the best arbiters of their own functional status. The patient self-rating may also be the most helpful piece of information we can offer to patients facing the uncertainties of treatment. In light of this, it is surprising how rarely the patient's opinion has been solicited. In some cases, it is even dismissed because it does not correlate with the objective findings.

Of 20 patients with T1 lesions treated with radiation, only 10% reported the absence of voice problems 1 to 7 years after treatment (37). Eighty percent of patients with T1 and T2 lesions reported voice fatigue (36). Neither of these two studies used validated outcomes instruments, like the Voice Handicap Index (VHI) (50) and the Voice-Related Quality of Life questionnaire (51), developed to facilitate reporting of comparable results. Behrman et al. (41) reported that VHI scores in radiated patients were not statistically distinct from those of patients diagnosed with age-related dysphonia. More standardized patient self-rating data may give a more realistic picture of voice outcomes following treatment of laryngeal cancer.

Because changes in vocal quality are common among patients following either radiation therapy or laser excision, voice therapy is probably useful to hasten recovery and maximize function. Adherence to a vocal hygiene program with daily exercises emphasizing proper tone focus, placement, and flexibility can result in more efficient, resonant voice. To date, the potentially helpful role of voice therapy in these patients has not been studied.

Supraglottic laryngectomy patients frequently experience dysphagia due to the combined effects of supraglottic sensory denervation, incomplete motion of the partially resected tongue base toward the posterior pharyngeal wall, restricted arytenoid motion, partial closure of the airway, and delays in bolus propulsion from narrowing at the esophageal entrance (52). These patients must avoid liquids and learn supraglottic (5,53) and supersupraglottic swallow (54,55) maneuvers to ensure feeding safety. Commercially available thickening agents may be used to thicken the consistency of thin liquids for safer swallowing. Supraglottic laryngectomy patients frequently experience breathiness and/or hoarseness that may respond to short-term voice therapy. They may also demonstrate an increase in fundamental frequency, which may result from added tension to the vocal cords, thought to be the result of forced adduction exercises (5).

Voice and swallowing problems following hemilaryngectomy vary according to the extent of surgery. If arytenoid resection is included, the risk for aspiration is greater. If the hemilaryngectomy is isolated to one true vocal fold, and one false vocal fold, the ventricle, and the epiglottis are preserved, swallowing may be improved with a chin tuck to assist in airway protection and head turning toward the operated side to direct food from the compromised area (5). Vocal characteristics of the hemilaryngectomee have been described as rough, low-pitch, breathy, and constricted, perhaps due to excessive supraglottic activity to achieve adequate glottal adduction (56). Therapy techniques such as forced adduction exercises, digital pressure to the thyroid ala, decreased speaking rate, and phrasing may decrease vocal strain, improve voice quality, and increase vocal intensity by reducing glottal opening (5). Surgical vocal augmentation techniques warrant consideration to improve glottal closure.

Although few laryngectomy patients complain about difficulty swallowing, 10% to 58% of laryngectomees experience dysphagia (57–59). Problems appear to center around the pharyngoesophageal (PE) segment (58). Total laryngectomy may produce increased resistance to bolus transfer from stenosis and decreased upper esophageal segment (UES) negative pressure. Resections of the hyoid bone and thyroid cartilage further aggravate this problem by allowing the pharyngeal lumen to collapse (60).

Traditionally, cricopharyngeal hypertonicity has been treated operatively by means of dilatation, pharyngeal plexus neurectomy, or cricopharyngeal myotomy (61,62). Botulinum toxin (BTX), an inhibitor of acetylcholine release at the neuromuscular junction that provided temporary muscle weakening, permits nonsurgical treatment of upper esophageal sphincter spasm. In noncontrolled prospective clinical studies, 70% to 100% of patients with dysphagia due to cricopharyngeal spasm benefited (63–65). Decreased spasm was confirmed by cineradiography, and sometimes by manometry. Treatment permitted the consumption of solid food, removal of feeding tubes, and weight gain. Benefit was greatest in patients who had cricopharyngeal spasm as the only abnormality, as opposed to those with associated dysmotility. Botulinum toxin injection can also be used as a diagnostic maneuver to identify patients who would benefit from myotomy (64). Of note, some cricopharyngeal spasm is caused or aggravated by reflux of gastric acid, and this must be treated before relaxing the sphincter. Heartburn has been reported as a complication of upper esophageal sphincter weakening (63). Botulinum toxin can be injected transcutaneously, with the aid of electromyography, or via flexible endoscope. Treatment must be repeated about every 3 months, but it offers a way to postpone and perhaps avoid myotomy altogether in the radiated neck or the debilitated patient.

In addition to dysphagia secondary to postsurgical changes, patients treated by chemotherapy, radiotherapy, and concomitant chemoradiation may experience dysphagia due to decreased salivary flow, edema, myositis, fibrosis, delayed triggering of the pharyngeal motor response, decreased laryngopharyngeal sensation, pharyngeal incoordination, and decreased laryngeal elevation (60,64). Patients in whom dysphagia is suspected should undergo objective assessment using MBS, FEES, or FEEST to identify the relevant factors and permit treatment. Van As et al. (66) used a quantitative videofluoroscopy protocol of the neoglottis in total laryngectomies during rest, swallowing, and speech to better evaluate the anatomy and morphology of the neoglottis during various tasks.

Hyposmia, a reduced sense of smell, which in one study was present immediately after total laryngectomy in approximately 94% of 49 patients, remained a long-term problem in 53% (26/49) due to the absence of nasal airflow (67,68). All patients with hyposmia reported dysgeusia or a reduced sense of odor-related flavor perception (68). Hilgers et al. (69) reported a 46% success rate in teaching patients "polite yawning," a technique in which patients learn to actively use their facial muscles to induce nasal airflow.

ARTIFICIAL LARYNGES

For some laryngectomy patients, concerns regarding loss of speech are more important than survival itself (70). Alternative voice sources for the laryngectomee include the use of a pneumatic or electronic speech aid, esophageal speech, or tracheoesophageal puncture (TEP) speech. Patients who have undergone a partial or total glossectomy with severely restricted tongue mobility will be unable to use these voice sources, and may be introduced to computerized speaking systems or talking keyboards.

A 1987 study of voice rehabilitation practices revealed that the use of an artificial larynx (AL) or electronic speaking device was widely recommended by 90% of 400 head and neck surgeons surveyed, in many cases as a temporary means of communication after total laryngectomy (71). These battery-operated or pneumatic devices simulate sound, are relatively inexpensive, are easy to operate, and can be used by a patient with intact articulation 1 to 2 days after surgery. These devices continue to serve a useful purpose, and surgeons and speech pathologists should encourage all patients to own an AL as a primary or auxiliary speech system. Pneumatic devices consist of a piece that fits over the tracheal stoma, a unit containing a reed that produces sound, and a tube that directs sound into the

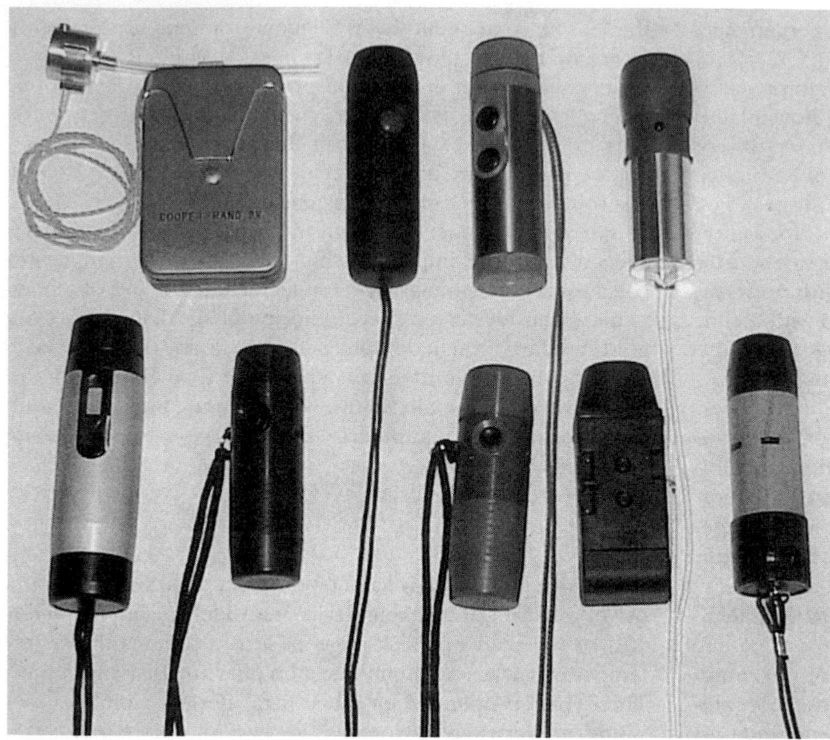

Figure 11.1 Various speech aids. **Top (left to right):** The Cooper-Rand Electronic Speech Aid (Luminaud Inc., Mentor, Oh.); the NuVois 2 (Mountain Precision Manufacturing, Boise, Id.); the Servox Inton (Siemens Hearing Instruments, Inc., Prospect Heights, Il.); the Romet (Romet, Inc., Las Vegas, Nv.). **Bottom (left to right):** The OptiVox (Bivona Medical Technologies, Gary, In.); the TruTone and SolaTone (Griffin Laboratories, Temecula, Ca.); the Denrick (Denrick, Inc., Honolulu, Hi.); and the Amplicord model 55 (Amplicord, Inc., Rome, Italy) (From Miller SD, Sessions R. Rehabilitation after treatment for head and neck cancer. In: De Vita VT, Hellman S, Rosenberg S, eds. *Cancer: principles & practice of oncology.* Philadelphia: Lippincott Williams & Wilkins, 2001, with permission.)

mouth to be articulated. Three pneumatic devices remain on the market: the Dutch Speech DSP8 Speech Aid available from Memacon in the Netherlands; the Taiwan tube popularized in Hong Kong (72); and the Tokyo Speech Aid, which is available from Clyde Welch, Harlan, Iowa. Pneumatic devices are much less expensive than battery-operated electronic devices and are more popular in Europe than in the United States.

A variety of hand-held battery-operated ALs or electrolarynges are currently available. Examples are illustrated in Figure 11.1. The Cooper-Rand Electronic Speech Aid (Luminaud Inc., Mentor, Oh.) is an electrolarynx that is used exclusively with an intraoral adapter. This adapter directs sound into the oral cavity through a tube placed in the mouth. The NuVois 1 and 2 (Mountain Precision Manufacturing, Boise, Id.), Servox Inton (Siemens Hearing Instruments, Inc., Prospect Heights, Il.), Romet (Romet, Inc., Las Vegas, Nv.), OptiVox (Bivona Medical Technologies, Gary, In.), TruTone and SolaTone (Griffin Laboratories, Temecula, Ca.), Denrick (Denrick, Inc., Honolulu, Hi.), SPKR (UNI Mfg. Co., Ontario, Or.) (not pictured), and Amplicord model 55 (Amplicord, Inc., Rome, Italy) are neck-type devices that transmit sound through the tissues of the neck into the oral cavity for speech production. These devices are activated with an on-off switch and are equipped with an adapter so they can be used as intraoral or neck-type devices. The availability of both options is extremely desirable, as patients use the intraoral adapter after surgery or radiation when the neck is edematous. Users of the TruTone (Griffin Laboratories) can set intonation sensitivity and vary intonation by pressure changes on the activator switch. The Amplicord model 95 is pressure activated as it contacts the neck rather than being activated by a switch. The UltraVoice (UltraVoice, Ltd., Paoli, Pa.) (Fig. 11.2) is an intraoral electrolarynx custom built into a denture or retainer and activated by a remote control switch.

ESOPHAGEAL SPEECH

Esophageal speech involves learning to inject or inhale air into the esophagus through the sphincter created by surgical closure of the PE segment or gullet after laryngectomy. The trapped air is then released through the PE segment, which is the vibratory source for sound in the laryngectomee (73–77).

Typically, the speech pathologist encourages the laryngectomee to attempt esophageal sound soon after the patient is able to swallow food comfortably. Patients learn to produce esophageal sound via injection (plosive, glossal press, and glos-

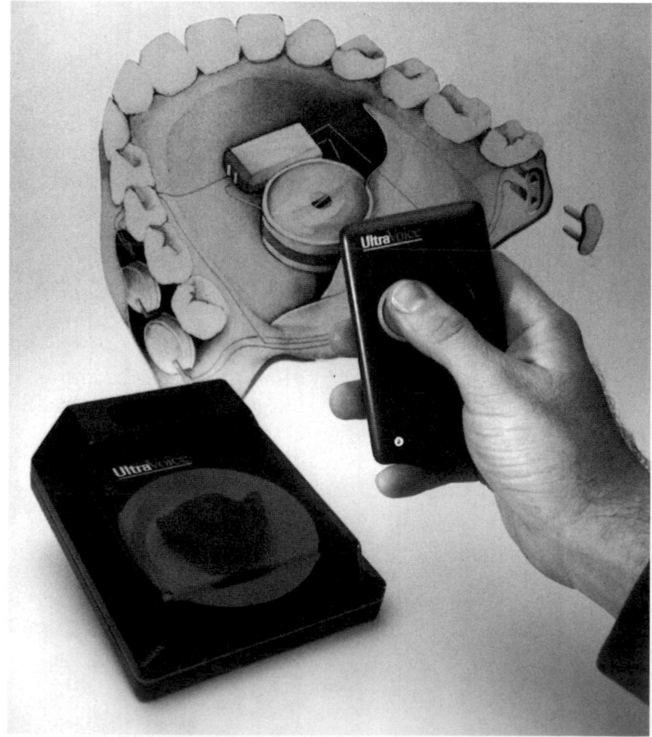

Figure 11.2 Ultra Voice. (Courtesy of UltraVoice, Ltd., Paoli, Pa.)

sopharyngeal press), inhalation, or a combination of both methods. Basically, injection methods involve the patient's learning to trap air in the mouth and forcing it into the esophagus. Some patients learn the inhalation method, in which a lowered pressure in the esophageal segment relative to atmospheric pressure allows air to enter the gullet. Patients then speak on the sound that is generated from the air in the esophagus. More extensive descriptions of these methods can be found in Diedrich and Youngstrom (74) and Gardner (75).

Even though esophageal speech can be introduced to the patient 1 or 2 weeks after the total laryngectomy, the development of functional capabilities with this method may take from 6 months to 1 year to learn; in fact, some patients never master it. Previous reports regarding the success rate in learning esophageal speech have varied from 26% to 55% (78–80); however, Fujii et al. (81) found that 74% (51 of 69) of their patients successfully used esophageal speech in daily communication. Age was the most important factor determining success and failure. Ninety percent of the patients in this study who were younger than 60 years were successful in learning esophageal speech, as compared with 10% of those older than 75 years (81). Although motivation and age appear to be important to the achievement of esophageal speech (79,82), abnormalities of the vibrating esophageal segment—tonic and hypertonic spasms—are the most commonly cited reasons for esophageal speech failure (83,84). Botulinum toxin has been used to reduce the cricopharyngeal muscle spasm sometimes responsible for failure of TEP patients to achieve satisfactory speech (85–87). Perhaps laryngectomees who cannot master esophageal speech may benefit from this same treatment.

In patients in whom esophageal speaking has failed, the tonicity or relaxation of the PE segment can be accurately evaluated by simultaneous use of videofluoroscopy and esophageal insufflation (88). This is not routinely performed in the postoperative laryngectomy patient. An easier and reliable way to assess initial opening pressures of the PE segment is a portable manometry system that can be used 4 weeks after laryngectomy (89). An initial opening pressure of between 15 and 20 mm Hg has been found to correlate with the production of a good esophageal voice (89,90).

TRACHEOESOPHAGEAL PUNCTURE

Most head and neck surgeons and most professionals who rehabilitate laryngectomees think that in properly selected patients the TEP, introduced by Singer and Blom (91) in 1980, is the standard of care for reconstitution of voice after laryngectomy. Rather than relying on the trapping of air in the esophagus, the creation of a permanent fistula through the tracheoesophageal wall permits the shunting of pulmonary air into and up the esophagus; thus, the basis for noise—vibration of the PE segment walls—is generated. Importantly, unlike esophageal speech, the reservoir of air does not depend on the gulping or trapping of air; instead, it is limited only by expiratory capacity, and, as such, more closely resembles normal voice. A valved prosthesis is placed into the puncture and, when the tracheal stoma is occluded, directs pulmonary air into the esophagus for speech. The one-way valve design of the prosthesis prevents aspiration from the esophagus into the trachea.

A device that contains a Silastic diaphragm fit into a peristomal housing permits normal respiration during silent periods; however, expiratory air for speech shuts off the pressure-sensitive diaphragm, thus diverting air through the tracheoesophageal fistula into the esophagus. This external device, called a tracheostoma breathing valve, was developed in 1982, and is of immeasurable value in rehabilitation because it eliminates the need for manual occlusion of the stoma during speech (92). However, success rates in achieving prolonged use of the breathing valve and varied housings, adhesives, and buttons have varied from 9% to 85% (93).

Initially, silicone-based glues were the only adhesives available to adhere the tracheostomal housing for the breathing valve to the patient's skin. Often, patients find the hypoallergenic glues irritating to the skin surrounding the stoma and report frustration because the housing seal leaks due to uneven stomal contours and/or the pulmonary pressures required to close the diaphragm (93,94). Self-adhesive discs are available from InHealth Technologies (Carpinteria, Ca.), Atos Medical Inc. (Milwaukee, Wi.), and Bivona Medical Technologies (Gary, In.) (Figs. 11.3 through 11.5). These flexible housings are more comfortable for the patient, although they adhere for varying amounts of time depending on the disk size, texture, and amount of pulmonary "back-pressure" needed to achieve speech (93). The Provox HandsFree HME Multi-Magnet Valve system (Atos Medical Inc., Milwaukee, Wis.) combines a heat and moisture exchange system with a tracheostoma speaking valve. This valve system fits into a self-adhesive housing; however, it is designed with a pressure release valve to reduce the problematic back-pressure generated during speech and a cough (Fig. 11.5).

The Barton button (Barton-Mayo, Rochester, Minn.) developed in 1988 (94) is a soft silicone rubber button that uses intraluminal rather than peristomal attachment for the housing (not pictured). Ideally, the button fits snuggly into the stoma, eliminating the need for peristomal adhesives; however, patients with irregular stomal contours, lack of a contiguous stomal tip, and improper button length experience air and mucus leakage around the button, expulsion of the button, and mucosal irritation. Lewin et al. (93) have reported increased success with use of a modified Barton button. Hilgers and Ackerstaff (95) propose that sectioning of the sternal heal of both sternocleidomastoid muscles be done during surgery to provide an optimal tracheostomal site.

Following total laryngectomy, patients frequently experience respiratory problems, including coughing, excessive sputum production, and shortness of breath (96). In addition, pulmonary physiology is negatively influenced by the decrease in airway resistance of the stoma (97). Many laryngectomy patients benefit from use of a heat and moisture exchange (HME) system, consisting of a removable plastic HME cartridge attached to a self-adhesive tape disk housing. The cartridge humidifies inspired air, permitting voicing when digitally occluded. Use of HME system improves pulmonary function by increasing airway resistance (98), tracheal temperature, and humidity, thus retaining 250 to 300 mL of the 500 mL of water lost by stomal breathing (99). InHealth Technologies, Bivona Medical Technologies, and Atos Medical Inc. provide HME cartridges for use with adhesive housings or as attachments to breathing valves (Figs. 11.3 through 11.5). For a historical review of the evolution of voice restoration procedures and prostheses, refer to Singer (100) and Singer and Blom (101).

Initially, TEP was performed as a second surgery in patients who had been laryngectomized; however, many surgeons and speech pathologists now prefer that the TEP be done at the time of the laryngectomy. Controversy as to the value of the secondary versus primary TEP is ongoing and is unlikely to end. In the past several years, the secondary TEP has been performed successfully as an outpatient office procedure using a flexible endoscope with local anesthesia and intravenous sedation (102,103). Some surgeons and speech pathologists prefer that the TEP be performed secondarily, at least 3 months following initial laryngectomy, so that factors such as stoma size, vibration of the PE segment, migration of the puncture site following radiation, and general health of the patient can be better controlled. Proponents of the primary

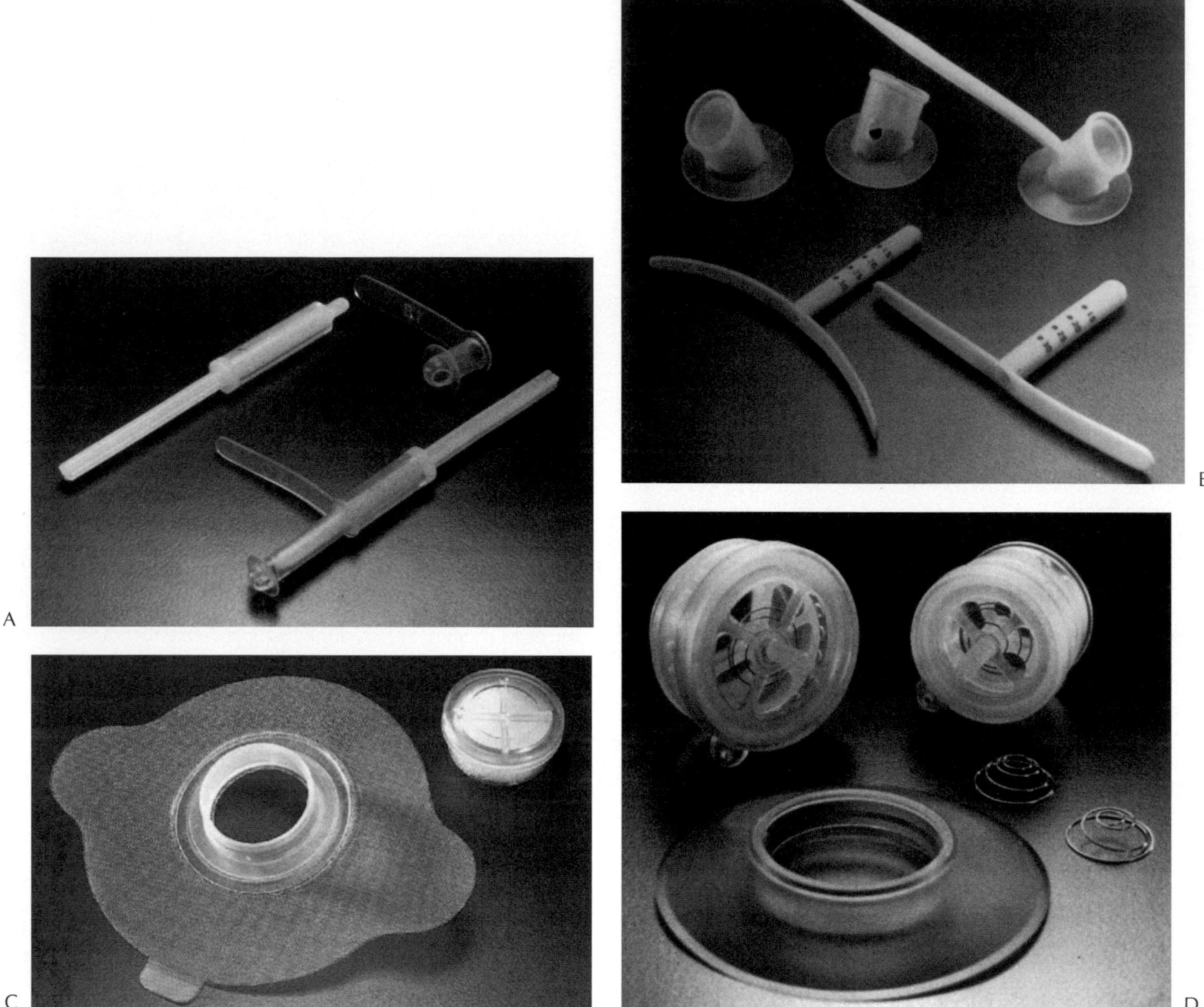

Figure 11.3 Bivona voice restoration products. **A:** Ultra-low-resistance prostheses and inserter. **B:** Bivona-Colorado button, Bivona-Colorado template, and Bivona-Colorado sizing devices. **C:** Self-adhesive tape disk housing and HME cartridge. **D:** Tracheostoma Valve II. (Courtesy of Bivona Medical Technologies, Gary, In.)

puncture argue that patients are psychologically uplifted (104) by the fact that they can speak 3 weeks after surgery. Furthermore, primary TEP proponents cite the value of technical simplicity, effectiveness, low morbidity, and cost-effectiveness of the one-stage procedure.

Success rates for both primary and secondary procedures are 73% to 95% (105–108). Regardless of time of puncture, an average of 7 hours of speech therapy is needed to learn to maintain the prosthesis and to obtain optimal communication using the TEP (105). Researchers have reported a decrease in TEP speech success rates from an initial 84% to 67% at 9 months (106) and 65% at 10 years (107) due to such patient factors as delays in seeking medical attention when the valve becomes dislodged and failure to care for the equipment properly. Saurajen et al. (109) reported that both primary and secondary TEP patients who attend voice restoration clinics and clean their prostheses regularly have significantly better voices than those who do not. Although the Blom-Singer technique is popular in the United States, specialists in other parts of the world favor different methods to restore phonation (110). Most interesting was a study by Quer et al. (111), who performed TEP at the time of the laryngectomy and also provided intensive esophageal speech instruction to 24 patients. Seventy percent of the patients (16 out of 23) later chose to use esophageal rather than TEP speech even though they agreed that TEP speech was superior to esophageal speech.

CANDIDACY FOR TRACHEOESOPHAGEAL PUNCTURE

The success of voice restoration depends on a multidisciplinary team committed to thorough patient assessment, consistent management, and flexibility in problem solving. Success with a TEP depends on good stoma construction, adequate stoma size, and accurate placement and angle of the tracheoesophageal puncture (112). The tracheal stoma should be at least 1.5 cm and not retracted behind the manubrium. If stomal stenosis is a problem, a Bivona-Colorado stent (Fig. 11.3) can be used by the surgeon to create the puncture. A Bivona-Colorado prosthesis, which is built into the tracheostoma vent, is inserted into the puncture.

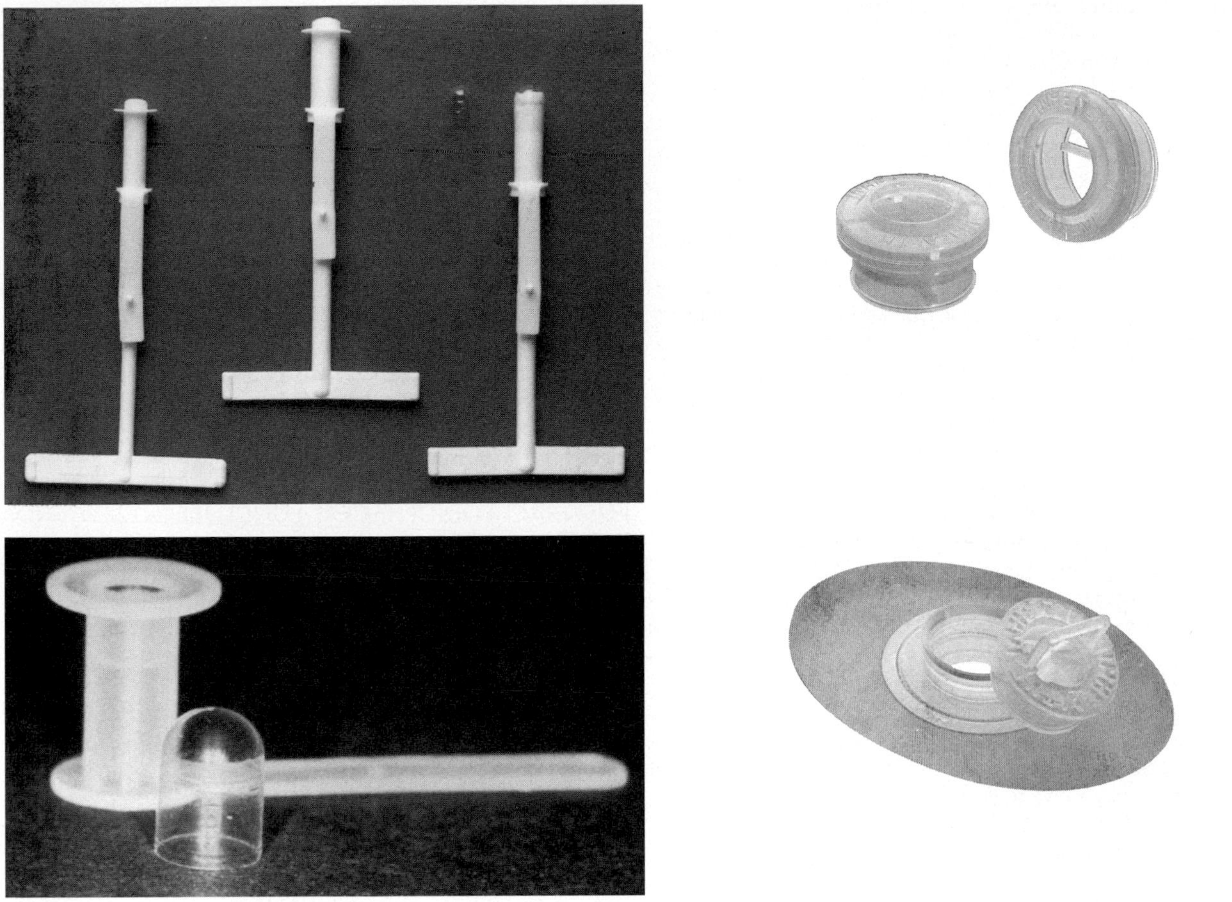

Figure 11.4 InHealth voice restoration products. **A:** No. 16 Fr and No. 18 Fr low-pressure prostheses, gel cap, and inserters. **B:** HME cartridge. **C:** Indwelling voice prosthesis and gel cap. **D:** Tracheostoma breathing valve and self-adhesive disk housing. (Courtesy of InHealth Technologies, Carpinteria, Ca.)

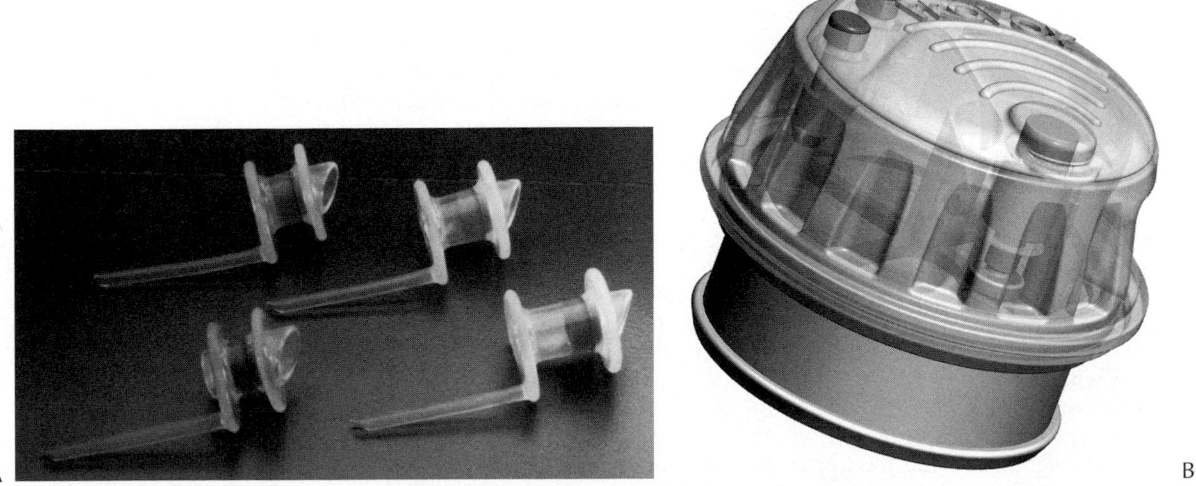

Figure 11.5 Atos voice restoration products. **A:** Atos Medical Provox 2 prostheses. **B:** Provox HandsFree HME System. (Courtesy of Atos Medical Inc., Milwaukee, Wis.)

Patients with emphysema, severe allergies, or pulmonary complications are generally not good TEP candidates due to copious amounts of secretions and reduced air volume associated with these conditions. The patient's cognitive status, financial condition, physical health, and desire for communication should be considered before TEP. The presence or absence of radiation therapy does not seem to have a significant relationship to the success or failure of TEP (113).

Because of the development of low-resistance, self-retaining prostheses inserted by the speech pathologist or surgeon (or both) and composed of materials designed to last approximately 3 to 6 months, manual dexterity and visual acuity are no longer essential for the use of this technology. These prostheses include the InHealth Indwelling (InHealth Technologies, Santa Barbara, Ca.) (Fig. 11.4); Provox 2 (114) (Atos Medical Inc., Milwaukee, Wis.) (Fig. 11.5); Voicemaster (115) (Amsterdam, Netherlands); and Nijdam (116) (Sweden) (not pictured:. The Provox (Atos Medical Inc.) and Groningen prostheses (Groningen, Holland) (not pictured) are popular indwelling prostheses in Europe. They are inserted only by a surgeon in a retrograde fashion through the mouth and out the puncture site. Ackerstaff et al. (117) report that 94% of patients and 97% of professionals prefer anterograde placement by the speech pathologist or surgeon to retrograde placement. No significant difference was noted in the device life of the Provox 2 and the Provox. These self-retaining prostheses last approximately 3 to 6 months (118–120); however, the median time for replacement is 89 days, with replacement primarily due to leakage through the prosthesis (108). An oral mycostatic solution may need to be used daily to prevent overgrowth of *Candida albicans,* which may grow onto the flap and prohibit complete closure of the flap for swallowing (117).

In following TEP patients over 13 years, Lavertu et al. (118) found that the absence of pharyngeal stricture was the only significant predictor of good to excellent speech. Because the tonicity of the PE segment in a primary puncture patient prior to the laryngectomy cannot be assessed, surgeons often perform a pharyngeal constrictor myotomy, a unilateral pharyngeal plexus neurectomy, or a unilateral pharyngeal plexus neurectomy with drainage myotomy limited to the cricopharyngeus at the time of surgery. Although all three methods are equally effective in preventing pharyngospasms, Singer et al. (61) advocate use of the pharyngeal plexus neurectomy because it preserves the vascular supply to the pharyngeal wall and preserves any residual resting tone in the PE segment, resulting in a higher speaking fundamental frequency compared with the other methods. Bastian and Muzaffar (119) report that cricopharyngeal myotomy for spasm of the cricopharyngeal muscle following a TEP can easily and effectively be performed by laser endoscopy.

Many speech pathologists perform air insufflation testing prior to a secondary puncture, although it has been challenged that failed air insufflation testing prior to the TEP does not predict successful TEP speech acquisition 6 months later (120). Lewin et al. (121) reported greater than 90% success in predicting TEP failures when intraesophageal peak pressures levels are obtained in conjunction with the air insufflation test. The air insufflation test is performed by insertion of a transnasal catheter approximately 25 cm into the upper thoracic esophagus. The catheter is attached to a circular tracheostomal housing, which is secured to the patient's skin by an adhesive. As air is insufflated into the catheter, patients are instructed to inhale, occlude the stomal assembly, and sustain a vowel sound for as long as they can. Success is determined by the patient's ability to sustain a vowel for 15 to 20 seconds and count from 1 to 15 (91). To ensure optimal results, it is important for the patient to feel relaxed and comfortable with the examiner. Multiple trials and a repeat visit are often necessary to confirm test results.

If insufflation testing fails but speech is achieved in a patient after a pharyngeal plexus nerve block with lidocaine, PE spasm is suspected. This should be confirmed via a videofluoroscopic MBS performed during rest, swallow, and during speech with air insufflation. If the PE segment is confirmed to be highly resistant to airflow, it may be treated similarly to dysphagia from PE segment hypertonicity, discussed above. Botulinum toxin has proved an effective alternative to pharyngeal constrictor myotomy or unilateral pharyngeal plexus neurectomy. The majority of patients so treated are able to achieve tracheoesophageal voice (85–87). If speech during the air insufflation test is faint or whispery, the PE segment may be hypotonic. Digital pressure on the outside of the neck may help to produce a stronger sound. The existence of hypotonicity is not a contraindication for TEP, although it may indicate the need for a neck band or digital pressure postoperatively to enhance contact of intraluminal vibratory surfaces.

POSTTRACHEOESOPHAGEAL PUNCTURE INTERVENTION

With primary TEP, a catheter is placed in the tracheoesophageal fistula, and fitting of the voice prosthesis in a primary TEP patient generally takes place from 10 to 21 days following surgery (122). If radiation therapy is planned, the patient should be advised that speech may diminish during the third to fourth week of radiation due to mucositis and radiation-induced edema. The secondary TEP patient is fit approximately 1 week after surgery. The size 14 french (Fr) catheter placed during surgery is removed, and the patency of the tract is assessed by asking the patient to take a breath and say "Ah" on exhalation while the speech pathologist or patient occludes the stoma. If the tract is patent, but sound cannot be attained, the patient can be fit with a prosthesis, but should be counseled that speech may not occur until there is further healing of the tissue tract. To determine the proper prosthesis size, the InHealth fistula measurement probe or the Bivona fitting kit (Fig. 11.3) are used to measure the length of the tissue tract. Once appropriate length has been determined, the patient is fit with a 16-Fr duckbill or 16-Fr or 20-Fr lower resistance prosthesis (Figs. 11.3 and 11.4). Gel caps are typically used to aid in the insertion of InHealth lower resistance prostheses (Fig. 11.4). Following insertion of the prosthesis into the fistula tract, the patient drinks water, which melts the gel cap, permitting the retention collar to expand into place. If leakage around the stoma occurs, a catheter may be inserted until the fistula narrows. If leakage occurs through the prosthesis, it may need to be downsized and/or replaced.

During this initial session, patients are taught to digitally occlude their stoma, being sure not to apply pressure to the vibrating segment. They are taught how to phrase their speech and to use appropriate abdominal support to initiate sound. Patients are also instructed regarding the possibility of fistula closure and how to manage the problem if the prosthesis becomes dislodged. It is essential that the speech pathologist be available for the first few days following fitting of a patient's prostheses should problems arise.

Swallowing and Speech After Extensive Reconstruction of the Pharynx or Cervical Esophagus

Researchers report that after extensive pharyngeal resection or cervical esophageal resection (or both), the tubed radial forearm free flap maximizes functional rehabilitation of the patient by providing the best swallowing and speech results (123–125). Free jejunal transfer also has gained wide acceptance in PE reconstruction because the jejunum is well vascularized and is associated with a low incidence of fistula formation and stricture. Voice restoration has been successfully achieved in these jejunal interpositions with the creation of either a primary tracheojejunal shunt at the time of the surgery (126,127) or a secondary procedure (128). Reconstruction with jejunal interposition and gastric pull-up have demonstrated better swallowing results than those with myocutaneous (pectoralis and latissimus dorsi) flaps, and colon interposition (104,127). Performance of a TEP in gastric pull-up patients has been successful in certain small heterogeneous patient groups (129,130), but this is unpredictable, and the overall experience is limited.

Dysphagia in jejunal interposition patients may occur from discoordination of jejunal peristalsis with occasional oral and nasal regurgitation. Regurgitation of food is frequently noted in the gastric pull-up patient, owing to an absent esophagogastric sphincter. These patients are encouraged to eat small meals throughout the day. From a functional point of view and from a morbidity standpoint, the jejunal interposition is generally considered to be a superior method of reconstruction compared with the gastric pull-up.

Patients undergoing total laryngopharyngectomy or laryngopharyngoesophagectomy with jejunal graft reconstruction experience a lack of innervation and muscle in the wall of the jejunum that causes hypotonicity. Therefore, sound may be easier to attain than esophageal speech; however, it is often softer in intensity and limited to fewer syllables per air charge than esophageal speech even with digital pressure (131). Voice quality is often described as wet due to mucus in the jejunum; however, the success rates of primary or secondary tracheojejunal/puncture are 72% to 93% (132–134).

Comparison of Esophageal, Tracheoesophageal Puncture, and Normal Speech

Acoustic and temporal studies indicate that TEP speech more closely approximates laryngeal speech in fundamental frequency, intensity, reading rate, percent silent time, and maximum phonation time (135,136). Significantly higher fundamental frequencies were found during reading in neurectomized primary TEP patients as compared with primary TEP patients receiving myotomy or a neurectomy with myotomy. In addition, TEP speakers using the tracheostoma breathing valve demonstrated faster speaking rates and fewer pauses. The valve prevents the escape of air sometimes observed with digital occlusion of the tracheostoma (122). Although TEP speech in general is more intelligible and preferred over esophageal speech, the monotonous tone, voicing errors, and fricative and affricate errors are similar in TEP and esophageal speakers (122). Prosthetic speech and esophageal speech differ primarily in maximum phonation times (13 seconds and 1.76 seconds, respectively; 26 seconds for normal speech) and the ability to voice without lag time (137). When TEP speech after a total laryngectomy is compared with TEP speech after a laryngopharyngectomy with pectoralis major flap reconstruction, no significant differences were noted for soft and loud intensity levels, fundamental frequency for soft voice, and jitter, although perceptual analysis revealed significant differences (138). Speech in the tracheojejunal/esophageal puncture patients has even less pitch variation, more noise in the signal, shorter mean phonation time, a wet quality, and a softer intensity voice than TEP speech (139).

Techniques such as digital high-speed imaging of the neoglottis have provided reliable information regarding the variety of vibratory patterns of the neoglottis in tracheoesophageal speakers (140), while standardized acoustic assessments using the Multi Dimensional Voice Program (MDVP; Kay Elemetrics Corp., Lincoln Park, NJ.) have demonstrated similarities and differences in the voices of tracheoesophageal and normal speakers (137). These strategies, coupled with quantitative videofluoroscopy (66), enable visual assessment of the vibratory neoglottis in relation to perceptual and acoustic evaluation of tracheoesophageal voice quality. Relations among these measurements may provide insight into the role of different neoglottic characteristics on alaryngeal voice quality.

The diagnosis and treatment of head and neck cancer may proceed quickly; however, a patient's adjustment to the diagnosis of a malignancy, its management, and the subsequent disability is not a short-term process (141,142). Patients and their families require different information and support at various times of the treatment process. A variety of resources are available to laryngectomees and their families.

Resources

Several good books are available for the laryngectomee and can be provided to the patient before or after surgery. These guides provide useful information regarding anatomic changes, stoma care, first aid, alternative communication options, practice exercises, and support groups. They include the following titles:

- *Self-Help for the Laryngectomee,* by Edmund Lauder
- *The Clinician's Guide of Alaryngeal Speech Therapy,* by Minnie S. Graham
- *A Handbook for the Laryngectomee,* by Robert L. Keith

INTERNET WEB SITES

The Larynx Link

The Larynx Link (*www.larynxlink.com*) is the official Internet site of the International Association of Laryngectomees (IAL), a voluntary, nonprofit organization dedicated to total rehabilitation of laryngectomees. The purpose of the IAL is to facilitate the formation of new laryngectomee clubs, foster improvement of hospital laryngectomee visitor programs, and upgrade standards for teachers of alaryngeal speech. This is an extensive resource site providing written information, videotapes, addresses of suppliers, a directory of certified speech instructors, and registration for the annual Voice Rehabilitation Institute.

Web Whispers Nu-Voice Club

This informative site (*www.webwhispers.org*), an affiliate of the IAL, is an excellent resource for laryngectomees and their families. It offers an easily accessible interactive chat room and a wealth of information.

Manufacturing and Product Information

The Web Sites for InHealth Technologies (*www.Inhealth.com*), Atos Medical Inc. (*www.Atosmedical.com*), and Bivona Medical Technologies (*www.Bivona.com*) provide helpful manufacturing and product information.

REFERENCES

1. Logemann JA. *Manual for the videofluorographic study of swallowing,* 2nd ed. Austin: PRO-ED, 1993.
2. Langmore S, Schatz K, Olson N. Fiberoptic endoscopic evaluation of swallowing safety: a new procedure. *Dysphagia* 1988;2:216.
3. Aviv J, Kim T, Goodhart M, et al. FEEST: a new bedside endoscopic test of the motor and sensory components of swallowing. *Ann Otol Rhinol Laryngol* 1998;107:378.
4. Lazarus C, Logemann J, Gibon P. Effects of maneuvers on swallowing function in a dysphagic oral cancer patient. *Head Neck* 1993;15:419.
5. Logemann JA. Speech and swallowing rehabilitation for head and neck tumor patients. In: Myers EN, Suen JY, eds. *Cancer of the head and neck,* 2nd ed. New York: Churchill Livingstone, 1989:1021.

6. Dios PD, Feijoo JF, Ferreiro MC, et al. Functional consequences of partial glossectomy. *Am Assoc Oral Maxillofac Surg* 1994;52:12.
7. Urken ML, Biller HF. A new bilobed design for the sensate radial forearm flap to preserve tongue mobility following significant glossectomy. *Arch Otolaryngol Head Neck Surg* 1994;120:26.
8. Urken ML, Moscoso JF, Lawson W, et al. A systematic approach to functional reconstruction of the oral cavity following partial and total glossectomy. *Arch Otolaryngol Head Neck Surg* 1994;120:589.
9. Heller SH, Levy J, Sciubba JJ. Speech patterns following partial glossectomy for small tumors of the tongue. *Head Neck* 1991:340.
10. Dios PD, Conley JJ. The crippled oral cavity. *Plast Reconstr Surg* 1962:469.
11. Yamamoto Y, Sugihara T, Furuta Y, et al. Functional reconstruction of the tongue and deglutition muscles following extensive resection of tongue cancer. *Plast Reconstr Surg* 1998;102:99.
12. Wheeler R, Logemann JA, Rosen M. Maxillary reshaping prosthesis: effectiveness in improving speech and swallowing of post-surgical oral cancer patients. *J Prosthet Dent* 1980;43:314.
13. Hirano M, Matsuoka H, Kuroiwa Y, et al. Dysphagia following various degrees of surgical resection for oral cancer. *Ann Otol Rhinol Laryngol* 1992;101:138.
14. Teichgraeber J, Bowman J, Geopfert H. Functional analysis of treatment of oral cavity cancer. *Arch Otolaryngol Head Neck Surg* 1986;112:9.
15. Rentschler GJ, Mann MB. The effects of glossectomy on intelligibility of speech and oral perception discrimination. *J Oral Surg* 1980;38:348.
16. Salibian AH, Allison GR, Armstrong WB, et al. Functional hemitongue reconstruction with the microvascular ulnar forearm flap. *Plast Reconstr Surg* 1999;104:654.
17. Lyos AT, Evans GR, Perez D, et al. Tongue reconstruction: outcomes with the rectus abdominis flap. *Plast Reconstr Surg* 1999;103:442.
18. Pompei S, Caravelli G, Vigili MG, et al. Free radial forearm flap and myocutaneous flaps in oncological reconstructive surgery of the oral cavity, comparison of functional results. *Minerva Chir* 1998;53:183.
19. Tiwari RM, Greven AJ, Karim ABMF, et al. Total glossectomy: reconstruction and rehabilitation. *J Laryngol Otol* 1989;103:917.
20. Tiwari RM, Karim ABMF, Greven AJ, et al. Total glossectomy with laryngeal preservation. *Arch Otolaryngol Head Neck Surg* 1993;119:945.
21. Urken ML, Vickery C, Weinberg H, et al. The neurofascicutaneous radial forearm free flap for functional reconstruction of near-total glossectomy defects. *Laryngocope* 1990;100:161.
22. Urken ML, Biller HF. A new bilobed design for the sensate radial forearm flap to preserve tongue mobility following significant glossectomy. *Arch Otolaryngol Head Neck Surg* 1994;120:589.
23. Aviv JE, Keen MS, Rodriquez HP, et al. Bilobed radial forearm free flap for functional reconstruction of near-total glossectomy defects. *Laryngoscope* 1994;104:893.
24. Hell B, Heissler E, Gath H, et al. The infrahyoid flap. A technique for defect closure in the floor of the mouth, the tongue, the buccal mucosa, and the lateral pharyngeal wall. *Int J Oral Maxillofac Surg* 1997;26:35.
25. Horwitz EM, Frazier AJ, Martinez AA, et al. Excellent functional outcome in patients with squamous cell carcinoma of the base of the tongue treated with external irradiation and interstitial iodine 125 boost. *Cancer* 1996;78:948.
26. Aviv JE, Hecht C, Weinberg H, et al. Surface sensibility of the floor of the mouth and tongue in healthy controls and in radiated patients. *Otolaryngol Head Neck Surg* 1992;107:418.
27. Neuschaefer-Rube C, Wein BB, Angerstein W, et al. Sector-related grey scale analysis of video ultrasound recorded tongue movements in swallowing. *HNO* 1997;45:556.
28. Krappen S, Remmert S, Gehrking E, et al. Cinematographic functional diagnosis of swallowing after plastic reconstruction of large tumor defects of the mouth cavity and pharynx. *Laryngorhinootologie* 1997;76:229.
29. Sommer K, Burk C, Sommer T, et al. Perfusion manometry in the evaluation of postoperative swallowing function following various reconstructive procedures of the upper aero-digestive tract. *Laryngorhinootologie* 1997;76:178.
30. McGuirt WF, Blalock D, Koufman JA, et al. Voice analysis of patients with endoscopically treated early laryngeal carcinoma. *Ann Otol Rhinol Laryngol* 1992:101:142–146.
31. Harrison LB, Solomon B, Miller S, et al. Prospective computer-assisted voice analysis for patients with early stage glottic cancer: a preliminary report of the functional result of laryngeal irradiation. *Int J Radiat Oncol Biol Phys* 1990;19:123–127.
32. Miller S, Harrison LB, Solomon B, et al. Vocal changes in patients undergoing radiation therapy for glottic carcinoma. *Laryngoscope* 1990;100:603–606.
33. Rovirosa A, Martinez-Celdran E, Ortega A, et al. Acoustic analysis after radiotherapy in T1 vocal cord carcinoma: a new approach to the analysis of voice quality. *Int J Radiat Oncol Biol Phys* 2000;47:73–79.
34. Verdonck-de Leeuw IM, Hilgers FJM, Keus RB, et al. Multidimensional assessment of voice characteristics after radiotherapy for early glottic cancer. *Laryngoscope* 1999;109:241–248.
35. Hirano M, Hirade Y, Kawasaki H. Vocal function following carbon dioxide laser surgery for glottic carcinoma. *Ann Otol Rhinol Laryngol* 1985;94:232–235.
36. Honocodeevar-Boltezar I, Zargi M. Voice quality after radiation therapy for early glottic cancer. *Arch Otolaryngol Head Neck Surg* 2000;126:1097–1100.
37. Lehman JJ, Bless DM, Brandenburg JH. An objective assessment of voice production after radiation therapy for stage I squamous call carcinoma of the glottis. *Otolaryngol Head Neck Surg* 1988;98:121–129.
38. Tsunoda K, Soda Y, Tojima H, et al. Stroboscopic observation of the larynx after radiation in patients with T1 glottic carcinoma. *Acta Otolaryngol* 1997; 527:165–166.
39. Dagli AS, Mahieu HF, Festen JM. Quantitative analysis of voice quality in early glottic laryngeal carcinomas treated with radiotherapy. *Eur Arch Otorhinolaryngol* 1997;254:78–80.
40. Benninger MS, Gillen J, Thieme P, et al. Factors associated with recurrence and voice quality following radiation therapy for T1 and T2 glottic carcinomas. *Laryngoscope* 1994;104:294–198.
41. Behrman A, Abramson AL, Myssiorek D. A comparison of radiation-induced and presbylaryngeal dysphonia. *Otolaryngol Head Neck Surg* 2001;125:193–200.
42. Woodson GE, Rosen CA, Murry T, et al. Assessing vocal function after chemoradiation for advanced laryngeal carcinoma. *Arch Otolaryngol Head Neck Surg* 1996;122:858–864.
43. Stewart MG, Chen AY, Stach CB. Outcomes analysis of voice and quality of life in patients with laryngeal cancer. *Arch Otolaryngol Head Neck Surg* 1998; 124:143–148.
44. McGuirt WF, Blalock D, Koufman JA, et al. Comparative voice results after laser resection or irradiation of T1 vocal cord carcinoma. *Arch Otolaryngol Head Neck Surg* 1994;120:951–955.
45. Sittel C, Eckel HE, Eschenburg C. Phonatory results after laser surgery for glottic carcinoma. *Otolaryngol Head Neck Surg* 1998;119:418–424.
46. Delsupehe KG, Zink I, Lejaegere M, et al. Voice quality after narrow margin laser cordectomy compared with laryngeal irradiation. *Otolaryngol Head Neck Surg* 1999;121:528–533.
47. Casiano RR, Cooper JD, Lundy DS, et al. Laser cordectomy for T1 glottic carcinoma: a 10-year experience and videostroboscopic findings. *Otolaryngol Head Neck Surg* 1991;104:831–837.
48. Colden D, Zeitels SM, Hillman RE, et al. Stroboscopic assessment of vocal fold keratosis and glottic cancer. *Ann Otol Rhinol laryngol* 2001;110:293–298.
49. Finizia C, Dotevall H, Lundstrom E, et al. Acoustic and perceptual evaluation of voice and speech quality. *Arch Otolaryngol Head Neck Surg* 1999;125:157–163.
50. Jacobson BH, Johnson A, Grywalski C, et al. The Voice Handicap Index (VHI): development and validation. *Am J Speech Lang Pathol* 1997;6:66–70.
51. Hogikyan ND, Sethuraman G. Validation of an instrument to measure voice-related quality of life (V-RQOL). *J Voice* 1999;13:557–569.
52. Logemann J, Gibbons P, Rademaker A, et al. Mechanisms of recovery of swallow after supraglottic laryngectomy. *J Speech Hear Res* 1993;37:965.
53. Martin B, Logemann J, Shaker R, et al. Normal laryngeal valving patterns during three breath hold maneuvers: a pilot investigation. *Dysphagia* 1993;8:11.
54. Omae Y, Logemann J, Haqnson D, et al. Effects of two breath-holding maneuvers on oropharyngeal swallow. *Ann Otol Rhinol Laryngol* 1996;105:123.
55. Kahrilas P, Logemann J, Gibbons P. Food intake by maneuver: an extreme compensation for impaired swallowing. *Dysphagia* 1992;7:155.
56. Leeper H, Heeneman H, Reynolds C. Vocal function following vertical hemilaryngectomy: a preliminary investigation. *J Otolaryngol* 1990;19:62.
57. Balfe DM, Koehler RE, Setzen M, et al. Barium examination of the esophagus after total laryngectomy. *Radiology* 1982;143:501.
58. McConnell FM, Mendelsohn MS, Logemann JA. Examination of swallowing after total laryngectomy using manofluorography. *Head Neck Surg* 1986;9:3.
59. Kirchner JA, Scatliff JH, Dey FL, et al. The pharynx after laryngectomy: changes in its structure and function. *Laryngoscope* 1963;73:18.
60. Broniatowski M, Sonies B, Rubin J, et al. Current evaluation and treatment of patients with swallowing disorders. *Otol Head Neck Surg* 1999;120:464.
61. Singer MI, Blom ED, Hamaker RC. Pharyngeal plexus neurectomy for alaryngeal speech rehabilitation. *Laryngoscope* 1986;96:50.
62. McKenna JA, Dedo HH. Cricopharyngeal myotomy: Indications and technique. *Ann Otol Rhinol Laryngol* 1992;101:216–21.
63. Schneider I, Thumfart WF, Pototschnig C, et al. Treatment of dysfunction of the cricopharyngeal muscle with botulinum A toxin: introduction of a new, noninvasive method. *Ann Otol Rhinol Laryngol* 1994;103:31–35.
64. Blitzer A, Brin MF. Use of botulinum toxin for diagnosis and management of cricopharyngeal achalasia. *Otolaryngol Head Neck Surg* 1997;116:328–330.
65. Ahsan SF, Meleca RJ, Dworkin JP. Botulinum toxin injection of the cricopharyngeus muscle for the treatment of dysphagia. *Otolaryngol Head Neck Surg* 2000;122:691–695.
66. Van As CJ, Op de Coul BMR, Van Den Hoogen FJA, et al. Quantitative videofluoroscopy. *Arch Otolarygol Head Neck Surg* 2001;127:161–169.
67. Ackerstaff HA, Hilgers FJM, Aaronson NK, et al. Communication, functional disorders and lifestyle changes after total laryngectomy. *Clin Otolaryngol* 1994;19:295–300.
68. Van Dam FSAM, Hilgers FJM, Emsbroek G, et al. Deterioration of olfaction and gustation as a consequence of total laryngectomy. *Laryngoscope* 1999;109: 1150–1155.
69. Hilgers FJM, Van Dam FSAM, Keyzers S, et al. Rehabilitation of olfaction after laryngectomy by means of a nasal airflow-inducing maneuver. *Arch Otolaryngol Head Neck Surg* 2000;126:726–733.
70. McNeil BJ, Weichselbaum R, Pauker, SG. Speech and survival: tradeoffs between quality and quantity of life in laryngeal cancer. *N Engl J Med* 1981; 305:982.
71. Davis R, Vincent M, Shapshay S, et al. The anatomy and complication of "T" versus vertical closure of the hypopharynx after laryngectomy. *Laryngoscope* 1982;92:16.
72. Chalstrey SE, Bleach NR, Cheung D, et al. A pneumatic artificial larynx popularized in Hong Kong. *J Laryngol Otol* 1994;108:852.
73. Damste PH. Some obstacles to learning esophageal speech. In: Keith RL, Darley FH, eds. *Laryngectomee rehabilitation*, 2nd ed. San Diego: College-Hill Press, 1986:85.
74. Diedrich WM, Youngstrom KA. *Alaryngeal speech.* Springfield, IL: Charles C Thomas, 1966.

75. Gardner WH. *Laryngectomee speech and rehabilitation*. Springfield, IL: Charles C Thomas, 1971.
76. Singer MI. The upper esophageal sphincter: role in alaryngeal speech acquisition. *Head Neck Surg* 1988;II(suppl):S118.
77. Gates GA, Ryan W Cooper JC Jr, et al. Current status of laryngectomee rehabilitation I. Results of therapy. *Am J Otolarngol* 1982;3:1.
78. Van Weissenbruch R, Albers FW. Vocal rehabilitation after total laryngectomy using Provox voice prosthesis. *Clin Otolaryngol* 1993;18:359.
79. Mjones AB, Olofsson J, Danbolt C, et al. Oesophageal speech after laryngectomy: a study of possible influencing factors. *Clin Otolaryngol* 1991;16:442.
80. Salmon SJ. Adjusting to laryngectomy. In: Perkins WH, Northern JL, eds. *Current strategies of rehabilitation of the laryngectomized patient: seminars in speech and language*. New York: Thieme Medical Publishers, 1986.
81. Fujii T, Sato T, Yoshino K, et al. Voice rehabilitation with esophageal speech in the laryngectomized. *Nippon Jibiinkoka Gakkai Kaiho* 1993;96:1086.
82. Shanks JC. Evoking esophageal voice. *Semin Speech Lang* 1986;7:1.
83. Cheeseman AD, Knight J, McIvor J, et al. Tracheo-oesophageal "puncture speech": an assessment technique for failed oesophageal speakers. *J Laryngol Otol* 1986;100:191.
84. Perry A, Cheesman AD, McIvor JL, et al. British experience of surgical voice restoration techniques as a secondary procedure following total laryngectomy. *J Laryngol Otol* 1987;101:155.
85. Blitzer A, Komisar A, Baredes S, et al. Voice failure after tracheoesophageal puncture: management with botulinum toxin. *Otolaryngol Head Neck Surg* 1995;113:668–670.
86. Hoffman HT, Fischer H, VanDenmark D, et al. Botulinum toxin injection after total laryngectomy. *Head Neck* 1997;17:92–97.
87. Zormeier MM, Meleca RJ, Simpson ML, et al. Botulinum toxin injection to improve tracheoesophageal speech after total laryngectomy. *Otolaryngol Head Neck Surg* 1999;120:314–319.
88. Sloane PM, Griffin JM, O'Dwyer TP. Esophageal insufflation and videofluoroscopy for evaluation of esophageal speech in laryngectomy patients: clinical implications. *Radiology* 1991;181:433.
89. Morgan DW, Hadley J, Willis G, et al. Use of a portable manometer as a screening procedure in voice rehabilitation. *J Laryngol Otol* 1992;106:353.
90. Baugh RF, Lewin JS, Baker SR. Preoperative assessment of tracheoesophageal speech. *Laryngoscope* 1987;97:461.
91. Singer MI, Blom ED. An endoscopic technique for restoration of voice after laryngectomy. *Ann Otol Rhinol Laryngol* 1980;89:529.
92. Blom ED, Singer MI, Hamaker R. Tracheostoma valve for postlaryngectomy voice rehabilitation. *Ann Otol Rhinol Laryngol* 1082;91:576.
93. Lewin JS, Lemon J, Bishop-Leone, et al. Experience with Barton button and peristomal breathing valve attachments for hands-free tracheoesophageal speech. *Head Neck* 2000;3:142.
94. Barton D, DeSanto L, Pearson BW, et al. An endostomal tracheostomy tube of leakproof retention of the Blom-Singer stomal valve. *Otolaryngol Head Neck Surg* 1988;99.38–41.
95. Hilgers FJM, Ackerstaff AH. Comprehensive rehabilitation after total laryngectomy is more than voice alone. *Folia Phoniatr Logop* 2000;52:65–73.
96. Ackerstaff AH, Hilgers FJM, Aaronson NK, et al. Heat and moisture exchangers as a treatment option in the post-operative rehabilitation of laryngectomized patients. *Clin Otolaryngol* 1995;20:504–509.
97. Ackerstaff AH, Hilgers FJM, Balm AJM, et al. Improvements in respiratory and psychosocial functioning following total laryngectomy by the use of a heat and moisture exchanger. *Ann Otol Rhinol Laryngol* 1993;102:878–883.
98. Macrae D, Young P, Hamilton J, et al. Raising airway resistance in laryngectomees increases tissue oxygen saturation. *Clin Otolaryngol* 1996;21:366–368.
99. Toremalm NG. Heat and moisture exchange for post-tracheotomy care. *Acta Otolaryngol (Stockh)* 1960;52:1–12.
100. Singer MI. Voice rehabilitation. In: Cummings CW, ed. *Otolaryngology—head and neck surgery*, 2nd ed. St. Louis: Mosby, 1993:2190.
101. Singer MI, Blom ED. Medical techniques for voice restoration after total laryngectomy. *CA Cancer J Clin* 1990;40:166.
102. Chan H, Mesko T, Fields K, et al. An improved method of flexible endoscopic creation of tracheoesophageal fistula for voice restoration. *Surg Endosc* 1997; 11:1034.
103. Desyatnikova S, Caro JJ, Andersen PE, et al. Tracheoesophageal puncture in the office setting with local anesthesia. *Ann Otol Rhinol Laryngol* 2000;110:613.
104. Yoshida GY, Hamaker RC, Singer MI, et al. Primary voice restoration at laryngectomy. *Laryngoscope* 1989;99:1093.
105. Izdebski K, Reed C, Ross J, et al. Problems with tracheoesophageal fistula voice restoration in totally laryngectomized patients. *Arch Otolaryngol Head Neck Surg* 1994;120:840.
106. Van Weissenbruch R, Albers FWJ. Vocal rehabilitation after total laryngectomy using the Provox voice prosthesis. *Clin Otolaryngol* 1993;18:359.
107. Lacau St Guily J, Angelard B, El-Bez M, et al. Postlaryngectomy voice restoration. *Arch Otolaryngol Head Neck Surg* 1992;118:252.
108. Op de Coul BMR, Hilgers FJM, Balm AJM, et al. A decade of postlaryngectomy vocal rehabilitation in 318 patients. *Arch Otolaryngol Head Neck Surg* 2000;126:1320–1328.
109. Saurajen AS, Chee NW, Siow JK, et al. Tracheoesophageal puncture outcomes and predictors of success in laryngectomised patients. *Ann Acad Med Singapore* 2000;29:452.
110. Mehta AR, Sarkar S, Mehta SA, et al. The Indian experience with immediate tracheoesophageal puncture for voice restoration. *Eur Arch Otorhinolaryngol* 1995;252:209.
111. Quer M, Burgues-Vila J, Garcia-Crespillo P. Primary tracheoesophageal puncture vs esophageal speech. *Arch Otolaryngol Head Neck Surg* 1992;118:252.
112. Schultz JR, Harrison J. Defining and predicting tracheoesophageal puncture success. *Arch Otolaryngol Head Neck Surg* 1992;102:704.
113. Artazkoz del Toro JJ, Lopez MR. Surgical voice rehabilitation: influence of postoperative radiotherapy on tracheoesophageal fistulas. Long-term follow-up study. *Acta Otorrhinolaringol Esp* 1997;48:299.
114. Hilgers FJ, Ackerstaff AH, Balm AJ, et al. Development and clinical evaluation of a second-generation voice prosthesis (Provox 2), designed for anterograde and retrograde insertion. *Acta Otolaryngol (Stockh)* 1997;117:889.
115. Schouwenburg PF, Eerenstein SE, Grolman W. The Voicemaster voice prosthesis for the laryngectomized patient. *Clin Otolaryngol* 1998;23:555.
116. Van den Hoogen FJA, Nijdam HF, Veenstr A, et al. The Nijdam voice prosthesis. A self-retaining valveless voice prosthesis for vocal rehabilitation after total laryngectomy. *Acta Otolaryngol (Stockh)* 1996;116:913.
117. Ackerstaff AH, Fhilgers FJM, Meeuwis CA, et al. Multi-institutional assessment of the Provox 2 voice prosthesis. *Arch Otolaryngol Head Neck Surg* 1999; 125:167–173.
118. Lavertu P, Guay ME, Meeker SS, et al. Secondary tracheoesophageal puncture: factors predictive of voice quality and prosthesis use. *Head Neck* 1996; 18:393.
119. Bastian RW, Muzaffar K. Endoscopic laser cricopharyngeal myotomy to salvage tracheoesophageal voice after total laryngectomy. *Arch Otolaryngol Head Neck Surg* 2001;127:691.
120. Callaway E, Truelson JM, Wolf GT, et al. Predictive value of objective esophageal insufflation testing for acquisition of tracheoesophageal speech. *Laryngoscope* 1992;102:704.
121. Lewin JS, Baugh RF, Baker SR. An objective method for prediction of tracheoesophageal speech production. *J Speech Hear Disord* 1990;52:212.
122. Paulowski BR, Blom ED, Logemann JA, et al. Functional outcome after surgery for prevention of pharyngospasms in tracheoesophageal speakers. Part II: swallow characteristics. *Laryngoscope* 1995;105:1104,
123. Anthony JP, Singer MI, Mathes SJ. Pharyngoesophageal reconstruction using the tubed free radial forearm flap. *Clin Plast Surg* 1994;21:137.
124. Kelly KE, Anthony JP, Singer M. Pharyngoesophageal reconstruction using the radial forearm fasciocutaneous free flap: preliminary results. *Otolaryngol Head Neck Surg* 1994;111:16.
125. Hussain A, Dolph JL, Padilla JF, et al. Tubed, folded radial forearm free flap for pharyngeal reconstruction and voice rehabilitation. *Ann Plast Surg* 1993; 30:541.
126. Kinishi M, Amatsu M, Tahara S, et al. Primary tracheojejunal shunt operation for voice restoration following pharyngolaryngoesophagectomy. *Ann Otol Rhinol Laryngol* 1991;100:435.
127. Matsuura K, Yamada A, Hashimoto S, et al. Simultaneous reconstruction of pharyngoesophagus and phonation following laryngopharyngoesophagectomy. *Nippon Jibiinkoka Gakkai Kaiho* 1999;102:208.
128. Bleach N, Perry A, Cheesman A. Surgical voice restoration with the Blom-Singer prosthesis following laryngopharyngoesophagectomy and pharyngogastric anastomosis. *Ann Otol Rhinol Laryngol* 1991;100:142.
129. Medina JE, Nance A, Burns L, et al. Voice restoration after total laryngectomy and cervical esophagectomy using the duckbill prosthesis. *Am J Surg* 1987;154:407.
130. Juarbe C, Sheman L, Wang R, et al. Tracheoesophageal puncture for voice restoration extended laryngopharyngectomy. *Arch Otolaryngol* 1989;115:356.
131. Wilson PS, Bruce-Lockhart FJ, Johnson AP, et al. Speech reconstruction following total laryngo-pharyngectomy with free jejunal repair. *Clin Otolaryngol* 1994;19:145.
132. Garth RJN, McRae A, Rhysevans PH. Tracheo-esophageal puncture: a review of problems and complications. *J Laryngol Otol* 1991;105:750.
133. Mendolsohn M, Morris M, Gallagher R. A comparative study of speech after total laryngectomy and total laryngopharyngectomy *Arch Otolaryngol Head Neck Surg* 1981;305:982.
134. Wenig BR, Mullooly V, Levy J, Abramson AL. Voice restoration following laryngectomy: the role of primary versus secondary tracheoesophageal puncture. *Ann Otol Rhinol Laryngol* 1989;98:70.
135. Robbins J, Fisher HB, Blom ED, et al. A comparative acoustic study of normal, esophageal, and tracheoesophageal speech production. *J Speech Hear Disord* 1984;49:202.
136. Casper J, Colton R. *Understanding voice problems; physiological perspective for diagnosis and treatment*.Baltimore: Williams & Wilkins, 1966
137. Van As CJ, Hilgers FJ M, Verdonck-de Leeuw IM, et al. Acoustical analysis and perceptual evaluation of tracheoesophageal prosthetic voice. *J Voice* 1998;2:239–248.
138. Deschler DB, Doherty ET, Reed CG, et al. Quantitative and qualitative analysis of tracheoesophageal voice following pectoralis major flap reconstruction of the neopharynx. *Otolaryngol Head Neck Surg* 1998;118:771.
139. Haughey BH, Fredrickson JM, Sessions DG, et al. A comparative study of speech after total laryngectomy and total laryngopharyngectomy. *Arch Otolaryngol Head Neck* 1993;119:487.
140. Van As CJ, Tigges M, Wittenberg T, et al. High-speed digital imaging of neoglottic vibration after total laryngectomy. *Arch Otolaryngol Head Neck Surg* 1999;125:891–897.
141. Blood GW, Luther AR, Stemple JC. Coping and adjustment in alaryngeal speakers. *Am J Speech Lang Pathol* 1992;1:63.
142. Doyle PC. *Foundations of voice and speech rehabilitation following laryngeal cancer*. San Diego: Singular, 1994.

CHAPTER 12

Ethical Considerations in Head and Neck Cancer

Edmund D. Pellegrino

Clinicians who care for cancer patients must be prepared to encounter the same range of ethical issues as their counterparts in other branches of medicine. What gives the care of cancer patients its special moral quality is the complexity and urgency of the physical, physiologic, and emotional potentials of a diagnosis of cancer. In the case of head and neck cancer, these ethical issues are accentuated by the real potentialities for disfigurement, the radical nature of some interventions, and the dying and death that may ensue when treatment fails (1,2). These factors deepen the patient's vulnerability and, correspondingly, the clinician's ethical obligations.

This chapter examines the major ethical issues in the care of head and neck cancer patients: (a) the source of ethical obligation, (b) autonomy and informed consent, (c) the anatomy of ethical decisions, (d) care of the dying patient, (e) team care, (f) experimental therapy, and (g) managed care.

SCOPE OF CLINICAL BIOMEDICAL ETHICS

Ethics in the health professions deals with two major kinds of issues. The first is the obligations of health professionals as health professionals (i.e., the ethics of professional life: the obligations entailed by the special social role of physician and nurse). The second set of issues comprises the entire spectrum of concrete ethical problems arising out of the expanded and unprecedented power of medical intervention into disease processes (e.g., the problems associated with abortion, euthanasia, withholding or withdrawing treatment, genetic manipulation, organ transplantation, human experimentation). Professional ethics deals with what it is to be a morally responsible doctor or nurse; clinical ethics deals with the ethical dilemmas involved in providing care in specific clinical situations. Both kinds of ethical issues are closely intertwined in any serious clinical decision; thus, they are discussed concurrently in this chapter (3–9).

FOUNDATION FOR CLINICAL ETHICS

The foundation for the ethical obligations of health professionals as professionals is set in the special nature of the relationship between the patient and the health professional (1). In that relationship, sick persons—those who are vulnerable, anxious, in need of help, and exploitable—present themselves to the health professional, who, by accepting the request for help, enters a relationship with ethical obligations. Sick persons are *patients,* persons bearing a burden, a problem; they are persons in need of relief from pain or suffering. Patients depend on the professional who has the knowledge to help and who promises to help by asking the patient, "How may I help you? What is wrong? What's troubling you?" The professional relationship hinges on a promise: to act in the patient's best interests and not to harm the patient. To be incompetent or to subvert the interests of the patient to one's own benefit or to the benefit of any person or thing other than that patient is to violate the trust that the professional promise generates.

To be faithful to this trust relationship first requires that the physician be competent; otherwise, the entire relationship is based on deception. Second, it requires that the physician's competence be used primarily in the interests of the patient, not those of the physician. As a result, there must be some suppression of physician self-interest when it conflicts with the good of the patient. At the bedside, the safest guideline to ethical decisions is the good of the patient as defined jointly by the patient or surrogates in collaboration with the physician.

Whatever physicians and other health professionals decide to do—whatever we propose, and the way in which we carry it out—must be tested against a moral "gold standard": Is it in the best interests of this patient? The good of the patient, however, is much more than the medical good we can achieve with our best evidence-based treatment. It must include three other levels of good: the patient's definition of that good, the patient's inherent good as a human being, and the patient's self-interpreted spiritual good (10).

This chapter discusses the application of this trust-based, or covenantal, model of medical ethics to clinical ethics, especially as it applies to patients with head and neck cancers.

AUTONOMY AND INFORMED CONSENT

Informed Consent

One essential facet of the trust relationship and of the good of the patient is respect for the patient's inherent dignity as a human being. Central to human dignity is the capacity for people to make their own decisions, to plan their lives, and to exert control within certain limits of the way they live their lives. This is the root of the principle of autonomy, which is of great importance in clinical medical ethics (11,12). Autonomy rests on patients' capacity for self-governance. Its most practical clinical expression is in the ethics of informed consent. This capacity provides the basis for the ethical obligation to obtain informed consent. This must be morally valid and is much more than a witnessed signature on a consent form (13–16).

For consent to be fully informed, certain requirements must be fulfilled. First, patients must be competent (i.e., must possess the capacity to make the decision in question). This capacity does not have to be global (e.g., the ability to sign over property or money or to enter legal contracts). Rather, clinical competence is a limited capacity confined to the choices surrounding a particular clinical decision. Therefore, there should be no impediments to reasoning, such as severe depression, physiologic disturbances of brain function, or significant barriers of language and culture (see later for the general criteria for clinical competence).

Second, the consent must be informed. The advantages, risks, short- and long-term effects on quality of life, and the consequences of nontreatment should be spelled out. The question of how much detail to provide often comes up (17); there is no formula for this. Generally, physicians are expected to provide the amount of detail a "reasonable" person would need. This requirement is loose enough so that in doubtful situations, more detail is better than less.

Third, consent must be free of coercion, overt or subtle. Deception, even though often practiced and even for the good end of treating the patient, is not defensible (18); neither is subtle coercion that arises from the way the physician selects or emphasizes the "facts." Physicians have great power to influence decisions, especially when patients are ill with cancer. Physicians can obtain almost any decision they wish. This fact imposes a special obligation not to abuse that power, even if coercion is presumed to be for the good of the patient. Rather, the vulnerability of the patient imposes the obligation to present the data as clearly and fairly as possible, even when the physician favors one course over another.

Under no circumstances does the requirement of informed consent imply that physicians should refrain from giving advice. While patients want to be given the facts and participate in decisions, they also want to know what the doctor thinks is the best course (19). Not to help the patient make a decision and not to tell the patient what the physician thinks best for the patient are forms of moral abandonment as blameworthy as manipulating the decision. The ethically sensitive physician is compelled to steer a careful course between coercion and gentle persuasion. This is a difficult but unavoidable duty for which the physician is accountable.

Fourth, an informed decision implies understanding, not merely being presented fairly with the facts. Educational, cultural, linguistic, and emotional barriers may impede understanding even when patients say or think they understand. One useful way to ascertain understanding is to ask patients to repeat what has been told them, to ask why they have decided for one option over another, and how they expect their choice to help them. Also, once a choice has been made, the matter is not closed. Patients often change their minds or their understandings about treatments, especially with complicated and long-term treatments, such as those involved in treatment of cancer. Periodic review and renewal of consent, especially when some new facet of treatment is introduced, are in order.

Fifth, informed consent should be authentic. It should be consistent with patients' history, values, or preferences to the extent that these are determinable. Any sharp break with authenticity warrants scrutiny. Patients may have changed their values consciously, but the change might also be the result of the emotional trauma of serious illness. It is the physician's responsibility to ascertain whether a sharp shift in values is permanent or temporary.

Sixth, after patients have been given the needed information and the opportunity to make their own decision or to transfer that authority to a surrogate, sometimes they ask the doctor to make the decision. The physician should respond but with caution. With proper safeguards, this is an option that patients should be able to elect. In responding, the physician must not suggest a personal preference but rather what would most clearly fit the patient's values.

Seventh, the person who is to perform the procedure must obtain the consent, as that person is the moral agent in whom the patient must trust. Medical students, residents, and nurses may and should participate, but they cannot substitute for the physician who performs the actual procedure and is morally accountable for the safety of the patient.

Truth Telling

Intimately related to both autonomy and informed consent is the issue of truth telling, especially in dealing with cancer patients. Two decades ago, physicians routinely withheld information for fear of harming the patient by disclosure of a diagnosis of cancer (20). The family was told instead. In recent years, this practice has been reversed (18,21). Physicians now disclose the diagnosis, prognosis, treatment options, and side effects to patients. This is almost always morally required if respect for autonomy, informed consent, patient participation, and compliance are to be realized.

Difficulties with this general rule arise in three situations. For example, a few patients might become so deeply distressed by knowledge of a diagnosis of cancer as to pose a suicide threat. Others, because of culture and customs, might not expect to be told. Still others may ask the physician to keep them ignorant if a diagnosis of cancer is made (22).

When there is incontrovertible, documented, and confirmed evidence that great harm might ensue, at least in theory, there is the possibility of ethically withholding all or some of the information. This so-called therapeutic privilege is rarely, if ever, justifiable in fact (23). Many experienced physicians and oncologists have never used this privilege. It may be justified as a temporary measure (24), but eventually patients must know the state of affairs they are confronting. When patients ultimately find out they have been deceived, even more harm is done, as the physician loses the patient's confidence in anything else that is done. Disclosure may even have some therapeutic effect (25).

Patients who specifically request that knowledge be withheld from them present a more difficult problem. To respect the patient's autonomy, a physician might want to comply, but this violates the requirements of informed consent and renders compliance and participation difficult or impossible. Often the desire for ignorance of the facts is a part of the denial process that merits attention of its own. In these circumstances, physicians might legitimately adopt two courses: one is to comply with the patient's request; the other is courteously to refuse to enter a therapeutic relationship under such conditions.

Truth telling is a more difficult issue as the United States and other countries become more culturally diverse (26). In some cultures and religious traditions, patients are not told unfavorable information so as not to deprive them of hope and its healing powers (27). Families and patients play out the drama of cancer or other serious illness in ways that may rely on deception, half-truth, or denial (28). Some argue that, even in such cultures, patients may want to know the truth. If this is really the case, the patient should be told. However, unless there is certitude on this point, it seems more respectful of the patient to handle the truth question within the cultural framework (29). Those physicians unwilling to respect such a cultural compromise should avoid caring for patients from cultures with values they may not share.

The key to avoidance of difficulties, however, lies in the manner in which the truth is communicated. Most of the harm attributed to truth telling arises from clumsy, insensitive, rushed, ill-informed, or ill-timed disclosures. There is no formula that will ensure nontraumatic truth telling when the news is bad (30). Some general guidelines are helpful in rendering an ethical obligation also psychosocially sensitive.

Disclosure must be fitted to the patient's educational, linguistic, and sociocultural background. Emphasis must be on understanding (i.e., on the patient's being able to repeat the essential information, to ask questions, and to repeat those questions, for better or worse, as the disease progresses). This requires time as well as timing. Some patients want all the truth at once; some will want it in graded doses; others, only when they ask for it. Knowing when to tell the truth, how much to tell at any one time, and how to help patients use it for themselves takes experience and training that must be carefully cultivated.

Oncologists who do not feel secure in adapting to the nuances of truth telling should recognize the immediate or subsequent harm their inability to adapt may inflict on the patient. Unlike the moral requirement that the person performing a procedure be the one who obtains consent, the duty of truth telling can be shared with others. Nurses may be more proficient than oncologists and should be encouraged to help in communicating with the patient. Indeed, all oncologists have an obligation to assess their personal capability and willingness to master the art of truth telling. If physicians find themselves wanting in this crucial aspect of care, there is a duty to enlist the aid of others more capable in this regard.

"ANATOMY" OF CLINICAL ETHICAL DECISIONS

Clinical ethics focuses on concrete and specific ethical questions about particular patients made by particular health professionals at particular times in the natural history of an illness. At the "moment of clinical truth," when the decision to act is actually made, there is a complex interaction of technical fact and concrete detail with moral principle and rules of procedure (31).

To simplify matters, the anatomy of clinical ethical decisions can be divided into a "fine" and a "gross" anatomy. This chapter focuses on the gross or skeletal anatomy, but it is appropriate first to delineate four broad categories of consideration that make up the fine anatomy, even though they cannot be examined in this chapter:

1. The clinical facts of the case (e.g., diagnosis, prognosis, expectations of treatment, side effects)
2. The values, beliefs, and preferences of the patient and the caregivers
3. The moral duties, principles, and rules by which the caregivers are guided and the way they interpret each
4. The ultimate source of morality for each decision maker, patient, family, or caregiver: simply personal preference, philosophy, religion, or social consensus

The positions patients and caregivers take on these four issues determine what they think to be right and good and also whether they will be in conflict with each other.

A full discussion of the fine anatomy of clinical ethical decisions is beyond the scope of this chapter. Concentration, therefore, is on four practical "bedside" questions that should help to foster orderly decision making (i.e., on the skeletal anatomy of the decision): (a) Who should make the decision? (b) By what criteria should the decision be made? (c) Are there conflicts among decision makers? (d) How should the conflicts be resolved and prevented?

Determining the Decision Maker

The ethical requirements for informed consent are applicable to patients, their surrogates, their living wills, their durable powers of attorney, and their physicians. However, the location of primary decision-making authority is often at issue in actual clinical practice, and some way of resolving conflicts among decision makers is essential. Figure 12.1 outlines the hierarchy of decision makers that this author uses as an algorithm to define the morally valid decision maker.

The first question in deciding who is the valid decision maker is the question of competence: Does the decision maker have the capacity for self-governance and self-authorization of a choice? This is a decision that clinicians make informally every day without reflecting much on it. Usually, a problem arises only when patients disagree with the physician's advice, question it, or have an obvious impediment to expression of

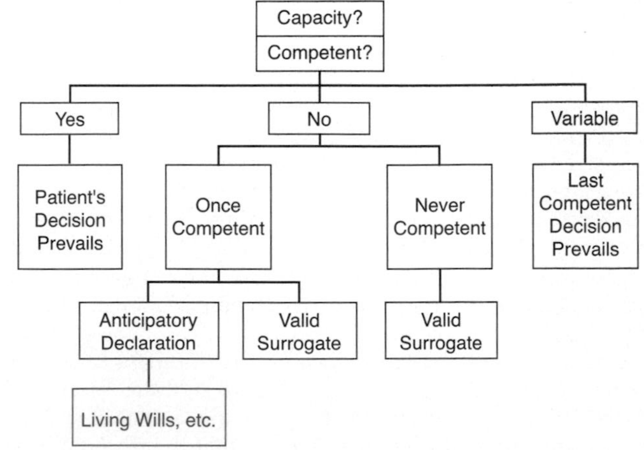

Figure 12.1 An algorithm to define the morally valid decision maker.

their choices. Determination of the capacity to make a decision (described previously) does not require psychiatric consultation, except when there is serious doubt, clinical depression, or emotional disorder of other types.

The criteria for clinical assessment of capacity to decide are several (14). First, the patient must have the ability to communicate with the physician by voice or sign (i.e., the ability to hear what is being said and respond to it in some detectable fashion). Second, the patient should understand the gravity of the decision being made, its alternatives, and its urgency. (See previous discussion of informed consent.) Third, a choice must be a reasoned judgment based on the patient's own values in some coherent way, regardless of whether those values are shared by the physician. For example, the Jehovah's Witness or the Christian Scientist makes reasoned judgments based in values that physicians may not share but that deserve respect in decision making. Fourth, there must be some constancy in the decision. Patients are free to change their minds when they are competent. However, if there is wide oscillation, frequent change of course, or varying justifications for a patient's choices, the patient's competence may be questioned.

If patients satisfy these criteria for capacity to decide, they are the morally valid decision makers whose self-governing authority takes precedence over that of the physician, family, surrogate, and the like. If patients are not now capable but once were, physicians must turn to some valid surrogate authority. This can be a valid living will or a durable power of attorney for health (i.e., persons legally designated as surrogates by patients to make health care decisions if and when the patients themselves no longer are competent). Under those circumstances, the patients' moral authority is vested in the surrogate or the living will, and these take precedence over the preferences of other decision makers. Other less formal living wills (e.g., a note left by the patient, a conversation with family) must be evaluated on their authenticity. In general, determination of decision-making capacity consists in finding the point on a continuum that extends from lack of, or complete capacity rather than an absolute yes or no that distinctly settles the issue.

However, neither patients' autonomy nor that of the patients' surrogates is absolute (32). Autonomy is limited under certain circumstances. Such is the case when there is a probable and serious identifiable threat of injury to an identifiable third party or parties. An example would be a demand for confidentiality when a patient testing seropositive for the human immunodeficiency virus (HIV) refuses to tell a sexual partner. Additionally, a situation might arise in which a patient requests something that violates the physician's personal moral beliefs. An example would be requesting active euthanasia from a Roman Catholic or Orthodox Jewish physician. When the patient requests a treatment that is outside the range of accepted medical practice or disproportionately risky autonomy is also restricted. Under each of these circumstances, physicians must respectfully refuse to comply. They must not impose their views of what is "good" for the patient, but neither should patients expect physicians to compromise their autonomy. Both physician and patient are autonomous persons; neither can submerge the autonomy of the other in the name of autonomy. If physicians in good conscience cannot comply with competent patients' requests, they should respectfully (and without rancor) withdraw from the relationship as soon as other physicians are found to whom they can transfer the case.

Decision-Making Criteria

Once the decision of who is the ethically valid decision maker is made, the focus must be centered on the validity of the criteria used to determine whether treatment should be initiated or withdrawn or whether a do-not-resuscitate (DNR) order should be written. A full discussion of these criteria and the complex interrelationships between them is beyond the scope of this chapter. An enumeration of the most important criteria that enter into a decision is in order, however. Among them are the diagnosis and prognosis; the state of brain function (impaired physiologic function, total brain death, or persistent vegetative state); the relationship among effectiveness (measurable change in outcome), benefit (some value perceived by the patient), and burdens (physical, emotional, and fiscal); quality of life as perceived by patients or their surrogates; costs of care as perceived by patients or their surrogates; age (to the extent that it modifies the outcome of treatment); and the determination of what is meant by futility. Discussion of each of these criteria and the moral weight each should carry in a particular case is beyond the scope of this chapter. However, a brief clarification of each, particularly of the central concept of clinical futility, is essential.

Diagnosis and prognosis are obvious starting points. They will of necessity define the other criteria. The physician's obligation here is clear. He or she must possess accurate factual knowledge about the natural history of the disease and its complications and individual variations. Clinical experience is essential, of course. However, there is also the obligation to keep one's information up-to-date, and this means a constant study of the literature to correct one's own observations. Nothing distresses families more, or more often confuses decision making than wavering, inaccurate, or idiosyncratic data about the future course of the patient.

Accuracy of diagnosis and prognosis are crucial in evaluating the central criterion, which is the judgment that a patient's treatment is futile. There is among ethicists and the lay public today much confusion about the concept of "futility." Some wish to do away with it entirely or, adversely, to give it mathematical precision. Others say it is the patient's prerogative, not the physician's. Others would, in the name of autonomy, require the physician to treat as long as the patient or family requires. Still others would make it a determination heavily dependent on age, quality of life, or economics.

Despite the debates, futility is an ineradicable criterion. As every physician knows, there comes a time in the natural history of any fatal illness when it is clear that the patient is beyond the help of medical technology. Further attempts can achieve no good for the patient. The patient is then "overmastered by the disease," to use Hippocrates' phrase (33). At this point there is no obligation to press onward; ineffective or nonbeneficial treatments on a dying patient are burdensome. To do so is no longer beneficence but malevolence. "Doing everything" in those circumstances is not noble but rather injurious to the sick person we are trying to help.

No mathematical equation can assure the clinician and family that future efforts are absolutely futile. Like other clinical decisions, futility is a matter of probabilities, weighing crucial factors and values peculiar to each patient against burdens. To this end three factors can be set in relation to each other: effectiveness, benefit, and burden.

Effectiveness is the assessment that a proposed treatment will or will not change the natural history of the disease. This assessment is based on the clinician's knowledge, diagnosis, prognosis, and therapeutic possibilities. *Benefit* is the patient's assessment that some good or value he or she cherishes can be achieved by the prolongation of the course of the illness, even when death is imminent, e.g., seeing a grandchild graduate from college, etc. *Burden* is the combined assessment by physician and family and/or patient of the physical, emotional, and spiritual suffering produced by the treatment effort itself.

When the relationship between these three, i.e., effectiveness, benefit, and burdens, is clearly negative, further medical efforts are no longer indicated. Morally, there is no obligation to offer or provide them. When the state of futility has been reached, the natural unfolding of the history of the disease should be impeded no longer. To ignore this point is to violate the first moral precept of medical ethics, to act in the patient's interests and do no harm.

Today there is a growing tendency to consider advanced age, costs of care, and quality of life as the sole determinants of futility. This is the consequence of a society focused on youth that is commercially driven and intolerant of any disability or discomfort. These three criteria can be used, but in a qualified manner. For example, age is a factor in prognosis, responsiveness to treatment, and the degree of burden a treatment might impose. The patient may use it as he sees fit. It may be used if stated in a living will or by a person with the patient's durable power of attorney.

Likewise, economics can be given significant weight by the competent patient, his valid surrogate, or living will. Quality of life in the same fashion can be invoked by the competent patient, his valid surrogate, or living will.

However, a treatment is not futile just because a patient is above a certain age or produces a quality of life caregivers do not find acceptable or costs society too much. The physician's covenant of trust is with the patient, and her clinical decision must be in the patient's interest. If there is to be rationing, it should be external to the physician–patient relationship and ordained by social or community policy. Then the physician can inform the patient about what he thinks is best and place the onus for rationing care where it belongs—on societal preferences and values, which may or may not be just.

A third subsidiary criterion used to evaluate futility is quality of life. The essential issue here is where the moral authority for such a determination should be located. Competent patients with the capacity to make autonomous decisions may decide that the quality of life they envision from a course of treatment may not be worthwhile for them. They can instruct their valid surrogate to make such decisions. Alternatively, they may make their choices regarding quality of life clear in a written advance directive.

However, physicians, nurses, and other health professionals may not use quality of life as a sole criterion. No one is qualified to determine the kind of life any other person may wish to lead, no matter how unsatisfactory it may appear to third parties. Disabled and handicapped individuals are very sensitive to judgments about the quality of their lives. For a health professional to say, "I would not want to live that way," is a gratuitous usurpation of moral authority.

At this point it is mandatory to insist that care itself is never futile. That is to say, the patient must never be abandoned. Futility does not mean that "nothing further can be done." Much more can, and must, be done. Comfort, relief of pain and suffering, emotional and social support, care of bodily needs, and visiting the patient are moral requirements for physicians, nurses, and family members. Palliative and hospice care are built on the obligations of those who attend the fatally ill person. We are never relieved of the ethical obligation to care, always for the human and humane dimensions of death and dying.

Head and neck physicians have special obligations to give of themselves in time, personal attention, and effort when their scientific and technologic capabilities are first applied, but even more so when they reach the limits of their effectiveness. This is not just a matter of the "art" of medicine. Nor is it a warrant for delegating all care to psychologists, nurses, social workers, families, or pastoral counselors. Important as they are, they do not replace the physician completely. The physician must assure the patient that he is committed to the course. He must not abandon the patient when his efforts to defeat the disease have failed. It is at this point that the physician becomes more truly a physician and a healer than when he uses his armamentarium of procedures, drugs, and medications.

Being present, visiting the patient, laying hands on the patient, and sitting at the bedside are not just psychological props. They are moral obligations. For skilled physicians this does not take time from other patients. Physicians who cannot give something of themselves this way, especially in head and neck surgery, should critically examine their fitness for the kinds of care as well as the kind of clinical procedure their specialty requires.

Clinicians and families use these criteria in varying combinations in their attempts to discern what is the right and good thing to do. All clinicians must, therefore, give thought to the moral weight and priority they assign to each of these criteria, especially when they are in conflict. In cancer patients, the interplay of these criteria for withholding and withdrawing treatment must be examined serially as the disease progresses. A good general set of guidelines is contained in a report on termination of life-sustaining treatment by the Hastings Center (34).

Conflict Resolution and Prevention

In the current climate of participation of interested parties in clinical decision, conflicts may arise between and among any of the following: physicians, patients, families, other health care team members, and institutional policies. The resolution of conflicts, like other aspects of ethical decision making, follows an orderly procedure. The first step is to ascertain the reason for the conflict. Is it due to differences in religious, philosophical, or cultural beliefs? Is it a matter of communication and understanding? Are there differences in interpretation of an advance directive? Is it a personality conflict? Are the identified differences irreconcilable? Are they negotiable (i.e., is compromise possible without loss of moral integrity)? Each reason or combination of reasons for conflict requires evaluation on its own merits. Resolution of conflict should focus on its cause or causes. It is important to recognize when conflict is irreconcilable.

Compromise is often possible without loss of moral integrity on the part of the decision makers. There are several ways to achieve it. First and most important is for all the participants in the decisions—patients (if possible), physicians, families, nurses, social workers, chaplains, and the like—to meet together. This happens far too infrequently. It is most easily accomplished under the aegis of an ethics committee, the purpose of which is not to make the decision or to decide who is right or wrong, but rather to clarify the issues, facilitate discussion, provide counsel, and assist the participants to make the best ethical decision possible given the difficulties and complexities the case may present (35,36). When all else fails and the issues remain irreconcilable, resorting to the courts may be necessary, remembering always that the courts can resolve only the legal questions, not the moral issues. Moreover, court-appointed proxies or guardians are neither necessarily competent to make moral decisions nor better at it than are the clinicians and families in the first place.

When surrogates disagree with one another, physicians must determine which of the surrogates most genuinely reflects the patient's interests and wishes. Many states have statutes that establish the order of surrogate authority. This may not parallel the physician's estimate of the order of moral authority based on which surrogate knows the patient's values best. Resolution of conflicts is complicated and difficult. Physicians cannot be expected to conduct a full-scale investigation into all the facts. This would leave little time for actual care of the patient. However, physicians and nurses are required to make the best effort the circumstances allow to act in accord with what they know of the patient's preferences and interests.

In an emergency, when surrogates are not available, physicians must act as *de facto* surrogates. Under such circumstances, prudence requires consultation with others on the scene: physicians, nurses, and chaplains. If there is time, an emergency ethics committee consultation may be helpful.

When all efforts to resolve ethical conflicts peaceably are unsuccessful, families may choose to discharge the physician. Also, for their part, physicians may decide that they cannot morally accept the conclusion of a negotiated resolution by an ethics committee or a court. They must then respectfully withdraw from the case, taking care always not to abandon the patient. This means making the orderly transferral of care to some other willing and competent physician. Opinions differ on whether it is morally required to refer the surrogates or patient to another physician who will provide what the patient or family requests. Some physicians find it morally repugnant to do so in certain cases (e.g., abortion or assisted suicide). For these physicians, this kind of assistance presents an unacceptable degree of moral complicity in acts they deem intrinsically wrong. Respect for the conscience of the physician is as integral to the principle of autonomy as is respect for the patient's moral values.

It is important to recognize as soon as possible when differences in moral beliefs among and between decision makers are irreconcilable. Not to do so is to make the process of care for patients with malignancies even more difficult than it is. Important decisions are delayed, and harm may come to the patient. Prevention of misunderstanding by anticipation and discussion of the ethical issues that may arise in the course of the disease are appropriate and necessary. Particular emphasis must be given to those things that physicians believe morally they ought never do.

Physicians who treat cancer patients (or any patient, for that matter) should consider preparing a leaflet outlining their personal beliefs. Critical issues about which there is apt to be strong disagreement with patients in our pluralistic society include withholding and withdrawing life-support measures, DNR orders, abortion, reproductive technologies, withholding nutrition and hydration, assisted suicide, euthanasia, and the use of embryonic stem cells. This leaflet should be provided before a formal physician-patient relationship is established.

The most important ways to prevent conflicts are as follows: (a) to anticipate the onset of the dying or terminal process, (b) to plan the timing of the discussion of patients' preferences regarding the way they wish to confront death and dying, and (c) to ensure continuing sharing of knowledge and participation of all important decision makers (patients, families, nurses, physicians, social workers, chaplains, and the like). Informed and involved decision makers can more easily discern and work out the sources of conflict than those who have not been working together in the last stages of a patient's life.

The Patient Self-Determination Act now requires that patients be asked whether they have an advance directive. They are not required to have one, but if they do, caregivers are required to respect it (37). An effective preventive against misunderstanding is participation of physicians in preparing an advance directive or counseling both patients and their durable powers of attorney. This is an opportunity for patients to explain what their wishes are, what they mean when they request doing everything, or doing nothing extraordinary, or not wanting any tubes or artificial means of treatment.

Without a clear understanding of patients' intentions in using these terms, the availability of a living will may create as many problems as it resolves. The mere presence of a living will does not ensure that incompetent patients' wishes will be carried out. There are too many possibilities for misunderstanding or disagreement about what patients actually mean by their instructions. In actual practice, too often the advance directive is ignored or not consulted, as one study showed (38). This is a situation that physicians must remedy if their ethical obligations to patients and families are to be fulfilled and ethical and legal conflicts are to be avoided.

In treating cancer patients, there is usually more opportunity to clarify these matters than with most patients. The possibility of death can and must be faced as the disease progresses. There is usually time to anticipate it and to learn about patients' values and emotional and spiritual resources. With proper sensitivity and timing, patients can more readily be prepared to confront dying and to prepare an advance directive, the intent of which can be made clearer to physician and family by fuller and more frequent discussion.

CARE OF THE DYING PATIENT

Care of terminally ill and dying patients is an obligation of every physician. The remarkable advances in treatment notwithstanding, oncologists face this obligation more frequently and over more extended periods than other specialists. Many of the chapters in this book deal with the relevant clinical details of terminal care. This chapter emphasizes only the ethical aspects: the obligations to relieve pain and suffering, the question of futility, cardiopulmonary resuscitation, euthanasia, and assisted suicide.

Pain and Suffering

Clearly, the relief of pain is a primary moral obligation, and this requires mastery of the many contemporary methods of pain relief. Not to use these measures optimally is a moral failure. Sooner or later, it becomes a matter for malpractice litigation. It is beyond the scope of this chapter to discuss the many details of proper pain management (39–41).

Relief of suffering is an equally compelling moral obligation. Pain is only one facet of the more complex clinical reality of suffering. Pain may occur without suffering if it is recognized as transient and without threat to life or of disability (e.g., stubbing one's toe). Conversely, suffering may occur without physical pain (e.g., the grief felt on the death of a loved one). Suffering is a highly personalized and complex response of a particular patient to the predicament of cancer, and is unique for each patient (42).

Suffering has many causes: clinical depression; a feeling of alienation or the actual facts of alienation from, and abandonment by, family, friends, or the physician; feelings of guilt or unworthiness; feelings of being a burden physically, emotionally, financially, and the like. For some, the source of suffering is a spiritual crisis: alienation from God or the need for reconciliation or atonement for a sinful life. For others, these factors do not apply. The physician's obligation is to discern the particular combination of factors that characterize suffering in each patient and to attend to each by drawing on appropriate resources of the health care team.

Treatment of suffering calls for the careful integration of psychological, social, and spiritual modalities, which, together with proper pain relief, constitute comprehensive palliative care. Few physicians can claim to be masters of all the requisite techniques. Therefore, it is mandatory that physicians recognize their strengths and limitations in this kind of care, whatever those might be. The moral obligation is to consult, to seek counsel, and to ask the assistance of other, better-qualified health professionals, and to recognize when this is necessary.

Euthanasia and assisted suicide have come to be regarded as ways to relieve suffering by an increasing number of patients and physicians. The moral dimensions of this topic are discussed later.

Futility

Inevitably, in the course of any serious illness (and often in cancer treatment), there occurs a point at which further treatment becomes totally ineffective or marginal as well as burdensome or nonbeneficial. This has been recognized clinically since the time of Hippocrates as a moral obligation not to treat patients "overmastered by their disease" (43). However, the concept of futility has been reexamined, and its utility has been questioned (44–46). The most useful fruit of this debate has been to broaden the concept beyond simple medical or physiologic futility to include futility as perceived by the patient.

Futility now must be defined in terms both medical and nonmedical. Many speak now of "objective" medical futility (i.e., that stage at which further treatment will not alter the downhill course of the disease) and of subjective, or patient-determined, futility (i.e., that point at which no benefit or value important to the patient is achievable). (See discussion earlier in this chapter.)

From the ethical point of view, futility is a mutually determined state in which patients or the patients' surrogates and physician mutually agree that the patients' good is no longer served by medical intervention. At this point, treatments may be withheld or withdrawn, even if they are life-sustaining. There is no formula by which this point of futility is precisely determined. In general, it is that point at which effectiveness and benefit are disproportionate to the burdens the treatment imposes. The futility criterion can be morally employed only when both physician and patient or surrogate agree that no patient good is served by further treatment.

Cardiopulmonary Resuscitation

Thirty-five years ago, closed-chest cardiopulmonary resuscitation (CPR) was introduced for a specific indication: restarting a heart that had a good myocardium but had suffered asystole or ventricular fibrillation (47). Properly administered and without delay under those circumstances, CPR has proved to be effective in preserving life. Lifesaving measures, however, such as CPR, have since come to be used every time cardiopulmonary arrest occurs, even when this is the terminating event of a long-drawn-out disease, such as cancer, or of multiple organ system failure (48). Under these circumstances, particularly with widespread malignancies or extensive cerebral damage, resuscitation is not indicated. Such patients usually do not survive to leave the hospital or may end up in a persistent vegetative state (49–51).

Yet, for a variety of reasons (e.g., patient or family requests to do everything possible or fear of litigation), there is now a widespread presumption that CPR is to be instituted unless there is a specific order to the contrary (i.e., the so-called DNR order). From the ethical viewpoint, DNR orders are justifiable when treatment is futile, when potential benefits are significantly overweighed by burdens, and when a mentally competent patient or morally valid surrogate requests it. To write a DNR order does not excuse physicians, nurses, and others from providing all necessary care, comfort, and symptom relief (52).

Difficulties arise when physicians believe resuscitation itself would be futile but patients or families want everything done. Opinion presently is divided: Some believe physicians should accede to a request for CPR even if they believe it is contraindicated; others hold that physicians may unilaterally write DNR orders; still others say that physicians need not offer CPR when it is not indicated (53). The current situation is too fluid to permit categorical statements; each case will have to be judged on its own merits. However, in general, the criterion of the relationship among effectiveness, benefit, and burdens (as discussed earlier) should be useful in making the decision to issue a DNR order.

Euthanasia and Assisted Suicide

A decade ago, euthanasia and physician-assisted suicide were considered categorically unethical and totally inconsistent with the physician's role as a healer. Today, however, judicial opinion, public opinion, "right-to-die" organizations, and a growing number of physicians are giving sanction to both practices (54–56). Either or both practices have been openly performed in the Netherlands (57,58), were given legal status in Australia (59), and have been legalized in Oregon (60).

Proponents of euthanasia and assisted suicide base their support on a presumed constitutional right to die, on patient autonomy, on compassion for the sufferer, on the lack of distinction between killing patients intentionally or letting them die by omission of treatment, and on a relativity of moral beliefs about the origins, meanings, and purposes of human life (53,60–63). Opponents contend, just as vigorously, that there is no constitutional right to die, and that both euthanasia and assisted suicide are acts of distorted compassion, are corrosive of the trust relationship between physicians and patient, and are of very dubious autonomy (64,65). Instead, they assert that euthanasia and assisted suicide expose vulnerable patients to subtle coercion and economic discrimination in an era of managed care. They find the "slippery slope" a reality in the growing laxity of the conditions originally intended to prevent abuses in the Netherlands, where voluntary euthanasia, euthanasia for nonterminal illnesses, and extension to minors are now practiced or advocated (66).

The outcome of the current controversy about legalization and ethical legitimization is uncertain at this writing. As a consequence, all physicians, particularly oncologists, are compelled to confront the question of whether physician-assisted suicide or euthanasia is to be classified as constituting a "good" death and, if so, in what form. Several forms apply: (a) active hastening of death at the request of a mentally competent patient, (b) involuntary euthanasia that hastens death intentionally without the patient's consent, and (c) involuntary euthanasia that hastens the death of patients unable to give consent. These are matters of the utmost moral consequence. How they are decided will determine the moral quality of the physician-patient interaction and of the society that tolerates and reports these practices. Head and neck cancer specialists will be confronted with these issues daily.

The author is opposed to all direct, intentional killing, on several grounds. If pain and suffering are treated adequately, (a) intentional killing is not necessary; (b) it undermines trust; (c) it is not compassionate; (d) it is dubiously autonomous; (e) it is socially disastrous, as the slippery slope is a reality; and (f) it is in direct violation of the physician's role as healer. In their final effects, the presumed beneficence of euthanasia and assisted suicide is illusory (65).

Opposition to euthanasia and assisted suicide does not require treating patients who are dying, when the burdens far outweigh the benefits, or when death is imminent and inevitable from other causes. There are valid reasons for withdrawing or witholding treatment of certain patients with head and neck cancer. These may be followed without compromise of the physician's primary obligation to the patient (67). Palliative care is an obligation because, in the long run, it offers assurance of a "good" death. It has its own ethical aspects, with which oncologists should be familiar (68).

TEAM CARE ETHICS

One element missing from the Hippocratic ethic and from subsequent traditional codes is the recognition of the ethics of team care. Today, team care is a reality in all fields of medicine and particularly in oncology. The ethics of collective decision making, therefore, must be better known to all clinicians (69). All team members share some responsibility for the ethical character of their collective decisions, although not all to the same degree. Physicians' ethical decisions—the central position of their roles notwithstanding—do not automatically bind other members of the team. All team members are moral agents accountable for their acts. One cannot invoke the team's decision as an excuse for ethically indefensible decisions or acts. On certain key issues—turning off a respirator, withdrawing a nasogastric tube, carrying out a DNR order—there may be serious conflicts among team members grounded in divergent religious, philosophical, or cultural value systems. Other conflicts may arise about what action to take when incompetence, dishonesty, or violations of patients' rights by other team members are observed. These and other intergroup conflicts can no longer be ignored as they were in the past. "Whistle blowing" may be morally mandatory if the harm to a patient is of a serious nature. Open discussion is essential between and among health care team members, patients, and families before decisions are made. When conflicts are unavoidable, ethics committee consultation may be necessary to permit patients and families and health care providers to respect one another's values, rights, and beliefs.

When conflicts among team members interfere in proper care, patients must be apprised of those differences so that they may change institutions, attending physicians, or nurses whenever this is possible.

EXPERIMENTAL THERAPY

In oncology, the intensive search for improved methods of therapy and disease containment and the necessity for controlled clinical trials result in frequent involvement with research protocols (70). In oncology, the dividing line between therapeutic and nontherapeutic and between experimental and "standard" treatment is often difficult to define. The well-established guidelines governing human investigation—satisfaction of the criteria for informed consent, approval by the institutional review board, and the like—apply as in all forms of therapeutic and nontherapeutic research (71,72).

Special problems in oncotherapy research include randomization when a new therapy seems promising, knowing when to discontinue a useless or harmful trial, and deciding when to treat "out of protocol." The eagerness of patients for cure and the physician's desire to cure may conspire, making both vulnerable to overly optimistic interpretations of marginal or null results of a therapeutic trial or to "fudging" data so that patients can enter a trial (73). In multicenter studies, major decisions about protocols are often made centrally and cooperatively (74,75). Decisions made at a distance may not be applicable to particular patients in a particular institution and pose an ethical problem for conscientious physicians. Here, the final test for clinicians is whether, in their best judgment, a treatment is in the patients' interests.

For many oncologists, randomized clinical trials pose serious personal ethical problems. This is particularly true when a clinician may be convinced that a treatment is effective yet she must recruit patients into a randomized study in which some patients do not receive this therapy. Another issue is acceptance of financial incentives for recruiting patients. The nature and extent of ethical issues in randomized trials has long been recognized (76). In randomized clinical trials involving comparisons of their therapeutic benefits and/or toxicity of different treatments, the principle of "equipoise" replaces responsibility on the clinical investigator for ensuring the principle is interpreted and applied (77). This is a topic that every oncologist must investigate on his own if he is to preserve his moral integrity as an investigator and a physician.

In oncology especially, the fusion of the role of the experimentalist and therapist, of investigator and personal physician, is the norm. Knowing how and when to separate those roles, always keeping the welfare of patients ahead of the welfare of the protocol, is a requisite but extremely complex moral obligation. The separation of those roles (i.e., dividing care between two physicians, the caregiver, and the investigator) has pros and cons worthy of more serious consideration than is often the case. The possibility of separating the roles of attending physician and clinical investigator is unsettled (78).

MANAGED CARE

All the ethical issues considered thus far are greatly complicated in the present era of managed care, wherein cost containment rather than the good of the patient is the primary aim (79,80). To the extent that managed care prevents unnecessary, unwanted, or therapeutically dubious treatment, it can be salubrious for the patient. By its nature, managed care, however, poses problems of divided loyalty, often forcing physicians to choose between what they think is optimal for their patients and the fiscal impact of an expensive treatment on others enrolled in the same plan or on society in general. This is especially the case with implicit rationing, in which the physician is given a fixed sum to cover needs of a fixed number of patients (81). Under this system, physicians must decide which patients receive priority for expensive treatments (82). More ominously, where financial incentives are offered for cost savings, physicians' self-interest is pitted against the interests of the patients.

Many forms of cancer therapy are expensive, especially those involving complicated serial procedures, as in head and neck cancer, chemotherapy, and surgery. The extent to which optimal (as opposed to acceptable or tolerable) treatment schedules are followed varies among both insurance plans and managed-care organizations. Referrals for complicated diagnostic procedures, follow-up care by oncologists, uses of expensive antineoplastic agents, bone marrow transplantations, and the like are subject to scrutiny and denial. The tendency to delay reference to the specialist, to engage in "watchful waiting" or inappropriate therapeutic trials, is fostered in managed care settings. Managed care poses ethical conflicts for both generalists and oncologists. More must be learned about the effects of different kinds of managed care on morbidity, mortality, and patient satisfaction before ethical guidelines can be more fully formulated. Suffice it to say once again, as this chapter has reiterated, that the moral test will be the good of patients, and the moral obligations of oncologists will depend on how every clinical decision affects the patient and on the trust relationship to which all physicians owe primary allegiance.

When all is said and done, the character of physicians is at the heart of medical ethics. Principles or rules are finally interpreted by them. Whatever action is taken that helps or injures patients comes through the physician's order. Physicians are unavoidably moral accomplices. They are the final safeguard of the patient's welfare. Character and virtue, therefore, are crucial as supplements and complements to any system of medical ethics, particularly in an era in which economic exigency conflicts with patient welfare. Physicians must always remember in the moment of clinical truth, when they decide what they will or will not do for a particular patient, that they cannot avoid accountability (83,84). It is this reality that makes it mandatory for all clinicians (and particularly oncologists) to study most carefully the ethical dimensions of their everyday clinical decisions.

REFERENCES

1. Conley J. Ethics in head and neck surgery. *Arch Otolaryngol* 1981;107:655–657.
2. Frank HA, Davidson TM. Ethical dilemmas in head and neck cancer. *Head Neck* 1989;11:22–26.
3. Beauchamp TL, Childress JF. *Principles of biomedical ethics,* 4th ed. New York: Oxford University Press, 1994.
4. O'Rourke KD, Ashley BM. *Health care ethics,* 2nd ed. St. Louis: Catholic Health Association of the United States Press, 1982.
5. Vanderpool HY, Weiss GB. Ethics and cancer: a survey of the literature. *South Med J* 1987;80:500–506.
6. Harrison D. Moral dilemmas in head and neck cancer. *Laryngoscope* 1990;100: 1191–1193.
7. Tristram Engelhardt H Jr. *The foundations of bioethics,* 2nd ed. New York: Oxford University Press, 1995.
8. Thomasma DC, Graber GC. *Theory and practice of medical ethics.* New York: Continuum, 1989.
9. Loewy E. *Textbook of medical ethics.* New York: Plenum, 1989.
10. Pellegrino ED, Thomasma DC. *For the patient's good: the restoration of beneficence in health care.* New York: Oxford University Press, 1987.
11. Dworkin G. *The theory and practice of autonomy.* New York: Cambridge University Press, 1988:9–11.
12. Veatch RM. *Patient physician relationship: the patient as partner.* Bloomington, IN: Indiana University Press, 1991.
13. Faden RR, Beauchamp TL. *A history and theory of informed consent.* New York: Oxford University Press, 1986.
14. Pellegrino ED. Informal judgments of competence and incompetence. In: Gardell Cutter MA, Shelp EE, eds. *Competency: a study of informal competency determinations in primary care. Philosophy and medicine series,* No. 39. Dordrecht, Holland: Kluwer Academic Publishers, 1991:29–45.
15. Brody H. Transparency: informed consent in primary care. *Hastings Cent Rep* 1989;19:5–9.
16. Ward PH. Informed consent in the patient with advanced cancer of the aerodigestive tract. *Head Neck* 1989;11:22–26.
17. Swisher KN. Informed consent does not require physician to disclose statistical life expectancy data to cancer patients (*Arato v. Avedon*). *J Health Care Risk Manage* 1994;14:38–40.
18. Novack DH, Detering BJ, Arnold R, et al. Physicians' attitudes toward using deception to resolve difficult problems. *JAMA* 1989;261:2980–2985.
19. Schneide C. *Anatomy in practice.* New York: Oxford University Press, 1998.
20. Oken D. What to tell cancer patients: a study of medical attitudes. *JAMA* 1961;175:1120–1128.
21. Novack DH, Freireich EJ, Vairub S. Changes in physicians' attitudes toward telling the cancer patient. *JAMA* 1979;241:897–900.
22. Pentz RD. The vagaries of informed consent: experiences in oncologic care. *Clin Ethics Rep* 1995;9:1–6.
23. President's Commission for the Study of Ethical Problems in Medicine and Biomedicine and Behavioral Research. *Making health care decisions: the ethical and legal implications of informed consent in the patient practitioner relationship,* vol 1. Washington: U.S. Government Printing Office, 1982:96.
24. Soule R. The case against total candor. *Med World News* 1979;20:94.
25. Wartman SA, Morlock LL, Malitz FE, et al. Do prescriptions adversely affect doctor-patient interactions? *Am J Public Health* 1981;71:1360.
26. Orona CJ, Koenig BA, Davis AJ. Cultural aspects of non-disclosure. *Comb Q Healthcare Ethics* 1994;3:338–346.
27. Blackhall LJ, Murphy ST, Frank G, et al. Ethnicity and attitudes towards patient autonomy. *JAMA* 1995;274:820–825.
28. Surbonne A. The information to the cancer patient: psychosocial and spiritual implications. *Support Care Cancer* 1993;1:89–91.
29. Pellegrino ED. Is truth telling to the patient a cultural artifact? *JAMA* 1992; 268:1734–1735.
30. Sardell AN, Trierweiler SJ. Disclosing the cancer diagnosis: procedures that influence patient hopefulness. *Cancer* 1993;72:3355–3365.
31. Pellegrino ED. Withholding and withdrawing treatments: ethics at the bedside. *Clin Neurosurg* 1989;35:164–184.
32. Pellegrino ED. Patient and physician autonomy: conflicting rights and obligations in the physician-patient relationship. *J Contemp Health Law Policy* 1994;10:47–68.
33. Hippocrates. On the Art. In: W.H. Jones, translator. Hippocrates, Vol. II. Loeb Classical Library, Cambridge, Harvard University Press, 1981:193.
34. Hastings Center. *Guidelines on the termination of life-sustaining treatment and the care of the dying. A report by the Hastings Center.* Briarcliff Manor, NY: Hastings Center, 1987.
35. Ross JW. *Health care ethics committees: the next generation.* Chicago: American Hospital Publishers, 1993.
36. Ethics Committees. *Core resources.* Briarcliff Manor, NY: Hastings Center, 1989.
37. United States Congress. *Patient Self Determination Act: Omnibus Budget Reconciliation Act of 1990.* Publication L 101–5084106, 4751. Washington, DC: U.S. Government Printing Office, 1990.
38. The SUPPORT Principal Investigators. A controlled trial to improve care of seriously ill, hospitalized patients: the Study to Understand Prognosis and Preferences to Outcomes and Risks of Treatment (SUPPORT). *JAMA* 1995;274:1591–1598.
39. Hammes BJ, Cain JM. The ethics of pain management for cancer patients: case studies and analysis. *J Pain Symptom Manage* 1994;9:166–170.
40. Brescia FJ. An overview of pain and symptom management in advanced cancer. *J Pain Symptom Manage* 1987;2:S7–S11.
41. Truog RD, Berde CB. Pain, euthanasia, and anesthesiologists. *Anesthesiology* 1993;78:353–360.
42. Cassell E. The nature of suffering and the goals of medicine. *N Engl J Med* 1982;306:639–645.
43. Hippocrates. The art. In: Hippocrates II, ed. *Loeb classical library,* No. 148. Jones WHS, translator. Cambridge, MA: Harvard University Press, 1981:193.
44. Lantos JD, Singer PA, Wacker RM, et al. The illusion of futility in clinical practice. *Am J Med* 1989;87:81–84.
45. Truog RD, Brett AS, Frader J. The problem with futility. *N Engl J Med* 1992;326: 1560–1564.
46. Jecker NS, Schneiderman LJ. The duty not to treat. *Camb Q Healthcare Ethics* 1993;2:151–159.
47. Ganz PA. Quality of life and the patient with cancer: individual and policy implications. *Cancer* 1994;74(suppl 4):1445–1452.
48. Kouwenhoeven W, Jude JR, Knickerbocker GG. Closed chest cardiac massage. *JAMA* 1960;173:1064.
49. Owen C, Tennant C, Levi J. Resuscitation in cancer: comparison of patient and health staff preferences. *Gen Hosp Psychiatry* 1994;16:277–285.
50. Multisociety Task Force on PVS. Medical aspects of the persistent vegetative state (2) [see comments]. *N Engl J Med* 1994;330:1572–1579.
51. Multisociety Task Force on PVS. Medical aspects of the persistent vegetative state (1) [see comments]. *N Engl J Med* 1994;330:1499–1508.
52. Faber-Langendoen K. Resuscitation of patients with metastatic cancer: is transient benefit still futile? *Arch Intern Med* 1991;151:235–239.
53. Sulmasy D, Geller G, Levine DM, et al. The quality of mercy: caring for patients with do-not-resuscitate orders. *JAMA* 1992;267:682–686.
54. Tomlinson T, Brody H. Futility and the ethics of resuscitation. *JAMA* 1990;264: 1276–1280.
55. *Quill v. Vacco* 80 F.3d 716 (2nd Cit. 1996).
56. *Compassion in Dying v. Washington,* 1995 WL 94679 at 4.
57. Royal Dutch Medical Association. *Euthanasia in the Netherlands,* 4th ed. Utrecht: Royal Dutch Medical Association, 1995.
58. Remmelink Commission. *Medical practice with regard to euthanasia and related medical decisions in the Netherlands: results of an inquiry and the government's view.* Netherlands: Ministry of Welfare, Health, and Cultural Affairs, 1991.
59. Northern Territory Rights of the Terminally Ill Act, No. 12. 1995.
60. State of Oregon. *Oregon Measure 16: Death with Dignity Act* in Oregon State Legislature, Official 1994 General Election Voter's Pamphlet: Statewide Measures. Salem, OR: State of Oregon, 1994:121–124.
61. Quill T. *Death and dignity: making choices and taking charge.* New York: Norton, 1993.
62. Kevorkian J. *Prescription medicine: the goodness of planned death.* Buffalo, NY: Prometheus Books, 1991.
63. Miller FG, Brody H. Professional integrity and physician-assisted death. *Hastings Cent Rep* 1995;25:5–8.
64. Wanzer SH, Federman DD, Edelstein ST, et al. The physician's responsibility toward hopelessly ill patients, a second look. *N Engl J Med* 1989;320:884–889.
65. Kass LR. Neither for love nor money: why doctors must not kill. *Public Interest* 1989;Winter:25–46.
66. Pellegrino ED. The false promise of euthanasia and assisted suicide. In: Emanuel L, ed. *Regulating how we die.* Cambridge, MA: Harvard University Press, 1998:71–91.
67. Young EWD. The ethics of nontreatment of patients with cancers of the head and neck. *Arch Otolaryngol Head Neck Surg* 1991;117:769–773.
68. Roy DJ. Ethical issues in the treatment of cancer patients: report and recommendations. *J Palliat Care* 1989;5:56–61.
69. Pellegrino ED. The ethics of collective judgments in medicine and health care. *J Med Philos* 1982;7:3–10.
70. Cowan DH. Research on the therapy of cancer, with comment on IRB review of multi-institutional trials. In: Greenwald RA, Ryan MK, Mulvihill JE, eds.

Human subjects research: a handbook for institutional review boards. New York: Plenum, 1982:151–167.

71. Levine R. *Ethics and regulation of clinical research.* Baltimore: Urban & Schwarzenberg, 1981.
72. Tobias JS, Houghton J. Is informed consent essential for all chemotherapy studies? *Eur J Cancer* 1994;30A:897–899.
73. Vanderpool HY, Weiss GB. False data and last hopes: enrolling ineligible patients in clinical trials. *Hastings Cent Rep* 1987;17:16–19.
74. Vanderpool HY. The ethics of clinical experimentation with anti-cancer drugs. In: Gross SC, Garb S, eds. *Cancer treatment and research in humanistic perspective.* New York: Springer-Verlag, 1985:16–46.
75. Shuster JJ, Krischer JP, Boyett JM. Ethical issues in cooperative cancer therapy trials from a statistical viewpoint. *Am J Pediatr Hematol Oncol* 1985;7(1–2): 57–63.
76. Levine R. *Ethics and regulation of clinical research.* Baltimore: Urban & Schwarzenberg, 1981:125–137.
77. Freedman B. Equipoise and the ethics of clinical research. *N Engl J Med* 1987;317:141–145.
78. Guttentag O. The physician's point of view. *Science* 1953;117:207–210.
79. Hainsworth JD. Treating advanced cancer in an era of increasing cost consciousness [Editorial]. *Arch Intern Med* 1995;155:2035–2036.
80. Markham M. Patient choice, cost and survival of critically ill cancer patients: a societal dilemma [Editorial]. *J Cancer Res Clin Oncol* 1993;120(1–2):3–4.
81. Sulmasy DP. Physicians, cost control and ethics. *Ann Intern Med* 1992;116: 920–926.
82. Stoll BA. Choosing between cancer patients. *J Med Ethics* 1990;16:71–74.
83. Pellegrino ED. The healing relationship: the architectonics of clinical medicine. In: Shelp E, ed. *The clinical encounter, the moral fabric of the patient physician relationship. Philosophy and medicine series,* No. 4. Dordrecht, Holland: D. Reidel, 1983:153–172.
84. Drane JR. *Becoming a good doctor—the place of virtue and character in medical ethics.* New York: Sheed & Ward, 1988.

PART II

Site-Specific Principles of Management of Head and Neck Cancer

CHAPTER 13

Surgical Management of Cervical Lymph Nodes

Jesus E. Medina and John R. Houck, Jr.

Treatment of the regional lymph nodes is an integral component of the management of patients with squamous cell carcinoma (SCC) of the head and neck region. For several decades since the beginning of the 20th century, surgical treatment of cervical metastases consisted of radical neck dissection (RND) as described by Crile (1) in 1906 and popularized by Martin et al. (2) during the 1950s. During the last 20 years, significant changes have occurred in the treatment of the neck. As a result, today RND is not the only operation used for surgical treatment of the neck, and surgery is not the only treatment for every patient with cervical lymph node metastases (Fig. 13.1).

More than ever before, appropriate management of the cervical lymph nodes requires a good understanding of the incidence, patterns, and prognostic implications of lymph node metastases and of the role of combined surgery, radiation therapy, and chemotherapy in the treatment of the neck in cancer patients.

INCIDENCE OF CERVICAL METASTASES

The propensity of SCCs of the upper aerodigestive tract to metastasize to the cervical lymph nodes varies depending on the site of origin of the lesions and on the size of tumor or tumor (T) stage. Lindberg's (3) classic incidence figures (based on the presence of palpable lymphadenopathy in more than 2,000 patients with SCC of the head and neck) have been refined by the studies of Byers et al. (4) and Shah (5), in which a large number of neck dissection specimens were evaluated (Tables 13.1, 13.2). From these observations, we have learned that carcinomas of the pharynx have a higher propensity to metastasize to the lymph nodes than do carcinomas of the larynx and oral cavity. In fact, this propensity is so high for carcinomas of the nasopharynx, tonsillar fossa, base of the tongue, and hypopharynx that the rate of occurrence of lymph node metastases in patients with small (Tl and T2) and large (T3 and T4) tumors is between 70% and 90%. On the other hand, the incidence of lymph node metastases for T1 carcinomas of the oral cavity ranges only between 2% and 25%, but it increases as T stage increases.

PATTERNS OF SPREAD

Anatomic and radiographic studies of the lymphatics of the head and neck have demonstrated that the lymphatic drainage of the different areas of the upper aerodigestive tract occurs along predictable pathways (6,7). Furthermore, multiple clinical studies (5,8) have demonstrated that tumors from these areas metastasize to the lymph nodes following the same pathways, at least as long as the neck has not been treated previously with surgery or radiation therapy (Tables 13.3, 13.4). A now commonly accepted concept is that the lymph node groups that harbor metastases most often in patients with carcinomas of the oral cavity are the submental (Ia), submandibular (Ib), upper jugular (II), and midjugular nodes (III), whereas in patients with tumors of the oropharynx, larynx, and hypopharynx, the lymph nodes along the jugular vein (II, III, and IV) are involved more frequently. These patterns of distribution have been shown convincingly to occur

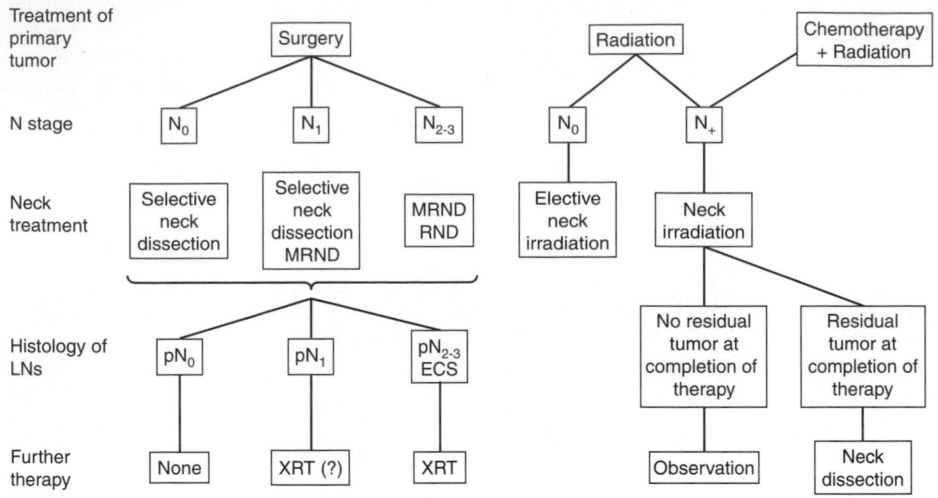

Figure 13.1 Treatment of the neck. Squamous cell carcinoma of the upper aerodigestive tract. ECS, extracapsular spread; p, pathologic; RND, radical neck dissection.

TABLE 13.1 Incidence of Lymph Node Metastases

	Percent of necks with nodal metastases			
Site of primary tumor	**T1**	**T2**	**T3**	**T4**
Oral cavity				
Oral tongue	14	30	47.5	76.5
Floor of mouth	11	29	43.5	53.5
Retromolar trigone	11.5	37.5	54	67.5
Oropharynx				
Tonsil	70.5	67.5	70	89.5
Base of tongue	70	71	74.5	84.5
Pharyngeal walls	25	30	67	76
Larynx				
Glottic				
Supraglottic	39	41.5	64.5	59
Hypopharynx	63	69.5	79	73.5
Nasopharynx	92.5	84.5	88.5	83

Data are based on physical examination.
Source: Modified from Lindberg R. Distribution of cervical lymph node metastases from squamous cell carcinoma of the upper respiratory and digestive tracts. *Cancer* 1972;29:1446–1449, with permission.

TABLE 13.2 Incidence of Histopathologic Lymph Node Metastases

	T stage	
Site of primary tumor	**T1–2**	**T3–4**
Oral cavity		
Oral tongue	18.6	31.6
Floor of mouth	18.6	26.3
Lower gum	11.5	13.3
Buccal mucosa	—	—
Retromolar trigone	36.4	33.3
Oropharynx		
Tonsil	—	—
Base of tongue	—	50.0
Pharyngeal walls	20.0	62.5
Larynx		
Glottic	21.4	14.0
Supraglottic	30.8	25.0
Hypopharynx		
Pyriform sinus	66.7	55.2

Source: Modified from Remmler D, Byers RM, Scheetz JE. A prospective study of shoulder disability resulting from radical and modified neck dissections. *Head Neck Surg* 1986;8:280–286, with permission.

TABLE 13.3 Pattern of Nodal Metastases

	Percentage of nodal involvement					
Primary site	**IA**	**IB**	**II**	**III**	**IV**	**V**
Oral tongue	3.3[a]	22.8	59.7	10.7	2.6	7.0
	9.0[b]	18.0	73.0	18.0	—	—
	—[c]	14.0	19.0	16.0	3.0	—
Floor of mouth	4.3[a]	43.1	37.1	9.5	4.3	1.7
	7.0[b]	64.0	43.0	—	—	—
	—[c]	16.0	12.0	7.0	2.0	—
Buccal mucosa	—[a]	—	—	—	—	—
	—[b]	—	—	—	—	—
	—[c]	44.0	11.0	—	—	—
Lower gum	—[a]	—	—	—	—	—
	—[b]	60.0	40.0	—	—	—
	—[c]	27.0	21.0	6.0	4.0	2.0
Retromolar trigone	0.6[a]	17.1	61.8	16.4	3.3	0.6
	—[b]	25.0	63.0	12.5	—	—
	—[c]	19.0	12.0	6.0	6.0	0.0
Supraglottic larynx	0.5[a]	1.0	47.6	34.0	10.7	6.3
	—[b]	—	48.0	38.0	5.0	—
	—[c]	6.0	18.0	18.0	9.0	1.5
Glottic larynx	—[a]	—	—	—	—	—
	—[b]	—	55.0	27.0	—	—
	—[c]	—	21.0	29.0	7.0	7.0

[a]Based on clinical examination (see ref. 3).
[b]Based on examination of selective neck dissections (see ref. 4).
[c]Based on examination of radical neck dissections (see ref. 5).

both in patients who are staged N0 clinically and are found to have occult metastases and in patients with palpable, histologically proved lymph node metastases (5,8). What must be kept in mind, however, is that skip metastases (i.e., direct metastases beyond the first or second echelon of expected lymphatic drainage) do occur (9).

The retropharyngeal nodes must be emphasized as a common site for metastases in tumors of the hypopharynx, tonsillar fossa, soft palate, posterior and lateral oropharyngeal walls, and paratracheal nodes—a common site of metastases for laryngeal carcinomas involving the subglottic region and for carcinomas of the cervical esophagus (10–12).

TABLE 13.4 Pattern of Nodal Metastases

	Percentage of nodal involvement					
Primary site	**IA**	**IB**	**II**	**III**	**IV**	**V**
Tonsil	0.6[a]	9.2	59.5	14.4	8.1	8.1
	—[b]	—	—	—	—	—
	—[c]	—	—	—	—	—
Base of tongue	0.8[a]	4.4	56.4	25.3	5.8	7.1
	—[b]	—	67.0	33.0	33.0	17.0
	—[c]	—	—	—	—	—
Pharyngeal wall	1.5[a]	3.6	56.9	22.6	5.10	10.2
	—[b]	20.0	80.0	40.0	40.0	—
	—[c]	—	—	—	—	—
Hypopharynx	0.3[a]	0.6	44.2	33.4	12.8	8.6
	—[b]	—	67.0	33.0	7.0	—
	—[c]	—	13.0	13.0	—	—
Nasopharynx	1.1[a]	2.6	44.8	16.8	8.6	26.1
	—[b]	—	—	—	—	—
	—[c]	—	—	—	—	—

[a]Based on clinical examination (see ref. 3).
[b]Based on examination of selective neck dissections (see ref. 4).
[c]Based on examination of radical neck dissections (see ref. 5).

PROGNOSTIC IMPLICATIONS OF NECK NODE METASTASES

The presence of clinically obvious, histologically proven lymph node metastasis is the single most important prognostic factor in patients with SCC of the head and neck. In general, it decreases the overall survival by at least one-half (13). However, the unfavorable impact on survival varies, depending on certain factors.

The presence of extracapsular spread (ECS) of tumor has been explored in numerous studies that demonstrated that tumor extension beyond the capsule of a lymph node worsens the prognosis. Johnson et al. (14) report that less than 40% of patients with histologic evidence of ECS were free of disease 24 months after therapy. Furthermore, the survival of these patients was significantly lower than that in comparable patients whose metastases were confined to the lymph nodes (15). Similarly, Steinhart et al. (16) found that the rate of ECS was especially high (70%) in patients with carcinomas of the hypopharynx and that the 5-year survival rate differed greatly for patients with ECS of tumor (28%) and patients with no metastases (77%). Interestingly, a correlation between the degree of ECS and prognosis has not yet been established clearly, though Carter et al. (17) have reported that macroscopically recognizable ECS carries a prognosis worse than that of microscopic spread.

In a study performed at the Mayo Clinic, a desmoplastic stromal pattern in the lymph nodes involved by tumor was associated with an almost sevenfold increase in the risk for recurrence in the neck. The study included 284 patients who had pathologically confirmed metastatic SCC, underwent neck dissection, and did not receive adjuvant therapy (18). This finding has not been reported previously.

The number of lymph nodes involved affects the survival of patients with histologically positive nodes; survival is significantly lower when multiple nodes are involved (13). A study by Leemans et al. (19) reports a 10.7% overall incidence of distant metastases in a group of 281 head and neck cancer patients who underwent a neck dissection, whereas it was 46.8% in the group of patients with three or more positive nodes.

The level of the neck metastases figures significantly. Several studies have suggested that survival decreases as lymph nodes in lower levels of the neck become involved (20–23). This tendency has been demonstrated best by Ho (24) and Teo et al. (25) for nasopharyngeal carcinoma: the lower the level, the worse the prognosis. Grandi et al. (26) have defined three levels in the neck (upper, middle, and lower), divided by two imaginary lines that pass through the hyoid bone and through the lower border of the thyroid cartilage. They found that the worst prognosis was associated with the presence of nodal metastases at the lower level. On the basis of these observations, a new staging system has been adopted for the neck in patients with nasopharyngeal carcinoma (26, 27).

The prognostic significance of nonpalpable (occult) metastases in the N0 neck is less clearly defined. Studying it is more difficult because the T stage also affects prognosis and may overshadow the effect of occult neck nodes (28). However, ECS has been shown to occur in nonpalpable lymph nodes (4). Also, as in patients with palpable nodal metastases, the number and location of involved nodes in the N0 neck appears to affect prognosis (21,29–31). For instance, Kalnins et al. (32) found that patients with SCC of the oral cavity and uninvolved neck nodes had a 75% 5-year survival. Survival decreased to 49% when one node was histopathologically involved, to 30% when two nodes were involved, and to 13% when three or more nodes were involved by tumor.

TYPES OF NECK DISSECTION

The six levels currently used encompass the complete topographic anatomy of the neck. Lymph nodes involving regions not located within these levels should be referred to by the name of their specific nodal group; examples of these are the superior mediastinum, the retropharyngeal, the periparotid, the buccinator, the postauricular, and the suboccipital lymph nodes. The concept of sublevels has been introduced into the classification since certain zones have been identified within the six levels, which may have significance. These are sublevels IA (submental nodes), IB (submandibular nodes), IIA and IIB (together comprising the upper jugular nodes), and VA (spinal accessory nodes) and VB (transverse cervical and supraclavicular nodes). The boundaries for each of these sublevels are defined in Table 13.5, and are visually demonstrated in Figure 13.2.

The definitions of types of neck dissection recently proposed by the American Head and Neck Society and the American Academy of Otolaryngology—Head and Neck Surgery remain unchanged as previously outlined in the 1991 classification report (32a). These are:

1. Radical neck dissection is considered to be the standard basic procedure for cervical lymphadenectomy. All other neck dissections represent one or more alterations of this procedure.
2. The operation is called modified radical neck dissection when the alteration involves preservation of one or more nonlymphatic structures routinely removed in the radical neck dissection.
3. The operation is called selective neck dissection when the alteration involves preservation of one or more lymph node groups/levels routinely removed in the radical neck dissection.
4. The operation is called extended neck dissection when the alteration involves removal of additional lymph node groups or nonlymphatic structures relative to the radical neck dissection.

The proposed new classification is essentially the same as the 1991 version with the exception that specific names for certain types of selective neck dissection should be de-emphasized. The rationale for this recommendation is based on the increased number of variations, which have been introduced over the past decade. A comparison of the two classifications is shown in Table 13.6.

Radical Dissection

Radical neck dissection consists of the removal of all five lymph node groups on one side of the neck, including the sternocleidomastoid muscle (SCM), the internal jugular vein (IJV), and the spinal accessory nerve (Fig. 13.3).

Modified Dissections

Modifications of RND were developed with the intention of reducing the morbidity of this operation by preserving one or more of the following structures: the spinal accessory nerve, the IJV, or the SCM. Like RND, the modified RNDs remove all five nodal groups on one side of the neck. The three neck dissections that can be included in this category differ from one another

TABLE 13.5 Lymph Node Levels and Sublevels

Lymph node level	Description
Level I	*Sublevel IA (Submental):* Lymph nodes within the triangular boundary of the anterior belly of the digastric muscles and the hyoid bone. *Sublevel IB (Submandibular):* Lymph nodes within the boundaries of the anterior belly of the digastric muscle, the stylohyoid muscle, and the body of the mandible.
Level II (upper jugular)	Lymph nodes located around the upper third of the internal jugular vein and adjacent spinal accessory nerve extending from the level of the skull base (above) to the level of the inferior border of the hyoid bone (below). The anterior (medial) boundary is the stylohyoid muscle (the radiologic correlate is the vertical plane defined by the posterior surface of the submandibular gland) and the posterior (lateral) boundary is the posterior border of the sternocleidomastoid muscle. *Sublevel IIA:* Nodes located anterior (medial) to the vertical plane defined by the spinal accessory nerve. *Sublevel IIB:* Nodes located posterior (lateral) to the vertical plane defined by the spinal accessory nerve.
Level III (midjugular)	Lymph nodes located around the middle third of the internal jugular vein extending from the inferior border of the hyoid bone (above) to the inferior border of the cricoid cartilage (below). The anterior (medial) boundary is the lateral border of the sternohyoid muscle, and the posterior (lateral) boundary is the posterior border of the sternocleidomastoid muscle.
Level IV (lower jugular)	Lymph nodes located around the lower third of the internal jugular vein extending from the inferior border of the cricoid cartilage (above) to the clavicle below.
Level V (posterior triangle)	This group is comprised predominantly of the lymph nodes located along the lower half of the spinal accessory nerve and the transverse cervical artery. The supraclavicular nodes are also included in posterior triangle group. The superior boundary is the apex formed by convergence of the sternocleidomastoid and trapezius muscles, the inferior boundary is the clavicle, the anterior (medial) boundary is the posterior border of the sterno-cleidomastoid muscle, and the posterior (lateral) boundary is the anterior boundary is the anterior border of the trapezius muscle. A horizontal plane marking the inferior border of the anterior cricoid arch separates sublevels. *Sublevel V-A:* Above this plane, includes the spinal accessory nodes. *Sublevel V-B:* Below this plane, includes the nodes that follow the transverse cervical vessels and the supraclavicular nodes (with the exception of the Virchow node which is located in level IV).
Level VI (anterior compartment)	Lymph nodes in this compartment include the pre- and paratracheal nodes, precricoid (delphian) node, and the perithyroidal nodes including the lymph nodes along the recurrent laryngeal nerves. The superior boundary is the hyoid bone, the inferior boundary is the suprasternal notch, and the lateral boundaries are the common carotid arteries.

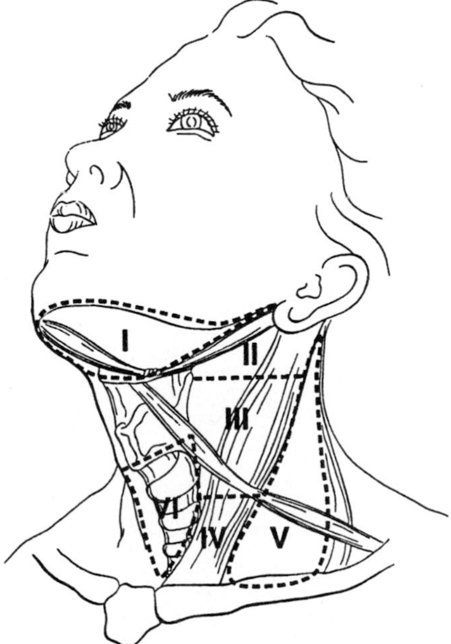

Figure 13.2 Schematic diagram indicating the location of the lymph node levels in the neck.

TABLE 13.6 Classification of Neck Dissection

1991 classification	2001 classification
1. Radical neck dissection	1. Radical neck dissection
2. Modified radical neck dissection	2. Modified radical neck dissection
3. Selective neck dissection	3. Selective neck dissection (SND):
a. supraomohyoid	a. SND (I–III/IV)
b. lateral	b. SND (II–IV)
c. posterolateral	c. SND (II–V, postauricular, suboccipital)
d. anterior	d. SND (level VI)
4. Extended neck dissection	4. Extended neck dissection

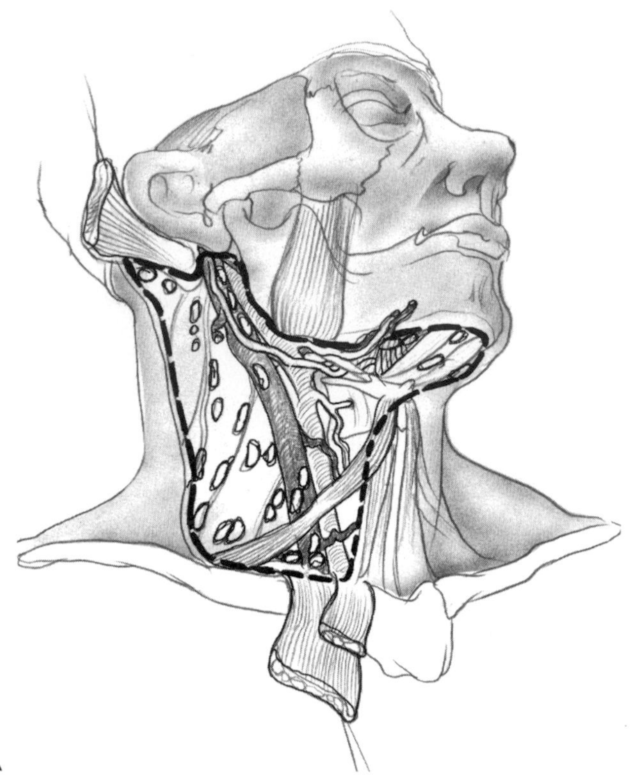
A

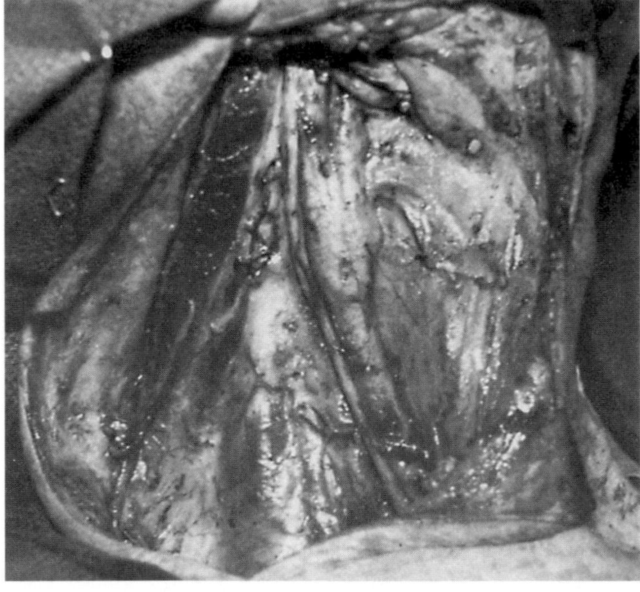
B

Figure 13.3 Schematic **(A)** and intraoperative photograph **(B)** of the radical neck dissection. (From Bailey BJ, et al., eds. *Head and neck surgery—otolaryngology.* Philadelphia: JB Lippincott, 1993:1200, with permission.)

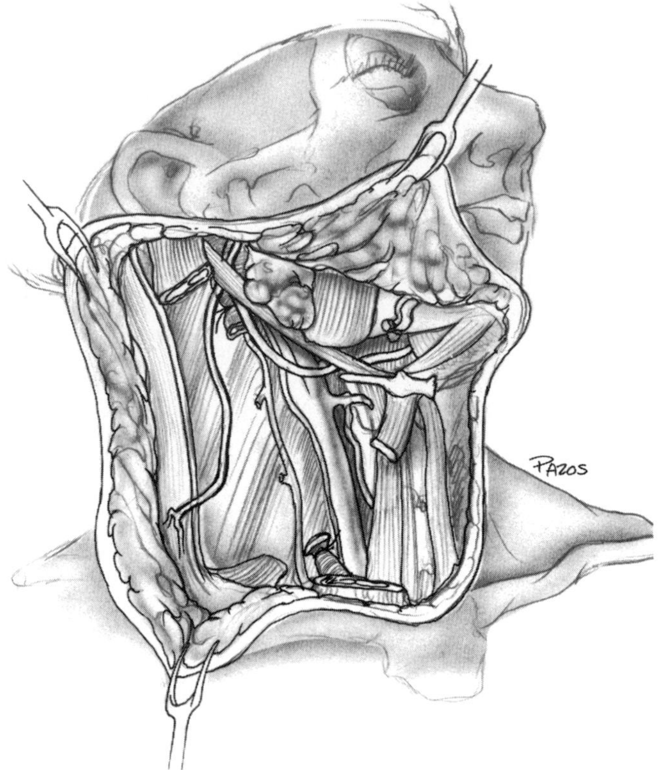

A

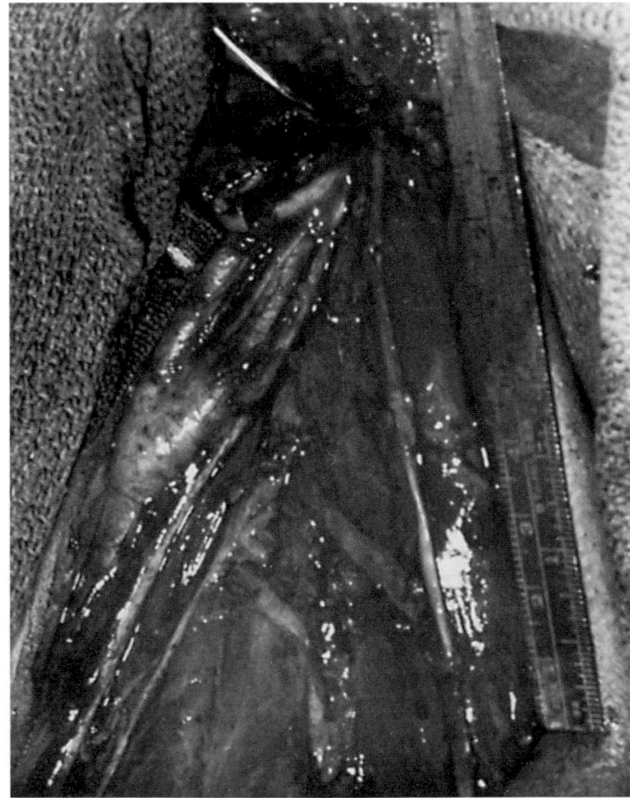
B

Figure 13.4 Schematic **(A)** and intraoperative photograph **(B)** of modified radical neck dissection (type I). (From Bailey BJ, et al., eds. *Head and neck surgery—otolaryngology.* Philadelphia: JB Lippincott, 1993:1202, with permission.)

TABLE 13.7 Classification of Modified Radical Neck Dissections

Type I	SCM, IJV (XI is preserved)
Type II	SCM (IJV and XI are preserved)
Type III	None (SCM, IJV, XI are preserved)

IJV, internal jugular vein; SCM, sternocleidomastoid muscle; XI, cranial nerve XI.

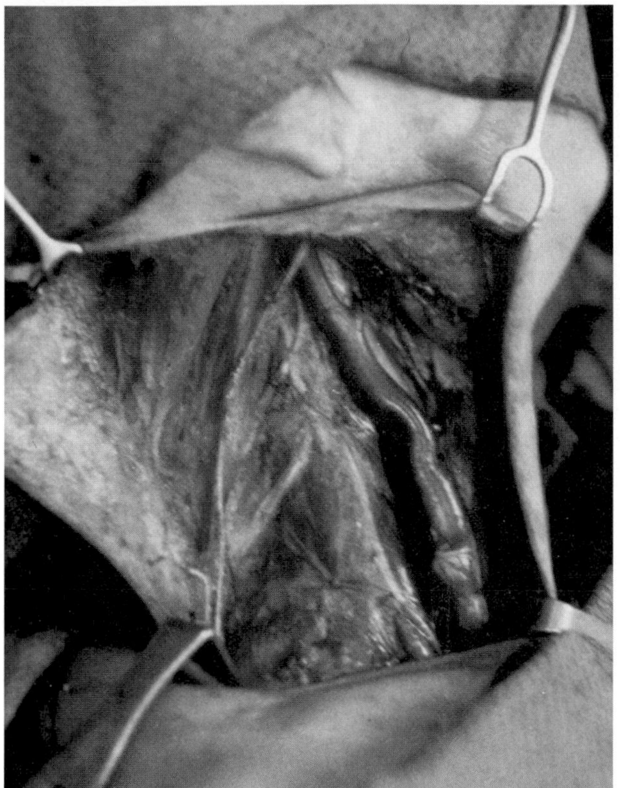

Figure 13.5 Intraoperative photograph of modified radical neck dissection (type II).

only in the number of neural, vascular, and muscular structures that are preserved. Therefore, Medina (33) suggests subclassifying these neck dissections (Table 13.7) as follows:

- type I, in which only one structure—the spinal accessory nerve—is preserved (Fig. 13.4)
- type II, in which two structures—the spinal accessory nerve and the IJV—are preserved (Fig. 13.5)
- type III, in which all three structures—the spinal accessory nerve, the IJV, and the SCM—are preserved (Fig. 13.6).

Selective Dissections

Selective neck dissections consist of the removal of only the lymph node groups that are at highest risk for containing metastases, according to the location of the primary tumor. The spinal accessory nerve, the IJV, and the SCM are preserved. Four different neck dissections can be included in this category: lateral neck dissection (lymph node groups II, III, and IV are removed; Fig. 13.7); supraomohyoid neck dissection (lymph node groups I, II, and III are removed; Fig. 13.8); posterolateral neck dissection (the suboccipital and retroauricular nodes are removed in addition to lymph node groups II, III, IV, and V; Fig. 13.9); and anterior neck dissection (the pretracheal and paratracheal nodes are removed; Fig. 13.10).

The term *extended neck dissection* is used, in addition to any of the foregoing designations, when a given neck dissection is extended to include either lymph node groups or structures of the neck that are not removed routinely. Such entities as the retropharyngeal nodes or the carotid artery are included.

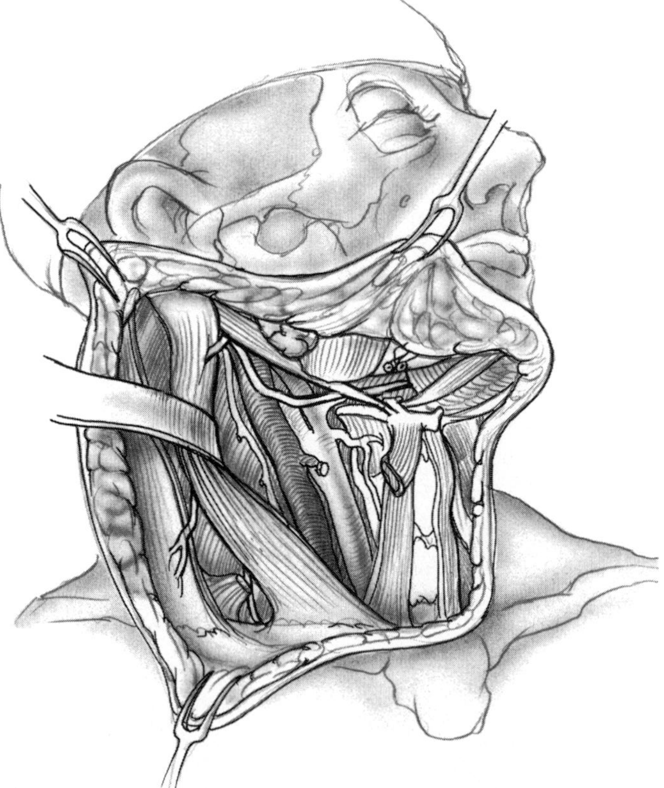

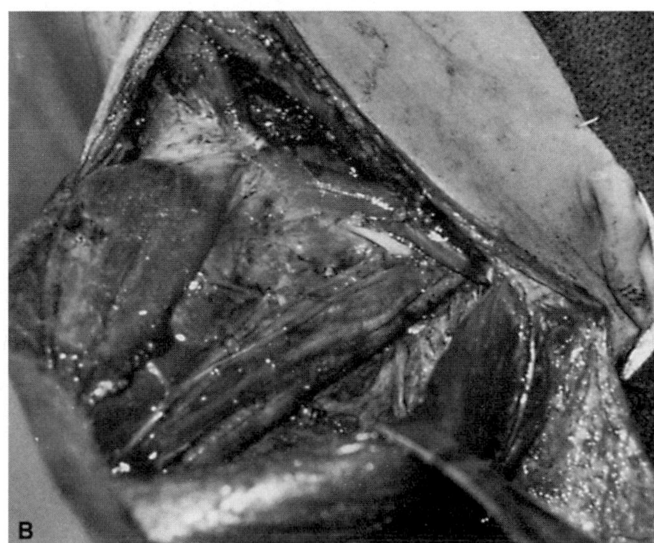

Figure 13.6 Schematic **(A)** and intraoperative photograph **(B)** of modified radical neck dissection (type III). (From Bailey BJ, et al., eds. *Head and neck surgery—otolaryngology.* Philadelphia: JB Lippincott, 1993:1204, with permission.)

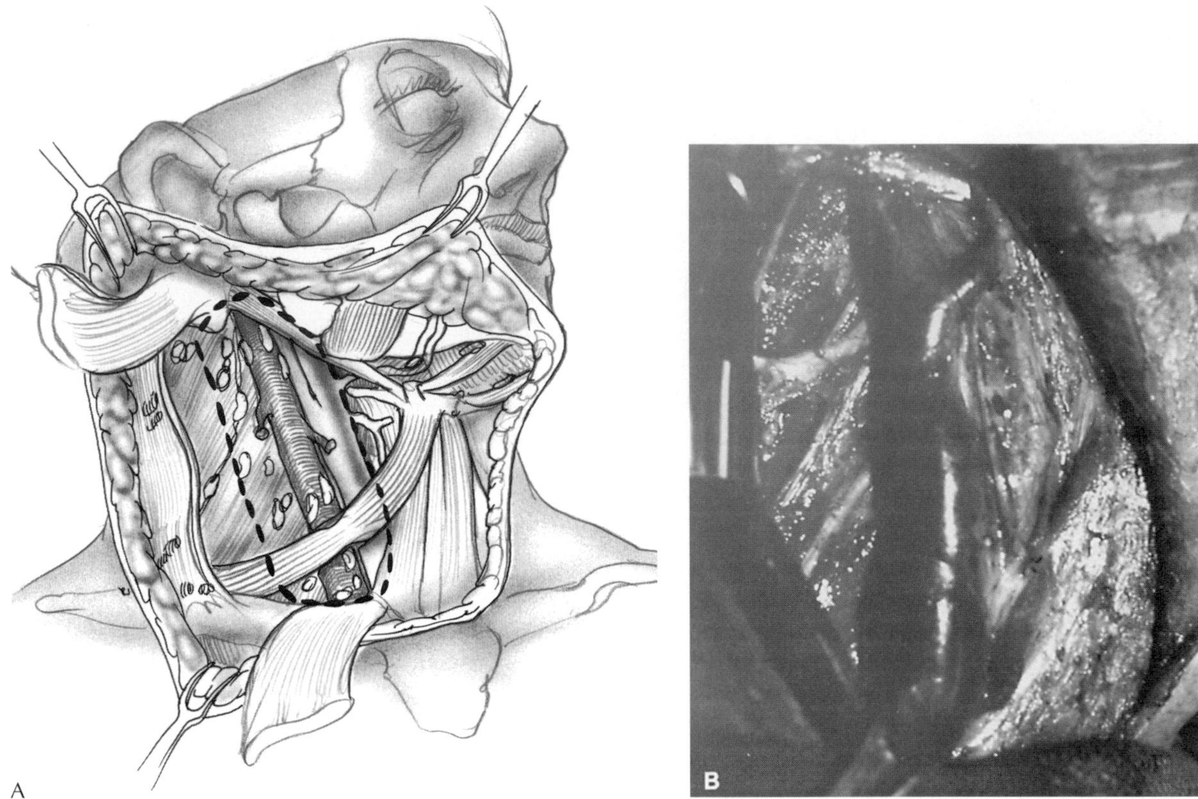

Figure 13.7 Schematic **(A)** and intraoperative photograph **(B)** of lateral neck dissection. (From Bailey BJ, et al., eds. *Head and neck surgery—otolaryngology.* Philadelphia: JB Lippincott, 1993:1207, with permission.)

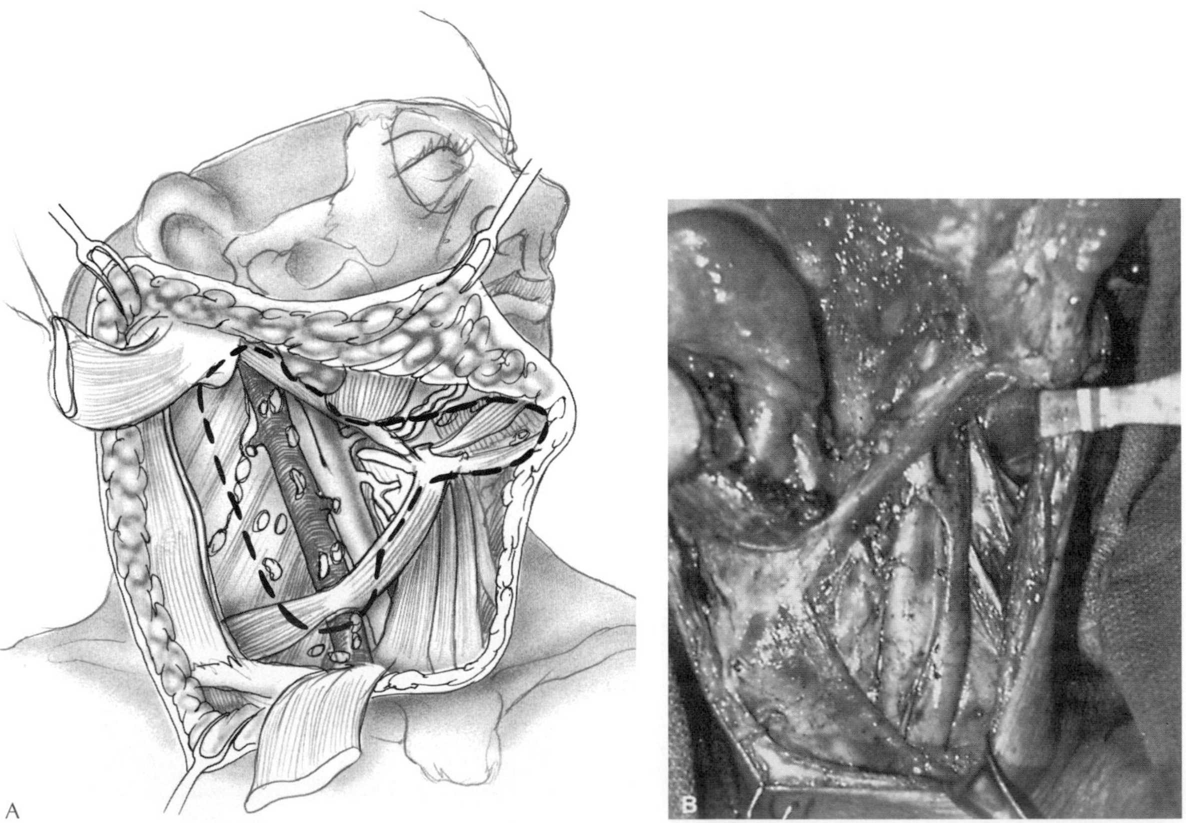

Figure 13.8 Schematic **(A)** and intraoperative photograph **(B)** of supraomohyoid neck dissection. (From Bailey BJ, et al., eds. *Head and neck surgery—otolaryngology.* Philadelphia: JB Lippincott, 1993:1206, with permission.)

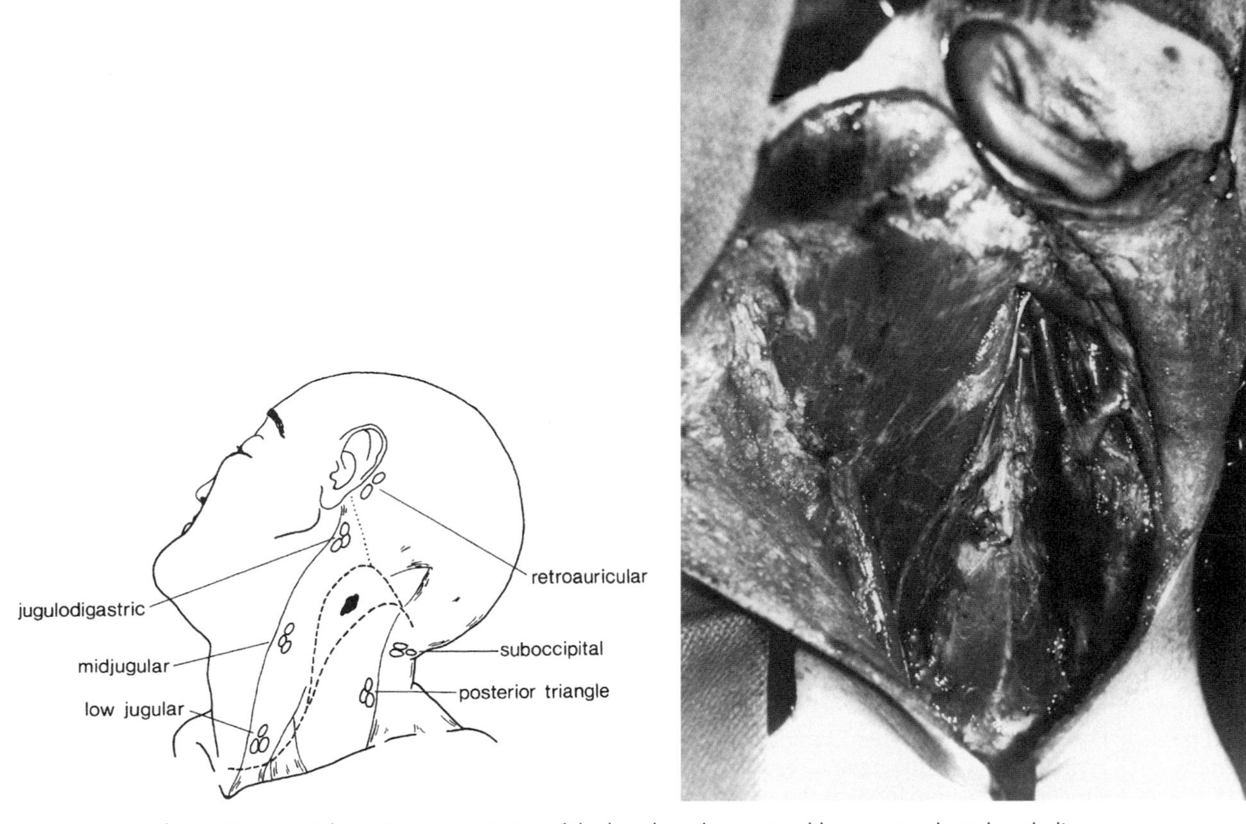

Figure 13.9 **A:** Schematic representation of the lymph nodes removed by a posterolateral neck dissection. **B:** Intraoperative photograph.

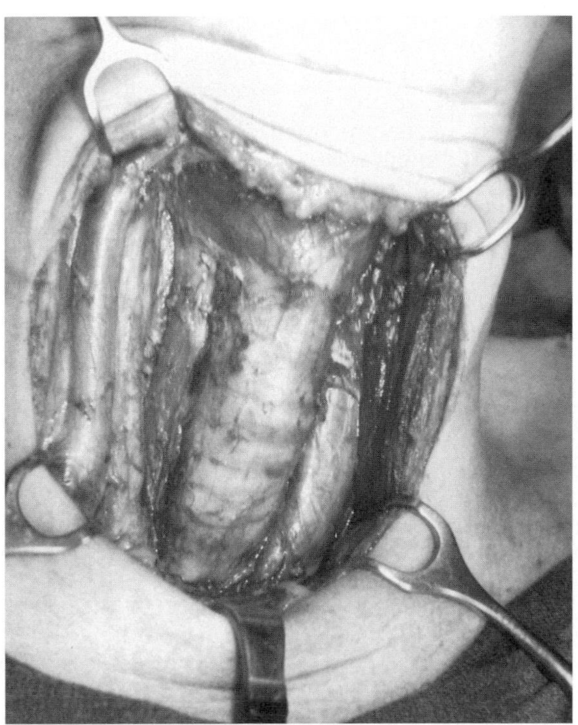

Figure 13.10 Intraoperative anterior neck dissection.

PRINCIPLES OF MANAGEMENT OF THE N0 NECK

Indications for Treatment

The clinically negative neck in patients with SCC of the upper aerodigestive tract can be treated with equal success using surgery or radiation therapy. In general, the decision to treat the neck and the choice of treatment modality are dictated by the likelihood of occult lymph node metastases associated with the primary tumor; the modality selected to treat the primary tumor; and, in some instances, the need to enter the neck for reasons of surgical access to the primary tumor.

Treatment of the N0 neck is considered warranted when the probability of occult metastases is greater than 20%. This belief, long held by head and neck surgeons, was reinforced by Weiss et al. (34) using decision analysis to determine the optimal strategy for treatment of the N0 neck as a function of the probability of occult cervical metastases.

Currently, determination of the probability of occult metastases in the lymph nodes is based on various indirect clinical and histopathologic parameters and, when appropriate, imaging studies. That molecular and genetic characteristics of tumors also may be useful in this regard is encouraging.

Imaging Studies

The advent of modern imaging technology brought hopes of reliably identifying metastasis in lymph nodes before they became palpable. Unquestionably, computed tomography (CT) and magnetic resonance imaging (MRI) have a sensitivity and specificity higher than clinical examination in the detection of lymph nodes larger than 1 or 1.5 cm in diameter (35–37). Their interpretation relies primarily on the size of the lymph nodes; they cannot distinguish reactive enlargement of a node from enlargement due to metastasis. Though a correlation exists between the size of a lymph node and the probability of its containing metastasis, not all enlarged lymph nodes contain metastatic deposits. Equally important is the observation that, in patients with SCC, a large number of nodes are found to contain metastatic tumor measure less than 1 cm (38). Furthermore, even the presence of a central area of lucency within a node shown on CT, once considered pathognomonic of tumor necrosis within a node (39), can be mimicked by an artery with plaque formation or a fatty inclusion in a lymph node (35). The short and the long axis diameters of enlarged lymph nodes appear to be valuable in differentiating benign and malignant enlargement in cervical lymphadenopathy. In a study by Steinkamp et al. (40), 730 enlarged cervical lymph nodes in 285 patients were examined using ultrasonography, and the long–short (l/s) ratio was calculated. Histologic examination after neck dissection revealed that 95% of enlarged cervical nodes shown ultrasonographically to have an l/s ratio of more than 2 were diagnosed correctly as benign. Nodes presenting with a more circular shape and an l/s ratio of less than 2 were diagnosed correctly as metastases, with 95% accuracy (40).

Multidirectional ultrasound scanning appears more promising for a better preoperative evaluation of the N0 neck (41). It can depict lymph nodes as small as 3 mm in diameter, from which material for cytopathologic examination can be obtained by directed fine-needle aspiration biopsy (35).

Predictors of Nodal Metastases

The incidence of occult lymph node metastases for the different tumors according to site of origin and T stage is outlined in Tables 13.2 through 13.4. Tumor site and stage are helpful general indicators of the likelihood of occult metastases for a given primary tumor, but they are not completely accurate; hence, the constant search for better ways to determine the presence or absence of metastatic deposits in the lymph nodes.

Available to clinicians today is an increasing number of clinical, histologic, biochemical, and genetic factors that may be useful predictors of the propensity of a tumor to metastasize to the lymph nodes, and these factors may be useful in treatment planning. For example, in one study of 126 patients who had SCC of the oral cavity and underwent neck dissection as part of their treatment, Martinez-Gimeno et al. (42) found a statistically significant association between lymph node metastasis and the presence of microvascular invasion, grade of differentiation, tumor thickness, inflammatory infiltration, tumoral interphase, and the presence of perineural spread. On the basis of their results, these investigators designed a scoring system with a range of points from a to d. Scoring was done as follows: a, 7 to 12 points; b, 13 to 16 points; c, 17 to 20 points; and d, 21 to 30 points. The respective risk for metastasis was: a, 0%; b, 20%; c, 63.6%; and d, 86.3%.

TUMOR THICKNESS

The incidence of nodal metastases in patients with SCC of the floor of the mouth and oral tongue appears to increase as a function of the thickness of the primary tumor. In 1986, Mohit-Tabatabai et al. (43) found a significant correlation between tumor thickness of greater than 1.5 mm and subsequent development of neck metastases in a series of patients with stage I and stage II carcinomas of the floor of the mouth. In the same year, Spiro et al. (44), in a study of 105 patients with oral and oropharyngeal carcinoma with N0 necks, found that lymph node metastases occurred more frequently in patients whose tumors measured at least 2 mm thick.

By the use of mathematic modeling, the estimated risk for cervical node metastasis relative to thickness of SCC of the oral cavity was found to be approximately 3.9% for cancers 1-mm thick, 17% for cancers 2-mm thick, and 25% for cancers 3-mm thick (45). Similar findings by Frierson and Cooper (46) in patients with carcinoma of the lower lip and by Rasgon et al. (47) in patients with oral and oropharyngeal carcinoma support the importance of thickness as a predictor of nodal metastases. However, its usefulness in planning treatment of the neck is limited by the difficulty in determining tumor thickness through inspection or in biopsy specimens.

HISTOLOGIC GRADE

Despite the absence of general agreement about the prognostic impact of histologic differentiation, several studies have demonstrated a higher incidence of neck node metastases in patients with poorly differentiated SCC (22,46, 48,49). In oral cavity tumors, a higher grade of malignancy in terms of degree of differentiation and character of the borders may increase risk for metastases beyond the first and second echelon of regional lymph nodes (50) and may increase the risk for occult metastases in lower levels of the neck.

INVASIVE MARGIN OF THE TUMOR

More recently, attention has focused on the "malignancy grading" and character of the invasive margin of the tumor (pushing vs. infiltrating). Bryne et al. (51) have shown that patients with oral cavity carcinomas that exhibit an infiltrating margin with abundant mitoses and nuclear polymorphism are associated with a dismal survival. Others have shown an increased risk for occult lymph node metastases for such tumors (46,48,50, 52,53).

VASCULAR INVASION

The role of vascular invasion as a risk factor for lymph node metastases is unclear. In a study of 43 patients, Close et al. (54) found lymph node metastases in 77% of the cases in which vascular invasion was present but in only 25% of the cases in which it was absent. Though Crissman et al. (53) and Poleksic and Kalwaic (55) have found a similar correlation, others have not (46,47).

PERINEURAL INVASION

Several studies have suggested a strong correlation between the presence of perineural invasion at the primary site and cervical lymph node metastases (46,48).

INFLAMMATORY INFILTRATE

A marked inflammatory infiltrate in the stroma surrounding the tumor has been found to correlate with a lower incidence of lymph node metastases in some studies (43,46,48). Other studies have not shown such correlation (49,53,54).

DNA PLOIDY

Data from the literature are contradictory concerning the therapeutic and prognostic implications of DNA content in tumors of the head and neck. On the one hand, several investigators have found that cervical lymph node metastases are more frequent in patients with DNA nondiploid tumors than in similar patients with diploid tumors (56,57). In a study of 94 cases with advanced laryngeal cancers, ploidy was determined by computerized cytomorphometry. A high adjusted DNA index was associated with a higher incidence of lymph node metastases and with a higher number of histologically positive nodes (58).

However, just as many investigators have not been able to demonstrate such clear correlations (59,60). These differences, most likely due to the varying methods used by the different laboratories, limit the clinical applicability of DNA content analysis in decisions concerning treatment of the N0 neck.

TUMOR ANGIOGENESIS

Tumor angiogenesis has been associated with metastasis in breast, prostate, and non-small cell lung cancers. For head and neck SCC, Williams et al. (61) report that angiogenesis as determined by immunostaining of endothelial cells for factor VIII-related antigen was related strongly to the probability of metastasis in a group of 66 patients with oral cavity tumors and N0 necks. However, Leedy et al. (62) report, in a series of 57 patients who had tongue tumors and both N0 and N+ necks, that tumor angiogenesis was of no predictive value.

INTEGRITY OF THE BASEMENT MEMBRANE

Continuity of the basement membrane appears to be a predictor of nodal metastases, independent of T stage and differentiation. Murakami et al. (63) have investigated the immunohistologic localization and continuity of type IV collagen in the basement membrane surrounding the "cancer nest" into the stroma. These authors found that membrane discontinuity (breaks or absence) correlated significantly with cervical lymph node metastasis, whereas intact membrane was associated with a low frequency of cervical lymph node metastasis.

Surgical Treatment

INDICATIONS

Surgical treatment of the N0 neck is preferred when surgery is selected for the treatment of the primary tumor, particularly when the expectations of controlling the primary tumor with surgery alone are reasonably good. In such cases (e.g., T2 and selected T3 tumors of the oral cavity, T1 and T2 tumors of the supraglottic larynx), appropriate dissection of the regional lymph nodes alone is, in most cases, sufficient to control the disease in the neck. However, postoperative radiation therapy may be beneficial when the following features are found on histopathologic examination of the node dissection specimen(s):

- Presence of tumor in more than two or three lymph nodes
- Presence of tumor in multiple node groups
- Presence of extracapsular extension of tumor

Surgical dissection of the cervical lymph nodes also is desirable to facilitate adequate resection of the primary tumor when the neck must be entered and certain structures, such as the hypoglossal nerve or the carotid artery, must be exposed.

TYPE OF NECK DISSECTION

Radical neck dissection and modified RNDs are being used by fewer surgeons for the treatment of the N0 neck. Instead, selective neck dissections increasingly are accepted in the surgical treatment of the N0 neck (Table 13.8). These neck dissections are predicated on the basis of several observations.

As shown in Tables 13.3 and 13.4 (3,4,64–66), nodal metastases are found in predictable regions of the neck, depending on the site of the primary tumor. In a retrospective study that included 914 patients who underwent a lymph node dissection, the sentinel nodes for well-lateralized oral cavity tumors were defined as the homolateral levels I, II, and III; for oropharyngeal, hypopharyngeal, and laryngeal tumors, the sentinel nodes were defined as levels II and III (66).

En bloc removal of only the lymph node groups at highest risk for harboring metastases appears to have the same therapeutic value and provides the surgeon with the same staging information as the more extensive RNDs and modified RNDs (67–69). The morbidity associated with these operations is minimal and potentially reversible (70,71).

Two operations are included in this category of neck dissections:

TABLE 13.8 Treatment of N0 Neck

		Oropharynx			
Location of primary	**Oral cavity**	**BOT**	**Tonsil pharyngeal walls**	**Hypopharynx**	**Larynx**
Type of neck dissection	SND I–III/IV	SND II–III (IV)	SND II–IV Retropharyngeal	SND II–IV Retropharyngeal	SND II–IV (Subglottic: level VI)

BOT, base of tongue; SND, selective neck dissection.

TABLE 13.9 Lateral Neck Dissection Recurrence within Dissected Side of the Neck (Primary Controlled, 2-Year Follow-up)

Pathologic staging	Medina[a] Surgery only (%)	Byers[b] Surgery only (%)	Medina Surgery + irradiation (%)	Byers Surgery + irradiation (%)
N0	0 of 15 (0)	10 of 130 (8)	1 of 19 (5.2)	1 of 126 (1)
N1	—	0 of 4 (0)	0 of 3 (0)	0 of 17 (0)
Multiple nodes; extracapsular extension	—	—	0 of 6 (0)	3 of 20 (15)

[a]University of Oklahoma experience.
[b]Data modified from Byers RM. Modified neck dissection: a study of 967 cases from 1970 to 1980. *Am J Surg* 1986;150:414–421.

1. The lateral neck dissection consists of the *en bloc* removal of nodal regions II, III, and IV. This procedure is indicated in patients with tumors of the larynx, oropharynx, and hypopharynx staged T2 through T4 N0. Because the lymphatic drainage of these regions is such that metastases frequently are bilateral, often the operation is performed on both sides of the neck. The results obtained with this operation are shown in Table 13.9.
2. The supraomohyoid neck dissection consists of the *en bloc* removal of nodal regions I, II, and III. It is the preferred procedure for the surgical management of patients with SCC of the oral cavity. The procedure is performed on both sides of the neck in patients with cancers of the anterior tongue and floor of the mouth. This type of dissection is also performed when an elective neck dissection is indicated in the management of patients who have SCC of the lip or skin in the midportion of the face.

A bilateral dissection is performed when the lesion is located at or near the midline.

Postoperative radiation therapy is used when metastases are found in multiple nodes at one level or in nodes at multiple levels or when ECS of tumor is present.

In a prospective analysis of our practice (70), the use of supraomohyoid and lateral neck dissections in this manner produced a rate of recurrence in the neck that ranged from 0% (when the removed nodes were histologically negative) to 12.5% (in the presence of multiple positive nodes or ECS) (Table 13.10). Similar results of 5% to 15% and 5% to 21% have been reported by Byers (65) and Spiro et al. (67), respectively. In a more recent prospective study, a recurrence in the neck after supraomohyoid neck dissection occurred in 4 of 34 patients (11.7%) with T1 to T2 SCC of the oral cavity (71). Others have reported similar results (72).

Intraoperative Staging of the N0 Neck

Incorrect clinical staging of the N0 occurs in approximately 20% of patients, even when imaging studies are used. Rassekh et al. (73) addressed the issue of intraoperative staging of the neck in a prospective study of 108 neck dissections. Intraoperative palpation and inspection did not significantly improve the surgeon's ability to predict nodal stage. Of 62 patients with clinical N0 necks on both sides, 26 were staged N+ by intraoperative node examination. Nineteen of these 26 were histologically negative (73% false-positive). Of the 36 patients intraoperatively staged as N0, 10 were histologically positive (28% false-negative). Thus, upstaging the neck without frozen-section examination of suspected lymph nodes is not reliable. Although these authors recommended converting the selective dissection to an RND or modified RND on the basis of the results of frozen sections, this route has not been found necessary in our experience. Removal of the SCM, the IJV, or the posterior triangle of the neck is not performed unless these areas are obviously involved by the tumor. The decision to extend a selective neck dissection to include the jugular vein, the spinal accessory nerve, or (occasionally) the hypoglossal or the vagus nerve is based on the findings at the time of surgery and on an objective assessment of the extent of nodal disease by the surgeon.

An anterior compartment dissection (removal of the pretracheal and paratracheal lymph nodes) seldom is performed alone. It is indicated as part of the surgical treatment of tumors of the thyroid, subglottic larynx, trachea, and cervical esophagus.

TABLE 13.10 Supraomohyoid Neck Dissection Recurrence within Dissected Side of the Neck (Primary Controlled, 2-Year Follow-up)

	Surgery only (%)		Surgery and postoperative radiation therapy (%)	
Pathologic staging	Medina[a]	Byers[b]	Medina	Byers
N0	0 of 51	7 of 30 (5)	1 of 29 (3.45)	2 of 24 (8)
N1	—	1 of 10 (10)	0 of 3	0 of 8
Multiple nodes, extracapsular extension	0 of 1	5 of 21 (24)	2 of 16 (12.5)	6 of 41 (15)

[a]University of Oklahoma experience.
[b]Data modified from Byers RM. Modified neck dissection: a study of 967 cases from 1970 to 1980. *Am J Surg* 1986;150:414–421.

TABLE 13.11. Recurrence Rates in the N1 Neck After Selective Neck Dissection

Neck dissection type	Total	Surgery (%)	Surgery + radiation (%)	Other (%)
Supraomohyoid	92	10 of 44 (23)	13 of 46 (28)	1 of 2 (50)
Lateral	26	3 of 8 (38)	2 of 18 (11)	—
Total	118	13 of 52 (25)	15 of 64 (23)	1 of 2 (50)

Source: Data from Houck JR, Medina JE. Management of cervical lymph nodes in squamous carcinomas of the head and neck. *Semin Surg Oncol* 1995;11:228–239.

Elective Neck Irradiation

The N0 neck is treated with radiation therapy in patients in whom the primary tumor is irradiated, and in whom the likelihood of occult nodal metastases is 20% or higher. Radiation therapy is also used in patients in whom postoperative treatment is indicated on the basis of the characteristics of the primary tumor alone (T4 and infiltrating T3 tumors) and when these can be resected adequately without entering the neck. Fletcher (74) and others have shown that the risk for developing clinically positive nodes in an N0 neck can be reduced to perhaps 5% with the use of comprehensive neck irradiation (75).

MANAGEMENT OF THE N+ NECK

Surgery continues to be the mainstay in the treatment of patients with palpable cervical lymph node metastases. A notable exception is the treatment of the neck in patients with nasopharyngeal carcinoma in which even large nodal metastases are controlled readily with radiation. A neck dissection is indicated only when radiation has controlled the primary tumor but has failed to control the tumor in the neck (76,77).

Imaging Studies

Preoperative imaging of extensive metastases in the neck with CT and MRI has focused mainly on assessment of resectability. A more recent and intriguing focus is the use of image analysis in predicting response to therapy. Nodal density, as compared with the density of nuchal muscles in contrasted CT scans, has been shown to have a strong correlation with response to cisplatin-based chemotherapy (78). This concept merits further evaluation.

In terms of assessing resectability, CT scanning and MRI enable surgeons to define more clearly the relationship of a metastatic tumor to such critical structures as the common and the internal carotid arteries, the cervical spine and the vertebral artery, and the brachial plexus. The advantages of having such information in advance are obvious, particularly when tumor involvement of the common or the internal carotid artery is suspected. Such a case renders it desirable to assess accurately the structural and functional status of the contralateral carotid and the collateral intracerebral circulation. Angiography now is complemented routinely by measuring carotid backpressure and using balloon occlusion techniques while monitoring the patient for evidence of neurologic deficits under normotensive and hypotensive conditions (79).

Surgical Treatment

As more surgeons accept the surgical and oncologic feasibility of removing involved lymph nodes along with surrounding fibrofatty tissue (but without removal of such important uninvolved structures as the spinal accessory nerve), the surgical management of the N+ neck is becoming a matter of judgment. In addition, with the judicious combination of surgery and radiation therapy, excellent tumor control in the neck can be obtained while preserving function and cosmesis (65). The main goal of neck dissection is, however, to adequately remove the tumor from the neck and not to rely on radiation therapy to compensate for poor surgical technique. Preservation of adjacent structures should be pursued only when a clearly identifiable plane exists between the tumor and that structure. Cutting into and spilling of tumor must be avoided.

The results obtained with selective neck dissection in patients with stage N1 disease, in which the node is less than 3 cm in diameter, is mobile, and is located in the first echelon of lymphatic drainage (80) are listed in Table 13.11. For more advanced nodal metastases, Tables 13.12 (81–87) and 13.13 (88–93) show the rates of tumor control in the neck reported

TABLE 13.12 Recurrence Rates in the Neck After Type I Modified Radical Neck Dissections

			Percentage of recurrence	
Study	No. of dissections	Follow-up (mos)	Elective procedure	Therapeutic procedure
Pearlman et al. (81)	56	18	7	20
Bradenburg and Lee (82)	65	60	5	11
	69	24	4	5
Roy and Beahrs (83)	89	40	4	17
Skolnik et al. (84)	42	—	0	0
Chu and Strawitz (85)	21	24	—	5
Carenfelt and Eliasson (86)	81	53	—	9
Andersen et al. (87)	132	38	—	8

TABLE 13.13 Recurrence Rates in the Neck with Type III Modified Radical Neck Dissection

Study	No. of dissections	Follow-up (mos)	Recurrence rate (%) for elective procedures	Recurrence rate (%) for therapeutic procedures		
			N0	N1	N+	N2
Lingeman et al. (88)	59	—	0	15.0	—	25
Molinari et al. (89)	128	36	1.3	—	3.7	—
Joseph et al. (90)	18	18	16.5	0	—	—
Gavilan and Gavilan (91)	242	60	8.9	7.9	—	20
Bocca et al. (92)	843	60	2.4	—	30.4	—
Calearo and Teatini (93)	258	36	3.2[a]	—	5.6[b]	—

[a]Clinically and histologically node-negative.
[b]Clinically and histologically node-positive. In these cases, authors did not distinguish between N1 and N2.

with modified RND. These results appear to be comparable to those obtained with RND. Andersen et al. (94) reviewed the results of 378 neck dissections performed in 366 patients with clinically and pathologically positive nodal metastases from SCC of the upper aerodigestive tract. The study compared survival and tumor recurrence in the neck in patients who had RND with those who had modified RND with preservation of the spinal accessory nerve. Preservation of the spinal accessory nerve did not affect survival and tumor control in the neck. Interestingly, the pattern of failure in the neck was similar for the two operations.

Postoperative Radiation Therapy

Numerous studies suggest that when multiple nodes are involved at multiple levels of the neck and when ECS of tumor is found, the rate of tumor recurrence in the neck is decreased by the addition of radiation therapy (13,15,17,95,96). The timing and the dose of radiation therapy are crucial if good regional control is to be achieved. Results of one prospective clinical trial provide the basis for the recommendation that patients with advanced head and neck cancer treated with daily fractions of 1.8 Gy should receive a minimum postoperative dose of 57.6 Gy to the entire operative bed. Sites of increased risk for recurrence, such as areas of the neck wherein ECS of tumor was found, should be boosted to 63 Gy. Radiation therapy should be started as soon as possible after surgery (97). Some studies have suggested that a delay in the initiation of radiation therapy beyond 6 weeks may compromise tumor control (96), but this caution has been disputed.

Large doses of radiation intraoperatively delivered to the neck may be useful in the treatment of patients with advanced cervical metastases. Freeman et al. (98) report one of the largest experiences with this technique. Seventy-five patients who had advanced cervical metastasis with possible invasion of the deep muscles or carotid artery were approached with aggressive resection and intraoperative radiation therapy (IORT). All metastatic nodes were greater than 3 cm, 65% were fixed on clinical examination, and 35% involved the carotid artery. Fifteen of the patients required extended neck dissections with carotid resections and grafting. After the resection, an average single dose of 2,000 cGy of electron beam IORT was delivered. At 2 years, the local control rate within the IORT port was 68% (98). This technique requires a sophisticated and expensive setup in the operating suite and requires cumbersome transport of an anesthetized patient with a large open wound to the radiation therapy facility.

SPECIAL ISSUES IN THE TREATMENT OF THE NECK

Resection of the Carotid Artery

The extent of the tumor in the neck may dictate the need to extend a neck dissection to include such structures as the hypoglossal nerve, the carotid, and the overlying skin, none of which normally is removed by this operation. The controversy about the advisability of resecting the common or the internal carotid artery has not been resolved. Some surgeons still believe that carotid resection in patients with advanced SCC of the neck does not improve long-term survival (102), even though improved techniques for vascular and soft-tissue reconstruction have rendered possible the resection of the carotid with acceptable morbidity (100,101).

Advanced Neck Metastases with a Small Primary Tumor

Advanced metastasis occurs more often with carcinomas of the oropharynx or hypopharynx. Treatment can consist of (a) excision of the primary tumor, concomitant neck dissection, and postoperative radiation or (b) radiation therapy to the primary tumor and the neck, followed by neck dissection 4 to 6 weeks later. The latter approach is preferred by some surgeons because the primary tumor is small and usually is located in an area in which preservation of function is more likely with radiation, such as the soft palate, base of the tongue, or hypopharynx. This approach, however, presents two significant drawbacks: (a) the uncertainty of tumor control at the primary site 4 to 6 weeks after completion of radiation therapy and (b) the intraoperative and postoperative consequences on tissue planes and healing of radiation.

A new treatment alternative to this problem was reported by the surgeons at the M. D. Anderson Cancer Center (102), where a neck dissection was performed first and was followed by radiation therapy (a postoperative dose to the neck and a definitive dose to the primary tumor). In a selected group of 35 patients with advanced neck disease (median size, 5 × 4 cm) and primary tumors thought to be amenable to treatment by radiation therapy, recurrence of tumor in the neck occurred in only 11% of the patients; the overall 5-year survival was 55%. Using a similar treatment approach in 65 patients with tumors of the larynx and hypopharynx, the French Head and Neck Study Group observed a rate of recurrence in the neck of 4.6% (103).

For this treatment approach to succeed, the resectability of the tumor in the neck must be assessed carefully, and the neck dissection must be performed meticulously, with care to avoid complications that may delay the initiation of radiation. Furthermore, the radiation oncologist must be willing to begin therapy as soon as a few days after surgery. In this study, delaying the start of radiation therapy for more than 2 weeks was associated with a significant decrease in survival.

Treatment of the Neck and Neoadjuvant Chemotherapy

Decisions about treatment of the neck deserve special consideration when neoadjuvant chemotherapy and radiation therapy are used for organ preservation in patients with palpable cervical lymph node metastases. In this regard, valuable information has been provided by an analysis of a subset of 92 patients who had laryngeal carcinoma and advanced neck disease (N2 or N3) and were treated as part of the Veterans Administration Cooperative Study (104) of induction chemotherapy (cisplatin and 5-fluorouracil) and definitive radiation (6,600–7,600 cGy). After chemotherapy and radiation, a neck dissection was necessary in 68% of the patients in whom the tumor in the neck exhibited less than a complete clinical response to the induction chemotherapy and in 28% of the patients in whom a complete response was observed. Armstrong et al. (105) have reported similar observations.

Though the authors of these studies recommend a neck dissection be performed only when less than a complete response to chemotherapy occurs, arguably a 28% probability of persistent tumor in the neck justifies also performing a neck dissection in patients who have a complete clinical response to chemotherapy. After all, most head and neck surgeons recommend treating the N0 neck when the probability of occult metastases is 20% or higher. This argument is strengthened by the fact that 60% of those patients died of uncontrolled disease in the neck, despite salvage neck dissection (104).

Sequelae of Neck Dissection

SCAPULAR DESTABILIZATION

The most troublesome sequelae after RND result from the removal of the spinal accessory nerve and denervation of the trapezius muscle. The resultant destabilization of the scapula leads to drooping and lateral and anterior rotation followed by progressive flaring away from the vertebral column posteriorly. The loss of the trapezius function decreases the patient's ability to abduct the shoulder above 90 degrees. These physical changes result in the recognized shoulder syndrome of pain, weakness, and deformity of the shoulder girdle commonly associated with RND (Fig. 13.11). These effects all are accentuated in patients who are overweight, in whom the weight of tissue anteriorly increases the anterior forces.

In the last few years, the literature has reflected debate over whether a significant difference is seen in postoperative shoulder function after an RND and the modifications of RND that preserve the spinal accessory nerve. Using patient questionnaires, Schuller et al. (106) compared symptomatology and the ability to return to preoperative employment in patients who underwent either an RND or a modified RND. Though they found no statistically significant difference between the two groups, Sterns and Shaheen (107) and others (108; R. Byers, personal communication, 1994), using methods similar to Schuller's, found that most patients who had a nerve-sparing procedure did not have postoperative pain or shoulder dysfunction.

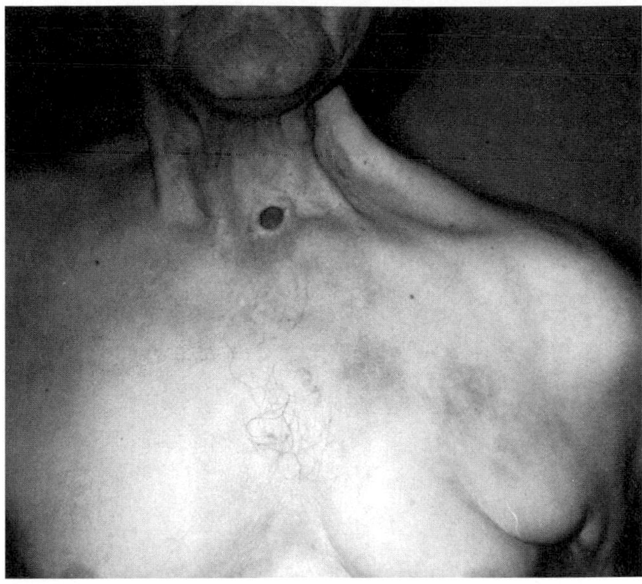

Figure 13.11 Shoulder deformity characteristic of denervation of the trapezius muscle.

Only recently have prospective objective data on shoulder dysfunction after neck dissection been gathered. Leipzig et al. (109) studied 109 patients who had undergone various types of neck dissections. They used the surgeon's preoperative and postoperative observations of shoulder movement rated by the degree of shoulder dysfunction. The authors concluded that any type of neck dissection could result in impairment of function of the shoulder. Dysfunction, however, occurred more frequently among those patients in whom the spinal accessory nerve was dissected or resected extensively.

In a 1986 prospective study, Sobol et al. (69) compared preoperative and postoperative measures of shoulder range of motion. In some patients, postoperative electromyograms (EMGs) also were obtained. Shoulder range of motion in patients who underwent a nerve-sparing procedure was better than in those who had an RND. Interestingly, however, the type of nerve-sparing procedure was found to affect the degree of shoulder disability. Sixteen weeks after surgery, patients who had undergone a modified RND (in which the entire length of the nerve was dissected) did not have shoulder range of motion better than that in patients who had a standard RND. However, patients who underwent a supraomohyoid neck dissection (embodying less extensive dissection of the spinal accessory nerve) performed significantly better ($p \geq 0.05$) than did either of the other two groups, both in terms of shoulder range of motion and EMG findings on the trapezius muscle. Importantly, at 16 weeks after surgery, moderate to severe EMG abnormalities were noted in as many as 65% of the patients in whom the spinal accessory nerve was dissected in its entire length (modified RND). Though no severe abnormalities were noted in the group undergoing supraomohyoid neck dissection, 22% of them showed moderate abnormalities.

Several patients from each group had repeat studies at 1 year after a surgery. Unlike the outcome in the patients who had had an RND, clear evidence of improvement in all parameters studied was seen in patients in whom the nerve was spared.

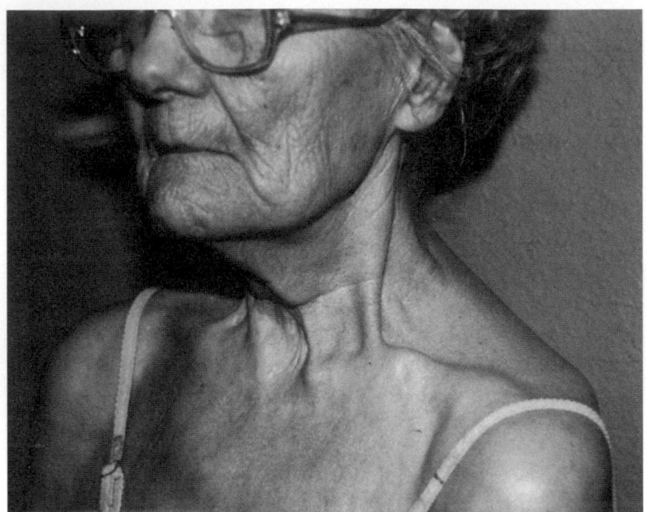

Figure 13.12 Patient with denervated trapezius and shoulder drooping several years after modified radical neck dissection with preservation of internal jugular vein, sternocleidomastoid muscle, and XI nerve (type III).

A more recent prospective study by Remmler et al. (68) also revealed that patients who had a nerve-sparing procedure experienced a significant but temporary phase of spinal accessory nerve dysfunction. In this study, preoperative strength, range-of-motion measures, and EMG of the trapezius muscle were compared with postoperative measures obtained at 1, 3, 6, and 12 months. The groups studied consisted of patients undergoing nerve-sparing procedures and those in whom the nerve was resected. Most of the patients in the nerve-sparing group had supraomohyoid neck dissections. Patients who underwent RND had a significant decrease in trapezius muscle strength and underwent denervation of the trapezius muscle on EMG at 1 month; these parameters did not improve with time. Interestingly, patients in the nerve-sparing group had a small but significant reduction in trapezius muscle strength and evidence of trapezius muscle denervation at 1 and 3 months, which improved by 12 months.

The last three studies have provided evidence that even procedures involving minimal dissection of the spinal accessory nerve can result in shoulder dysfunction (Fig. 13.12). Although this outcome appears to be reversible, every effort should be made to avoid undue trauma to the nerve (particularly stretching) during any neck dissection in which the nerve is preserved. Furthermore, every patient who undergoes neck dissection must be questioned about the function of the shoulder and must be evaluated by a physical therapist early in the postoperative period. Should any deficit be detected, the patient should be counseled and coached properly to ensure proper rehabilitation of the shoulder.

Surgical Complications

In addition to the medical complications that can occur after any surgical procedure in the head and neck region, several surgical complications can be related solely or in part to the neck dissection.

AIR LEAKS

Circulation of air through a wound drain is a common complication usually encountered during the first postoperative day. The point of entrance of air may be located somewhere along the skin incision. However, if the drains are connected to suction in the operating room just before the completion of the wound closure, such an air leak usually becomes apparent at that time and can be corrected. Other points of entrance may not become apparent until after surgery, when the position of the neck changes or the patient begins to move. The typical example of this situation is the improperly secured suction wound drain that becomes displaced, thus exposing one or more of the drain vents.

Air leaks with potentially more serious consequences are those that occur through a communication of the neck wound with the tracheostomy site or through a mucosal suture line. In these, air and contaminated secretions enter the neck wound. Early identification of the site of leakage, therefore, is desirable. Doing so may not be a simple task, however, and correction may require revision of the wound closure in the operating room.

BLEEDING

Postoperative hemorrhage usually occurs immediately after surgery. External bleeding through the incision without distortion of the skin flaps often originates in a subcutaneous blood vessel. In most instances, this effect can be controlled readily by ligation or infiltration of the surrounding tissues with an anesthetic solution containing epinephrine. On the other hand, pronounced swelling or ballooning of the skin flaps during the immediate postoperative period must be attributed to a hematoma in the wound, even if bleeding is not obvious. If the swelling or ballooning is detected early, manipulating the drains occasionally results in evacuation of the accumulated blood and resolves the problem; however, if this is not accomplished immediately or if blood reaccumulates quickly, the best response is to return the patient to the operating room to explore the wound under sterile conditions, to evacuate the hematoma, and to control the bleeding. Attempting to do this in the recovery room or at the bedside usually is ill advised because lighting may be inadequate, surgical equipment may have to be improvised, and sterile conditions can be compromised. Failure to recognize or to manage a postoperative hematoma properly may predispose the patient to the development of wound infection. Although bulky pressure dressings may be useful in curtailing postoperative edema, they do not prevent hematomas and may, in fact, delay their recognition.

Jugular vein rupture should be considered in patients who have undergone primary tumor excision with modified RND and in whom the procedure is complicated by a pharyngocutaneous fistula. In this circumstance, the bleeding is venous and occurs repeatedly (110).

CHYLOUS FISTULA

Despite the best efforts of surgeons, a postoperative chylous fistula occurs after 1% to 2% of neck dissections (111). Spiro et al. (112) reviewed 823 neck dissections that included removal of the lymph nodes in level IV. They found that in most patients who developed a chylous fistula, a chylous leak had been identified intraoperatively but was thought to be under control intraoperatively in most patients who developed a chylous fistula (111,112). It behooves the surgeon, therefore, to avoid injury to the thoracic duct proper and also to ligate or clip even potential lymphatic tributaries in the area of the thoracic duct. This precaution may be accomplished with relative ease if the operative field is kept bloodless during dissection in this area of the neck. Furthermore, as soon as the dissection of this area is completed and again before closing the wound, the area is observed for 20 or 30 seconds while the anesthesiologist increases the intrathoracic pressure.

Even the smallest leak of chylous material must be pursued seriously until it is arrested. Direct clamping and ligating may be difficult and sometimes counterproductive, owing to the fragility of the lymphatic vessels and the surrounding fatty tissue. Hemoclips are ideal to control a source of leakage that is visualized clearly. Otherwise, use of suture ligatures is preferable (with pliable material, such as 5-0 silk). They should be tied over a piece of hemostatic sponge to avoid tearing.

Management of this complication depends on the time of onset of the leak and the amount of chyle drainage in a 24-hour period and on the ability of the physician to prevent accumulation of chyle under the skin flaps. When the daily output of chyle exceeds 500 mL to 600 mL, especially when the chyle fistula becomes apparent immediately after surgery, conservative closed-wound management is unlikely to succeed. In such cases, we prefer early surgical exploration, before the adjacent tissues become markedly inflamed and before the fibrinous material that coats these tissues becomes adherent, thus obscuring and jeopardizing such important structures as the phrenic and the vagus nerves. Chylous fistulae that become apparent only after enteral feedings are resumed—and particularly those that drain less than 600 mL of chyle per day—initially are managed conservatively with closed wound drainage and low-fat nutritional support.

FACIAL AND CEREBRAL EDEMA

Synchronous bilateral RNDs in which both IJVs are ligated can result in the development of facial edema, cerebral edema, or both. Sometimes, the facial edema can be severe (Fig. 13.13). This effect appears to be a mechanical problem of venous drainage, which resolves to a variable extent with time as collateral circulation is established. Such swelling is more common and more severe in patients who had previous radiation to the head and neck and in those patients in whom the resection includes large segments of the lateral and posterior pharyngeal walls.

We have been able to prevent massive facial edema by preserving at least one external jugular vein whenever a bilateral RND is anticipated. The external jugular vein usually is separated from the tumor in the neck by the SCM and can be dissected free between the tail of the parotid and the subclavian veins (Fig. 13.14). Others recommend grafting of one of the IJVs.

After bilateral RND, the development of cerebral edema may cause impaired neurologic function and even coma. Ligation of the IJVs leads to increased intracranial pressure (113,114). In a study by Weiss et al. (34), four patients who had staged bilateral RNDs underwent placement of a subarachnoid bolt for direct monitoring of intracranial pressure. Marked elevations of pressure were noted immediately after ligation of the IJV, with a maximum peak at 30 minutes. Furthermore, systemic hypertension was observed in response to elevated intracranial pressure (Cushing reflex). Also, the increased cerebral venous pressure that occurs as a result of ligating both IJVs in dogs has been shown experimentally to be associated with inappropriate secretion of antidiuretic hormone (115). One then can speculate that the resulting expansion of extracellular fluids

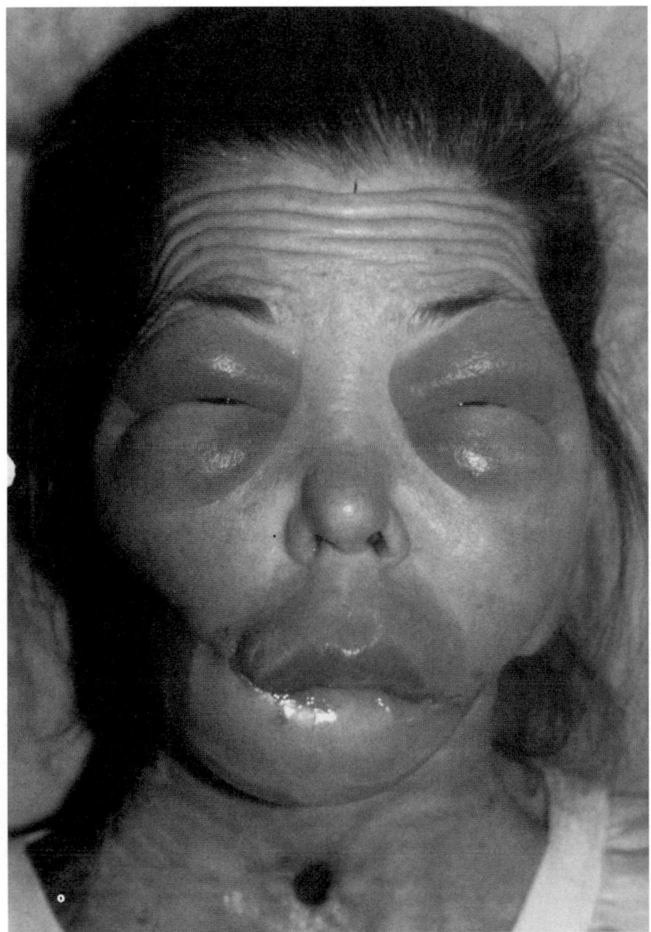

Figure 13.13 Severe facial edema that can occur after bilateral neck dissection.

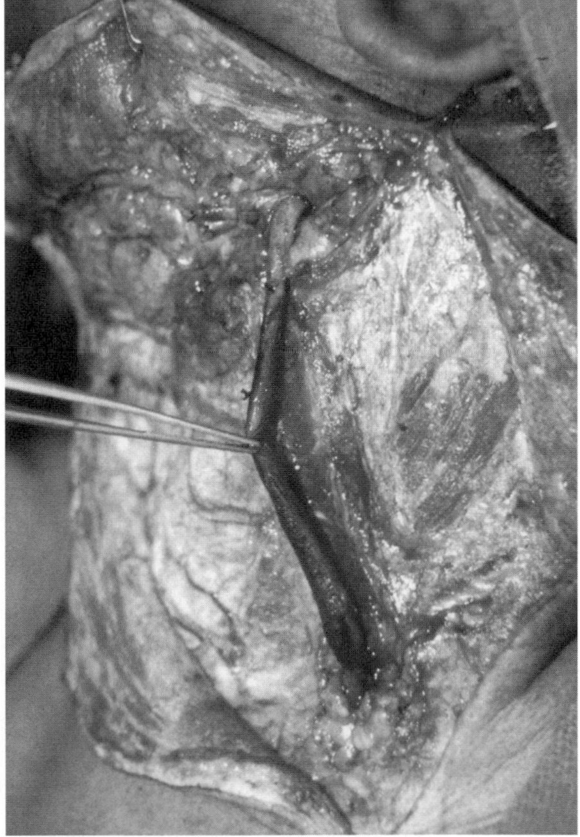

Figure 13.14 Dissection of the external jugular vein from the parotid to the supraclavicular region before performing a radical neck dissection.

and dilutional hyponatremia could aggravate cerebral edema, creating a vicious cycle.

In practice, these observations behoove the surgeon and the anesthesiologist to curtail the administration of fluids during and after bilateral RNDs (116). Furthermore, perioperative management of fluid and electrolytes in these cases should not be guided solely by the patient's urine output but additionally by monitoring of central venous pressure, cardiac output, serum, and urine osmolarity. Also interesting to note is that after bilateral neck dissection, some patients may lose their hypoxic ventilatory responses, owing to carotid body denervation (117).

BLINDNESS

Blindness after bilateral RND is a rare but catastrophic complication. To date, five cases have been reported in the literature (118). Posterior ischemic optic neuropathy after bilateral RND may be related to hypotension. In one report, histologic examination revealed intraorbital optic nerve infarction, suggesting as possible etiologic factors intraoperative hypotension and severe venous distention. Thus, avoiding drug-induced hypotension is important for preventing this complication (119).

JUGULAR VEIN THROMBOSIS

Preservation of the IJV during neck dissection does not ensure its postoperative patency, particularly when radiation therapy also is used. In a retrospective study using cervical duplex and pulsed Doppler imaging to determine IJV patency after modified RND, the rate of patency of the IJV was found to be 87% (120). Cotter et al. (121) used preoperative and postoperative CT or MRI on 69 patients undergoing 79 vein-sparing neck dissections. Sixty-eight veins (86%) were patent after surgery (121). Interestingly, radiation therapy appears to influence patency of the IJV. Through noninvasive color Doppler ultrasonography scan, the IJVs were found to be normal bilaterally in 18% of patients who had undergone a modified RND and radiation therapy, in 88% of patients who had undergone a neck dissection alone, and in 57% of patients who had undergone radiation therapy alone (122).

RADIOLOGIC IMAGING CONCERNS

Bernard B. O'Malley and Suresh K. Mukherji

The main roles for imaging of the neck for surgical management include confirming the N0 status of the neck, excluding nodal metastases contralateral to clinically palpable disease, the extent of bulky adenopathy, and evaluation of the posttreatment neck. Imaging the neck for metastatic disease is an adjunct to clinical palpation. Imaging is especially important in obese patients or patient with thick necks. Diagnosing adenopathy in the neck is based on morphology by CT (Fig. 13.15), MRI, or ultrasonography (126–128). Computed tomography imaging requires intravenous contrast. Contrast is also beneficial in MRI for evaluating central areas of low attenuation, which may represent small focal metastases. Other imaging modalities, which may also be used to evaluate the neck, include radioimmunoscintigraphy, positron emission tomography scanning (129), and iron–dextran enhanced MRI (130,131). These latter methods along with Doppler ultrasonography provide a more accurate physiologic evaluation of lymph nodes. Sonography adds little to the work-up if contrast CT has been performed except for higher specificity when used to guide fine-needle aspiration (132).

Computed tomography and MRI (Fig.13.16) are the primary diagnostic modalities used in North America for staging the neck. The slice thickness should not exceed 5 mm with either modality, and many institutions prefer 3-mm thick sections for CT. The imaging should begin at the skull base and extend inferiorly to the level of the head of the clavicles (Fig. 13.17). To obtain adequate vascular opacification with CT prior to imaging, approximately 30 to 50 cc are required prior to acquiring the first image. The exact timing of the bolus and the delay in imaging varies with specific types of CT scanners (Fig. 13.18). No such delay is required with MRI after contrast administration.

Standard cross-sectional CT and MRI are based on lymph node morphology size and enhancement features. Adjunctive methods can be applied with better accuracy when scans are equivocal. Doppler analysis of the intrinsic blood flow has been shown to be beneficial in characterizing suspicious nodes even before they are enlarged (133). Conventional sonography is less sensitive than CT, MRI, or fluorodeoxyglucose-positron emission tomography (FDG-PET) (134). The benefit of sonography is the convenience of performing a fine-needle aspiration if the node remains suspicious. Fine-needle aspiration is an efficient and highly accurate method for confirming or excluding nodal metastases (135). Nuclear imaging with thallium-201 (136) can help reduce the false-positive cross-sectional results. The use of FDG-PET is now established as a very powerful adjunct to staging the head and neck (137).

Accurate staging of the neck opposite to the side of palpable nodal disease is essential for proper treatment of the neck. The risk for contralateral nodal metastases contributes to the morbidity of bilateral neck treatment. Careful analysis will help to differentiate among the subgroups of N2 disease (138). One must be familiar with the typical lymphatic drainage patterns for the various primary sites so as to avoid false-positive lymph node staging (Fig. 13.19). On a similar theme, one must be aware of the typical neck dissections associated with the various primary sites and should bring to the surgeon's attention any suspicious lymph node findings that may fall out of that standard operative approach (139). Among the adverse prognostic factors of cervical nodal metastases is the number of levels involved and ECS. Extracapsular penetration can be diagnosed by obliteration of the normal fat plane surrounding a metastatic lymph node. Tumors that have imaging evidence of extending across midline or those arising from midline structures such as palate, tongue base and supraglottic, are at greater risk for metastases to the contralateral neck.

Another important role of neck imaging is the regional evaluation of a known aggregate nodal mass relative to the adjacent neurovascular structures and to evaluate invasion of deep neck muscle before invasion. This information is important as the presence of carotid encasement or invasion of the deep neck muscles renders patients unresectable at many institutions. Carotid invasion can be suggested if a tumor surrounds the carotid artery by more than 270 degrees. Invasion of the deep neck musculature can be suggested on imaging if there is direct evidence of tumor extension in the paraspinal musculature.

Follow-up scanning for recurrent adenopathy after irradiation or neck dissection is a challenging but very important task. There is a growing trend to image patients prior to planned neck dissection. Recent investigations have questioned the need for planned neck dissection if there is complete radiographic resolution following combined chemotherapy and radiation therapy. Recent studies have suggested that a greater than 90% reduction in the volume of a metastatic node following combined therapy compared with a pretreatment study predicts eradication of tumor within the node (140). Film interpretation requires familiarity with the appearance of the neck after irradiation and the degrees of neck dissection: limited and comprehensive (141). Imaging of the postsurgical neck is even more challenging. A typical problem area is the infiltrated appearance of the high carotid sheath after dissection that included sacrifice of the jugular vein. This is an infrequent site for recurrence and such a diagnosis should be made with caution, particularly in the absence of a developing lower cranial neuropathy. Flap reconstructions must be interpreted carefully because of local distortion at the reconstructed site (Fig. 13.20) and the distortion related to the dissection for the attachment of the vascular pedicle (142,143). Usually, some degree of redundancy occurs (related to the positioning of the flap) and often gives rise to the imaging appearance of a pseudomass (see Fig. 19.9). This effect is typical on follow-up of the interposed jejunum after laryngopharyngectomy.

Turn to imaging atlas beginning on the next page.

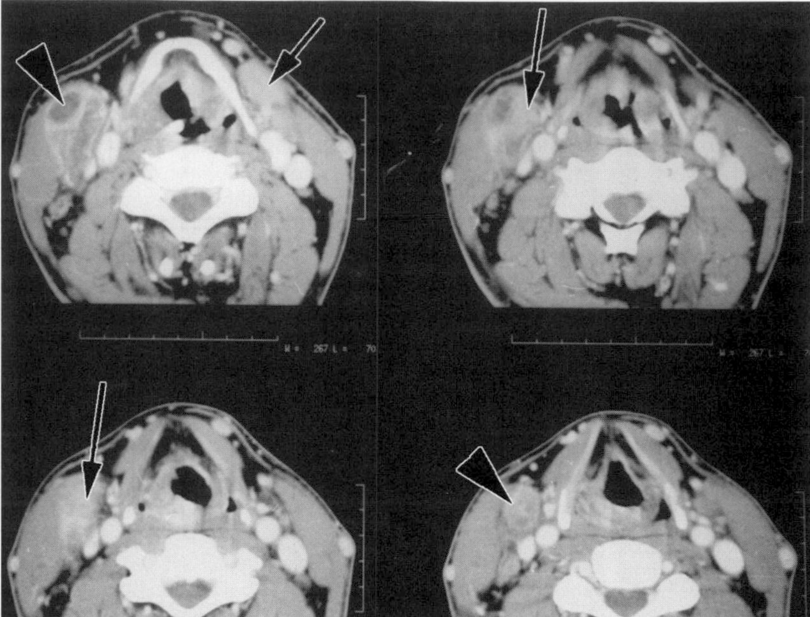

Figure 13.15 Metastatic squamous cancer. Serial enhanced axial computed tomography images show typical pattern of moderately enhancing pathologic lymph nodes (*arrows*) mixed with necrotic nodes (*arrowheads*) in a patient with a supraglottic primary tumor. Contrast this with the more homogeneous pattern of lymph nodes despite varied sizes in lymphoma (see Fig. 34.3).

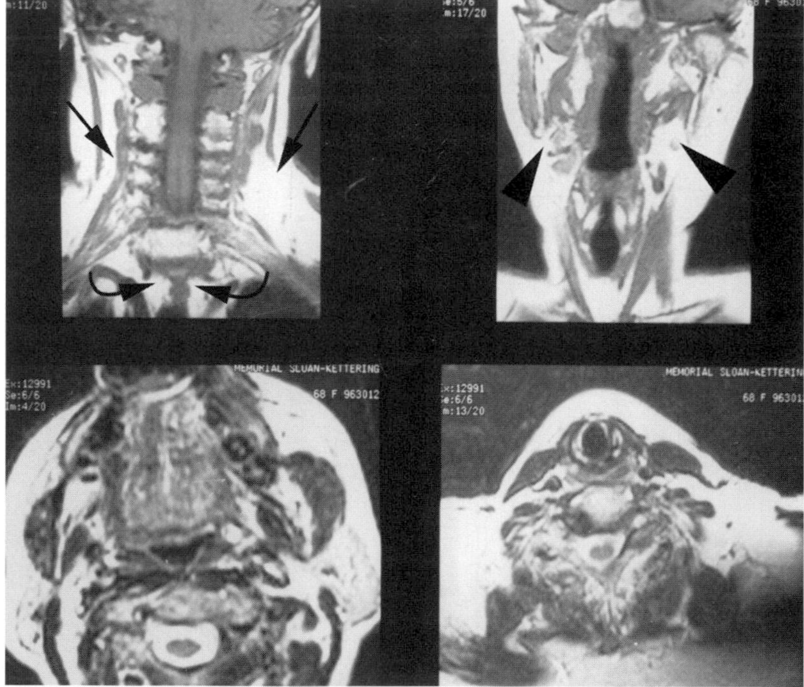

Figure 13.16 Neck magnetic resonance imaging survey. Direct coronal T1 view (**top**) of posterior chain (**left**) and anterior chain (**right**) show no pathologic nodes (*arrows*). Coronal view also covers the tracheoesophageal grooves in the superior mediastinum (*curved arrows*). Selected axial T2 views of suprahyoid and infrahyoid neck confirm N0 status.

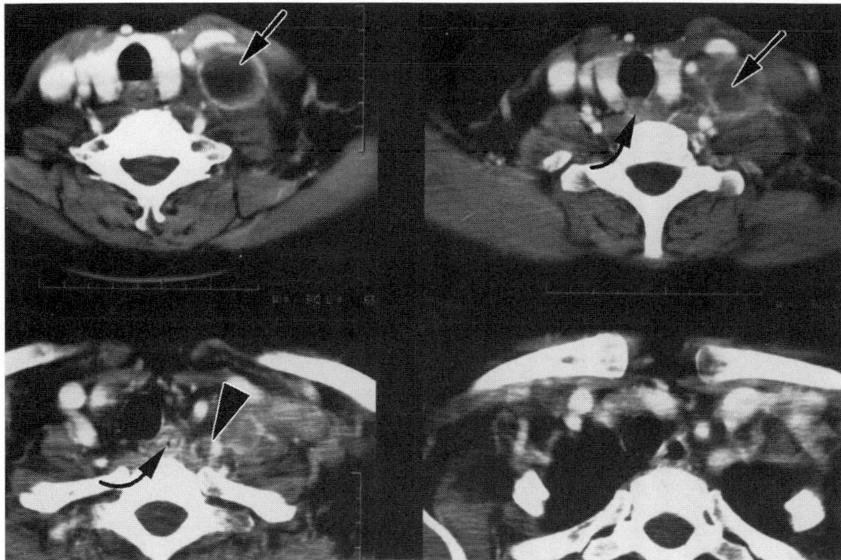

Figure 13.17 Virchow lymph node. Enhanced serial axial computed tomography images through the lower neck. A necrotic lymph node at the left venous angle (*arrows*) and a smaller pathologic lymph node (*arrowhead*) due to a clinically occult primary squamous cancer of the esophagus (*curved arrow*) are shown.

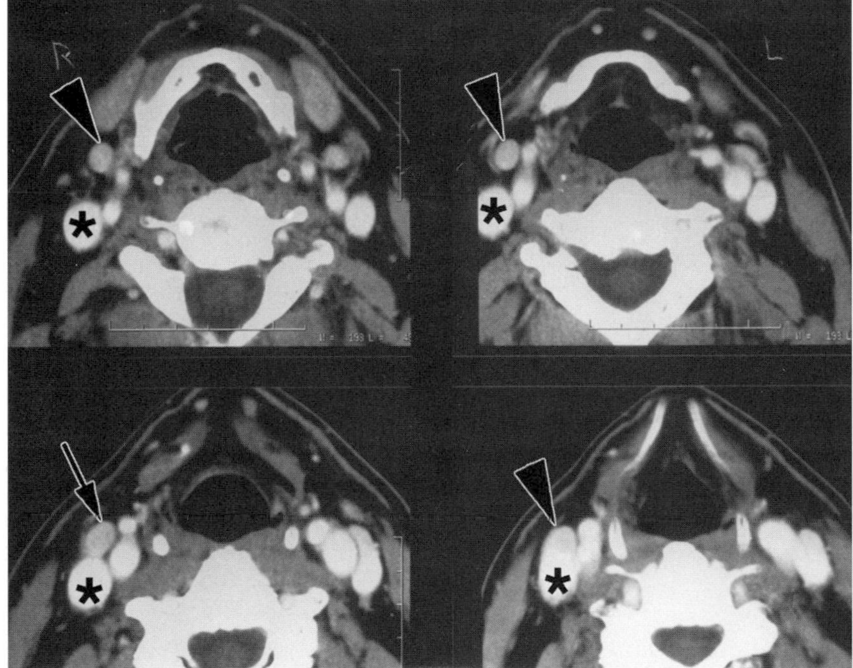

Figure 13.18 Serial enhanced axial computed tomography images show the value of 5-mm thick sections at the suprahyoid neck. The differential venous opacification results in the appearance of a suspicious lymph node in the anterior chain (*arrow*) on one section. Inspection of serial sections confirms the facial vein (*arrowheads*) draining into the internal jugular vein (*asterisk*).

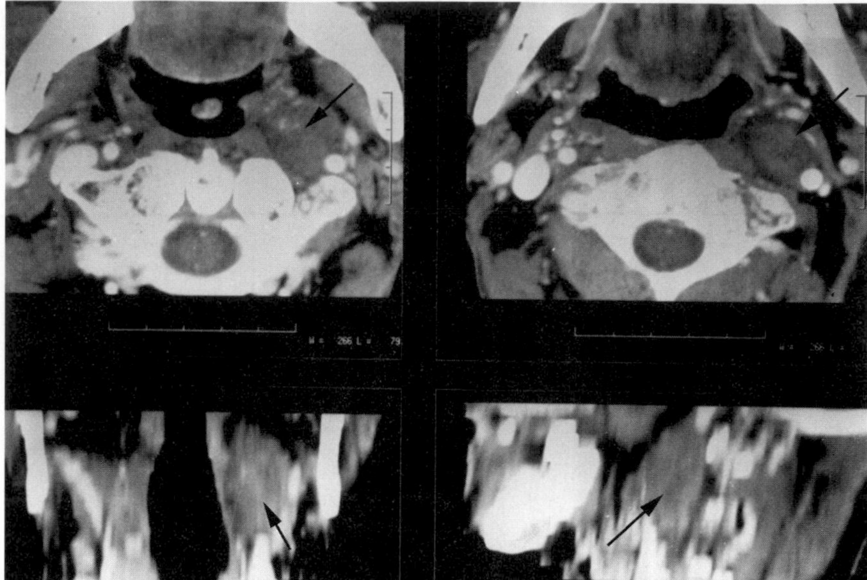

Figure 13.19 False-positive lymph node staging. Enhanced axial computed tomography (**top**) and reformatted coronal and parasagittal views (**bottom**) show a lesion in the carotid space (*arrows*) suspected to be adenopathy. Percutaneous computed tomography-guided biopsy yielded neuroma.

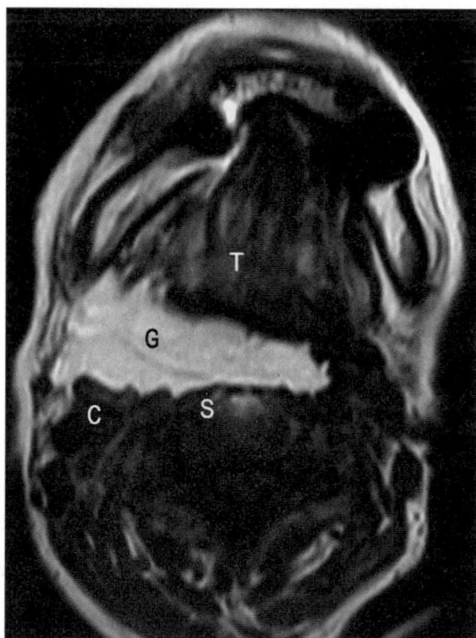

Figure 13.20 Flap reconstruction. Axial T1-weighted magnetic resonance image of a reconstructed pharynx. Distortion of the tongue base (*T*) related to position of myocutaneous graft (*G*), which is applied to the carotid space (*C*) and prevertebral plane of the spine (*S*).

REFERENCES

1. Crile G. Excision of cancer of the head and neck. *JAMA* 1906;47:1780–1786.
2. Martin H, Del Valle B, Erhlich H, et al. Neck dissection. *Cancer* 1951;4:441–449.
3. Lindberg R. Distribution of cervical lymph node metastases from squamous cell carcinoma of the upper respiratory and digestive tracts. *Cancer* 1972;29: 1446–1449.
4. Byers RM, Wolf PF, Ballantyne AJ. Rationale for elective modified neck dissection. *Head Neck Surg* 1988;10:160–167.
5. Shah JP. Patterns of cervical lymph node metastasis from squamous carcinomas of the upper aerodigestive tract. *Am J Surg* 1990;160: 405–409.
6. Fisch UP, Sigel ME. Cervical lymphatic system as visualized by lymphography. *Ann Otol Rhinol Laryngol* 1964;73:869–882.
7. Tobias MI. Lymphatics of the larynx, the trachea, and the oesophagus. In: Rouviere H, ed. *Anatomy of the human lymphatic system: a compendium.* Ann Arbor, MI: Edwards Brothers, 1938:57–62.
8. Skolnik EM. The posterior triangle in radical neck surgery. *Arch Otolaryngol Head Neck Surg* 1976;102:1–4.
9. Toker C. Some observations on the distribution of metastatic squamous carcinoma within cervical lymph nodes. *Ann Surg* 1963; 157:419–426.
10. Ballantyne AJ. Significance of retropharyngeal nodes in cancer of the head and neck. *Am J Surg* 1964;108:500–503.
11. Hasegawa Y, Matsuura H. Retropharyngeal node dissection in cancer of the oropharynx and hypopharynx. *Head Neck* 1994;16:173–180.
12. McLaughlin MP, Mendenhall WM, Mancuso A, et al. Retropharyngeal adenopathy as a predictor of outcome in squamous cell carcinoma of the head and neck. *Head Neck* 1995;17:190–198.
13. O'Brien CJ, Smith JW, Soong SJ, et al. Neck dissection with and without radiotherapy—prognostic factors, patterns of recurrence and survival.*Am J Surg* 1986;152:456–463.
14. Johnson JT, Barnes EL, Myers EN. The extracapsular spread of tumors in cervical node metastasis. *Arch Otolaryngol Head Neck Surg* 1981;107:725–728.
15. Johnson JT, Myers EN, Bedetti CD, et al. Cervical lymph node metastases. *Arch Otolaryngol Head Neck Surg* 1985;111:534–537.
16. Steinhart H, Schroeder HG, Buchta B, et al. Prognostic significance of extracapsular invasion in cervical lymph node metastases of squamous epithelial carcinoma. *Laryngorhinootologie* 1994;73:620–625.
17. Carter RL, Barr LC, O'Brien CJ. Transcapsular spread of metastatic squamous cell carcinoma. *Am J Surg* 1985;150:495–499.
18. Olsen KD, Caruso M, Foote RL, et al. Primary head and neck cancer. Histopathologic predictors of recurrence after neck dissection in patients with lymph node involvement. *Arch Otolaryngol Head Neck Surg* 1994;120: 1370–1374.
19. Leemans CR, Tiwari R, Nauta JJ, et al. Regional lymph node involvement and its significance in the development of distant metastases in head and neck carcinoma. *Cancer* 1993; 71:452–456.
20. Spiro RH, Alfonso AE, Farr HW, et al. Cervical node metastasis from epidermoid carcinoma of the oral cavity and oropharynx. A critical assessment of current staging. *Am J Surg* 1974;128:562–567.
21. Tulenko J, Priore RL, Hoffmeister FS. Cancer of the tongue. *Am J Surg* 1966; 112:562–568.
22. Mendelson BC, Woods JE, Beahrs OH. Neck dissection in the treatment of carcinoma of the anterior two thirds of the tongue. *Surg Gynecol Obstet* 1976; 143:75–80.
23. Shah JP, Tollefsen HR. Epidermoid carcinoma of the supraglottic larynx. *Am J Surg* 1974;128:494–500.
24. Ho JHC. An epidemiological and clinical study of nasopharyngeal carcinoma. *Int J Radiat Oncol Biol Phys* 1978;4:183–198.
25. Teo PML, Leung SF, Yu P, et al. A comparison of Ho's, International Union against Cancer, and American Joint Committee Stage Classifications for nasopharyngeal carcinoma. *Cancer* 1991;67:434–439.
26. Grandi C, Boracchi P, Mezzanotte G, et al. Analysis of prognostic factors and proposal of a new classification for nasopharyngeal cancer. *Head Neck Surg* 1990;12:31–40.
27. Greene F, Page D, Fleming I, et al. *AJCC cancer staging manual,* 6th ed. New York: Springer Verlag, 2002.
28. Baatenburg de Jong RJ, Gullane PG, Freeman JL. The significance of false positive nodes in patients with oral cancer. *J Otolaryngol* 1993;22:154–159.
29. DeSanto LW, Holt JJ, Beahrs OH. Neck dissection: is it worthwhile? *Laryngoscope* 1982;92:502–509.
30. Fall HW, Goldfarb PM, Farr CW. Epidermoid carcinoma of the mouth and pharynx at Memorial Sloan Kettering Cancer Center. *Am J Surg* 1980;140: 563–567.
31. Shaba AR, Spiro RH, Shah JP, et al. Squamous carcinoma of the floor of the mouth. *Am J Surg* 1984;148:455–459.
32. Kalnins IK, Leonard AG, Sako K. Correlation between prognosis and degree of lymph node involvement in carcinoma of the oral cavity. *Am J Surg* 1977; 134:450–454.

32a. Robins KT, Medina JE, Wolfe GT. Standardizing neck dissection terminology. *Arch Otolaryngol Head Neck Surg* 1991;117:604–605.

33. Medina JE. A rational classification of neck dissections. *Otolaryngol Head Neck Surg* 1989;100:169–176.
34. Weiss MH, Harrison LB, Isaacs RS. Use of decision analysis in planning a management strategy for the stage N0 neck. *Arch Otolaryngol Head Neck Surg* 1994;120:699–702.
35. Close L, Merkel M, Vuitch ME, et al. Computed tomographic evaluation for regional lymph node involvement in cancer of the oral cavity and oropharynx. *Head Neck Surg* 1989;11:309–317.
36. Friedman M, Mafee MF, Pacella BL, et al. Rationale for elective neck dissection in 1990. *Laryngoscope* 1990;100:54–59.
37. Friedman M, Shelton VK, Mafee MM. Metastatic neck disease: evaluation by computed tomography. *Arch Otolaryngol Head Neck Surg* 1984;110:443–447.
38. Cachin Y. Management of cervical nodes in head and neck cancer. In: Evans PH, Robin PE, Fielding JW eds. *Head and neck cancer.* New York: Alan R. Liss, 1983.
39. Mancuso A, Hanafee WN. *Computed tomography and magnetic resonance imaging of the head and neck.* Baltimore: Williams & Wilkins, 1985.
40. Steinkamp HJ, Cornehl M, Hosten N, et al. Cervical lymphadenopathy: ratio of long- to short-axis diameter as a predictor of malignancy. *Br J Radiol* 1995;68:266–270.
41. Van den Brekel MW, Castelijns JA, Stel HV, et al. Modern imaging techniques and ultrasound guided aspiration cytology for the assessment of neck node metastases: a prospective comparative study. *Eur Arch Otorhinolaryngol* 1993; 250:11–17.
42. Martinez-Gimeno C, Rodriguez RM, Navarro C, et al. Squamous cell carcinoma of the oral cavity: a clinicopathologic scoring system for evaluating risk of cervical lymph node metastasis. *Laryngoscope* 1995;105:728–733.
43. Mohit-Tabatabai MA, Sobel HJ, Rush BF, et al. Relation of thickness of floor of mouth stage I and II cancers to regional metastasis. *Am J Surg* 1986;152: 351–353.
44. Spiro RH, Huvos AG, Wong GY, et al. Predictive value of tumor thickness in squamous cell carcinoma confined to the tongue and floor of the mouth. *Am J Surg* 1986;152:345–350.
45. Long JP, Schechter GL, Nettleton JM, et al. Correlating primary head and neck cancer thickness, growth and treatment delay with the risk of cervical nodal metastasis. Final Program and Abstract Book. Fourth International Conference on Head and Neck Cancer, July 28–August 1, 1996. 1996;80(abst).
46. Frierson HF, Cooper PH. Prognostic factors in squamous cell carcinoma of the lower lip. *Hum Pathol* 1986;17:346–354.
47. Rasgon BM, Cruz RM, Hilsinger RL, et al. Relation of lymph node metastasis to histopathologic appearance in oral cavity and oropharyngeal carcinoma: a case series and literature review. *Laryngoscope* 1989;99:1103–1110.
48. Willen R, Nathanson A, Moberger C, et al. Squamous cell carcinoma of the gingiva: histological classification and grading of malignancy. *Acta Otolaryngol* 1975;79:146–154.
49. McGavran MH, Bauer WC, Ogura JH. The incidence of cervical lymph node metastases from epidermoid carcinoma of the larynx and their relationship to certain characteristics of the primary tumor: a study based on the clinical and pathological findings for 96 patients treated by primary en bloc laryngectomy and radical neck dissection. *Cancer* 1961;14:55–65.
50. Umeda M, Yokoo S, Take Y, et al. Lymph node metastasis in squamous cell carcinoma of the oral cavity: correlation between histologic features and the prevalence of metastasis. *Head Neck Surg* 1992;14:263–272.
51. Bryne M, Koppang HS, Lilleng R, et al. Malignancy grading of the deep invasive margins of oral squamous cell carcinomas has high prognostic value. *J Pathol* 1992;166:375–381.
52. Yamamoto E, Miyakawa A, Kohama G. Mode of invasion and lymph node metastasis in squamous cell carcinoma of the oral cavity. *Head Neck Surg* 1984;6:938–947.
53. Crissman JD, Liu WY, Gluckman JL, et al. Prognostic value of histopathologic parameters in squamous cell carcinoma of the oropharynx. *Cancer* 1984; 54:2995–3001.
54. Close LG, Burns DK, Reisch J, et al. Microvascular invasion in cancer of the oral cavity and oropharynx. *Arch Otolaryngol Head Neck Surg* 1987;113: 1191–1195.
55. Poleksic S, Kalwaic HJ. Prognostic value of vascular invasion in squamous cell carcinoma of the head and neck. *Plast Reconstr Surg* 1978;61:234–240.
56. Tytor M, Olofsson J, Ledin T, et al. Squamous cell carcinoma of the oral cavity. A review of 176 cases with application of malignancy grading and DNA measurements. *Clin Otolaryngol* 1990;15:235–252.
57. Hemmer J, Schon E, Kreidler J, et al. Prognostic implications of DNA ploidy in squamous cell carcinoma of the tongue assessed by flow cytometry. *J Cancer Res Clin Oncol* 1990;116:83–86.
58. Wolf GT, Fisher SG, Truelson JM, et al. DNA content and regional metastases in patients with advanced laryngeal squamous carcinoma. Department of Veterans Affairs Laryngeal Study Group. *Laryngoscope* 1994;104:479–483.
59. Franzen G, Olofsson J, Tytor M, et al. Malignancy grading and cytophotometric evaluation of T1 lip carcinomas. *Clin Otolaryngol* 1987;12:81–87.
60. Lampe HB, Flint A, Wolf GT, et al. Flow cytometry: DNA analysis of squamous cell carcinoma of the upper aerodigestive tract. *J Otolaryngol* 1987;16: 371–375.
61. Williams JK, Carlson GW, Cohen C, et al. Tumor angiogenesis as a prognostic factor in oral cavity tumors. *Am J Surg* 1994;168:373–380.
62. Leedy DA, Cohen JI, Trune DR, et al. Tumor angiogenesis, the p53 antigen, and cervical metastasis in squamous cell carcinoma of the oral tongue. *Otolaryngol Head Neck Surg* 1994;111(abst):417–422.
63. Murakami M, Mimaki S, Saitou Y, et al. Immunohistological investigation of the type IV collagen in the basement membrane surrounding the cancer nest (cancer nest membrane) of head and neck squamous cell carcinoma—its relation to frequency of cervical lymph node metastasis. *J Otorhinolaryngol Soc Jpn* 1992;95:1773–1784.

64. Mamelle G, Pampurik J, Luboinski B, et al. Lymph node prognostic factors in head and neck squamous cell carcinomas. *Am J Surg* 1994;168:494–498.
65. Byers RM. Modified neck dissection: a study of 967 cases from 1970 to 1980. *Am J Surg* 1986;150:414–421.
66. Medina JE, Byers RM. Supraomohyoid neck dissection: rationale, indications and surgical technique. *Head Neck Surg* 1989;11:111–122.
67. Spiro JD, Spiro RH, Shah JP, et al. Critical assessment of supraomohyoid neck dissection. *Am J Surg* 1988;156: 286–289.
68. Remmler D, Byers RM, Scheetz JE. A prospective study of shoulder disability resulting from radical and modified neck dissections. *Head Neck Surg* 1986;8:280–286.
69. Sobol S, Jensen C, Sawyer W II, et al. Objective comparison of physical dysfunction after neck dissection. *Am J Surg* 1985;150:503–509.
70. Medina JE, Johnson D. Selective neck dissection. Paper presented at the 33rd Annual Meeting of the American Society for Head and Neck Surgery, Waikoloa, Hawaii, May 7–9, 1991.
71. Kligerman J, Lima RA, Scares JR, et al. Supraomohyoid neck dissection in the treatment of T1/T2 squamous cell carcinoma of the oral cavity. *Am J Surg* 1994;168(abst):391–397.
72. Pradhan SA, D'Cruz AK, Gulla RI. What is optimum neck dissection for T3/4 buccal-gingival cancers? *Ear Arch Otorhinolaryngol* 1995;252:143–145.
73. Rassekh C, Johnson J, Myers E. Accuracy of intraoperative staging of the N0 neck in squamous cell carcinoma. *Laryngoscope* 1995;105: 1334–1336.
74. Fletcher GH. Elective irradiation of subclinical disease in cancers of the head and neck. *Cancer* 1972;29:1450–1454.
75. Mendenhall WM, Million RR, Cassissi NJ. Elective neck irradiation in carcinoma of the head and neck. *Head Neck Surg* 1980;3:15–20.
76. Mesic JB, Fletcher GH, Goepfert H. Megalovoltage irradiation of epithelial tumors of the nasopharynx. *Int J Radiat Oncol Biol Phys* 1981;7:447–453.
77. Chen WZ, Zhou DL, Luo KS. Long term observation after radiotherapy for nasopharyngeal carcinoma (NPC). *Int J Radiat Oncol Biol Phys* 1989;16: 311–314.
78. Janot F, Cvitkovic E, Piekarski J, et al. Correlation between nodal density in contrasted scans and response to cisplatin-based chemotherapy in head and neck squamous cell cancer: a prospective validation. *Head Neck Surg* 1993; 15:222–229.
79. De Vries EJ, Sekhar LN, Janecka IP, et al. Elective resection of the internal carotid artery without reconstruction. *Laryngoscope* 1988;98:960–966.
80. Houck JR, Medina JE. Management of cervical lymph nodes in squamous carcinomas of the head and neck. *Semin Surg Oncol* 1995;11:228–239.
81. Pearlman NW, Meyers AD, Sullivan WG. Modified radical neck dissection for squamous cell carcinoma of the head and neck. *Surg Gynecol Obstet* 1982; 154:214–216.
82. Brandenburg JH, Lee CY. The XI nerve in radical neck surgery. *Laryngoscope*1981;91:1851–1859.
83. Roy PH, Beahrs OH. Spinal accessory nerve in radical neck dissections. *Am J Surg* 1969;118:800–804.
84. Skolnik EM, Tenta LT, Wineinger DM, et al. Preservation of XI cranial nerve in neck dissection. *Laryngoscope* 1967;77:1304–1314.
85. Chu W, Strawitz JG. Results in suprahyoid, modified radical, and standard radical neck dissections for metastatic squamous cell carcinoma: recurrence and survival. *Am J Surg* 1978;136:512–515.
86. Carenfelt C, Eliasson K. Cervical metastases following radical neck dissection that preserved the spinal accessory nerve. *Head Neck Surg* 1980;2:181–184.
87. Andersen PE, Shah JP, Cambronero E, et al. The role of comprehensive neck dissection with preservation of the spinal accessory nerve in the clinically positive neck. *Am J Surg* 1994;168:499–502(abst).
88. Lingeman RE, Stephens R, Helmus C, et al. Neck dissection: radical or conservative. *Ann Otol Rhinol Laryngol* 1977;86: 737–744.
89. Molinari R, Chiesa F, Cantu G, et al. Retrospective comparison of conservative and radical neck dissection in laryngeal cancer. *Ann Otol Rhinol Laryngol* 1980;89:578–581.
90. Joseph CA, Gregor RT, Davidge-Pitts KJ. The role of functional neck dissection in the management of advanced tumors of the upper aerodigestive tract. *S Afr J Surg* 1985;23:83–87.
91. Gavilan C, Gavilan J. Five-year results of functional neck dissection for cancer of the larynx. *Arch Otolaryngol Head Neck Surg* 1995;115:1193–1196.
92. Bocca E, Pignataro O, Oldini C. Functional neck dissection: an evaluation and review of 843 cases. *Laryngoscope* 1984;94:942–945.
93. Calearo CV, Teatini G. Functional neck dissection: anatomical grounds, surgical technique, clinical observations. *Ann Otol Rhinol Laryngol* 1983;89:215–222.
94. Andersen PE, Shah JP, Cambronero E, et al. The role of comprehensive neck dissection with preservation of the spinal accessory nerve in the clinically positive neck. *Am J Surg* 1994;168:499–502.
95. Marcial UA, Pajak TF. Radiation therapy alone or in combination with surgery in head and neck cancer. *Cancer* 1985;255:2259–2269.
96. Vikram B, Strong EW, Shah JP, et al. Failure in the neck following multimodality treatment for advanced head and neck cancer. *Head Neck Surg* 1984;6:724–729.
97. Peters LJ, Goepfert H, Kiang AK, et al. Evaluation of the dose for postoperative radiation therapy of head and neck cancer: first report of a prospective randomized trial. *Int J Radiat Oncol Biol Phys* 1993;26:3–11.
98. Freeman SB, Hamaker RC, Rate WR, et al. Management of advanced cervical metastasis using intraoperative radiotherapy. *Laryngoscope* 1995;105:575–578.
99. Brennan JA, Jafek BW. Elective carotid artery resection for advanced squamous cell carcinoma of the neck. *Laryngoscope* 1994;104: 259–263.
100. McIver NP, Willinsky RA, Terbrugge KG, et al. Validity of test occlusion studies prior to internal carotid artery sacrifice. *Head Neck Surg* 1994;16:11–16.
101. Reilly MK, Perry MO, Netterville JL, et al. Carotid artery replacement in conjunction with resection of squamous cell carcinoma of the neck: preliminary results. *J Vasc Surg* 1992;15: 324–330.
102. Byers RM, Clayman GL, Guillamondegui OM, et al. Resection of advanced cervical metastasis prior to definitive radiotherapy for primary squamous carcinomas of the upper aerodigestive tract. *Head Neck Surg* 1992;14:133–138.
103. French Head and Neck Study Group. Early pharyngolaryngeal carcinomas with palpable nodes. *Am J Surg* 1991;162:377–380.
104. Wolf GT, Fisher SG. Effectiveness of salvage neck dissection for advanced regional metastases when induction chemotherapy and radiation are used for organ preservation. *Laryngoscope* 1992;102: 934–939.
105. Armstrong J, Pfister D, Strong E, et al. The management of the clinically positive neck as part of a larynx preservation approach. *Int J Radiat Oncol Biol Phys* 1993;26:759–765.
106. Schuller DE, Reiches NA, Hamaker RC. Analysis of disability resulting from treatment including radical neck dissection or modified neck dissection. *Head Neck Surg* 1983;6:551–558.
107. Sterns MP, Shaheen OH. Preservation of the accessory nerve in neck dissections. *J Otol Rhinol Laryngol* 1981;95:1141–1148.
108. Short SO, Kaplan JN, Laramore GE, et al. Shoulder pain and function after neck dissection with or without preservation of the spinal accessory nerve. *Am J Surg* 1984;148:478–482.
108a. Weitz JW Weitz SL, McElhinney AJ. A technique for preservation of spinal accessory nerve function in radical neck dissection. *Head Neck Surg* 1982;5: 75–78.
109. Leipzig B, Suen JY, English JL, et al. Functional evaluation of the spinal accessory nerve after neck dissection. *Am J Surg* 1983;146:526–530.
110. Timon CV, Brown D, Gullane P. Internal jugular vein blowout complicating head and neck surgery. J Laryngol Otol 1994;108:423–425.
111. Crumley RL, Smith JD. Postoperative chylous fistula prevention and management. *Laryngoscope* 1976;86:804–816.
112. Spiro JD, Spiro RH, Strong EW. The management of chyle fistula. *Laryngoscope* 1990;100:771–774.
113. Sugarbaker ED, Wiley HM. Intracranial pressure studies incident to the resection of the internal jugular vein. *Cancer* 1951;4:242–250.
114. Royster MP. The relation between internal jugular vein pressure and CSF pressure in the operation of radical neck dissection. *Ann Surg* 1953;137:826–831.
115. Wenig BL, Heller KS. The syndrome of inappropriate secretion of antidiuretic hormone (SIADH) following neck dissection. *Laryngoscope* 1987;97:467–470.
116. McQuarrie DG, Mayberg M, Faerguson M. A physiologic approach to the problem of simultaneous bilateral neck dissection. *Am J Neurosurg* 1977;134: 455–460.
117. Moorthy S, Sullivan T, Fallon JH, et al. Loss of hypoxic ventilatory response following bilateral neck dissection. *Anesth Analg* 1993;76:791–794.
118. Marks SC, Jaques DA, Hirata RM, et al. Blindness following bilateral radical neck dissection. *Head Neck* 1990;12:342–345.
119. Schobel GA, Schmidbauer M, Millesi W, et al. Posterior ischemic optic neuropathy following bilateral radical neck dissection. *Int J Oral Maxillofac Surg* 1995;24:283–287.
120. Zohar Y, Strauss M, Sabo R, et al. Internal jugular vein patency after functional neck dissection: venous duplex imaging. *Ann Otol Rhinol Laryngol* 1995;104:532–536.
121. Cotter CS, Stringer SP, Landau S, et al. Patency of the internal jugular vein following modified radical neck dissection. *Laryngoscope* 1994;104:841–845.
122. Docherty JG, Carter R, Sheldon CD, et al. Relative effect of surgery and radiotherapy on the internal jugular vein following functional neck dissection. *Head Neck* 1993;15:553–556.
123. Shah JP, Candela FC, Poddar AK. The patterns of cervical lymph node metastases from squamous carcinoma of the oral cavity. *Cancer* 1990;66:109–113.
124. Candela FC, Kothari K, Shah JP. Patterns of cervical node metastases from squamous carcinoma of the oropharynx and hypopharynx. *Head Neck Surg* 1990;12:197–203.
125. Candela FC, Shah J, Jaques DP, et al. Patterns of cervical node metastases from squamous carcinoma of the larynx. *Arch Otolaryngol Head Neck Surg* 1990;116:432–435.

Radiologic Imaging Concerns

126. Som PM. Detection of metastasis in cervical lymph nodes: CT and MR criteria and differential diagnosis [Review]. AJR Am J *Roentgenol* 1992;158:961–969.
127. van den Brekel MW, Castelijns JA, Snow GB. Detection of lymph node metastases in the neck: radiologic criteria [Editorial; Comment]. *Radiology* 1994;192: 617–618.
128. Baatenburg de Jong RJ, Knegt P, Verwoerd CD. Reduction of the number of neck treatments in patients with head and neck cancer [Review]. *Cancer* 1993;71:2312–2318.
129. Braams JW, Pruim J, Freling NJ, et al. Detection of lymph node metastases of squamous-cell cancer of the head and neck with FDG-PET and MRI. *J Nucl Med* 1995;36:211–216.
130. Anzai Y, Blackwell KE, Hirschowitz SL, et al. Initial clinical experience with dextran-coated superparamagnetic iron oxide for detection of lymph node metastases in patients with head and neck cancer [see Comments]. *Radiology* 1994;192:709–715.

131. Anzai Y, Prince MR. Iron oxide-enhanced MR lymphography: the evaluation of cervical lymph node metastases in head and neck cancer [Review]. *J Magn Reson Imag* 1997;7:75–81.
132. Takes RP, Righi P, Meeuwis CA, et al. The value of ultrasound with ultrasound-guided fine-needle aspiration biopsy compared to computed tomography in the detection of regional metastases in the clinically negative neck. *Int J Radiat Oncol Biol Phys* 1998;40:1027–1032.
133. Ariji Y, Kimura Y. Power Doppler sonography of cervical lymph nodes in patients with head and neck cancer. *AJNR Am J Neuroradiol* 1998;19:303–307.
134. Adams S, Baum RP, Stuckensen T, et al. Prospective comparison of 18F-FDG PET with conventional imaging modalities (CT, MRI, US) in lymph node staging of head and neck cancer. *Eur J Nucl Med* 1998;25:1255–1260.
135. Boland GW, Lee MJ, Mueller PR, et al. Efficacy of sonographically guided biopsy of thyroid masses and cervical lymph nodes. *AJR Am J Roentgenol* 1993;161:1053–1056.
136. Gregor RT, Valdes-Olmos R, Koops W, et al. Preliminary experience with thallous chloride T1 201-labeled single-photon emission computed tomography scanning in head and neck cancer. *Arch Otolaryngol Head Neck Surg* 1996;122:509–514.
137. Stokkel MP, ten Broek FW, Hordijk GJ, et al. Preoperative evaluation of patients with primary head and neck cancer using dual-head 18fluorodeoxyglucose positron emission tomography. *Ann Surg* 2000;231:229–234.
138. Fleming I, Cooper J, Henson D, eds. *AJCC cancer staging manual,* 5th ed. Philadelphia: Lippincott-Raven, 1997.
139. Kraus DH, Rosenberg DB, Davidson BJ, et al. Supraspinal accessory lymph node metastases in supraomohyoid neck dissection. *Am J Surg* 1996;172:646–649.
140. Labadie RF, Yarbrough WG, Weissler MC, et al. Nodal volume reduction after concurrent chemo- and radiotherapy: correlation between initial CT and histopathologic findings. *AJNR Am J Neuroradiol* 2000;21:310–314.
141. Som PM, Urken ML, Biller H, et al. Imaging the postoperative neck [Review]. *Radiology* 1993;187:593–603.
142. Hudgins PA, Burson JG, Gussack GS, et al. CT and MR appearance of recurrent malignant head and neck neoplasms after resection and flap reconstruction. *AJNR Am J Neuroradiol* 1994;15:1689–1694.
143. Wester DJ, Whiteman ML, Singer S, et al. Imaging of the postoperative neck with emphasis on surgical flaps and their complications. *AJR Am J Roentgenol* 1995;164:989–993.

CHAPTER 14

Radiation Therapy and Chemotherapy Management of Cervical Lymph Nodes*

Harry Quon and Louis B. Harrison

The management of cervical lymph node metastases represents an integral component in the successful management of head and neck squamous cell carcinomas (HNSCC). This is due to the consistent, progressive, and predictable metastatic spread of HNSCC into cervical lymph nodes in the nonviolated neck and the adverse prognostic impact of patients with cervical nodal metastases. Despite this, the potential for cure and salvage in patients with cervical nodal metastases exists. Several factors influence the treatment strategies for the neck both in the definitive and in the recurrent setting necessitating an individualized approach for each patient. In particular, considerations of the management strategy for the primary site are paramount. This review will focus on these management issues with an emphasis on issues pertinent to the nonsurgical management of neck metastases and its integration with the surgical management of neck metastases. The therapeutic approaches for both clinically node-negative and node-positive non-nasopharyngeal HNSCC and nasopharyngeal squamous cell carcinomas are summarized in Figures 14.1 and 14.2, respectively.

DEFINITIVE MANAGEMENT OF THE CLINICALLY N0 NECK

Definitive treatment of HNSCC with no clinically evident cervical nodal metastases must consider the necessity for elective treatment of microscopic nodal metastases when deciding on the treatment strategy for the primary tumor site. Where primary radiotherapy or chemoradiation is indicated, elective nodal irradiation (ENI) must be considered. Issues of its timing, indications, efficacy, and the nodal basins that require irradiation have not been systematically evaluated. Current practice has evolved from careful clinical observation and conclusions about efficacy such that further rigorous study is no longer possible due to the loss of clinical equipoise. However, guidance may be derived from limited randomized surgical data on elective neck dissection and an observational approach (1,2).

Management options for the N0 neck may include observation or elective therapy. Nonsurgical elective therapy of the neck involves ENI. To date, no randomized or comparative studies of observation (reserving therapeutic neck irradiation for salvage) versus ENI have been reported. In general, the basis for ENI has been extrapolated from several limited comparative studies of elective neck dissection and postoperative radiotherapy as indicated compared with neck observation and therapeutic neck dissection (1–4).

Vandenbrouck et al. report on a limited randomized trial of 75 patients with T1 to T3 N0 oral cavity carcinomas randomized to elective neck dissection or neck observation (1). Of 39 patients receiving an elective neck dissection, 49% had pathologic nodal metastases with 26% of these (5 of 19) patients having evidence of extracapsular extension. Of the 36 patients randomized to neck observation, 53% subsequently developed neck relapses with 17 of 19 (89%) patients having resectable disease and able to undergo salvage neck dissection. This revealed pathologic nodes in 15 of 17 (88%) patients with 60% having extracapsular extension. Overall survival was not significantly different with mature follow-up. It is unclear if this trial was sufficiently powered to demonstrate a meaningful difference that was further compromised by a disproportionate number of patients in the elective neck dissection cohort experiencing intercurrent deaths.

A second prospective randomized trial comparing elective versus therapeutic neck dissection in early squamous cell carcinoma of the oral tongue was reported by Fakih et al. (2). With a median follow-up of 20 months, the disease-free survival was 52% in the group treated with hemiglossectomy and 63% in the group receiving hemiglossectomy and radical neck dissection (p = NS). No significant differences were noted with regard to survival for both of these cohorts. On the basis of increased nodal metastases with tumor depths greater than 4 mm, the investigators suggest that this subgroup may be more likely to benefit from further study with elective neck dissection.

Piedbois et al. report a retrospective comparative study of 233 patients with early stage oral cavity carcinoma with the primary site treated with an interstitial iridium-192 (^{192}Ir) implant but

*Please refer to the Appendix, Imaging Considerations for Radiation Therapy Treatment Planning. This section shows the important radiologic anatomy that allows the radiation oncologist to design the target volumes for treatment planning.

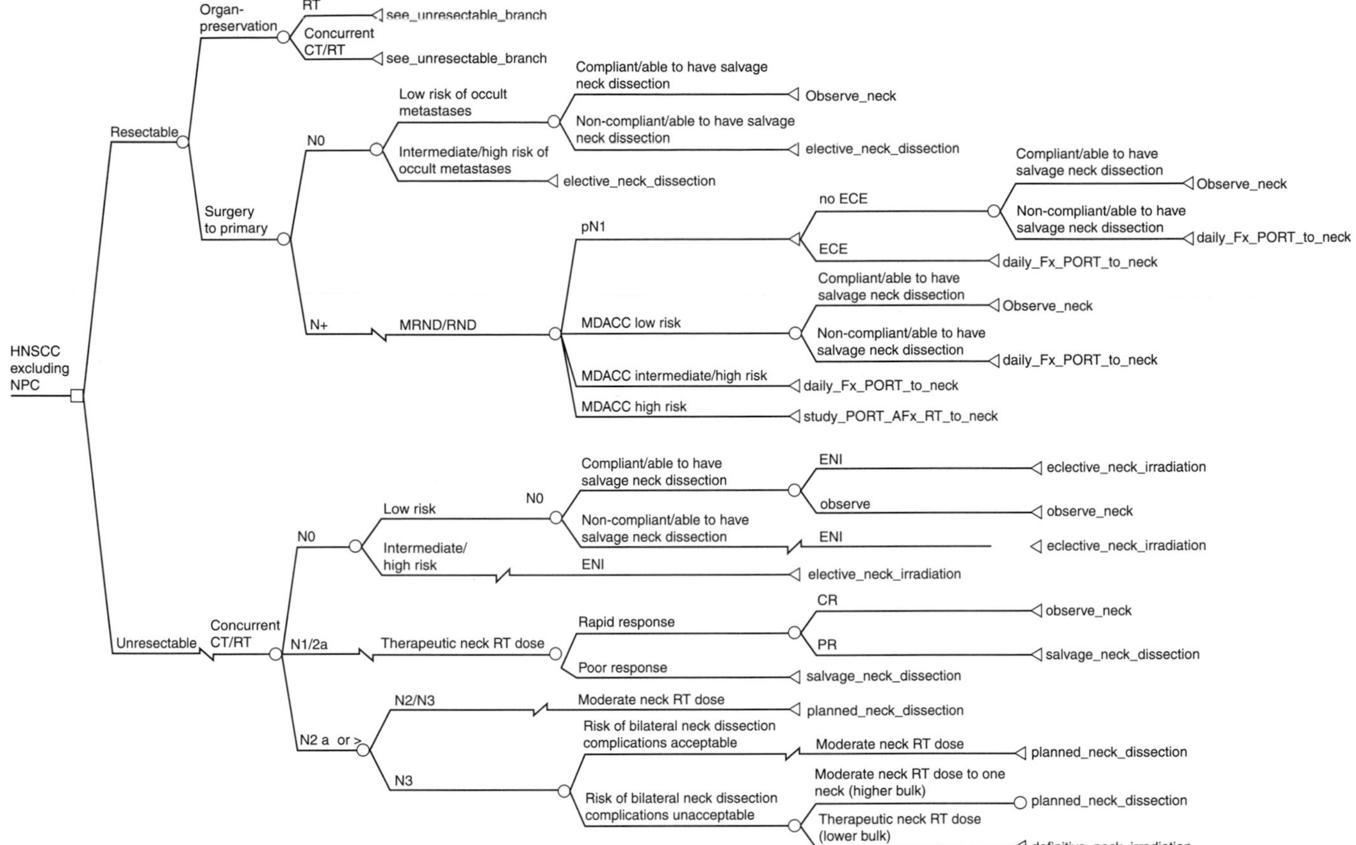

Figure 14.1 Treatment algorithm for head and neck squamous cell carcinomas other than nasopharyngeal carcinoma. *HNSCC,* head and neck squamous cell carcinoma; *NPC,* nasopharyngeal carcinoma; *Rx,* treatment; *N0,* node-negative; *N+,* node-positive; *MRND,* modified radical neck dissection; *RND,* radical neck dissection; *END,* elective neck dissection; *NE,* neck dissection; *RT,* radiation therapy; *CTRT,* chemoradiation; *AFx,* accelerated fractionation; *ENI,* elective neck irradiation; *PORT,* postoperative radiation therapy; *CR,* complete response; *PR,* partial response.

with either elective neck dissection or neck observation resulting in two cohorts of patients for analysis (3). This resulted from a change in departmental policies minimizing the impact of potential selection biases. Neck dissection revealed metastases in 25% of the neck specimens and received postoperative radiotherapy. In comparison, 17% developed a neck relapse with neck observation with salvage surgery successful in 62%. The 10-year survival was 37% and 31%, respectively, with regression analysis demonstrating that neck observation was associated with an adverse risk for disease-related mortality ($p < 0.04$).

Haddadin et al. report on a retrospective analysis of 137 patients with T1 to T2 N0 oral tongue carcinomas with at least

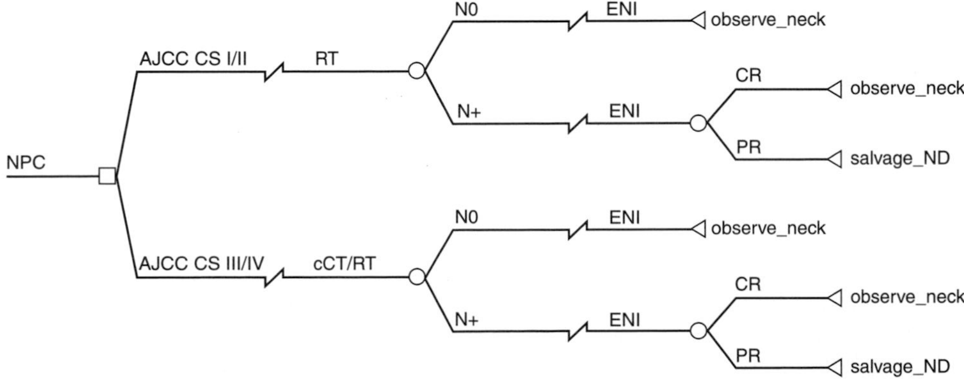

Figure 14.2 Treatment algorithm for squamous cell carcinoma of the nasopharynx. *N0,* node-negative; *N+,* node-positive; *ENI,* elective neck irradiation; *CR,* complete response; *PR,* partial response; *ND,* neck dissection.

2 years of follow-up who either received an elective neck dissection, neck observation with salvage therapeutic neck dissection, or no neck surgery at all (4). The cohort receiving elective neck dissection had a superior 5-year cause-specific survival compared with the two other groups despite a negative bias due to a greater proportion of pathologic upstaging of the primary tumor and clinical T2 lesions.

Indications for elective irradiation of the neck are based on an assessment of the risk for occult nodal metastases that is, in turn, principally a function of the primary tumor site location and clinical features of the primary tumor. Conceptually, the former has generally been interpreted to reflect anatomic differences with respect to the prevalence of lymphatics and the presence of anatomic barriers to invasion into the lymphatic system. In practice, the influence of the primary tumor on the risk for metastasis is summarized by the T stage that reflects size and involvement of anatomic subsites at greater risk for lymphatic invasion. Promising work with sentinel lymph node biopsies may provide the promise of further selecting patients in whom elective neck irradiation may not be required. In turn, this would reduce the morbidity associated with ENI. Currently, this remains an experimental therapeutic option.

The risk for occult nodal metastasis has largely been derived from the frequency of clinically evident nodal metastasis at presentation or from surgical series in which patients with N0 necks are subjected to an elective neck dissection. The former patient cohort provides an estimation of this risk but is potentially confounded by the association between T and N stage. That is, patients presenting with clinically evident nodal metastases may have T-stage tumors that are more biologically malignant than in the patient cohort presenting with N0 neck disease. Several reports have summarized the risk for metastases (5–9). Mendenhall et al. provide an operative definition dividing risk stratification into low-, intermediate-, and high-risk groups reflecting a risk for occult neck disease in less than 20%, 20% to 30%, and more than 30%, respectively (Table 14.1) (7).

No comparative or efficacy study exists to guide the decision of what risk for occult neck disease warrants ENI. The rationale for elective therapy versus neck observation recognizes the false-negative rate of clinical and radiologic evaluation of the neck and the recognition that occult nodal metastases invariably progress to become clinically apparent with the risk for extracapsular extension (ECE) related to the nodal size (1). These considerations are significant as the risk for distant metastasis is related to not only the presence of ECE but also the level of cervical lymph node involvement and the duration of harboring cervical metastases. Ambrosch and Brinck report a 7.9% incidence of micrometastases in an otherwise N0 neck specimen with further serial sectioning and immunohistochemical analysis highlighting the potential magnitude for false-negative assessment of the neck even with routine pathologic evaluation (10).

In the absence of randomized data, Weiss et al. have used decision-analysis techniques with a measure of quality-adjusted survival as the principal utility to guide the decision of elective versus deferred neck management (11). The authors have suggested that neck management offers greater utility when the probability of occult nodal metastases is 20% or greater. Although this finding is consistent with the majority of clinical practice, other investigators have argued that the threshold for therapy should be lower in light of the potential adverse consequences (9). A treatment threshold of 5% to 10% has been proposed (9). Although this decision analysis is noteworthy, the validity of its conclusions is largely dependent on an invalidated measure for quality-adjusted survival. Further studies validating or refuting these conclusions are warranted. In practice, the accepted risk must consider the morbidity of neck relapses, the probability of a salvageable relapse, and the patient's compliance to close surveillance in the absence of ENI.

The efficacy of ENI is largely based on retrospective studies demonstrating reduced neck relapses (12,13). Mendenhall et al. report a retrospective review of 159 patients with squamous cell carcinoma of the oral cavity, oropharynx, nasopharynx, hypopharynx, and supraglottic larynx with a clinically negative neck (stage N0) to determine the value of ENI (13). The primary cancer was controlled in 125 patients. Among these patients the neck failure rate was 1.9% with ENI and 18% without ENI. Among a group of patients expected to have a less than 20% risk for occult nodal metastases, the neck relapse rate was 13% in patients who did not receive ENI versus 6% in patients who received ENI. Similarly, among a group of patients with an expected risk for occult nodal metastases greater than 20%, the neck relapse rate was 31% and 5%, respectively.

The optimal dose for treating subclinical disease has largely been accepted to be 45 to 50 Gy in 2 Gy per fraction based on work summarized by Fletcher (12). Fletcher summarizes the incidence of neck relapses in a contralateral, initially clinically negative neck for tumors of the floor of mouth, oral tongue, and faucial arch. The incidence of neck relapses decreased from 9% to 10.5% to 0% when delivered doses of 30 cGy for 3 weeks to 40 cGy for 4 weeks were compared with the delivery of 50 cGy for 5 weeks, respectively. However, it is clear that the burden of

TABLE 14.1 University of Florida Risk Group Definitions for Subclinical Neck Disease

Risk group	Risk of subclinical neck disease	T stage	Tumor site
Low risk	<20%	T1	Floor of mouth, oral tongue, retromolar trigone, gingiva, hard palate, buccal mucosa
Intermediate risk	20%–30%	T1	Soft palate, pharyngeal wall, supraglottic larynx, tonsil
		T2	Floor of mouth, oral tongue, retromolar trigone, gingiva, hard palate, buccal mucosa
Higher risk			
A	>30%	T1–4	Nasopharynx, pyriform sinus, base of tongue
		T2–4	Soft palate, pharyngeal wall, supraglottic larynx, tonsil
		T3–4	Floor of mouth, oral tongue, retromolar trigone, gingiva, hard palate, buccal mucosa
B	>30%		Any site with clinically positive upper neck nodes

Source: Adapted from Mendenhall WM, Parsons JT, Million RR. Elective lower neck irradiation: 5000 cGy/25 fractions versus 4050 cGy/15 fractions. *Int J Radiat Oncol Biol Phys* 1988;15:439–440, with permission.

cells in a subclinical neck may range from 1 to M, where M represents the number of cells that are just clinically undetectable. This would suggest that a dose–response relationship likely exists. This hypothesis was supported in a review by Withers et al. of the incidence of subsequent overt metastases following elective irradiation to potential sites of metastatic disease for various tumor sites (14). This analysis would suggest a linear dose–response relationship with no threshold dose indicating that even with doses less than 45 to 50 Gy meaningful control of subclinical disease may be achieved depending on the metastatic burden present. This is further supported by the observations of Mendenhall et al. who demonstrated 100% disease control of clinically uninvolved low neck following elective irradiation with either 50 Gy in 25 fractions or 40.5 Gy in 15 fractions both given as daily fractions (7). The latter fractionation schedule is less biologically effective. These investigators stratified the analysis by the risk for occult subclinical neck disease based on the T stage and tumor site but not the presence of clinical neck disease. The latter was not specified. The absence of statistical testing and an underpowered analysis limit the significance of these conclusions. It may be demonstrated that with a neck control rate of 98% to 100% with 50 Gy in 25 fractions, the ability to detect even a generous meaningful difference of 15%, more than 50 patients would be required in each fractionation schedule.

The issue of risk-appropriate dosing for subclinical disease is particularly relevant for T2 N0 tumors of the oral tongue treated with combination external beam and an implant. Several independent retrospective reports have observed a greater rate of local control when a greater proportion of the dose delivered to the primary site was given by brachytherapy, suggesting that a lower elective external beam dose to the neck may be effective (15–17). In fact, several investigators have recommended a brachytherapy implant alone to the primary site with the neck managed by an elective neck dissection (18,19). Although these retrospective series are not without methodologic concern, it is nevertheless compelling that a consistent conclusion has been made by multiple independent institutions. Hence, a comparable neck control rate may ultimately be realized with reduced doses that are associated with a reduced probability of neck control due to a lower baseline risk for subclinical neck disease. Unfortunately, the ability to precisely and reproducibly quantitate the burden of subclinical neck disease limits this therapeutic approach.

Recently, Gregoire et al. have reported an invaluable systematic review of the literature regarding the delineation of lymph node target volumes indicated for head and neck radiation therapy. This summary is particularly invaluable for axial-based image treatment planning that is used for conformal irradiation and intensity modulated radiotherapy techniques (9). In general, most tumor sites are associated with a sufficient risk for occult nodal metastases that warrants a recommendation for ENI to nodal groups that are at risk based on the tumor site and specific primary features. Gregoire et al. provide a summary recommendation of the nodal groups that should receive ENI in the neck without altered lymphatic flow (Table 14.2) (9). These recommendations do not address specific presentations that may modulate the risk for occult metastases. It has been accepted in practice that a risk for less than 20% warrants at least a deliberation for ENI considering the competing issues of potential benefit and toxicities and risk for secondary HNSCC requiring further therapy. Some general recommendations can be made.

Nodal metastases are typically seen in levels I to III for oral cavity tumors and in levels II to IV for oropharyngeal, hypopharyngeal, and laryngeal tumors. Bilateral ENI should be considered for tumors arising from or extending to midline structures such as the soft palate, base of tongue, and pharyngeal wall. The tumor sites such as the nasopharynx and hypopharynx are associated with a high risk for nodal metastases, typically seen in 80% and 70%, respectively, warranting therapeutic or ENI regardless of the specific tumor presentation. Similarly, tumors of the base of tongue and supraglottic larynx necessitate neck management irrespective of the specific tumor presentation. In contrast, tumor involvement of ipsilateral structures such as the parotid warrants consideration of ipsilateral ENI (20). Elective nodal irradiation including the retropharyngeal lymph nodes is often preferred for primary tumors involving the nasopharynx, pharyngeal wall, and the soft palate, as surgical management typically does not address this echelon of nodes. Elective nodal irradiation including level IV lymph nodes should be considered due to the risk for skip metastases that bypass the orderly contiguous progression in the anterior cervical nodes, especially for anteriorly located oral tongue lesions (8,21). Involvement of the ipsilateral level V lymph nodes in oral cavity tumors is rare, occurring in less than 1%, and does not warrant ENI. However, with increasing involvement of levels I to III or the involvement of level IV, the

TABLE 14.2 Guidelines for Neck Treatment in Patients with Head and Neck Squamous Cell Carcinomas

	Eschelons of lymph nodes to be treated	
Primary tumor site	**Stage N0–N1**	**Stage N2b**
Oral cavity	I, II, III, and IV (for anterior tongue tumors only)	I, II, III, IV, and V (may omit if only levels I–III are involved)
Oropharynx	II, III, IV and retropharyngeal nodes (for posterior pharyngeal wall tumors only)	I, II, III, IV, V and retropharyngeal nodes
Hypopharynx	II[a], III, IV, and VI (for esophageal extension only)	I, II, III, IV, V, retropharyngeal nodes, and VI (for esophageal extension only)
Larynx[b]	II[a], III, IV, and VI (for transglottic and subglottic tumors)	I, II, III, IV, V, VI (for transglottic and subglottic tumors)
Nasopharynx	II, III, IV, V, and retropharyngeal nodes	II, III, IV, V, and retropharyngeal nodes

[a]May exclude level IIB for N0 patients.
[b]Excludes T1 N0 glottic carcinomas.
Source: Adapted from Gregoire V, Coche E, Coshard G, et al. Selection and delineation of lymph node target volumes in head and neck conformal radiotherapy. Proposal for standardizing terminology and procedure based on the surgical experience. *Radiother Oncol* 2000; 56:135–150, with permission.

risk for level V involvement increases warranting ENI. In contrast, involvement of only the true vocal cords does not warrant ENI due to the paucity of lymphatic drainage. Several recent reports addressing nodal groups warranting ENI for specific circumstances warrant further elaboration.

It has generally been regarded that maxillary sinus carcinomas do not require ENI due to the low incidence of neck metastases at presentation and subsequent relapse. Several investigators have recently suggested the potential efficacy of ENI for locally advanced N0 squamous cell carcinoma of the maxilla (22–24). Le et al. report a retrospective review of 97 patients with maxillary sinus carcinoma treated with primary radiotherapy (24). The majority (58/97) had a diagnosis of squamous cell carcinoma. Eleven patients presented with nodal metastases typically to the ipsilateral level I and II nodal groups. An additional 25 patients received bilateral ENI. The 5-year actuarial risk for nodal relapse was 0% in patients receiving ENI and 20% for those not receiving ENI. The most common site of nodal relapse was in the ipsilateral level I and II nodal groups with relapses occurring only in T3 and T4 lesions. The influence of selection bias with regard to these results is unclear. However, it is likely to have biased against the efficacy of ENI because those patients receiving ENI were likely to have had more advanced disease. Only 1 of 10 patients with neck relapse was salvaged. Of greater significance was the observation that the 5-year actuarial risk for distant metastases was 29% for patients with neck control and 81% for patients with neck failure. Multivariate analysis demonstrated that T stage, N stage, and regional nodal control (HR = 4.5, $p = 0.006$) independently influenced this risk. The 5-year survival was 37% and 0% for patients with neck control and neck relapse, respectively ($p = 0.3$). Late complications arising from neck irradiation occurred in 1 of 36 patients who developed ipsilateral brachial plexopathy and severe neck fibrosis. In light of the relapse pattern, the investigators concluded that ipsilateral ENI to only the upper neck (levels I and II) be considered for patients with T3 and T4 N0 squamous cell carcinoma of the maxillary sinus. Similar conclusions were reached by other investigators (23,25). In a smaller study, Paulino et al. note that the risk for neck relapses was strongly influenced by T stage and was paradoxically greater for T1 and T2 lesions than for T3 and T4 lesions (22). These investigators note that the significance of these findings may be spurious due to the small number of patients with early T lesions and conclude by recommending that ipsilateral ENI be delivered for patients with T1 to T4 squamous cell carcinomas of the maxillary antrum.

Recently, O'Sullivan et al. reported the results of a large retrospective review of 228 patients treated with ipsilateral radiotherapy for squamous cell carcinoma of the tonsil with the majority (133/228) having N0 disease (26). It was concluded that contralateral ENI was not required for N0 patients as no patients demonstrated a contralateral neck failure. However, both the presence of ipsilateral neck metastases at presentation and increasing medial tumor extension were associated with increasing risks of contralateral neck failure. For patients with ipsilateral node metastases with no involvement of the soft palate or base of tongue, the risk for contralateral neck failure was 3.8% (crude). In the presence of ipsilateral node metastases, the risk for contralateral neck failure was 9.5%, 14%, and 21% (all crude rates) for involvement of the soft palate, base of tongue, and both structures, respectively. However, the authors appropriately note the limitations of these observations as they included patients with uncontrolled primaries and involved a total of only eight patients with contralateral neck failures. Despite this, the report provides confidence in the selection of patients with T1 N0 tonsil carcinomas (as well as selected patients with more advanced disease) for only ipsilateral ENI. Similar observations were also reported by Jackson et al., further supporting these observations (27).

DEFINITIVE MANAGEMENT OF THE N+ NECK

Management Options

The management of clinically evident neck metastases, particularly advanced neck disease, includes several established treatment strategies. Treatment options may include preoperative radiation followed by surgery, radiotherapy followed by planned or salvage neck dissection, surgery followed by postoperative radiation, concurrent chemoradiation followed by planned or salvage neck dissection, and neoadjuvant chemotherapy followed by radiation and neck dissection with reports of neck dissection preceding or following radiation to the neck. The former treatment approach is largely of historical interest and is distinguished conceptually by the use of low to moderate doses of radiation before surgery; doses intended to address subclinical tumor disease in patients who are deemed to have resectable disease prior to any therapy. This strategy will not be discussed and has largely been abandoned due to concerns of potential increased surgical complications without the benefit of pathologic evaluation to facilitate patient selection for radiotherapy. No published randomized data exist comparing the therapeutic efficacy of a surgical approach to an organ-preserving strategy. Several issues guide the treatment decision-making process. These include the resectability of the primary and neck disease, the functional morbidity incurred with surgical resection at the primary site, and the appropriateness of the primary lesion for potential organ-preserving therapy with either radiation alone or in combination with chemotherapy. When unresectable disease exists, the use of chemoradiation strategies has largely been favored. Although the optimal chemoradiotherapy regimen for both organ preservation and unresectable disease remains to be defined, preliminary data from a recent Intergroup trial comparing a neoadjuvant chemoradiation to a concurrent chemoradiation strategy would favor the latter with regard to the probability of primary organ preservation (28). Following these therapeutic considerations for the primary lesion, the principal issue with regard to neck management has been the role of adjuvant therapy, be it postoperative radiotherapy or post-radiotherapy neck dissection.

SURGERY AND POSTOPERATIVE RADIATION

Surgery and postoperative radiation remains a common strategy for the management of locally advanced but resectable HNSCC. Indications requiring postoperative radiotherapy (PORT) have been reported in several retrospective reviews. Significant factors reported have included the primary tumor site (29–31), the status of the resection margins (32–34), the presence of perineural invasion (35), and the presence of ECE in nodal metastases (32,36,37). Carter et al. report an extensive analysis of 250 radical neck specimens and their clinical significance (37). Both the presence and the extent of ECE was found to be the most important factor predicting for neck relapse with a distinction between macroscopic and microscopic ECE emphasized with the former having a worse prognosis (37). Prospective validation of these primary and regional clinicopathologic risk factors are available from two large randomized trials (38,39). Peters et al. report the results of a dose-finding study whereby 302 patients were stratified into risk groups based on an empiric scoring system for primary and regional risk factors selected from a review of the reported literature

(38). The study failed to validate this scoring system but did demonstrate the strong adverse prognostic influence of ECE in lymph nodes on the risk for locoregional relapse. Unfortunately, prognostic analysis was not performed for regional control alone. It also provided evidence of a progressive increasing risk for locoregional relapse in patients demonstrating two or more risk factors. These included the presence of a primary oral cavity site, close or positive surgical resection margins, perineural invasion, two or more metastatic lymph nodes, the largest metastatic lymph node being greater than 3 cm, a treatment delay to PORT greater than 6 weeks and a Zubrod performance status of ≥2. A subsequent mature multi-institutional randomized trial reported by Ang et al. stratified patients requiring PORT again based on clinicopathologic risk stratification (39). Patients with no adverse pathologic factors were deemed low risk and were not given PORT. Patients with one of the previously noted pathologic risk factors were deemed intermediate risk and those with ECE or the presence of ≥2 risk factors were deemed high risk. With a median follow-up of 59 months, a significant inverse relationship between risk groups and both actuarial locoregional control (LRC) and overall survival was observed with the exception of comparable LRC rates for low-risk and intermediate-risk patients (5-year actuarial LRC 90% vs. 94%, respectively). This was suggested to reflect the efficacy of PORT in the latter cohort of patients. High-risk patients had a 5-year actuarial LRC and survival rate of 68% and 42%, respectively. These results confirmed that in the absence of adverse pathologic factors, as studied, low-risk patients do not require PORT. In contrast, high-risk patients as identified warrant further investigation.

Although the study by Ang et al. provides the strongest evidence with regard to indications for PORT, it does not address the presence of a solitary pathologic lymph node (39). In the study by Carter et al., where ECE is present even in a solitary lymph node, the 3-year neck relapse rate was found to be 25% (37). Where no ECE is present, Barkley et al. note neck relapse in 5 of 47 (11%) patients with N1 disease treated with surgery alone compared with a comparable retrospective cohort of 21 patients that received PORT with no neck relapse observed (40). Hence, neck irradiation is commonly recommended in the setting of ECE, reserving neck observation where no ECE is present and the patient is likely to remain compliant to a course of close observation.

Evidence supporting the therapeutic efficacy of postoperative irradiation to the neck specifically is difficult to discern as most comparative studies typically report on PORT for both primary and regional indications. The efficacy of PORT is predominantly based on retrospective comparative analyses and limited randomized trials that have not conclusively established its therapeutic efficacy (41). Mishra et al. report on the randomization of 140 patients with stage III and IV (T3–T4, N0–N2B) buccal mucosa carcinoma to PORT (mean dose 60 Gy) or observation following surgical resection (42). A significant improvement in the disease-free survival was observed in favor of PORT (68% vs. 8%, $p < 0.005$) following a minimum follow-up of 36 months. This observation is noteworthy given the selection bias against the PORT arm that resulted from a biased randomization process due to surgeon preference, yielding a greater proportion of advanced node-positive disease in the PORT arm. Kokal et al. report the preliminary results of a potentially underpowered randomized trial of 51 patients with stage III and IV squamous cell carcinoma arising from the oral cavity, larynx, and pharynx treated with surgery or surgery and adjuvant PORT (50 Gy) (43). The surgery also included an ipsilateral radical neck dissection. The study excluded randomizing patients in the postoperative setting if the resection margins were positive or there was clinical evidence of nodal metastases, hence, largely evaluating the role of PORT for pathologic nodal metastases. A median follow-up of 30 months was reported. Not surprisingly, no significant differences in disease-free or overall survival were observed. Fewer nonsignificant contralateral undissected neck recurrences (5.3% vs. 14.8%, crude rates) and fewer distant metastases (5.3% vs. 14.8%, crude rates) were observed in favor of the cohort receiving PORT. This resulted in a nonsignificant difference in the actuarial relapse rate and 3-year overall survival rate (37% vs. 68%, $p = 0.16$ and 58.5% vs. 46.5%, $p = 0.31$, respectively) in favor of the irradiated group.

Several retrospective comparative studies exist to support the therapeutic efficacy of PORT, particularly in patients with nodal ECE. However, accurate interpretation is limited by the potential influence resulting from a lack of control for local disease recurrence potentially reseeding the neck and the reporting of contralateral neck control. Lundahl et al. report a retrospective matched-pair analysis of 95 consecutively treated patients with PORT (bilateral neck irradiation; median dose 56 Gy) matched to a historical cohort treated with a neck dissection alone (44). Patients with unilateral N1 or N2 neck disease were matched with regard to several clinical parameters including the number of metastatic lymph nodes. Extracapsular extension was not controlled for in this matched- pair analysis, although the authors did match for a desmoplastic lymph node pattern that they observed to be strongly correlated with the risk for ECE (45). Patients not receiving PORT were found to have nearly a sixfold (RR 5.82, $p = 0.0002$) risk for recurrence in the dissected neck, nearly a fivefold risk for relapse in the neck overall (RR 4.72, $p < 0.0001$), and more than a twofold risk for a cancer-related death (RR 2.21, $p = 0.0052$). These findings are particularly significant in light of the limited number of matched pairs. Frank et al. also report an improvement in both overall survival and disease-free survival in a retrospective comparative review of 110 patients with carcinoma of the hypopharynx treated with either surgery alone or followed by PORT (46). Despite the presence of more advanced disease, the cohort receiving PORT was demonstrated to have a superior locoregional relapse rate (14% vs. 57%, $p < 0.0001$), disease-free survival, and adjusted 5-year survival (48% vs. 18%, $p = 0.029$). Treatment with PORT was an independent prognostic factor in multivariate analysis for both disease-free survival ($p = 0.0009$) and overall survival ($p = 0.0289$).

Data also exist suggesting efficacy in high-risk patients with nodal ECE. In a retrospective review of 405 patients treated at the Netherlands Cancer Institute, Bartelink et al. conclude that PORT was favored when compared with surgery alone due to reduced regional relapses only in the cohort of patients with ECE but no preoperative fixation of lymph nodes (47). Similarly, Huang et al. report superior survival rates in a retrospective review of a more homogeneous cohort of 125 patients with high-risk features (ECE or positive resection margin) treated with either surgery and PORT or surgery alone (48). Factors demonstrated to independently influence survival included the use of PORT ($p = 0.0001$) and the number of lymph nodes with ECE ($p = 0.0001$). Despite the use of PORT, the number of lymph nodes with ECE remained significant attesting to the adverse influence of this pathologic feature. This study is significant because the two study populations resulted from the management bias of the operating surgeons to prefer or not to prefer PORT. This clearly defined treatment selection limits the selection bias that often confounds retrospective analyses.

Several studies are noteworthy with regard to the optimal delivery of PORT to the neck. In their dose-finding randomized trial, Peters et al. observed an increased risk for primary site failures in low-risk patients (defined by a scoring system for pathologic factors) receiving ≤54 Gy (52.2–54 Gy) on interim analysis (38). This prompted an increase in the total dose to 57.6 Gy in this randomized arm. There did not appear to be a comparable increased risk for neck relapses (neck control: ≤54 Gy, 89%; 57.6 Gy, 86%; 63 Gy, 89%) although it is unclear what proportion of the small number of patients evaluated at these dose levels were treated for regional risk factors. For patients stratified to the high-risk group, there did not appear to be any significant benefit with regard to both primary site (89% vs. 81%) and neck control rates (84% vs. 77%) when the 63 Gy dose level was compared with the 68.4 Gy dose level. Although these observations may reflect an underpowered analysis, it has been concluded that a dose of at least 63 Gy is warranted to postoperative sites at greatest risk. These investigators postulated that the lack of significant benefit with further dose escalation might be secondary to the adverse effects of accelerated tumor clonogen repopulation resulting from daily fractionated radiotherapy.

Recently, a follow-up multi-institutional prospective randomized trial of 288 consecutively registered (before surgery) patients with 213 patients deemed to require PORT was reported (39). The authors hypothesized that patients with high-risk features as defined by the presence of ECE itself or two or more risk factors, based on the study by Peters et al. (38), would benefit with an accelerated radiotherapy schedule. In total, 151 patients were subsequently randomized to either 63 Gy in 5 weeks (M. D. Anderson Cancer Center delayed concomitant boost radiotherapy schedule) or to a traditional schedule of 7 weeks. A nonsignificant improvement in LRC ($p = 0.11$) and survival ($p = 0.08$) in favor of the accelerated radiotherapy schedule was noted. The nonsignificant differences in LRC and survival are best interpreted as insufficient evidence to conclude that a difference exists between the two schedules. However, the results reported might provide early suggestion that a difference may exist in favor of the experimental arm but has not been conclusively demonstrated, as the authors appropriately discuss. In further subgroup analysis, a significant difference in the LRC ($p = 0.03$) and survival rates ($p = 0.01$) was observed when the high-risk cohort treated with the conventional fractionation schedule was partitioned according to the treatment interval between surgery and the start of PORT with a 6-week cutoff. No such differences were observed in the cohort randomized to the accelerated schedule for either end point. However, significance for these subgroup analyses may require a lower significant p-value criterion to minimize the risk for a false-positive conclusion. Hence, these observations may not be as significant as reported. Similarly, the demonstration of a significant adverse impact on both LRC and survival rates when analyzed by the overall treatment time must be carefully regarded as evidence to support the use of an accelerated fractionated regimen. However, it does indicate the potential adverse impact of treatment delays and interruptions, particularly in patients at high risk for relapse. This observation is further supported by a retrospective review of PORT in 135 patients with oral cavity carcinomas where a significant difference in LRC was demonstrated in high-risk patients, necessitating PORT for multiple indications when analyzed by the overall treatment time (49). Patients receiving surgery and PORT in ≤100 days had a significantly higher LRC rate (60% vs. 14%, $p = 0.04$).

A recently reported large retrospective review of 214 patients demonstrated in a multivariate analysis for LRC that the time interval to PORT was of greater significance than the overall irradiation time (50). This further underscores the importance of up-front multidisciplinary preoperative planning. The strength of this analysis lies in the large study population permitting the modeling of a large number of clinical and treatment factors. Hence, the use of an accelerated PORT schedule to compensate for prolonged delays to PORT in high-risk patients may be limited and should remain the subject of further study (51–55). Caution to adopt such an accelerated PORT schedule is also appropriate in light of a mature phase I to II study reporting on possibly a higher rate of consequential late toxicity with the use of a comparable accelerated PORT schedule (54). It is also advisable that prolonged treatment interruptions should also be avoided. Amdur et al. report adverse LRC rates (5-year: 80% vs. 44%, $p = 0.002$), cause-specific survival (5-year: 57% vs. 37%, $p < 0.001$), and overall survival (5-year: 33% vs. 15%, $p = 0.005$) when a continuous course PORT schedule was compared with a split-course PORT schedule (56).

Similarly, the use of concurrent chemoradiation should remain the subject of ongoing studies in light of the potential risk for increased acute toxicities and subsequent adverse treatment interruptions. A French cooperative study of weekly 50-mg cisplatin and conventional daily radiotherapy in 83 patients with nodal ECE suggests that this strategy is potentially promising (57). These investigators report significant improvements in the 5-year overall survival (36% vs. 13%, $p < 0.01$), cause-specific survival (47% vs. 23%, $p < 0.05$), and borderline significant improvement in the 5-year survival without locoregional relapse (70% vs. 55%, $p = 0.05$). The trial was closed prematurely due to poor patient accrual. However, these results are potentially confounded by the range of doses permitted to metastatic nodal sites with ECE (65–74 Gy). This observation was further supported by a multivariate analysis demonstrating that total radiation dose to ipsilateral cervical nodes and T stage (with chemotherapy losing significance) were the only factors demonstrated to have a significant influence on the occurrence of locoregional relapse.

Lastly, concern regarding the potential underdosing of subcutaneous neck tissues with the use of higher photon radiation (≥6 mV) has been supported in a recently reported large retrospective review of 1,452 consecutively treated patients (58). Treatment was delivered with either 6 mV photons or cobalt-60 (^{60}Co) photon irradiation resulting from a departmental change in treatment machines. Regional neck control was found to be superior with the use of ^{60}Co photon irradiation (79% vs. 60%, $p = 0.03$) in patients at high-risk as defined by the presence of ECE, more than two metastatic nodes, or T4 primary lesions.

In summary, the use of PORT remains an important component in the management of locally advanced resectable HSNCC with pathologic high-risk features for relapse. Of these, the presence of nodal ECE is a dominant factor influencing the risk for regional relapse. There is persuasive retrospective evidence and limited definitive prospective data (38) supporting reduced regional relapse with the delivery of PORT. The issue of survival benefit remains more controversial, particularly in patients with ECE due to the competing risk for distant metastases (59). Patients undergoing surgical resection, in which PORT is deemed to be likely, should be jointly evaluated prior to surgery so that expeditious treatment planning can be properly organized. Standard PORT remains with a daily fractionated schedule to at least one dose of 63 Gy to high-risk areas with the use of accelerated schedules or concurrent chemotherapy remaining promising but requiring further study.

A role for PORT following a lymph node excision for a solitary lymph node has also been reported, addressing the adequacy of radiotherapy in the management of a neck with potentially a higher burden of residual microscopic disease (60,61). Mack et al. (61) report on 41 patients referred for irradiation following excision of a solitary neck metastasis with no gross residual disease. The N stage was Nx (n = 7 patients), N1 (n =

15 patients), N2A (n = 18 patients), and N3A (n = 1 patient). Neck irradiation was administered with doses ranging from 5,485 cGy to 8,100 cGy (median dose, 6,675 cGy). A planned neck dissection was administered in two patients. Actuarial neck control was 95% at both 5 and 10 years. Distant metastasis was observed in 0 of 36 patients with disease controlled above the clavicles versus 3 of 5 patients with relapse above the clavicles. Hence, this report would support the efficacy of post-excision radiotherapy to the neck for most patients presenting with solitary N1 or N2A disease without an increased risk for distant metastasis. The efficacy of post-excision radiotherapy for N3A disease is unclear given the higher risk for residual microscopic disease in the neck. A neck dissection would appear to be warranted. Ellis et al. confirm that the potential adverse effects of violating the neck with an open neck biopsy, on both the probability of neck control and the risk for distant metastasis, could not be demonstrated in a regression analysis when radiotherapy was subsequently delivered to the neck (62). In a separate report from the same institution, Parsons et al. also report on the neck control rates following an open neck node biopsy resulting in patients with or without gross residual disease (60). Gross residual neck disease remained in 55 patients. A neck control rate of 64% was observed when the neck treatment was predominantly with radiotherapy alone. The subsequent consistent addition of a planned neck dissection improved the neck control rates. For N1 to N2 disease, the neck control rate was 65% with irradiation alone and for N2 disease 86% with the addition of a neck dissection. For N3A disease, the neck control rate increased from 29% (2/7) to 63% (5/8) supporting the need for a neck dissection where the burden of residual microscopic disease is increased.

RADIATION ALONE AND RADIATION WITH PLANNED NECK DISSECTION

Primary radiotherapy alone, or as part of a combination chemoradiotherapy strategy, may be used for organ preservation or unresectable disease. Conventional daily fractionated radiotherapy would appear to be appropriate for low-intermediate bulk primary lesions with N1 nodal disease, although these lesions have been included in chemoradiotherapy trials. However, it is unclear if the benefits observed to date with concurrent chemoradiation exist for this specific subgroup of patients at the expense of increased toxicity. For low-intermediate bulk primary lesions presenting with more advanced neck disease, organ-preserving management options may include daily fractionated radiotherapy with or without a brachytherapy implant (for appropriate tumor sites) with planned neck dissection, altered fractionation radiotherapy, or a chemoradiation strategy with or without neck dissection. The latter two options, including combination chemotherapy and altered fractionated radiotherapy, have been used in the management of more advanced resectable or unresectable primary lesions. The relative efficacy of these different strategies with regard to regional control is unclear. Typically, a planned neck dissection has been incorporated in the regional management of at least N2 and N3 disease. However, it has been argued that a planned neck dissection may not be required in patients treated with definitive doses to the nodal disease and in whom a complete clinical response has been achieved (63). In these patients, the ability to detect a complete clinical response, and the efficacy and toxicities associated with salvage neck dissection become relevant considerations. The role of positron emission testing imaging with its increased negative predictive power to detect a complete clinical response allowing for further refined patient selection remains a promising and active area of investigation. An understanding of the relative risks and benefits of these various regional management strategies is therefore important in the decision-making process.

The management of non-nasopharyngeal HNSCC nodal metastases has been rooted in the belief that surgical resection was required with increasing size of nodal metastases and the concern of such metastases being more radioresistant. Fletcher recognized that nodal radiocurability was inversely related to the size of the metastases and the need to deliver higher doses to achieve radiocurability (12). As a result, MacComb and Fletcher (64) introduced the concept of moderate doses of radiotherapy combined with a planned neck dissection that was further supported by Barkley et al. (40). This combined modality approach has further evolved to treatment of nodal metastases greater than 3 cm, typically N2 and N3 disease, with daily fractionated radiotherapy alone yielding high regional control rates for N1 disease. However, in light of the adverse impact of regional relapses, it has been argued that even the low risk for neck relapse for N1 disease treated with radiotherapy alone should be improved on with a planned neck dissection (65). This approach must weigh the relative benefits of reduced regional relapses with the risk for complications arising from a planned neck dissection and the type of neck dissection used. The latter issue will not be discussed in this chapter.

In a retrospective review of 110 patients, where primary lesions were controlled, Mendenhall et al. demonstrated an inverse relationship between the size of the lymph node and its subsequent control rate (66). For lymph nodes 1.5 to 2 cm, 2.5 to 3 cm, 3.5 to 6 cm, ≥7 cm, the regional control rates were 88%, 74%, 70%, and 0%, respectively. These authors also demonstrated a marked influence of treatment time and total dose for lymph nodes 2.5 cm to 6 cm, implying that a more accelerated schedule while delivering a sufficient cytotoxic dose may be particularly important for regional control. In a follow-up retrospective review, Mendenhall et al. confirmed a high regional control rate of 92% in an updated cohort of patients with a single lymph node less than 3 cm treated with daily fractionated radiotherapy alone (67). There was no apparent difference in regional control when compared with a cohort of patients treated with radiation and a planned neck dissection (91%) confirming the adequacy of radiotherapy alone for N1 disease (67). However, other investigators have suggested that a planned neck dissection may further reduce the approximately 10% neck relapse expected with radiotherapy alone (65,68).

The adverse impact of multiple nodes treated with daily fractionated radiotherapy on regional control rate was further elaborated in the review by Mendenhall et al. (67). In their analysis, the addition of a neck dissection appeared to increase the regional control rate although statistical significance was not reported and was confounded by limited numbers of patients with larger lymph nodes treated with radiotherapy alone (67). For patients treated with neck irradiation, the risk for neck failure increased with the presence of more than one clinically positive lymph node and with increasing maximum lymph node size. In contrast, for patients treated with radiation and planned neck dissections the risk for neck failure did not differ with the presence of increasing numbers of clinically positive lymph nodes. These investigators also demonstrated that for nodes less than 6 cm, a dose of 50 Gy appeared to be sufficient when combined with a neck dissection and recommended at least 60 Gy for nodes greater than 6 cm. However, the risk for post-neck dissection wound complications was increased when maximum subcutaneous doses ≥60 Gy were delivered (17% vs. 6%) with a suggestion that most of the increased complications occurred when the neck dissection was performed more than 6 weeks after radiotherapy (29% vs. 14%). Again, this observation may be inherently confounded by patients with more aggressive disease possibly requiring more extensive surgery with inherent increased risk for complications and delay to radiotherapy. Further analysis noted a dose-dependent relationship for neck dissection wound complications for doses 45 to 90 Gy (69). Typically, 60 Gy is delivered to nodal metastases with a planned neck dissection.

Other retrospective reviews have consistently reported efficacy of a planned neck dissection for advanced neck disease (65,68,70–75). In general, high regional control rates have been reported that are discordant with the rate of positive pathologic neck specimens suggesting therapeutic benefit. Typically, positive neck specimens have been seen in 30% to 50% of cases (65,70,71,74,76,77). Lee et al. report on a cohort of 68 patients with base of tongue carcinoma treated uniformly with 60 Gy delivered to palpable nodal disease followed by a planned neck dissection for all patients with N1 to N3 neck disease (65). As a brachytherapy implant was used to boost the primary, the use of a neck dissection was readily incorporated during the general anesthesia required for the implant. A mature actuarial regional control rate of 100% was observed despite 30% of the neck dissections demonstrating histologic disease. In contrast, an actuarial regional control rate of 86% was noted in a cohort of patients treated with radiotherapy alone to the neck before the institutional policy of planned neck dissections was employed. All neck relapses occurred in patients with N0 to N1 disease. Neck morbidity from the combined modality therapy was noted to be limited to only two patients. It is also noteworthy that a clinical complete response lacked sufficient predictive power for a pathologic complete response. Discordant results were observed with not only patients with clinical complete responses demonstrating persistent pathologic disease but also patients with clinical partial responses having a negative pathologic specimen. Hence, the authors concluded that despite the potential of over-treatment in possibly 70% of treated patients, systematic planned neck dissection was recommended given the favorable therapeutic ratio. Other comparable retrospective series reporting the results of comparable strategies in the treatment of base of tongue carcinomas have demonstrated high regional control rates (76,78,79). Lusinchi et al. report 3-year neck control of 69% for patients treated with planned neck dissection and 71.3% for those who received definitive doses of radiation (80). However, these investigators selected patients for a neck dissection based on the presence of persistent neck disease after 45 Gy, potentially creating a negative bias against the neck dissection cohort.

Narayan et al. report the results of a planned neck dissection for N2 and N3 disease in 52 patients treated with a definitive course of radiotherapy delivered to both the primary and nodal sites of gross disease (71). Five-year actuarial neck control was 83% with no difference in regional control rates by N stage (N1: 100%, N2: 87%, N3: 86%), an observation also noted by Lee et al. (65). Isolated neck failure was observed in 8% of patients. It is unclear whether the increased dose to the neck nodes combined with a neck dissection increases the regional control rates, especially for more advanced nodal disease. As would be expected with higher doses delivered to the neck prior to the neck dissection, 17% of patients sustained a significant complication related to the neck dissection. Davidson et al. also observed a dose-dependent relationship for post-radiotherapy neck dissection complications (81).

Erkal et al. report the results of 107 patients with carcinoma of the soft palate with neck management consisting of definitive irradiation or with a planned neck dissection (27 patients) (75). Multivariate analysis revealed that overall treatment time (p = 0.003) and a planned neck dissection (p = 0.001) significantly influenced LRC. Neck stage did not impact on LRC likely because of the influence of a planned neck dissection in the model. More significantly, overall treatment time and a planned neck dissection also affected cause-specific survival (p = 0.005 and p = 0.0003, respectively) and overall survival (p = 0.04 and p = 0.05, respectively) with overall stage also affecting overall survival (p = 0.0001). Complications related to the neck dissection occurred in 11% compared with 3% of patients experiencing a late radiotherapy complication.

Byers et al. have reported on the results of initial neck dissection prior to a definitive course of radiotherapy to the primary site that included postoperative neck radiotherapy (82). Typically, this strategy was undertaken to minimize the overall treatment time for early primary lesions with advanced resectable unilateral nodal disease where a general anesthetic was thought to be required for dental extractions with the advantage of avoiding a second anesthetic. These investigators demonstrated that the success of this strategy necessitated meticulous attention and skill to minimize any delay to start radiotherapy. In patients with a delay greater than 14 days, overall survival was demonstrated to be adversely affected (p = 0.01). This strategy also poses the potential for altered lymphatics and a necessity to irradiate the surgical scar and drainage sites with increased irradiated normal tissues. Although the sequencing of a planned neck dissection after definitive radiotherapy is not without disadvantages (82), the use of an upfront neck dissection does not appear to provide any significant benefit, and may be a disadvantage in certain circumstances.

Hence, the use of a planned neck dissection is associated with a high regional control rate, especially for N2 and N3 neck disease. Neck failures typically less than 10% have been reported despite most reports not controlling for primary relapses. Evidence exists to suggest that the regional control benefits of a planned neck dissection may also translate into improvements in cause-specific survival. This systematic strategy may potentially overtreat 50% to 70% of patients and expose them to the complications related to a neck dissection. Appropriate planning to minimize the dose delivered to the neck and to ensure that the neck dissection is not unduly delayed will minimize the risk for neck dissection complications. This strategy has also been advocated given the few patients who recur with potentially salvageable disease (83) and the low probability of successful salvage (14%–22%) of subsequent neck relapses (66,84).

Despite the high regional control rates associated with a planned neck dissection, it is not without complications (71,75, 81). In this regard, the analysis by Prada Gomez et al. is relevant in providing insight into the factors influencing the radiocurability of lymph nodes thereby possibly further selecting patients requiring a neck dissection (85). These investigators report the results of a multivariate analysis for regional control rates in a cohort of 313 patients treated predominantly with daily fractionated radiotherapy. This study is significant for the size of the study population permitting multiple patient- and treatment-related factors to be modeled. Although the dose delivered varied between 50 and 80 Gy, this factor was accounted for in the model. Significant independent factors included lymph node response to radiation (p = 0.0000), lymph node size (p = 0.0000), radiotherapy dose (p = 0.0037), control of the primary lesion (p = 0.0015), and treatment of recurrent nodal metastases following prior definitive surgery (p = 0.0286). With the primary controlled, regional control for lymph nodes less than 3 cm and for nodes greater than 3 cm was 89% and 32%, respectively. Bartelink confirms the prognostic value of the regression rate of nodal metastases in a small cohort of 27 patients treated to 70 Gy in 7 weeks using bi-dimensional measurements of index lymph nodes (86). Only 1of 12 patients with a fast regression rate developed a neck recurrence. In contrast, neck recurrence was significantly different in 7 of 15 patients with a slow regression rate failing as defined by a time of more than 20 days to half the volume of an index lymph node followed throughout the course of the radiotherapy. Bartelink indicates that the prognostic distinction could be made as early as day 28 after the start of the radiotherapy (86). Bartelink et al. also demonstrate a significant correlation between the risk for regional relapse and the presence of residual palpable neck disease at 6 weeks after completing a course of definitive daily fractionated radiotherapy to the neck (87).

In light of recent interests in altered fractionated radiotherapy schedules, it is of value to review its impact on regional control rate and the potential to further select lesions suitable for radiotherapy alone. Both hyperfractionated and accelerated fractionation regimens have been studied. A recent multi-institutional randomized trial indicated a modest advantage with the use of both a hyperfractionated schedule and a delayed concomitant boost accelerated schedule (88). Unfortunately, the impact on regional control was not specifically reported in this first report as patients with N2 and N3 disease were permitted treatment with a neck dissection. However, Parsons et al. report the impact of the same high-dose hyperfractionated radiotherapy schedule studied on regional control rates censoring for primary failures due to the possibility of reseeding (89). In this retrospective review, a small subgroup of patients with advanced neck disease (based on the 1983 American Joint Committee on Cancer system) did not receive a planned neck dissection as per specific departmental policies. For patients with solitary large nodal metastases (N2A and N3A) treated with radiation and a neck dissection (17 patients) or definitive hyperfractionated radiotherapy (9 patients), the 5-year actuarial regional control rate was 74% versus 41% ($p = 0.036$), respectively. The proportion of patients with N2A and N3A was noted to be virtually identical between these two patient cohorts. Similar observations were noted when comparing patients with multiple advanced neck nodes (N2B and N3B) with 5-year actuarial regional control rates of 85% (39 patients) and 68% (43 patients) ($p = 0.03$) for patients treated with a planned neck dissection or definitive radiotherapy, respectively. The authors noted reservations regarding the use of high-dose definitive radiotherapy for large-volume N2 to N3 neck disease due to inferior regional control rates and increased neck fibrosis with increased surgical wound complications. The results with irradiation alone were not distinguished based on the response rate of the neck to irradiation alone.

The impact of an accelerated radiotherapy schedule on regional control rates has also been studied. A recent retrospective comparative review of 121 patients with stage III and IV supraglottic carcinoma treated with primary radiotherapy is noteworthy for its analysis of factors including different fractionation schedules impacting on regional control (90). Patients were treated with either conventionally fractionated (n = 45) or split-course accelerated fractionated radiotherapy schedules with definitive doses delivered to nodal metastases due to a sequential departmental policy change. Patients treated with daily fractionated radiotherapy received 58 to 70.2 Gy (median dose, 65 Gy) in 1.8 to 2 Gy per fraction. Patients treated with split-course radiotherapy received a total dose of 60.8 Gy to 73.6 Gy (median dose, 67.2 Gy) in 1.6 Gy per fraction twice a day. Various twice-daily regimens reflecting sequential treatment policies were analyzed. From 1979 to 1982, 1.6 Gy twice daily for 12 days was followed by 7 to 14 days of planned treatment interruption with treatment resuming with 1.8 Gy daily for a median total dose of 65 Gy. After 1982, 1.6 Gy twice daily was delivered to a total dose of 66 Gy or 70 Gy maintaining the planned treatment break. Patients with a nodal complete response were observed. At 4 to 6 weeks, a complete response and a partial response were observed in 71% and 29%, respectively, with the probability of a complete response greater with pretreatment nodal sizes less than 3 cm. Of the 80 patients followed, the rate of isolated regional relapse was 7.5% (6 of 80). In multivariate analysis, the risk for regional relapse in patients with a complete response demonstrated no relationship to the pretreatment nodal size in contrast to those with a partial response ($p = 0.004$). In the latter cohort, the risk for regional relapse was 1.9 per cm increase in pretreatment nodal size. Hence, while the probability of achieving a complete response is related to the pretreatment nodal size, once a complete response has been achieved, the risk for regional relapse is unrelated to the pretreatment nodal size. Other investigators have also confirmed this observation with an accelerated radiotherapy schedule (84,91,92). Multivariate analysis of regional control of all patients demonstrates that factors associated with a favorable regional control rate include female sex (85% vs. 50%, $p = 0.025$), accelerated fractionation (75% vs. 50%, $p = 0.005$), and complete response (77% vs. 35%, $p = 0.008$). That the radiotherapy schedule was independent of the influence of a complete response would support the use of an accelerated schedule even for larger nodal disease.

Several investigators have further elaborated on the use of an accelerated radiotherapy schedule alone for larger nodal metastases (84,91,92). Bataini et al. report the results of a large retrospective review of 708 patients with squamous cell carcinoma of the oropharynx or the pharyngolarynx with clinical nodal metastases treated with accelerated concomitant boost radiotherapy to the neck (91). More than two thirds of patients received greater than 70 Gy over 6 weeks. At the completion of the radiotherapy, one-third (247/759) of metastatic nodes had demonstrated a complete response. With further follow-up, 72% (546/759), 77% (586/759), and 79% (597/759) of lymph nodes had demonstrated a complete response at 2, 4, and 6 months, respectively. At 2 months, 83%, 63%, and 45% of lymph nodes less than 3 cm, 3 to 6 cm, and greater than 6 cm had demonstrated a complete response, respectively. The significant differences in complete response rates continued at 4 and 6 months (Fig. 14.3). The mean time to complete response for lymph nodes less than 3 cm, 3 to 6 cm, and greater than 6 cm was 40, 51, and 62 days, respectively, with greater variability demonstrated for lymph nodes ≥3 cm. For complete neck responses, the regional relapse rate remained less than 8% with no significant differences according to pretreatment lymph node sizes. For persistent lymph nodes, regional control rates were adversely affected by larger pretreatment lymph node sizes. At 6 months, regional control was 31% and 12% for lymph nodes ≤6 cm and ≥6 cm, respectively. Regional control for all patients with lymph nodes less than 3 cm, 3 to 6 cm, and greater than 6 cm was 90%, 85%, and approximately 75%, respectively. A dose–response relationship was observed for lymph nodes ≥3 cm (93) with a dose of 65 Gy, 70 to 75 Gy, and 75 Gy recommended for lymph nodes less than 3 cm, 3 to 6 cm, and greater than 6 cm, respectively (91). Multivariate analysis demonstrated that lymph node size was the most significant factor associated with regional control (94). Moderate to severe complications were reported in 9% of patients (crude) with 3% of patients with complications related to neck irradiation (93). The majority of these complications were noted to be cervical fibrosis associated with entrapment and paralysis of the hypoglossal nerve (93).

The observation of an isolated regional relapse occurring in less than 10% of neck nodes achieving a complete response to definitive radiotherapy doses has been consistently observed

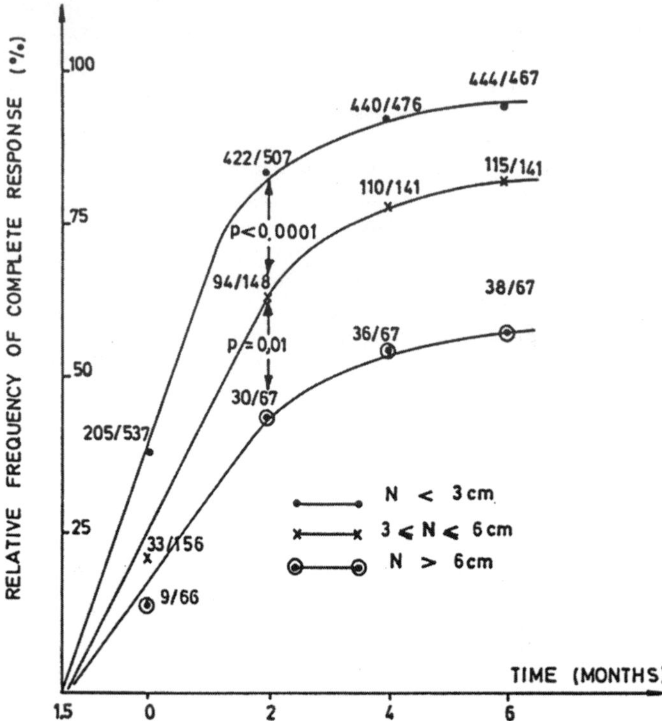

Figure 14.3 Complete response rate for cervical lymph nodes treated with definitive accelerated radiotherapy by lymph node size. (Adapted from Bataini JP, Bernier J, Jaulerry C, et al. Impact of neck node radioresponsiveness on the regional control probability in patients with oropharynx and pharyngolarynx cancers managed by definitive radiotherapy. *Int J Radiat Oncol Biol Phys* 1987;13:817–824.)

and reported by several independent investigators (84,90–92). Peters et al. report an isolated crude regional failure rate of 4.8% (3/62), 0% (0/13), and 20% (5/25) in 100 patients with advanced oropharyngeal carcinoma treated with delayed concomitant boost accelerated radiotherapy alone (with neck observation), radiotherapy with a planned neck dissection, and in patients with neck surgery prior to radiotherapy, respectively (84). Similarly, in the subgroup of complete responders, there was no difference in regional control between lymph nodes ≤3 cm and those greater than 3 cm. Neck failure was greater in nodes larger than 3 cm, demonstrating an incomplete response. In patients treated with radiotherapy alone, the risk for neck fibrosis increased with increasing neck node size. Johnson et al. also report an isolated regional failure rate of 5% in patients with stage III and IV HNSCC treated with a concomitant boost accelerated hyperfractionated radiotherapy schedule and neck observation for a complete neck disease response (92).

Patients treated with definitive doses of radiation but where residual neck disease remains require a neck dissection. Only approximately 45% to 60% of such residual abnormalities will be demonstrated to have residual histologic disease with the majority being salvaged. However, the vast majority of patients with residual neck abnormalities do not undergo salvage neck surgery. Peters et al. report on 13 of 59 patients requiring surgery for clinical residual neck disease. Only 6 of 13 (46%) were pathologically positive with no subsequent neck relapses and no regional relapses noted. Chan et al. (90) report 35 patients with residual neck disease with 25 of 35 (71%) receiving a neck dissection. The remaining patients did not undergo a neck dissection due to patient refusal or the presence of unresectable disease either at the primary or neck. The number of patients with residual neck abnormalities undergoing neck surgery when stratified by their original neck staging suggests comparable rates of regional control for N1 to N2b disease. However, the small numbers of patients in these subgroups precludes any definitive assessment of the significance of any differences noted. Johnson et al. note 18 patients with residual neck abnormalities with only 5 of 18 (28%) undergoing salvage neck surgery. Similar reasons for those patients not undergoing neck surgery were also described. Residual tumor was observed in 3 of 5 patients (60%), with no regional failure observed in 4 of 5 (80%) patients. The only patient with recurrence in the neck had gross residual disease in the neck specimen.

Although it remains unclear if a neck dissection can further reduce the risk for regional relapse in complete neck responses, it is clear that for this subgroup of patients, the risk for surgical complications (81) may offset any additional benefit that may exist. At 2 to 4 months following definitive neck irradiation, approximately 70 of every 100 patients treated would be spared the risks associated with neck dissection at the expense of an increased risk for radiation-induced neck fibrosis. This strategy also comes at the expense of potentially increasing the risk for surgical neck complications for the approximately 30 patients with an incomplete response and the 5 to 6 patients subsequently relapsing in the neck with a controlled primary.

Hence, several investigators have advocated that systematic planned neck dissections should be reevaluated with selection of patients based on nodal response to radiotherapy (63,84). However, it is important to emphasize that this strategy necessitates the delivery of definitive doses with an accelerated schedule likely preferred for more advanced nodal disease. Daily fractionated radiotherapy to definitive doses appears sufficient for nodal masses less than 3 cm. This strategy should not be confused with the delivery of suboptimal doses where a complete response has been observed. In this situation, despite the presence of a complete response, microscopic residual disease may not be sufficiently eradicated with doses regarded suboptimal for pretreatment gross disease. Clearly, definitive irradiation to lymph nodes is a reasonable therapeutic option for larger nodal metastases in which a planned neck dissection is not possible. When considered, it is important to select patients where the primary lesion is likely to be associated with a high probability of control to primary irradiation. It is important to balance this strategy with the increased neck fibrosis that is particularly problematic when irradiating large neck volumes and in critical locations where entrapment and paralysis of the brachial plexus and CN XII may be of concern.

Neck management for nasopharyngeal carcinoma (NPC) has typically been with primary radiation or chemoradiation for more advanced stages of disease, recognizing more radioresponsive and radiocurable neck disease. The role of neck dissection has typically been reserved for management of residual or recurrent neck disease. Chow et al. present the results of the only retrospective comparative matched-pair analysis providing support for this therapeutic paradigm (95). A total of 104 patients with NPC and 104 patients with non-nasopharyngeal HNSCC were selected based on a desire to achieve sufficient statistical power, detecting for a clinically significant difference of 30% in regional control rates (80% NPC vs. 50%). Rigorous study methodology was employed in this retrospective review. All patients were uniformly treated with definitive radiotherapy alone with cases matched according to the largest nodal size to the nearest centimeter. Multiple (>1) metastatic lymph nodes were found in 70 of the 104 patients with NPC compared with 44 of the 104 patients who were non-NPC matched cases. The difference was nonsignificant. The mean nodal size in both groups was 4.1 cm. The 3-year and 5-year nodal recurrence-free rates were 71% versus 43% in the NPC group and 62% versus 43% in the matched control group ($p < 0.0001$). Patients with non-NPC HNSCC nodal metastases were three times more likely to have a nodal failure with no difference in this relative risk even after excluding cases of preceding primary failures. Significant differences with regard to the nodal recurrence rate remained in favor of the NPC cohort even after excluding lymphoepithelial NPC histologies that have been suggested to be more radiosensitive.

CHEMOTHERAPY AND RADIATION WITH OR WITHOUT A NECK DISSECTION

Various strategies integrating chemotherapy with a definitive course of radiotherapy have been studied. These include neoadjuvant chemotherapy followed by radiation, concurrent chemoradiation including intraarterial chemotherapy, and concurrent but alternating chemotherapy and radiation strategies. The role of a neck dissection has generally been accepted for similar indications as in patients treated with radiotherapy alone. Accepted indications have included N2 or N3 neck disease and the presence of residual neck disease. Experience to date has demonstrated that response rates are increased, particularly for concurrent chemoradiation strategies that have been exploited for primary organ preservation (96). In this regard, it is reasonable to question if the addition of chemotherapy may in turn increase the nodal complete response and regional control rate and what impact its use has on the risk for neck dissection complications.

Induction chemotherapy has been employed as a strategy to select for favorable responsive tumors that may be appropriately treated with organ-preserving primary radiation. An extensive body of literature exists demonstrating that local and regional control and survival are not improved but that distant metastasis is reduced (97–102). In general, several retrospective reviews have examined the role of a neck dissection, particularly where a complete nodal response has been achieved following the induction chemotherapy (103,104). Several small series suggest that in complete neck responses following induction chemoradiation, neck dissection may be omitted (103,105). This is contrary to the results of a larger retrospective multivariate analysis of 350 patients that demonstrated that the addition of a neck dissection was beneficial even for complete nodal responses (104). Incomplete nodal responses should undergo a neck dissection with evidence supporting improved regional control (104) and survival (105).

A recently completed Intergroup (91-11) randomized trial has demonstrated that concurrent chemoradiation is superior to induction chemotherapy as a strategy for larynx preservation (28). More significantly, a small randomized trial that compared concurrent chemoradiation versus neoadjuvant chemotherapy and radiotherapy with both arms receiving cisplatin and 5-fluorouracil (5-FU), demonstrates superior regional control with the concurrent chemoradiation (106). Hence, neck management issues following induction chemotherapy are of limited therapeutic relevance.

Lavertu et al. report on the comparative results of neck management resulting from a randomized trial of concurrent cisplatin and 5-FU (two cycles) and daily fractionated radiotherapy versus daily fractionated radiotherapy alone (96). Treatment response was assessed at both the primary and the neck after 50 to 55 Gy with nonresponders (<50% response) and those with disease-progression proceeding to surgery. Otherwise, radiotherapy continued to 65 to 72 Gy followed by a planned neck dissection after evaluation at 4 to 6 weeks for residual disease or for N2 and N3 disease regardless of the response. The addition of chemotherapy was observed to increase the clinical complete response rates in the neck compared with treatment with radiotherapy alone. For reasons unstated, 18 patients with N2 to N3 disease did not undergo a planned neck dissection with 3 of 12 patients with a complete response experiencing a neck relapse. In contrast, for patients with N2 to N3 disease undergoing a planned neck dissection, no recurrences were noted in 18 of 35 patients with a complete response despite 4 of 18 specimens being pathologically positive (22%). It is also noteworthy that of the 17 patients who underwent a neck dissection for persistent adenopathy with 8 of the 17 (47%) being pathologically positive, only 1 of the 8 relapsed in the neck. In a separate study, Lavertu et al. report on the surgical complications prospectively documented (107). Major complications occurred in 12% in both groups. The incidence of major wound complications related to the planned neck dissection was 7% and 0% for patients treated with radiation and chemoradiation, respectively. These findings are noteworthy given that primary boosts and selected electron nodal boosts to 66 to 72 Gy were permitted. Despite observing no significant differences in survival for a planned neck dissection (which likely reflected an underpowered analysis), these investigators continued to advocate a planned neck dissection for N2 and N3 disease irrespective of treatment response and for persistent adenopathy.

Stenson et al. report on 69 of 237 patients treated on several concurrent chemoradiation protocols undergoing a planned neck dissection for N2 or N3 neck disease or for residual neck adenopathy (108). Planned neck dissection was recommended based on 35% of the neck specimens being pathologically positive (N2: 36%, N3: 50%, $p = 0.09$) with a 26% and 10% incidence of total complications and wound complications, respectively. Although consistent with the previously mentioned findings of Lavertu et al., it is unclear to what extent selection bias may have influenced these results as 177 patients were noted to have N2 and N3 disease with only the results of 69 patients reported.

Several reports have suggested comparable if not improved regional control rates with concurrent weekly intraarterial cisplatin radiosensitization based on the pioneering work of Robbins (109–111). In an analysis of 52 patients with N2 and N3 disease, a 59% complete response was observed with approximately half of these patients undergoing a planned neck dissection (109). No pathologic disease was observed and no regional relapses occurred in this cohort. For those with a partial response the majority underwent a neck dissection yielding pathologic disease in 14 of 18 specimens (78%) with 1 of 14 failing in the neck. Overall regional control rate was 91%. The wound complication rate was 17%. Samant et al. report a nodal complete response rate of 76% with a regional control rate of 96% in 25 patients with advanced piriform sinus carcinoma (110). Ahmed et al. report on the results of this strategy for a subgroup of 31 patients with N3 disease (111). The complete response rate was 74%. Neck dissection was performed in 19 of 31 patients with 26% demonstrating histologic disease with no neck recurrences noted in this cohort. Of the 12 patients followed, only 4 were evaluable with the remaining patients dying of intercurrent disease or not completing treatment. No neck relapses were observed.

Several concurrent chemoradiation randomized trials have been reported permitting an evaluation of the impact of chemoradiation on regional control. Calais et al. also demonstrated an improvement in regional control with concurrent chemoradiation in 224 patients with oropharyngeal carcinomas randomized to concurrent 5-FU and cisplatin with daily fractionated radiotherapy or radiotherapy alone (112). In contrast, Jeremic et al. report no difference in regional control rate treated definitively with concurrent daily low-dose cisplatin or carboplatin and daily fractionated radiotherapy compared with daily radiotherapy alone (113). These findings suggest that radiosensitization of advanced nodal disease is possible and that a dose-intensive relationship may exist.

In summary, improved regional control rates appear to be possible due to chemotherapy radiosensitization with neck dissection specimens suggesting improved eradication of microscopic disease. However, a policy of planned neck dissection is likely to still improve regional control rates in approximately 20% to 35% of patients despite a complete nodal response. Despite the risk for over treating a greater proportion of patients with this policy, surgical complications do not appear to be unacceptably increased.

MANAGEMENT OF RECURRENT NECK DISEASE

Patients recurring with neck disease unfortunately are associated with a poor prognosis for several reasons. These include the frequent relapse of unresectable disease often due to its proximity or encasement of the carotid vessels, the frequent recurrence with local disease, the high risk for distant metastases, the selection of more biologically aggressive and treatment-resistant clonogens, and the therapeutic limitations due to prior surgery or irradiation to the neck. Management of patients with such poor prognosis presents a therapeutic dilemma, as even palliation often requires effective neck disease control with the therapeutic ratio often limited by prior neck treatment.

In a retrospective analysis of 139 patients with neck disease treated with radiotherapy, Mendenhall et al. note that the majority of patients failing in the neck did not undergo an attempt for salvage due to unresectable disease at the primary site or the presence of distant metastases (66). In total, only nine patients underwent an attempted salvage. Although the details were not provided, of 25 patients failing in a solitary lymph node, 6 underwent attempted salvage with only 2 being successful. Ten patients failed with ≥2 neck nodes and three received attempted salvage with none being salvaged. Similarly, Peters et al. describe only one of seven attempted salvage neck surgeries being successful (84).

Despite these dismal salvage rates, several retrospective series report on the efficacy of an interstitial brachytherapy implant in combination with salvage neck dissection typically in necks previously irradiated and dissected. Typically, these reports have included neck disease resected with either gross or microscopic residual disease. The extent to which selection bias impacts on the outcomes reported is difficult to discern. Often these series mix primary and neck recurrences and treatment of nonrecurrent lesions, which makes an accurate review difficult (114–117). Three studies treated exclusively recurrent disease (115,118,119). Despite these limitations, this treatment strategy does appear to be able to afford potentially meaningful control of neck relapses. Although no comparative studies have been reported, efficacy has been inferred based on clinical experience expecting further neck relapse within the first 1 to 2 years with the majority of patients receiving an implant showing at least a delay to progression (115). Although a brachytherapy implant permits sufficient cytotoxic doses to be delivered at a defined volume that limits the risk for complications, the risk for wound complications may be further reduced by a planned coordinated introduction of nonirradiated tissue flaps. Both pedicle myocutaneous flaps (120) and microvascular free flaps have been described (121). In turn the introduction of nonirradiated skin and soft-tissue further serves to minimize the risk for carotid exposure and rupture and may facilitate further external beam irradiation to be delivered. Typically, low dose rate implants used either iodine-125 (^{125}I) (Fig. 14.4) or ^{192}Ir (Fig. 14.5). The former is typically used as a permanent interstitial implant with advantages of reduced radiation exposure. The latter is advantageous as it provides more generous coverage of the tumor bed, has the ability to after-load providing an opportunity for dosimetric optimization, and permits sufficient wound fibrogenesis minimizing the risk for wound dehiscence (122). In general, control rates of approximately 40% to 80% have been reported with complication rates of 20% to 50%. Hence, patient selection is particularly important for this indication.

Chen et al. report on 24 patients with advanced recurrent HNSCC, using salvage surgery and intraoperative ^{125}I implantation delivering a minimum dose of 100 Gy to the tumor bed with a pedicle myocutaneous flap covering the carotid artery (119). Neck failure was the sole or at least one component of the relapse in 19 patients. Local disease control was 42%. Two-year overall and cause-specific survivals were 29% and 50%, respectively, with a major complication rate of 21% and an overall complication rate of 50%. Two patients developed carotid rupture but in the presence of further neck recurrent disease. Ultrasound studies were performed on average 30 months after treatment with no patient demonstrating signs of carotid artery occlusive disease. The contralateral carotid artery was used as a control.

Park et al. report on 39 ^{125}I implants in 35 patients with extensive recurrent HNSCC following salvage surgery with indications of either a close or positive resection margin (118). The neck was implanted in 44% of the cases. The average dose delivered was 82.8 Gy. The 5-year local control rate, disease-free survival, and overall survival were 29%, 41%, and 29%, respectively. Significant complications occurred in 36% of all cases. Major complications included flap necrosis in 26%, fistula formation in 8%, carotid rupture in 5%, osteoradionecrosis in 3%,

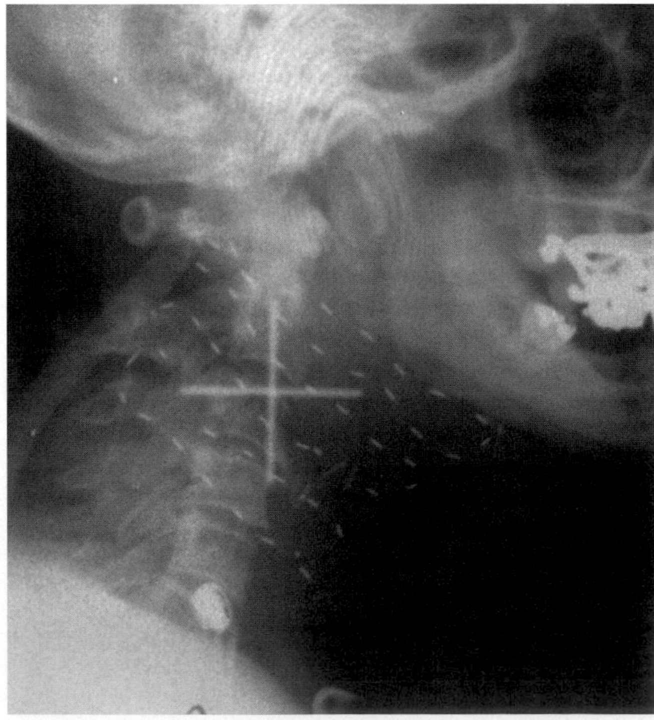

Figure 14.4 Permanent iodine-125 implant in the neck of a patient with recurrent disease in the neck following complete surgical resection.

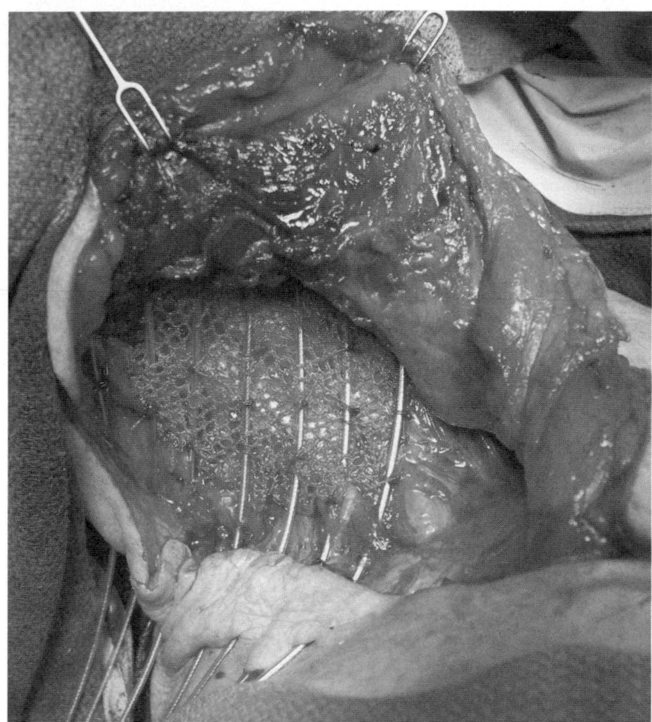

Figure 14.5 Temporary iridium-192 implant in the neck of a patient with recurrent disease in the neck following complete surgical resection and reconstruction with a pedicled pectoralis major flap.

and death due to sepsis in 3%. Two patients experienced a carotid rupture that occurred in the context of recurrent neck disease.

Vikram et al. report on 21 patients with recurrent HNSCC (115). Neck implantation was the most common indication in eight patients (38%). All gross tumor could not be removed in 15 patients, whereas satisfactory margins could not be obtained in 6. In 11 patients, a temporary implant of ^{192}Ir (median dose 48 Gy in 6 days) was used with a permanent ^{125}I implant used in the remaining patients. The actuarial 2-year local control and survival rate was 81% and 55%, respectively. Complications developed in four patients (19%) and proved fatal in one patient.

Fee et al. report on 29 patients with large masses attached to the carotid artery undergoing surgical resection with preservation of the artery and intraoperative ^{125}I with an absorbable suture (114). Nine patients with gross residual disease that was implanted were excluded from analysis with four of the nine recurring in the implanted volume. All nine patients died within 12 months. Eighteen patients (64%) were treated for recurrent neoplasms with neck masses ≥4 cm, having failed prior surgery or radiation. A mean dose of 163 Gy was delivered to the implant volume over 1 year for this cohort. With a minimum follow-up of 1 year, 76% of patients were disease-free in the implant volume and 62% were disease-free in the entire neck for the entire group. Mean survival was 15 months (2–50 months) in the primary group and 12 months (4–26 months) in the recurrent group. Neck recurrence occurred in 39% of those treated for recurrent disease with 22% occurring within the implant. Distant metastases occurred in 39% of those treated for recurrent disease. The overall and major complication rate was 41% and 28%, respectively. Two carotid rupture complications were noted again in the context of recurrent neck disease.

Paryani et al. (116) report on 38 patients with locally advanced head and neck cancer attached to the carotid artery treated with resection and ^{125}I Vicryl suture implant. Most patients had neck masses that were greater than 6 cm without clinically evident distant metastases. Twenty-six patients (68%) had recurrent disease. For the cohort with recurrent disease, local control within the implant volume was observed in 81%. Distant relapses were also observed in 50% of patients treated for recurrent disease. Mean survival was 9 months. The overall complication rate was 26% with most complications involving wound breakdown or flap necrosis. Once again, three patients developed a carotid rupture in the context of biopsy-proven recurrent disease.

The role of intraoperative radiotherapy, with either intraoperative electron beam radiotherapy or temporary surface mold brachytherapy using commercially available applicators and standard HDR after-loaders (HDR-intraoperative radiation therapy) (Fig. 14.6), also has been studied in the management of recurrent neck disease failing following prior neck radiotherapy (123–128). To date, only retrospective series have been reported with heterogeneous patient and tumor selection criteria, the extent of surgical resection, and the volume of intraoperative irradiation limiting an accurate analysis of the efficacy of this treatment strategy. Complete surgical resection remains an important determinant for subsequent neck control (123,127). However, these reviews do establish the feasibility and provide insight into the spectrum of toxicities and doses that may be delivered safely. Doses ranging from 10 to 30 Gy or 7 to 12 Gy have been delivered as the sole treatment or when combined with repeat external beam radiotherapy. Complications appear to be acceptable and may include wound complications, osteoradionecrosis (~5%), and carotid rupture (<5%) that also appear to be related to progressive or recurrent disease. This technique is particularly attractive for several conceptual reasons, warranting continued investigation to include the prompt delivery of radiotherapy before the adverse impact of postoperative surgical bed hypoxia is established and the accurate delivery of large doses of radiotherapy. The delivery of large doses of radiotherapy may be particularly advantageous in overcoming radioresistant recurrent disease.

In summary, the use of either brachytherapy or intraoperative techniques may afford a meaningful delay in the time to progression or salvage of neck relapses. Although no studies with quality-of-life end points or comparative analysis have been performed to validate the observations noted in retrospec-

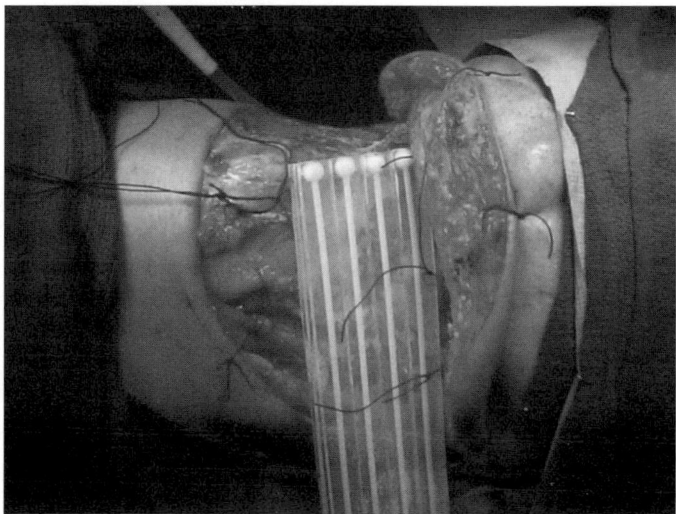

Figure 14.6 Intraoperative high dose rate brachytherapy to the neck in a patient with recurrent neck disease following complete surgical resection.

tive reviews, in light of the morbidity associated with neck recurrences, its application in selected patients may be appropriate.

REFERENCES

1. Vandenbrouck C, Sancho-Gamier H, Chassagne D, et al. Elective versus therapeutic radical neck dissection in epidermoid carcinoma of the oral cavity: results of a randomized clinical trial. *Cancer* 1980;46:386–390.
2. Fakih AR, Rao RS, Borges AM, et al. Elective versus therapeutic neck dissection in early carcinoma of the oral tongue. *Am J Surg* 1989;158:309–313.
3. Piedbois P, Mazeron JJ, Haddad E, et al. Stage I-II squamous cell carcinoma of the oral cavity treated by iridium-192: is elective neck dissection indicated? *Radiother Oncol* 1991;21:100–106.
4. Haddadin KJ, Soutar DS, Oliver RJ, et al. Improved survival for patients with clinically T1/T2, N0 tongue tumors undergoing a prophylactic neck dissection. *Head Neck* 1999;21:517–525.
5. Lindberg R. Distribution of cervical lymph node metastases from squamous cell carcinoma of the upper respiratory and digestive tracts. *Cancer* 1972;29: 1446–1449.
6. Bataini JP, Bernier J, Brugere J, et al. Natural history of neck disease in patients with squamous cell carcinoma of oropharynx and pharyngolarynx. *Radiother Oncol* 1985;3:245–255.
7. Mendenhall WM, Parsons JT, Million RR. Elective lower neck irradiation: 5000 cGy/25 fractions versus 4050 cGy/15 fractions. *Int J Radiat Oncol Biol Phys* 1988;15:439–440.
8. Shah JP. Patterns of cervical lymph node metastasis from squamous carcinomas of the upper aerodigestive tract. *Am J Surg* 1990; 160:405–409.
9. Gregoire V, Coche E, Cosnard G, et al. Selection and delineation of lymph node target volumes in head and neck conformal radiotherapy. Proposal for standardizing terminology and procedure based on the surgical experience. *Radiother Oncol* 2000;56:135–150.
10. Ambrosch P, Brinck U. Detection of nodal micrometastases in head and neck cancer by serial sectioning and immunostaining. *Oncology (Huntingt)* 1996;10:1221–1226; discussion 1226, 1229.
11. Weiss MH, Harrison LB, Isaacs RS. Use of decision analysis in planning a management strategy for the stage N0 neck. *Arch Otolaryngol Head Neck Surg* 1994;120:699–702.
12. Fletcher GH. Elective irradiation of subclinical disease in cancers of the head and neck. *Cancer* 1972;29:1450–1454.
13. Mendenhall WM, Million RR, Cassisi NJ. Elective neck irradiation in squamous-cell carcinoma of the head and neck. *Head Neck Surg* 1980;3:15–20.
14. Withers HR, Peters LJ, Taylor JM. Dose-response relationship for radiation therapy of subclinical disease. *Int J Radiat Oncol Biol Phys* 1995;31:353–359.
15. Fu KK, Chan EK, Phillips TL, et al. Time, dose and volume factors in interstitial radium implants of carcinoma of the oral tongue. *Radiology* 1976; 119:209–213.
16. Mendenhall WM, Parsons JT, Stringer SP, et al. T2 oral tongue carcinoma treated with radiotherapy: analysis of local control and complications. *Radiother Oncol* 1989;16:275–281.
17. Wendt CD, Peters LJ, Deiclos L, et al. Primary radiotherapy in the treatment of stage I and II oral tongue cancers: importance of the proportion of therapy delivered with interstitial therapy [see Comments]. *Int J Radiat Oncol Biol Phys* 1990; 18:1287–1292.
18. Benk V, Mazeron JJ, Grimard L, et al. Comparison of curietherapy versus external irradiation combined with curietherapy in stage II squamous cell carcinomas of the mobile tongue [see Comments]. *Radiother Oncol* 1990;18: 339–347.
19. Pernot M, Malissard L, Aletti P, et al. Iridium-192 brachytherapy in the management of 147 T2NO oral tongue carcinomas treated with irradiation alone: comparison of two treatment techniques. *Radiother Oncol* 1992;23:223–228.
20. Armstrong JG, Harrison LB, Thaler HT, et al. The indications for elective treatment of the neck in cancer of the major salivary glands. *Cancer* 1992;69: 615–619.
21. Byers RM, Weber RS, Andrews T, et al. Frequency and therapeutic implications of "skip metastases" in the neck from squamous carcinoma of the oral tongue. *Head Neck* 1997;19:14–19.
22. Paulino AC, Fisher SG, Marks JE. Is prophylactic neck irradiation indicated in patients with squamous cell carcinoma of the maxillary sinus? *Int J Radiat Oncol Biol Phys* 1997;39:283–289.
23. Jeremic B, Shibamoto Y, Milicic B, et al. Elective ipsilateral neck irradiation of patients with locally advanced maxillary sinus carcinoma. *Cancer* 2000;88: 2246–2251.
24. Le QT, Fu KK, Kaplan MJ, et al. Lymph node metastasis in maxillary sinus carcinoma. *Int J Radiat Oncol Biol Phys* 2000;46:541–549.
25. Jiang GL, Ang KK, Peters LJ, et al. Maxillary sinus carcinomas: natural history and results of postoperative radiotherapy. *Radiother Oncol* 1991;21: 193–200.
26. O'Sullivan B, Warde P, Grice B, et al. The benefits and pitfalls of ipsilateral radiotherapy in carcinoma of the tonsillar region. *Int J Radiat Oncol Biol Phys* 2001;51:332–343.
27. Jackson SM, Hay JH, Flores AD, et al. Cancer of the tonsil: the results of ipsilateral radiation treatment. *Radiother Oncol* 1999;51:123–128.
28. Wolf GT. Commentary: phase III trial to preserve the larynx: induction chemotherapy and radiotherapy versus concurrent chemotherapy and radiotherapy versus radiotherapy—intergroup trial R91-11. *J Clin Oncol* 2001; 19:28S–31S.
29. Kramer S, Gelber RD, Snow JB, et al. Combined radiation therapy and surgery in the management of advanced head and neck cancer: final report of study 73-03 of the Radiation Therapy Oncology Group. *Head Neck Surg* 1987; 10:19–30.
30. Amdur RJ, Parsons JT, Mendenhall WM, et al. Postoperative irradiation for squamous cell carcinoma of the head and neck: an analysis of treatment results and complications. *Int J Radiat Oncol Biol Phys* 1989;16:25–36.
31. Farr HW, Arthur K. Epidermoid carcinoma of the mouth and pharynx 1960–1964. *J Laryngol Otol* 1972;86:243–253.
32. Shah JP, Cendon RA, Farr HW, et al. Carcinoma of the oral cavity. Factors affecting treatment failure at the primary site and neck. *Am J Surg* 1976; 132:504–507.
33. Pfreundner L, Willner J, Marx A, et al. The influence of the radicality of resection and dose of postoperative radiation therapy on local control and survival in carcinomas of the upper aerodigestive tract. *Int J Radiat Oncol Biol Phys* 2000;47:1.287–297.
34. Looser KG, Shah JP, Strong EW. The significance of "positive" margins in surgically resected epidermoid carcinomas. *Head Neck Surg* 1978;1:107–111.
35. Carter RL, Tanner NS, Clifford P, et al. Perineural spread in squamous cell carcinomas of the head and neck: a clinicopathological study. *Clin Otolaryngol* 1979;4:271–281.
36. Johnson JT, Barnes EL, Myers EN, et al. The extracapsular spread of tumors in cervical node metastasis. *Arch Otolaryngol* 1981;107:725–729.
37. Carter RL, Bliss JM, Soo KC, et al. Radical neck dissections for squamous carcinomas: pathological findings and their clinical implications with particular reference to transcapsular spread. *Int J Radiat Oncol Biol Phys* 1987;13: 825–832.
38. Peters LJ, Goepfert H, Ang KK, et al. Evaluation of the dose for postoperative radiation therapy of head and neck cancer: first report of a prospective randomized trial. *Int J Radiat Oncol Biol Phys* 1993;26:3–11.
39. Ang KK, Trotti A, Brown BW, et al. Randomized trial addressing risk features and time factors of surgery plus radiotherapy in advanced head-and-neck cancer. *Int J Radiat Oncol Biol Phys* 2001;51:571–578.
40. Barkley HT Jr, Fletcher GH, Jesse RH, et al. Management of cervical lymph node metastases in squamous cell carcinoma of the tonsillar fossa, base of tongue, supraglottic larynx, and hypopharynx. *Am J Surg* 1972;124:462–467.
41. Peters LJ. The efficacy of postoperative radiotherapy for advanced head and neck cancer: quality of the evidence. *Int J Radiat Oncol Biol Phys* 1998;40: 527–528.
42. Mishra RC, Singh DN, Mishra TK. Post-operative radiotherapy in carcinoma of buccal mucosa, a prospective randomized trial. *Eur J Surg Oncol* 1996;22: 502–504.
43. Kokal WA, Neifeld JP, Eisert D, et al. Postoperative radiation as adjuvant treatment for carcinoma of the oral cavity, larynx, and pharynx: preliminary report of a prospective randomized trial. *J Surg Oncol* 1988;38:71–76.
44. Lundahl RE, Foote RL, Bonner JA, et al. Combined neck dissection and postoperative radiation therapy in the management of the high-risk neck: a matched-pair analysis. *Int J Radiat Oncol Biol Phys* 1998;40:529–534.
45. Olsen KD, Caruso M, Foote RL, et al. Primary head and neck cancer. Histopathologic predictors of recurrence after neck dissection in patients with lymph node involvement. *Arch Otolaryngol Head Neck Surg* 1994;120: 1370–1374.
46. Frank JL, Garb JL, Kay S, et al. Postoperative radiotherapy improves survival in squamous cell carcinoma of the hypopharynx. *Am J Surg* 1994;168:476–480.
47. Bartelink H, Breur K, Hart G, et al. The value of postoperative radiotherapy as an adjuvant to radical neck dissection. *Cancer* 1983;52:1008–1013.
48. Huang CJ, Chao KS, Tsai J, et al. Cancer of retromolar trigone: long-term radiation therapy outcome. *Head Neck* 2001;23:758–763.
49. Parsons JT, Mendenhall WM, Stringer SP, et al. An analysis of factors influencing the outcome of postoperative irradiation for squamous cell carcinoma of the oral cavity. *Int J Radiat Oncol Biol Phys* 1997;39:137–148.
50. Muriel VP, Tejada MR, de Dios Luna del Castillo J. Time-dose-response relationships in postoperatively irradiated patients with head and neck squamous cell carcinomas. *Radiother Oncol* 2001;60:137–145.
51. Awwad HK, Khafagy Y, Barsoum M, et al. Accelerated versus conventional fractionation in the postoperative irradiation of locally advanced head and neck cancer: influence of tumour proliferation. *Radiother Oncol* 1992;25:261–266.
52. Trotti A, Klotch D, Endicott J, et al. A prospective trial of accelerated radiotherapy in the postoperative treatment of high-risk squamous cell carcinoma of the head and neck. *Int J Radiat Oncol Biol Phys* 1993;26:13–21.
53. Sanguineti G, Corvo R, Vitale V, et al. Postoperative radiotherapy for head and neck squamous cell carcinomas: feasibility of a biphasic accelerated treatment schedule. *Int J Radiat Oncol Biol Phys* 1996;36:1147–1153.
54. Trotti A, Klotch D, Endicott J, et al. Postoperative accelerated radiotherapy in high-risk squamous cell carcinoma of the head and neck: long-term results of a prospective trial. *Head Neck* 1998;20:119–123.
55. Shah N, Saunders MI, Dische S. A pilot study of postoperative CHART and CHARTWEL in head and neck cancer. *Clin Oncol (R Coll Radiol)* 2000; 12: 392–396.
56. Amdur RJ, Parsons JT, Mendenhall WM, et al. Split-course versus continuous-course irradiation in the postoperative setting for squamous cell carcinoma of the head and neck. *Int J Radiat Oncol Biol Phys* 1989;17:279–285.

57. Bachaud JM, Cohen-Jonathan E, Alzieu C, et al. Combined postoperative radiotherapy and weekly cisplatin infusion for locally advanced head and neck carcinoma: final report of a randomized trial. *Int J Radiat Oncol Biol Phys* 1996;36:999–1004.
58. Fortin A, Allard J, Albert M, Roy J. Outcome of patients treated with cobalt and 6 MV in head and neck cancers. *Head Neck* 2001;23:181–188.
59. O'Brien CJ, Smith JW, Soong SJ, et al. Neck dissection with and without radiotherapy: prognostic factors, patterns of recurrence, and survival. *Am J Surg* 1986; 152:456–463.
60. Parsons JT, Million RR, Cassisi NJ. The influence of excisional or incisional biopsy of metastatic neck nodes on the management of head and neck cancer. *Int J Radiat Oncol Biol Phys* 1985;11:1447–1454.
61. Mack Y, Parsons JT, Mendenhall WM, et al. Squamous cell carcinoma of the head and neck: management after excisional biopsy of a solitary metastatic neck node. *Int J Radiat Oncol Biol Phys* 1993;25:619–622.
62. Ellis ER, Mendenhall WM, Rao PV, et al. Incisional or excisional neck-node biopsy before definitive radiotherapy, alone or followed by neck dissection. *Head Neck* 1991;13:177–183.
63. Corry J, Smith JG, Peters LJ. The concept of a planned neck dissection is obsolete. *Cancer J* 2001;7:472–474.
64. MacComb WS, Fletcher GH. Planned combination of surgery and radiation in treatment of advanced primary head and neck cancer. *Am J Roentgenol* 1957;77:397–415.
65. Lee HJ, Zelefsky MJ, Kraus DH, et al. Long-term regional control after radiation therapy and neck dissection for base of tongue carcinoma. *Int J Radiat Oncol Biol Phys* 1997;38:995–1000.
66. Mendenhall WM, Million RR, Bova FJ. Analysis of time-dose factors in clinically positive neck nodes treated with irradiation alone in squamous cell carcinoma of the head and neck. *Int J Radiat Oncol Biol Phys* 1984;10:639–643.
67. Mendenhall WM, Million RR, Cassisi NJ. Squamous cell carcinoma of the head and neck treated with radiation therapy: the role of neck dissection for clinically positive neck nodes. *Int J Radiat Oncol Biol Phys* 1986;12:733–740.
68. Foote RL, Parsons JT, Mendenhall WM, et al. Is interstitial implantation essential for successful radiotherapeutic treatment of base of tongue carcinoma? *Int J Radiat Oncol Biol Phys* 1990;18:1293–1298.
69. Taylor JM, Mendenhall WM, Parsons JT, et al. The influence of dose and time on wound complications following post-radiation neck dissection. *Int J Radiat Oncol Biol Phys* 1992;23:41–46.
70. Boyd TS, Harari PM, Tannehill SP, et al. Planned postradiotherapy neck dissection in patients with advanced head and neck cancer. *Head Neck* 1998;20: 132–137.
71. Narayan K, Crane CH, Kleid S, et al. Planned neck dissection as an adjunct to the management of patients with advanced neck disease treated with definitive radiotherapy: for some or for all? *Head Neck* 1999;21:606–613.
72. Smeele LE, Leemans CR, Reid CB, et al. Neck dissection for advanced lymph node metastasis before definitive radiotherapy for primary carcinoma of the head and neck. *Laryngoscope* 2000;110:1210–1214.
73. Newkirk KA, Cullen KJ, Harter KW, et al. Planned neck dissection for advanced primary head and neck malignancy treated with organ preservation therapy: disease control and survival outcomes. *Head Neck* 200 1;23: 73–79.
74. Somerset JD, Mendenhall WM, Amdur RJ, et al. Planned postradiotherapy bilateral neck dissection for head and neck cancer. *Am J Otolaryngol* 2001; 22:383–386.
75. Erkal HS, Serin M, Amdur RJ, et al. Squamous cell carcinomas of the soft palate treated with radiation therapy alone or followed by planned neck dissection. *Int J Radiat Oncol Biol Phys* 2001;50:359–366.
76. Horwitz. EM, Frazier AJ, Vicini FA, et al. The impact of temporary iodine-125 interstitial implant boost in the primary management of, squamous cell carcinoma of the oropharynx. *Head Neck* 1997; 19:219–226.
77. Wang SJ, Wang MB, Calcaterra TC. Radiotherapy followed by neck dissection for small head and neck cancers with advanced cervical metastases. *Ann Otol Rhinol Laryngol* 1999;108:128–131.
78. Housset M, Baillet F, Dessard-Diana B, et al. A retrospective study of three treatment techniques for T1-T2 base of tongue lesions: surgery plus postoperative radiation, external radiation plus interstitial implantation and external radiation alone. *Int J Radiat Oncol Biol Phys* 1987;13:511–516.
79. Crook J, Mazeron JJ, Marinello G, et al. Combined external irradiation and interstitial implantation for T1 and T2 epidermoid carcinomas of base of tongue: the Creteil experience (1971–1981). *Int J Radiat Oncol Biol Phys* 1988; 15:105–114.
80. Lusinchi A, Eskandari J, Son Y, et al. External irradiation plus curietherapy boost in 108 base of tongue carcinomas. *Int J Radiat Oncol Biol Phys* 1989; 17:1191–1197.
81. Davidson BJ, Newkirk KA, Harter KW, et al. Complications from planned, posttreatment neck dissections. *Arch Otolaryngol Head Neck Surg* 1999; 125: 401–405.
82. Byers RM, Clayman GL, Guillamondequi OM, et al. Resection of advanced cervical metastasis prior to definitive radiotherapy for primary squamous carcinomas of the upper aerodigestive tract. *Head Neck* 1992; 14:133–138.
83. Mabanta SR, Mendenhall WM, Stringer SP, et al. Salvage treatment for neck recurrence after irradiation alone for head and neck squamous cell carcinoma with clinically positive neck nodes. *Head Neck* 1999;21:591–594.
84. Peters LJ, Weber RS, Morrison WH, et al. Neck surgery in patients with primary oropharyngeal cancer treated by radiotherapy. *Head Neck* 1996;18: 552–559.
85. Prada Gomez PJ, Rodriguez R, Rijo GJ, et al. Control of neck nodes in squamous cell carcinoma of the head and neck by radiotherapy: prognostic factors. *Clin Otolaryngol* 1992; 17:163–169.
86. Bartelink H. Prognostic value of the regression rate of neck node metastases during radiotherapy. *Int J Radiat Oncol Biol Phys* 1983;9:993–996.
87. Bartelink H, Breur K, Hart G. Radiotherapy of lymph node metastases in patients with squamous cell carcinoma of the head and neck region. *Int J Radiat Oncol Biol Phys* 1982;8:983–989.
88. Fu KK, Pajak TF, Trotti A, et al. A Radiation Therapy Oncology Group (RTOG) phase III randomized study to compare hyperfractionation and two variants of accelerated fractionation to standard fractionation radiotherapy for head and neck squamous cell carcinomas: first report of RTOG 9003. *Int J Radiat Oncol Biol Phys* 2000;48:7–16.
89. Parsons JT, Mendenhall WM, Cassisi NJ, et al. Neck dissection after twice-a-day radiotherapy: morbidity and recurrence rates. *Head Neck* 1989; 11: 400–404.
90. Chan AW, Ancukiewicz M, Carballo N, et al. The role of postradiotherapy neck dissection in supraglottic carcinoma. *Int J Radiat Oncol Biol Phys* 2001;50: 367–375.
91. Bataini JP, Bernier J, Jaulerry C, et al. Impact of neck node radioresponsiveness on the regional control probability in patients with oropharynx and pharyngolarynx. Cancers managed by definitive radiotherapy. *Int J Radiat Oncol Biol Phys* 1987;13:817–824.
92. Johnson CR, Silverman LN, Clay LB, et al. Radiotherapeutic management of bulky cervical lymphadenopathy in squamous cell carcinoma of the head and neck: is postradiotherapy neck dissection necessary? *Radiat Oncol Invest* 1998;6:52–57.
93. Bernier J, Bataini JP. Regional outcome in oropharyngeal and pharyngolaryngeal cancer treated with high dose per fraction radiotherapy. Analysis of neck disease response in 1646 cases. *Radiother Oncol* 1986;6:87–103.
94. Bataini JP, Bernier J, Asselain B, et al. Primary radiotherapy of squamous cell carcinoma of the oropharynx and pharyngolarynx: tentative multivariate modeling system to predict the radiocurability of neck nodes. *Int J Radiat Oncol Biol Phys* 1988;14:635–642.
95. Chow E, Payne D, Keane T, et al. Enhanced control by radiotherapy of cervical lymph node metastases arising from nasopharyngeal carcinoma compared with nodal metastases from other head and neck squamous cell carcinomas. *Int J Radiat Oncol Biol Phys* 1997;39:149–154.
96. Lavertu P, Adelstein DJ, Saxton JP, et al. Management of the neck in a randomized trial comparing concurrent chemotherapy and radiotherapy with radiotherapy alone in resectable stage III and N squamous cell head and neck cancer. *Head Neck* 1997; 19:559–566.
97. Martin M, Hazan A, Vergnes L, et al. Randomized study of 5 fluorouracil and cis platin as neoadjuvant therapy in head and neck cancer: a preliminary report. *Int J Radiat Oncol Biol Phys* 1990;19:973–975.
98. The Department of Veterans Affairs Laryngeal Cancer Study Group. Induction chemotherapy plus radiation compared with surgery plus radiation in patients with advanced laryngeal cancer. *N Engl J Med* 1991;324:1685–1690.
99. Jaulerry C, Rodriguez J, Brunin F, et al. Induction chemotherapy in advanced head and neck tumors: results of two randomized trials. *Int J Radiat Oncol Biol Phys* 1992;23:483–489.
100. Paccagnella A, Orlando A, Marchiori C, et al. Phase III trial of initial chemotherapy in stage III or IV head and neck cancers: a study by the Gruppo di Studio sui Tumori della Testa e del Collo. *J Natl Cancer Inst* 1994; 86:265–272.
101. Lefebvre JL, Chevalier D, Luboinski B, et al. Larynx preservation in pyriform sinus cancer: preliminary results of a European Organization for Research and Treatment of Cancer phase III trial. EORTC Head and Neck Cancer Cooperative Group. *J Natl Cancer Inst* 1996;88:890–899.
102. Lewin F, Damber L, Jonsson H, et al. Neoadjuvant chemotherapy with cisplatin and 5-fluorouracil in advanced squamous cell carcinoma of the head and neck: a randomized phase III study. *Radiother Oncol* 1997;43:23–28.
103. Armstrong J, Pfister D, Strong E, et al. The management of the clinically positive neck as part of a larynx preservation approach. *Int J Radiat Oncol Biol Phys* 1993;26:759–765.
104. Leon X, Quer M, Orus C, et al. Treatment of neck nodes after induction chemotherapy in patients with primary advanced tumours. *Eur Arch Otorhinolaryngol* 2000;257:521–525.
105. Clayman GL, Johnson CJ 2nd, Morrison W, et al. The role of neck dissection after chemoradiotherapy for oropharyngeal cancer with advanced nodal disease. *Arch Otolaryngol Head Neck Surg* 2001;127:135–139.
106. Taylor SGT, Murthy AK, Vannetzel JM, et al. Randomized comparison of neoadjuvant cisplatin and fluorouracil infusion followed by radiation versus concomitant treatment in advanced head and neck cancer. *J Clin Oncol* 1994;12:385–395.
107. Lavertu P, Bonafede JP, Adelstein DJ, et al. Comparison of surgical complications after organ-preservation therapy in patients with stage III or IV squamous cell head and neck cancer. *Arch Otolaryngol Head Neck Surg* 1998; 124: 401–406.
108. Stenson KM, Haraf DJ, Pelzer H, et al. The role of cervical lymphadenectomy after aggressive concomitant chemoradiotherapy: the feasibility of selective neck dissection. *Arch Otolaryngol Head Neck Surg* 2000;126:950–956.
109. Robbins KT, Wong FS, Kumar P, et al. Efficacy of targeted chemoradiation and planned selective neck dissection to control bulky nodal disease in advanced head and neck cancer. *Arch Otolaryngol Head Neck Surg* 1999;125: 670–675.

110. Samant S, Kumar P, Wan J, et al. Concomitant radiation therapy and targeted cisplatin chemotherapy for the treatment of advanced pyriform sinus carcinoma: disease control and preservation of organ function. *Head Neck* 1999; 21:595–601.
111. Ahmed KA, Robbins KT, Wong F, et al. Efficacy of concomitant chemoradiation and surgical salvage for N3 nodal disease associated with upper aerodigestive tract carcinoma. *Laryngoscope* 2000;110:1789–1793.
112. Calais G, Alfonsi M, Bardet E, et al. Randomized trial of radiation therapy versus concomitant chemotherapy and radiation therapy for advanced-stage oropharynx carcinoma. *J Natl Cancer Inst* 1999;91:2081–2086.
113. Jeremic B, Shibamoto Y, Stanisavljevic B, et al. Radiation therapy alone or with concurrent low-dose daily either cisplatin or carboplatin in locally advanced unresectable squamous cell carcinoma of the head and neck: a prospective randomized trial. *Radiother Oncol* 1997;43:29–37.
114. Fee WE Jr, Goffinet DR, Paryani S, et al. Intraoperative iodine 125 implants. Their use in large tumors in the neck attached to the carotid artery. *Arch Otolaryngol* 1983; 109:727–730.
115. Vikram B, Strong EW, Shah JP, et al. Intraoperative radiotherapy in patients with recurrent head and neck cancer. *Am J Surg* 1985;150:485–487.
116. Paryani SB, Goffinet DR, Fee WE Jr, et al. Iodine 125 suture implants in the management of advanced tumors in the neck attached to the carotid artery. *J Clin Oncol* 1985;3:809–812.
117. Lee DJ, Liberman FZ, Park RI, et al. Intraoperative I-125 seed implantation for extensive recurrent head and neck carcinomas. *Radiology* 1991;178: 879–882.
118. Park RI, Liberman FZ, Lee DJ, et al. Iodine-125 seed implantation as an adjunct to surgery in advanced recurrent squamous cell cancer of the head and neck. *Laryngoscope* 1991;101:405–410.
119. Chen KY, Mohr RM, Silverman CL. Interstitial iodine 125 in advanced recurrent squamous cell carcinoma of the head and neck with follow-up evaluation of carotid artery by ultrasound. *Ann Otol Rhinol Laryngol* 1996;105: 955–961.
120. Stafford N, Dearnaley D. Treatment of "inoperable" neck nodes using surgical clearance and postoperative interstitial irradiation. *Br J Surg* 1988;75:62–64.
121. Moscoso JF, Urken ML, Dalton J, et al. Simultaneous interstitial radiotherapy with regional or free-flap reconstruction, following salvage surgery of recurrent head and neck carcinoma. Analysis of complications. *Arch Otolaryngol Head Neck Surg* 1994;120:965–972.
122. Harrison LB, Zelefsky MJ, Armstrong JG, et al. Brachytherapy and function preservation in the localized management of soft tissue sarcomas of the extremity. *Semin Radiat Oncol* 1993;3:260–269.
123. Schleicher UM, Phonias C, Spaeth J, et al. Intraoperative radiotherapy for pre-irradiated head and neck cancer. *Radiother Oncol* 2001;58:77–81.
124. Martinez-Monge R, Azinovic I, Alcalde J, et al. IORT in the management of locally advanced or recurrent head and neck cancer. *Front Radiat Ther Oncol* 1997;31:122–125.
125. Coleman CW, Roach M 3rd, Ling SM, et al. Adjuvant electron-beam IORT in high-risk head and neck cancer patients. *Front Radiat Ther Oncol* 1997;31: 105–111.
126. Toita T, Nakano M, Takizawa Y, et al. Intraoperative radiation therapy (IORT) for head and neck cancer. *Int J Radiat Oncol Biol Phys* 1994;30:1219–1224.
127. Rate WR, Garrett P, Hamaker R, et al. Intraoperative radiation therapy for recurrent head and neck cancer. *Cancer* 1991;67:2738–2740.
128. Garrett P, Pugh N, Ross D, et al. Intraoperative radiation therapy for advanced or recurrent head and neck cancer. *Int J Radiat Oncol Biol Phys* 1987; 13:785–788.

CHAPTER 15

Metastatic Cancer to the Neck from an Unknown Primary Site

Bruce J. Davidson and K. William Harter

The diagnosis, evaluation, treatment, and follow-up of a patient with cervical metastases from an unknown primary neoplasm involve a wide spectrum of topics in oncology. These include the application of known patterns of spread in an effort to locate a primary squamous cell carcinoma (SCC) as well as an appreciation for spontaneous regression of primary disease and early metastatic potential. More complicated concepts must be applied, and more complex techniques, such as immunohistochemistry and cytogenetics, may be required when metastatic nodes are poorly differentiated or demonstrate a nonsquamous histology. Though well-founded treatment philosophies for SCC exist, other approaches may be required in adenocarcinoma or melanoma from an unknown primary.

Even for SCCs from an unknown primary lesion, controversies remain with regard to the workup and treatment of tumors of various stages. It must be recognized that these patients are at risk for a delayed presentation of their original occult tumor in addition to their risk, like others with head and neck SCC, of second primary lesions. They require a treatment and follow-up plan that addresses the neck disease as well as these risks. This chapter is an overview of cervical metastases from occult primary SCCs, and it describes a viable treatment philosophy for its various clinical presentations. In addition, other histologies that may present with neck metastases and an unknown primary tumor are discussed briefly.

It is helpful to be oriented to the general category of unknown primary cancer before focusing on unknown primary SCC to cervical nodes. There is decreasing incidence of unknown primary cancers recorded by the Surveillance, Epidemiology and End Results program cancer registry, a fact that perhaps reflects improved diagnostic capabilities. Of the more than 1 million cancer cases recorded in this registry from 1973 to 1987, 2% were unknown primary cancers. Of these 26,000 cancers, 55% were adenocarcinomas, whereas only 14% were epidermoid carcinomas (1). The University of Kansas has reported a 25-year registry experience with 21,000 patients. In this study, 4% were unknown primary neoplasms, only 10% of which were SCCs (2). When all body areas and sites are considered, unknown primary cancer usually presents as a bone, lung, or liver lesion. Carcinoma in cervical nodes represents less than 10% of all unknown primary neoplasms.

Thus, SCC in cervical lymph nodes with no detectable primary tumor contributes to a small subset of patients with unknown primary cancer. Table 15.1 shows the array of histologies that may present as unknown primary cancer (3). We point this out to demonstrate the perspective of medical oncologists who may become involved in the treatment of patients with unknown primary cancers. Squamous cell neck metastases from an unknown primary tumor represent a distinct subgroup of cancer patients. The workup and treatment of these patients is distinct from that for most other patients with unknown primary cancers, and their prognosis usually is better.

DEFINITION

What is meant by *unknown*? In point of fact, what is unknown to the generalist may be easily discoverable by a thorough head and neck examination, with the availability of enhanced optics and multiple methods of office endoscopy. A classic reference

TABLE 15.1 Unknown Primary Carcinoma: Diagnostic Subgroups

Light-microscopic diagnosis	Final diagnosis	Percentage of cases
Adenocarcinoma (60%)	Specific subgroup	6
	No subgroup	54
PDC/PDA (30%)	Lymphoma, melanoma, sarcoma	3
	Specific carcinoma	1
	PDC/PDA	26
PDMN	Lymphoma	3
	PDC/PDA	1
	Melanoma, sarcoma, other	1
Squamous cell carcinoma	Specific subgroup	4
	No subgroup	1

PDC/PDA, poorly differentiated carcinoma or adenocarcinoma; PDMN, poorly differentiated malignant neoplasm.
Source: Adapted from Hainsworth JD, Greco FA. Treatment of patients with cancer of an unknown primary site. *N Engl J Med* 1993;329:257–263.

addressing this issue describes patients referred to Memorial Hospital with cancer presenting in a cervical lymph node and no identified primary lesion (4). In more than half of these patients, the primary lesion was found by the admitting physician or by the head and neck specialist within 2 weeks of presentation (4). More recently, the University of Liverpool reported a series of patients who had been referred to the head and neck unit with SCC presenting in a lymph node but without primary tumor apparent to the referring physician. The primary lesion was found by history or office examination in 56% of the cases. Chest radiography located an additional 4% (5). This series effectively demonstrated that a primary tumor that is "unknown" to the referring physician can be quickly redefined. The primary lesion was located by panendoscopy in an additional 16% (5), underscoring the importance of establishing a standard definition in discussing cervical metastases from an unknown primary tumor.

A suitable definition of neck carcinoma of unknown primary origin should include the following (6):

- No history of previous malignancy or cancer ablation of any indeterminate lesion
- No history of definite symptoms related to a specific organ system
- No clinical or laboratory evidence of a primary neoplasm
- One or more cervical masses proved histologically or cytologically to be carcinoma.

Fundamental in this definition of SCCs is the need for a thorough examination of the head and neck that includes office endoscopy as well as the added stipulation that examination under anesthesia and panendoscopy be negative for any evidence of a primary lesion. Controversy exists about the role of "blind" or "random" biopsies in these patients, an area discussed in detail later. As part of this definition, we do not suggest that multiple biopsies of clinically normal mucosa are needed to establish the diagnosis of unknown primary SCC. Adherence to this definition of cervical metastases from an unknown primary malignancy prevents premature classification of patients and places the defining time point at the transition between diagnostic evaluation (including panendoscopy) and any therapeutic intervention.

RELEVANT ANATOMY

The anatomy that is relevant to a discussion of cervical metastases from an unknown primary SCC is primarily that of the cervical lymphatics and associated structures in the neck. This section highlights features that affect the presentation, diagnosis, and management of cervical metastases from unknown primary carcinomas. In addition to the importance of cervical lymphatics in unknown primary cancers, the anatomy of several mucosal sites in the upper aerodigestive tract increases the likelihood that small primary lesions in these areas will be either asymptomatic or occult on examination. A description of these sites is included.

The anatomy of the cervical lymphatics can be divided broadly into superficial and deep lymph nodes. The superficial nodes are part of a collar of lymphatics that drain the lower lip, facial skin and buccal mucosa, parotid gland, pinna, and posterior scalp. The nodal groups include submental, facial, submandibular, parotid, and occipital nodes. These are easily palpable and clinically are found frequently to be enlarged by regional inflammation. The more anterior of these superficial nodes drain into deep lymphatics at the level of the omohyoid muscle, which is in the midjugular region. Facial, submandibular, and parotid nodes drain into deep lymphatics of the upper jugular chain, whereas occipital nodes drain into the deep lymphatics of the spinal accessory chain.

The deep cervical lymphatics follow two main pathways. The predominant path of drainage—and the most frequent area to manifest metastatic nodal disease—is along the jugular vein. Nodal groups along this chain include the jugulodigastric and jugulo-omohyoid nodes. The jugulodigastric group receives drainage from superficial nodes of the submandibular triangle and the parotid gland as well as from multiple pharyngeal and laryngeal mucosal sites, rendering this area a frequent site of metastatic nodal disease. The jugulo-omohyoid nodes receive lymphatics from the submental triangle, direct lymphatics from oral cavity sites, and drainage from the adjacent hypopharynx and larynx. The lower nodes of the jugular chain drain the glottic and subglottic larynx, the hypopharynx, and the thyroid. In addition, these nodes receive lymphatic drainage from more cephalad nodes in the jugular system.

The second pathway of deep cervical lymphatics follows the course of the spinal accessory nerve. The nodes at the superior aspect of this chain lie in the area of the jugular foramen and drain nasopharyngeal sites and retropharyngeal lymphatics. From this area, the spinal accessory lymphatics follow the course of the nerve into the posterior triangle. The posterior triangle nodes receive lymphatic drainage from the posterior scalp and posterior aspect of the pinna and receive drainage from lymphatics higher in the accessory chain.

In the region of the posterior belly of the digastric, the pathways of the jugular and accessory lymphatic chains are not distinguished easily. Clinically, this overlap of the jugular and accessory chains is addressed in selective neck dissections that include level II. The supraomohyoid neck dissection used to stage N0 necks in oral cavity carcinoma removes both the upper jugular and the upper spinal accessory nodes in this region. Whereas this junctional area frequently is found to contain metastatic nodes in head and neck carcinoma, a relatively low incidence of posterior triangle (lower spinal accessory) nodal metastases is seen (7,8). This finding would indicate that the majority of lymphatic drainage from this area courses along the jugular chain.

Crossing the lower neck, a group of nodes follows the course of the transverse cervical artery. This group provides additional communication between the spinal accessory and the jugular chain of lymphatics. The transverse cervical chain lies in close proximity to the thoracic duct at the medial aspect of the left neck, and an accessory thoracic duct may be present in the right neck as well. The watershed of nodes in the supraclavicular and low medial neck includes structures drained via the thoracic duct and associated collateral lymphatics. Nodal disease presenting in these areas often ensues from infraclavicular and even subdiaphragmatic primary lesions. Thus, as compared with higher nodes in the neck, cervical metastases to the supraclavicular area from an unknown primary tumor are less often suspected to arise from an occult upper aerodigestive tract primary tumor.

Other neck anatomy relevant to cervical lymphatics relates to structures in proximity that may become involved as metastatic nodes enlarge and develop extracapsular spread and local infiltration. Upper jugular nodes lie in close association with the jugular vein, the sternocleidomastoid muscle, the posterior belly of the digastric, the external and internal carotid arteries, and the vagus, spinal accessory, and hypoglossal nerves. Of these structures, the jugular vein most commonly is infiltrated with tumor. Massive nodal metastases may involve any of the structures just listed. Additionally, disease of this magnitude may infiltrate overlying skin and may extend through deep cervical fascia to infiltrate the splenius capitis, levator scapulae, or scalene muscles.

Surgeons who developed the classic radical neck dissection recognized the potential for infiltration of the internal jugular vein, the sternocleidomastoid muscle, and the spinal accessory nerve, and were aware of the relatively low morbidity from sacrifice of these structures. What has become apparent more recently, however, is that the spinal accessory nerve, like the other cranial nerves in this area, usually can be preserved without jeopardizing the oncologic soundness of the operation (9–11). This finding reduces the incidence of postoperative morbidity from sacrifice of the spinal accessory nerve (12). Exceptions to spinal accessory nerve preservation are situations in which the nerve is surrounded or is immediately adjacent to tumor.

The anatomy of several regional mucosal sites, such as the nasopharynx, tonsil, and base of tongue, must be considered in evaluating a patient for an unknown primary SCC. These sites represent the components of Waldeyer's ring and contain a variable amount of lymphoid tissue. The irregularities of the mucosa over underlying lymphoid tissue result in mucosal crypts, and a significant portion of the mucosa in these areas may not be visible by inspection clinically. Thus, the natural variability and the potential for subsurface mucosa unavailable for inspection create a greater likelihood that an early carcinoma will remain occult in these areas.

Two of the areas of Waldeyer's ring—the nasopharynx and the base of tongue—and the hypopharynx are notorious for the development of clinically asymptomatic lesions. Perhaps owing to a dearth of sensory nerves in these zones, symptoms of pain or dysphagia tend to appear late. The "silence" of these areas, especially for the base of tongue and hypopharynx, is perplexing. Both areas are crucial to normal swallowing, and their insensitivity to mucosal neoplastic disease may be related in part to a natural redundancy in the swallowing mechanism.

NATURAL HISTORY AND PATTERNS OF SPREAD

The anatomic reasons why primary lesions at certain sites of the upper aerodigestive tract might be asymptomatic or occult on head and neck examination have been discussed. One would expect that, left untreated, these mucosal primary lesions ultimately would become clinically apparent. However, several series of patients who were treated solely by surgery to the neck have been reported. In these series, primary tumors in the head and neck become evident in only 2% to 28% of patients (13–16). This low incidence of primary disease does not appear to be a consequence of short follow-up or frequent failure in the neck.

How can the majority of patients with untreated aerodigestive tract lesions never develop a primary lesion? One possibility is that the neck metastases originate from an infraclavicular primary tumor. Other possibilities are that the neck mass is the only site of carcinoma, that no primary tumor ever existed, and that disease developed in an epithelial rest or branchiogenic cyst. A third explanation is that spontaneous regression of the primary tumor occurs after metastatic disease has become established.

In a study by Jones et al. (5), the prevalence of infraclavicular primary tumors in those patients presenting with squamous cell metastases in cervical nodes was 30 of 267 (11%). This finding compares with 174 of 267 (65%) who were found to have head and neck primary tumors. The majority (83%) of these infraclavicular primary lesions were in the lung. History, examination, radiography, and endoscopy were responsible for identifying 15 of 25 lung cancers; the remaining 10 were discovered in follow-up or at autopsy. Thus, of the 65 patients with no primary tumor identified after panendoscopy, 10 (15%) were found ultimately to have lung primary tumors. These figures are in agreement with several series of unknown primary squamous carcinomas to cervical nodes. These series report the late presentation of an infraclavicular primary tumor in 2% to 12% of patients (16–18), and 3% to 8% of all patients are reported to present lung primaries (13,19).

These data may have to be regarded as overestimates of the role of infraclavicular primary tumors resulting in cervical metastases. From prospective follow-up of patients treated for head and neck SCC, the incidence of second primary tumors is 4% per year (20,21). Lung and esophageal carcinomas frequently are identified as the sites of these second primary carcinomas (22). Thus, it is difficult to discern a delayed presentation of an original infraclavicular primary tumor from a second primary cancer.

The location of the neck node gives an indication of the likelihood of an infraclavicular primary tumor. Supraclavicular nodal metastases of SCC are associated with infraclavicular primary neoplasms in 63% of cases, whereas only 5% of patients with jugular chain nodes are found to have infraclavicular primary tumors (5). Thus, whereas infraclavicular primary tumors may be discovered during the evaluation or follow-up of patients with cervical metastases, this outcome accounts for only a small proportion of these patients. Jugular nodal metastases, in particular, are unlikely to be the result of an occult infraclavicular primary tumor.

Benign rests of nonlymphoid tissue occasionally are found in otherwise normal lymph nodes. Rests of thyroidal or salivary tissue can be found in cervical or mediastinal lymph nodes and are presumed to be embryologically incorporated when located in close proximity to the thyroid or salivary glands. Collections of benign nevus cells can be found in otherwise normal cervical and axillary lymph nodes (23). They may represent benign metastases from dermal nevi, developmental anomalies, or glomangiomatous hamartomas (23). With regard to SCC arising in a cervical lymph node, neither epithelial rests nor metastases of benign squamous epithelium are reported to occur in normal nodes. This phenomenon, therefore, does not appear to be a viable explanation for SCC in cervical nodes with no known primary tumor.

The theory that cervical neoplastic disease has developed in a branchial cleft remnant or a branchiogenic carcinoma was discussed first in 1882 by von Volkmann (cited in ref. 4). Much controversy has surrounded this concept over the years, but the weight of evidence argues against it as an explanation for malignant cervical masses. First, clinically apparent branchial cleft abnormalities must be acknowledged to be relatively uncommon. Unless a great number of patients have subclinical branchial cleft cysts that never become clinically detectable, the existence of an adequate pool of patients who could develop neoplastic disease within their branchial cleft cysts seems highly unlikely.

Martin and Morfit (4) discussed the issue of branchiogenic carcinoma and concluded that the majority of reported cases did not meet criteria necessary to support a branchiogenic origin. Their criteria were admittedly strict and included (a) the patient must have survived at least 5 years free of disease; (b) treatment must have been directed only to the cervical tumor situated along the line of the embryologic branchial clefts; and (c) histologically, the tumor must have been squamous or epidermoid carcinoma.

Using these criteria, Martin and Morfit (4) found that of 55 patients presenting with cancer in a neck mass and no obvious primary tumor, only 8 fulfilled criteria for a branchiogenic carcinoma. These authors pointed out, however, that radiation was used in some of these patients, and thus an occult primary tumor within the field may have been treated (4).

A more recent discussion of cancer arising in apparent branchial cleft cysts during a 30-year period was reported at the University of Liverpool. Here, 9 of 270 cancers presenting as neck masses were cystic squamous cell metastases (24). Primary carcinomas subsequently were discovered in the tonsils of six patients and in the base of tongue in one patient. Two primary tumors remained occult. The same institution noted that in a 5-year period, 25 branchial cleft cyst excisions revealed 4 patients (16%) with SCC (24). The University of Pittsburgh reported a 10% incidence of metastatic carcinoma in lateral cervical cysts, half of which were found to have origin in the pharynx (25). Apparently this experience suggests that cystic metastases may appear clinically similar to branchial cleft cysts, but when SCC is discovered in such a cyst, a pharyngeal or lingual tonsillar primary tumor should be suspected.

Spontaneous regression of primary malignancies has a rich history of documentation, primarily by case reports. Approximately 20 cases per year have been reported in the literature (26); however, few cases of head and neck SCC have been described. A review of all cases of spontaneous regression reported from 1966 to 1987 found 504 cases (26). In order of decreasing frequency, the majority of these tumors were malignant melanoma, renal cell carcinoma, lymphoma, leukemia, retinoblastoma, and breast cancer. Only 13 cancers from the head and neck were reported (five adenoid cystic, four larynx, one pharynx, and three others). Reported in addition were 10 unknown primary carcinomas whose metastases underwent spontaneous regression, but the histology of these neoplasms was not described. Host–tumor interactions mediated by humoral or cellular immunologic mechanisms have been suggested to be responsible for spontaneous regression, but precise mechanisms are not yet known.

Evidence of spontaneous regression of aerodigestive tract mucosal lesions can be found in reports of oral leukoplakia. What should be pointed out, however, is that this diagnosis is clinical and does not identify a histologically malignant or even premalignant lesion in most cases. *Leukoplakia* is defined clinically as a white patch of mucosa, at least 5 mm in diameter, not removed by rubbing, and not meeting criteria for any diagnosable oral condition (e.g., lichen planus). Observation of leukoplakia without surgical removal reveals disappearance or regression in 37% to 44% of lesions (27,28). Though this regression rate is a significant proportion of all leukoplakias, these studies do not report changes in tobacco or alcohol use or other habits; nutritional improvements; or other nonsurgical measures that might play a role in regression of these lesions.

What also must be realized is that biopsies reveal dysplasia in only approximately 12% of leukoplakic oral lesions (27). When patients with dysplastic oral lesions are identified, lesions are more likely to be excised or otherwise treated definitively, so finding observational studies is difficult. However, these lesions, too, may show disappearance or regression in some 10% of patients (29). These estimates of spontaneous regression are contrasted with a 0% to 4% incidence of malignant transformation in oral leukoplakia (27,28) and an 11% incidence of transformation in oral cavity dysplasia (29). Though these reports of regression in clinical leukoplakia and oral dysplasia support the concept of spontaneous regression, they do not describe regression of invasive SCC after it has acquired metastatic potential. Such evidence would give stronger support for the role of spontaneous regression in SCC cervical metastases of unknown primary tumor.

The scant evidence for spontaneously regressing SCCs does not support this mechanism as a likely explanation for the lack of a primary tumor in patients with SCC in the neck attributed to an unknown primary lesion. Though spontaneous regression of the primary tumor may occur in many unknown primary SCCs, one would expect to see more evidence of spontaneous regression of known tumors to support this effect as a frequent phenomenon.

Another concept that arises in a discussion of the natural history of these cancers addresses the observation that they show phenotypic characteristics of aggressive behavior (i.e., metastasis) though their primary lesions remain subclinical. The specific molecular alterations that might allow such behavior still are poorly understood but perhaps involve aberrant regulation of enzymes important in digestion of basement membrane, cellular motility, and cellular attachment. Although research continues to attempt to describe the relationship between the altered expression of such enzymes and the metastatic phenotype, matrix metalloproteinases, collagenases, and stromolysins are believed to be involved in this process. No research describes the properties of these enzymes in SCC of unknown primary. However, some evidence does suggest that, in oral cavity carcinoma, increased expression of metalloproteinase-2 is correlated with the presence of lymph node metastases (30). When applied to a small series of hypopharyngeal carcinomas, however, this marker failed to correlate with lymph node metastases (31).

A common molecular event in head and neck SCC is mutation of the tumor suppressor gene *p53*. An investigation of a series of tumors presenting as cervical lymph node metastases of unknown primary failed to identify mutations within exons 4–9 of *p53* in 23 tumors (32). In contrast, however, researchers at Johns Hopkins have shown identical genetic events at 17p13 (the *p53* locus) from nodal and benign mucosal tissue in 5 of 18 patients tested (33).

At this point, no specific or nonspecific molecular abnormalities appear to correlate with the phenotype seen in SCC from an unknown primary tumor. Apparently, these metastases are derived from subclinical tumors. Despite acquiring the metastatic capability at an early primary tumor stage, these primary lesions are not necessarily locally aggressive and may follow one of several courses. They may regress spontaneously, remain stable (and occult), or increase in size and become apparent in subsequent follow-up. Treatment recommendations and decisions may be affected by a perceived risk for developing a clinically apparent primary tumor that is not supported in the literature.

The natural history of the "primary tumor" is a major consideration, but as with many head and neck SCCs, the extent of metastatic cancer in cervical nodes determines locoregional control and survival. By definition, patients with such metastases have at least regional disease at presentation (assuming an upper aerodigestive tract occult primary tumor). The natural history of patients with regional metastases includes progression of neck disease, erosion of overlying skin, and, ultimately, a significant risk for major vessel erosion and hemorrhage.

The likelihood of clinically evident distant metastases in head and neck cancer increases as neck disease progresses (34). Although few distant metastases can be found at presentation, follow-up reveals that N1 disease is associated with distant metastases in 26% of patients (34). N3 neck metastases are associated with distant metastasis in 52% (34). Lower neck metastases are associated with distant metastasis in 27%, whereas patients with upper neck nodes have only a 13% incidence of distant metastases (35). When locoregional disease is controlled by initial treatment, the rate of distant metastases is 12% at 3 years. However, when locoregional control was not obtained, distant metastases develop in 32% (34). Distant metastases most often detected are in the lungs, but bone, liver, and various other sites also may be involved.

CLINICAL PRESENTATION

The typical patient presenting with cervical metastases from an unknown primary tumor reports a unilateral, painless neck mass of several weeks' to months' duration. Workup includes a history pertaining to the mass, including the time of onset, progression or fluctuation in size since first detection, and such symptoms as pain in the area of the mass. History of a previous carcinoma or new symptoms may elucidate diagnosis of the primary lesion and result in appropriate classification and treatment of the patient with a detectable primary lesion. History of tobacco and alcohol use may direct suspicions toward an SCC of mucosal origin, whereas excessive sun exposure would raise suspicions for a skin primary tumor. A history of radiation exposure may indicate a thyroid, salivary, or skin primary tumor.

Once an adequate history is obtained, an examination should be carried out and should include a careful survey of the head and neck. This examination should include the skin of the scalp and neck. A comb may be helpful in examining the scalp with thick hair. Examination should focus next on the ears, nasal cavity, and oral cavity. The oropharynx is a critical area in searching for an occult primary SCC. Extensive lymphoid tissue may obscure a small lesion within palatine or lingual tonsillar crypts. Clinical examination of patients with a strong gag reflex may be difficult, but in cooperative patients clinical examination of the pharynx often is superior to that obtained at examination under anesthesia and panendoscopy. In addition to providing for careful inspection of the tonsillar tissue for any asymmetry, the clinical examination should include both a mirror and a digital examination of the base of tongue. Not uncommonly, a subtle area of induration of the base of tongue may be the only sign of a primary lesion. Mirror examinations of the nasopharynx, hypopharynx, and larynx remain important despite advances in office endoscopy, and such examinations should be attempted. The neck examination should precede office endoscopy. Attention should be directed to the thyroid and salivary glands in addition to the nodal mass under consideration. An accurate measure of any palpable lymph nodes should be recorded, and the extent of neck disease should be described by neck level as well as by N staging. Fixation of the mass to overlying skin or underlying structures and any evidence of cranial nerve weakness (cranial nerves VII, X, XI, and XII) should be noted, as these conditions may dictate the necessary extent of subsequent neck dissection.

Office endoscopy produces several options in examining the patient with neck metastases from an unknown primary tumor. Rigid nasal endoscopes provide excellent optics for viewing the nasopharynx, and, under topical anesthesia, biopsy of a potential nasopharyngeal primary tumor is possible at the initial visit. Owing to fewer secretions and the tone of pharyngeal musculature in the awake patient, this office view of the nasopharynx often is superior to that obtained when the patient is supine and under general anesthesia for panendoscopy. Though rigid nasopharyngoscopy could be followed by rigid laryngoscopy to survey the potential primary tumor sites in the upper aerodigestive tract, flexible nasopharyngoscopy is our examination of choice in office endoscopy. This provides an adequate view of the nasopharynx and of the hypopharynx and larynx with a single passage of the scope. If any suspicious areas in the nasopharynx are visualized, a rigid nasal endoscope can be used immediately to assess this area. Flexible nasopharyngoscopy is less efficient in the oropharynx, because neither the tonsillar fossae nor the base of tongue is visualized well by this technique. An advantage of flexible nasopharyngoscopy is seen in examination of the hypopharynx. By use of a modified Valsalva maneuver (asking the patient to blow out his cheeks), the hypopharynx becomes distended, and the view into the piriform sinuses is enhanced greatly. The larynx can be surveyed also using the flexible scope; if any suspicious area is noted, the improved optics of rigid laryngoscopy are brought into play.

At all points in the history or examination of the patient with a neck mass, a differential diagnosis should be kept in mind. The various congenital, infectious, inflammatory, traumatic, and neoplastic causes of neck masses are not listed here, but several points can be made. Rapidly growing or painful neck masses often are found to be inflammatory in nature, but a squamous cell metastasis with cystic degeneration may present as a neck mass of rather sudden onset. Congenital cysts first may become apparent after upper respiratory infections and may fluctuate in size. Tuberculosis presenting as a neck mass often is insidious in onset, with a long history of painful neck mass or masses. Multiple bilateral nodes often indicate a nonneoplastic condition, but lymphoma must be considered in these cases in which nodes are rubbery and mobile. Nodes in the submental triangle rarely are an indication of metastatic malignant neoplasms. Nodes in the posterior triangle in a young patient often are benign. When malignant nodes are

TABLE 15.2 Unknown Primary Malignancies Presenting in Cervical Lymph Nodes

			Histology (%)					
Study (year)	Reference	No. of patients	SCC	Anapl/Undiff	Adeno	Mucoep	Melanoma	Other
Weir (1995)	18	144	62	30	8[a]			
Davidson (1994)	36	115	63	11	7	4	10	4[b]
Spiro (1983)	37	157	60	10	22		8	
Jesse (1973)	38	210	62	28	10			

Adeno, adenocarcinoma; Anapl/Undiff, anaplastic or undifferentiated carcinoma; Mucoep, mucoepidermoid carcinoma; SCC, squamous cell carcinoma.
[a]Includes adenocarcinoma, mucoepidermoid carcinoma, and lymphoepithelioma.
[b]Includes three lymphoepitheliomas and one small-cell carcinoma.

TABLE 15.3 Unknown Primary Squamous Cell Carcinoma: Nodal Status at Presentation

			N Stage						
Study (year)	Reference	No. of patients	NX	N1	N2	N2a	N2b	N2c	N3
Weir (1995)	18	144	30	6	33			28	
Davidson (1994)	36	79		29	41	25	12	4	30
Maulard (1992)	40	113		21	48	40	8		26
Marcial-Vega (1990)	41	72		17		19	25	17 (3b)	22 (3a)
Harper (1990)	42	69		26		16	22	12 (3b)	25 (3a)
Wang (1990)	13	157	38	14		13	9	11 (3b)	15 (3a)

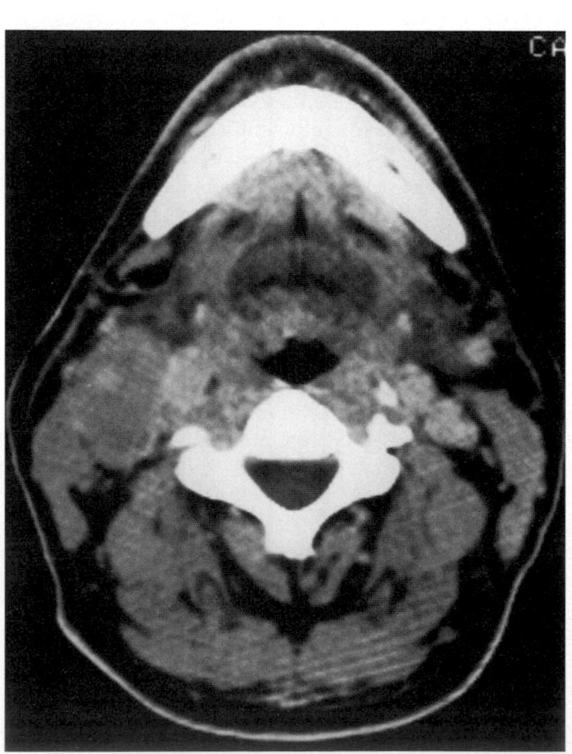

Figure 15.1 Neck computed tomography showing a right level II, 4 × 5 cm metastasis in T0N2aM0 squamous cell carcinoma of unknown primary.

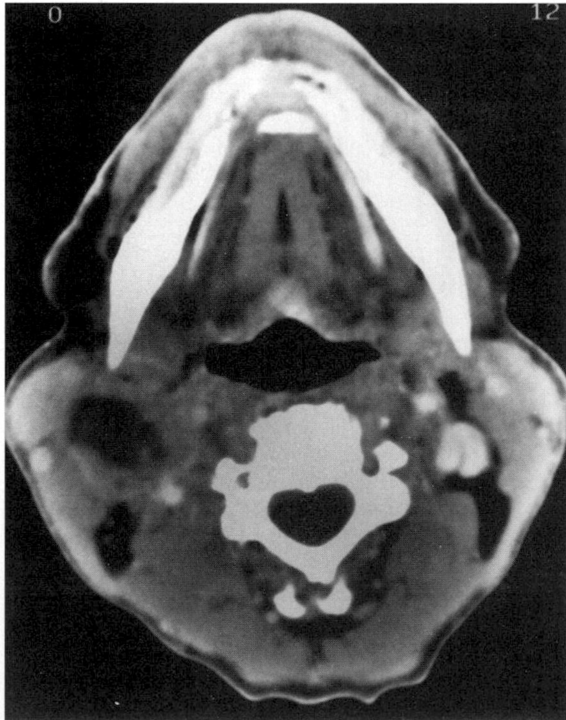

Figure 15.2 Neck computed tomography in a patient who presented with a mass in the right infraauricular area. Fine-needle aspiration biopsy showing admixture of tumor cells. Normal salivary acini led to suspicion of salivary gland malignancy. Panendoscopy was negative. Pathology after resection showed moderately differentiated squamous cell carcinoma in periparotid lymph node and multiple cervical nodes.

found in this area, a nasopharynx or scalp primary tumor should be sought.

Finally, patients are often referred for evaluation by a head and neck specialist after a course of oral antibiotics has failed to resolve a neck mass of recent onset. Though we acknowledge that our perspective is biased by a referral practice, we discourage the routine use of antibiotics for neck masses unless evidence or history of an infectious cause exists.

Of those patients who ultimately prove to have a malignant neck node, the majority will have an SCC histologically. However, malignancies of other histology do present in the neck, and this should be considered. Series reporting unknown primary cervical metastases consist of SCC in about 60% of cases (Table 15.2) (18,36–38). Anaplastic or undifferentiated carcinomas, melanomas, and adenocarcinomas contribute equally to the remaining group of malignant masses. Though carcinoma classified as anaplastic, undifferentiated, or lymphoepithelioma requires an approach that remains focused on the upper aerodigestive tract as the most likely source of a primary lesion, the diagnoses of adenocarcinoma or melanoma each require distinct approaches in the evaluation and treatment. These histologies are discussed later in this chapter.

In the circumstance of nodal metastases that ultimately proves to be SCC, the most common clinical presentation is a single unilateral neck mass at level II in a patient 50 to 70 years old. Approximately 80% of patients are men, and most will have a significant history of tobacco and alcohol use. Though these parameters give an impression of the typical patient, the age distributions reported in recent series include patients in their twenties, and one report includes a 15-year-old patient (39).

The clinical staging of patients with unknown primary SCC is shown in Table 15.3 (13,18,36,40–42). In these series, patients who presented either NX after biopsy, N1, or N2a make up the largest group of patients (36% to 69%). Presentation with multiple nodes occurred in 16% to 42%, and massive adenopathy was seen at presentation in 26% to 39%.

The predominant location of neck metastases in these patients is level II (Fig. 15.1). Considering all patients, regardless of whether metastases are single or multiple, level II nodal disease is present in more than half (37,41). When single-node disease is considered, level II metastases present in 44% to 52% (13,14). After level II, levels I and III are the most likely sites for cervical metastases from unknown primary SCC. Lower neck metastases and posterior triangle metastases make up a small fraction of these cases and usually are seen in patients with multiple neck nodes. In a series from the University of Texas M. D. Anderson Cancer Center, 10 of 108 patients (9%) presented with single-node metastasis to level V (13). Parotid node metastases also may present and may be the sole nodal disease in some 4% of patients (Fig. 15.2) (13).

DIAGNOSTIC EVALUATION AND STAGING

Clinical Investigation

The credo of otolaryngologists and head and neck surgeons long has been that no neck mass should undergo biopsy before a complete head and neck examination. This philosophy initially was formulated as a response to the injudicious use of open biopsy of neck masses without previous examination and panendoscopy. Many of the patients subjected to open biopsy in the past had discoverable aerodigestive tract lesions, and open biopsy was thought to compromise subsequent control of neck disease and survival. Despite wide awareness of this standard of care, the number of patients referred for treatment of cervical squamous cell metastases of unknown primary tumor after open biopsy remains fairly high. In the more recent series from U.S. cancer centers, 64% to 74% of patients presented after open biopsy (13,36).

A complete head and neck examination before biopsy is important because the examination may reveal mucosal irregularities that are suspicious for carcinoma and, depending on the location and the nature of these areas, a mucosal biopsy in clinic may be the most expeditious and inexpensive way to obtain a diagnosis. Easily accessible areas include sites in the oral cavity, nasopharynx, and oropharynx (except for base of tongue).

Assuming that a neoplastic neck mass is suspected and no accessible mucosal lesion is identified on clinical examination, we recommend fine-needle aspiration of the mass as the next step in the workup. Many surgeons choose to perform this procedure during the same visit. We agree with this approach but usually involve the cytopathologist at the time of aspiration to ensure that an adequate cytologic sample has been obtained. If a lymphoma or other nonsquamous histology is suspected by the cytopathologist on cursory review of the slides, additional material can be obtained for any appropriate immunohistochemical and molecular diagnostic studies required.

Laboratory and radiologic studies may be helpful in the workup of neoplastic neck masses. No laboratory tests are sensitive or specific for SCC; however, if other neck mass etiologies are to be ruled out, a complete blood cell count, thyroid function tests, and calcitonin levels may be indicated in selected patients. Except for calcitonin testing in medullary thyroid carcinoma, none of these blood tests is specific for neck metastasis. Serologic studies for Epstein-Barr virus usually are abnormal in nasopharyngeal carcinomas (43), but in nonendemic populations are unlikely to be helpful in discovering an occult primary carcinoma. A Sequential Multiple Analysis of 20 chemical constituents (SMA-20) long has been regarded as an essential screen for liver and bone enzyme abnormalities that may indicate distant metastases. However, work from the University of Iowa demonstrates abnormal liver function tests in one half of all head and neck cancer patients but no correlation with liver metastases (44).

Often, confusion surrounds the use of radiologic studies in the evaluation of neck masses. Chest radiography, though not required for nonneoplastic neck masses, is an inexpensive screen for primary, metastatic, and second primary lung lesions. Computed tomography (CT) or magnetic resonance imaging (MRI) of the neck has a role in SCC cervical metastases of unknown origin for two reasons: such imaging enhances the assessment of neck disease, and helps to detect the primary lesion. Up to 30% of neck nodes judged to be pathologic are not palpable (45), and necks are upstaged by CT in 20% to 30% (46). In attempting to detect the occult primary tumor, CT or MRI may direct attention at endoscopy to subclinical abnormalities that otherwise may be overlooked. In support of this, CT was used in 17 patients who had malignant neck masses by fine-needle aspiration but no primary tumor by clinical examination and office endoscopy. Suspicious abnormalities were detected by CT in 10 patients, and primary tumors subsequently were confirmed by biopsy in 4 patients (47). Though the role and use of CT and MRI are discussed further, we mention them here to emphasize that these investigations should precede panendoscopy, not only because the information can be used to direct biopsies but also so that postbiopsy edema does not compromise the specificity of these studies. Fine-needle aspiration, on the other hand, causes minimal tissue-plane disruption and edema, and may be pursued safely before CT scan.

Fine-needle aspiration of a neck mass may reveal any of several malignant histologies, and special studies using immunohistochemical or molecular diagnostics may be helpful in characterizing poorly differentiated neoplasms. These modalities are reviewed elsewhere in this chapter. Unless results are firmly diagnostic of a nonepithelial malignancy (confirmation of which is difficult by cytology alone), the upper aerodigestive tract should be investigated for a primary malignant lesion. As indicated, this evaluation may include radiologic studies. Panendoscopy is the next step in management and should precede open biopsy for lesions that are equivocal by cytologic analysis.

An algorithm for diagnosis of suspicious neck mass is presented in Figure 15.3.

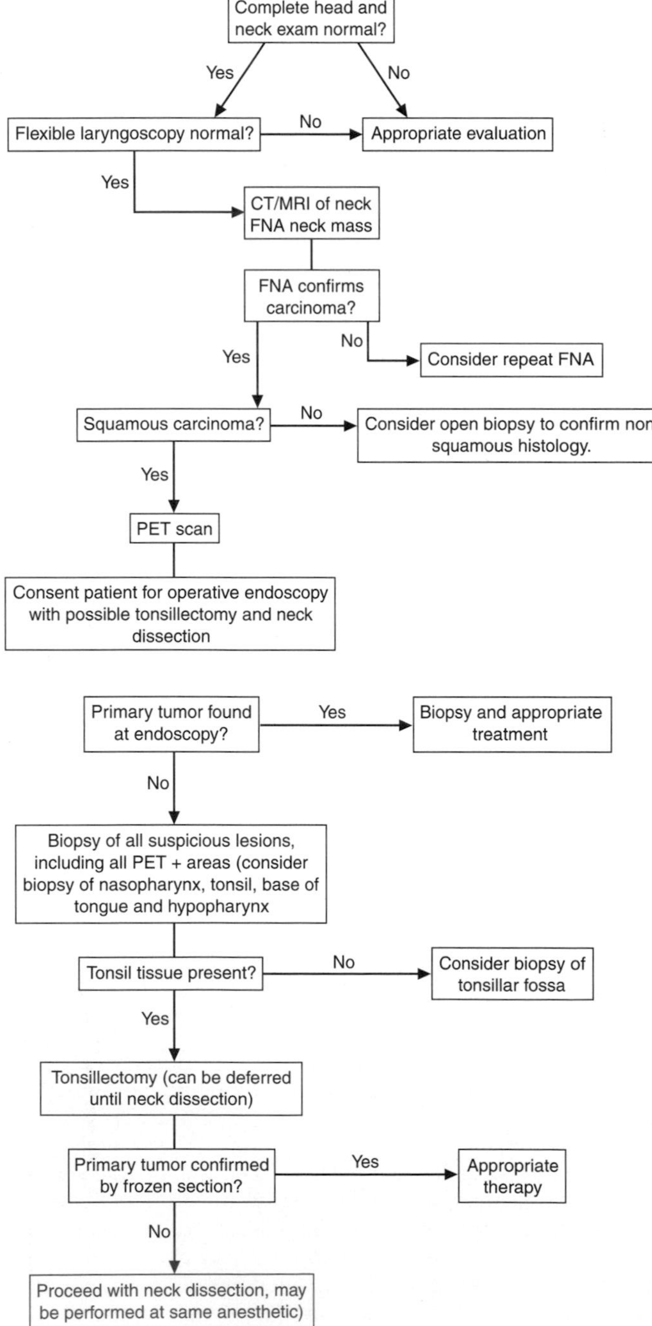

Figure 15.3 Algorithm for diagnosis of a neck mass suspicious for carcinoma.

Panendoscopy

Panendoscopy is an imprecise term that may include assessment of the nasopharynx, oral cavity and oropharynx, hypopharynx, larynx, esophagus, and tracheobronchial tree. The primary focus is on the upper aerodigestive tract, and (as indicated) several of these sites will have been assessed clinically by head and neck examination and office endoscopy. With operative endoscopy and examination under anesthesia, the nasopharynx, tonsils, and base of tongue can be palpated for signs of induration. Biopsies can be obtained from any suspicious areas. If not previously visualized in the clinic, the examination should include rigid nasal endoscopy to view the nasopharynx. Direct laryngoscopy allows visualization of the oropharynx, hypopharynx, and larynx, and attention should focus on the tonsil, base of tongue, and piriform sinus for subtle evidence of a primary lesion. Rigid cervical esophagoscopy is useful to visualize the esophageal inlet, an area poorly seen by flexible esophagoscopy.

Flexible esophagoscopy and bronchoscopy provide improved optics compared with their rigid counterparts, and (except for the esophageal inlet) both allow more complete surveys for possible primary lesions. However, the likelihood that upper and middle jugular adenopathy is metastatic from an occult primary tumor from these areas appears to be fairly low. Use of these modalities in attempting to discover a primary carcinoma should be individualized. One or both flexible examinations may be needed in assessment of a metastatic node in the supraclavicular fossa, lower jugular chain, or tracheoesophageal groove, but they may be omitted in most patients with upper or middle jugular metastases and no known primary tumor. In support of this treatment policy, Table 15.4 describes the late presentation of lung and esophageal primary tumors in six series of unknown primary SCC (13,17–19, 36,40,41). Despite variations in the use of bronchoscopy and esophagoscopy, these series report that lung cancers became manifest in 1% to 8% and esophageal cancers in 0% to 2%. This low incidence of such lesions, the possibility that these "late" primary tumors may represent second primary lesions, and the low likelihood that asymptomatic and radiologically occult esophageal or lung cancers would present with jugular nodes lead us to conclude that the use of esophagoscopy and bronchoscopy should be individualized in this group of patients.

Random Biopsy

During endoscopy, all suspicious lesions should be biopsied. The role of biopsy is controversial in evaluating apparently normal mucosa from the nasopharynx, tonsil, base of tongue, and piriform sinus in an effort to discover the primary tumor. These efforts are termed *random, random-guided, directed,* or *blind* biopsies by various authors. Some centers suggest biopsy of all of these areas and include bilateral tonsillectomy, whereas other centers at the opposite end of the spectrum advocate biopsy only of suspicious areas of mucosa.

Analysis of these retrospective data is inherently difficult because the philosophy of each center may have influenced which patients were ultimately classified as unknown primary cancers. Centers that do not routinely perform biopsy of all areas may report a series that mixes patients who have subclinical but histologically discoverable lesions with patients who have histologically normal mucosal sites and cervical metastases. Centers that routinely perform multiple biopsies may report series selected against those with subclinical primary tumors and report a more homogeneous group of patients. To test the value of multiple biopsies would require a prospective study in which all patients underwent the same series of biop-

TABLE 15.4 Incidence of Late Presentation of Infraclavicular Primaries in Unknown Primary Squamous Cell Carcinoma

				Late primary tumors	
Study (year)	**Reference**	**No. of patients**	**Endoscopy**	**Esophageal (%)**	**Lung (%)**
Weir (1995)	18	144	EUA head and neck	[a]	10 (7)[a]
Davidson (1994)	36	73	B 38%, E 48%	0 (0)	1 (1)
Maulard (1992)	40	113	Selected B and E	0 (0)	3 (3)
Wang (1990)	13	157	Selected B and E	1 (1)	4 (3)
Marcial-Vega (1990)	41	72	B 60%, E 71%	0 (0)	5 (7)
Glynne-Jones (1990)	19	87	Not stated	2 (2)	7 (8)
LeFebvre (1990)	17	190	Panendoscopy	1 (1)	3 (2)

B, bronchoscopy; E, esophagoscopy; EUA, examination under anesthesia.
[a]Reported as lung and esophageal.

sies. This format would avoid the selection bias inherent in retrospective reviews.

A small series of patients reported from Johns Hopkins University Medical Center was evaluated in a systemic fashion from 1976 to 1982 (48). The philosophy used at this institution was that if panendoscopy revealed a suggestive lesion, biopsy was obtained, often with frozen section. If no abnormalities were detected (or if frozen sections were negative), biopsies from the nasopharynx, tonsil, base of tongue, and piriform sinus were obtained. Adenoidectomy or ipsilateral tonsillectomy was performed when significant lymphoid tissue was present. Of 33 patients referred with unknown primary SCC, 11 had lesions discovered before panendoscopy. Primary tumors were discovered at panendoscopy and were confirmed by biopsy in 4 of the remaining 22 patients. Random biopsies were performed in the 18 remaining patients, and these revealed two nasopharyngeal and one tonsillar primary tumor (48). This 17% yield from random biopsy was felt to warrant such an approach.

The utility of random biopsies should be measured by the applicability of the information obtained. An N2 to N3 neck will certainly require postoperative radiation therapy for adequate control of neck disease, and neck portals will place the oropharynx (and hypopharynx if desired) within the radiated field. In contrast, an N1 neck could be controlled with surgery alone if pathologic findings are favorable (i.e., single node without extracapsular spread). Though N2 to N3 neck radiation portals conceivably could omit the nasopharynx if negative biopsies were obtained, it appears to us that the N1 subset of patients with favorable surgical pathology would benefit most from negative biopsies of all sites, or from the finding of a small cryptic tonsillar primary removed with negative margins at tonsillectomy.

Tonsillectomy

The adequacy of biopsy samples obtained by cup forceps has been questioned by centers advocating tonsillectomy in assessment of these patients. With significant amounts of tonsil mucosa lying in crypts, random biopsies may not be adequate to assess the patients for a subclinical tonsillar primary lesion. At the University of Vermont, a series of 19 patients with unknown primary SCC was found to include 6 (32%) with tonsillar primary tumors discovered at tonsillectomy (49). Clinical findings were "absent or inconclusive" for tonsillar abnormalities, and CT scanning was negative before tonsillectomy. However, patient evaluations varied in this series. Not all 19 patients underwent tonsillectomy, and no description of the examination under anesthesia (e.g., induration or asymmetry) was given. Other series have also reported positive biopsies through the use of tonsillectomy in 18% to 39% of patients evaluated for unknown primary SCC (50–52). Though this high prevalence of tonsillar primary tumors is noteworthy, it is not consistent with data from reports describing the course of patients treated by neck surgery alone. These series show only a 3% to 4% incidence of tonsillar primary tumors arising in follow-up (14,53).

The appropriate use of tonsillectomy remains controversial. Experience from the University of Florida would indicate that the likelihood of cancer in tonsillectomy specimens is low (10%) when examination and CT/MRI scans are negative (51). In contrast, surgeons at Johns Hopkins argue in favor of bilateral (not simply ipsilateral) tonsillectomy due to the finding that 10% of patients undergoing tonsillectomy have bilateral or contralateral disease (54). It is the authors' opinion that tonsillectomy is an appropriate investigation in this population of patients, but, due to the postoperative discomfort of tonsillectomy, we choose to perform the tonsillectomy at the time of neck dissection.

Metabolic Imaging

Efforts to identify a primary neoplasm in patients presenting with SCC in a cervical lymph node have used the fact that tumors have an increased metabolic activity with respect to surrounding normal aerodigestive mucosa. The isotope ^{18}F-fluorodeoxyglucose (FDG), a glucose analog, enters cells using normal transport mechanisms. The application of FDG uses the fact that glucose metabolism (and therefore FDG uptake) is increased in malignant cells, but FDG cannot be further metabolized and remains concentrated in tumor tissues.

Imaging modalities using FDG include positron emission tomography (PET) and single photon emission computed tomography (SPECT). Positron emission tomography scans are considered to have superior spatial resolution and count sensitivity. The limitation of detection is from 5 to 10 mm for PET scans and about twice that for SPECT scans. Initial reports of the use of FDG in the detection of unknown primary carcinomas involved the use of SPECT scans and resulted in the detection of 11 primaries in 10 of 18 patients with squamous cancer of unknown primary. Sensitivity and specificity were 80% and 38%, respectively (55). Subsequent reports using PET scans have reported the detection of unknown primary lesions in 13% to 38% (56–60) of patients evaluated. This is further described in Table 15.5. It would appear that less than a third of patients will have a detectable primary lesion by PET scan, and when CT or MRI or prior random biopsies are negative, the yield for PET scan is approximately 20%.

TABLE 15.5. Positron Emission Tomography (PET) Scan Assessment in Carcinoma of Unknown Primary Site

Institution (year)	Reference	Patients	Primary found on PET	Notes (SCC neck unless noted)
Hamburg (2000)	56	53	20 (38%)	44 neck; 9 other
UCLA (1999)	57	14	3 (21%)	PET after CT and random biopsy
UCSF (1999)	58	14	7 (50%)	2/9 (22%) with negative MRI/CT
Wake Forest (1999)	59	13	1 (8%)	6 (46%) false-positive PET
Groningen (1998)	60	11	2 (18%)	
Total		105	33 (31%)	

CT, computed tomography; MRI, magnetic resonance imaging; SCC, squamous cell carcinoma.

Open Biopsy

If the neck is suspicious for metastatic cancer, fine-needle aspiration is nondiagnostic, and panendoscopy is negative, an open biopsy may be required. It is performed best with preparations in place to treat the neck definitively should a malignant diagnosis be obtained on frozen section. The biopsy incision should be designed carefully such that it can be incorporated into a neck dissection incision if required later.

The influence of node biopsy on disease control is controversial. Based on experience at the University of Iowa, McGuirt and McCabe (61) recommended against open biopsy, showing worse outcome in patients who had squamous cell metastases and who underwent cervical node biopsy before referral for definitive treatment of the neck. These patients were found to have a significantly increased risk for neck recurrence and distant metastases. A matched-pair analysis controlling for age, sex, histology, site, stage, and treatment protocol showed a significantly increased risk for distant metastases in the node biopsy group (61). However, survival was not addressed by these data.

Other series do not demonstrate a detrimental effect of open biopsy. In a University of Florida study very similar in size to the Iowa study, patients treated with radiation therapy and surgery with and without previous node biopsy were compared with respect to outcome. No difference was seen in overall neck control, distant metastases, or cause-specific survival (62). Two subgroups, those with N1 and N2a neck disease, actually had significantly improved cause-specific survival when pretreatment node biopsy was used (62). These data do not suggest that open biopsy is advocated; it is not. However, the treatment of patients after open biopsy does not appear to have the grave consequences previously reported as long as radiation therapy is included in the subsequent management of the malignancy.

Staging

The staging for SCC metastatic to the neck from an unknown primary tumor follows tumor, node, metastasis (TNM) guidelines established for neck and distant metastases in other head and neck SCCs. All patients, by definition, are classified as T0 in the absence of evidence of unknown primary tumors, and all are termed N+. In this chapter, various N stages are defined as outlined in guidelines from the American Joint Committee on Cancer (fifth edition) (63). However, the sixth edition has recently been introduced (63a). There have not been any changes in the N staging, except that the descriptors "U" and "L" have been added to denote whether the nodal disease is confined to the upper neck (above the cricoid) or extends into the lower neck. All available clinical information (including CT or MRI findings) should be used to define the stage. M1 denotes patients with distant metastases. Because all patients are deemed N+, stage I and II cancers do not exist. Patients with N1 neck disease and no distant metastases are designated stage III, but all other patients are stage IV at diagnosis.

MANAGEMENT OF UNKNOWN PRIMARY TUMORS

A discussion of unknown primary tumor management broken down by stage of disease is relatively simple because (as was stated) stages I and II do not exist. Patients are either stage III or IV, with only one fourth of patients with N1 disease falling into the former category. Management, for the most part, is a discussion of the treatment of advanced SCC. As with other sites in the head and neck, most patients with advanced disease should be treated with combined-modality therapy, in this case using surgery and radiation. There is some controversy regarding the extent of surgery and the radiation portals required in the treatment of these tumors. In addition, possible exceptions to combined use of surgery and radiotherapy are discussed below.

An algorithm for treatment of unknown primary carcinoma is presented in Figure 15.4.

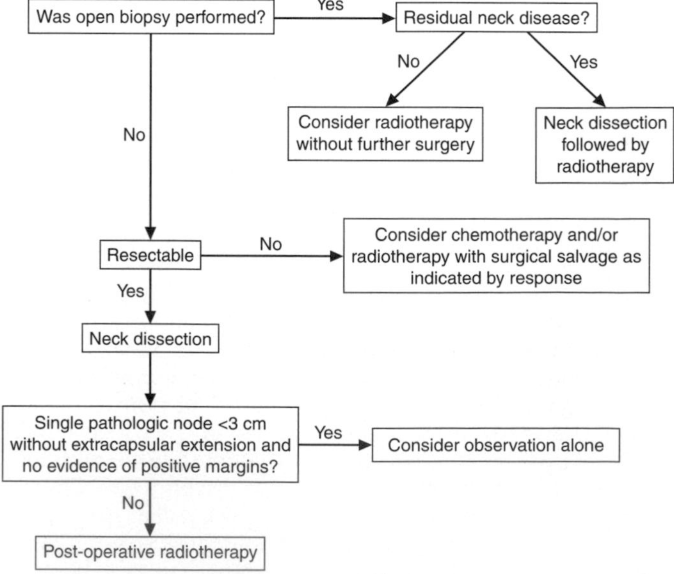

Figure 15.4 Algorithm for treatment of an unknown primary carcinoma.

Stage III (N1)

Patients present with N1 disease in 17% to 29% of cases with unknown primary SCC (see Table 15.3). This minority of patients may be eligible for single-modality treatment. However, combined treatment using surgery and radiation therapy is indicated in most patients because of the inaccuracy of clinical staging to predict microscopic disease; the frequent occurrence of extracapsular spread in N1 necks, which can impact neck control; and the concern for development of a late primary tumor within the head and neck.

Clinical neck staging and pathologic staging can differ considerably. In unknown primary neck disease that is clinically N1, 45% of patients are found to have multiple nodes (pathologically N2b) at surgery (36; unpublished data). Similar discrepancies have been reported in comparing single-node disease (N1 or N2a) and pathologic findings. Here, 57% of patients have multiple nodes on neck dissection (17).

The finding of extracapsular spread or connective tissue disease in metastatic SCC to the neck is an ominous finding that is associated with an increase in neck failure and distant metastases and decreased disease-free survival (64). Even those who remain free of disease locoregionally have a higher incidence of distant metastases when extracapsular spread is detected (64). In unknown primary cancers, the finding of extracapsular disease is reported in 35% of patients with clinical N1 neck disease (36) and in 28% of patients with pathologic N1 disease (13). Clinically uninvolved areas of the neck have been reported to harbor foci of cancer with extracapsular extension in 39% of patients with unknown primary cancer (17). These high rates of extracapsular extension are reflective of the findings in patients with known primary tumors (64). The addition of radiation therapy reduces the risk for neck failure (65). Patients with unknown primary cancer and multiple nodes or extracapsular spread, therefore, merit the addition of radiation therapy to control their neck disease and to improve survival.

The third issue to be addressed in considering surgery alone to treat SCC of unknown primary tumor is the risk for missing a subclinical primary tumor in the head and neck. Though omission of radiation therapy often has been assumed to result in an increased risk for manifesting a head and neck primary tumor in follow-up, the available data do not support this. Fu (66) compared series using surgery alone to series using surgery plus ipsilateral radiation therapy and to those using surgery plus bilateral radiation therapy. She found a 16% incidence of late primary tumors presenting above the clavicles in the surgery-alone group versus a 9% and a 10% incidence, respectively, in the other groups. These data would suggest that mucosal radiation therapy would be required in some 14 patients to prevent one mucosal primary tumor. Thus, the available data do not support strongly the need for radiation therapy to all head and neck mucosal sites in an effort to reduce the likelihood that a head and neck primary tumor will present later. However, when radiation therapy is indicated for control of neck disease in patients with unknown primary SCC, the neck portals will incidentally include a significant portion of the oropharynx and a portion of the nasopharynx, thereby providing some therapy to these areas. This is discussed later (see "Radiation Therapy Technique"). Specific efforts to enlarge the field and cover all mucosal sites are probably not warranted.

The other choice in single-modality therapy in these patients is radiation therapy alone. The University of Florida has reported neck control rates of 92% and 91%, respectively, whether radiation alone or radiation therapy plus neck dissection is used for cervical metastases less than 3 cm in diameter (67). The University of Virginia, however, showed increased neck control when combined-modality therapy is used even for N1 neck disease, although the differences did not reach statistical significance (68). Neither of these series focused on cervical metastases from unknown primary cancers, and the use of radiation alone to treat SCC of unknown primary tumor is biased by inclusion of patients in whom nodes were not assessable (NX) at the time of radiation therapy due to previous node biopsies. Thus, information on the treatment of stage III SCC of unknown primary tumor using radiation alone is limited, and the potential impact of previous node biopsy in these patients may influence reported results.

Surgery for squamous cell metastases to the neck should include a comprehensive neck dissection (levels I to V) in most cases. The choice of whether this dissection is radical or modified is left to the surgeon's discretion, but, in most neck dissections, the spinal accessory nerve can be spared without compromising neck control (11). Other modifications, such as sparing the sternocleidomastoid muscle or internal jugular vein, can be more challenging technically and may be riskier oncologically. For N1 disease in the upper neck, a supraomohyoid neck dissection may be considered in selected patients.

With pathologic findings obtained at surgery, advice regarding the need for radiation therapy can be given to the patient. Extracapsular spread or multiple positive nodes require radiation therapy for neck control. Absence of these findings leads us to conclude that radiation therapy is not essential for neck control but may be used in selected patients for its association with fewer late mucosal primary tumors. This decision must be made by the well-informed patient, taking into account the patient's age and reliability for follow-up.

RADIATION DOSE AND TECHNIQUE

Comprehensive Irradiation

We recognize the controversy that exists with regard to radiating the necks alone versus the necks plus the potential mucosal primary sites. In this section we do not declare a right or wrong approach, but merely describe the available techniques and doses. A further discussion about technique appears at the end of this chapter (see "Radiation Therapy Technique").

The standard technique for comprehensive nodal irradiation is opposed lateral fields matched to anterior yoke field (to include the low neck and supraclavicular fossae). These portals allow inclusion of potential mucosal primary tumor sites, with little additional technical difficulty. Our protocol for such patients is to begin with opposed lateral fields shaped to include the upper jugular, subdigastric, midjugular, and posterior cervical lymph nodes and the appropriate potential primary tumor sites (with or without the nasopharynx, depending on nodal presentation). Then these fields are matched with a single anterior yoke field encompassing the lower jugular nodes bilaterally and the bilateral low posterior cervical and bilateral supraclavicular lymph nodes. A half-beam block is employed on the yoke field to minimize divergence at the junction. Additionally, a match-line spinal cord block also is added to eliminate the risk for divergent overlap in the spinal cord. Because of the sensitivity of the normal tissues to daily radiation, dose is kept at 180 cGy per day. At 4,500 cGy, full spinal cord blocking is added to the lateral photon fields. Then the nodal volumes underneath the spinal cord block are treated bilaterally with custom electron fields. Both photon fields and each electron field are treated to an additional 900 cGy in 180-cGy fractions, typically employing 6- to 9-MeV electrons for the posterior fields. At 5,040 cGy, a final electron boost to previous sites of gross adenopathy is designed and carried to between

5,580 and 5,940 cGy, depending on previous extent of disease. The University of Florida (42) advocates slightly higher doses: 5,500 to 6,000 cGy to the nodal areas and aerodigestive sites, with a 500- to 1,000-cGy boost to any suspected primary tumor site. Their data show a 93% mucosal control rate (13 of 14 patients) with 5,500 to 6,000 cGy. However, the control rate for 5,000 to 5,500 cGy was 89% (8 of 9 patients). A falloff in mucosal control appears to occur for doses of less than 5,000 cGy to 81% (13 of 16) (42). Wang (69) advocates 5,000 cGy, with an additional boost of 1,500 cGy if a primary lesion is detected. He makes the important point that serial examinations of the entire aerodigestive mucosa must be made during the initial 2,000 cGy to attempt to identify an area of mucosal inflammation, which might indicate an occult primary lesion.

Limited Radiotherapy

Although the comprehensive irradiation of both necks and the potential mucosal primary sites has been widely practiced, the use of more limited radiotherapy fields has been evaluated. In an effort to reduce the impact of radiotherapy, modifications have included bilateral radiotherapy with the reduction of mucosal site irradiation. Other options include unilateral radiotherapy with or without unilateral mucosal irradiation. The improvements in endoscopic evaluation, diagnostic imaging, and metabolic imaging should make the detection of a primary tumor increasingly likely and should enhance the safety of omitting potential mucosal sites from the field of radiation therapy.

Inclusion of Potential Aerodigestive Tract Potential Primary Sites

If radiotherapy were effective in reducing the emergence of mucosal primaries, one would expect this to be demonstrated when comparing patients undergoing surgery alone to those undergoing surgery and radiotherapy. The meta-analysis described previously noted a statistically significant reduction in mucosal primaries from 16% in the surgery alone group to 10% in those treated with surgery and radiotherapy (66). This modest effect must be weighed against the impact of radiotherapy.

The potential mucosal primary tumor sites in the upper aerodigestive tract are anatomically quite disparate (nasopharynx, tonsillar fossae, base of tongue, supraglottic larynx, and hypopharynx), and their uniform inclusion in radiation portals entails a large volume of sensitive normal tissues. Such comprehensive therapeutic portals produce a large-volume mucositis acutely during treatment and result in the likely destruction of the bulk of salivary gland tissue, with the consequence of a permanent xerostomia. Less common potential complications of aerodigestive tract irradiation include laryngeal edema, mandibular radionecrosis, masseter fibrosis, and temporomandibular joint dysfunction.

A review of the typical sites of presentation of late mucosal primary disease can support the elimination of specific mucosal sites from inclusion in radiation portals. In the M. D. Anderson Cancer Center series (38), 21 of 104 patients (20%) managed with surgery alone subsequently manifested a primary lesion. However, only 2 of the 21 metachronous primary tumors were found in the nasopharynx, whereas the overwhelming majority (16 of 21) was found to arise in the tonsil, base of tongue, or hypopharynx. Thus, depending on the nodal location, the nasopharynx may not need to be included in the radiation portal. The oropharynx, on the other hand, would appear to merit inclusion within the radiation portals when radiation is utilized in the neck. The tonsillectomy data alluded to previously in this chapter (49,51,54) also support inclusion of at least a portion of the oropharynx.

Studies comparing variations in the extent of radiotherapy reveal conflicting data. The Princess Margaret Hospital has reported on 144 patients with unknown primary carcinoma of whom 85 received radiotherapy to nodal tissue alone whereas 59 underwent nodal and mucosal radiotherapy. Head and neck mucosal disease presented in 7% of those undergoing radiotherapy to nodal tissue alone but in 2% of those receiving nodal and mucosal radiotherapy (18). Conversely, data from Loyola University has compared bilateral radiotherapy including mucosal sites to unilateral radiotherapy. Of 36 patients treated with bilateral radiotherapy, 3 (8%) developed a subsequent primary whereas 7 (44%) of 16 in the unilateral group revealed a mucosal primary in follow-up (70). Including these results along with 12 other case series, one finds that mucosal primaries are detected in 5% to 44% (median 8%) of cases undergoing unilateral radiotherapy and in 2% to 13% (median 9.5%) of cases undergoing bilateral radiotherapy (71). Thus, the impact of radiotherapy portal selection on the likelihood of presentation of a late mucosal primary is not clearly defined in the literature. Furthermore, given the tendency of these patients to develop metachronous head and neck primary cancers, it is absolutely unclear whether these primaries are new or are related to the prior presentation. This factor significantly compromises the analysis.

When considering the use of radiotherapy to prevent the presentation of a late mucosal primary, it cannot be shown to benefit the majority of patients (i.e., the majority would not develop a primary tumor if simply observed). Thus, considering the morbidity (both acute and late) of full aerodigestive tract irradiation and considering the anatomic primary tumor site data noted above, individualization of therapeutic volumes should be possible, thus limiting toxicity. Conversely, cancers of the nasopharynx very rarely spread to either midjugular or lower jugular nodes. Patients presenting with adenopathy at these sites who have no clinically or radiologically suspicious findings in the nasopharynx can certainly be treated without inclusion of the nasopharynx.

Ipsilateral versus Bilateral Radiation Therapy

The limitation of radiotherapy to ipsilateral portals provides the benefits of combined modality therapy in the clinically positive neck while eliminating the impact of radiotherapy on the contralateral neck and the majority of aerodigestive mucosa. The use of unilateral radiotherapy has been shown to provide equivalent control in the treated neck. The impact of this approach on the possible emergence of a mucosal primary is discussed above. The choice of unilateral over bilateral radiotherapy may reduce the disease control rates in the contralateral neck. Overall disease control and survival have also been compared using these modalities of radiotherapy.

Similar to the assessment of the effects of radiotherapy on mucosal disease, evaluating the impact of radiotherapy on the contralateral neck may involve a comparison of patients treated with surgery alone and those undergoing surgery and radiotherapy. In a series of 164 patients from M. D. Anderson Cancer Center with ipsilateral neck disease, metachronous recurrence in the contralateral neck area was a significant problem when radiotherapy was not used. Surgery alone resulted in a 16% failure rate (16 of 97 patients), compared with 0% after combined-modality treatment (0 of 28) and 0% in patients with radiation alone (0 of 39) (13).

When unilateral radiotherapy was compared with bilateral radiotherapy in a series from Loyola University, contralateral failure was significantly more common in patients receiving unilateral radiotherapy, 44% versus 14% (70). No differences in survival were noted between the two groups. A series of 352 patients over a 20-year period has been reported by the Danish Society of Head and Neck Oncology (72). Although the majority of patients were treated using bilateral radiotherapy, 10% of cases were treated by unilateral radiotherapy. Five-year disease control was significantly better in the bilateral radiotherapy group (51%) than the unilateral group (27%). Similar differences in survival were reported, 45% and 28% respectively, but did not reach significance ($p = 0.1$).

No randomized series and few balanced case series have been reported that compare bilateral and unilateral radiotherapy. The above data would suggest a worse outcome with respect to contralateral metastases and disease control when unilateral radiotherapy is utilized.

A recent review reported the neck relapse rate to be 31% to 63% (median 52%) when unilateral radiotherapy was used and 8% to 48% (median 19%) when comprehensive radiotherapy was used (71). This same review reported overall survival to be 22% to 41% (median 37%) with unilateral radiotherapy and 34% to 63% (median 50%) with bilateral therapy (71). Although these data cannot uncover biases that may have led to the selection of particular radiotherapy approaches, they would appear to support bilateral fields when radiotherapy is utilized in squamous carcinoma of unknown primary.

RADIATION THERAPY AFTER NODE BIOPSY

Support has been shown for the use of radiation therapy after excisional node biopsy without a formal (or even limited) neck dissection. A retrospective review of patients treated at the University of Florida has reported a 95% control rate in the treated neck (73). These 41 patients included 22 with unknown primary tumors. The patients were mostly N1 and N2a before node biopsy and had no evidence of disease after excision. Median radiation therapy dose was 6,600 cGy in this heterogeneous group. These data lend support to the use of radiation therapy alone in a patient who has no palpable adenopathy after undergoing previous node biopsy for metastatic SCC. The radiation dose required may need to be increased in these cases. Our recommendation usually is to proceed with comprehensive neck dissection and determine radiotherapy dosing based on the final pathologic findings in the neck. As noted earlier, favorable pathologic findings might allow the avoidance of radiation therapy, but this decision becomes much more difficult when a previous surgeon has violated the neck.

Stage IV

Stage IV SCC of unknown primary tumor is found in a broad collection of patients, from those with a single mass 3 to 6 cm (N2a), to those with multiple nodes (N2b or N2c), to those with massive adenopathy (N3), to those with distant metastases at presentation. All patients who are stage IV due to neck disease should receive combined-modality treatment, whereas those with distant metastases at presentation warrant consideration for palliative treatment.

N2 and N3 diseases warrant a comprehensive neck dissection in almost all cases. Though sparing the spinal accessory may be possible in these patients, many will require radical neck dissections. Extensions of the neck dissection to include overlying skin, digastric muscle, hypoglossal nerve, vagus nerve, and even carotid artery may be needed in patients with N3 disease.

Radiation therapy may be given before or after surgery. However, when surgery is planned from the outset, a theoretical advantage is found in performing surgery first. In this way, pathologic findings from surgery can be considered and addressed in radiation therapy planning and administration.

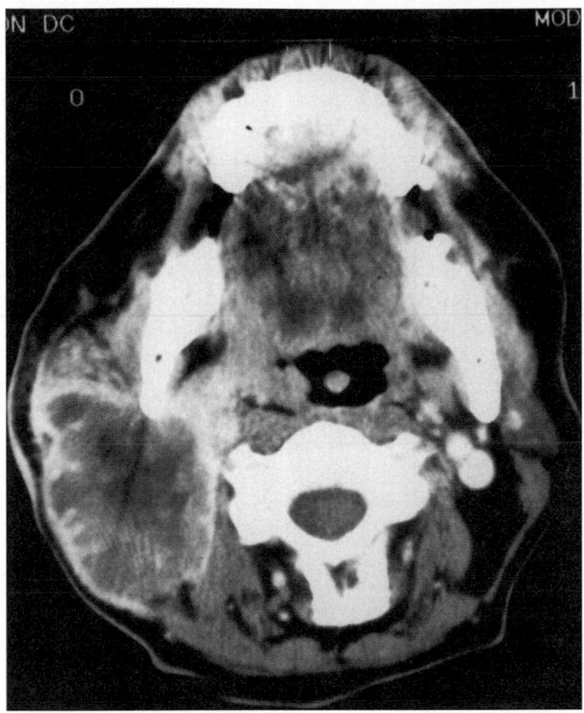

Figure 15.5 T0N3M0 squamous cell carcinoma. Patient refused surgical intervention. Tumor was treated with concomitant cisplatin and radiation therapy, with partial response.

This consideration may influence total dose required and may direct areas of the neck for treatment boosts.

Neck disease may be deemed unresectable, owing to its relationship to the carotid artery; invasion of deep muscles of the neck, brachial plexus, and visceral structures; or extension to high retropharyngeal nodes (Fig. 15.5). In these cases, chemotherapy or radiation therapy may be used to reduce neck disease. Borderline resectable lesions may be rendered resectable by such an approach, but the extent of surgery required after such treatment is not defined clearly.

The use of chemotherapy in combination with radiation therapy (either sequentially or concomitantly) has been advocated for advanced neck squamous cell metastases of unknown primary tumor. This protocol has been reported to result in increased disease control and survival, but the comparison group received predominantly radiation therapy alone rather than combined-modality therapy, as would be suggested in N2 and N3 neck disease (64).

When metastatic disease to distant sites is found at presentation, treatment should be considered palliative. The role for aggressive treatment to the neck in these cases must be individualized. The emotional and physical impact of uncontrolled neck disease must be considered in recommending treatment to these patients. If neck disease is resectable and the metastatic disease burden is minimal, neck dissection and even adjuvant radiation therapy may be indicated. Treatment of the neck may improve quality of life for these patients, but decisions should be balanced against the short overall survival expected in this subgroup.

Results

NECK CONTROL

Control of neck disease is the primary determinant of survival in many head and neck cancers and, in unknown primary cancer, it is even more central to disease control, as usually it is the only focus of disease at presentation. Neck control has been reported to be 75% to 87% in patients with clinical N1 disease using surgery alone (14,16,74) and 82% to 88% in patients receiving combined surgery and radiation therapy (36,40). Excellent control also has been reported for N1 disease using radiation therapy alone, but, as indicated earlier, these data are influenced by the inclusion of patients having undergone previous excisional node biopsies (42). Thus, for N1 disease, surgery alone and combined-modality therapy appear equivalent. The finding that, in 3 neck failures of 21 clinical N1 necks treated, 2 had been upstaged pathologically to N2b (36; and unpublished data) lends support to the use of neck dissection first, followed by radiation therapy as indicated by the pathologic assessment of the neck. For N2 disease, neck control using neck dissection and radiation therapy is 70% to 94%; control of N3 disease is 50% to 69% (36,40,42) using surgery and radiation therapy, a significant improvement over previous results using surgery alone (36).

APPEARANCE OF A PRIMARY LESION

Appearance of a primary lesion in the head and neck after treatment for SCC of unknown primary tumor can be anticipated in 5% to 15% of patients (13,18,19,36,42). Finding statistical evidence that the use of radiation therapy is effective in preventing the appearance of mucosal primary tumors is difficult. When Fu (66) combined results from multiple series, she found head and neck primary tumors in 33 of 211 (16%) treated with surgery alone and in 63 of 620 (10%) treated with surgery and bilateral neck irradiation. Chi-square testing reveals a significant difference here ($p = 0.043$) but, as noted previously, some 14 patients at risk would need to be treated with radiation therapy to prevent one additional primary cancer. The comparison of unilateral and bilateral radiotherapy reported in the recent review by Nieder et al. (71) found considerable variation in the incidence of late primary disease in patients in that mucosal primaries were shown in 5% to 44% of patients undergoing unilateral versus 2% to 13% for comprehensive radiotherapy. However, the median incidence was similar at 8% and 9.5%, respectively. Also, as mentioned earlier, it is impossible to differentiate the true primary versus a second primary cancer. Finally, modern examination and imaging should significantly enhance the detection of a primary, making it potentially safer to exclude mucosal sites from the fields of radiation therapy.

A relationship between radiation dose and the likelihood of primary tumor development also has been suggested. Primary lesions presented in 19% when less than 5,000 cGy was given, 11% when 5,000 to 5,500 cGy was used, and 7% when the dose was more than 5,500 cGy (42). However, this trend did not reach statistical significance, owing to small patient numbers. Thus, these results support the use of radiation therapy to reduce the incidence of primary lesions in the head and neck, but the data are not so compelling that the side effects of radiation therapy should be overlooked. The low rate of primary tumors in the surgery-alone group allows for consideration of withholding radiation therapy in selected patients. The use of unilateral radiotherapy has some support in the literature with respect to primary disease, but the data on contralateral neck failure remains of concern (70). Therefore, bilateral neck radiation therapy is preferred.

DISTANT METASTASES

Distant metastases occur in 13% to 33% of patients with SCC from an unknown primary tumor (13,18,36). Even patients with N1 disease have a 14% incidence of distant failure (B. J. Davidson, unpublished data). Two of three patients with distant metastases will have failed treatment in the head and neck (18), but even that group of patients with control of disease in the head and neck has a small risk for developing distant metastases (36). Median survival in patients identified with distant metastases is 4 to 6 months.

SURVIVAL

Overall survival at 5 years from SCC of unknown primary tumor ranges from 19% to 55% (13,17,18,36,40). When neck dissection and radiation therapy are used, this range is 35% to 63% (13,17,39). The use of radiation as the initial treatment modality has been reported from the Princess Margaret Hospital, with overall 5-year survival of 41%, despite the fact that 47% of patients so treated experienced failure within the treated neck (18). Whether the neck alone or the neck and potential primary tumor sites are included in the radiation portal does not appear to influence overall survival (18,41). The disease-specific survival ranges from 45% to 75% (13,36,40,41). Regardless of the treatment chosen, the factor that appears most strongly to predict survival is N stage (13,18,36,40). Survival for NX to N1 disease is 62% to 86% (13,36,40). For N2 disease, survival is 40% to 50% (36,40,41). For N3 disease, survival is 19% to 38% (36,40,41). Other factors that appear to predict survival are complete resection (36), complete response after radiation therapy (41), and radiation therapy dose of more than 5,000 cGy (18). Presentation of a primary tumor during follow-up has been correlated with worse survival in multivariate analyses (36,41). This finding may be related to the previous use of radiation therapy and the resulting compromise in treatment options available for these patients. Not all series include patients who present with supraclavicular metastases, but, for those that do, this is shown to be a very poor prognostic category, with 5-year survival of less than 10% (19).

FUNCTIONAL RESULTS AND QUALITY OF LIFE

Function and quality-of-life factors in patients with SCC of unknown primary tumor are relevant to two main issues: the impact of neck dissection and the effects of radiation therapy. The absence of a primary lesion produces a corresponding absence of functional morbidity related to resection of an upper aerodigestive site. Radiation consequences in this group of patients are no different from those for head and neck cancer in general and depend on the choice of treatment portals. Chemotherapy in these patients remains experimental, and little available information addresses the consequences of chemotherapy in this population of patients.

The impact of standard radical neck dissection is primarily on shoulder function. Resection of the sternocleidomastoid muscle causes a cosmetic defect in the operated neck, and whereas resection of the internal jugular vein and cervical lymphatics may cause facial edema that is aggravated by radiation therapy, these effects usually are temporary and of little functional significance unless symptomatic laryngeal edema develops. Resection of the spinal accessory nerve, however, results in loss of trapezius muscle innervation. This leads to limitation of rotation of the scapula, abduction of the shoulder, and shoulder flexion. Patients develop drooping of the involved shoulder and complain of stiffness and dull pain. These findings are termed the *shoulder syndrome.* Evidence of shoulder dysfunction can be seen in almost all patients who have undergone radical neck dissection, and approximately 60% complain of moderate to severe pain in reaching above the level of the shoulder or lifting (12). This limitation results in moderate to severe impairment in strength and range of motion in 100% of these patients (75).

With the advent of more evidence recently that sparing of the spinal accessory nerve does not have an impact on survival, improvements in shoulder morbidity for this population of patients is anticipated. However, preservation of the nerve during surgery does not ensure perfect function, as dissection requires manipulation that can affect the blood supply to the nerve or can result in direct injury to the nerve, owing to stretching. The functional outcomes research in this group of patients shows moderate to severe pain in 35% (12) with shoulder rotation or lifting. Moderate to severe limits on strength and range of motion have been shown in 65% (75) at 16 weeks after surgery. However, longer-term follow-up has shown improvements in electrodiagnostic testing and middle trapezius muscle strength (but not range of motion or upper trapezius strength) for up to 1 year in patients undergoing modified or selective neck dissections (76).

The finding of significant shoulder dysfunction when the spinal accessory nerve is spared may be explained by onset of a secondary syndrome in these patients: adhesive capsulitis (77). This syndrome is associated with limits of shoulder abduction and forward flexion but also includes loss of external and internal rotation and pain in lying on the affected side. The pathology here involves capsular thickening, loss of synovial fluid, and synovial adhesions. Patten and Hillel (77) described a series of neck dissection patients in whom the symptoms of adhesive capsulitis were present at 1 month after surgery and were the predominant findings by 12 months. The patients also showed persistent shoulder symptoms despite return of electromyographic stimulation of the spinal accessory nerve in perhaps 90% of them. Immobilization is believed to play a major role in the development of adhesive capsulitis. As efforts at prevention are thought to be critical, owing to a lack of effective treatment options (77), patient education is essential, and formal physical therapy should be considered in all patients undergoing neck dissection.

The lasting effects of radiation therapy include loss of taste and salivary function, loss of hair follicles in the treated field, and fibrosis of connective tissue. Loss of salivary function usually is the most troublesome side effect. This loss begins early in the course of radiation therapy and, after 6 weeks of conventional treatment, resting and stimulated salivary flow has dropped to 0% to 20% of pretreatment levels (78). Serous acinar cells appear to be the most vulnerable, and the resulting changes in salivary composition include increased viscosity; decreased pH; increased sodium, chloride, calcium, magnesium, and protein; and decreased bicarbonate and immunoglobulin A (IgA) (79). Xerostomia requires some dietary change in most patients.

Xerostomia appears to be related to radiation therapy dose, but dose levels in excess of 50 Gy are associated with severe xerostomia and little recovery over time in the majority of patients (80). In addition to dose, the other important factor in predicting xerostomia is the amount of parotid tissue irradiated (78,81). Unilateral radiation therapy results in slight to no oral dryness in most patients (80). Omission of the nasopharynx from the field and use of fields that are tailored to the necks should also decrease the dose to the major and minor salivary gland tissue, which should help reduce xerostomia.

The consequences of xerostomia include radiation-induced dental caries, which appears to be the result of alterations in oral microflora and reduced salivary pH. These dental caries combined with microvascular alterations in the mandible can result in development of osteonecrosis. Osteonecrosis occurs in 4% to 22% of patients receiving radiation therapy for head and neck cancer (79). Osteonecrosis may occur in any patient after radiation therapy, although most cases occur in patients who have undergone dental extractions after treatment.

Most patients complain of taste alterations during the acute phases of radiation therapy; many report slow improvement over time. Long-term quality-of-life information describes significant taste alterations in approximately 20% of patients (82). However, separating taste alterations caused by direct damage from those symptoms secondary to xerostomia often is difficult.

Fibrosis of submucosal and cervical soft tissues occurs in many patients after radiation therapy. Submucosal fibrosis manifests as mucosal pallor, thinning, and loss of pliability. These effects usually are asymptomatic and require no intervention. Ulceration and necrosis may occur and can result in bone exposure, thus raising the risk for osteonecrosis. Fibrosis of cervical soft tissues may cause similar thinning and loss of pliability. McGuirt et al. (83) have suggested an increased risk for carotid artery atherosclerosis in irradiated patients, presumably due to endothelial proliferation and collagen deposition.

Complications

Many reports of complication rates after neck dissection are confounded by the inclusion of patients having simultaneous surgery on a primary lesion. A Medline search of articles published between 1966 and 1996 reveals only one study reporting all complications in patients undergoing isolated neck dissections. Nonfatal complications were seen in 50 of 132 patients (38%), and perioperative mortality was observed in 6 of 132 (5%). The most common complications were seromas, wound infections, and skin necrosis, occurring in 24% of all patients (84). Other complications include marginal mandibular nerve weakness, chyle leaks, and hematomas. Vagal and hypoglossal nerve injuries seldom are seen after neck dissection. These structures may require resection, however, in extended radical neck dissections when tumor infiltration is noted.

Complications of radiation therapy may include dental caries and osteoradionecrosis (noted earlier). Other complications after radiation therapy to the neck include laryngeal edema and hypothyroidism. Spinal cord necrosis and transverse myelitis are very rare but potentially lethal complications of neck irradiation. If the necks are treated alone, then the larynx will be blocked and laryngeal edema will not occur.

MANAGEMENT OF RECURRENCE

Recurrence after treatment of SCC of unknown primary tumor may include several manifestations of disease. A primary tumor noted after treatment, a second primary tumor, neck recurrence, or contralateral neck recurrences all require roughly the same decision process. Distant metastases require an approach that is palliative.

When recurrence occurs at a mucosal site in the head and neck, it may represent the initial occult primary tumor or a second primary tumor. If radiation was not given during treatment of the initial neck disease, likelihood of controlling the mucosal recurrence is greater than if this modality has been used. If radiation therapy has been used, the patients should be assessed for possible resection. Though margins of less than 1 cm may be adequate in nonirradiated tissue, the irradiated patient may have insidious spread of mucosal or submucosal disease, and surgical resection may require significantly more than 1-cm margins. This fact may influence the impact of resection on quality of life and on the patient's decision as to whether surgery is acceptable. The preparation for reconstruction should take these potentially extended margins into account. Contralateral neck recurrence merits neck dissection in resectable patients. Once again, previous radiation therapy may influence the pattern of spread of this recurrent neck disease.

Ipsilateral neck recurrence after neck dissection is rarely treatable by further surgery. This type of recurrence and that of distant metastases likely will require consideration of palliative treatment. Response rates for disease that recurs within an irradiated field are lower than those for isolated distant metastases. The reason for this effect is that isolated distant metastases may have been seeded before locoregional treatment and would be less likely to be derived from clones that are radioresistant.

SPECIAL ISSUES

Adenocarcinoma

When adenocarcinoma occurs in the neck from an unknown primary tumor, the results of treatment are far less favorable than those for squamous carcinoma. A large series treated at the M. D. Anderson Cancer Center has been reported. Of these 223 patients, 76% presented with nodes in the supraclavicular fossa, and metastatic disease outside of the neck was present in 86% on referral (85). Survival was less than 10% at 5 years, and the various combinations of surgery, radiation therapy, and chemotherapy used did not reveal any one treatment modality to be superior. Increased survival was noted for patients with unilateral neck disease and for those with nodes above the level of the cricoid. However, even those patients with superior neck nodes were found to have only a 20% 5-year survival.

Current recommendations regarding workup of the patient with unknown primary adenocarcinoma do not favor an exhaustive search for a primary lesion. Recommendations are for a chemistry profile, complete blood cell count, prostate-specific antigen in men, chest radiograph, mammography in women, and a CT of the abdomen in addition to investigation of any symptoms (86). An assessment of the biopsy specimen appears to be one of the most useful efforts. Poorly differentiated tumors may represent a treatable malignancy, such as lymphoma or a germ-cell tumor. If fine-needle biopsy has been performed and any question exists concerning the pathology, panendoscopy followed by excisional biopsy is suggested.

Malignant Melanoma

Approximately 4% of all cases of malignant melanoma present with an unidentified primary tumor site. As 20% of all malignant melanomas occur in the head and neck, the head and neck cancer specialist should be familiar with malignant melanoma of unknown primary tumor. The clinical course of 46 patients with malignant melanomas was reviewed (87). These patients presented with cervical or parotid masses. After surgical resection by parotidectomy or neck dissection, approximately two thirds had adjuvant treatment with radiation therapy, chemotherapy, or immunotherapy. Survival in this group of patients was 56% at 5 years and did not appear to be related significantly to extent of surgical treatment or to the use of adjuvant therapy. Number of positive lymph nodes was correlated with the risk for distant metastases but not with survival in this series. Survival in this series of stage II melanoma patients of unknown primary tumor appears more favorable than do those with a known primary tumor and neck disease. Reasons for this outcome may include differences in host immune response, leading to spontaneous regression of the primary tumor, and an antitumor response, influencing control of the cervical metastases.

RADIOLOGIC IMAGING CONCERNS: THE UNKNOWN PRIMARY

Bernard B. O'Malley and Suresh K. Mukherji

Imaging of the head and neck to locate an occult primary SCC of the aerodigestive tract is requested much less often now with the advancement of office instrumentation. Very necrotic lymph nodes can also be seen in metastatic thyroid cancers. Unilateral cystic lesions in the anterior neck when solitary are often presumed to be a swollen branchial cleft cyst. Endoscopy and ipsilateral tonsillectomy are advocated by some for this imaging finding (88). Cross-sectional imaging occasionally reveals areas suspicious enough to warrant directed biopsy or repeat biopsy (Fig. 15.6). Laser-induced fluorescence (LIF) has been shown to be twice as productive as imaging in locating potential sites for biopsy (89).

Either CT or MRI may be used to evaluate potential locations for unknown primary tumors. The additive yield of performing both studies is small and likely does not warrant the cost. The intent of the study should be to increase the diagnostic yield of endoscopic biopsies by identifying areas of asymmetric soft tissue. The most common reported locations are the nasopharynx (Fig. 15.7), tonsil (Fig. 15.8), tongue base, and pyriform sinus. In our experience, the most common locations of endoscopically occult lesions evaluated by experienced clinicians tend to be in the far lateral glossotonsillar sulcus/lateral tongue base area and pyriform sinus. All focal areas of asymmetric soft tissue thickening should be considered suspicious.

Identifying the location of the metastatic lymph nodes can increase the degree of suspicion of asymmetric areas. Occult nasopharyngeal carcinomas should be expected if patients have positive retropharyngeal lymph nodes or bilateral lymph nodes, especially levels IV and V (90). An occult tumor in the glossotonsillar sulcus/lateral tongue base region or pyriform sinus should be considered if the ipsilateral level II and III lymph nodes are involved. The possibility of an ipsilateral pyriform sinus should be strongly considered if there is an additional retropharyngeal lymph node involved.

Positron emission tomography imaging using FDG has been shown to improve the diagnostic yield of identifying unknown primary tumors (91,92). We feel that best use of PET is to improve the diagnostic yield of speculative biopsies (93). This can be accomplished by obtaining more tissue from sites that are known to harbor unknown primary tumors that demonstrate focally increased uptake compared with the contralateral side. Positron emission tomography will not be able to identify all unknown primary tumors but studies reported and increase in the diagnostic yield by 30% to 50% (94). The best results of PET in this specific clinical scenario will be obtained if it is performed prior to aggressive biopsies, and postsurgical inflammation has the potential to increase the false-positive rate (95). Imaging with more conventional nuclear agents such as Tl-201 with SPECT has also been shown to be productive in the setting of SCC of unknown primary (96).

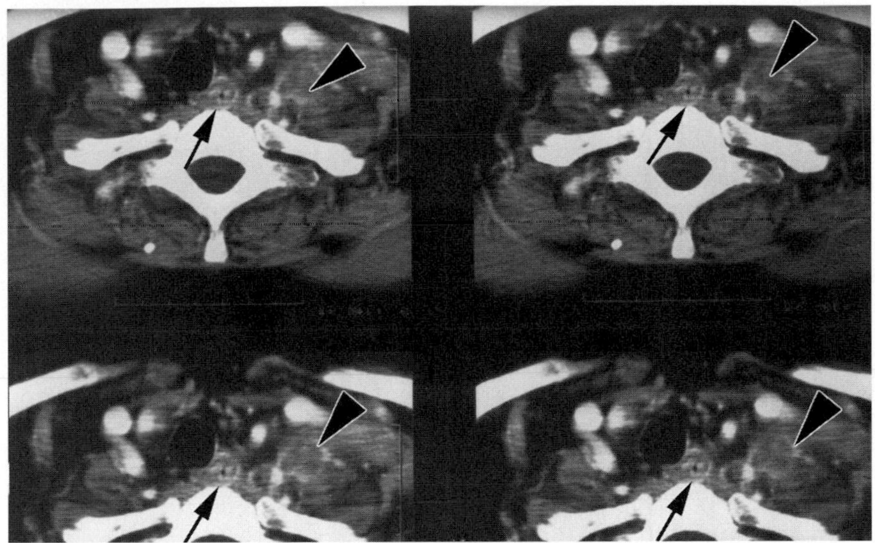

Figure 15.6 Serial enhanced axial computed tomographic images at the thoracic inlet. Images show left supraclavicular (Virchow) adenopathy (*arrowheads*) related to an occult esophageal squamous cancer (*arrows*).

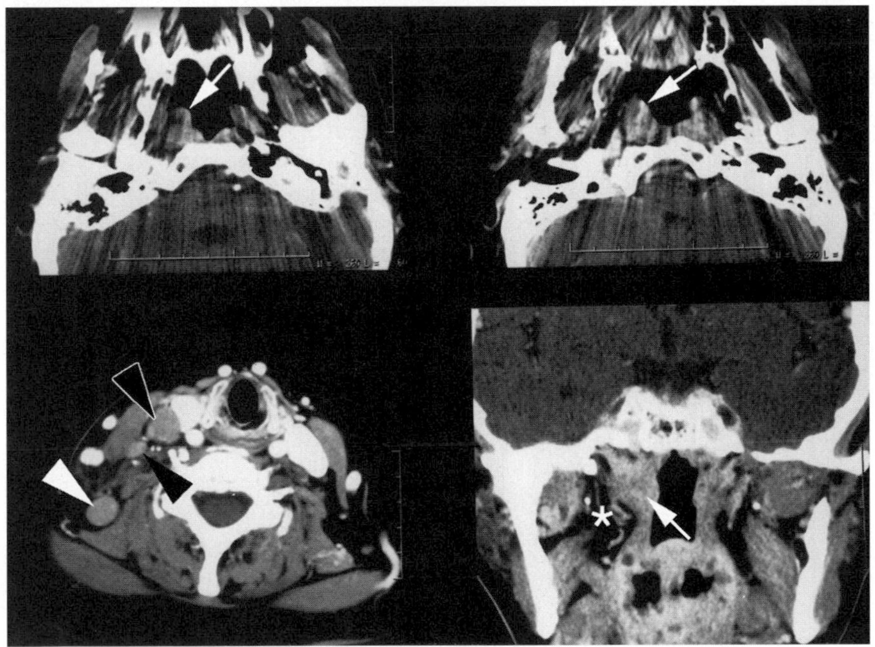

Figure 15.7 Early nasopharyngeal cancer. Enhanced axial computed tomography and direct coronal view (bottom right) show several pathologic right-sided neck nodes (*arrowheads*) in a patient with squamous cell carcinoma of unknown primary. Axial and coronal views show a T1-stage lesion of the right nasopharynx (*arrows*). The parapharyngeal space is normal (*asterisk*).

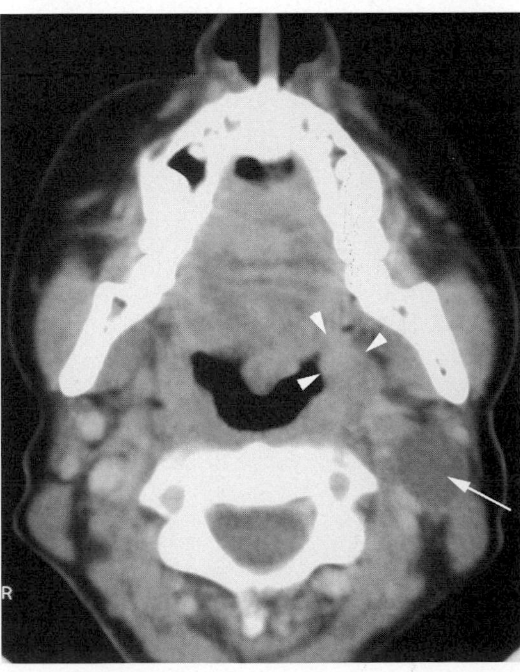

Figure 15.8 Adenopathy from occult tonsil squamous cell carcinoma. Enhanced axial computed tomography scan of the neck at the level of the oropharynx shows the tonsil mass (*arrowheads*) and necrotic lymph node metastasis (*arrow*).

RADIATION THERAPY TECHNIQUE

Louis B. Harrison, Rudolph Woode, and William M. Mendenhall

As outlined in this chapter, there is some controversy as to the optimal fields for radiation therapy in the situation of an unknown primary cancer. If there is no obvious primary site after a diligent search that has included proper radiologic imaging, PET scan, direct laryngoscopy and examination under anesthesia, tonsillectomy (usually), and directed biopsies, then it is our preference to provide radiation therapy to the necks alone, without making a specific effort to irradiate all of the mucosal surfaces of the head and neck. In treating both sides of the neck, including retropharyngeal nodes, a significant portion of the base of tongue, nasopharynx, and tonsil will be in the field. However, the fields are designed to be comprehensive with respect to the neck. By doing this, there will be incidental coverage of these other structures. The larynx and the hypopharynx are blocked. The oropharynx is covered by this approach, as well as a portion of the nasopharynx. If clinically wise in a particular circumstance, the field can be slightly enlarged to include the entire nasopharynx.

The upper neck, including retropharyngeal nodes, is treated with opposed lateral fields. After approximately 4,500 cGy, a spinal cord block is added. The upper neck and retropharyngeal nodes are then treated with 5,400 cGy. At that point, the retropharyngeal nodes can be blocked. The remainder of the upper neck is treated with a total dose of 6,300 cGy. Electrons are used posterior to the block, to complete the treatment to the posterior cervical lymph nodes. On the side of the neck that is involved, those lymph nodes are generally treated with 6,300 cGy. On the contralateral side, those lymph nodes are treated with approximately 5,400 cGy, thereby completing the elective irradiation to the contralateral side.

The upper neck fields are junctioned above the larynx, but below the hyoid bone. The low neck is treated with a single anteroposterior (AP) field, with a block in the upper midline. This block protects the larynx and the spinal cord. Infraclavicular blocks are also added. The fields come low enough to include the insertion of the sternocleidomastoid muscle. We treat this field with 5,000 cGy in 5 weeks, with the dose calculated at the D_{max} point. A point is chosen to represent the level of the low neck nodes. The dose is prescribed at the depth of maximal dose, at that point.

Either cobalt 60 or 6 Mv photons are usually used. If we use 6 Mv photons, we place 5 mm of bolus over the dissected neck.

Case Study

A 52-year-old man presented with a 2-cm left neck mass (Fig. 15.9). He was seen by a local otolaryngologist, who excised a lymph node. Pathology was SCC, metastatic to a lymph node, which was apparently completely excised. At that time, he was referred to us for further evaluation. Complete head and neck examination, CT scan, and PET scan, as well as an examination under anesthesia, failed to reveal any primary site. There was no clear evidence of other disease activity. His PET scan was negative. After much deliberation, and although neck dissection was discussed, we abided by the patient's preference and treated him with external beam irradiation alone.

The initial bilateral opposed fields included the upper neck and retropharyngeal area. As is seen on the simulation film (Fig. 15.9A), a scar was placed on the excision site in the left neck. The patient received 4,500 cGy in 5 weeks, after which a spinal cord block was added. The upper neck and retropharyngeal nodes were treated with 5,400 cGy; at that point, the retropharyngeal nodes were blocked, and both upper necks were treated with 6,300 cGy in 7 weeks. The posterior necks were treated with electron beam. An additional 1,800 cGy was given on the left, bringing the total to 6,300 cGy. An additional 900 cGy was given on the right, bringing the total to 5,400 cGy. Bolus was placed on the scar (5 mm), and the patient was treated with 6 Mv photons.

As can be seen in Figure 15.9A, a portion of the nasopharynx, base of tongue, pharyngeal wall, and tonsil are all in the upper neck field. The larynx/hypopharynx is blocked, both on the lateral and AP fields. Modification of these fields can be made to suit specific circumstances. For example, in a Chinese male with an elevated Epstein-Barr virus titre, one might include the entire nasopharynx. If there is a particular concern about the oropharynx, the field can be a little more generous with respect to the tonsil and anterior base of tongue. These fields are shown to represent guidelines, and we encourage individualization as clinically indicated. This issue continues to evolve.

In Figure 15.9B, the low neck was treated with a single AP field. A total of 5,000 cGy was given in 5 weeks, with a block in the upper midline. There was also an infraclavicular block.

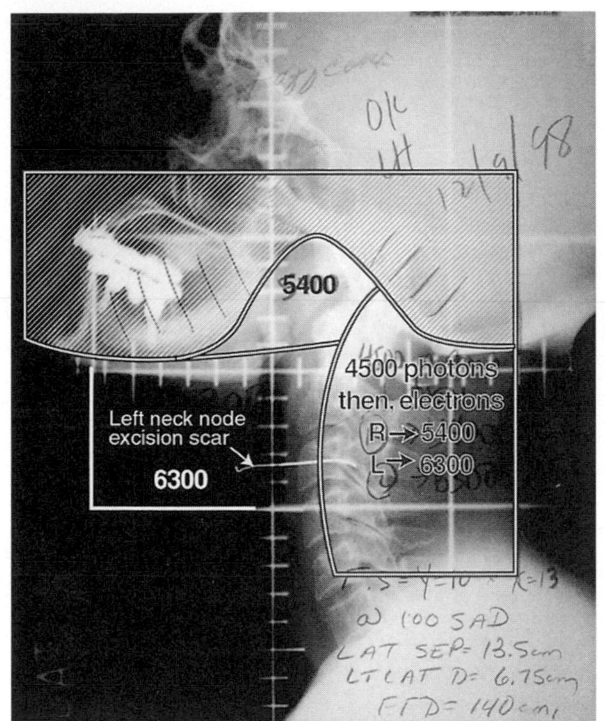

A

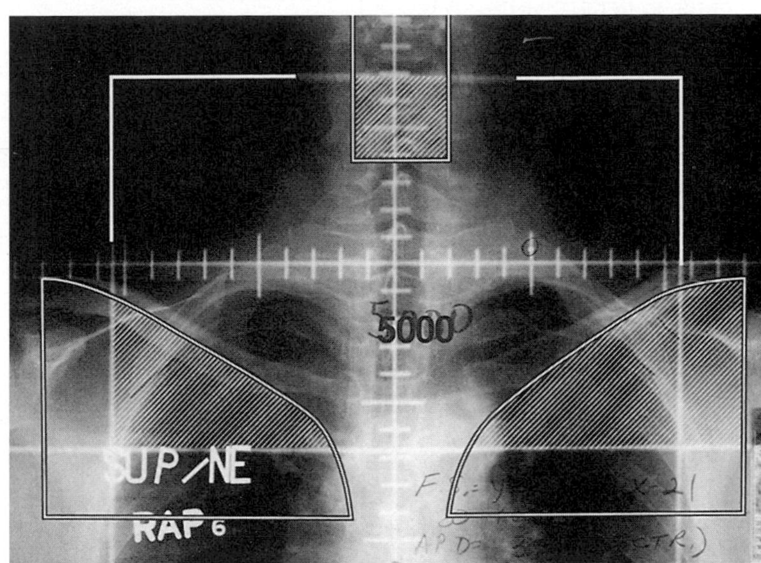

B

Figure 15.9 A 52-year-old man with a 2-cm left neck mass. **A:** A scar is placed on the excision site in the left neck. **B:** The low neck was treated with a single anteroposterior field.

REFERENCES

1. Muir C. Cancer of unknown primary site. *Cancer* 1995;75(suppl 1):353–356.
2. Holmes FF, Fonts TL. Metastatic cancer of unknown primary site. *Cancer* 1970; 26:816–820.
3. Hainsworth JD, Greco FA. Treatment of patients with cancer of an unknown primary site. *N Engl J Med* 1993;329:257–263.
4. Martin H, Morfit HM. Cervical lymph node metastasis as the first symptom of cancer. *Surg Gynecol Obstet* 1944;78:133–159.
5. Jones AS, Cook JA, Phillips DE, et al. Squamous carcinoma presenting as an enlarged cervical lymph node. *Cancer* 1993;72:1756–1761.
6. Comess MS, Beahrs OH, Dockerty MB. Cervical metastases from occult carcinoma. *Surg Gynecol Obstet* 1957;104:607–617.
7. Schuller DE, Platz CE, Krause CJ. Spinal accessory lymph nodes: a prospective study of metastatic involvement. *Laryngoscope* 1978;88:439–449.
8. Davidson BJ, Kulkarny V, Delacure MD, et al. Posterior triangle metastases of squamous cell carcinoma of the upper aerodigestive tract. *Am J Surg* 1993;166: 395–398.
9. Khafif RA, Gelbfish GA, Asase DK, et al. Modified radical neck dissection in cancer of the mouth, pharynx, and larynx. *Head Neck* 1990;12:476–482.
10. Byers RM. Modified neck dissection. *Am J Surg* 1985;150:414–421.
11. Anderson PE, Shah JP, Cambronero E, et al. The role of comprehensive neck dissection with preservation of the spinal accessory nerve in the clinically positive neck. *Am J Surg* 1994;168:499–502.
12. Leipzig B, Suen JY, English JL, et al. Functional evaluation of the spinal accessory nerve after neck dissection. *Am J Surg* 1983;146:526–530.
13. Wang RC, Goepfert H, Barber AE, et al. Unknown primary squamous cell carcinoma metastatic to the neck. *Arch Otolaryngol Head Neck Surg* 1990;116: 1388–1393.
14. Jesse RH, Perez CA, Fletcher GH. Cervical lymph node metastasis: unknown primary cancer. *Cancer* 1973;4:854–859.
15. Leipzig B, Winter ML, Hokanson JA. Cervical metastases of unknown origin. *Laryngoscope* 1981;91:593–598.
16. Nordstrom DG, Tewfik HH, Latourette HB. Cervical metastases from an unknown primary. *Int J Radiat Oncol Biol Phys* 1979;5:73–76.
17. Lefebvre J, CocheDequeant B, Ton Van J, et al. Cervical lymph nodes from an unknown primary tumor in 190 patients. *Am J Surg* 1990;160:443–446.
18. Weir L, Keane T, Cummings B, et al. Radiation treatment of cervical lymph node metastases from an unknown primary: an analysis of outcome by treatment volume and other prognostic factors. *Radiother Oncol* 1995;35:206–211.
19. Glynne Jones RGT, Anand AK, Young TE, et al. Metastatic carcinoma in the cervical lymph nodes from an occult primary: a conservative approach to the role of radiotherapy. *Int J Radiat Oncol Biol Phys* 1990;18:289–294.
20. Hong WK, Lippman SM, Itri LM, et al. Prevention of second primary tumors with isotretinoin in squamous carcinoma of the head and neck. *N Engl J Med* 1990;323:795–801.
21. Benner SE, Pajak TF, Lippman SM, et al. Prevention of second primary tumors with isotretinoin in patients with squamous cell carcinoma of the head and neck: longterm followup. *J Natl Cancer Inst* 1994;86:140–141.
22. Haughey BH, Gates GA, Arfken CL, et al. Metaanalysis of second malignant tumors in head and neck cancer: the case for an endoscopic screening protocol. *Ann Otol Rhinol Laryngol* 1992;101:105–112.
23. Kant JA, Jaffe ES. The interpretation of nonlymphoid elements in lymph node biopsy specimens. In: Jaffe ES, ed. *Surgical pathology of the lymph nodes and related organs.* Philadelphia: WB Saunders, 1985:412–437.
24. Flanagan PM, Roland NJ, Jones AS. Cervical node metastases presenting with features of branchial cysts. *J Laryngol Otol* 1994;108:1068–1071.
25. Gourin CG, Johnson JT. Incidence of unsuspected metastases in lateral cervical cysts. *Laryngoscope* 2000;110:1637–1641.
26. Challis GB, Stam HJ. The spontaneous regression of cancer. *Acta Oncol* 1990; 29:545–550.
27. Mehta FS, Daftary DK, Shroff BC, et al. Clinical and histologic study of oral leukoplakia in relation to habits. *Oral Pathol* 1969;28:372–388.
28. Pindborg JJ, Joist O, Renstrup G, et al. Studies in oral leukoplakia: a preliminary report on the period prevalence of malignant transformation in leukoplakia based on a followup study of 248 patients. *J Am Dent Assoc* 1968;76: 767–771.
29. Minzer HH, Coleman SA, Hopkins KR. Observations on the clinical characteristics of oral lesions showing histologic epithelial dysplasia. *Oral Surg* 1972; 33:389–399.
30. Kusakawa J, Sasaguri Y, Shima I, et al. Expression of matrix metalloproteinase-2 related to lymph node metastasis of oral squamous cell carcinoma. *Am J Clin Pathol* 1993;99:18–23.
31. Miyajima Y, Nakano R, Morimatsu M. Analysis of expression of matrix metalloproteinases 2 and 9 in hypopharyngeal squamous cell carcinoma by *in situ* hybridization. *Ann Otol Rhinol Laryngol* 1995;104:678–684.
32. Gottschlich S, Schuhmacher O, Gorogh T, et al. Analysis of the p53 gene status of lymph node metastasis in the head and neck region in occult primary cancer. *Laryngorhinootologie* 2000;79:434–437.
33. Califano J, Westra WH, Koch W, et al. Unknown primary head and neck squamous cell carcinoma: molecular identification of the site of origin. *J Natl Cancer Inst* 1999;91:599–604.
34. Leibel SA, Scott CB, Mohiuddin M, et al. The effect of local regional control on distant metastatic dissemination in carcinoma of the head and neck: results of an analysis from the RTOG head and neck database. *Int J Radiat Oncol Biol Phys* 1991;21:549–556.
35. Ellis ER, Mendenhall WM, Rao PV, et al. Does node location affect the incidence of distant metastases in head and neck squamous cell carcinoma? *Int J Radiat Oncol Biol Phys* 1989;17:293–297.
36. Davidson BJ, Spiro JH, Patel S, et al. Cervical metastases of occult origin. The impact of combined modality therapy. *Am J Surg* 1994;168:395–399.
37. Spiro RH, DeRose G, Strong EW. Cervical node metastasis of occult origin. *Am J Surg* 1983;146:441–446.
38. Jesse RH, Perez CA, Fletcher GH. Cervical lymph node metastasis of unknown primary cancer. *Cancer* 1973;31:854–859.
39. Bataini JP, Rodriguez J, Jaulerry C, et al. Treatment of metastatic neck nodes secondary to an occult epidermoid carcinoma of the head and neck. *Laryngoscope* 1987;97:1080–1084.
40. Maulard C, Housset M, Brunel P, et al. Postoperative radiation therapy for cervical lymph node metastases from an occult squamous cell carcinoma. *Laryngoscope* 1992;102:884–890.
41. Marcial Vega VA, Cardenes H, Perez CA, et al. Cervical metastases from unknown primaries: radiotherapeutic management and appearance of subsequent primaries. *Int J Radiat Oncol Biol Phys* 1990;19:919–928.
42. Harper CS, Mendenhall WM, Parsons JT, et al. Cancer in neck nodes with unknown primary site: role of mucosal radiotherapy. *Head Neck* 1990;12: 463–469.
43. Neel HB, Taylor WE. New staging system for nasopharyngeal carcinoma. *Arch Otolaryngol Head Neck Surg* 1989;115:1293–1303.
44. Korver KD, Graham SM, Hoffman HT, et al. Liver function studies in the assessment of head and neck cancer patients. *Head Neck* 1995;17:531–534.
45. Dillon WP, Harnsberger HR. The impact of radiologic imaging on staging of cancer in the head and neck. *Semin Oncol* 1991;18:64–79.
46. Stevens MH, Harnsberger HR, Mancuso AA, et al. Computed tomography of cervical lymph nodes. Staging and management of head and neck cancer. *Arch Otolaryngol* 1985;111:735–739.
47. Murakai AS, Mancuso AA, Harnsberger HR. Metastatic cervical adenopathy from tumors of unknown origin: the role of CT. *Radiology* 1984;152:749–753.
48. Lee D, Rostock RA, Harris A, et al. Clinical evaluation of patients with metastatic squamous carcinoma of the neck with occult primary tumor. *South Med J* 1986;79:979–983.
49. Righi P, Sofferman RA. Screening unilateral tonsillectomy in the unknown primary. *Laryngoscope* 1995;105:548–550.
50. McQuone SJ, Eisele DW, Lee D-J, et al. Occult tonsillar carcinoma in the unknown primary. *Laryngoscope* 1998;108:1605–1610.
51. Mendenhall WM, Mancuso AA, Parsons JT, et al. Diagnostic evaluation of squamous cell carcinoma metastatic to cervical lymph nodes from an unknown head and neck primary site. *Head Neck* 1998;20:739–744.
52. Randall DA, Johnstone PAS, Foss RD, et al. Tonsillectomy in diagnosis of the unknown primary tumor of the head and neck. *Otolaryngol Head Neck Surg* 2000;122:52–55.
53. Barrie JR, Knapper WH, Strong EW. Cervical nodal metastases of unknown origin. *Am J Surg* 1970;120:466–470.
54. Koch WM, Bhatti N, Williams MF, et al. Oncologic rationale for bilateral tonsillectomy in head and neck squamous cell carcinoma of unknown primary source. *Otolaryngol Head Neck Surg* 2001;124:331–333.
55. Mukherji SK, Drane WE, Mancuso AA, et al. Occult primary tumors of the head and neck: detection with 2-[F-18] fluoro-2-deoxy-D-glucose SPECT. *Radiology* 1996;199:761–766.
56. Bohuslavizki KH, Klutmann S, Kroger S, et al. FDG PET detection of unknown primary tumors. *J Nucl Med* 2000;41:816–822.
57. Safa AA, Tran LM, Rege S, et al. The role of positron emission tomography in occult primary head and neck cancers. *Cancer J Sci Am* 1999;5:214–218.
58. Aassar OA, Fischbein NJ, Caputo GR, et al. Metastatic head and neck cancer: role and usefulness of FDG PET in locating occult primary tumors. *Radiology* 1999;210:177–181.
59. Greven KM, Keyes JW, Williams DW, et al. Occult primary tumors of the head and neck: lack of benefit from positron emission tomography imaging with 2-[F-18]fluoro-2-deoxy-D-glucose. *Cancer* 1999;86:114–118.
60. Kole AC, Nieweg OE, Pruim J, et al. Detection of unknown occult primary tumors using positron emission tomography. *Cancer* 1998;82:1160–1166.
61. McGuirt WE McCabe BF. Significance of node biopsy before definitive treatment of cervical metastatic carcinoma. *Laryngoscope* 1978;88:594–597.
62. Ellis ER, Mendenhall WM, Rao PV, et al. Incisional or excisional neck node biopsy before definitive radiotherapy, alone or followed by neck dissection. *Head Neck* 1991;13:177–183.
63. Fleming ID, Cooper JS, Henson DE, et al. *AJCC cancer staging manual,* 5th ed. Philadelphia: American Joint Committee on Cancer, Lippincott, 1997.

63a. Greene F, Page D, Fleming I, et al. *AJCC cancer staging manual,* 6th ed. New York: Springer-Verlag, 2002.

64. Johnson JT, Myers EN, Bedetti CD, et al. Cervical lymph node metastasis: incidence and implications of extracapsular spread. *Arch Otolaryngol* 1985;111: 534–537.
65. Huang DT, Johnson CR, Schmidt Ullrich R, et al. Postoperative radiotherapy in head and neck carcinoma with extracapsular lymph node extension and/or positive resection margins: a comparative study. *Int J Radiat Oncol Biol Phys* 1992;23:737–742.
66. Fu KK. Neck node metastases from unknown primary. *Front Radiat Ther Oncol* 1994;28:66–78.

67. Mendenhall WM, Million RR, Cassisi NJ. Squamous cell carcinoma of the head and neck treated with radiation therapy: the role of neck dissection for clinically positive neck nodes. *Int J Radiat Oncol Biol Phys* 1986;12:733–740.
68. Spaulding CA, Hahn SS, Constable WC. The effectiveness of treatment of lymph nodes in cancers of the pyriform sinus and supraglottis. *Int J Radiat Oncol Biol Phys* 1987;13:963–968.
69. Wang CC. Management of squamous cell carcinoma in cervical nodes with an "unknown primary." In: Wang CC, ed. *Radiation therapy for head and neck neoplasms.* Chicago: Yearbook Medical Publishers, 1990:330–339.
70. Reddy SP, Marks JE. Metastatic carcinoma in the cervical lymph nodes from and unknown primary site: results of bilateral neck plus mucosal irradiation vs ipsilateral neck irradiation. *Int J Radiat Oncol Biol Phys* 1997;37:797–802.
71. Nieder C, Gregoire V, Ang KK. Cervical lymph node metastases from occult squamous cell carcinoma: cut down a tree to get an apple? *Int J Radiat Oncol Biol Phys* 2001;50:727–733.
72. Grau C, Johansen LV, Jakobsen J, et al. Cervical lymph node metastases from unknown primary tumors. Results from a national survey by the Danish Society for Head and Neck Oncology. *Radiother Oncol* 2000;55:121–129.
73. Mack Y, Persons JY, Mendenhall WM, et al. Squamous cell carcinoma of the head and neck: management after excisional biopsy of a solitary metastatic neck node. *Int J Radiat Oncol Biol Phys* 1993;25:619–622.
74. Coster JR, Foote RL, Olsen KD, et al. Cervical nodal metastasis of squamous cell carcinoma of unknown origin: indications for withholding radiation therapy. *Int J Radiat Oncol Biol Phys* 1992;23:743–749.
75. Sobol S, Jenson C, Sawyer W, et al. Objective comparison of physical dysfunction after neck dissection. *Am J Surg* 1985;150:503–509.
76. Remmler D, Byers R, Scheetz J, et al. A prospective study of shoulder disability resulting from radical and modified neck dissections. *Head Neck* 1986;8: 280–286.
77. Patten C, Hillel AD. Accessory nerve palsy of adhesive capsulitis? *Arch Otolaryngol Head Neck Surg* 1993;119:215–220.
78. Leslie MD, Dische S. The early changes in salivary gland function during and after radiotherapy given for head and neck cancer. *Radiother Oncol* 1994;30: 26–32.
79. Cooper JS, Fu K, Marks J, et al. Late effects of radiation therapy in the head and neck region. *Int J Radiat Oncol Biol Phys* 1995;31:1141–1164.
80. Franzen L, Funegard U, Ericson T, et al. Parotid gland function during and following radiotherapy of malignancies in the head and neck. *Eur J Cancer* 1992; 28:457–462.
81. Liu RP, Fleming TJ, Toth BB, et al. Salivary flow rates in patients with head and neck cancer 0.5 to 25 years after radiotherapy. *Oral Surg Oral Med Oral Path Oral Radiol Endod* 1990;70:724–729.
82. Bjordal K, Freng A, Thorvik J, et al. Patient self-reported and clinician-rated quality of life in head and neck cancer patients: a cross-sectional study. *Eur J Cancer B Oral Oncol* 1995;31:235–241.
83. McGuirt WF, Feehs RS, Bond G, et al. Irradiation-induced atherosclerosis: a factor in therapeutic planning. *Ann Otol Rhinol Laryngol* 1992;101:222–228.
84. Bland KI, Klamer TW, Polk HC, et al. Isolated regional lymph node dissection. *Ann Surg* 1981;193:372–376.
85. Lee NK, Byers RM, Abbruzzese JL, et al. Metastatic adenocarcinoma to the neck from an unknown primary source. *Am J Surg* 1991;162:306–309.
86. Greco FA, Hainsworth JD. Cancer of unknown primary site. In: Devita VT, Hellman S, Rosenberg SA, eds. *Cancer: principles and practice of oncology,* 4th ed. Philadelphia: JB Lippincott, 1993:2540–2546.
87. Nasri S, Namazie A, Dulguerov P, et al. Malignant melanoma of cervical and parotid lymph nodes with an unknown primary site. *Laryngoscope* 1994;104: 1194–1198.

Radiologic Imaging Concerns

88. Flanagan PM, Roland NJ, Jones AS. Cervical node metastases presenting with features of branchial cysts. *J Laryngol Otol* 1994;108:1068–1071.
89. Kulapaditharom B, Boonkitticharoen V, Kunachak S. Fluorescence-guided biopsy in the diagnosis of an unknown primary cancer in patients with metastatic cervical lymph nodes. *Ann Otol Rhinol Laryngol* 1999;108(7 pt 1): 700–704.
90. Shah JP. Patterns of cervical lymph node metastasis from squamous carcinomas of the upper aerodigestive tract. *Am J Surg* 1990;160:405–409.
91. Mukherji SK, Drane WE, Mancuso AA, et al. Occult primary tumors of the head and neck: detection with 2-[F-18] fluoro-2-deoxy-D-glucose SPECT. *Radiology* 1996;199:761–766.
92. Braams JW, Pruim J, Kole AC, et al. Detection of unknown primary head and neck tumors by positron emission tomography. *Int J Oral Maxillofacial Surg* 1997;26:112–115.
93. Safa AA, Tran LM, Rege S, et al. The role of positron emission tomography in occult primary head and neck cancers. *Cancer J Sci Am* 1999;5:214–218.
94. Bohuslavizki KH, Klutmann S, Kroger S, et al. FDG PET detection of unknown primary tumors. *J Nucl Med* 2000;41:816–822.
95. Greven KM, Keyes JW Jr, Williams DW 3rd, et al. Occult primary tumors of the head and neck: lack of benefit from positron emission tomography imaging with 2-[F-18]fluoro-2-deoxy-D-glucose. *Cancer* 1999;86:114–118.
96. Valdes Olmos RA, Balm AJ, Hilgers FJ, et al. Thallium-201 SPECT in the diagnosis of head and neck cancer. *J Nucl Med* 1997;38:873–879.

CHAPTER 16

Cancer of the Oral Cavity

Jatin P. Shah and Michael J. Zelefsky

INCIDENCE, ETIOLOGY, AND WORLD DISTRIBUTION

Cancer of the oral cavity comprises approximately 30% of all malignant tumors of the head and neck. Nearly 95% of these are squamous cell carcinomas (SCCs). The American Cancer Society projected approximately 32,300 new cancers in the oral cavity and pharynx, and approximately 9,000 deaths attributable to these cancers in 2002 (1). Worldwide, head and neck cancer is the sixth most common human cancer. In Southeast Asia and particularly in India, cancer of the oral cavity is the most common cancer, comprising 35% of all cancers in men and 18% of all cancers in women. This high incidence of cancer is attributable largely to the habit of chewing betel nuts, tobacco, and pan (a mixture of tobacco, betel nut, lime, and other substances wrapped in a vegetable leaf), a very common practice in Southeast Asia.

Although no specific etiology has been established as yet, numerous risk factors contribute to the genesis of oral cancer. Certain patients have a high genetic and familial predisposition to the development of cancer; this tendency is evidenced by mutations through an autosomal-dominant inheritance of one allele of the *p53* tumor suppressor gene, as seen in Li-Fraumeni syndrome (2).

Fanconi anemia (FA) is an autosomal-recessive chromosomal instability syndrome characterized by progressive lethal pancytopenia, skeletal abnormalities, chromosomal instability, and hypersensitivity to DNA cross-linking agents such as mitomycin C and to ionizing radiation. The hematologic abnormalities associated with the disease generally present early in childhood as transfusion-dependent aplastic anemia and bone marrow failure. Bone marrow transplantation currently offers the only chance for cure, and although hematologic malignancies such as leukemia are more frequent, the susceptibility of these patients to solid tumors is being increasingly appreciated as treatment results for hematologic disease improve. The median survival in over 700 patients in the International Fanconi Anemia Registry is only 24 years, and the cumulative incidence of developing a solid tumor by age 40 is approximately 30% (David Kutler, M.D., personal communication). Most of these tumors are located in either the anogenital or upper aerodigestive tract. Bloom syndrome also is an autosomal-recessive growth disorder that subjects individuals to an increased incidence of cancer at a young age, including carcinomas in the head and neck region (3). However, the exceedingly strong influence of tobacco and alcohol exposure on the genesis of SCCs of the upper aerodigestive tract obscures the underlying genetic predisposition that may exist.

Dietary factors do not play a direct role in the genesis of SCCs of the oral cavity. However, alcohol is a risk factor in many patients, and nutritional deficiency commonly is associated with severe alcohol consumption. Other dietary deficiencies, such as iron deficiency, are associated with development of

Plummer-Vinson syndrome, wherein SCC of the hypopharynx and oral cavity frequently is observed (4). Although no direct evidence substantiates the development of SCC of the oral cavity attributable to dietary factors, the recent endeavors in chemoprevention using vitamin A analogs may provide indirect evidence suggesting nutritional influences on carcinogenesis in the oral cavity. Prostaglandins (PGs) are thought to play a role in pathogenesis of cancer through modulation of various events such as cell proliferation, apoptosis, angiogeneses, and immune surveillance. This observation is also supported by epidemiologic and experimental evidence that nonsteroidal antiinflammatory drugs (NSAIDs), which are inhibitors of PG biosynthesis, reduce the risk for tumorigenesis. Cyclooxygenase (COX) catalyzes the synthesis of PGs from arachidonic acid, and there is accumulating evidence for a cause-effect relationship between overexpression of COX-2, an inducible form of COX, and development of cancer. Selective inhibition of COX-2, therefore, presents an attractive method for chemoprevention of upper aerodigestive tract carcinoma. The role of selective COX-2 inhibitors is being evaluated in clinical trails in patients with oral leukoplakia and Barrett's esophagus.

Social factors and lifestyle habits have a major impact on development of oral cancer. Most patients with SCCs of the oral cavity provide a history of tobacco and alcohol consumption. Use of either substance alone increases the risk for development of head and neck carcinoma; however, when both tobacco and alcohol are used, a synergistic effect increases the relative risk severalfold for development of cancer compared with that in nonusers (Fig. 16.1) (5). Alcohol may act as a promoter, an irritant, or a solvent to increase the solubility of carcinogens from tobacco, leading to development of cancer. Experimental evidence suggests that alcohol suppresses the efficiency of DNA repair after exposure to nitrosamine compounds (6). Other forms of tobacco use also contribute to oral cancer. These include, as mentioned earlier, chewing of pan. Chronic use of pan is associated with a high incidence of carcinoma of the cheek mucosa, retromolar trigone, and base of the tongue in India. Increasing use of chewing tobacco has led to a 50-fold increased risk for oral cancer in chronic snuff users in the United States (7).

Although viral factors may play a role in the genesis of cancer of the head and neck, direct linkage between human papillomavirus (HPV) and oral cancer remains to be established. Human papillomavirus can be detected by molecular means in 60% to 90% of oral cavity SCCs (8). However, establishing its role in the etiology of development of cancer is difficult, as HPV is present in nearly 40% of normal oral mucosa (9).

Poor dental hygiene is associated with a higher incidence of oral cancer. Chronic irritation from repeated and prolonged episodes of dental sepsis and chronic irritation from ill-fitting dentures have been implicated in the genesis of carcinoma of the gum and hard palate. In general, the risk for oral cancer is increased significantly in individuals with poor dental hygiene, compared with those with healthy dentition. Chronic irritation from ill-fitting dentures leads to development of epulis fissuratum and (eventually) epithelial dysplastic changes leading to hyperkeratosis, dysplasia, and SCC. The recent increase of development of tongue cancer in nonsmoking young adults in the United States is disturbing. Clearly, genetic factors may play an important role in these individuals; however, no specific etiology has been established as yet. Finally, the incidence of tongue carcinoma in women is rising in the United States. Over the last 50 years, it has more than doubled, increasing from 15% of all tongue cancers in the 1930s to 40% in the 1980s (10).

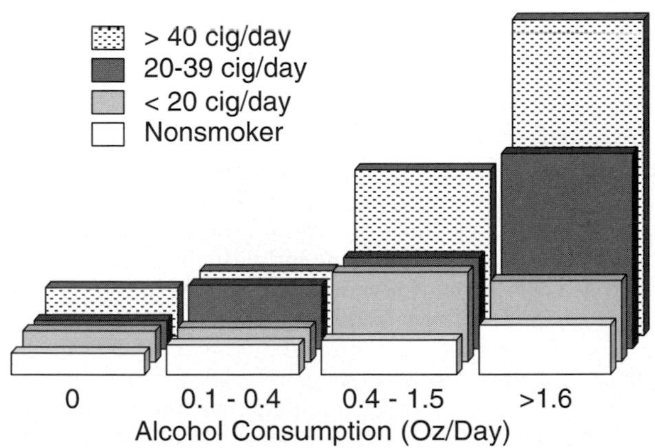

Figure 16.1 Relative risk of oropharyngeal cancer in relation to smoking and alcohol consumption. (Data prepared from Rothman K, Keller A. The effect of joint exposure to alcohol and tobacco on risk of cancer of the mouth and pharynx. *J Chron Dis* 1972;25:711–716.)

ANATOMY

The anterior limit of the oral cavity is the junction of the skin and vermilion border of the lip. The posterior limit is at the junction of the hard and soft palate superiorly, the circumvallate papillae inferiorly, and the anterior tonsillar pillars laterally. This anatomic region embryologically conforms to those sites lined by the ectoderm of the stomodeum, with contributions from the first and second branchial arches. The mucosa of the oral cavity is lined largely by squamous epithelium interspersed by minor salivary glands that range up to 1,000 in number. Although the minor salivary glands are distributed throughout the oral cavity, they are particularly concentrated in the hard and soft palate. The various sites in the oral cavity designated by the American Joint Committee for Staging on Cancer are shown in Figure 16.2. The buccal mucosa represents the epithelial lining beginning at the commissure of the oral cavity anteriorly and extends up to the retromolar gingiva posteriorly. Superiorly and inferiorly, it extends up to the gingivobuccal junction.

The alveolar ridge is composed of an osseous alveolar process that supports dentition and its overlying mucosa or gingiva. The ridge extends from the gingivobuccal sulcus laterally

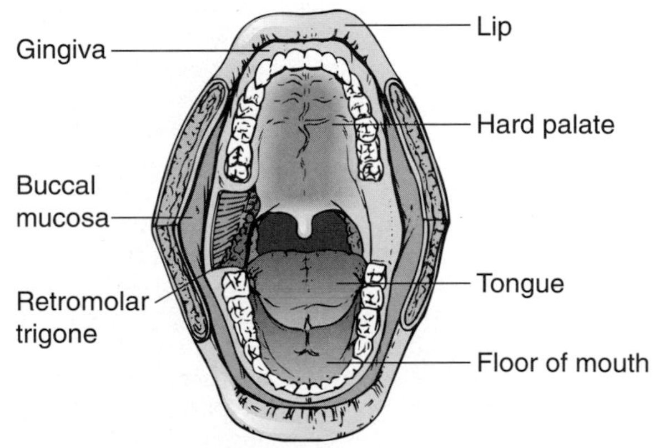

Figure 16.2 Primary sites in the oral cavity.

to the junction of the gum and the floor-of-mouth mucosa or hard palate medially. The posterior limit of the lower alveolus is the retromolar trigone. The maxillary tubercle is the posterior limit of the upper alveolus.

The retromolar trigone, an area posterior to the last mandibular molar tooth, extends superiorly up to the maxillary tubercle. It is defined laterally by the buccal mucosa and medially by the anterior tonsillar pillar.

The floor of the mouth is a semilunar area extending from the inner margin of the lower alveolus to the ventral surface of the oral tongue. It extends posteriorly to the base of the anterior tonsillar pillars. The mucosa of the floor of the mouth is supported by the mylohyoid, geniohyoid, and genioglossus muscles. Between the mucosa and this muscular diaphragm are located the sublingual salivary gland, Wharton's duct, and numerous minor salivary glands.

The hard palate is defined by the upper alveolus anteriorly and by the junction of the hard and soft palates posteriorly. Laterally, it is defined by the alveolar ridge.

The oral tongue is the freely mobile anterior two thirds of the tongue lined by squamous epithelium, which composes its dorsal and undersurface. The epithelium of the dorsum of the tongue consists of fungiform, filiform, and circumvallate papillae. The tongue is composed of an intrinsic, complex, and unique consortium of musculature that traverses three planes. These muscles are separated in the midline by the median raphae. The intrinsic muscles of the tongue produce changes in its shape during speech and swallowing. The extrinsic muscles of the tongue (genioglossus, hyoglossus, styloglossus, and palatoglossus), on the other hand, not only modify the shape of the tongue but also assist in the movement of the tongue backward, forward, upward, downward, and sideways.

Blood supply to the oral cavity is provided largely by branches of the external carotid artery. Lingual arteries provide blood supply to the tongue and literally are end arteries leading to the possibility of necrosis of the tongue by their ligation. Blood supply to the lips and the cheek mucosa is provided through the facial arteries, and blood supply to the alveolar ridges is provided by the internal maxillary and inferior alveolar arteries.

Lymphatics of the oral cavity drain through regional lymphatic channels, culminating in submental, submandibular, and upper jugular-jugulodigastric lymph nodes that form the first-echelon nodal sites for most primary tumors in the oral cavity. Direct lymphatic channels extend from the tongue to lower jugular lymph nodes, occasionally leading to the development of skip metastasis. Lymph nodes located in the soft tissues of the cheek (buccinator lymph node) occasionally are at risk for involvement from carcinomas of the upper alveolar ridge and cheek mucosa. Lymphatic dissemination of primary epithelial cancers of the oral cavity usually occur in a predictable and sequential progressive fashion.

Three types of nerves provide physiologic function to the oral cavity. The sensory nerve supply to the oral cavity is provided by the sensory component of the second and third divisions of the trigeminal nerve, through the superior and inferior alveolar and lingual nerves. Special senses of taste and secretomotor functions to the salivary glands are provided through chorda tympani traversing along the lingual nerve and providing secretomotor fibers to the submandibular salivary gland. Motor control of the lips and cheek (orbicularis oris and buccinator) is provided by the facial nerve. The hypoglossal nerve is the motor nerve for the intrinsic and extrinsic muscles of the tongue. Movements of the mandible are performed by the masseter, temporalis, and medial and lateral pterygoid muscles. Their actions are controlled by the motor components of the second and third divisions of the trigeminal nerve.

The most important functions of the oral cavity are mastication, deglutition, maintenance of oral competency, and articulation of speech. The ability to masticate food depends on the integrity of the alveolar ridges to support the patient's teeth or dentures. The tongue is the most vital component of the oral phase of deglutition. It distributes the food for mastication in the oral cavity, produces an admixture of saliva and the food to form a bolus, and advances that bolus to the oropharynx for the pharyngeal phase of swallowing. Thus, alteration in the functional integrity of the tongue leads to difficulty with mastication, speech, and swallowing. Composed of buccinator muscles, the cheeks are important for holding food in position against the prime masticators and working in concert with the lips to help retain saliva within the oral cavity by maintaining its competence. Functional loss of cheek or lip may cause drooling of saliva and inability to produce effective chewing. Although the tongue is the primary articulator in the upper phonatory system, loss of lips also causes inability to produce effective articulation.

The anatomic disposition of the various structures of the oral cavity in part determines local progression and extension of disease from the primary site. Thus, tumors of the cheek mucosa often spread along the surface plane but may penetrate through the underlying musculature and perforate overlying skin. Lesions of the gingiva extend to the periosteum and, through the dental sockets, may involve the underlying mandible. Once lingual tumors penetrate the intrinsic musculature, they may spread along the intermuscular planes and render assessment of the third dimension of the tumor difficult. Tumors of the floor of the mouth may extend inferiorly and involve the muscular diaphragm and the soft tissues in the submental region.

NATURAL HISTORY AND PATTERNS OF SPREAD

Due to the high association of alcohol and tobacco abuse and the genesis of SCC of the oral cavity, very often premalignant changes are visible or present before the development of invasive carcinoma. These changes relate to epithelial and subepithelial anatomic and histomorphologic disturbances. Epithelial changes include disturbances in the keratin content of the epithelial layer and cellular cytoplasmic changes that may be detectable by measuring fluorescent changes in the emitting and transmitting patterns of light. Distinct fluorescent patterns have been reported in normal mucosa, premalignant mucosa at risk, and in patients with carcinoma (11). This interesting field of investigation requires further work to establish the clinical application of measurements of autofluorescence in detecting premalignant epithelial changes in the population at risk.

Progressive epithelial changes lead to development of hyperkeratosis, parakeratosis, dyskeratosis, carcinoma *in situ*, and, eventually, invasive carcinoma. This continuum of progression of epithelial transformation from a normal to a malignant cell may take years in some individuals. But such sequential progressive cytologic changes are not observed in all patients and indeed may be absent in some patients with invasive SCC. Most epithelial premalignant changes present as white discoloration (leukoplakia). The risk for development of leukoplakia into invasive carcinoma has been estimated at approximately 4% to 6% (12–14). Some patients may manifest premalignant changes by red discoloration (erythroplakia).

The risk for development of invasive carcinoma in erythroplakia is as high as 30% (15). In the South Asian population, submucous fibrosis is quite common. This reaction is fibrotic, leading to atrophic changes in the epithelium but exhibiting significant fibrosis and contracture formation in a submucosal plane in the region of the retromolar trigone, which gives rise to trismus. Although no direct evidence is linked to the genesis of epithelial carcinoma, submucous fibrosis indeed is present in the Indian subcontinent in a great majority of patients developing oral carcinoma.

A varying degree of keratinization usually is present on the surface of a primary tumor. The extent of keratinization is a reflection of the degree of differentiation of the underlying malignant process. Highly keratinized tumors usually are well differentiated and may manifest as low-grade keratinizing SCC or verrucous carcinoma. In contrast, poorly differentiated SCCs show very little or no keratinization and may present as poorly differentiated SCCs. Although the current staging system takes into account only the surface dimensions of the tumor, the third dimension (depth of invasion or thickness of the tumor) is important in terms of the risk for regional lymphatic dissemination and prognosis (16). Local extension by spread to adjacent structures may lead to invasion of the underlying soft tissues and muscles, bone, or neurovascular structures. The spread of the tumor may also occur through lymphatics to regional lymph nodes or via bloodstream dissemination to distant sites.

Local Spread

Local invasion of primary SCCs of the oral cavity may extend to the adjacent mucosa, manifesting a zone of invasion with progressive changes demonstrating carcinoma *in situ* and dysplasia in adjacent mucosa. Molecular changes in adjacent mucosal margins may precede cytologic changes discernible by light microscopy as atypia or carcinoma *in situ* (17). Extension of epithelial tumor into the depth of the underlying tissues may cause invasion of the intrinsic and extrinsic musculature of the tongue by primary carcinomas of the oral tongue and floor of mouth, or to the muscles of the floor of mouth, the buccinator muscle, and muscles of the lip for floor-of-mouth, cheek mucosa, and lip tumors, respectively. Further progression of local tumor spread may trigger invasion of neurovascular structures, causing vascular invasion and perineural invasion. Although neurotropism is not a classic character of oral SCCs, some patients with SCCs of the lip do manifest neurotropism with extension of tumor along the inferior alveolar nerve into the mandibular canal (Fig. 16.3). Such neurotropic spread to the inferior alveolar nerve may occur from SCC and melanomas of the lower lip. Neurotropism of adenoidcystic carcinoma is well known. Adenoidcystic carcinoma of minor salivary gland origin in the oral cavity may involve the lingual, hypoglossal, inferior alveolar, superior alveolar infraorbital, or facial nerves (18).

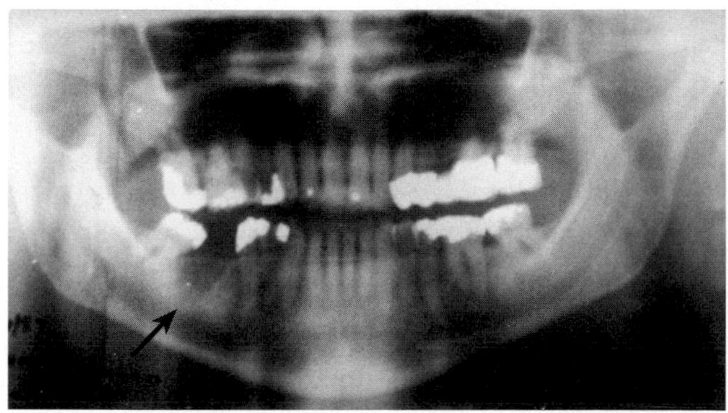

Figure 16.3 Panoramic roentgenogram of the mandible. Shown is expansion of the inferior alveolar canal due to neurotropic spread of squamous cell carcinoma of the lower lip.

Bone invasion by tumors of the hard palate and upper alveolus can take place by direct infiltration of the surface lesion into the underlying palatal bone and upper alveolar ridge or maxillary antrum. Similarly, invasion of the mandible by carcinomas of the lower alveolus occurs by direct penetration. Lesions of the gingiva can extend directly into the cancellous part of the mandible and mandibular canal through the dental sockets. In edentulous patients, such direct spread may occur through "dental pores" on the edentulous alveolar ridge. Conversely, extension of tongue and floor-of-mouth tumors occurs in a predictable progressive fashion through the alveolar process. Direct extension through an intact periosteum and lingual cortex of the mandible is not seen. Whole-organ section studies performed by several investigators have demonstrated a predictable pathway of extension of lingual and floor-of-mouth tumors to the mandible (19–21). These lesions extend along the floor of the mouth to the attached lingual gingiva and proceed to the socket of the adjacent tooth. Migration of malignant cells then proceeds along the root of the tooth into the cancellous part of the mandible and thence along the mandibular canal. Once tumor invasion extends to the mandibular canal, it can proceed distally or proximally along the mandibular canal and the inferior alveolar nerve (Fig. 16.4). Understanding of the mechanism of progression of oral cancer and invasion of the mandible has permitted the development of mandible-sparing approaches in surgical treatment of oral cancers in which the mandible is at risk for invasion.

Another phenomenon unique to the mucosa of the upper aerodigestive tract is field cancerization. Patients with significant exposure to tobacco and alcohol often demonstrate the milieu of "condemned mucosa" that is highly susceptible to the development of multiple primary cancers. In such patients, varying degrees of epithelial changes may be present, reflecting neocarcinogenesis at different stages of development of invasive cancers (22). This process eventually leads to the development of multiple synchronous or metachronous primary carcinomas in the mucosa at risk. The incidence of multifocal changes, however, is seen in the pharynx more often than in the oral cavity.

A peculiar variant of multifocal oral cancers is observed in elderly women without significant history of tobacco or alcohol consumption. These multiple primary tumors usually are low-grade, well-differentiated keratinizing SCCs. Often these lesions are accompanied by multiple areas of hyperkeratosis or dyskeratosis. Nearly always, these lesions are confined to the oral cavity and are not seen in the oropharynx, hypopharynx, or larynx.

Lymphatic Spread

The risk for dissemination to regional lymphatics is related to the site of the primary tumor, its surface dimensions, the depth of invasion, and its histologic grade. Certain primary sites have a high predilection for dissemination to regional lymphatics, such as the tongue and the floor of the mouth, compared with the hard palate, wherein regional dissemination to lymphatics is infrequent. Larger primary lesions have an increased risk for dissemination to regional lymphatics, compared with that in smaller tumors. Similarly, thicker tumors carry a higher risk than do thin tumors (Fig. 16.5). The factors that increase the risk for lymphatic dissemination from a primary cancer of the oral cavity are listed in Table 16.1.

Once lymphatic permeation occurs, malignant cells travel through the lymphatics in the floor of the mouth to first-echelon lymph nodes situated in the submental, submandibular, and jugulodigastric region of cervical lymphatics. Usually,

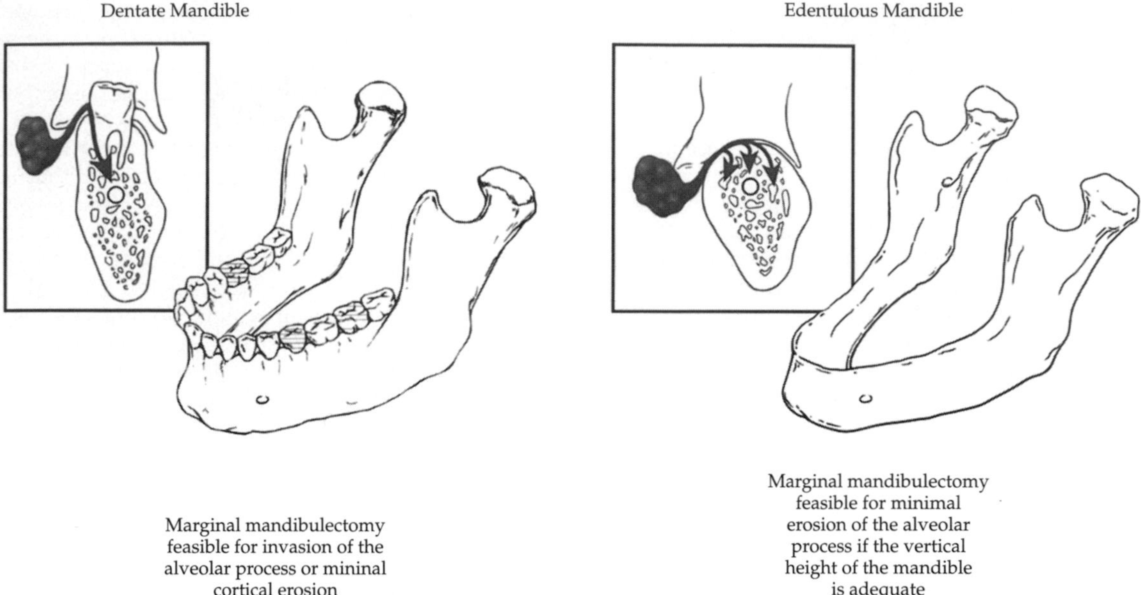

Figure 16.4 Routes of spread to mandible from oral cancer in dentate and edentulous mandible.

the first-echelon lymph nodes for each primary site are predictable. Although in-transit metastases are rare, radioisotope studies have shown the presence of in-transit lymphatic deposits from cancers of the tongue and the floor of the mouth (23). The patterns of regional dissemination of lymphatics from oral carcinomas have been well documented (24–27). The first-echelon lymph nodes for primary carcinomas of the oral cavity are located in the supraomohyoid triangle of the neck and cover the lymph nodes in the submental, submandibular, upper jugular, and midjugular lymph nodes (Fig. 16.6). Skip metastases from primary carcinomas of the oral tongue have been reported in as many as 15% of patients without involvement of the first-echelon lymph nodes (28). However, generally the risk is in the 2% to 4% range. These skip metastases usually occur to level IV (lower jugular) lymph nodes. Dissemination to lymph nodes in the posterior triangle of the neck in the absence of disease in the anterior triangle of the neck, however, is exceedingly rare (29). Thus, regional lymphatic dissemination from primary carcinomas of the oral cavity occur in a predictable and sequential fashion. Understanding of the lymphatic progression of metastatic tumor in this manner permits the development of function-sparing surgical approaches to management of regional lymphatic metastasis.

Distant Dissemination

Distant metastases from primary SCCs of the oral cavity at the time of initial diagnosis are exceedingly rare. Dissemination to distant sites without local progression or regional spread usually does not occur. However, patients with advanced-stage lymph node metastasis (N2 or N3 disease) are at a significant risk for dissemination to distant sites. The most frequent sites for distant metastases are lung and bones, and metastases usually occur in patients with locally advanced or regionally advanced disease or those with recurrent disease.

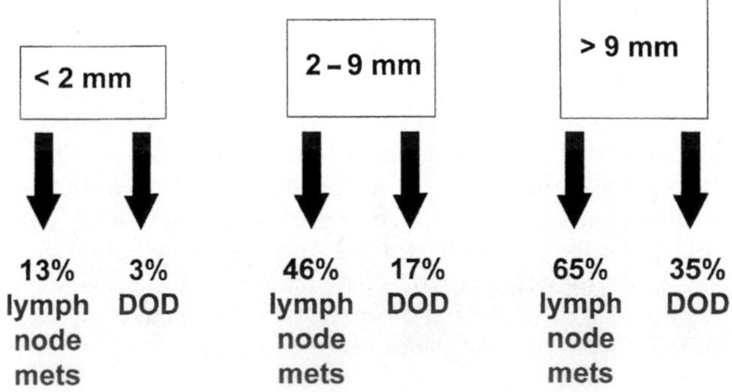

Figure 16.5 Risk for regional lymph node metastasis and death from oral cancer in relation to measured thickness of the primary tumor. DOD, dead of disease; mets, metastasis.

TABLE 16.1 Factors that Influence the Risk for Lymph Node Metastasis

Site
Size
T stage
Location (anterior vs. posterior)
Histomorphologic features
Endophytic vs. exophytic
Tumor thickness
Differentiation (well differentiated vs. poorly differentiated)

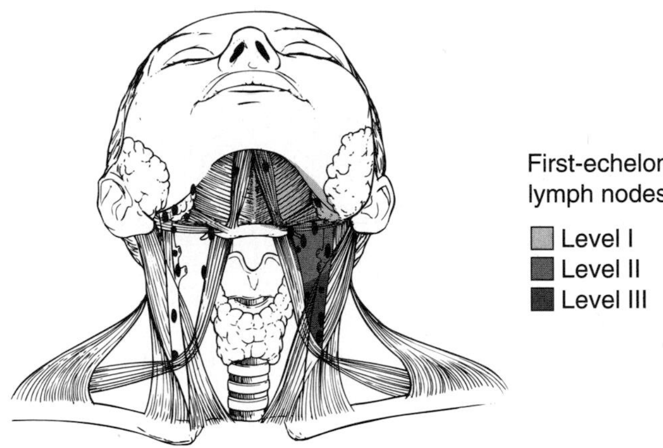

Figure 16.6 First-echelon lymph nodes at risk for metastasis from carcinoma of the oral cavity are located in the supraomohyoid triangle.

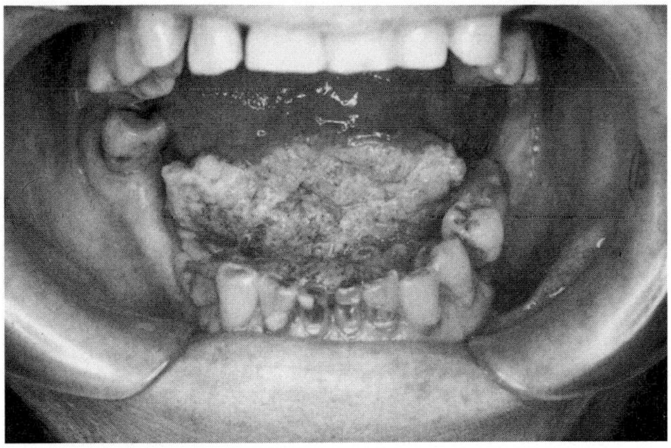

Figure 16.8 Exophytic cauliflower-like carcinoma of the anterior floor of the mouth.

CLINICAL PRESENTATION

The clinical characteristics of primary carcinomas arising on the mucosal surface of the oral cavity vary. The tumor may be ulcerative, exophytic, or endophytic, or it may manifest as a superficial proliferative lesion. Occasionally, papillary fronds are present, and a keratotic verrucous appearance is manifested by varying amounts of keratin content on the superficial layers of the tumor. Usually, the clinical characteristics of the lesion are sufficient to raise the index of suspicion regarding the possibility of a malignant neoplasm and the need to establish tissue diagnosis by a biopsy. Usually, ulcerative lesions are accompanied by an irregular edge and induration of the underlying soft tissues (Fig. 16.7). Exophytic lesions may present either as a cauliflower-like irregular growth, or as a flat, pink to pinkish white proliferative lesion (Fig. 16.8). Occasionally, a pink, velvety, flat lesion is the only manifestation of a superficially invasive or carcinoma *in situ* (Fig. 16.9). Squamous cell carcinomas with excessive keratin production and verrucous carcinomas present as white, heaped-up lesions with varying degrees of keratin debris on the surface (Fig. 16.10). Tumors that usually are preceded by a squamous papilloma manifest papillary projections on the surface (Fig. 16.11). Bleeding from the surface of the lesion is a sign highly indicative of malignancy and should raise suspicion for a neoplastic process. Endophytic lesions have a small surface component but a substantial amount of soft tissue induration beneath the surface. Pain is associated with those lesions that usually are ulcerated and located on the more sensitive part of the oral cavity, such as the lateral border of the tongue and adjacent floor of the mouth.

Leukoplakia and erythroplakia (as discussed) confer a variable risk for transformation into carcinoma. Speckled leukoplakia represents a particularly high incidence of malignant transformation. Multiple primary cancers occur synchronously in approximately 4% of patients with primary cancers of the oral cavity (30). Therefore, a thorough examination of the oral cavity and the remaining upper aerodigestive tract should be performed in every case.

Most primary SCCs of the oral cavity are located in those areas of the oral mucosa that constantly are exposed to saliva. Thus, a majority of oral cancers are located on the lateral border and undersurface of the tongue and on the floor of the mouth. The distribution of various sites in the oral cavity for primary SCCs in the U.S. is shown in Figure 16.12.

Clinical Staging

The American Joint Committee on Cancer (AJCC) and the International Union Against Cancer (UICC) (31) take into consideration the surface dimensions of primary tumors of the oral cav-

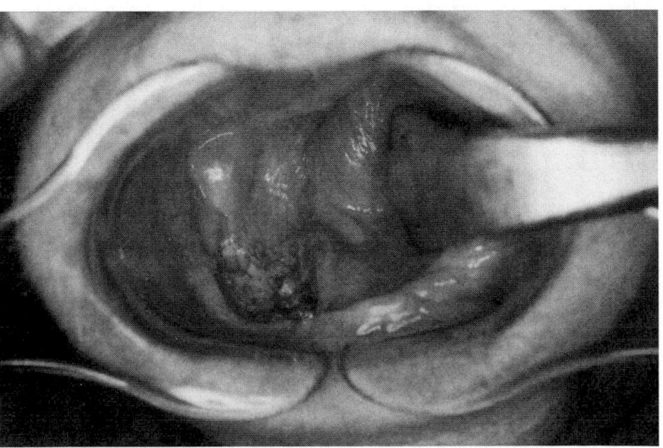

Figure 16.7 Ulcerated carcinoma of the floor of the mouth involving lower gum.

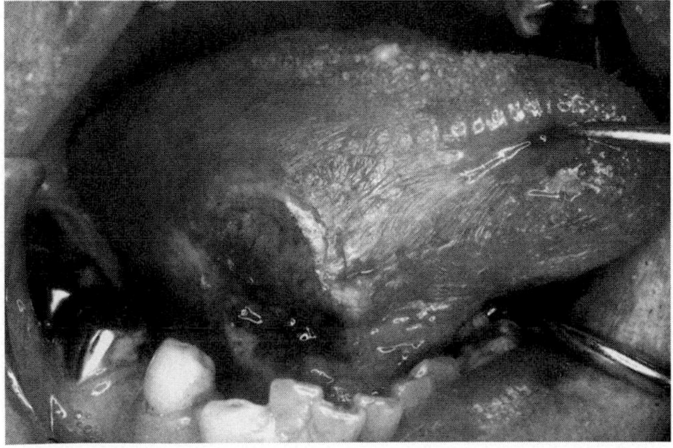

Figure 16.9 Ulcerated, flat, mostly endophytic carcinoma of the lateral border of the tongue.

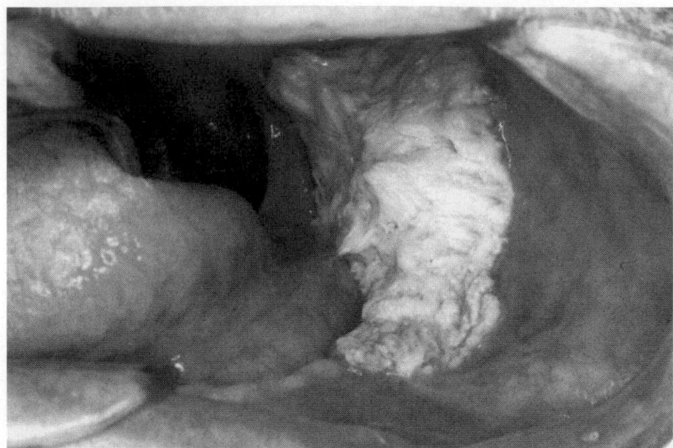

Figure 16.10 Verrucous carcinoma of the edentulous lower gum.

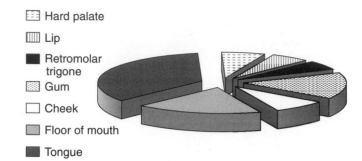

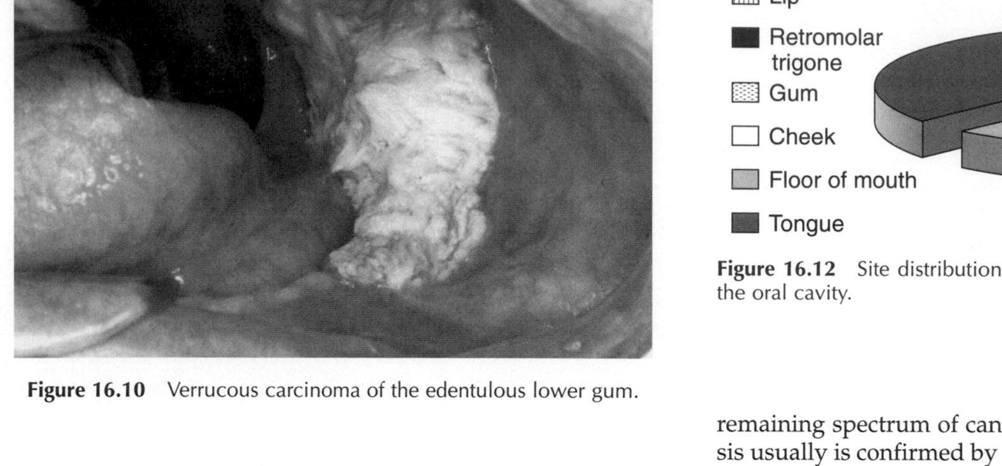

Figure 16.12 Site distribution of primary squamous cell carcinomas of the oral cavity.

ity in the tumor staging system. Lesions less than 2 cm in their maximum surface dimension are staged as T1, 2 to 4 cm as T2, more than 4 cm as T3. The most recent AJCC revision (31) has subdivided T4 oral cavity lesions into T4a (resectable) and T4b (unresectable), which leads to the division of stage IV into stage IVa (advanced, resectable), IVb (advanced, unresectable), and IVc (advanced, metastatic) (31). T4 lip lesions are unchanged from the previous description. In the oral cavity, T4a now includes tumors that invade adjacent structures, e.g., cortical bone, deep tongue muscles, maxillary sinus, or skin of face. T4b includes tumors of more severe extension, i.e., invading the masticator space, pterygoid plates, or skull base, or encasing the carotid artery. It should be noted that superficial bone or tooth-socket erosion is still classified as T3. The node staging system is uniform for all primary sites and is described in Chapter 13. The stage groupings are shown in Table 16.2. In patients without evidence of regional lymph node metastasis, lesions generally are called *early-stage oral carcinomas,* and, in those with nodal metastasis, lesions usually are termed *advanced-stage oral cancers.*

More than 90% of primary carcinomas arising in the oral cavity are of squamous cell origin (Fig. 16.13). The degree of differentiation varies; however, most of the patients have moderately differentiated keratinizing SCCs. Minor salivary gland carcinomas and melanomas and other rare tumors comprise the remaining spectrum of cancer of the oral cavity. Tissue diagnosis usually is confirmed by a wedge or a punch biopsy obtained (preferably) from the periphery of the lesion to demonstrate a zone of invasion. However, adequate tissue sample from the center of the tumor often is sufficient to establish tissue diagnosis. Biopsy from the surface of the lesion in highly keratinizing SCCs and verrucous carcinomas may not provide a representative sample, and often the diagnosis of invasive carcinoma can be missed. Therefore, in such situations wherein excessive keratin deposit is seen on the surface of an exophytic lesion, the biopsy should be obtained from the periphery of the lesion or from the depth of the tumor to secure a representative sample to establish tissue diagnosis.

Diagnostic Evaluation

The diagnostic evaluation of a patient suspected of having a primary SCC of the oral cavity requires documentation of the patient's demographic characteristics and lifestyle habits, particularly with reference to consumption of tobacco and alcohol and other irritating agents that may play an etiologic role in the genesis of the primary oral cancer. A complete history also should include the history of dental hygiene and that of exposure to any other known carcinogens. Family history should be elicited to rule out any predisposing syndromes with genetic alterations increasing the risk for a primary oral cancer.

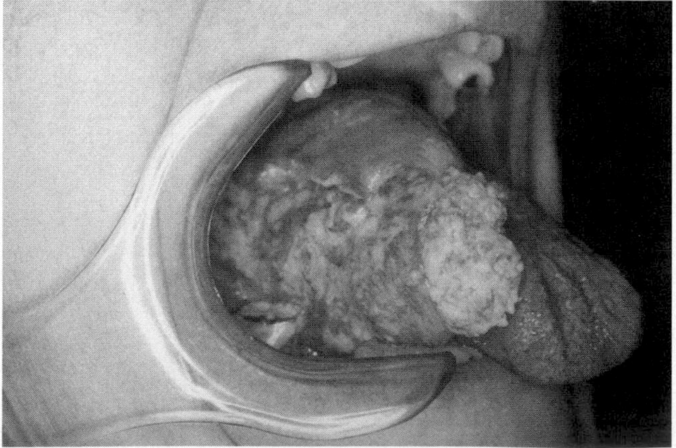

Figure 16.11 Exophytic, papillary, well-differentiated squamous cell carcinoma of the oral tongue.

TABLE 16.2 2002 American Joint Committee on Cancer (AJCC) Stage Groupings for Squamous Cell Carcinoma of the Oral Cavity

Stage 0	Tis	N0	M0
Stage I	T1	N0	M0
Stage II	T2	N0	M0
Stage III	T3	N0	M0
	T1	N1	M0
	T2	N1	M0
	T3	N1	M0
Stage IV	T4a	N0	M0
	T4a	N1	M0
	T1	N2	M0
	T2	N2	M0
	T3	N2	M0
	T4a	N2	M0
Stage IVb	Any T	N3	M0
	T4b	Any N	M0
Stage IVc	Any T	Any N	M1

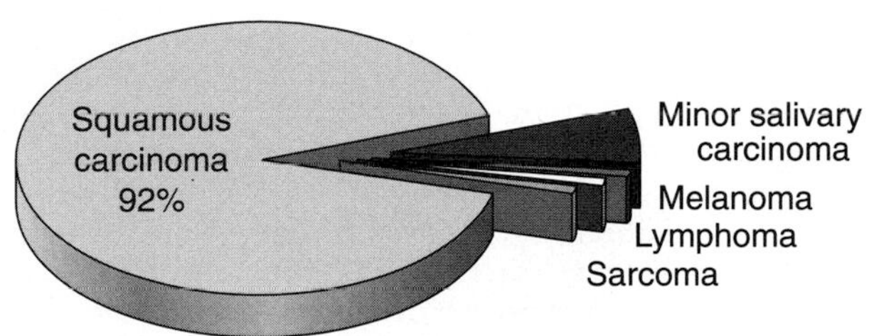

Figure 16.13 Histologic distribution of primary malignant tumors of the oral cavity.

A complete head and neck examination is essential not only to assess the extent of the primary tumor and regional lymph nodes but also to rule out the possibility of synchronous multiple primary carcinomas in the upper aerodigestive tract. Examination of the primary lesion requires adequate lighting and occasionally the use of a magnifying glass to study accurately the surface characteristics of the lesion. Inspection and palpation are essential to appreciate the surface dimension and the third dimension of the presenting lesion. Of particular importance is the proximity of the primary tumor to the adjacent bone, such as mandible or maxilla. Patients with painful lesions might not permit adequate palpation without anesthesia. Thus, satisfactory examination under anesthesia, particularly with reference to the third dimension of the primary tumor and its proximity to bone, should be performed carefully in such patients so as to facilitate treatment planning. Deeply invasive tumors with infiltration of the intrinsic and extrinsic muscles of the tongue may reduce the mobility of the tongue, signifying a massive primary lesion.

Systematic palpation of regional cervical lymph nodes is essential to accurately assign a clinical stage to the cancer. Bimanual palpation of the floor of the mouth is required to assess adequately the clinical characteristics of submental and submandibular group of lymph nodes. After adequate assessment of the primary tumor, regional lymphatics, and the remaining head and neck region, a biopsy is performed to confirm tissue diagnosis. At that point, a clinical diagnosis and stage assignment is ascribed to the lesion.

The current staging system proposed by the AJCC and the UICC (31) is deficient in assessing the third dimension of the primary lesion in determining prognosis. For example, the primary tumor staging system does not take into consideration the thickness of the primary tumor. Surface dimensions are well known to be only one parameter of the primary tumor and reflect its behavior with relation to its risk for dissemination to regional lymph nodes and relation to eventual survival after appropriate treatment (16). It is also well known that exophytic tumors generally have a favorable prognosis compared with endophytic tumors. This parameter is also not included in the current staging system. In addition, such biomarkers as molecular and genetic abnormalities, which may have prognostic importance, also are not included in the tumor staging system. Similarly, the current staging system for regional lymph nodes considers only the size, number, and laterality of lymph nodes but does not consider, for example, the location of the lymph nodes. In addition, extranodal spread is not factored into the nodal staging system. Thus, the clinical staging system should consider other parameters in future revisions of the staging system.

In addition to the evaluation of the primary lesion and assignment of a clinical stage and confirmation of tissue diagnosis, pretreatment dental evaluation is vitally important in treatment planning. Patients with loose teeth within the center of the tumor or in the proximity of the tumor should not have any dental extractions prior to surgical intervention. Premature extraction of teeth opens up new tissue spaces and raises the risk for further local progression of disease by exposing dental sockets and opening up the mandibular canal for potential tumor implantation and progression.

MANAGEMENT

Factors Affecting Choice of Treatment

The factors that influence the choice of initial treatment are those related to the characteristics of the primary tumor (tumor factors), those related to the patient (patient factors), and those related to the treatment delivery team (physician factors). In the selection of optimal therapy, therefore, one should consider these three sets of factors for treatment planning. Clearly, the goals of treatment for cancer of the oral cavity are (a) curing the cancer, (b) preserving or restoring form and function, (c) minimizing the sequelae of treatment, (d) delivering the optimal treatment in a cost-effective and expeditious manner, and (e) preventing second primary tumors. To achieve these goals, the currently available therapeutic modalities include surgery, radiation therapy, chemotherapy, and combinations of the foregoing treatment modalities for the control of the presenting tumor and for primary and secondary prevention strategies, with lifestyle changes for reducing the risk for multiple primary tumors.

TUMOR FACTORS

The tumor factors that influence the choice of initial treatment are related to site, size (T stage), location (anterior versus posterior), proximity to bone (mandible or maxilla), status of cervical lymph nodes, and pathology of the primary tumor (histologic type, grade, and depth of invasion). In addition, any previous treatment rendered to the lesion will influence the choice of therapy.

The size of the primary tumor clearly has a heavy impact on the decision regarding the choice of initial therapy. Small and superficial primary tumors are easily accessible for a relatively simple surgical excision through the open mouth. Larger tumors require more extensive surgical approaches for exposure and excision. Conversely, certain primary sites in the oral cavity are readily suitable for initial treatment by radiation therapy, such as primary tumors of the mobile tongue, in contrast to those situated in proximity to bone, such as a lesion of the lower gum. In addition, with increasing size and the depth of infiltration of the primary lesion, the risk for regional lymph node metastasis increases, bringing into consideration the need for elective treatment of the clinically negative neck at risk for having micrometastasis. Also, certain primary sites have a higher risk for nodal metastasis than other primary sites in the oral cavity.

For example, primary tumors of the oral tongue and floor of mouth have a higher risk for regional dissemination to lymph nodes than similar staged lesions of the hard palate or upper gum. Primary tumors located anteriorly in the oral cavity have a lesser risk for dissemination to regional lymph nodes than similarly staged lesions in the posterior part of the oral cavity or oropharynx.

Clinically palpable cervical lymph node metastasis requires the need for neck dissection as an integral part of surgical treatment planning. The extent of neck dissection, however, depends on the extent of nodal metastasis and the location of palpable metastatic lymph nodes. Though detailed discussion regarding the management of cervical lymph node metastasis is presented elsewhere, it is appropriate here to mention that a comprehensive neck dissection, excising lymph nodes at levels I to V, is indicated in patients with clinically palpable lymph node metastasis in the neck. The spinal accessory nerve usually can be spared unless it is grossly involved by cancer (32). In contrast, a supraomohyoid neck dissection encompassing levels I to III is considered adequate in most patients with a clinically negative neck in whom a significant risk (more than 15%) exists for microscopic dissemination to regional lymph nodes (33). An exception to this rule may be primary SCCs of the lateral border of the tongue, in which an elective dissection of the clinically negative neck should include levels I through IV (28). Similarly, when radiation therapy is used as a single modality to treat lymph node disease, similar technical factors are critical to achieving a high rate of regional control.

The histology of the primary tumor is an important parameter that has an impact on selection of initial treatment. Though most SCCs are radioresponsive, those with excessive keratin deposits and verrucous carcinomas are relatively less radioresponsive. The histologic grade of the lesion generally reflects the aggressiveness of the tumor. Both poorly differentiated and undifferentiated carcinomas are predictably more aggressive in comparison to moderately well- and well-differentiated carcinomas. However, the most crucial pathologic feature of the primary tumor having an impact on selection of initial therapy and eventual prognosis is its depth of infiltration. Thin and superficially invasive lesions have a lower risk for regional lymph node metastasis, are highly curable, and offer an excellent prognosis. Thicker lesions that deeply infiltrate the underlying soft tissues have a significantly increased incidence of regional lymph node metastasis, with its adverse impact on prognosis. Though it would be ideal to know the thickness of the lesion before surgical intervention, in most instances securing that information prior to surgical excision of the primary tumor is clinically impractical. Therefore, thickness of the lesion, as appreciated by palpation, generally is reasonably effective in distinguishing deeply invasive lesion from superficial lesion, in estimating the extent of soft tissue or bone resection for the primary tumor, and in deciding on the need for elective dissection of regional lymph nodes at risk in the clinically negative neck.

Patients with advanced stage of disease (i.e., those presenting with spread to regional cervical lymph nodes or with large primary tumors, such as T3 and T4) are candidates for combined modality treatment. Currently, surgical resection followed by postoperative radiation therapy is considered standard treatment for most patients with stage III and resectable stage IV SCCs of the oral cavity.

PATIENT FACTORS

Several patient factors are important in the selection of initial treatment. These are patient's age, general medical condition, occupation, tolerance to treatment, acceptance and compliance with the recommended therapy, lifestyle (smoking and drinking), and socioeconomic considerations. Older age generally is not considered to be a contraindication for implementation of adequate initial surgical treatment for oral carcinoma. However, with advancing age, intercurrent disease, and debility secondary to associated cardiopulmonary conditions, the implementation of extensive surgical intervention poses increased risk. The ability of the patient to tolerate an optimal therapeutic program is similarly an important factor that can influence the choice of initial therapy. The patient's occupation and acceptance of and compliance with the proposed treatment program are similarly important considerations in planning optimal therapy for the tumor. The patient's lifestyle, particularly regarding smoking and drinking, has a heavy impact on the selection and tolerance of the treatment offered. Unwillingness on the part of the patient to give up smoking and drinking further complicates the administration of adequate treatment and increases the risk for multiple primary tumors. Finally, socioeconomic considerations have started playing an increasing role in the selection and implementation of initial therapy in a cost-effective manner. Allocation of resources required to deliver therapy have to be judged on the basis of outcomes analysis of a particular treatment program. Previous treatment for other lesions in the same area also will influence the decision regarding selection of treatment. For example, radiation therapy previously delivered to the same area for a different lesion may not be available to treat a second tumor in the same area.

PHYSICIAN FACTORS

Several physician- and provider-related factors also are important in the selection of initial therapy. These factors are related to the technical and professional skills in surgery, radiation therapy, chemotherapy, rehabilitation services, dental and prosthetic services, and psychosocial support services. Management of oral cancer is a multidisciplinary team effort, and technical capabilities and support services from various disciplines are essential for a successful outcome. A comprehensive head and neck disease management team consists of the head and neck surgeon combined with other surgical specialties—microsurgery, neurosurgery, vascular surgery, plastic and reconstructive surgery, and dental surgery—and prosthetics. Similar expertise in radiation oncology (including brachytherapy) is essential for integration of combined treatment programs of external, interstitial, and altered fractionation schemes as well as familiarity with three-dimensional and intensity-modulated treatment programs. A well-organized team of medical oncologists expert in administration of chemotherapeutic drugs and the management of chemotherapy-related complications is essential in the management of patients with advanced disease and recurrent tumors. Experience with the complexities of concurrent chemoradiotherapy programs is essential.

In addition to these factors, physical and psychosocial rehabilitation services are vitally important for long-term restoration of the quality of life after treatment of oral cancer. Thus, a multidisciplinary head and neck oncology team should include the services of a psychologist, social worker, and family support groups to provide the patient with all essential services.

Selection of Initial Treatment

Both surgical resection and radiation therapy are applicable, either singly or in combination, in the treatment of cancer of the oral cavity. The role of chemotherapy, however, in the management of oral cancer remains investigational. Small and superficial tumors of the oral cavity are equally amenable for cure by surgical resection or radiation therapy. Therefore, a single modality is preferred as definitive treatment in early-stage tumors (T1 and T2) of the oral cavity. When the end point of treatment (i.e., cure of cancer) is comparable, other factors must play a role in the selection of initial treatment. These factors include complications, cost, convenience, compliance, and long-term sequelae of treatment (Fig. 16.14).

Generally, the choice of initial treatment for early-stage oral cancer (T1 and T2) is surgery. Usually, surgical excision of primary tumor can be accomplished through the open mouth with minimal functional disability. Surgical resection is expeditious and cost-effective and has the advantage of allowing repeated interventions in patients who develop multiple primary lesions. The long-term sequelae of surgical treatment for early-stage

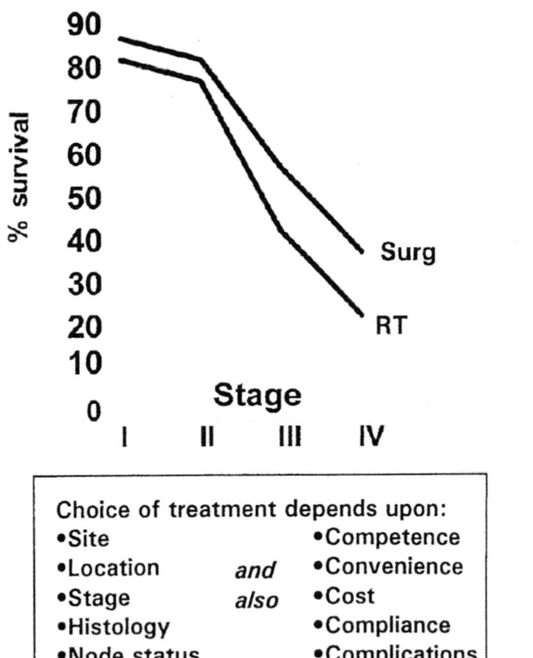

Figure 16.14 Survival with single-modality treatment in relation to stage of disease and factors affecting choice of initial treatment for squamous cell carcinoma of the oral cavity.

oral cancer are related to only minor and transient functional disturbance of clarity of speech and mastication.

Radiation therapy as initial definitive treatment for early-stage oral cancer (T1 and T2) generally is not preferred. In most instances, both external and interstitial treatment are required for maximal therapeutic effect. The treatment requires several weeks to deliver the necessary dose. Although functional disability due to loss of tissue is not seen, the long-term sequelae of treatment are significant. Permanent xerostomia, the lifelong need for fluoride prophylaxis, and the long-term risk for dental caries and possible development of osteoradionecrosis of the mandible render definitive radiation therapy an unattractive choice of initial treatment for early-stage oral cancer. However, in patients who are prohibitive surgical risks or in whom significant functional loss is anticipated after surgery, radiation therapy may be considered as definitive treatment with comparable cure rates.

Patients with advanced-stage tumors clearly require combined-modality treatment for successful outcome. Radiation therapy in combination with surgery can be employed either before or after surgery. Obvious advantages and disadvantages accrue to preoperative as opposed to postoperative radiation therapy.

Preoperative radiation therapy produces delay in the implementation of the surgical treatment by several weeks. However, this time can be employed gainfully in improvement of nutrition of the patient either by nasogastric tube feedings or by supplemental nutrition through a gastrostomy tube. The employment of preoperative radiation therapy has been claimed to enhance resectability. However, what must be borne in mind is that tumor response with shrinkage of the primary tumor should not influence the extent of surgical resection. It is well known that tumors do not shrink concentrically, and viable islands of tumor cells still may be present in grossly normal-appearing tissues adjacent to the residual tumor after preoperative radiation therapy. Therefore, the extent of surgical resection should be essentially the same as that assessed initially prior to preoperative irradiation. In the past, patients who required multiple stages of reconstructive procedures were considered candidates for preoperative radiation therapy because it did not pose any conflict with staged reconstructive procedures. However, contemporary surgical techniques attain primary reconstruction in one stage, due to the availability of regional cutaneous, myocutaneous, and microvascular free flaps. Therefore, that argument no longer is applicable. Conversely, preoperative irradiation may pose a problem with healing of tissue and might increase the risk for local wound complications. In addition, an important disadvantage of preoperative radiation therapy is its dose limitation. Increasing the dose of preoperative radiation therapy increases wound complications from surgery.

For locally advanced disease, postoperative radiation therapy offers significant advantages over preoperative radiation therapy and offers better or comparable local and regional control rates of cancer (34,35). No delay occurs in implementation of surgical resection, and no dose limitations are imposed on postoperative radiation therapy. What must be borne in mind, however, is that postoperative wound complications can delay early implementation of postoperative radiation therapy. Postoperative radiation therapy does not influence the extent of surgical resection, and healing and wound complications are not a factor, because irradiation is given after surgery. Currently, doses in the range of 6,000 cGy or more to the primary site and to the neck are recommended, with a boost to areas at increased risk for local recurrence. Thus, for patients with advanced-stage resectable disease (stages III and IV), surgical resection with immediate appropriate reconstruction followed by postoperative radiation therapy is considered the preferred sequence of a combined-modality treatment program. Currently, advanced unresectable disease is managed by a multidisciplinary treatment program of concurrent chemo/radiotherapy with or without hyperfractionation, keeping surgery in reserve for salvage.

The factors that influence the choice of a surgical approach for a primary tumor of the oral cavity or oropharynx are the size of the primary tumor, its depth of infiltration, its site (i.e., anterior versus posterior location), and its proximity to the mandible or maxilla. Therefore, thorough clinical assessment of the primary tumor is mandatory for selecting the appropriate surgical procedure. Examination under anesthesia often is indicated to accomplish this goal. The proximity of the tumor to the maxilla or mandible mandates the need for clinical and radiographic assessment for ruling out the possibility of bone invasion. Radiographic assessment with computed tomography (CT) scans or magnetic resonance imaging (MRI) also may provide information regarding the extent of soft tissue involvement by tumor.

Surgical Approaches

A variety of surgical approaches are available, as shown in Figure 16.15. Small superficial primary lesions located in the anterior oral cavity can be excised via an oral approach. A lower cheek flap, however, is required for adequate exposure for resection of larger primary tumors or those located posteriorly and in considering resection of any part of the mandible. Larger primary tumors located further posteriorly in the oral cavity without proximity to the mandible can be resected via a mandibulotomy approach (36). An upper cheek flap is required for resection of tumors of the palate or upper gum, and a visor flap approach may be employed both to avoid an incision in the midline of the lower lip and chin and to provide exposure of the anterior aspect of the oral cavity for a monoblock composite resection.

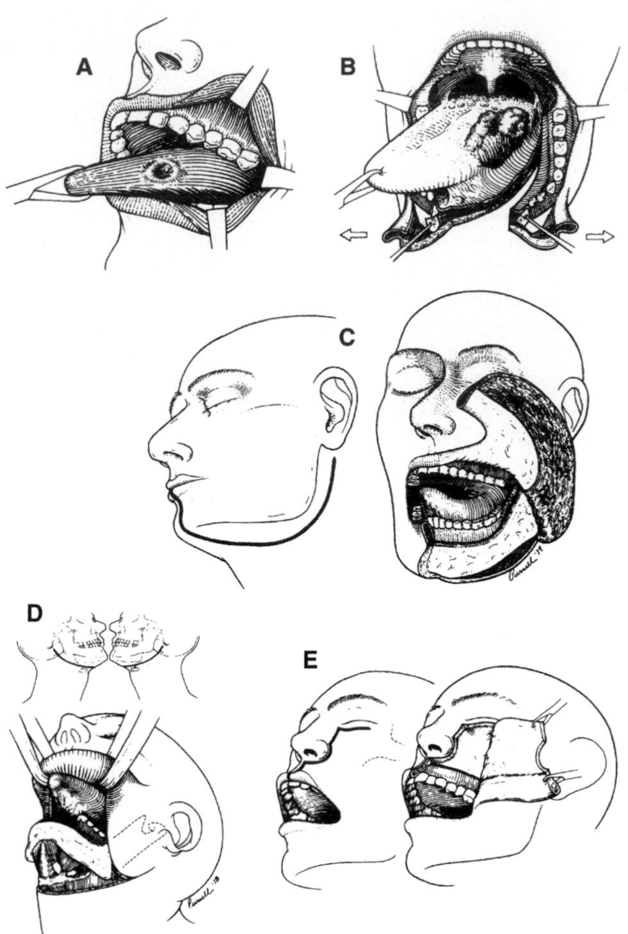

Figure 16.15 Surgical approaches to carcinoma of the oral cavity. **A:** Oral approach. **B:** Mandibulotomy approach. **C:** Lower cheek flap approach. **D:** Visor flap approach. **E:** Upper cheek flap approach. (From Shah JP. *Head and neck surgery,* 2nd ed. London: Mosby-Wolfe, 1996, with permission.)

MANAGEMENT OF THE MANDIBLE

Adequate assessment of the mandible for tumor invasion is essential for appropriate surgical treatment planning (37). The mandible is considered at risk when the primary tumor overlies the mandible, is adherent to the mandible, or is in the proximity of the mandible. In addition to careful examination under anesthesia by bimanual palpation, radiographic evaluation of the mandible with a panoramic roentgenogram or a CT scan is essential for satisfactory treatment planning.

As mentioned, primary carcinomas of the oral cavity extend along the surface mucosa and the submucosal soft tissues and approach the attached lingual, buccal, or labial gingiva. From this point onward, the tumor does not extend directly through intact periosteum and cortical bone toward the cancellous part because the periosteum acts as a significant protective barrier. Instead, the tumor advances along the attached gingiva toward the alveolus. In patients with teeth, the tumor extends through the dental socket into the cancellous part of the bone. In edentulous patients, the tumor extends up to the alveolar process, infiltrates the dental pores in the alveolar process, and then extends to the cancellous part of the mandible. Therefore, in patients with tumors near the mandible (or even those demonstrating early invasion of the mandible), marginal mandibulectomy is feasible, as the lower cortex of the mandible inferior to the roots of the teeth remains uninvolved and can be spared. In edentulous patients, however, the feasibility of marginal mandibulectomy depends on the vertical height of the mandible. With aging, the alveolar process recedes, and the mandibular canal gets closer and closer to the alveolar surface. Resorption of the alveolar process eventually leads to a "pipestem mandible" in very elderly patients. The ability to perform a satisfactory marginal mandibulectomy in such patients is nearly impossible, owing to the risk for iatrogenic fracture intraoperatively or spontaneous fracture in the postoperative period due to avascularity of the residual mandible.

When tumor extension involves the cancellous part of the mandible, a segmental mandibulectomy must be performed. Segmental mandibulectomy also may be required in patients who have massive primary tumors adjacent to the mandible with significant soft tissue disease adherent to or surrounding the mandible. However, segmental mandibulectomy should never be considered simply to gain access to the primary oral cavity tumor that is not in the vicinity of the mandible. The concept of the "commando operation" needs to be redefined, as no lymphatic channels pass through the mandible, therefore not warranting the need for an in-continuity composite resection of the uninvolved mandible.

MANDIBLE-SPARING APPROACHES

The understanding of tumor progression leading to invasion of the mandible has enabled the development of mandible-sparing approaches that include marginal mandibulectomy and mandibulotomy (Fig. 16.16). Marginal mandibulectomy is indicated in the following situations: (a) to obtain satisfactory three-dimensional margins around the primary tumor, (b) when the primary tumor approximates the mandible, and (c) when minimal cortical erosion or minimal erosion of the alveolar process of the mandible is present. Marginal mandibulectomy is contraindicated in the presence of massive soft tissue disease or of gross invasion into the cancellous part of the mandible, or in patients with previously irradiated edentulous mandibles or patients with pipe-stem mandible.

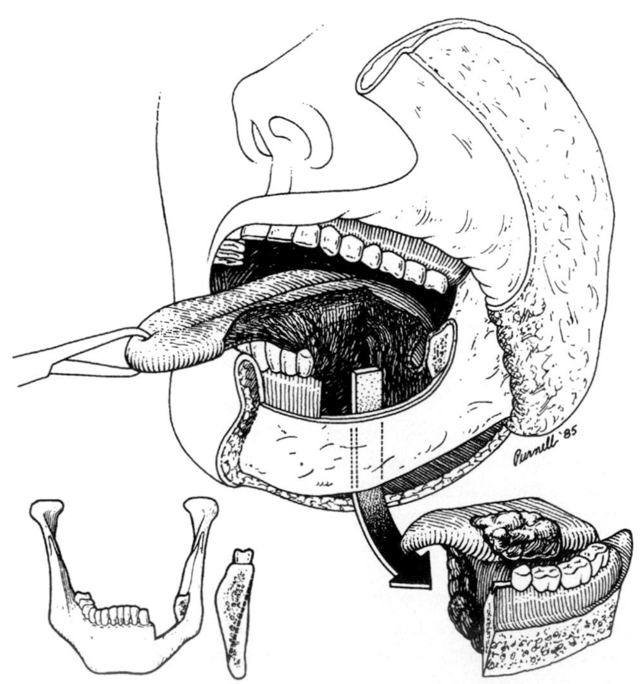

Figure 16.16 Marginal mandibulectomy. (From Shah JP. *Head and neck surgery,* 2nd ed. London: Mosby-Wolfe, 1996, with permission.)

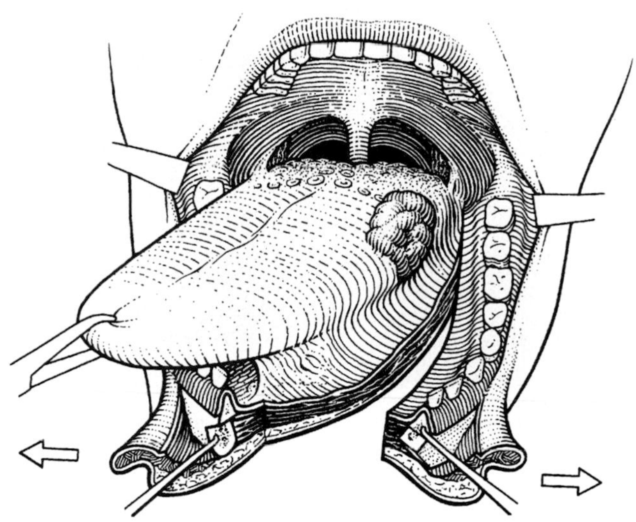

Figure 16.17 Mandibulotomy. (From Shah JP. *Head and neck surgery,* 2nd ed. London: Mosby-Wolfe, 1996, with permission.)

Mandibulotomy or mandibular osteotomy is an excellent mandible-sparing surgical approach designed to gain access to the oral cavity or oropharynx for resection of primary tumors not accessible through the open mouth or through the lower cheek-flap approach (Fig. 16.17) (34,36). Mandibulotomy can be performed in the lateral location, anterior midline, or paramedian position. Lateral mandibulotomy has several anatomic, physiologic, and functional disadvantages and therefore generally is not recommended. Midline mandibulotomy avoids all the disadvantages of lateral mandibulotomy but often causes loss of one or both central incisors and also disturbs the geniohyoid and genioglossus muscles. A paramedian mandibulotomy between the lateral incisor and canine tooth avoids all the disadvantages of the lateral and midline mandibulotomy and provides satisfactory wide exposure with minimal functional debility.

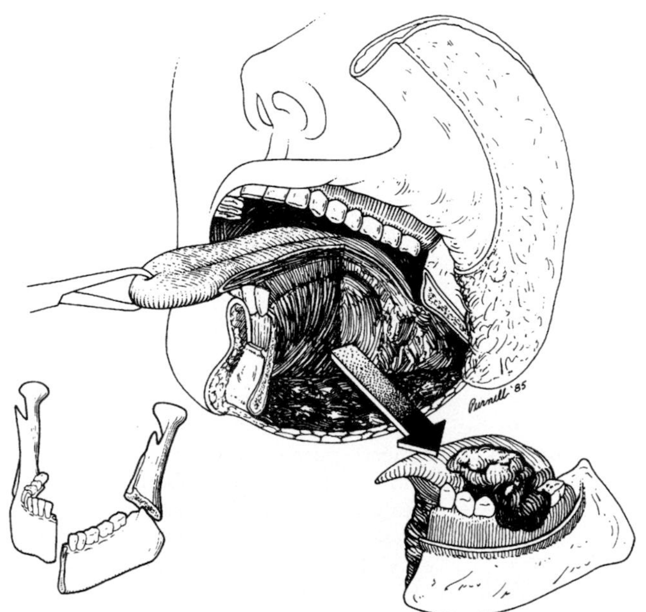

Figure 16.18 Segmental mandibulectomy. (From Shah JP. *Head and neck surgery,* 2nd ed. London: Mosby-Wolfe, 1996, with permission.)

A segmental mandibulectomy is required in the presence of gross invasion of the cancellous part of the mandible or invasion of the alveolar canal by perineural spread. Segmental mandibulectomy is required also for primary malignant tumors of the mandible (Fig. 16.18). The location of segmental mandibulectomy significantly affects the aesthetic and functional outcome of surgery. The aesthetic impact of resection of the ascending ramus and the posterior part of the body of the mandible is not severe, but its functional impact is significant. Loss of the mandibular segment produces unbalanced jaw movements, owing to unequal pull of contralateral extrinsic muscles of mastication and significant malocclusion, and renders the patient unable to chew and consume solid food. Resection of the anterior part of the body of the mandible and its anterior arch produces the most crippling aesthetic and functional disability if the mandible is not reconstructed. These patients are unable to consume solid food, have significant speech impairment, drool saliva, and display an unacceptable "Andy Gump" type of aesthetic deformity.

Mandible reconstruction, therefore, should be considered in surgical treatment planning for all patients requiring segmental mandibulectomy. Although metallic plates are employed in reestablishing the continuity of the resected part of the mandible, they are far from ideal and are associated with a significant risk for exposure, requiring eventual removal. Microvascular free-flap reconstruction of the mandible currently is considered state-of-the-art. Fibula free flap is the ideal donor site and offers outstanding aesthetic and functional results with minimal complications. Osseointegrated dental implants are considered in selected patients as a secondary procedure for total reconstruction and rehabilitation of a teeth-bearing mandible.

RESULTS OF TREATMENT

The single most important factor affecting long-term results after treatment of carcinoma of the oral cavity is the stage of disease at the time of presentation. For early-stage tumors, excellent cure rates are achieved. The 5-year survival rates for patients with oral cancer treated at Memorial Sloan-Kettering Cancer Center between 1986 and 1995 are shown in Figure 16.19. The overall survival is stage- and site-dependent (37). With the employment of adjuvant postoperative radiation therapy, significant improvement in survival for patients with advanced-stage oral carcinoma is observed compared with single-modality treatment (38). Combination of treatment modalities in that manner also has altered the patterns of treatment failure, such that nearly one third of patients now develop dis-

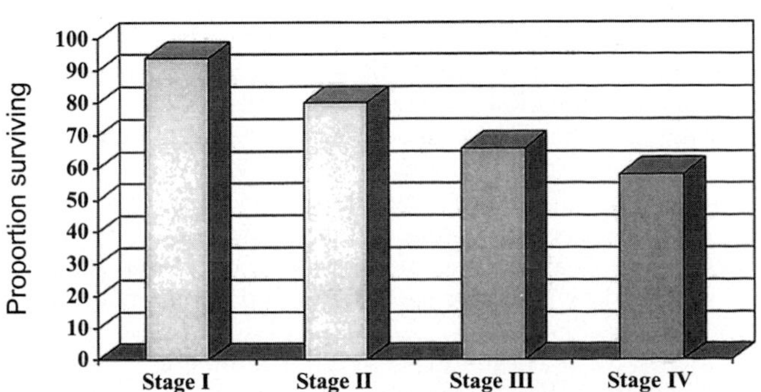

Figure 16.19. Five-year disease-specific survival in patients with squamous cell carcinoma of the oral cavity by stage of disease at Memorial Sloan-Kettering Cancer Center (1986–1995).

tant metastases that eventually lead to demise. In approximately one third of patients, multiple primary tumors develop, either in the upper aerodigestive tract or lung or in other sites. Long-term prognosis in these patients clearly depends on the stage and extent of the subsequent primary lesions. A continued improvement in survival for oral cancer has been observed over the last 40 years, owing to improvements in surgical techniques, combination of treatment modalities, increasing use of elective treatment of the negative neck, and employment of adjuvant postoperative radiation therapy in patients with advanced-stage disease (10).

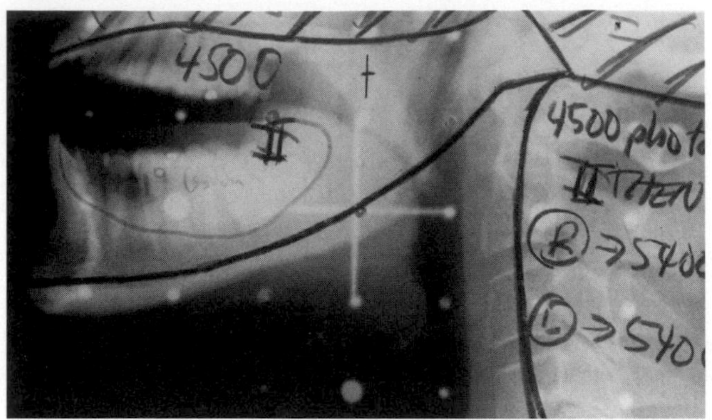

Figure 16.20 A simulation portal for a patient with T2N0 tongue cancer. (Courtesy of Louis Harrison, M.D.)

Radiation Therapy for Oral Cavity Cancers

In general, the outcome for patients with oral cavity cancers treated with radiation therapy is similar to that for surgical approaches for comparably staged patients. Patients with early-stage lesions (T1 to T2 and selected T3 lesions) can be treated effectively with external radiation therapy or interstitial implantation. Patients with more advanced disease often require combined-modality approaches to achieve a higher likelihood of locoregional control. Selection criteria for a particular treatment modality depend on many factors, including the extent of disease, degree of disease infiltration, location of the primary disease, and medical comorbidities of the patient and other variables.

Compared with those in other sites in the head and neck, oral cavity tumors have a higher observed rate of local recurrence after definitive therapy (35,38,39). Several investigators have noted that outcome for oral cavity cancer depends on the particular subsite involved. Patients with oral tongue tumors, in particular, may have a higher propensity for local recurrence than those with floor-of-mouth cancers (40). Though the radiosensitivity of tumor clonogens may be similar within the oral cavity, the patterns of local spread and possible underestimation of the true extent of disease may be considerations in explaining the higher observed rates of local failure for the oral tongue subsite.

ORAL TONGUE TREATMENT APPROACHES

Radiation Therapy With or Without Neck Dissection

The optimal radiation therapy approach for most T1 lesions is brachytherapy alone, which is accomplished most often with an Iridium-192 (^{192}Ir) temporary implantation. Depending on the location of the tumor within the oral tongue, the catheters can be inserted under general anesthesia via a submental or intraoral approach. The iridium then is loaded 1 to 2 days after surgery after completion of localization and computerized dosimetry. The usual dose range achieved is 40 to 50 cGy per hour, and the total dose delivered is 50 to 60 Gy. For infiltrating T1 lesions or stage T2 disease, we prefer delivering initially with external-beam radiation therapy (EBRT) approximately 30 to 40 Gy, followed by an interstitial implantation boost.

Although patients with node-negative disease can be treated with radiation therapy alone, patients with palpable lymphadenopathy often are treated with a neck dissection at the time of the tongue implantation. Our policy is to wait approximately 3 weeks after the completion of the external radiation phase of therapy before proceeding with the implantation and possible neck dissection.

Patients treated with EBRT require simulation with bite-block immobilization. A customized mask is used to enhance immobilization further and to reduce potential setup errors. Because of the rich vascular and lymphatic supply of the tongue, even lateralized lesions require inclusion of the majority of the tongue within the initial treatment portals and on both sides of the neck. Opposing portals are used to encompass the tongue and upper neck bilaterally. Figure 16.20 illustrates a typical simulation portal for a patient with a T2N0 oral tongue cancer. The inferior border of the lateral portal is matched at the level of the hyoid bone to a low anterior neck field. The spinal cord is blocked on the low neck, the block also functioning to shield the glottic larynx and to minimize potential for laryngeal edema. The use of a bite block is helpful also for depressing the tongue and separating it from the palate, where it can be shielded more easily. For anterior tongue and floor-of-mouth lesions, care should be taken to avoid unnecessary irradiation of the lip. Devices fabricated to interpose between the lip and gingiva can increase effectively the distance of the lip from the tumor volume at risk and can decrease the severity of acute reactions.

RESULTS OF RADIATION THERAPY FOR ORAL TONGUE CANCERS

One of the largest experiences using radiation therapy for cancers of the oral tongue was reported by Decroix and Ghossein (41). In that report, 602 patients were treated with EBRT and interstitial implantation, and excellent control rates and outcomes were noted. The local recurrence rates were 14%, 22%, and 29% for T1, T2, and T3 tumors, respectively, comparing favorably to results reported for similarly staged patients undergoing partial glossectomy. The authors noted that one third of patients failed at the periphery of the implant, and that a higher percentage of patients with T1 lesions failed outside of the high-dose region of the implanted volume. These data underscore the insidious growth patterns of oral tongue tumors and the neck in incorporating larger margins of apparently normal tissue in close proximity to palpable disease.

Especially for oral tongue tumors, the brachytherapy procedure represents a critical aspect of the radiotherapeutic management of the disease, and the dose contributed by the implant must represent the major part of the cumulative prescription dose (42–44). In one series reported by Pernot et al. (42), 181 patients were treated with brachytherapy alone for oral tongue lesions, and 267 were treated with combined EBRT and implantation. The 5-year actuarial local control rate for all 448 patients was 93% for T1, 65% for T2, and 49% for T3 lesions. When patients with T2 lesions were analyzed separately, the control rates were 90% for those treated with implantation alone, compared with 50% for those treated with the combined-modality approach. Similar results have been reported by Mendenhall et al. (43) for T2 lesions of the oral tongue. In that study, among patients treated for T2 lesions, local control was achieved more often when a greater component of the dose was delivered via the implant than via the EBRT. The authors recommend at least 35 Gy from the implant in addition to 20 to 30 Gy from the EBRT. Investigations from the M. D. Anderson Cancer Center also correlated the contribution of implant dose with local control for patients with T1 to T2 oral tongue cancers (44). Among patients who were treated with combination EBRT and interstitial implantation, the local control rate was 92% for those who received lower external radiation doses (less than 40 Gy) and higher brachytherapy doses, compared with a 65% control rate for patients who received lower implant doses. However, given the retrospective nature of these reports, these data must be interpreted with caution, as selection factors likely played a significant role in choosing favorable, smaller T2 lesions for implantation alone rather than a combined-modality approach for more advanced or infiltrative lesions.

Although for many years radiation therapy alone (brachytherapy with or without EBRT) has been the accepted treatment approach at the University of Florida for early-stage cancer of the oral tongue, beginning in 1985 investigators from that institution introduced a change in treatment policy in favor of primary surgical treatment (45). This shift in treatment approach was made secondary to the observation that 14 of 42 patients (33%) with T1 to T2 oral tongue cancers experienced soft tissue necrosis or bone exposure after definitive radiation therapy. Fein et al. (45) reported the outcome of this recently adopted surgical approach compared with results achieved with radiation therapy alone. In that series, most patients treated with radiation therapy alone underwent combined EBRT and interstitial implantation. The actuarial local control rates at 2 years for T1 tumors were 79% and 76%, respectively, for patients in the radiation therapy and surgery groups ($p = 0.76$). Similarly, the actuarial local control rates at 2 years for T2 tumors were 72% and 76%, respectively, for the radiation therapy and surgery groups ($p = 0.86$). When the incidence of treatment-related complications was analyzed by T stage, a significantly higher complication rate was noted for locally advanced tumors treated with radiation therapy compared with surgery (31% and 5%, respectively). The incidence of severe treatment-related complications for T1 to T2 lesions, however, was similar for patients treated with radiation therapy to those treated with surgery (11% and 11%, respectively).

High dose rate brachytherapy (HDR-BRT) has become an attractive means of delivering a concentrated dose of radiation for oral cavity lesions. Recently, encouraging results have been reported using HDR-BRT for early-stage oral tongue cancers. Inoue et al. (46) reported the results of a phase III randomized trial comparing the outcome of HDR and low dose rate (LDR) interstitial implantation for T1-T2 oral tongue cancers. In that trial 25 patients were treated with HDR-BRT using a submental approach and received twice daily fractions of 6 Gy for a cumulative dose of 60 Gy. In the LDR group, the median tumor dose was 70 Gy delivered over a median of 117 hours. The median follow-up times in the HDR and LDR groups were 78 and 85 months, respectively. The 5-year actuarial local control rates for the HDR and LDR groups were similar (87% and 84%, respectively). Leung et al. (47) reported on 19 patients with T1-T2 oral tongue cancer treated with HDR-BRT as the definitive management for their disease. These investigators reported a 95% control rate at 4 years. Five patients developed soft tissue ulceration.

In general, outcome for patients treated with radiation therapy alone for locally advanced disease is poor. Local failure rates are in excess of 60% to 70%, and 5-year survival rates are approximately 25% to 30% (48–50). Combined-modality therapy in the form of surgery and postoperative radiation therapy is used commonly in the setting of stage III and stage IV disease. Zelefsky et al. (40) reported the outcome of patients with oral tongue carcinomas treated with surgery and postoperative radiation therapy. The local control was 62% at 5 years, and the overall survival in this group was 55%. Local control for oral tongue tumors was significantly lower than that achieved for patients with floor-of-mouth tumors. A multivariate analysis confirmed these findings. The margin status did not influence the local control outcome.

Because of inherent problems in assessing the true extent of the tumor intraoperatively, the surgeon may have difficulty in achieving negative surgical margins for oral tongue cancers. In many cases, frozen-section margins are obtained to determine the need for further resection before completion of the operation. The prognosis for an initially negative margin in the oral tongue may be different from that for the patient with an initially positive but subsequently negative margin. Investigators from the M. D. Anderson Cancer Center reported a 13% local failure rate with initially negative surgical margins compared with 22% local failure for ultimately negative but initially positive margins (51). These differences may have significant implications for selecting high-risk patients who may benefit from adjunctive postoperative radiation therapy. Caution should be exercised in making the decision to use postoperative radiation therapy on the sole basis of the final pathology findings. Close multidisciplinary interaction is essential to make the most prudent decision for adjuvant radiation therapy. In the setting of an ultimately negative margin that initially required additional intraoperative excisions to achieve a negative margin status, consideration should be given for postoperative radiation therapy, especially in the presence of other advanced prognostic factors. Because of the relatively poor local control rates achieved with conventional fractionation for oral cavity cancers with high-risk features for failure (positive or close margins, multiple neck nodes, vascular or perineural invasion), some are employing twice-daily fractionation schemes in the postoperative setting.

The need for adjuvant postoperative radiotherapy for patients who underwent resection for T1-T2 oral tongue cancers with close or positive margins represents a challenging management problem. In general, such patients can be treated with postoperative EBRT to most, if not all, of the oral cavity with expected posttreatment sequelae. Lapeyre et al. (52) reported the results of adjuvant postoperative brachytherapy for oral cavity tumors who had documented positive or close margins after surgery. Thirty-six patients were treated with ^{192}Ir to a mean dose of 60 Gy. With a median follow-up time of 80 months, local control and disease-free survival rates was 89% and 85% at 5 years. Five patients developed soft tissue necrosis and two patients developed bone exposure after this procedure.

FLOOR-OF-MOUTH TUMORS

Surgical Therapy With or Without Radiation Therapy

Early floor-of-mouth lesions are treated more often with surgery. In cases where radiation therapy is used, improved outcome has been noted when interstitial therapy is added (43,50). For lesions in close proximity to the mandible, brachytherapy should be avoided because of the high risk for osteonecrosis.

For more advanced disease, surgery and postoperative radiation therapy are recommended. The general treatment approach includes the use of opposing lateral portals to treat the primary site and upper neck, which form a junction to a low neck field at the level of the thyroid notch (Fig. 16.21). A midline

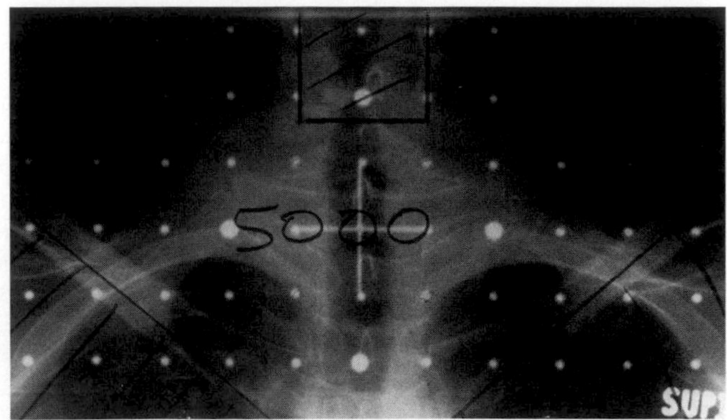

Figure 16.21 Lower neck field for treatment of cervical lymph nodes. Notice that the larynx is blocked, as well as the lung in the infraclavicular area. (Courtesy of Louis Harrison, M.D.)

block is used for the low neck field to protect the larynx and the spinal cord. The dose to the low neck region is 50 Gy in 5 weeks. The upper neck and primary site generally are treated to 45 Gy, after which a spinal cord block is placed. The primary site and neck then are treated to 54 Gy and with a final boost that results in a cumulative tumor dose of 63 Gy. Especially in the setting of pathologically confirmed disease in the neck, electron fields are used posterior to the spinal cord block to treat the posterior cervical lymph nodes (level V) as needed.

Results of Radiation Therapy for Floor-of-Mouth Cancers

Wang et al. (53) reported the results of external radiation with and without intraoral cone therapy. The 3-year disease-free survival rates were 85% and 58% for T1 and T2 lesions, respectively. For selected patients in that experience, in whom treatment was amenable to intraoral cone therapy, the control rates were 13 of 13 (100%) and 19 of 20 (95%) for T1 and T2 lesions, respectively. Similar outcome for early-stage disease has been reported by investigators from the University of Florida (43).

Mazeron et al. (54) reported the outcome of 79 patients treated with brachytherapy alone or in combination with EBRT for early-stage floor-of-mouth lesions. Most patients were treated with 65 Gy using ^{192}Ir. The control rates for T1 and T2 lesions were 94% and 74%, respectively. Factors that were predictive of tumor control included the size of the lesion and the absence of gingival extension. Similar findings were reported by Matsumoto et al. (55). In their analysis of 90 patients with stage T1 and stage T2 floor-of-mouth lesions treated with brachytherapy (mostly using ^{198}Au), local control depended on tumor size and the presence of gingival extension of disease. The local control rates using this treatment approach for lesions measuring 0 to less 2 cm, 2 to 3 cm, and more than 3 cm were 89%, 76%, and 56%, respectively. Furthermore, the incidence of local control for T1 to T2 lesions without gingival involvement was 82%, compared with 55% for patients with gingival disease extension. The incidence of moderate complications was 26%, and the incidence of severe complications necessitating surgical intervention was 5%. Nevertheless, because of the close proximity to the mandible, caution must be exercised in performing an implant, especially for disease with gingival extension, because of an increased risk for osteonecrosis.

An update of the Gustave-Roussy Institute experience with brachytherapy for early-stage floor-of-mouth cancers was recently reported (56). Brachytherapy delivered a median dose of 70 Gy via ^{192}Ir using the Paris system rules. Follow-up times ranged from 9 to 19 years. The local control rates for T1 and T2 lesions were 93% and 88%, respectively. Grade 2 to 3 bone exposure was noted in 18% of treated patients, yet this complication was less often observed among patients with better dental hygiene and those who were treated with a custom intraoral dental shield.

The results with radiation therapy alone for T3 and T4 lesions are less favorable. Rodgers et al. (57) reported 55% and 40% control rates with radiation therapy alone for T3 and T4 lesions, respectively. Advanced-stage tumors can be treated more effectively with surgery and postoperative radiation therapy. When retrospectively compared with results for similarly staged patients treated in the same institution with surgery and radiation therapy, the results were better with the combined modality.

COMPLICATIONS

The complications of treatment of oral cancer are related largely to the treatment modality employed and the functional sequelae of such therapy. Therefore, complications can be related to surgery or radiation therapy.

Surgical Complications

Complications after surgery for oral cancer include both early complications in the immediate postoperative period and late complications related to functional and aesthetic sequelae of surgery. The early complications are related to the operative procedures and include hemorrhage, aspiration pneumonia, and wound breakdown with resultant fistula formation. Development of these complications increases morbidity, prolongs hospitalization, increases the cost of therapy, and produces an adverse impact on long-term functional outcome. Delayed complications of surgery include alteration in the clarity of speech, mastication, and swallowing. They are related largely to the loss of the mobile portion of the tongue and lack of clarity of articulation and bolus transport and mastication in the oral cavity. With loss of the mandible or dentition, the function of mastication is significantly altered. Fortunately, contemporary reconstructive techniques establish the continuity of the mandible when segmental mandibulectomy is performed, and the technical advances in osseointegration have permitted restoration of the dentition to rehabilitate the function of mastication and speech. The aesthetic sequelae of surgical treatment are related to external appearance and wound contracture. Again, these effects are largely of historical importance, as contemporary surgical techniques avoid unpleasant incisional scars and soft tissue and bone loss, owing to the availability of immediate reconstructive techniques.

Radiation Therapy Complications

As noted with surgery, the complications of radiation therapy also are early and late. The early complications are related to development of acute mucositis and its sequelae. Acute mucositis in the oral cavity produces painful ulceration, thus impairing the patient's ability to swallow and speak, and requires the need for pain control. Prolonged mucositis may lead to development of fungal infection requiring appropriate antifungal treatment. Generally, the early complication of mucositis can be ameliorated with maintenance of optimal oral hygiene and frequent oral irrigations. Loss of taste, although not permanent, is a disabling symptom that may last from several weeks to several months after radiation therapy. However, in most patients, the function of taste returns to near-normal level, although some patients continue to complain about a metallic taste in the mouth.

Xerostomia is the most disabling complication and is a permanent sequela of radiation therapy. Every patient receiving radiation therapy to the oral cavity will have varying degrees of xerostomia. The lack of saliva causes significant discomfort and debility with speech, mastication, and swallowing. Many patients require the use of a bottle of water to maintain moisture in the oral cavity. Although artificial sialogogues are commercially available, their efficacy is not predictable, and they are not a satisfactory solution to the disabling problem of xerostomia. A randomized trial has demonstrated subjective improvement of symptoms of xerostomia in approximately 50% of patients treated with pilocarpine (58).

Dental caries and osteoradionecrosis also are serious late complications of radiation therapy. Appropriate preradiation dental evaluation and fluoride prophylaxis reduce the risk for dental caries. Presence of dental sepsis and introduction of a septic focus through dental extraction initiate the process of osteoradionecrosis. Therefore, if dental extraction or any endodontic manipulation is to be undertaken in a patient who has received previous radiation therapy for oral cancer, both the patient and the dentist should be aware of the potential risk for osteoradionecrosis and its prevention by appropriate antibiotic coverage in the perioperative period, atraumatic manipulation during extraction of the tooth, filing of sharp spicules of exposed bone, and, when feasible, closure of the dental socket with sutures is desirable. If significant dental sepsis is present, increasing the risk for radionecrosis, hyperbaric oxygen treatment should be considered before and after extractions. With these precautions, the risk for osteoradionecrosis is reduced. If radionecrosis ensues in spite of these precautions, its appropriate management should be undertaken. With the availability of microvascular composite free-flap techniques, an aggressive approach is now recommended for management of osteoradionecrosis of the mandible. The osteoradionecrotic segment of mandible is resected until healthy bone stumps are demonstrated. The surgical defect usually is repaired with a microvascular free flap of fibula. With the aggressive management of osteoradionecrosis, the long-term morbidity of this complication is reduced, and progressive bone loss is minimized.

MANAGEMENT OF RECURRENCE

Recurrent disease after initial treatment may develop at the primary site, at regional lymph nodes, or at distant sites. Management of recurrence is described for each of these locations.

Local Recurrence

Local recurrence at any site after initial successful treatment of oral cancer can be managed either by surgery or radiation therapy. If a satisfactory surgical resection is technically feasible and functionally suitable, that procedure remains the preferred modality of treatment. However, if surgical resection is thought to be technically impossible or is held to be functionally crippling, nonsurgical management includes implementation of external or interstitial radiation therapy for control of recurrent disease. An imperative reminder is in order: *Retreatment of oral cancer produces further functional debility and affects the quality of life.* If further surgery and external or interstitial radiation therapy are not feasible, palliative treatment with systemic chemotherapy is considered. The response rates in the recurrent setting are low (15% to 20%), and the duration of response is approximately 5 to 7 months.

Regional Recurrence

If recurrent disease develops in the regional lymph nodes in a previously undissected neck, patients are offered an appropriate comprehensive neck dissection followed by postoperative radiation therapy. If recurrent disease occurs in a previously dissected and irradiated neck, consideration is given to further surgical resection. That course depends on the availability of interstitial implantation of the surgical bed and appropriate coverage of the surgical defect using nonirradiated regional cutaneous, myocutaneous, or microvascular free flaps. Regional control after such treatment attempts is respectable, and significant palliation is obtained by such aggressive intervention. Significant palliation can also be achieved by interstitial implantation alone of unresectable recurrent disease in the neck in selected patients.

Distant Recurrence

Development of metastatic disease to lungs or bone requires consideration of systemic treatment. Currently, none of the available chemotherapeutic drugs offers a predictable tumor response of long-lasting duration. Methotrexate, cisplatin, 5-fluorouracil, and Taxol are the drugs of choice. Cisplatin and 5-fluorouracil in combination are given every 3 weeks for up to four to six cycles, depending on treatment response. Weekly methotrexate may be continued for several months and for up to 2 to 3 years if continued tumor response is demonstrated and patient tolerance is observed. However, the indications for systemic chemotherapy in the absence of symptoms from metastatic disease are debatable. In general, response of metastatic deposits to systemic treatment is manifested in approximately 15% to 20% of patients, and the duration of response is approximately 5 to 7 months.

PAIN CONTROL

When local, regional, or distant recurrence of oral cancer produces symptoms with pain, control of pain becomes an issue of high priority. Appropriate consultation with pain management teams for pain control—with an analgesic effect lasting several hours—is desirable. Consonant with pain control is maintenance of nutrition, which may require the use of a percutaneous gastrostomy. Eventually, patients with terminal disease require hospice care in a home setting. Involvement of psychosocial services at this juncture is vitally important in maintaining continued home-environment care for these patients until a peaceful and painless demise occurs in the comfort of family and friends.

SPECIAL ISSUES

The most important advances in the management of oral cavity over the last 25 years are related to the development of microvascular free-flap surgery for reconstruction of the mandible and the development of osseointegrated implants for restoration of dentition. A high degree of technical skill is required with expertise in microsurgery for reconstruction of the mandible. The current choice of mandible reconstruction is a free flap of fibula. Restoration of the continuity of the arch of the mandible thus is achieved in a single operation. Consideration is given for osseointegrated implants to restore dentition to patients who remain free of disease for at least 1 year after mandible reconstruction. Thus, total rehabilitation of the patient undergoing composite resection for advanced oral cancer can now be achieved in a satisfactory fashion.

Another important advance over the last 10 years is the general interest in chemoprevention of oral cancer. Several analogs of vitamin A, such as beta-carotene and 13-cisretinoic acid, have demonstrated preventive effects for genesis of epithelial cancers in various tumor systems in the laboratory and in animal models. Clinical trials are under way for prevention of multiple primary cancers in patients who remain clinically free from any evidence of persistent or recurrent disease at least 6 months after definitive treatment for early-stage oral carcinomas. Similar trials of chemoprevention using NSAIDs, acting as COX-2 inhibitors, are also currently active.

RADIOLOGIC IMAGING CONCERNS

Bernard B. O'Malley and Suresh K. Mukherji

Imaging of the mouth is a challenging experience, even with the first diagnosis of a lesion in a virgin oral cavity. Before cross-sectional techniques, radiographic evaluation added little to the clinical evaluation. Early computed axial tomography scan improved on the evaluation of osseous involvement at the mandible and maxilla (59), albeit providing simple binary information. Thin (3 mm) sections through the jaw with appropriate postprocessing of the scan data can provide accurate detection of mandible involvement (60). Some would advocate use of radionuclide bone scanning to improve the sensitivity and specificity of bone invasion to 100% and 86%, respectively, when combined with orthopantomography (61). Improvements in technical CT factors, particularly reduction in scan time per section, have allowed more accurate evaluation of the regional soft tissues, especially when intravenous contrast is used. The advancement in computer technology has moved complex multiplanar reformatting and curved rendering from "off-board" after-market devices to built-in system features. Magnetic resonance imaging, first clinically introduced for brain imaging, has advanced oral cavity imaging further by providing even greater soft tissue information (Fig. 16.22) without the requirement for intravenous contrast. However, MRI may be overly sensitive to regional soft tissue abnormalities without adequate specificity (62). This is particularly problematic for MRI in the posttreatment setting (63). Some degree of overestimation of the regional extent of a primary lesion probably is acceptable, and each institution functions with an understanding of the relative weight of imaging information impact on upstaging of lesions.

Panoramic radiographs of the mandible (and maxilla) currently are relegated to the role of evaluation of the status of fixation plates and healing of reconstructions (Fig. 16.23). Panoramic radiographs can demonstrate bone invasion (Fig. 16.24) with advanced lesions, but evaluation of the cancellous and cortical bone for early erosion (Fig. 16.25), destruction, or osteitis is better performed with cross-sectional imaging. Oblique radiographs are helpful for evaluation of either side of the body mandible when artifact distorts the panoramic view. Spot-occlusal radiographs are required for detailed evaluation of the alveolus, particularly at the symphysis, incisors, and canines. X-ray tomography remains the only technique not degraded by artifact from dental amalgam. Magnetic resonance imaging has supplanted tomography of the temporomandibular joint if no metallic endoprostheses (which severely degrade images of the region) are present.

Evaluation for the extent of mandibular involvement would fall ideally between the sensitivity of CT and that of MRI (64). The value of MRI is its strong negative predictive value for bone involvement (64,65). Reportedly, normal cortical bone with a clinically fixed lesion indicates occult periosteal involvement or bone infiltration. The extent of anticipated marginal or segmental resection in this setting, however, may be overestimated by MRI, which cannot always resolve reactive changes within the cancellous bone related to the tumor or to prior dental disease (65). Fat-suppression MRI techniques are helpful for evaluation of cancellous bone if a homogeneous saturation can be achieved and if local distortion due to dental amalgam is limited (66). Overall, the combination of exquisite soft tissue detail and reasonably accurate evaluation of the status of bone margins makes MRI the study of choice for most subsites of the oral cavity. Artifact from dental work compromises both MRI and CT. Nuclear techniques may provide information that is adjunctive to cross-sectional imaging if the spatial resolution is acceptable relative to lesion size. Imaging of the various subsites of the oral cavity is discussed below. Table 16.3 is a checklist for a comprehensive imaging evaluation of those subsites.

TABLE 16.3 Oral Cavity Imaging Checklist

Lip carcinomas
Bone erosion
Soft tissue invasion
Floor of mouth (FOM) carcinomas
Extent of bone erosion
Deep invasion along the mylohyoid and hyoglossus muscles
Relationship to ipsilateral lingual neurovascular bundle
Extension across midline and relationship to contralateral neurovascular bundle
Tongue base invasion
Extension into the soft tissues of the neck
Oral tongue
Invasion of ipsilateral lingual neurovascular bundle
Extension across midline and relationship to contralateral neurovascular bundle
Invasion of the floor of mouth and associated bone erosion
Buccal mucosa
Submucosal extension
Bone erosion
Gingiva and hard palate
Bone erosion
Perineural invasion of the incisive canal, greater and lesser palatine foramen
Retromolar trigone
Bone erosion
Submucosal spread
Perineural invasion

Oral Tongue

The AJCC staging of tumor in the oral cavity is a function of size (67). Invasion of an adjacent structure designates a lesion categorically T4. Imaging of the oral tongue rarely is needed for size determination. Furthermore, the substance of the tongue is heterogeneous, which limits exact sizing of a lesion. Correctly performed imaging in a cooperative patient, however, can determine the presence or absence of extension across the midline lingual septum (Fig. 16.26). Axial or direct coronal views can exclude extension to the floor of mouth (Fig. 16.27) or involvement of the glossotonsillar sulcus. This determination is made more accurately by correlating various MRI sequences and planes than by CT (62). Both axial and direct coronal CT scans often are degraded by streak artifact from dental amalgam. However, CT does offer shorter imaging time for patients with oral pain and difficulty with secretions. Ultrasonography can be used by experienced operators to evaluate the tongue but is very dependent on operator skills. Although ultrasound can depict local extension, it is less suitable for follow-up for differentiation of residual disease versus treatment fibrosis in the radiated cohort (68). Follow-up imaging is very instrumental after multimodality treatment. Imaging can reveal abnormalities that are not visible under well-healed flaps or fibrosed tissues (see Fig. 4.29).

Gingiva

Evaluation of the alveolus for carcinoma of the gingiva rarely is performed for early disease. Imaging of advanced disease may be productive, especially for the maxillary alveolus (Fig. 16.28) and for the retromolar trigone (Figs. 16.29 and 16.30). Estimation of the extent of disease on the alveolus is limited because of extreme tissue density differences between air, tissue, and bone-teeth, even in those with preserved dentition. Accurate diagnosis is particularly difficult in those with relative permeative-appearing bone, as in the edentulous patient, or with irregularity in those with recent extractions. Magnetic resonance imaging is particularly weak in determining bone invasion related to lesions arising in the gingiva (69). In the mandible, proximity of disease to the nerve of the alveolar canal can be estimated by reformatted views, including the widely used Denta Scan® (G.E. Medical Systems, Milwaukee, Wi.). In the maxilla, the degree of involvement of the base of the antrum is readily shown. Lateral extension to the gingivobuccal sulcus is better estimated clinically, but posterior submucosal extension to the pterygoid processes can be shown in the axial plane, which is particularly helpful in the patient with trismus. Medial extension to the floor of mouth should be excluded for lesions of the lingual plate (Fig. 16.31).

Floor of Mouth

The floor-of-mouth lesion is well imaged in the conventional axial (Fig. 16.32) or direct coronal plane. Posterior extension to the hypoglossal-lingual neurovascular pedicle can be demonstrated (70). Inferior extension to and through the mylohyoid is shown best with fat-suppressed MRI or direct coronal contrast CT. Simple obstruction of Wharton's duct should be differentiated from infiltration of the submandibular gland (Fig. 16.33).

Palate

Squamous cancer of the palate rarely presents at advanced stages. Early lesions usually are managed through the open mouth, with low risk for involvement of the underlying palatine bone (Fig. 16.34). Minor salivary lesions and invasive SCC of the hard and soft palate require careful multiplanar imaging at (and particularly above) the level of the palate (Fig. 16.35) (71). Accurate preoperative estimation of disease facilitates early prosthesis planning and rehabilitative efforts. Careful evaluation of the palatine canal and adjacent pterygopalatine fossa (Fig. 16.36) in the setting of minor salivary gland lesions facilitates proper preoperative planning of extent of resection and consideration of immediate reconstructive options. Follow-up scanning is performed readily with CT as an adjunct to the clinical examination. Although a clinically apparent lesion may be obvious, the deep perineural component cannot be seen (Fig. 16.37).

Buccal Mucosa

Squamous buccal lesions rarely require imaging of the primary site. Recurrent or advanced lesions occasionally invade the masticators (primarily the masseter muscle) or gingivobuccal sulcus (72). Imaging of the buccal mucosa is difficult, as it is collapsed against the teeth. Modified imaging performed in either axial or coronal projections with the cheeks (73) distended may help estimate regional extension within the oral cavity (Figs. 16.38 and 16.39). Mucosal lesions of minor salivary origin require careful combination of clinical and imaging evaluation, particularly when the lesion is reported to be long-standing (Fig. 16.40).

Jaw Lesions

Lesions of the mandible and maxilla include locally infiltrating mucosal lesions, primary osseous and dentigerous lesion, and (less commonly) lymphoproliferative malignancy, metastatic disease, or systemic metabolic disorders. (The locally infiltrative primary mucosal lesions were discussed in the preceding section.) The mandible (and maxilla) rarely is the presenting site of a previously undiagnosed metabolic disorder or systemic malignancy.

Epithelial and other lesions of dental origin may require cross-sectional imaging if they appear suspicious on x-ray views (74). Most lesions that appear lytic radiographically are related to simple cystic lesions of dentigerous origin. However, the grade of a malignant jaw lesion cannot be predicted from a single imaging study or group of imaging studies obtained at one point. Aggressive-appearing lesions may not be malignant (or neoplastic). Lesions that appear well circumscribed may be very biologically aggressive or have high local recurrence rates (Fig. 16.41). The role of imaging is to outline the lesion with respect to the mandibular nerve, extraosseous extension, and remaining teeth. Computed tomography evaluates cortical bone well and should be designed to highlight spatial resolution (Fig. 16.42). Magnetic resonance imaging can assess the cancellous bone better than can CT if field distortion from dental amalgam does not produce artifact that disturbs the post-contrast series, especially in attempting fat suppression. Computed tomography is very useful in the serial evaluation of the osseous integrity of composite grafts for jaw reconstruction (Fig. 16.43).

Osteonecrosis of the mandible occurs at predictable sites under certain treatment protocols. The diagnosis is made on clinical grounds, therefore, and radiographic or tomographic findings lag behind the onset and recovery of osteonecrosis. The appearance on radiographs is a permeative radiolucency compared with the typical appearance of diffuse sclerosis of radiation osteitis. The difficulty is ruling out the possibility of local tumor recurrence.

Turn to imaging atlas beginning on the next page.

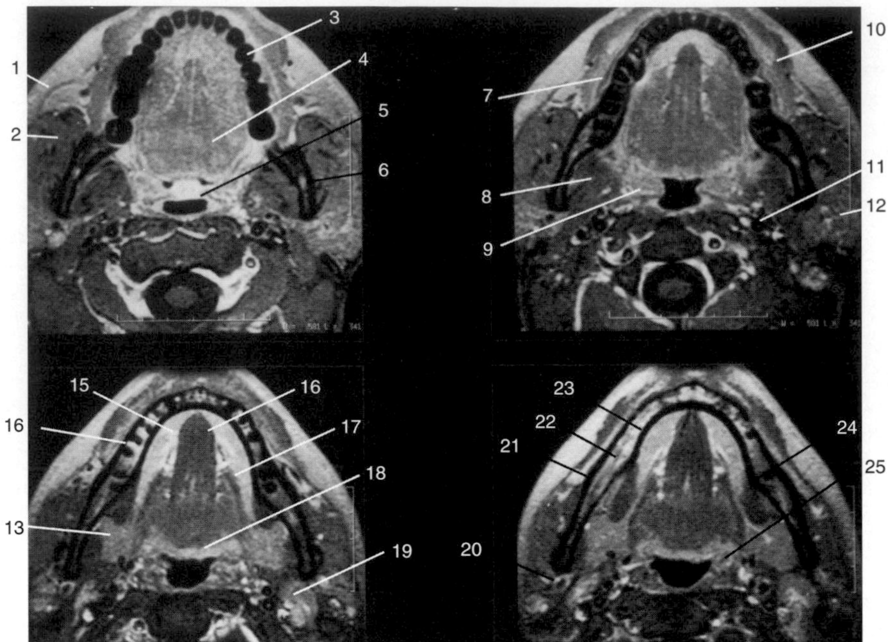

Figure 16.22 Magnetic resonance imaging of oral cavity: normal. *1,* Wharton's duct; *2,* masseter; *3,* mandibular tooth; *4,* intrinsic tongue muscles; *5,* uvula; *6,* mandibular foramen; *7,* buccal mucosa; *8,* medial pterygoid; *9,* tonsillar pillar; *10,* buccinator muscle; *11,* internal carotid; *12,* superficial lobe parotid; *13,* hilum of submandibular gland; *14,* molar tooth root; *15,* sublingual glands; *16,* genioglossus; *17,* palatoglossus; *18,* mucosa tongue; *19,* internal jugular view; *20,* retromandibular vein; *21,* lingual plate of mandible; *22,* alveolus segment of V^2; *23,* buccal plate of mandible; *24,* mylohyoid; *25,* oropharynx.

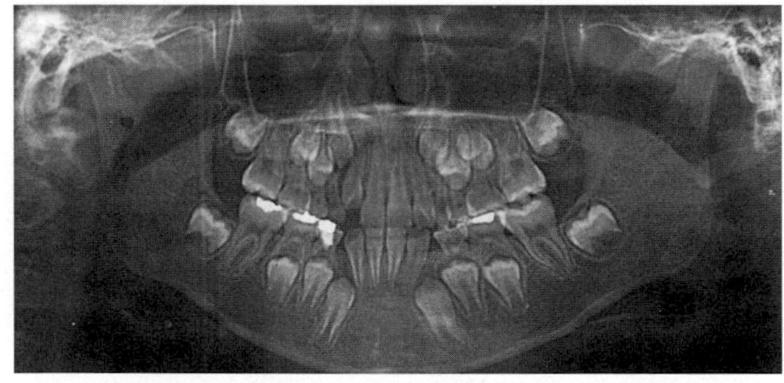

Figure 16.23 Panoramic mandible. Panoramic radiograph of the mandible provides a survey of the mandible and maxilla with overlying artifacts. Digital processing reduces distracting density variations due to the airway and spine.

A

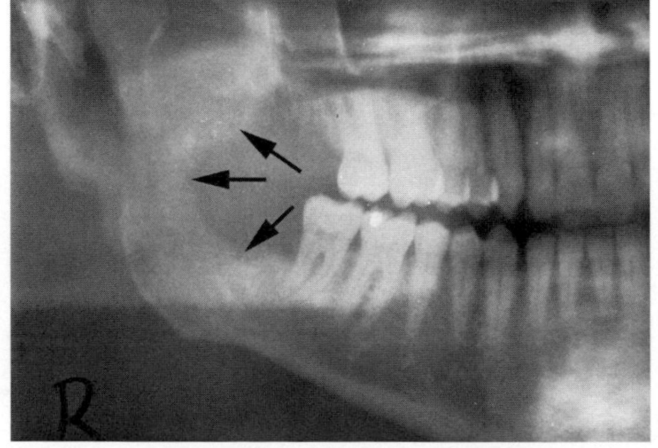

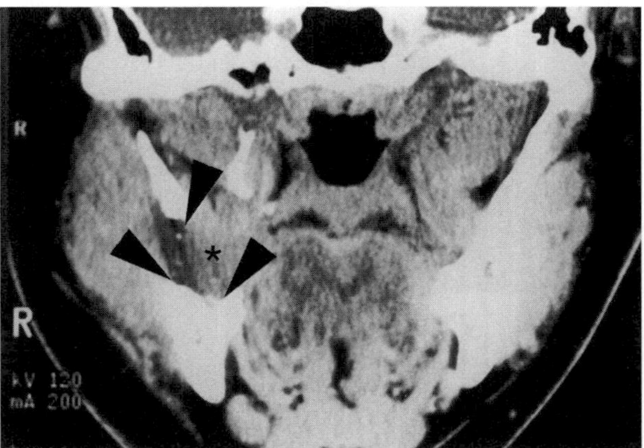

B

Figure 16.24 Panoramic mandible. **A:** Magnified image from a conventional panoramic view of the mandible shows erosive changes of the retromolar bone and coronoid process (*arrows*). **B:** Direct coronal enhanced computed tomogram of the same patient shows the enhancing retromolar squamous cancer (*asterisk*) and the corresponding bone erosion (*arrowheads*).

A,B
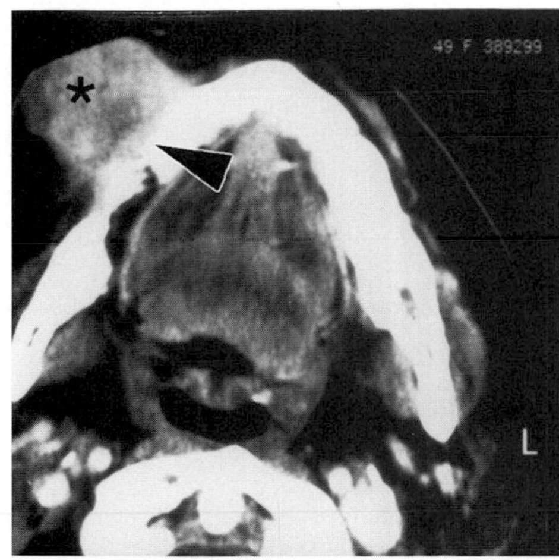

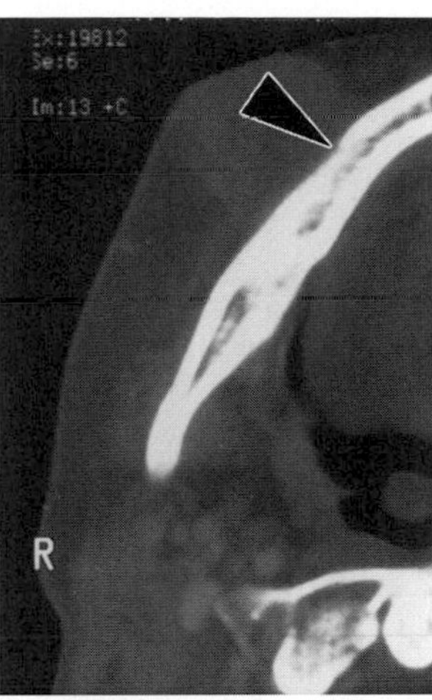

Figure 16.25 Bone erosion. Enhanced axial computed tomogram of soft tissue **(A)** and bone-window views **(B)**, which demonstrate a large squamous cell cancer of the gingivobuccal sulcus (*asterisk*) with corresponding erosion of the buccal plate of the mandible (*arrowheads*).

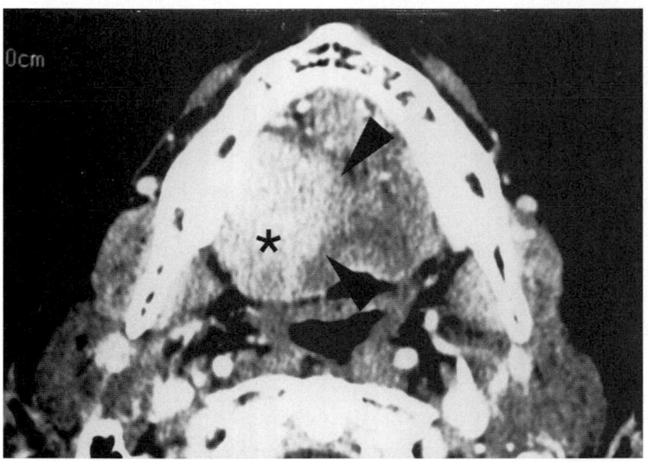

Figure 16.26 Advanced oral tongue cancer. Enhanced axial computed tomogram of large oral tongue cancer (*asterisk*) involving the midline (*arrowheads*).

A
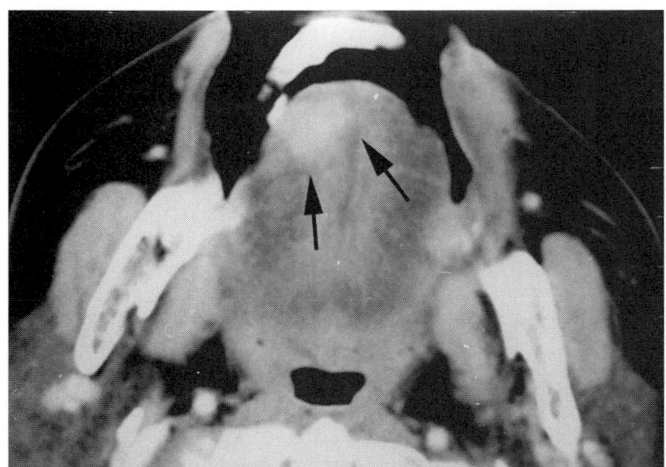
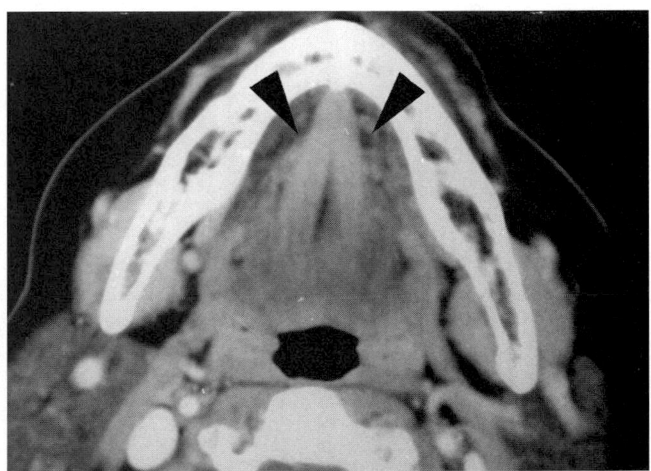
B

Figure 16.27 Early oral tongue cancer. Enhanced axial computed tomogram of tongue **(A)** and floor of mouth **(B)** shows a small but ill-defined lesion of the right side of oral tongue (*arrows*) with no involvement of subjacent floor of mouth (*arrowheads*).

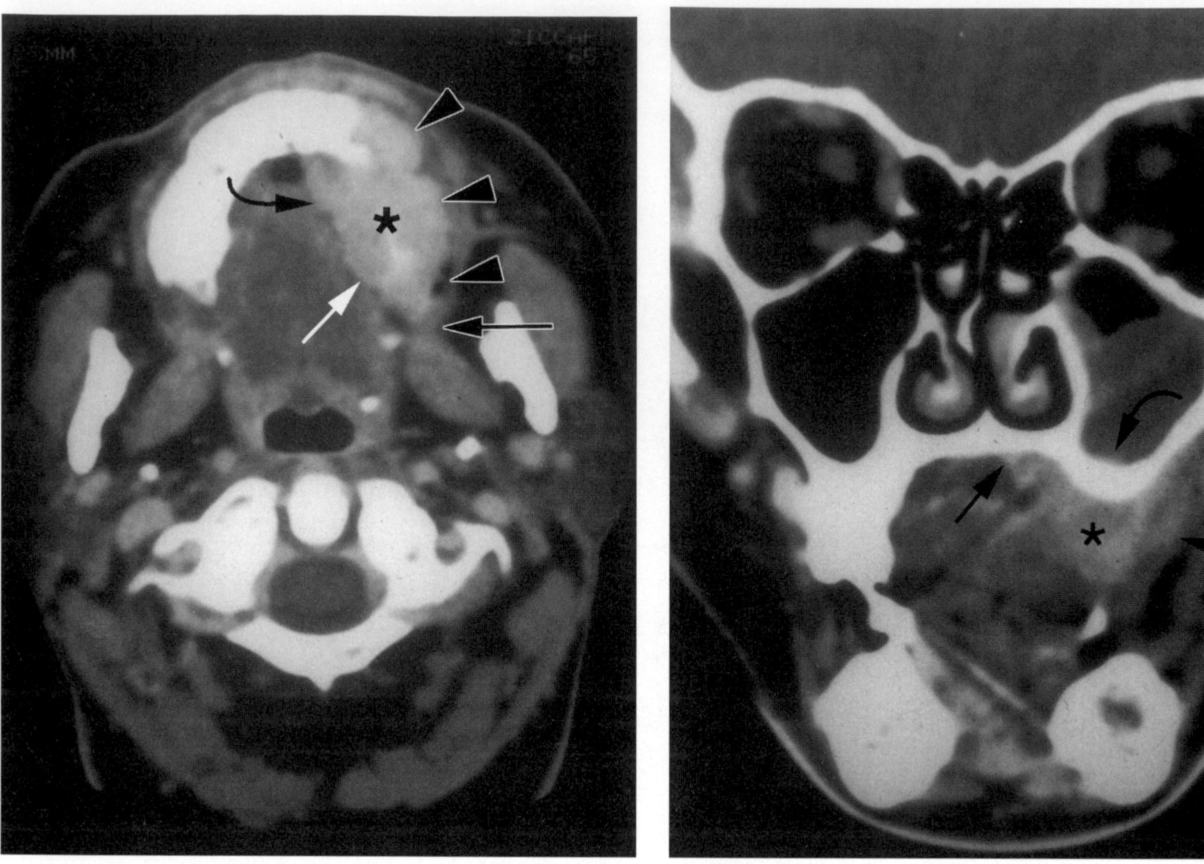

Figure 16.28 Advanced gingival cancer. Enhanced **(A)** axial and **(B)** direct coronal computed tomographic views of a large squamous cell cancer (*asterisk*) of the maxillary alveolus, with medial (*arrow*) and lateral (*arrowheads*) extent well outlined. Early antral invasion (*curved arrow*) surrounded by reactive secretions. Note preserved pterygomaxillary raphe (*long arrow*).

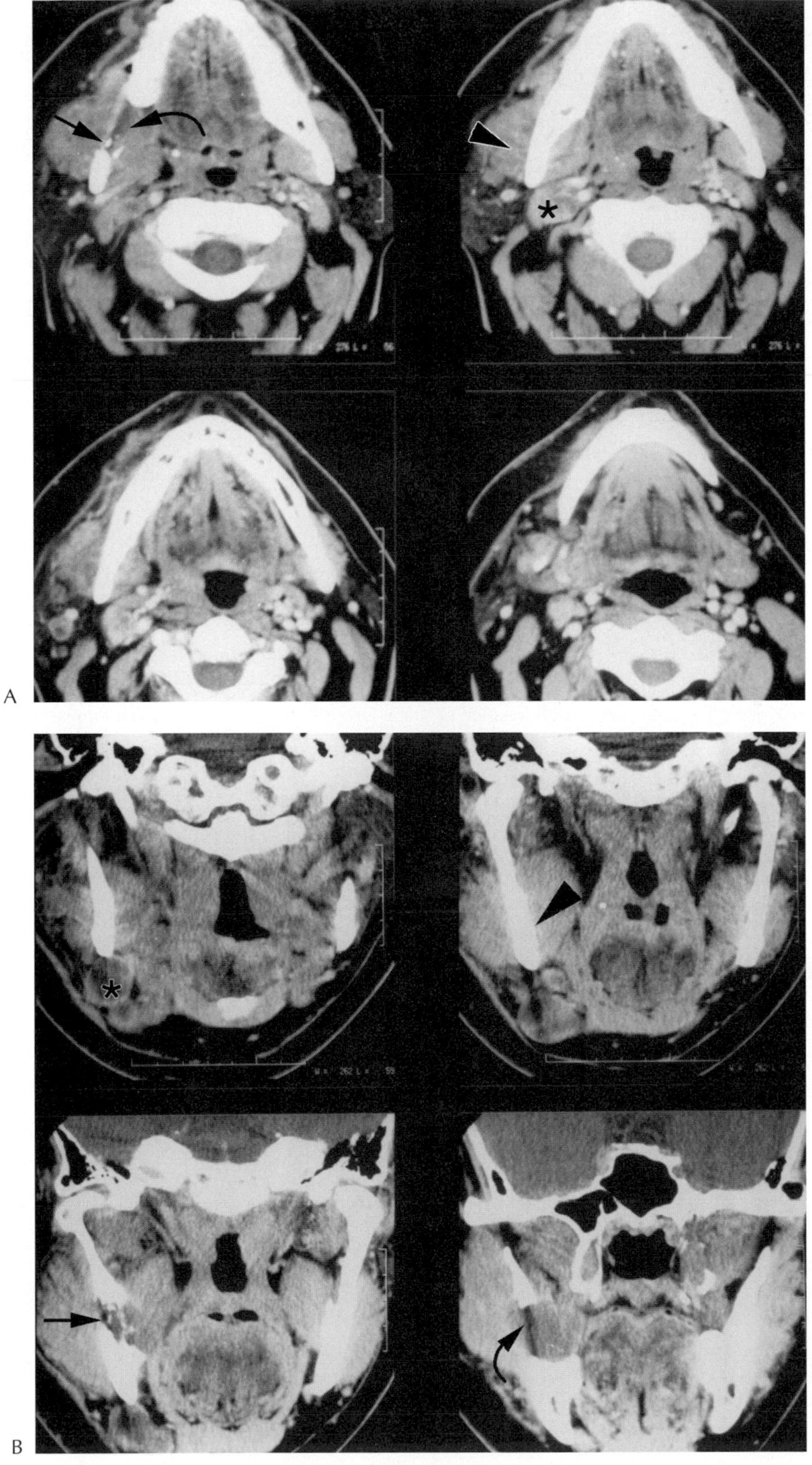

Figure 16.29 Advanced retromolar cancer. Enhanced axial **(A)** and coronal **(B)** views of oral cavity show retromolar mass (*curved arrow*) with bone destruction (*arrow*), muscle infiltration (*arrowhead*), and regional adenopathy (*asterisk*).

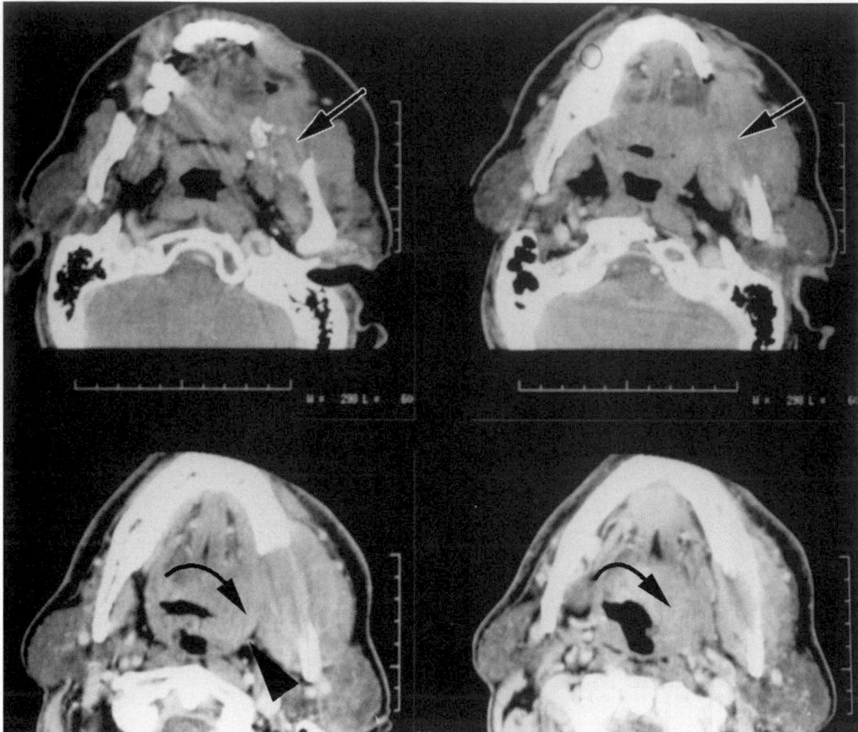

Figure 16.30 Advanced retromolar cancer. Enhanced axial computed tomogram shows large retromolar squamous cell cancer (*arrow*) with invasion of lateral tongue base (*curved arrow*) and oropharyngeal wall (*arrowhead*).

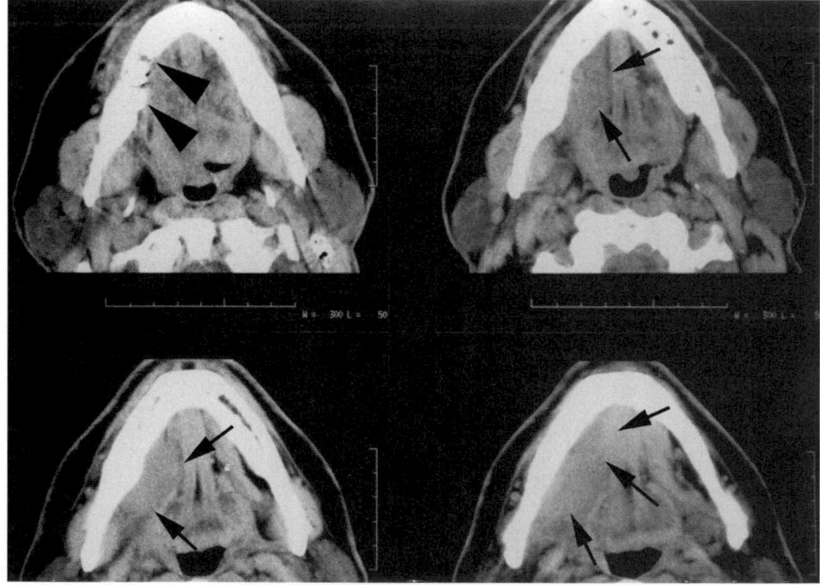

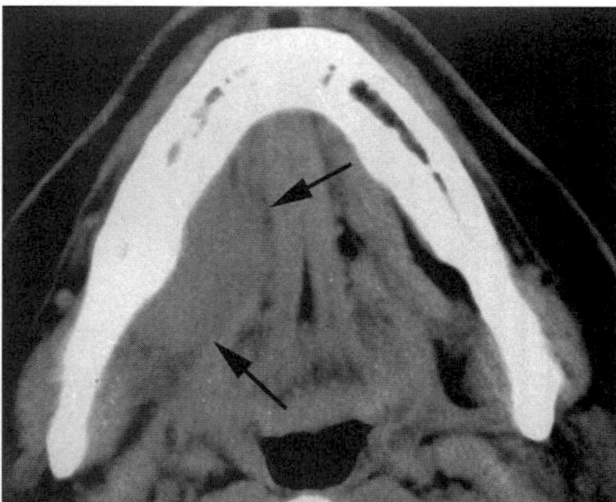

Figure 16.31 Extensive carcinoma of gingiva. Serial non–contrast-enhanced axial computed tomogram of oral cavity shows erosive changes of lingual plate of right mandible (*arrowheads*) secondary to large carcinoma of alveolus, extending through the right floor of mouth (*arrows*).

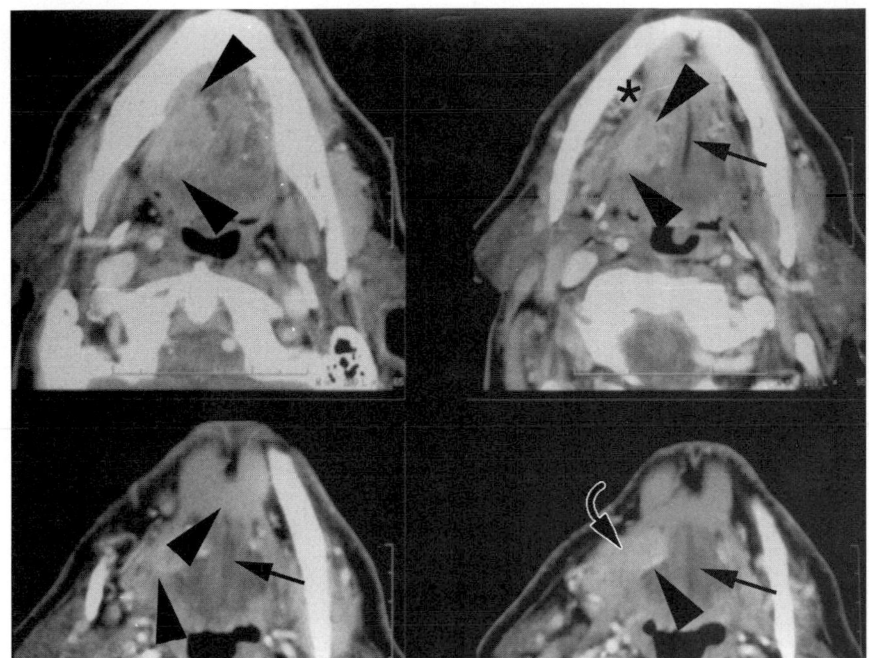

Figure 16.32 Floor-of-mouth cancer. Serial enhanced axial computed tomographic images through the oral cavity show an enhancing lesion (*arrowheads*). Note preservation of the lingual septum (*arrows*) despite the invasion of the tongue. Extension through the mylohyoid muscle (*curved arrow*) into the submental compartment and suspicious lymph node (*asterisk*).

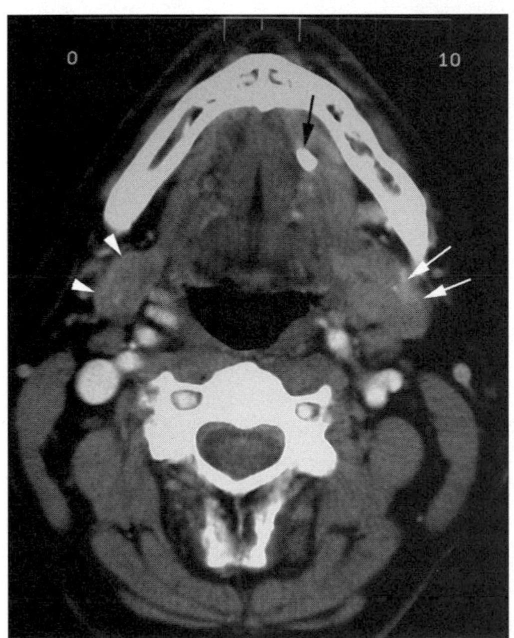

Figure 16.33 Pseudomass of the neck. The left submandibular gland (*white arrows*) is swollen compared with the right (*white arrowheads*) due to an obstructing calculus (*black arrow*) within the Wharton duct.

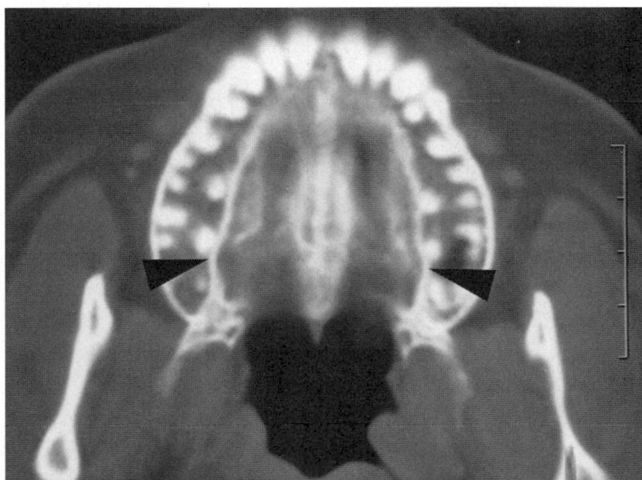

Figure 16.34 Normal hard palate. Axial bone-window view of hard palate showing normal symmetric greater palatine foramina (*arrowheads*).

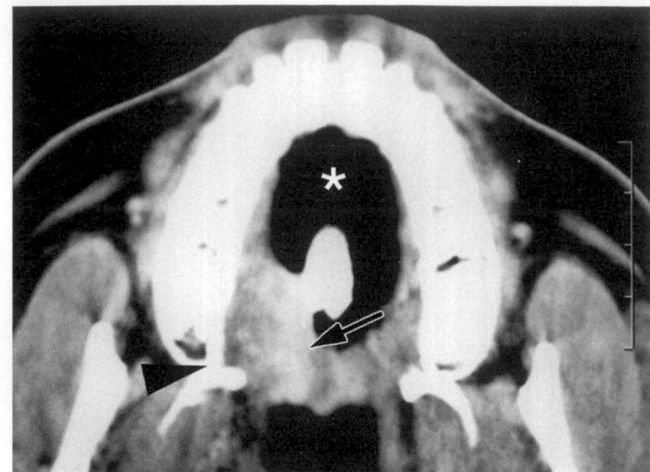
A

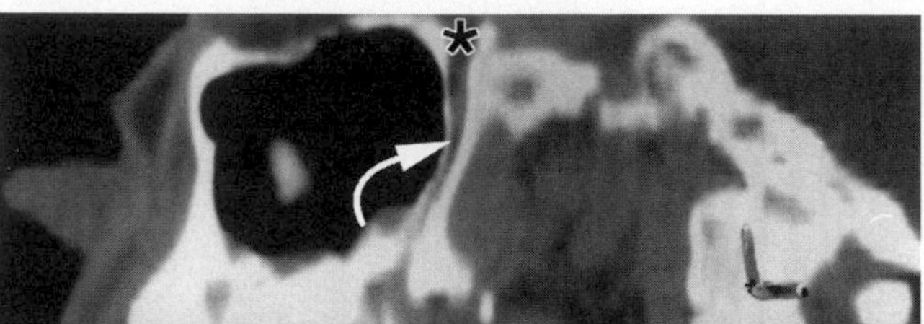
C

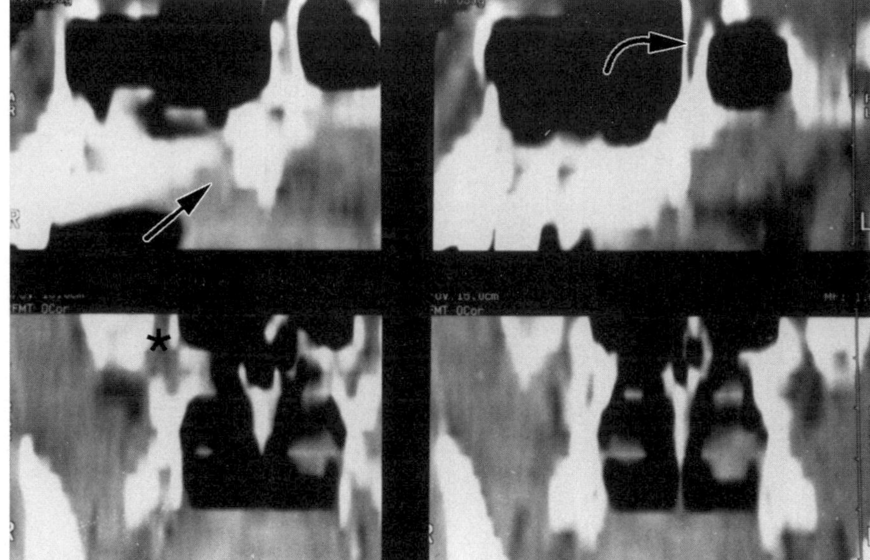
B

Figure 16.35 Early palate cancer. Enhanced axial computed tomogram **(A)** and reformatted sagittal (upper) and coronal (lower) views **(B)** of minor salivary gland cancer (*arrow*) approaching but not including greater palatine foramen (*arrowhead*). **C:** The palatine canal (*curved arrow*) and pterygopalatine fossa are normal.

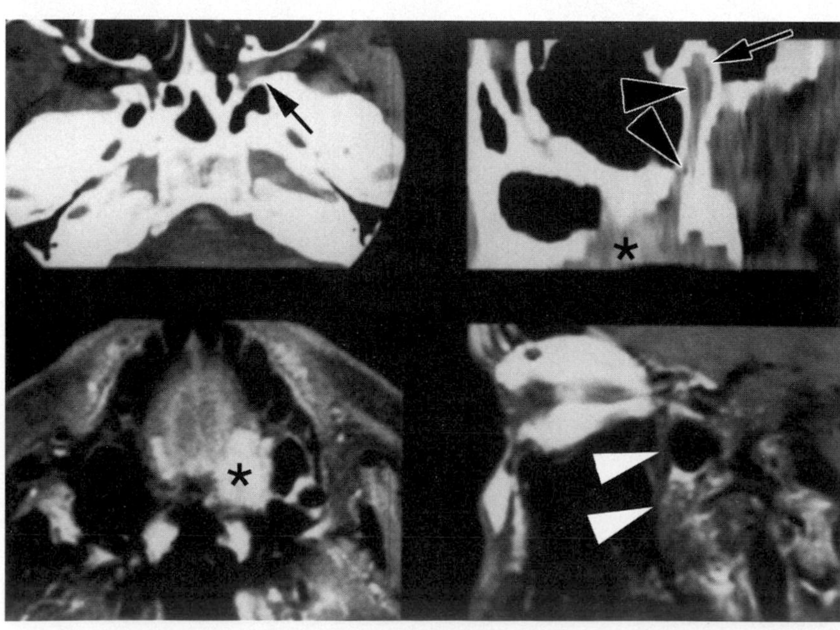

Figure 16.36 Neurotropic palate cancer. (Clockwise from top left) Enhanced axial computed tomogram (CT) of pterygopalatine fossa, parasagittal reformatted CT, and corresponding sagittal and axial magnetic resonance imaging (MRI) show the unanticipated extension to pterygopalatine fossa (*arrow*) along palatine canal (*arrowheads*) from the small posterior hard palate primary tumor (*asterisk*), which is better seen on MRI than on CT.

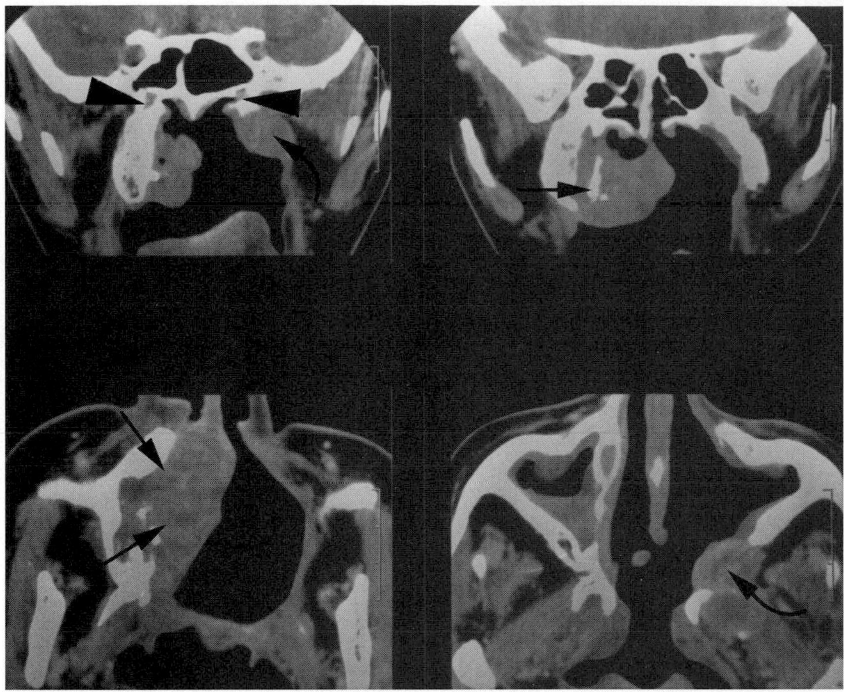

Figure 16.37 Recurrent palate cancer. Direct coronal (top) and axial enhanced computed tomographic images showing multifocal recurrence at the right maxillary margin (*arrows*) and left pterygoid suprastructure (*curved arrows*) and involvement of both pterygopalatine fossae (*arrowheads*).

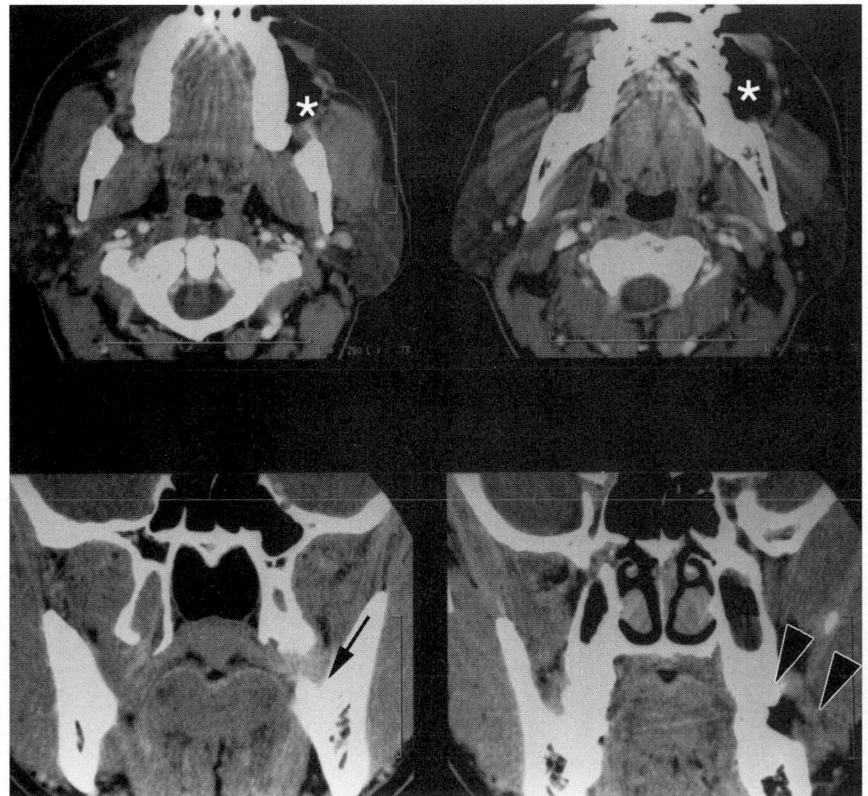

Figure 16.38 Retromolar cancer. **A:** Gauze placed in gingivobuccal sulcus creates air space (*asterisk*) that separates mucosa from retromolar lesion (*arrow*) and spreads out mucosa, revealing true thickening **(B)**, which indicates lateral tumor infiltration (*arrowheads*). *(continued on next page)*

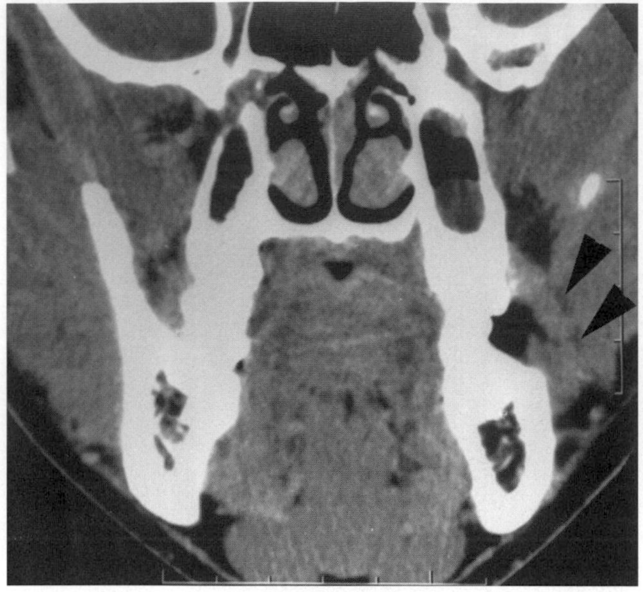

B

Figure 16.38 *(continued)*

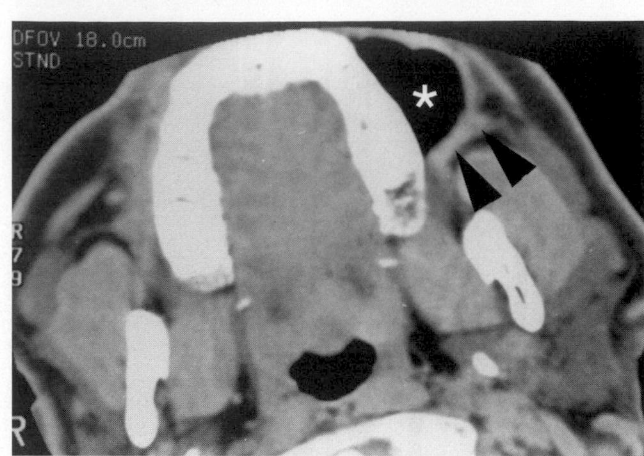

Figure 16.39 Buccal cancer. Gauze placed in gingivobuccal sulcus creates air space (*) and stretches out mucosa, revealing submucosal extension of squamous cell cancer of buccal mucosa (*arrowheads*).

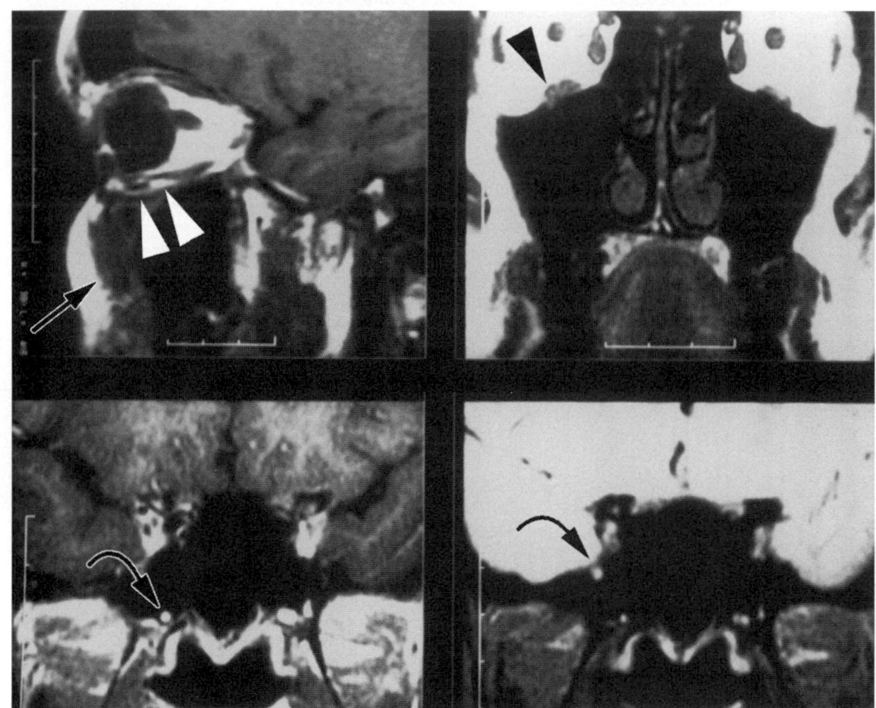

A

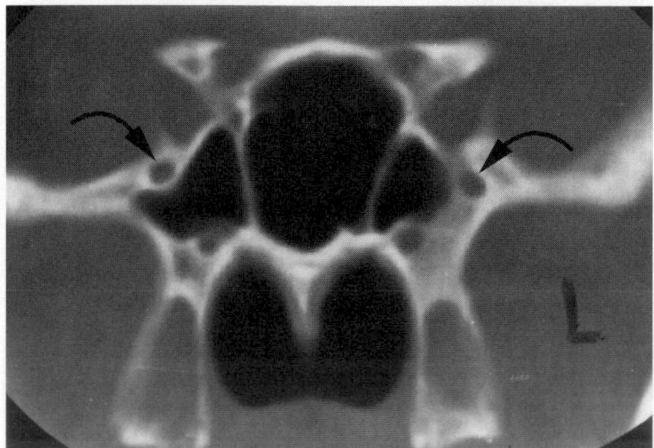

B

Figure 16.40 Neurotropic buccal cancer. **A:** (Clockwise from top left) Sagittal T1, coronal T1, and coronal T2 views show a small premaxillary lesion of minor salivary origin that arose at the mucosa of the gingivobuccal sulcus (*arrow*), extending through infraorbital foramen, along the inferior orbital groove (*arrowheads*), through pterygopalatine fossa to the pterygoid canal (*curved arrow*) at the skull base. **B:** Note the lack of structural widening of the pterygoid canal (*curved arrows*) despite the abnormality on the coronal magnetic resonance image.

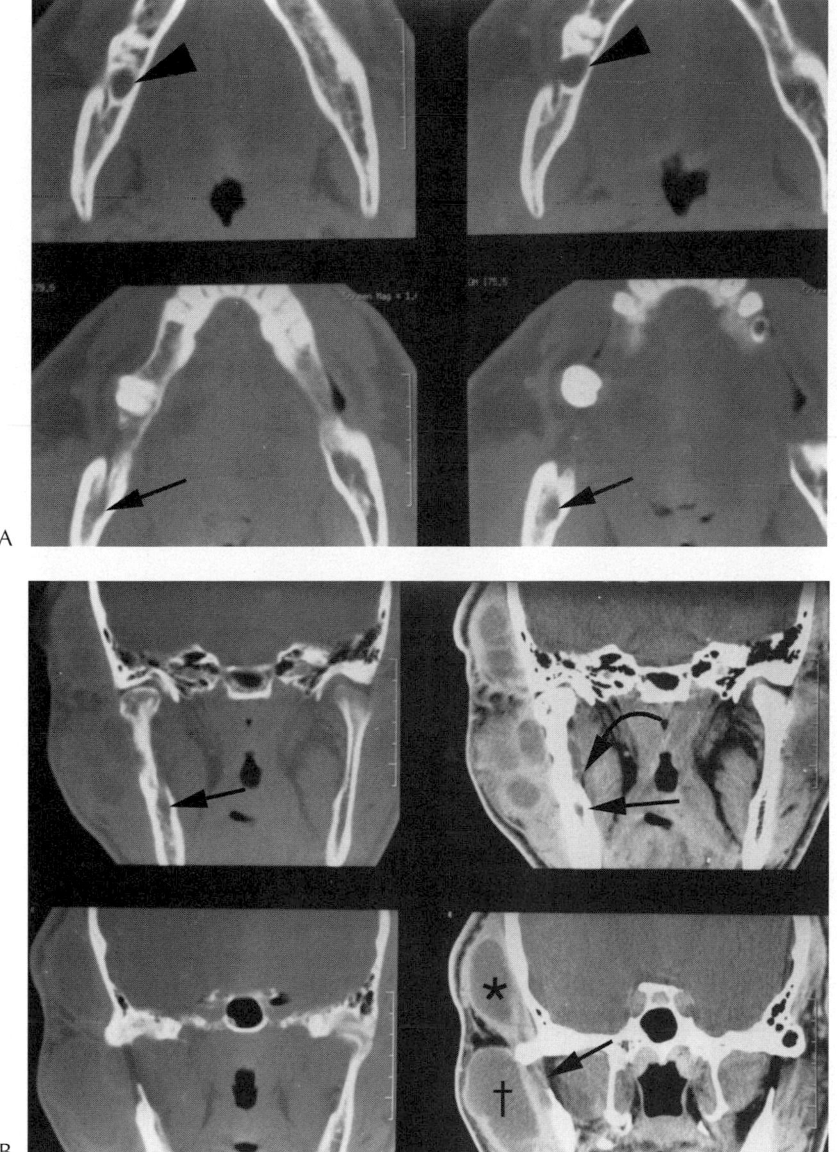

Figure 16.41 Recurrent keratocyst. **A:** Serial axial bone-window views show intraosseous recurrence (*arrowheads*), which tracks upward along the alveolar canal (*short arrows*). **B:** Bone and soft tissue windows from enhanced direct coronal views show suprazygomatic (*asterisk*) and infrazygomatic (†) keratocyst herniating through the coronoid notch (*long arrow*), growing out of mandibular foramen (*curved arrows*).

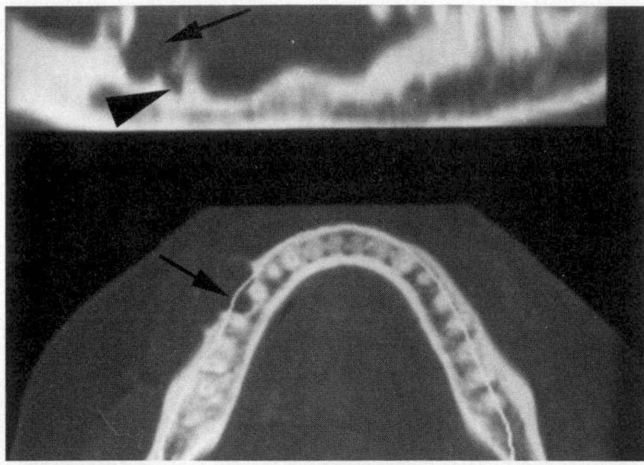

Figure 16.42 Computed tomographic reformatted view of mandible. Curved reformatted bone-window view of small lytic lesion (*arrows*) of buccal plate that approximates the mental foramen (*arrowhead*).

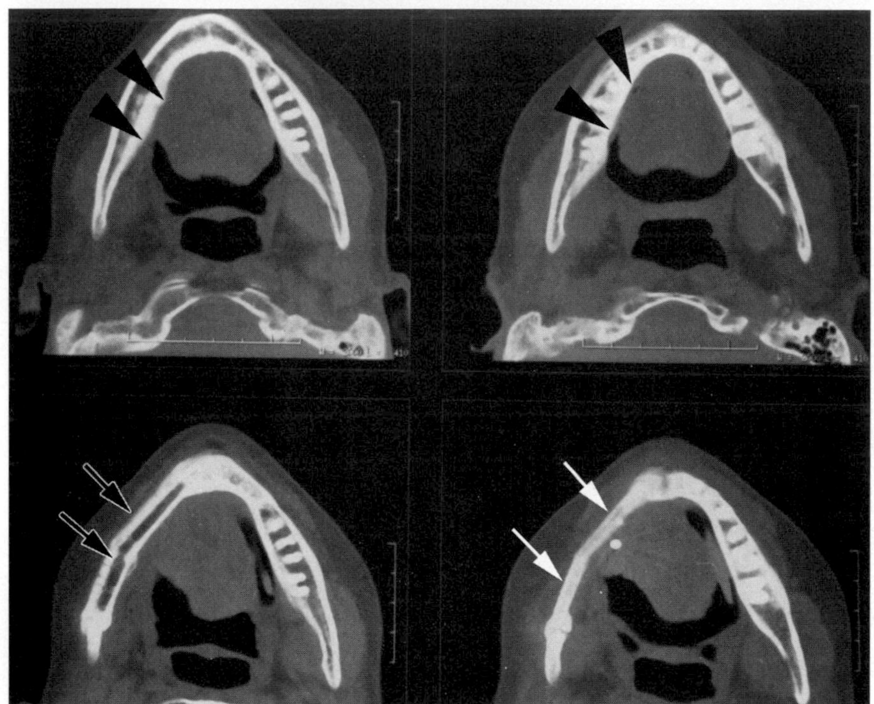

A

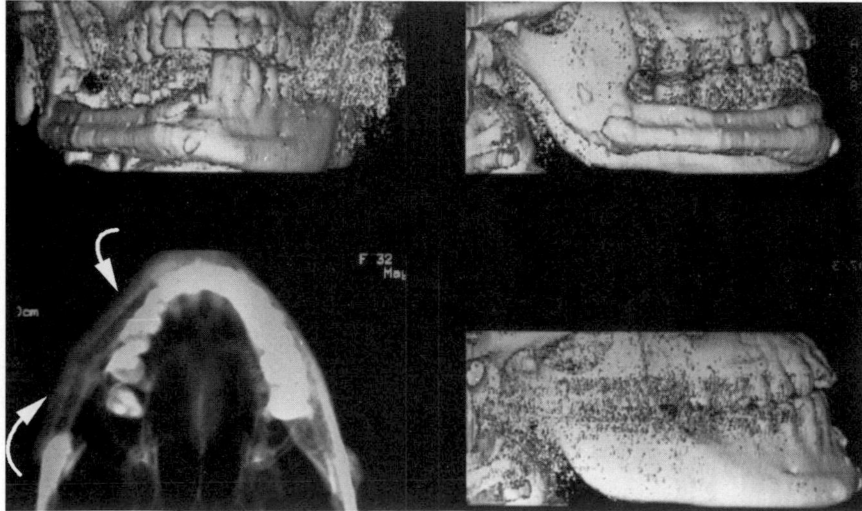

B

Figure 16.43 Preoperative and postoperative mandible. Top panel of axial bone-window views **(A)** shows sclerotic reaction (*arrowheads*) to infiltrating squamous cell cancer of gingiva. Bottom panel shows same view of segmental mandibulectomy and fibular free flap (*arrows*). **B:** Postoperative frontal and lateral three-dimensional surface rendering of reconstructed mandible (top panel), compared with preoperative lateral three-dimensional rendering (bottom right). Bottom left is base view of "ray-sum" projection from three-dimensional data, showing cortical and cancellous components of reconstruction (*curved arrows*).

RADIATION THERAPY TECHNIQUE*

William M. Mendenhall and Louis B. Harrison

The most common sites treated with radiation therapy include the lip, floor of mouth, and oral tongue. Lesions of the retromolar trigone are treated with techniques similar to those used for the anterior tonsillar pillar, which are described elsewhere. Patients are often treated surgically followed by postoperative irradiation, depending on stage and pathologic findings, or by irradiation alone.

Lip

Lesions of the upper lip are uncommon; the treatment techniques described hereafter apply primarily to the lower lip, but can be modified to treat the upper lip. Patients with superficial, well-differentiated SCC of the lip have a low risk for cancer in the neck nodes and may be irradiated with brachytherapy alone or EBRT alone. A short course of EBRT precedes the interstitial implant if the lesion is too thick to be adequately encompassed in a single-plane implant (>1 cm). External beam irradiation may be given with either *en face* electrons or orthovoltage irradiation with a lead mask to collimate the beam on the skin surface and a lead shield behind the lip to reduce the exit dose to the oral cavity. Orthovoltage irradiation is preferred at the University of Florida because the dose distribution is superior to that achieved with electron beam. Although it is possible to adequately treat patients with electrons, it is easier to underdose part of the tumor because of the lower surface dose and the beam constriction, and because the dose distribution is more affected by an irregular surface contour than in the case with 250 kVp x-rays.

Interstitial irradiation may be accomplished with rigid needles containing cesium or afterloaded ^{192}Ir using the plastic tube technique. The advantage of the rigid needles is that they may be mounted in a nylon bar to maintain optimal spacing between the sources. The plastic tube technique is often preferred because the length of sources can be more varied depending on the location and extent of the tumor. Rigid needles are placed perpendicular to the surface of the lip, whereas plastic tubes are placed parallel to the lip with crossers added as necessary. An example of a patient with a T2N0 squamous cell carcinoma of the lower lip treated with limited-field orthovoltage irradiation followed by an interstitial implant is depicted in Figure 16.44 (75).

Patients who have lesions that are larger and/or poorly differentiated and are thought to have a high likelihood of spread to the neck nodes (usually levels 1 and 2) receive treatment with parallel-opposed fields with the inferior border at the thyroid notch, the posterior border 2 to 3 cm behind the posterior edge of the cervical vertebral bodies, the superior border 2 cm above the lip lesion, and the anterior border 2 cm anterior to the lip lesion. A cork is placed in the mouth to displace the upper lip superiorly and the oral tongue posteriorly and superiorly. After approximately 45 Gy with once-daily fractionation, or its radiobiologic equivalent, the dose to the primary lesion is boosted with an interstitial implant.

Floor of Mouth

Superficial (<4 mm thick), well-differentiated, T1N0 floor of mouth cancers may be treated with an interstitial implant alone or intraoral cone irradiation.

Brachytherapy is accomplished with either rigid cesium needles or ^{192}Ir sources afterloaded into plastic tubes. The cesium needles may be mounted in a customized nylon template to maintain optimal (1 cm) spacing (Figs. 16.45 and 16.46) (75,76). Implantation as well as removal of the cesium needles is also much faster if they are mounted in a template. A suture is placed through the submentum and tied to a cotton "cigarette" to anchor the template in place (77). Interstitial implantation follows EBRT when the two are combined so that the lesion regresses and is more likely to be adequately encompassed by the implant.

Intraoral cone irradiation may be given successfully with either orthovoltage irradiation or electron beam (78). The cone is placed into the mouth by the attending physician; the cone abuts the mucosa and is centered over the lesion. Placement of the cone is easier in patients who are edentulous and those who do not have a very brisk gag reflex. The position of the cone is verified before treatment with the use of a periscope (Fig. 16.47) (79). Intraoral cone irradiation is performed before megavoltage EBRT so that the lesion can be easily visualized and there is no radiation mucositis that would render cone placement more difficult because of patient discomfort.

External beam portals for floor-of-mouth cancers are usually parallel opposed and weighted 1:1, or 3:2 to the side of the tumor, if it is lateralized. The field borders are similar to those used for more advanced lower lip cancers, except that the lip and anterior skin of the chin and submentum are not tangentially irradiated and placement of the cork or intraoral stent depends on whether the ventral tongue is involved (Figs. 16.48 and 16.49) (80). The low neck is irradiated with a separate anterior field with a tapered midline larynx block.

Oral Tongue

Superficial (<4 mm), well-differentiated, T1N0 oral tongue cancers can be treated with an interstitial implant alone or intraoral cone irradiation (78,81). It is more difficult to treat oral tongue cancers with the intraoral cone because of the mobility of the tongue; for this reason we usually prefer brachytherapy.

Interstitial implantation is accomplished with cesium needles in a rigid nylon bar for superficial lesions (Fig. 16.50) (82). Alternatively, ^{192}Ir sources may be afterloaded into plastic tubes. The latter technique is preferred for larger lesions. The dose to the mandible can be reduced by inserting a pack to move the mandible medially (Fig. 16.51) (75). Alternatively, a customized lead-lined dental appliance can be placed between the sources and the alveolar ridge (83).

More advanced T1-T2N0 oral tongue cancers are treated with brachytherapy and an elective neck dissection. In less advanced cases, EBRT precedes the interstitial implant to treat the neck electively along with the primary cancer. It is imperative to treat the patient in as short an overall time as possible to optimize the likelihood of local control (81,84). The portals used to treat the oral tongue are similar to those used for the floor of mouth, except that an intraoral stent is used to displace the tongue inferiorly and posteriorly (Fig. 16.52) (80). The low neck is treated with a separate anterior field.

The treatment techniques employed for postoperative irradiation are similar to those employed for irradiation alone, except that brachytherapy is rarely used for a boost dose and the portals are often larger because patients have more advanced disease with positive margins and/or multiple involved lymph nodes (Figs. 16.53 and 16.54) (85). The portals are parallel opposed and weighted 3:2 to the side of the tumor, if it is lateralized.

*Please refer to the Appendix, Imaging Considerations for Radiation Therapy Treatment Planning. This section shows the important radiologic anatomy that allows the radiation oncologist to design the target volumes for treatment planning.

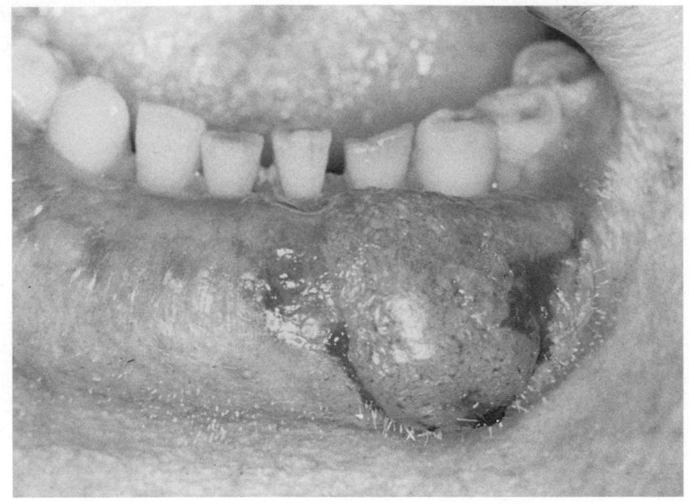
A

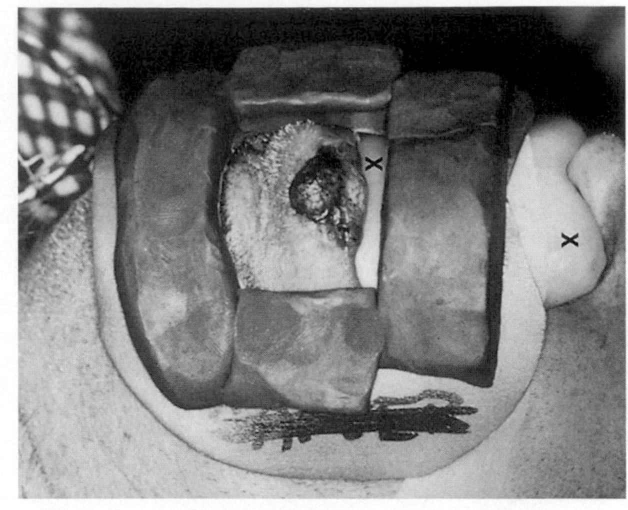

B

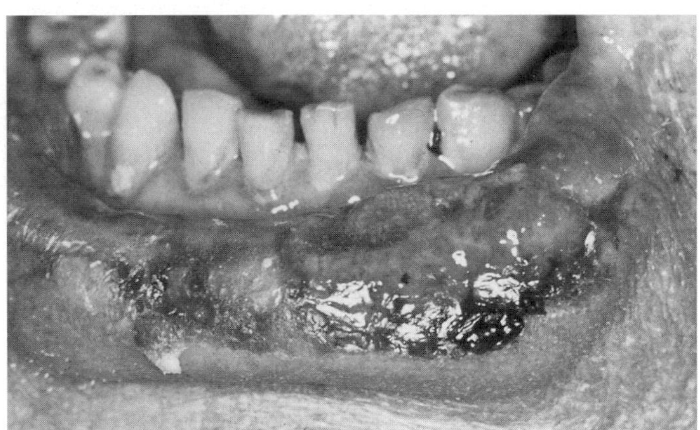
C

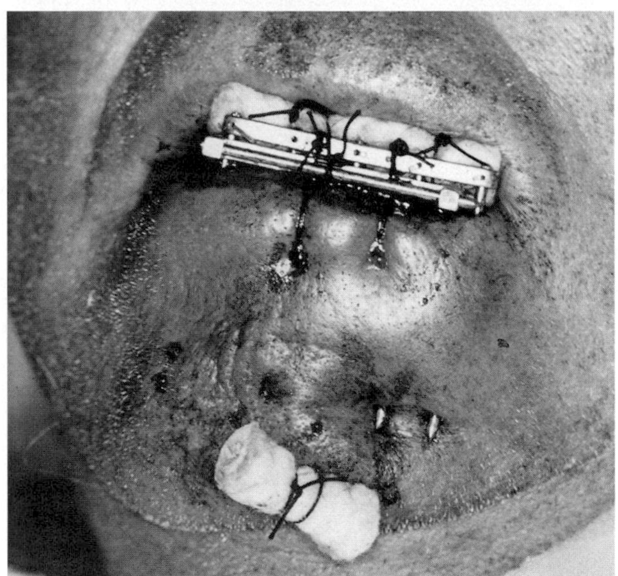
D

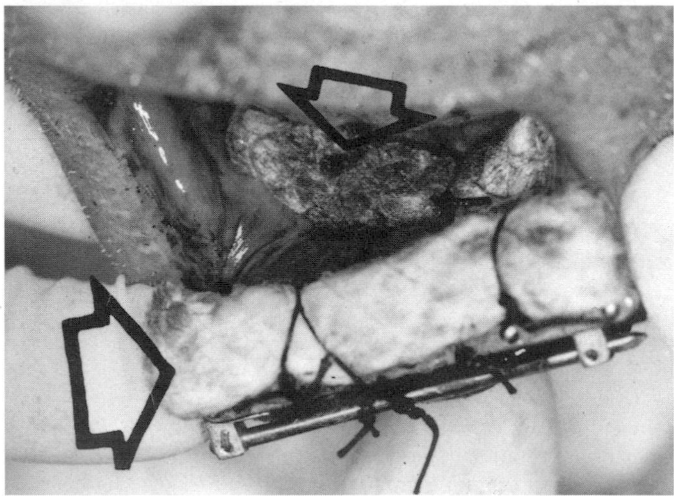
E

Figure 16.44 A 67-year-old man had T2N0 squamous cell carcinoma of the lower lip. **A:** Lesion measured 3.0 × 2.0 × 1.5 cm. Radiation therapy was elected because of functional deficit likely to result from excision of large lesion. **B:** Lead mask (2-mm-thick) designed to outline portal. Lead putty was added to the shield to reduce transit irradiation to less than 1%. Separate lead shield covered with beeswax was inserted behind lower the lip (*X*). Patient received 30 Gy over 2 weeks, 3 Gy per fraction, 250 kV (0.5 mm^3). **C:** By completion of 3 Gy, the patient had brisk mucositis of lip and approximately 60% to 70% regression of obvious tumor. **D:** Single-plane radium needle implant with double crossing. Pack was tied to top of bar to displace upper lip away from radiation, and chin pack anchored gingivolabial pack in place (see **E**). **E:** Gauze pack (*arrows*) sewn into gingivolabial gutter to displace radium from mandible, teeth, and gums.

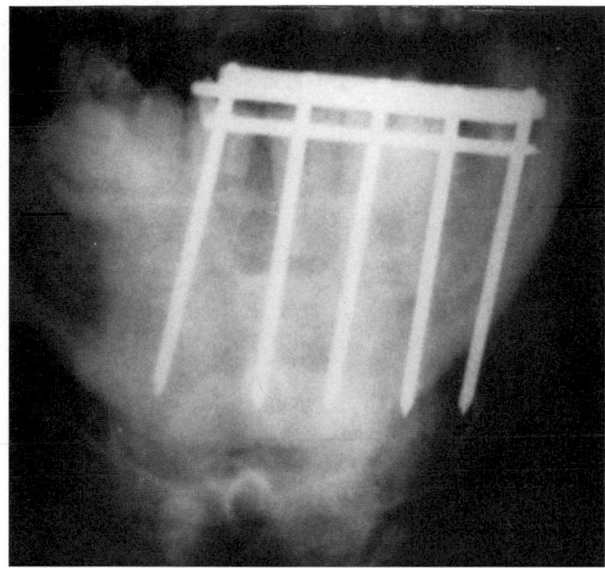
F

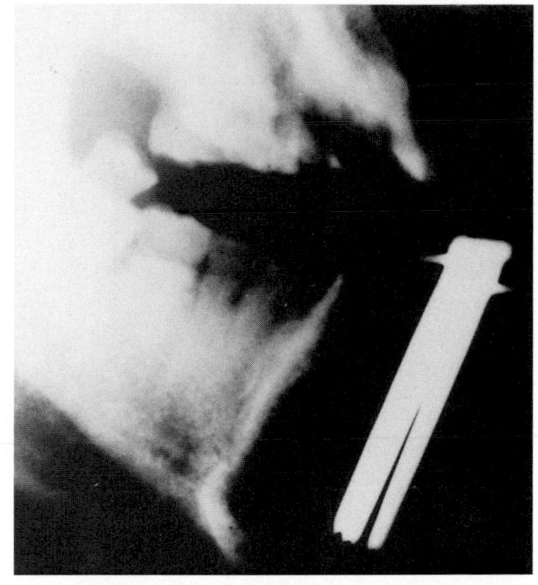
G

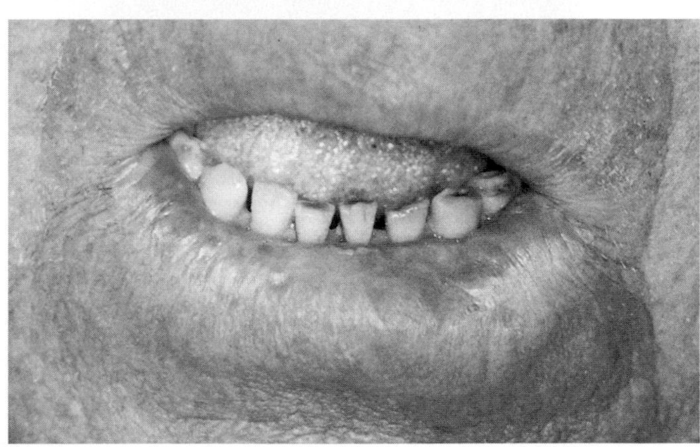
I

H

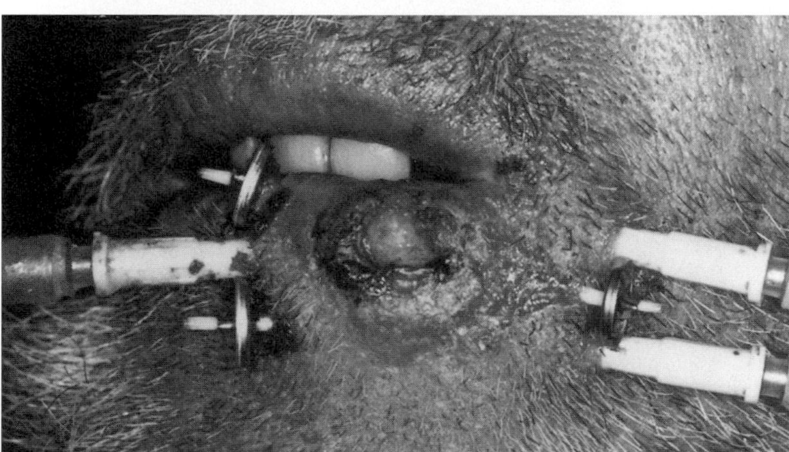
J

Figure 16.44 ***(continued)*** **F,G:** Anteroposterior and lateral views of implant. Implant added 35 Gy at 0.5 cm. **H:** At 2.5 weeks after implantation. Note superficial ulceration. **I:** At 22 months after treatment. No evidence of disease, and lip was completely healed. Nine-year follow-up revealed no evidence of disease. **J:** ^{192}Ir implant used for a T1N0 squamous cell carcinoma of the lip. Patient received 65 Gy in 6.5 days. Angiocatheters were used to introduce the sources. (**A–I:** From Million RR, Cassisi NJ, Mancuso AA. Oral cavity. In: Million RR, Cassisi NJ, eds. *Management of head and neck cancer: a multidisciplinary approach,* 2nd ed. Philadelphia: Lippincott, 1994:321–400, with permission; **J:** Courtesy of Louis B. Harrison, M.D.)

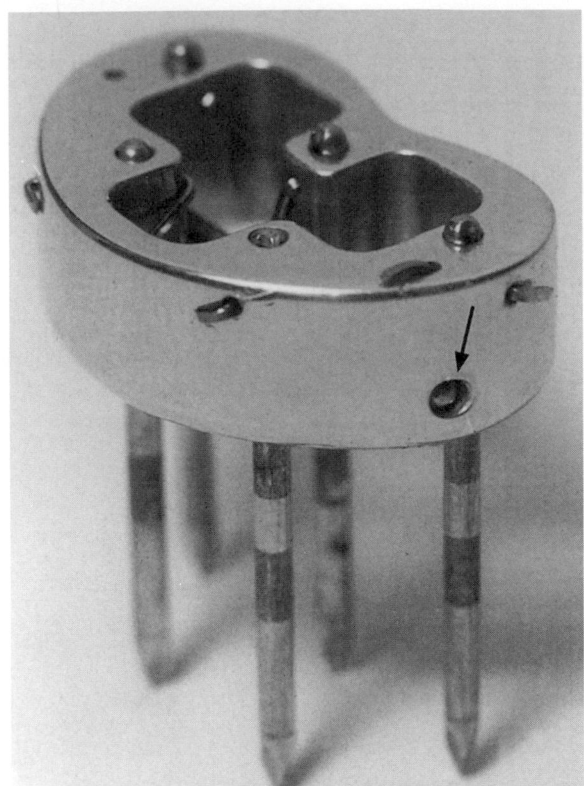

Figure 16.45 Custom-made implant device for stage T1-T2 cancers of floor of mouth. Note single crossing needle (*arrow*) through center. Devices machined from nylon also are available. Cesium needles usually are used (2.0 cm active length, 3.2 cm actual length). Intensity of needles is adjusted so dose rate is approximately 0.4 Gy per hour to area of gross disease. To ensure adequate surface dose, height of implant device (9 mm) is such that 3 mm of active ends of cesium needles extend above mucosal surface. Crossing needle is also 3 mm above mucosal surface (i.e., at active ends of needles). (From Marcus RB Jr, Million RR, Mitchell TP. A preloaded, custom-designed implantation device for stage T1–T2 carcinoma of the floor of mouth. *Int J Radiat Oncol Biol Phys* 1980;6:111–113, with permission.)

A 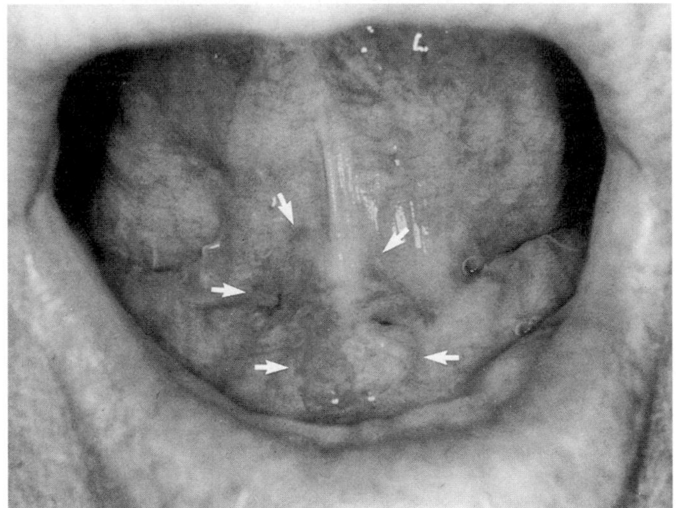

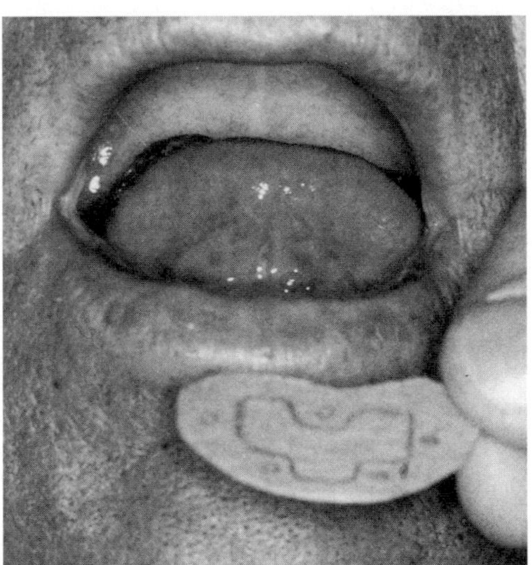 B

Figure 16.46 Radiation treatment technique for squamous cell carcinoma of floor of mouth (T2N0). **A:** Lesion measuring 2.5 × 2.5 cm (*arrows*), including induration, and tethered to periosteum at midline. Treatment plan is 50 Gy over 5 weeks with parallel-opposed portals that include submandibular and subdigastric lymph nodes. Midjugular lymph nodes are treated with anterior portal. Implant is planned to add 15 Gy. **B:** Cardboard template for design of radium needle holder. Cesium needles are currently used rather than radium needles.

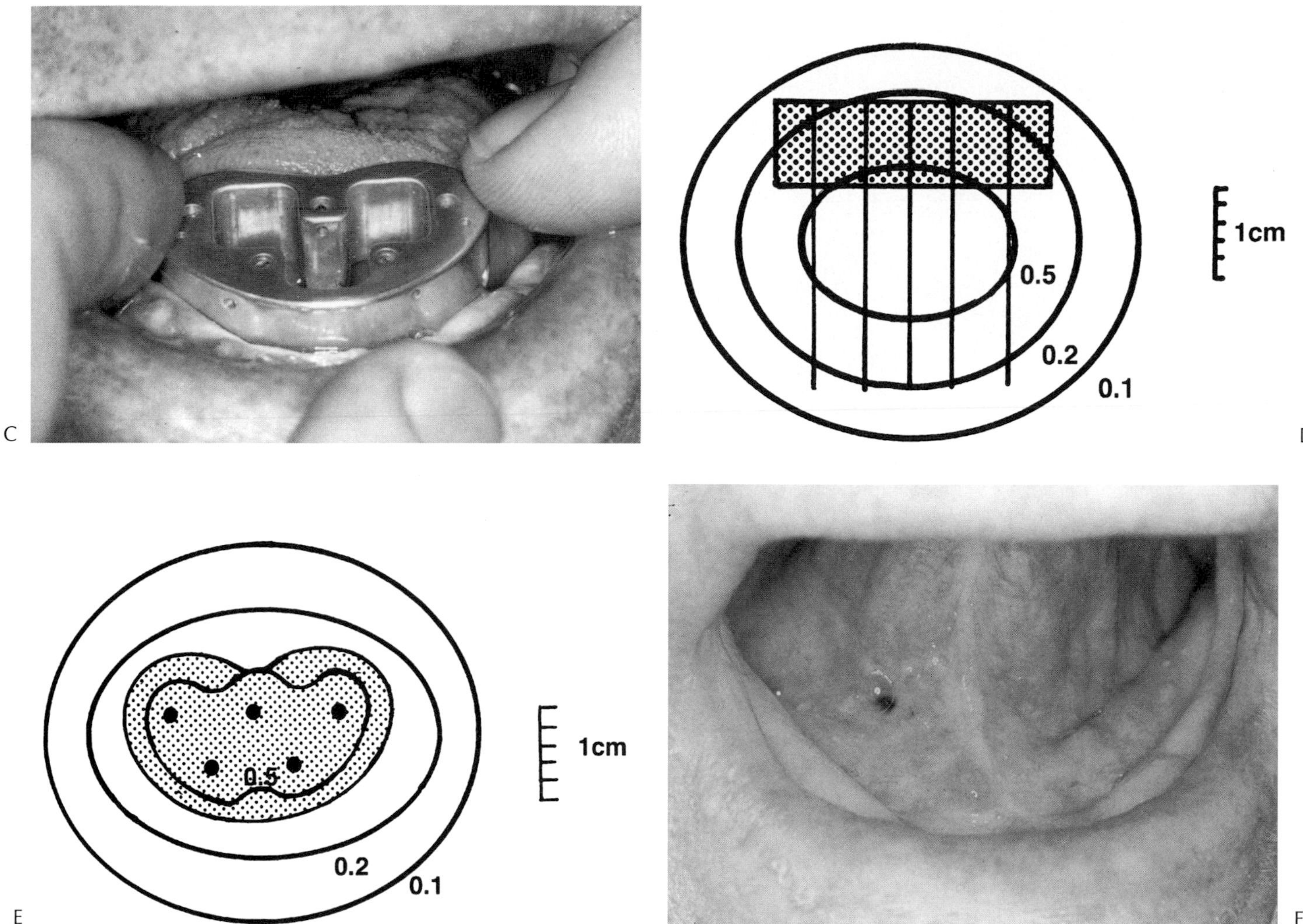

Figure 16.46 ***(continued)*** **C:** One day before surgery, before securing radium needles to implant device, implant holder is placed into floor of mouth to ensure adequate fit and check adequacy of tumor coverage. At surgery, device is sutured with two 1–0 silk sutures passed on long curved needle through submentum into floor of mouth. Five, 2.0 cm active length, full-intensity radium needles without crossing are used. **D:** Coronal isodose distribution. The 0.5 Gy per hour line is selected for specification of dose; implant remains in place for 30 hours. *Stippled area,* implant device. **E:** Transverse isodose distribution through middle of needles. The 0.5 Gy per hour isodose line is approximately 2 mm outside needles. Highest dose rate to anterior lingual gingiva would be about 0.3 to 0.35 Gy per hour, or at least 4.5 Gy less than minimum tumor dose. **F:** Patient is free of disease at 4 years, 8 months with no complications. (From Million RR, Cassisi NJ, Mancuso AA. Oral cavity. In: Million RR, Cassisi NJ, eds. *Management of head and neck cancer: a multidisciplinary approach,* 2nd ed. Philadelphia: Lippincott, 1994:321–400, with permission.)

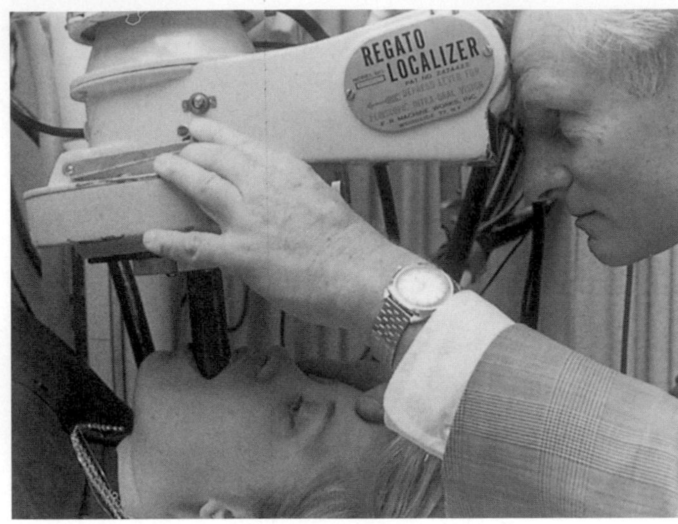

Figure 16.47 Positioning of lead cone used for orthovoltage intraoral therapy is checked each day by physician. A good localizer is essential for final positioning. (From Million RR, Cassisi NJ. General principles for treatment of cancers in the head and neck: Radiation therapy. In: Million RR, Cassisi NJ, eds. *Management of head and neck cancer: a multidisciplinary approach.* Philadelphia: Lippincott, 1984:77–90, with permission.)

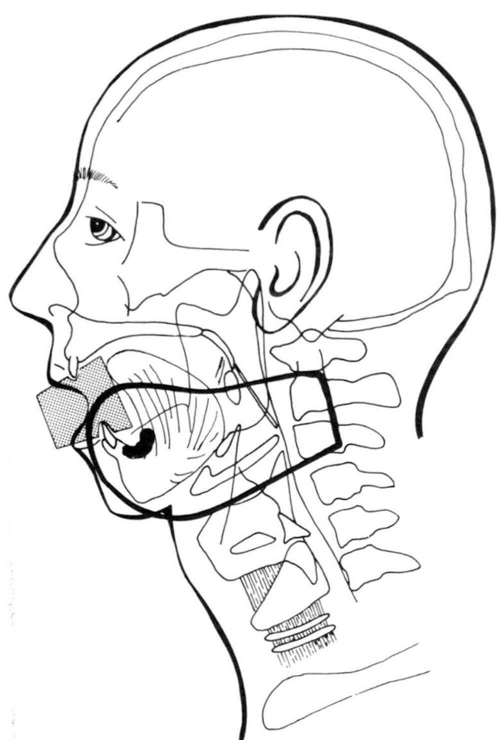

Figure 16.48 Portal for irradiation of limited anterior floor of mouth carcinoma (no tongue invasion; N0 or N1 neck disease) by parallel-opposed ^{60}Co fields. Two notches on a cork ensure it is held in the same position between upper and lower incisors during every treatment session; tip of tongue is displaced from treatment field. Anterior border of field covers full thickness of mandibular arch. Lower field edge is at the thyroid cartilage, ensuring adequate coverage of submandibular lymph nodes. Subdigastric lymph nodes are covered adequately by including entire width of vertebral bodies posteriorly. Superior border is shaped so the oropharynx, much of oral cavity, and parotid glands are out of portal. Minimum tumor dose is specified at primary site (i.e., not along central axis of portal) with aid of computer dosimetry. (From Parsons JT, Million RR. Radiotherapy of tumors of the oral cavity. In: Thawley SE, Panje WR, Batsakis JG, et al., eds. *Comprehensive management of head and neck tumors,* 2nd ed. Philadelphia: WB Saunders, 1999:695–719, with permission.)

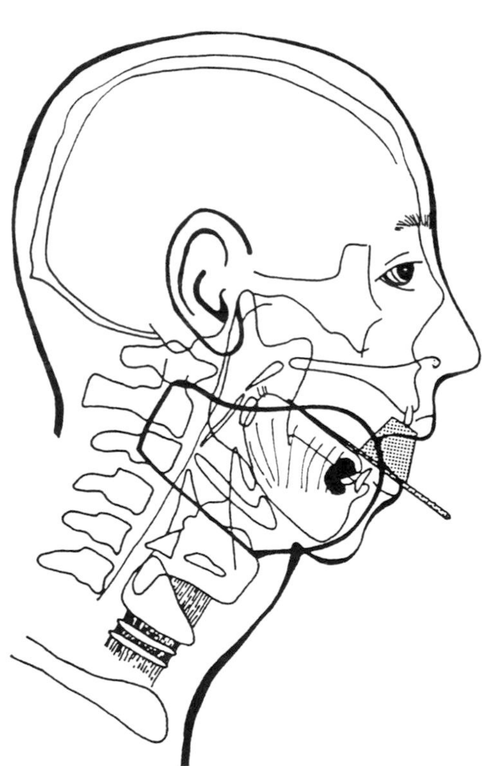

Figure 16.49 Treatment portal for carcinoma of floor of mouth with tongue invasion. Tongue is depressed into floor of mouth with tongue blade and cork. (From Parsons JT, Mendenhall WM, Million RR. Radiotherapy of tumors of the oral cavity. In: Thawley SE, Panje WR, Batsakis JG, et al., eds. *Comprehensive management of head and neck tumors,* 2nd ed. Philadelphia: WB Saunders, 1999:695–719, with permission.)

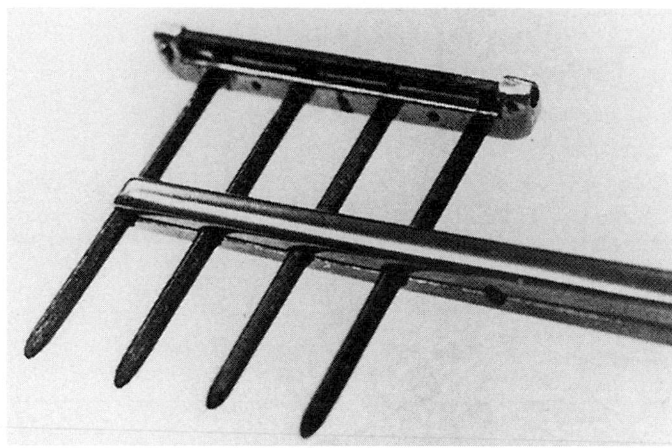

Figure 16.50 Cesium needles mounted in rigid device for single-plane implantation oral tongue cancer. Note single crossing needle. Holders originally were of stainless steel or aluminum; nylon has proved more satisfactory. Needles are secured to bar with half-hard stainless steel wire passed through eyelets. Allen forceps has been drilled at 1-cm intervals to grasp needles during surgery. (From Ellingwood KE, Million RR, Mitchell TP. A preloaded radium needle implant device for maintenance of needle spacing. *Cancer* 1976;37:2558–2860, with permission.)

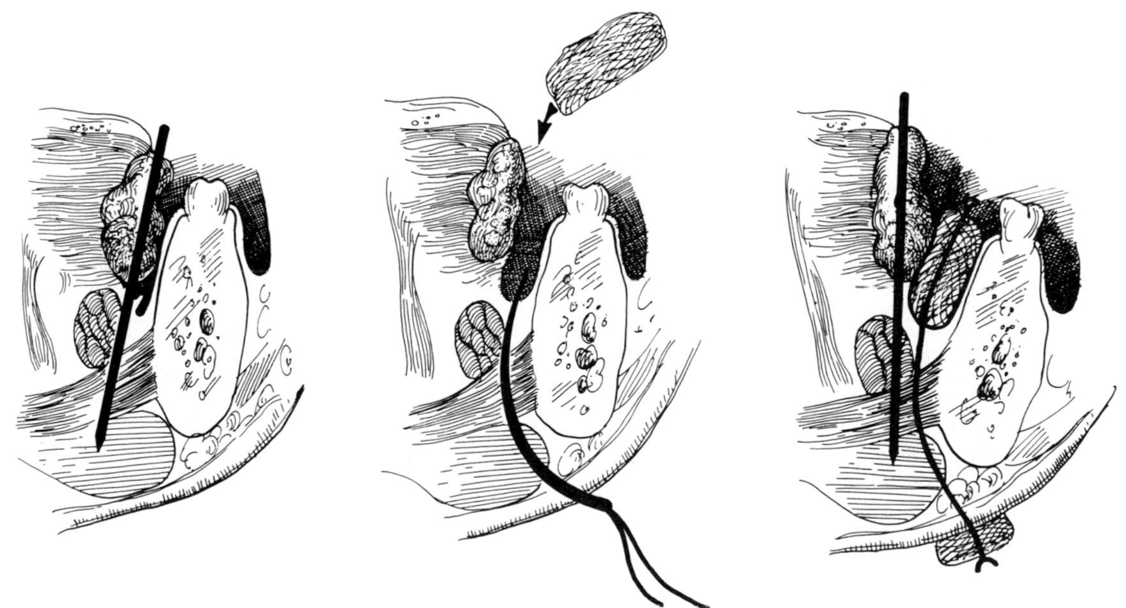

Figure 16.51 Cesium needle implant for cancer of lateral border of oral tongue. Gauze packing displaces tongue from mandible and thus reduces dose to bone. Large curved needle inserted through skin into lateral floor of mouth. Gauze pack tied to suture and secured between mandible and tongue after implant is completed. (From Million RR, Cassisi NJ, Mancuso AA. Oral cavity. In: Million RR, Cassisi NJ, eds. *Management of head and neck cancer: a multidisciplinary approach,* 2nd ed. Philadelphia: Lippincott, 1994:321–400, with permission.)

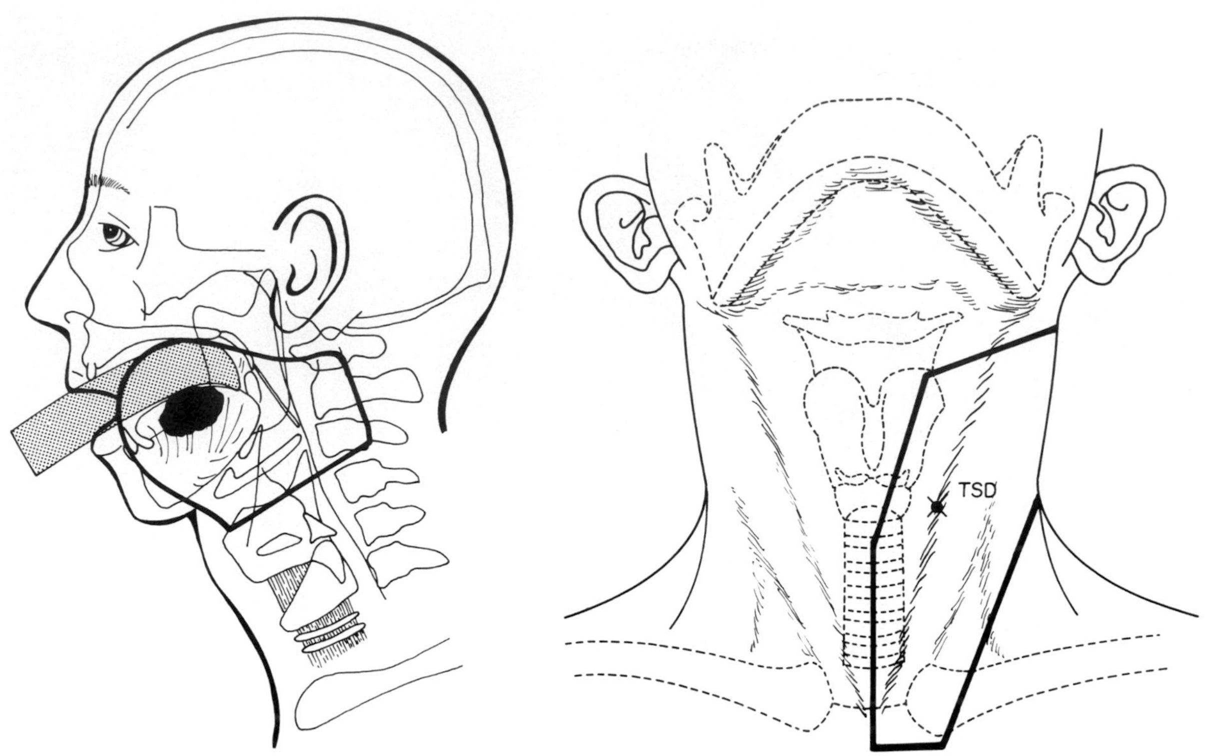

Figure 16.52 Well-lateralized squamous cell carcinoma of the tongue (neck stage N0). **A:** A single ipsilateral field is used. The field encompasses the submaxillary and subdigastric lymph nodes; the entire width of the vertebral body is included to ensure adequate posterior coverage of the subdigastric lymph nodes. Stainless steel pins are usually inserted into the anteriormost and posteriormost aspects of the lesion to aid in localizing the cancer of the treatment planning (simulation) roentgenogram and to confirm coverage by the interstitial implant. For superficial lesions smaller than 2.0 cm in diameter, the low neck is not irradiated (unless the histology is poorly differentiated squamous cell carcinoma). The larynx is excluded from the radiation field. The anterior submental skin and subcutaneous tissues are shielded, when possible, to reduce submental edema and late development of fibrosis. The upper border is shaped to exclude most of the parotid gland. An intraoral lead block (*stippled area*) shields the contralateral mucosa. The block is coated with beeswax to prevent a high-dose effect on the adjacent mucosa resulting from scattered low-energy electrons from the metal surface. The usual preinterstitial tumor dose is 30 Gy in 10 fractions using ^{60}Co. For larger lesions that extend near the midline, treatment is applied by means of parallel-opposed portals with no intraoral lead block. **B:** For well-lateralized lesions greater that 2.0 cm in patients with stage N0 neck, only the ipsilateral low neck is irradiated. (From Parsons JT, Mendenhall WM, Million RR. Radiotherapy of tumors of the oral cavity. In: Thawley SE, Panje WR, Batsakis JR, et al., eds. *Comprehensive management of head and neck tumors,* 2nd ed. Philadelphia: WB Saunders, 1999:695–719, with permission.)

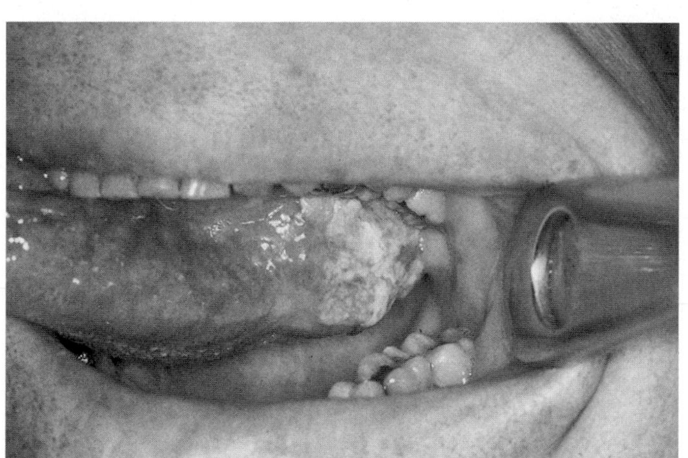

A

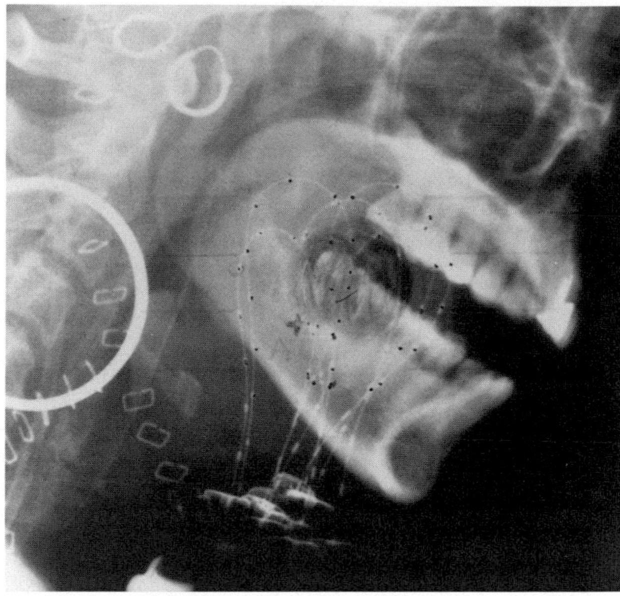

B

Figure 16.53 **A:** Well lateralized squamous cell cancer of the left side of the posterior aspect of the oral tongue. **B:** Patient had a looping ^{192}Ir implant delivering 65 Gy in 6.5 days and a neck dissection. (Courtesy of Louis B. Harrison, M.D.)

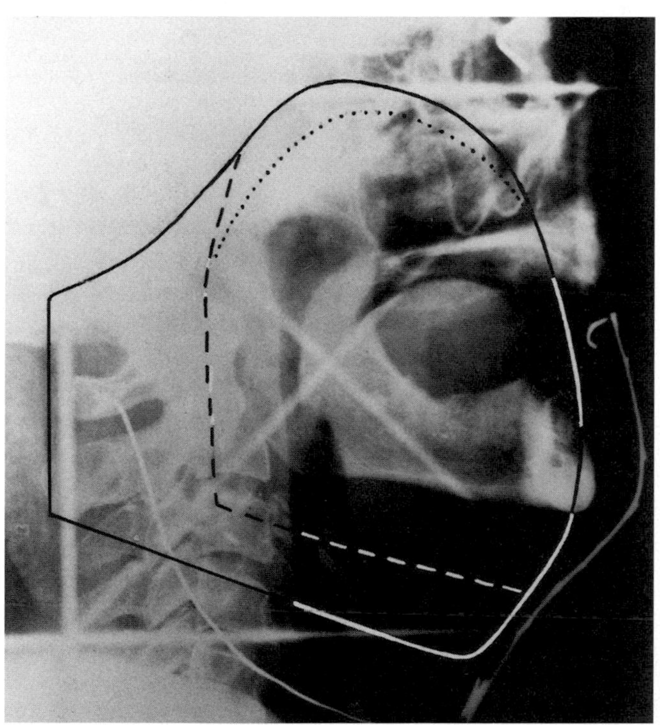

A

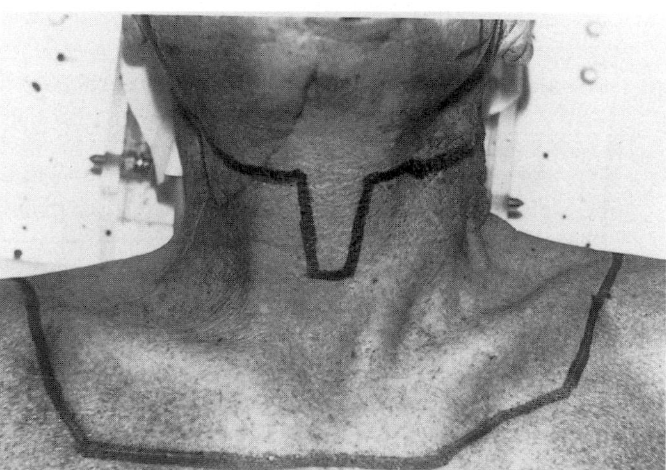

B

Figure 16.54 Typical portal for irradiation after hemimandibulectomy, partial maxillectomy, and radical neck dissection for pathologic stage T4N0 retromolar trigone lesion. **A:** Field reductions made at 45 Gy (*dashed line*) and 60 Gy (*dotted line*). **B:** Low neck receives 50 Gy given dose (at D_{max}) in 25 fractions. Larynx and a segment of spinal cord are shielded by tapered midline block. (From Amdur RJ, Parsons JT, Mendenhall WM, et al. Postoperative irradiation for squamous cell carcinoma of the head and neck: an analysis of treatment results and complications. *Int J Radiat Oncol Biol Phys* 1989;16:25–36, with permission.)

REFERENCES

1. Jemal A, Thomas A, Murray T, et al. Cancer Statistics, 2002. *CA Cancer J Clin* 2002;52:23–47.
2. Li FP, Correa P, Fraumeni JF. Testing for germ line p53 mutations in cancer families. *Cancer Epidemiol Biomarkers Prev* 1991;1:91–94.
3. Berkower AS, Biller HE. Head and neck cancer associated with Bloom's syndrome. *Laryngoscope* 1998;98:746–748.
4. Ahlbom HE. Simple achlorhydric anemia. Plummer-Vinson syndrome and carcinoma of the mouth, pharynx and esophagus in women. *BMJ* 1936;2:331.
5. Rothman K, Keller A. The effect of joint exposure to alcohol and tobacco on risk of cancer of the mouth and pharynx. *J Chronic Dis* 1972;25:711–716.
6. Mufti S, Salvagnini M, Lieber C, et al. Chronic ethanol consumption inhibits repair of dimethylnitrosamine induced DNA alkylation. *Biochem Biophys Res Commun* 1988;152:423–431.
7. Winn D, Blot W, Shy C. Snuff dipping and oral cancer among women in the southern United States. *N Engl J Med* 1981;304:745–749.
8. Watts SL, Brewer EE, Fry TL. Human papillomavirus DNA types in squamous cell carcinomas of the head and neck. *Oral Surg Oral Med Oral Fathol Oral Radial Endod* 1991;71:701–707.
9. Woods KV, Shilltoe EJ, Spitz MR, et al. Analysis of human papillomavirus DNA in oral squamous cell carcinomas. *J Oral Pathol* 1993;22:101–108.
10. Franceschi D, Gupta R, Spiro RH, et al. Improved survival in the management of squamous carcinoma of the oral tongue. *Am J Surg* 1993;166:360–365.
11. Kolli VR, Shaba AR, Savage HE, et al. Native cellular fluorescence can identify changes in epithelial thickness in-vivo in the upper aerodigestive tract. *Am J Surg* 1994;170:495–498.
12. Pindborg JJ. Studies in oral leukoplakia. *J Am Dent Assoc* 1968;76:767–770.
13. Silverman S, Rozen RD. Observations on the clinical characteristics and natural history of oral leukoplakia. *J Am Dent Assoc* 1968;76:772–776.
14. Waldron CA, Shafer WG. Leukoplakia revisited: a clinicopathologic study of 3256 oral leukoplakias. *Cancer* 1975;36:1386–1392.
15. Mashberg A, Morrissey JB, Garfinkel L. A study of the appearance of early asymptomatic oral squamous cell carcinoma. *Cancer* 1973;32:1436.
16. Spiro RH, Huvos AG, Wong GY. Predictive value of tumor thickness in squamous carcinoma confined to the tongue and floor of mouth. *Am J Surg* 1986; 152:420–423.
17. Brennan JA, Mao L, Hruban RH, et al. Molecular assessment of histopathologic staging in squamous cell carcinoma of the head and neck. *N Engl J Med* 1995;332:429–435.
18. Batsakis JG. *Tumors of the head and neck.* Baltimore: Williams & Wilkins, 1979.
19. McGregor AD, MacDonald DG. Patterns of spread of squamous cell carcinoma to the ramus of the mandible. *Head Neck* 1993;15:440–444.
20. O'Brien CJ, Carter RL, Soo KC, et al. Invasion of the mandible by squamous carcinomas of the oral cavity and oral pharynx. *Head Neck Surg* 1986;8:247–256.
21. McGregor AD, MacDonald DG. Patterns of spread of squamous cell carcinoma within the mandible. *Head Neck Surg* 1989;11:457–461.
22. Slaughter DP, Southwick HW, Smejkal W. "Field cancerization" in oral stratified squamous epithelium. Clinical implications of multicentric origin. *Cancer* 1953;6:963–968.
23. Virag MM, Bunavrevic A, Aljinovic N. Recurrence of oral cancer due to discontinuous periosteal involvement. *Am J Surg* 1991;162:388–392.
24. Shah JP Patterns of cervical lymph node metastases from squamous carcinoma of the upper aerodigestive tract. *Am J Surg* 1990;160:405–409.
25. Shah JP, Candela FC, Poddar AK. The patterns of cervical lymph node metastases from squamous carcinoma of the oral cavity. *Cancer* 1990;66:109–113.
26. Byers RM, Wolf PE, Ballantyne AJ. Rationale for elective modified neck dissection. *Head Neck Surg* 1988;10:160–167.
27. Lindberg RD. Distribution of cervical lymph node metastases from squamous cell carcinoma of the upper respiratory and digestive tract. *Cancer* 1972;29: 1446–1449.
28. Byers RM, Weber RS, Andrews T, et al. Frequency and therapeutic implications of "skip metastases" in the neck from squamous carcinoma of the oral tongue. *Head Neck* 1997;19:14–19.
29. Davidson BJ, Kulkarny V, Delacure MD, et al. Posterior triangle metastases of squamous cell carcinoma of the upper aerodigestive tract. *Am J Surg* 1993;166: 395–398.
30. Leipzig B, Zellmer JE, Klug D. The role of endoscopy in evaluating patients with head and neck cancer. *Arch Otolaryngol* 1985;111:589–594.
31. Greene F, Page D, Fleming I, et al. *AJCC cancer staging manual,* 6th ed. New York: Springer-Verlag, 2002.
32. Andersen PE, Shah JP, Cambronero E, et al. The role of comprehensive neck dissection with preservation of the spinal accessory nerve in the clinically positive neck. *Am J Surg* 1994;168:499–502.
33. Shah JP, Andersen PE. The impact of patterns of neck metastases on modifications of neck dissection. *Ann Surg Oncol* 1994;1:521–532.
34. Vikram B, Strong EW, Shah JP, et al. Elective postoperative radiotherapy in stages III and IV epidermoid carcinoma of the head and neck. *Am J Surg* 1980;140:580–584.
35. Kramer S, Gelber RD, Snow JB, et al. Combined radiation therapy and surgery in the management of advanced head and neck cancer: final report of study 73-03 of the Radiation Oncology Group. *Head Neck Surg* 1987;10:19–30.
36. Spiro RH, Gerald F, Shah JP, et al. Mandibulotomy approach to oropharyngeal tumors. *Am J Surg* 1985;150:460–469.
37. Shah JP. *Head and neck surgery,* 2nd ed. London: Mosby-Wolfe, 1996:189–196.
38. Zelefsky MJ, Harrison LB, Armstrong JG. Long term treatment results of postoperative radiation therapy for advanced stage oropharyngeal carcinoma. *Cancer* 1992;70:2388–2395.
39. Bamberg M, Schulz U, Scherer E. Postoperative split course radiotherapy of squamous cell carcinoma of the oral tongue. *Int J Radiat Oncol Biol Phys* 1979; 5:515–519.
40. Zelefsky MJ, Harrison LB, Fass DE, et al. Postoperative radiotherapy for oral cancers: impact of anatomic subsite on treatment outcome. *Head Neck* 1990;12: 470–475.
41. Decroix Y, Ghossein NA. Experience of the Curie Institute in the treatment of cancer of the mobile tongue. *Cancer* 1981;47:496–502.
42. Pernot M, Malissard L, Hoffstetter S, et al. The study of tumoral, radiobiological and general health factors that influence the results and complications in a series of 448 oral tongue carcinomas treated exclusively by irradiation. *Int J Radiat Oncol Biol Phys* 1994;29:673–679.
43. Mendenhall WM, Cise WSV, Bova FG, et al. Analysis of time dose factors in squamous cell carcinoma of the oral tongue and floor of mouth treated with radiotherapy alone. *Int J Radiat Oncol Biol Phys* 1981;7:1005–1011.
44. Ange D, Lindberg R, Guillamondegui O. Management of squamous cell carcinoma of the oral tongue and floor of mouth after excisional biopsy. *Radiology* 1975;116:143–146.
45. Fein DA, Mendenhall WM, Parsons JT, et al. Carcinoma of the oral tongue: a comparison of results and complications of treatment with radiotherapy and/or surgery. *Head Neck* 1994;16:358–365.
46. Inoue T, Inoue T, Yoshida K, et al. Phase III trial of high vs low dose-rate interstitial radiotherapy for early mobile tongue cancer. *Int J Radiat Oncol Biol Phys* 2001;51:171–175.
47. Leung T, Wong V, Kwan K, et al. High dose rate brachytherapy for early stage oral tongue cancer. *Head Neck* 24:274–281,2002.
48. Fu K, Ray JW, Chan EK, et al. External and interstitial radiation therapy for the oral tongue: a review of 32 years of experience. *Am J Roentgenol Radium Ther Nucl Med* 1976;127:107–115.
49. Gilbert EH, Goffinet DR, Bagshaw MA. Carcinoma of the oral tongue and floor of mouth: fifteen years of experience with linear accelerator therapy. *Cancer* 1975;35:1517–1524.
50. Chu A, Fletcher GH. Incidence and causes of failures to control by irradiation the primary lesions in squamous cell carcinomas of the anterior two-thirds of the tongue and floor of mouth. *AJR* 1973;117:502–508.
51. Scholl P, Byers RM, Batsakis JG, et al. Microscopic cut through of cancer in the surgical treatment of squamous carcinoma of the tongue: prognostic and therapeutic implications. *Am J Surg* 1987;152:354–360.
52. Lapeyre M, Hoffstetter S, Peiffert D, et al. Postoperative brachytherapy alone for T1–T2 NO squamous cell carcinomas of the oral tongue and floor of mouth with close or positive margins. *Int J Radiat Oncol Biol Phys* 2000;48: 37–42.
53. Wang CC, Doppke K, Biggs P. Intra-oral cone radiation therapy for selected carcinomas of the oral cavity. *Int J Radiat Oncol Biol Phys* 1983;9:1185.
54. Mazeron J, Grimard L, Raynal M, et al. Iridium-192 curietherapy for T1 and T2 epidermoid carcinomas of the floor of mouth. *Int J Radiat Oncol Biol Phys* 1990; 18:1299–1306.
55. Matsumoto S, Takeda M, Shibuya H, et al. T1 and T2 squamous cell carcinomas of the floor of the mouth: results of brachytherapy mainly using 98 AU grains. *Int J Radiat Oncol Biol Phys* 1996;34:833–841.
56. Marsiglia H, Haie-Meder C, Sasso G, et al. Brachytherapy for T1–T2 floor of mouth cancers: the Gustave-Roussy institute experience. *Int J Radiat Oncol Biol Phys* 2002;52:1257–1263.
57. Rodgers LW Jr, String SP, Mendenhall WM, et al. Management of squamous cell carcinomas of the floor of mouth. *Head Neck* 1993;15:16–19.
58. Johnson JT, Ferretti GA, Nethrey WJ, et al. Oral pilocarpine for postirradiation xerostomia in patients with head and neck cancer. *N Engl J Med* 1993;329: 390–395.

Radiologic Imaging Concerns

59. Ord RA, Sarmadi M, Papadimitrou J. A comparison of segmental and marginal bony resection for oral squamous cell carcinoma involving the mandible. *J Oral Maxillofac Surg* 1997;55:470–477; discussion 477–478.
60. Mukherji SK, Isaacs DL, Creager A, et al. CT detection of mandibular invasion by squamous cell carcinoma of the oral cavity. *AJR* 2001;177:237–243.
61. Lewis-Jones HG, Rogers SN, Beirne JC, et al. Radionuclide bone imaging for detection of mandibular invasion by squamous cell carcinoma. *Br J Radiol* 2000;73:488–493.
62. Brown JS, Griffith JF, Phelps PD, et al. A comparison of different imaging modalities and direct inspection after periosteal stripping in predicting the invasion of the mandible by oral squamous cell carcinoma. *Br J Oral Maxillofacial Surg* 1994;32:347–359.
63. Leslie A, Fyfe E, Guest P, et al. Staging of squamous cell carcinoma of the oral cavity and oropharynx: a comparison of MRI and CT in T- and N-staging. *J Comput Assist Tomogr* 1999;23:43–49.
64. Campbell RS, Baker E, Chippindale AJ, et al. MRI T staging of squamous cell carcinoma of the oral cavity: radiological-pathological correlation. *Clin Radiol* 1995;50:533–540.

65. Chung TS, Yousem DM, Seigerman HM, et al. MR of mandibular invasion in patients with oral and oropharyngeal malignant neoplasms. *AJNR* 1994;15: 1949–1955.
66. Heissler E, Steinkamp HJ, Heim T, et al. Value of magnetic resonance imaging in staging carcinomas of the oral cavity and oropharynx. *Int J Oral Maxillofac Surg* 1994;23:22–27.
67. Fleming I, Cooper J, Henson D, eds. *AJCC cancer staging manual,* 5th ed. Philadelphia: Lippincott, 1997.
68. Narayana HM, Panda NK, Mann SB, et al. Ultrasound versus physical examination in staging carcinoma of the mobile tongue. *J Laryngol Otol* 1996;110:43–47.
69. Nagata Y, Ohba T, Tahara T, et al. Advanced imaging of carcinoma of the mandibular gingiva. *Dentomaxillofac Radiol* 1997;26:192–194.
70. Mukherji SK, Weeks SM, Castillo M, et al. Squamous cell carcinomas that arise in the oral cavity and tongue base: can CT help predict perineural or vascular invasion? *Radiology* 1996;198:157–162.
71. Rypens R, Lemort M, Dor P, et al. Vidian metastasis of adenoid cystic carcinoma. *J Neuroradiol* 1991;18:286–289.
72. Tart RP, Kotzur IM, Mancuso AA, et al. CT and MR imaging of the buccal space and buccal space masses [Review]. *Radiographics* 1995;15:531–550.
73. Weissman JL, Carrau RL. "Puffed-cheek" CT improves evaluation of the oral cavity. *AJNR* 2001;22:741–744.
74. Weber AL. Imaging of cysts and odontogenic tumors of the jaw. Definition and classification. *Radiol Clin North Am* 1993;31:101–120.

Radiation Therapy Technique

75. Million RR, Cassisi NJ, Mancuso AA. Oral cavity. In: Million RR, Cassisi NJ, eds. *Management of head and neck cancer: a multidisciplinary approach,* 2nd ed. Philadelphia: Lippincott, 1994:321–400.
76. Marcus RB Jr, Million RR, Mitchell TP. A preloaded, custom-designed implantation device for stage T1-T2 carcinoma of the floor of mouth. *Int J Radiat Oncol Biol Phys* 1980;6:111–113.
77. Parsons JT, Palta JR, Mendenhall WM, et al. Head and neck cancer. In: Levitt SH, Khan FM, Potish RA, et al., eds. *Levitt and Tapley's technological basis of radiation therapy: clinical applications,* 3rd ed. Baltimore: Lippincott Williams & Wilkins, 1999:269–299.
78. Wang CC. Intraoral cone for carcinoma of the oral cavity. *Front Radiat Ther Oncol* 1991;25:128–131.
79. Million RR, Cassisi NJ. General principles for treatment of cancers in the head and neck: Radiation therapy. In: Million RR, Cassisi NJ, eds. *Management of head and neck cancer: a multidisciplinary approach,* 1st ed. Philadelphia: Lippincott, 1984:77–90.
80. Parsons JT, Mendenhall WM, Million RR. Radiotherapy of tumors of the oral cavity. In: Thawley SE, Panje WR, Batsakis JG, et al., eds. *Comprehensive management of head and neck tumors,* 2nd ed. Philadelphia: WB Saunders, 1999: 695–719.
81. Mendenhall WM, Van Cise WS, Bova FJ, et al. Analysis of time-dose factors in squamous cell carcinoma of the oral tongue and floor of mouth treated with radiation therapy alone. *Int J Radiat Oncol Biol Phys* 1981;7:1005–1011.
82. Ellingwood KE, Million RR, Mitchell TP. A preloaded radium needle implant device for maintenance of needle spacing. *Cancer* 1976;37:2858–2860.
83. Pierquin B, Wilson JF, Chassagne D. *Modern brachytherapy*. New York: Masson Publishing USA, 1987.
84. Mendenhall WM, Parsons JT, Stringer SP, et al. T2 oral tongue carcinoma treated with radiotherapy: analysis of local control and complications. *Radiother Oncol* 1989;16:275–281.
85. Amdur RJ, Parsons JT, Mendenhall WM, et al. Postoperative irradiation for squamous cell carcinoma of the head and neck: an analysis of treatment results and complications. *Int J Radiat Oncol Biol Phys* 1989;16:25–36.

CHAPTER 17

Cancer of the Oropharynx

Kenneth S. Hu, Louis B. Harrison, Bruce Culliney, Adam P. Dicker, and Roy B. Sessions

Tumors of the oropharynx comprise approximately 5,000 new cases each year in the United States (1). Patients with a history of tobacco or alcohol use are at increased risk for these tumors. Such a history can also be associated with other metachronous or synchronous tumors of the aerodigestive tract. The prognosis for oropharyngeal carcinoma depends on the location of the primary tumor and the stage at presentation. The most important cause of death is locoregional recurrence, which, if it occurs, usually manifests itself within 2 years. Patients who survive are at risk for developing a second or third primary cancer in the upper aerodigestive tract or in the lower respiratory tract. The treatment strategies are numerous for these patients, and advances in organ preservation with attention to quality of life will be among the major issues for oncologists in the next decade.

ANATOMY OF THE OROPHARYNX

The pharynx is divided into the nasopharynx, oropharynx, and hypopharynx (Fig. 17.1). The oropharynx is located between the soft palate superiorly and the hyoid bone inferiorly. It is continuous with the oral cavity anteriorly and communicates with the nasopharynx above and the supraglottic larynx and hypopharynx below. Within the oropharynx are four different sites: soft palate, tonsillar region (fossa and pillars), base of tongue, and posterior and lateral pharyngeal wall between the nasopharynx and the pharyngoepiglottic fold (Fig. 17.2).

Soft Palate

The soft palate includes the uvula and incompletely separates the oral cavity and oropharynx from the nasopharynx. It is continuous laterally with the tonsillar pillars and attaches anteriorly to the hard palate. It forms both the roof of the oropharynx and the floor of the nasopharynx. The soft palate demarcates the oral cavity from the oropharynx as well as the oropharynx from the nasopharynx. Tumors arising from the oropharyngeal surface are far more common than are those arising from the nasopharyngeal surface.

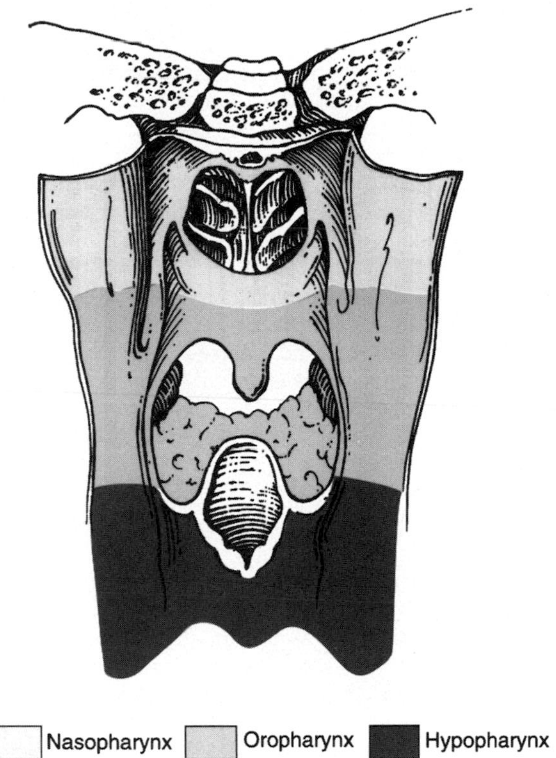

Figure 17.1 Regions of the pharynx.

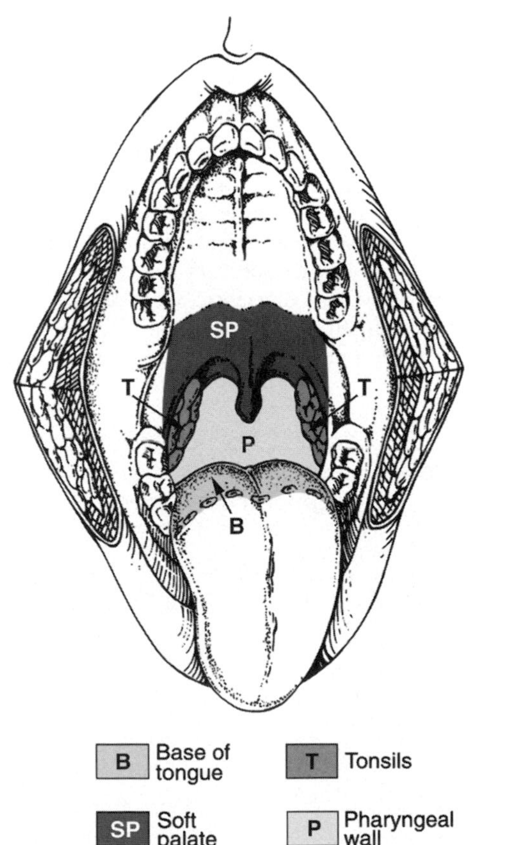

Figure 17.2 Topographic surface anatomy of the oropharynx; view from oral cavity.

Tonsillar Region

The palatine (or faucial) tonsils, located posteriorly on the lateral wall of the oropharynx, are almond-shaped structures of largely lymphoid tissue embedded in a fibrous capsule. The tonsillar fossa, which encases the palatine tonsil, is bounded by an anterior and posterior portion, commonly called the pillars. These contain the palatoglossus and palatopharyngeus muscles, respectively, and converge superiorly to join with the soft palate. The inferior portion of the fossa is the glossopalatine sulcus.

Base of Tongue

The base of tongue is defined as the tissue that extends inferiorly from the circumvallate papilla to the vallecula (base of the epiglottis) and encompasses the pharyngoepiglottic and glossoepiglottic folds. Laterally, it extends to the glossopalatine sulcus. The tongue musculature is composed of the genioglossus, styloglossus, palatoglossus, and hypoglossus muscles. The blood supply is identical to that of the oral tongue, and innervation is through the hypoglossal nerve.

Pharyngeal Wall

The posterior pharyngeal wall starts at the inferior aspect of the nasopharynx in the region of the soft palate and extends to the level of the epiglottis inferiorly. It comprises the posterolateral surfaces of the oropharynx. The pharyngeal constrictor muscles constitute the framework of the pharyngeal wall. The wall is related to the second and third cervical vertebrae and contains the mucosa, submucosa, pharyngobasilar fascia, underlying superior constrictor muscle, and buccopharyngeal fascia. The lateral aspect of the pharyngeal wall is continuous with the pharyngoepiglottic fold and continues into the lateral aspect of the piriform sinus. Nerve supply is from cranial nerves IX and X. The pharyngeal wall is rich in lymphatics, the primary drainage being directed to the retropharyngeal nodes and levels II and III.

Lymphatics of the Oropharynx

The lymphatic drainage of the neck was described in a classic paper by Rouviere (2) in 1938 and has been refined by others (3,4). The lymph node groups are described by clinical levels I to V as depicted in Figure 17.3.

The primary drainage of the oropharynx is to the jugulodigastric (level II) node(s) located in the upper deep jugular chain. The tonsillar region, pharyngeal portion of the soft palate, lateral and posterior oropharyngeal walls, and base of tongue also are drained by the retropharyngeal and parapharyngeal nodes. These nodes are located in the retropharyngeal and parapharyngeal space that is closely related to cranial nerves IX through XII, the internal jugular vein, and the internal carotid artery at the base of skull. The parapharyngeal lymph nodes are known also as the junctional nodes, owing to the junction of the spinal accessory (level V) and upper internal jugular lymphatic chains.

The probability of lymphatic metastasis is related to size and location of the primary tumor within the oropharynx. The order of progression of lymph node metastases usually proceeds superiorly, from the high cervical first-echelon nodes (level II) inferiorly to the midcervical and lower cervical nodes (levels III and IV). Skip metastasis can occur in which a particular lymph node level is bypassed, but this is very unusual. Candela et al. (5), from 1965 to 1986, evaluated 333 previously untreated patients with primary squamous cell carcinoma (SCC) of the

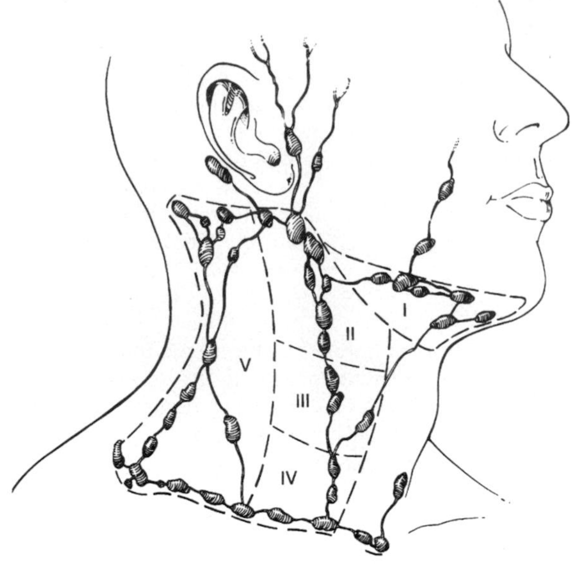

Figure 17.3 Anatomic lymph node levels of the neck.

oropharynx or hypopharynx to ascertain the prevalence of neck node metastases by neck level. The patients underwent classic radical neck dissections. Isolated skip metastases outside of level II, III, or IV occurred in only one patient (0.3%). Otherwise, level I or V involvement always was associated with nodal metastases at other levels (5).

Tumors located in the midline (base of tongue, soft palate, and posterior pharyngeal wall) exhibit a higher propensity for bilateral lymphadenopathy. The probability of cervical node metastases, as demonstrated by clinical examination of the soft palate, tonsillar fossa, base of tongue, and oropharyngeal wall, is shown in Table 17.1 (6).

TABLE 17.1 Percentage Incidence of Cervical Lymph Node Metastasis as Determined by Clinical Examination

Location	N0	N1	N2
Oropharyngeal wall			
T1	75	0	25
T2	70	10	20
T3	33	23	45
T4	24	24	52
Soft palate			
T1	92	0	8
T2	64	12	25
T3	35	26	39
T4	33	11	56
Tonsillar fossa			
T1	30	41	30
T2	33	14	54
T3	30	18	52
T4	11	13	77
Base of tongue			
T1	30	15	55
T2	29	15	57
T3	26	23	52
T4	16	9	76

Source: Adapted from Lindberg R. Distribution of cervical lymph node metastases from squamous cell carcinoma of the upper respiratory and digestive tracts. *Cancer* 1972;29:1446–1449.

PATHOLOGY

More than 90% of tumors of the oropharynx are SCC, the remainder being malignant melanomas, minor salivary gland tumors, sarcomas, plasmacytomas, lymphomas, and other rare tumors (7). Benign and malignant tumors that can be found in the oropharynx are listed in Table 17.2. Metastases to the oropharynx do occur (8–11). Lymphoepithelioma is more common in the tonsillar region and base of tongue. The distinction between lymphoepithelioma and SCC is important, with the former likely to be particularly radiosensitive (12). Non-Hodgkin lymphoma is seen in approximately 5% of tonsillar malignancies and rarely is encountered in the base of tongue.

CLINICAL PRESENTATION, PATHOGENESIS, AND PATTERNS OF SPREAD

Patients with primary tumors of the oropharynx frequently are asymptomatic until their primary tumors reach a significant size or metastasize to a lymph node in the neck. The usual complaints are that of vague discomfort, irritation, or a mass in the neck. The manifestation of symptoms depends on the location of the primary tumor within the oropharynx. Some tumors are visualized easily and frequently are found by dentists and physicians (e.g., tonsil), whereas others are not visualized as easily. The most common complaint is of pain, which can be attributed either to deep infiltration of tumor or to referred pain. The following sections list some of the possible clinical scenarios based on the site of the primary tumor within the oropharynx.

Soft Palate

Tumors of the soft palate are almost exclusively found on the anterior surface (the oropharynx portion as opposed to the nasopharynx portion) (Fig. 17.4). In a study of 359 male U.S. military veterans diagnosed with 424 cancers of the oral cavity and oropharynx, tobacco smoking was found to be more strongly associated with soft palate lesions than with lesions in more anterior sites (13). Tumors can extend to involve the tonsillar pillars and the base of tongue. Occasionally, these lesions may extend laterally and superiorly as far as the nasopharynx. Involvement of the palatine nerve can result in tumor tracking

TABLE 17.2 Differential Diagnosis of an Oropharyngeal Mass

Malignant
- Squamous cell carcinoma
- Minor salivary gland tumor
- Lymphoma
- Sarcoma
- Melanoma
- Plasmacytoma
- Other

Benign
- Papilloma
- Retention cyst
- Fibroma
- Lipoma
- Hemangioma
- Lymphangioma
- Neuroma
- Other

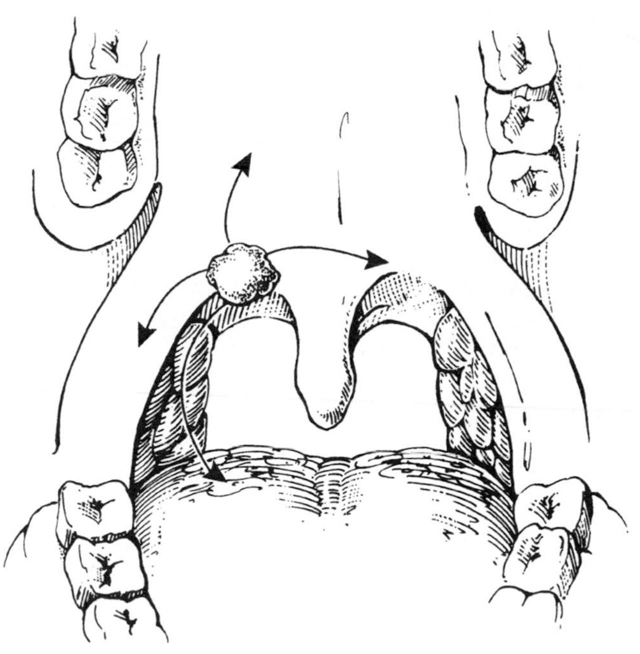

Figure 17.4 Patterns of tumor spread in soft palate.

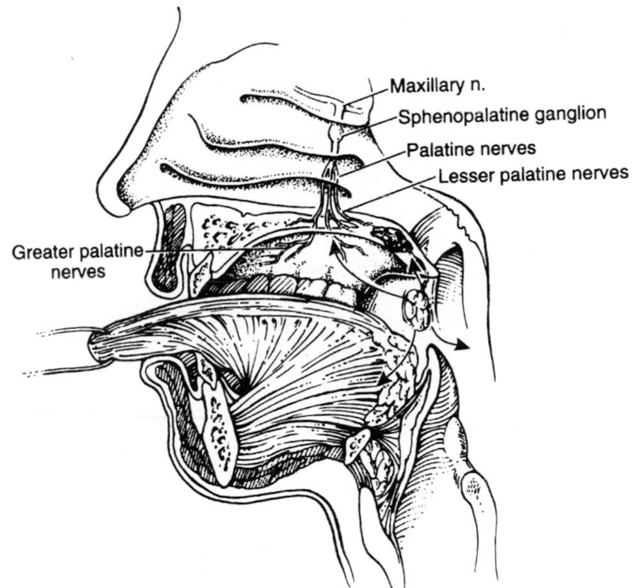

Figure 17.5 Patterns of spread of tonsillar carcinoma.

along this pathway, with extension into the cranium. Lymphatic involvement is primarily to level II. Lesions of the midline and uvula can result in bilateral nodal metastases more frequently than do lateralized lesions.

Tonsil

The most common location for a primary tumor of the oropharynx is the anterior tonsillar pillar and tonsil. Common presenting symptoms are ipsilateral referred otalgia, discomfort, poorly fitting dentures, or a sensation of a lump or foreign body in the throat. Lesions involving the anterior tonsillar pillar can appear as areas of dysplasia, inflammation, or a superficial spreading or exophytic lesion. Frequently, these lesions become endophytic, ulcerate, and can spread laterally to the buccal mucosa and directly to the retromolar trigone II (Fig. 17.5). Inferior extension to the base of tongue is common. Perez et al. (14) report that of 218 patients presenting with SCC of the tonsillar region, the soft palate was involved in 131 (60%) and extension to the base of tongue occurred in 120 (55%). Superior extension can involve the soft and hard palate. Medial extension can involve the oral tongue. The close proximity of the anterior tonsillar pillar to the mandible places the periosteum and bone at risk in advanced cases. Posterior extension with destruction of the tonsillar pillars can involve the pterygoid muscles, with subsequent trismus and pain. The lymphatic drainage is primarily to level II but can involve level I and the retropharyngeal and parapharyngeal nodes.

Tumors of the tonsillar fossa (in contrast to those of the tonsillar pillar) are either exophytic or ulcerative and present in more advanced stages than do tumors of the pillars or soft palate. Approximately 75% of patients will present with stage III or IV disease, for which the patterns of extension are similar to those of the tonsillar pillar. In addition, lateral extension can involve the parapharyngeal space toward the base of skull, causing neurologic signs and symptoms. Tumors of the posterior tonsillar pillar can extend inferiorly and involve the pharyngoepiglottic fold and the posterior aspect of the thyroid cartilage. These lesions also more frequently involve the level V nodes, owing to extension to the spinal accessory chain group.

The probability of clinical lymph node involvement is greater with tumors of the tonsillar fossa, especially contralateral involvement, in contrast to that of the tonsillar pillar. The lymphatic drainage depends on the location of the primary tumor. Lindberg (6) describes nodal metastases in 76% of patients with tonsillar fossa tumors. The most common nodal group was level II. Contralateral lymph nodes were detected in 11% of patients. In contrast, tumors of the anterior tonsillar pillar or retromolar trigone region have an incidence of ipsilateral lymph node metastases of 45%, level II being the most common node-bearing region. Contralateral adenopathy was present in only 5% of patients.

Base of Tongue

Squamous cell carcinoma of the base of tongue is highly insidious. The base of tongue is almost devoid of pain fibers, and frequently these tumors are asymptomatic until they have progressed significantly. Many who present with a neck node are found, on examination, to have a base-of-tongue lesion. Visualization of this area on physical examination is difficult, and so a lesion often is missed (15). Patients may experience the sensation of a mass or discomfort in the throat, with bleeding and pain at later stages. Patients also might experience difficulty in swallowing or with speech. Occasionally, referred otalgia is the first symptom. If the size of the primary tumor increases such that it involves the pterygoid muscles, trismus can result.

Extension anteriorly can involve the oral tongue, superior and lateral extension can involve the tonsil, and inferior extension can involve the vallecula, epiglottis, and preepiglottic space (Fig. 17.6). Locally advanced base-of-tongue tumors can infiltrate the deep muscle and cause fixation.

Lymph node metastasis is common, owing to the rich lymphatic drainage of the base of tongue. The most common first-echelon nodal region is level II, though involvement of levels III and IV is also seen. Approximately 70% of patients or more will present with ipsilateral metastases, and 10% to 20% will present with bilateral nodal metastases.

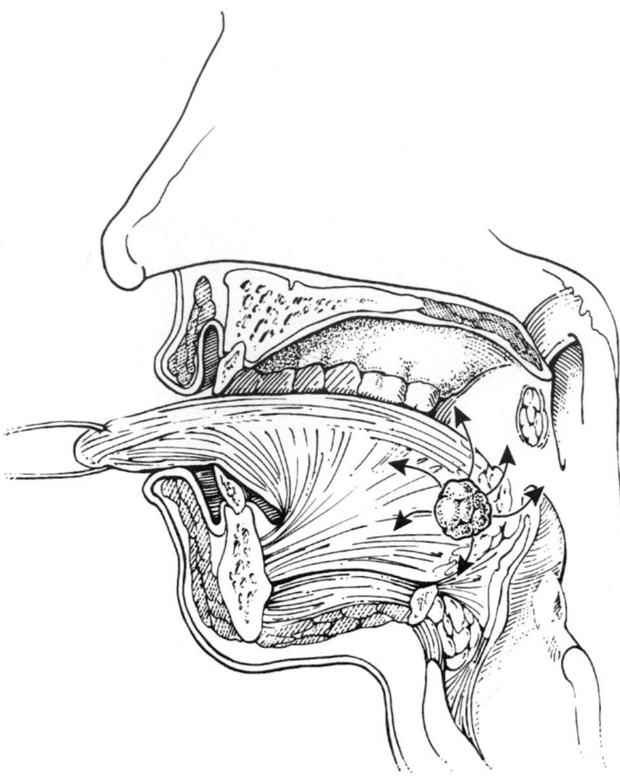

Figure 17.6 Patterns of spread of base-of-tongue cancer.

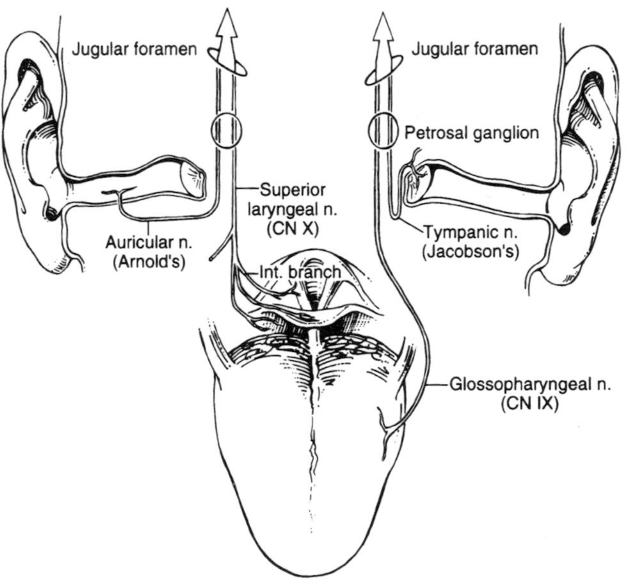

Figure 17.7 Neural pathways of referred otalgia. For pain sensed in the front of the helix and tragus, the skin of the anterior wall of the external auditory canal, the tympanic membrane, and the temple, pain is referred through the auriculotemporal nerve, which joins the lingual nerve, where the two become the mandibular nerve and enter the foramen ovale. The sensation of deep ear pain is through the tympanic nerve (Jacobson), which joins the glossopharyngeal nerve (cranial nerve IX) as the two traverse the jugular foramen. These general somatic afferent fibers innervate the base of tongue, the inner surface of the tympanic membrane, and the upper pharynx. For pain sensed in the back of the pinna, the posterior wall of the external auditory canal, and the external surface of the tympanic membrane, pain is referred through the auricular nerve (Arnold), which joins the superior laryngeal nerve (cranial nerve X), which in turn innervates the larynx, pharynx, and epiglottis as it traverses the jugular foramen.

Pharyngeal Wall

Tumors of the pharyngeal wall region generally are diagnosed in an advanced stage due to the silent location in which they develop. Symptoms can include pain and bleeding and a mass in the neck. Disease involvement can extend to the nasopharynx superiorly, the prevertebral fascia posteriorly, and piriform sinuses and hypopharyngeal wall inferiorly. Clinically palpable cervical lymph node metastases are present in 25% of patients with T1 lesions, 30% of those with T2 lesions, 66% of patients with T3 lesions, and more than 75% of patients with T4 disease. Because most pharyngeal wall tumors extend past the midline, bilateral cervical metastases are common.

Referred Otalgia

Referred otalgia can be one of the first symptoms that a patient experiences with a mass in the oropharynx. The pathway for this referred pain is mediated by cranial nerves IX and X. The pathophysiology for otalgia depends on the site of pain (Fig. 17.7).

DIAGNOSTIC EVALUATION

History

The history should be part of a comprehensive evaluation of any patient with head and neck cancer. Patients usually present with pain and dysphagia and, occasionally, referred otalgia. If the history strongly reveals tobacco and alcohol use, efforts should be made to determine whether the patient is an alcoholic and continues to smoke. Alcoholic smokers are at risk for other chronic diseases of the heart, lung, peripheral vascular system, and liver, and may present with signs of malnutrition. Before the institution of any therapeutic modality, patients should cease alcohol and tobacco use. It may be necessary to guide the patient toward cessation programs. Clearly, those who discontinue smoking will better tolerate treatment and obtain a better result (16).

Physical Examination

The details of the physical examination are discussed in Chapter 1. Specific aspects of the physical examination should include evaluation of the lesion (exophytic or infiltrative), tongue mobility, and palatal motion. Fixation of the tongue will result in incomplete protrusion or deviation of the tongue to the side of tumor involvement. In patients with a smoking and drinking history, three sites have a greater propensity for developing carcinoma than do others in the oral cavity and oropharynx: floor of mouth, ventrolateral tongue, and lingual aspect of the retromolar trigone and the anterior tonsillar pillar (17,18).

For tumors of the tonsil or lateral pharyngeal wall, the examiner should test for anesthesia in the distribution of the ipsilateral mental nerve (V3). Any abnormality might suggest involvement of the inferior alveolar nerve in its pathway as it courses through the mandible or the base of skull and may direct the appropriate imaging study (12). The tonsil is adjacent to the ascending ramus of the mandible, and posterolateral to the tonsil is the parapharyngeal space. Tumors may extend into this area and be palpable in the neck on bimanual palpation. Owing to the relationship of the anterior tonsil (palatoglossus muscle) and the base of tongue, tonsillar cancers frequently extend into this region.

After the direct visual examination has been completed, indirect mirror examination followed by indirect fiberoptic nasopharyngoscopy is performed. We photograph or extensively diagram the physical findings in every patient. This often includes a videotape. Such records are an excellent means of documenting the physical findings and of comparing future examination results to the initial presentation; they also serve as a teaching tool.

At the conclusion of the examination of the oral cavity and oropharynx, bimanual palpation of the floor of mouth, mandible, and base of tongue should be performed. In selected cases, an examination under anesthesia is recommended as a means of obtaining information that is not completely accessible during office examination.

Initial Workup and Radiographic Evaluation

In addition to a history and physical examination, a complete blood cell count, screening profile, and chest roentgenogram are recommended (Fig. 17.8). Biopsy of a suspicious lesion is necessary to confirm the diagnosis (19). A more detailed metastatic workup is indicated only when strong clinical or laboratory suspicion of metastatic disease exists. See Chapter 4 for radiographic evaluation.

Staging

The current staging criteria for tumors of the oropharynx, as defined by the American Joint Committee on Cancer (AJCC) (20), are listed in Table 17.3. This is a clinical staging system and not a pathologic staging system. If radiographic information reveals a discrepancy from clinical staging, this should be noted (e.g., clinical—cT2, N2b; radiographic—rN2c). Current staging allows the radiographic findings to factor into the staging designation.

Dental Evaluation and Prophylaxis

Treatment of the oropharynx by external beam radiation therapy (EBRT) can result in a number of temporary and permanent effects on the oral cavity and oropharynx. Among these are mucositis, xerostomia, and infections. Dentulous patients are at increased risk for dental caries owing to the reduction in salivary flow, pH, and proliferation of bacteria believed to be responsible for caries. A complete dental evaluation should be performed before any therapy is undertaken (see Chapter 6 for further details).

MANAGEMENT STRATEGIES, RESULTS, AND OUTCOMES

Treatment decisions depend both on the ability of a particular modality to control the primary tumor and on the state of the neck and its associated morbidity. In general, early stage disease can be treated by either radiation therapy (RT) or surgery, whereas more advanced lesions often are treated by combinations of these methods. Radiation therapy is chosen more often than surgery for most early lesions because the cure rates are high and the functional outcome is better. Chemotherapy generally is reserved for patients with very advanced disease or for certain organ-sparing protocols. In the following sections, the

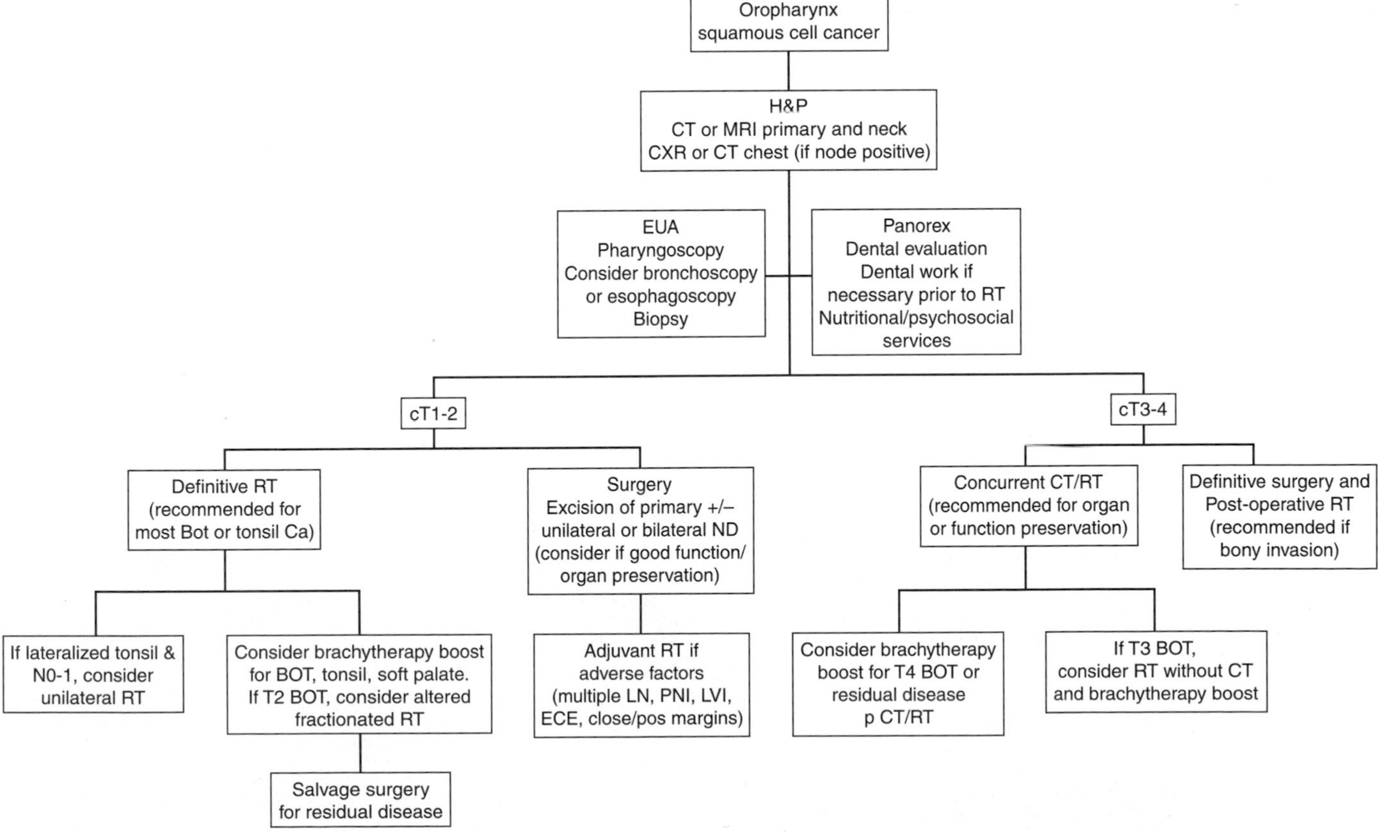

Figure 17.8 Algorithm for the workup and diagnosis of oropharynx carcinomas. BOT, base of tongue; CT, computed tomography; CXR, chest x-ray; ECE, extracapsular extension; H&P, history and physical; LN, lymph node; LVI, lymph vessel invasion; MRI, magnetic resonance imaging; ND, neck dissection; PNI, perineural invasion RT, radiation therapy.

TABLE 17.3 2002 American Joint Committee on Cancer Classification of Oropharyngeal Cancer

Primary tumor (T)	
T1	Tumor ≤2 cm in greatest dimension
T2	Tumor >2 cm but not >4 cm in greatest dimension
T3	Tumor >4 cm in greatest dimension
T4a	Tumor invades the larynx, deep/extrinsic muscle of the tongue, medial pterygoid, hard palate, or mandible
T4b	Tumor invades lateral pterygoid muscle, pterygoid plates, lateral nasopharynx, or skull base or encases carotid artery
Regional lymph nodes (N)	
N0	No regional lymph node metastasis
N1	Metastasis in a single ipsilateral node, ≤3 cm
N2a	Metastasis in a single ipsilateral node, >3 cm but <6 cm
N2b	Metastasis in multiple ipsilateral nodes, >3 cm but <6 cm
N2c	Metastasis in bilateral or contralateral lymph nodes, none >6 cm
N3	Metastasis in a lymph node >6 cm
Distant metastasis (M)	
M0	No distant metastasis present
M1	Distant metastasis present

Stage			
Stage 0	Tis	N0	M0
Stage I	T1	N0	M0
Stage II	T2	N0	M0
Stage III	T3	N0	M0
	T1-3	N1	M0
Stage IVa	T4a	N0	M0
	T4a	N1	M0
	T1-3	N2	M0
	T4b	Any N	M0
Stage IVb	Any T	N3	M0
Stage IVc	Any T	Any N	M1

Source: Greene F, Page D, Fleming I, et al. *AJCC cancer staging manual,* 6th ed. New York: Springer-Verlag, 2002.

management guidelines, outcomes, and results will be reported by subsite of the oropharynx (Figs. 17.9, 17.10).

Soft Palate

SELECTION OF THERAPEUTIC MODALITY

Early Disease

For early stage lesions of the soft palate, either surgical resection or RT has provided excellent local control. Most patients will be treated with RT because the results are excellent and the functional result probably is better (Fig. 17.11). Also, because many lesions are near the midline, radiation treatment of the primary site and both sides of the neck is easy. In general, more morbidity ensues with surgical therapy to these same areas, especially if postoperative radiation becomes necessary.

Advanced Disease

Patients with advanced soft-palate disease usually will receive combined surgery and postoperative RT. The use of RT alone has been reported, and the results for advanced stage lesions are suboptimal (21). However, increasing evidence demonstrates that concurrent chemoradiation improves locoregional control (LRC) and survival compared with radiation alone and

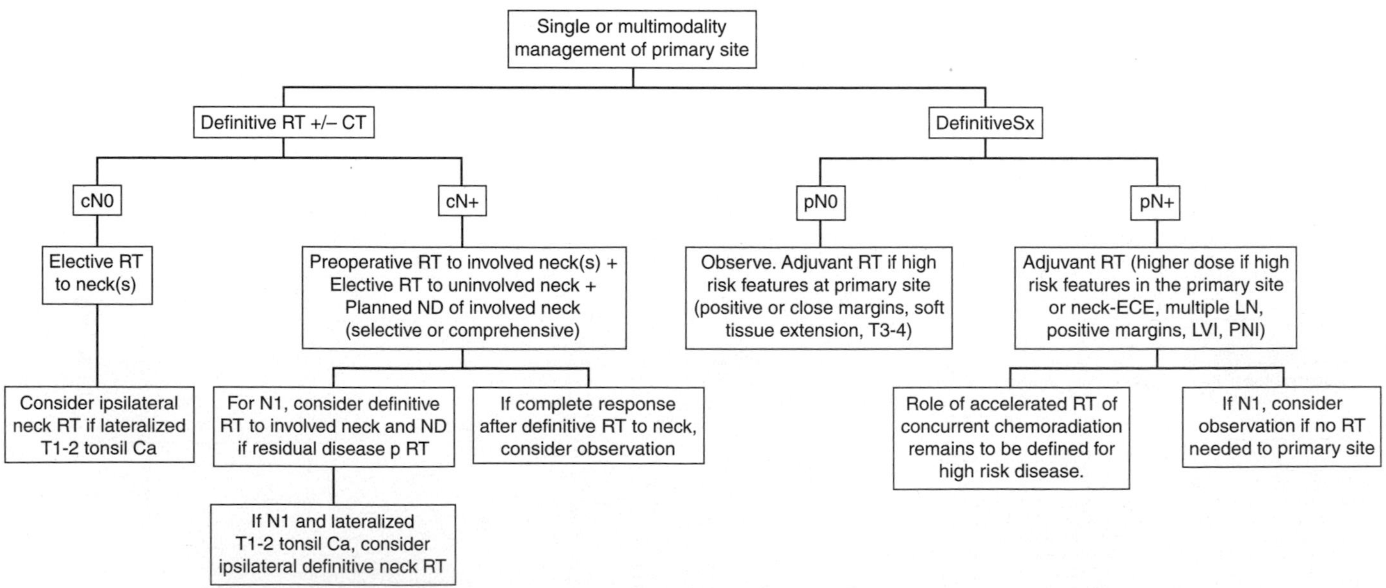

Figure 17.9 Algorithm for the management of the neck in patients with oropharyngeal carcinomas. CT, computed tomography; ECE, extracapsular extension; LN, lymph node; LVI, lymph vessel invasion; ND, neck dissection; PNI, perineural invasion; RT, radiation therapy.

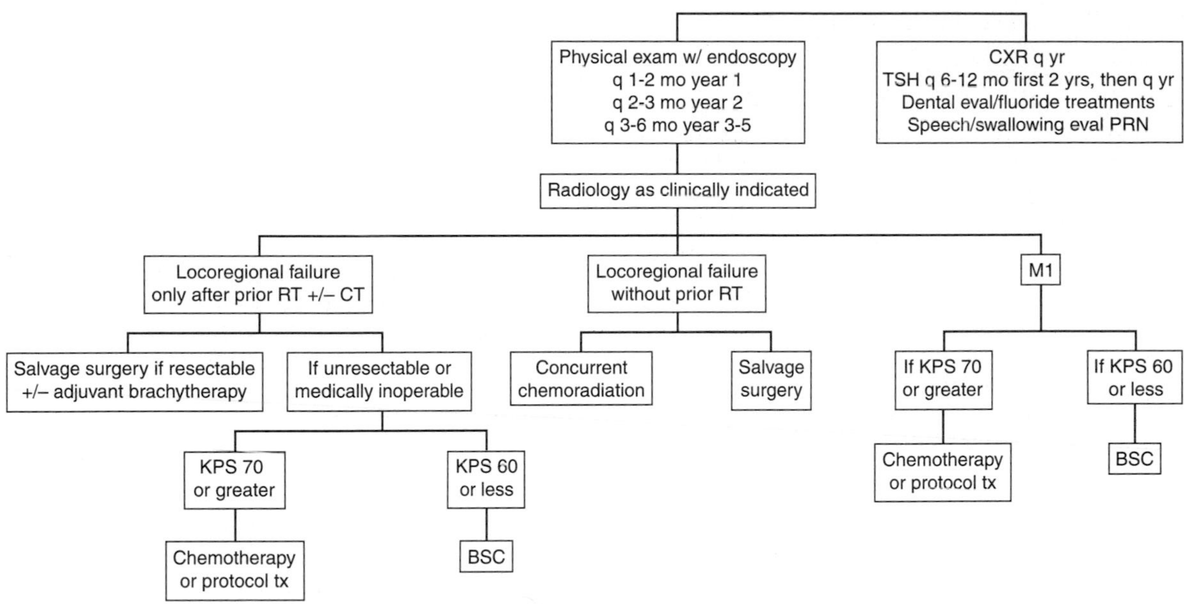

Figure 17.10 Algorithm for followup after treatment of oropharyngeal carcinomas. BSC, best supportive care; CT, computed tomography; CXR, chest x-ray; KPS, Karnofsky performance status; PRN, as needed; RT, radiation therapy; TSH, thyroid-stimulating hormone.

therefore is gaining wider acceptance as an alternative treatment option for advanced oropharynx cancers (22–24).

Neck

The application of elective neck treatment is not well defined. Even with small tumors (<2 cm in diameter), approximately 50% of patients with soft palate lesions will have clinical or radiographic evidence of neck disease on presentation. Of patients with a clinically negative neck, a significant percentage were found eventually to have neck disease (25).

For clinically negative neck nodes, all patients receive 5,000 to 5,400 cGy in 5 to 6 weeks. For clinically positive lymph nodes, this should be followed by either an additional boost to therapeutic doses to the neck or by neck dissection (26). For patients with palpable nodes, our preference is to perform neck dissection.

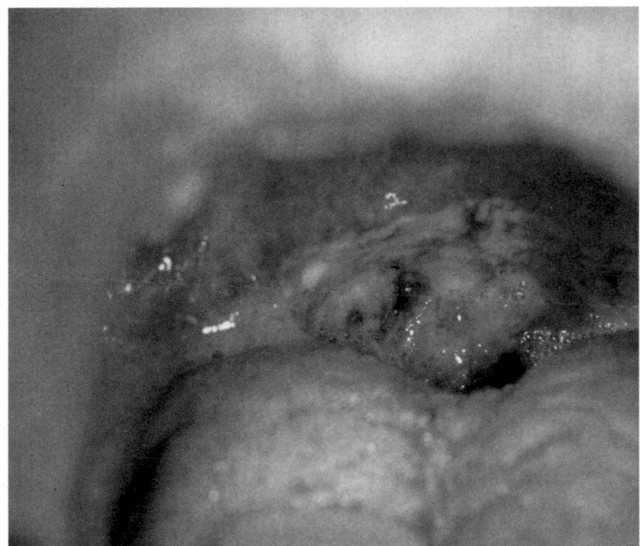

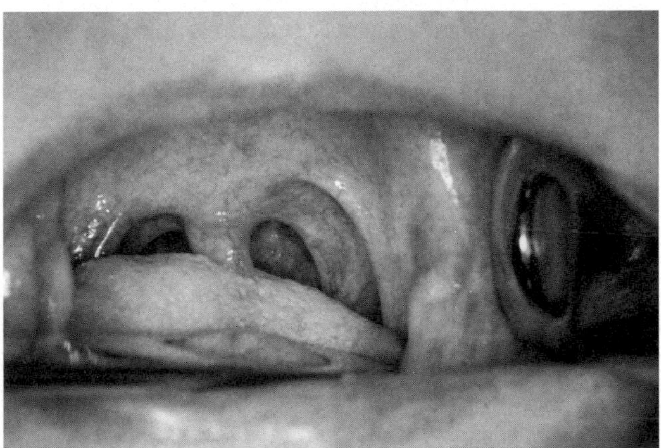

Figure 17.11 A patient with a T2N0 squamous cell cancer of the soft palate prior to and after radiation therapy. This patient was treated with external beam radiation therapy to the primary site and both sides of the neck. Opposed lateral portals were used in conjunction with a low anterior neck field. The primary site and low neck regions received 4,500 cGy, after which a spinal cord block was placed. The primary site and upper neck regions, including the retropharyngeal nodes, then were treated to 5,400 cGy. The final dose to the primary site was 6,840 cGy. Fraction size is 180 cGy per day. The lower neck is treated with an anterior portal to 5,000 cGy over 5 weeks. The posterior neck regions are boosted with electrons to protect the spinal cord to 5,400 cGy. The spinal cord is protected at the junction of the lateral and low anterior fields by a midline block in the low neck field. The block also protects the larynx. On setup, the field junction is placed above the thyroid notch but below the hyoid bone. The patient currently has no evidence of disease.

OUTCOME AND RESULTS: EARLY DISEASE

Definitive External Beam Radiotherapy

Two major series examine the use of EBRT alone or in conjunction with planned neck dissection. Amdur et al. (21) analyzed 75 patients with SCC of the soft palate or uvula (or both). Patients received between 6,000 and 7,000 cGy. The ultimate local control rates after surgical salvage of irradiation failures for T1 through T4 lesions were 100%, 84%, 45%, and 25%, respectively. Overall, 13% of patients treated with continuous-course irradiation experienced irradiation-related bone or soft tissue complications. Weber et al. (27) reviewed the experience at the University of Texas M. D. Anderson Cancer Center. Treatment to the primary site consisted of RT for 150 patients, surgery alone for 28 patients, and combined therapy for 10 patients. Local control rates for T1 through T4 lesions were 91%, 77%, 77%, and 35%, respectively. Local control was obtained in 88% of patients with N0 necks and in 77% of patients with nodal involvement. In addition, these investigators found that patients with tumor extension to the tongue base, midline tumors, or tumors that extended across the palatine arch had inferior survival compared with those who did not exhibit those features ($p < 0.05$) (27).

Combined External Beam Radiation Therapy and Brachytherapy Implant

The use of a brachytherapy implant for small soft palate lesions has been reported extensively by French investigators. Esche et al. (28) describe 43 patients with carcinoma of the soft palate and uvula who were treated by interstitial implant and EBRT. Patients received 5,000 cGy external irradiation to the oropharynx and neck, followed by 2,000 to 3,500 cGy delivered by a low-dose rate (40–100 cGy/hour) interstitial iridium-192 (^{192}Ir) implant. This therapy yielded a local control of 92%, with no local failures in 34 T1 primary tumors. One serious complication was seen. Overall actuarial survival was 60% at 3 years and 37% at 5 years, but cause-specific survivals were 81% and 64%, respectively. The leading cause of death was other aerodigestive cancers, with an actuarial rate of occurrence of 10% per year after treatment of a soft palate cancer.

Mazeron et al. (29) report on a subset of patients with early stage tumors who received EBRT to the primary tumor and neck nodes to a dose of 4,500 cGy, followed by 3,000 cGy delivered by a ^{192}Ir implant to the primary tumor. Local control was 85% for soft palate tumors. Regional control was 97% for patients with N0 disease and 88% for patients with N1 through N3 disease. Soft tissue ulceration occurred in 17 patients, all of whom healed spontaneously.

Pernot et al. (30) report on 277 patients with velotonsillar cancer (oropharyngeal cancer excluding base of tongue and valleculae) who were treated by brachytherapy either alone (14 patients) or combined with external beam irradiation (263 patients) using an after-loading ^{192}Ir technique. Thirty-five percent of the patients had soft palate lesions. Of the patients treated for early lesions in the soft palate, the local control rates for T1 to T2N0 and T1 to T2N1 to N3 were 90% and 86%, respectively. No local recurrence was detected after 3 years.

External Beam Radiation Therapy versus External Beam Radiation Therapy plus Brachytherapy

The need for an implant was analyzed retrospectively by Mazeron et al. (26), who report T1 and T2 carcinomas of the soft palate and uvula treated definitively by EBRT alone (16 patients), ^{192}Ir implant alone (14 patients), or a combination of the two methods (29 patients). Two techniques of implantation were used: the guide-gutter technique (33 patients) and the plastic-tube technique (10 patients). Local failure was 25% after EBRT alone, 0% after ^{192}Ir implant alone, and 18% after combined therapy. No local failures were seen with the plastic tube technique compared with 15% for guide gutters. Only two nodal failures were observed (3%). Crude 5-year disease-free survival (DFS) was 33%. Severe complications were limited to one incident of osteonecrosis, one soft-tissue necrosis, and one case of partial palatal incompetence. Xerostomia was reduced when implantation was used for part or all of the treatment. This is not conclusive proof that an implant is required, and these results may be difficult to duplicate without the requisite expertise in brachytherapy. Clearly, patient selection factors are important in these results.

Fractionated High-Dose Rate or Pulsed-Dose Rate Brachytherapy

In an effort to minimize occupational radiation exposure and decrease the patient isolation period while minimizing normal tissue complications, Levendag et al. report an initial experience combining EBRT with high-dose rate (HDR—100 cGy/minute) or pulsed-dose rate (PDR) brachytherapy in 38 patients—19 soft palate tumors (14 T1–2) and 19 tonsillar cancers (31). Twice-a-day fractions of 3.0 to 5.4 Gy HDR to a dose of 15 to 27 Gy or 4×2 Gy to 8×1 Gy per day of PDR to a dose of 20 to 28 Gy was delivered within 1 to 2 weeks after completion of EBRT (46–50 Gy, median cumulative dose of 66 Gy). At a mean follow-up of 2.6 years, 87% of soft palate tumors were locally controlled. The incidence of grade 3 mucositis or ulceration was no different between patients treated with PDR versus HDR and similar to those reported after low dose-rate brachytherapy.

Clearly, RT is very effective for patients with early disease but is suboptimal for patients with advanced disease. The need for a brachytherapy implant has not been proven. However, there are anecdotal comments related to improved salivary function in those patients who received an implant, due to the decreased external beam dose to the major salivary glands. Patient selection is important, and a radiation oncologist with experience in palatal implants must perform the therapy.

ADVANCED DISEASE

Most advanced soft palate tumors should be treated with combined surgery and postoperative RT. Radiation therapy alone has been reported to offer suboptimal results (21).

RECURRENT DISEASE AND SALVAGE

The treatment strategy for recurrence relates to tumor resectability. In those patients who have resectable disease, surgery should precede RT. If prior RT was undertaken, then "adjuvant" brachytherapy to the tumor bed may be considered if there are concerns about the margins of resection.

Patients who have previously received "full-tolerance" RT and who later develop either a second primary tumor or recurrence can be salvaged with a brachytherapy implant. Maulard et al. (32) report on 28 patients with prior irradiation of the oropharynx who underwent salvage brachytherapy for an SCC of the tonsil or soft palate. The patients had no evidence of regional metastatic disease. Salvage brachytherapy consisted of two split-course implantations performed 1 month apart, delivering 3,500 and 3,000 cGy, respectively. Fifteen patients (54%) were disease-free before the second implant, and 23 (82%) were clinically disease-free at the end of treatment. Five local failures have been observed, without any influence of the tumor size, the topographic site of the tumor, or the histology. Of the four patients in whom EBRT had failed previously, three were disease-free after salvage brachytherapy. The overall local control rate was 68%, with a mean follow-up of 41 months. Soft tissue necrosis was observed in four cases and, in all patients, the interval between previous RT and salvage treatment was short (mean, 7 months).

Brachytherapy implant is a reasonable option for salvage therapy in patients with recurrent and second cancers occurring in the oropharynx. However, as with any re-treatment situation, the complication rate will be higher than it is with primary therapy.

Tonsillar Region

SELECTION OF THERAPEUTIC MODALITY

Early Disease

Early lesions in the tonsillar region can be treated by RT or surgery. Radiation generally is preferred because the results are excellent and the functional outcome is better. Treatment entails portals that include the primary site and ipsilateral neck, including the retropharyngeal nodes. Care is taken to avoid irradiating the contralateral parotid gland to reduce the incidence of xerostomia. For those patients treated surgically, either a transoral or mandibulotomy approach generally is used for the primary site. When better exposure is required, a combined lip-splitting incision with an anterior midline or lateral mandibulotomy is used. If there is superficial extension to the periosteum of the mandible, a partial mandibulectomy may be performed. For clinically negative necks, a modified supraomohyoid neck dissection, as a staging procedure, often is performed. If nodes are positive, postoperative radiation is added.

Advanced Disease

Patients with stage III and IV tonsillar disease can be managed in several ways. Definitive radiation with the addition of a neck dissection for node-positive patients often is used. However, for locally advanced lesions, combined-modality treatment consisting of surgery followed by RT more commonly is applied. This is especially true for tumors that are infiltrative rather than exophytic in nature. Surgery for advanced disease generally entails a segmental mandibulectomy. Definitive concurrent chemoradiation to the primary with planned neck dissection in patients with advanced neck disease is a reasonable treatment option in view of recent studies (22–24).

Radiation Therapy

The use of RT as the definitive treatment for tumors of the tonsillar fossa is appropriate for T1, T2, and T3 (exophytic) tumors. For infiltrative or endophytic T3 or T4 lesions, either surgery combined with postoperative RT or an organ-preserving approach involving chemotherapy should be used. The target volume of the ipsilateral treatment should include the primary lesion with at least 2-cm margins, the ipsilateral jugular vein, and retropharyngeal lymph nodes. If disease extends to the base of tongue, then EBRT alone is not as effective as EBRT plus implant to the tongue (33). In this case, full-dose EBRT is delivered, followed by an interstitial ^{192}Ir implant as a boost to the tongue portion of the target.

For ipsilateral lesions, radiation is given through a wedged pair that incorporates the primary site and the ipsilateral neck. The upper neck is treated in the same portals as is the primary site; the lower neck is treated with a single anteroposterior field, with the larynx and the spinal cord protected at the field junction. In general, most T1 to T2 lesions in patients with an N0 or N1 neck can be treated with ipsilateral fields (Fig. 17.12). Lesions that cross the midline, involve the tongue base, or involve N2 or more advanced neck disease should be treated with bilateral opposed portals and a low neck field that protects the larynx and spinal cord at the field junction. At the time of simulation, a bite block is used and all scars are marked with wire. A computed tomographic (CT) scan is performed to assist in treatment planning for lesions treated unilaterally. For patients who will receive bilateral radiation, a planning CT scan generally is not required.

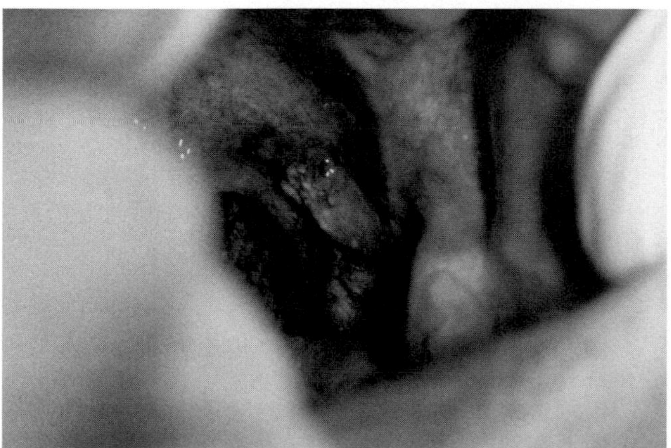

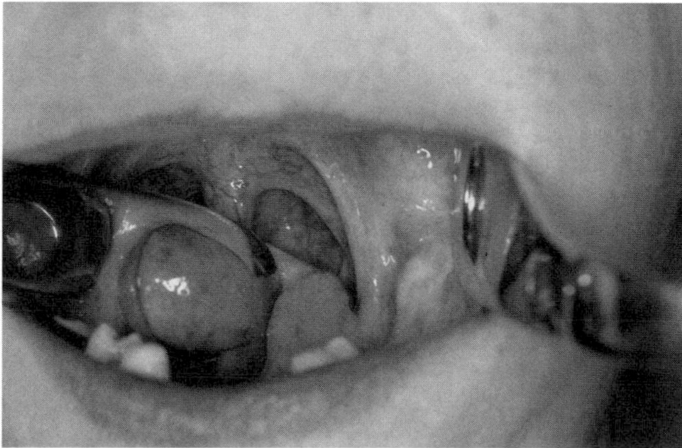

Figure 17.12 A patient with a T2N0 squamous cell cancer of the tonsil before and after radiation therapy. This patient was treated with external beam radiation therapy to the primary site and ipsilateral neck using an ipsilateral wedge pair beam arrangement in conjunction with an ipsilateral low anterior neck field (see Fig. 17.14). The final dose to the primary site was 7,020 cGy. Fraction size is 180 cGy per day. The lower neck was treated with an anterior portal to 5,000 cGy over 5 weeks.

OUTCOME AND RESULTS

Early Disease

Surgery Alone. The use of surgery as the sole treatment for early tonsillar disease is not reported frequently. However, excellent local control rates ranging from 80% to 90% have been reported (30,34,35). When there is extension to the lateral pharyngeal wall or base of tongue, local recurrence approaches 33% and 47%, respectively (36–38). The degree to which local control can be obtained depends on the extension of disease outside the tonsillar fossa.

External Beam Radiation Therapy Alone. No definitive randomized studies comparing surgery versus EBRT have been reported. However, no obvious differences between these modalities in LRC or absolute survival can be determined based on the reported literature (34,39–50). If local control is maintained in patients by EBRT alone, the greatest risk to these patients is the development of future aerodigestive malignancies (51). In general, the results using conventionally fractionated EBRT alone (1.8–2.0 Gy/dose over 6.5 to 7 weeks to doses of 65–70 Gy) are excellent for early stage tumors (35,43–45,52).

Mendenhall updated the University of Florida experience where definitive radiation to the primary site is the institutional policy for treatment of 400 tonsillar cancers over a 23-year period with a minimum 2-year follow-up (39). Patients were treated with continuous course radiation (n = 160, median total dose 66 Gy) or using hyperfractionation (n = 240, median total dose 77 Gy). Only 18 patients received chemotherapy, 147 underwent planned neck dissection, and 107 underwent an interstitial brachytherapy boost. Five-year rates of local control were as follows: T1 (n = 56) 83%; T2 (n = 150) 81%; T3 (n = 126) 74%; and T4 (n = 68) 60%. Of the 83 local recurrences, 36 underwent salvage therapy and 17 were successfully salvaged. The ultimate local control rates were T1 92%, T2 89%, T3 77%, and T4 65%. Five-year disease-specific survivals by 1998 AJCC stage (fifth edition) were as follows: I 100%, II 86%, III 82%, IVa 63%, and IVb 22%. Absolute overall survival (OS) at 5 years was as follows: I 51%, II 60%, III 57%, IVa 47%, and IVb 14%. No severe acute radiation-related complications were reported; however, 5% (19/400) developed severe late complications including osteoradionecrosis requiring mandibulectomy (n = 8), dysphagia requiring gastrostomy (n = 6), bone exposure necessitating debridement and hyperbaric treatment (n = 3), orocutaneous fistula (n = 1), and fatal aspiration pneumonia (n = l).

Remmler et al. (36) report the results in 160 patients in whom EBRT was the sole therapy for the majority of patients. Primary tumor control rates were 100% for T1 lesions, 89% for T2, 68% for T3, and 24% for T4. In addition, radiation therapeutic control of cervical metastases in patients was excellent (95%). When a planned neck dissection was performed 5 weeks after RT, the control of cancer in the neck was 100%. The incidence of distant metastases was 10% and was not affected by the selection of therapy. The 2- and 5-year determinate survival figures for 112 patients treated with RT alone were 67% and 48%, respectively, whereas 31 patients treated with RT followed by neck dissection achieved a 5-year survival rate of 48% (Table 17.4).

Lower doses or split-course radiation results in poorer LRC (131). Using RT alone, Bataini et al. (43) report that in tumors arising from the glossopalatine sulcus, characterized by involvement of the tongue, inferior local control is achieved as compared with similar therapy for tumors arising from other sites within the tonsillar region.

IPSILATERAL EXTERNAL BEAM RADIATION THERAPY. For patients with T1 and T2 lesions, treatment of the ipsilateral neck alone usually is possible without having to irradiate the contralateral neck, which minimizes irradiation to the contralateral salivary gland and reduces the incidence of xerostomia. Eisbruch has demonstrated that patients treated unilaterally report less xerostomia and better quality of life compared with those treated with intensity-modulated RT delivery of bilateral radiation with contralateral parotid sparing (53). However, careful patient selection is required to minimize the risk for contralateral neck failure. Two recent major series document excellent outcomes using ipsilateral neck EBRT.

O'Sullivan et al. report the results of 228 tonsillar carcinomas treated with ipsilateral RT over a 20-year period at Princess Margaret Hospital (54). Eligible patients typically had T1 or T2 tumors (191 T1–2, 30 T3, 7 T4) with N0 (133 N0, 35 N1, 27 N2–3) disease. During this period, only 16 patients were treated surgically. Radiation was typically delivered with wedged-pair cobalt beams and ipsilateral low anterior neck field delivering 50 Gy in 4 weeks (90% isodose line) to the primary volume. At a median follow-up of 5.7 years, the 3-year local control rate was 77%, regional control was 80%, and cause-specific survival

TABLE 17.4 Tonsillar Carcinoma: Local Control and Survival with External Beam Radiation Therapy with or without Brachytherapy Implant

				Percentage local control				Percentage local control				5-year survival (%)	
Study and institution	No. of patients	Median follow-up (mos)	Percentage stage T3–4	T1	T2	T3	T4	N0	N1	N2	N3	DFS	Overall
Remmler et al., M. D. Anderson Cancer Center (36)	112	50	63	100	89	68	24	95	95	95	95	48	85
Wong et al., M. D. Anderson Cancer Center (44)	174	36	50	94	79	59	50	100	100	100	68	—	—
Bataini et al., Institut Curie (43)	698	60	72	89	84	63	43	NS	NS	NS	NS	NS	NS
Pernot et al., Centre Alexis[a] (30)	277	36	36	89	86	69	—	NS	NS	NS	NS	62	NS
Mazeron et al.,[a] Henri Mondor (57)	165	60	0	100	94	—	—	NS	NS	NS	NS	71	53

DFS, disease-free survival; NS, not significant.
[a]With implant.

was 76%. Contralateral neck failure occurred in 3% (8/228). All patients with T1 lesions or N0 neck status had 100% contralateral neck control. Patients with a 10% or greater risk for contralateral neck failure included those with T3 lesions, lesions involving the medial one third of the soft hemipalate, tumors invading the middle third of the ipsilateral base of tongue, and patients with N1 disease.

Jackson et al. report an 18-year experience of 178 patients receiving ipsilateral treatment using limited fields for tonsillar cancers (55). Patients presented primarily with T1 to T2 (117/178—66%) and N0 (101/178—57%) disease, but 29% (52/178) had T3 tumors and 30% had N1 disease, with 63% presenting with stage III to IV disease. Sixty Gy per 25 fxns (50–66 Gy) was delivered to gross tumor volume with a 1-cm margin and first echelon lymph nodes using 2 or 3 wedged fields. The length of follow-up was not stated. The rates of LRC and contralateral neck recurrence by stage were as follows after ipsilateral RT: I (n = 23), 91%, 0%; II (n = 43), 74%, 2%; III (n = 82), 51%, 4%; IV (n = 30), 53%, 0%. Patients with N0 (n = 101) or N1 (n = 54) disease had contralateral failure rates of 0% and 4%, respectively. None of the 23 patients with N2 to N3 disease had contralateral failure; however, the determinate risk for contralateral failure may have been obscured by the 52% incidence of ipsilateral failure. The authors were unable to relate the risk for contralateral neck failure according to the degree of tumor extension along the glossopalatine fold due to the retrospective nature of the study. The overall rate of local control was 75% (T1–2, 84% and T3–4, 58%) and OS was 56%.

External Beam Radiation Therapy and Brachytherapy. The goal of implantation when combined with EBRT is to improve local control of the tumor while preserving salivary function and lessening muscular fibrosis.

Pernot et al. (30) report on 277 patients, 101 of whom had advanced disease (T3). The 5-year local control, disease-specific survival, and OS rates by T stage (T1, T2, T3) were as follows: local control, 89%, 86%, and 69%, respectively; disease-specific survival, 78%, 62%, and 46%, respectively; and OS, 62%, 53%, and 43%, respectively. No local recurrence was detected after 3 years. In a later update of 361 cases, the 5-year outcomes of patients with tonsil, posterior pillar, or soft palate cancers (group A) were compared with those involving the anterior pillar and glossopharyngeal sulcus (group B) (42). Local control was better in group A patients compared with those in group B as follows: T1 94% vs. 75%; T2 93% vs. 67%; and T3 71% vs. 51%; respectively. Disease-specific survival and OS was also better in group A as follows: T1: 88%, 65% vs. 55%, 48%; T2 78%, 63% vs. 43%, 38%; and T3 53%, 49% vs. 27%, 27%, respectively. Multivariate analysis revealed that a treatment interval of less than 20 days between EBRT and brachytherapy and an overall treatment time of less than 55 days yielded better outcomes. Complications in this patient population appeared to be related to a total dose greater than 80 Gy, dose rate greater than 70 cGy per hour, treated surface area greater than 12 cm^2, treatment volume greater than 30 cc, and absence of leaded protection (56).

External Beam Radiation Therapy versus External Beam Radiation Therapy plus Brachytherapy. Mazeron et al. (57) report on 165 T1 to T2 SCCs of the faucial arch. Because of institutional policy changes, these authors were able to compare patients who received EBRT alone with those with EBRT and implantation. Those who received an implant were first treated by EBRT to the tumor site and neck areas (4,500 cGy in 25 fractions over 5 weeks) and then received a 3,000-cGy low-dose-rate iridium implant. For patients with clinically positive nodes, either additional 2,500- to 3,000-cGy electron beam irradiation to the nodes or neck dissection was added. Both local control (77% vs. 94% at 5 years; $p < 0.01$) and DFS (56% vs. 71%; $p = 0.03$) were improved for the implant group. No randomized study has shown whether this combined approach is superior to EBRT alone. Nonetheless, even advocates of the use of EBRT alone agree that the addition of an implant can improve local control when disease extends into the tongue (33).

High-Dose-Rate Brachytherapy. High-dose-rate brachytherapy (HDR-BT) as boost treatment with external beam radiation has been reported in two small series to offer excellent local control for early stage tonsil, base of tongue, and soft palate tumors with local control of 83% to 87% but lower with T3 to T4 tumors, 42% to 47% (31,58). Fractionated HDR-BT using b.i.d. treatments of 1.2 to 3.0 Gy fractions was combined with EBRT to total cumulative doses of 66 to 72 Gy. Successful surgical salvage was 50% to 60% among those who failed locally with no obvious increase in surgical complications such as fistula or flap necrosis. Rates of serious complications (primarily soft tissue ulcer and mandibular osteoradionecrosis) were reported in 10% to 16% of patients and were similar to those reported by low-dose-rate brachytherapy reports.

Advanced Disease

The management of patients with advanced tonsillar lesions is more complex and controversial. Some argue for RT alone, reserving surgery for salvage (59,60). Others advocate surgery and postoperative RT (61,62). Definitive chemoradiation also represents a treatment option to be considered in eligible patients, particularly those with locally advanced and deeply infiltrating primary tumors.

Surgery and Postoperative Radiation. Traditionally, definitive resection is recommended in patients with advanced disease. Hicks reported on the Roswell Park Cancer Institute experience of 76 patients with tonsillar cancer treated with single modality therapy—surgery (56 patients) and radiation (20 patients) (40). Among stage III to IV patients (n = 52), surgery resulted in better 5-year DFS (47% vs. 27%, $p < 0.05$) compared with radiation alone, although a greater percentage of patients were stage IV in the RT cohort (75% vs. 44%, $p < 0.05$) and split-course treatment was delivered to about half those receiving radiation.

Surgery frequently results in close or positive margins and multiple positive neck nodes. Two reports highlight the importance of postoperative adjuvant RT in advanced cases. The first, by Zelefsky et al. (62), reported the long-term treatment results for advanced oropharyngeal carcinomas treated with surgery and postoperative RT at the Memorial Sloan-Kettering Cancer Center. Twenty patients with SCC of the tonsillar fossa were treated with surgery plus RT. The 7-year actuarial local control rate for tonsillar fossa lesions was 83%. Local control was achieved in 94% of patients with T3 lesions and in 75% of patients with T4 lesions. Among patients with positive or close margins who received postoperative doses of 6,000 cGy or more, the long-term control rate was 93%. At 7 years, the OS for all patients was 52%, and the DFS was 64%. The actuarial incidence of neck failure was 18%. For all patients, the likelihood of having distant metastasis at 7 years was 30%.

The second study, by Foote et al., evaluated 72 patients who had surgery either with or without postoperative adjuvant RT for advanced disease (34). These investigators note that the main pattern of treatment failure was above the clavicles. This occurred in 39% of patients treated with surgery alone compared with 31% of patients undergoing surgery and postoperative adjuvant RT (despite the more advanced neck disease of the surgery and RT group) and was significantly related ($p = 0.002$)

to the overall clinical tumor, node, metastasis (TNM) stage. Five-year OS rates for patients with clinical stage III and IV disease who were treated with surgery and postoperative adjuvant RT were 100% and 78%, compared with 56% and 43%, respectively.

Perez et al. (63) analyzed 296 patients with histologically proved epidermoid carcinoma of the tonsillar fossa: 127 were treated with irradiation alone (5,500–7,000 cGy), 133 received preoperative RT (2,000–3,000 cGy) or were planned initially for preoperative irradiation but were treated with RT alone, and 36 received postoperative irradiation (5,000–6,000 cGy). The primary tumor recurrence rate in the T1 to T2 groups was approximately 20% for patients treated with irradiation and surgery and 30% for those treated with irradiation alone (difference not statistically significant), 30% in patients with stage T3 lesions in all treatment groups, and 33% in patients with T4 disease treated with surgery and postoperative irradiation, compared with 52% for patients treated with irradiation alone ($p = 0.03$). Dasmahapatra et al. (61) likewise report for stage III disease that the 5-year survival after RT and surgery was 31%, compared with 11% for radiation alone; and for stage IV disease, the respective 3- and 5-year survival rates for RT and surgery were 24% and 15%, compared with 6% and 0%, respectively, for RT alone.

In contrast, Spiro and Spiro (64) reviewed 162 patients with carcinoma of the tonsillar fossa treated between 1969 and 1983. Combined surgery and RT were used in 29% of patients with stage II disease, 40% of patients with stage III disease, and 67% of patients with stage IV disease. The 3-year determinate local control rates were 89%, 83%, 58%, and 49% for stages I through IV, respectively. The overall 2-year crude survival is 58%. A 60% 2-year survival for T3 lesions compares favorably with other series for treatment of T3 lesions. No survival benefit was seen in advanced stage disease, but this might reflect a selection bias against combined modality treatment compared with those receiving RT alone.

A number of retrospective reports have examined preoperative RT (4,500–5,000 cGy over 5 weeks) versus definitive RT or neck dissection (48,49,65). No advantage to preoperative RT was seen. Thus, preoperative RT for resectable lesions for which surgery is planned is no longer used as a strategy for the primary site. Patients with early stage primary lesions but advanced neck disease are often treated with definitive RT to the primary with preoperative radiation to the neck followed by planned neck dissection.

External Beam Radiation Therapy and Brachytherapy. The use of a combination of external megavoltage irradiation and interstitial ^{192}Ir implants for T3 lesions has been reported by Puthawala et al. (66). Local control of disease in patients with T3 and T4 lesions was 79%, compared with 95% for T1 and T2 lesions. Treatment-related complications such as soft tissue necrosis or osteoradionecrosis occurred in 6% of patients in the primary group and in 23% in the recurrent group. No significant functional or aesthetic impairments were reported.

A number of investigators have reported that patients with tumor that extends to the tongue have an inferior outcome compared with patients with no tongue extension. However, when an implant is used, this difference is negated. In the retrospective report of Leborgne et al. (67), local relapse was 64% and the 3-year DFS rate was 23% in 39 patients with tongue extension who were treated with EBRT alone, as compared with 33% and 43%, respectively, for 90 patients with no tongue extension. However, in those treated with EBRT plus brachytherapy, the local relapse rate was 40% and the 3-year survival rate 60%.

Recurrent Disease and Salvage

Surgical salvage of recurrent disease after RT has a greater chance of success for tumors of the anterior tonsillar pillar than for those in the tonsillar fossa. Gehanno et al. (38) report on salvage surgery for 50 patients with tumors of the tonsillar region. The actuarial survival rates at 3 and 5 years after salvage surgery were 38% and 24%, respectively. Compared with primary surgery, a higher postoperative mortality (8% vs. 1.4%) also was seen. Tumor extension that required resection into the tongue base was found to be a negative prognostic factor; survival declined dramatically in such cases.

Peiffert et al. (68) report on using brachytherapy salvage (6,000 cGy) in 73 patients who presented with velotonsillar SCC in a previously irradiated area. The 5-year actuarial local control rates for T1N0 and T2N0 disease were 80% and 67%, respectively. The regional relapse rate was 10% in both groups. Grade 2 complications occurred in 13% of patients, and these were not related to the volume treated or to the dose rate. No grade 3 or 4 complications occurred. The 5-year specific survival rate is 64%. Of note, 42% of the patients in this series died from another carcinoma.

Puthawala et al. (66), using implantation alone, obtained a 75% local control rate in patients with recurrent disease, with a 2-year absolute DFS rate of 42%. Treatment-related complications such as soft tissue necrosis or osteoradionecrosis occurred in 23% of these patients who had received previous RT.

Base of Tongue

SELECTION OF THERAPEUTIC MODALITY

Early Disease

Early stage base-of-tongue disease is successfully treated with either surgery or definitive RT. The results are equivalent for local control and survival. The morbidity of a surgical procedure must be weighed against the morbidity of RT. In the overwhelming majority of cases, RT is selected because it provides a better functional result and quality-of-life (QOL) outcome.

Advanced Disease

Major resection has traditionally been recommended in patients with advanced base-of-tongue disease. This often entails a total laryngectomy as well as a bone or tongue resection followed by postoperative RT. Although significant advances have been made for the laryngectomies, a significant rehabilitation process ensues for all patients, and some never regain the ability to communicate orally. In an effort to improve QOL, other approaches such as the combined use of chemotherapy and RT for organ preservation are now considered appropriate treatment options. Radiation therapy alone (with the addition of neck dissection for patients with palpable nodes at presentation) also is used for certain moderately advanced lesions. Most patients, even those with advanced disease, can be offered nonsurgical options that provide local control equivalent to that achieved surgically and better QOL. Primary surgery is not commonly employed in most centers, including our own.

Radiation Therapy. Primary RT is the preferred definitive treatment for most tumors of the base of tongue. It is the sole primary therapy for most T1, T2, and many T3 (exophytic) tumors. For infiltrative or endophytic T3 or T4 lesions, either surgery combined with postoperative RT or an organ-preservation approach using RT and chemotherapy should be used. The target volume of the parallel opposed fields should include the base of tongue and margin that will incorporate a portion of the oral tongue, vallecula, pharyngeal walls, and suprahyoid epiglottis, as well as the superior portion of the preepiglottic space. Owing to the high probability of lymph node metastasis, these portals also will include the bilateral regional and retropharyngeal lymph node groups. This is also true in the case of the patient with a clinically negative neck.

Our preferred strategy entails EBRT followed by an interstitial ^{192}Ir implant as a boost to the base of tongue. We believe that this offers the most consistent excellent local control and best function results compared with either EBRT alone or to primary surgery. External beam radiation is delivered to a dose of 5,400 cGy in 30 fractions (180 cGy/fraction). The spinal cord is shielded after 4,500 cGy. At that point, photons are used to treat the tongue and the anterior upper neck to 5,400 cGy, and electrons are used to treat the posterior neck to 5,400 cGy. We generally boost the area of palpable nodes with an additional 600 cGy with electrons, bringing the total to 6,000 cGy. Either 4-mV or 6-mV energies of cobalt-60 (^{60}Co) are used. An example of three treatment borders and fields is shown in Figure 17.13.

A brachytherapy boost to the tongue base (2,000–3,000 cGy) is performed approximately 3 weeks after EBRT (5,000–5,400 cGy). The implant consists of ^{192}Ir after-loading catheters placed with a looping technique (69,70), which involves the percutaneous introduction of curved trocars by means of a submental approach through the base of tongue. The catheter is threaded through the trocar and looped back through an adjacent trocar, creating a loop in the tongue. For patients with disease extension toward the pharyngoepiglottic fold, lateral loops are added to encompass this region (69). Both ends exit the skin of the neck. An array of loop is fashioned to encompass the target volume plus a 1.0- to 1.5-cm margin. The spacing between each end of the loop is 1 cm and between each plane is 1.0 to 1.5 cm (Fig. 17.14). As a safety precaution, a temporary tracheostomy is performed in patients immediately before the implantation. A temporary nasogastric feeding tube is placed at the completion of the procedure. The neck is managed by elective RT in the patient with N0 disease and by combined surgery and RT in patients with palpable disease. When a neck dissection is planned, the implantation and dissection are performed during the same anesthetic period. Patients are loaded several days after the procedure, after the majority of swelling has subsided and patients are able to suction themselves and perform tracheostomy care. Efforts are made to protect the palate by use of a customized shield that is under patient control.

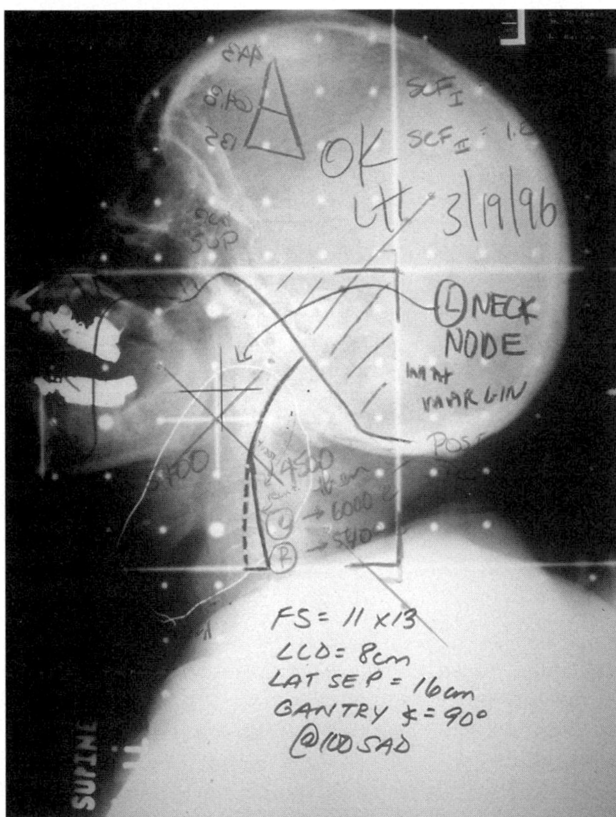

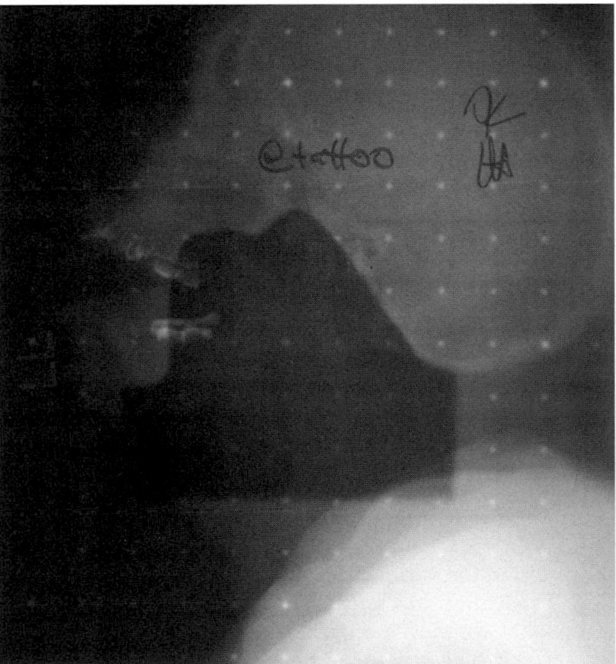

Figure 17.13 Simulation film of a patient with base-of-tongue cancer. All patients are immobilized using custom-designed 2.4-mm-thick Aquaplast masks and a bite block. The superior border includes the retropharyngeal and upper jugular lymph nodes (levels I and II). The inferior border is at the hyoid bone, which clinically lies just above the thyroid notch and can be palpated. The posterior border is placed at the posterior aspect of the spinal process. The anterior border is approximately 2 cm from the primary tumor. Even in the case of a small primary tumor, both necks are treated. The field should include levels I, II, III, and V. There should be generous coverage of the retropharyngeal nodes (region of C2). For patients who will receive a brachytherapy implant, no other reduction in the field is made. If a lymph node is bisected or lies at the junction of the lateral and anterior neck field, we do not change the fields, as this is a "hot match" and will not be underdosed. The larynx is not included in the treatment portal except in the case of a patient receiving chemoradiation for larynx preservation, where the larynx itself may be involved.

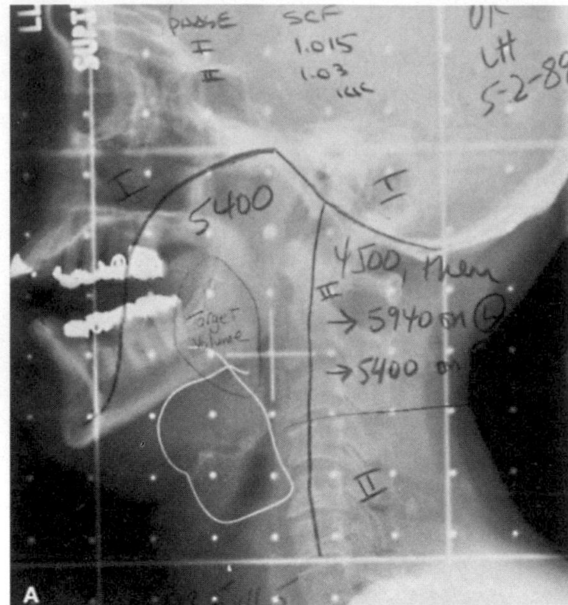

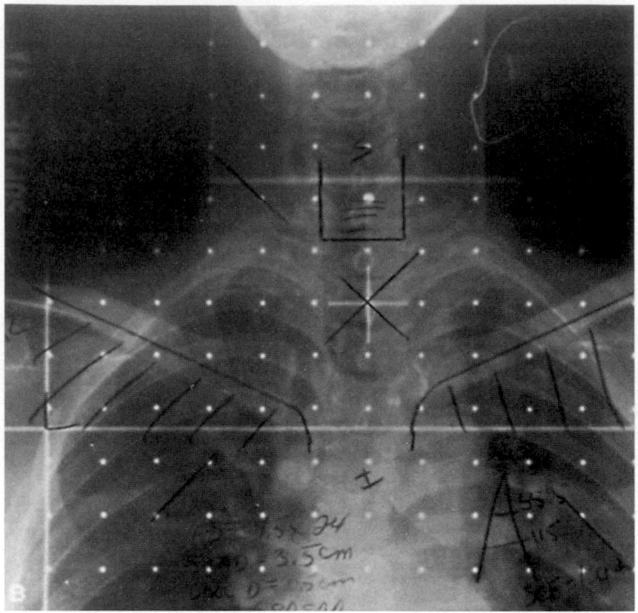

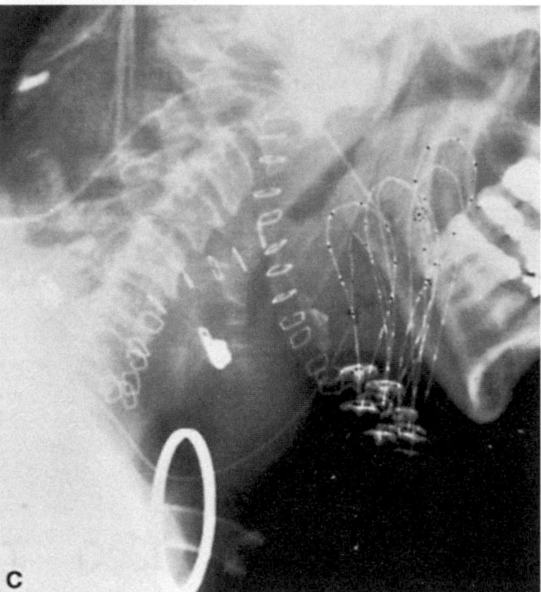

Figure 17.14 A patient with a T2N2 squamous cancer of the left side of the base of the tongue. The treatment plan consisted of initial external beam radiation therapy to the primary site and the entire neck bilaterally. This was followed by a left radical neck dissection and an implant, both done with the same anesthesia. **A:** The simulation film shows the primary site outlined and the neck node with wire around it. A bite block is in place. A total of 4,500 cGy was given to the primary site and both upper necks, after which a spinal cord block was placed. The primary and upper neck was then treated with 5,400 cGy. Fraction size was 180 cGy per day. After that, the bed of the lymph node in the left neck was boosted on the right and to 5,940 cGy on the left. **B:** The low neck was treated with a single anterior field to 5,000 cGy per 5 weeks. A midline block protects the spinal cord at the field junction. **C:** Approximately 3 weeks after the external radiation was completed, the patient was taken to the operating room and a left radical neck dissection and an iridium-192 implant were done. The figure shows the catheters looped through the base of the tongue by the submental approach. Also visible are the skin staples from the neck surgery. The implant delivered an additional 2,800 cGy. The neck specimen was histologically negative. The patient had no evidence of disease at 6 years. He had a soft tissue ulcer in the tongue that healed with conservative management.

In general, our patients are treated with a three-field technique that uses isocentrically opposed lateral fields matched to a lower anterior neck field. For these fields, our patients generally are treated in the supine position, with the neck maximally extended. To facilitate neck extension, we use a headrest and cloth straps that are placed around the patient's wrists and are attached by Velcro to a wooden board that is by the patient's feet. This aids in pulling the shoulders inferiorly to maximize exposure of the head and neck.

We generally use a bite block in the treatment of oropharyngeal cancers, both to facilitate immobilization and to reduce the amount of normal tissue situated in the treatment field. In the case of base-of-tongue tumors, the bite block keeps the primary tumor within the field, whereas for a soft-palate tumor it helps to reduce the amount of tongue that would be unnecessarily treated. After construction of the mask, a custom bite block is constructed by molding the 2.4-mm Aquaplast around a tongue depressor blade and inserting it into the patient's mouth while the patient is in the desired treatment position. The bite block must be placed as far posteriorly as possible to ensure that it functions properly. If dental fluoride trays were made to be worn during treatment, they should be in place during the simulation. The setup is performed under radiographic guidance.

Surgical Therapy. Selected patients with small base-of-tongue lesions and a negative neck can be managed with primary resection and elective neck dissection. A significant percentage will be found to harbor positive microscopic nodes, thereby necessitating postoperative RT. Therefore, for purposes of maximizing functional outcome and using only one modality, primary RT is the preferred strategy. Surgery generally is reserved for patients who cannot receive RT or for those with particularly endophytic, locally advanced lesions that are difficult to control with RT alone.

In contrast, patients with nodal metastases routinely will undergo a surgical procedure in the neck if the primary tumor is being treated by radiation alone. The neck dissection preferably is performed at the completion of RT. If the primary tumor is being managed surgically, surgery followed by RT is preferred. In our practice, patients generally undergo a combination of EBRT and a brachytherapy implant (discussed later in the chapter). In this setting, the implant and the neck dissection are carried out during the same anesthetic period, approximately 3 weeks after the EBRT is completed. Andersen et al. (71) have shown that preservation of the spinal accessory nerve in a modified neck dissection in patients with clinically evident nodal metastases was not associated with increased risk for treatment failure in the dissected neck.

Base-of-tongue tumors may be resected transorally or through a mandibulotomy and transhyoid pharyngotomy. The transoral approach is indicated only for small, well-circumscribed lesions that are located superficially. The mandibulotomy technique allows superior access and frequently is combined with a graft (72). When a patient has evidence of bone invasion or close encroachment of tumor to bone, frequently a mandibulectomy is performed. The use of a flap or plate with this procedure depends on the age of the patient, the amount of tissue resected, and the anticipated functional or cosmetic outcome.

Patients with advanced tumors usually will require a major or total glossectomy. In addition, some patients may require a total glossectomy owing to local extension of their tumor. The need for laryngeal resection (either subtotal supraglottic resection or total laryngectomy) depends on the extent of disease and the risk for aspiration. In most patients in whom a laryngectomy is deemed necessary for base-of-tongue cancer, the indication is for prevention of chronic aspiration, not for oncologic purposes.

After surgery, patients will spend a great deal of time learning to swallow and avoiding aspiration. If the dysfunction is significant, the patient may require placement of a percutaneous endoscopic gastrostomy (PEG), which can be performed at the time of surgery (73). A prosthesis may have to be constructed to aid speech and swallowing. Speech rehabilitation is started as soon as possible while the patient is still in the hospital.

Postoperative Adjuvant Radiation Therapy. After careful examination of the resected specimen by the pathologist, attention should be paid to the size of the primary tumor, histology, surgical margins, evidence of perineural extension, and lymph nodes. Patients with small tumors (stage T2), clear negative margins, no evidence of perineural extension, and histologically negative lymph nodes do not require postoperative RT. Radiation therapy generally is used when the surgical wound is seeded, when close or positive margins are present, and in the presence of extranodal tumor spread (extracapsular extension), multiple positive nodes, or extensive vascular or perineural invasion (74). Because larger primary tumors are poorly controlled locally with surgery alone, postoperative RT is suggested in this group of patients. The retropharyngeal lymph nodes are included in the treatment of the primary tumor (62). Owing to the high probability for bilateral neck disease, RT is used electively to control the area of unoperated contralateral neck.

The interval between surgery and RT was examined by Vikram (75), who reports that a delay of 7 weeks or more was associated with increased locoregional failure and decreased survival. The neck disease recurrence rate was 2% if the postoperative RT was started within 6 weeks compared with 22% at later than 6 weeks. A reanalysis by Schiff et al. (76) suggest that a prolonged delay in postoperative RT does not have a negative impact on LRC as long as appropriate tumoricidal doses of more than 6,000 cGy are employed. Seventy-three percent in the delayed treatment group received doses less than 56 Gy, accounting for their increased risk for locoregional failure. Bastit et al. report no difference in LRC or survival in a retrospective study of 420 oropharyngeal and hypopharyngeal carcinomas who were treated with similar doses (59 Gy/6 weeks) either within (n = 219) or after 30 days (n = 201) from surgery (77). However, Ang et al. report that among high-risk patients (positive margins, extracapsular nodal extension, or multiple lymph nodes), a duration of less than 11 weeks from the end of surgery to the end of radiation resulted in better LRC and survival compared with those treated over a longer period (78). We recommend starting radiation as soon as possible (76).

OUTCOME

Early Disease

Surgery Alone versus Radiotherapy. Surgical results for early base-of-tongue tumors reflect relatively high local control rates—from 75% to 85% (77,78). Primary EBRT, alone or followed by a planned neck dissection, also has a high local control rate of approximately 80% to 90% for T1 to T2 lesions and 70% to 85% for T3 tumors (Table 17.5). Survival for RT is similar to that after surgery, but with a lower risk for severe complications than surgery (79). Of interest, tumor growth patterns

TABLE 17.5 Base-of-Tongue Carcinoma: Local Control and Survival with External Beam Radiation Therapy Alone

				Percentage local control				Percentage local control				5-year overall survival (%)			
Study and institution	No. of patients	Median follow-up (yrs)	Percentage stage T3–4	T1	T2	T3	T4	N0	N1	N2	N3	T1	T2	T3	T4
Jaulerry, Institut Curie (17)	166	5	58	96	57	45	23	86	79	58	61	49	29	23	16
Spanos, M. D. Anderson Cancer Center (154)	174	10[a]	54	91	71	78	52	NS	NS	NS	NS	100	58	38	20
Foote, University of Florida (172)	84	8	54	89	88	77	36	NS	NS	NS	NS	100	86	56	36[b]
Houssett et al., Hospital Necker (70)	54	8	0	78	47	—	—	4	9	—	40	17	17	—	—

NS, not significant.
[a]Extrapolated.
[b]Average of stages IVa and Nb.

TABLE 17.6 Base-of-Tongue Carcinoma: Local Control and Survival with External Beam Radiation Therapy and Brachytherapy Implant Boosts

				Percentage local control				Percentage local control				5-year survival (%)	
Study and institution	No. of patients	Median follow-up (mos)	Percentage stage T3–4	T1	T2	T3	T4	N0	N1	N2	N3	DFS	Overall
Harrison et al., MSKCC (80–82)	36	22	31	100	100	80	100	100	100	100	100	NS	85
Housset et al., University of Paris (70)	29	96	All T1–T2	100	80	—	—	94	100	—	94	NS	52
Puthwala et al., Long Beach (84)	70	60	74	100	88	75	67	84[a]	81	78	50	67	35
Goffinet et al., Stanford University (69)	14	32	50	71[b]	—	—	—	NS	NS	NS	NS	76	NS

DFS, disease-free survival; MSKCC, Memorial Sloan-Kettering Cancer Center; NS, not significant.
[a]Without salvage.
[b]Not broken down.

were predictive of the response to RT (Table 17.5). The primary control rate at 2 years for patients with exophytic tumors was 84%, as opposed to 58% for patients with ulcerative or infiltrative tumors ($p = 0.04$).

Data from numerous authors have shown that the local control for early stage tumors is in the range of 80% to 100% when treated with combined EBRT and brachytherapy implantation (Table 17.6). Pernot et al. report a 5-year respective local control of 93% and 72% for T1 (n = 14) and T2 (n = 27) base-of-tongue tumors treated with a combined EBRT and brachytherapy approach. Corresponding 5-year disease-specific survivals were 76% and 62%, respectively (42).

Houssett et al. (70) have evaluated a comparison among surgery plus postoperative RT, EBRT plus implantation, and EBRT alone for a series of patients with T1 to T2 base-of-tongue lesions. This series is unique in that it attempts to address the issue of which management strategy is optimal. Demographic and oncologic characteristics of the patients were well balanced except that, among the EBRT-alone group, there were significantly more patients with exophytic (more favorable) lesions. Despite this imbalance, the patients who received EBRT alone had approximately twice the local failure rate as those in the other two groups (40% vs. 20%). This study suggests that EBRT plus implantation is certainly oncologically equivalent to surgery plus postoperative RT and that EBRT alone is inferior.

Advanced Disease

Advanced base-of-tongue tumors are poorly controlled with one treatment modality. The natural history of advanced tumors of the base of tongue can be gleaned from Dupont et al. (79a), who report on 34 patients with advanced SCC of the base of tongue (20 with T3 and 14 with T4 lesions) treated by surgical resection. These patients underwent an operative procedure as the sole definitive form of treatment. Twenty-eight patients (82%) presented with clinically positive cervical nodal metastases. The local control at 2 years was 27% (n = 9) and the OS was 20% (n = 7). Of note, 44% of patients (n = 15) required laryngectomy as part of the primary surgical treatment and 15% (n = 5) required laryngectomy owing to chronic aspiration, resulting in a total of 59% of patients who required total laryngectomy. Of the 19 patients who had a unilateral neck dissection, failure in the neck was experienced by 53% (70% contralateral, 30% ipsilateral).

Information regarding definitive EBRT for carcinomas of the base of tongue spans at least five decades. Data are typically from single institutions and do not take into account developments in diagnostic radiology and radiation oncology. For advanced tumors, definitive RT produced a local control rate of approximately 50%, as compared with 75% to 90% for surgery and postoperative RT (77).

The series reported by Harrison et al. (80) involves mainly patients with stage III and IV disease who were treated with EBRT plus implantation and neck dissection. Patients who would have required laryngectomy had they undergone primary surgery received neoadjuvant chemotherapy followed by EBRT and implantation as part of a larynx preservation study. Sixty-eight patients were managed by this approach between 1981 and 1995. The range of follow-up was 1 to 151 months, with a median follow-up of 36 months. In this series, the actuarial local control rate at both 5 and 10 years was 88%, regional control was 96% at both 5 and 10 years, distant metastasis-free survival rates were 91% and 76%, respectively, DFS rates were 80% and 67%, respectively, and OS rates were 86% and 52%, respectively. After EBRT, 78% of dissected necks were pathologically negative. With surgical salvage, the local control rate was 94% (80–83). Almost identical results have been reported by Goffinet et al. (69) and Puthawala et al. (84). A dose–response effect appears to occur, with higher local control being associated with doses of at least 7,500 cGy (85).

In the opinion of the authors, the treatment of choice for patients with SCC of the base of the tongue is definitive RT, including a brachytherapy implant. The overwhelming majority of patients present with stage III or IV disease. In general, treatment consists of 5,000 to 5,400 cGy with EBRT and a 2,000- to 3,000-cGy boost to the base of tongue through a ^{192}Ir implant using after-loading catheters. Necks are managed with elective radiation alone in the N0 group or with radiation plus neck dissection in the group with palpable neck node metastases. The data make clear that most patients' disease will be controlled with this strategy. We believe that this approach should be considered the treatment of choice whenever feasible. For those few advanced stage patients who cannot be managed with an organ-preserving approach, surgery followed by RT generally is used.

Surgery and Postoperative Adjuvant Radiotherapy. Recognizing that advanced carcinomas treated surgically will need postoperative RT, Zelefsky et al. (62) report the long-term treatment results for base-of-tongue and tonsillar fossa carcinomas treated at the Memorial Sloan-Kettering Cancer Center. Between 1973 and 1986, 51 patients were treated with surgery plus RT. Indications included advanced disease (stage T3 or T4, 66%); close or positive margins (64%), and multiple positive neck nodes (84%). The 7-year actuarial local control rates are impressive: 81% for carcinomas of the base of tongue. Local control was achieved in 94% and 75% of patients with T3 and T4 lesions, respectively. For patients with positive or close margins who received postoperative doses of 6,000 cGy or more, the long-term control rate was 93%. The authors also examined the influence of treatment interruptions. The actuarial control rate among patients who required a treatment break was 64%, in contrast to those who did not require interruption of their treatment, in whom the actuarial control rate was 93% ($p = 0.05$). At 7 years, the OS for all patients was 52%, and the DFS was 64%. For all patients, the likelihood of having distant metastasis at 7 years was 30%.

Two randomized trials have examined preoperative versus postoperative RT, and the results appear to be better with postoperative therapy. Although no trials address tumors of the oropharynx specifically, it is reasonable to infer from data on other head and neck sites. The Radiation Therapy Oncology Group (RTOG) trial 73-03 randomized patients with advanced operable tumors of the supraglottic larynx or hypopharynx to 5,000 cGy before surgery or 6,000 cGy after surgery, and patients with tumors of the oral cavity or oropharynx were assigned to preoperative, postoperative, or definitive RT (86). The LRC rate at 4 years was superior in the postoperative groups (58% vs. 48%, respectively; $p = 0.04$). The Gustav-Roussy trial (87) randomized patients with primary tumors of the hypopharynx to preoperative or postoperative RT. A statistically significant difference ($p < 0.01$) in survival rates, complications, and QOL existed in favor of postoperative RT. The postoperative RT group had a superior 5-year survival rate of 56% compared with 20% in the preoperative group (87). In the modern era, preoperative radiation no longer is used for lesions that are resectable and for which resection will be part of the planned management strategy.

In an attempt to reduce the probability of tumor repopulation during a long course of treatment, investigators have used the concomitant radiation boost schedule in a postoperative setting. The regimen is characterized by delivering the boost (10 fractions) as second daily treatments at a time when accelerated repopulation is theorized to occur (78,88). Ang et al. report a multi-institutional randomized trial prospectively randomizing 213 patients who underwent surgical treatment to adjuvant radiation based on previously defined pathologic risk factors (78). Low-risk patients (n = 31) were observed, intermediate-risk patients (n = 31) received 57.6 Gy in 6.5 weeks, and high-risk patients were randomized to 63 Gy in 7 weeks (n = 75) or in 5 weeks (n = 76) using the delayed concomitant boost schedule. Locoregional control was similar between low-risk patients who received no adjuvant radiation and intermediate-risk patients who received conventionally fractionated radiation to 57.6 Gy (5-year LRC 90% vs. 94%, respectively). High-risk patients treated with delayed concomitant boost showed a trend toward improved LRC and survival compared with those treated with conventional fractionation ($p = 0.11$, $p = 0.08$, respectively). This benefit was postulated to be due to the shortening of treatment duration between surgery and the end of radiation, thereby overcoming tumor repopulation. Among high-risk patients, shorter treatment duration significantly improved LRC (5-year LRC was follows: 76% for <11 weeks, 62% for 11–13 weeks, and 38% > 13 weeks). Moreover, among high-risk patients treated with conventionally fractionated radiation those treated below the median treatment duration had a higher 5-year LRC (71% vs. 50%, $p = 0.03$, estimated from graph) and survival (45% vs. 12%, $p = 0.01$, estimated from graph) compared with those whose treatment duration exceeded the median time. Acute toxicity was increased in the delayed concomitant boost arm compared with conventionally fractionated (confluent mucositis 62% vs. 36%) but late grade 3 to 4 chronic toxicity was no different (38% vs. 42%, respectively at 5 years).

Bernier et al. report preliminary results of the European Organization for the Research and Treatment of Cancer 22931 phase III multicenter randomized trial demonstrating the benefit of concurrent chemoradiation compared with conventional radiation as postoperative adjuvant treatment (90). Three-hundred thirty-four patients with resected advanced head and neck cancers were randomized to conventional fractionated radiation (2 Gy up to 66 Gy) or to cisplatinum (100 mg/m^2/cycle on weeks 1, 4, and 7) concurrent with the same radiation regimen. At a median follow-up of 34 months, patients receiving postoperative chemoradiation had better 3-year DFS (59% vs. 41%, $p = 0.0096$), 3-year OS (65% vs. 49%, $p = 0.0057$), and improved local control ($p = 0.0014$). The data regarding distant metastases or secondary primary tumors were not reported. Patients receiving concurrent chemoradiation had increased grade 3 or 4 toxicities, including mucositis (44% vs. 21%, $p = 0.0004$), granulocytopenia in 11%, and thrombocytopenia in 2%. No obvious differences in chronic toxicities were reported.

Recurrent Disease and Salvage

The approach to the patient with recurrent base-of-tongue disease depends on the initial therapy the patient received. The use of surgery alone as the salvage procedure in cases of base-of-tongue cancer that were treated previously with RT was reported by Pradhan et al. (91). In approximately one third of the patients local control was achieved for at least 1 year. Thirty-five patients required a total glossectomy, of whom 26 did not undergo removal of the larynx. Only 13 patients were alive more than 3 years after salvage.

Others have used ^{192}Ir after-loading techniques in patients who received full-tolerance radiation (with or without previous surgery). Langlois et al. (92) report on 123 patients treated for recurrence or new cancer of the tongue or oropharynx arising in previously irradiated tissues. The actuarial local control rate was 67% at 2 years and 59% at 5 years. Local control of the tumor was achieved in most of these patients, though the actuarial survival was only 48% at 2 years and 24% at 5 years. The complication rate was slightly higher; 28 patients developed mucosal necrosis.

Mazeron et al. (93) had similar results: actuarial local control was 72% at 2 years and 69% at 5 years. Although local control of the tumor was achieved in the majority of these patients, only 14% remained alive at 5 years. The best results were achieved in patients with lesions of the faucial arch and posterior pharyngeal wall; local control was achieved in 100% of these patients. Patients with lesions of the base of tongue and of the glossotonsillar sulcus had suboptimal results; local control was achieved in only 61%.

Owing to the high complication rates, Housset et al. (94) compared two techniques of iridium implantation for salvage. Patients received either single-course implants, delivering 6,000 cGy, or split-course implants with a source shift, the goal being to decrease treatment complications. The first and second course of the split-course implants delivered 3,500 and 3,000 cGy, respectively, at a 1-month interval. The active lines of the second implant were placed parallel to and between the lines of the first implant. This shift in the source position resulted in a more uniform dose within the treated volume, with a 60% reduction in the high-dose sleeves. The overall local failure rate was 45.5% (25 of 55). The difference between the local failure rate after single-course implants

(52%) and after split-course implants (37.5%) was not statistically significant. The only complication noted in the 40 patients in whom immediate local control was achieved after either implantation technique was mucosal necrosis. Of note, the split-course implants were associated with a 2.5-fold decrease in the incidence of necrosis: 43% (9 of 21) in the single-course group and 16% (3 of 19) in the split-course group ($p = 0.05$).

Pharyngeal Wall

SELECTION OF THERAPEUTIC MODALITY

Early Disease

Early lesions of the pharyngeal wall can be treated by RT or surgery. Radiation therapy generally is preferred because the results are good to excellent and confer less functional impairment than is likely after surgery. Treatment portals are the primary site and bilateral neck, including the retropharyngeal nodes. For those treated surgically, a transhyoid approach or anterior pharyngotomy generally is used for the primary site. A bilateral modified neck dissection often is performed. If nodes are positive, postoperative RT is added.

Advanced Disease

Definitive radiation with the addition of a neck dissection for node-positive patients rarely is used. Most locally advanced lesions are best approached with combined-modality treatment consisting of surgery followed by RT or an organ-preservation strategy. A number of different surgical approaches can be used, among them a circumferential pharyngectomy, pharyngoesophagectomy, pharyngolaryngectomy, or pharyngolaryngoesophagectomy (95). When primary repair is not possible, a number of reconstructive options are available: pectoralis major myocutaneous flap, free revascularized radial forearm flap, transposed stomach (96), or free revascularized jejunum (97). Owing to the high incidence of retropharyngeal and cervical lymph node involvement, postoperative RT is recommended.

Radiation Therapy. For pharyngeal wall tumors, radiation treatment planning is more complicated owing to the technical problem of the close proximity of the spinal cord to the primary lesion. With doses in excess of 4,500 cGy, when the spinal cord is blocked, the posterior edge of the treatment field is extremely close to the posterior aspect of the tumor. A number of strategies have been suggested to overcome this problem (98). First, the sharpest beam edge must be used to avoid underdosing the posterior aspect of the tumor. This is accomplished by the use of a 6-mV or 4-mV accelerator beam and by avoiding the use of ^{60}Co. Second, custom Cerrobend blocks should be used to define the posterior border. Third, the posterior border should be placed at the most anterior aspect of the spinal cord. Finally, frequent portal films throughout treatment are necessary to ensure proper setup and spinal cord protection.

Another method of addressing pharyngeal wall tumors that wrap around the spine has been described by Grimard et al. (99), who use an asymmetric arc technique consisting of two posterior arcs with closure of one jaw beyond the central axis. Each arc delivers the total dose to each ipsilateral side, whereas the median region of the U-shaped volume is treated by the summation of both arcs.

RESULTS AND OUTCOME

Surgery Alone

The use of surgical resection alone for pharyngeal wall tumors has been reported by Guillamondegui et al. (100). Twenty-eight percent of patients had recurrent tumors above the clavicles. Salvage in the form of RT or surgery was successful in less than one third of those patients. Patients with positive retropharyngeal nodes had an increased rate of distant metastases (22%) compared with those who did not have positive nodes (15%).

Definitive Radiation Therapy Alone

Fein et al. (98), from the University of Florida, retrospectively compared the effect of the use of once-daily to twice-daily fractionation on local control in 99 patients with carcinomas of the hypopharyngeal or oropharyngeal wall or both. The local control rates for patients treated with once-daily versus twice-daily fractionation were, for T1 lesions, 100% vs. 100%; for T2 lesions, 67% vs. 92%; for T3 lesions, 43% vs. 80%; and for T4 lesions, 17% vs. 50%. These investigators also examined their former technique (posterior border placed at middle of the vertebral body when the portals were reduced off the spinal cord) compared with their current, modified technique (posterior border placed at posterior edge of the vertebral body). The local control rates were 100% each for T1 lesions; 57% vs. 100% for T2 lesions; 46% vs. 73% for T3 lesions; and 29% vs. 75% for T4 lesions (83).

Meoz-Mendez et al. (101) report on 164 patients treated at the M. D. Anderson Cancer Center for carcinomas of the hypopharynx and pharyngeal walls. Local control rates for T1 through T4 lesions were 71%, 73%, 61%, and 37%, respectively. For patients with T3 and T4 tumors, the combination of surgery and RT was superior to RT alone (75% local control versus 51%).

Surgery and Radiation Therapy

Marks et al. (102) retrospectively compared the results of treatment in 51 patients after low-dose (2,500 to 3,000 cGy) preoperative RT and surgery to the results in those who had definitive RT. No difference was found in local control or survival (17%); however, the surgery plus RT group experienced a significant number of complications (fistula, 31%; carotid rupture, 14%; operative mortality, 14%). The same authors updated their experience with a group consisting of 89 patients (86,103). These patients were treated with high doses of radiation (5,000–7,200 cGy) either for preoperative intent or for definitive therapy. Treatment outcome, survival, and tumor and nodal control were better for the RT-plus-surgery group than for the RT-alone group. The patterns of relapse differed for the two groups, with low-dose preoperative irradiation and surgery offering greater control of the primary tumor and high-dose irradiation achieving better control of nodal disease. To draw any conclusions from this article is difficult, as the reported study spanned almost 20 years, during which time many technologic advances were made in radiation oncology, anesthesia, and surgery.

Spiro et al. (95) reviewed a 12-year experience with 295 patients treated for SCC of the pharynx at the Memorial Sloan-Kettering Cancer Center. Of these patients, 78 patients had lesions in the posterior wall. Surgery was the definitive therapy for the primary tumor in 73%. A second group of 21 patients with more extensive tumors required a laryngectomy and complex reconstruction, often with postoperative RT, and five had lesions that were implanted after access was provided by a mandibulotomy. The cumulative 5-year survival for the entire group was 32% and ranged from 44% in those with favorable lesions to 15% in those with extensive tumors. The overall complication rate was 50%. For the group that received an implant, local control was excellent.

The use of a brachytherapy implant [either ^{192}Ir or iodine-125 (125I)] and EBRT was reported by Son and Kacinski (104) for a small group of patients. The local control rate was 86% and actuarial survival was 82% at 5 years. These results are impressive but must be confirmed. In general, results in patients with extensive lesions still leave much to be desired, despite radical surgery and aggressive RT, and creative brachytherapy techniques warrant further investigation.

SPECIAL ISSUES AND FUTURE DIRECTIONS

Organ Preservation in Advanced Oropharyngeal Cancer: Role of Chemotherapy and Altered Fractionated Radiation

Patients with advanced tumors of the oropharynx who require extensive surgery with or without total laryngectomy typically have experienced suboptimal results. Owing to the size and location of these tumors, primary surgery can have a significant impact on the functional, psychological, and cosmetic consequences for these patients. The previous standard for organ preservation was established by the Veterans Affairs (VA) Laryngeal Cancer Study Trial (105,106) in which induction chemotherapy plus conventionally fractionated EBRT (which allowed preservation of the larynx in 66%) produced survival rates equivalent to those undergoing total laryngectomy with postoperative EBRT. However, recent studies and meta-analyses have demonstrated that a concurrent chemoradiation appears superior to the VA regimen or to EBRT alone and have brought into question the benefit of induction chemotherapy (22–24,107–112). Forastiere et al. report the preliminary results of RTOG 91-11, demonstrating that in patients with larynx cancer requiring total laryngectomy and randomized to (a) conventional fractionated EBRT (70 Gy/7 weeks) alone, (b) the VA regimen, or (c) concurrent cisplatin (100 mg/m^2 weeks 1, 4, and 7) with conventional fractionated EBRT (70 Gy/7 weeks), those in arm C had superior laryngectomy-free survival compared with the other arms (108). A number of trials restricted to oropharynx cancers have demonstrated similar findings.

A French randomized multicenter study of strictly oropharyngeal cancers tested the benefit of adding induction chemotherapy to definitive locoregional treatment (107). Three hundred eighteen patients were randomized to three cycles of cisplatinum/5-fluorouracil (5-FU) (100 mg/m^2 and 1,000 mg/m^2/day × 5 days, respectively on weeks 1, 4, and 7 followed by locoregional treatment (n = 157) within 2 to 3 weeks versus locoregional treatment alone (n = 161). About 75% were stage III or IV (49% stage III) and the remainder stage II. Patients underwent either definitive RT (70 Gy/7 weeks, n = 174) or radical resection followed by postoperative radiation (50–65 Gy/5–6.5 weeks, n = 142). The target enrollment was 760 patients, but the study was closed due to poor accrual near the end of the 6-year period. Among those receiving chemotherapy, the response rate was 56% (20% complete) with grade 3 or 4 toxicity in 16%, primarily of hematologic, gastrointestinal, and mucositis origin. At a median follow-up of 5 years, OS was higher (estimated 5-year actuarial OS 52% vs. 42%, p = 0.03, respectively) but no statistically significant difference was found in locoregional failure (25% vs. 30%), distant metastasis rate (8% vs. 12%), or DFS in those receiving chemotherapy. The survival benefit appeared independent of the type of locoregional treatment received. However, the authors concluded that no definitive statement could be made about the role of neoadjuvant chemotherapy in oropharyngeal cancer as the data were not "convincing enough" and the target accrual incomplete.

Calais et al. report a landmark French intergroup (GORTEC) phase III randomized trial designed to test whether the addition of concurrent chemotherapy to conventionally fractionated RT improves outcome compared with conventionally fractionated RT alone for patients with advanced stage oropharynx carcinoma (22–24). Two hundred and twenty-six patients with stage III (32%) and IV (68%) tumors were randomized to 70 Gy per 7 weeks or 70 Gy with 3 cycles of concurrent carboplatin (70 mg/m^2/day × 4) and 5-FU (600 mg/m^2/day × 4) (weeks 1, 4, and 7). The arms were balanced with regard to stage, sex, tumor site, performance status age, and histology. Acute toxicities were increased in the concurrent arm including grade 3 or 4 mucositis (71% vs. 39%, p = 0.005), dermatitis (67% vs. 59%, p = 0.02), and need for feeding tube (36% vs. 15%, p = 0.02) compared with the control arm. However, the incidence of treatment-related mortality [1% (1/109) vs. 0%], overall treatment duration (52 vs. 50 days, respectively), and treatment interruption ≥3 days (19% vs. 16%, respectively) were similar. Severe cervical fibrosis was increased in the combined modality treatment group (12% vs. 3%, p = 0.08, respectively) but the overall rate of severe chronic toxicity was 14% versus 9%, respectively. At a median follow-up of 35 months, patients in the combined modality arm had a higher 3-year LRC (66% vs. 42%, p = 0.03), DFS (42% vs. 20%, p = 0.04), and OS (51% vs. 31%, p = 0.02) but no difference in rate of distant metastases (11% vs. 11%, respectively). The approximately 20% improvement in survival and LRC argues for the addition of concurrent chemotherapy in patients with advanced oropharynx cancer treated with definitive radiation. However, the optimal chemoradiotherapy regimen with regard to fractionation scheme and chemotherapy agents remains to be defined.

Altered Fractionated Radiation

Withers et al. analyzed outcomes from nine centers using widely different dose-fractionation radiation regimens treating a total of 676 tonsil carcinomas (range of total dose 50–72 Gy, dose per fraction 1.8–3.3 Gy, and overall treatment time 3–8 weeks) (88). Total dose and treatment duration were significant treatment parameters which impacted on local control, but dose per fraction was not important. The data were most consistent with the model of delayed accelerated tumor repopulation occurring 30 days after the beginning of treatment with a compensatory dose of 0.73 Gy per day of treatment prolongation. Thus, shortening treatment duration to minimize accelerated repopulation or increasing total dose without adding to late complications have become important areas of investigation. Attempts to improve LRC with altered fractionation have seemed promising in single-institution studies (39,46,113–117).

Based on such evidence, the RTOG conducted a landmark trial (RTOG-90-03) comparing the leading U.S. altered fractionated regimens for multiple head and neck cancer sites, including oropharynx cancers (60%) (118). One-thousand and seventy-three patients with primarily advanced SCCs of the head and neck were randomized to four arms:

1. Conventional fractionation (CF) 2 Gy daily, 5 days a week to 70 Gy over 7 weeks
2. Split-course accelerated fractionation (S-AF) with 1.6 Gy b.i.d. to 67.2 Gy over 6 weeks with an intentional 2-week break after 38.4 Gy and an interfraction interval of 6 hours
3. Delayed concomitant boost (DCB) with daily morning 1.8 Gy treatments and a 1.5 Gy afternoon concomitant boost for the last 12 days of treatment with a 6-hour interfraction interval and a total dose of 72 Gy over 6 weeks
4. Pure hyperfractionation (HF) with 1.2 Gy twice daily with an interfraction interval of 6 hours to a dose of 81.6 Gy per 7 weeks.

Eligible sites included oropharynx, oral cavity, hypopharynx, and supraglottic larynx with stage III or IV disease or stage II if hypopharynx or base of tongue was the tumor origin. In a preliminary analysis with a median follow-up of 23 months for all analyzable patients, the DCB and HF arms had significantly better 2-year LRC compared with CF (54.5% vs. 54.4% vs. 46%, respectively, $p = 0.05$ DCB vs. CF and $p = 0.045$ HF vs. CF) and trend toward improved DFS (39.3% vs. 37.6% vs. 31.7%, respectively, $p = 0.054$ DCB vs. CF and $p = 0.067$ DCB vs. CF) were seen in the both the DCB radiation arm and HF arms compared with CF. Overall survival was no different. Acute grade 3 to 4 toxicity was increased compared with CF (59% vs. 55% vs. 35%, respectively). Chronic grade 3 to 4 toxicity was increased at 3 months for the delayed concomitant boost arm (37% vs. 27%) but was no different by 6 to 24 months compared with the control arm. There was no difference in chronic grade 3 to 4 toxicity in the HF arm (28% vs. 27%) compared with CF.

Horiot et al. report results of the EORTC 22791 randomized trial comparing an HF regimen of 1.15 cGy b.i.d. (4–6 hours between fractions) to 80.5 Gy over 7 weeks versus CF of 1.8 to 2.0 Gy to 70 Gy over 7 to 8 weeks in the treatment of 356 patients with T2–T3N0–1 oropharyngeal cancers excluding the base of tongue (119). With a mean follow-up of about 4 years, HF improved 5-year actuarial LRC compared with CF (59% vs. 40%, respectively $p = 0.02$) with a trend toward improved survival (38% versus 29%, respectively, $p = 0.08$). T3 tumors benefited from HF but T2 lesions did not. More severe acute mucositis occurred in the HF, but did not increase the incidence of treatment interruption. The incidence of grade 2 or 3 late effects was no different between the two arms.

Combining Chemotherapy with Altered Fractionated Radiation

As both the addition of concurrent chemotherapy and altered fractionated radiation have been have been shown independently to improve outcome for head and neck cancer patients, the present challenge is to find the optimal chemoradiation regimen(s) that offer high rates of LRC, are not unduly morbid, offer maximal preservation of organ function, and may be integrated with new biologic agents (22–24,108,118). Multiple phase II and randomized studies have reported possible regimens. The benefit of induction chemotherapy remains to be defined.

PHASE II STUDIES

Our group published the results of a phase II trial that treated 82 patients with unresectable head and neck cancer using the delayed concomitant boost technique radiation (70 Gy/6 weeks, b.i.d. RT last 2 weeks) with concurrent cisplatin (100 mg/m^2) given every 3 weeks for 2 cycles (120).

Adjuvant chemotherapy was given in 68%. Although 40% had initial skull base invasion, the response rate was 94% with 60% complete responses. Oropharynx cancers comprised 23% of all tumors treated. For all patients at a minimal follow-up of 3 years, the 3-year local control, OS, and distant-metastasis-free survival was 58%, 36%, and 58%, respectively. Seventy percent of patients with base of skull invasion were locally controlled. The treatment was reasonably well tolerated. The 3-year local control for oropharynx cancers was 64%. All patients experienced grade 3 acute mucositis usually during the concomitant boost phase. Twenty-four percent required a treatment break, the majority requiring less than one week. Two deaths due to sepsis occurred during treatment. Severe chronic toxicity occurred in three patients with one osteoradionecrosis, one frontal lobe necrosis, and one case of lung toxicity secondary to adjuvant chemotherapy. Given the especially poor prognosis of this group, the local control was good and survival better than expected with such an aggressive chemoradiation program.

A modified version of delayed concomitant boost radiation was reported by Bieri et al. in which a planned total dose of 69.6 Gy was shortened to total of 5.5 weeks and one third of the patients received primarily concurrent cisplatin-based chemotherapy (121). Among the 55 patients with oropharynx carcinoma (76% stage III/IV), LRC at 3 years was 69.5% at a median follow-up of 32 months. Eighty-two percent experienced grade 3 or 4 mucositis. Patients receiving chemotherapy had a greater rate of grade 3 dysphagia (68% vs. 25%, $p = 0.003$), hospitalization (37% vs. 14%, $p = 0.08$), and need for nasogastric tube (68% vs. 22%, $p = 0.001$). Late RTOG grade 3/4 complications occurred in 12% of patients and consisted of laryngeal edema, mucosal necrosis, and mandibular osteoradionecrosis.

Induction chemotherapy followed by RT was used in the treatment of patients with T4 (AJCC, 2nd edition) oropharyngeal carcinomas at the University of Florida (122). Chemotherapy consisted of cisplatinum (100 mg/m^2) and 5-FU (1,000 mg/m^2/day × 5 days) every 3 to 4 weeks for several cycles (63% received 3 cycles) followed by definitive RT (83% received hyperfractionated RT to 74.4– 81.75 Gy). Twenty-six patients were able complete the chemotherapy and high-dose radiation. The major response rate after induction chemotherapy was 97% (35% complete response [CR] and 62% partial response [PR]). These rates were compared with a similar group of 34 patients with T4 oropharyngeal tumors treated with a comparable radiation regimen without chemotherapy during the same time period and also to 83 patients with T4 tumors treated with RT alone over a three-decade time span. All patients were followed for a minimum of 1 year and none were lost to follow-up until death from 1964 to 1996. On multivariate analysis, no difference in local failure (37% vs. 62% vs. 52%, respectively) or regional or distant failure (13% vs. 27% vs. 24%, respectively) was detected in those receiving induction chemotherapy compared with patients treated with RT alone. However, disease-specific survival and OS were improved in those who received induction chemotherapy (58% vs. 27% vs. 37% and 42% vs. 17% vs. 23%, respectively). Due to the nonrandomized nature of the study and the lack of statistically significant improvement in parameters of tumor control, the authors cautioned against any conclusions regarding the benefit of induction chemotherapy.

A phase II study using induction chemotherapy followed by concurrent chemoradiation was reported by Vokes et al. (123). Sixty-one patients with advanced oropharyngeal carcinomas (97% IV, 82% T3–4, and 85% N2–3) were treated with three cycles of cisplatinum (100 mg/m^2), 5-FU (640 mg/m^2/days × 5 days), leucovorin (300–600 mg/m^2/day × 6 days), and interferon-α (2 million U/m^2/day × 6 day) for three cycles then proceeded to concurrent chemoradiotherapy if at least a near complete response was obtained. This consisted of split courses of weekly concurrent hydroxyurea (2,000 mg/day × 5 days) and 5-FU (800 mg/m^2 × 5 days) with 900 to 1,000 cGy per 5 days given every other week to a total dose of 68 to 75 Gy for gross disease. Neck dissections (n = 35) were performed for N2 to N3 disease. After induction chemotherapy, 65% obtained a complete response and 34% a partial response. Sixteen patients underwent resection of the primary tumor (11 organ-sparing and 13 after induction chemotherapy). At a median follow-up of 39 months (68 months among survivors), LRC was 70%, distant-metastasis-free survival 89%, DFS 64%, and OS 51%. Locoregional control was 100% in patients with T1 to T2 (n = 11) or N0 (n = 1), 81% for T3 (n = 16), 53% for T4 (n = 34), and 67% to 69% N1 to N3 (n = 60). No difference was noted in local control among those undergoing surgery of the primary site versus those treated with chemoradiation alone (5-year LRC 66% vs. 72%). Regional control was obtained in 98%. An update with 93 patients showed similar results (124). Acute toxicity was substantial with severe or life-threatening mucositis in 57% and leukopenia in 65% during the induction phase, whereas 81% had grade 3 or 4 mucositis during the concurrent chemoradiation. The authors concluded that the treatment sequence of induction chemotherapy followed by concurrent chemoradiation and optional organ-preservation surgery is promising but that less toxic regimens need to be identified (124).

Bensadoun et al. report on 54 patients with unresectable oropharynx and hypopharynx carcinoma treated with concomitant hyperfractionated radiation (75.6–80.4 Gy) and three cycles of 5-FU/cisplatin (CDDP) (750 mg/m^2/day or 750 mg/day × 5 days and 100 mg/m^2, respectively on weeks 1, 4, and 7) (125). The regimen was acutely toxic (4% mortality from treatment-related septicemia, 86% grade 3/4 mucositis by cycle 2 of chemotherapy, grade 3 or 4 neutropenia in 43% by cycle 2) but no patient required a treatment break greater than 4 days due to mucositis. No grade ≥3-late toxicities were reported; grade 2 xerostomia was reported in 70% and grade 2 cervical fibrosis in 45%. At a median follow-up of 16 months, LRC was 67% at 6 months and disease-specific survival 72% at 2 years. Other chemoradiation regimens for oropharyngeal carcinomas with encouraging LRC rates but short-term follow-up or small patient numbers include those using concurrent weekly paclitaxel (30–50 mg/m^2/week) (126) and the use of induction chemotherapy with preoperative concurrent chemoradiation followed by organ-preserving surgery (127).

RANDOMIZED TRIALS

Concurrent chemotherapy with hyperfractionated radiation was explored by Brizel et al. in a phase III randomized trial (128). One hundred and sixteen patients with advanced head and neck cancer were randomized to hyperfractionated radiation alone treated with 1.25 Gy b.i.d. (6-hour interfraction interval) 5 days per week to 75 Gy over a 6-week period versus a concurrent chemoradiation arm consisting of 5-FU/CDDP given on weeks 1 and 6 of split-course hyperfractionated radiation. In contrast to the control arm, an intentional 1-week treatment break was required in the experimental arm and the total dose was slightly lower (70 Gy). Both groups received two adjuvant courses of 5-FU/CDDP after completion of radiation. At a median follow-up of 41 months, the chemoradiation showed improved LRC (70% vs. 44%, p = 0.01) and a trend toward improved 3-year OS (55% vs. 34%, p = 0.07) and relapse-free survival (61% vs. 41%, p = 0.08). However, patients in the chemoradiation arm developed more acute toxicity including the requirement for more feeding tubes (44% vs. 29%) and worse hematologic suppression. Three fourths of patients in both arms experienced confluent mucositis. Chronic toxicity was no different, with about a 10% incidence of necrosis of the skin or bone in both arms. The trial has been criticized, not only for the added toxicity, but also because of the imbalance in the proportion of advanced neck disease (44% vs. 63%) treated in the concurrent chemoradiation which may have accounted for the difference in LRC.

Jeremic et al. report a phase III randomized study testing whether daily low-dose cisplatin improved outcome for patients undergoing hyperfractionation radiation compared with those treated with the same hyperfractionated radiation alone in locally advanced head and neck SCCs (37% were oropharynx) (129). One hundred and thirty patients with stage III or IV disease were randomized to 1.1 Gy b.i.d. to 77 Gy per 7 weeks alone or with cisplatin (6 mg/m^2/day). At a median follow-up of 79 months, the investigational arm showed improved LRC (50% vs. 36% at 5 years, p = 0.041), progression-free survival (46% vs. 25% at 5 years, p = 0.0068 and OS (46% vs. 25% at 5 years, p = 0.0075), and fewer distant metastases (14% vs. 43% at 5 years, p = 0.0013). The latter result was unexpected and raised the possibility that concurrent daily cisplatin may impact on incidence of distant metastases by a direct systemic effect or secondarily through improved LRC. Daily concurrent chemotherapy was well tolerated with no increase in acute grade 3 mucositis and esophagitis. There were no increases in late skin or severe effects to bone or salivary gland.

A German multicenter randomized trial tested whether the combination of hyperfractionated accelerated radiation (69.6 Gy/5 5.5 weeks) with carboplatin (70 mg/m^2) and 5-FU (600 mg/m^2/day × 5 days) on weeks 1 and 5 of RT improved outcome compared with the same radiation regimen alone (130). Two hundred and forty patients with stage III (4%) to IV (96%) oropharyngeal (n = 178) and hypopharynx (n = 62) tumors were entered in a 2 × 2 study randomizing patients to receive radiation with or without chemotherapy and then again to receive granulocyte colony-stimulating factor (G-CSF) or not. G-CSF was administered to determine its effect on mucositis. Treatment was tolerable in both study arms with higher mucosal and hematologic toxicity in the chemotherapy/RT arm but no difference in duration of treatment (41 vs. 42 days) or total radiation dose delivered (68.5 Gy vs. 69.9 Gy) in the chemotherapy/RT vs. RT arms, respectively. Response rates at 6 weeks after treatment were similar 92% (CR = 40%) after chemotherapy/RT and 88% (CR = 34%) after RT alone. At a median follow-up of 22 months, the 1- and 2-year respective rates of LRC were 69% and 51% after chemotherapy/RT compared with 58% and 45% after RT (p = 0.14). On subset analysis, patients with oropharyngeal carcinomas had l-year improved survival with local control after chemoradiation (60% vs. 40%, p = 0.01) and trend toward improved LRC (70% vs. 58%, l-year and 51% vs. 42% 2-year, p = 0.07) compared with RT alone. Patients receiving chemotherapy/RT had increased grade 3 and 4 toxicities including mucositis (68% vs. 52%, p = 0.01), vomiting (8% vs. 2%, p = 0.02), and hematologic toxicity (neutropenia, 18% vs. 0%) with similar rates of dermatitis (30% vs. 28). Patients receiving chemotherapy/RT had more swallowing problems and continuous need for feeding tube (51% vs. 25%, p = 0.02). Interestingly, patients receiving G-CSF had reduced LRC (55 vs. 38%, p = 0.0072) and decreased mucositis (p = 0.06). This raises the issue of possible tumor radioprotection and certainly deserves further evaluation.

Prognostic Factors

Commonly reported prognostic factors for LRC, disease-free survival, or OS include T stage, N status, and gender and performance status (35,131). Multiple studies have investigated various radiographic parameters and molecular markers as potential predictive factors in patients treated definitely for oropharynx cancers. In contrast to cancers involving the larynx (132), hypopharynx (133), and nasopharynx (134), pretreatment chemotherapy-determined primary tumor volume is not predictive for local control after definitive RT alone using conventional (135) or altered fractionated radiation (136). Encouraging results from single institution studies have reported that a high intratumoral microvessel density predicts for poorer local control and worse OS after definitive radiation of oropharynx carcinoma (137) and that a high Ki-67 labeling index is associated with local relapse (138) and shorter mean time to relapse (139) after definitive resection and postoperative radiation. Overexpression of proliferating cell nuclear antigen (PCNA; an estimate of growth fraction), (139,140), vascular endothelial growth factor (VEGF), or thrombospondin-1 (both markers of angiogenesis) have shown no predictive value in patients with oropharynx cancer treated with either definitive RT or combined surgery and radiation (137,139,140). Studies that have reviewed *p53* overexpression have yielded conflicting results regarding its prognostic value for this tumor site (137–139). Hypoxia as detected by Eppendorf measurement of cervical lymph nodes involved with head and neck cancer has been associated with worse radiation (141–143) or chemoradiation response (144) of the involved lymph node. Anemia has also been associated with poor outcome after radiation (131,145) and its correction may improve outcome (146). Overexpression of a hypoxia-induced transcription factor, hif-l-α (hypoxia-inducible factor-1α), was shown in a study of 98 patients with oropharyngeal cancers treated with definitive radiation correlated with the chance of complete response at the primary and nodal sites after treatment as well as local failure-free, disease-free, and overall survival on multivariate analysis (147). These markers remain to be validated in larger, multi-institutional trials.

TREATMENT SEQUELAE AND COMPLICATIONS

Surgical Resection

Sequelae related to surgery can be grouped into intraoperative, immediate, and delayed postoperative complications. Operative mortality for either primary tumor resection or neck dissections should be less than 5%. Among the intraoperative complications are damage to nerves (including cranial nerves V, VII, and XI), and vascular, lymphatic, and pulmonary complications (148,149). Delayed complications include fistula, dysarthria, mandibular necrosis, trismus, exposure of the carotid artery (150), lymphedema, and decreased function of muscle groups after a neck dissection. Even after preservation of the spinal accessory nerve, signs of muscle dysfunction can be seen (151). Extensive resections can affect speech and swallowing. Often, to prevent aspiration, a laryngectomy is performed (152), causing additional functional morbidity.

The base of tongue propels food past the larynx. Any reconstruction of the anterior floor of mouth that inhibits tongue-tip and lateral movement will reduce a patient's ability to chew, to control foods in the mouth, and to initiate the swallow. The more tongue that is tethered or restricted in its motion after resection, the more severe will be the swallowing disorder. Surgical reconstruction that creates the greatest range of back and base-of-tongue movement will result in the best tongue control for swallowing (152).

Salvage surgical procedures performed after induction chemotherapy and definitive RT have been reported to be associated with a higher rate of major wound complications (153). In a review of 96 patients, surgical salvage within 1 year of initial treatment resulted in a 77% incidence of major wound complications, compared with a 20% incidence if surgical salvage was performed 1 year after initial treatment (153). The mean time to resolution of fistulae and flap necrosis was 7.7 months. Two deaths were attributed to major wound complications: one patient had a carotid blowout, and another died of postoperative pneumonia.

Radiation Therapy

The major sequelae of RT can be divided into acute and chronic side effects. These depend on total dose, fraction size, fractionation, prior or concomitant therapy (i.e., surgery or chemotherapy), and target volume. The potential acute effects on the oral cavity and pharynx after approximately 1 week of RT include mucositis, sore throat, loss of taste, and xerostomia (if any of the major salivary glands are in the treatment portal). The decrease in saliva changes the microflora in the mouth and can dramatically increase the number of dental caries in the patient. Fluoride gel treatments are effective in reducing the subsequent incidence of dental caries. Approximately 5% of patients develop sialadenitis within 24 hours of the first irradiation treatment, and this resolves within 24 to 48 hours. The skin experiences erythema, peeling, and tanning. If the capacity of the basal cell layer to repopulate the epidermis is overwhelmed, the result is moist desquamation. Likewise epilation of hair-bearing areas with accompanying loss of sweat and sebaceous gland function occurs.

The late effects of RT after approximately 3,500 to 4,000 cGy can include xerostomia and altered sense of taste. Potential long-term complications at doses exceeding 6,000 cGy include soft-tissue and bone ulceration and necrosis. Radiation is believed to exert an avascular effect on tissues and epithelia that are thinner and more susceptible to injury. The process usually starts with ulceration of soft tissues, which can progress to bone exposure. If bone is then injured, bone necrosis or osteoradionecrosis can result. Treatment of this latter process is frustrating and difficult. For minor bone exposures, conservative measures are used, debridement being performed when indicated. For refractory cases, hyperbaric oxygen treatment has been advocated. Factors that can influence osteoradionecrosis include elective dental extraction after RT and treatment of tumors near bone (154,155). In the modern era, osteonecrosis should be an uncommon event (<5%) (156).

The use of brachytherapy implants also can contribute to osteoradionecrosis. Harrison et al. (82) point out that the patients who develop complications usually received the brachytherapy implant as the initial mode of therapy and the entire tumor bed was implanted. When EBRT was used for initial treatment, the boost was administered to the smaller volume of residual disease and the incidence of soft-tissue ulceration and osteoradionecrosis was reduced greatly. Technique also plays a role. The nonlooping technique is associated with a higher reported injury rate than the looping technique (80,82).

QUALITY OF LIFE

A great deal of interest has been expressed in patient QOL since the turn of the millennium. Oncologists are recognizing that a cured patient who is disabled as a result of treatment is not the same as a patient who requires significant intervention by the health care system or dependence on society for social services. Measures of QOL, although still evolving, are now important parts of research protocols. We currently use a number of tools to study this process. One such tool is the Memorial Symptom Assessment Scale (MSAS), a comprehensive symptom measure that records (a) prevalence of 32 physical and psychological symptoms commonly experienced by cancer patients, (b) symptom characteristics, and (c) measures of symptom distress (157). Another such tool is the Functional Assessment of Cancer Therapy (FACT), a multidimensional 33-item QOL instrument. A study in a mixed cancer population (n = 545) demonstrated the internal consistency and validity of the total and subscale scores for various domains of well-being (158). Each score is calculated as the sum of the responses given to specific groups of questions relating to physical, emotional, social, and functional well-being.

A third QOL evaluation tool is the head and neck performance status scale (PSS). The PSS is an interviewer-rated head and neck cancer performance status scale that yields separate scores reflecting a patient's ability to eat in public, comprehensibility of a patient's speech, and normalcy of diet. The scale has been validated and used in prior surveys of patients with base-of-tongue cancer. Each score corresponds to a description of the functional capability that attends it. The higher the score, the better is the function. A score of 100 indicates normal function and is the best possible score (159).

Harrison et al. (160) retrospectively examined patients with SCC of the base of tongue who were treated with primary RT or primary surgery, comparing the QOL and functional outcome. Patients had been treated primarily either by RT or surgery depending on the philosophy of their primary physician. Primary RT consisted of 4,500- to 5,400-cGy EBRT followed by a ^{192}Ir implant that delivered an additional 2,000 to 3,000 cGy over 2 to 3 days. In those with involved lymph nodes, a neck dissection was performed at the same time as the implantation. Primary surgery consisted of resection of the base-of-tongue lesion, neck dissection, and postoperative RT. Both groups had similar local control (80%–90%). A subjective performance status scale for head and neck cancer patients was used to assess the QOL in these patients (0 to 100, where 0 = worst function and 100 = normal function), measuring the patient's ability to eat in public, comprehensibility of the patient's speech, and normalcy of diet (Fig. 17.15) (158). Patients treated with RT had consistently better performance status and QOL scores. This was true for those with early (T1–2) as well as more advanced (T3–4) disease. In addition, comparison of scores for early and advanced disease treated by primary RT revealed no difference in all three functional categories for T1 to T2 as compared with T3 to T4 disease ($p = 0.84$), showing that QOL scores remain high for all stages. For surgery, functional status deteriorated significantly when comparing T1 to T2 and T3 to T4 lesions ($p = 0.0014$), consistent with the fact that larger tumors require more extensive operations. The investigators' results show that RT provides a better performance status than surgery for base-of-tongue cancer, whether the patient exhibits early or advanced disease. Functional scores remained high for all T stages treated with irradiation but deteriorated with more advanced T stages for patients treated surgically (160).

Patients with advanced oropharyngeal cancer who underwent induction chemotherapy followed by RT as a means of organ function preservation and whose appropriate surgical management would have required a tongue procedure and potential total laryngectomy were evaluated for QOL.

In addition to QOL issues, Harrison et al. (160–162) have examined the long-term socioeconomic outcomes for patients with cancer of the base of tongue who were treated with an organ preservation approach. At the time of follow-up (median, 5 years), patients' annual incomes were similar to those at the time of presentation (89% exceeding \$20,000; 52% exceeding \$60,000). Of those working full-time, 72% were still in full-time work, and 83% of those working part-time were in part-time work.

Quality of life has recently been recognized as an issue of paramount importance in the decision analysis for managing patients with head and neck cancer, and confirmatory studies that use

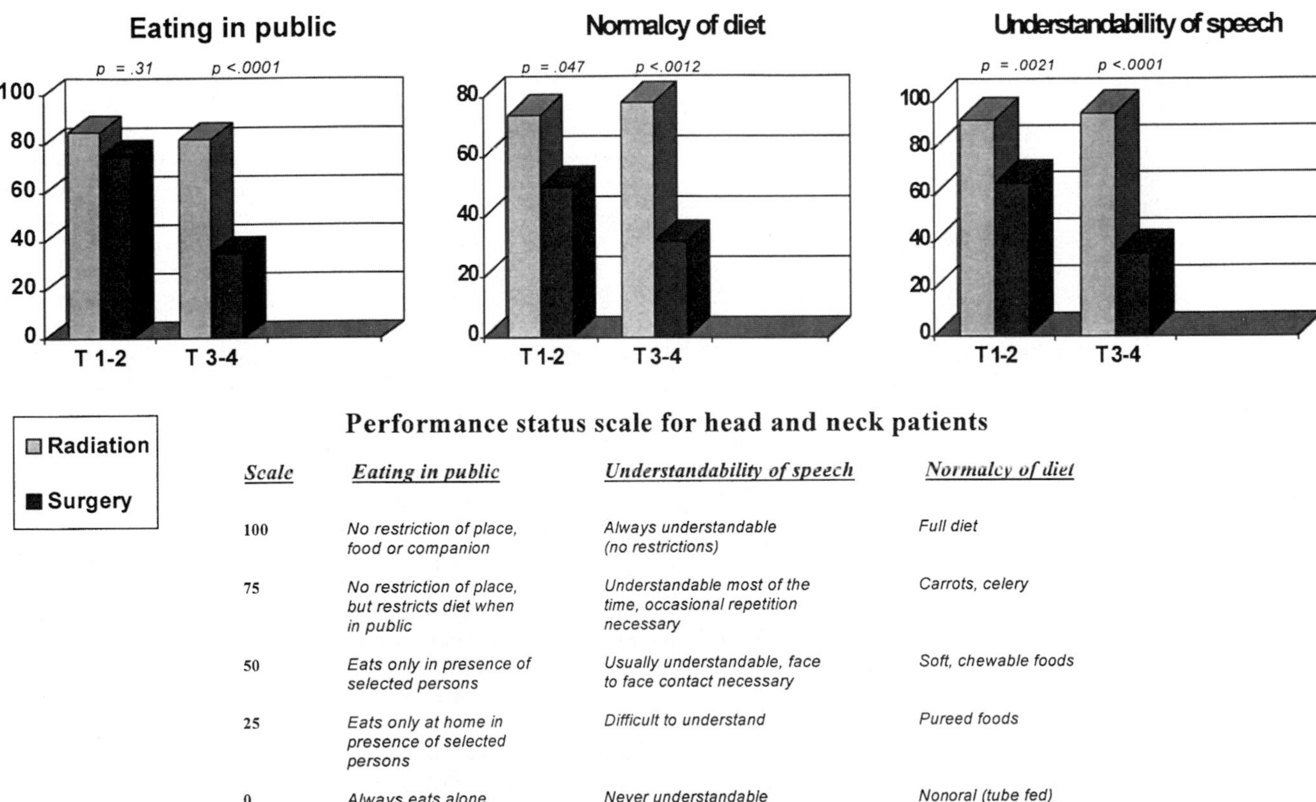

Performance status scale for head and neck patients

Scale	Eating in public	Understandability of speech	Normalcy of diet
100	*No restriction of place, food or companion*	*Always understandable (no restrictions)*	*Full diet*
75	*No restriction of place, but restricts diet when in public*	*Understandable most of the time, occasional repetition necessary*	*Carrots, celery*
50	*Eats only in presence of selected persons*	*Usually understandable, face to face contact necessary*	*Soft, chewable foods*
25	*Eats only at home in presence of selected persons*	*Difficult to understand*	*Pureed foods*
0	*Always eats alone*	*Never understandable*	*Nonoral (tube fed)*

Figure 17.15 Performance status scales for normalcy of diet, eating in public, and comprehensibility of speech after treatment for squamous cell cancer of the base of tongue: a comparison of primary radiation therapy and primary surgery. (Adapted from Harrison LB, Zelefsky MJ, Armstrong JG, et al. Performance status after treatment for squamous cell cancer of the base of tongue—a comparison of primary radiation therapy versus primary surgery. *Int J Radiat Oncol Biol Phys* 1994;30:953–957.)

objective criteria are needed to compare in more detail the various treatment modalities for oropharyngeal cancers. Clearly, QOL issues must factor strongly into the decision-making process and selection of the appropriate management strategy.

RADIOLOGIC IMAGING CONCERNS

Bernard B. O'Malley and Suresh K. Mukherji

The oropharynx provides a challenge to imaging for several reasons. The undulating mucosal surfaces have varied contours among different patients. Most of these surfaces contain lymphoid or minor salivary tissue, which enhances normally with intravenous contrast, obscuring early lesions. Furthermore, many of these surfaces appose one another within the various sulci, which complicates determining the number of subsites involved. Fluoroscopy can still provide complementary information to the clinical examination in patients who are difficult to examine. Computed tomography imaging is a reliable method for preoperative staging but is not used to detect mucosal primary lesions (163). Additional unpredictable factors include swallowing motion and streak artifact. Because of the presence of painful lesions in the oropharynx, patients habitually swallow to reduce discomfort. This is accentuated by the warm sensation many patients feel in the throat during the bolus phase of intravenous CT contrast infusion. These motion-degraded images can simply be repeated at the necessary levels.

Streak artifacts related to dental amalgam and permanent dental appliances vary among patients. Simple re-angling of the scan plane around the amalgam can reduce the degree to which the oropharyngeal subsites are obscured and will permit adequate visualization of the majority of oropharyngeal subsites. In those few patients who have extensive dental amalgam, one alternative is to perform direct coronal views through the oropharynx after repositioning the head or to employ magnetic resonance imaging (MRI). The amalgam does cause minor local artifact on MRI scans. Permanent appliances cause serious MRI degradation, particularly on the important fat-suppressed series.

The *tongue base* enhances moderately intensely owing to normal lymphoid tissue. The degree of lymphoid tissue varies among patients and is often asymmetric, thus limiting the diagnostic value of detection of mucosal lesions and their local superficial extent (Fig. 17.16). This is especially problematic for excluding extension across the valleculae (Fig. 17.17) and laterally across the glossotonsillar sulcus (Fig. 17.17). Direct invasion of the intrinsic tongue and penetration of the pre-epiglottic space can readily be identified with MRI (164) or CT (Fig. 17.18). In patients who cannot receive intravenous contrast, MRI may be the better examination for deep extension.

Posterior and lateral *pharyngeal wall* lesions are easily overlooked radiographically, and imaging is not a substitute for an adequate clinical examination. Even when a mucosal lesion is known to be present, the full superficial extent is not estimated accurately by cross-sectional imaging (Fig. 17.19). Computed tomography scanning and MRI are both useful for detecting clinically occult parapharyngeal extension (Fig. 17.20) but not highly specific for deep prevertebral extension (Fig. 17.21). The trend toward limited neck dissections for clinical N0 necks (165) means that the entire retropharyngeal lymph node group must be carefully examined in addition to the jugular chain.

Patients with lesions of the *soft palate* cannot be staged completely without coronal views, because of their ready access to so many adjacent tissue planes (Fig. 17.22) which must extend to the skull base. The imaging study must extend to the skull base and be reconstructed in bone algorithm to exclude skull base invasion. In high-risk patients, MRI is the preferred modality as it is superior to CT for identifying tumor spread along the tensor and levator palatini muscle and skull base involvement. Retropharyngeal lymph nodes are also more easily assessed with MRI than compared with CT (166).

The normal thickness of the faucial tonsil limits delectability of early lesions. The deep extent of advanced lesions, however, can be tracked carefully with multiplanar CT scanning or MRI. Extension to the palate (Fig. 17.23), tongue base, masticator space (Fig. 17.24), and mandible (Fig. 17.25) should be excluded. Parapharyngeal extension and lateral retropharyngeal adenopathy (Fig. 17.26) are seen only on imaging and must be emphasized in the report. Contiguous extension to the preepiglottic space can be evaluated with MRI (Fig. 17.27).

Follow-up imaging includes two main categories of patients: those being evaluated for estimation of treatment response and those who have responded and are being followed with clinical and imaging surveillance. Although follow-up imaging has not yet proven to be useful in patient survival (167) it may help select patients for an alternate pathway on a disease management algorithm when partial response or nonresponse is detected early. Surveillance scanning is especially challenging because of the structural deformity of the combined modality treatment results (Fig. 17.28). Immediate postoperative imaging is not recommended unless gross residual disease is known to be present. Most practitioners wait for at least 6 weeks if not 3 months for an initial baseline posttreatment scan. Imaging is particularly important in treated patients, as conducting a clinical examination becomes more difficult due to scarring. Computed tomography can confirm removal or reduction of masses from surgical or nonsurgical groups, respectively. It efficiently includes the primary site and nodal response, which are not always congruent. Neck dissection can be recommended for insufficient response at involved lymph node stations (168). Magnetic resonance imaging has been shown to be more accurate in differentiating fibrosis from residual tumor (169). Magnetic resonance imaging is most accurate when disease can be detected extending into additional or adjacent compartments. Positron emission tomographic scanning will play an increasingly useful role in the evaluation of treated patients because of the aforementioned limitations of other modalities.

Posttreatment imaging for oropharyngeal carcinomas must be specifically evaluated for clinically occult recurrent or persistent disease (Fig. 17.29). Common sites of recurrence that cannot be detected on clinical examination are direct spread to the carotid space and involvement of the retropharyngeal lymph nodes. Consistent imaging protocols are vital for patients being followed after nonoperative combined chemoirradiation treatment (Fig. 17.30).

Ultimately, metabolic imaging will provide the most useful information for managing patients in treatment algorithms (Fig. 17.31). Fluorodeoxyglucose-positron emission tomography (FDG-PET) activity is elevated in most neoplastic and intense inflammatory processes. Very high FDG activity at the primary site on pretreatment PET scans portends a poor survival (170). Fluorodeoxyglucose-positron emission tomography scans will usually show moderate activity in the treatment bed due to inflammation. The value of a posttreatment scan hinges on the presence of a baseline pretreatment PET scan. If activity diminishes toward background or shows at least a 50% decline, then a treatment response has occurred. Some nonsquamous neoplasms show limited FDG activity. For this reason, a posttreatment-only FDG-PET scan with low metabolic activity should be interpreted with caution. Fortunately, most squamous neoplasms are very metabolically active.

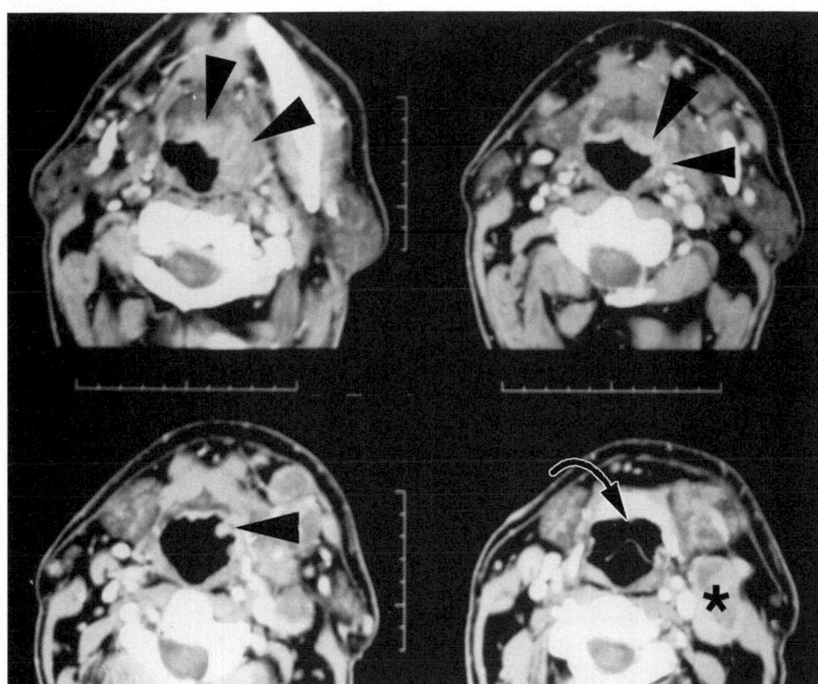

Figure 17.16 Localized base-of-tongue lesion. Enhanced axial computed tomographic scan of tongue base shows moderately sized lesion at mucosa of left side of base of tongue with minimal involvement of substance of tongue (*arrowheads*). Ipsilateral submental and level II through III adenopathy is seen (*asterisk*). Note that the hyoid bone is intact (*curved arrow*).

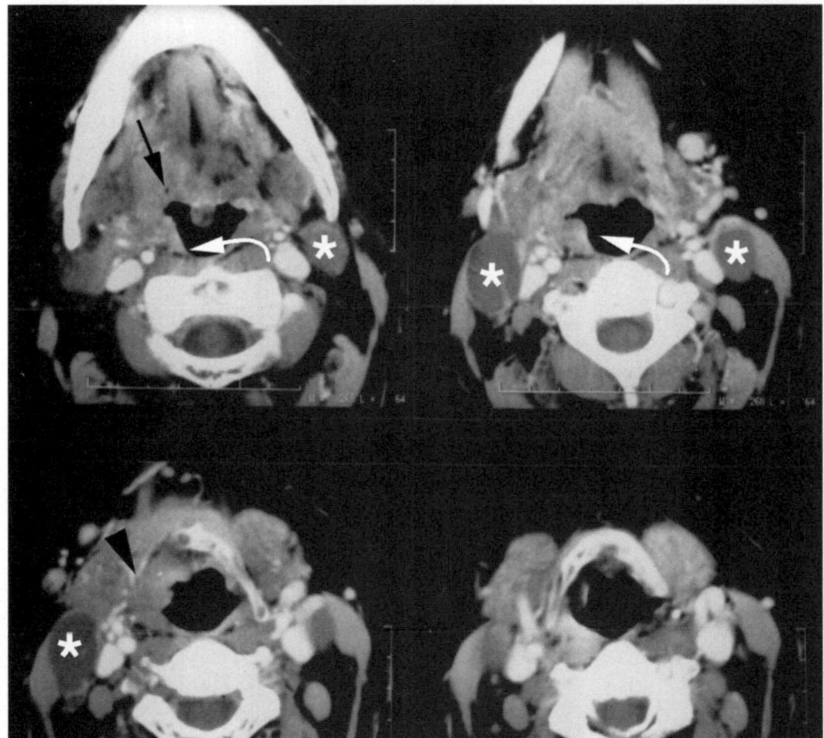

Figure 17.17 Base of tongue to vallecula. Enhanced axial computed tomographic views show right-sided base-of-tongue lesion infiltrating the glossotonsillar sulcus (*arrow*), along the lateral pharyngeal wall (*curved arrows*), and across the vallecula (*arrowhead*). Note necrotic bilateral adenopathy (*asterisk*).

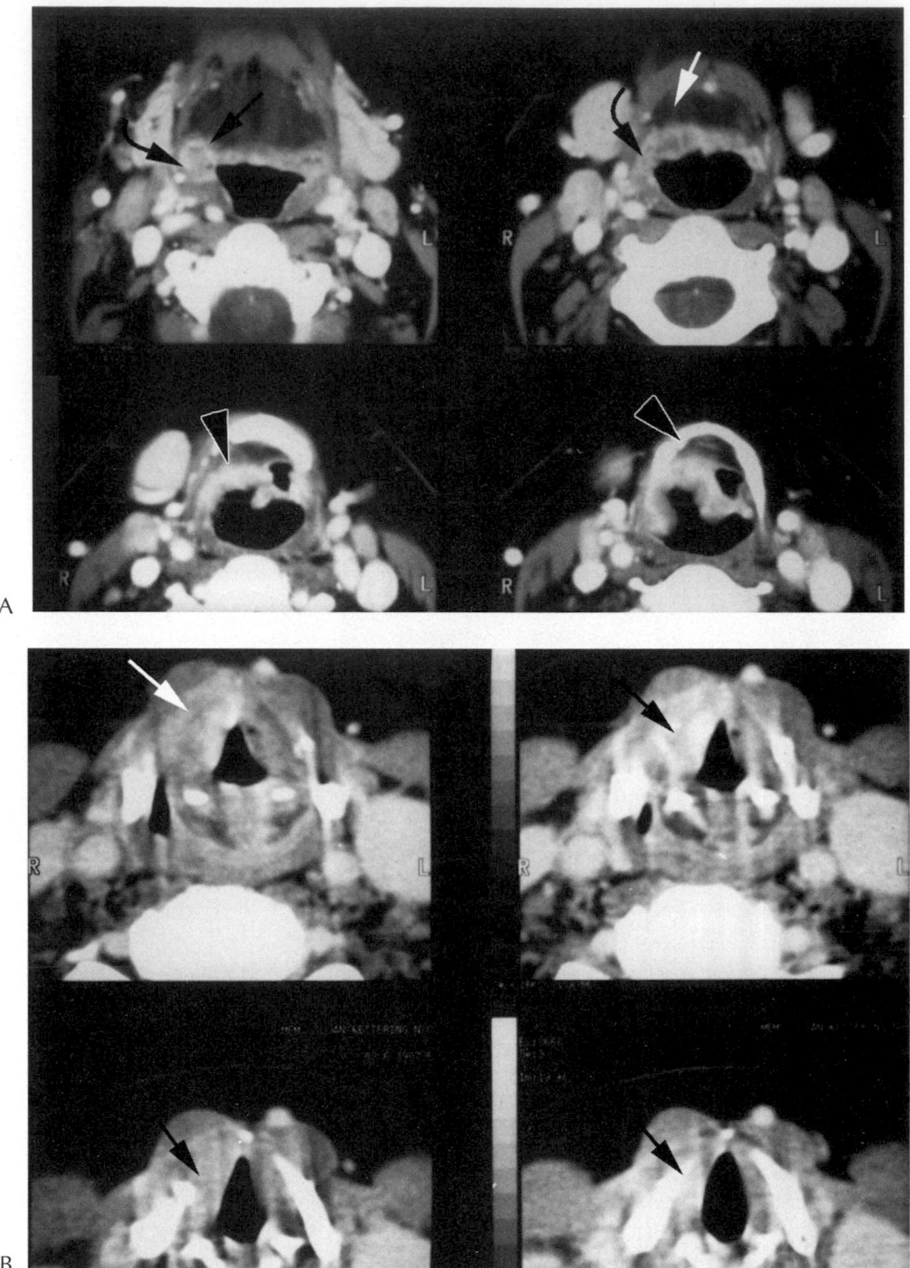

Figure 17.18 Base of tongue to larynx. Right-sided base-of-tongue lesion (*arrow*) extending **(A)** into the glossotonsillar sulcus (*curved arrows*) and **(B)** into larynx through the preepiglottic space (*arrowheads*) into the paraglottic space (*long arrows*).

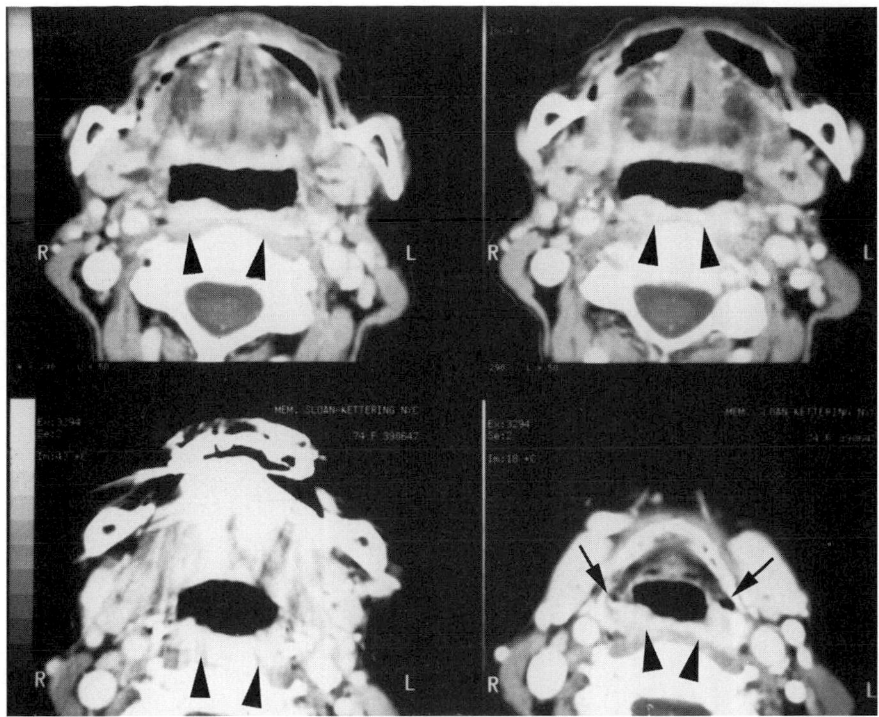

Figure 17.19 Posterior pharyngeal wall lesion. Enhanced axial computed tomographic views show intensely enhancing lesion of posterior oropharyngeal wall (*arrowheads*) approaching the piriform aperture bilaterally (*arrows*). No lateral retropharyngeal adenopathy is noted.

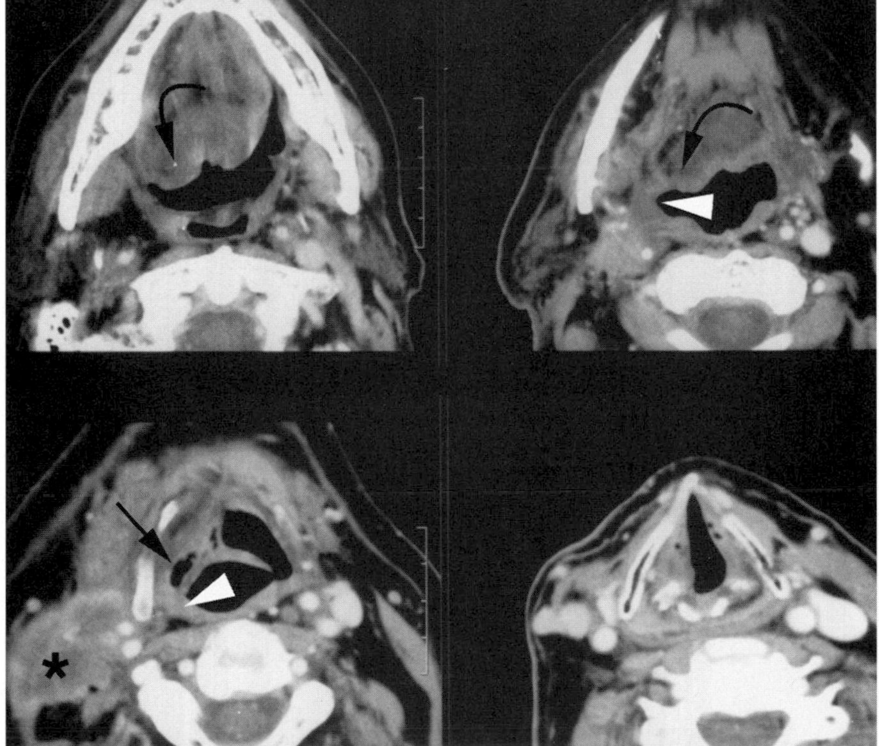

Figure 17.20 Pharyngeal wall lesion. Enhanced axial computed tomographic scan shows right lateral wall lesion (*arrowheads*) extending to vallecula (*arrow*) with necrotic ipsilateral adenopathy (*asterisk*). Note laxity of right side of base of tongue (*curved arrows*) due to recent neoplastic involvement of cranial nerve XII by matted adenopathy.

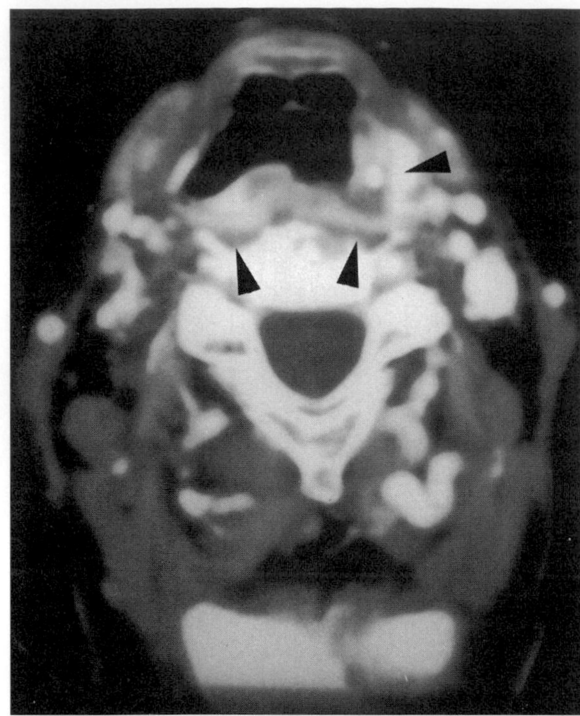

Figure 17.21 Posterolateral pharyngeal wall lesion. Enhanced axial computed tomographic scan shows posterior and left lateral pharyngeal wall cancer (*arrowheads*) poorly marginated with the prevertebral fascia.

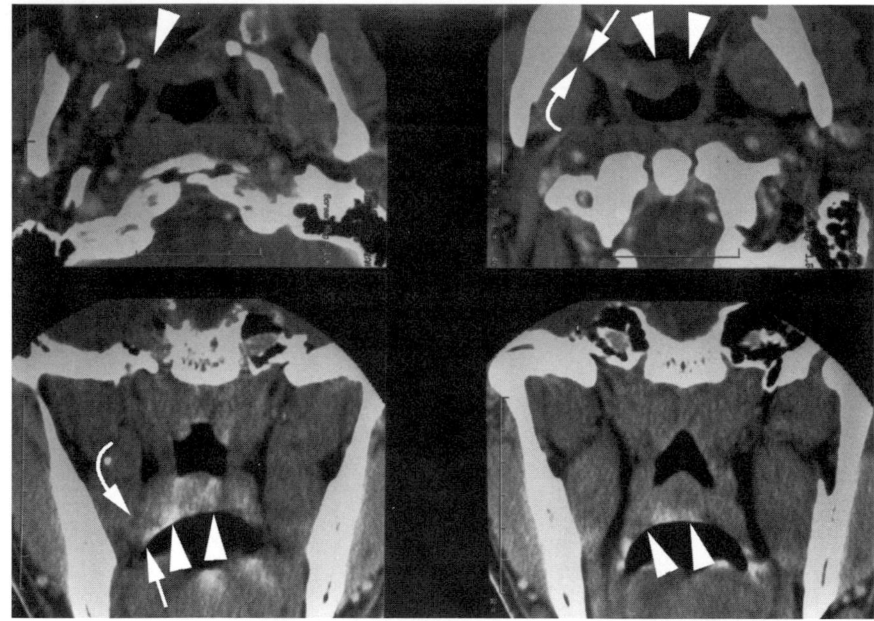

Figure 17.22 Soft palate cancer. Enhanced axial (**top**) and direct coronal (**bottom**) computed tomographic views of a carcinoma of the soft palate (*arrowheads*) extending to the tonsil (*arrows*), poorly marginated with the medial pterygoid muscle (*curved arrow*).

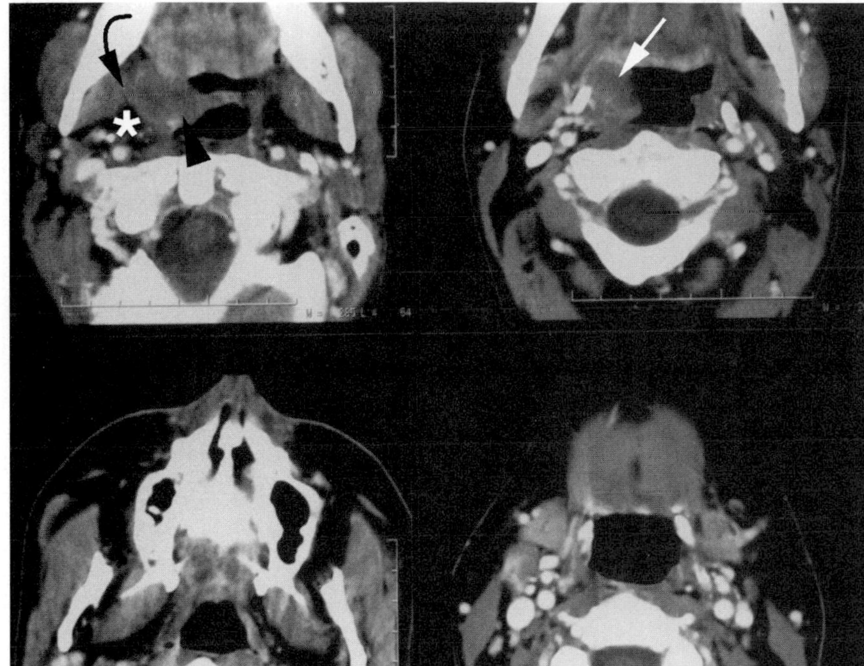

Figure 17.23 Tonsil to palate. Enhanced axial computed tomographic scan shows early right tonsillar cancer (*arrow*) extending up to soft palate (*arrowhead*) without parapharyngeal (*asterisk*) or masticator (*curved arrow*) involvement.

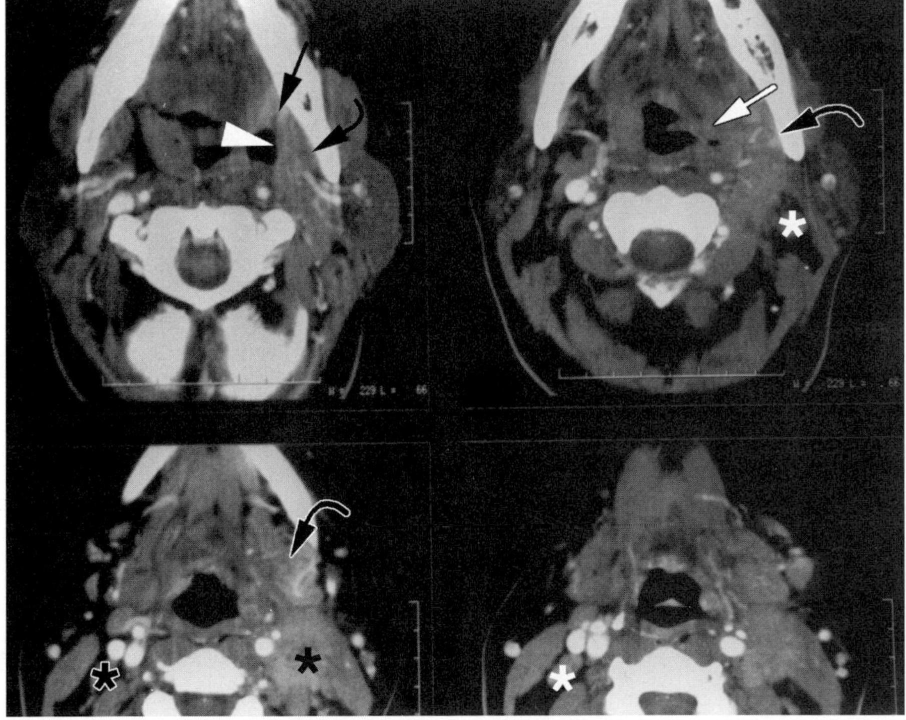

Figure 17.24 Extensive tonsillar cancer. Enhanced axial computed tomographic scan through oropharynx shows left tonsillar lesion (*arrows*) with extensive ulceration (*arrowhead*) approaching the mandible (*curved arrow*). Note extensive bilateral adenopathy.

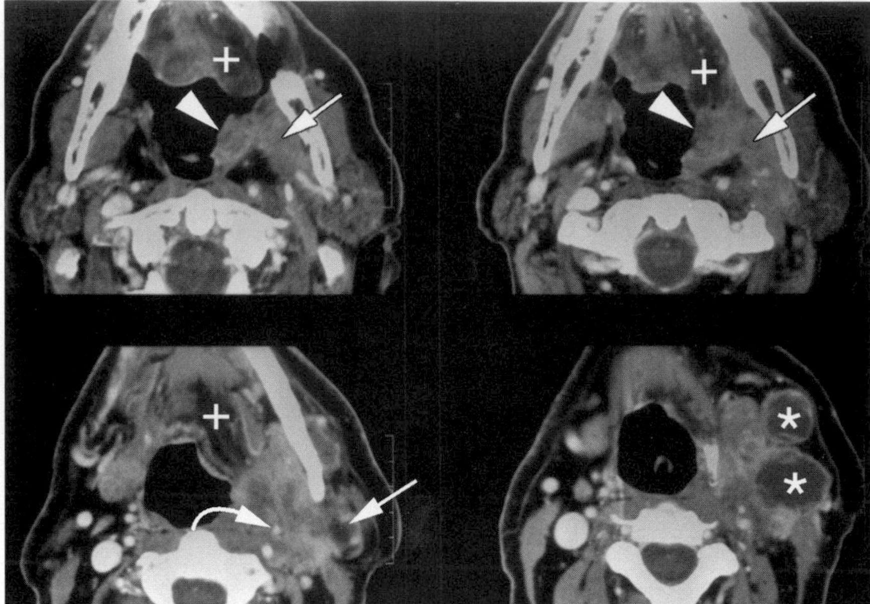

Figure 17.25 Progressive tonsillar cancer. Enhanced axial computed tomographic scan shows large left tonsillar lesion (*arrowheads*) infiltrating through the medial pterygoid (*arrows*) to the mandible and parapharyngeal space (*curved arrow*). Note necrotic ipsilateral adenopathy (*asterisk*) and chronic denervation atrophy of left cranial nerve XII (+).

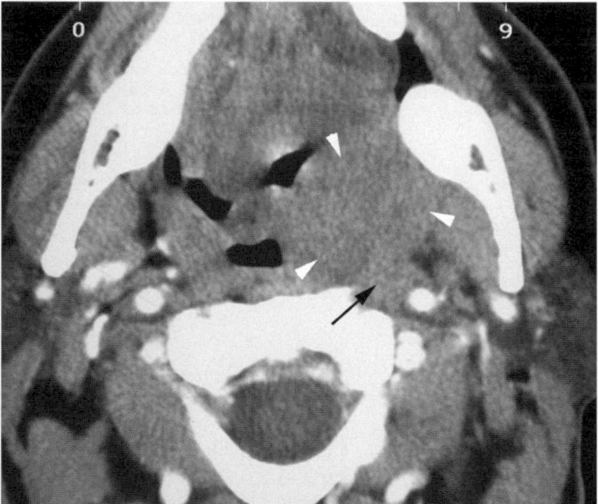

Figure 17.26 Lateral retropharyngeal adenopathy. Enhanced axial computed tomographic scan through the upper oropharynx shows a pathologic left lateral retropharyngeal node (*arrow*) due to a large tonsil squamous cell carcinoma antigen (*arrowheads*).

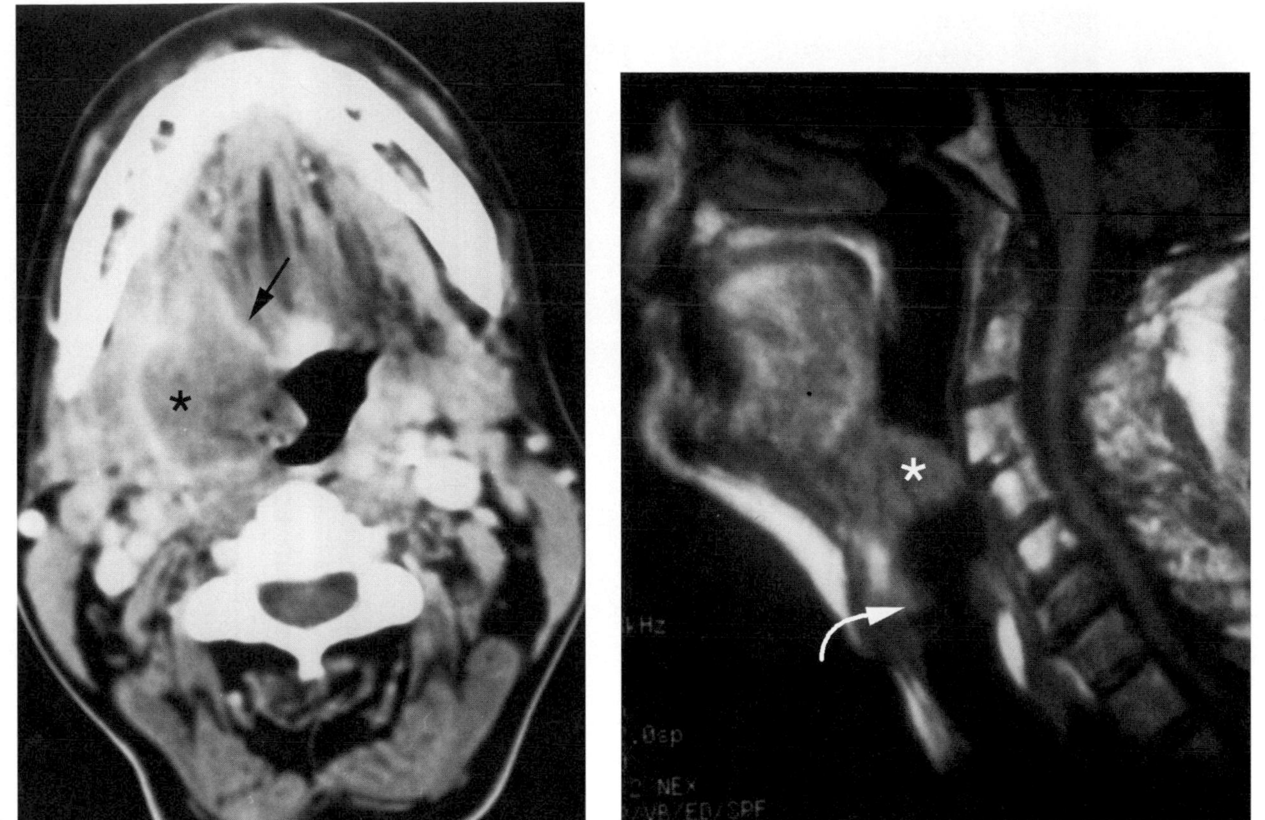

Figure 17.27 Tonsil to preepiglottic space. **A:** Enhanced axial computed tomographic scan shows bulky right tonsillar cancer (*asterisk*) involving the right side of base of tongue (*arrow*). **B:** Sagittal T1 magnetic resonance image shows extension to most of the preepiglottic space (*asterisk*). Note false cord level (*curved arrow*).

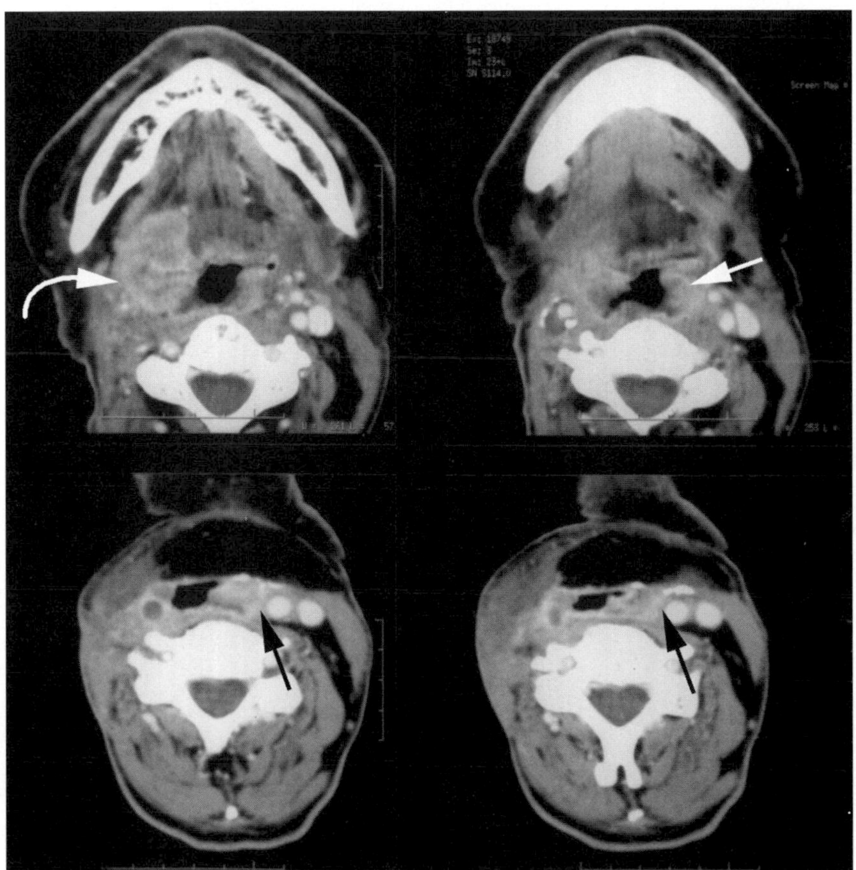

Figure 17.28 Recurrent pharyngeal wall cancer. Enhanced axial computed tomographic views show recurrent left lateral pharyngeal wall lesion (*arrows*) and developing contralateral (**right**) pharyngeal wall disease (*curved arrow*) after prior laryngopharyngectomy for left lateral pharyngeal wall cancer.

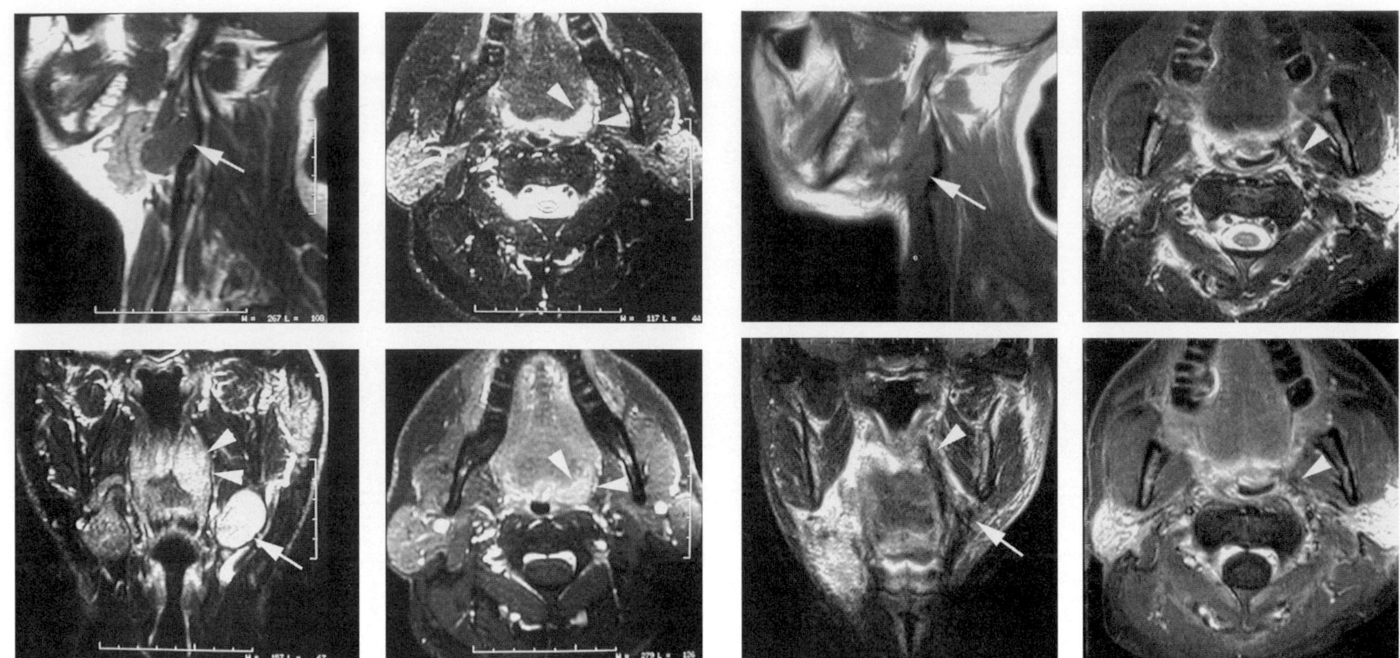

Figure 17.29 Tonsil squamous cell carcinoma antigen (SCCA) pre- and postoperative magnetic resonance imaging (MRI). **A:** Preoperative MRIs clockwise from top left include: sagittal T1, axial T2, enhanced axial T1, and coronal T2. Primary SCCA of the left palatine tonsil (*arrowheads*) and ipsilateral level II adenopathy (*arrows*). **B:** Postoperative MRIs in exact same format show value in standard imaging protocols with collapsed operative bed left tonsil (*arrowheads*) and operative change left neck dissection.

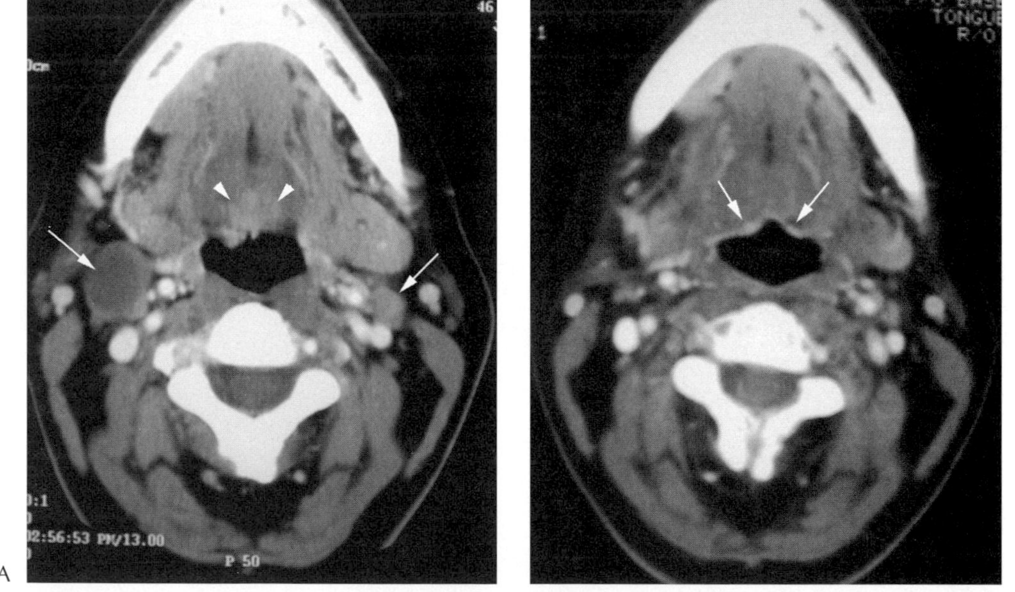

Figure 17.30 Nonsurgical management follow-up base-of-tongue squamous cell carcinoma (SCC). **A:** Enhanced axial computed tomography shows endophytic base-of-tongue SCC (*arrowheads*) with bilateral adenopathy (*arrows*) typical for midline lesions. **B:** Post–chemo-irradiation scan shows defect at tongue base (*arrows*) indicating complete radiographic response including lymph nodes.

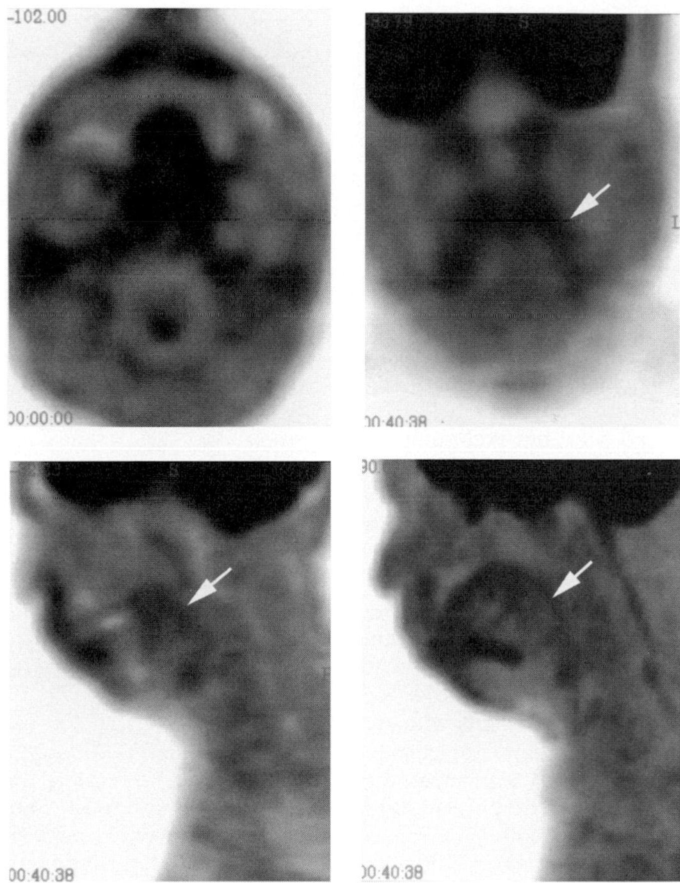

Figure 17.31 Tonsil squamous cell carcinoma fluorodeoxyglucose-positron emission tomography (FDG-PET) scan, postoperative scan of patient shown in Fig. 17.29. **Clockwise from top left:** axial, coronal, parasagittal, and composite lateral FDG-PET images show symmetric physiologic distribution on axial view and no hypermetabolic activity in operative bed (*arrows*) to indicate residual disease after surgery and radiation.

RADIATION THERAPY TECHNIQUE*

Louis B. Harrison, Rudolph Woode, and William M. Mendenhall

Tonsil

The chapter has provided extensive discussion about the relative indications for unilateral neck treatment versus bilateral neck treatment for patients with carcinoma of the tonsil. We will review the technique for each of these situations (Figs. 17.32 and 17.33).

In the situation of bilateral neck treatment, the patient is generally treated with lateral opposed fields for the primary site and upper neck, which are matched with a low neck field. The field is junctioned just below the hyoid bone, but excluding the glottic larynx. The larynx is protected with a midline block in the upper midline of the low neck field.

The initial field arrangement generally covers the primary site and the upper neck nodes. The retropharyngeal nodes are included in the fields. The spinal cord is protected after 4,400 or 4,500 cGy, depending on whether 200 cGy or 180 cGy fractions are used. Once the spinal cord block is placed, the primary site and neck nodes continue to be treated. After 5,000 to 5,400 cGy, clinically negative sites can be further protected. All gross disease is then taken to the total prescription dose. In patients who are going to receive a planned neck dissection, it is our practice to treat the involved neck to approximately 60 Gy. After that, the primary site alone is boosted to the prescription dose. Early stage lesions are generally treated to approximately 6,600 cGy, whereas more advanced lesions are treated to approximately 7,000 cGy. For more advanced lesions, a concomitant boost technique is often used. Sometimes a lymph node may be located in such a way as to be directly in the beam for the primary boost. In that situation, the node receives full doses. If the node resolves completely, it is sometimes possible to avoid neck dissection.

Once the spinal cord block is added, the posterior neck is treated with appropriate energy electron beams. Again, if gross disease exists in the posterior neck, the region is taken to the prescription dose. If not, it is taken to a dose that is appropriate for microscopic disease (5,000–5,400 cGy).

There are certain technical details that should be considered. Many patients have significant metallic dental fillings. As much as possible, care should be taken to avoid irradiating these areas. If that is not possible, heavily reinforced dental trays can be used to absorb much of the scatter and minimize the mucositis that often develops adjacent to these metallic fillings. Also, attempts should be made to avoid irradiating the external auditory canal, the roots of the teeth, and the anterior portion of the oral cavity. A bite block is always used, which helps to spare a portion of the tongue and the hard palate.

Base of Tongue

Patients with cancer of the base of tongue (Fig. 17.34) are usually treated at the primary site and both sides of the neck. There are no situations where ipsilateral neck treatment is offered. The treatment technique involves bilateral opposed fields for the primary site and upper neck, matched to a low neck field. The patient is simulated with head extension and a bite block. The upper neck fields include the primary site and upper neck. The field is junctioned above the larynx, so as to eliminate the glottic larynx from RT. The low neck field has a block in the upper midline for protection of the spinal cord and the larynx.

Our practice is to use an implant for the boost treatment. In centers that use a concomitant boost technique, a field reduction will be designed to incorporate the base of tongue, with adequate margin.

Soft Palate

Patients with soft palate cancer are treated at the primary site and both sides of the neck (Fig. 17.35). As with base of tongue, there are no data to support the concept of ipsilateral neck irradiation in these patients.

The fields are very similar to the conventional techniques used for base of tongue and tonsil. The treatment begins with opposed lateral fields for the primary site and upper neck. These fields are junctioned above the larynx, so as to protect the glottic larynx. The low neck field has a block in the upper midline, protecting the spinal cord and the larynx.

The patient is simulated with head extension, and a bite block. The field design includes the retropharyngeal nodes, which are at risk for all oropharyngeal cancers. Care is usually taken to block the roots of the teeth, and the external auditory canal.

*Please refer to the Appendix, Imaging Considerations for Radiation Therapy Treatment Planning. This section shows the important radiologic anatomy that allows the radiation oncologist to design the target volumes for treatment planning.

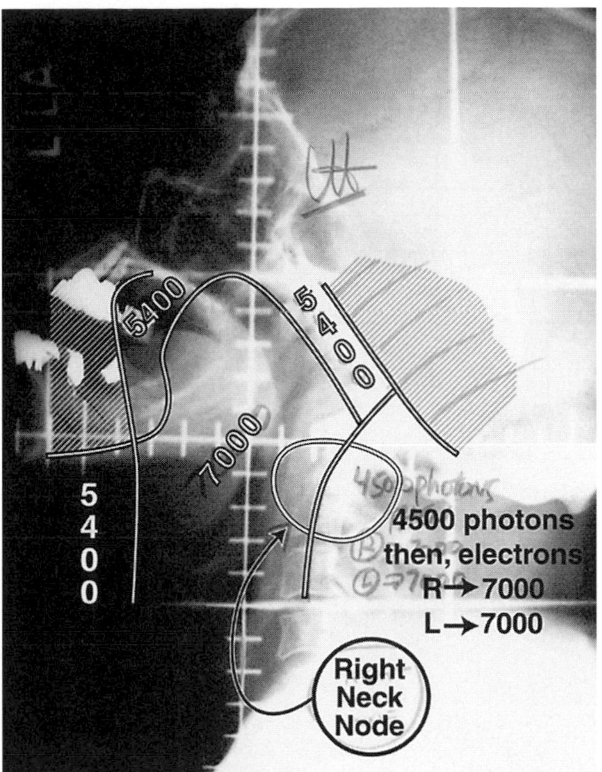

Figure 17.32 Tonsil cancer. Bilateral neck treatment technique. The bilateral opposed portals for a patient treated with this technique. This patient is a 60-year-old woman who has a T2N2c squamous cell carcinoma of the tonsillar fossa. There were palpable lymph nodes in the right neck, and radiologically evident lymph nodes in the left upper neck. The patient was simulated with his head extended and a bite block. Wire was placed around the palpable right neck node. The patient was treated with 180 cGy fractions. The initial field covers the primary site, upper neck, including the upper jugular chain, and the retropharyngeal nodes. Level 1 lymph nodes were also included. The field is junctioned to avoid radiation therapy to the larynx. The field comes to the posterior aspect of the spinous processes, which properly incorporates the entire posterior neck. This field is treated to 4,500 cGy, after which a spinal cord block is added. The primary site and upper neck nodes are continued to 5,400 cGy. At that point, treatment is confined to the primary site and areas of clinically involved disease in the neck. The gross disease is treated to a total of 7,000 cGy. A concomitant boost technique is used. There are several fractionation schemes that can be used. In this case, the patient receives a total of 7,000 cGy in 6 weeks. During the last 2 weeks of the treatment, the patient receives a second daily fraction approximately 5 to 6 hours after the morning fraction. This treatment encompasses the entire boost volume, and received 160 cGy per fraction. Therefore, this area receives 10 afternoon fractions in the last 2 weeks of treatment, providing a 1,600 cGy boost. When added to the 5,400 cGy that has been delivered, the total dose becomes 7,000 cGy in 6 weeks. In this patient, because there is disease involving the posterior necks on both sides, the electron fields are also treated to 7,000 cGy using a similar technique.

A

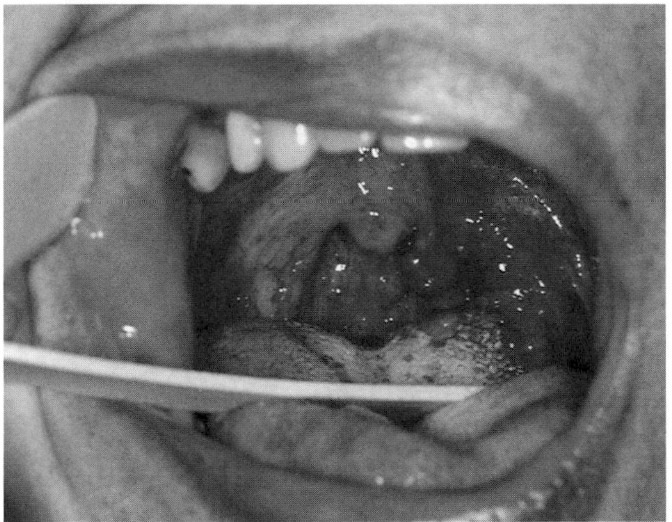

B

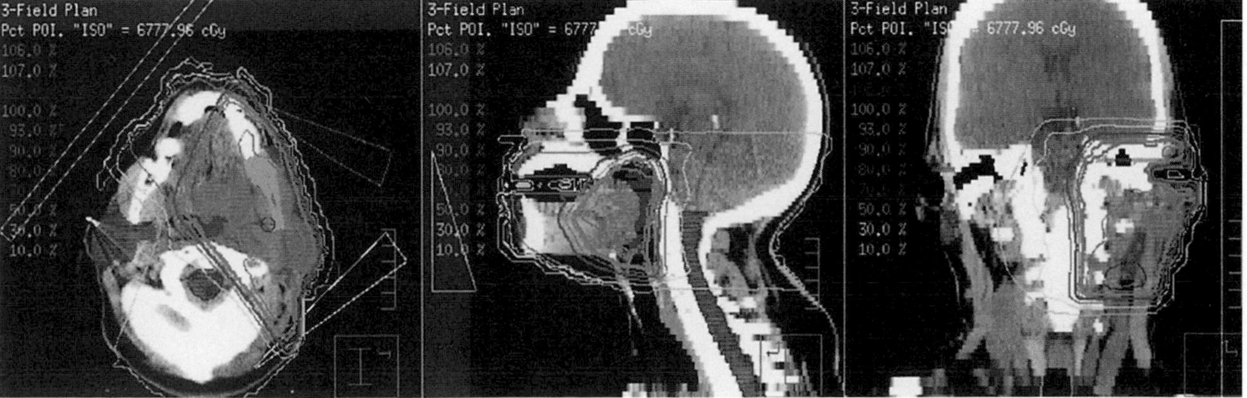

Figure 17.33 Tonsil cancer. Unilateral neck treatment technique. A patient treated with unilateral fields. This patient is a 50-year-old woman with a T2N0 squamous cell carcinoma of the left tonsil. Our plan is to treat this patient with definitive radiation therapy. **A:** This is a photograph of the primary lesion. It involves the tonsillar fossa, with involvement of the anterior tonsillar pillar, and superficial involvement of base of tongue. **B:** This patient was treated with a three-field plan. This involves a wedged-pair plan, with a low-weighted right anterior oblique field, to help cover the tongue extension without overdosing the spinal cord. The planning tumor volume (PTV) is contoured. The primary site, extension along the soft palate, extension into the base of tongue, upper neck nodes, and retropharyngeal nodes are all included. An axial, sagittal, and coronal dose distribution shows that the PTV is well covered. The salivary gland tissue of the contralateral neck, especially the parotid gland, is well protected. *(continued on next page)*

C

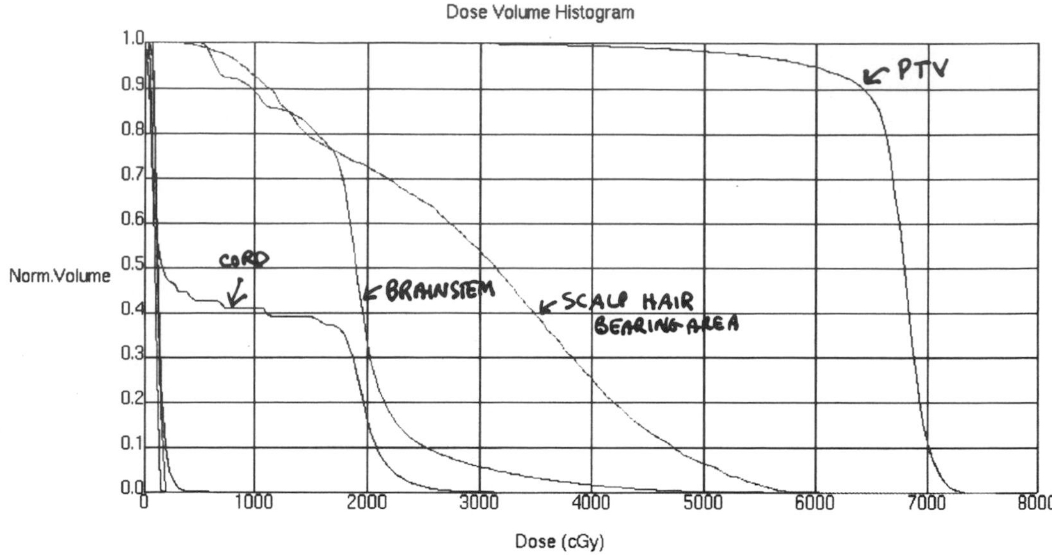

D

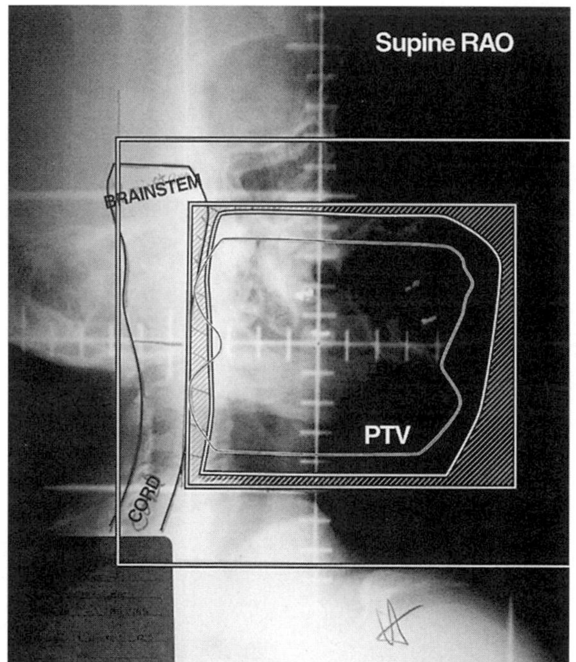

E

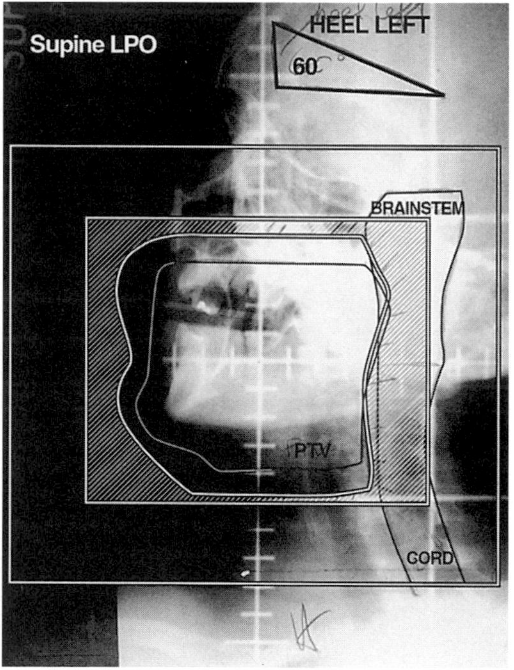

F

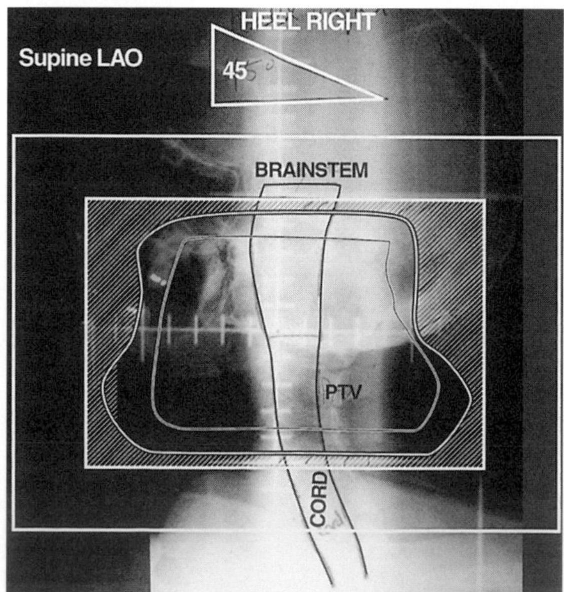

Figure 17.33 ***(continued)*** **C:** Dose-volume histogram of this plan showing good coverage of the target volume and adequate protection of the surrounding normal tissue. The curves are depicting extremely low doses to the right parotid as well as the right and left retina. **D–F:** The simulation films showing the fields that were used. As mentioned previously, these consisted of a left anterior oblique (LAO), a left posterior oblique (LPO), and a lightly weighted right anterior oblique (RAO).

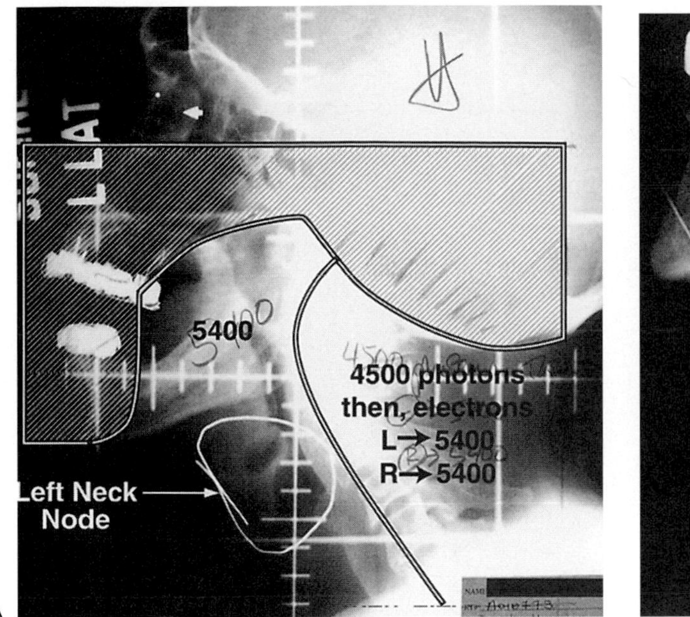

A

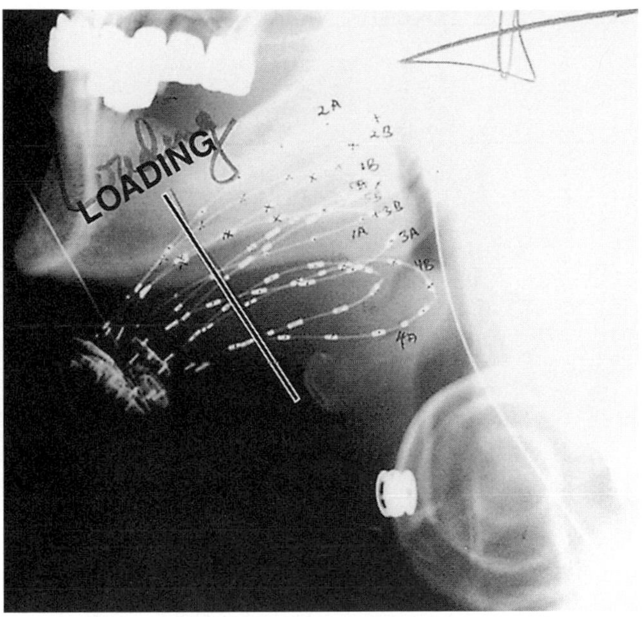

B

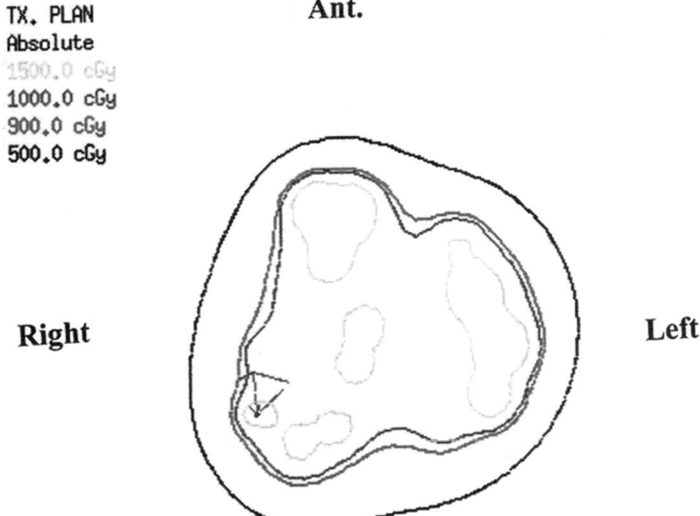

C

Post.

Figure 17.34 Base of tongue carcinoma. Technique using external beam plus brachytherapy. This patient had a T2N2a squamous cell carcinoma of the base of tongue with a left cervical lymph node metastasis. Our treatment plan involved external beam radiation therapy, followed by implant and neck dissection. **A:** The patient was simulated with his head extended, and a bite block. Wire was placed around the left neck node. The initial fields include the primary site with adequate margin, and the upper neck nodes. The field was junctioned at the level of the thyroid notch, so as to avoid laryngeal irradiation. However, the vallecula is completely encompassed in the field. The patient is treated at 180 cGy per day to a total dose of 4,500 cGy. At that point, a spinal cord block is added. The primary site and upper neck is then treated to a total of 5,400 cGy. The posterior lymph nodes are treated to a dose of 5,400 cGy, using appropriate energy electron beams. After 5,400 cGy a clinically designed electron field is used to boost the involved neck node up to 60 Gy. **B:** Approximately 3 weeks after the completion of external beam, the patient is brought to the operating room for a planned neck dissection and a brachytherapy procedure. This is a localization film from the implant. It is a looping implant, where several rows of catheters are looped through the submental approach. Several rows of catheters are placed. The catheters are placed in loops, as shown on the localization film. The loops are approximately 1 to 1.5 cm. in breadth. Sequential loops are situated throughout the base of tongue, so as to encompass the bed of the original tumor. A 1.5- to 2-cm margin is generally placed within the confines of the anatomic space of the base of tongue. Usually, the glossotonsillar sulcus is incorporated into the implant, especially for lateralized lesions. Because the hypoglossal nerve runs through the glossotonsillar sulcus, care is taken not to insert trocars directly through the sulcus. Catheters are looped over the sulcus, thereby minimizing traumatic injury to the hypoglossal nerve. A line that denotes the extent of the loading is shown on the radiograph. This should conform to the location of the lesion. Generally, an attempt is made to spare the skin in the loading schema. It is usually technically feasible to include the vallecula in the implant, as shown in this particular patient. For T1 to T2 lesions, an additional 2,000 to 2,500 cGy is delivered; for T3 to T4 lesions, an additional 2,500 to 3,000 cGy is delivered. The general attempt is to cover the target area with the 900 to 1,000 cGy per day isodose contour. **C:** Isodose contours showing a relatively homogeneous dose distribution. The patient received 2,500 cGy prescribed to the 1,000 cGy per day isodose line.

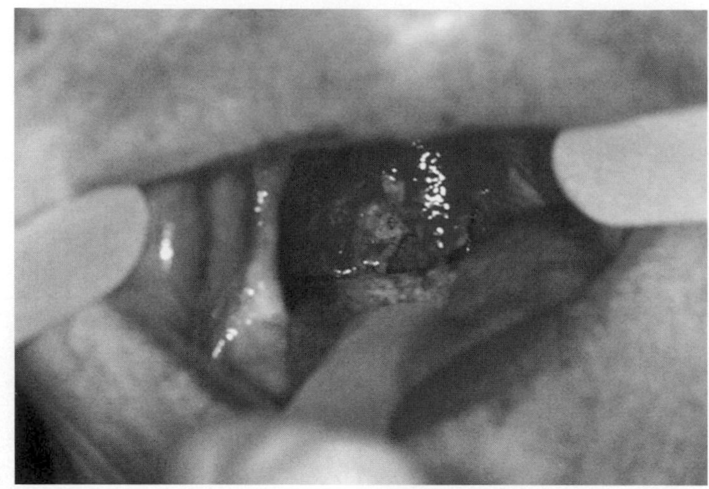

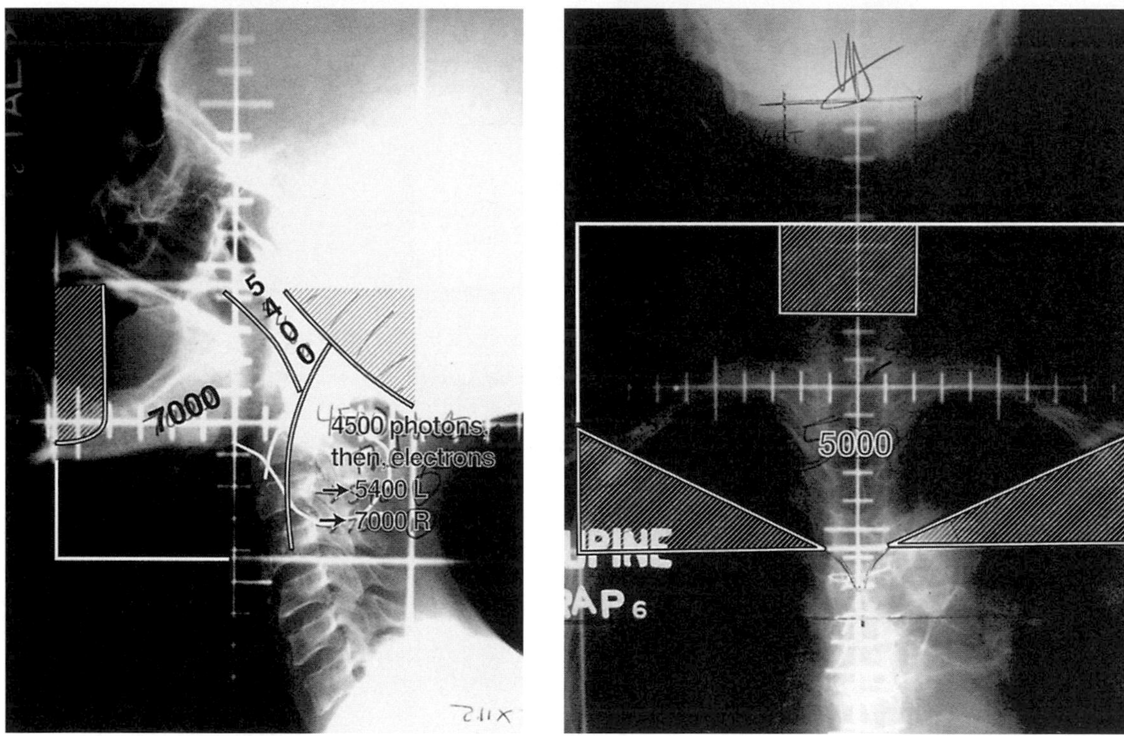

Figure 17.35 Technique for treating carcinoma of the soft palate. This patient had a T3N1M0 squamous cell carcinoma of the soft palate. She had a right neck node enclosed in wire. She was treated with definitive radiation therapy. **A:** This is a photograph of her lesion prior to therapy. It involves the medial right soft palate extending into the uvula. **B:** The patient was treated with opposed lateral fields to the primary site and upper neck. She was treated with 180 cGy per fraction. After 4,500 cGy, the spinal cord was blocked. The primary site, retropharyngeal nodes, and upper neck nodes were treated to 5,400 cGy. The boost field includes the primary site alone. This patient was treated with a concomitant boost technique. Therefore, the boost field was treated as a second daily fraction during weeks 5 and 6 of the radiation therapy. The timing of the second daily fraction was 5 to 6 hours after the morning fraction. A dose of 160 cGy was used for the afternoon fraction, thus giving a total dose of 7,000 cGy in 6 weeks to the primary site, as well as the uninvolved right neck, including the right posterior neck. The entire upper neck was included in the field due to concern about small nodes on the computed tomogram that were not definitely palpable. For the posterior neck, after the spinal cord block is added and appropriate energy electron fields are used. The posterior necks were treated to 5,400 cGy on the clinically negative left side, and to 7,000 cGy on the clinically positive right side. **C:** The low neck field was treated to 5,000 cGy in 5 weeks. Blocks were placed to protect the spinal cord and larynx in the upper midline. Infraclavicular blocks were also placed to shield the underlying lung tissue.

SURGICAL APPROACHES FOR THE RESECTION OF TUMORS OF THE OROPHARYNX

Roy B. Sessions

Tumors of the oropharynx often require either a mandibulotomy or a pharyngotomy for adequate surgical exposure. Resection of tumors of this region is technically challenging and, even when properly performed, can result in serious morbidity associated with swallowing disability and aspiration. These resections may jeopardize the integrity of the lingual arteries, the hypoglossal nerves, or both, and thus endanger the viability and function of the remaining tongue.

The first step in the surgical procedure consists of securing the airway. A tracheostomy using local anesthesia is preferable because instrumental trauma can cause tumor bleeding and difficult intubation. Before selecting the exact approach, the surgeon should carefully access the posterior, anterior, and lateral extent of the tumor. Those that are clearly anterior to the valleculae and tumors of the posterior oropharyngeal wall may be resected through a transhyoid pharyngotomy. Otherwise, a lateral pharyngotomy is a safer route to approach the pharynx, provided the tumor is at or near the midline and does not extend laterally into the glossopharyngeal fold or the lateral pharyngeal wall. When the lateral extent of the tumor is questionable, a mandibulotomy and "mandibular swing" may be necessary to adequately expose the tumor.

The surgical procedure illustrated in Figure 17.36A demonstrates an approach to the right side of the pharynx. This illustration shows a completed neck dissection and the pertinent neurovascular structures in the area where the pharyngotomy is to be performed. The hypoglossal nerve is mobilized and retracted upward and the superior laryngeal nerve retracted downward. Figure 17.36B demonstrates the pharyngeal entry through a vertical incision that is placed between those two nerves. Palpation of the base of the tongue with the index finger ensures proper placement of the pharyngotomy in the lateral pharyngeal wall and grossly away from the tumor. At this point, it may be necessary to remove a lateral segment of the hyoid bone. The pharyngotomy is extended superiorly and inferiorly, with the base of the tongue and the tumor under direct vision. Additional exposure may be gained by extending the pharyngotomy through the glossopharyngeal and glossopalatine folds and into the lateral floor of the mouth (Fig. 17.36C).

With the tumor adequately exposed, the resection proceeds, leaving around it a margin of grossly normal tissue. Closure of the surgical defect is not begun until all the margins have been examined by frozen section. In most instances, primary closure can be easily accomplished. Otherwise, a pectoralis muscle flap or a free flap transfer are used. If the lateral pharyngotomy approach does not afford adequate exposure of the base of the tongue and the tumor, a mandibular split with "swing" approach may be necessary. In that circumstance, the superior flap is divided in the midline and the incision is extended up through the lower lip. At either the mandibular midline or a point 3 cm lateral to the midline, an osteotomy is performed, and then the alveolar ridge mucosa is incised posteriorly. The mandible is then retracted or "swung" laterally and superiorly. The base of the tongue, valleculae, and the epiglottis are thus exposed, and with the tumor now under direct vision, its excision proceeds as is shown in Figure 17.37A.

After the adequacy of the margins of resection are confirmed by histologic examination, the surgical defect is repaired primarily (Fig. 17.37B), and the osteotomy is stabilized with appropriate plates and screws.

In cases in which the tumor extends laterally and involves the mandible, a composite resection that includes mandible may be necessary (Fig. 17.37C).

Retropharyngeal Node Dissection

Metastases to the retropharyngeal lymph nodes can occur from carcinomas of the oropharynx, particularly those arising from the tonsil and the lateral and posterior oropharyngeal walls. Therefore, when these tumors are treated surgically, it is advisable to remove the retropharyngeal fat pad and nodes on one or both sides. The technique of elective removal of these nodes is relatively simple. After the neck dissection is completed, and often after the primary tumor has been excised, the retropharyngeal space is exposed by either retracting or dividing the posterior belly of the digastric muscle and, to a variable extent, the styloid muscles (Fig. 17.38). The identification of the internal carotid artery and the cervical sympathetic chain are critical to performing this operation safely. The fascia is incised medially to the carotid bifurcation and a thin retropharyngeal fat pad is easily identified. This pad contains one to three lymph nodes scattered between the level of the carotid bifurcation and the base of the skull. The medial extent of the pad is usually readily identifiable and thus is easily dissected free. Laterally, it is somewhat less defined, and therefore, the surgeon must follow the internal carotid artery and cervical sympathetic chain, as the dissection proceeds superiorly. The superior cut is best done from lateral to medial to avoid injury to the carotid artery.

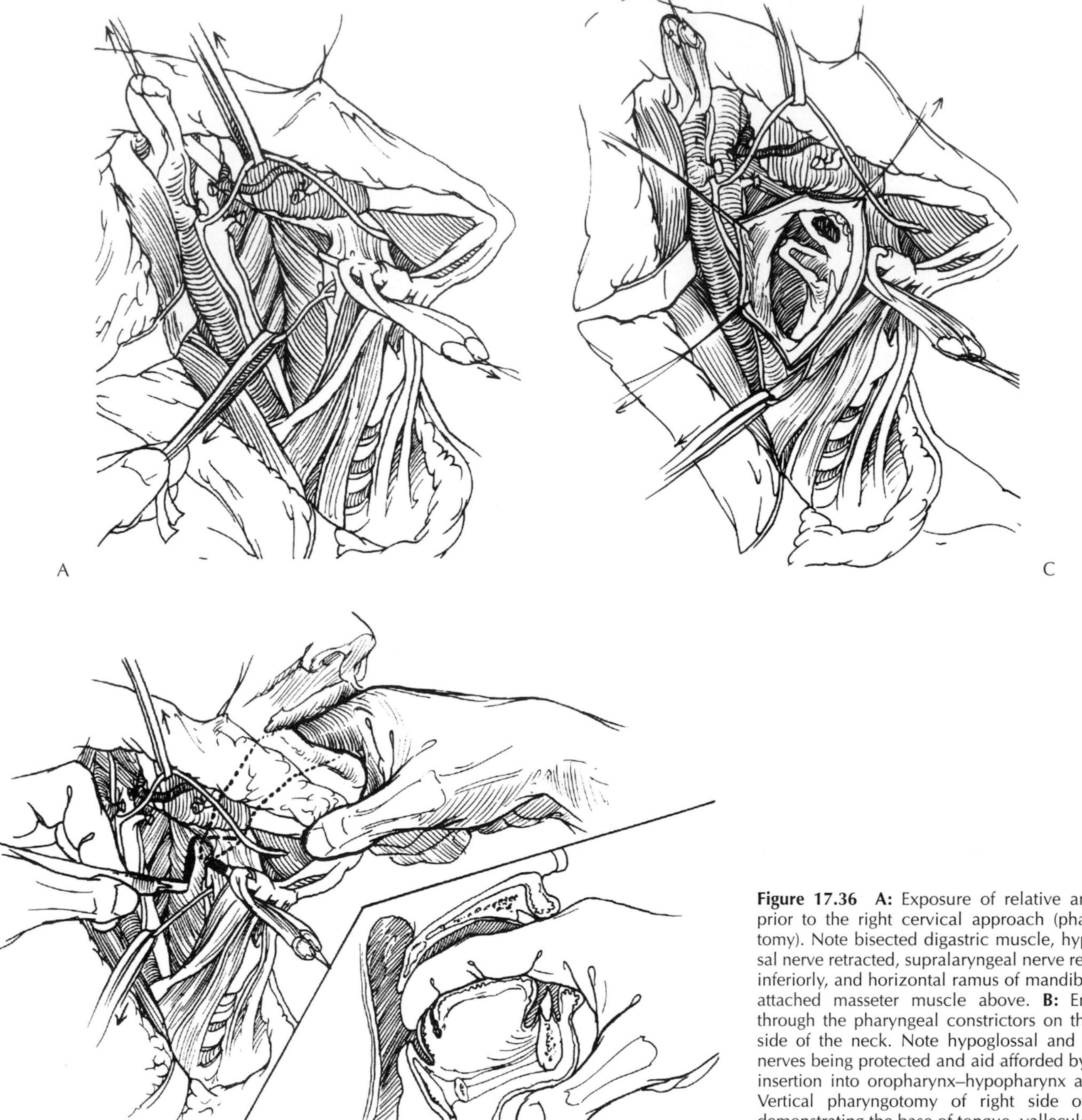

Figure 17.36 **A:** Exposure of relative anatomy prior to the right cervical approach (pharyngotomy). Note bisected digastric muscle, hypoglossal nerve retracted, supralaryngeal nerve retracted inferiorly, and horizontal ramus of mandible with attached masseter muscle above. **B:** Entrance through the pharyngeal constrictors on the right side of the neck. Note hypoglossal and lingual nerves being protected and aid afforded by finger insertion into oropharynx–hypopharynx area. **C:** Vertical pharyngotomy of right side of neck demonstrating the base of tongue, valleculae, and epiglottis thus exposed.

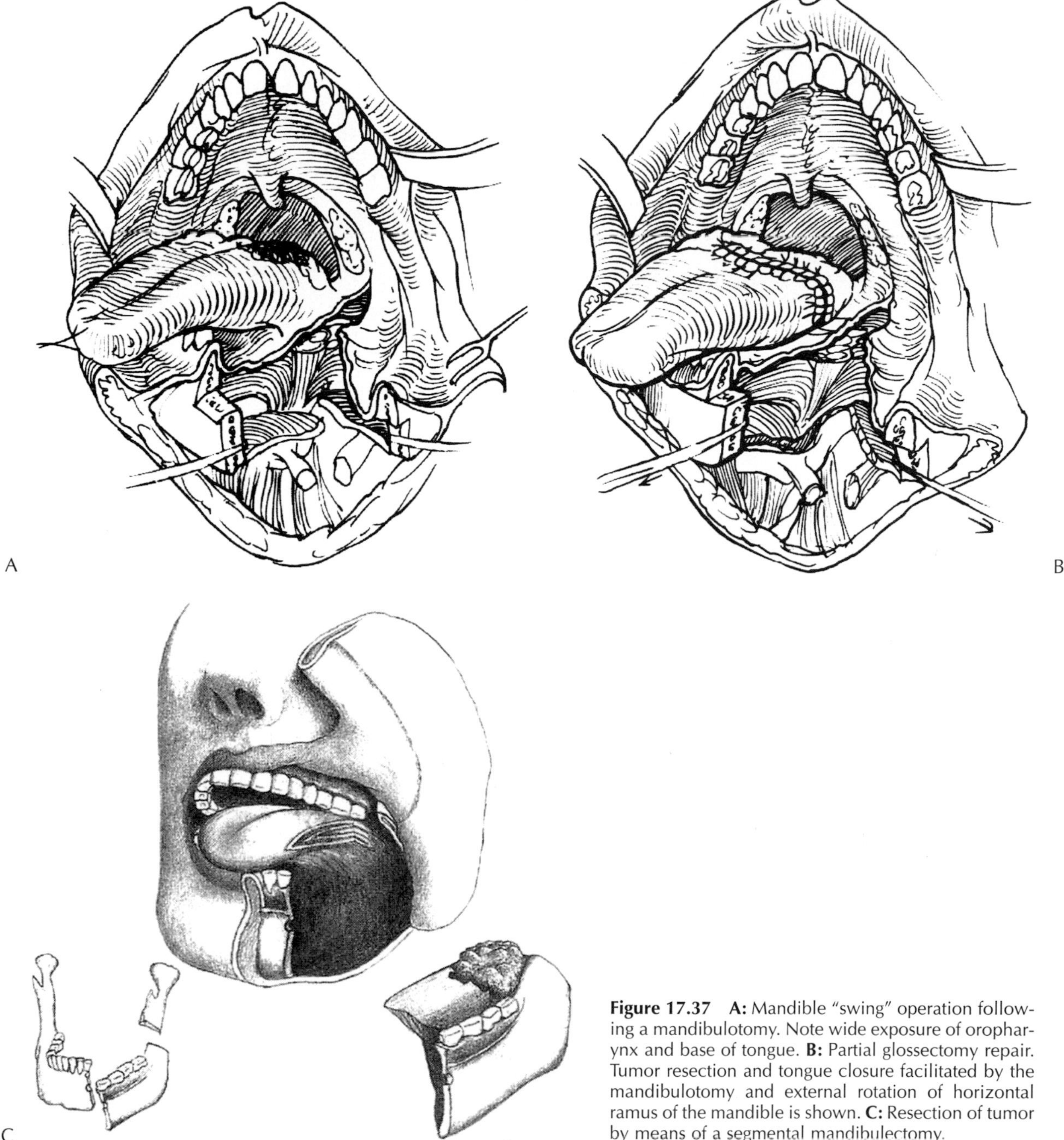

Figure 17.37 **A:** Mandible "swing" operation following a mandibulotomy. Note wide exposure of oropharynx and base of tongue. **B:** Partial glossectomy repair. Tumor resection and tongue closure facilitated by the mandibulotomy and external rotation of horizontal ramus of the mandible is shown. **C:** Resection of tumor by means of a segmental mandibulectomy.

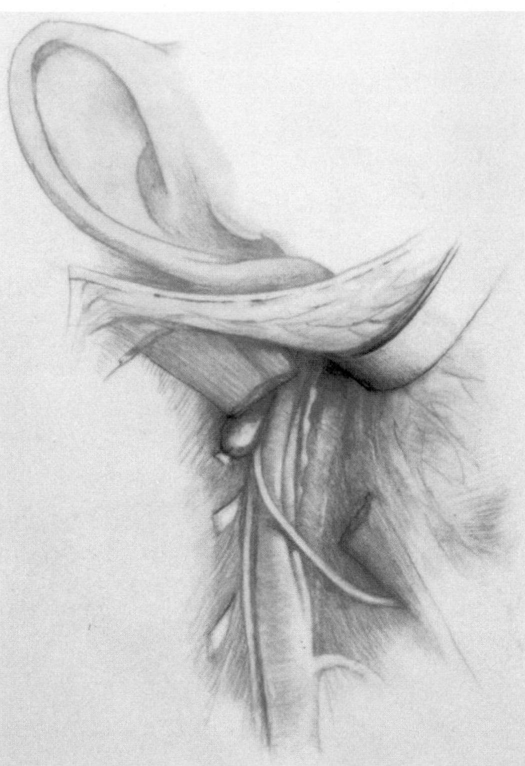

Figure 17.38 Retropharyngeal node dissection of right side. Note past neck dissection status and carotid bifurcation and diagastric muscle.

REFERENCES

1. Wingo PA, Tong T, Bolden S. Cancer statistics, 1996. *CA Cancer J Clin* 1996; 46:5–27.
2. Rouviere H. *Anatomy of the human lymphatic system.* Ann Arbor, MI: Edwards Brothers, 1938.
3. Fisch UP. Cervical lymphography in cases of laryngopharyngeal carcinoma. *J Laryngol Otol* 1964;78:715–726.
4. Haagensen CD, et al. *The lymphatics in cancer.* Philadelphia: WB Saunders, 1972.
5. Candela FC, Kothari K, Shah JP. Patterns of cervical node metastases from squamous carcinoma of the oropharynx and hypopharynx. *Head Neck* 1990; 12:197–203.
6. Lindberg R. Distribution of cervical lymph node metastases from squamous cell carcinoma of the upper respiratory and digestive tracts. *Cancer* 1972;29:1446–1449.
7. Crawford BE, Callihan MD, Corio RL, et al. Oral pathology. *Otolaryngol Clin North Am* 1979;12:29–43.
8. Low WK, Sng I, Balakrishnan A. Palatine tonsillar metastasis from carcinoma of the colon. *J Laryngol Otol* 1994;108:449–451.
9. Mochimatsu I, Tsukuda M, Furukawa S, et al. Tumours metastasizing to the head and neck—a report of seven cases [Review]. *J Laryngol Otol* 1993;107: 1171–1173.
10. Tesei F, Farneti G, Cavicchi O, et al. A case of Merkel-cell carcinoma metastatic to the tonsil. *J Laryngol Otol* 1992;106:1100–1102.
11. Asami K, Yokoi H, Hattori T, et al. Metastatic gall bladder carcinoma of the palatine tonsil [Review]. *J Laryngol Otol* 1989;103:211–213.
12. Johnson J. Oropharynx. In: Gluckman JL, Gullane P, Johnson J, eds. *Practical approach to head and neck tumors.* New York: Raven Press, 1995:91–104.
13. Boffetta P, Mashberg A, Winkelmann R, et al. Carcinogenic effect of tobacco smoking and alcohol drinking on anatomic sites of the oral cavity and oropharynx. *Int J Cancer* 1992;52:530–533.
14. Perez CA, Purdy JA, Breaux SR, et al. Carcinoma of the tonsillar fossa: a nonrandomized comparison of preoperative radiation and surgery or irradiation alone: long-term results. *Cancer* 1982;50:2314–2322.
15. Shugar MA, Nosal P, Gavron JP. Technique for routine screening for carcinoma of the base of tongue. *J Am Dent Assoc* 1982;104:646–647.
16. Brownian GP, Wong G, Hodson I, et al. Influence of cigarette smoking on the efficacy of radiation therapy in head and neck cancer [see Comments]. *N Engl J Med* 1993;328:159–163.
17. Mashberg A, Meyers H. Anatomical site and size of 222 early asymptomatic oral squamous cell carcinomas: a continuing prospective study of oral cancer: II. *Cancer* 1976;37:2149–2157.
18. Mashberg A, Samit AM. Early diagnosis of asymptomatic oral and oropharyngeal squamous cancers. *CA Cancer J Clin* 1995;45:328–351.
19. Shaha AR, Shah JP. Biopsy techniques in head and neck. *Surg Oncol Clin North Am* 1995;4:15–28.
20. Greene F, Page D, Fleming I, et al. *AJCC cancer staging manual,* 6th ed. New York: Springer-Verlag, 2002.
21. Amdur RJ, Mendenhall WM, Parsons JT, et al. Carcinoma of the soft palate treated with irradiation: analysis of results and complications. *Radiother Oncol* 1987;9: 185–194.
22. Calais G, et al. Randomized trial of radiation therapy versus concomitant chemotherapy and radiation therapy for advanced-stage oropharynx carcinoma. *J Natl Cancer Inst* 1999; 91:2081–2016.
23. Calais G, et al. [Stage III and IV cancers of the oropharynx: results of a randomized study of Gortec comparing radiotherapy alone with concomitant chemotherapy]. *Bull Cancer* 2000;87:48–53.
24. Calais G, et al. Radiation (RT) alone versus RT with concomitant chemotherapy (CT) in stages III and IV oropharynx carcinoma. Final results of the 94-01 GORTEC randomized study. *Int J Radiat Oncol Biol Phys* 2001;51[3, Suppl 1]:1.
25. Har-El G, Shaha A, Chaudry R, et al. Carcinoma of the uvula and midline soft palate: indication for neck treatment. *Head Neck* 1992;14:99–101.
26. Mazeron JJ, Marinello G, Crook J, et al. Definitive radiation treatment for early stage carcinoma of the soft palate and uvula: the indications for iridium 192 implantation. *Int J Radiat Oncol Biol Phys* 1987;13:1829–1837.
27. Weber RS, Peters LJ, Wolf P, et al. Squamous cell carcinoma of the soft palate, uvula, and anterior faucial pillar. *Otolaryngol Head Neck Surg* 1988;99:16–23.
28. Esche BA, Haie CM, Gerbaulet AP, et al. Interstitial and external radiotherapy in carcinoma of the soft palate and uvula. *Int J Radiat Oncol Biol Phys* 1988;15: 619–625.
29. Mazeron JJ, Crook J, Martin M, et al. Iridium 192 implantation of squamous cell carcinomas of the oropharynx [Review]. *Am J Otolaryngol* 1989;10: 317–321.
30. Pernot M, Malissard L, Taghian A, et al. Velotonsillar squamous cell carcinoma: 277 cases treated by combined external irradiation and brachytherapy—results according to extension, localization, and dose rate. *Int J Radiat Oncol Biol Phys* 1992;23:715–723.
31. Levendag PC, et al. Fractionated high-dose-rate and pulsed-dose-rate brachytherapy: first clinical experience in squamous cell carcinoma of the tonsillar fossa and soft palate. *Int J Radiat Oncol Biol Phys* 1997;38:497–506.
32. Maulard C, Housset M, Delanian S, et al. Salvage split course brachytherapy for tonsil and soft palate carcinoma: treatment techniques and results. *Laryngoscope* 1994;104:359–363.
33. Million RR. Squamous cell carcinoma of the head and neck: combined therapy: surgery and post-operative irradiation. *Int J Radiat Oncol Biol Phys* 1979;5:2161–2162.
34. Foote RL, et al. Tonsil cancer. Patterns of failure after surgery alone and surgery combined with postoperative radiation therapy. *Cancer* 1994;73: 2638–2647.
35. Perez CA, et al. Carcinoma of the tonsillar fossa: prognostic factors and long-term therapy outcome. *Int J Radiat Oncol Biol Phys* 1998;42:1077–1084.
36. Remmler D, Medina JE, Byers RM, et al. Treatment of choice for squamous carcinoma of the tonsillar fossa. *Head Neck Surg* 1985;7:206–211.
37. Weichert KA, Aron B, Maltz R, et al. Carcinoma of the tonsil: treatment by a planned combination of radiation and surgery. *Int J Radiat Oncol Biol Phys* 1976;1:505–508.
38. Gehanno P, Depondt J, Guedon C, et al. Primary and salvage surgery for cancer of the tonsillar region: a retrospective study of 120 patients [see Comments]. *Head Neck* 1993;15:185–189.
39. Mendenhall WM, et al. Radiation therapy for squamous cell carcinoma of the tonsillar region: a preferred alternative to surgery? *J Clin Oncol* 2000;18: 2219–2225.
40. Hicks WL Jr, et al. Surgery versus radiation therapy as single-modality treatment of tonsillar fossa carcinoma: the Roswell Park Cancer Institute experience (1971–1991). *Laryngoscope* 1998;108:1014–1019.
41. Mizono GS, et al. Carcinoma of the tonsillar region. *Laryngoscope* 1986;96: 240–244.
42. Pernot M, et al. Role of interstitial brachytherapy in oral and oropharyngeal carcinoma: reflection of a series of 1344 patients treated at the time of initial presentation. *Otolaryngol Head Neck Surg* 1996;115:519–526.
43. Bataini JP, Asselain B, Jaulerry C, et al. A multivariate primary tumour control analysis in 465 patients treated by radical radiotherapy for cancer of the tonsillar region: clinical and treatment parameters as prognostic factors [see Comments]. *Radiother Oncol* 1989; 14:265–277.
44. Wong CS, et al. Definitive radiotherapy for squamous cell carcinoma of the tonsillar fossa. *Int J Radiat Oncol Biol Phys* 1989;16:657–662.
45. Amornmarn R, et al. Radiation management of carcinoma of the tonsillar region. *Cancer* 1984;54:1293–1299.
46. Gwozdz JT, et al. Concomitant boost radiotherapy for squamous carcinoma of the tonsillar fossa. *Int J Radiat Oncol Biol Phys* 1997;39:127–135.
47. Gluckman JL, Black RJ, Crissman JD. Cancer of the oropharynx. *Otolaryngol Clin North Am* 1985;18:451–459.
48. Givens CD Jr, Johns ME, Cantrell RW. Carcinoma of the tonsil. Analysis of 162 cases. *Arch Otolaryngol* 1981;107:730–734.
49. Rabuzzi DD, et al. Treatment results of combined high-dose preoperative radiotherapy and surgery for oropharyngeal cancer. *Laryngoscope* 1982;92: 989–992.
50. Garrett PG, et al. Carcinoma of the tonsil: the effect of dose-time-volume factors on local control. *Int J Radiat Oncol Biol Phys* 1985;11:703–706.
51. Garrett PG, Beale FA, Cummings BL, et al. Cancer of the tonsil: results of radical radiation therapy with surgery in reserve. *Am J Surg* 1983;146:432–435.
52. Shukovsky LJ, Fletcher GH. Time-dose and tumor volume relationships in the irradiation of squamous cell carcinoma of the tonsillar fossa. *Radiology* 1973;107:621–626.
53. Eisbruch A, et al. Xerostomia and its predictors following parotid-sparing irradiation of head-and-neck cancer. *Int J Radiat Oncol Biol Phys* 2001;50:695–704.
54. O'Sullivan B, et al. The benefits and pitfalls of ipsilateral radiotherapy in carcinoma of the tonsillar region. *Int J Radiat Oncol Biol Phys* 2001;51:332–343.
55. Jackson SM, et al. Cancer of the tonsil: the results of ipsilateral radiation treatment. *Radiother Oncol* 1999;51:123–128.
56. Pernot M, Luporsi E, Hoffstetter S, et al. Complications following definitive irradiation for cancers of the oral cavity and the oropharynx (in a series of 1134 patients). *Int J Radiat Oncol Biol Phys* 1997;37:577–585.
57. Mazeron JJ, Belkacemi Y, Simon JM, et al. Place of iridium 192 implantation in definitive irradiation of faucial arch squamous cell carcinomas. *Int J Radiat Oncol Biol Phys* 1993;27:251–257.
58. Rudoltz MS, et al. High-dose-rate brachytherapy for primary carcinomas of the oral cavity and oropharynx. *Laryngoscope* 1999;109:1967–1973.
59. Mendenhall WM, Parsons JT, Cassisi NJ, et al. Squamous cell carcinoma of the tonsillar area treated with radical irradiation. *Radiother Oncol* 1987;10: 23–30.
60. Kaplan R, Million RR, Cassisi NJ. Carcinoma of the tonsil: results of radical irradiation with surgery reserved for radiation failure. *Laryngoscope* 1977;87: 600–607.
61. Dasmahapatra KS, Mohit-Tabatabai MA, Rush BF Jr, et al. Cancer of the tonsil. Improved survival with combination therapy. *Cancer* 1986;57:451–455.
62. Zelefsky MJ, Harrison LB, Armstrong JG. Long-term treatment results of postoperative radiation therapy for advanced stage oropharyngeal carcinoma. *Cancer* 1992;70:2388–2395.
63. Perez CA, Carmichael T, Devineni VR, et al. Carcinoma of the tonsillar fossa: a nonrandomized comparison of irradiation alone or combined with surgery: long-term results. *Head Neck* 1991;13:282–290.
64. Spiro JD, Spiro RH. Carcinoma of the tonsillar fossa. An update. *Arch Otolaryngol Head Neck Surg* 1989;115:1186–1189.
65. Quenelle DJ, Crissman JD, Shumrick DA. Tonsil carcinoma—treatment results. *Laryngoscope* 1979;89:1842–1846.
66. Puthawala AA, Syed AM, Gates TC. Iridium-192 implants in the treatment of tonsillar region malignancies. *Arch Otolaryngol* 1985;111:812–815.
67. Leborgne JH, Leborgne F, Barlocci LA, et al. The place of brachytherapy in

the treatment of carcinoma of the tonsil with lingual extension. *Int J Radiat Oncol Biol Phys* 1986;12:1787–1792.
68. Peiffert D, Pernot M, Malissard L, et al. Salvage irradiation by brachytherapy of velotonsillar squamous cell carcinoma in a previously irradiated field: results in 73 cases [see Comments]. *Int J Radiat Oncol Biol Phys* 1994;29: 681–686.
69. Goffinet DR, Fee WE Jr, Wells J, et al. 192Ir pharyngoepiglottic fold interstitial implants. The key to successful treatment of base tongue carcinoma by radiation therapy. *Cancer* 1985;55:941–948.
70. Housset M, Baillet F, Dessard-Diana B, et al. A retrospective study of three treatment techniques for T1-T2 base of tongue lesions: surgery plus postoperative radiation, external radiation plus interstitial implantation and external radiation alone. *Int J Radiat Oncol Biol Phys* 1987;13:511–516.
71. Andersen PE, Shah JP, Cambronero E, et al. The role of comprehensive neck dissection with preservation of the spinal accessory nerve in the clinically positive neck. *Am J Surg* 1994;168:499–502.
72. Spiro RH, Gerold FP, Strong EW. Mandibular "swing" approach for oral and oropharyngeal tumors. *Head Neck Surg* 1981;3:371–378.
73. Shike M, Bemer YN, Gerdes H, et al. Percutaneous endoscopic gastrostomy and jejunostomy for long-term feeding in patients with cancer of the head and neck. *Otolaryngol Head Neck Surg* 1989;101:549–554.
74. Byrd SE, Richardson M, Gil G, et al. The spread of carcinoma of the base of the tongue as detected by computer tomography. *Rev Laryngol Otol Rhinol (Bord)* 1983;104:247–250.
75. Vikram B. Importance of the time interval between surgery and postoperative radiation therapy in the combined management of head and neck cancer. *Int J Radiat Oncol Biol Phys* 1979;5:1837–1840.
76. Schiff PB, Harrison LB, Strong EW et al. Impact of the time interval between surgery and postoperative radiation therapy on locoregional control in advanced head and neck cancer. *J Surg Oncol* 1990;43:203–208.
77. Bastit L, et al., Influence of the delay of adjuvant postoperative radiation therapy on relapse and survival in oropharyngeal and hypopharyngeal cancers. *Int J Radiat Oncol Biol Phys* 2001;49:139–146.
78. Ang KK, et al., Randomized trial addressing risk features and time factors of surgery plus radiotherapy in advanced head-and-neck cancer. *Int J Radiat Oncol Biol Phys* 2001; 51:571–578.
79. Hinerman RW, Parsons JT, Mendenhall WM, et al. External beam irradiation alone or combined with neck dissection for base of tongue carcinoma: an alternative to primary surgery. *Laryngoscope* 1994;104:1466–1470.
79a. Dupont JB, Guillamondegui OM, Jesse RH. Surgical treatment of advanced carcinomas of the base of tongue. *Am J Surg* 1978;136:501–503.
80. Harrison LB, Zelefsky MJ, Sessions RB, et al. Base-of-tongue cancer treated with external beam irradiation plus brachytherapy: oncologic and functional outcome. *Radiology* 1992;184:267–270.
81. Harrison LB, Lee H, Kraus DH, et al. Long term results of primary radiation therapy for squamous cancer of the base of tongue. *Radiother Oncol* 1996;39: S6(abst).
82. Harrison LB, Sessions RB, Strong EW, et al. Brachytherapy as part of the definitive management of squamous cancer of the base of tongue. *Int J Radiat Oncol Biol Phys* 1989;17:1309–1312.
83. Harrison LB, Kraus DH, Zelefsky MJ, et al. Long term results of primary radiation therapy for squamous cell cancer of the base of tongue. *Proc Int Mtg Head Neck Cancer* 1996;71(abst).
84. Puthawala AA, Syed AM, Eads DL, et al. Limited external beam and interstitial 192iridium irradiation in the treatment of carcinoma of the base of the tongue: a ten year experience. *Int J Radiat Oncol Biol Phys* 1988;14:839–848.
85. Crook J, Mazeron JJ, Marinello G, et al. Combined external irradiation and interstitial implantation for T1 and T2 epidermoid carcinomas of base of tongue: the Creteil experience (1971–1981). *Int J Radiat Oncol Biol Phys* 1988;15:105–114.
86. Kramer S, Gelber RD, Snow JB, et al. Combined radiation therapy and surgery in the management of advanced head and neck cancer: final report of study 73-03 of the Radiation Therapy Oncology Group. *Head Neck Surg* 1987;10:19–30.
87. Vandenbrouck C, Sancho H, LeFur R, et al. Results of a randomized clinical trial of preoperative irradiation versus postoperative in treatment of tumors of the hypopharynx. *Cancer* 1977;39:1445–1449.
88. Withers HR, et al, Local control of carcinoma of the tonsil by radiation therapy: an analysis of patterns of fractionation in nine institutions. *Int J Radiat Oncol Biol Phys* 1995;33:549–562.
89. Peters LJ, Goepfert H, Ang KK, et al. Evaluation of the dose for postoperative radiation therapy of head and neck cancer: first report of a prospective randomized trial [see Comments]. *Int J Radiat Oncol Biol Phys* 1993;26:3–11.
90. Bernier J, et al. Chemoradiotherapy as compared to radiotherapy alone significantly increases disease-free and OS in head and neck cancer patients after surgery: results of EORTC phase III trial 22931. *Int J Radiat Oncol Biol Phys* 2001;51[3, Suppl 1]: 1.
91. Pradhan SA, Rajpal RM, Kothary PM. Surgical management of postradiation residual/recurrent cancer of the base of the tongue. *J Surg Oncol* 1980; 14:201–206.
92. Langlois D, Hoffstetter S, Malissard L, et al. Salvage irradiation of oropharynx and mobile tongue about 192 iridium brachytherapy in Centre Alexis Vautrin. *Int J Radiat Oncol Biol Phys* 1988;14:849–853.
93. Mazeron JJ, Langlois D, Glaubiger D, et al. Salvage irradiation of oropharyngeal cancers using iridium 192 wire implants: 5-year results of 70 cases. *Int J Radiat Oncol Biol Phys* 1987;13:957–962.
94. Housset M, Baillet F, Delanian S, et al. Split course interstitial brachytherapy with a source shift: the results of a new iridium implant technique versus single course implants for salvage irradiation of base of tongue cancers in 55 patients. *Int J Radiat Oncol Biol Phys* 1991;20:965–971.
95. Spiro RH, Kelly J, Vega AL, et al. Squamous carcinoma of the posterior pharyngeal wall. *Am J Surg* 1990;160:420–423.
96. Spiro RH, Bains MS, Shah JP, et al. Gastric transposition for head and neck cancer: a critical update. *Am J Surg* 1991;162:348–352.
97. Michiwaki Y, Schmelzeisen R, Hacki T, et al. Functional effects of a free jejunum flap used for reconstruction in the oropharyngeal region. *J Craniomaxillofac Surg* 1993;21:153–156.
98. Fein DA, Mendenhall WM, Parsons JT, et al. Pharyngeal wall carcinoma treated with radiotherapy: impact of treatment technique and fractionation. *Int J Radiat Oncol Biol Phys* 1993;26:751–757.
99. Grimard L, Szanto J, Girard A, et al. Asymmetric arc technique for posterior pharyngeal wall and retropharyngeal space tumors. *Int J Radiat Oncol Biol Phys* 1995;31:611–615.
100. Guillamondegui OM, Meoz R, Jesse RE. Surgical treatment of squamous cell carcinoma of the pharyngeal walls. *Am J Surg* 1978;136:474–476.
101. Meoz-Mendez RT, Fletcher GH, Guillamondegui OM, et al. Analysis of the results of irradiation in the treatment of squamous cell carcinomas of the pharyngeal walls. *Int J Radiat Oncol Biol Phys* 1978;4:579–585.
102. Marks JE, Freeman RB, Lee F, et al. Pharyngeal wall cancer: an analysis of treatment results, complications, and patterns of failure. *Int J Radiat Oncol Biol Phys* 1978;4:587–593.
103. Marks JE, Smith PG, Sessions DG. Pharyngeal wall cancer. A reappraisal after comparison of treatment methods. *Arch Otolaryngol* 1985;111:79–85.
104. Son YH, Kacinski BM. Therapeutic concepts of brachytherapy/megavoltage in sequence for pharyngeal wall cancers. Results of integrated dose therapy. *Cancer* 1987;59:1268–1273.
105. The Department of Veterans Affairs Laryngeal Cancer Study Group. Induction chemotherapy plus radiation compared with surgery plus radiation in patients with advanced laryngeal cancer. *N Engl J Med* 1991;324:1685–1690.
106. Spaulding MB, Fischer SG, Wolf GT. The Department of Veterans Affairs Cooperative Laryngeal Cancer Study Group. Tumor response, toxicity, and survival after neoadjuvant organ-preserving chemotherapy for advanced laryngeal carcinoma. *J Clin Oncol* 1994;12:1592–1599.
107. Domenge C, et al. Randomized trial of neoadjuvant chemotherapy in oropharyngeal carcinoma. French Groupe d'Etude des Tumeurs de la Tete et du Cou (GETTEC). *Br J Cancer* 2000;83:1594–1598.
108. Forastiere AA, et al., Phase III trial to preserve the larynx: induction chemotherapy and radiotherapy versus concomitant chemoradiotherapy versus radiotherapy alone, Intergroup Trial R91-11. *Proc ASCO* 2001;20:2a.
109. Pignon JP, Bourhis J. Meta-analysis of chemotherapy in head and neck cancer: individual patient data vs. literature data. *Br J Cancer* 1995;72:1062–1063.
110. Pignon JP, et al. Chemotherapy added to locoregional treatment for head and neck squamous-cell carcinoma: three meta-analyses of updated individual data. MACH-NC Collaborative Group. Meta-Analysis of Chemotherapy on Head and Neck Cancer. *Lancet* 2000;355:949–955.
111. El-Sayed S, Nelson N. Adjuvant and adjunctive chemotherapy in the management of squamous cell carcinoma of the head and neck region. A meta-analysis of prospective and randomized trials. *J Clin Oncol* 1996;14:838–847.
112. Munro AJ. An overview of randomised controlled trials of adjuvant chemotherapy in head and neck cancer. *Br J Cancer* 1995;71:83–91.
113. Ang KK, Peters LJ, Weber RS, et al. Concomitant boost radiotherapy schedules in the treatment of carcinoma of the oropharynx and nasopharynx. *Int J Radiat Oncol Biol Phys* 1990;19:1339–1345.
114. Wang CC. Local control of oropharyngeal carcinoma after two accelerated hyperfractionation radiation therapy schemes. *Int J Radiat Oncol Biol Phys* 1988;14:1143–1146.
115. Ang KK. Altered fractionation trials in head and neck cancer. *Semin Radiat Oncol* 1998;8:230–236.
116. Cummings BJ. Benefits of accelerated hyperfractionation for head and neck cancer. *Acta Oncol* 1999;38:131–136.
117. Million RR, Parsons JT, Cassisi NJ. Twice-a-day irradiation technique for squamous cell carcinomas of the head and neck. *Cancer* 1985;55 (Suppl):2096–2099.
118. Fu KK, et al. A Radiation Therapy Oncology Group (RTOG) phase III randomized study to compare hyperfractionation and two variants of accelerated fractionation to standard fractionation radiotherapy for head and neck squamous cell carcinomas: first report of RTOG 9003. *Int J Radiat Oncol Biol Phys* 2000;48:7–16.
119. Horiot JC, et al. Hyperfractionation versus conventional fractionation in oropharyngeal carcinoma: final analysis of a randomized trial of the EORTC cooperative group of radiotherapy. *Radiother Oncol* 1992;25:231–241.
120. Harrison LB, et al. A prospective phase II trial of concomitant chemotherapy and radiotherapy with delayed accelerated fractionation in unresectable tumors of the head and neck. *Head Neck* 1998;20:497–503.
121. Bieri S, et al. Concomitant boost radiotherapy in oropharynx carcinomas. *Acta Oncol* 1998;37:687–691.
122. Nathu RM, et al. Induction chemotherapy and radiation therapy for T4 oropharyngeal carcinoma. *Radiat Oncol Invest* 1999;7:98–105.
123. Vokes EE, et al. Induction chemotherapy followed by concomitant chemoradiotherapy for advanced head and neck cancer: impact on the natural history of the disease. *J Clin Oncol* 1995;13:876–883.
124. Kies MS, et al. Induction chemotherapy followed by concurrent chemoradi-

ation for advanced head and neck cancer: improved disease control and survival. *J Clin Oncol* 1998;16:2715–2721.
125. Bensadoun RJ, et al. Concomitant b.i.d. radiotherapy and chemotherapy with cisplatin and 5-fluorouracil in unresectable squamous-cell carcinoma of the pharynx: clinical and pharmacological data of a French multicenter phase II study. *Int J Radiat Oncol Biol Phys* 1998;42:237–245.
126. Machtay M, et al. Pilot study of organ preservation multimodality therapy for locally advanced resectable oropharyngeal carcinoma. *Am J Clin Oncol* 2000;23: 509–515.
127. Giralt JL, et al. Preoperative induction chemotherapy followed by concurrent chemoradiotherapy in advanced carcinoma of the oral cavity and oropharynx. *Cancer* 2000; 89:939–945.
128. Brizel DM, et al. Hyperfractionated irradiation with or without concurrent chemotherapy for locally advanced head and neck cancer. *N Engl J Med* 1998;338:1798–804.
129. Jeremic B, et al. Hyperfractionated radiation therapy with or without concurrent low-dose daily cisplatin in locally advanced squamous cell carcinoma of the head and neck: a prospective randomized trial. *J Clin Oncol* 2000;18:1458–1464.
130. Staar S, et al. Intensified hyperfractionated accelerated radiotherapy limits the additional benefit of simultaneous chemotherapy—results of a multicentric randomized German trial in advanced head-and-neck cancer. *Int J Radiat Oncol Biol Phys* 2001;50:1161–1171.
131. Johansen LV, Grau C, Overgaard J. Squamous cell carcinoma of the oropharynx—an analysis of treatment results in 289 consecutive patients. *Acta Oncol* 2000;39:985–994.
132. Pameijer FA, et al. Can pretreatment computed tomography predict local control in T3 squamous cell carcinoma of the glottic larynx treated with definitive radiotherapy? *Int J Radiat Oncol Biol Phys* 1997;37:1011–21.
133. Pameijer FA, et al. Evaluation of pretreatment computed tomography as a predictor of local control in T1/T2 pyriform sinus carcinoma treated with definitive radiotherapy. *Head Neck* 1998;20:159–168.
134. Chua DT, et al. Volumetric analysis of tumor extent in nasopharyngeal carcinoma and correlation with treatment outcome. *Int J Radiat Oncol Biol Phys* 1997;39:711–719.
135. Hermans R, et al. The relation of CT-determined tumor parameters and local and regional outcome of tonsillar cancer after definitive radiation treatment. *Int J Radiat Oncol Biol Phys* 2001;50:37–45.
136. Nathu RM, et al. The impact of primary tumor volume on local control for oropharyngeal squamous cell carcinoma treated with radiotherapy. *Head Neck* 2000;22:1–5.
137. Aebersold DM, et al. Intratumoral microvessel density predicts local treatment failure of radically irradiated squamous cell cancer of the oropharynx. *Int J Radiat Oncol Biol Phys* 2000;48:17–25.
138. Grabenbauer GG, et al. Squamous cell carcinoma of the oropharynx: Ki-67 and p53 can identify patients at high risk for local recurrence after surgery and postoperative radiotherapy. *Int J Radiat Oncol Biol Phys* 2000;48:1041–1050.
139. Sittel C, et al. Ki-67 (MIB1), p53, and Lewis-X (LeuMI) as prognostic factors of recurrence in T1 and T2 laryngeal carcinoma. *Laryngoscope* 2000;110:1012–1017.
140. Jaskulski D, et al. Inhibition of cellular proliferation by antisense oligodeoxynucleotides to PCNA cyclin. *Science* 1988;240:1544–1546.
141. Nordsmark M, Overgard M, Overgaard J. Pretreatment oxygenation predicts radiation response in advanced squamous cell carcinoma treated by radiation therapy. *Radiother Oncol* 1996;41:31–39.
142. Nordsmark M, Overgard J. A confirmatory prognostic study on oxygenation status and loco-regional control in advanced head and neck squamous cell carcinoma treated by radiation therapy. *Radiother Oncol* 2000;57:39–43.
143. Brizel DM, et al. Tumor hypoxia adversely affects the prognosis of carcinoma of the head and neck. *Int J Radiat Oncol Biol Phys* 1997;38:285–289.
144. Vanselow B, et al. Oxygenation of advanced head and neck cancer: prognostic marker for the response to primary radiochemotherapy. *Otolaryngol Head Neck Surg* 2000;122:856–862.
145. Overgaard J, et al. A randomized double-blind phase III study of nimorazole as a hypoxic radiosensitizer of primary radiotherapy in supraglottic larynx and pharynx carcinoma. Results of the Danish Head and Neck Cancer Study (DAHANCA) Protocol 5-85. *Radiother Oncol* 1998;46:135–146.
146. Glaser CM, et al. Impact of hemoglobin level and use of recombinant erythropoietin on efficacy of preoperative chemoradiation therapy for squamous cell carcinoma of the oral cavity and oropharynx. *Int J Radiat Oncol Biol Phys* 2001;50:705–715.
147. Aebersold DM, et al. Expression of hypoxia-inducible factor-1 alpha: a novel predictive and prognostic parameter in the radiotherapy of oropharyngeal cancer. *Cancer Res* 2001;61:2911–2916.
148. Rhys Evans PH. Complications in head and neck surgery and how to avoid trouble [Review]. *J Laryngol Otol* 1989;1103:926–929.
149. Coleman JJ III. Complications in head and neck surgery [Review]. *Surg Clin North Am* 1986;66:1.49–167.
150. Sanders EM, Davis KR, Whelan CS, et al. Threatened carotid artery rupture: a complication of radical neck surgery. *J Surg Oncol* 1986;33:190–193.
151. Saunders JR Jr, Hirata RM, Jaques DA. Considering the spinal accessory nerve in head and neck surgery. *Am J Surg* 1985;150:491–494.
152. Logemann JA. Deglutition disorders in cancer of the head and neck. In: Kagan AR, Miles J, eds. *Head and neck oncology, clinical management.* New York: Pergamon Press, 1989:155–161.
153. Sassler AM, Esclamado RM, Wolf GT. Surgery after organ preservation therapy. Analysis of wound complications. *Arch Otolaryngol Head Neck Surg* 1995; 121:162–165.
154. Spanos WJ Jr, Shukovsky LJ, Fletcher GH. Time, dose, and tumor volume relationships in irradiation of squamous cell carcinomas of the base of the tongue. *Cancer* 1976;37:2591–2599.
155. Bedwinek JM, Shukovsky LJ, Fletcher GH, et al. Osteonecrosis in patients treated with definitive radiotherapy for squamous cell carcinomas of the oral cavity and naso- and oropharynx. *Radiology* 1976;119:665–667.
156. Parsons JT, Million RR, Cassisi NJ. Carcinoma of the base of the tongue: results of radical irradiation with surgery reserved for irradiation failure. *Laryngoscope* 1982;92:689–696.
157. Portenoy RK, Thaler HT, Kornblith AB, et al. The Memorial Symptom Assessment Scale: an instrument for the evaluation of symptom prevalence, characteristics and distress. *Eur J Cancer* 1994;30A:1326–1336.
158. Cella DF, Tulsky DS, Gray G, et al. The Functional Assessment of Cancer Therapy scale: development and validation of the general measure. *J Clin Oncol* 1993;11:570–579.
159. List MA, Ritter-Sterr C, Lansky SB. A performance status scale for head and neck cancer patients. *Cancer* 1990;66:564–569.
160. Harrison LB, Zelefsky MJ, Armstrong JG, et al. Performance status after treatment for squamous cell cancer of the base of tongue—a comparison of primary radiation therapy versus primary surgery. *Int J Radiat Oncol Biol Phys* 1994; 30:953–957.
161. Harrison LB, Zelefsky MJ, Pfister D, et al. Detailed quality of life assessment in patients treated with primary radiotherapy for squamous cell cancer of the base of the tongue. *Head Neck* 1997;19:169–175.
162. Harrison LB, Zelefsky MJ, Pfister D, et al. Detailed quality of life assessment on long term survivors of primary radiation therapy for cancer of the base of tongue. *Head Neck* 1997;19:169–175.

Radiologic Imaging Concerns

163. Keberle M, Kenn W, Tschammler A, et al. Current value of double-contrast pharyngography and of computed tomography for the detection and for staging of hypopharyngeal, oropharyngeal and supraglottic tumors. *Eur Radiol* 1999;9:1843–1850.
164. Loevner LA, Yousem DM, Montone KT, et al. Can radiologists accurately predict preepiglottic space invasion with MR imaging? *AJR Am J Roentgenol* 1997;169:1681–1687.
165. Spiro RH, Morgan GJ, Strong EW, Shah JP. Supraomohyoid neck dissection. *Am J Surg* 1996;172:650–653.
166. Casselman JW. The value of MRI in the diagnosis and staging of nasopharynx tumors. *J Belge Radiol* 1994;77:67–71.
167. Cooney TR, Poulsen MG. Is routine follow-up useful after combined-modality therapy for advanced head and neck cancer? *Arch Otolaryngol Head Neck Surg* 1999;125:379–382.
168. Clayman GL, Johnson CJ 2nd, Morrison W, et al. The role of neck dissection after chemoradiotherapy for oropharyngeal cancer with advanced nodal disease. *Arch Otolaryngol Head Neck Surg* 2001;127:135–139.
169. Glazer HS, Lee JK, Levitt RG, et al. Radiation fibrosis: differentiation from recurrent tumor by MR imaging. *Radiology* 1985;156:721–726.
170. Minn H, Lapela M, Klemi PJ, et al. Prediction of survival with fluorine-18-fluoro-deoxyglucose and PET in head and neck cancer. *J Nucl Med* 1997; 38:1907–1911.
171. Jaulerry C, Rodriguez J, Brunin F, et al. Results of radiation therapy in carcinoma of the base of the tongue. The Curie Institute experience with about 166 cases. *Cancer* 1991;67:1532–1538.
172. Foote RL, Parsons JT, Mendenhall WM, et al. Is interstitial implantation essential for successful radiotherapeutic treatment of the base of tongue carcinoma? *Int J Radiat Oncol Biol Phys* 1991;21:868.

CHAPTER 18

Early Stage Cancer of the Larynx

William M. Mendenhall, Lucian Sulica, and Roy B. Sessions

Cancer of the larynx represented about 0.7% of the total cancer risk in 2001 and is the most common head and neck cancer, if one excludes skin malignancies (1). In the United States, 10,000 new cases of cancer of the larynx (8,000 men and 2,000 women) and about 4,000 deaths from laryngeal cancer were predicted for 2001 (1). It is infrequent relative to cancers of the breast, lung, and prostate, yet a substantial amount of literature has been published regarding this disease. This apparently disproportionate body of writing reflects the perceived importance of this neoplasm, which is in turn related to its potential impact on people's communicative ability; the threat to a patient's vocal organ is associated with profound psychological and socioeconomic overtones.

Curing the cancer at any cost no longer is accepted casually. More than ever before, a premium is placed on return to a productive and useful life after cancer treatment. Originally, larynx cancer treatment focused predominantly on cure by relentless and aggressive surgery. That era was followed by the emergence of conservative partial laryngeal operations, the development of sophisticated radiation methods, and, most recently, organ-sparing strategies in which chemotherapeutic, radiotherapeutic, and surgical methods are used in a variety of combinations (2–4). The overall 5-year cure rate for patients with laryngeal squamous cell carcinoma (SCC) is almost 70%. Though those data have not changed dramatically over the past 25 years (5–7), the treatment options and their sequencing have, and a higher percentage of patients with laryngeal cancer are retaining their larynx as a result.

EPIDEMIOLOGY AND ETIOLOGY OF LARYNGEAL CANCER

Although considerable variation in the incidence of larynx cancer differences exists between countries, its distribution within a given population is consistent. Regardless of the culture, the disease most commonly affects middle-aged or older men who have smoked tobacco and have consumed excessive alcohol (8–10); laryngeal cancer rarely occurs in people who have not engaged in either practice. The risk for tobacco-related cancers of the upper alimentary tract declines among ex-smokers after 5 years, and is said to approach the risk for nonsmokers after 10 years of abstention (11). The peak incidence of larynx cancer is in the sixth decade. The disease occurs only rarely in young people (12). Compared with whites, blacks in America have a significantly higher incidence of larynx cancer (13). This disease always has been more common in men but, because of the long-term effects of changing smoking patterns, the male-to-female ratio has changed dramatically during the last 40 years. In 1956, the ratio was 15:1, whereas current studies show a 5:1 ratio of men to women.

In addition to tobacco, etiologic factors that have been suggested in laryngeal cancer are voice abuse and generalized inflammation from chronic laryngitis (8,14), certain dietary factors (15–17), chronic gastric reflux (18,19), and exposure to wood dust, nitrogen mustard, asbestos, and ionizing radiation (20–22). The carcinogenic effect on the larynx that results from smoking tobacco—whether by pipe, cigarette, or cigar—is, however, the cause most widely held responsible for this malignancy. Some evidence exists that heavy marijuana smoking may be associated with laryngeal cancer in young patients. Larynx cancer occasionally does occur in patients who have never smoked (20). Possibly, human papilloma virus (HPV) is an important cofactor in aerodigestive carcinogenesis in general, especially in the larynx (23–30). Undoubtedly, the etiology of larynx cancer is multifactorial.

ANATOMY

The larynx is a uniquely complicated organ strategically located at the division of the upper aerodigestive tract into the gastrointestinal tract and the airway. Alteration of its function by either surgery or disease can have a significant impact on vocal, digestive, and respiratory physiology. The outside framework of the larynx is formed by the hyoid bone, thyroid cartilage, and cricoid cartilage. The cricoid cartilage, which forms the base of the larynx, is the only complete ring in the entire airway which makes it especially important in maintaining airway patency. The thyroid cartilage rests atop the cricoid, articulating with it posteriorly, and envelops the soft tissues of the glottis. The hyoid bone lies superiorly, connected to the thyroid by the thyrohyoid membrane and the strap muscles, and in turn suspended from another series of muscular and ligamentous slings.

The more mobile interior framework is composed of the leaf-shaped epiglottis and the arytenoid cartilages. The paired arytenoid cartilages each lie on the posterior cephalic rim of the cricoid cartilage. Each vocal cord stretches from an anterior projection of the arytenoid known as the vocal process to the anterior midline of the inside of the thyroid cartilage. The arytenoid cartilages move in both a rocking and sliding manner on the cricoid abducts and adduct the true vocal cords. The corniculate and cuneiform cartilages are sesamoid cartilages that rest atop the arytenoids, producing small, rounded bulges at the posterior aspect of each aryepiglottic fold. They appear to serve no important purpose. The thyroid and cricoid cartilages and a portion of the arytenoid cartilage are hyaline cartilage and may partially ossify with age, particularly in men, a phenomenon that appears to invite invasion by adjacent tumor. The epiglottis is elastic cartilage; ossification does not occur, and even focal calcification is rare (31).

The thyrohyoid, cricothyroid, and cricotracheal membranes link together the external laryngeal framework. The epiglottis is joined superiorly to the hyoid bone by the midline hyoepiglottic ligament, and inferiorly to the thyroid cartilage by the thyroepiglottic ligament at a point just below the thyroid notch and above the anterior commissure. The arrangement of the ligaments and membranes that connect the lower portion of the framework is complicated and physiologically important. This structure as a whole is called the conus elasticus. It functions as a Venturi tube, affecting the flow of expired air to and through the glottis. Its base is a ring attached to the upper interior of the cricoid cartilage. As it rises, it tapers to a slitlike opening created by its upper borders, which are thickened into the vocal ligament on each side.

The intrinsic muscles of the larynx control the movement of the vocal cords. All but the cricothyroid muscle are innervated by the ipsilateral recurrent laryngeal nerve, a branch of the vagus. This includes the posterior cricoarytenoid muscle, the only abductor of the vocal fold. All muscles except for the cricothyroid move the arytenoid cartilage in relation to the rest of the laryngeal framework to produce vocal cord adduction or abduction. The cricothyroid muscle produces tension and elongation of the vocal cords by rocking the thyroid cartilage on the cricoid in a visorlike fashion, and is innervated by the ipsilateral superior laryngeal nerve, which also carries all of the afferent fibers of the larynx above the glottis. In general, both the motor and sensory innervations of the larynx are strictly lateralized; that is, there is no cross-innervation. The interarytenoid muscle may be an exception to this.

For the purposes of assessment and treatment of neoplastic disease, it is useful to divide the larynx into three subsites: the supraglottis, the glottis, and the subglottis. Different embryonic development of these subsites establishes distinct lymphatic drainage patterns and thus, markedly different clinical behavior of cancers of each location. Knowledge of these patterns has substantial impact on our ability to predict the likelihood of occult metastases to various parts of the neck and on planning of the various partial laryngectomies. Discussion of larynx cancers without reference to their exact location can lead to inaccurate and inadequate treatment.

All structures superior to a line drawn horizontally along the apex of the laryngeal ventricle lie in the supraglottis. These include the epiglottis, the false vocal folds, and the aryepiglottic folds. The lymphatics of the supraglottic larynx are profuse, and consequently, metastases occur frequently and on both sides of the neck (32). From the standpoint of lymphatic drainage, the supraglottic larynx is independent of the structures below. Lymphatic spread from the epiglottis is directed bilaterally to the false cords. The drainage from the false cords and the remainder of the supraglottic larynx is lateral and superior, and these channels exit the larynx through the thyrohyoid membrane and the preepiglottic space to the adjacent deep cervical nodes, principally the subdigastric lymph nodes, but also the middle internal jugular chain nodes. The crest of the aryepiglottic folds forms the boundary between the larynx and the hypopharynx, such that the medial wall of the aryepiglottic fold lies within the endolarynx, and its lateral wall makes up the medial wall of the adjacent pyriform sinus (Fig. 18.1). Lesions that arise on the rim of the aryepiglottic folds, therefore, have been appropriately termed marginal cancers. Marginal lesions that extend predominantly into the larynx behave more as supraglottic neoplasms, whereas those that spill into the pyriform sinus tend to follow the natural history of hypopharyngeal cancer.

The subglottis is considered to begin 5 mm below the free margin of the vocal cords and extend to the inferior border of the cricoid cartilage. The subglottic area has relatively few capillary lymphatics. The lymphatic trunks pass through the cricothyroid membrane to the pretracheal, or delphian lymph nodes, so-called because, like the ancient Greek oracle of the same name, they give warning of bad news. The subglottic area also drains posteriorly through the cricotracheal membrane, with some trunks going to the paratracheal lymph nodes and others continuing to the inferior jugular chain.

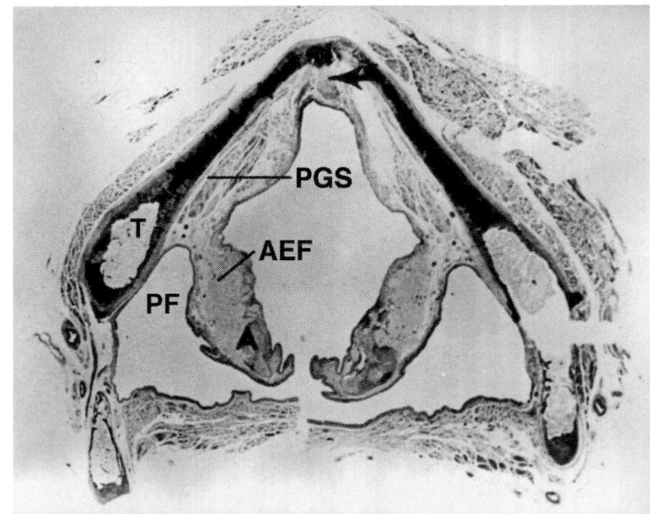

Figure 18.1 Human larynx whole-organ section. Axial section through larynx and hypopharynx at the level of the cephalic portion of the arytenoids cartilages (*A*) and aryepiglottic folds (*AEF*). Note paraglottic space (*PGS*) and ossified thyroid cartilage (*T*) immediately adjacent to the lateral wall of the pyriform fossa (*PF*). Note the proximity of the anterior wall of the pyriform fossa to the paraglottic space. *Dark arrow* at the top of figure is on a ligamentous portion of the petiole just under the lower tip of the epiglottis and just cephalic to the anterior commissure ligament of Broyle. (Courtesy of John Kirchner, M.D., Division of Otolaryngology, Yale University School of Medicine, New Haven, CT).

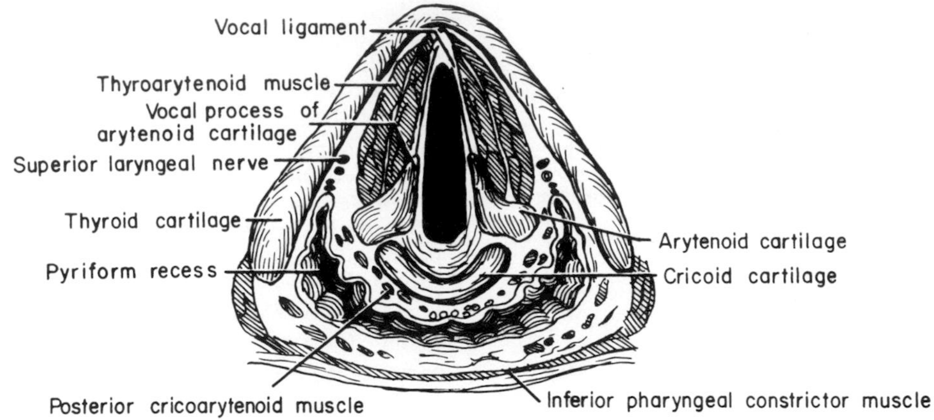

Figure 18.2 Cross-section of larynx at the level of the vocal folds. (Redrawn from Sabotta J. *Atlas der Anatomie des Menschen* in two volumes, 20th ed. Munich: Urban & Fischer Verlag, 1975, with permission.)

The glottis consists of the paired vocal cords (Fig. 18.2). Each spans the distance from the anterior midline of the thyroid cartilage to the vocal process of its arytenoid cartilage. The vocal cords are somewhat misnamed. They really are reflections of mucosa draped over the underlying muscles and projection of the conus elasticus, rather than cordlike structures. The term "vocal folds" is more accurate than "vocal cords" and has essentially replaced the latter term among laryngologists. The vocal folds proper are essentially devoid of lymphatic channels. Thus, cervical metastases from glottic carcinoma suggest spread outside of or deep to the superficial portion of the glottis. Lymphatic drainage of the deep part of the glottic larynx is largely lateralized, so that the left side is essentially independent of the right, in contrast to the bilaterally draining supraglottic larynx.

Unlike the rest of the larynx, which is lined with respiratory epithelium, the vocal folds are covered by nonkeratinizing pseudostratified squamous epithelium. Underlying this is a three-layered lamina propria of unique biochemical composition that allows free movement of the overlying mucosa over the vocal ligament, critical to normal voice production. During phonation, the vocal folds adduct until their mucosal surfaces are just touching. Air actively expelled from the lungs passes between them and causes the mucosal membranes of each to vibrate, generating the so-called mucosal wave. The vibratory mechanism that produces the voice is therefore due to the mobility of the mucous membrane relative to the underlying musculature of the vocal fold. It is important to appreciate that this is a passive motion, and that this mucosal motion is altogether different from the gross vocal fold motion discussed in the tumor, node, metastasis (TNM) staging system. It is the compromise of mucosal mobility, and not a deficit of gross motion, which causes the hoarseness that is the hallmark sign of early glottic carcinoma. Further, it is the preservation or restoration of this mobility that ensures a good voice quality in the treatment of early laryngeal cancer.

The division of the larynx into three subsites applies primarily to mucosal disease. Between the external framework of the thyroid cartilage and hyoid bone and the inner muscular framework, the preepiglottic and paraglottic fat spaces form, for practical purposes, one continuous space occupying the entire cephalic-to-caudal laryngeal length (Figs. 18.3 and 18.4). Once a tumor penetrates into the depths of the larynx, it no longer should be considered early disease. Lam and Wong (33) showed that the thin, membranous septa located between the paraglottic and preepiglottic space are capable of holding a tumor in check, but only to a very limited degree. The space is traversed by blood and lymphatic vessels and nerves. Because few capillary lymphatics arise in this area, invasion of the fat space should only indirectly be associated with lymph node metastases. The space is limited by the conus elasticus inferiorly; the thyroid ala, the thyrohyoid membrane, and the hyoid bone anterolaterally; the hyoepiglottic ligament superiorly; and the fascia of the intrinsic muscles on the medial side. Posteriorly, it is adjacent to the anterior wall of the pyriform sinus. Once an early cancer enters into the paraglottic space, it can extend cau-

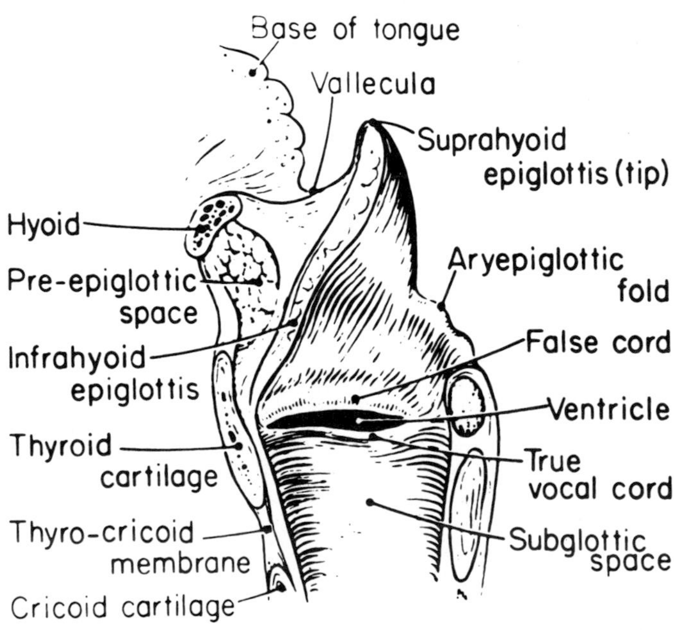

Figure 18.3 Diagram of the sagittal section of the larynx. Note adjacency of the epiglottis to the preepiglottic space, and note also the proximity of the cephalic extent of this space to the base of the tongue. Finally, note intimate relationship of the subglottic mucosa to the cricothyroid membrane anteriorly. This is the point of exit for anterior cancers that are diverted caudally from the glottic level. (Redrawn from Sabotta J. *Atlas der Anatomie des Menschen* in two volumes, 20th ed. Munich: Urban & Fischer Verlag, 1975, with permission.)

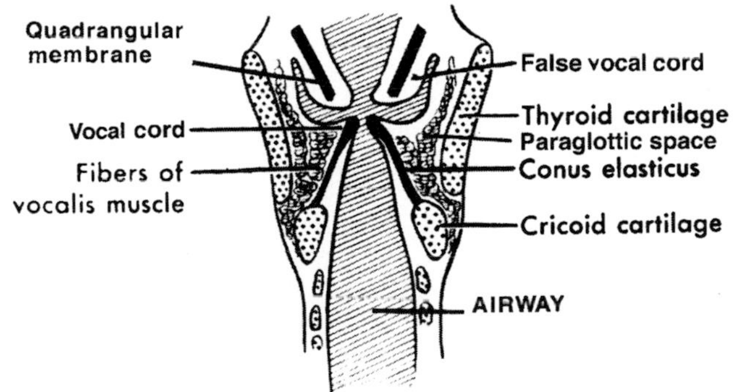

Figure 18.4 Diagram of coronal section of the larynx. This rendition is taken through the middle one third of the larynx, showing the fibrous barriers in both the supraglottic and the lower larynx, the intrinsic laryngeal muscles, and the thyroid and cricoid cartilages.

dally into the cricothyroid area, from which point it can exit directly into the cervical soft tissue. Cephalic extension can lead to the preepiglottic space and hence into the tongue base, or exit from the larynx by way of the thyrohyoid membrane.

PATHOLOGY AND PATTERNS OF SPREAD

Pathology

Nearly all malignant tumors of the larynx arise from the surface epithelium and therefore are SCC or one of its variants such as spindle cell or verrucous carcinoma. Sarcomas, adenocarcinomas, neuroendocrine tumors, and other unusual neoplasms account for the balance of tumors that arise in the larynx. Although some variability exists between series, more than 50% of laryngeal SCCs present as localized disease without metastasis, 25% present as local disease with regional metastasis, and 15% are seen first at an advanced stage with or without distant metastasis. As with other aerodigestive carcinomas, metachronous and synchronous disease are important considerations in developing appropriate diagnostic and therapeutic strategies. Overall, the incidence of metachronous tumors (i.e., second primary aerodigestive SCCs) is reported to be between 5% and 35% of all aerodigestive cases (34–37), with the esophagus being the most common second site (36,37). The larynx, however, seems to demonstrate a more frequent association with lung rather than esophageal carcinoma. This is a logical consequence of the impact of inhaling rather than ingesting carcinogenic substances.

Epithelial Disease

The mucosal changes that lead to cancer take years to develop, and that evolution likely follows a fairly consistent pattern. Most laryngeal SCCs result from prolonged exposure to recognized carcinogens that stimulate mucosal hyperplasia and metaplasia. Some of these changes are associated with keratosis, and others are not. In some situations, epithelial atypia or dysplasia may exist, and the degree of cellular disturbance probably determines whether a lesion is destined to become malignant (38–40). The degree of dysplasia is graded as mild, moderate, or severe, depending on the extent of involvement of the thickness of the surface epithelium. In general, the less the degree of dysplasia, the less likely is the transformation to invasive carcinoma. Conversely, the higher the grade of dysplasia, the more likely is such a progression. In one large study by Slamniker et al. (41), 3% of patients who demonstrated vocal fold keratosis without atypia and 7% with mild atypia ultimately developed invasive carcinoma; however, in those patients with moderate and severe atypia, 18% and 24%, respectively, developed carcinoma. Another study by Hjslet et al. (42) showed a similar probability of cancer evolution in the group with less dysplasia and a strikingly higher probability in those patients with severe atypia.

At best, the gross appearance of a lesion of the mucosal surface is an inconsistent indicator of its potential for harboring malignancy. The term leukoplakia describes a white lesion, usually appearing as such because of keratinization. Erythroplakia, also a clinical term, describes a red lesion on a mucous membrane. Many investigators believe that the risk for cancer development is substantially higher in lesions that are soft and red (40). Without histologic study, however, even the most experienced diagnostician cannot predict consistently the presence of cancer or the likelihood of its evolution in any of these surface lesions. Furthermore, any given spot within a lesion is not necessarily representative of the rest of that lesion. The fact that carcinoma *in situ* (CIS) often is surrounded by dysplastic epithelium and that many areas of invasive carcinoma are surrounded by zones of CIS and dysplastic epithelium (43) suggest that each of these morphologic categories of epithelial disturbance is but part of a dynamic spectrum of disorders, each perhaps related and representing different stages of the same process. This line of thinking would suggest that dysplasia leads to CIS, which leads to invasive carcinoma.

This concept is challenged vigorously in some quarters. Contrary thought suggests that the spectrum of abnormal epithelial maturation and individual cellular aberrations can occur in circumstances that may or may not precede an invasive carcinoma. In the opinion of some investigators, severe dysplasia, especially in the larynx, is not a prerequisite for the development of an invasive SCC. In fact, invasive carcinoma can develop in an epithelium with only mild or partial thickness and dysplastic changes. As classically defined, CIS represents full-thickness mucosal epithelial dysplastic change without violation of the basement membrane. For all intents and purposes, severe dysplasia can be synonymous with CIS. However, CIS is known to arise from the basal epithelial layer in the absence of overlying dysplastic changes. In this setting, therefore, the definition of CIS can be expanded to include those lesions in which the mucosal alterations are so severe as to signal a high probability for progression to an invasive carcinoma if left untreated. Extension of the dysplastic process to involve the mucoserous glands still is considered CIS and not invasive carcinoma. Such is not the case with violation of the basement membrane, at which point CIS becomes invasive carcinoma.

Cellular characteristics vary by site; in the supraglottis, lesions are more likely to be nonkeratinizing and poorly differentiated, and generally they demonstrate more aggressive local behavior (44). Those lesions of the true vocal folds, on the other hand, more often are well differentiated and tend to be less locally aggressive. Although the degree of cellular differentiation is not thought to be the most significant factor in tumor grading, it does seem to correlate with the probability of cervical metastasis (45–47), which in turn creates a strong impact on survival (48,49). Finally, the actual tumor thickness and depth of invasion almost certainly have an influence on metastasis and, ultimately, on survival.

A variety of studies have attempted to standardize the predictive value of thickness in SCCs of the upper aerodigestive tract with the probability of cervical metastasis and, therefore, the prognosis (50–54). Though intuitively one might expect a direct correlation between the two, a number of studies have found no statistically significant association between tumor thickness and nodal metastasis (55–57). Also, it should be noted that those studies that do demonstrate a correlation between thickness and metastasis generally focused on sites other than the larynx. Because of the anatomic complexity and embryologic uniqueness of the larynx, one cannot necessarily transpose such data from other organs.

As is true in other aerodigestive sites, a multifactorial analysis of a variety of parameters, including patient performance status, may produce a more predictable prognostic indicator than the standard TNM staging outlined by the American Joint Committee on Cancer (AJCC), as shown in Table 18.1.

TABLE 18.1 Staging

Tumor stage	Characteristics
Supraglottis	
T1	Tumor limited to one subsite of supraglottis with normal vocal cord mobility
T2	Tumor invades mucosa of more than one adjacent subsite of supraglottis or glottis or region outside the supraglottis (e.g., mucosa of base of tongue, vallecula, medial wall of pyriform sinus) without fixation of the larynx
T3	Tumor limited to larynx with vocal cord fixation or invades any of the following: postcricoid area, preepiglottic tissues, or [a]minor thyroid erosion (inner cortex)
T4	Tumor invades through the thyroid cartilage, or extends into soft tissues of the neck, thyroid, or esophagus T4a[a]: Resectable (e.g., tumor invades trachea, soft tissues of neck, strap muscles, thyroid, or esophagus) T4b[a]: Unresectable (e.g., tumor invades prevertebral space, encases carotid artery, or invades mediastinal structures)
Glottis	
T1	Tumor limited to vocal cord(s) (may involve anterior or posterior commissure) with normal mobility T1a: Tumor limited to one vocal cord T1b: Tumor involves both vocal cords
T2	Tumor extends to supraglottis or subglottis, or with impaired vocal fold mobility
T3	Tumor limited to the larynx with vocal fold fixation, or [a]invades paraglottic space, or minor thyroid cartilage erosion (inner cortex)
T4	Tumor invades through the thyroid cartilage or to other tissues beyond the larynx (e.g., trachea, soft tissues of neck including thyroid, pharynx) T4a[a]: Resectable, see above T4b[a]: Unresectable, see above
Subglottis	
T1	Tumor limited to the subglottis
T2	Tumor extends to vocal fold(s) with normal or impaired mobility
T3	Tumor limited to larynx with vocal fold fixation
T4	Tumor invades through cricoid or thyroid cartilage or extends to other tissues beyond the larynx (e.g., trachea, soft tissues of neck including thyroid, esophagus) T4a[a]: Resectable. Tumor invades criciod or thyroid cartilage or invades tissues beyond the larynx (e.g., trachea, soft tissues of neck, strap muscles, thyroid, or esophagus) T4b[a]: Unresectable. Tumor invades prevertebral space, encases carotid artery, or invades mediastinum

[a]Changes that are now included in the 6th edition of the American Joint Committee on Cancer: *Cancer staging manual,* by Greene F, et al. New York: Springer Verlag, 2002:47–57.
Source: Modified from American Joint Committee on Cancer: *Manual for staging of cancer,* 5th ed. Philadelphia: Lippincott Williams & Wilkins, 1998:45–55.

Local Spread

SUPRAGLOTTIS

Lesions of the supraglottic larynx tend to spread locally. Most supraglottic lesions arise on the epiglottis; fewer are seen on the false vocal folds and aryepiglottic folds. Those lesions that occur on the suprahyoid or upper part of the epiglottis are usually exophytic, whereas those that occur on the lower portion of that structure are likely to be endophytic or ulcerative (44,58). Endophytic growth is especially significant in this particular area of the epiglottis because foramina here lead directly through the cartilage into the preepiglottic space, which in turn lead out of the larynx into the tongue base. What may appear to be a localized tumor in the endolarynx, therefore, actually can extend unrecognized out of the larynx (47). Such tumors may also present in the vallecula and base of tongue without involving the suprahyoid epiglottis. Tumors are confined initially to the preepiglottic space by the ligamentous boundaries of that compartment but, once those barriers are overcome, the loosely arranged skeletal muscle fibers of the tongue provide no restriction to further tumor extension (59,60). Modern imaging, especially by magnetic resonance imaging (MRI), has greatly improved the ability to recognize tumor extension into the preepiglottic space and base of tongue. Certain circumstances in which the condition of the preepiglottic space is unclear may offer a role for fine-needle aspiration and cytologic evaluation of the tissue extracted from that area.

Those lesions that occur on the laryngeal surface of the epiglottis are capable of invading and destroying that structure. Conversely, supraglottic lesions almost never destroy the thyroid cartilage (60,61). This feature has an influence on the design of treatment plans. For example, an ossified and invaded thyroid cartilage poses a substantial problem for surgeons attempting to perform partial laryngectomy and also probably for radiation and medical oncologists employing strategies designed for organ preservation. True "early laryngeal cancer" (i.e., the primary focus of this chapter) is not always clearly definable. Understaging can easily occur in such circumstances as unrecognized preepiglottic space involvement or cartilage invasion masks the distinction between early and late disease.

Identifying laryngeal cartilage invasion, whether from glottic or supraglottic carcinoma, is important in treatment planning. However, this has always been difficult because the patchy ossification that occurs in the laryngeal framework frequently presents an ambiguous radiologic and clinical picture. Generally, cartilage is more vulnerable to tumor invasion in those areas where it is ossified, most commonly in the region of the anterior commissure tendon or the junction of the anterior one fourth and the posterior three fourths of the thyroid lamina. Healthy, nonossified cartilage provides a fairly resistant natural barrier to cancer invasion.

Aryepiglottic fold cancers behave somewhat differently from their counterparts in the endolarynx. The evolution of these so-called marginal lesions is similar to pyriform sinus cancers, which spread in a more diffuse fashion and metastasize more frequently. Though some investigators believe aryepiglottic cancers are somewhat distinct biologically, their particularly ominous natural history probably relates as much to regional anatomy (i.e., the abundant and multidirectional lymphatic drainage of the area) as to anything else (62).

The quadrangular membrane within the aryepiglottic fold probably serves an important role of diverting the leading edge of tumors. Those lesions that begin on the portion of the false vocal fold visible to office examination initially are contained medial to the quadrangular membrane and are diverted onto the laryngeal surface of the epiglottis, at which point they can extend through foramina into the preepiglottic space as previously discussed. Lesions on this area of the epiglottis also can extend inferiorly across the glottic anterior commissure and into the subglottic larynx, from where they can escape the larynx into the anterior neck and to the delphian node. Infrahyoid lesions that extend onto or below the vocal folds are at high risk for thyroid cartilage invasion, even if the folds themselves are mobile (63).

Supraglottic cancers that begin on the underside of the false vocal folds or the laryngeal ventricle itself are usually diverted by the quadrangular membrane laterally into the paraglottic space early in their development, from which they can extend cephalically or caudally. Submucosal spread can progress for a considerable distance without producing physical signs. Also as a result of invasion into the paraglottic compartment, these carcinomas extend to the perichondrium of the thyroid cartilage quite early. Frank cartilage invasion, however, is usually a delayed phenomenon. Extension to the lower portion of the infrahyoid epiglottis and invasion of the preepiglottic space are common. True vocal fold invasion is often associated with thyroid cartilage invasion.

Because of the profuse lymphatic network of the area, supraglottic carcinomas frequently metastasize to the cervical lymph nodes, and failure of treatment usually occurs in the neck rather than at the primary site (32,64–67). The incidence of patients demonstrating clinically positive lymph nodes at the time of diagnosis is 23% to 50% for supraglottic carcinoma of all stages (58,68–72). If a neck dissection is performed, a substantial number of those patients with clinically negative necks tumors are found to have histologically identifiable disease. If left untreated, this progresses to gross disease (64,65). In supraglottic cancers, the probabilities of cervical metastasis and of delayed contralateral metastasis increase in direct proportion to the size of the primary (i.e., the T stage) (44,62,73). Lindberg (32) reports impressively high overall metastatic rates with various supraglottic carcinomas: T1 had 63%, T2 had 70%, T3 had 79%, and T4 had 73%.

In that group of patients who have supraglottic lesions and present with a clinically positive cervical node 2 cm in diameter or more, the possibility for contralateral neck metastasis is 40% or higher (74). The epiglottis is particularly prone to produce bilateral metastasis and, even in smaller lesions of that site, the incidence of contralateral metastasis is more than 20% (73). Many of the data on clinically positive necks and on occult metastasis were compiled before the routine employment of computed tomography (CT) and MRI of the neck. With the employment of these more sophisticated staging methods added to the current 75% to 85% accuracy of physical examination (75,76), the overall incidence of metastasis noted at the time of diagnosis probably is higher than what has been reported previously.

GLOTTIS

Glottic or true vocal fold carcinoma is the laryngeal cancer most commonly encountered in the United States. Although these lesions usually are well differentiated, often they demonstrate an infiltrative growth pattern, even when they appear exophytic and well organized. When diagnosed, about two thirds are confined to the vocal folds, usually one fold. Most true vocal fold cancers occur on the anterior two thirds of that structure; a small percentage of them are isolated to the anterior commissure, but they only rarely occur on the posterior commissure (77).

As in other laryngeal tumors, the growth characteristics and natural history of glottic carcinomas are determined by the unique local anatomy. First, the sparseness of the lymphatic drainage of the true vocal folds in all areas other than near the posterior commissure renders metastasis of early lesions extremely unlikely. Second, the elastic layers (conus elasticus and thyroglottic ligament) within the vocal fold tend to divert free-edge vocal fold lesions from continuing into the underlying vocalis muscle and paraglottic space.

The anterior commissure ligament (Broyle's ligament) is another anatomic factor that influences growth pattern. This ligament is a blending point, joining the vertical fibers from the inferior tip of the epiglottis with the horizontal fibers of the vocal ligament. In effect, it forms the bridge between the anterior ends of the respective true vocal folds. As no actual internal perichondrium exists at the anterior aspect of the thyroid cartilage, this ligament lies immediately against the inner lamina of that cartilage: it serves as the perichondrium. The presence of the anterior commissure ligament initially retards penetration of cancers, often probably causing their diversion cephalically onto the epiglottis or caudally onto the cricothyroid membrane (63). If the cancer overcomes the ligamentous barrier at the anterior commissure, the cartilage is penetrated (78). This event is particularly likely in thyroid cartilages that are ossified and, when this does occur, therapeutic choices for both the radiation oncologist and the surgeon are substantially limited (79,80).

When caudal extension does occur, these lesions readily can escape the larynx into the anterior neck, either into the soft tissue or to the delphian lymph node (81). The exit of anterior subglottic cancers is facilitated by the location of the mucosa of that area directly against the cricothyroid membrane. One centimeter of subglottic extension anteriorly or 4 to 5 mm of subglottic extension posteriorly brings the border of the tumor to the upper margin of the cricoid, exceeding the anatomic limits for conventional hemilaryngectomy.

As vocal fold lesions enlarge, they extend to the false fold, vocal process of the arytenoid, and subglottic region. Infiltrative lesions invade the vocal ligament and muscle and eventually reach the paraglottic space and the perichondrium of the thyroid cartilage. Advanced glottic lesions eventually penetrate through the thyroid cartilage or via the cricothyroid space to enter the neck, where they may invade the thyroid gland.

With penetration through the mucosa into the underlying tissues, all degrees of motion impairment—from subtle membrane stiffness to frank fixation of the vocal fold—can follow. These can be caused by invasion of the vocal fold muscle, of the cricoarytenoid joint, or, very rarely, of the recurrent laryngeal nerve. Perineural spread is uncommon in laryngeal malignancies. Impairment of motion has a telling effect on local control and on survival data, a fact reflected in AJCC staging designations. Much discussion continues about vocal fold mobility change and the associated therapeutic implications; the clinical judgment of the oncologist is tested most in this group of glottic cancers.

SUBGLOTTIS

Carcinomas that arise in the subglottic larynx are unusual, making up only 1% to 8% of all laryngeal cancers (77). These lesions tend to be poorly differentiated and often demonstrate an infiltrative growth pattern unrestricted by tissue barriers. Because of this, and because they are often diagnosed late, they frequently are circumferential and can extend downward, along the tracheal wall. They involve the cricoid cartilage early because there is no intervening muscle layer. The incidence of cervical metastasis of subglottic cancers is reported to be 20% to 30%, but that figure is obscured somewhat by the fact that the primary drainage pattern of these lesions is to the less detectable pretracheal and paratracheal nodes. The actual incidence of metastasis therefore may be significantly higher (82,83).

Lymphatic Spread

The location and stage of neck nodes detected on admission for previously untreated patients with SCC of the supraglottic larynx are given in Figure 18.5 (32). The disease spreads mainly to the subdigastric nodes. The submandibular area is rarely involved, and there is only a small risk for spinal accessory lymph node involvement. The incidence of clinically positive nodes is 55% at the time of diagnosis; 16% are bilateral (32). Elective neck dissection shows pathologically positive nodes in 16% of cases; observation of initially node-negative necks eventually identifies the appearance of positive nodes in 33% of cases (84,85). Spread to the pyriform sinus, vallecula, and base of the tongue increases the risk for lymph node metastases. The risk for late-appearing contralateral lymph node metastasis is 37% if the ipsilateral neck is pathologically positive, but the risk is unrelated to whether the nodes in the ipsilateral neck were palpable before neck dissection.

In carcinoma of the vocal fold, the incidence of clinically positive lymph nodes at diagnosis approaches zero for T1 lesions and 1.7% for T2 lesions (86). The incidence of neck metastases increases to 20% to 30% for T3 and T4 lesions. Supraglottic spread is associated with metastasis to the jugulodigastric nodes. Anterior commissure and anterior subglottic invasion are associated with involvement of the delphian node.

Lederman (87) reports a 10% incidence of positive lymph nodes in 73 patients with subglottic carcinoma.

Extraordinary Cancers

The pathology and pathogenesis of verrucous carcinoma is unique and deserves special consideration. This unusual tumor is poorly understood, and its etiology, classification, and response to treatment are all controversial (88,89). Verrucous carcinoma is described as a distinct neoplastic entity of squamous origin that occurs in the oral cavity, larynx, esophagus, and sinonasal tract and on the genitalia (34,90–94). It probably is virally induced.

Despite views to the contrary, many investigators consider verrucous carcinoma to be an entity unto itself (95). The finding that some tumors originally thought to be verrucous carcinoma are discovered to have features of SCC and can metastasize does not, in their opinion, justify combining the two diagnoses. These investigators argue that such tumors always were low-grade squamous cell rather than verrucous carcinomas (92). Other investigators, though conceding that verrucous carcinoma is unique, believe it to be only a variant of well-differentiated SCC. Different authors believe that because verrucous carcinomas neither fulfill the histologic and cytologic criteria of malignancy nor possess the capability to metastasize, they should be renamed verrucous acanthomas (96).

Diagnosing verrucous carcinoma is difficult, even when the clinical index of suspicion is high. This relates to the fact that it demonstrates an exuberant and keratinizing hyperplasia that is benign by pure histologic and cytologic criteria (97). When this lesion does occur in the larynx, usually it is observed on the true vocal fold (34,89,93), where it grows slowly and can cause significant local destruction by relentless expansion. Even though these lesions often destroy cartilage, they do not tend to metastasize, and aggressiveness characteristically occurs locally. The diagnosis is largely a clinical one, achieved most effectively by a pathologist and surgeon acting in concert, but usually only after multiple biopsies have been obtained and the clinical judgment and the self-confidence of the surgeon have been tested. The typical verrucous carcinoma is slow-growing but relentless, appears exophytic and warty, is broad-based at its interface with the mucosa, and is either tan or white. The surface often is necrotic and infected, and the associated inflammation of adjacent tissues frequently is remarkable. This tendency to cause inflammation can influence treatment planning erroneously. For example, a patient with verrucous carcinoma can demonstrate enlarged, worrisome adjacent cervical lymph nodes when, in fact, the adenopathy is only secondary to the inflammatory process. Even though this phenomenon has been described in other aerodigestive tumors (98), it can be particularly problematic in verrucous carcinomas (94,99). The mere presence of lymphadenopathy in the drainage area of an impressive primary tumor is worrisome, no matter how benign-appearing the histology. In such a circumstance, clinical judgment is enhanced greatly by modern imaging and cytologic techniques.

This debate about the nature of verrucous carcinoma has therapeutic implications, especially when the lesion occurs in the larynx. Essentially, SCC is a radiosensitive cancer, a fact that

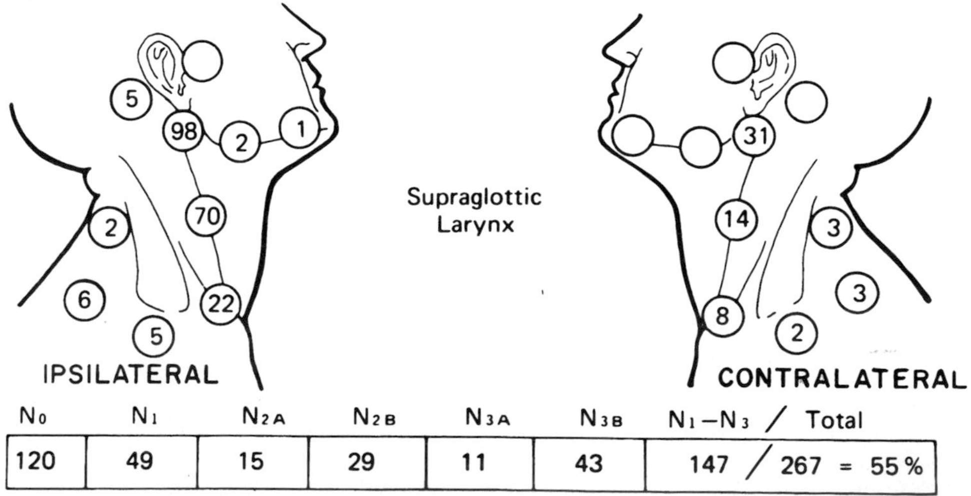

N_0	N_1	N_{2A}	N_{2B}	N_{3A}	N_{3B}	N_1-N_3 / Total
120	49	15	29	11	43	147 / 267 = 55 %

Figure 18.5 Cervical nodal distribution of supraglottic carcinoma on admission to the M.D. Anderson Cancer Center, 1948–1965. (From Lindberg RD. Distribution of cervical lymph node metastases from squamous cell carcinoma of the upper respiratory and digestive tracts. *Cancer* 1972;29:1446–1449, with permission.)

offers treatment options to the physician. Conversely, verrucous carcinoma has been regarded as somewhat radioresistant, whether found in the mouth or in the larynx (88). Additionally, both anecdotal information and dogma in the literature suggest a potential for radiation-induced dedifferentiation of these tumors into anaplastic cancer. This is reported to occur in 7% to 30% of verrucous carcinomas, depending on the study cited (68,88,90,100–105), and the alteration of the DNA facilitating the integration of the HPV into host cells has been proposed as an explanation for this change (106). Both the concept of radiation resistance and the transformation into anaplastic cancers are disputed vigorously, however, and especially in the case of anaplastic transformation, there is reason to raise doubt about the validity of the concept in this particular neoplasm (92–94,107–109). Batsakis et al. (92) find the descriptions and illustrations in those studies identifying anaplastic transformation inadequate. Essentially, though partial laryngeal surgery generally is considered the preferred strategy for verrucous larynx cancers, radiation is recommended if a total laryngectomy would be required for complete tumor removal (110). We have observed typical verrucous lesions that have disappeared with radiation therapy and not recurred. O'Sullivan et al. (111) have also made this observation. Radiation failure obviously dictates total laryngectomy.

Knowledge and understanding of the neuroendocrine family of tumors is evolving as a result of recent diagnostic techniques that allow pathologists to label a variety of previously undefined cancers as specifically neuroendocrine. Almost certainly, an immunohistochemical reexamination of laryngeal cancers previously diagnosed as atypical or undifferentiated malignancies would result in the reclassification of many as neuroendocrine in origin. These small-cell tumors look and act much like their counterpart oat-cell lung lesions and, as such, generally are managed by chemotherapy and radiation therapy (3,112,113). Surgical procedures do not seem to enhance the likelihood of survival in patients with these tumors (113,114). Carcinoids and paragangliomas are the other neuroendocrine tumors that occur in the larynx. These rare tumors seem to be managed best surgically (115).

Cartilaginous malignancies (116), adenocarcinomas, sarcomas, malignant fibrous histiocytomas, plasmacytomas, granular cell tumors, and primary lymphomas have been reported but are rare (115–120). Primary melanomas of the larynx are equally rare. For example, of all the larynx cancers reported from Memorial Sloan-Kettering Cancer Center between 1949 and 1983, only three were melanomas (121). Melanomas, like renal cell carcinomas and others, can metastasize to the larynx.

DIAGNOSIS AND EVALUATION OF LARYNGEAL CANCERS

Cancers of the supraglottic larynx usually do not produce early symptoms or signs, so the first hint of such a cancer commonly is cervical adenopathy. When symptoms do occur, often they are subtle; pain perceived in the primary site or referred to the ear by way of a branch of the vagus known as the Arnold nerve, a scratchy sensation when swallowing, or merely an alteration of one's tolerance for hot or cold foods may be all that is noticeable. Airway alteration, hoarseness, or the tendency to aspirate liquids occur with more advanced lesions.

Cancers of the glottis, on the other hand, often are detected early in the course of the disease because even a slight alteration of the vibratory dynamics of the true vocal fold mucosa produces voice change. Smokers often are chronically hoarse, however, and such alteration of the voice may go unnoticed for weeks or even months. Anyone with a voice change that persists beyond 2 or 3 weeks should be urged to have a laryngeal examination. For patients with cancer of the glottis to seek medical attention because of cervical adenopathy is unusual. With such lesions, metastasis generally occurs late in the course of the disease, long after the early warning signals.

Subglottic cancers are uncommon, but when they do occur, they are somewhat silent and fail to produce early symptoms. The disease is, therefore, often advanced by the time of diagnosis.

Diagnostic procedures for laryngeal cancer at the University of Florida are summarized in Figure 18.6. Examining the larynx in the upright and awake patient is essential to fully appreciate the natural position and relaxed motion of the larynx. Subtle motion changes are visualized only in an awake patient. Certain subtleties of contour, such as bulging and tethering, also are not visually appreciable under anesthesia.

Almost all larynx cancers are squamous carcinomas and, as such, are surface lesions. Most are visible by routine laryngeal mirror inspection, but a small percentage are located in obscure areas and require more sophisticated technology, such as the modern generation of flexible endoscopes. These instruments have become essential to a broad range of physicians in providing the capability of detailed laryngeal examination. The optical resolution of these instruments has enhanced the process of tumor mapping before, during, and after treatment. Importantly, these methods allow the occasional laryngeal examiner to visualize areas that previously have been hidden.

Laryngeal stroboscopy, which allows examination of mucosal wave integrity, is important for evaluation of surface lesions of the vocal folds. In cases in which a very small glottic carcinoma is suspected, this technique has the potential to reveal tethering of the mucosal surface, and in fact, preliminary investigations suggest that it may be able to offer insight into the depth of histologic invasion (122,123). According to the body-cover mucosal wave theory of voice production, normal phonation is a product of unimpeded passive motion of vocal fold mucosa, propelled by expired air, over a more rigid underlying structure. This mucosal mobility depends on the unique layered microstructure of the vocal folds. As a malignant lesion

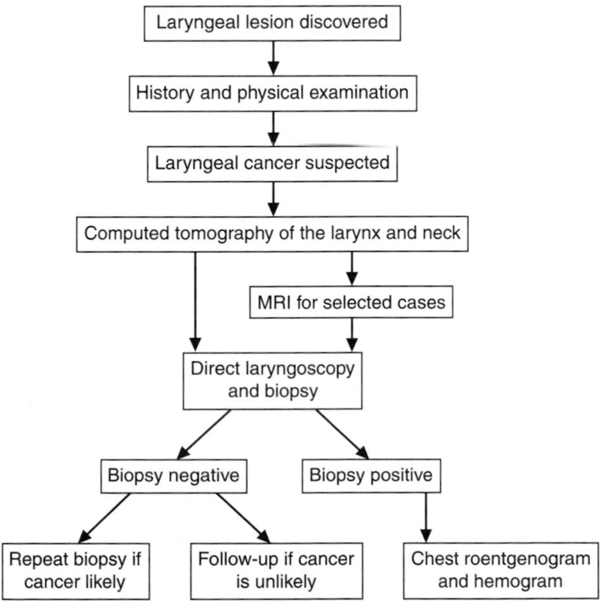

Figure 18.6 Algorithm for diagnostic evaluation of a laryngeal lesion.

invades across these layers, the mucosal surface would be expected to become less pliable. In more recent investigative work, stroboscopy has not proved to be consistently predictive. A study of 62 lesions in 52 patients revealed that stroboscopically observed abnormalities of mucosal wave correlate neither with histologic diagnosis (atypia vs. carcinoma) nor with depth of invasion (124). The majority of lesions, regardless of microscopic characteristics, showed abnormalities in the mucosal wave. Occasionally these were surprisingly pronounced, even when only intraepithelial atypia was present. Edema from perilesional inflammatory infiltrate and subepithelial fibrosis from phonotrauma caused by the mucosal alterations may account for the unexpected stiffness observed. More disturbing, one carcinoma invading the vocal ligament was associated with an intact mucosal wave. Very limited invasion evidently can leave enough intact superficial lamina propria to preserve the mucosal wave. Thus, the surgeon should not place undue faith in preoperative stroboscopic evaluation, and must be ready to alter plans according to intraoperative information provided by the pathologist.

Computed tomography scan with contrast enhancement is the radiographic method of choice for studying the larynx. The CT scan should precede biopsy so that tissue trauma caused by biopsy is not confused with tumor. Computed tomography is preferred to MRI because the longer scanning time for MRI results in motion artifact (125). Computed tomography slices, 3-mm-thick, are obtained at 3-mm intervals through the larynx and at 5-mm intervals for the remainder of the study. The gantry is angled so that the scan slices are parallel to the plane of the true vocal folds. It is also necessary to obtain a CT scan of the entire neck to detect positive, nonpalpable lymph nodes. Malignant retropharyngeal adenopathy may be present at diagnosis in patients with laryngeal cancer who have advanced neck disease (126). Retropharyngeal adenopathy is often not apparent on physical examination but can usually be seen on CT scan.

Contrast enhancement helps to delineate the blood vessels and thyroid gland. The tumor itself often enhances, probably because of reactive inflammatory changes. In addition to CT, MRI may be obtained to define subtle extralaryngeal spread or early cartilage destruction. The value of MRI for detecting early cartilage destruction remains open for discussion. Sagittal MRI may be useful to examine the base of the tongue for tumor invasion.

Computed tomography does not show minimal mucosal lesions and is sometimes not indicated for well-defined, easily visualized T1 vocal fold carcinomas. However, CT is excellent for determining subglottic extension and extension anterior to the anterior commissure. In fact, CT is often used in selected T1 and most T2 lesions for these reasons alone. Computed tomography scanning is also useful in the diagnosis of moderately advanced and advanced lesions; it is excellent for demonstrating extension outside the larynx into the soft tissues of the neck and has potential for determining thyroid or cricoid cartilage invasion. Early cartilage involvement is difficult to detect with axial scans, but it may be demonstrated by coronal or sagittal scanning techniques. If the low-density plane of the paraglottic space is intact, cartilage is probably not invaded by tumor.

The CT scan provides an excellent means for viewing the preepiglottic and paraglottic fat spaces. Soft tissue extension into the neck or base of the tongue also can be seen. The CT scan is also useful for determining extension to the subglottic areas (31).

Direct laryngoscopy, under microscopy if the subtlety of the lesions warrants, is the final diagnostic step. At this time biopsy and detailed examination of the region takes place. The ventricles, subglottis, apex of the pyriform sinus, and postcricoid area must be carefully inspected because these areas are not consistently seen in office examination of the awake patient. A biopsy specimen is taken from the obvious lesion; additional specimens may be obtained from suspicious areas. When performing a biopsy of the mucosa of the true vocal fold, every effort should be taken to preserve noninvolved mucosa. The procedure of mucosal stripping compromises posttreatment voice results for both radiation and surgery (127,128) and is acceptable today only in the case of diffuse lesions involving the overwhelming majority of the vocal fold surface. Microexcisional techniques yield ample tissue for diagnosis without the negative impact on voice.

STAGING

The 1998 AJCC staging system for laryngeal primary cancer is listed in Table 18.1 (129) and is the staging system used in this chapter. In 2002, the AJCC issued the 6th edition of its cancer staging manual (30), which is largely the same as the 5th edition. The only significant change relates to T4 lesions. T4 lesions have now been divided into T4a (resectable) and T4b (unresectable), leading to the division of stage IV into stage IVA (locally advanced resectable), IVB (locally advanced unresectable), and IVC (M1 disease).

Staging provides a commonality of language essential for effective outcomes analysis. It should be remembered that the staging cited (and that reported by the AJCC) is clinical, and is based on ultimate tumor performance. The accuracy of clinical staging methods has been updated periodically on the basis of better recognition of performance. For example, Pillsbury and Kirchner (131) studied this question by comparing whole-organ sections of nonirradiated larynges and compared the actual pathologic findings with the preoperative staging. They found that 40% had been categorized incorrectly and that most inaccuracies consisted of understaging. Most commonly, the depth of invasion had been underestimated, and the frequency of cartilage invasion was much higher than had been realized previously. Certainly, as imaging technology continues to improve, so will the accuracy of staging.

Only in the early T stages can one identify the specific site of origin with certainty. As the lesion enlarges, the site of origin is an educated guess based on the location of the greatest bulk of tumor. The major difference between the 1992 and 1998 staging systems is that a supraglottic cancer that invades the mucosa of the base of tongue or medial wall of the pyriform sinus can be staged as a T2 lesion. This has resulted in a negative stage migration such that the likelihood of local control for supraglottic cancer will likely be lower within each T stage while remaining the same overall.

Increasing stage is associated with diminishing survival. The most remarkable change occurs between stages II and III, the zone that generally represents the appearance of cervical metastasis. This chapter is written with the awareness of the absence of an exact definition of "early" cancer; however, metastasis, no matter how slight, is recognized commonly to represent an advanced state of disease.

TREATMENT AND OUTCOMES

Important advances have been made in the development of chemotherapy–radiation therapy strategies for larynx preservation in patients who would otherwise have required total laryngectomy. Our focus on early laryngeal cancer is designed to address malignancies of less tumor volume and specific locations within the larynx that lend themselves to one of several treatment methods:

- Surgical removal alone: conservation (partial) laryngeal operations or endoscopic tumor removal
- Radiation therapy alone
- Conservation laryngeal surgery plus elective regional radiation to the neck areas.

A detailed description of the various partial laryngeal operations used to manage both supraglottic and glottic cancer is beyond the scope of this chapter, but the student of this aspect of head and neck oncology should at the least have a summary knowledge of the methods known collectively as *conservation laryngeal surgery*.

The compartmentalization of the larynx and the directional drainage patterns of the lymph channels that result from embryologic and anatomic factors provide the surgeon with an opportunity to carry out oncologically sound resections without removing the entire organ, and thus preserve swallowing and vocal function. The so-called partial or conservation laryngectomies are associated with the same cure rates as a total laryngectomy in the same lesion. A variety of conservation surgery procedures can be applied to variations of laryngeal cancer and, although a description of them is not provided here, a classification of each, developed in 1988 by Sessions et al. (132), should be helpful to the reader in placing this important surgical methodology into the proper perspective. Since that publication, the development of supracricoid laryngectomy and its variations have further expanded surgical options.

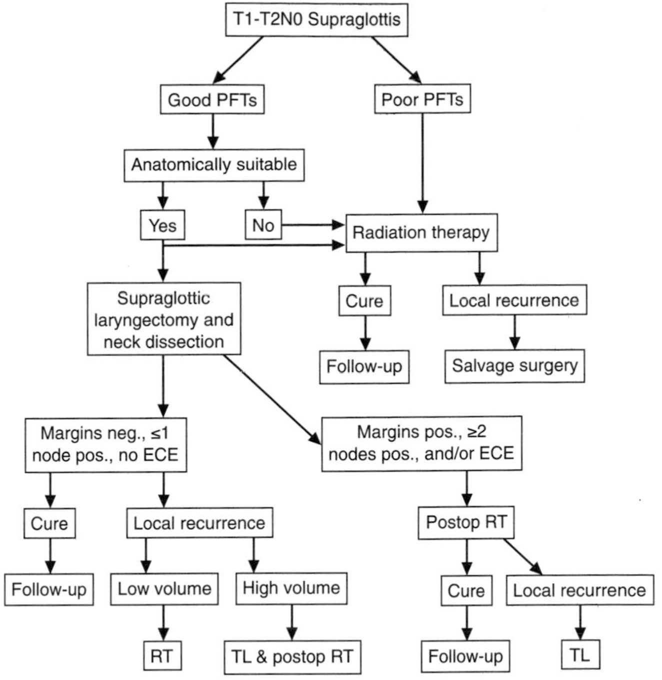

Figure 18.7 Treatment algorithm for T1N0 and T2N0 squamous cell carcinoma of the supraglottis. PFTs, pulmonary function tests; ECE, extracapsular extension; TL, total laryngectomy; RT, radiation therapy.

Supraglottic Cancers

Early stage primary supraglottic disease is highly curable by radiation therapy or by partial laryngeal surgery with or without adjuvant irradiation. However, more advanced lesions usually require treatment with combined modalities, often including total laryngectomy. The decision to use radiation therapy or partial laryngeal surgery depends on several factors including the anatomic extent of the tumor, medical condition of the patient, philosophy of the treating physicians, and the inclination of the patient and family (Fig. 18.7).

Unlike glottic cancer, where cervical metastases are uncommon for early stage disease, the potential for nodal spread in supraglottic lesions is substantial (44,133). A significant probability of contralateral metastasis exists as well, and increases with primary size (81). This is especially true for epiglottic lesions, which make up most of the supraglottic carcinomas. Furthermore, because many epiglottic cancers are midline, both sides of the neck are at risk for metastasis, and this should be addressed in any treatment program. The site of treatment failure in supraglottic cancer is usually the neck; therefore, treatment strategies require neck management for virtually all lesions. For the N0 neck, this implies selective neck dissection or elective radiation. For patients with a clinically positive neck, it implies neck dissection, occasionally therapeutic radiation only, or a combination of both.

Overall, approximately 80% of patients are treated initially by radiation. Approximately half of patients seen at the University of Florida whose lesions are technically amenable to supraglottic laryngectomy have prohibitive medical comorbidities, principally compromised pulmonary function; these patients are necessarily treated by irradiation. Analysis of local control by anatomic site within the supraglottic larynx reveals no obvious differences in local control for stage-matched lesions. However, primary tumor volume as assessed by CT is inversely related to local tumor control after radiation therapy (135,136). A large, bulky lesion is a common reason to select supraglottic laryngectomy.

The so-called supraglottic laryngectomy (horizontal hemilaryngectomy, see Fig. 19.19) allows retention of vocal and swallowing functions. Because of the unique lymphatic drainage patterns of the larynx and the presence of natural anatomic barriers to tumor spread, this operation is oncologically sound, yielding the same local control rates as those achieved by total laryngectomy in comparable lesions (58,137–139).

A supraglottic laryngectomy is essentially a horizontally directed hemilaryngectomy in which the surgeon removes the upper half of the thyroid cartilage and its contents: the false vocal folds, the epiglottis, and the aryepiglottic folds. The superior boundary of the resection lies in the valleculae or even more anteriorly, according to the extent of tumor. A portion of the base of the tongue may be resected if there is question of preepiglottic involvement. The superior edge of the thyroid cartilage remnant is approximated to the remaining base of the tongue. Because the motor nerve supply of the vocal folds comes from below, through the recurrent laryngeal nerves, glottic abduction and adduction are retained and, as a result, voice and the critical ability to close the glottis are preserved. Even with the retention of glottic closure, however, the supraglottic laryngectomy is physiologically challenging: patients with chronic pulmonary disease do not tolerate the aspiration that sometimes follows the operation. The appropriate use of the supraglottic laryngectomy is accomplished only by surgeons properly trained in its technique and, more importantly, experienced and informed enough to select suitable candidates. A succinct discussion of the method of selection for suitability for conservation procedures was developed by Sessions et al. (132), and even though new overall treatment strategies have been developed since its publication, the fundamental decision-making principles remain the same and can still be applied. As alternative treatment schemata are implemented more frequently, fewer supraglottic laryngectomies will be performed; thus, the number of surgeons experienced in these methods inevitably will diminish. Though the idea of saving more larynges without compromising cure certainly is worthwhile, those subtle skills necessary for achieving excellent functional results with partial laryngectomies are to some extent being lost by the new generation of head and neck surgeons.

The complications reported for supraglottic laryngectomy include fistula (8%), carotid artery exposure or blowout (3%–5%), infection or wound sloughing (3%–7%), and other fatal complications (3%) (140). The risk for complication appears increased if tumor margins are involved by tumor.

Supraglottic laryngectomy usually is not recommended in patients who have had full-course radiation therapy because of frequently associated persistent swelling, compromised wound healing, and challenging swallowing rehabilitation. Essentially, the decision to radiate a supraglottic laryngeal lesion should be made with the realization that treatment failure almost always mandates total laryngectomy. Supraglottic laryngectomy, however, does not necessarily prohibit subsequent irradiation. At the University of Florida, approximately 50% of supraglottic laryngectomies have been followed by postoperative irradiation because of neck disease and, less often, positive margins.

Definitive external beam radiation therapy is fairly effective for the management of early supraglottic cancers. As stated earlier, the neck must be treated electively in all cases. Therefore, the treatment technique must include both the primary site (treated definitively) and the neck areas (treated electively). For early stage primary disease that presents with palpable neck metastases, primary radiation often is used at the primary site and the neck areas, followed by a neck dissection to the involved neck region.

In patients irradiated for supraglottic carcinoma, sore throat persists until 3 to 4 weeks after completion of treatment. There is an associated dry mouth from irradiation of the salivary and parotid glands, a loss of taste, and a sensation of a lump in the throat. It is unusual for patients to require a tracheotomy before irradiation unless severe lymphedema develops at the time of direct laryngoscopy and biopsy. However, in patients who have recovered from the direct laryngoscopy and biopsy without obstruction, a tracheotomy has rarely been required during a fractionated course of radiation therapy.

Examples of acute chondritis requiring discontinuation of treatment have not been seen, although most epiglottic lesions exhibit cartilage invasion. The epiglottis remains thicker than normal for long periods of time, but this is not often associated with difficulty in swallowing, respiratory obstruction, or aspiration. The patient is cautioned to eat and drink slowly until the edema resolves. The false fold and arytenoids may develop some edema.

Lesions of the suprahyoid epiglottis frequently destroy the tip of the epiglottis, and it may require some time for the exposed cartilage to heal. Successful irradiation of infrahyoid epiglottis tumors is not associated with a high rate of necrosis, even though most of these lesions penetrate the porous epiglottic cartilage.

Shukovsky (141) analyzed the risk for severe complications for 114 patients with SCC of the supraglottic larynx. Necrosis developed in five patients, and severe edema developed in seven patients. All but one of these complications appeared with doses in excess of 70 Gy delivered over 7 weeks or with larger treatment volumes. At the University of Florida, the incidence of severe complications in 209 patients treated with radiation therapy alone or combined with neck dissection was 0 of 18 (0%) for T1 cancers and 4 of 81 (5%) for T2 lesions (135).

TREATMENT RESULTS

In research dating back to 1972, Wang et al. (143) reported an extensive experience with radiating early lesions. They reported 5-year actuarial disease-free survivals of 73% and 50%, respectively, for T1 and T2 lesions. When surgical salvage was added, this survival increased to 80% and 58%, respectively. A total of 92% of T1 patients and 86% of T2 patients survived with their larynx intact. Mendenhall et al. (144) reported local control of 100% of T1 and 81% of T2 supraglottic lesions. When surgical salvage was added, local control for T2 cancers increased to 88%. Importantly, this study revealed no significant differences in local control by anatomic subsite. These data were fortified when Mendenhall et al. (144) later reported on 209 patients with a minimum 2-year follow-up after radiation therapy with or without neck dissection. Local control was 100% for T1 lesions and 83% for T2 lesions. In the T2 group, local control was 80% for once-daily radiation versus 90% for twice-daily treatment. A further update of the University of Florida series of 274 patients treated with radiation therapy revealed the following 5-year local control rates: T1, 100%, and T2, 86% (Table 18.2) (145). The patients in this recent update were staged according to the 1998 AJCC staging, which produced some negative stage migration. The local tumor control rate after radiation therapy is inversely related to the CT-calculated primary tumor volume (136).

The 3-year cause-specific survival rates for patients with supraglottic carcinoma treated by supraglottic laryngectomy at Washington University were 64 of 78 (82%) for patients with T1N0 cancers and 23 of 34 (68%) for those with T2N0 malignancies (147). Low-dose preoperative irradiation was given to some patients. Bocca (148) reports 250 cases of T1 and T2 supraglottic carcinoma treated by supraglottic laryngectomy and bilateral elective or therapeutic neck dissection. The local recurrence rate was 11%, and the neck recurrence rate was 5%; in 9 patients, salvage was achieved by further therapy. The 5-year survival rate was 80%.

MANAGEMENT OF THE NECK

Evaluation and management of the neck are critical to successful therapy of supraglottic cancer. Levendag and Vikram (67) studied elective surgical management of the neck in a group of patients with stage I and stage II supraglottic carcinomas treated with surgery alone at the Memorial Sloan-Kettering Cancer Center. Of those patients who underwent elective neck dissection (i.e., the group with clinically negative neck areas), 32% were found to have histologically positive cervical lymph nodes. This metastasis rate in clinically negative neck areas is similar to time-honored data first published in conjunction with the early literature on supraglottic laryngectomy. In the study by Levendag and Vikram (67), treatment eventually failed in the dissected neck in half of the patients. Additionally,

TABLE 18.2 Supraglottic Squamous Cell Carcinoma: Locoregional Control and Cause-Specific Survival After Radiation Therapy at the University of Florida (n = 91)

1998 AJCC stage	Locoregional control (%)	Cause-specific survival (%)
I	100	100
II	86	93

AJCC, American Joint Committee on Cancer.
Source: Hinerman RW, Mendenhall WM, Amdur RJ, et al. Carcinoma of the supraglottic larynx: treatment results with radiotherapy alone or with planned neck dissection. *Head Neck* 2001.

treatment in 19% of patients with negative elective neck dissections failed in the contralateral neck. Finally, in a group of 48 patients who did not have elective neck dissection, treatment in 29% failed in the neck. Essentially, therefore, a total of 35% of the T1 to T2N0 patients ultimately developed cervical lymph node metastases. Importantly, nearly two thirds of those with relapses in the neck eventually died from their cancer. Conversely, none of the patients without neck relapse died from supraglottic cancer. These investigators compared their experiences with a similar patient group from the other studies that showed similar neck failure rates with surgery alone and when radiation therapy was administered to the neck areas. Harwood et al. (149) reports a 3% failure rate in the electively radiated neck. Therefore, recommending elective neck management seems intuitively correct for even the smallest supraglottic cancer.

A relative advantage of radiation therapy in the treatment of the primary site of early stage supraglottic disease is that bilateral elective neck treatment can be included with minimal morbidity in the radiation plan. If an adequate dose of elective neck radiation is given, neck relapse should be less than 5%. If, however, surgery is chosen as the treatment for a T1 or T2 supraglottic lesion, the supraglottic laryngectomy should be combined with bilateral staging selective neck dissections. The consistent drainage patterns of supraglottic lesions allow the surgeon to tailor the dissection to harvest those specific nodes at high risk for the particular lesion. This capability allows the surgeon to minimize the morbidity associated with the operation. The value of this principle is demonstrated vividly by the fact that supraglottic carcinomas rarely metastasize to level I. Dissection of level I, therefore, generally is deleted from any selective neck dissection performed for these primary tumors.

Postoperative radiation therapy is added in the patients in whom metastatic disease or involved margins is found at surgery. In treating the neck, however, consideration should be given to protecting the remaining larynx because of the morbidity associated with treating the post-supraglottic laryngectomy with radiation. Laryngeal edema and the need for prolonged tracheostomy or laryngectomy are potential problems in this situation.

Supraglottic laryngectomy is followed by local failure only rarely. In those surgical patients in whom staging neck surgery yields histologically negative neck regions, usually no need is found for postoperative radiation therapy. The accuracy of well-performed staging neck dissections in predicting cervical metastasis, though not perfect, is high. The obvious disadvantage to this approach is that in those patients who do demonstrate histologically positive neck areas and in whom radiation then is employed, two different treatment modalities have been expended. This approach stands in contrast to the strategy in which radiation therapy is employed initially to the primary tumor and neck regions. The disadvantage of the "radiation only" plan is that when failure occurs, total rather than partial laryngectomy is required. Also to be pointed out, however, is that in the rare local recurrence after supraglottic laryngectomy, total laryngectomy also becomes necessary for salvage. With this type of treatment strategy planning, as much as in any area of cancer treatment, continuous interdisciplinary communication and cooperation are essential.

In early supraglottic cancer, therefore, the decision of what approach to use on the neck is not based on rigid criteria but instead on a variety of considerations, not the least of which is the planned treatment for the primary site. If, for example, a supraglottic primary tumor with clinically negative neck areas is scheduled for definitive radiation, the treatment portals usually are designed to treat both primary and the neck regions. In the circumstance in which the primary tumor is to be treated surgically, the neck should be staged with the appropriate neck dissection. If the nodes harvested in the dissection are histologically negative, one can avoid postoperative radiation, assuming, of course, that the operation on the primary tumor successfully encompassed it. On the other hand, if the neck contains metastases, our belief is that postoperative radiation should be employed. If the initial plan of attack for the primary tumor is surgical, it is important that the selection process be based on those time-honored selection principles outlined in 1988 by Sessions et al. (132). These selection factors will help to avoid the need for postoperative radiation and to maximize the chance for surgical cure. Furthermore, the pathologic analysis of the margin in supraglottic laryngectomy must be undertaken carefully because postoperative radiation of the primary site in this operation is fraught with significant complications, in both the short and the long term.

Glottic and Subglottic Cancers

CARCINOMA *IN SITU*

Carcinoma *in situ* of the true vocal fold is highly curable, and this goal can be achieved equally well by microlaryngoscopic excision, laser vaporization, or radiation therapy (150–153). Pure CIS lesions probably are unusual; frequent association with invasive carcinoma is seen. Those series in which recurrences were observed after CIS treated by stripping of the vocal fold mucosa almost certainly consisted of a heterogeneous group of lesions that included some containing areas of overlooked invasive cancer. Microscopic foci of cancer probably remained after instrumentation, hence the somewhat high failure rate. By definition, true CIS remains superficial to the basement membrane and mucosal removal, whether by stripping, excision or laser vaporization, and should yield the same cure rate as that of any other treatment method, including radiation therapy. In fact, radiation therapy has certain advantages for these lesions: radiation is a more definitive treatment for unrecognized invasive cancer; general anesthesia is not required; and when treatment fails, a voice-saving surgical procedure still can salvage some vocal capacity for most patients. Microlaryngoscopic surgical techniques, on the other hand, offer simple, one-step removal in the course of the same operation required for diagnosis, and radiation therapy remains in reserve should there be recurrence. Considering the significant incidence of second primary tumors in this family of tumors, this latter advantage is not irrelevant in the development of treatment strategy. Also noteworthy is that as long as the integrity of the submucosal tissues is not violated, the voice quality after microexcision is comparable to that achieved with radiation.

Submucosal infusion during direct laryngoscopy is a potentially useful tool for evaluation of early invasive lesions. Infusion of saline, epinephrine, or lidocaine into the superficial lamina propria has occasionally been used in microlaryngoscopic surgery for hemostasis or supplementary anesthesia, or to minimize trauma during dissection. The dimpling of the mucosa at sites of tethering to the underlying ligament is a familiar phenomenon to the phonosurgeon, and helps to reveal the extent and depth of a small invasive carcinoma hidden among CIS (154). Prospective investigation remains to be done, but submucosal infusion may aid intraoperative decision making.

Wherever possible, so-called stripping of the vocal fold mucosa should be avoided because of its adverse effect on voice. The more precise microexcision, on the other hand, is followed by minimal impact on vocal function if performed judiciously. Additionally, microexcision has the advantage over

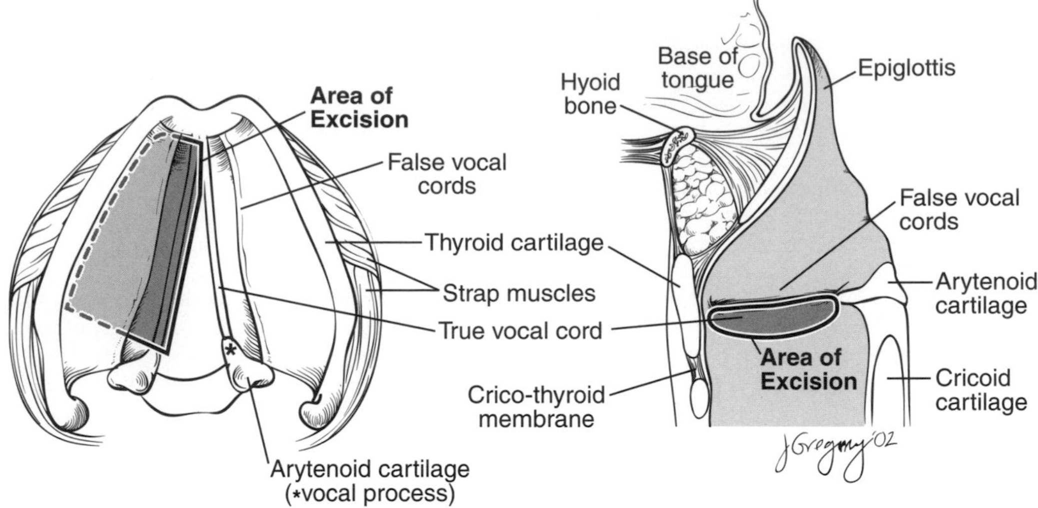

Figure 18.8 Cordectomy. The procedure has very limited applicability. It can be done endoscopically using cutting or laser techniques. Opening the larynx from the front also allows the surgeon to view the interior of the larynx directly. In this procedure, only the vocal cord is removed.

both laser vaporization and radiation therapy of providing the pathologist with a specimen that preserves the histologic appearance of the lesion, perhaps revealing small areas of microinvasion that otherwise would have gone unappreciated.

Radiation therapy may be used as the definitive treatment of CIS when microexcision is either impractical or unacceptable to the patient. Pêne and Fletcher (155) describe the results for 79 patients with CIS and 7 patients with dysplasia. The local failure rate was 11% for lesions with a T1 anatomic distribution and 26% for T2 lesions. Elman et al. (156) report similar results. Nineteen patients with CIS were treated at the University of Florida, and the disease was locally controlled in 18 (95%), with a minimum follow-up of 2 years (157).

Radiation also is used as a salvage treatment for patients with recurrent CIS after prior surgical procedures. Some disagreement exists among laryngologists on this point; some believe that endoscopic cordectomy (Fig. 18.8) is the superior method of addressing this problem, from both a curative and an economic standpoint (150). In cases of early glottic carcinoma, as indeed in all cases of head and neck cancer with good cure rates, functional outcome—voice quality in this context—must be a primary consideration. It is clear that voice generally tends to be superior following radiation (158,159). Nevertheless, surgery can achieve good oncologic results without compromise of vocal function in carefully selected lesions, namely, unilateral disease sparing the anterior commissure, subglottis, and arytenoid (160,161). In addition, voice quality deteriorates in proportion to the amount of vocalis muscle resected (162). It follows, then, that in general, pure CIS is extremely amenable to microexcision. The difficulty remains in predicting histology before surgery. As we have seen, strobo-videolaryngoscopy is not a reliable tool in this endeavor (124).

T1 AND T2 LESIONS

For early glottic cancer (T1 to T2), excellent local control is achieved by radiation or partial laryngectomy, or even endoscopic resection in some lesions. The relative advantage of radiation over surgery relates to vocal function. From the point of view of vocal function, the limitations for endoscopic resection of CIS described previously remain the same for T1 and T2 glottic lesions. By virtue of their larger size, however, these lesions are less likely to satisfy these criteria. Radiation offers better voice quality than that achieved with hemilaryngectomy or cordectomy. Near-normal vocalization can be expected in most cases managed by radiation therapy. A complete review of relevant studies is available in the rehabilitation chapter. Another advantage to radiating early glottic cancer is that hemilaryngectomy can be used successfully for salvage in many patients in whom radiation has failed (86,163–166). Thus, in a carefully selected subset of patients, even the second line of defense against glottic cancer does not involve sacrifice of the entire larynx. Beyond this, total laryngectomy sometimes offers still a

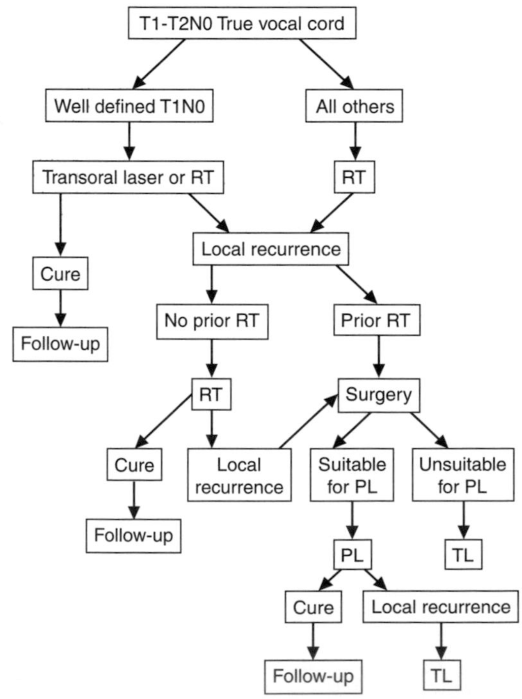

Figure 18.9 Treatment algorithm for T1N0 and T2N0 squamous cell carcinoma of the true vocal fold. RT, radiation therapy; PL, partial laryngectomy; TL, total laryngectomy.

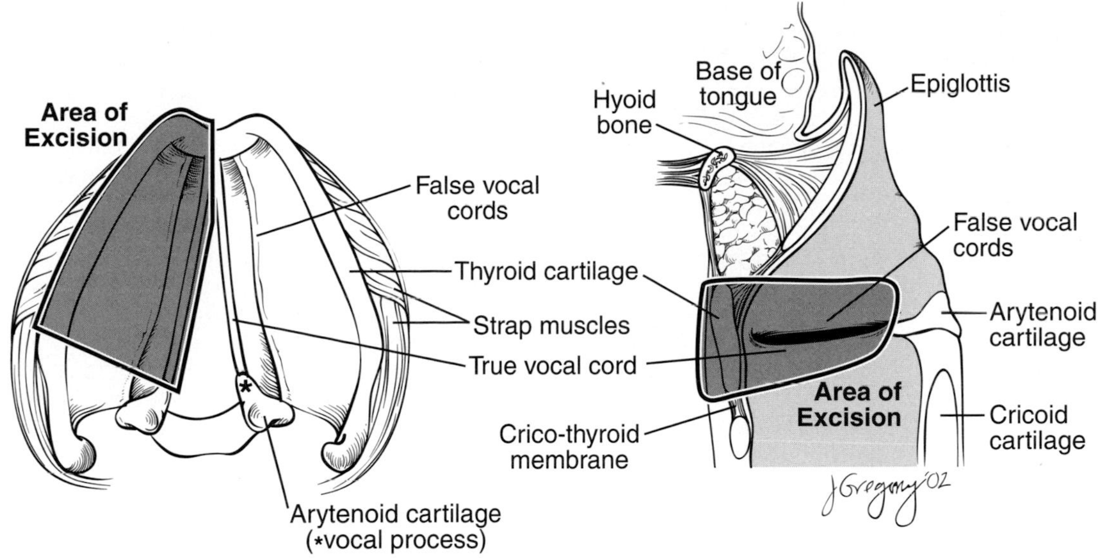

Figure 18.10 Hemilaryngectomy. The classic hemilaryngectomy is employed for true vocal cord tumors. Note that the remaining half of the larynx is unimpaired and voice production can continue.

third chance at salvage (167). A seamless and continuous interdisciplinary interaction in the management and follow-up of these patients is essential (Fig. 18.9).

When used in properly selected cases, conservation surgical procedures for glottic cancer consistently yield excellent functional and oncologic results. The procedure most commonly employed is the vertical hemilaryngectomy in which the surgeon bisects the larynx and removes a variable portion or all of the true and false vocal folds along with the respective half of the thyroid cartilage (Figs. 18.10, 18.11). Given the standards of current treatment strategies, the majority of vertical hemilaryngectomies are performed for patients in whom radiation treatment has failed. Vertical hemilaryngectomy can be employed effectively in a high percentage of radiation-failure glottic lesions. Because most of the lesions for which vertical hemilaryngectomy is employed are located on the anterior two thirds of the vocal fold, the most posterior resection line usually lies in front of the arytenoid cartilage. In those circumstances in which the cancer extends onto the posterior larynx, this cartilage can be resected. By using the perichondrium from the external surface of that half of the thyroid cartilage that has been removed, the operated side of the larynx heals in the midline, forming a firm buttress (pseudocord) against which the remaining (i.e., normal) true vocal fold can close the glottic gap and thus vibrate for phonation. The postoperative complications and sequelae of hemilaryngectomy include chondritis, wound slough, inadequate glottic closure, and anterior commissure webs (140).

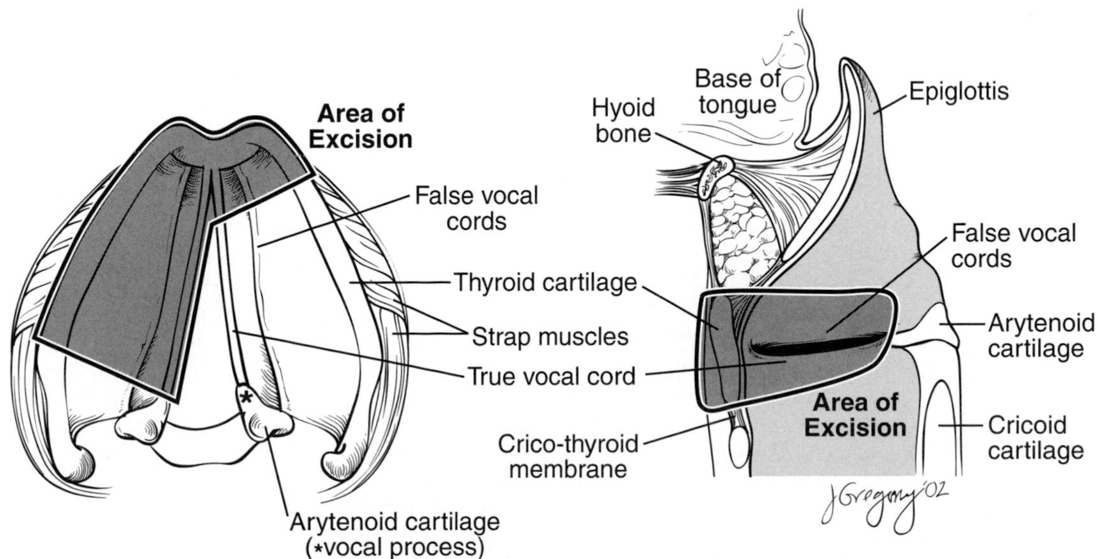

Figure 18.11 Extended frontolateral laryngectomy. Diagrammatic representation of the removal of the hemilarynx (i.e., half the larynx plus a portion of the contralateral vocal cord and thyroid cartilage). Area of excision is shaded.

Supracricoid laryngectomy, as reported by Laccourreye et al. (169), is a procedure designed to remove moderate-sized cancers involving the supraglottic and glottic larynx. The majority of the larynx may be removed with preservation of the cricoid and one arytenoid with its neurovascular supply. The defect is closed by approximating the base of the tongue to the laryngeal remnant. The oncologic and functional results of this procedure in selected patients are reported to be excellent.

In most centers, irradiation is the initial treatment prescribed for T1 and T2 lesions, with surgery reserved for salvage after radiation therapy failure (86,170–172). The acute reactions from the treatment of early vocal fold cancer are relatively mild. During the first 2 to 3 weeks, the voice may improve as the tumor regresses. The voice generally becomes hoarse again because of radiation-induced changes, even though the tumor continues to regress. A sore throat develops beginning at the end of the second week, but medication is often not required. The voice begins to improve approximately 3 weeks after completion of treatment. Patients with extensive lesions often recover a near-normal voice, although not as frequently as those with small tumors.

Edema of the larynx is the most common sequela after irradiation for glottic or supraglottic lesions. The rate of clearance of the edema is related to the radiation dose, volume of tissue irradiated, addition of a neck dissection, continued use of alcohol and tobacco, and size and extent of the original lesion. Edema may be accentuated by a radical neck dissection and may require 6 to 12 months to subside. Corticosteroids such as dexamethasone have been used to reduce radiation-induced edema after recurrence has been ruled out by biopsy. If ulceration and pain occur, administration of an antibiotic such as tetracycline may help.

Soft tissue necrosis leading to chondritis occurs in less than 1% of patients, usually in those who continue to smoke. Soft tissue and cartilage necroses mimic recurrence, with hoarseness, pain, and edema; a laryngectomy may be recommended as a last resort for fear of recurrent cancer, even though biopsy specimens show only necrosis.

Of 519 patients with T1N0 or T2N0 vocal fold cancer treated at the University of Florida, 5 (1%) experienced severe complications (173). These included total laryngectomy for a suspected local recurrence (1 patient), permanent tracheostomy for edema (3 patients), and a pharyngocutaneous fistula following a salvage total laryngectomy (1 patient).

TREATMENT RESULTS

The actual survival results for primary surgery for T1 glottic cancer are 84% to 98% with laryngofissure and cordectomy, respectively (150,174–177). Neel et al. (178) report results for 182 patients with early vocal fold carcinoma who were suitable for cordectomy; 177 had lesions that were confined to one fold. The lesions were 2 to 25 mm in length. The follow-up was less than 3 years in 18% of the cases. Laryngeal recurrence developed in four patients, and neck recurrence developed in three patients. Only three patients (2%) died of vocal fold cancer. Various series have reported similar results with hemilaryngectomy, which is considered to be oncologically and functionally a better operation than cordectomy. Essentially, the 5-year survival rates for primary surgery and primary radiation in T1 lesions are comparable (179–183). Local control obtained in the T1 glottic group using conservation surgical procedures is reported to be 78% by Kirchner and Owen (68) and 87% by Ogura et al. (185).

Thomas et al. (186) report on 159 patients who underwent open partial laryngectomy for T1 glottic cancers at the Mayo Clinic between 1976 and 1986. Seventeen of 159 patients had *in situ* lesions; the remainder were invasive. Local recurrence developed in 11 patients (7%), and 9 patients eventually required laryngectomy. Disease recurrence in the neck was reported in 10 patients, and distant metastases were noted in 10 patients. Ogura et al. (187) describe a 3-year disease-free survival rate of 91% for 281 patients treated by hemilaryngectomy. The local recurrence rate was 4%, and the neck recurrence rate was 1.5%; 74% of the treatment failures were controlled by salvage therapy. Bauer et al. (188) analyzed the significance of the surgical margins in 111 hemilaryngectomy specimens. Thirty-nine patients (35%) had involved margins (usually the anterior margin). The local recurrence rate was 10% with 5-year minimum follow-up. Only 7 of 39 patients (18%) with an involved margin experienced recurrence, compared with 6% with uninvolved margins. Another 5% had recurrence evident in the cervical lymph nodes. Four patients eventually died of cancer.

Results obtained for comparable (T1) lesions treated by radiation therapy show local control of 91% by Harwood (152) and 93% by Pellitteri et al. (183). As is true with any treatment the local control rate decreases with increasing tumor bulk. Dickens et al. (189) have reported the results for such tumors of various sizes and extent. The lesions were categorized by the type of surgical procedure that would have been necessary had surgery been used. This type of analysis provides an excellent basis for comparing the results of surgery and radiation. The local control with radiation alone in patients suitable for cordectomy was 97%; in patients who needed hemilaryngectomy, it was 94%. In both categories, local control increased to 100% when surgical salvage was added. Extension of these glottic carcinomas onto the anterior and posterior aspects of the larynx lessens the local control rates achieved with radiation therapy, and the surgical procedure required for salvage often was a total laryngectomy rather than a hemilaryngectomy (189).

With anterior commissure involvement, Sessions et al. (190) report a 5-year survival with surgical treatment of 74% for T1 and T2 lesions. These authors found that survival and recurrence rates of anterior commissure lesions correlate with the size and stage of the tumor (191). Results with radiation therapy for early stage glottic carcinomas that involve the anterior commissure are reported by Olofsson (192) to be 80% survival at 5 years (including those recurrences salvaged by surgery) and by Kirchner and Fischer (78), who report a local control rate of 85%. Those anterior commissure lesions that are thin and of lesser volume and that do not have substantial subglottic extension probably are treated with equal efficiency by partial laryngectomy or radiation therapy. As lesions become more advanced, the natural barrier of the anterior commissure ligament is overcome, and the thyroid cartilage is invaded (192); therefore, radiation therapy becomes less appealing than surgery as the initial treatment. Most tumors involving the anterior commissure occur as a result of spread from the true vocal fold. Lesions actually arising in the anterior commissure are unusual, making up only 1% to 2% of glottic cancers (191,192).

The management of T2 glottic lesions is more complicated because this group is more heterogeneous. Surgical management usually consists of vertical hemilaryngectomy, and 83% and 82% 3-year survival rates have been reported in two major series (185,190). Hemilaryngectomy including the ipsilateral arytenoid was reported by Som (195) for 130 cases of vocal fold carcinoma extending posteriorly to the vocal process and face of the arytenoid. The cure rate was 74% for 104 patients with T2 lesions. Primary radiation therapy plus surgical salvage yielded a net 5-year survival rate of 92% in the series by Pellitteri et al. (183), 72% in Wang's series (181), 90% in the series by Fletcher et al. (179), and 72% in Jorgensen's series (182). Because of the heterogeneity of the T2 group of larynx cancer patients, Wang (181) has suggested subdividing these lesions into those with

TABLE 18.3 T1 and T2 Carcinoma of the Glottic Larynx Treated with Radiation Therapy

Investigation	No. of patients		Local control[a] (%)		Ultimate local control (%)	
	T1	T2	T1	T2	T1	T2
Princess Margaret Hospital, Toronto, Canada (195)	333	244	86	69	—	—
M. D. Anderson Cancer Center, Houston, Tx. (196)	332	275	89	74	98	94
University of Maryland, Baltimore (197)	86	34	92	88	99	94
University of California at San Francisco (199)	315	83	85	70	96[b]	91[b]
University of Florida, Gainesville (170)	291	228	94/93[c]	80/72[d]	98/98[c]	96/96[d]

[a]No exclusions.
[b]10-year locoregional control.
[c]T1a/T1b.
[d]T2a/T2b.

Source: Modified from Mendenhall WM, Parsons JT, Million RR, et al. T1–T2 squamous cell carcinoma of the glottic larynx treated with radiation therapy: relationship of dose-fractionation factors to local control and complications. *Int J Radiat Oncol Biol Phys* 1988;15: 1267–1273.

normal mobility (T2a) and those with impaired mobility (T2b). He showed that local control was obtained in 86% of the former and 63% of the latter when primary radiation was used. Similar observations were made by Harwood (152), whose series yielded 77% and 51% local control rates for T2a and T2b lesions, respectively. Essentially, T2b lesions seem to behave more as T3 lesions than as T2 lesions.

Radiation therapy usually is recommended as the primary treatment modality for T2 lesions with normal vocal fold mobility (i.e., T2a). In those lesions that demonstrate motion impairment and thus are classified as T2b, hemilaryngectomy usually is preferred. These criteria can vary, depending on tumor bulk, and some of these T2b lesions with less bulky disease can be irradiated successfully. Also noteworthy is that when vocal fold motion is restricted by surface tumor bulk rather than by invasion of the underlying muscle, radiation often is effective. The overall 5-year survival for T1 glottic carcinomas is 82% to 96%; for T2 lesions, it is 51% to 85% (174,196–198).

The local tumor control rates reported from several institutions for invasive SCC are in the range of 90% for T1 and 70% for T2 disease (173,199–203). The surgical salvage rate is 90% to 95% for patients with T1 or T2 lesions that recur after irradiation (Table 18.3) (166,173,199–203). The local tumor control and survival rates according to stage for 519 patients with SCC of the vocal fold who were treated by radiation therapy at the University of Florida are given in Tables 18.4 and 18.5 (173). Most patients with T1 lesions were irradiated once daily at 2.25 Gy per fraction; those with T2 cancers received 2.25 Gy per fraction once daily or 1.2 Gy per fraction twice daily.

Based on our data and the literature, there is a direct relationship between the rate of local tumor control and overall treatment time (which is related to dose per fraction) with poor results obtained particularly in the T2 lesions treated at 1.8 to 1.9 Gy per fraction to similar or higher total doses (166,173,203). Schwaibold et al. (205) report on 56 evaluable patients treated with irradiation for T1N0 glottic carcinoma. Twenty-eight patients were treated at 1.8 Gy per fraction with a local tumor control rate of 75%, which was compared with 100% local control for 28 patients treated at 2 Gy or higher per fraction. Kim et al. (206) also note a relationship between local control and dose per fraction.

The 5-year rates of neck recurrence after irradiation of the primary site alone in patients whose disease was locally controlled after treatment were as follows: T1, 0%; T2a, 3%; and T2b, 8% (173). However, if the cancer recurred at the primary site after irradiation for T1 and T2 cancers, the risk for recurrence in the neck nodes was approximately 20% to 25% (207).

Verrucous lesions have the reputation of being unresponsive to radiation therapy and, in some instances, converting into invasive, often anaplastic, metastasizing lesions. Partial laryngectomy is recommended for early verrucous carcinoma of the glottis, but irradiation is recommended if the alternative is total laryngectomy (110). We have observed typical verrucous lesions that have disappeared with radiation therapy and not recurred. O'Sullivan et al. (111) also have made this observation. Additionally, a variety of tumors that recur after unsuccessful treatment (with surgery, radiation therapy, or chemotherapy) are more likely to exhibit more aggressive behavior.

TABLE 18.4 T1 and T2 Carcinoma of the Glottic Larynx: Local Control at 5 Years After Irradiation (519 Patients)

Stage	No. of patients	Local control after initial therapy (%)	Ultimate local control (%)	Ultimate local control with larynx preservation (%)
T1a	230	94	98	95
T1b	61	93	98	98
T2a	146	80	96	82
T2b	82	72	96	76

Source: Mendenhall WM, Amdur RJ, Morris CG, et al. T1-T2N0 squamous cell carcinoma of the glottic larynx treated with radiation therapy. *J Clin Oncol* 2001;19:4029–4036.

TABLE 18.5 T1 and T2 Carcinoma of the Glottic Larynx: 5-Year Survival Rates (519 Patients)

Stage	No. of patients	Absolute survival (%)	Cause-specific survival (%)
T1a N0	230	82	98
T1b N0	61	79	98
T2a N0	146	77	95
T2b N0	82	77	90

Source: Mendenhall WM, Amdur RJ, Morris CG, et al. T1-T2N0 squamous cell carcinoma of the glottic larynx treated with radiation therapy. *J Clin Oncol* 2001;19:4029–4036.

Management of Recurrence

FOLLOW-UP POLICY

Follow-up of patients with early lesions is planned for every 4 to 8 weeks for 2 years, every 3 months for year 3, every 6 months for years 4 and 5, and then annually for life. Follow-up of these patients is as important as the treatment itself because early detection of recurrence usually results in salvage that may include cure with voice preservation (208).

If recurrence is suspected but biopsy is negative, patients are reexamined at 2- to 4-week intervals until the matter is settled. The value of follow-up CT scans for detecting early local recurrence remains to be determined.

Wagenfeld et al. (209) studied 740 cases of glottic larynx cancer treated from 1965 to 1974 to determine the incidence of second respiratory tract malignancies. With a minimum follow-up of 5 years, 48 second respiratory tract malignancies occurred, although only 14 were expected. Twenty-five were in the lung, and 23 were scattered among other head and neck sites. Only 7 of the 23 second head and neck primary lesions resulted in death; these second lesions were frequently diagnosed in an early stage during routine follow-up for the glottic lesion. Because the risk for a lethal lung primary lesion is nearly as great as that of dying of an early glottic carcinoma, annual chest roentgenograms are obligatory.

Most recurrences of early glottic carcinoma appear within 18 months, but late recurrences may appear after 5 years (140). With careful follow-up, recurrence is sometimes detected before the patient notices a change of voice. There is often lymphedema for 1 to 2 months after irradiation, which usually subsides or stabilizes. An increase in edema, particularly if associated with hoarseness or pain, suggests recurrence, even if there is no obvious tumor. Fixation of a previously mobile vocal fold also implies local recurrence, but we have occasionally observed a patient who has experienced a fixed fold with an otherwise normal-appearing larynx and who has not shown evidence of recurrence. It may be difficult to diagnose recurrence if the tumor is submucosal. Generous deep biopsies are required. If recurrence is strongly suspected, laryngectomy may rarely be advised without biopsy-confirmed evidence of recurrence.

Recurrence following radiation therapy may be salvaged by cordectomy, hemilaryngectomy, or total laryngectomy. Biller et al. (210) report a 78% salvage rate by hemilaryngectomy for 18 selected patients in whom irradiation failed; total laryngectomy was eventually required in two patients. Only two patients died of cancer. These investigators offered criteria for using hemilaryngectomy: a mobile index vocal fold, a contralateral vocal fold unaffected by disease, an uninvolved arytenoid, and subglottic extension limited to 5 mm. In our experience, 10 patients irradiated for T1 or T2 vocal fold cancers underwent a hemilaryngectomy following a local recurrence, and 6 were successfully salvaged (86).

The rate of salvage by irradiation for recurrences or new tumors that appear after initial treatment by hemilaryngectomy is about 50% (211).

The overall likelihood of successful salvage after a local recurrence of supraglottic cancer is about 50%; it is probably somewhat better for patients who initially have stage I or II disease (208). Low-volume local recurrence may sometimes be successfully treated with radiation therapy. Patients with high-volume recurrences are best managed with a total laryngectomy and postoperative irradiation; very few are suitable for a voice-sparing procedure. Approximately one third of patients sustain a major complication secondary to salvage surgery, usually related to poor wound healing. When an isolated recurrence develops in the neck, patients have a 50% to 60% chance of cure by means of a salvage neck dissection (213). There is no possibility of cure after development of distant metastases, and management is palliative with either supportive care or chemotherapy.

SPECIAL ISSUES AND FUTURE DIRECTIONS

Limited data are available pertaining to the use of chemotherapy alone as the initial step in treatment of patients with early stage laryngeal cancer (214,215). A small subset of patients may be cured with chemotherapy alone, thus sparing them the morbidity of irradiation or partial laryngectomy. A caveat is that the cure rates for patients with early stage disease are already very high, the morbidity of chemotherapy may be more severe than that associated with conventional treatment, and over 90% of patients must proceed to irradiation or surgery despite the chemotherapy (which probably does not enhance the likelihood of cure).

CONCLUSION

The overwhelming majority of early stage glottic and supraglottic cancers are curable. Precise evaluation of the extent and stage of disease is essential to achieving the best outcomes. Because these cancers can have a major impact on voice and on the ability to communicate, the ability to eat, and the general quality of life, optimal care requires an experienced team of physicians, nurses, and voice specialists. Only by combining sophisticated surgical and radiotherapeutic management will the highest cure rates and functional results be realized.

ACKNOWLEDGMENT

We thank the research support staff of the University of Florida Health Science Center's Department of Radiation Oncology for their help with statistics, editing, and manuscript preparation.

RADIOLOGIC IMAGING CONCERNS

Bernard B. O'Malley and Suresh K. Mukherji

The choice of modality between CT and MRI depends on multiple variables (216). The most important variable is patient condition (Fig. 18.12). Throat discomfort due to local or referred symptoms and difficulty in managing secretions limit the application of MRI for detailed laryngeal imaging. Patients experiencing these symptoms of locally aggressive disease are the worst candidates for imaging. Reducing scan time always compromises the quality of the image. Computed tomography is faster but is limited to one (axial) plane and essentially one "series," compared with the multiple sequences and planes available with MRI. Magnetic resonance imaging is more sensitive to early infiltration of tissue planes and would be preferred for staging of the endolarynx (217). Another variable is imaging equipment. High-speed CT is requisite for that modality. This latest generation of CT technology is "helical" (or "spiral") CT, which avoids the staggered motion of the body through the scanner by using slip-ring technology. This advance allows for greater detail and is less susceptible to patient motion and respiratory artifacts (218). Because of the ability of a helical scanner to scan an organ into one contiguous data set, the quality of subsequent reformatted coronal and sagittal views is improved (218). Another advantage of CT is that it is technically a very reproducible method of scanning the neck. The resulting images also have a very acceptable interobserver and intraobserver variability in interpretation (219).

The most important imaging landmarks of the larynx are the paraglottic space, the anterior commissure, the subglottic extent, and the preepiglottic space. Very early vocal cord lesions rarely come to imaging. Imaging of early lesions that meet the threshold for suspicion of risk for submucosal involvement require thin-section examination with CT (1–1.5 mm) or MRI (2–3 mm). Axial images should be obtained parallel to the plane of the true cords. This view is the best plane for clearing the anterior and posterior commissures. Direct coronal MRI or reformatted CT images are helpful for tracking disease within the paraglottic space (Fig. 18.13). The preepiglottic space is best evaluated in the axial plane or by direct sagittal MRI (Fig. 18.14) or reformatted CT (Fig. 18.15). Noncontrast MRI can evaluate the critical preepiglottic space landmark for supraglottic tumor (220).

Given that the patient with early squamous cancer of the larynx has multiple treatment options, imaging of the organ requires careful planning (221) and analysis despite the early stage. Clinical evaluation best determines the mucosal extent of the lesion. The primary role of imaging is to confirm that the lesion is early stage (T1 or T2) and exclude significant submucosal extension or early cartilage invasion. In our experience, imaging upstages clinically T1 and T2 lesions to T4 in 10% to 20% of cases. Imaging studies should be specifically evaluated for:

1. Early cartilage invasion (thyroid, arytenoid, cricoid)
2. Anterior extension to the anterior commissure and possible early thyroid cartilage invasion along the Broyle's ligament
3. Posterior extension into the interarytenoid posterior commissure
4. Transglottic extension
5. Subglottic extension.

This information must be specifically assessed on each imaging study to confirm that the tumor is an early lesion. Tumors centered in the anterior commissure may be primary anterior commissure tumors. These tumors are often best identified on imaging due to their characteristic pattern of extent. Proper identification of these tumors is important due to their propensity for early thyroid cartilage invasion and because of their very anterior location, the potential geographic inhomogeneity of dose distribution that may lead to under dosing. Gross morphologic changes to the larynx such as laryngocele are occasionally caused by squamous cancer. Images of any laryngocele should be examined for the possibility of a causative tumor (Fig. 18.16).

Occasionally, tumors are associated with sclerotic changes of the cartilage. Pathologic studies have revealed a 50% likelihood of microscopic cartilage invasion in a single sclerotic cartilage directly adjacent to tumor. There is a much greater likelihood (>90%) of cartilage invasion if more than two adjacent cartilages are sclerotic next to tumor. As a result, cartilage sclerosis has been correlated with a poorer local control rate with radiation therapy (222). Initial studies suggested that CT has a higher specificity for cartilage invasion (223) than MRI despite CT's lower sensitivity. However, more recent investigations suggest a similar diagnostic accuracy for both imaging modalities for detecting cartilage invasion.

Supraglottic lesions are analyzed in a similar fashion, with particular attention to the preepiglottic and paraglottic spaces (Fig. 18.17). Because of the variable size and undulating contours of the aryepiglottic folds, detecting and outlining lesions are difficult at that site. Early extension into the pyriform aperture and medial wall of the sinus is better excluded clinically. Tumor volume has been shown to be a significant independent pre-treatment indicator of prognosis for local control at all subsites of the larynx including the glottis (224) and supraglottis (136,225,226). The influence is less significant in cases treated surgically (228).

Follow-up posttreatment imaging has a limited role and is not obtained routinely in the absence of clinically suspicious signs of recurrence or progression. Early follow-up CT may be under utilized, however, as CT can show early treatment failure before clinically suspected (229). Irradiation produces generalized increase in the mucosal thickness and enhancement (230). Confirming resolution of an index lesion or excluding superficial recurrence is difficult against those background changes (Fig. 18.18). This edema resolves and leaves the mucosa with a thickened appearance on follow-up imaging (Fig. 18.19). Surgical deformities produce a unique appearance in individual patients requiring carefully reproduced imaging protocols to detect recurrence at an early stage. Treatment necrosis is clinically problematic, and cross-sectional imaging is nonspecific in this setting (Fig. 18.20). Even in the presence of necrotic-appearing soft tissue, the possibility of residual underlying tumor cannot be excluded with certainty. Solid areas of new or recurrent enhancement may be suggested as productive biopsy targets. Pameijer et al. (231) outlined a scoring system to create a risk profile on treated patients based in (contrast) CT features. Focal mass greater than 1 cm or residual mass not less than 50% of original tumor volume predicted poorer prognosis. The modality of choice in this setting is fluorodeoxyglucose-positron emission tomography (FDG-PET) imaging (232). The hypermetabolism of neoplastic cells is greater than that of the surrounding inflammation and low-level mucosal activity. It was initially thought that PET scanning should be postponed for months after treatment. Earlier short-term evaluation may in fact be a method to determine if the treatment plan is effective in a given patient allowing a faster track to salvage treatment before long-term treatment effects make further treatment less attractive. The scans, when negative, can obviate the need for posttreatment biopsy or encourage further biopsy when suggestive of persistent or recurrent disease (233). These scans should be interpreted in correlation with cross-sectional images from CT or MRI. Positron emission tomography scans do have a false-positive rate because of treatment-related inflammatory activity. A method to improve specificity that has been used for lung nodules has been shown to be helpful in the head and neck. If the patient is re-scanned through the neck primary site following a brief delay after the initial scan, the inflammatory lesions are more likely to show a decline in activity than tumor (234).

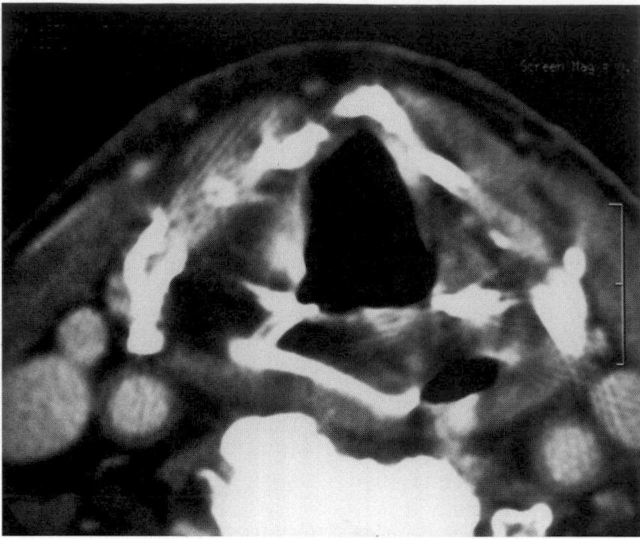

Figure 18.12 Patient motion. Enhanced axial computed tomography scan through the glottis. Figure shows patient swallowing (or respiratory) motion, which degrades image quality even at 2 seconds per scan.

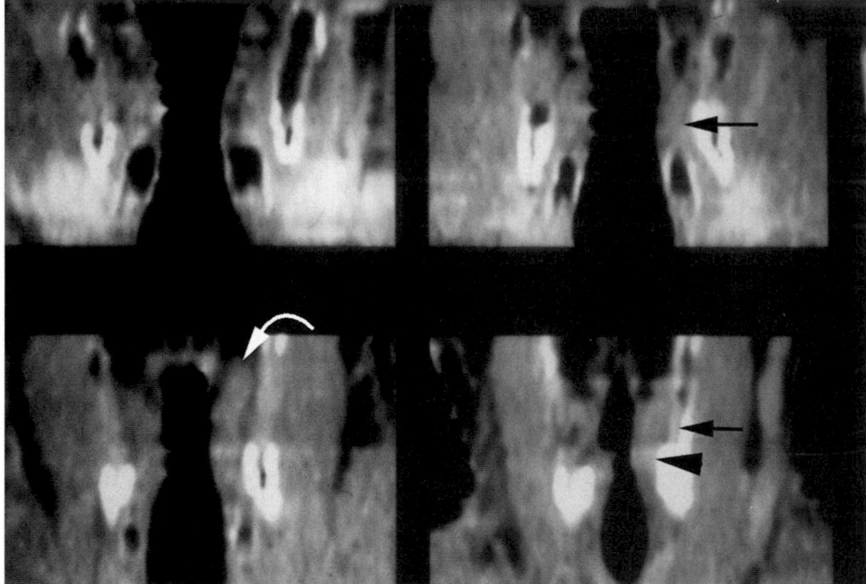

Figure 18.13 Transglottic lesion. Coronal reformatted contrast computed tomographic images show lesion of the left true cord (*arrowhead*) tracking upward through the paraglottic space (*arrows*) toward the preepiglottic space (*curved arrow*).

A 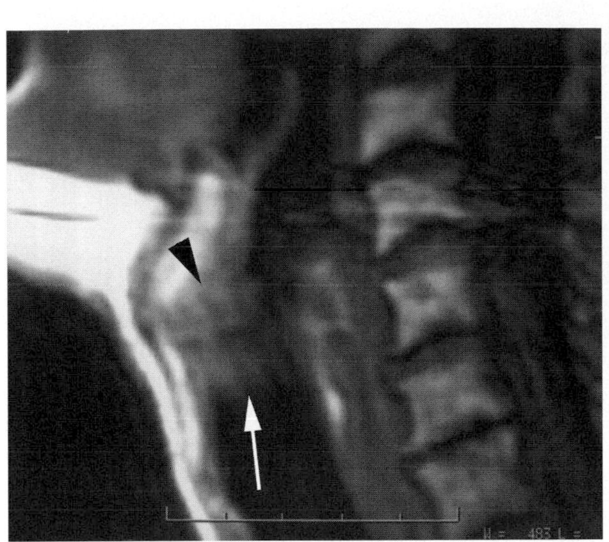

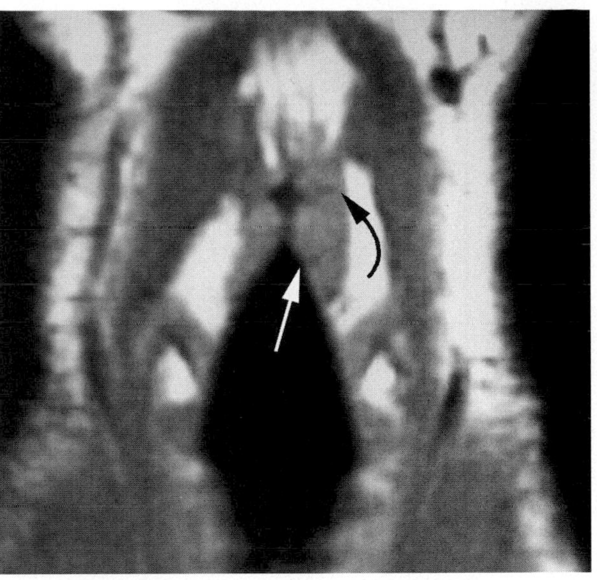 B

Figure 18.14 Preepiglottic space magnetic resonance imaging. Parasagittal **(A)** and coronal **(B)** magnetic resonance imaging views of a left true cord lesion (*arrow*) shown in the paraglottic space on the coronal view (*curved arrow*) but limited to the lower preepiglottic space by the sagittal view (*arrowhead*).

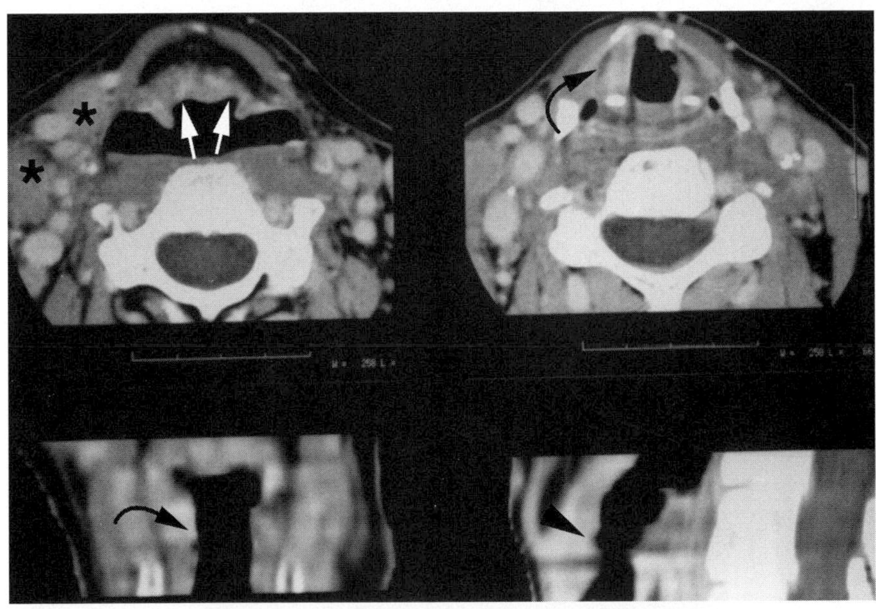

Figure 18.15 Advanced supraglottic carcinoma-epiglottis. Adjacent enhanced axial views show moderately thick lesion arising from laryngeal surface of epiglottis (*arrows*), with extensive involvement of lower preepiglottic space on sagittal reformatted image (*arrowhead*) and right paraglottic space (*curved arrow*) on coronal reformatted image (lower left). *Asterisks* indicate pathologic lymph nodes.

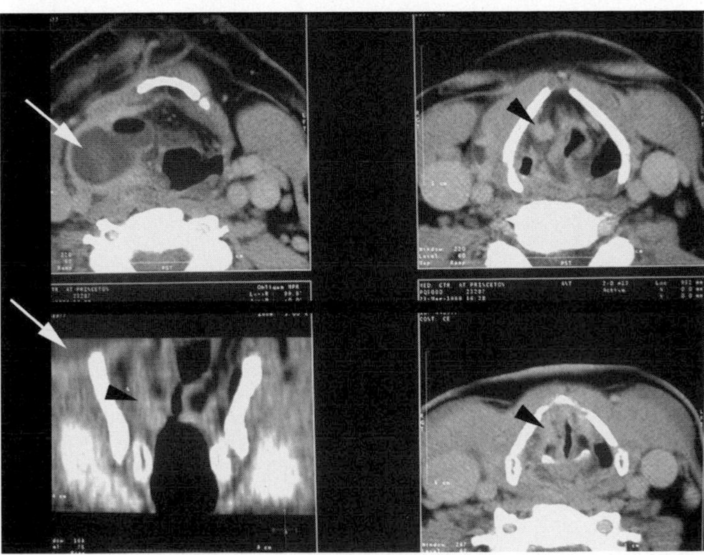

Figure 18.16 Laryngocele. Enhanced computed tomographic scan of the head and neck. **Clockwise from top left:** Axial supraglottic level, false cord level, true cord level, and reformatted coronal views show a large laryngocele (*arrows*) connected to the laryngeal ventricle through a tract (*arrowhead*). This patient never manifested an obstructing tumor.

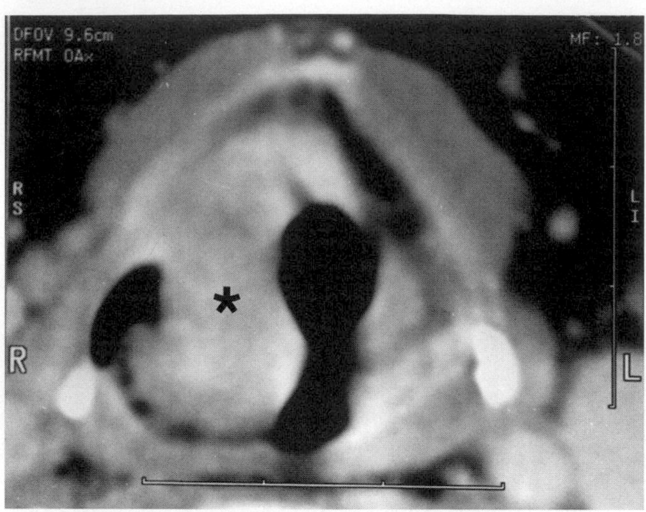

A

Figure 18.17 Bulky supraglottic lesion—aryepiglottic fold. **A:** Selected axial computed tomographic view through the larynx shows bulky tumor of aryepiglottic fold (*asterisk*) with involvement of right paraglottic space. **B:** Reformatted sagittal (top left) and serial coronal views show epiglottic component at the midline (*arrow*) and paraglottic involvement (*arrowhead*) and extralaryngeal extension (*curved arrow*).

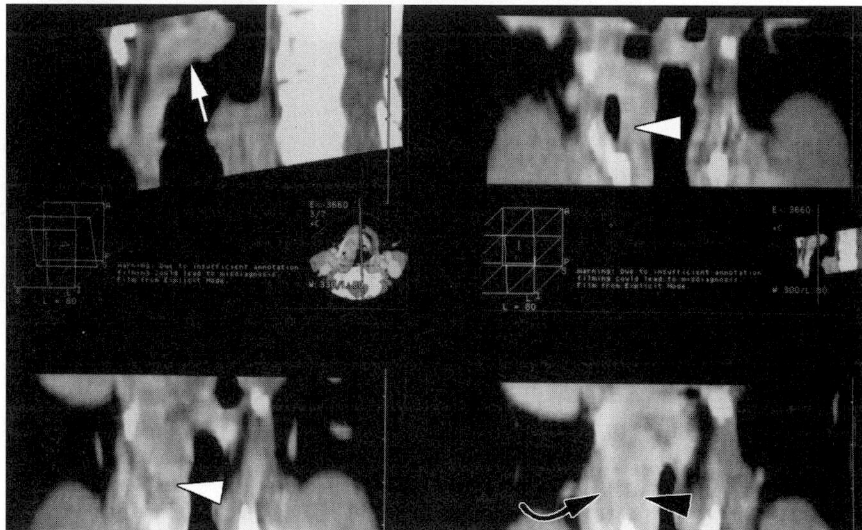

B

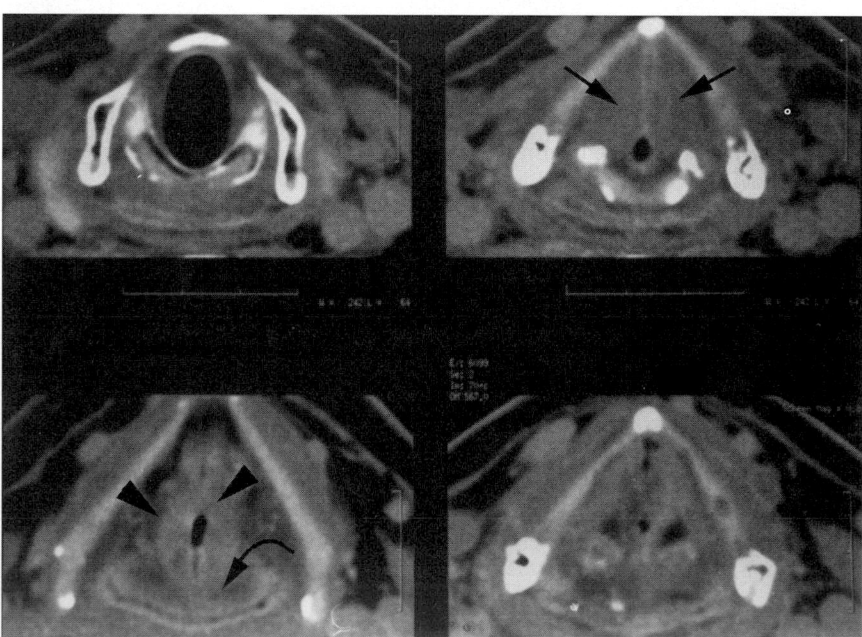

Figure 18.18 Acute treatment changes. **Clockwise from top left:** Enhanced thin axial computed tomographic sections of a treated T1 glottic lesion from subglottic to false cord level show edema of paraglottic space (*arrows*) and generalized increased enhancement of the mucosal surfaces at the false cord level (*arrowheads*) and hypopharynx (*curved arrow*).

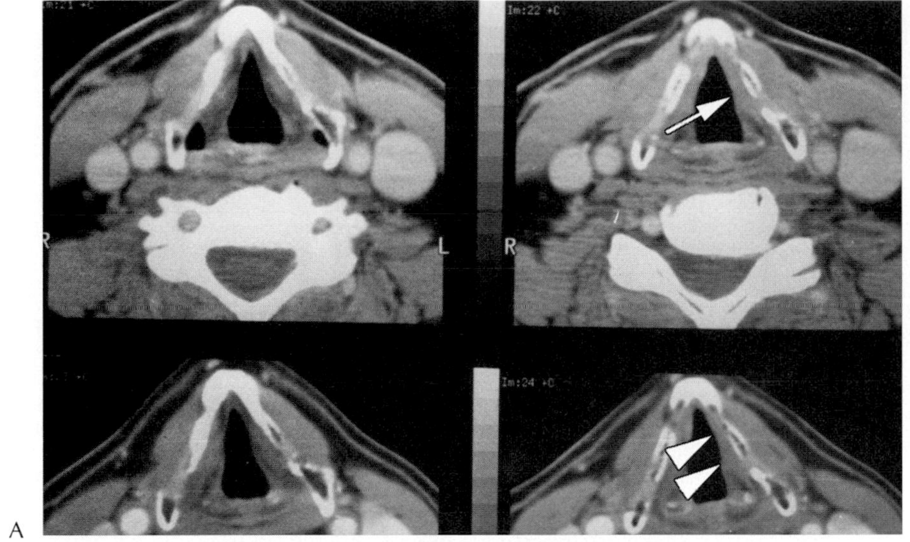

Figure 18.19 Pretreatment **(A)** and posttreatment **(B)** enhanced axial computed tomography sections through the glottis. Figure shows residual thickening of left true vocal cord (*arrowhead*) after irradiation for early vocal cord cancer (*arrow*), clinically reported as no evidence of disease.

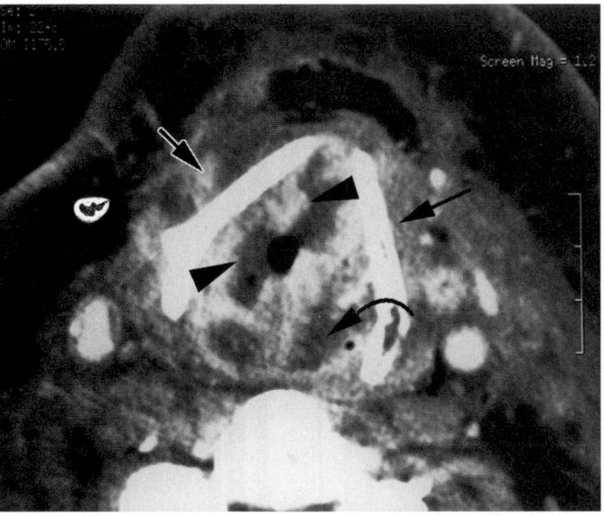

Figure 18.20 Treatment necrosis. Enhanced axial computed tomography of T2 lesion shows foci of necrotic larynx (*arrowheads*), with intense edema of the postcricoid region (*curved arrow*) and edema of the strap muscles (*arrows*).

RADIATION THERAPY TECHNIQUE*

William M. Mendenhall

T1N0 and T2N0 Glottic Larynx

The portals used to treat T1N0 and T2N0 glottic carcinomas are limited to the primary lesion. The risk for occult disease in the neck nodes is very low, even for patients with T2b tumors, and elective neck irradiation is not indicated.

Patients may be treated either in the lateral decubitus position, with the fields set up daily by the physician using anatomic landmarks, or in the supine position with a mask of low-temperature thermoplastic (WFR/Aquaplast Corp., Wyckoff, N.J.) to ensure accurate repositioning. The former has been our practice at the University of Florida because it has been our bias that the field sizes may be smaller if the fields are set up according to the anatomic landmarks, and these landmarks (particularly the posterior edge of the thyroid ala) are easier to palpate with the patient in the lateral decubitus position. Parallel-opposed fields are used and weighted 3:2 toward the side of the cancer, if it is lateralized. Weighting the fields reduces the dose to the contralateral posterior larynx. The field borders for a T1N0 cancer involving the anterior two-thirds of the cord are the middle of the thyroid notch, the bottom of the cricoid cartilage, 1 cm posterior to the thyroid lamina, and 1.5 cm anterior fall off (Fig. 18.21) (235,236). The fields are enlarged for T2 cancers depending on the sites of disease extension. Approximately 5% of the dose may be delivered with an anterior field centered over the tumor, with the patient supine, to reduce the dose laterally. Patients are treated with ^{60}Co, 4-mV x-rays, or 6-mV x-rays; the dose delivered to the tumor is similar for these beams (237). Patients with cancers that invade the anterior commissure and extend anteriorly though the cricothyroid membrane into the soft tissues of the neck may be under dosed with 6-mV x-rays. However, these lesions are T4 by definition, and the treatment techniques are addressed elsewhere.

A commonly used dose-fractionation schedule at many institutions is 66 Gy for T1 lesions and 70 Gy for T2 cancers given in 2-Gy fractions. Evidence suggests that increasing the dose per fraction may improve the likelihood of local control (199–202,205,206,238). Ample data suggest that 1.8 Gy once daily results in significantly lower local control rates compared with 2 Gy once daily (206). Patients with T1 or T2 vocal cord cancer treated with once-a-day fractionation at the University of Florida are irradiated with 2.25-Gy fractions to 63 Gy for T1 and T2a cancers and 65.25 Gy for T2b lesions (239,240).

T1N0 and T2N0 Supraglottic Larynx

The risk for occult disease in the neck nodes is relatively high, even for early stage lesions; therefore, the nodes at risk are treated bilaterally in conjunction with the primary malignancy. For patients with a clinically negative neck, the nodes at highest risk are those in levels 2, 3, and 4. Nodes in levels 1, 5, and 6 and the retropharyngeal lymph nodes are unlikely to harbor metastatic disease, and the fields are not enlarged to include these areas.

Patients are treated with parallel-opposed fields weighted to the side of the cancer, if it is lateralized. The fields usually extend from the bottom of the cricoid cartilage to 1 to 2 cm above the angle of the mandible, to the posterior edge of the spinous processes, and fall off 1.5 cm anteriorly if the cancer extends to the anterior commissure or petiole. If not, a strip of anterior skin may be spared (Fig. 18.22) (241). The low internal jugular lymph nodes are included in a tight low-neck field with a small, tapered midline block (Fig. 18.23) (241). The fields are reduced off of the spinal cord at approximately 45 Gy, and a second mucosal reduction is performed at 60 Gy to encompass the initial gross disease with a 1.5- to 2.0-cm margin.

Most patients treated at the University of Florida are currently irradiated twice a day at 1.2 Gy per fraction with a minimum 6-hour interfraction interval, in a continuous course. The dose for T1 and T2 lesions is 74.4 Gy. The total doses for patients irradiated once daily at 2 Gy per fraction are 60 Gy for T1 cancers and 64 to 66 Gy for T2 cancers. All patients are treated with the continuous-course technique (242).

*Please refer to the Appendix, Imaging Considerations for Radiation Therapy Treatment Planning. This section shows the important radiologic anatomy that allows the radiation oncologist to design the target volumes for treatment planning.

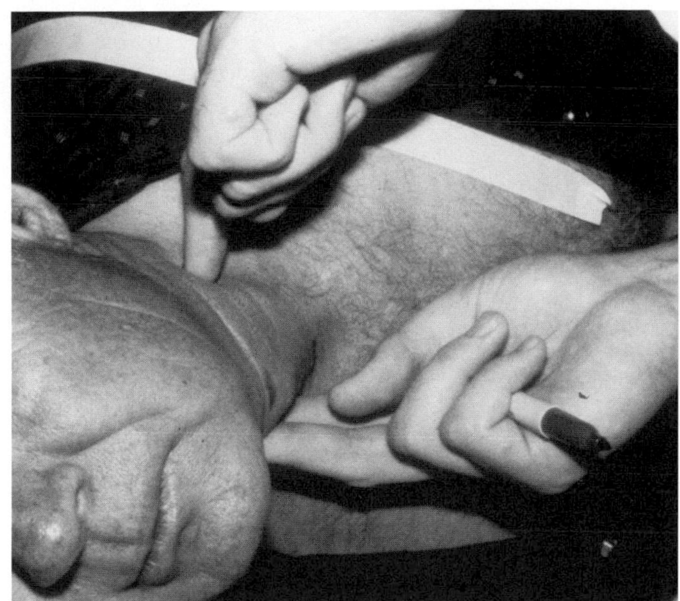

A

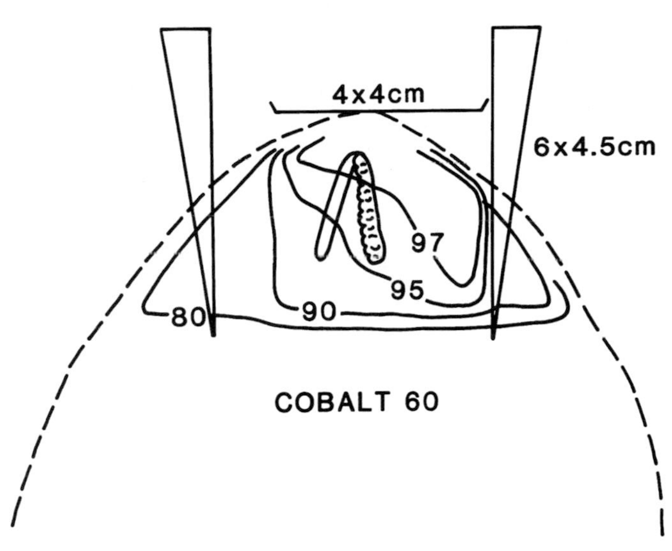

C

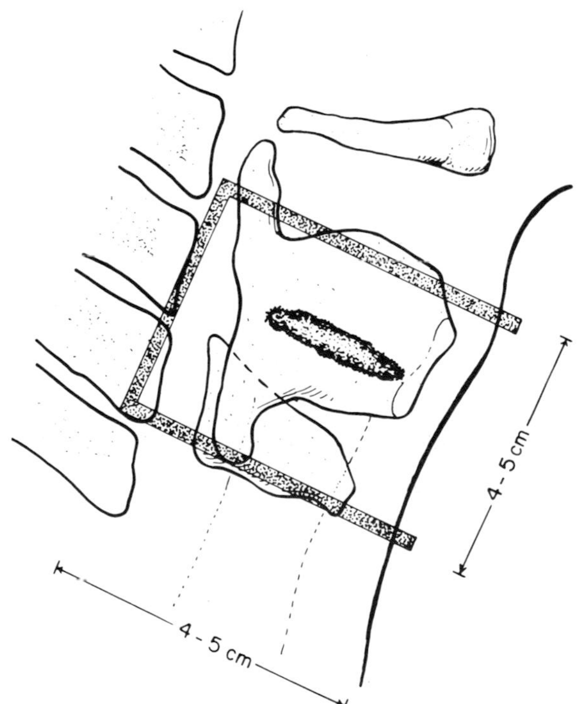

B

Figure 18.21 Radiation treatment technique for carcinoma of the glottic larynx, stage T1 to T2. **A:** Patient is in the lateral decubitus position. To locate the posterior border of the thyroid cartilage, the fingers of one hand are positioned under the patient's neck and the larynx is lifted gently a few millimeters while the index finger of the other hand simultaneously locates the posterior edge of the thyroid lamina. **B:** For T1 cancer, the superior border of the field usually is at the midthyroid notch (height of the notch typically is about 1 cm or slightly more in men); for minimal lesions (e.g., carcinoma *in situ*), the bottom of the thyroid notch is chosen. If the ventricle or false vocal cords are minimally involved, the top of the notch (which corresponds to the cephalad portion of the thyroid lamina as palpated just off midline) is often selected; more advanced lesions call for greater superior coverage. If only the anterior half of the vocal cord is involved, the posterior border is placed at the back of the midportion of the thyroid lamina. If the posterior portion of the cord is involved, the border is 1 cm behind the lamina. If the anterior face of the arytenoid is also involved, the posterior border is placed 1.5 cm behind the cartilage. If no subglottic extension is detected, the inferior border of the radiation portal is at the bottom of the cricoid arch as palpated at midline. If computed tomography demonstrates subglottic extension, the portal is adjusted accordingly. Anteriorly, the beam falls off (by 1.5 cm) over the patient's skin. **C:** A three-field technique (two lateral wedge fields and an anterior open field) is used commonly to treat vocal cord cancer at the University of Florida. Lateral fields are differentially weighted to the involved side. The anterior field, which usually measures 4 cm × 4 cm, is centered approximately 0.5 cm lateral to the midline in patients with one cord involved and typically delivers about 5% of the total tumor dose (usually on the last two treatment days) after treatment from the lateral portals is completed. The anterior portal is essentially a reduced portal that centers the high dose to the tumor. The isodose line at which the dose is specified is that which covers gross disease. By appropriate field weightings, encompassing the tumor within the 95% to 97% of maximum isodose line is virtually always possible. (**A,C:** From Parsons JT, Palta JR, Mendenhall WM, et al. Head and neck cancer. In: Levitt SH, Khan FM, Potish RA, et al., eds. *Levitt and Tapley's technological basis of radiation therapy: practical clinical applications,* 3rd ed. Baltimore: Lippincott Williams & Wilkins, 1999, with permission; **B:** From Million RR, Cassisi NJ, Mancuso AA. Larynx. In: Million RR, Cassisi NJ, eds. *Management of head and neck cancer: a multidisciplinary approach,* 2nd ed. Philadelphia: JB Lippincott, 1994, with permission.)

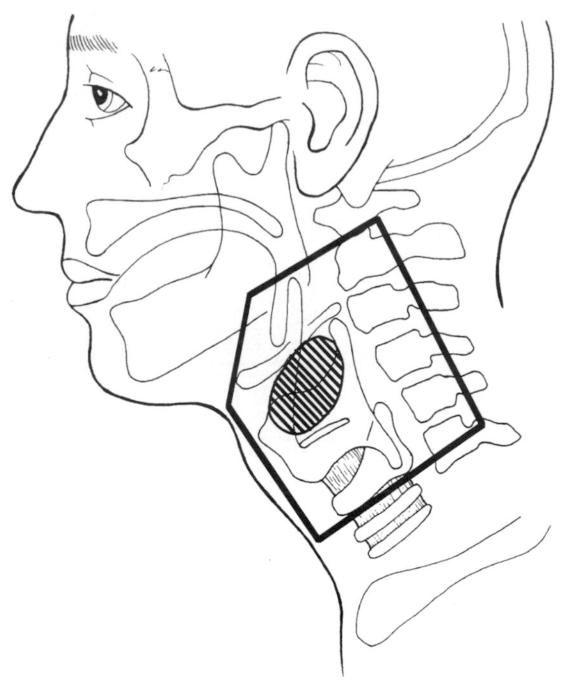

Figure 18.22 Example of a portal for a lesion of the lower epiglottis or false vocal cord and a clinically negative neck. The subdigastric nodes are included but not the junctional nodes. Depending on the anatomy and tumor extent, the anterior border may fall off (i.e., "flash") or a small strip of skin may be shielded. (From Million RR, Cassisi NJ, Mancuso AA, et al. Management of the neck for squamous cell carcinoma. In: Million RR, Cassisi NJ, eds. *Management of head and neck cancer: a multidisciplinary approach,* 2nd ed. Philadelphia: JB Lippincott, 1994, with permission.)

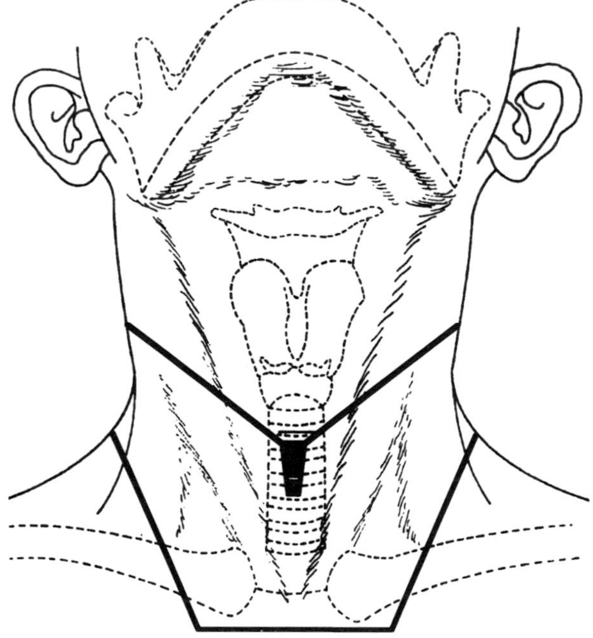

Figure 18.23 Example of a low neck portal for a T1 to T2 supraglottic carcinoma. The main nodes at risk are in the low jugular. A very narrow and short midline shield is used. (From Million RR, Cassisi NJ, Mancuso AA, et al. Management of the neck for squamous cell carcinoma. In: Million RR, Cassisi NJ, eds. *Management of head and neck cancer: a multidisciplinary approach,* 2nd ed. Philadelphia: JB Lippincott, 1994, with permission.)

REFERENCES

1. Greenlee RT, Hill-Harmon MB, Murray T, et al. Cancer statistics, 2001. *CA: Cancer J Clin* 2001;51:15–36.
2. Karp D, Vaughan C, Carter R, et al. Larynx preservation with induction chemotherapy plus radiation as an alternative to laryngectomy. *Am J Clin Oncol* 1991;14:273.
3. Hong W O'Donoghue G, Sheetz S. Sequential response patterns to chemotherapy and radiotherapy in head and neck cancer. In: Wagener D, Bligham G, Sweetz V, et al., eds. *Primary chemotherapy in cancer medicine,* Vol 201. New York: Alan R. Liss, 1985:191.
4. Pfister D, Strong E, Harrison L. Larynx preservation with combined chemo and radiotherapy in advanced head and neck cancer. *J Clin Oncol* 1991;9:830.
5. Cann CI, Fried MP, Rothman KJ. Epidemiology of squamous cell cancer of the head and neck. *Otolaryngol Clin North Am* 1985;18:367.
6. Gloecker Ries LA, Miller BA, Hankey BF, et al. *SEER cancer statistics review, 1973–1991.* Washington, DC: Surveillance Program, Division of Cancer Prevention and Control, National Cancer Institute, 1992.
7. Barclay T, Rao N. The incidence and mortality rates for laryngeal cancer from total cancer registries. *Laryngoscope* 1975;83:254.
8. Krajina Z, Kucar Z, Zonic-Carnelutti V. Epidemiology of laryngeal cancer. *Laryngoscope* 1975;85:11.
9. Iwai H, Koike Y. Primary laryngoplasty. *Laryngoscope* 1975;85:929.
10. Lowry W. Alcoholism in cancer of the head and neck. *Laryngoscope* 1975;85: 1275.
11. Wynder EL. The epidemiology of cancers of the upper alimentary and upper respiratory tracts. *Laryngoscope* 1978;88:50–51.
12. Austen D. Larynx. In: Schottenfeld P, FR Aumeni J, eds. *Cancer epidemiology and prevention.* Philadelphia: WB Sanders, 1982:554.
13. Iwamoto H. An epidemiological study of laryngeal cancer in Japan (1960–1969). *Laryngoscope* 1975;85:1162.
14. Hiranandani L. Panel on epidemiology and etiology of laryngeal carcinoma. *Laryngoscope* 1975;85:1197.
15. DeStefani E, Correa P, Oreggia F. Risk factors for laryngeal cancer. *Cancer* 1987;60:3087.
16. Graham S, Mettlin C, Marshall J. Dietary factors in the epidemiology of cancer of the larynx. *Am J Epidemiol* 1981;113:675.
17. Morrison M. Is chronic gastroesophageal reflux a causative factor in glottic carcinoma? *Otolaryngol Head Neck Surg* 1988;99:370.
18. Wynder E, Bross I, Day E. Epidemiological approach to the etiology of cancer of the larynx. *JAMA* 1956;160;1384.
19. Koufman JA, Cummins MM. Reflux and early laryngeal carcinoma: a prospective study using pH monitoring. Presented at: Southern Section of the American Laryngological, Rhinological, and Otological Society; January 1995; Key West, FL.
20. Kurozumi S, Harada Y, Sugimoto Y, et al. Airway malignancy in poisonous gas workers. *J Laryngol Otol* 1977;91:217.
21. Morgan R, Shettigara P. Occupational asbestos exposure, smoking, and laryngeal carcinoma. *Ann N Y Acad Sci* 1976;271:308.
22. Goolden A. Radiation cancer of the pharynx. *BMJ* 1951;2:1110.
23. Doyle DJ, Henderson LA, LeJeune FE, et al. Changes in human papillomavirus typing of recurrent respiratory papillomatosis progressing to malignant neoplasm. *Arch Otolaryngol Head Neck Surg* 1994;120:1273.
24. Fouret P, Dabit D, Sibony M, et al. Expression of p53 protein related to the presence of human papillomavirus infection in precancerous lesions of the larynx. *Am J Pathol* 1995;146:599.
25. Gissman L, Wolnik W Ikenberg H, et al. Human papilloma virus types 6 and 11 DNA sequences in genital and laryngeal papillomas and in some cervical cancers. *Proc Natl Acad Sci U S A* 1983;80:560.
26. Howley PM. The human papillomaviruses. *Arch Pathol Lab Med* 1982;106:429.
27. Kashima H, Tzyy-Choou W Mounts P, et al. Carcinoma ex-papilloma: histologic and virologic studies in whole-organ sections of the larynx. *Laryngoscope* 1988;98:619.
28. Kashima HK, Kutcher M, Kessis T, et al. Human papillomavirus in squamous cell carcinoma, leukoplakia, lichen planus and clinically normal epithelium of the oral cavity. *Ann Otol Rhinol Laryngol* 1990;99:55.
29. Lynch P. Warts and cancer. *Am J Dermatopathol* 1982;4:55.
30. Son YH. *Radiation carcinogenesis.* Cancer 1975;37:941.
31. Mancuso AA, Hanafee WN. *Computed tomography and magnetic resonance imaging of the head and neck,* 2nd ed. Baltimore: Williams & Wilkins, 1985.
32. Lindberg R. Distribution of cervical lymph node metastases from squamous cell carcinoma of upper respiratory and digestive tracts. *Cancer* 1972;29: 1446–1449.
33. Lam KH, Wong J. The preepiglottic and paraglottic spaces in relation to spread of carcinoma of the larynx. *Am J Otolaryngol* 1983;4:81–91.
34. Luna MA, Tortoledo ME. Verrucous carcinoma. In: Gnepp DR, ed. *Pathology of the head and neck.* New York: Churchill Livingstone, 1988:497.
35. Mansel RH, Vermeersch H. Panendoscopies for second primaries in head and neck cancer. Presented at: American Laryngological Society Meeting; May 1981; Vancouver, BC.
36. McGuirt WE, Matthews B, Koufman JA. Multiple simultaneous tumors in patients with head and neck cancer. *Cancer* 1982;50:1195.
37. Shapshay SM, Hong WK, Fried MP, et al. Simultaneous carcinomas of the esophagus and upper aerodigestive tract. *Otolaryngol Head Neck Surg* 1980;88: 373.
38. Crissman J. Laryngeal keratosis preceding laryngeal carcinoma. *Arch Otolaryngol* 1982;108:445.
39. Crissman J. Laryngeal keratosis and subsequent carcinoma. *Head Neck Surg* 1979;1:386.
40. Hellquist H, Lundgren J, Olofsson J. Hyperplasia, keratosis dysplasia and carcinoma in-situ of the vocal cords. *Clin Otolaryngol* 1982;7:11.
41. Slamniker B, Bauer W Painter C, et al. The transformation of laryngeal keratosis into invasive carcinoma. *Am J Otolaryngol* 1989;10:42.
42. Hjslet P, Nielsen P, Palvio P. Premalignant lesions of the larynx. *Acta Otolaryngol* 1989;107:130.
43. Bauer W. Concomitant carcinoma in situ and invasive carcinoma of the larynx. In: Alberti P, Bryce D, eds. *Workshops from the Centennial Conference on laryngeal cancer.* East Norwalk, CT: Appleton-Century-Crofts, 1976:127.
44. McGavran M, Bauer w, Ogura J. The incidence of cervical lymph node metastases from epidermoid carcinoma of the larynx and their relationship to certain characteristics of the primary tumor. *Cancer* 1961;14:55.
45. Kashima H. The characteristics of laryngeal cancer correlating with cervical lymph node metastasis. In: Alberti P, Bryce D, eds. *Workshops from the Centennial Conference on laryngeal cancer.* East Norwalk, CT: Appleton-Century-Crofts, 1976:855.
46. Reid A, Robin P, Poewll J, et al. Staging carcinoma: its value. *J Laryngol Otol* 1991;105:456.
47. Hirabayshi H, Koshi K, Uno K. Extracapsular spread of squamous carcinoma in neck nodes: prognostic factors in laryngeal cancer. *Laryngoscope* 1991;101: 502.
48. Spiro R, Alfonso A, Farr H, Strong E. Cervical node metastases for epidermal carcinoma: a critical assessment of current staging. *Am J Surg* 1974;128:566.
49. Molinari R. Clinical classification of laryngeal carcinoma: critique of existing classifications and proposals of a new working classification. *Acta Otorhinolaryngol* 1991;10:579.
50. Mohit-Tabatabai M, Sobel H, Rush B, et al. Relationship of thickness of floor of mouth stage I and II cancers to regional metastasis. *Am J Surg* 1986;152:351.
51. Spiro RH, Huvos AG, Wong GY, et al. Predictive value of tumor thickness in squamous carcinoma confined to the tongue and floor of the mouth. *Am J Surg* 1986;152:345.
52. Rasgon BM, Cruz RM, Hilsinger RL, et al. Relation of lymph node metastasis to histopathologic appearance in oral cavity and oropharyngeal carcinoma: a case series and literature review. *Laryngoscope* 1989;99:1103.
53. Platz H, Fries R, Hudeo M, et al. The prognostic relevance of various factors at the time of first admission of the patient. *J Maxillofac Surg* 1983;11:3.
54. Baredes S, Leeman DJ, Chen TS, et al. Significance of tumor thickness in soft palate carcinoma. *Laryngoscope* 1993;103:389.
55. Ravasz LA, Hordijk GJ, Slootweg PJ, et al. Uni- and multivariate analysis of eight indications for post-operative radiotherapy and their significance for local-regional cure in advanced head and neck cancer. *J Laryngol Otol* 1993;107:437.
56. Close LG, Brown PM, Vuitch MF, et al. Microscopic invasion and survival in cancer of the oral cavity and oropharynx. *Arch Otolaryngol Head Neck Surg* 1989;115:1304.
57. Morton RP, Ferguson CM, Lambie NK, et al. Tumor thickness in early tongue cancer. *Arch Otolaryngol Head Neck Surg* 1994;120:717.
58. Kirchner J, Cornog J, Holmes R. Transglottic cancer: its growth and spread within the larynx. *Arch Otolaryngol* 1974;99:247.
59. Micheau C, Luboinski B, Sancho H, et al. Modes of invasion of cancer of the larynx: a statistical, histological and radioclinical analysis of 120 cases. *Cancer* 1976;38:346.
60. Kirchner J. One hundred laryngeal cancer studies by serial section. *Ann Otol Rhinol Laryngol* 1969;78:689.
61. Olofsson J, Lord I, VanNostrand A. Vocal cord fixation in laryngeal carcinoma. *Acta Otolaryngol (Stockh)* 1973;75:486.
62. Ogura J, Spector G, Sessions D. Conservation surgery for carcinoma of the marginal area. *Laryngoscope* 1975;85:1801.
63. Kirchner JA. Staging as seen in serial sections. *Laryngoscope* 1975;85: 1816–1821.
64. Ogura J, Biller H, Wette R. Elective neck dissection for pharyngeal and laryngeal cancers. *Ann Otol Rhinol Laryngol* 1971;80:646.
65. Putney F. Elective versus delayed neck dissection in cancer of the larynx. *Surg Gynecol Obstet* 1961;112:736.
66. Fletcher G. Elective irradiation of subclinical disease in cancers of the head and neck. *Cancer* 1972;29:1450.
67. Levendag P, Vikram B. The problem of neck relapse in early-stage supraglottic cancer—results of different treatment modalities for the clinically negative neck. *Int J Radiat Oncol Biol Phys* 1987;13:1621.
68. Kirchner J, Owen J. Five hundred cancers of the larynx and pyriform sinus. *Laryngoscope* 1977;87:1288.
69. Ogura J, Sessions D, Spector G. Conservation surgery for epidermoid carcinoma of the supraglottic larynx. *Laryngoscope* 1975;85:1808.
70. Fayos J. Carcinoma of the endolarynx: results of irradiation. *Cancer* 1975;35: 1525.
71. Hansen H. Supraglottic carcinoma of the aryepiglottis fold. *Laryngoscope* 1975;85:1667.
72. Shah J, Tollefsen H. Epidermoid carcinoma of the supraglottic larynx. *Am J Surg* 1974;128:494.

73. Biller H, Davis W, Ogura J. Delayed contralateral cervical metastasis with laryngeal and laryngopharyngeal cancers. *Laryngoscope* 1971;81:1499.
74. Som M. Conservation surgery for carcinoma of the supraglottis. *J Laryngol Otol* 1970;84:655.
75. Sako K. Fallibility of palpation in diagnosis of metastasis to nodes. *Surg Gynecol Obstet* 1964;118:989.
76. Spiro R. Cervical node metastasis from epidermoid carcinoma of the oral cavity and oropharynx. *Am J Surg* 1974;128:562.
77. Lawson W, Biller H, Suen J. Cancer of the larynx. In: Myers G, Suen J, eds. *Cancer of the head and neck,* 2nd ed. New York: Churchill Livingstone 1989:533.
78. Kirchner J, Fischer J. Anterior commissure cancer. In: Alberti P, Bryce D, eds. *Workshops from the Centennial Conference on laryngeal cancer.* East Norwalk, CT: Appleton-Century-Crofts, 1976:679.
79. Jesse R, Lindberg R, Horiot J. Vocal cord cancer with anterior commissure extension: choice of treatment. *Am J Surg* 1971; 122:437.
80. Sessions D, Ogura J, Fried M. Laryngeal carcinoma involving anterior commissure and subglottis. In: Alberti P, Bryce D, eds. *Workshops from the Centennial Conference on laryngeal cancer.* East Norwalk, CT: Appleton-Century-Crofts, 1976:674–678.
81. Olofsson J, van Nostrand AWP. Growth and spread of laryngeal and hypopharyngeal carcinoma with reflections on the effect of preoperative irradiation: 139 cases studied by whole organ serial sectioning. *Acta Otolaryngol Suppl (Stockh)* 1973;308:1–84.
82. Stell P. The subglottic space. In: Alberti P, Bryce D, eds. *Workshops from the Centennial Conference on laryngeal cancer.* East Norwalk, CT: Appleton-Century-Crofts, 1976:682.
83. Harrison D. The pathology and management of subglottic cancer. *Ann Otol Rhinol Laryngol* 1971;80:6.
84. Fletcher GH. Elective irradiation of subclinical disease in cancers of the head and neck. *Cancer* 1972;29:1450–1454.
85. Ogura JH, Biller HF, Wette R. Elective neck dissection for pharyngeal and laryngeal cancers: an evaluation. *Ann Otol Rhinol Laryngol* 1971;80:646–650.
86. Mendenhall WM, Parsons JT, Stringer SP, et al. T1-T2 vocal cord carcinoma: a basis for comparing the results of radiotherapy and surgery. *Head Neck Surg* 1988;10:373–377.
87. Lederman M. [The place of radiotherapy in the treatment of cancer of the larynx]. *Ann Radiol (Paris)* 1961;4:443.
88. Kraus F, Perez-Mesa C. Verrucous carcinoma: clinical and pathological study of 105 cases involving oral cavity, larynx, and genitalia. *Cancer* 1966; 19:26.
89. VanNostrand A, Olofsson J. Verrucous carcinoma of the larynx. *Cancer* 1972; 30:691.
90. Biller H, Ogura J, Bauer W. Verrucous cancer of the larynx. *Laryngoscope* 1971; 81:1323.
91. Ackerman L. Verrucous carcinoma of the oral cavity. *Surgery* 1948;23:670.
92. Batsakis J, Hybels R, Crissman J, Rice D. The pathology of head and neck tumors: verrucous carcinoma: XV. *Head Neck Surg* 1982;5:29.
93. Ferlito A, Recher G. Ackerman's tumor (verrucous carcinoma) of the larynx. A clinicopathologic study of 77 cases. *Cancer* 1980;46:1517.
94. Medina JE, Dichtel W, Luna MA. Verrucous-squamous carcinomas of the oral cavity. A clinicopathologic study of 104 cases. *Arch Otolaryngol* 1984;110:437.
95. Abramson AL, Brandsma JL, Steinberg BM, et al. Verrucous carcinoma of the larynx: possible human papillomavirus etiology. *Acta Otolaryngol (Stockh)* 1985;111:709.
96. Glanz H, Kleinasser O. Verrucous carcinoma of the larynx—a misnomer. *Arch Otorhinolaryngol* 1987;244:108.
97. Myers E, Sobol S, Ogura H. Hemilaryngectomy for verrucous carcinoma of the glottis. *Laryngoscope* 1980;90:693.
98. Sessions R, Hudkins C. Malignant cervical adenopathy. In: Cummings C, ed. *Otolaryngology: head and neck surgery,* 2nd ed. St. Louis: Mosby, 1992:1605.
99. Vidyasagar MS, Fernandes DJ, Pai Kasturi D, et al. Radiotherapy and verrucous carcinoma of the oral cavity. A study of 107 cases. *Acta Oncologica* 1992;31:43.
100. Fonts E, Greenlaw R, Rush B, et al. Verrucous squamous cell carcinoma of the oral cavity. *Cancer* 1969;23:152.
101. Perez CA, Kraus FT, Evans JC, et al. Anaplastic transformation in verrucous carcinoma of the oral cavity after radiation therapy. *Radiology* 1966;26:108.
102. Elliot G, MacDougall J, Elliot J. Problems of verrucous squamous carcinoma. *Ann Surg* 1973;177:21.
103. Hagen P, Lyons GD, Haindel C. Verrucous carcinoma of the larynx: role of human papillomavirus, radiation and surgery. *Laryngoscope* 1993;103:253.
104. Demian SDE, Bushkin FL, Echevarria RA. Perineural invasion and anaplastic transformation of verrucous carcinoma. *Cancer* 1973; 32:395.
105. Tharp ME II, Shidnia H. Radiotherapy in the treatment of verrucous carcinoma of the head and neck. *Laryngoscope* 1995;105:391.
106. Vesely J, Sibl O, Kudrmann J, et al. Verrucous carcinoma of the larynx. *Otolaryngology* 1989;38:284.
107. Rider W. Toronto experience of verrucous carcinoma of the larynx. In: Alberti P, Bryce D, eds. *Workshops from the Centennial Conference on laryngeal cancer.* East Norwalk, CT: Appleton-Century-Crofts, 1976:460.
108. Burns H, VanNostrand A, Bryce D. Verrucous carcinoma of the larynx: management by radiotherapy and surgery. *Ann Otol Rhinol Laryngol* 1976;85:538.
109. McDonald JS, Crissman JD, Gluckman JL. Verrucous carcinoma of the oral cavity. *Head Neck* 1982;5:22.
110. Burns HP, van Nostrand AW, Bryce DP. Verrucous carcinoma of the larynx: management by radiotherapy and surgery. *Ann Otol Rhinol Laryngol* 1976;85: 538–543.
111. O'Sullivan B, Warde P, Keane T, et al. Outcome following radiotherapy in verrucous carcinoma of the larynx. *Int J Radiat Oncol Biol Phys* 1995;32:611–617.
112. Myerowitz R, Barnes E, Myers E. Small cell anaplastic (oat cell) carcinoma of the larynx. *Laryngoscope* 1978;88:1697.
113. Gould V, Linnoila R, Memoli V, Warren W. Neuroendocrine components of the bronchopulmonary tract. *Lab Invest* 1983;49:519.
114. Mullins J, Newman R, Coltman C. Primary oat cell carcinoma of the larynx. *Cancer* 1979;43:711.
115. Goldman N, Hood C, Singleton G. Carcinoid of the larynx. *Arch Otolaryngol* 1969;90:90.
116. Huizenga C, Balogh K. Cartilaginous tumors of the larynx. *Cancer* 1970;26: 201.
117. Blitzer A, Lawson W, Biller H. Malignant fibrous histiocytoma of the head and neck. *Laryngoscope* 1977;87:1479.
118. Maniglia A, Xue J. Plasmacytoma of the larynx. *Laryngoscope* 1983;93:741.
119. Booth J, Osborn D. Granular cell myoblastoma of the larynx. *Acta Otolaryngol* 1970;70:279.
120. Anderson H, Maisel R, Cantrell R. Isolated laryngeal lymphoma. *Laryngoscope* 1976;86:1251.
121. Reuter V, Woodruff J. Melanoma of the larynx. *Laryngoscope* 1986;96:389.
122. Sessions RB, Miller SD, Martin GF, et al. Videolaryngostroboscopic analysis of minimal glottic cancer. *Trans Am Laryngol Assoc* 110;1989:56–59.
123. Zhao R, Hirano M, Tanaka S, et al. Vocal fold epithelial hyperplasia: vibratory behavior versus extent of lesion. *Arch Otolaryngol Head Neck Surg* 1999; 117:1015–1018.
124. Colden D, Zeitels SM, Hillman RE, et al. Stroboscopic assessment of vocal fold keratosis and glottic cancer. *Ann Otol Rhinol Laryngol* 110;2001: 293–298.
125. Mancuso AA. Imaging in patients with head and neck cancer. In: Million RR, Cassisi NJ, eds. *Management of head and neck cancer: a multidisciplinary approach,* 2nd ed. Philadelphia: JB Lippincott Co, 1994:43–59.
126. McLaughlin MP, Mendenhall WM, Mancuso AA, et al. Retropharyngeal adenopathy as a predictor of outcome in squamous cell carcinoma of the head and neck. *Head Neck* 1995;17:190–198.
127. Verdonck-de Leeuw IM, Hilgers FJM, Keus RB, et al. Multidimensional assessment of voice characteristics after radiotherapy for early glottic cancer. *Laryngoscope* 1999:109:241–248.
128. Benninger MS, Gillen J, Thieme P, et al. Factors associated with recurrence and voice quality following radiation therapy for T1 and T2 glottic carcinomas. *Laryngoscope* 1994;104:294–198.
129. American Joint Committee on Cancer. *AJCC cancer staging handbook.* Philadelphia: Lippincott-Raven, 1998:45–49.
130. Greene F, Page D, Fleming I, et al. *AJCC cancer staging manual,* 6th ed. New York: Springer Verlag, 2002.
131. Pillsbury H, Kirchner J. Clinical vs. histologic staging in laryngeal cancer. *Arch Otolaryngol* 1979;105:157.
132. Sessions R, Parish R. How are patients chosen for conservation surgery of the larynx? In: Harrison DFN, ed. *Dilemmas in otorhinolaryngology.* London: Churchill Livingstone, 1988:283.
133. Gissman L, Wolnik W, Ikenberg H, et al. Human papilloma virus types 6 and 11 DNA sequences in genital and laryngeal papillomas and in some cervical cancers. *Proc Natl Acad Sci U S A* 1983;80:560.
134. Reference deleted in proof.
135. Mendenhall WM, Parsons JT, Mancuso AA, et al. Radiotherapy for squamous cell carcinoma of the supraglottic larynx: an alternative to surgery. *Head Neck* 1996;18:24–35.
136. Mancuso AA, Mukherji SK, Schmalfuss I, et al. Preradiotherapy computed tomography as a predictor of local control in supraglottic carcinoma. *J Clin Oncol* 1999;17:631–637.
137. Jankovic I, Merkas Z. Radiotherapy as the primary approach in the treatment of laryngeal cancer. In: Alberti P, Bryce D, eds. *Workshops from the Centennial Conference on laryngeal cancer.* East Norwalk, CT: Appleton-Century-Crofts, 1976:881.
138. Reference deleted in proof.
139. Ogura J, Biller H. Conservative surgery in cancer of the head and neck. *Otolaryngol Clin North Am* 1969;2:641.
140. Gall AM, Sessions DG, Ogura JH. Complications following surgery for cancer of the larynx and hypopharynx. *Cancer* 1977;39:624–631.
141. Shukovsky LJ. Dose, time, volume relationships in squamous cell carcinoma of the supraglottic larynx. *Am J Roentgenol Radium Ther Nucl Med* 1970;108:27–29.
142. Reference deleted in proof.
143. Wang CC, Schulz M, Miller D. Combined radiotherapy and surgery for carcinoma of the supraglottis and pyriform sinus. *Am J Surg* 1972;124:551.
144. Mendenhall W Parsons J, Stringer S. Carcinoma of the supraglottic larynx: a basis for comparing the results of radiotherapy and surgery. *Head Neck* 1990; 12:204.
145. Hinerman RW, Mendenhall WM, Amdur RJ, et al. Carcinoma of the supraglottic larynx: treatment results with radiotherapy alone or with planned neck dissection. *Head Neck* 2001.
146. Reference deleted in proof.
147. Ogura JH, Sessions DG, Spector GJ. Conservation surgery for epidermoid carcinoma of the supraglottic larynx. *Laryngoscope* 1975;85:1808–1815.
148. Bocca E. Supraglottic cancer. *Laryngoscope* 1975;85:1318–1326.
149. Harwood A, Beale F, Cummings B. Supraglottic laryngeal carcinoma: an analysis of dose-time-volume factors in 410 patients. *Int J Radiat Oncol Biol Phys* 1983;9:311.

150. Strong M. Laser management of premalignant lesions of the larynx. In: Alberti P, Bryce D, eds. *Workshops from the Centennial Conference on laryngeal cancer.* East Norwalk, CT: Appleton-Century-Crofts, 1976:154.
151. McGuirt WF, Kaufman JA. Endoscopic laser surgery: an alternative to laryngeal cancer treatment. *Arch Otolaryngol Head Neck Surg* 1987;113:501.
152. Harwood A. Cancer of the larynx—the Toronto experience. *J Otolaryngol* 1982;11:1.
153. Ellman A, Goodman M, Wang C, et al. In situ carcinoma of the vocal cords. *Cancer* 1979;43:2422.
154. Kass ES, Hillman RE, Zeitels SM. Vocal fold submucosal infusion technique in phonomicrosurgery. *Ann Otol Rhinol Laryngol* 1996;105:341–347.
155. Pêne F, Fletcher GH. Results in irradiation of the in situ carcinomas of the vocal cords. *Cancer* 1976;37:2586–2590.
156. Elman AJ, Goodman M, Wang CC, et al. In situ carcinoma of the vocal cords. *Cancer* 1979;43:2422–2428.
157. Fein DA, Mendenhall WM, Parsons JT, et al. Carcinoma in situ of the glottic larynx: the role of radiotherapy. *Int J Radiat Oncol Biol Phys* 1993;27: 379–384.
158. Woodson GE, Rosen CA, Murry T, et al. Assessing vocal function after chemoradiation for advanced laryngeal carcinoma. *Arch Otolaryngol Head Neck Surg* 1996;122:858–864.
159. Stewart MG, Chen AY, Stach CB. Outcomes analysis of voice and quality of life in patients with laryngeal cancer. *Arch Otolaryngol Head Neck Surg* 124; 1998:143–148
160. McGuirt WF, Blalock D, Koufman JA, et al. Comparative voice results after laser resection or irradiation of T1 vocal cord carcinoma. *Arch Otolaryngol Head Neck Surg* 1994:120:951–955.
161. Sittel C, Eckel HE, Eschenburg C. Phonatory results after laser surgery for glottic carcinoma. *Otolaryngol Head Neck Surg* 1998:119:418–424.
162. Hirano M, Hirade Y, Kawasaki H. Vocal function following carbon dioxide laser surgery for glottic carcinoma. *Ann Otol Rhinol Laryngol* 1985;94:232–235.
163. Biller H, Barnhill F, Ogura J, Perez C. Hemilaryngectomy following radiation failure for carcinoma of the vocal cords. *Laryngoscope* 1970;80:249.
164. Sorenson H, Hansen H, Thomsen K. Partial laryngectomy following irradiation. *Laryngoscope* 1980;90:1344.
165. Reference deleted in proof.
166. Mendenhall WM, Parsons JT, Million RR, et al. T1-T2 squamous cell carcinoma of the glottic larynx treated with radiation therapy: relationship of dose-fractionation factors to local control and complications. *Int J Radiat Oncol Biol Phys* 1988;15:1267–1273.
167. Biller HF, Ogura JH, Pratt LL. Hemilaryngectomy for T2 glottic cancer. *Arch Otolaryngol* 1971;93:238–243.
168. Reference deleted in proof.
169. Laccourreye H, Laccourreye O, Weinstein G, et al. Supracricoid laryngectomy with cricohyoidoepiglottopexy: a partial laryngeal procedure for glottic carcinoma. *Ann Otol Rhinol Laryngol* 1990;99:421–426.
170. Fein DA, Mendenhall WM, Parsons JT, et al. T1-T2 squamous cell carcinoma of the glottic larynx treated with radiotherapy: a multivariate analysis of variables potentially influencing local control. *Int J Radiat Oncol Biol Phys* 1993;25:605–611.
171. Mendenhall WM, Parsons JT, Stringer SP, et al. Management of Tis, T1, and T2 squamous cell carcinoma of the glottic larynx. *Am J Otolaryngol* 1994;15: 250–257.
172. O'Sullivan B, Mackillop W, Gilbert R, et al. Controversies in the management of laryngeal cancer: results of an international survey of patterns of care. *Radiother Oncol* 1994;31:23–32.
173. Mendenhall WM, Amdur RJ, Morris CG, et al. T1-T2 N0 squamous cell carcinoma of the glottic larynx treated with radiation therapy. *J Clin Oncol* 2001; 19:4029–4036.
174. Daly C, Strong E. Carcinoma of the glottic larynx. *Am J Surg* 1975;130:489.
175. Leroux-Robert J. A statistical study of 620 laryngeal carcinomas of the glottic region personally operated upon more than five years ago. *Laryngoscope* 1975;85:1440.
176. Sessions D, Maness G, McSwain B. Laryngofissure in the treatment of carcinoma of the vocal cord. *Laryngoscope* 1964;75:490.
177. Southwick H. Cancer of the larynx: surgical management. In: *Seventh National Cancer Conference proceedings.* Philadelphia: JB Lippincott Co, 1973.
178. Neel HB III, Devine KD, DeSanto LW. Laryngofissure and cordectomy for early cordal carcinoma: outcome in 182 patients. *Otolaryngol Head Neck Surg* 1980;88:79–84.
179. Fletcher G, Lindberg R, Hamberger H, et al. Reasons for irradiation failure in squamous cell carcinoma of the larynx. *Laryngoscope* 1975;85:987.
180. Constable WC, White R, El-Mahdi AM, et al. Radiotherapeutic management of cancer of the glottis. University of Virginia, 1956–1971. *Laryngoscope* 1975; 85:1494.
181. Wang CC. Treatment of glottic carcinoma by megavoltage radiation therapy and results. *Am J Roentgenol Radiol Ther Med* 1974; 120:157.
182. Jorgensen K. Carcinoma of the larynx: III. Therapeutic results. *Acta Radiol* 1974;13:446.
183. Pellitteri P, Kennedy T, Vrabec D, et al. Radiotherapy, the mainstay in the treatment of early glottic carcinoma. *Arch Otolaryngol Head Neck Surg* 1991; 117:297.
184. Reference deleted in proof.
185. Ogura J, Sessions D, Spector G. Analysis of surgical therapy for epidermoid carcinoma of the laryngeal glottis. *Laryngoscope* 1975;85:1522.
186. Thomas JV, Olsen KD, Neel HB III, et al. Early glottic carcinoma treated with open laryngeal procedures. *Arch Otolaryngol—Head Neck Surg* 1994;120: 264–268.
187. Ogura JH, Sessions DG, Spector GJ. Analysis of surgical therapy for epidermoid carcinoma of the laryngeal glottis. *Laryngoscope* 1975;85:1522–1530.
188. Bauer WC, Lesinki SG, Ogura JH. The significance of positive margins in hemilaryngectomy specimens. *Laryngoscope* 1975;85:1–13.
189. Dickens W Cassisi N, Million R, et al. Treatment of early vocal cord carcinoma: a comparison of apples and apples. *Laryngoscope* 1983;93:216.
190. Sessions D, Ogura J, Fried M. The anterior commissure in glottic carcinoma. *Laryngoscope* 1974;85:1624.
191. Olofsson J, Williams G, Rider W Bryce D. Anterior commissure carcinoma: primary treatment with radiotherapy in 57 patients. *Arch Otolaryngol* 1972; 95:230.
192. Oloffson J. Specific features of laryngeal carcinoma involving the anterior commissure and subglottic region. In: Alperti P, Bryce D, eds. *Workshops from the Centennial Conference on laryngeal cancer.* New York: Appleton-Century-Crofts, 1976.
193. Reference deleted in proof.
194. Reference deleted in proof.
195. Som ML. Cordal cancer with extension to vocal process. *Laryngoscope* 1975; 85:1298–1307.
196. Ennuyer H, Bataini P. Laryngeal carcinomas: VI. *Laryngoscope* 1975;85:1467.
197. Hawkins N. The treatment of glottic carcinoma: an analysis of 800 cases: VIII. *Laryngoscope* 1975;85:1485.
198. Stewart J, Brown J, Palmer M, et al. The management of glottic carcinoma by primary irradiation with surgery in reserve: VII. *Laryngoscope* 1975;85:1 477.
199. Harwood AR, Beale FA, Cummings BJ, et al. T2 glottic cancer: an analysis of dose-time-volume factors. *Int J Radiat Oncol Biol Phys* 1981;7:1501–1505.
200. Fletcher GH, Goepfert H. Larynx and pyriform sinus. In: Fletcher GH, ed. *Textbook of Radiotherapy,* 3rd ed. Philadelphia: Lea & Febiger, 1980:330–363.
201. Amornmarn R, Prempree T, Viravathana T, et al. A therapeutic approach to early vocal cord carcinoma. *Acta Radiol Oncol* 1985;24:321–325.
202. Woodhouse RJ, Quivey JM, Fu KK, et al. Treatment of carcinoma of the vocal cord: a review of 20 years experience. *Laryngoscope* 1981;91:1155–1162.
203. Le Q-TX, Fu KK, Kroll S, et al. Influence of fraction size, total dose, and overall time on local control of T1-T2 glottic carcinoma. *Int J Radiat Oncol Biol Phys* 1997;39:115–126.
204. Reference deleted in proof.
205. Schwaibold F, Scariato A, Nunno M, et al. The effect of fraction size on control of early glottic cancer. *Int J Radiat Oncol Biol Phys* 1988;14:451–454.
206. Kim RY, Marks ME, Salter MM. Early-stage glottic cancer: importance of dose fractionation in radiation therapy. *Radiology* 1992;182:273–275.
207. Mendenhall WM, Parsons JT, Brant TA, et al. Is elective neck treatment indicated for T2N0 squamous cell carcinoma of the glottic larynx? *Radiother Oncol* 1989;14:199–202.
208. Parsons JT, Mendenhall WM, Stringer SP, et al. Salvage surgery following radiation failure in squamous cell carcinoma of the supraglottic larynx. *Int J Radiat Oncol Biol Phys* 1995;32:605–609.
209. Wagenfeld DJ, Harwood AR, Bryce DP, et al. Second primary respiratory tract malignancies in glottic carcinoma. *Cancer* 1980;46:1883–1886.
210. Biller HF, Barnhill FR Jr, Ogura JH, et al. Hemilaryngectomy following radiation failure for carcinoma of the vocal cords. *Laryngoscope* 1970;80: 249–253.
211. Lee F, Perlmutter S, Ogura JH. Laryngeal radiation after hemilaryngectomy. *Laryngoscope* 1980;90:1534–1539.
212. Reference deleted in proof.
213. Mendenhall WM, Parsons JT, Million RR. Elective lower neck irradiation: 5000 cGy/25 fractions versus 4050 cGy/15 fractions. *Int J Radiat Oncol Biol Phys* 1988;15:439–440.
214. Laccourreye O, Diaz EM Jr, Bassot V, et al. A multimodal strategy for the treatment of patients with T2 invasive squamous cell carcinoma of the glottis. *Cancer* 1999;85:40–46.
215. Mendenhall WM, Tannehill SP, Hotz MA, et al. Should chemotherapy alone be the initial treatment for glottic squamous cell carcinoma? [Review]. *Eur J Cancer* 1999;35:1309–1313.

Radiologic Imaging Concerns

216. Katsounakis J, Remy H, Vuong T, et al. Impact of magnetic resonance imaging and computed tomography on the staging of laryngeal cancer. *Eur Arch Otorhinolaryngol* 1995;252:206–208.
217. Curtin HD. Importance of imaging demonstration of neoplastic invasion of laryngeal cartilage. [Editorial; Comment]. *Radiology* 1995;194:643–644.
218. Korkmaz H, Cerezci NG, Akmansu H, et al. A comparison of spiral and conventional computerized tomography methods in diagnosing various laryngeal lesions. *Eur Arch Otorhinolaryngol* 1998;255:149–154.
219. Hermans R, Van der Goten A, Baert AL. Image interpretation in CT of laryngeal carcinoma: a study on intra- and interobserver reproducibility. *Eur Radiol* 1997;7:1086–1090.
220. Loevner LA, Yousem DM, Montone KT, et al. Can radiologists accurately predict preepiglottic space invasion with MR imaging? *AJR Am J Roentgenol* 1997;169:1681–1687.
221. Hermans R, Van den Bogaert W, De Vuysere S, et al. Computed tomography

of laryngeal carcinoma: technique, imaging findings and implications for radiation therapy. *J Belg Radiol* 1998;81:190–198.

222. Mendenhall WM. T3-4 squamous cell carcinoma of the larynx treated with radiation therapy alone. *Semin Radiat Oncol* 1998;8:262–269.
223. Amilibia E, Juan A, Nogues J, et al. [Neoplastic invasion of laryngeal cartilage: diagnosis by computed tomography]. *Acta Otorhinolaringol Esp* 2001;52: 207–210.
224. Hermans R, Van den Bogaert W, Rijnders A, et al. Predicting the local outcome of glottic squamous cell carcinoma after definitive radiation therapy: value of computed tomography-determined tumour parameters. *Radiother Oncol* 1999;50:39–46.
225. Hermans R, Van den Bogaert W, Rijnders A, et al. Value of computed tomography as outcome predictor of supraglottic squamous cell carcinoma treated by definitive radiation therapy. *Int J Radiat Oncol Biol Phys* 1999;44: 755–765.
226. Mukherji SK, O'Brien SM, Gerstle RJ, et al. The ability of tumor volume to predict local control in surgically treated squamous cell carcinoma of the supraglottic larynx. *Head Neck* 2000;22:282–287.
227. Reference deleted in proof.
228. Lo SM, Venkatesan V, Matthews TW, Rogers J. Tumour volume: implications in T2/T3 glottic/supraglottic squamous cell carcinoma. *J Otolaryngol* 1998; 27:247–251.
229. Hermans R, Pameijer FA, Mancuso AA, et al. Laryngeal or hypopharyngeal squamous cell carcinoma: can follow-up CT after definitive radiation therapy be used to detect local failure earlier than clinical examination alone? *Radiology* 2000;214:683–687.
230. Mukherji SK, Mancuso AA, Kotzur IM, et al. Radiologic appearance of the irradiated larynx. Part II. Primary site response. *Radiology* 1994;193:149–154.
231. Pameijer FA, Hermans R, Mancuso AA, et al. Pre- and post-radiotherapy computed tomography in laryngeal cancer: imaging-based prediction of local failure. *Int J Radiat Oncol Biol Phys* 1999;45:359–366.
232. Greven KM, Williams DW 3rd, Keyes JW Jr., et al. Distinguishing tumor recurrence from irradiation sequelae with positron emission tomography in patients treated for larynx cancer. *Int J Radiat Oncol Biol Phys* 1994;29: 841–845.
233. Kim HJ, Boyd J, Dunphy F, et al. F-18 FDG PET scan after radiotherapy for early-stage larynx cancer. *Clin Nucl Med* 1998;23:750–752.
234. Hustinx R, Smith RJ, Benard F, et al. Dual time point fluorine-18 fluorodeoxyglucose positron emission tomography: a potential method to differentiate malignancy from inflammation and normal tissue in the head and neck. *Eur J Nucl Med* 1999;26:1345–1348.

Radiation Therapy Technique

235. Parsons JT, Palta JR, Mendenhall WM, et al. Head and neck cancer. In: Levitt SH, Khan FM, Potish RA, et al., eds. *Levitt and Tapley's technological basis of radiation therapy: clinical applications,* 3rd ed. Baltimore: Lippincott Williams & Wilkins, 1999:269–299.
236. Million RR, Cassisi NJ, Mancuso AA. Larynx. In: Million RR, Cassisi NJ, eds. *Management of head and neck cancer: a multidisciplinary approach,* 2nd ed. Philadelphia: JB Lippincott, 1994; 431–497.
237. Sombeck MD, Kalbaugh KJ, Mendenhall WM, et al. Radiotherapy for early vocal cord cancer: a dosimetric analysis of 60Co versus 6 MV photons. *Head Neck* 1996;18:167–173.
238. Harwood AR, Hawkins NV, Rider WD, et al. Radiotherapy of early glottic cancer—I. *Int J Radiat Oncol Biol Phys* 1979;5:473–476.
239. Million RR, Cassisi NJ, Clark JR. Cancer in the head and neck. In: DeVita VT Jr, Hellman S, Rosenberg SA, eds. *Cancer: principles and practice of oncology,* 3rd ed. Philadelphia: JB Lippincott Co, 1989:488–580.
240. Parsons JT. Time-dose-volume relations in radiation therapy. In: Million RR, Cassisi NJ, eds. *Management of head and neck cancer: a multidisciplinary approach,* 2nd ed. Philadelphia: JB Lippincott Co, 1994:203–243.
241. Million RR, Cassisi NJ, Mancuso AA, et al. Management of the neck for squamous cell carcinoma. In: Million RR, Cassisi NJ, eds. *Management of head and neck cancer: a multidisciplinary approach,* 2nd ed. Philadelphia: JB Lippincott Co, 1994:75–142.
242. Parsons JT, Bova FJ, Million RR. A re-evaluation of split-course technique for squamous cell carcinoma of the head and neck. *Int J Radiat Oncol Biol Phys* 1980;6:1645–1652.

CHAPTER 19

Advanced Stage Cancer of the Larynx

Gary L. Clayman, Douglas K. Frank, Adam S. Garden, and Merrill S. Kies

Because of the prominent role that the larynx plays in communication, respiration, and protection of the lower airway, the treatment of advanced laryngeal cancer presents formidable functional consequences. Unique to this particular site of head and neck cancer, quality-of-life issues have been incorporated into treatment decision making more extensively than for other cancer sites (1). Squamous cell carcinoma (SCC) of the larynx generally is diagnosed at an earlier stage of development than other head and neck sites, primarily owing to early manifestation of symptoms. As a result, cure rates generally are higher than for other sites. Some functional integrity often is preserved in these early stage lesions, regardless of treatment modality. In some circumstances, however, laryngeal SCC may present at an advanced stage (T3, T4), either primarily or as recurrent disease. The evaluation, functional considerations, and management options for laryngeal T3 and T4 SCCs are the focus of this chapter. Attention will be given to laryngeal preservation concepts.

RELEVANT ANATOMY

Three subdivisions—supraglottic, glottic, and subglottic—form the basis for classifying cancers that arise at different sites within the larynx. The supraglottic larynx includes the epiglottis, aryepiglottic folds, false vocal folds, and roof of the ventricles. The glottic larynx includes the floor of the ventricles, the anterior and posterior commissure areas, and the true vocal folds. The subglottic larynx generally is accepted to begin at a point 5 mm below the free edge of the true vocal folds and extends to the bottom of the cricoid cartilage.

The three laryngeal subdivisions are clinically important in embryonic development, vascular and lymphatic anatomy, and patterns of tumor growth. The frequency of regional lymph node metastases is determined largely by the laryngeal subdivisions, with glottic lesions having the lowest incidence and supraglottic lesions the highest incidence (2). The characteristics used in clinical staging of primary tumors arising in the supraglottic, glottic, and subglottic larynx are listed in Table 19.1. These characteristics conform to the staging system outlined by the American Joint Committee on Cancer (AJCC) in 1997 (3). The 5th edition of the AJCC staging manual (3) was recently updated with the 6th edition (3a). The editions are basically the same except for T4 lesions, which are now divided into T4a (resectable) and T4b (unresectable). This leads to the division of stage IV into IVA (locally advance, resectable), IVB (locally advanced, unresectable), and IVC (M1 disease). Examination of this staging system makes clear that there is significant anatomic overlap with regard to the three laryngeal subdivisions for T3 and T4 lesions. Thus, the exact laryngeal subsite of origin may not be clear in some advanced lesions.

NATURAL HISTORY AND PATTERNS OF SPREAD

Considerable attention has been devoted to anatomic studies of the vascular and lymphatic compartments of the larynx (4–6). These studies have formed the basis for defining natural anatomic barriers to cancer spread within the larynx. Furthermore, these studies have contributed to the development of precise partial laryngeal resections for small cancers and for certain more advanced lesions. Perhaps some of the most elegant studies on the anatomic barriers to spread of laryngeal cancer, by subsite, have been carried out by Kirchner and Carter (7).

Advanced Supraglottic Cancer

Supraglottic primary tumors account for 25% to 50% of all laryngeal cancers (8). A knowledge of the laryngeal compart-

TABLE 19.1 Tumor (T) Staging System for Laryngeal Cancer

Supraglottis	
Tis	Carcinoma *in situ*
T1	Tumor confined to site of origin with normal vocal fold mobility
T2	Tumor involving more than one supraglottic subsite or glottis without fixation of the glottis
T3	Tumor limited to larynx, with fixation or extension (or both) to involve postcricoid area, preepiglottic space, or [a]paraglottic space or minor thyroid cartilage erosion (e.g., inner cortex) or through the thyroid cartilage
T4	Massive tumor extending beyond larynx to involve oropharynx and soft tissues of neck or destruction of thyroid cartilage
	T4a[a]: Resectable (e.g., tumor invades trachea, soft tissues of neck including deep extrinsic muscle of the tongue, strap muscles, thyroid, or esophagus)
	T4b[a]: Unresectable (e.g., tumor invades prevertebral space, encases carotid artery, or invades mediastinal structures)
Glottis	
Tis	Carcinoma *in situ*
T1	Tumor confined to vocal cords, with normal mobility (includes involvement of anterior or posterior commissures)
	T1a[a]: Tumor limited to one vocal cord
	T1b[a]: Tumor involves both vocal cords
T2	Supraglottic or subglottic extension of tumor (or both) with normal or impaired vocal cord mobility
T3	Tumor confined to the larynx, with vocal cord fixation, or [a]invades paraglottic space or minor thyroid cartilage invasion (inner cortex)
T4	Massive tumor with thyroid cartilage destruction or extension beyond confines of larynx, or both
	T4a[a]: Resectable. Tumor invades through thyroid cartilage or invades tissues beyond larynx (e.g., trachea, soft tissues of neck, strap muscles, thyroid, or esophagus)
	T4b[a]: Unresectable. Tumor invades prevertebral space, encases carotid artery or invades mediastinal structures
Subglottis	
Tis	Carcinoma *in situ*
T1	Tumor confined to the subglottic region
T2	Tumor extension to vocal cords, with normal or impaired vocal cord mobility
T3	Tumor confined to the larynx, with vocal cord fixation
T4	Massive tumor, with cartilage destruction or extension beyond confines of larynx, or both
	T4a[a]: See above, same as glottis and supraglottis
	T4a[a]: See above, same as glottis and supraglottis

[a]Denotes new classification included in 6th ed. of the American Joint Committee on Cancer: *Cancer staging manual* by Greene F, et al. New York: Springer-Verlag, 2002.
Source: McNeil BJ, Weichselbaum R, Parker SG. Speech and survival: tradeoffs between quality and quantity of life in laryngeal cancer. *N Engl J Med* 1981;305:982.

ments aids in understanding the spread of SCC in this area. Supraglottic cancer originating on the false vocal folds or above this region may be limited by the quadrangular membrane. If this membrane is breached, the next anatomic barrier would be the internal perichondrium of the thyroid lamina. Extralaryngeal spread may occur through the thyroid lamina. Epiglottic tumors initially are impeded by the epiglottic perichondrium and the thyroepiglottic ligament (7). This barrier is breached by extension of tumor through the fenestra of the epiglottic cartilage (9), ultimately allowing entrance into the preepiglottic space, where tumor growth can be limited by additional elastic tissue. Once in the preepiglottic space, tumor may extend to the thyroid cartilage or through the thyrohyoid membrane.

Some advanced supraglottic lesions may involve the piriform sinus (Table 19.1). A propensity to invade the thyroid cartilage, involve the cricoarytenoid and interarytenoid muscles, and extend anteriorly into the paraglottic space has been demonstrated in these lesions. Transglottic spread is facilitated by paraglottic space involvement. Extension through the cricothyroid membrane ultimately may occur (10). Some supraglottic tumors may extend superiorly to involve the tongue base and other oropharyngeal structures.

In considering the natural history of advanced supraglottic cancer, the incidence of regional lymph node metastases must be considered. The supraglottic larynx is rich in lymphatics. The frequency of neck node metastases is high with T2 or higher stage tumors. Of patients with T3 and T4 lesions, 39% to 65% have clinically palpable neck lymph nodes at the time of diagnosis (11–13). The supraglottic larynx is a midline structure; thus, a high rate of palpable bilateral lymphatic metastases occurs (12). Lee et al. (14) have reported a 32% (28/87 patients) incidence of pathologically confirmed nodal disease in the clinically N0 neck, whereas Shah and Tollefsen (13) note a 34% (22/65 patients) incidence of occult nodal disease in all supraglottic tumors staged as N0. The rate of distant metastases approaches 30% in patients with stage IV disease (15). Favored sites of distant metastases include the lung, liver, and bone (16).

Advanced Glottic Cancer

The true vocal folds, vocal ligament, and anterior commissure tendon present initial barriers to the local spread of glottic cancer. With further growth, glottic cancers may be impeded by the conus elasticus and the thyroid lamina internal perichondrium. The most advanced lesions ultimately will breach the thyroid lamina or cricothyroid membrane (or both) and extend outside the larynx (7).

A transglottic cancer is one that crosses the ventricle in a vertical direction. Such a tumor may arise in either the glottic or supraglottic larynx. These lesions, as well as those that involve the anterior commissure, are associated with invasion of the thyroid cartilage in 40% to 60% of cases (17). Transglottic tumors also have a propensity to enter the paraglottic space. Once in the paraglottic space, tumors may travel inferiorly and laterally, escaping from the larynx through the cricothyroid membrane in some cases (4).

These tumors also are associated with a 30% to 50% incidence of regional metastases, as well as a high incidence of vocal fold paralysis (2,4,18). Skolnik et al. (19) have reported an incidence of palpable cervical metastases of 25% and 65% for T3 and T4 glottic lesions, respectively. Rates of occult metastases may approach 20% in the clinically N0 neck (20). One may expect the incidence of occult nodal disease to be higher in those lesions that cross the ventricle (transglottic) to involve the lymphatically rich supraglottic larynx. Distant metastases can appear with advanced glottic disease, with favored sites similar to those for advanced supraglottic disease (16).

Advanced Subglottic Cancer

Subglottic lesions are usually the result of contiguous spread from tumors originating from more superior laryngeal sites. Primary carcinoma in this region of the larynx is relatively rare. Approximately 1% to 8% of all laryngeal cancers originate at this site (21,22). These lesions usually are advanced at diagnosis, and regional lymph node metastases occur frequently (22). Harrison (23) notes that the incidence of nodal metastases in subglottic cancer may be underestimated as many of the draining lymphatics of this region cannot be adequately palpated. He reports that 50% of larynges with primary subglottic cancer, when examined by serial section, contained paratracheal lymph node metastases. Fixation of the true vocal folds is frequent, as is circumferential spread, invasion of the laryngotracheal cartilage, and extralaryngeal spread. Tumors in this region may invade the cricoid cartilage, the trachea, or the thyroid gland and anterior neck soft tissues via extension through the cricothyroid membrane (17,21,22,24). Tumors may come to involve the cervical esophagus by extending posteriorly below the cricoid cartilage (23).

CLINICAL PRESENTATION

Early diagnosis of laryngeal SCC is critical for achieving high survival rates and laryngeal preservation (25). Most cancers that are diagnosed at an early stage arise in the glottic larynx. Minimal changes in the mass of the vibrating vocal fold due to tumor growth result in changes in the fold's vibrating characteristics, which are evident as dysphonia or hoarseness. More advanced glottic lesions may present with frank airway compromise or regional lymph node metastases, the frequency of which was pointed out earlier.

Supraglottic cancers usually are more advanced than glottic cancers at the time of diagnosis. SCCs arising in the supraglottic larynx generally do not produce early symptoms of hoarseness. Rather, the earliest symptoms of a supraglottic cancer are sore throat and dysphagia (20). Referred otalgia, or development of a neck mass representing regional metastases also may occur as a presenting sign. Airway compromise may be an early symptom of a more advanced subglottic malignancy. Hoarseness from extension to the true vocal folds and hemoptysis are other presenting symptoms of advanced subglottic lesions (21–23).

DIAGNOSTIC EVALUATION AND STAGING

The history and physical examination are the cornerstones of the initial comprehensive evaluation of any patient with SCC of the larynx. Many individuals with laryngeal cancer will relate a history of smoking, often in association with alcohol consumption. In addition to palpation of the laryngeal cartilaginous framework, the physical examination should include evaluation of the cervical lymphatics including thyroid compartments.

Modern clinical evaluation of laryngeal cancer begins with indirect mirror-assisted or fiberoptic laryngoscopy (important in evaluating for vocal fold paralysis) and, ultimately, direct laryngoscopy. Computed tomography (CT), magnetic resonance imaging (MRI) of the larynx and neck, and videostroboscopic analysis are important adjunctive diagnostic tests. These radiologic assessments are of value in assessing direct extension of tumor to the preepiglottic and paraglottic spaces of the larynx, detecting cartilage invasion, and evaluating the soft tissues and lymph nodes of the neck. These studies have replaced conventional tomography and contrast laryngograms. Angiography and CT play a role in evaluating the cervical vasculature in patients with advanced disease thought to involve the great vessels. Distant metastatic disease often is sought via CT evaluation of the chest.

Precise evaluation of tumor extent demands direct laryngoscopy under anesthesia. For large obstructive tumors, this may necessitate prior tracheotomy. In some patients with large obstructive lesions, debulking the tumor mass at the time of direct laryngoscopy can obviate the need for tracheotomy and thereby reduce the potential risk for tumor seeding of the tracheostomy site. Even with precise clinical evaluation, inaccurate estimation of tumor extent (usually underestimation) occurs in 30% to 40% of cases (26). Most often, this involves failure to identify invasion of the laryngeal cartilaginous framework. Nevertheless, if clinical examination confirms normal vocal fold function and absence of anterior commissure involvement, radiologic imaging of the larynx has no clear role in assessment of a patient.

The staging of advanced laryngeal SCC conforms to the system outlined by the AJCC in 2002 (7) (Table 19.1) (3). Tumor staging of supraglottic cancers is based on the subsite or region of the supraglottic larynx involved by cancer. Subsites include the false vocal folds, arytenoids, lingual and laryngeal surfaces of the epiglottis, and aryepiglottic folds. Regarding advanced supraglottic lesions, those that cause fixation of the vocal fold or involve the postcricoid region, medial wall of the piriform sinus, or preepiglottic space are classified as T3. Those that extend beyond the larynx or invade the thyroid cartilage are classified as T4.

Glottic carcinomas also are staged according to subsites involved. Lesions with vocal fold fixation are classified as T3, whereas those with cartilage involvement or extension outside the larynx are classified as T4. Advanced subglottic cancers cause fixation of the vocal fold (T3) or invade cartilage or extend outside the larynx (T4).

MANAGEMENT AND RESULTS

The treatment of more advanced laryngeal cancers (T3 and T4) has historically included radical surgery with or without radiation therapy. Often this surgery and subsequent therapy resulted in loss of voice, compounding the effects of the disease process. In recent years, the treatment of more advanced laryngeal cancers has become controversial as larynx-preserving approaches have developed. In this section, we highlight the current overall management of laryngeal cancers by stage and subsite, emphasizing the situations in which preservation techniques have been applied. The results of the outlined therapeutic endeavors will also be highlighted.

Advanced Supraglottic Cancer

T3 supraglottic cancer, by definition, need not involve the glottis. Recall from Table 19.1 that such lesions may involve the preepiglottic space or the medial wall of the piriform sinus with or without vocal fold fixation. Thus, some advanced supraglottic lesions are amenable to conservation surgical techniques. The surgical treatment options for supraglottic cancer at all stages are multiple and controversial and include surgery alone, surgery combined with preoperative or postoperative radiation therapy, induction chemotherapy (protocol studies) followed by surgical approaches and primary radiation therapy with surgical salvage if needed (8,11,14,27–29). Following completion of the cooperative group trial 91-11 (30), possible treatment algorithm for advanced supraglottic cancer is demonstrated in Figure 19.1. The appropriate modality of treatment depends on the size and location of the tumor, whether or not the vocal folds are involved, the status of the cervical lymphatics, and patient characteristics such as age and pulmonary reserve. Laryngeal preservation should be the goal whenever technically feasible.

T3 lesions without vocal fold fixation may be treated with supraglottic laryngectomy (Fig. 19.19). This modality of treatment mandates the satisfaction of strict preoperative criteria. Mendenhall et al. (31) have outlined the contraindications for supraglottic laryngectomy, including tumor extension anterior to the circumvallate papillae, involvement of both arytenoids, significant extension to the piriform sinus, vocal fold fixation, and thyroid or cricoid cartilage invasion. Extension of tumor to the preepiglottic space is not a contraindication to supraglottic laryngectomy. When these criteria are met, disease-free survival of approximately 75% at 3 years can be expected (14,29,32). The local recurrence rate is typically low at 10% (29). Results of the supraglottic operation approximate those of total laryngectomy (27). Vermund (33) reports an absolute survival of 45% (14/31 patients) in those individuals with T3 N0 supraglottic disease treated surgically. Patients with vocal fold fixation, as well as those who received total laryngectomy, were included in these statistics. Some more advanced lesions, such as those involving the vallecula or tongue base, may be surgically treated by an expansion of the supraglottic laryngectomy technique, as outlined by Bocca et al. (32). Lee et al. (14) and Goepfert et al. (34) have advocated postoperative radiation therapy for the primary lesion for positive surgical margins and significant extralaryngeal extension into the tongue base, pharyngeal wall, or soft tissues of the neck. In every patient undergoing supraglottic laryngectomy, preoperative permission must be obtained for total laryngectomy (see Fig. 19.18) in case the surgical findings dictate that more extensive surgery is needed to extirpate the cancer.

Radical radiation with surgical salvage for failure has been evaluated in the management of moderately advanced supraglottic cancer (some T3 and T4 lesions) that is amenable to supraglottic laryngectomy. Supraglottic laryngectomy may offer better survival and local control in appropriate lesions than radical radiation therapy with surgical salvage (8,27,28, 35,36). Marks et al. (28) reports 30% (6/20 patients) of patients irradiated for cure of resectable supraglottic cancer experienced local failure. All local failures required total laryngectomy. Eighty-seven percent (100/119 patients) in the primarily surgically treated group (supraglottic laryngectomy) in this study had voice preservation. Vermund (33) notes a 36% (43/120 patients) absolute 5-year survival in patients with T3 N0 supraglottic lesions treated with primary radiation therapy, including those with fixation of the vocal folds. All T3 lesions and node-positive disease negatively affected survival, regardless of treatment, in Vermund's (33) review.

Because supraglottic laryngectomy is associated with variable degrees of postoperative aspiration, adequate pulmonary status is a prerequisite for this surgery (27), as is intact mobility of the true vocal folds. Approximately 20% of patients require prolonged tracheotomy, a condition that may be related to edema secondary to postoperative radiation, which often is employed as part of the combined therapy of advanced lesions. The rates of persistent swallowing difficulties are low, however, and the need for completion laryngectomy for persistent aspiration is only about 5% (14). In general, the quality of voice after supraglottic laryngectomy has been rated as good or satisfactory by most patients undergoing this procedure (36–38). Similar voice results have been reported after primary radiation therapy for the treatment of laryngeal cancer (37).

The T3 supraglottic cancer involving the upper medial wall of the piriform sinus may be managed using conservation surgical techniques. Partial laryngopharyngectomy, which is essentially an extended supraglottic laryngectomy, adequately addresses this tumor as long as the vocal folds, arytenoids, and apex of the piriform sinus are free of disease (39). The thyroid cartilage cannot be invaded by tumor. Surgical management of such lesions should probably be followed by postoperative radiation therapy following the guidelines outlined earlier.

Supraglottic lesions that cause vocal fold fixation (T3), involve the postcricoid region (T3), or invade the laryngeal cartilage or extralaryngeal sites (T4) can be effectively managed with total laryngectomy and postoperative radiation therapy. Organ-preserving therapeutic modalities for these clinical situations are discussed later in relation to glottic carcinomas that would otherwise require total laryngectomy.

The frequency of palpable and occult neck node metastases is high with T2 or higher stage supraglottic tumors, as was detailed previously. The potential for bilateral cervical metastases with advanced supraglottic lesions has already been mentioned. Neck recurrence probably represents the greatest cause of failure in the overall management of supraglottic cancer (8, 27,28). For these reasons, treatment of the cervical lymphatics,

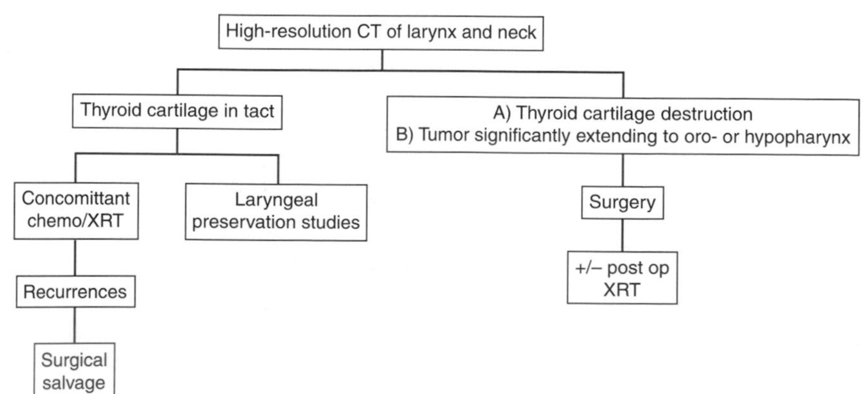

Figure 19.1 Possible treatment algorithm for advanced supraglottic cancer. *CT,* computed tomography; *XRT,* x-ray therapy; *chemo,* chemotherapy.

usually bilaterally, should be performed. Selective neck dissection addressing levels II, III, and IV is likely adequate in the N0 neck, but more comprehensive neck dissections should be carried out in patients with N+ disease. Level I need not be dissected unless clinically or radiographically involved. Whereas most authors advocate elective bilateral neck dissections in the clinically N0 neck (14,27,32), others do not believe that such a procedure offers a survival advantage (13). Some authors argue that neck dissection can be delayed until clinically evident metastases occur (40,41). Although the issue of optimal management for the patient with N0 disease has not been settled, we advocate the approach in which bilateral selective node dissections are performed and postoperative radiation is reserved for patients with proven regional metastases (14,29).

Advanced Glottic Cancer

The treatment of glottic cancer, like that of supraglottic cancer, is influenced greatly by the secondary goal of voice preservation. As with supraglottic cancers, careful clinical tumor staging is necessary as underestimation of tumor extent is common (26). A treatment algorithm for advanced glottic cancers is given in Figure 19.2.

Management of advanced T3 and T4 glottic cancers historically has consisted of total laryngectomy with or without radiation therapy (18,42–46). Overall disease-free survival with this therapy varies depending on the study, with 5-year rates for T3 lesions ranging from 49% to 80% (19,33,46) and 5-year rates for T4 lesions ranging from 32% to 63% (33,46). Jesse (44) reports a 4-year disease-free survival of 54% (26/48 patients) in his series of T4 lesions.

The addition of radiation therapy to total laryngectomy for localized T3 lesions has not been clearly demonstrated to contribute significant increases in local control or survival. However, in patients with regional nodal metastases, significant subglottic extension of tumor, tracheotomy before definitive treatment, or extension of tumor to the pharyngeal wall, the addition of postoperative radiation therapy seems to offer a survival advantage (44,46). These tumor characteristics may be representative of more aggressive behavior. Patients with T3 transglottic lesions may also benefit from adjuvant radiation therapy (18).

Because of a relatively high rate of occult regional metastases, patients with advanced glottic cancers may be considered for elective selective neck dissections for staging purposes when surgery is performed for primary disease. Radical neck

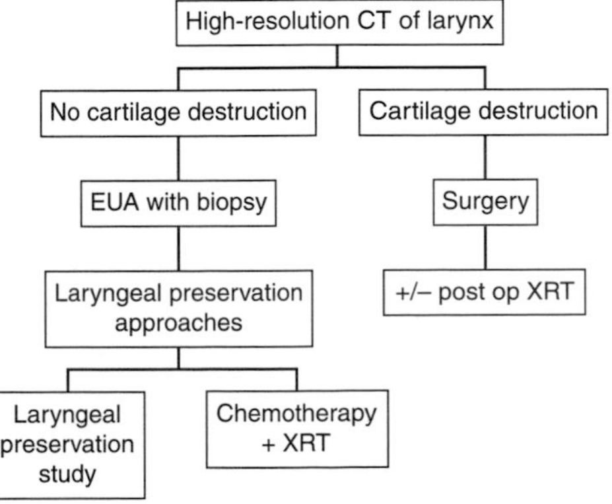

Figure 19.2 Possible treatment algorithm for advanced glottic cancer. *CT,* computed tomography; *EUA,* endoscopy of the upper aerodigestive tract; *XRT,* x-ray therapy.

dissection (RND)[1] or modified radical neck dissection (MRND)[2] should be performed in the instance of N+ disease. Such lesions often require adjuvant radiation therapy (as discussed previously). For lesions that cross the ventricle to involve the supraglottic larynx (transglottic), consideration of the cervical lymphatics becomes similar to that for primary supraglottic lesions. For very localized T3 lesions, prophylactic neck dissection may not be necessary at the time of the initial operation, as the risk for occult metastases is low (45).

In terms of primary surgical management, we should point out that not all advanced glottic cancers require total laryngectomy. Certain T3 glottic tumors may be amenable to conservation surgical techniques such as the subtotal laryngectomy with cricohyoidoepiglottopexy (47) (see Fig. 19.20). Appropriate candidates for this procedure should have mobile arytenoids and less than 7 mm of subglottic tumor extension. This procedure is associated with 75% (78/104 patients) survival at 5 years and a 5% local recurrence rate. In 1980, Pearson et al. (48) described the extended hemilaryngectomy for the treatment of certain glottic cancers staged as T3. This procedure involves the creation of a tracheopharyngeal shunt, which allows for phonation during expiration. Deglutition is not impeded by this procedure, as the shunt closes during swallowing.

Controversy continues to surround the use of definitive radiation with surgical salvage in patients with advanced (T3, T4) but localized glottic cancers. Reported overall survival rates at 5 years range widely from 8% to 87% (33,44–51) in patients with T3/T4N0 disease, with larynx preservation in approximately 60% to 70% of these patients (16,47,48). A large, long-term British study demonstrated that salvage laryngectomy was possible in fewer than 50% of patients for tumor recurrence after definitive radiation therapy (52). Complication rates have been previously reported to increase with surgical salvage of radiation treatment failures (49), and survival may be compromised following primary radiotherapy. Moreover, the management of advanced larynx cancer may be substantially changed with the advent of chemoradiation strategies.

In 1985 the Veterans Affairs Cooperative Studies Program (56) initiated a multiinstitutional, randomized, prospective trial in which more than 300 patients with stage III or IV squamous cell carcinoma were randomly assigned to receive induction chemotherapy with cisplatin and infusional 5-fluorouracil followed by radiotherapy or total laryngectomy and postoperative radiation. In the experimental chemotherapy arm, surgery was reserved for salvage in patients with inadequate response to the induction chemotherapy or those with persistent or recurrent disease after completing the entire treatment program. There was no difference in survival between the treatment arms, approximately 70% at two years. Laryngeal preservation was achieved in 62% of surviving patients treated with chemotherapy and radiation. Patients with locally advanced disease (T4 N2/3) required salvage laryngectomy in greater than 50% of cases. The chemotherapy arm was found to have a decreased risk of distant disease as a first site of recurrence. A subsequent trial similar in design to the VA larynx study (56), focused on patients with cancers of the hypopharynx and again yielded no statistically significant survival difference between the experimental induction chemotherapy and radiation group versus patients undergoing more standard local therapy, surgical resection and post operative radiation. These trials have led to the acceptance of induction chemotherapy with cisplatin and

[1]RND is a classic procedure that includes removal of the internal jugular vein, sternocleidomastoid muscle, and the spinal accessory nerve.
[2]MRND is a technical variation of the RND that spares one or more of the involved structures.

infusional 5-fluorouracil followed by radiation therapy as a reasonable alternative for patients with intermediate stage cancers of the larynx and hypopharynx.

In follow-up to the VA study, the Head and Neck Intergroup (30) has conducted a prospective 3-arm study comparing induction chemotherapy with cisplatin and 5-FU followed by radiotherapy; radiotherapy alone; and radiotherapy with concomitant cisplatin. For entry, patients had stage III/IV disease but T1 and advanced T4 lesions conferred ineligibility. Infiltrating tumor greater that 1 cm into the tongue base or the demonstration of thyroid cartilage destruction was not allowed. Five hundred ten patients were entered; 65% of them had stage III disease. Two thirds of patients had supraglottic primary sites. No unexpected toxicity was observed. With no difference in overall survival, the concomitant treatment arm resulted in superior larynx preservation, 88% compared to 74% with sequential chemotherapy and radiation and 69% with radiotherapy alone. Risk of distant disease recurrence was reduced in both of the chemotherapy arms. The results of this study indicate that concomitant chemoradiation is an effective therapeutic approach allowing for larynx preservation in a high percentage of patients without a sacrifice in overall survival. Notably, patients with destructive T4 primary tumors were excluded from this study. Long-term outcomes including quality of life and functional data are awaited.

Advanced Subglottic Cancer

Subglottic cancer tends to present late in its course, usually as T3 and T4 lesions (22). The management of this disease has largely stressed radical surgical extirpation through wide-field laryngectomy. The importance of paratracheal lymph node dissection and isthmusectomy versus partial or total thyroidectomy as part of the initial surgical procedure has also been mentioned (21–23). Shaha and Shah (22), in their series of patients with subglottic cancer, recommend postoperative radiation therapy for those with advanced disease. These authors further stated that elective dissection of the N0 neck may not be warranted. Harrison (23) has emphasized the rather low survival rate for primary subglottic cancers, regardless of treatment, whereas Shaha and Shah (22) report a 5-year cure rate of 70% (10/14 patients) in their series in which most of their patients had advanced disease. Vermund (33), in his comparative review of the treatment of laryngeal cancer, found an overall 5-year survival of 42% (24/58 patients) for primary surgical treatment of subglottic cancer.

The experience of treating primary subglottic cancer using radiation therapy as the primary modality has been somewhat limited. In the comparative study by Vermund (33), the 5-year survival rate for patients with subglottic cancer treated with radiation was 36% (46/127 patients). Outcomes with respect to specific stage of disease and functional data were not mentioned. Guedea et al. (59) studied the results of radical radiation therapy on a small group of patients with primary subglottic carcinoma. Three of their patients had T4N0 disease. One patient was without disease at 4 years but required a temporary tracheotomy. Another patient died of intercurrent disease at 4 years, though the patient's cancer was controlled locally. The third patient required salvage laryngectomy at 6 months and ultimately died of recurrent disease at 2.5 years.

COMPLICATIONS

A complete discussion of advanced laryngeal cancer must pay particular attention to complications of management. Specific complications often are related to the treatment modality employed: surgery, radiation therapy, chemotherapy, or any combination thereof. Certain patient factors, such as age and general health, often dictate the therapeutic regimen to be employed, as potential morbidities of a given treatment may be contraindicated in a particular patient.

The need for adequate pulmonary reserve for conservation surgical techniques, specifically supraglottic laryngectomy, has been mentioned. Besides aspiration leading to pneumonia, these patients are at risk for postoperative fistula, infection, vocal fold paralysis, prolonged dysphagia, and prolonged dyspnea (14,28,60). Postoperative supraglottic swelling may contribute to respiratory and swallowing complications of this procedure and can significantly delay tracheotomy decannulation. Gastrostomy tube insertion sometimes is needed. These more severe complications have been encountered with a combined modality (surgery with preoperative or postoperative radiation therapy) approach (14,28,61), as well as with radiation therapy as a single modality (11,15,31,62). Chondritis and cartilage necrosis have been noted as a potential complication of curative doses of radiation therapy in patients with advanced supraglottic disease (31,62). With intractable aspiration and gastrostomy dependence, conversion to total laryngectomy may be required.

Management of the most advanced laryngeal lesions presently involves combinations of surgery, radiation therapy, and chemotherapy. Total laryngectomy alone may be associated with wound infection, pharyngocutaneous fistula, skin necrosis, esophageal stenosis, and carotid rupture (18,19,63,64). Hypothyroidism is to be expected if the thyroid gland is removed as part of the surgical management. Mucositis, skin changes, cartilage necrosis, fistula, esophageal stenosis, and hypothyroidism have been associated with curative radiation therapy for advanced laryngeal cancer (18,33,49). The incidence of complications may be increased with surgery (salvage) after radiation therapy, which may be related to the timing of operative intervention (33). Carotid rupture, pharyngocutaneous fistula, and tissue necrosis have been reported in this situation (49). The introduction of chemotherapy into the management armamentarium of advanced laryngeal cancer is associated with treatment-limiting toxicities and even death (55,56), a fact that must be remembered when a patient is being considered for organ preservation. Free tissue transfer reconstruction may be used for hypopharyngeal repair to minimize complications following aggressive chemotherapy and radiotherapy efforts in organ preservation approaches (57).

MANAGEMENT OF RECURRENCE

Recurrent disease can manifest itself at the primary site (including peristomal recurrence), in the regional lymphatics, or in distant sites. The sites of distant metastases of advanced laryngeal cancer were discussed earlier. This discussion focuses largely on local and regional recurrence.

In the surgical management of advanced supraglottic cancer, recurrent disease in the neck continues to be a significant problem (8,27–29,32). Overall, most recurrences are seen within the first posttreatment year (32). Although the incidence of local recurrence in surgically treated patients is typically less than that of regional recurrence, local recurrence often warrants total laryngectomy. Survival statistics after local recurrence and salvage total laryngectomy have been variable, ranging from 41% to 66% at 5 years in those patients who were candidates for the procedure (29,32). Bocca et al. (32), in their large series of patients with supraglottic laryngectomy, noted that most neck recurrences in surgically treated necks were seen in patients with N2 and N3 disease. DeSanto (8) notes the uniformly poor survival among those patients who experienced recurrence in a previously dissected neck. Soo et al. (29) were able to successfully manage 53% of their patients with supraglottic laryngectomy who experienced regional recurrence. Management consisted of surgery (neck dissection) or surgery with radiation therapy.

The management of advanced supraglottic cancer with primary radiation therapy may offer an advantage in terms of decreased neck recurrence; however, an increase in local recurrence may be appreciated (8,31). Total laryngectomy may be required as part of the management plan for recurrent disease in this situation.

In cases of advanced cancer originating in the glottic larynx, just as in the supraglottic larynx, recurrence at the primary site and neck must be considered. Patients treated with total laryngectomy primarily also must be observed for tracheal stomal recurrence. In a study of patients with advanced glottic cancer treated surgically, Yuen et al. (46) reports, 18% (28/155 patients) of T3 patients and 32% (12/37 patients) of T4 patients experienced treatment failure above the clavicles. Failure in the neck occurred predominantly on the nondissected side. These authors note uniformly poor survival in those patients with locoregional or stomal recurrence. Stomal recurrence, a very poor prognostic sign, was noted to occur in a large percentage of patients with subglottic tumor extension in this series. Mittal et al. (18), in their review of patients with transglottic cancer, were able to salvage only 26% (10/38 patients) of their locoregional failures with surgery or radiation. Hyperthermia also was employed. None of their patients with stomal recurrence survived. In the series by DeSanto (43), 7% (6/88 patients) of patients with T3 nontransglottic cancer died of uncontrolled primary disease. Most of these patients were treated initially with total laryngectomy. In this series, neck recurrence in nondissected necks could usually be treated with neck dissection. Most of these patients survived.

In the series reported by Harwood et al. (50), which explored the role of radical radiation therapy with surgical salvage for failures in the management of advanced glottic cancer, 49% (55/112 patients) of individuals experienced local recurrence. Two patients experienced disease recurrence in the neck. Most local recurrences required total laryngectomy. Of patients salvaged in this manner, 65% (31/48 patients) survived. Croll et al. (49) found a 33% (19/58 patients) local recurrence rate and a 9% (5/58 patients) nodal recurrence rate in their patients who were treated with radical radiation therapy for advanced laryngeal cancer. Local recurrence warranted total laryngectomy, which yielded more cures in the patients who were staged initially as T3. N+ nodal status in this series, as with others, was a poor prognostic sign, being associated with an increased locoregional recurrence rate.

Primary subglottic cancer may recur locally, in the paratracheal nodes, in the mediastinum, at the tracheal margin, or at the stoma (23,58). Treatment in these circumstances should include salvage laryngectomy, when possible, in the initially irradiated patient. Appropriate neck or mediastinal dissection should be employed for recurrence at these sites. Poor prognosis should be expected under these circumstances.

Peristomal recurrence after total laryngectomy is a dreaded outcome of the disease process. The development of peristomal recurrence has been reported to be related to tracheotomy before treatment of the cancer, as well as to subglottic extension of tumor. Peristomal recurrences are most consistent with recurrence in paratracheal lymphatic basins with extracapsular extension into the stoma and trachea. Prevention seems to be the best treatment for this problem, therefore, postoperative radiation therapy is advocated to the stomal area in patients at risk (65,66). Radiation alone offers little hope for success in the event of peristomal recurrence. Combination induction chemotherapy with full-course radiation therapy or surgery (including mediastinal dissection) has been recommended in this situation (65).

RADIOLOGIC IMAGING CONCERNS

Bernard B. O'Malley and Suresh Mukherji

Awareness of the treatment options for patients presenting with advanced laryngeal cancer determines the style of scanning and the tempering of comments in one's image interpretation (67–80). Whether the patient is a candidate for total laryngectomy, near-total laryngectomy, radiation therapy, or combined chemotherapy–radiation therapy requires knowledge of an institution's treatment protocols and eligibility criteria. The interpretation of each imaging study should comment on the presence of:

1. Cartilage invasion
2. Exolaryngeal spread
3. Transglottic extension
4. Subglottic spread

Advanced supraglottic carcinomas should be specifically evaluated for preepiglottic spread (T3) and tongue base invasion (T4). Natural variability of cartilage calcification of the thyroid lamina hinders evaluation for cartilage invasion (Fig. 19.3).

Either CT or MRI can provide the aforementioned information. In general, CT is often better tolerated than MRI, due to the propensity of airway compromise and pooled secretions in patients with advanced laryngeal carcinoma (72). Direct coronal views lay out the degree of subglottic extension (Fig. 19.4), which is important for surgical decision making or radiation portal planning. Direct coronal MRI or reformatting of axial CT image data are the best methods of obtaining such views (Fig. 19.5). The degree of hypopharyngeal involvement is best determined clinically but can be estimated with axial CT or MRI sections (Fig. 19.6). Paraglottic space is readily evaluated in the axial CT plane (Fig. 19.7). Preepiglottic space can be assessed with either CT or magnetic resonance sagittal plane with MRI (74) or reformatted CT; these views show the proximity of disease to the hyoid bone and lower preepiglottic space (Fig. 19.8).

Exolaryngeal extension is easily identified on the standard axial projection (Fig. 19.9). This view also shows the degree of involvement of the carotid sheath and the integrity of the prevertebral plane from extralaryngeal disease or adenopathy. Accuracy of these latter findings depends on the use of intravenous contrast. Lymph node staging requires particular attention to the tracheoesophageal grooves caudad into the superior mediastinum and lateral retropharyngeal stations cephalad up to the skull base (Fig. 19.10). All of the aforementioned anatomic structures can be visualized with standard 5-mm-thick scans of the neck and 3-mm sections of the larynx. Thinner sections may be appropriate for production of more realistic three-dimensional renderings.

Follow-up imaging of the neck is important, given the clinical distortion of the alimentary tract after laryngectomy or swelling of the larynx during and after radiation therapy or chemotherapy. Surgical salvage is important in the T3 and T4 patient group and survival is not compromised when local recurrence is detected early (75). Attempts to reconstruct an extended partial laryngectomy with tracheal transposition require familiarity with the novel imaging appearance of this reconstruction (76). In the laryngectomy cohort, CT is an efficient evaluative modality for the primary site, stomal region (Fig. 19.11), and lymph nodes. Enhanced axial views are obtained of the entire pharynx down to the upper mediastinum. A small amount of dilute barium is administered to outline the "neopharynx" or "pull-up" to eliminate the pseudomass appearance of the native asymmetries of the reconstructed segment (Fig. 19.12). Contrast-enhanced CT performed in contiguous axial 3-mm sections is helpful for evaluating for recurrent disease in patients with both surgical and nonsurgical organ preservation techniques (Fig. 19.13). Either CT or MRI can be performed. We prefer CT for its technical consistency in patients prone to motion artifact following treatment.

Eventually fluorodeoxyglucose-positron emission tomography (FDG-PET) imaging may become the initial follow-up imaging study now that its high diagnostic accuracy has been determined and cost reimbursement has been settled (Fig. 19.14) (79). Positron emission tomography results in this population are typically not negative but are instrumental in demonstrating a trend from high to lower standardized uptake values. This group of patients therefore would benefit from a baseline pretreatment examination. Although FDG-PET suffers from a limited specificity, it has a high sensitivity and strong negative predictive value in the organ preservation population (80). The technology uses a generic agent in FDG, which contributes to its limited specificity when there is associated inflammation. Eventually more specific ligands will be developed for wide clinical use. For now, attempts at improving specificity include scanning the patient and then re-scanning after at least a 30-minute delay. The metabolic activity of the inflammatory tissue fades relative to neoplastic tissue. All nuclear images should be correlated with cross-sectional examinations to determine the subsites involved.

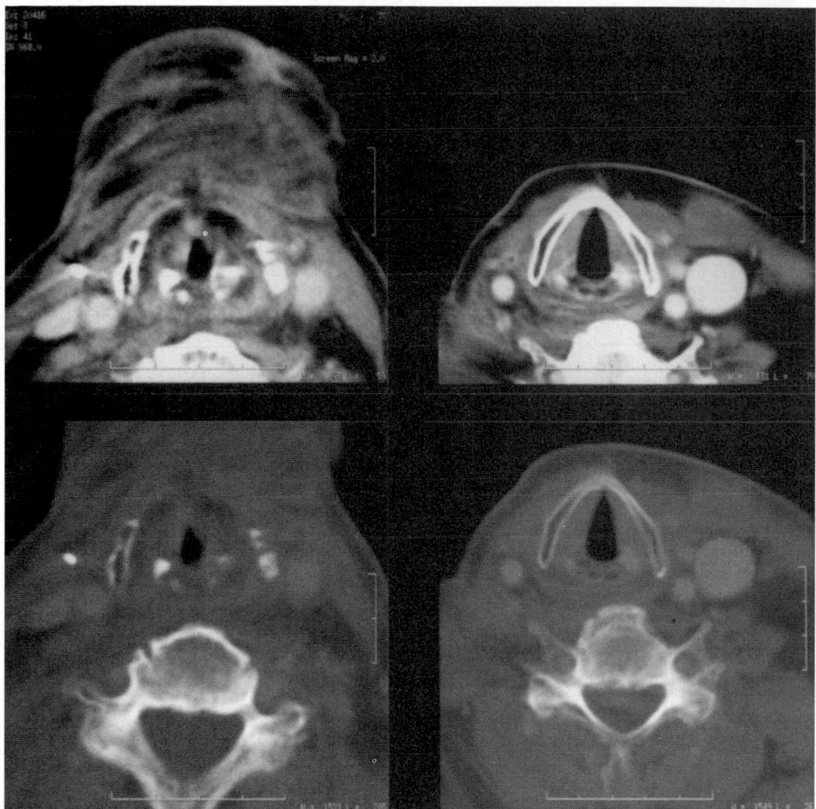

Figure 19.3 Variable cartilage calcification. Matched soft tissue (top) and bone (bottom) type windows of two different patients (right and left) show the variability of calcification between patients and between two sides of the same patient (left).

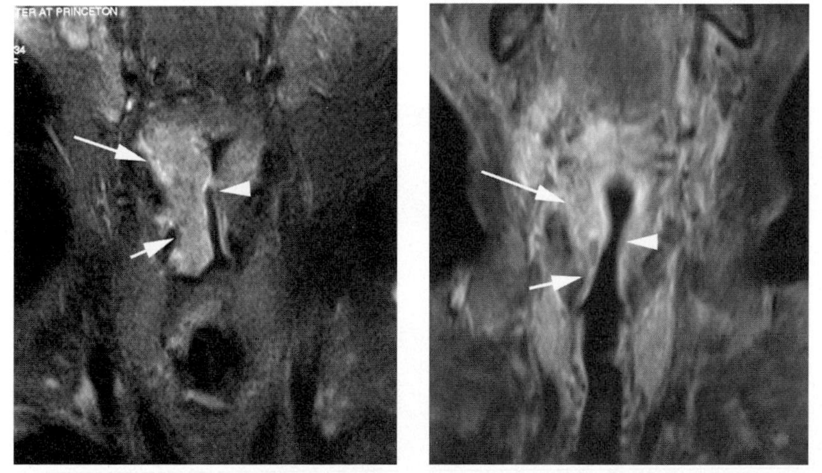

Figure 19.4 Transglottic squamous cell carcinoma treatment follow-up. **A:** Pretreatment coronal magnetic resonance image (MRI) with contrast shows the large transglottic mass (*long arrow*) straddling the plane of the ventricle (*arrowhead*) with extensive subglottic component (*short arrow*). **B:** Posttreatment coronal MRI with contrast shows marked reduction of subglottic component (*short arrow*). *Arrowhead* defines level of ventricle.

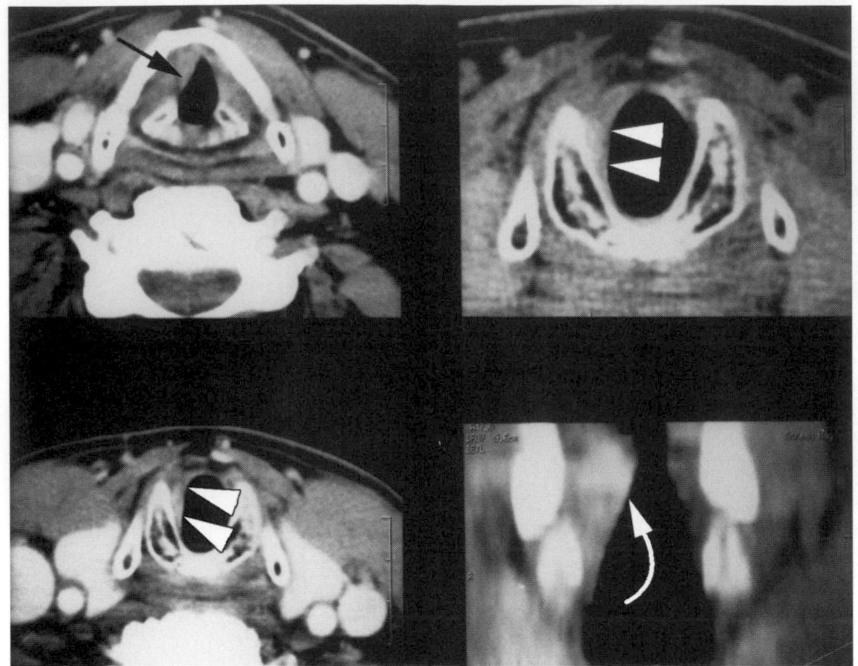

Figure 19.5 Subglottic extension. Serial enhanced axial and single reformatted coronal views of a right glottic lesion (*arrow*). The subglottic component is shown better on the lower right reformatted coronal view (*curved arrow*) than on the axial source images (*arrowheads*).

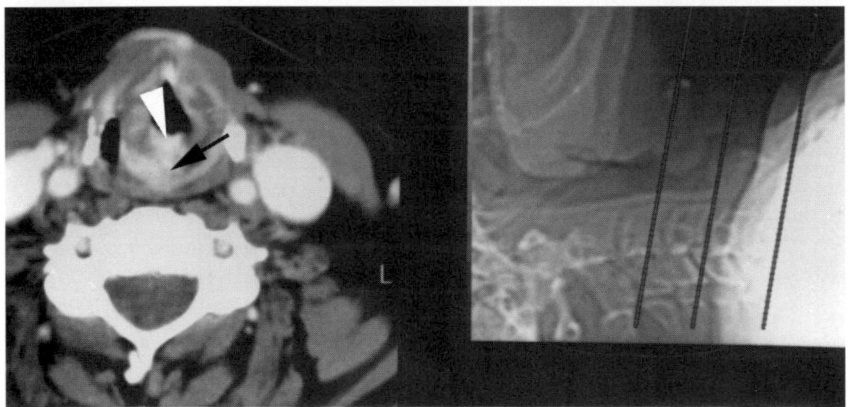

Figure 19.6 Hypopharyngeal extension. Enhanced axial computed tomogram of glottis **(A)** and corresponding cross-reference view **(B)** show lesion at the posterior commissure (*arrowhead*) extending into the hypopharynx (*arrow*).

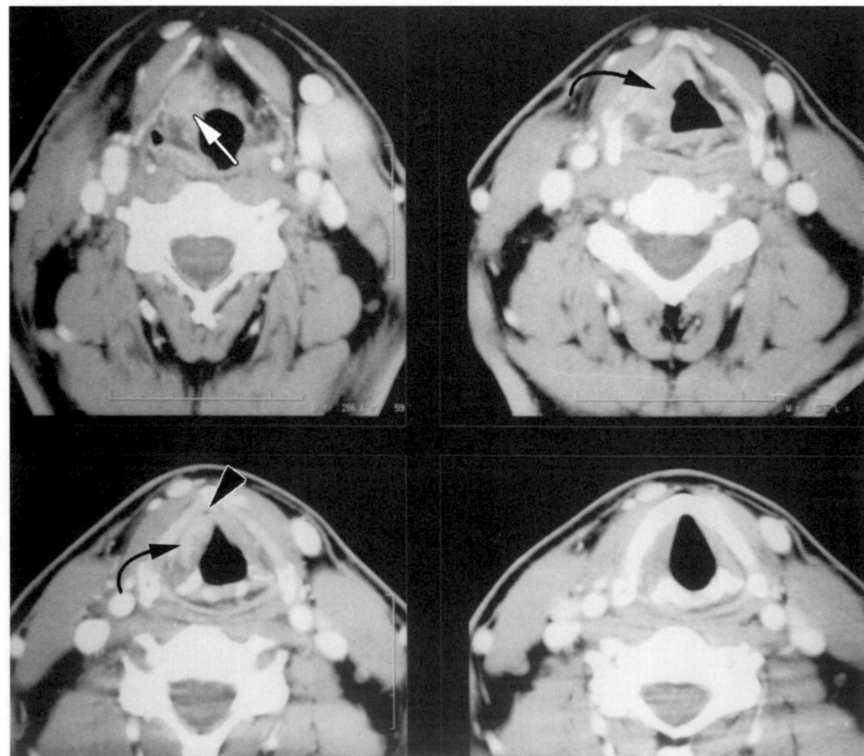

Figure 19.7 False cord lesion. Enhanced serial axial computed tomogram images show large tumor of right false cord (*arrow*) involving the paraglottic space (*curved arrow*) and approaching the anterior commissure (*arrowhead*). Thyroid lamina is intact.

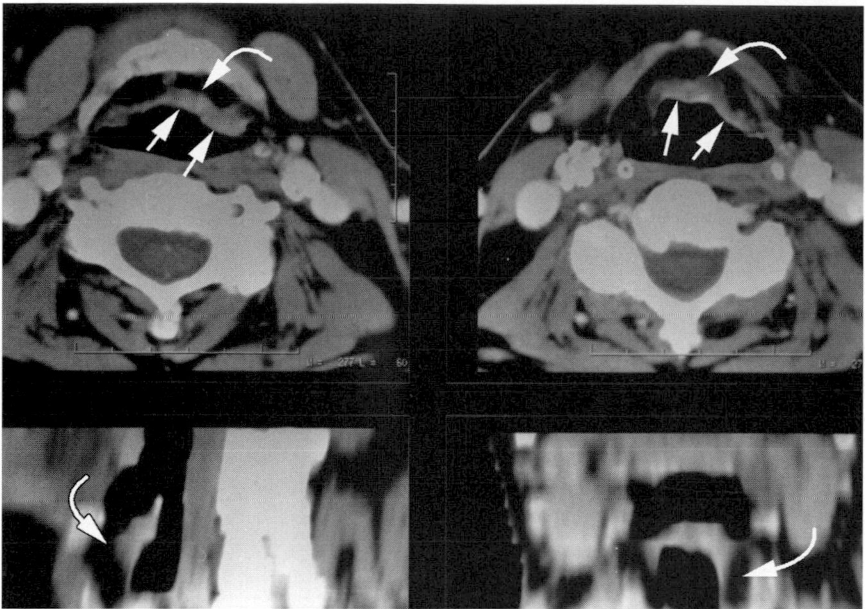

Figure 19.8 Early supraglottic carcinoma epiglottis. Adjacent enhanced axial sections (top) through epiglottis show plaque of tumor on laryngeal surface (*arrows*), with infiltration of the preepiglottic space (*curved arrows*). Sagittal (left) and coronal (right) reformatted projections show limited extent of preepiglottic space involvement (*curved arrows*).

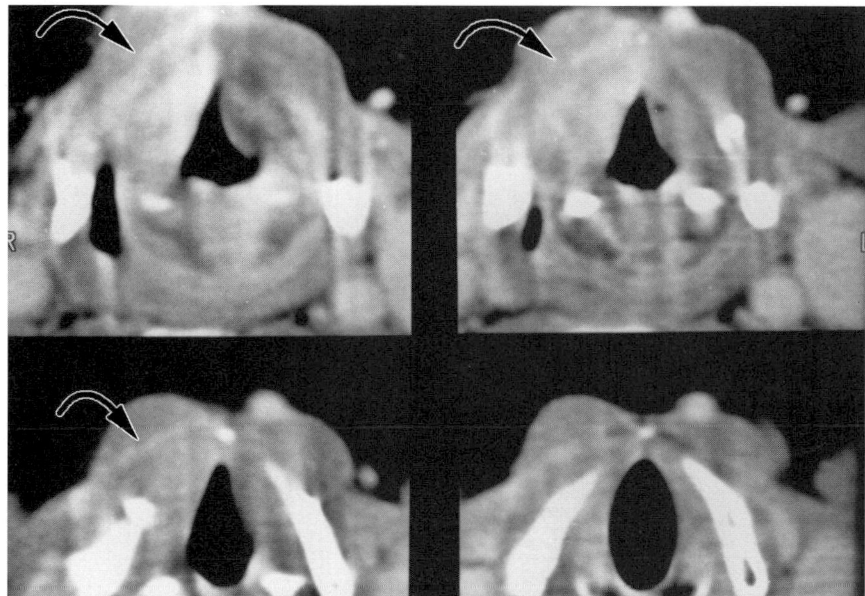

Figure 19.9 Extralaryngeal extension. Selected enhanced axial computed tomographic sections through the larynx show early extralaryngeal extension of a right glottic lesion through the thyroid lamina (*curved arrow*).

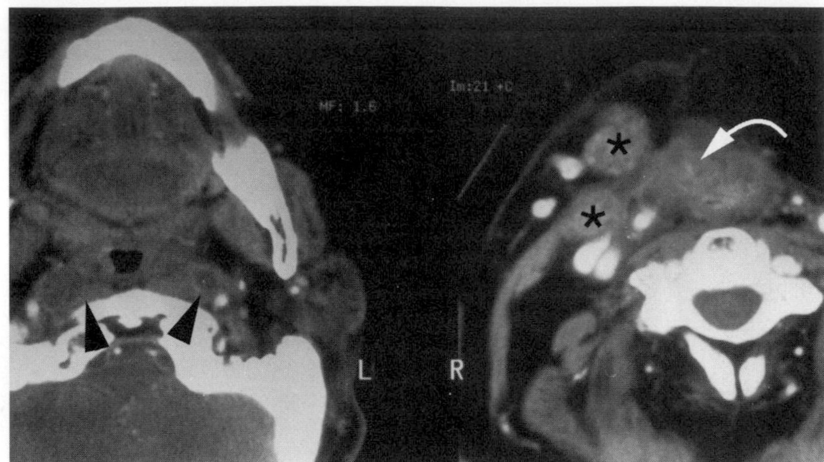

A

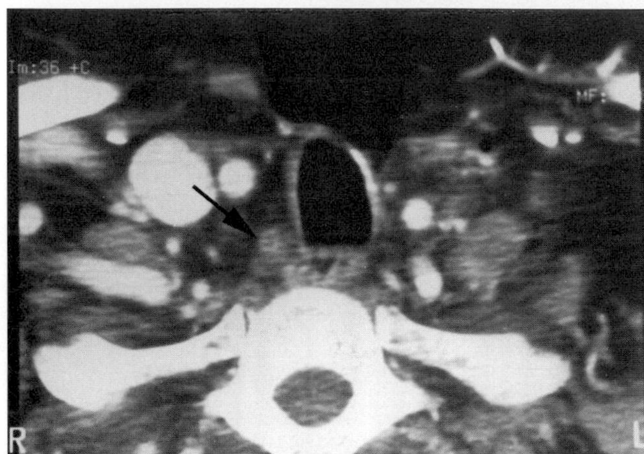

B

Figure 19.10 Adenopathy. Selected enhanced axial computed tomographic images in a patient with recurrence at the tongue base anastomosis (*curved arrow*). Upper neck images **(A)** show right cervical adenopathy (*asterisk*) and bilateral lateral retropharyngeal adenopathy at the C1 level (*arrowheads*). The lower image through the inlet **(B)** shows a pathologic right tracheoesophageal lymph node (*arrow*).

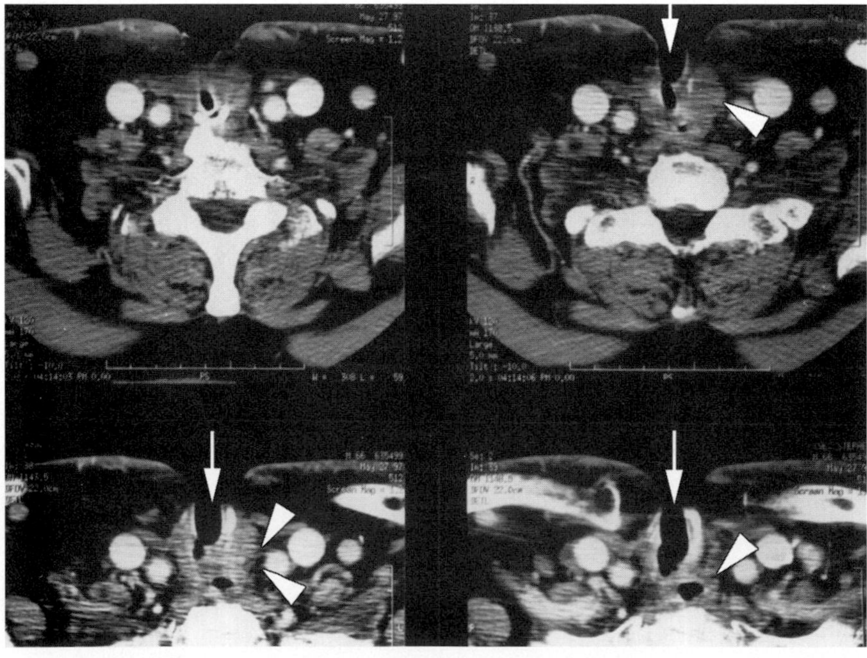

Figure 19.11 Early left parastomal recurrence. Serial enhanced axial computed tomographic images through the stoma (*arrow*) show recurrence (*arrowheads*) in the tracheoesophageal groove in a laryngectomy patient whose tracheoesophageal puncture device began to malfunction.

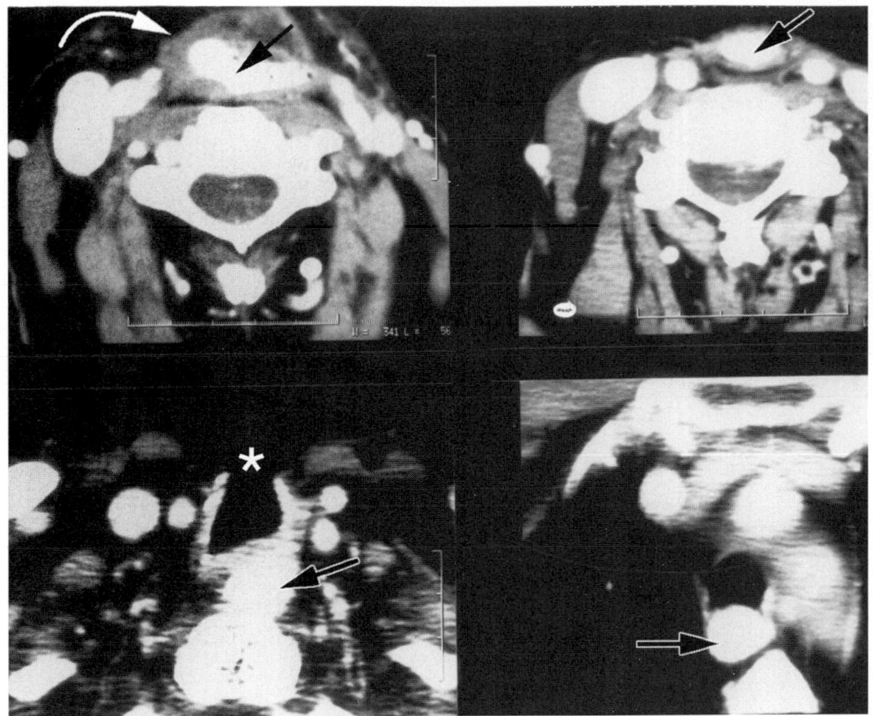

Figure 19.12 Negative follow-up scans of postlaryngectomy. Serial enhanced axial computed tomographic images from level of base-of-tongue anastomosis (top left) through to the upper mediastinum. Note normal asymmetry of the graft. Barium paste outlines the reconstructed alimentary tract (*arrows*). Normal stoma is indicated with an *asterisk*.

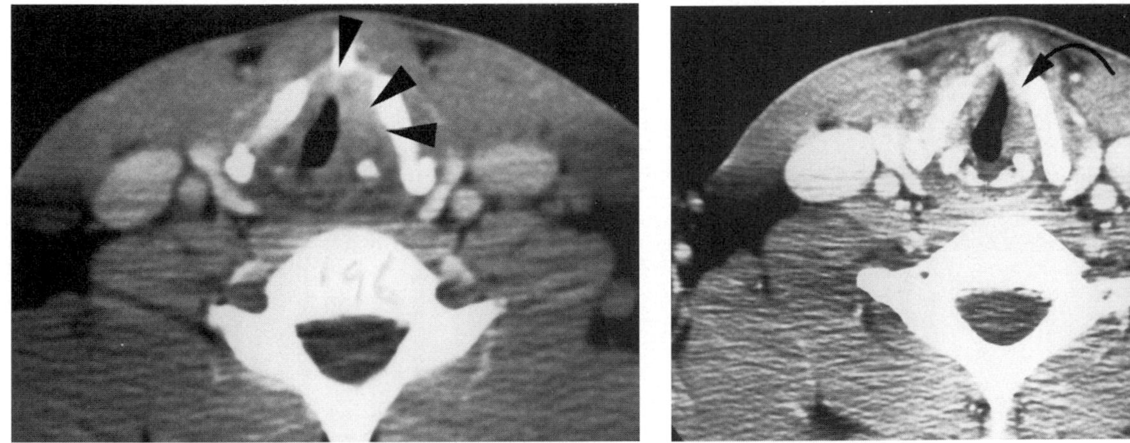

Figure 19.13 Follow-up larynx preservation protocol. Matched **(A)** pretreatment and **(B)** posttreatment views of a T3 to T4 lesion of glottis (*arrowheads*), with minimal residual thickening of the anterior one third of the true cord on follow-up (*curved arrow*).

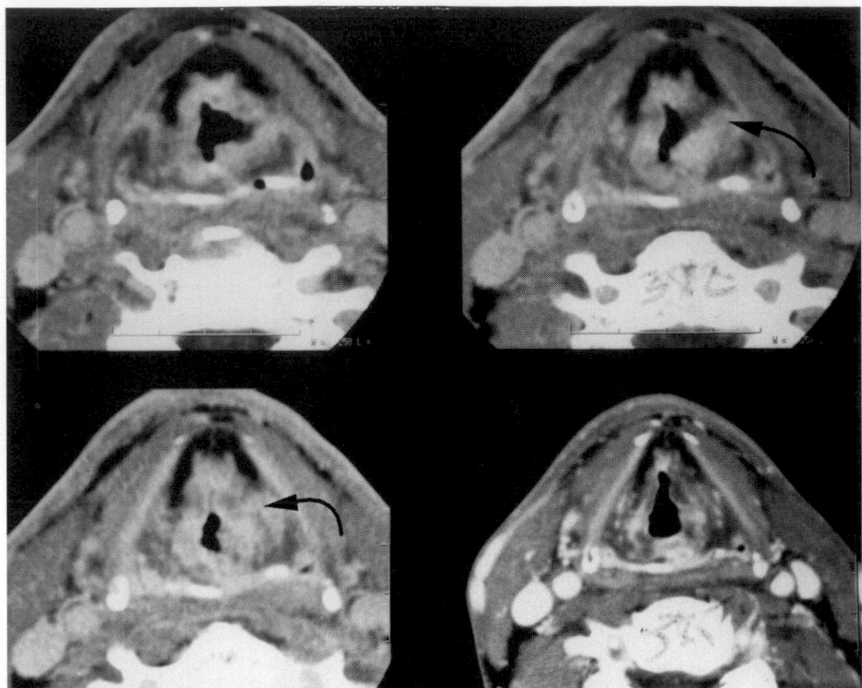

A

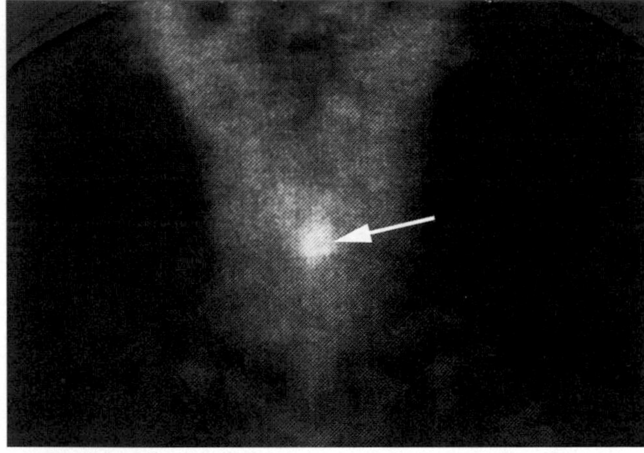

B

Figure 19.14 Persistent disease. **A:** Serial detailed enhanced axial sections of the larynx showing residual fullness of the supraglottic mucosa, with a focal residual component at the left paraglottic space (*curved arrow*) after irradiation for a T3 lesion. **B:** Coronal fluorodeoxyglucose-positron emission tomography view shows hypermetabolic focus of active tumor that corresponds to the computed tomographic abnormality (*arrow*).

RADIATION THERAPY TECHNIQUE

William M. Mendenhall

Patients with T3 and T4 laryngeal cancers are treated with parallel-opposed portals weighted 3:2 to the side of the lesion unless the cancer is midline or significantly crosses the midline necessitating 1:1 weighting. The initial portals extend from 2 cm above the angle of the mandible to the bottom of the cricoid cartilage, 1.5 cm anterior to the skin of the anterior neck, and to the posterior aspect of the spinous processes of the cervical vertebrae. The posterior border may be tight for patients with node-negative glottic cancer where the risk for level 5 node involvement is minimal (Fig. 19.15) (81). A strip of skin may be spared for patients with supraglottic cancers depending on the anterior extent of the tumor. The fields are enlarged depending on the location of the primary tumor and neck disease. For example, the inferior edge of the field may be placed 1 to 2 cm below the bottom of the cricoid cartilage if there is subglottic extension. Because patients with positive neck nodes have an increased risk for retropharyngeal lymph node involvement, it is necessary to include the retropharyngeal lymph nodes at the level of the C1-C2 vertebral bodies in the initial portals. The fields are reduced off of the spinal cord at approximately 45 Gy, and a second mucosal reduction usually occurs at about 60 Gy. If necessary, electron beam may be used to treat the posterior strip after reducing off the cord. The low neck is treated with an anterior field with a small, tapered midline block.

The portals used to treat patients after surgery, which would usually entail a total laryngectomy and neck dissection for patients with an advanced primary cancer, are depicted in Figure 19.16 (82). The anterior field edge allows tangential irradiation of the skin of the anterior neck. The neck nodes are often positive, necessitating inclusion of the retropharyngeal and junctional nodes in the initial portals. The lower border of the lateral fields slants superiorly from anterior to posterior, and the central axis of the anterior low neck field is placed at the field junction so that dose to the spinal cord at the junction is low (Fig. 19.17) (83). This field-matching technique has been used for almost four decades at the University of Florida with a very low risk or radiation myelitis and a low risk for failure in the neck at the junction. Patients are treated with cobalt-60 or 6-mV x-ray; we prefer the former if available. Vaseline gauze bolus is placed in the incision to ensure an adequate surface dose. The low neck node is given 50 Gy in 25 fractions specified at D_{max}, after which the dose to the stoma may be boosted with an electron beam (usually 12 MeV) if there is subglottic extension.

The technique employed for preoperative irradiation is the same as that used for patients treated with irradiation alone.

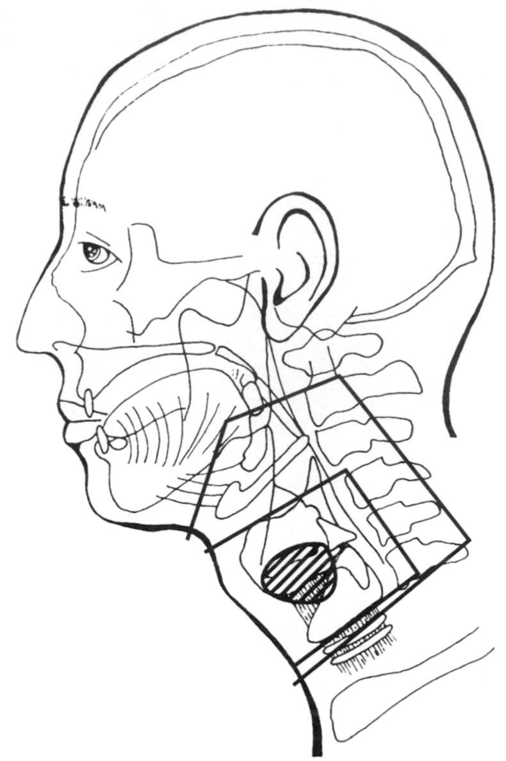

Figure 19.15 Portals for T3 and T4 lesions. The initial portal includes the jugulodigastric and midjugular lymph nodes. In the N0 patient, the highest jugular lymph nodes near the base of the skull are at little risk for involvement. To ensure adequate coverage of the midjugular lymph nodes, it is necessary to include the spinal cord in the treatment volume. The placement of the inferior border depends on the presence and degree of subglottic extension as determined by direct laryngoscopy and computed tomography and is commonly 1 to 2 cm below the inferior border of the cricoid cartilage; this line is slanted to facilitate matching with the anterior low neck portal. Anteriorly, the beam is allowed to "fall off" over the skin and subcutaneous tissues. The entire preepiglottic space is included within the initial treatment volume. (From Parsons JT, Mendenhall WM, Mancuso AA, et al. Twice-a-day radiotherapy for T3 squamous cell carcinoma of the glottic larynx. *Head Neck* 1989;11:123–128, with permission.)

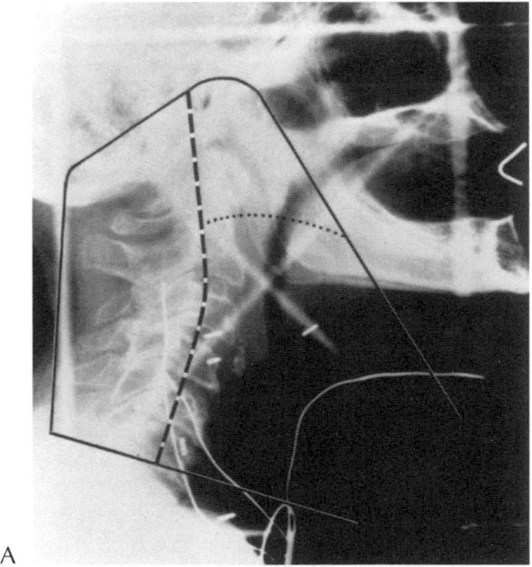

A

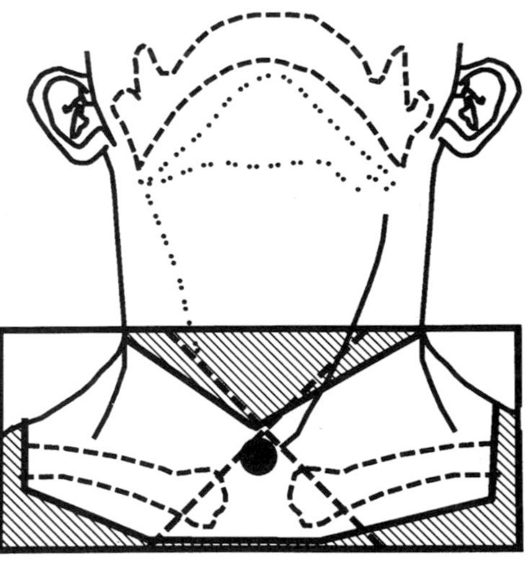

B

Figure 19.16 University of Florida three-field technique for laryngeal irradiation. **A:** Typical simulation field for laryngopharyngeal irradiation. An initial off-cord reduction executed at 50 Gy is indicated by the *dashed lines,* whereas the second reduction (60 Gy) is indicated by the *dotted lines*. The slanting inferior border reduces the length of spinal cord in the primary field, avoids irradiating the shoulders, and facilitates avoidance of a field overlap with the low neck match field. **B:** Schematic diagram of the low neck field. The *solid line rectangle* represents the setting of the machine collimators, whereas the *shaded areas* represent the portions of the field that are blocked using full-height hand blocks made of Lipowitz metal. The superior border of the low neck field is common with the inferior borders of the primary fields. Because of the hand blocking of the low neck field, the superior border of the field assumes a V shape. Therefore, a short segment of the spinal cord remains untreated at the match line between fields. (From Amdur RJ, Parsons JT, Mendenhall WM, et al. Postoperative irradiation for squamous cell carcinoma of the head and neck: an analysis of treatment results and complications. *Int J Radiation Oncol Biol Phys* 1989;16:25–36, with permission.)

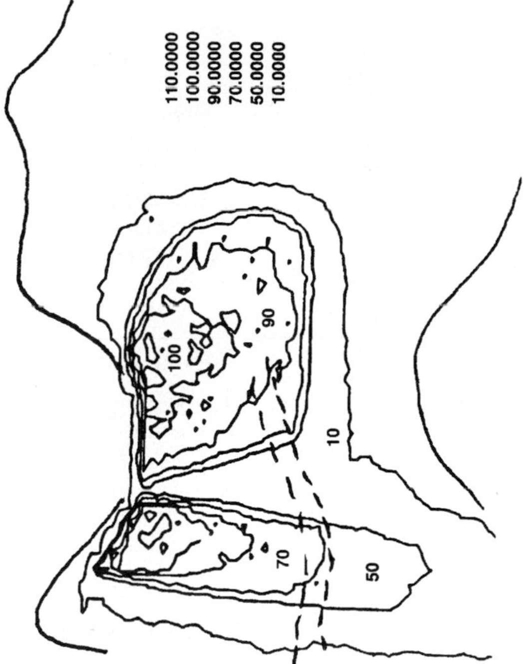

Figure 19.17 Averaged cobalt-60 distribution for larynx primary field with low neck match and trachea block removed. The dose distribution was obtained using a TLD sheet, and the doses are normalized to the central axis dose. (From Meeks SL, Williams RO, Bova FJ, et al. The midline dose distribution for a three-field radiotherapy technique. *Med Dosim* 1999;24:91–98, with permission.)

SURGICAL TECHNIQUE

Jesus E. Medina

Total Laryngectomy

A tracheostomy can be performed under local or general anesthesia, depending on the state of patency of the airway prior to laryngectomy (Fig 19.18). The creation of the permanent tracheal stoma can be at that site or lower, depending on the location and extent of the tumor.

The appropriate skin incision for a total laryngectomy depends on the surgeon's intention for the neck, and varies from the simple midline vertical if no neck dissection is planned, to a mastoid to mastoid apron flap in which bilateral neck surgery is required, to a more unilaterally oriented incision with a horizontal limb across the neck, with a vertical limb for exposure of the posterior triangle of the neck. If a neck dissection is done in conjunction with the laryngectomy, the neck specimen should be left attached to the larynx along the lateral aspect of the thyroid and cricoid cartilages. The thyroid gland isthmus is divided in the midline and the lobe ipsilateral to the pathology is generally left with the to-be-removed larynx, irrespective of whether or not there is an associated neck dissection. The pharyngeal constrictors are divided at their attachment to the posterior border of the thyroid cartilage, and those transected muscles are dissected free from the larynx, thus exposing the external surface of the piriform sinus mucosa. This isolation of the cartilaginous component of the larynx is accomplished bilaterally. The trachea is transected between the 2-3 or lower (depending on the location of the laryngeal tumor). When the trachea is entered, inspection of the internal trachea is done to ensure adequate distance below the tumor. The trachea and larynx are separated from the esophagus until the posterior cricoarytenoid muscles are visualized. The pharynx is then entered in one of two ways: through the piriform sinus opposite the side of the lesion, or through the vallecula. The vallecula is transected at a level immediately above the hyoid bone, which is always included in the resected specimen. After entry and vallecula incision, the mucosa of the piriform sinus opposite the lesion and the postcricoid mucosa are incised, under direct vision, preserving as much mucosa as possible. Margin analysis under frozen section is done on appropriate sites.

The neopharynx can be repaired in one of several ways, all of which have as the common denominator mucosal inversion to minimize the occurrence of a pharyngeal–cutaneous fistula. The various repairs can be accomplished in a straight vertical fashion, a horizontal, or a "T" closure, which combines both the vertical and the horizontal methods. After the first layer (mucosal) is closed, many surgeons recommend saline injection into the mouth and pharynx with moderate pressure from a bulb syringe; thus the pharyngeal closure is observed for leakage. The second layer of sutures is placed through and approximating the edges of the inferior constrictors to each other. A cricopharyngeal myotomy or a pharyngeal plexus neurectomy is preformed to prevent postoperative pharyngeal constrictor spasm, which might hinder vocal rehabilitation. The reader is referred to the chapter on rehabilitation (Chapter 11) for details of this important aspect of laryngectomy.

Permanent tracheal stomal construction is accomplished by suturing cervical skin to the tailored transected end of the trachea.

Partial Laryngectomy

The supraglottic laryngectomy is a partial laryngectomy that removes the part of the larynx above the true vocal cords up to the base of the tongue. The remaining lower half of the larynx, which contains the voice production part of the larynx, is reattached to the base of the tongue (Fig. 19.19). Certain selective supraglottic laryngeal cancers are thus removed, while the physiologic functions of the larynx are retained.

The principles of partial laryngectomy are also demonstrated by the supracricoid partial laryngectomy (SCPL), which is designed to retain the functional cricoarytenoid unit and is designed for certain supraglottic and transglottic carcinomas. In this operation, the entire thyroid cartilage (rather than the upper half described in the standard supraglottic laryngectomy), the paraglottic spaces, the epiglottis and the preepiglottic space are removed, while one or both arytenoid cartilages, the cricoid cartilage, and the hyoid bone are preserved (Fig. 19.20). The cricoid cartilage is then suspended by suturing it to the hyoid bone and the base of the tongue. Essentially, this procedure is advocated by some as the surgical treatment of tumors that extend beyond the limits of a supraglottic laryngectomy. Examples of these circumstances might be supraglottic tumors that invade the ventricle, extend to the glottis, or impair the motility of the true vocal cord. It is also sometimes indicated for the treatment of transglottic and supraglottic tumors with minimal invasion of the thyroid cartilage, as well as those with vocal cord fixation, preepiglottic space involvement, or both. The procedure can also sometimes be employed by tumors that originate in the anterior commissure. Key to the performance of SCPL is the absence of arytenoid fixation due to tumor involving either the cricoarytenoid musculature or the cricoarytenoid joint due to the proximity of the cricoid cartilage to these structures. Therefore, arytenoid fixation is a contraindication for this operation. Other contraindications include subglottic extension of tumor beyond 10 mm anteriorly or 5 mm posteriorly, cricoid cartilage invasion, and tumor extension beyond the larynx. Notably, these various partial laryngectomy operations are contraindicated when the patient has severe respiratory insufficiency.

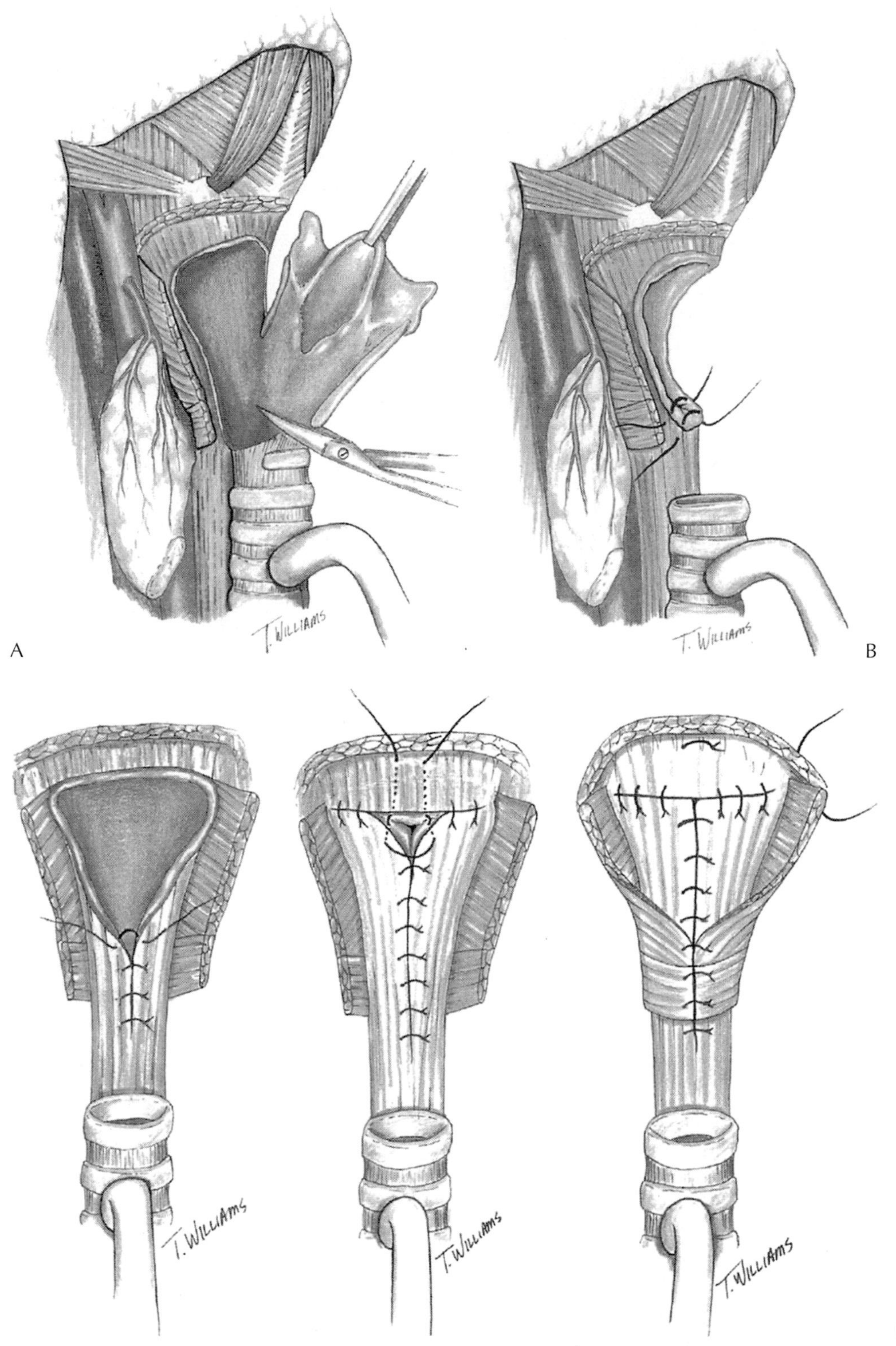

Figure 19.18 **A:** Excision of the larynx from the pharynx. Note scissors transecting the airway, well above the tracheotomy site. Note the thyroid gland that has been transected (frequently, part of the thyroid gland is removed with the larynx). **B:** Right lateral view of the neopharynx following removal of the larynx. The pharyngeal mucosa is ready for closure, using inverting suture techniques. **C:** Frontal view of the neopharynx, partially closed in a vertical, mucosal inversion method. This is one of several methods of closure; the horizontal method, the vertical method, and the "T" method, which combines the vertical and horizontal methods. **D:** Near completion of vertical method of pharyngeal reconstruction, (i.e., closure) following laryngectomy. Note that at this stage the airway is completely separate from the digestive system (i.e., the neopharynx). **E:** Postlaryngectomy pharyngeal reconstruction in which the "T" method of closure was used and horizontal and vertical methods were combined. Note that the transected edges of the pharyngeal constrictor muscles are being sutured over the primary mucosal closure. Thus, a second layer is imposed on the primary wound surface.

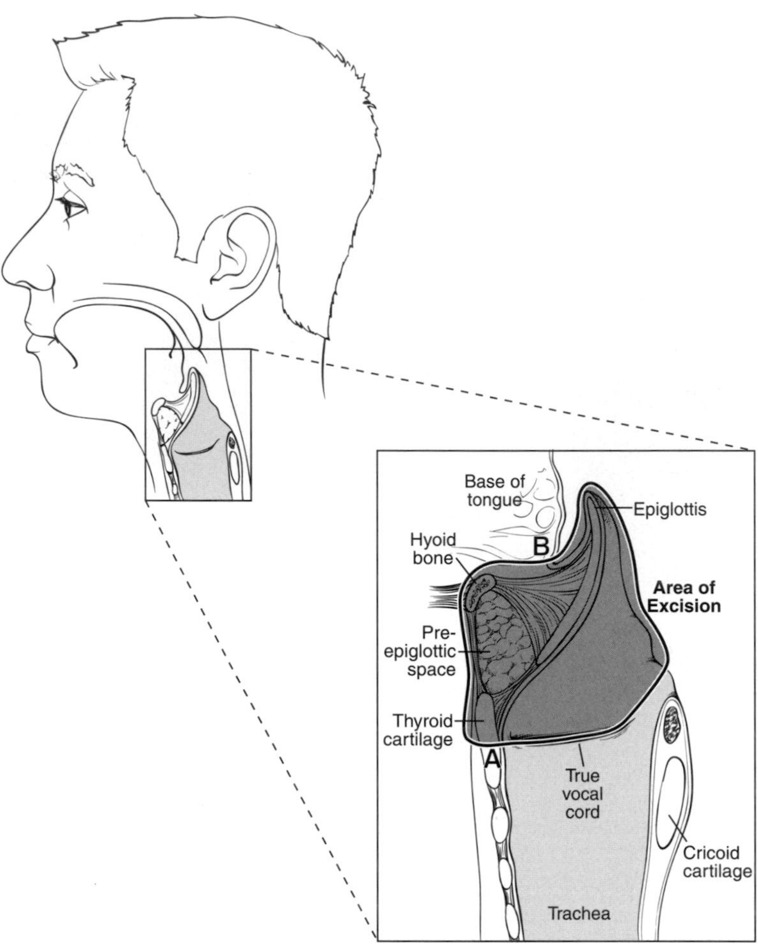

Figure 19.19 Supraglottic laryngectomy. **Inset:** Note the relative position of the entire larynx between the base of the tongue above and the trachea below. Detail seen in lower right. *Shaded area* includes the areas to be removed (i.e., hyoid bone and supraglottic larynx, including epiglottis and false vocal cords). The glottic level of the larynx (*A*), which is surgically approximated to the base of the tongue (*B*). The vocal production part of the larynx is preserved.

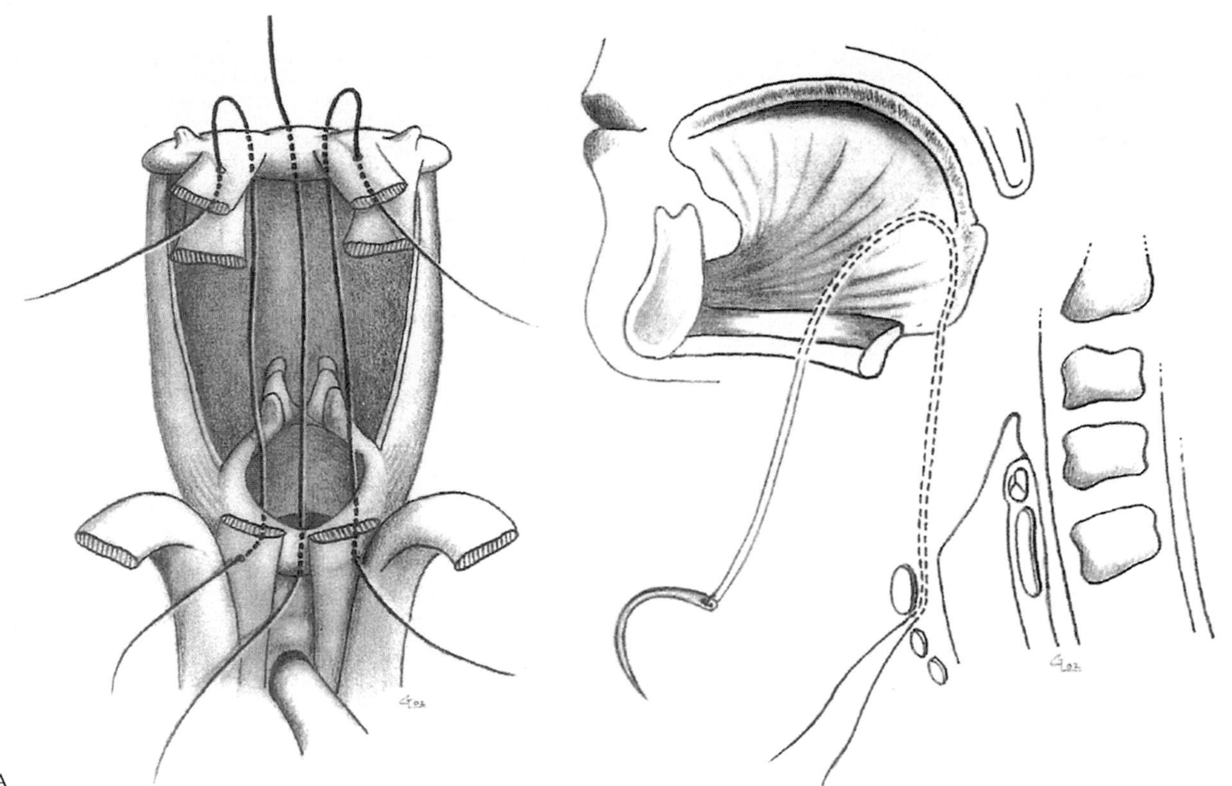

Figure 19.20 **A:** Supracricoid partial laryngectomy, frontal view. Drawing depicts the anatomic defect following the removal of certain laryngeal components. In this frontal view, note the remaining structures—cricoid cartilage, arytenoid cartilages, hyoid bone, and overlying strap muscles. Note the "impaction sutures" that have been looped around the cricoid cartilage and the hyoid bone. Ultimately, after tracheal release below, the sutures are tightened to impact the hyoid against the cricoid. Typically, three sutures are employed. **B:** Supracricoid partial laryngectomy, lateral view. Left lateral view of diagram showing anatomic defect following a supracricoid partial laryngectomy. Note the "impaction suture" in place around the hyoid bone and into the tongue base above, and around the cricoid cartilage below. The sutures serve to pull together the separated parts, thus reconstructing a vocal unit.

REFERENCES

1. McNeil BJ, Weichselbaum R, Parker SG. Speech and survival: tradeoffs between quality and quantity of life in laryngeal cancer. *N Engl J Med* 1981; 305:982.
2. McGavran MH, Bauer WC, Ogura JH. The incidence of cervical lymph node metastases from epidermoid carcinoma of the larynx and their relationship to certain characteristics of the primary tumor. *Cancer* 1961;14:55.
3. Beahrs OH, Hensen DE, Hunter RVP, et al, eds. *Manual for staging of cancer,* 3rd ed. Philadelphia: JB Lippincott Co, 1988.

3a. Greene F, Page D, Fleming I, et al. *AJCC cancer staging manual,* 6th ed. New York: Springer Verlag, 2002.

4. Kirchner JA, Cornog JL, Holmes RE. Transglottic cancer. Its growth and spread within the larynx. *Arch Otolaryngol* 1974;99:247.
5. Pressman JJ, Dowdy A, Libby M. Further studies upon the submucosal compartments and lymphatics of the larynx by the injection of dye and radioisotopes. *Ann Otol Rhinol Laryngol* 1956;65:963.
6. Welsh LW, Welsh JJ, Rizzo TA Jr. Laryngeal spaces and lymphatics: current anatomic concepts. *Ann Otol Rhinol Laryngol Suppl* 1983;105:19.
7. Kirchner JA, Carter D. Intralaryngeal barriers to the spread of cancer. *Acta Otolaryngol (Stockh)* 1987;103:503.
8. DeSanto LW. Cancer of the supraglottic larynx: a review of 260 patients. *Otolaryngol Head Neck Surg* 1985;93:705.
9. Bocca E, Pignataro O, Mosciaro O. Supraglottic surgery of the larynx. *Ann Otol Rhinol Laryngol* 1968;77:1005.
10. Kirchner JA. One hundred laryngeal cancers studied by serial section. *Ann Otol Rhinol Laryngol* 1969;78:689.
11. Fu KK, Eisenberg L, Dedo HH, et al. Results of integrated management of supraglottic carcinoma. *Cancer* 1977;40:2874.
12. Lindberg R. Distribution of cervical lymph node metastases from squamous cell carcinoma of the upper respiratory and digestive tracts. *Cancer* 1972;29: 1446.
13. Shah JP, Tollefsen HR. Epidermoid carcinoma of the supraglottic larynx. *Am J Surg* 1974;128:494.
14. Lee NK, Goepfert H, Awendt CD. Supraglottic laryngectomy for intermediate stage cancer: UTMD Anderson Cancer Center experience with combined therapy. *Laryngoscope* 1990;100:831.
15. Spaulding CA, Krochak RJ, Hahn SS, et al. Radiotherapeutic management of cancer of the supraglottis. *Cancer* 1986; 57:1292.
16. Kotwall C, Sako K, Razack MS, et al. Metastatic patterns in squamous cell cancer of the head and neck. *Am J Surg* 1987;154:439.
17. Kirchner JA. Two hundred laryngeal cancers: patterns of growth and spread as seen in serial sections. *Laryngoscope* 1977;87:474.
18. Mittal B, Marks JE, Ogura JH. Transglottic carcinoma. *Cancer* 1984;53:151.
19. Skolnick EM, Yee KF, Wheatley MA, et al. Carcinoma of the laryngeal glottis therapy and end results. *Laryngoscope* 1975;85:1453.
20. Bryce DP. The management of laryngeal cancer. *J Otolaryngol* 1979;8:105.
21. Hanna EYN. Subglottic cancer. *Am J Otolaryngol* 1994;15:322.
22. Shaha AR, Shah JP. Carcinoma of the subglottic larynx. *Am J Surg* 1982;144: 456.
23. Harrison DFN. The pathology and management of subglottic cancer. *Ann Otol Rhinol Laryngol* 1971;80:6.
24. Saleh EM, Mancuso AA, Alhussaini AA. Computed tomography of primary subglottic cancer: clinical importance of typical spread pattern. *Head Neck* 1992;14:125.
25. DeSanto LW. The options in early laryngeal carcinoma. *N Engl J Med* 1982;306: 910.
26. Pillsbury HR, Kirchner JA. Clinical vs histopathologic staging in laryngeal cancer. *Arch Otolaryngol* 1979;105:157.
27. Coates HL, DeSanto LW, Devine KD, et al. Carcinoma of the supraglottic larynx. A review of 221 cases. *Arch Otolaryngol* 1976;102:686.
28. Marks JE, Freeman RB, Lee F, et al. Carcinoma of the supraglottic larynx. *Am J Roentgenol* 1979;132:255.
29. Soo KC, Shah JP, Gopinath KS, et al. Analysis of prognostic variables and results after supraglottic partial laryngectomy. *Am J Surg* 1988;156:301.
30. Forastiere AA, Berkey B, Maor M, et al. Phase III trial to preserve the larynx: induction chemotherapy and radiation therapy versus concomitant chemoradiation therapy versus radiotherapy alone or Intergroup Trial R91-11. *Proceedings of the American Society of Clinical Oncology* 2001(20):2a.
31. Mendenhall WM, Parsons IT, Stringer SP, et al. Carcinoma of the supraglottic larynx: a basis for comparing the results of radiotherapy and surgery. *Head Neck* 1990;12:204.
32. Bocca E, Pignataro O, Oldini C. Supraglottic laryngectomy: 30 years of experience. *Ann Otol Rhinol Laryngol* 1983;92:14.
33. Vermund H. Role of radiotherapy in cancer of the larynx as related to the TNM system of staging. *Cancer* 1970;25:485.
34. Goepfert H, Jesse RH, Fletcher GH, et al. Optimal treatment for technically resectable squamous cell carcinoma of the supraglottic larynx. *Laryngoscope* 1975;85:14.
35. Fletcher GH, Jesse RH, Lindberg RD, et al. The place of radiotherapy in the management of squamous cell carcinoma of the supraglottic larynx. *Am J Radiol* 1975;108:19.
36. Maceri DR, Laupe HB, Makielski KH, et al. Conservation laryngeal surgery. A critical analysis. *Arch Otolaryngol* 1985;111:361.
37. Schuller DE, Metch B, Stein DW, et al. Preoperative chemotherapy in advanced resectable head and neck cancer: final report of the Southwest Oncology Group. *Laryngoscope* 1988;98:1205.
38. Strijbos M, Van Den Broek P, Manni JJ, et al. Supraglottic laryngectomy: short and long term functional results. *Clin Otolaryngol* 1987;12:265.
39. Ogura JH, Mallen RW. Partial laryngopharyngectomy for supraglottic and pharyngeal carcinoma. *Trans Am Acad Ophthalmol Otolaryngol* 1965;69:832.
40. Nadol JB Jr. Treatment of carcinoma of the epiglottis. *Ann Otol Rhinol Laryngol* 1981;90:442.
41. Shah JP, Anderson PE. The impact of patterns of nodal metastasis on modifications of neck dissection. *Ann Surg Oncol* 1994;1:521.
42. Arriagada R, Eschwege F, Cachin Y, et al. The value of combining radiotherapy with surgery in the treatment of hypopharyngeal and laryngeal cancers. *Cancer* 1983;51:1819.
43. DeSanto LW. T3 glottic cancer options and consequences of the options. *Laryngoscope* 1984;94:1311.
44. Jesse RH. The evaluation and treatment of patients with extensive squamous cancer of the vocal cords. *Laryngoscope* 1975;85:1424.
45. Leroux RJ. A statistical study of 620 laryngeal carcinomas of the glottic region personally operated upon more than 5 years ago. *Laryngoscope* 1985;85:1440.
46. Yuen A, Medina JE, Goepfert H, et al. Management of stage T3 and T4 glottic carcinomas. *Am J Surg* 1984;148:467.
47. Piquet JJ, Chevalier D. Subtotal laryngectomy with cricohyoidoepiglottopexy for the treatment of extended glottic carcinomas. *Am J Surg* 1991;162:357.
48. Pearson BW, Woods RD II, Hartman DE. Extended hemilaryngectomy of T3 glottic carcinoma with preservation of speech and swallowing. *Laryngoscope* 1980;90:1950.
49. Croll GA, Gerritsen GJ, Tiwari RM, et al. Primary radiotherapy with surgery in reserve for advanced laryngeal carcinoma: results and complications. *Eur J Surg Oncol* 1989;15:350.
50. Harwood AR, Bryce DP, Rider WD. Management of T3 glottic cancer. *Arch Otolaryngol* 1980;106:697.
51. Kazem I, van den Broek P. Planned preoperative radiation therapy vs definitive radiotherapy for advanced laryngeal carcinoma. *Laryngoscope* 1984;94:1355.
52. Wiernik G, Bates TD, Bleehen MN, et al. Final report of the general clinical result of the British Institute of Radiology fractionation study of the 3F wk versus 5F wk in radiotherapy of carcinoma of the laryngopharynx. *Br J Radiol* 1990;63:169.
53. Ensley JF, Jacobs JR, Weaver A, et al. Correlation between response to cisplatinum combination chemotherapy and subsequent radiotherapy in previously untreated patients with advanced squamous cell cancers of the head and neck. *Cancer* 1984;54:811.
54. Jacobs C, Goffinet DR, Goffinet L, et al. Chemotherapy as a substitute for surgery in the treatment of advanced resectable head and neck cancer: a report from the Northern California Oncology Group. *Cancer* 1987;60:1178.
55. Karp D, Vaughan C, Carter R, et al. Voice preservation using induction chemotherapy (CT) plus radiation therapy (RT) as an alternative to laryngectomy in advanced head and neck cancer: long term follow up. *Am J Clin Oncol* 1991;14:273.
56. VA Laryngeal Cancer Study Group. Induction chemotherapy plus radiation compared with surgery plus radiation in patients with advanced laryngeal cancer. *N Engl J Med* 1991;324:1685.
57. Teknos TN, Myers LL, Bradford CR, et al. Free tissue reconstruction of the hypopharynx after organ preservation therapy: analysis of wound complications. *Laryngoscope* 2001;111:1192–1196.
58. Martin M, Gehanno P, Depondt J, et al. A phase III study: induction carboplatin and 5-fluorouracil before locoregional treatment versus locoregional treatment alone in head and neck carcinomas. *Proc Am Soc Clin Oncol* 1994;13: A906(abst).
59. Guedea F, Parsons JT, Mendenhall WM, et al. Primary subglottic cancer: results of radical radiation therapy. *Int J Radiat Oncol Biol Phys* 1991;21:1607.
60. Bocca E. Supraglottic cancer. *Laryngoscope* 1975;85:1318.
61. Goepfert H, Lindberg RD, Jesse RH. Combined laryngeal conservation surgery and irradiation: can we expand on the indications for conservative therapy? *Otolaryngol Head Neck Surg* 1981;89:974.
62. Issa PY. Cancer of the supraglottic larynx treated by radiotherapy exclusively. *Int J Radiat Oncol Biol Phys* 1985;15:843.
63. Daly CJ, Strong EW. Carcinoma of the glottic larynx. *Am J Surg* 1975;130:489.
64. Norris CM. Laryngectomy and neck dissection. *Otolaryngol Clin North Am* 1969;69:667.
65. Davis RK, Shapshay SM. Peristomal recurrence, pathophysiology, prevention and treatment. *Otolaryngol Clin North Am* 1980; I 3:499.
66. Schneider JJ, Lindberg RD, Jesse RH. Prevention of tracheal stoma recurrences after total laryngectomy by postoperative irradiation. *J Surg Oncol* 1975;7:187.

Radiologic Imaging Concerns

67. Ang KK, Trotti A, Brown BW, et al. Randomized trial addressing risk features and time factors of surgery plus radiotherapy in advanced head-and-neck cancer. *Int J Radiat Oncol Biol Phys* 2001;51:571–578.
68. Nakayama M, Brandenburg JH. Clinical underestimation of laryngeal cancer. Predictive indicators. *Arch Otolaryngol Head Neck Surg* 1993;119:950–957.
69. Amilibia E, Juan A, Nogues J, et al. [Neoplastic invasion of laryngeal cartilage: diagnosis by computed tomography]. *Acta Otorhinolaringol Esp* 2001;52:207–210.
70. Curtin HD. Importance of imaging demonstration of neoplastic invasion of laryngeal cartilage. [Editorial; Comment]. *Radiology* 1995;194:643–644.

71. Lee WR, Mancuso AA, Saleh EM, et al. Can pretreatment computed tomography findings predict local control in T3 squamous cell carcinoma of the glottic larynx treated with radiotherapy alone? *Int J Radiat Oncol Biol Phys* 1993;25: 683–687.
72. Katsounakis J, Remy H, Vuong T, et al. Impact of magnetic resonance imaging and computed tomography on the staging of laryngeal cancer. *Eur Arch Otorhinolaryngol* 1995;252:206–208.
73. Schmalfuss IM, Mancuso AA, Tart RP. Arytenoid cartilage sclerosis: normal variations and clinical significance. *AJNR Am J Neuroradiol* 1998;19:719–722.
74. Loevner LA, Yousem DM, Montone KT, et al. Can radiologists accurately predict preepiglottic space invasion with MR imaging? *AJR Am J Roentgenol* 1997; 169:1681–1687.
75. Clayman GL, Weber RS, Guillamondegui O, et al. Laryngeal preservation for advanced laryngeal and hypopharyngeal cancers. *Arch Otolaryngol Head Neck Surg* 1995;121:219–223.
76. Delaere P, Vander Poorten V, Guelinckx P, et al. Progress in larynx-sparing surgery for glottic cancer through tracheal transplantation. *Plast Reconstr Surg* 1999;104:1635–1641.
77. Lee JH, Sohn JE, Choe DH, et al. Sonographic findings of the neopharynx after total laryngectomy: comparison with CT. *AJNR Am J Neuroradiol* 2000;21: 823–827.
78. Mukherji SK, Mancuso AA, Kotzur IM, et al. Radiologic appearance of the irradiated larynx. Part II. Primary site response. *Radiology* 1994;193:149–154.
79. Greven KM, Williams DW 3rd, Keyes JW Jr, et al. Positron emission tomography of patients with head and neck carcinoma before and after high dose irradiation [see Comments]. *Cancer* 1994;74:1355–1359.
80. Fischbein NJ, OS AA, Caputo GR, et al. Clinical utility of positron emission tomography with 18F-fluorodeoxyglucose in detecting residual/recurrent squamous cell carcinoma of the head and neck. *AJNR Am J Neuroradiol* 1998; 19:1189–1196.

Radiation Therapy Technique

81. Parsons JT, Mendenhall WM, Mancuso AA, et al. Twice-a-day radiotherapy for T3 squamous cell carcinoma of the glottic larynx. *Head Neck* 1989;11: 123–128.
82. Amdur RJ, Parsons JT, Mendenhall WM, et al. Postoperative irradiation for squamous cell carcinoma of the head and neck: an analysis of treatment results and complications. *Int J Radiat Oncol Biol Phys* 1989;16:25–36.
83. Meeks SL, Williams RO, Bova FJ, et al. The midline dose distribution for a three-field radiotherapy technique. *Med Dosim* 1999;24:91–98.

CHAPTER 20

Cancer of the Hypopharynx and Cervical Esophagus

David G. Pfister, Kenneth S. Hu, and Jean-Louis Lefebvre

Cancers of the hypopharynx and cervical esophagus pose many therapeutic challenges. Despite diagnostic and therapeutic advances, overall survival rates remain disappointing. Locoregional control of these tumors is difficult to attain, being complicated by their frequent multicentricity, remarkable tendency to spread submucosally, and high likelihood of advanced primary stage or nodal disease at presentation, such that control may necessitate total laryngectomy with its related sequelae. Patients with these cancers are typically older, frequently malnourished from tumor-related dysphagia and poor dietary habits (1), and have associated tobacco and alcohol use lifestyle factors that contribute to a high rate of second primary tumors and other medical comorbidities (1–4). These issues further complicate treatment choice, patient management, and rehabilitation. Consequently, multidisciplinary, individualized approaches to management are required. Head and neck, reconstructive, plastic, and thoracic surgeons, radiation therapists, medical oncologists, along with speech and swallowing pathologists, symptom management specialists, and nutritionists must work in concert and share the goals of both cure and functional rehabilitation of the patient.

Further complicating matters is that the available data to guide management of these diseases has many limitations. The two sites are often considered together because of their shared histology, anatomic proximity, and frequent extension between the sites (Table 20.1) (1), as well as similar clinical presentation and management issues. Nonetheless, the hypopharynx and cervical esophagus are technically separate sites and are staged using different tumor, node, and metastasis (TNM) criteria (5). In treatment studies, hypopharynx tumors are generally considered with other upper aerodigestive tract cancers, the cervical esophagus with other esophageal tumors, and thus are frequently reported separately. Because of the relatively small numbers of patients, randomized trials are limited in number, site-specific random assignment studies are rare, and clinical series frequently span multiple years. Data on therapy for hypopharyngeal cancer is often weighted toward or limited to tumors of the piriform sinus, given its predominance as a subsite (6–8); the cervical esophagus is a rare primary site in phase III esophageal trials. Available studies either provide limited data on quality of life and functional outcomes, or lack such data altogether. Thus, delineating patient selection issues and comparing outcomes for alternative treatments in these patients can be difficult.

In the context of this background information, the management of hypopharyngeal and cervical esophageal cancers is reviewed. The results of available randomized trials are emphasized. However, the data for the cervical esophagus are much more limited, as the breakdown of numbers shown in Table 20.1 would suggest.

TABLE 20.1 Hypopharyngeal–Cervical Esophageal Cancer: Incidence by Site and Stage[a]

		Stage			
Site	No. of patients (%)	I	II	III	IV
Posterior hypopharynx	13 (8)	2	11	—	—
Hypopharynx with oropharyngeal extension	24 (16)	—	—	20	4
Hypopharynx with esophageal extension	51 (33)	—	—	39	12
Piriform fossa	23 (15)	2	17	4	—
Piriform fossa with esophageal extension	36 (24)	—	—	28	8
Cervical (postcricoid esophagus)	6 (4)	—	2	1	3
Total number	153	4	30	92	27
Total percentage	100	3	19	60	18

[a]Experience with 153 patients, Department of Otolaryngology, Head and Neck Surgery of the Eastern Virginia Medical School.
Source: Schecter GL, Kalafsky JT. Cancer of the hypopharynx and cervical esophagus: management concepts. *Oncology* 1988;2:17, with permission.

INCIDENCE, ETIOLOGY, AND EPIDEMIOLOGY

Carcinomas of the hypopharynx or cervical esophagus are uncommon diseases, collectively representing approximately 10% of all upper aerodigestive tract tumors and far less than 1% of all cancer diagnosed in the United States each year (9). Squamous cell carcinoma (SCC) is by far the most frequent histologic type of cancer in the hypopharynx and cervical esophagus. As such, most of the described incidence and risk factor information applies to this cell type. Overall, the incidence of these cancers is generally higher in men than in women. However, there is reported geographic variation with regard to tumor location and patient sex, with cancers of the lower hypopharynx/posterior cricoid area being more common in women, particularly in Scandinavia (10–12). Also, the incidence over time may change with evolution in smoking habits. These tumors typically occur in individuals over 50 years of age, with a peak incidence in the sixth and seventh decades, and at an approximate rate of 1 in 100,000 persons per year. In the United States, the most common site of origin in the hypopharynx is the piriform sinus (66%–75%), followed by the posterior pharyngeal wall and postcricoid region (20%–25%) (13).

Excessive tobacco and alcohol consumption contribute to the development of SCC in the upper aerodigestive tract and particularly in the pharynx and cervical esophagus (14,15), and represent the primary risk factors for these diseases. Though not carcinogenic alone, ethanol acts as a promoter to the mutagenic effects of tobacco-derived substances and thereby contributes to the carcinogenic synergy seen with concurrent tobacco and alcohol use. Both the high incidence of second primary tumors and the concomitant mucosal dysplasia frequently found surrounding primary tumors suggest the presence of a regional field effect (16), which is consistent with widespread exposure to carcinogens.

Multistep carcinogenesis and field carcinogenesis are important concepts in discussing hypopharyngeal and esophageal cancers, as the carcinogens that initiate tumorigenesis also affect the nontransformed surrounding tissues. Mutations in the tumor suppressor gene *p53*, which occur at a rate of approximately 40% to 70% (17) in head and neck cancers, are the most frequent molecular abnormalities observed in these cancers at present. Premalignant lesions, including carcinoma *in situ* and moderate to severe dysplasia, in contrast, have been found to contain mutations in *p53* in only perhaps 20% of cases (18). Experimental evidence shows more frequent mutations of *p53* in smokers than in nonsmokers. Further supporting the field hypothesis are chromosome labeling and loss of heterozygosity (LOH) studies showing that LOH at 9p and abnormalities in chromosome 11 are present in histologically normal mucosa adjacent to these tumors (19). Further understanding of the progression to malignancy and identification of putative tumor suppressor genes in these malignancies may come as studies like these are pursued.

The role of human papilloma virus (HPV) as a contributing factor to carcinogenesis, particularly of SCC, is an area of active investigation. Immunohistochemical stains show the presence of the genome of the oncogenic high-risk HPV type 16 in a significant minority of head and neck cancers, including 19% of the hypopharynx cancers investigated (20). Human papilloma virus DNA sequences are also found in esophageal SCCs (21). The pathogenic and prognostic implications of finding HPV and its interaction with other risk factors like tobacco and alcohol are still being defined (22,23).

Dietary deficiencies may also contribute to the development of neoplasms in this region (10,12). The Plummer-Vinson (Paterson-Kelly) syndrome, for instance, is characterized by hypopharyngeal webs, dysphagia, weight loss, and iron-deficiency anemia. It is usually recognized among nonsmoking women between 30 and 50 years of age. Failure to recognize and treat this syndrome has historically been associated with a high incidence of postcricoid carcinomas in nonsmoking northern European women. If it is diagnosed and treated early with bougienage, iron, and vitamin B supplements, however, the disease process may be reversed. In addition, vitamin A and its analogs, including 13-*cis*-retinoic acid, promote the normal maturation of squamous epithelium. Insufficient dietary vitamin A might, therefore, contribute to the persistence of immature basal cell types. The roles of vitamin and other nutritional deficiencies in the pathogenesis and progression of hypopharyngeal and cervical esophageal cancers merit further investigation (24–26), especially because malnutrition is common at presentation (1).

Our understanding of the initiation and progression of carcinogenic processes continues to evolve as advances in molecular biology and biotechnology continue. Genetic deficiencies in the metabolism of tobacco-related and other carcinogens, aberrations in DNA repair mechanisms, and defects in cell-cycle regulation mechanisms may all also be involved in the development of pharyngeal and esophageal cancers, and elucidation of these mechanisms awaits further study.

RELEVANT ANATOMY

The hypopharynx (laryngopharynx) extends from the level of the hyoid bone down to the esophageal introitus. It is contiguous with the oropharynx and lies behind the larynx, partially surrounding it on either side. The hypopharynx encompasses three regions: the piriform sinuses, the pharyngeal wall, and the postcricoid area. The distal end of the hypopharynx corresponds approximately to the level of the sixth cervical vertebra. The cervical esophagus extends from the lower edge of the cricoid cartilage to the thoracic inlet.

The anterior wall of the hypopharynx opens directly into the larynx, and the posterior surfaces of the arytenoid cartilages form the upper boundary of the postcricoid area. The lumen formed by these walls is cone-shaped, with the wider opening superior, funneling into the postcricoid and cervical esophageal area.

The wall of the hypopharynx is composed of four layers. The innermost layer is a mucosal lining of stratified squamous epithelium over a loose stroma. The next layer is fibrous and is formed by the pharyngeal aponeurosis. The third is a muscular layer that is composed of the inferior constrictor muscle and, in the upper portion, of the distal aspect of the middle constrictor. The most distal fibers of the inferior constrictor condense into the cricopharyngeus muscle, and just proximal to this muscle is an area of relative weakness known as the Killian triangle. The outermost layer is a fascial layer, derived from the buccopharyngeal fascia.

The piriform sinuses arise at the level of the pharyngoepiglottic fold, with the anterior, lateral, and medial walls narrowing inferiorly to form the apices. The tips of the inverted pyramids extend just slightly below the cricoid cartilage.

Laterally, the superior aspects of the piriform sinuses are bordered by the thyrohyoid membrane, through which passes the internal branch of the superior laryngeal nerve. The sensory axons of this nerve synapse superiorly in the jugular ganglion along with nerves of the external auditory canal (Arnold nerve). The remainder of sensation is derived from fibers of the glossopharyngeal nerve. The terminal branches of the recurrent laryngeal nerve pass through and supply nerve impulses to the fibers of the cricopharyngeus muscle and the posterior cricoarytenoid muscles of the larynx. Completing the motor supply of the hypopharynx is the pharyngeal plexus. The arterial supply is derived from branches of the superior thyroid arteries to the larynx and from lingual and ascending pharyngeal collateral arteries.

The cricopharyngeus, which makes up the narrowest portion of the upper alimentary tract, is the junction between the postcricoid area and the cervical esophagus. The Lanier triangle is the muscular aponeurosis between the cricopharyngeus and the upper portion of the esophageal musculature.

The esophagus is lined by nonkeratinizing squamous epithelium over loose areolar tissue with a muscular coat consisting of an inner circular and an outer longitudinal layer that is covered by a fascial sheath. The outermost layer of the cervical esophagus, as with the hypopharynx, is continuous with the buccopharyngeal fascia. This layer separates the esophagus posteriorly from the retroesophageal space, which is continuous with the retropharyngeal space above and the posterior mediastinum below. The cervical esophagus is in direct apposition to the trachea anteriorly, although it deviates slightly to the left of this organ. In the tracheoesophageal groove bilaterally the recurrent laryngeal nerves and the paratracheal nodes are found. The lateral lobes of the thyroid gland are related to the cervical esophagus and may be involved in neoplasms originating there. The carotid sheaths and their contents are found more laterally.

The nerve supply for the cervical esophagus is provided by branches of the recurrent laryngeal nerves and sympathetic trunks. The arterial supply is provided by branches of the inferior thyroid arteries and ascending vessels from the thoracic esophagus; the venous drainage is primarily to the inferior thyroid veins.

The hypopharynx and cervical esophagus have extensive lymphatic drainage systems. Major lymphatic drainage channels terminate in the lymph nodes along the jugular chain (27). The subdigastric, upper, and midjugular nodes form the primary echelon of lymphatic drainage. Lymphatic drainage from the posterior pharyngeal wall also includes the retropharyngeal lymph nodes and the node of Rouviere at the skull base (Fig. 20.1) (28).

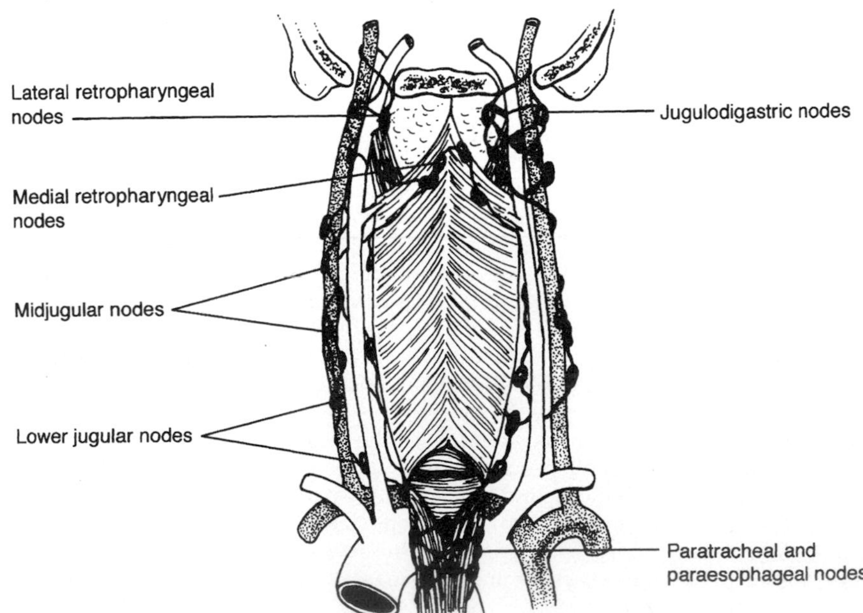

Figure 20.1 Principal nodal groups that receive lymphatic drainage from the hypopharynx and cervical esophagus.

The lymphatics from the piriform sinuses travel along with the recurrent laryngeal nerves through the cricothyroid membrane. Inferiorly, lymph nodes along the recurrent laryngeal nerves and the paratracheal nodes are sentinel nodes to the inferior hypopharynx and the cervical esophagus.

The basins of lymphatic drainage for the larynx and the anterior and posterior pharynx may be divided into two groups (27). The anterior channels drain the piriform sinuses and pierce the thyrohyoid membrane along with the superior laryngeal artery. These vessels, which number between three and five, are joined by the channels draining the supraglottic larynx. The vessels may take separate courses, with some draining to the subdigastric, midjugular, or anterior nodes below the common facial vein. The posterior group drains the pharyngeal wall and passes through the inferior constrictor muscle to the retropharyngeal or upper internal jugular chain of nodes.

The lymphatic drainage of the cervical esophagus is related intimately to that of the pharynx and larynx (27). Lymphatic collecting vessels traverse the mucosa and deeper muscular layers draining to the recurrent laryngeal or paratracheal nodes. Alternatively, they may pass superiorly to join the lymphatic trunks of the larynx or pharynx and may terminate in the internal jugular chain of nodes. The lymphatics of the cricopharyngeus muscle may pass to the lower retropharyngeal nodes, and subsequently to the recurrent laryngeal nodes, within the paratracheal and esophageal grooves. Besides these nodal groups, the lymph nodes in the upper mediastinum also may be a drainage portal for tumors of the cervical esophagus.

NATURAL HISTORY, PATHOLOGY, PATHOGENESIS, AND PATTERNS OF SPREAD

Upward of 95% of tumors of the hypopharynx or cervical esophagus are SCC or a variant (1); poorly differentiated tumors predominate. Accordingly, reported data on natural history and patterns of spread focus on tumors of this histologic type. Malignant tumors of salivary gland origin are encountered occasionally. Benign or malignant mesenchymal tumors in these locations are rare (29,30).

Submucosal extension should be anticipated in essentially all tumors of the hypopharynx and cervical esophagus. It is not unusual to have 10 mm of tumor extension beyond the visible disease process (31,32). Postcricoid lesions often exhibit 5 mm of submucosal extension and may spread to the recurrent laryngeal nerve, causing a unilateral vocal cord paralysis. Skip lesions are not uncommon with tumors of the postcricoid area extending into the cervical esophagus (33). Esophageal primary tumors may grow transmurally to involve the tracheal wall and the tissues in the thoracic inlet. Tumors arising on the pharyngeal walls more often are ulcerated and infiltrate into the underlying pharyngeal musculature.

These neoplasms may spread along regional nerves, such as the cervical sympathetic nerves, vagus, and glossopharyngeal nerves (34). Piriform sinus cancer may spread medially, displacing and fixing the lateral wall of the larynx with extension into the subglottic area. Involvement of the cricoarytenoid joint, cricoarytenoid muscle, or recurrent laryngeal nerve may cause a loss of vocal cord mobility (35,36). As the tumor enlarges, it may extend along the lateral or posterior pharyngeal wall to the contralateral piriform sinus. Postcricoid extension is known to occur, but growth into the cervical esophagus is rare.

Piriform sinus carcinomas with lateral extension frequently destroy the posterolateral portion of the thyroid cartilage, but invasion of the cricoid cartilage is uncommon. Direct extension to the superior lobe of the thyroid gland is not infrequent. Likewise, perithyroid and intrathyroid lymphatic tumor emboli are seen as well (35).

Posterior pharyngeal wall cancers usually become large before diagnosis. Invasion into the prevertebral fascia is a late sequela; however, superior extension to the base of the tonsil and the oropharyngeal wall and inferior spread to the postcricoid hypopharynx are not uncommon.

Postcricoid tumors usually are advanced on presentation and tend to grow circumferentially, invading the cricoid cartilage and cricoarytenoid muscle. As the tumor progresses, growth inferiorly leads to involvement of the cervical esophagus. With anterior tumor spread, extension into the common party wall may occur.

Sixty percent of patients having tumors arising on the posterior pharyngeal wall will have regional lymph node metastasis (frequently bilateral) (37). Retropharyngeal nodal metastases are present in 44% of these patients with pharyngeal wall primaries (38). Forty percent of patients with postcricoid tumors will have regional disease and, in those with piriform fossa primary tumors, the incidence is 75% (33,39,40). The paratracheal lymph nodes commonly are seeded with metastatic deposits from these tumors (41). It is important to note that 50% to 80% of patients who have primary tumors of the hypopharynx will have occult cervical nodal disease, with frequent involvement of the contralateral neck (42–44).

With cervical esophageal cancers, there is a high incidence of cervical and mediastinal lymph node metastases, especially in the jugular and paratracheal lymph nodes (41,45,46). Approximately 80% of these patients will have pathologic lymph node metastasis in the paratracheal basins (41). Kelly et al. demonstrated involvement of the upper, middle, and lower jugular lymph nodes in 14%, 18%, and 18% of cases, respectively, whereas paratracheal involvement occurred in 32%; however, the incidence of posterior cervical triangle lymph nodes was low at 4.5% (46).

Distant metastases occur more often with these primary sites both at presentation and with follow up compared with other cancers of the upper aerodigestive tract. Distant spread occurs in up to 60% of hypopharynx cancers (47). The most common sites of metastases are lung, mediastinal lymph nodes, liver, and bone. In one autopsy series of squamous cell esophageal cancers not limited to the cervical esophagus, up to 85% of patients had metastatic disease, with the most common metastatic sites being lymph nodes, lung, and liver (48).

Once a tumor has developed, its capacity to grow, invade, and metastasize depends on interactions within a complex biologic microenvironment. Growth and invasiveness are affected by environmental components such as degradative enzymes, including collagenases, plasminogen activators, and cathepsins; by angiogenic factors; by cell-surface properties and motility factors; by growth factors, cytokines, and their receptors; and by interactions with stromal cells and local nerve fibers. Furthermore, the general nutritional and medical status of the patient as well as attendant pharmacologic interventions may play important roles in tumor growth. A complex host immunosurveillance system may either promote or retard tumor growth. Although investigation into the role of tumor-infiltrating lymphocytes, natural killer cells, T-cell–mediated immunity, and activated cellular immunity continue in pharyngeal and other head and neck cancers, the complexity of the tumor microenvironment has made it increasingly difficult to characterize the impact of the immune system on the course of these malignancies (49–53).

CLINICAL PRESENTATION

Patients are typically older and provide a history of significant tobacco or alcohol use. Symptoms related to locoregional disease spread predominate. Most patients with these tumors present with symptoms of sore throat, dysphagia/odynophagia with weight loss, hoarseness, a neck mass, or referred otalgia (6). The last symptom, frequent in patients with cancers of the piriform sinus, reflects that sensory axons of the superior laryngeal nerve synapse with nerves of the external auditory canal. Early tumors often cause vague unilateral throat pain and progress to severe dysphagia. Development of such laryngeal symptoms as hoarseness is indicative of more advanced lesions. Careful review of symptoms often will reveal that the patient has difficulty in swallowing (even liquids), repeatedly clears the throat, and experiences a foreign-body sensation in the throat. Progressive dysphagia, initially for solid foods and later for liquids, is a hallmark symptom for tumors of the lower hypopharynx and cervical esophagus. Depending on the rate of growth, patients may simply modify their diets to accommodate the dysphagia, and further delay diagnosis. For tumors arising in the piriform sinus, hoarseness may be secondary either to direct laryngeal invasion or to recurrent laryngeal nerve involvement by tumor extension into the postcricoid or cervical esophageal regions.

Patients with hypopharyngeal and cervical esophageal cancers often have an impaired nutritional status with weight loss secondary to inadequate diet or excessive alcohol intake. This may compound their debilitation. In patients with circumferential lesions, weight loss may be pronounced. Drooling, when present, may be blood-tinged and is indicative of a more advanced tumor.

Palpable cervical adenopathy on initial clinical examination is common, whereas a mass in the neck is the presenting complaint in approximately 25% of patients. Occasionally, patients with large retropharyngeal nodal metastasis report a characteristic pain pattern originating in the occipital area and radiating to a point behind the eye.

DIAGNOSTIC EVALUATION AND CLINICAL STAGING

Examination of the hypopharynx and larynx with the indirect mirror usually reveals tumors of the posterior pharyngeal wall or upper piriform sinus. The apex of the piriform sinus may be obscured by pooled secretions. Thus, tumors in this location may escape detection. Tumors of the postcricoid region are similarly difficult to visualize; however, arytenoid edema, erythema, and loss of laryngeal crepitus are important signs of tumors in this location.

Careful assessment of laryngeal function and vocal cord mobility are imperative because involvement of the larynx indicates more advanced disease and has significant therapeutic implications. Direct extension of the cancer into the tissues of the neck and into the prevertebral fascia can be assessed by careful physical examination and appropriate diagnostic imaging.

As patients may present with a cervical metastasis of unknown primary origin, careful clinical examination with topical anesthesia is critical to finding an occult primary tumor. The fiberoptic laryngoscope is often invaluable for evaluation of the hypopharynx. Eliciting a Valsalva maneuver during fiberoptic examination frequently facilitates the delineation of superficial tumor extension. In addition, videostroboscopic examination has enhanced the ability to monitor and photographically document these neoplasms.

Tumors located more inferiorly will require examination under anesthesia for visualization. Due to the high incidence of multiple primary tumors, a thorough evaluation of the entire upper aerodigestive tract including the esophagus, trachea, and bronchi is recommended at this time. A panendoscopy under general anesthesia allows the examiner to explore all of these sites and to better define the macroscopic limits of the primary. A barium swallow may be helpful and is frequently performed as part of the evaluation of these patients. Depending on how early in the workup it is performed, the test may or may not provide useful additional information.

Assessment should be made of the patient's nutritional status based on the patient's ideal weight and the degree of recent weight loss. The nutritionist is an important member of the multidisciplinary head and neck cancer treatment team, and early correction of deficits should begin while the patient's workup is in progress.

The American Joint Committee for Cancer (AJCC) has set forth the current clinical staging system (5), which was most recently revised in 2002. Clinical staging expresses an estimation of disease extent and facilitates treatment selection and the comparison of outcomes. Assessment is based primarily on inspection, including both direct and indirect examinations. Palpation of neck nodes is essential. Imaging studies including computed tomography (CT) or magnetic resonance imaging (MRI) are helpful to define the extent of the primary tumor and for complete nodal evaluation, especially of the retropharyngeal lymph nodes, which are at risk in these tumor sites. A Valsalva maneuver during CT scan, if feasible during imaging, may facilitate visualization of the hypopharyngeal structures. Magnetic resonance imaging may define soft tissue extension more accurately than CT scan, but this is offset by longer scanning time and related motion-induced artifacts. Routinely doing both scans is not indicated. Extending cross-sectional imaging to include the chest often clarifies the inferior extent of disease, mediastinal spread, and also evaluates for distant metastases, as the lung is a common site of distant spread, as well as second lung primaries. Fluorodeoxyglucose-positron emission tomography (FDG-PET) scans may be helpful in clarifying equivocal findings short of biopsy. The clinical stage frequently does not correlate with pathologic staging. This effect results from clinical underestimation secondary to the extensive submucosal growth, cartilage invasion, and the deeply invasive characteristics of these tumors.

Classification of primary lesions of the hypopharynx and cervical esophagus is given in Table 20.2; nodal classification is given in Table 20.3. For lesions of the cervical esophagus, the recommended staging of the primary site is identical to that for the intrathoracic esophagus. However, the lymph nodes considered regional for the cervical esophagus are considered distant metastases for intrathoracic lesions.

Clinical staging permits an estimation of prognosis, but has its limitations. Clinical staging is a two-dimensional, static measurement based on volume, for which it is an imperfect measure, and anatomic location of disease. It does not take into account the ability of the host organism to enhance or suppress tumor growth or the progression of disease based on tumor heterogeneity (54). Tumors are composed of a heterogeneous clonogenic population of cells having different biologic potential for metastasis, neural, vascular, and lymphatic invasion. Tumor heterogeneity leads to a variable response to therapeutic modalities, such as ionizing radiation and chemotherapeutic agents.

Variations in genotype and phenotypic expression among tumor cells are being studied to determine their impact on

TABLE 20.2 Staging of Primary Tumors of the Hypopharynx and Cervical Esophagus

Hypopharynx	
Tis	Carcinoma *in situ*
T1	Tumor limited to one subsite of hypopharynx and ≤2 cm in greatest dimension
T2	Tumor invades more than one subsite of hypopharynx or an adjacent site, or measures >2 cm but ≤4 cm without fixation of hemilarynx
T3	Tumor >4 cm or with fixation of hemilarynx
T4a	Tumor invades thyroid/cricoid cartilage, hyoid bone, thyroid gland, esophagus, or central compartment soft tissue. Central compartment soft tissue includes prelaryngeal strap muscles and subcutaneous fat
T4b	Tumor invades prevertebral fascia, encases carotid artery, or involves mediastinal structures
Cervical esophagus	
Tx	Primary tumor cannot be assessed
T0	No evidence of primary tumor
Tis	Carcinoma *in situ*
T1	Tumor invades lamina propria or submucosa
T2	Tumor invades muscularis propria
T3	Tumor invades adventitia
T4	Tumor invades adjacent structures

Source: Adapted from Greene F, Page D, Fleming I, et al. *AJCC cancer staging manual,* 6th ed. New York: Springer-Verlag, 2002.

tumor progression. Key pieces of the puzzle may include oncogene expression, tumor suppressor gene mutations, the accumulation of multiple genetic events, DNA-repair defects, differential expression of cell-surface antigens, growth factors and their receptors, autocrine and paracrine regulatory factors (e.g., degradative enzymes, angiogenic factors, immune modulators, growth factors), and tumor glycoprotein content. For example, tumor cell lines that over express epidermal growth factor receptor may be more tumorigenic than cell lines that express less of this receptor (55). Recent molecular studies have shown that the accumulation of genetic mutations may compromise survival among head and neck cancer patients. However, studies to date of a variety of potential genetic markers, including the tumor suppressor gene *Rb* and such oncogenes as *ras, myc, int-2, bcl-1,* and *C-erbneu* have yielded no reliable predictors of response of the tumor to therapy, phenotypic behavior, or patient survival that are now used in standard clinical practice.

TABLE 20.3 Nodal Staging for Tumors of the Hypopharynx and Cervical Esophagus

Hypopharynx	
NX	Regional lymph nodes cannot be assessed
N0	No regional lymph node metastasis
N1	Single ipsilateral lymph node metastasis ≤3 cm in greatest dimension
N2a	Single ipsilateral lymph node metastasis >3 cm but ≤6 cm
N2b	Multiple ipsilateral lymph node metastasis none >6 cm
N2c	Bilateral or contralateral lymph node metastasis none >6 cm
N3	Lymph node metastasis >6 cm in greatest dimension
Cervical esophagus	
NX	Regional lymph nodes cannot be assessed
N0	No regional lymph node metastasis
N1	Regional lymph node metastasis involving cervical, scalene, internal jugular, peri-esophageal, and supraclavicular areas

Source: Adapted from Greene F, Page D, Fleming I, et al. *AJCC cancer staging manual,* 6th ed. New York: Springer-Verlag, 2002.

MANAGEMENT STRATEGIES AND TREATMENT PLANNING GUIDELINES

The management of patients with cancers in the hypopharynx and cervical esophagus depends on several factors. The physician must be aware of the natural history of these tumors and take into consideration the patient's performance status, extent of disease, and the presence and extent of lymph node metastases. Surgery and radiation therapy, either alone or in combination, have historically been the standard therapeutic modalities for tumors of these areas. The minority of patients who present with early and less invasive tumors may be considered for laryngeal conservation surgical procedures or primary radiation, but must be carefully selected. Patients with more advanced disease typically require combined modality therapy, and surgery, if pursued at the primary site, will jeopardize the larynx. Figures 20.2 and 20.3 contain a summary treatment algorithm for each site. A more detailed review follows.

Hypopharyngeal Cancer

T1 AND T2 DISEASE

Early stage patients constitute approximately 20% of all those who present with hypopharynx cancers (56). Important goals in patients with T1 and T2 resectable disease are to obtain local control while optimizing functional outcome, which can be accomplished with either conservation surgery or radiation therapy (57–64). Neck management is also indicated, as even clinically N0 patients will have a 30% to 40% risk for occult neck metastases (65). If anticipated disease control is equivalent for conservation surgery or radiation therapy, generally radiation is preferred for two reasons. First, the functional outcome will likely be superior, as sacrifice of the superior laryngeal nerve can lead to laryngopharyngeal dyssynergia and chronic aspiration (6,58,66,67). Second, postoperative radiation therapy, with its related morbidity, is often necessary even after conservation surgery because of submucosal spread of tumor (especially for pharyngeal wall and postcricoid lesions), positive margins, or adjuvant neck management. However, rigorous studies that assess and compare functional differences between conservation surgery and definitive radiation therapy in this group of patients have not been performed.

The appropriate management of early stage cancers of the hypopharynx requires the treating physician to consider many different factors, and deciding between primary conservation surgery and definitive radiation is often not straightforward. In general, most patients with stage I and low-bulk, exophytic, stage II disease will receive primary radiation therapy, with conservation surgery being considered, if feasible, for other lesions, especially if T2 (68). Another commonly applied rule of thumb is that surgery generally is preferred when feasible for tumors of the "cartilaginous" portion of the pyriform sinus (i.e., behind the thyroid ala), whereas primary radiation is preferred for tumors of the membranous region (i.e., superiorly, behind the thyrohyoid membrane).

Conservation Surgery

Eligibility for conservation surgery requires careful patient selection and considerable surgical expertise to optimize outcome. Otherwise, a high likelihood of local disease failure or chronic aspiration and its long-term sequelae may result. Simply because the primary lesion is T1 or T2 does not mean that a conservation surgical option is appropriate. Even though the current edition of the TNM staging system incorporates both the number of involved subsites and the greatest dimension of

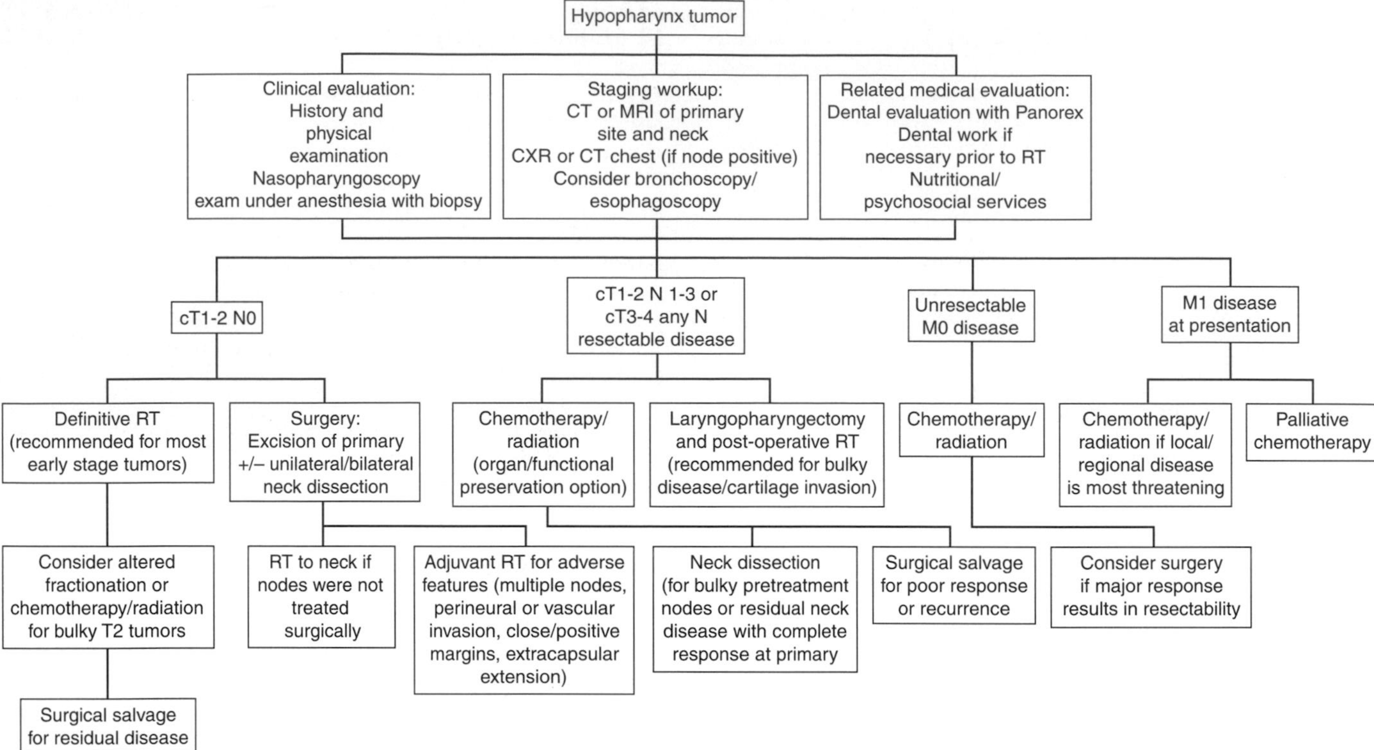

Figure 20.2 Workup and management of hypopharynx cancer. *c,* clinical; *CT,* computed axial tomography; *CXR,* chest x-ray; *MRI,* magnetic resonance imaging; *RT,* radiation therapy.

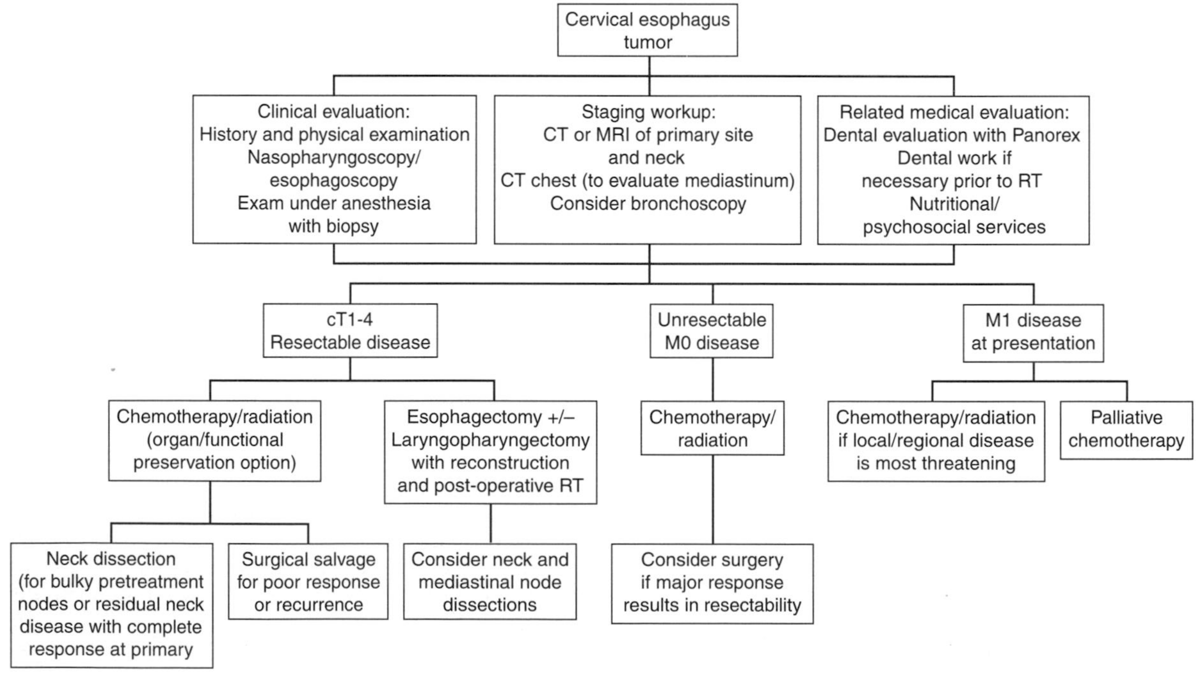

Figure 20.3 Workup and management of cervical esophageal cancer. *CT,* computed axial tomography; *MRI,* magnetic resonance imaging; *RT,* radiation therapy.

the primary tumor, clinical assessment of T stage can be misleading in that many T2 lesions are deceptively bulky and infiltrative despite their T2 status. This finding is relevant vis-à-vis the anticipated disease control with radiation therapy alone and the feasibility of conservation surgery. Tumor location and patient comorbidity must also be considered. As outlined by Ogura and Sessions, tumors involving the piriform apex, anterior wall ("anterior angle"), or postcricoid area, causing any impairment in vocal cord mobility, or showing evidence of bulky lymph node spread, or even a favorable tumor in a patient with poor lung function often will require total laryngectomy (69). In fact, the majority of T2 tumors, especially of the piriform sinus and postcricoid area, if managed surgically, would require total laryngectomy (7). In practice, therefore, many patients with T2 hypopharyngeal cancers are best considered, for management purposes, with the T3 to T4 resectable disease group.

In selected patients, however, with T1 and T2 tumors of the medial wall of the piriform sinus or of the hypopharyngeal aspect of the aryepiglottic fold, a supracricoid hemilaryngopharyngectomy has been advocated (58,70). Patients who are candidates for this procedure must have good pulmonary reserve and a tumor that does not extend to the apex of the piriform sinus. Patients may have limited mobility of the cricoarytenoid joint, but vocal cord mobility must be present. The surgical resection involves the supracricoid hemilarynx and medial aspect of the piriform sinus as well as the ipsilateral arytenoid. A bipedicle flap consisting of the external thyroid perichondrium and strap muscles is used to reconstruct the hemilarynx. In addition, patients undergo dissection of the ipsilateral neck (levels II–IV), the paratracheal lymphatics, and the ipsilateral thyroid lobe. After this procedure, patients are able to phonate with the remaining contralateral vocal cord, and in most cases, swallowing rehabilitation is feasible. In a variant of the procedure, the medial wall is removed above the level of the true vocal cord, and the anticipated functional outcomes are superior.

The technique of partial pharyngectomy through a lateral approach is indicated for T1 and T2 lesions of the lateral wall of the piriform fossa, provided that they do not reach the anterior wall or its apex (tumors involving the postcricoid area and the intrinsic larynx being excluded), or for similarly staged lesions of the external half of the posterior wall of the hypopharynx that do not reach the postcricoid area or fix the prevertebral fascia. Primary closure rarely is feasible.

Partial pharyngectomy through a lateral pharyngotomy or transhyoid pharyngotomy or posterior pharyngectomy is indicated for T1 and small T2 lesions (no larger than 3 cm in diameter) of the posterior wall of the hypopharynx, provided that they are well delimited and without extension to the postcricoid area or fixation to the prevertebral fascia. The main challenges are how to get satisfactory margins and how to reconstruct the posterior wall defect, the latter being typically done with a skin graft. Median labiomandibular glossotomy also can be employed for small lesions of the posterior pharyngeal wall, but can result in significant temporomandibular joint morbidity.

Dissection of the cervical lymphatics should be performed at the time of definitive surgery due to the high incidence of occult cervical metastasis (42,43,65). Midline lesions, or those approaching the midline, require treatment of bilateral regional lymph node basins, including the superior, middle, and inferior jugular lymphatics. Management of the retropharyngeal nodes must also be considered as these nodes contain disease in almost half of patients with primary tumors of the pharyngeal wall (34). Nevertheless, complete dissection of the retropharyngeal nodes rarely is required in the management of hypopharyngeal cancers unless there is radiographic evidence of metastases in these nodes. In those cases in which only the neck is being dissected and the primary tumor will be treated by definitive radiation therapy, the retropharyngeal nodes are resected only if clinical or radiographic disease exists. At the time of total or subtotal pharyngectomy, the retropharyngeal nodes, if encountered, are resected in the surgical vicinity of the primary tumor. Surgical removal of the retropharyngeal nodes above the level of the soft palate is not necessary unless the nodes are clinically or radiographically involved with disease as shown by cross-sectional imaging. If combined surgery and radiation therapy are planned, radiation portals must address the superior, middle, and inferior jugular lymphatics as well as the entire retropharyngeal nodal basins.

The main concern after conservation surgery of the hypopharynx is the extent to which normal swallowing has been impaired. When irradiation has been used after surgery, swallowing incompetence is further exacerbated by treatment-related edema. If a cricoid resection is necessary, the postoperative functional results are highly compromised. Converting a partial laryngectomy to a total procedure may be the only solution for patients who have significant aspiration or poor lung function and are plagued by recurrent bouts of aspiration pneumonia. Longer-term, there is also a risk for pharyngeal stenosis.

Radiation Therapy

Early hypopharyngeal SCCs may be effectively treated with irradiation, especially when the tumors are exophytic and do not involve the apex (7,71–75). When conventional fractionation is used with curative intent, the dose per fraction is 180 to 200 cGy per day to a total dose of 6,600 to 7,020 cGy delivered through opposing lateral portals matched to a low anterior neck field. To maximize dose homogeneity throughout the portal (and, in particular, at the level of the larynx), larynx compensators are routinely used. The clinically negative neck at risk should receive 5,000 to 5,400 cGy using similar fractionation. Bilateral neck management is necessary. Especially for bulkier T2 lesions, data from single arm studies suggest an advantage with selected hyperfractionated radiation schedules (76,77) and should be particularly considered for this group.

Radiation has the advantage of sterilizing occult and early cervical metastases, thereby obviating the need for extensive nodal dissections and their associated morbidity. As most early lesions of the hypopharynx will require postoperative irradiation, we believe that single-modality therapy is superior to resection of the primary tumor followed by postoperative irradiation. Surgical salvage, despite increased complication rates, is possible after irradiation failures (7,72,73). However, this surgery will typically require total laryngectomy, even if a function-preserving procedure might have been possible previously.

T3 AND T4 RESECTABLE DISEASE

Most patients will present with advanced stage disease and if managed surgically, will require total laryngectomy. For patients seeking to avoid this procedure, or with unresectable disease, the integration of chemotherapy with radiation therapy has been evaluated in randomized trials and represents a treatment option that should routinely be considered.

Surgery and Radiation

The historical standard treatment for patients with T3 and T4 resectable disease is total laryngectomy and partial pharyngectomy to achieve adequate surgical margins, as well as to prevent the morbidity associated with chronic aspiration of food and saliva. A simultaneous neck dissection to clear nodal disease is often performed. The potential for submucosal disease extension and adjacent mucosal dysplasia or carcinoma *in situ* must be considered when planning surgical margins. The closure of the surgical defect may be primary or involve some type of reconstruction (myocutaneous flap, gastric pull-up, or microvascular-free tissue transfer). Surgical management is followed by postoperative radiation therapy in patients with bulky T-stage disease, positive or close surgical margins, or lymph node involvement. The preference for postoperative rather than preoperative radiation was established in view of several issues. With planned preoperative irradiation, tumor margins may be obscured and the potential for increased postoperative complications exists. The advantages of planned postoperative irradiation are that the true tumor extent is known and that higher radiation doses may be delivered to the regional lymphatics. Non–site-specific randomized data suggest that local control is superior with postoperative application of radiation therapy (73,78). The weight of evidence, mainly derived from non–site-specific randomized studies, fails to support a role for induction/neoadjuvant or adjuvant chemotherapy in the setting of a planned resection (79–83).

When postoperative radiation is administered, a typical dose and fractionation schedule would be 6,300 cGy to the primary tumor bed and 5,400 cGy to low-risk regions of the neck (in 180–200 cGy fractions). The low anterior neck is treated with a dose of 5,000 cGy; the stoma (when present) often is boosted with electrons to 6,000 cGy. Bilateral neck management is necessary.

Chemoradiotherapy

The use of chemotherapy in conjunction with radiation therapy represents a legitimate treatment alternative to immediate surgery in patients with advanced hypopharyngeal cancer seeking to avoid total laryngectomy. A sequential approach of chemotherapy followed by definitive radiation in patients with a significant response is supported by a randomized trial by the European Organization for the Research and Treatment of Cancer (EORTC) (84), where equivalent survival to that obtained with primary surgery and postoperative radiation therapy was demonstrated. Patients received three cycles of standard cisplatin/infusional 5-fluorouracil. If a complete response including normalization of vocal cord motion was achieved, the patient proceeded to definitive dose radiation. The timing of neck dissection, if indicated, was left to the discretion of the treating surgeon. Surgery was reserved for inadequate response to chemotherapy, disease persistence, or relapse.

A

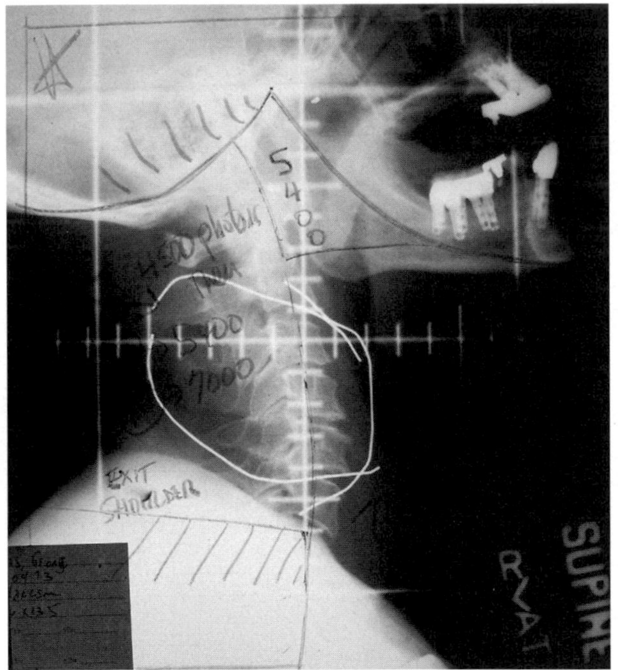

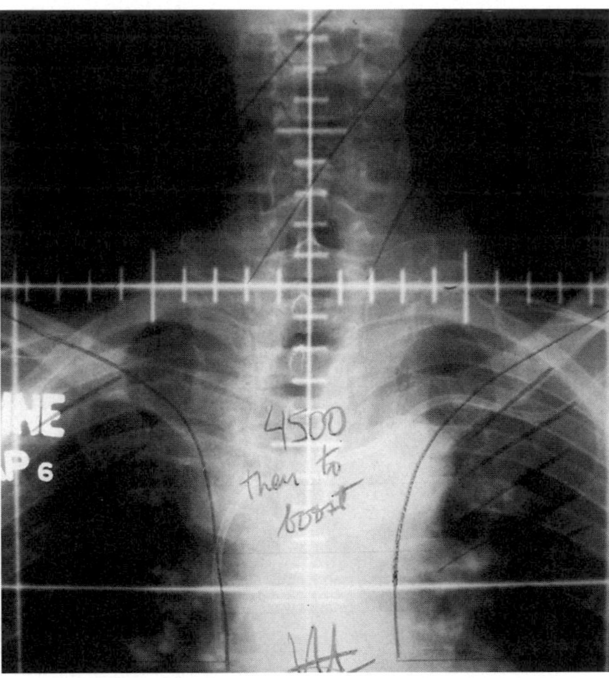

B

Figure 20.4 Sample portal films from a patient with hypopharyngeal/cervical esophageal cancer: The patient is a 63-year-old smoker and drinker who presented with sore throat and a right neck lump. Workup revealed a bulky squamous cell carcinoma involving the left piriform sinus invading the cervical esophagus with multiple bilateral lymph nodes at levels II, III, and IV. Computed tomography (CT) of the chest revealed multiple bilateral pulmonary nodules making the patient a stage IV (T4 N2c M1) by American Joint Committee on Cancer standards. Given the patient's excellent performance status, a course of concurrent cisplatin-based chemotherapy with radiation was recommended. A dose of 70-Gy with standard fractionation was prescribed to the entire primary tumor volume and involved lymph nodes. The upper portion of the target was treated with opposed lateral fields and the lower half was treated with a three-dimensional (3D) plan. The patient had a complete response at the primary site and continued with further chemotherapy for the lung disease. **A:** Typical portal for hypopharyngeal carcinoma. The superior border should generously encompass the retropharyngeal region above the level of C1 to C2. The posterior border of the lateral field generally is placed behind the spinous processes of the vertebral bodies. In cases of lymph node involvement, the posterior border is appropriately placed to encompass those lymph nodes with adequate margins, as denoted by the wires. The anterior border can be placed to exclude the submental region at level I, as this area rarely is involved for this subsite. The inferior border of this field is matched well below the cricoid cartilage, to encompass the entirety of the hypopharynx. **B:** A low anterior neck portal is matched to the lateral portals to treat electively the supraclavicular nodal regions. Note that the spinal cord block is placed at the inferior aspect of the lateral fields (see **A**).

Although the EORTC study demonstrated that some patients could retain a functional larynx with an overall survival similar to that for surgery and radiation, the actual reported organ preservation and survival rates leave much room for improvement. Other laryngeal preservation approaches exist, but experience with them is either limited or a definitive comparison to surgery and radiation therapy has not yet been accomplished for this site (85,86). In hopes of improving locoregional control, the optimal way to integrate chemotherapy with radiation is being evaluated as well as the role for altered fractionation radiation schedules for the hypopharynx and other sites (82,87–90). Representative port films are shown in Figure 20.4.

UNRESECTABLE M0 DISEASE, M1 DISEASE

Although resectability is a subjective assessment, tumor fixed to the cervical spine, massive T4 disease, or bulky lymphadenopathy fixed to the neurovascular bundle generally indicates that the disease is unresectable, or at least not resectable for cure. Affected patients will often be severely debilitated at presentation, further complicating their management and prognosis.

The historical management has used radiation therapy as a single modality, with palliative versus definitive dosing based on the radiation oncologist's clinical assessment. The radiation therapy literature is compromised for this group of patients in that published reports often fail to clearly define the resectability or operability of their patients (91). Nonetheless, there is little argument that disease control is poor.

Attempts to improve locoregional control have generally pursued one of two approaches. Altered fractionation radiation schedules have seemed promising in single-institution studies (Table 20.4), and a recently reported, large non–site-specific randomized trial demonstrated an improvement in local control with concomitant boost and continuous hyperfractionated radiation therapy schedules compared with standard once-daily radiation (90). Additionally, the integration of chemotherapy with radiation therapy has also received increased attention as an approach to unresectable disease (92,93). Concomitant therapy appears to have a more promising track record than a sequential approach (94–97). Locoregional toxicity typically is enhanced with the concomitant addition of chemotherapy (87, 94,97,98). It should be emphasized that this literature is often difficult to interpret, as a variety of different drug/radiation therapy schedules are used, the studies are generally not site-specific, and several of the trials show no difference in survival.

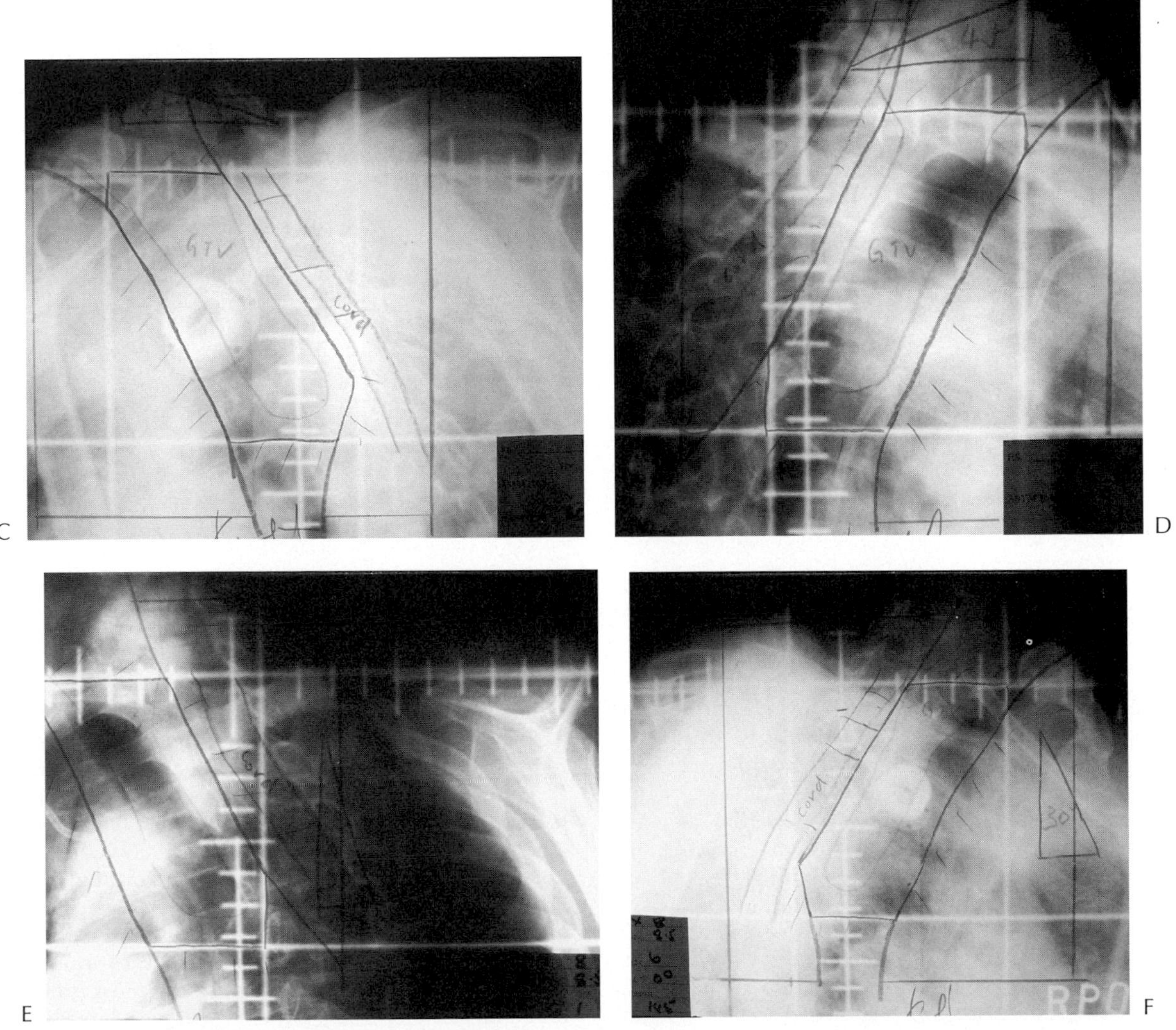

Figure 20.4 ***(continued)* C–F:** Due to tumor extension to the cervical esophagus, a CT-based 3D boost to consolidate the inferior portion of the tumor was necessary, with special attention to come off the spinal cord. In this plan, a four-field approach using paired obliques was implemented.

TABLE 20.4 Hypopharyngeal Cancer: Local Control and Survival for Patients Treated with External Beam Radiation Therapy (Selected Studies)

Series	T stage[a] and site	No. of patients	RT dose	Fractionation	Local control[b] (%)	5-year DFS (%)	5-year survival (%)
Bataini et al. (57)	T1–T2/PS	90	6,500–7,500 cGy planned	Conventional	32/62 (52)	T1 (49) T2 (48)	T1 (21) T2 (28)
	T3/PS	344			87/228 (38)	T3 (17)	T3 (17)
Dubois et al. (60)	T1–T2/PS	61	5,500–6,000 cGy	Conventional	45/61 (74)	NS	T1, T2 (11) (50 if N0)
	T3–T4/PS	148			51/148 (35)		T3, T4 (2)
Mendenhall et al. (61)	T1/PS	11	5,700–8,040 cGy (estimated from figure)	Conventional (except 11 patients) received twice-daily 120 cGy/fraction	8/9 (89)	I: 1/1 (100)	I: 1/1 (100)
	T2/PS	30			18/20 (90)	II: 3/3 (100)	II: 3/5 (60)
	T3/PS	7			3/5 (60)	III: 5/8 (63)	III: 5/13 (38)
	T4/PS	6			0/4 (0)	IVa: 7/12 (58) IVb: 2/8 (25)	IVa: 7/17 (41) IVb: 2/10 (20)
Garden et al. (62)	T2–T3/ hypopharynx	70[c]	7,180–7,970 cGy	HFX	33/39 (85)	NS for hypopharynx	NS for hypopharynx
Parsons et al. (63)	T2/PS	9	≥7,440 cGy	HFX	9/9 (100)	NS for PS or PW	NS for PS or PW
	T3/PS	3			2/3 (67)		
	T4/PS	1			0/1 (0)		
	T2/PW	10			8/10 (80)		
	T3/PW	12			8/12 (67)		
	T4/PW	3			1/3 (33)		
Fein et al. (64)	T1/PW	8	Conventional: 6,600–7,600 cGy HFX: 7,730–7,972 cGy (both depending on T stage)	Mixture of conventional and HFX	100%	I: 100%	I: 50%
	T2/PW	33			74%	II: 72%	I: 36%
	T3/PW	47			49%	III: 56%	III: 26%
	T4/PW	11			36%	IVa: 75% IVb: 29%	IVa: 28% IVb: 5%
Amdur et al. (131)	T1/PS	22	5,650–7,500 cGy	Conventional (54%)	19/22 (86)	I–II: N=25 (96)	I: N=7 (57)
	T2/PS	79	or 6,960–7,920 cGy	Twice daily 120 cGy/fraction (47%)	65/79 (82)	III: N=20 (62) IVa: N=44 (49) IVb: N=12 (33)	II: N=18 (61) III: N=20 (41) IVa: N=44 (29) IVb: N=12 (25)
Johansen et al. (137)	T1	27	5,700–6,800 cGy	Conventional	56%		37% (39% if N0)
	T2	34			41%		22% (29% if N0)
	T3	42			36%		19%
	T4	17			0%		0%

DFS, disease-free survival; HFX, hyperfractionated; NS, not stated; PS, piriform sinus; PW, pharyngeal wall; RT, radiation therapy.
[a]Tumor, node, metastases system used varies with time of publication.
[b]Excluded were those patients who died less than 2 yrs from treatment and who were continuously disease-free for the Mendenhall (61), Parsons (63), and Fein (64) series.
[c]Twenty-seven patients received induction chemotherapy.

The treatment for patients with unresectable, hypopharyngeal cancer is evolving. It remains defensible to treat such patients with conventionally fractionated radiation therapy alone. However, especially among good performance status patients who can tolerate the additional morbidity of combined-modality treatment, available data support the off-protocol use of chemotherapy with radiation, with data that are strongest for concomitant therapy.

The question of "downsizing" unresectable disease with neoadjuvant radiation therapy or chemotherapy to make it resectable often is asked. Given that the randomized data with induction chemotherapy prior to a planned resection did not demonstrate a survival advantage, this approach with chemotherapy is not recommended. For unresectable neck disease, there is a precedent for initial conventionally fractionated radiation: 5,000 cGy to the primary site, 6,000 cGy to the neck, followed by surgery 4 to 8 weeks later if there was sufficient regression of the neck disease off the neurovascular bundle (99).

Patients presenting with distant metastatic disease overall have a poorer prognosis than M0 patients. Because chemotherapy by itself is not generally a curative modality, most of these patients will have incurable disease. Accordingly, the benefits of aggressive multimodality treatment to the primary site and neck in the hope of obtaining locoregional control need to be balanced against the potential morbidities in a setting where cure is likely not possible. Because the most prominent symptoms for many of these patients will be related to the primary site or neck, aggressive combined modality therapy, often with chemotherapy and radiation, can still be justified. Alternatively, especially when locoregional symptoms are less compelling, initial chemotherapy can be pursued, and subsequent locoregional treatment tailored to the patient's clinical and performance status and response to chemotherapy.

Cervical Esophageal Cancer

Although surgical resection or radiation therapy have historically been the main treatment options, a 1992–1994 Patterns of Care (PCS) study of 400 patients sponsored by the National Cancer Institute and an American Cancer Society study of over 5,000 cases accrued in the National Cancer Data Base in 1993 showed that the most common treatment approach for esophageal cancer is definitive concurrent chemoradiation (100). Similarly, an extensive "patterns of practice" survey of 26 Canadian radiation oncology centers treating cervical esophageal cancers showed that concurrent chemoradiation was the most frequently used nonsurgical regimen, usually 60 Gy per 6 weeks with concurrent cisplatin-based chemotherapy (101). Management has been significantly influenced by the results of a phase III Radiation Therapy Oncology Group (RTOG) study in which concomitant radiotherapy and chemotherapy has been shown to be superior to radiotherapy alone (102). As is typical of such randomized studies, however, the cervical esophagus is an infrequently entered subsite.

T1 TO T3 AND SELECTED T4 RESECTABLE DISEASE

Surgery

Because of extensive local extramural extension and submucosal spread in those patients undergoing surgical management, a cervical or total esophagectomy with laryngopharyngectomy is generally necessary, even for what initially appears to be early stage disease. In a series of 67 cervical esophageal cancers seen at Memorial Sloan-Kettering Cancer Center (MSKCC), 22 of 36 surgically resectable lesions underwent resection. Margins were positive in 36%, and 55% had extraesophageal extension primarily to the neck, trachea, and larynx (46). In certain instances, exploration of the thoracic inlet may be necessary before resectability can be determined. Extensive tumors in this area that involve the great vessels or membranous trachea are not meaningfully resectable. Reconstruction most often entails gastric or jejunal interposition. Limited evidence suggests that the interposed jejunum or stomach may tolerate postoperative radiation doses of 60 to 65 Gy. However, intermittent hemorrhage from gastric grafts has been reported after postoperative radiation (103).

As part of surgical management, unilateral or bilateral neck dissection is necessary. Dissection of the superior mediastinal lymph nodes should be considered depending on the extent of disease at the primary site and neck, to clear the regional lymphatics. A unilateral lobectomy or total thyroidectomy is done to remove the gland, which may be directly invaded by tumor (31,104). Special attention is needed to preserve at least one parathyroid gland to prevent persistent postoperative hypocalcemia. Synchronous or metachronous aerodigestive primaries are frequent and should be ruled out.

Infrequently, tumors of the cervical esophagus that are well below the cricopharyngeus may be amenable to a larynx-sparing resection and repair by either free jejunal transfer or gastric pull-up (Fig. 20.5). The superior margin must be carefully examined, however, and found to be free of tumor. If the cricopharyngeus is involved, the larynx must be removed to prevent aspiration.

With regard to surgery, preoperative chemotherapy has not been shown to be of survival benefit to patients undergoing planned esophagectomy (105). Similarly, adjuvant chemotherapy in this treatment setting is of unproven benefit (106).

Radiation Therapy

Radiation therapy either alone or combined with chemotherapy represents the alternative approach to surgery. Treatment planning for carcinoma of the cervical esophagus is challenging due to the large target area (neck and upper thorax), the widely varying contour and thicknesses, the adjacent normal structures (especially the spinal cord), and the varying course of the esophagus. Various techniques have been used including wedge anterior, three-field (anterior and posterior obliques), and four-field (anterior, posterior and laterals) (Fig. 20.4). Three-dimensional treatment planning has improved the accuracy and positioning of beams and blocking. A 5-cm margin is placed superiorly and inferiorly. The target dose to gross tumor disease is 70 to 75 Gy when radiation alone is considered with field reductions at 45 to 50 Gy and 60 Gy. When administered before surgery, 45 to 50 Gy is delivered with surgery 4 to 6 weeks later. Postoperative doses of 60 to 70 Gy are prescribed depending on the margin status.

If chemotherapy is to be given concurrently, the final total dose is reduced to 50 to 60 Gy. Regimens using cisplatin or mitomycin with 5-fluororuacil have been best studied historically, although taxane-based schedules are receiving increased attention (107). The previously mentioned RTOG randomized study included two cycles of adjuvant cisplatin/infusional 5-fluorouracil (102), but this can be poorly tolerated and adjuvant chemotherapy is not routine in all chemotherapy/radiation schedules.

UNRESECTABLE M0, M1 DISEASE

The management of unresectable cervical esophageal cancer is influenced by the results of the RTOG randomized study (102). Combined modality chemotherapy and radiation is the preferred approach in patients with adequate performance and clinical status. Two randomized trials have evaluated a strategy of concomitant chemotherapy/radiation therapy versus radiation therapy alone in patients with unresectable esophageal cancer (108,109). Although interpretation of results is limited by small sample size, neither study demonstrated an improvement in overall survival. The study using concomitant cisplatin and split-course radiation, however, demonstrated a significant improvement in both local control and first progression-free survival with the addition of chemotherapy (109).

Patients with distant metastases at presentation are considered to have incurable disease because currently available systemic chemotherapies, while providing palliation, do not generally offer potential cure. The decision to pursue initial palliative chemotherapy versus an aggressive locoregional treatment is based on the presenting symptoms, the patient's clinical status, and the expected morbidities and benefits of the proposed intervention. In patients with adequate performance status, in whom the local disease is causing significant distress or is more immediately life-threatening, aggressive combined modality chemotherapy and radiation may be justified. However, when locoregional symptoms are less compelling, initial chemotherapy is usually pursued to spare the patient the increased morbidity of combined modality treatment at a time when there is little anticipation of long-term benefit.

Reconstruction

The optimal reconstructive technique after hypopharyngeal or cervical esophageal surgery includes one-stage reconstruction, use of tissue from outside the field of irradiation, and rapid healing without excessive morbidity. It is important for healing to occur rapidly so that timely postoperative irradiation may be administered. Unfortunately, major ablative surgery is required

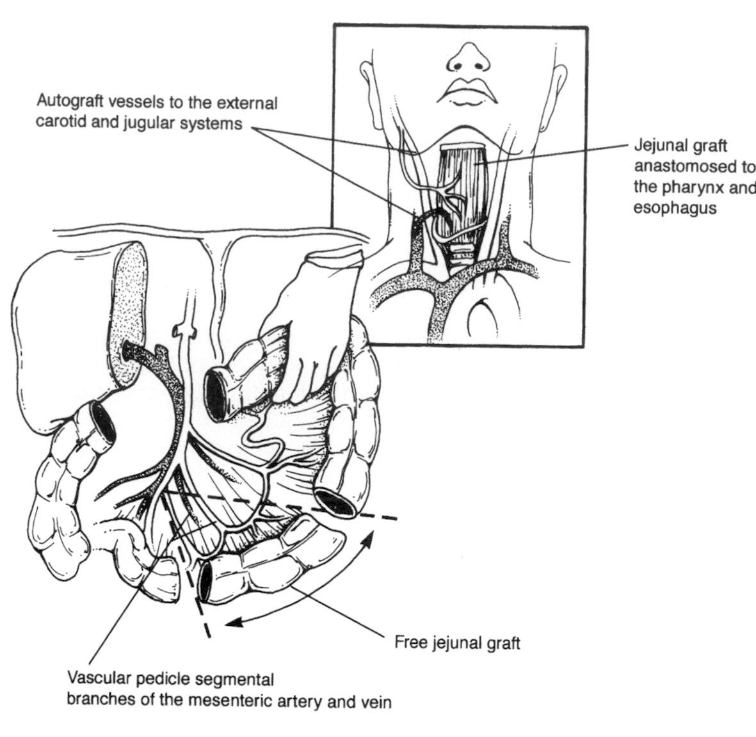

A

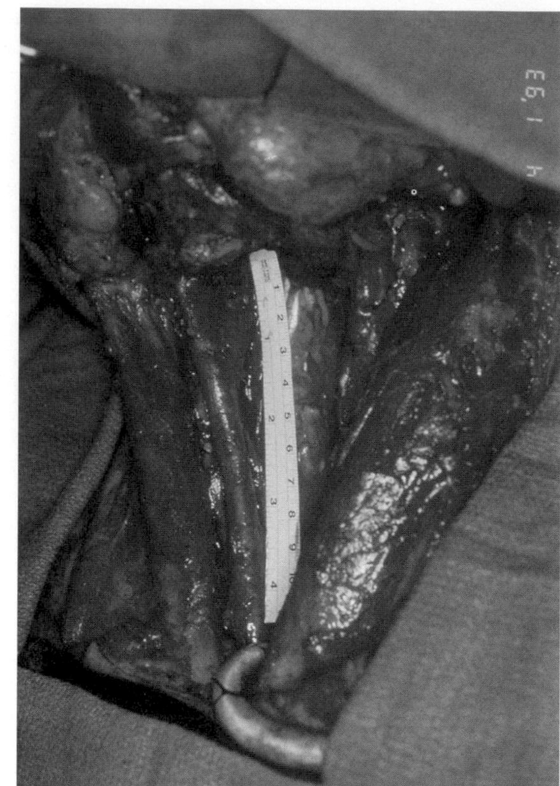

B

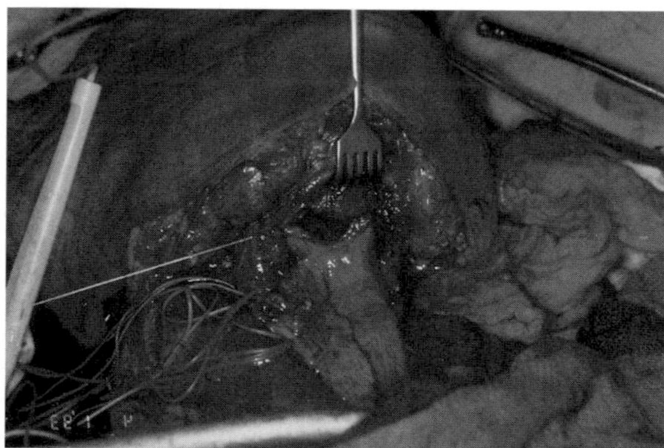

C

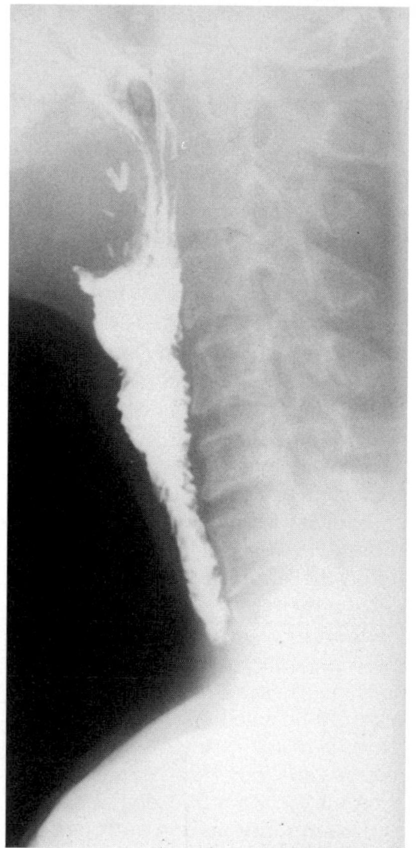

D

Figure 20.5 **A:** A 20- to 25-cm segment of jejunum harvested for total pharyngeal and cervical esophagus replacement. The autograft vessels are anastomosed to the external carotid and jugular systems. **B:** Defect (measuring 15 cm) after total laryngopharyngectomy. **C:** Jejunal flap sewn in place. Remaining sutures are used to close the upper pharynx. **D:** Barium swallow demonstrating free transit of contrast material through the jejunal segment.

for extensive tumors, and no reconstructive technique completely fulfills all these criteria (110).

Primary closure or skin grafts are sufficient for small defects; however, the degree of tissue loss rarely permits application of these methods. Posterior pharyngeal wall defects can, at times, be repaired by skin grafting. Flaps based on pedicles and colonic interpositions are mainly of historical interest. Current methods of hypopharyngeal reconstruction often employ the jejunal free flap with microvascular anastomosis or the gastric pull-up procedure for reestablishing continuity and function.

PECTORALIS MAJOR MYOCUTANEOUS FLAP AND RADIAL FOREARM PATCH GRAFTS

A pectoralis major myocutaneous flap and free tissue transfer (radial forearm flap) (Fig. 20.6) may be used for subtotal hypopharyngeal defects in which a posterior strip of mucosa remains (111,112). The use of radial forearm "patch grafts" instead of circumferential jejunal reconstruction may significantly improve swallowing (113). One must not, however, compromise total tumor extirpation, including the need to remove areas of submucosal and lymphatic spread in these cancers. The pectoralis flap is associated with a higher incidence of fistulae and stenosis and, because of its lack of pliability, is difficult to form into a tube. It is not useful in women with pendulous breasts. If a myocutaneous flap is necessary for total hypopharyngeal reconstruction, a trapezius myocutaneous flap is chosen, because its thinner skin and subcutaneous tissue allow it to be more easily shaped as needed (110,114). Technical complexities that necessitate a longer operating time and the variability of blood supply are potential drawbacks of this flap.

FREE JEJUNAL GRAFT

A free jejunal graft with microvascular anastomosis is an excellent method of reconstruction and probably is the reconstructive method of choice for lesions of the hypopharynx that require total pharyngectomy. Defects from the level of the nasopharynx to the thoracic inlet may be reconstructed with this technique. The free jejunal graft allows for early deglutition, is associated with a low incidence of stenosis and fistula, and, similar to the gastric interposition, tolerates postoperative irradiation relatively well (115–117). Care must be taken to fashion the jejunal interposition to the appropriate length, as the conduit may kink if it is too long, leading to dysphagia and stasis.

GASTRIC PULL-UP

Another reconstructive option, the feasibility of the gastric pull-up is significantly affected by the superior extent of resection. Persistent dysphagia afterward is uncommon, but patients may have symptoms of gastric dumping and reflux. The fistula rate afterward may approximate 20%.

Free jejunal transfer may be preferred to gastric pull-up due to better radiation tolerance of the jejunal graft. There is limited evidence that the transposed stomach tolerates postoperative radiation to doses of 60 to 65 Gy (118). However, Spiro et al. report several patients who experienced intermittent hemorrhage after postoperative radiation to the gastric graft (103). Extirpation of extensive disease, from nasopharynx through to thorax, may require both methods of reconstruction.

GASTRIC INTERPOSITION

When total pharyngoesophagectomy is required, gastric interposition is the method of choice for reconstruction. Advantages include a lower incidence of fistulae and strictures and allowance for a greater margin of resection than the pectoralis flap. However, major abdominal surgery and posterior mediastinal dissection are required to allow the stomach to be passed into the neck. Operative morbidity approaches 50%, and mortality rates are nearly 10% (119). Gastric outlet obstruction and stasis with regurgitation occur in a large percentage of patients, but the risk for this may be reduced if a pyloroplasty is performed at the time of surgery. Pharyngogastric anastomoses reportedly have a lower incidence of stenosis and leakage than do pedicle flaps (114,120).

Rehabilitation

Changes in deglutition, speech, and appearance after surgery should be included in a comprehensive program of postoperative education by the physician and staff. The patient must be taught self-care and be motivated to continue this care after hospital discharge. The more aggressive the postoperative education, the more a patients are able to participate in their own rehabilitation. When total laryngectomy is required, early speech rehabilitation is essential to help the patient gain the best form of alaryngeal communication.

With larynx preservation by either conservation surgery or radiation-based treatment, normal swallowing is altered and aspiration becomes a possibility. The speech pathologist, nurse, or physical therapist should begin the patient's deglutition training after laryngopharyngeal edema has subsided. The modified barium swallow or video cine-esophagogram can yield valuable information regarding anatomic and physiologic changes in the swallowing mechanism. Armed with this information, the therapist can better assist in the patient's return to normal deglutition.

In patients who have undergone laryngectomy, there are three main options for voice rehabilitation. The first is the classic esophageal voice that consists of swallowing air and bringing up wind. Sound is generated by the vibration of the pharyngoesophageal junction mucosa and is thereafter modulated by the tongue, teeth, and lips. In the case of hypopharyngeal or pharyngoesophageal surgery, the mucosa resection is larger than it is for laryngeal surgery with sectioning of the recurrent nerves lower in the neck. As a result, the quality of this type of voice rehabilitation in hypopharyngeal cancer is quite disappointing, belches being hardly controlled by patients. Voice is frequently interrupted and monotone. The second option is the placement of a voice prosthesis through a tracheoesophageal puncture. The results are much better with this option because the vibration of the mucosa is generated by air produced from the lungs and is better controlled by the patients. Voice is quite fluent and may be modulated in intensity. Data suggest that only one third of patients rehabilitating from hypopharynx cancer are able to attain satisfactory esophageal speech; with tracheoesophageal puncture, this rate will be approximately 70% (8). The main concern for these voice prostheses is their maintenance. Additionally, if patients have undergone reconstruction that required free tissue transfer or intestinal interposition, tracheoesophageal puncture may not be attainable. The third option is an electrolarynx, which is almost always usable, but produces a metallic voice and may be unacceptable to many patients.

Tobacco and alcohol use are risk factors for tumors of the hypopharynx and cervical esophagus, as well as for a variety of other primary sites. These lifestyle factors also contribute to the development of a spectrum of other medical morbidities. Although cessation or significant reduction of these behaviors during treatment is typical, their resumption after acute toxicity has resolved is common. Part of the rehabilitation process should include state of the art counseling and treatment to address these problems.

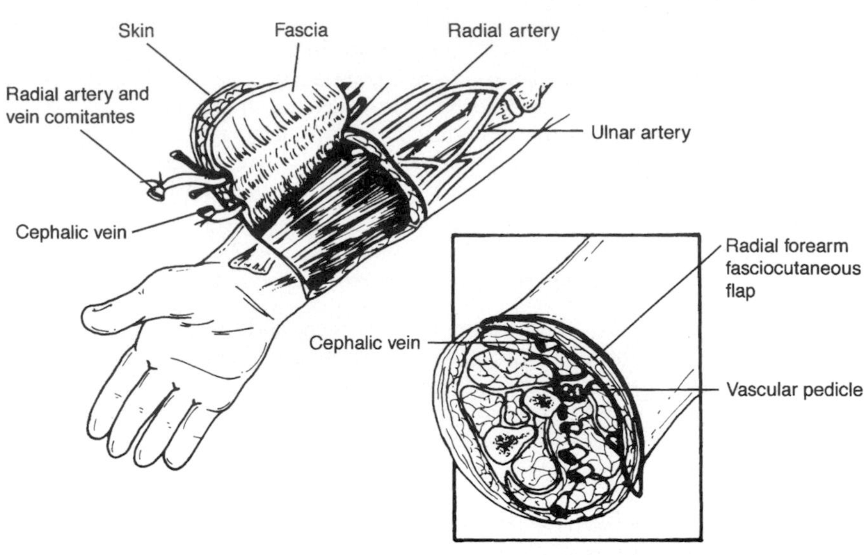

Figure 20.6 A: Radial forearm flap with skin island based on the distal radial artery. This flap may be tubed for total pharyngeal reconstruction or used as a patch for less-than-circumferential defects. **B:** Tubed radial forearm flap before inset into the defect. **C:** Close-up view showing the upper portion that will be sutured to the base of tongue and pharynx. **D:** Patient after inset and anastomosis of tubed radial forearm flap for total pharyngeal reconstruction. **E:** Radial forearm flap donor site resurfaced with a split-thickness skin graft.

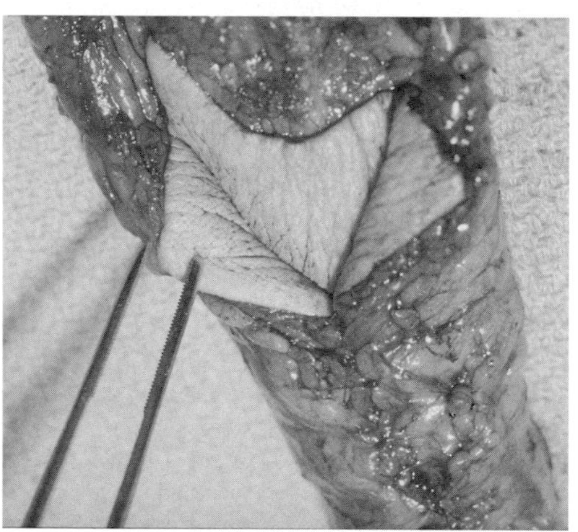

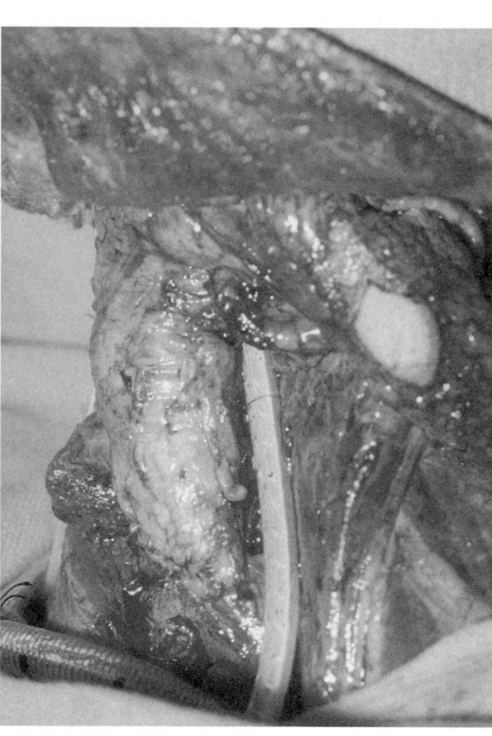

C,D

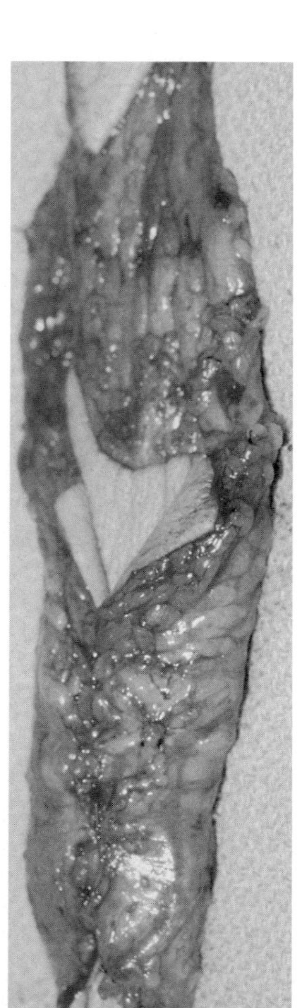

B

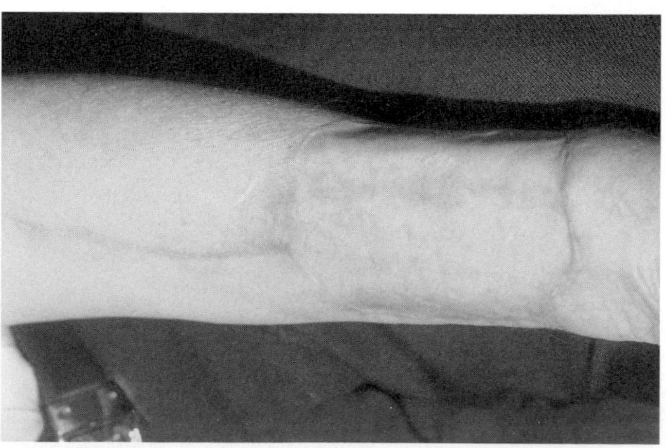

E

Follow-up

Despite advances in radiation, surgery, and chemotherapy as well as multidisciplinary care, overall survival at 5 years for hypopharynx and cervical esophageal cancers are disappointing, and for patients with advanced disease, survival rarely exceeds 30%. Death from locoregional recurrence is the primary reason, but distant metastases, second cancers, and intercurrent disease remain significant contributors to mortality in 30% to 40% of deaths (7,57,60,121–123). Relapse after 2 years is common (56), although the odds of relapse progressively decrease with time.

Posttreatment surveillance is primarily intended to identify locoregional failure and second primary cancers that are amenable to curative therapy, provide supportive care, and facilitate rehabilitation. Accordingly, symptom review, careful clinical examination of the primary site and neck by an experienced health care professional, supplemented with appropriate imaging based on patient symptoms or examination findings represent the cornerstones of follow-up. Depending on tumor location and potential limitations on visualization caused by posttreatment edema or retained secretions, flexible fiberoptic instruments with photographic or video capability are routinely used, and examination/endoscopy under anesthesia may be necessary, especially for more inferior lesions. The frequency of visits will vary depending on perceived risk for relapse and patient reliability, but generally starts with evaluations every 1 to 2 months during the first year with progressive decreases in frequency annually thereafter if the patient remains disease-free and without other significant health problems (Fig. 20.7).

Historically, an annual chest radiograph is performed as a screen for lung metastases and second primary cancers, although the extent to which this testing improves survival outcomes is difficult to demonstrate. Chest films have not been proven to be of benefit as a screening tool for lung cancer (124). Successful salvage of patients with distant metastases is infrequent. Randomized trials in other solid tumors have failed to demonstrate a significant improvement in survival improvement from aggressive imaging strategies for distant metastases (125,126) so aggressive surveillance for them is not routinely performed. Advances in newer imaging modalities, such as low-dose chest CT scans may affect this strategy in the future.

Among patients who received surgery or radiation to the thyroid gland, annual testing of thyroid-stimulating hormone levels is recommended. In this setting, the development of hypothyroidism on follow-up is common, and periodic testing facilitates the timely institution of thyroid supplementation. Although chemopreventive measures are an active area of investigation (127) and potentially important randomized trials are in progress, no drug is considered a standard treatment option at present for this purpose. Encouraging the patient to alter tobacco and alcohol habits associated with the development of these and other tumors remains the cornerstone of decreasing the risk for second primary cancers.

OUTCOMES AND RESULTS

The analysis of reported results for the treatment of carcinomas of the hypopharynx and cervical esophagus is complicated by:

1. The inclusion of these tumors with other head and neck or esophageal subsites
2. Unclear reporting of the resectability of tumors
3. Comorbidities and second primaries that impair survival and make it more difficult to demonstrate a beneficial treatment effect
4. Slow accrual to trials that may span a time period with changing methods of treatment and disease evaluation

Other confounding factors may include selection bias, variability of follow up, and different outcome measures. The majority of data are single-institutional studies, which are retrospective and often report results favoring the treatment preferred by the reporting author. In the context of these mitigating factors, published reports will be reviewed with an emphasis on randomized data, when available.

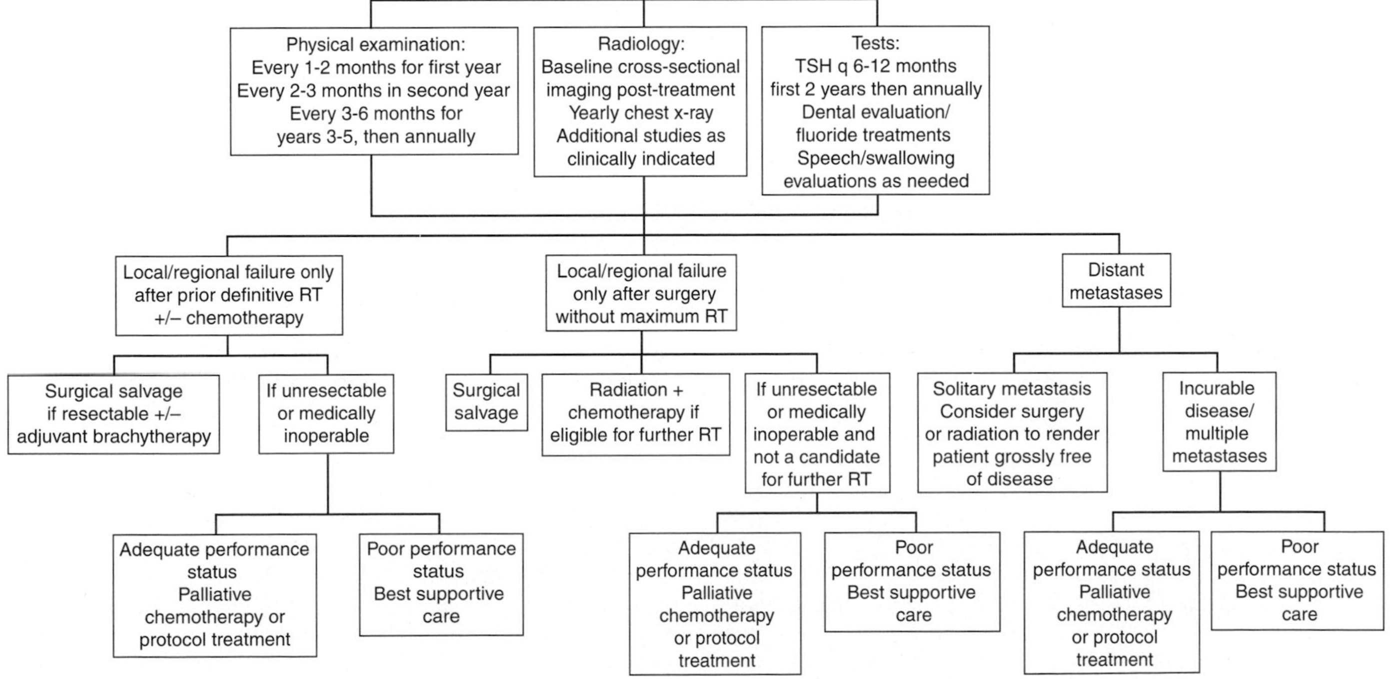

Figure 20.7 Follow-up and salvage therapy. *RT,* radiation therapy; *TSH,* thyroid stimulating hormone.

Hypopharyngeal Cancer

A large national survey conducted under the auspices of the American College of Surgeon's Commission on Cancer and the American Cancer Society compared treatment practices and outcomes involving over 1,300 hypopharynx cancers treated at 769 acute care hospitals throughout the United States between 1980 and 1985 (128). Three fourths of patients were diagnosed with stage III to IV disease. Overall 5-year disease-specific survival was 33% with about one third showing persistent disease after treatment and a similar proportion showing recurrence, two thirds of which were locoregional. In general, patients treated with surgery alone or surgery and radiation did better than patients treated with radiation alone or chemoradiation with 5-year disease-specific survivals of 50%, 48%, 26%, and 15%, respectively. It should be emphasized that these data were largely derived from retrospective, nonrandomized, and community-based practices and subject to a variety of biases. In addition, over the past two decades significant advances in all modalities have been made that may make such results out of date. However, the study suggests that surgery remains a standard treatment to which the various nonsurgical approaches should be compared.

A significant proportion of patients presenting with hypopharynx cancers may not be eligible for surgery. Eckel et al. report on 228 consecutive patients (129). Forty percent were unable to undergo surgery due to inability to achieve a curative resection; 15% had technically unresectable disease; 6% had distant metastases; 10% were medically unstable; 6% refused treatment; and 4% had synchronous secondary primaries that prevented an oncologically complete resection. Of those able to undergo surgery, only one third were eligible for larynx-preserving surgeries. Thus, multiple treatment approaches must be available for those patients who are not resectable, as well as for those who wish to pursue organ-sparing and function-preserving alternatives.

T1 AND T2 DISEASE

Single-institution retrospective data indicate comparable outcomes for patients with early lesions of the hypopharynx, particularly the piriform sinus, when treated either by surgery, either standard or larynx-sparing, or irradiation.

Surgery

Analysis of the results with surgery by stage is difficult due to the different end points reported (local control vs. locoregional control, disease-free vs. overall survival), the various proportion treated with larynx-conserving surgery vs. total laryngectomy, differing lengths of follow up, variable use of adjuvant radiation or even chemotherapy, as well as reporting of results by groups rather than by specific T or N stage (Table 20.5). Several authors report a high rate of local control (63%–97%) for surgically treated, early stage hypopharynx cancers (7,58,60,71). Disease-free survival ranged from 43% to 56% (6,130), whereas overall survivals from 37% to 74% were reported, with different authors using different lengths of follow up (37,58,60,71).

El Badawi et al. report a locoregional control rate of 82% for T1 to T2 disease (75). Dubois et al. report local control, locoregional control, and overall survival rates of 63%, 43%, and 37% at 5 years, respectively, after resection of T1 to T2 lesions (60). Vandenbrouk et al. report a local control of 89% for 18 patients with T1 to T2 lesions of the piriform sinus treated by conservative surgery alone (7). Marks et al. report the 5-year disease-free survival to be 43% (6), and Wang reports a 3-year disease-free survival of 56% for T1 to T2 lesions treated by surgery (130). Guillamondegui et al. report a 41% 2-year survival rate for patients with cancer of the pharyngeal walls treated by surgery alone (37). Ho et al. report results of surgical treatment and the causes of recurrence or death in 109 patients with SCC of the hypopharynx (71). The 5-year survival rates were related to the stage of the disease (stage I, 74%; stage II, 63%; stage III, 32%; stage IV, 14%). The local control rate was 86%, with no significant difference between those patients who underwent pharyngolaryngectomy and those who underwent pharyngolaryngoesophagectomy. Harrison and Thompson report a 3-year survival rate of 37% for patients with postcricoid cancers treated by pharyngolaryngoesophagectomy and gastric pull-up (119). The latter two reports support the opinion that total esophagectomy, though recommended for cervical esophageal cancers, is not necessary for cancers of the hypopharynx having minimal cervical esophageal extension.

Laccourreye et al. report the results of 34 patients treated with supracricoid hemilaryngopharyngectomy for T2 carcinomas involving the membranous portion of the piriform sinus (58). Tumors with vocal fixation or involving the apex, postcricoid area, posterior pharyngeal wall, or preepiglottic space were excluded. Postoperative radiation therapy routinely was given (45–70 Gy) in 91% and preoperative chemotherapy was given in 91%. The local control was 97% and overall survival was 56%. Decannulation was possible in 97% of patients, physiologic phonation was achieved in 94%, and deglutition was preserved in 31 of 34 patients at a median interval of 19 days. In this same cohort, aspiration pneumonia was noted in seven patients (20%), two of whom required a laryngectomy for severe aspiration. Chondroradionecrosis occurred in four patients resulting in one death and one patient requiring permanent tracheostomy. Dysphagia related to esophageal stricture occurred in three patients.

Radiation Therapy

With appropriate radiation treatment dose and technique, outcomes for early stage lesions are comparable to that for surgery. The local control rates for T1 to T2 lesions treated with radiation therapy alone are summarized in Table 20.4. Taken together, local control varies between 52% and 100%, and 5-year disease-free survival varies from 48% to 100%. Variability may be attributed to radiation technique/dose, patient selection factors, and neck staging (57,60,61,64).

Among 90 patients with T1 and T2 tumors of the piriform sinus treated with radiation therapy alone at the Institut Curie, local control and locoregional control at 2 years was 67% and 56%, respectively. Among determinant cases (patients who were followed for 2 years but had no evidence of distant metastases, neck-only failures, second primaries, or died of complications), the local control was 52% (57). However, some patients in this series received less than the planned total dose due to poor medical condition. Local control was only 36% for T1 to T2 tumors treated with up to 65 Gy, but improved to 65% among patients who received more than this dose.

Dubois et al. report a local control rate of 74% for T1 to T2 tumors after radiotherapy alone. This compared favorably to patients treated with surgery (either total or partial pharyngolaryngectomy) and postoperative radiation for which local control was 63% (60).

Mendenhall et al. published a 79% crude local control rate for 23 of 29 patients with T1 and T2 lesions of the piriform sinus treated at the University of Florida (UF) (61). Amdur et al. updated the UF experience with 101 T1 or T2 lesions involving the piriform sinus (131). Patients with stage III and IV overall stage by virtue of neck node involvement were included. Conventional fractionation using once-daily radiation to a mean dose of 67 Gy was given in 54 patients, whereas the oth-

TABLE 20.5 Early Stage Hypopharyngeal Cancer: Local Control and Survival for Patients Treated with Surgery (Selected Studies)

Series	T stage[a] and site	No. of patients	Type of surgery	Local control	Locoregional control	5-year DFS survival (%)	5-year overall survival (%)
El Badawi et al. (75)	T1–T2	20	Total laryngectomy	NS	82% (2-year)	NS Reported by technique not stage	NS
Dubois et al. (60)	T1–T2/PS (all N+)	54	Hemilaryngopharyngectomy or total pharyngolaryngectomy with postoperative XRT	63%	43%	NS	37%
	T3–T4/PS	100		46%	32%		30%
Vandenbrouk et al. (7)	T1–T2/PS	18	Conservative	89%			
Marks et al. (6)	T1–T2/PS	57	Preoperative radiation and partial laryngopharyngectomy	NS (Results reported by technique grouped early and advanced lesions)	NS	43%	NS
Wang (133)	T1–T2					56% (3-year)	
Guillamondegui et al. (37)	T1/PW	5	Surgery not otherwise specified	NS	75%	60% (after salvage)	80% (2-year)
	T2/PW	22 (18 N0)			70%	64%	72% (2-year)
Ho et al. (71)	T1N0	9	Pharyngolaryngoesophagectomy or total laryngectomy with circumferential or partial pharyngectomy and postoperative radiation	86%	80%	NS	74%
	T2N0	17		(Grouped by technique with more advanced lesions)		NS	63%
Harrison and Thompson (119)	PC		Pharyngolaryngoesophagectomy and gastric pull-up				37% (3-year)
Laccourreye et al. (58)	T2/PS	34	Neoadjuvant chemotherapy, supracricoid hemilaryngopharyngectomy, ipsilateral neck dissection, and postoperative radiation	97%	94%	NS	56%

DFS, disease-free survival; NS, not stated; PC, postcricoid; PS, piriform sinus; PW, pharyngeal wall; XRT, external beam radiation therapy.
[a]Tumor, node, metastases system used varies with time of publication.

ers in the study group received 1.2 Gy twice daily to a mean dose of 75 Gy. With a minimum follow-up of 5 years in 87% of patients, the 5-year actuarial local control for T1 and T2 was 90% and 80%, respectively. Local control with larynx preservation was 91% and 73%, respectively, at 5 years. Among the 14 local failures, salvage surgery was successful in 7 of 8 patients where it was attempted, so that the ultimate local control at 5 years for T1 and T2 disease was 95% and 91%, respectively, for the overall group. Univariate analysis showed apical involvement by tumor resulted in lower control for T1 lesions [33% (1/3) vs. 100% (14/14), $p = 0.02$], whereas there was a possible improvement in local control for T2 lesions with hyperfractionation compared with conventional fractionation [89% (33/37) vs. 73% (22/30), $p = 0.09$)]. Actuarial disease-specific survival was 96%, 62%, 49%, and 33% for patients with AJCC (1992) stage I to II, III, IVa and IVb disease. The corresponding rates of overall survival were 57%, 61%, 41%, 29%, and 25% for patients with AJCC (1992) stage I, II, III, IVa, and IVb disease. Severe late complications related to radiotherapy or salvage surgery occurred in 12% (12/101). Total laryngectomy was performed in three patients with no evidence of tumor in the specimen: two for chondronecrosis precipitated by biopsy and the other for clinical signs of suspected local failure. Two patients died of carotid blowout after undergoing surgery following conventional radiotherapy. Five required a permanent gastrostomy after radiotherapy, whereas one required permanent tracheostomy and another was needed transiently for one year. One patient developed an esophageal stricture, which was successfully dilated.

The published experience is more limited for other hypopharyngeal sites. Fein et al. report the UF experience in 99 patients with T1 to T4 pharyngeal wall tumors, of which 75 (76%) were characterized as hypopharyngeal primary tumors (64). Five-year local control rates for T1 and T2 patients were 100% and 74%, respectively. The radiation therapy technique changed during the time of the series. Before 1978, once-daily fractionation was used, and the posterior border of the field was placed at the midline of the vertebral body. Subsequently, twice-daily fractionation schemes were progressively employed, and the posterior border of the field was placed at the anterior aspect of the spinal cord. On multivariate analysis T stage (less advanced), fractionation schedule (hyperfractionated), and primary site (oropharynx) predicted for better control. Parsons et al. report an approximate 20% improvement in local control when hyperfractionated schedules were employed, compared with their historical experience with conventional fractionation therapy (63). The extent to which the change in the posterior border of the field explains this finding is difficult to assess.

Garden et al. report on 82 patients with early stage lesions (T1 = 19, T2 = 63) treated with definitive radiation at the M. D. Anderson Cancer Center (132). About half (52%) were node-positive. Patients received conventional (n = 38) or hyperfractionated radiation (n = 44) to doses of 60 to 79 Gy and 28% (n = 23) had neck dissection. At a minimum follow-up of 2 years among surviving patients, the 2-year local control rates were 89% and 77%, respectively. T2 patients treated with hyperfractionation (n = 40) had improved local control compared with conventional fractionation (n = 23) (86% vs. 60%, p = 0.004). Five-year survival for all patients was 52% (132).

Wang also reports better results with an altered fractionated scheme (133). The 3-year disease-free survival was 52% for patients with early lesions involving the hypopharynx. For all T1 to T4 lesions receiving 65 Gy, local control appeared improved with split-course, accelerated radiation (n = 54) compared with conventional fractionation (n = 28) (61% vs. 44% p = 0.09). In a major randomized non–site-specific study however, this approach proved no more efficacious than a once-daily, standard fractionation therapy (90).

In selected patients with small primary tumors that are amenable to definitive irradiation but in whom bulky cervical metastases are present, curative irradiation to the primary tumor and neck, followed by neck dissection, has been used and function has been preserved. Mendenhall et al. report a 2-year control rate of 80% for disease above the clavicles in patients with advanced neck disease and early primary tumors treated in this fashion (74). Dubois et al. (60) report that locoregional control was comparable in patients with low N-stage T1 to T2, N1b disease (locoregional control 68% vs. 69%, respectively), but worse with extensive neck disease, T1 to T2, N3 (locoregional control 11% vs. 34%, respectively), after treatment with radiotherapy alone compared with combined treatment.

Salvage Surgery

When radiation therapy fails, salvage surgery will typically require total laryngectomy, even if a function-preserving procedure might have been possible previously. Salvage surgery after definitive radiation therapy can be associated with significant morbidity, including tissue breakdown, chronic fistulae, and hemorrhage (134). Davidson et al. report on 88 patients with advanced larynx (n = 58) or hypopharynx (n = 30) cancers failing radiotherapy with or without chemotherapy who underwent salvage surgery (134). Among hypopharynx cancers, the rate of attempted salvage was 55% with success in 47%. The overall survival was 35% at 5 years, which is similar to those undergoing up-front surgery. The survival was related to the stage of the recurrent tumor rather than to the initial lesion. Complications occurred in 48% (42/88) and consisted primarily of fistula (n = 24), delayed wound healing (n = 4), and flap necrosis (n = 2). If patients are able to undergo salvage surgery with primary tumor and nodal excision, Dubois et al. show that the 5-year survival rates are comparable to patients with newly diagnosed lesions undergoing upfront surgery and radiation; however, the number who underwent such a procedure was small (17 of 157 total locoregional failures) (60). It should be emphasized that among all patients failing radiation therapy, multiple other series report that, at best, about half are eligible for salvage surgery; many are excluded because they present with even more advanced disease than at initial presentation. Even among those undergoing salvage surgery the overall survival is poor (20%–23% at 5 years) (135,136).

T3 AND T4 RESECTABLE DISEASE

Although early stage hypopharynx cancers may be treated by the selective application of either surgery or radiation alone, locally/regionally advanced disease requires a combined modality approach.

Surgery and Radiation

The historical standard treatment for patients with T3 and T4 resectable disease is total laryngectomy with partial pharyngectomy, often with neck dissection, followed by postoperative radiation therapy in patients with bulky T-stage disease, positive or close surgical margins, or lymph node involvement.

The results with radiation therapy as a single modality in the advanced disease setting—the historical larynx preservation option—are disappointing (60), especially in terms of obtaining local control (Table 20.4). Among 344 patients with T3 hypopharynx tumors treated with definitive, conventionally fractionated radiation therapy at the Institut Curie, determinate local control at 2 years was only 38% and 5-year survival was 17% (57). Johansen et al. report the Aarhus University experience of 138 consecutive patients with hypopharynx SCCs, of whom 120 were treated with radical radiotherapy out of 124 treated with curative intent (137). In this group, in which three-fourths of the patients were stage III to IV, 5-year overall survival, disease-specific survival, and locoregional control were 21%, 28%, and 23%, respectively. Five-year local and nodal failure was 61% and 48%, respectively. No T4 or N3 patients had tumor control. The results reported by Mendenhall et al. were little better (61). In the series of pharyngeal wall tumors described by Fein et al., the 5-year local control rates for T3 and T4 disease were 49% and 36%, respectively (64).

The use of adjuvant radiation therapy for hypopharyngeal cancer is heavily influenced by single-institution studies (Table 20.6) that suggest an improvement of approximately 28% to 43% in locoregional control when radiation therapy is combined with surgery, compared with historical results (75, 138–140). Despite locoregional control up to 89%, overall survival remains poor at 40% to 58% due to distant metastases and competing causes of mortality.

Several authors have shown the feasibility of combining surgery with radiation. Vandenbrouck et al. report on 199 patients treated with nonconservation surgery and postoperative radiation (50–65 Gy) (7). The majority had stage III to IV tumors (88% T3 or T4 and 73% node-positive). Locoregional control was 83% (local control 88%, regional control 92%), with a 5-year survival of 33%. Distant metastases occurred in 28%. Kraus et al. report on 132 patients undergoing combined surgery, three fourths of whom received radiation therapy (141). Seventy-eight percent had stage III to IV tumors. Locoregional control was obtained in 61%. Five-year overall survival and disease-free survival were 30% and 41%, respectively.

Retrospective comparisons from several authors suggest the superiority of the combined approach in patients with advanced disease. Dubois et al. report a 5-year local control, locoregional control, and overall survival of 46%, 32%, and 30%, respectively, in 100 patients with T3 to T4 disease treated with surgery and postoperative radiotherapy (60). In 148 patients treated with radiation alone, local control, locoregional control, and overall survival were 35%, 13%, and 2%, respectively. Meoz-Mendez et al. report a 25% failure rate for T3 and T4 tumors of the pharyngeal walls 1 year after treatment with surgery and postoperative irradiation and a 49% failure rate for similar lesions treated by irradiation alone (142). These authors concluded that for advanced lesions, combined therapy was superior.

Table 20.6 Hypopharyngeal Cancer: Comparison of Radiation vs. Surgery plus Radiation

Series	T stage[a] and site	No. of patients	Treatment	Local control	Locoregional control	5-year survival (%)
Van den Bogaert et al. (139)	T3–T4	66	Radiation	22%	NS	18%
	T3–T4	22	Surgery + radiation	51%	NS	18%
Mendenhall et al. (61)	T1–T2	35	Radiation	74%	NS	60%
	T3–T4	15		27%	NS	23%
	T1–T2	6	Surgery + radiation	67%	NS	33%
	T3–T4	47		72%	NS	30%
Dubois et al. (60)	T1–T2	61 (24 N0)	Radiation	74%	54%	11% (50% N0)
	T3–T4	148		35%	13%	2%
	T1–T2	54	Surgery + radiation	63%	43%	37%
	T3–T4	100		46%	32%	30%
Slotman et al. (140)	T3–T4	22	Radiation	NS	64%	22%
	T3–T4	32	Surgery + radiation	NS	97%	22%
Pingree et al. (149)	Stage I/II	78	Radiation	NS	NS	41%
	Stage III/IV	168				12%
	Stage I/II	46	Surgery + radiation	NS	NS	40%
	Stage III/IV	285				32%

NS, not stated.
[a]Tumor, node, metastases system used varies with time of publication.

Regional control according to N-stage varies from 77% to 96% for N0, 43% to 95% for N1, 50% to 80% for N2, and 42% to 90% for N3 (7,60,143). Five-year survival rates are a disappointing 11% to 35% (6,7,143) and are influenced by N stage: 33% to 40% for N0, 28% to 40% for N1, 20% to 24% for N2, and 9% to 24% for N3. Distant metastases are a common problem as is death from comorbid disease or second primaries.

El Badawi et al. reviewed the M. D. Anderson Cancer Center experience comparing 125 patients treated by total pharyngolaryngectomy, neck dissection, and postoperative radiation (60 Gy) to 203 similarly staged patients (T3–4 in 94% vs. 90%, and N2–3 58% and 52%, respectively) treated with surgery alone (75). Only patients with microscopic disease and those who received radiation within 3 months of surgery were included. Locoregional recurrence was 39% at 1 year after surgery alone, as opposed to 11% after combined therapy. Five-year local control and survival (40% vs. 25%, respectively) were superior in those patients receiving adjuvant radiation. Complications in the postoperative radiation group occurred in 31% (39/125) and consisted primarily of pharyngeal stenosis (n = 17), subcutaneous or muscle fibrosis, soft tissue necrosis (n = 6), and radiation myelitis (n = 2, both due to junctional overlap). Pharyngeal stenosis occurred in 8% in those undergoing surgery only.

Others have also demonstrated the survival benefit of radiation with surgery (144–147), whereas some have reported worse outcome (13,148,149). The conflicting reports are likely the result of the inherent selection bias against those receiving radiation, because these patients tend to have poorer prognostic features. Overall, there is enough data to suggest a benefit from radiation in this setting.

Adjuvant radiotherapy has been used either before surgery to doses ranging from 30 Gy to greater than 55 Gy (6,73,121), but more often after surgery to doses of 44 to 75 Gy (60,121,143). Two randomized studies show that postoperative radiation therapy yields superior locoregional control, compared with preoperative therapy. Vandenbrouck et al. report a randomized clinical trial of preoperative versus postoperative radiation therapy in 49 patients with tumors of the piriform sinus, aryepiglottic fold, or the arytenoid area and treated during the late 1960s (73). The preoperative group (n = 25) received 5,500 cGy to the tumor bed and lymph nodes prior to surgery. The postoperative group (n = 24) received 5,500 cGy within 4 weeks after surgery. The surgical procedure in both arms included total laryngectomy, partial pharyngectomy, and ipsilateral radical neck dissection. Primary site distribution was balanced between the arms, although there were more T4 (8 vs. 5) and N3 (11 vs. 8) tumors on the preoperative arm. Eight of 25 patients (32%) on the preoperative arm did not undergo surgery because of subsequently discovered surgical contraindications (n = 5), patient refusal (n = 2), and patient death (n = 1). The trial had to be terminated prematurely because of an unacceptably high incidence of fatal carotid rupture in the preoperative arm (5 vs. 1). The 5-year survival rate was statistically superior in the postoperative arm (56% vs. 20%, respectively). Fistulae took longer to heal in the preoperative versus postoperative group (mean of 98 vs. 23 days).

The Radiation Therapy Oncology Group (RTOG) conducted a similar study on 277 patients with locally advanced head and neck cancers at multiple sites including the hypopharynx (n = 73, 26%) (78). Patients were assigned randomly to one of three arms: preoperative radiation therapy (5,000 cGy in 180–200 cGy fractions over 5–6 weeks) followed 4 to 6 weeks later by surgery; surgery followed 4 weeks later by postoperative radiation therapy (6,000 cGy); or definitive radiation therapy (6,500–7,000 cGy) with surgery for salvage. Patients with hypopharyngeal cancer were not eligible for the third arm. Locoregional control was superior with postoperative treatment ($p = 0.04$), which translated into a trend in overall survival improvement ($p = 0.15$). Subset analysis for the hypopharynx group was not reported. The rates of severe surgical and radiation therapy complications were no different between the arms.

Reconstruction

Because surgery frequently requires some type of flap reconstruction, functional outcome after these more extensive procedures is particularly relevant. Available studies are typically retrospective in design with associated inherent limitations. Single-stage reconstruction appears feasible and decreases morbidity. Postoperative irradiation can be pursued in a timely way after these techniques.

Free jejunal transfer for repair of circumferential hypopharyngeal defects at the M. D. Anderson Cancer Center was reviewed (150). Among 93 patients who underwent 96 such procedures, the success rate was 97%. All three failures were repaired successfully with a repeat free jejunal transfer. The overall complication rate was 57% (55/96), with fistula and stricture occurring most commonly at rates of 19% and 15%, respectively. The perioperative mortality was 2%. Eighty percent of patients tolerated an oral diet; factors predicting an inability to swallow included superior extent of resection within the nasopharynx and a greater overall length of reconstruction. Postoperative radiation did not appear to increase the incidence of dysphagia.

Barrett et al. report the results of 17 patients undergoing hypopharyngeal resection with jejunal interposition grafts followed by high doses of postoperative radiotherapy [median dose of 5,940 cGy (3,960–6,660 cGy)] (151). At a median follow up of 4.5 years, 13 of the 17 patients had swallowing function good enough to maintain or increase their weights with G-tube removal, whereas 4 never regained adequate swallowing function and remained dependent on the G-tube after receiving doses of 3,960 to 5,940 cGy (151). Five of the 13 required intermittent dilations to maintain good swallowing function. Cole et al. report their experience with 29 patients who were treated to a median dose of 63 Gy after receiving jejunal interposition grafts. At a median follow up of 20 months, all except one were able to maintain an oral diet (152). Thiele et al. report on 201 patients treated with jejunal interposition after pharyngolaryngectomy (117). In this report, 172 patients received postoperative radiotherapy and 92% of the 201 patients maintained good swallowing function with maintenance of weight. These studies indicate that a segment of jejunum may be transferred and irradiated to therapeutic doses with acceptable morbidity.

Induction/Adjuvant Chemotherapy When Surgical Resection Is Planned

Treatment with cisplatin-based combination chemotherapy will yield a major response in 60% to 80% of patients with local/regionally advanced, previously untreated SCC of the upper aerodigestive tract (153,154). A number of randomized trials have attempted to evaluate whether chemotherapy administered as induction neoadjuvant, or adjuvant therapy, or some combination of these (collectively termed *sequential chemotherapy*) with standard surgery and radiation therapy improves outcome in resectable patients compared with locoregional treatment alone. These studies are typically not site-specific and often are hampered by sample size issues and lack of standardization of locoregional treatment (154). Nonetheless, they have been used to define the role of these systemic approaches in patients with hypopharyngeal cancer as well as other head and neck sites. The randomized studies discussed here will further illustrate our current understanding of sequential chemotherapy.

The Head and Neck Contracts Program evaluated both an induction strategy (one cycle of cisplatin, 100 mg/m^2 intravenously on day 1; and bleomycin, 15 mg intravenous push on day 3, followed on days 3–7 by a 15-mg/m^2 infusion), as well as induction combined with adjuvant chemotherapy (6 planned cycles of cisplatin, 80 mg/m^2) (79). The Intergroup Adjuvant Study 0034 sandwiched three cycles of cisplatin and 5-fluorouracil (4-day infusion at standard doses) between surgery and radiation (80). A study by Paccagnella et al. evaluated an induction strategy 4 cycles of cisplatin/5-fluorouracil (5-day infusion at standard doses) and, unlike the prior studies (which were limited to patients with resectable disease), included unresectable patients as well (81). Locoregional treatment involved surgery and postoperative radiation therapy in all three studies, with the exception of the unresectable patients in the last study who underwent radiation therapy plus neck dissection (the latter if clinically indicated). The percentages of patients with hypopharyngeal cancer randomized in each study were 19%, 17%, and 27%, respectively. All these studies demonstrated no difference in survival or locoregional control; yet there was evidence of chemotherapy effect in that the incidence of distant metastases was significantly decreased in all three.

A subsequent multivariate analysis of the Head and Neck Contracts Program's data demonstrated that the subset of patients with N2 disease benefited the most from an induction-adjuvant strategy; however, no marked improvement for patients with hypopharyngeal cancer was shown (155). Large meta-analyses also have not shown any benefit on survival or for sequential chemotherapy (82,83). On the basis of such data, the use of sequential chemotherapy therapy in the setting of a planned resection is not recommended outside the protocol setting.

Chemoradiotherapy

The organ preservation concept using induction chemotherapy followed by definitive radiotherapy has been shown to be feasible by a number of pilot studies (Table 20.7) (156–161). The general approach was that patients were given two to three cycles of induction chemotherapy followed by definitive radiation therapy, with surgery reserved for nonresponse to induction chemotherapy, persistent disease after radiation, or relapse. Laryngeal preservation received the greatest attention, and the need for total laryngectomy often defined the study population. As such, patients with laryngeal, hypopharyngeal and, at times, advanced oropharynx cancers were often combined (153,162).

Karp et al. used induction cisplatin-based chemotherapy followed by conventionally fractionated radiation (65–75 Gy) for 35 patients with larynx or hypopharynx cancers requiring total laryngectomy (160). Among the 21 patients with hypopharynx cancer treated in this manner, local control was 33% at 2 years with a median survival of 12 months. Outcomes were better in patients with larynx cancer (77% 2-year local control and minimum survival of 39 months, $p = 0.009$).

Shrinian et al. report the M. D. Anderson Cancer Center experience using induction cisplatin-based chemotherapy followed by hyperfractionated radiation to 74.2 to 76.6 Gy in 64 patients with locally advanced hypopharynx (n = 29), larynx (n = 26), or oropharynx (n = 9) cancer (163). With regard to the hypopharynx cancer subset, complete response after chemotherapy was 15%, which increased to 83% at the end of radiation. At a follow up of 15 to 54 months, the 2-year larynx preservation rate was 28%, and overall survival was 46%. In a retrospective comparison reported by Clayman et al., survival appeared to be comparable with a similar cohort of patients treated with standard surgery and radiation (157).

In the Memorial Hospital series, 26 patients with resectable, locally advanced hypopharynx cancers requiring total laryngectomy were treated with induction, cisplatin-based chemotherapy followed by conventionally fractionated radiotherapy (66–70 Gy), if a partial or complete response at the primary was obtained (156). The response rate to induction chemotherapy was 69% (complete response—CR 46%, partial response—PR 23%), whereas 19% underwent salvage surgery and postoperative radiotherapy. At a median follow-up of 5 years, larynx preservation with local control was obtained in 52%, local control in 58%, regional control in 47%, disease-free survival in 30%, and overall survival in 15%. Regional failure was 73% among N2 and N3 patients and incidence of 5-year distant metastases was 33%. These results were comparable to those obtained in a similar group of 30 patients treated with surgery and postoperative radiotherapy at the same institution (5-

TABLE 20.7 Larynx Preservation in Hypopharyngeal Cancer: Single-Arm Induction Chemotherapy Studies

Series	Total no./ hypopharynx no.	Disease extent[a]	Survival (criteria)	Larynx preservation (criteria)	Comments
Zelefsky et al. (156)	26	T3, T4: 69% N2, N3: 50% ST III, ST IV: 92%	15% (actuarial 5-year)	52% local control (no TL at 5 years)	Survivorship comparable to historical controls treated with surgery and RT
Clayman et al. (157)	55/29	T4, T4 100%	55% (actuarial 2-year)	69% (no salvage TL)	Survival similar to matched historical controls; local failure higher, but fewer distant metastases
Denard et al. (158)	81/31	T3, T4: 71% ST III, ST IV: 54%	29% (crude rate)	7 of 10: 70% (sub-group with initial indication for TL, CR to CT, no TL)	Some patients would not have required TL as standard treatment
Fountzilas et al. (159)	154/12	T3, T4: 75% N2, N3: 50% (oropharynx and hypopharynx combined)	30% (actuarial 2-year, estimated from curve)	6 of 12: 50% (sub-group of all pharynx tumors, CR to CT-RT, no TL)	No separate data for hypopharyngeal cancer
Karp et al. (160)	35/21	T3, T4: 67% N2, N3: 57% ST III, ST IV: 90%	12 months (median)	33% (2-year local control with CT–RT)	Survival (p = 0.009) and local control inferior to larynx group

CR, complete response; CT, chemotherapy; RT, radiation therapy; ST, stage; TL, total laryngectomy.
[a]Tumor, node, metastases system used varies with time of publication.

year local control 59%, regional control 69%, disease-free survival 42%, and overall survival 22%).

Kim et al. retrospectively reviewed 37 hypopharynx cancers treated with cisplatin/5-fluorouracil followed by 65 to 70 Gy (164). The major response rate to chemotherapy was 86% (CR 24%). Among the nine patients achieving CR, seven were without evidence of any recurrence, one had regional recurrence but was successfully salvaged, and one was lost to follow-up. Among the 23 patients with PR, 18 proceeded to radiation, three underwent resection, and two received no treatment. Six of the 18 receiving radiation after PR were without evidence of disease at 3 years. Of the five nonresponders, three underwent radiotherapy but only one was successfully controlled. In total, 20 patients achieved a CR after having received both chemotherapy and radiation. Median follow-up was 35 months. Comparison of the 20 patients achieving CR after chemotherapy and radiation to a similar group of patients treated with resection and postoperative radiation demonstrated no statistically significant difference in local control (85% vs. 94%), regional failure (10% vs. 6%), 3-year disease-free survival (52% vs. 61%), and 3-year overall survival (65% vs. 72%). Larynx preservation was achieved in 43% at 3 years.

Studies like these (Table 20.7) provided observations that served as the basis for the development of organ preservation programs (162), and in particular, the design of a landmark randomized controlled trial conducted under the auspices of the EORTC (84). In the EORTC larynx preservation trial, patients with locally advanced, hypopharyngeal cancer (limited to the piriform sinus or hypopharyngeal aspect of the aryepiglottic fold), whose standard management would have necessitated total laryngectomy (T2 to T4, any N, M0, but excluding T2 exophytic lesions of the membranous piriform sinus or the aryepiglottic fold, or N2c neck disease) were randomly assigned between June 1986 to June 1993 to one of two treatment arms. Of the 202 patients studied, 194 were eligible for treatment.

One arm (n = 94) consisted of standard surgery and radiation therapy treatment: immediate total laryngectomy with partial pharyngectomy, neck dissection, and postoperative irradiation (5,000–7,000 cGy, 200 cGy fractions). The second arm (n = 100) involved chemotherapy and radiation therapy: induction chemotherapy with up to three cycles of cisplatin and 5-fluorouracil (5-day infusion at standard doses), followed by irradiation (7,000 cGy, 200 cGy fractions) in patients with a clinical complete response at the primary site; or standard surgery and radiation therapy in patients with less than a complete response at the primary site. Complete response was defined as total resolution of all macroscopic disease and complete return of laryngeal mobility. In patients with persistent neck disease after induction chemotherapy, the timing of neck dissection (before or after radiation therapy) was left to the discretion of the treating institution.

Baseline prognostic factors and treatment results are summarized in Table 20.8. Eight enrolled patients were not evaluable, owing to distant metastases (n = 1), tumor of the anterior epilarynx (n = 1), history of cancer (n = 1), N2c nodal disease (n = 3), or lack of information (n = 2). Stage and disease-site factors were balanced. Most patients were male (186/194; 96%), and the median age was 55 years (range, 35–70 years). With a median follow-up of 51 months (3–106 months), there was no statistical difference between the arms in either the rates of local and regional failures or in the appearance of second primary cancers. However, there were fewer distant metastases in the chemotherapy/radiation therapy arm (25% vs. 36%, $p = 0.041$). The median (25 vs. 44 months) and 3-year survival rates (43% vs. 57%) also favored the larynx preservation arm. However, this survival difference was not maintained at 5 years (34% vs. 29%), suggesting that the impact of chemotherapy on distant metastases may have been a delay rather than a decrease in absolute terms of distant failure.

With regard to larynx preservation, a functional larynx required that there was local disease control and no tracheostomy or feeding tube. For patients enrolled in the induction arm who were alive and disease-free, the 3-year rate of a functional larynx was 28%. This rate increased to 42% (35% at 5 years) if patients who died of regional or distant disease or

TABLE 20.8 EORTC Hypopharynx Larynx Preservation Study

	Surgery–RT, n (%)	Chemotherapy–RT, n (%)
Randomized	99	103
Eligible	94	100
Site		
Piriform sinus	74 (79%)	78 (78%)
Aryepiglottic fold	20 (21%)	22 (22%)
Stage		
II	6 (6%)	7 (7%)
III	51 (54%)	59 (59%)
IV	37 (39%)	34 (34%)
T3, T4	78 (83%)	78 (78%)
N2, N3	31 (33%)	31 (31%)
Patient deaths: causes	57 (61%)	59 (59%)
Hypopharyngeal cancer	40	35
Second primary cancer	8	7
Treatment-related death	0	2
Noncancer death	6	8
Unknown	3	7
Median survival	25 mos	44 mos
3- and 5-year survival		
Overall survival	43%/35%	57%/30%
Disease-free survival	32%/27%	43%/25%
3- and 5-year laryngeal preservation	—/—	42%/35%

EORTC, European Organization for Research and Treatment of Cancer; RT, radiation therapy.
Source: Adapted from Lefebure J-L, Chevalier D, Leboinski B, et al. Larynx preservation in pyriform sinus cancer: preliminary results of a European Organization for Research and Treatment of Cancer phase III trial. *J Natl Cancer Inst* 1996;88:890.

unrelated causes, but with local control and a functional larynx without surgery to the primary site, were counted as having successful larynx preservation. If only complete responders to induction chemotherapy at the primary site are considered in the denominator, the rate further increased to 64%. Among patients currently alive (n = 41) who were treated on the chemotherapy/radiation therapy arm, 19 (46%) had a functional larynx.

One of the concerns surrounding this approach is that for patients who are nonresponders to chemotherapy, outcome may be impaired by the delay in definitive treatment. At least one uncontrolled study suggested that durable long-term surgical salvage in this setting was disappointing (165). Thirty-four patients (33%) with an inadequate response to chemotherapy subsequently underwent surgical salvage and postoperative radiation therapy per protocol. The outcome of these patients was not different from that observed on the standard surgery/radiation therapy treatment arm.

Parallels are commonly drawn between the Department of Veterans Affairs (VA) (166) and the EORTC (84) laryngeal preservation studies. Although the conclusions from these landmark trials are similar, three important differences deserve emphasis. In the VA study, all patients had advanced laryngeal cancer; patients with a complete or partial response at the primary site were candidates for definitive radiation therapy, and the neck dissection, when indicated on the chemotherapy/radiation therapy arm, was performed after radiation therapy. The EORTC study, on the other hand, was limited to patients with piriform sinus cancer or the hypopharyngeal aspect of the aryepiglottic fold; only patients with a clinical, complete response to induction chemotherapy were candidates for definitive radiation therapy; and the timing of the neck dissection on the experimental arm, when indicated, was left to the discretion of the treating institution.

One randomized study is difficult to interpret in that it apparently contradicts the EORTC larynx preservation trial, as well as prior induction chemotherapy studies showing no survival benefit of sequential chemotherapy in the setting of a planned resection. A French randomized trial compared surgery and postoperative radiation to radiation therapy alone after induction chemotherapy (167). Ninety-two patients with locally advanced resectable hypopharynx cancer (T3–T4, N0–3, all in the piriform sinus) received three courses of neoadjuvant chemotherapy of 5-fluorouracil (1,000 mg/m^2 × 4 days) and cisplatin (100 mg/m^2) every 2 weeks and were then randomized to total laryngopharyngectomy and postoperative radiation (50–60 Gy) (n = 47, arm A) or to conventionally fractionated radiation alone, 70 to 75 Gy (n = 45, arm B), with salvage surgery if required and possible. Response rates at the tumor and nodal sites were better in arm B than arm A (79% vs. 67%, 73% vs. 54%, respectively), but were not significantly so by statistical testing. Compliance with chemotherapy was similar as were grade 3 and 4 chemotherapy-associated toxicities. At a mean follow up of 92 months, 5-year overall survival and median survival were better in arm A (37% vs. 19% and 40 months vs. 20 months, $p = 0.04$, respectively) with better local control (63% vs. 39%, $p < 0.01$, respectively). The larynx preservation rate in arm B was not mentioned. In comparison to the EORTC, patients with less than a complete response to induction chemotherapy including nonresponders continued on to radiotherapy, which may account for the differences in outcome. Also, other different eligibility criteria and policies regarding the incorporation of salvage surgery of the primary site and neck may also be important factors in attempting to reconcile the results of this study with the EORTC larynx preservation trial.

Efforts to improve on organ preservation results with chemotherapy/radiation in head and neck cancers have mainly focused on changes either to the radiation fractionation, the chemotherapy sequencing or both. The more important randomized trials are not site-specific to the hypopharynx.

Single-institution studies demonstrated promising improvements in locoregional control with the use of altered fractionated radiation schedules (Table 20.4) (76,77,168). Based on such evidence, the RTOG conducted a landmark trial (RTOG 90-03) comparing the leading altered fractionated regimens for multiple head and neck cancer sites, including hypopharynx cancers (13%). This study randomized 1,073 patients with primarily advanced squamous cell cancers of the head and neck to one of four arms: (a) conventional fractionation (CF) 2 Gy daily, 5 days a week to 70 Gy over 7 weeks; (b) split-course, accelerated fractionation (S-AF) with 1.6 Gy twice daily to 67.2 Gy over 6 weeks with an intentional 2-week break after 38.4 Gy and an interfraction interval of 6 hours; (c) delayed concomitant boost (DCB) with daily morning 1.8-Gy treatments and 1.5-Gy afternoon concomitant boost for the last 12 days of treatment with a 6-hour interfraction interval and a total dose of 72 Gy over 6 weeks; and (d) pure hyperfractionation (HF) with 1.2 Gy twice daily with an interfraction interval of 6 hours to a dose of 81.6 Gy per 7 weeks. Eligible sites included the oral cavity, oropharynx, hypopharynx, and supraglottic larynx with stage III to IV disease, or stage II if hypopharynx or base of tongue. In a preliminary analysis with a median follow up of 23 months for all analyzable patients, there was significantly better 2-year, locoregional control for DCB (54.5%) and HF (54.4%) vs. CF (46%), $p = 0.05$ and 0.045, respectively, and a trend toward improved disease-free survival that favored DCB (39.3%) and HF (37.6%) vs. CF (31.7%) ($p = 0.054$ and 0.067, respectively) (90). Of note, overall survival was not significantly different among the four arms of the study. Acute grade 3 to 4 toxicity was increased compared with CF (59% vs. 55% vs. 35%, respectively). Chronic grade 3 to 4 toxicity was increased at 3 months for the DCB arm (37% vs. 27%), but was no different by 6 to 24 months compared with the control arm. There was no difference in chronic grade 3 to 4 toxicity in the HF arm (28% vs. 27%) compared with CF.

In studies not site-specific to the hypopharynx, others have shown in randomized studies that adding chemotherapy to conventionally fractionated radiation (87,88) or altered fractionated radiation (169) improves outcome in the treatment of head and neck cancers compared with radiation alone. Furthermore, when chemotherapy and radiation are combined, the concurrent integration of the modalities appears superior to a sequential approach (94–97). Although not all studies have shown a survival advantage with a concurrent strategy (170), available meta-analyses also demonstrate improvement in survival when chemotherapy is added concurrently to radiation (82,83), with superiority to sequential chemotherapy/radiation or to radiation alone. It should be emphasized that local acute toxicity is generally increased with the concurrent integration of the modalities, and that among resectable patients, when the contribution of salvage surgery is included, overall survival may not be improved by the integration of chemotherapy (87,89). The overwhelming majority of these concurrent studies infuse chemotherapy intravenously, although dose-intensive chemotherapy using targeted intraarterial chemotherapy concurrent with definitive radiotherapy have also shown encouraging preliminary results for hypopharynx cancers (171) as well as other head and neck cancers.

A randomized study addressing the management of advanced laryngeal cancer with larynx preservation intent is particularly relevant to future investigations of management strategies for advanced hypopharynx cancer. Forastiere et al. showed the superiority of adding chemotherapy concurrently rather than as induction to optimize larynx preservation in the preliminary analysis of the landmark RTOG 91-11, a three-arm study of patients with larynx cancers deemed to need total laryngectomy. Patients were randomized to three nonsurgical approaches: (a) conventionally fractionated radiation alone (70 Gy/7 weeks); (b) induction chemotherapy (standard cisplatin/infusional 5-fluorouracil) followed by 70 Gy per 7 weeks; or (c) cisplatin 100 mg/m^2 on days 1, 22, and 43 concurrent with 70 Gy per 7 weeks (89). At a minimum follow-up of 2 years, 2-year laryngectomy-free survival was best in the concurrent chemoradiation arm compared with arms B and A, respectively (66% vs. 58% vs. 52%). Median time to laryngectomy was also longest on the concurrent arm. Overall survival, however, was no different among the arms. A major EORTC study (No. 24 954) that is comparing sequential and concurrent chemotherapy/radiation strategies in patients with advanced larynx or hypopharynx cancer is in progress.

Given the concurrent chemotherapy/radiation data described here, the use of this approach in an adjuvant fashion is of great interest. A recently reported non–site-specific study done by the EORTC randomized 334 patients with locally advanced, poor-risk head and neck cancer to postoperative radiation (66 Gy in 33 fractions over 6.5 weeks) versus the same radiation program with cisplatin 100 mg/m^2 every 3 weeks for three cycles (172). Functional mucosal reactions were significantly more common with the addition of chemotherapy, although by objective criteria, these reactions were more similar. Locoregional control, disease-free survival, and overall survival were all significantly improved on the chemotherapy/radiation arm. The preliminary results of a similarly designed RTOG study failed to show improvements of similar magnitude (173). Further follow-up and analysis of these studies will be of great interest and may affect the adjuvant treatment recommendations for poor-risk patients.

UNRESECTABLE DISEASE M0, M1 DISEASE

In patients with surgically unresectable, locally advanced disease, the prognosis is dismal, with 5-year survival rates of 10% to 25% after treatment with definitive radiotherapy alone. Conventional management with radiation therapy as a single modality has yielded disappointing outcomes. For example, Mendenhall et al. report local control after initial radiation therapy in only one of eight patients with T4 piriform sinus cancer (61). With conventional fractionation for T4 pharyngeal wall tumors, the group at Massachusetts General Hospital reports a local control rate of 20% and a 3-year disease-free rate of 0% (133).

The integration of chemotherapy with radiation therapy is being pursued as an approach to unresectable disease (92,93), and the preceding discussion regarding chemoradiotherapy for advanced T3 to T4 disease is applicable here as well. Of interest, on subset analysis of the Paccagnella study (81), patients with unresectable tumors experienced improvement in survival, locoregional control, and distant control with induction chemotherapy. Concomitant therapy appears to have a more promising track record than a sequential approach (82,83,94–97). Improved control in the unresectable setting would have obvious implications for potential organ preservation strategies.

Perhaps the most publicized trial addressing the role of concomitant chemotherapy and radiation therapy in this setting was published by Merlano et al. (174). One hundred and fifty-seven patients with unresectable head and neck cancer were randomly assigned to radiation therapy alone (7,000 cGy in 180–200 cGy fractions) or to four courses of cisplatin (20 mg/m^2 intravenously) and 5-fluorouracil (200 mg/m^2 intravenously) for 5 consecutive days every 3 weeks, alternating with 2,000 cGy in 200 cGy fractions (total dose of 6,000 cGy). Eighteen percent of the randomized patients had hypopharyngeal cancer. The complete response rate (22% vs. 43%), 5-year locoregional relapse-free rate (32% vs. 64%), progression-free rate (9% vs. 21%), and overall survival (10% vs. 24%) all significantly favored the chemotherapy/radiation therapy arm. An update confirmed these results with longer term follow-up (175). A major concern surrounding this study was that the control rate with radiation therapy alone was poorer than expected, possibly reflecting treatment interruptions (>1 week in 25% of patients) and the relatively low mean radiation dose (6,560 cGy). A more recently repeated non–site-specific study performed through the cooperative group mechanism in the United States compared radiation alone (70 Gy, 2 Gy/day) to the same radiation schedule with concurrent cisplatin, or a split-dose radiation schedule with concurrent cisplatin and 5-fluorouracil with possible surgical resection depending on response. Chemotherapy/radiation proved superior to radiation alone, and the more complicated split-dose combination chemotherapy arm offered no advantage compared with the single-agent cisplatin/radiation arm (176).

Overall, the prognoses for patients with M1 disease at presentation are worse than for individuals with disease limited above the clavicles, and likely incurable. Patients with distant metastases are often lumped for study purposes with individuals having recurrent disease, in whom median survivals of less than one year are typical (177–180). Because patients presenting with M1 disease initially are untreated, the anticipated response rate to chemotherapy may be higher, and the application of a local modality such as radiation with or without chemotherapy to facilitate locoregional control is potentially feasible. As a result, some of these patients may have more prolonged survivals.

Cervical Esophageal Cancer

Efforts to evaluate management results for this site are hampered by its rarity, grouping of results with thoracic esophageal cancers or hypopharynx cancers, the wide variety of surgical and adjuvant approaches, and lack of accurate clinical staging. Available data however indicate that outcomes are disappointing regardless of treatment approach with 5-year survival rates ranging from 12% to 27% (181–183). Given this worrisome prognosis, optimizing palliation becomes an important goal.

Surgery

Surgery, usually in combination with postoperative radiation, is the historic standard approach. Collins and Spiro report on 71 patients with cervical esophageal cancers treated at MSKCC (184). Thirty-five patients underwent curative resection with primarily gastric transposition (n = 17), colonic interposition (n = 7), or deltopectoral flaps (n = 4). Twenty-six percent (9/35) had a positive microscopic margin. Fifty-four percent received adjuvant therapy consisting of radiation in 37% (13/35), chemoradiation 11% (4/35), or chemotherapy 6% (2/35). Postoperative complications occurred in 62%. Among those curatively resected, the primary complications were wound sepsis (20%), tracheal necrosis (13%), pharyngeal fistula/anastomotic leak (13%), and hemorrhage (4%). Perioperative mortality was 11%. The median duration of local response after surgery was 9 months. The median survival was 15 months. For all patients, the 5-year actuarial survival rate was 10%. Tracheal invasion and vocal cord paralysis were predictive of poorer survival. Locoregional failure occurred in 88% of the evaluable patients.

In a later report of 67 cervical esophageal cancers, 36 were considered resectable and managed with a variety of approaches intended for cure (46). Twenty-two underwent resection, ten were treated with primary radiotherapy with or without chemotherapy, and four received chemotherapy alone. Seven surgically treated patients received postoperative radiotherapy. Outcome was best in surgically treated patients with a mean survival of 45 months compared with 18 months for the 14 patients treated nonsurgically, and 17 months for all 67 patients in the study. Fifty percent of patients treated surgically were dead of disease and 50% were without disease. This compared with 79% who were dead of disease in the nonsurgically treated group. Locally persistent disease was present in 27% vs. 50%, respectively, for patients undergoing radical resection vs. radiotherapy. Swallowing assessment available in 40 patients showed that 12 of 19 treated surgically (63%) and 6 of 11 (55%) treated nonsurgically were able to eat by mouth. The authors concluded that a primary surgical approach offered better locoregional control and survival compared with nonsurgically treated patients with better palliation of dysphagia. However, it is difficult to determine how selection bias influenced outcome among the 36 patients who were considered resectable.

Griffiths and Shaw report that 34% of their patients with carcinoma of the cervical esophagus who were treated by resection and colon interposition were alive at last contact; however, the length of follow-up was brief (185). The two long-term survivors were treated by resection and postoperative irradiation. Preoperative irradiation did not render effective palliation, but did increase the risk for postsurgical complications. Kato et al. report that nine of 13 patients treated with esophageal reconstruction after surgery for carcinoma were alive and free of disease, whereas three died of recurrent carcinomas (116). Significant palliation was accomplished as all patients were able to swallow at the time they were discharged from the hospital. Resection followed by immediate reconstruction achieves the goals of reestablishing the ability to swallow, the timely administration of radiotherapy, and rapid healing (186).

The experience at the M. D. Anderson Cancer Center with cervical esophageal carcinoma treated by aggressive multimodality therapy, including surgery and postoperative radiation therapy, was similarly disappointing. Among 95 patients treated from 1965 to 1988, the 5-year disease-specific survival rate was 31%; however, overall survival was only 15% (187).

Bardini et al. report on 291 cervical esophageal and hypopharynx cancers, of which 187 originated in the cervical region (188). Fifty-three percent (n = 153) underwent resection (188). Five-year overall survival was 18% among those with cervical esophageal cancers. Among 24 patients with cervical esophageal carcinoma undergoing larynx-sparing surgery, none were cured. Various anastomotic methods were used including pharyngogastric (n = 95), colonic interposition (n = 11), or jejunal loop (n = 18). Anastomotic leaks occurred in 23%, 18%, 6%, respectively; and hospital mortality occurred in 15%, 18%, and 0%, respectively.

Radiation Therapy

Mendenhall et al. report the University of Florida experience of 34 patients with cervical esophageal cancer treated with definitive radiotherapy (189). Patients were treated to a dose of up to 70 Gy with conventional fractionation or 74.4 to 76.8 Gy with hyperfractionation. At a minimum follow-up of 5 years, the 5-year locoregional control, disease-specific survival, and overall survival rate were 25%, 22%, and 15%, respectively. The crude rate of distant metastases was 26%. Newaishy et al. report the Edinburgh experience, which treated 444 esophageal cancers with primary radiotherapy over a 19-year period; 37 of which were located in the cervical esophagus (190). Radiation therapy consisted of 50 to 55 Gy in 4 weeks. The 5-year crude survival was 19% and appeared better compared with those located in the thoracic esophagus (5-year crude survival 8%). Other series of radical radiotherapy report 5-year survival rates of 25% to 32% without reporting local control (182,191).

Brachytherapy is a possible option to boost the radiation dose to cervical esophageal lesions. However, its use has been discouraged by the American Brachytherapy Society due to the possibility of severe complications such as tracheoesophageal fistula formation (192).

Chemoradiation

An Intergroup study demonstrated the superiority of chemoradiation (cisplatin/5-fluorouracil × 4 cycles with 50 Gy/5 weeks concurrent with cycles 1 and 2) versus radiotherapy alone (64 Gy/6.5 weeks) for esophageal lesions (102,193). Most patients in this study had SCCs, but of 121 evaluable patients only one had cervical esophageal cancer. At last report with a minimum follow up of 5 years, the 5-year actuarial survival was 25% in the chemoradiation arm compared with 0% in patients treated with radiotherapy only (193). Locoregional persistent disease or failure was decreased by 20% in the chemoradiation patients (46% vs. 68%, respectively), but remained the primary source of failure. Treatment-related acute toxicity was increased in the combined modality arm (RTOG grade 4, 8% vs. 2% and treatment-related deaths, 2% vs. 0%), but no differences were detected in chronic toxicity. Improvements in dysphagia were no different between the arms. The results were reproduced in a subsequently accrued cohort treated with chemoradiation. However, all cases involved the thoracic esophagus, some of which were adenocarcinomas.

Concurrent chemoradiation for cervical esophageal cancers has been reported in multiple single-institution studies. Burmeister et al. report promising results on 34 cervical esophageal patients treated with primary chemoradiation (194). The majority of patients were early or intermediate stage [UICC I–IIB (31/34)]. Chemotherapy consisted primarily of cisplatin and 5-fluorouracil (n = 32) or 5-fluorouracil alone (n = 2) given concurrently on weeks 1 and 4 of conventional fractionated radiation to a mean dose of 61 Gy (50–65 Gy). Local complete response was 91% based on follow-up endoscopy. At a median follow-up of 55 months, local control was 88% and actuarial 5-year survival was 55%. Acute toxicities included need for tube feeding in 15% (5/34), grade 3+ myelosuppression in 12% (4/34), aspiration pneumonia in 6% (2/34), and cardiac failure in 3% (1/34). Chronic toxicities included primarily stricture formation in 44% (15/34), 4 of which required dilation. Nearly all patients were reported to maintain acceptable speech capacity. Two patients died of complications related to stricture formation including hemorrhage and tracheoesophageal fistula.

Soto Parra et al. report on 37 patients with more advanced cervical esophageal carcinoma (54% were stage III) also treated with cisplatin and 5-fluorouracil concurrent with radiation doses of 50 to 60 Gy (195). More advanced lesions were treated in this study. The complete response rate was 65% (24/37) and 5-year survival was 32%. One treatment-related death was reported. The rate of stricture was not reported. Santoro et al. report on 27 patients treated with 4 cycles of cisplatin/5-fluorouracil and split-course radiotherapy to 50 Gy (30 Gy during cycle 1 and 20 Gy at cycle 3 of chemotherapy). One-fourth of advanced stage lesions appeared cured by this approach; however, 64% eventually failed locally (196). The four patients with stage I disease were alive and disease-free at minimum follow-up of 43 months without requiring laryngectomy or esophagectomy.

Other approaches have modified the sequence of chemotherapy and radiation but without obvious improvement in survival. Stuschke et al. report on 17 locally advanced cervical esophageal cancers treated with induction chemotherapy followed by concurrent chemoradiation (197). Induction chemotherapy consisted of two to three courses of 5-fluorouracil/leucovorin/cisplatin with or without etoposide followed by concurrent cisplatin/etoposide and conventionally fractionated radiotherapy to 60 to 66 Gy. At a median follow-up of 37 months, 3-year survival was 24%. After treatment, 47% and 35% had a complete and partial response, respectively. Two-year locoregional failure was 67% and distant metastases 39%. The three long-term survivors had normal swallowing without severe chronic side effects.

A rapidly alternating regimen of chemotherapy with accelerated radiation was investigated in 47 patients with esophageal (n = 24) or hypopharynx cancers (n = 23) (123). The esophageal tumors were primarily of the upper or middle third in 75% (18/24) and squamous cell histology in 88% (21/24). Three cycles of cisplatin/5-fluorouracil were given on weeks 1, 4, and 7, whereas twice daily accelerated radiation was given on weeks 2, 5, and 8 delivering a total of 60 Gy. Acute toxicity was severe with 29% (7/24) treatment-related deaths, the majority related to sepsis, whereas 8% discontinued therapy due to toxicity. Among the 17 patients with evaluable cervical esophageal cancers, 94% had a complete response (confirmed pathologically in 14 of 17), whereas one patient had a partial response. Late toxicities included a chronic radiation pneumonitis, prolonged neutropenia, and esophageal fibrosis. At a median follow-up of 2 years, the 2-year locoregional control was 94% and distant metastases rate was 25%. Death due to esophageal cancer occurred in 17% (4/24), whereas an additional 7 patients died of other causes without cancer such that the 2-year actuarial survival was 28%. The authors concluded that although the rapidly alternating regimen produced high rates of locoregional control, considerable efforts, possibly including growth factor or peripheral stem cell support, would be needed to reduce toxicity to acceptable levels.

Although toxicity is significant, and outcomes have definite room for improvement, concurrent chemoradiation appears to represent the optimal nonsurgical approach with 5-year survival varying from 25% to 55%, probably reflecting the different proportions of advanced stage patients.

Trimodality Therapy

In an effort to address the high locoregional failure rates after concurrent chemoradiation, an important issue is the value of esophagectomy following chemoradiation. The outcomes of 400 patients with esophageal cancers treated in 63 institutions and studies in a 1992 to 1994 Patterns of Care survey showed that patients receiving trimodality treatment of preoperative chemoradiation followed by esophagectomy demonstrated a higher 2-year survival compared with chemoradiation (63% vs. 39%, $p = 0.11$) (100).

Randomized trials, primarily enrolling patients with thoracic esophageal cancers, have largely shown no survival benefit from preoperative chemotherapy or chemoradiation (198–202). The only trial that did show a survival benefit was reported by Walsh et al., and involved 113 patients with adenocarcinomas of the esophagus randomized to cisplatin/5-fluorouracil concurrent with 40 Gy in 3 weeks followed by surgery vs. resection alone (203). The trimodality arm showed an improvement in median survival (16 vs. 11 months) and 3-year survival (32% vs. 6%). However, survival in the control arm was lower than expected based on other large randomized studies. Limited observations using preoperative radiotherapy followed by surgery for cervical esophagus tumors have shown no obvious survival benefit with this approach (204).

A University of Michigan trial randomized patients with either cervical or thoracic esophageal carcinoma to a preoperative hyperfractionated chemoradiation regimen compared with surgery alone (205). One hundred patients received either chemotherapy (cisplatin, 5-fluorouracil, and vinblastine) concurrent with 1.5-Gy twice daily radiotherapy to 45 Gy all over 3 weeks followed 3 weeks later by transhiatal esophagectomy and gastric pull-up or colon interposition versus surgery alone.

Eight percent of patients on both arms had cancers located in the cervical esophagus, and three fourths overall were adenocarcinomas. At a median follow-up of 8.2 years, there was no significant difference in median survival (17.5 vs. 16.9 months) between surgery or preoperative chemoradiation followed by surgery. On multivariate analysis, SCCs and tumor size greater than 5 cm were poor prognostic factors for survival. However, there was no detectable difference between cervical versus thoracic esophageal lesions. Among patients receiving combined modality therapy, those with a pathologic complete response (28% of patients) had a better median overall survival compared with those with residual disease in the resected specimen (50 months vs. 12 months, respectively, $p = 0.01$).

UNRESECTABLE M0, M1

Two randomized trials have evaluated a strategy of concomitant chemotherapy/radiation therapy versus radiation therapy alone in patients with unresectable esophageal cancer (108,109). Neither study demonstrated an improvement in overall survival that remains at less than 12 months, on average.

Patients with distant metastases at presentation have incurable disease because currently available systemic chemotherapy is not predictably curative. These patients are often grouped with patients with incurable recurrent disease for chemotherapy treatment studies. As with the hypopharynx, combination chemotherapy may increase response rate, but the minority of patients will have a major response and the impact on survival is disappointing, with 1-year survival rates less than 50%. One randomized study has compared the efficacy of cisplatin with 5-fluorouracil to single-agent therapy (cisplatin). Eighty-nine patients with unresectable esophageal SCC were randomly chosen. The combined regimen doubled the response rate (36% vs. 11%). However, there was no significant difference in 1-year survival rates (38% vs. 28%; $p = 0.43$), although the number of patients randomized was too small to rule out a false-negative result (206).

Newer chemotherapy agents, including the taxanes (paclitaxel and docetaxel) as well as irinotecan have shown promising single-agent activity in esophageal cancer, although these studies were not limited to the cervical esophagus, or to squamous histology (207–210). Multimodality trials of paclitaxel incorporated into chemoradiation regimens show encouraging rates of pathologic complete responses (211,212). The appropriate means for incorporating these newer agents as well as biologically targeted agents that are currently in development remains investigational for cervical esophageal cancers.

Quality of Life

The effects of therapy for cancers of the hypopharynx and cervical esophagus must be considered beyond the disease process itself. Treatment results in profound effects on speech, swallowing, cosmetic appearance, social acceptance, and ability to return to the workplace.

Data quantitating the functional and quality-of-life outcomes of these patients are limited, especially in older studies. Unlike information regarding local control, survival, and toxicity, these outcomes are more difficult, if not impossible, to quantitate retrospectively. Most of the data are not site-specific.

Lefebvre et al. assessed function preservation in the EORTC hypopharynx study (84). Lack of requirement of a tracheostomy or a feeding tube was the primary criterion used. The authors highlighted the manner in which the laryngeal preservation rate can vary simply because of varying criteria. Certain studies have addressed the impact of total laryngectomy and other surgical procedures (213), including application of speech and swallowing physiologic measures (214). Coia et al. evaluated swallowing function after chemotherapy/radiation therapy in patients with esophageal cancer using a swallowing-function scoring system (215). Distal tumors had more improvement than those in the upper two thirds of the esophagus. Only the minority of patients in this series had cervical esophageal cancer. Bradford et al. evaluated functional results after free jejunal flap reconstruction in a series of 20 patients who underwent the procedure (216). Successful swallowing was retained in 58%, with a median time to success of 14.5 days.

Prospective clinical studies are investigating the subjective and objective effects on quality of life of these patients as a result of their disease and its treatment. A number of validated instruments now exist to obtain such information (FACT, EORTC-QLQ-C30, List scale) (217,218). However, these tools are generally applied to a cross-section of primary cancers, so site-specific data are very limited. Still, a clearer understanding of these issues, as well as relevant psychosocial issues, patient motivation, and coexisting medical problems, will allow physicians to educate and care for their patients in the most appropriate manner. It should be emphasized that physicians and other health care professionals may prioritize outcomes very differently than patients, and that patient input is extremely important (219–222).

COMPLICATIONS

Surgery

HYPOPHARYNX

Most early complications after laryngopharyngectomy result from leakage at the site of the pharyngeal closure. A common technical cause of fistulization is a tight closure, wherein inadequate mucosa is available. Another common etiology of fistulization is presence of tumor at the margins of resection. Patients, especially malnourished patients, who receive preoperative radiation, will experience the highest incidence of wound breakdown. Complications such as chronic aspiration and repeated pulmonary infections after partial laryngectomy may necessitate a completion laryngectomy. Stricture formation is a potential late complication.

CERVICAL ESOPHAGUS

Significant complications may occur after radical resection and depend on the extent of resection, method of reconstruction, performance status of the patient, and surgical experience. Operative mortality was reported as 11% in a MSKCC study with postoperative complications in 62% (184). Surgical complications occurred in over 50% of patients in a later MSKCC series, including perioperative death (4.5%), fistula (27%), wound infection (18%), pneumonia (4.5%), deep vein thrombosis (4.5%), and sepsis (4.5%) (46).

Radiation Therapy

Acute radiation toxicity is mainly related to mucositis within the field. Enteral nutrition through some type of feeding tube is often necessary. Laryngeal edema occurs but will necessitate a tracheostomy in less than 10% of patients. Xerostomia and change in taste generally occur at standard radiation doses. Possible late effects primarily include fibrosis of the esophagus, which may develop into a stricture or fistula. Tracheoesophageal fistula may result after tumor regression and radiation effect and can result in a mediastinitis or aspiration pneumonia. Hypothyroidism is another common late effect that may require hormone replacement. Laryngeal chondronecrosis or soft-tissue necrosis of the pharyngeal wall occurs in 2% to 4% of patients. Ongoing inability to swallow, requiring permanent gastrostomy occurs in 2% to 7% of patients treated with radiation therapy alone and increases to 16% in the postoperative setting. There is an approximate 10% incidence of severe fibrosis of the soft tissues in the neck (57,61,74,75).

Fibrosis of the lung within the field rarely results in symptoms. Lhermitte sign can occur 2 to 3 months after treatment and last several weeks to months.

Chemotherapy

Potential side effects of chemotherapy depend on the specific agents used. Although current antiemetic regimens using 5-hydroxytryptamine receptor antagonists with steroids can control nausea and vomiting in the majority of patients receiving a cisplatin-based regimen (223), other potential dose-related and cumulative toxicities from cisplatin most commonly include: ototoxicity with tinnitus or high frequency hearing loss, peripheral neuropathy, nephrotoxicity which can manifest as renal insufficiency or electrolyte wasting, and myelosuppression (224). Carboplatin has a lower risk for renal and neurologic sequelae, which is balanced by more dose-limiting marrow suppression. The agent 5-flourouracil also causes hematologic toxicity in addition to mucositis, diarrhea, and vascular irritation, which may uncommonly result in coronary artery spasm. The most common adverse effects of paclitaxel include peripheral neuropathy, myelosuppression, and alopecia at higher doses. In addition, there is a significant risk for hypersensitivity reactions to the Cremophor diluent.

When administered concomitant with radiation, any of the previously described chemotherapeutic agents can magnify the local toxicity. In the short run, this may manifest as increased mucositis with dysphagia requiring percutaneous feeding tubes to facilitate nutritional support or enhanced skin breakdown within the radiation field.

MANAGEMENT OF RECURRENCE

In patients with local and regional recurrence only, the feasibility of further surgery and radiation therapy is an important initial consideration for both sites, as these modalities offer the potential for more durable disease control. Most of these patients have received prior radiation therapy either as definitive or adjuvant treatment, which typically limits radiation therapy options. Nonetheless, there is an evolving literature of integrated chemotherapy/radiation therapy in selected patients. Although the average survival results in these series appear little better than those obtained with chemotherapy alone, durable responses in selected patients are well documented (225). Further improvement in targeted radiation techniques should increase the feasibility of such approaches.

Hypopharyngeal Cancer

When operable, recurrences, especially when local, generally will require extensive surgery, including partial or circumferential pharyngectomy and total laryngectomy. Depending on the inferior extent of disease, a gastric pull-up or jejunal interposition may be necessary. The exact procedure will depend on the locoregional extension, general condition of the patient and patient compliance, the quality of the skin and connective tissues after irradiation, and surgical expertise. As there is often no adjuvant therapy, preoperative assessment must ensure that an extensive resection is feasible. Given the risk for postoperative complications in the post-radiation therapy setting (134), the most reliable surgical repair must be selected to minimize the risk for fistula or wound breakdown. Judicious use of myocutaneous or other flaps is useful. In one series of 160 patients with hypopharyngeal cancer operated on after radiation therapy (mean dose, 7,200 cGy), such an approach decreased the postoperative death rate from 23% to 10% (226). For neck recurrences, the incision should not coincide with the arterial axis. Whenever possible, complete neck dissection rather than adenectomy should be done.

When surgery and radiation therapy are no longer feasible in the recurrent disease setting or there are distant metastases, chemotherapy is the historical palliative option. Studies evaluating the role of chemotherapy in this context are not site-specific. There are a number of active drugs. The most widely used are methotrexate, cisplatin-carboplatin, 5-fluorouracil, and more recently, paclitaxel, docetaxel, or gemcitabine (227). The activity of these agents is disappointing, and, even with therapy, patients typically live less than 1 year. Several randomized studies have compared single-agent versus combination chemotherapy (177–179). Combination chemotherapy with regimens like cisplatin/5-fluorouracil may increase the response rate, but the minority of patients will still have a major response, toxicity is increased, and there is no significant improvement in overall survival. Available data fail to support the routine initial use of combination chemotherapy in such patients, and emphasize the importance of new drug development. Adjunctive palliative measures, such as narcotic analgesics and nerve blocks for pain control or gastrostomy tubes to facilitate hydration and nutrition, are extremely important.

Cervical Esophageal Cancer

Although surgery or radiation-based treatment is initially considered for local and regional recurrence only, the odds of long-term salvage is low given the disappointing results in patients who are previously untreated. Many of these patients have received prior radiation therapy either as definitive or adjuvant treatment, so radiation therapy options are limited. Salvage surgery for local failure will jeopardize the larynx if present.

Incurable local disease is associated with debilitating dysphagia. A gastrostomy may bypass the problem and address related issues of nutrition and hydration but will not address the swallowing difficulty. Palliative bypass procedures can be performed, but operative mortality as high as 30% has been reported (228). External beam radiation therapy with or without chemotherapy will lead to improvement in 80% of appropriately selected patients, with palliation of the symptom until death in half of these responders. Improvement with radiation therapy generally takes 2 to 4 weeks, and the approach may not work as well in the setting of complete obstruction (215,229). Intraluminal brachytherapy, esophageal dilation, stent placement, tumor fulguration, and laser and photodynamic therapy have been used in this context (230,231). Cervical esophageal lesions are often too proximal for stent placement.

Chemotherapy as a single modality is not curative and associated with median survivals of less than a year, with approximately 30% of patients surviving 1 year. Besides the drugs listed for hypopharyngeal cancer, mitomycin C and the vinca alkaloids also are frequently used (107). As with hypopharynx cancer, a survival benefit with combination chemotherapy compared with a single agent is difficult to demonstrate (206). Novel investigational options deserve careful consideration for these patients.

FUTURE DIRECTIONS

Although many advancements have been made in the treatment of hypopharyngeal and cervical esophageal tumors, the outcomes, especially for patients with locally advanced and metastatic disease, remain disappointing. There are multiple opportunities for future investigation. Some of these apply or involve surgical therapies as well. Central to all such initiatives will be close interdisciplinary cooperation.

As most patients currently present with advanced disease, novel screening strategies will potentially increase the odds of early detection. Given the known role of tobacco and alcohol use as risk factors, developing optimal strategies to change high-risk behaviors is crucial, as are chemoprevention initiatives. Preliminary studies assessing the efficacy of oral administration of 13-*cis*-retinoic acid to reduce the incidence of second primaries in head and neck cancer patients are encouraging (127). This treatment and other promising chemopreventive agents deserve further evaluation in clinical trials given the risk among these patients of second primary tumors.

More work is needed to facilitate prognostication and therapeutic development, including the development and application of newer biomolecular tools. Our evolving understanding of the molecular biology of these tumors is already being applied to the clinical setting (232). New therapeutic agents that target specific molecular pathways in tumors, such as angiogenesis or the epidermal growth factor receptor pathway (233–235), are under development. The role of these novel strategies in the treatment of head and neck cancers is still being elucidated. We may be able to use genetic markers to differentiate between the clonal origin and heterogeneity of tumors, to better identify precancerous conditions for preventive screening, to distinguish new primary from recurrent tumors, and to detect cancerous cells in surgical margins and lymph nodes with greater sensitivity. For example, Koch et al. demonstrated the potential use of tumor-specific mutant oligomer probes for detecting rare cancer cells within surgical margins and lymph nodes (236). Although molecular probes may improve our pathologic analysis of head and neck neoplasms, further work is necessary to devise and implement alterations in therapeutic strategy that may be generated by these advances.

Improved locoregional control is central to increased survival in these diseases. The optimal integration of the various modalities to achieve this goal has yet to be defined. Organ and function preservation studies should remain a priority. Drugs with promising efficacy will require further assessment in the combined-modality/primary treatment setting as well as in the adjuvant setting to reduce the rate of distant failure. Follow-up of recent studies evaluating adjuvant concurrent chemotherapy with radiation is potentially important (172,173), as these studies may impact on the standard of care and treatment recommendations in the short run. Given the grim prognosis of patients with recurrent and metastatic disease, the development of better systemic therapies is sorely needed.

Well-done, randomized, site-specific studies will remain central to resolving many questions. Because of the relative rarity of these tumors and cost of such trials, however, single-arm studies will remain important sources of information. The quality of these studies need to be optimized to facilitate comparisons of treatment results among centers and to identify promising new approaches that warrant further evaluation in a random assignment trial.

Validated methodologies are available to quantitate function and quality of life in these patients. There is also an increasing interest in the relative costs of supposedly equivalent therapies. Such assessments will be crucial when comparing therapies that yield comparable local control and survival.

RADIOLOGIC IMAGING CONCERNS

Bernard B. O'Malley and Suresh K. Mukherji

The hypopharyngoesophageal complex is a continuum along which disease can arise or spread. Each subsegment, however, entails different clinical and imaging considerations. The lumen of this segment of the alimentary tract is best evaluated with oral contrast fluoroscopy (Fig. 20.8) (237). The hypopharynx and upper esophagus should be evaluated with air and contrast techniques in dynamic and static modes. Mural abnormalities need confirmation in the distended and collapsed phases, preferably in two different projections (Fig. 20.9). The swallowing mechanism should be studied with videofluoroscopy or high-speed camera attachments to the fluoroscope. In addition to outlining exophytic and obstructing lesions (Fig. 20.10), the fluoroscopic examination can reveal segmental motility disorders, which indicate infiltrating components of the lesion. Unfortunately, dysphagia is a late-presenting symptom of advanced tumor. Fluoroscopic examinations are helpful on follow-up during treatment to demonstrate treatment response, rule out fistulization, and differentiate recurrence from stricture in the reconstructed pharyngoesophageal segment.

Given the fact that most lesions present at advanced stages, cross-sectional imaging is useful for staging the extramural extension within and, occasionally, beyond the central compartment of the neck and mediastinum (Fig. 20.11). Either CT or MRI is adequate for lymph node staging and local extramural extension. Diluted oral contrast, not usually applied to neck imaging protocols, is used to locate the lumen (Fig. 20.12) and to help distinguish between contour abnormalities of the esophagus and pathologic tracheoesophageal nodes. Tumors of the cervical esophagus should be scanned by CT, with the patient in the (arms down) neck CT position (Fig. 20.13); such positioning reduces beam hardening artifact. Magnetic resonance imaging is also useful in locoregional staging of these lesions (238) but provides benefits that may not affect the patient's prognosis. Direct coronal and sagittal views give a panoramic layout of the lesion's cephalocaudal extent in a zone that too often is obscured by beam hardening with CT, due to the shoulder complex. In addition MRI provides excellent vascular outline even with conventional spin-echo sequences, which is helpful for patients with CT contrast contraindications. Cross-sectional imaging alone cannot exclude early esophageal cancer because of the normal variability of the thickness of the resting esophagus. Such evaluation becomes especially difficult when the neck has been irradiated for a prior condition (Fig. 20.14).

Endoscopic sonography of the esophagus provides a more accurate evaluation of the degree of mural involvement than does MRI or CT (239). High-resolution probes can differentiate individual layers of the esophageal wall from mucosa to adventitia. The technique would have greater overall impact if a larger proportion of patients presented at earlier histologic tumor stages (Fig. 20.15). The trade-off for high-resolution images is a limited sonographic field of view. Both CT and MRI provide more comprehensive regional staging and more accurate lymph node staging.

Clinical inspection of the hypopharynx is the leading method for detecting lesions of the piriform sinus. Fluoroscopic examinations of the hypopharynx are no longer necessary for diagnosing or staging advanced mucosal lesions (Fig. 20.16), but the piriform sinuses should be cleared, given the opportunity, in the cohort of patients at risk for (multiple) primary tumors of the aerodigestive tract. Because the status of the larynx often dictates the management of hypopharyngeal lesions, these patients are scanned with a larynx-style imaging protocol (Fig. 20.17). Thin-section CT or MRI scans are necessary to resolve tissue planes. One swallow of oral contrast helps to outline the mucosa and its recesses in this complex region (Fig. 20.18). Intravenous CT contrast is necessary for lymph node staging and helps to determine the status of the prevertebral margin (Fig. 20.19). Computed tomography has a strong negative predictive value for tumor invasion of the prevertebral muscle plane (240). Although it may overestimate the extent of disease (241), MRI adds to the accuracy of CT and helps to stratify patients within treatment algorithms (238), particularly with early hypopharyngeal lesions (242). Local control is influenced by the degree of involvement of the apex of the piriform sinus by T1 tumors (243) that can be cleared with CT.

Follow-up imaging after laryngopharyngectomy or an organ-preservation protocol should be dictated by clinical findings. Careful interpretation of the thickening of the alimentary tract in the irradiated patient is vital to avoid unnecessary endoscopic investigation. Sonography of the neopharynx with jejunal interposition allows one to follow up carefully for early local recurrence (244). This would be helpful in patients who cannot tolerate intravenous contrast or position supine for MRI or CT. Tumor volume reduction is the leading morphologic indicator for treatment response as in other sites of the neck (Fig. 20.20). One must also appreciate the lack of *dramatic* shrinkage of endophytic tumors despite symptomatic improvement. An MRI may have an advantage over CT by revealing persistent T2 signal abnormality despite the diminishing contrast enhancement usually ascribed to treatment response. Positron emission tomography scanning after treatment would be useful if a pretreatment scan were available to document the degree of decreased glucose metabolism.

Postlaryngectomy patients require detailed imaging of the neck down to and including the parastomal region. The reconstructed "neopharynx" often is redundant, particularly at the upper anastomosis, and one should be cautious in interpreting this pseudomass. Eccentric enhancement also persists along the pedicle side of the graft or pull-up, giving the impression of unilateral local recurrence. Generalized apparent fullness of the oropharynx also develops in the tracheostomy population due to chronically relaxed pharyngeal constrictors, which no longer contribute to breathing. The remainder of the mediastinum should be surveyed to rule out recurrence within or outside of the treatment portal.

In the larynx, preservation cohort cross-sectional imaging (CT or MRI) is the standard adjunct to the clinical examination. Decrease in tumor volume predicts likelihood of local control as in other subsites. Endoscopic sonography has been shown to be a reliable indicator of tumor size reduction of hypopharyngeal tumor (245). Hypopharynx tumors have a more infiltrating pattern on imaging than other sites in the neck. Imaging estimates of the anatomic borders of these lesions are challenging and become more difficult to determine after treatment. Functional imaging is instrumental in the initial staging as well as during the assessment of treatment response. Standardized uptake values (SUV) indicate the degree of hypermetabolic activity in the lesion. This absolute value portends poor risk for the patient when it is markedly elevated (246). The activity usually declines under treatment after a brief rise due to nonspecific activity related to local treatment-induced inflammation. A decline of the SUV predicts the degree of treatment effect and corresponds with local control (247). Lack of a significant response portends a poor prognosis and may indicate a need to rethink the patient's treatment options.

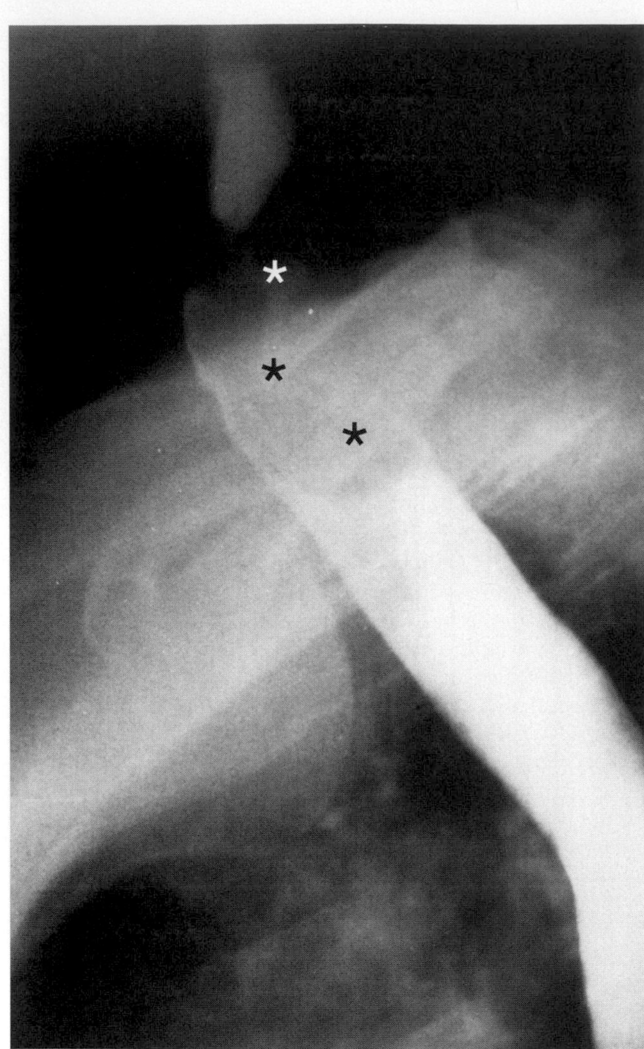

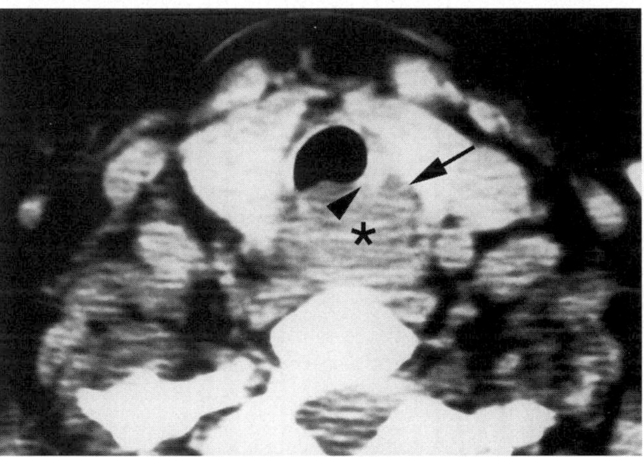

Figure 20.8 Exophytic esophageal cancer. Lateral esophagogram **(A)** shows a bulky, exophytic, partially obstructing esophageal lesion (*asterisk*) at the thoracic inlet. Enhanced axial computed tomogram at the inlet **(B)** of the low neck confirms the mass (*asterisk*) that infiltrates the tracheal cartilage (*arrowhead*) and thyroid bed (*arrow*).

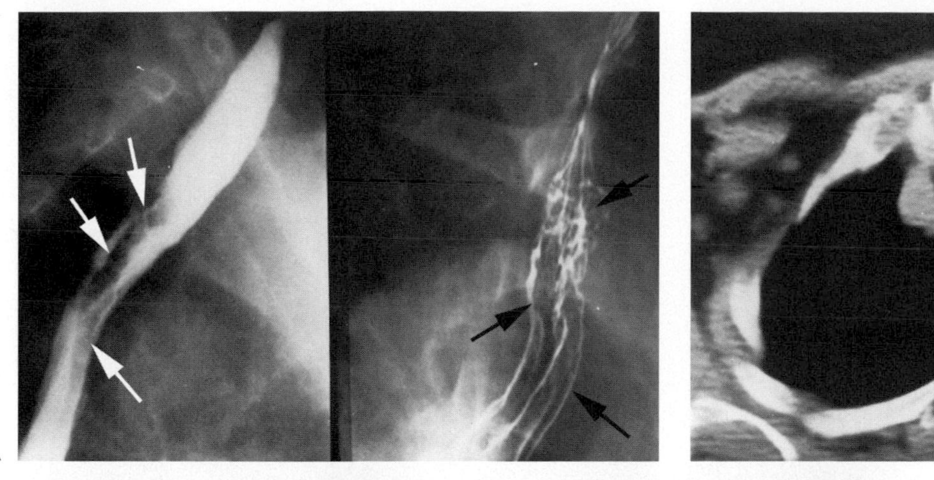

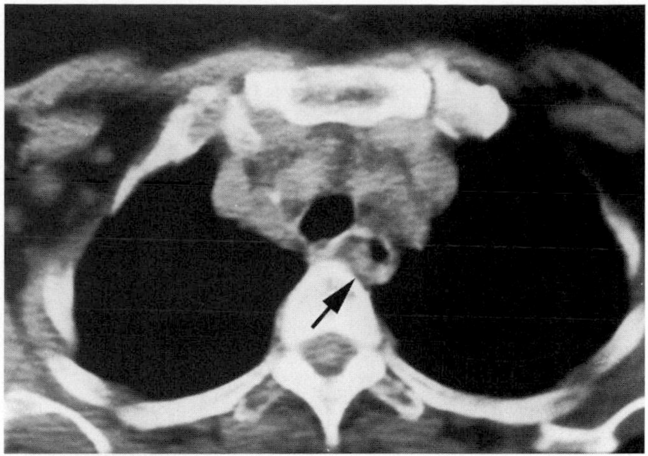

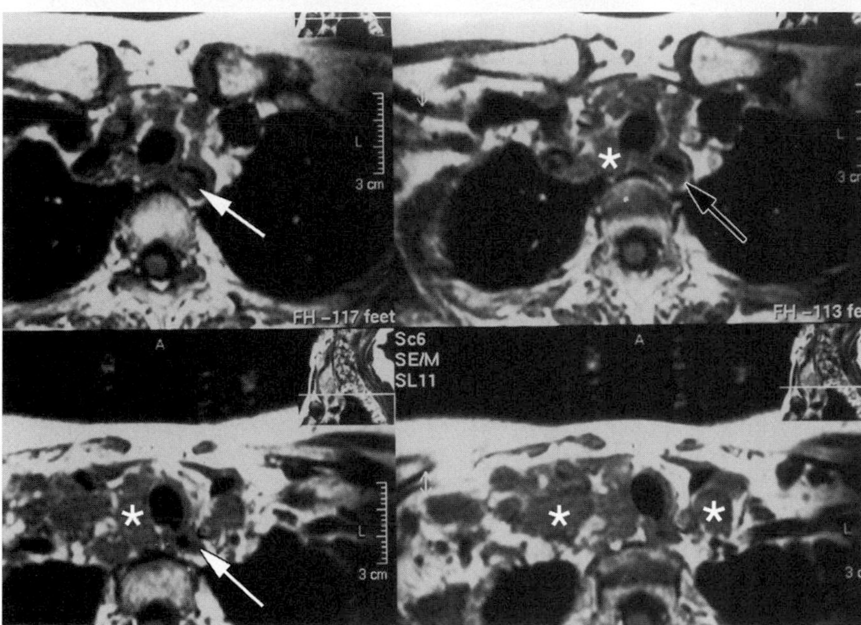

Figure 20.9 Varicoid-type esophageal cancer. **(A)** Oblique esophagogram shows mural lesion (*arrows*) on the distended (left) and collapsed (right) phases of the examination. This abnormality is easily overlooked on preceding cross-sectional magnetic resonance imaging **(B)** and computed tomographic examinations **(C),** which were obtained for cervical adenopathy (*asterisk*). Thickening of the esophagus (*arrows*) is often incidental but was pursued because of the regional adenopathy.

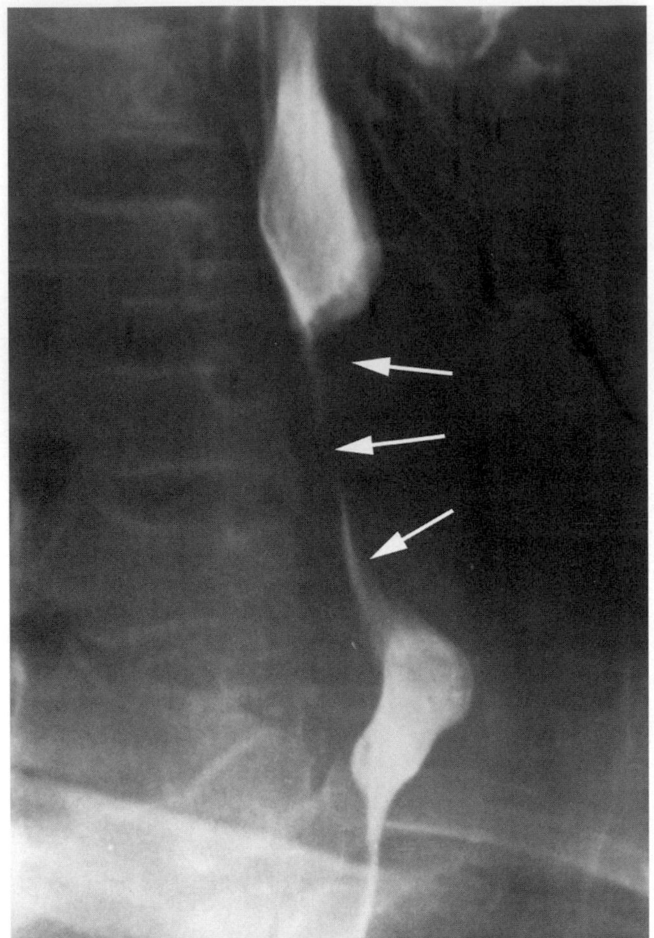

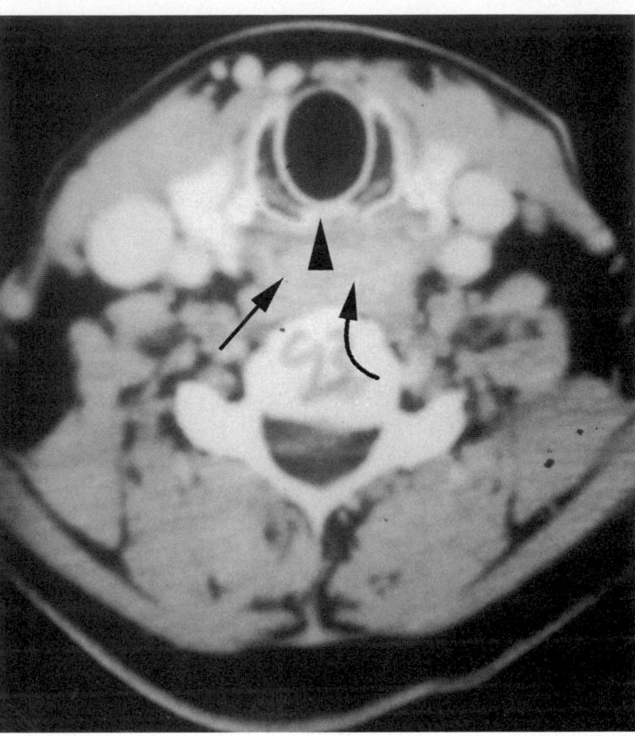

Figure 20.10 Carcinoma of the origin of the cervical esophagus. Lateral esophagogram **(A)** shows high-grade, subtotal obstruction of the cervical esophagus (*arrows*), seen here as a bulky lesion on contrast computed tomography (**B;** *arrow*). Note indistinct prevertebral fascia (*curved arrow*). Normal defect at the base of the cricoid (*arrowhead*) should not be misinterpreted as cartilage invasion.

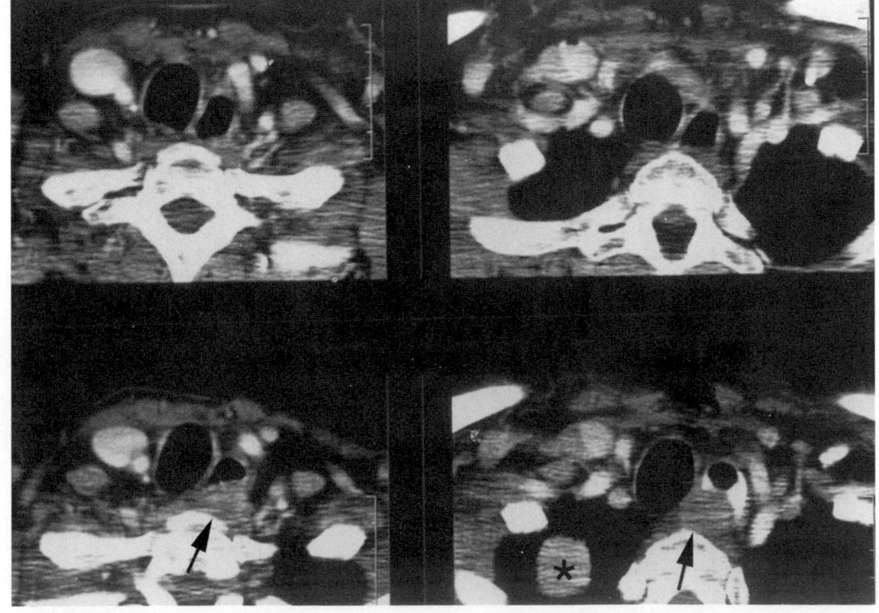

Figure 20.11 Nodal metastatic esophageal cancer. Serial enhanced computed tomographic images at the inlet show eccentric mural thickening at cervicothoracic esophageal junction (*arrows*). Barium paste outlines the mass. Pulmonary metastasis at right apex (*asterisk*).

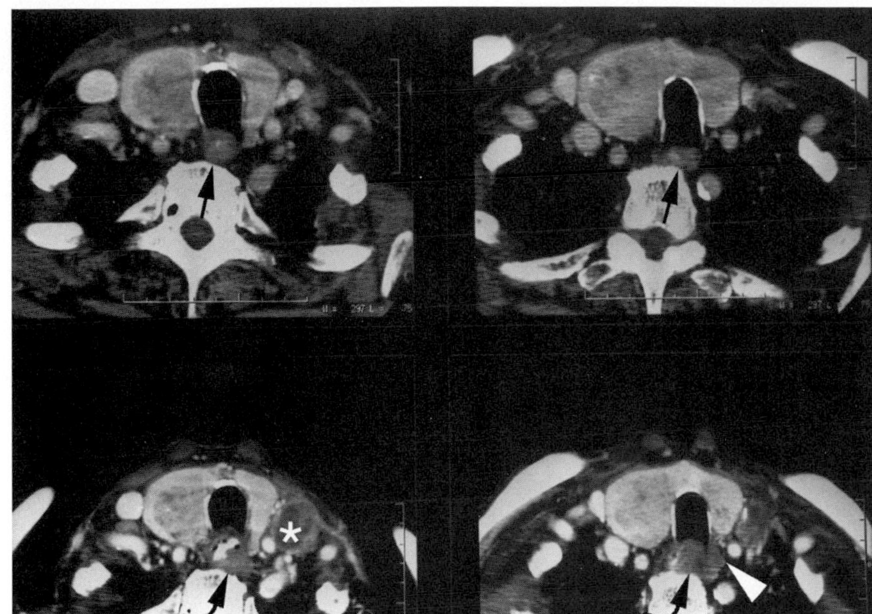

Figure 20.12 Systemic metastatic esophageal cancer. Serial enhanced axial computed tomographic images through inlet show thickened esophagus (*arrows*) with eccentric mass (*curved arrows*) at left posterior wall. Note pathologic (Virchow) node at the left supraclavicular fossa (*asterisk*). Barium paste outlines the lumen, showing a separate lesion to be a tracheoesophageal groove node (*arrowhead*).

A

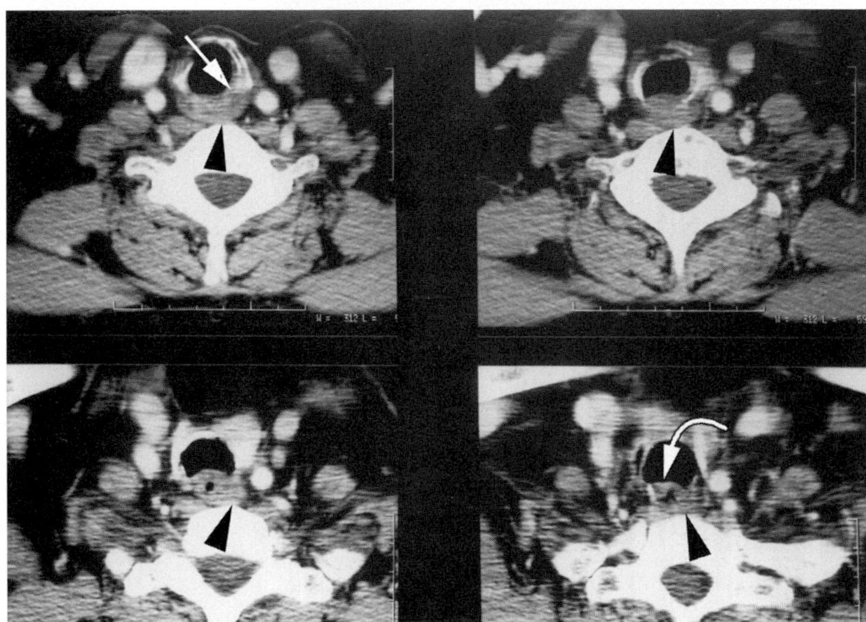

B

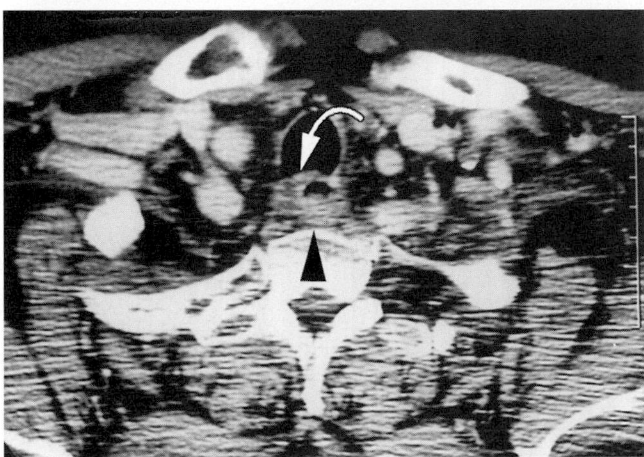

Figure 20.13 Carcinoma of cervical esophagus. **A:** Serial enhanced axial computed tomographic views of low neck show thickening of the cervical esophagus (*arrowheads*) from junction with hypopharynx (upper left) to inlet (lower right). Note infiltration of base of cricoid (*arrow*) and **(B)** membranous portion of trachea (*curved arrow*). Note that the contrast bolus technique does not obscure inlet, allowing evaluation of the prevertebral plane.

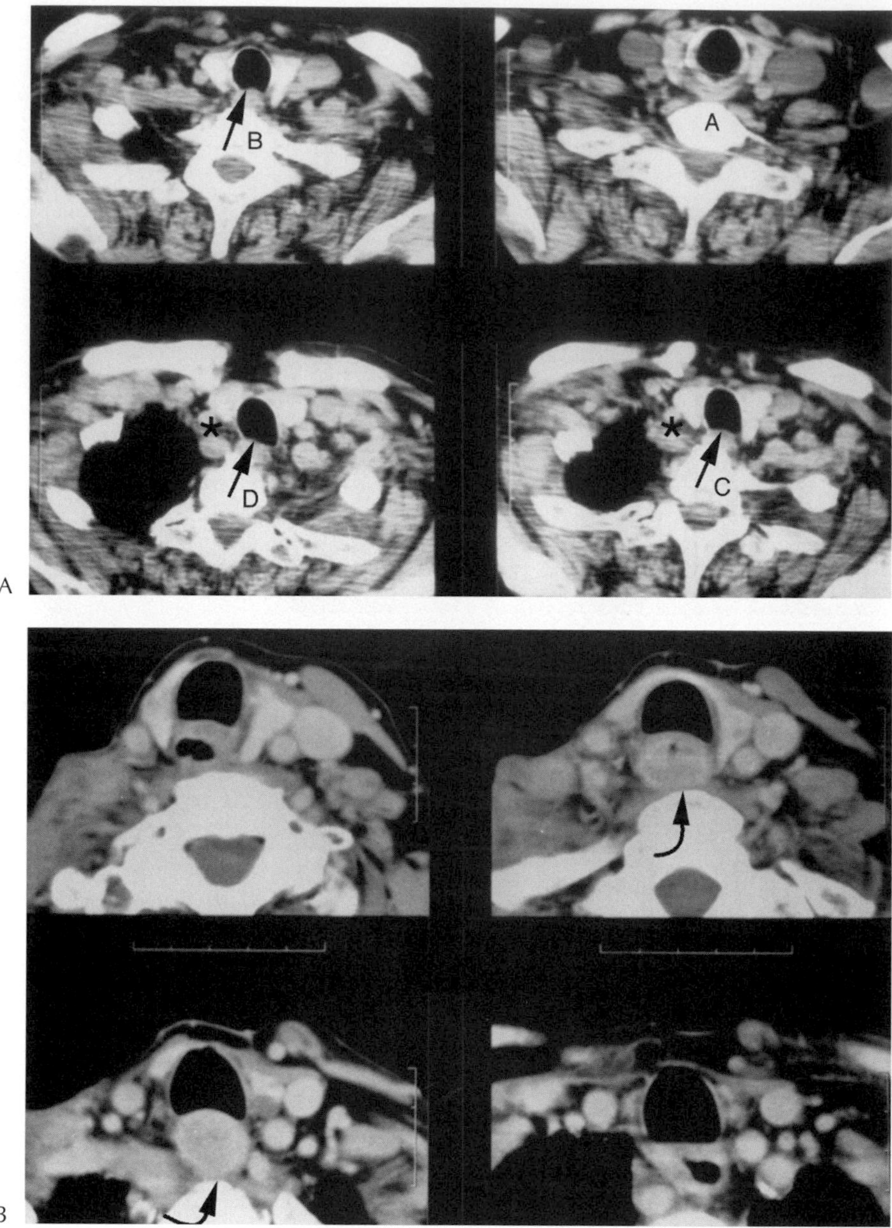

Figure 20.14 Developing esophageal cancer. **A:** Serial enhanced axial images through inlet before neck dissection for metastatic oral cavity cancer show normal thickness of esophagus (*arrows*). Incidental aberrant right subclavian artery (*asterisk*). (*A–D* in **A** represent a sequence of images.) **B:** Follow-up scan with serial enhanced axial computed tomography through inlet shows interval masslike thickening of cervical esophagus (*curved arrows*) greater than expected after neck irradiation.

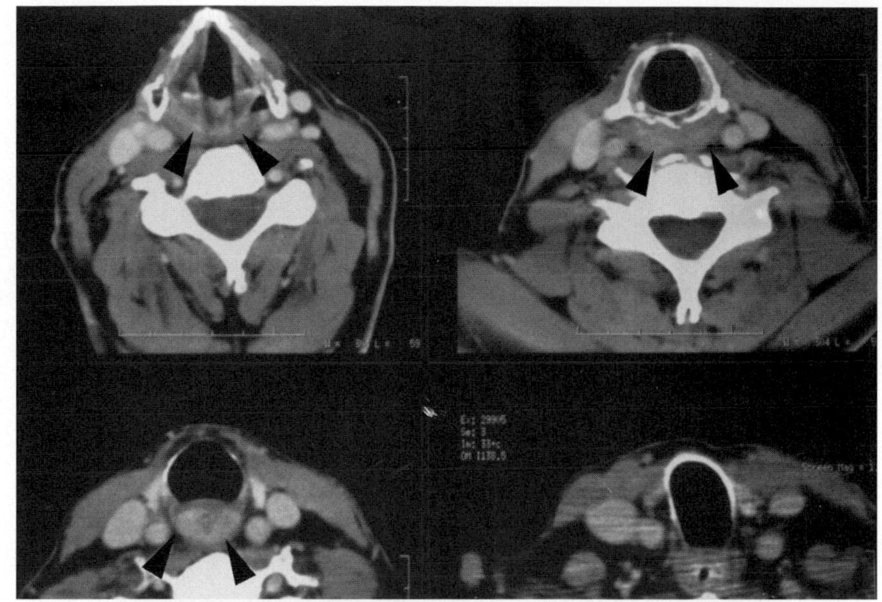

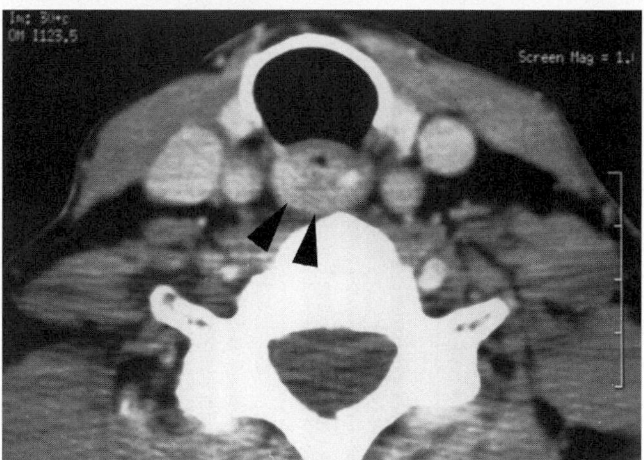

Figure 20.15 Hypopharyngeal carcinoma. Serial enhanced axial computed tomographic images show moderately thick lesion (*arrowheads*) of the low hypopharynx **(A)** involving the hypopharyngoesophageal junction **(B)**.

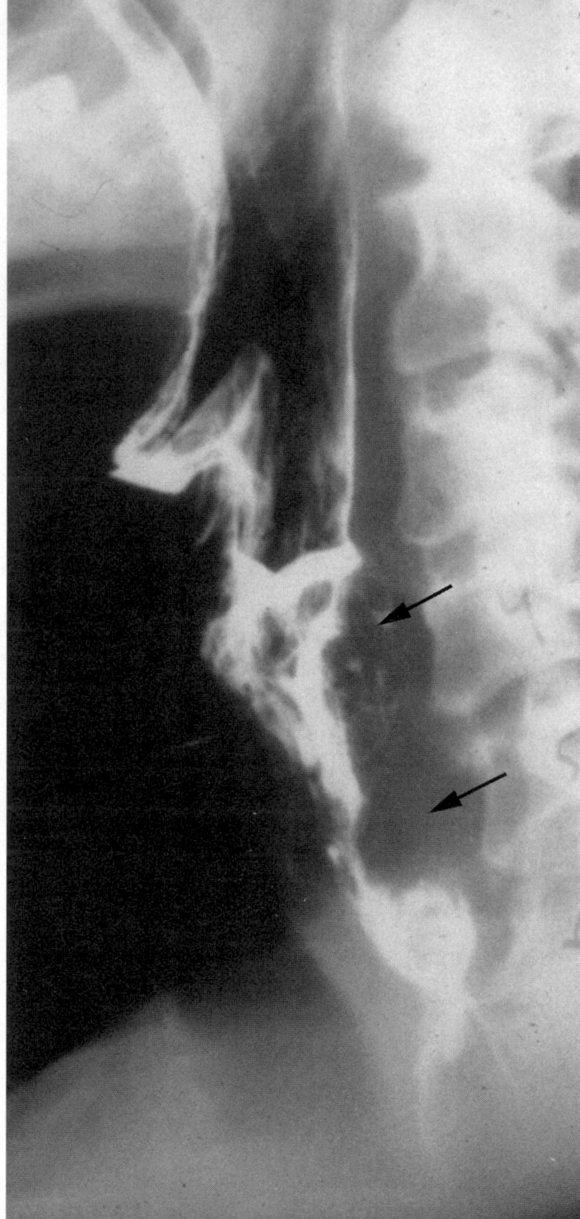

Figure 20.16 Large piriform cancer. **A:** Enhanced axial computed tomogram at larynx shows advanced left piriform lesion (*asterisk*) with cartilaginous involvement (*arrowhead*), extrapharyngeal extension (*arrows*), and paraglottic involvement (*curved arrow*). **B:** Lateral esophagogram shows extensive thickening of pharyngeal wall (*arrows*).

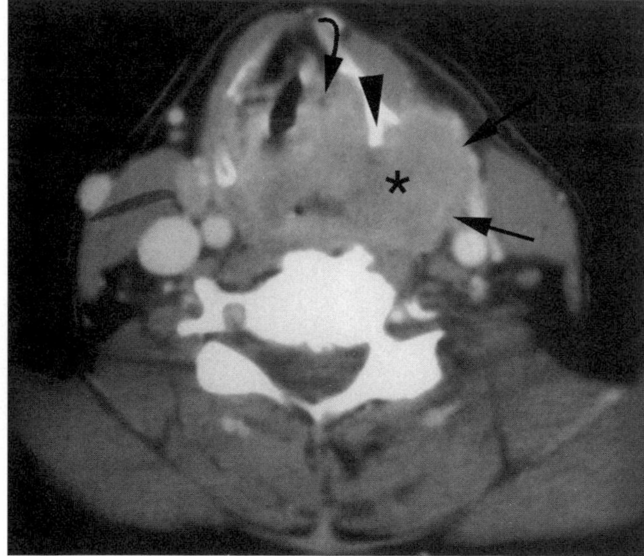

A

B

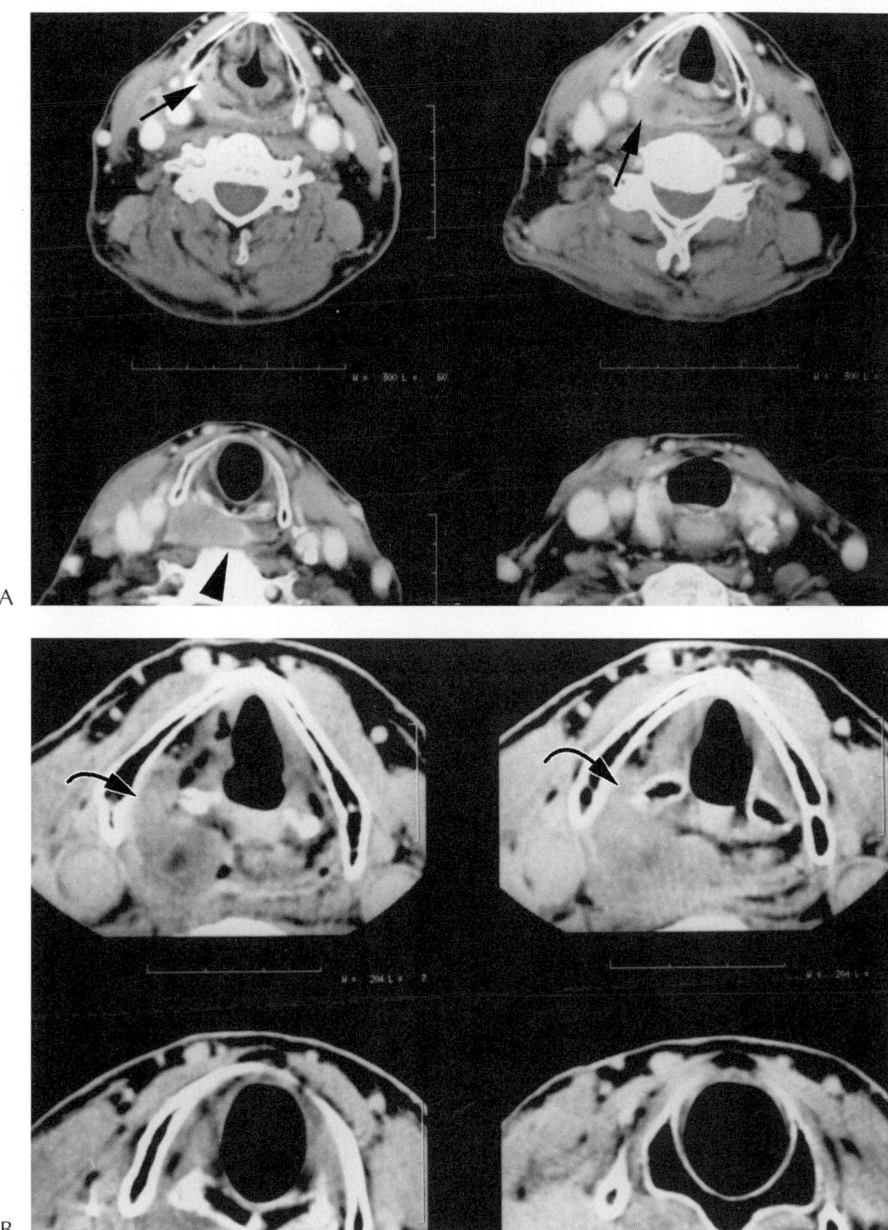

Figure 20.17 Localized right piriform lesion. **A:** Serial axial views show lesion of right piriform sinus (*arrows*), with extension just past midline (*arrowhead*). **B:** High-resolution views better show early involvement of adjacent right paraglottic space (*curved arrow*).

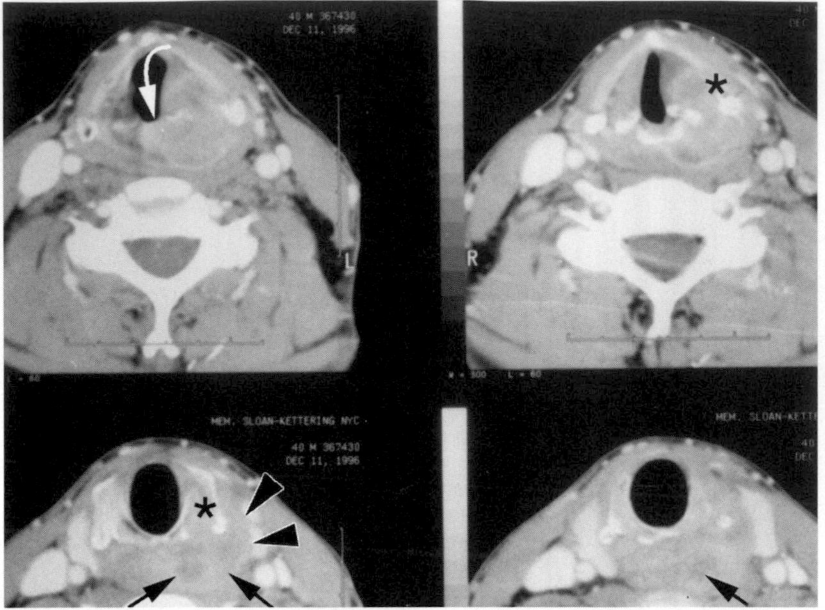

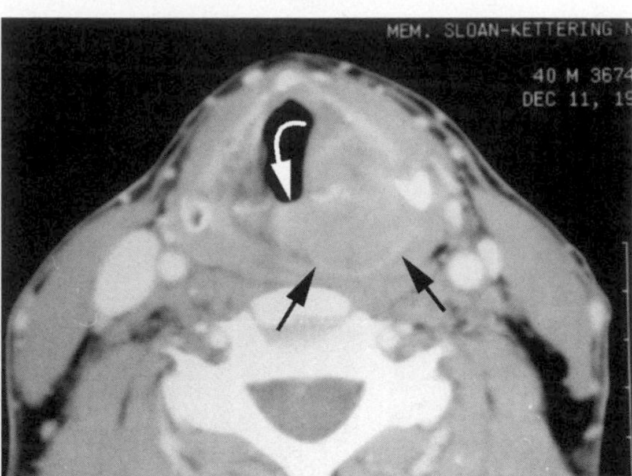

Figure 20.18 Advanced left piriform lesion. **A:** Serial enhanced axial views of larynx show large lesion arising in left piriform sinus (*arrows*), with extrapharyngeal extension (*arrowhead*) and cartilage invasion (*asterisk*). **B:** Note involvement of posterior commissure (*curved arrow*).

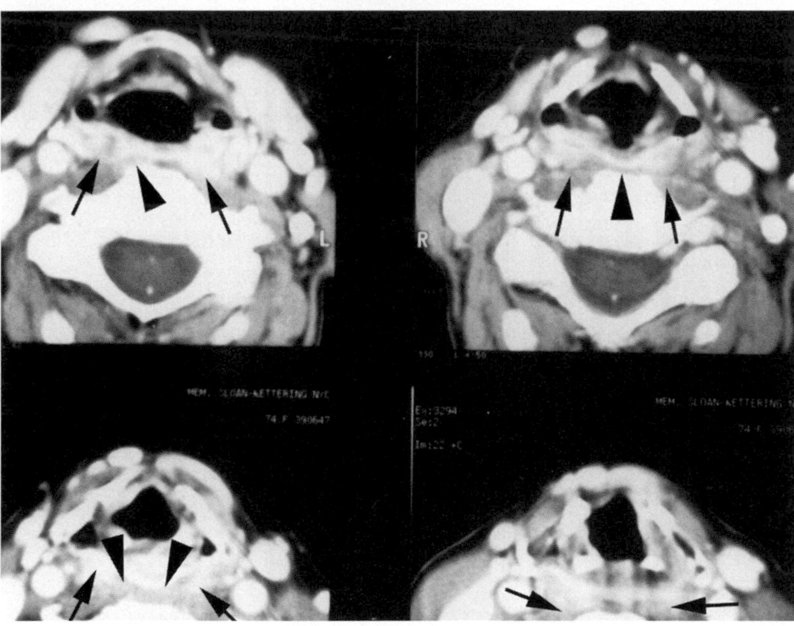

Figure 20.19 Treated hypopharyngeal cancer. Serial enhanced axial computed tomographic images of hypopharynx show irregularly enhancing lesion involving posterior pharyngeal wall bilaterally (*arrows*). The prevertebral margin is indistinct (*arrowheads*). No endolaryngeal involvement is noted.

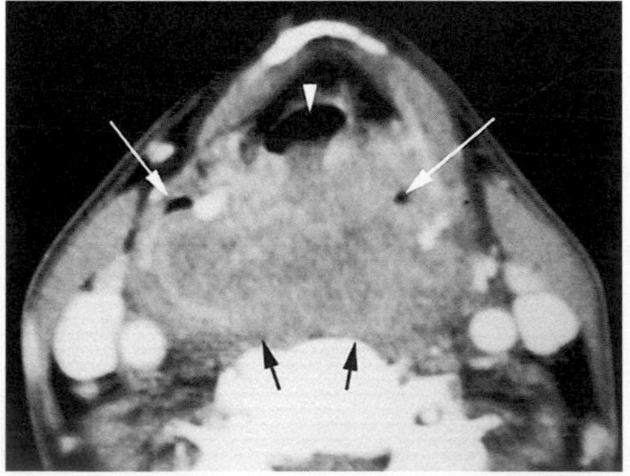

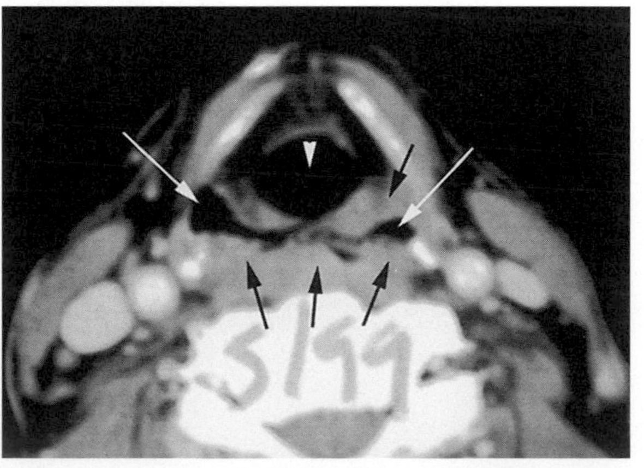

Figure 20.20 Hypopharynx squamous cell carcinoma follow-up. **A:** Enhanced axial computed tomography (CT) image shows bulky posterior wall hypopharynx mass displacing the piriform sinuses (*arrows*) and glottic airway (*arrowhead*). The prevertebral plane is invaded. **B:** Enhanced axial CT image after combined treatment shows dramatic shrinkage of mass with reconstitution of the glottic airway (*arrowhead*), re-aeration of piriform sinuses (*arrows*), and residual mucosal irregularity of posterior wall and left piriform sinus (*black arrows*).

RADIATION THERAPY TECHNIQUE*

William M. Mendenhall

Piriform Sinus

Parallel-opposed portals are used to treat the primary cancer and both sides of the neck to include lymph nodes in levels 2, 3, 4, and 5 and the retropharyngeal nodes at the level of the C1 to C2 vertebral bodies. It is difficult to detect subclinical disease at the piriform sinus apex, which is located somewhere between the top and bottom of the cricoid cartilage, even at direct laryngoscopy. Therefore, the inferior border of the initial portals is located 2 cm below the bottom of the cricoid cartilage. It may be difficult to obtain this margin if the patient has large shoulders and a low-lying larynx. If this is the case, the lateral portals are angled approximately 10 degrees inferiorly, and the anterior portal used to treat the low neck is eliminated. The anterior field border may be placed just behind the skin of the anterior neck to avoid tangentially irradiating this area for patients with T1 to T2 cancers and early stage neck disease. The superior border is placed at, or just below, the jugular foramen, and the posterior border is placed just posterior to the spinous processes of the vertebral bodies (Fig. 20.21) (248). Reduction off the spinal cord is performed at approximately 45 Gy, and a second mucosal reduction occurs at 60 Gy. Electron beam is used to treat the posterior strips, if necessary, after reduction off of the spinal cord.

The radiation therapy treatment technique after surgery that entails partial laryngectomy is as previously described. The technique employed after a total laryngectomy is the same as that described in Chapter 19.

Pharyngeal Wall

Because SCCs of the pharyngeal wall tend to spread submucosally, wide margins for the primary cancer are initially used. The portals are parallel opposed and usually weighted 1:1. The field margins for the initial fields usually extend to the bottom of the cricoid cartilage, 0.5 to 1.0 cm behind the skin of the anterior neck, the posterior processes of the vertebral bodies, and to (or just below) the jugular foramen. Because large tumors tend to extend posterolaterally around the vertebral bodies, the posterior border of the off-cord reductions is placed at the anterior edge of the spinal cord (Fig. 20.22) (249). The low neck is treated with an anterior field with a thin, tapered midline tracheal block. Electrons are used to treat the posterior strips after reduction off of the spinal cord, if necessary.

Cervical Esophagus

Anteroposterior-opposed portals weighted anteriorly are used to treat the primary cancer, upper mediastinum, and neck if moderate-dose irradiation is planned prior to definitive surgery. The superior border is placed at mid-mandible and splits the tragus; the neck is extended. The lateral borders include the supraclavicular fossae, and the inferior border is placed 5 cm below the inferior border of the primary cancer.

Treatment with high-dose irradiation alone or combined with adjuvant chemotherapy is more problematic because of the change in contour from the neck to the shoulders. Several options exist depending on the treatment planning and delivery system available. The initial target volume includes the primary lesion with 5-cm distal and proximal esophageal and hypopharyngeal margins, respectively. The lymph nodes included are levels 2, 3, 4, and 6 and the superior mediastinal lymph nodes. We currently use intensity modulated radiation therapy with inverse treatment planning. Subclinical disease is treated to approximately 45 to 50 Gy, and gross disease receives approximately 70 Gy. Alternatively, three-dimensional conformal radiation therapy may be used with a mono-isocentric technique. The inferior part of the treatment volume is treated with anterior and posterior portals or an anterior and two posterior oblique fields. The superior part of the treatment volume is treated with lateral parallel-opposed fields; the match line is changed twice. Finally, if neither of these techniques is possible, a four-field technique is used with a beeswax bolus to compensate for the change in contour of the shoulders (Fig. 20.23) (250). The disadvantage of this technique is that the shoulders are treated, the dose distribution is less homogeneous, and the skin receives a high dose of radiation.

*Please refer to the Appendix, Imaging Considerations for Radiation Therapy Treatment Planning. This section shows the important radiologic anatomy that allows the radiation oncologist to design the target volumes for treatment planning.

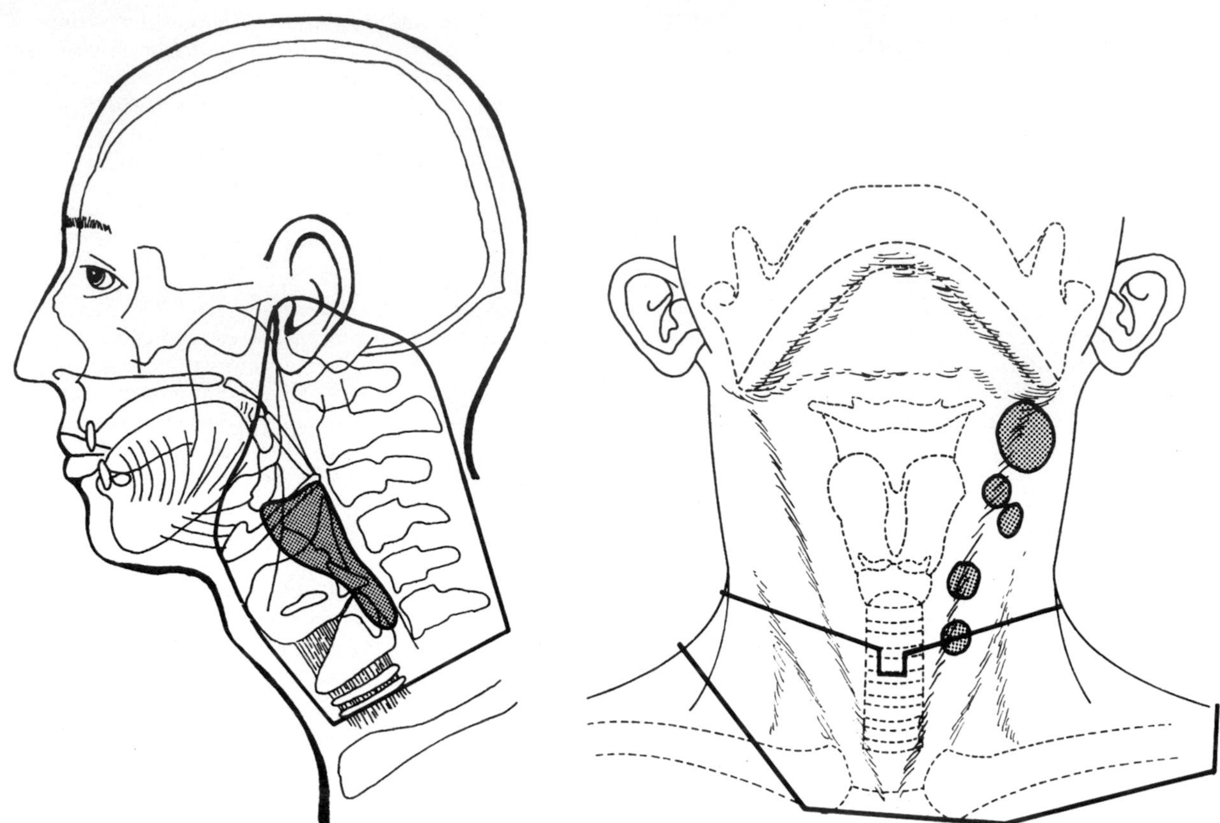

Figure 20.21 **A:** Portals used for the initial treatment volume in a patient with carcinoma (*stippled area*) of the piriform sinus and a clinically negative neck. Superiorly, the portal covers the junctional and retropharyngeal lymph nodes. The submandibular nodes are not included, but the spinal accessory chain is included. Anteriorly, at least 1 cm of skin and subcutaneous tissues (as viewed from the lateral projection) are usually spared. The inferior border is 2 to 3 cm below the bottom of the cricoid cartilage and is slanted to facilitate matching with the low neck portal and to avoid irradiating the shoulders. The posterior field edge usually encompasses the spinous processes of the vertebral bodies. As treatment progresses, portal reductions are made to shield the spinal cord and to limit the volume of mucosa that receives high-dose irradiation. **B:** Anterior portal for treatment of low neck in patients with hypopharyngeal or laryngeal cancer. Low neck is irradiated bilaterally. Match line is treated in primary portals but excluded from low neck field. Usually, a 1 × 1-cm midline block is introduced at the upper edge of the field, except in postoperative patients in whom tracheal stoma is at risk (see ref. 251). Each side of the low neck portal is individualized according to risk or presence of lymph node metastases on that side. (From Parsons JT, Palta JR, Mendenhall WM, et al. Head and neck cancer. In: Levitt SH, Khan FM, Potish RA, et al., eds. *Levitt and Tapley's technological basis of radiation therapy: clinical applications,* 3rd ed. Baltimore: Lippincott Williams & Wilkins, 1999:269–299, with permission.)

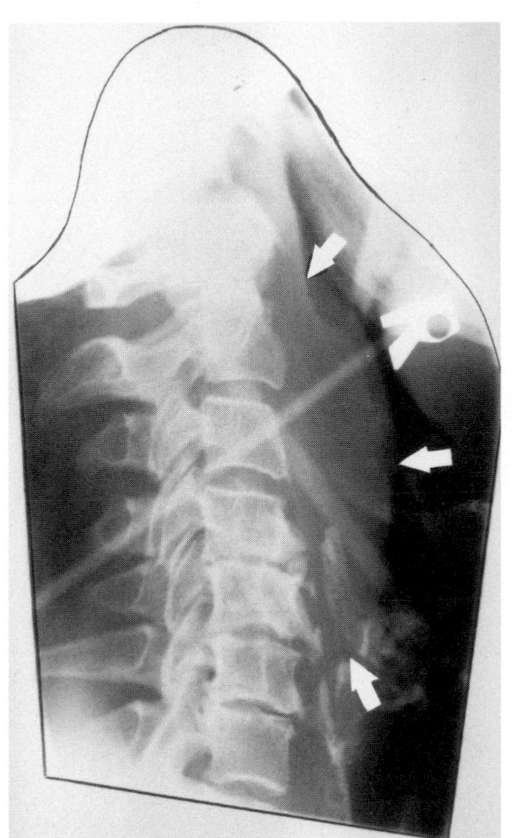

A

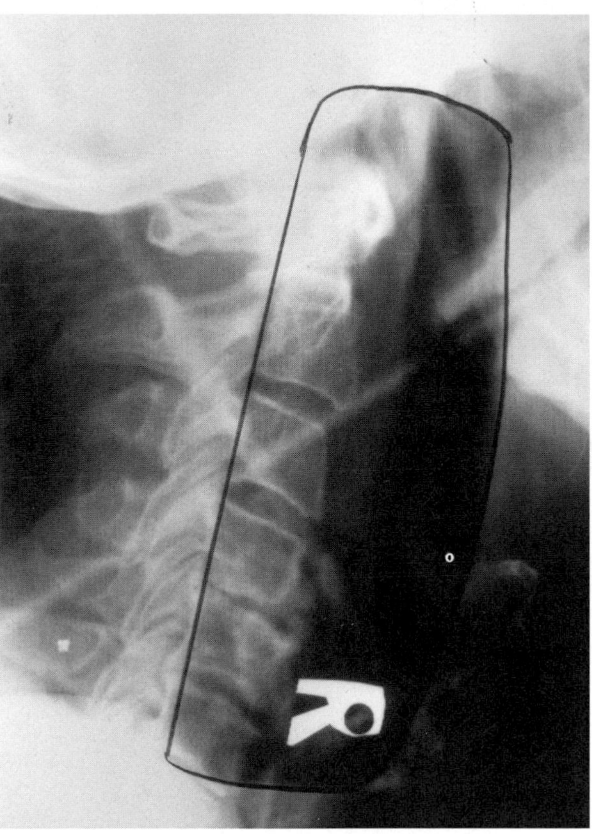

B

Figure 20.22 **A:** Initial treatment fields for a T3 N2b squamous cell carcinoma of the posterior pharyngeal wall. *Arrows* indicate the superior and inferior margins of the tumor. The anterior border of the field does not flash the skin of the anterior aspect of the neck, thus sparing the anterior portion of the larynx. **B:** Treatment field after reducing off the spinal cord. Note that the posterior edge of the field is at the posterior aspect of the vertebral bodies.

(continued on next page)

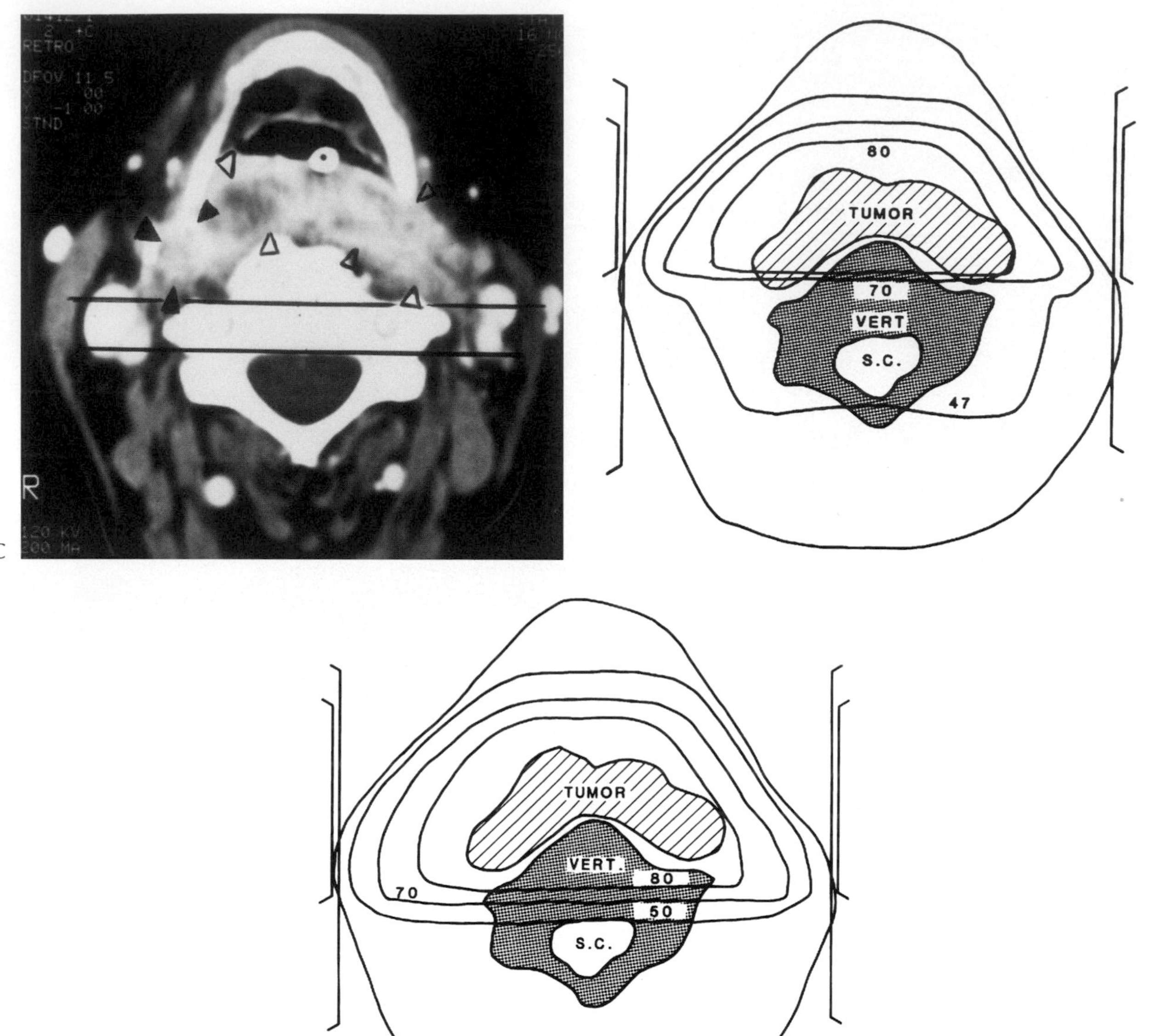

Figure 20.22 ***(continued)*** **C:** Computerized tomogram prior to treatment. The *open arrowheads* denote the primary tumor and the *closed arrowheads* indicate a retropharyngeal node. Note that there is tumor extending posterior to the anterior surface of the vertebral body. The anterior line indicates the posterior edge of the reduced field if it is designed to split the vertebral bodies. Note that tumor is on the edge of the field. The posterior line indicates the field margin if it is placed at the posterior edge of the vertebral bodies. These lines do not account for beam divergence and are drawn as if the central axis of the beam is placed at the posterior edge of the field. **D:** Computerized dosimetry for 45.6 Gy, 8 mV x-ray, weighted 1:1, followed by reduction off of the spinal cord and 33.6 Gy, 17 mV x-ray, weighted 1:1 (specified total dose = 79.2 Gy). The posterior edge of the reduced field is placed at the anterior aspect of the spinal cord. **E:** As in **(D),** except that the posterior edge of the reduced field splits the vertebral bodies. (From Mendenhall WM, Parsons JT, Mancuso AA, et al. Squamous cell carcinoma of the pharyngeal wall treated with irradiation. *Radiother Oncol* 1988;11:205–212, with permission.)

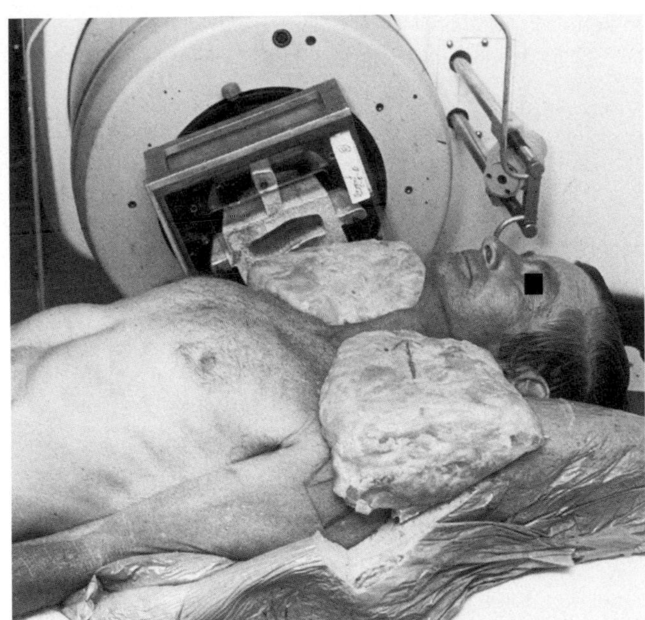

A

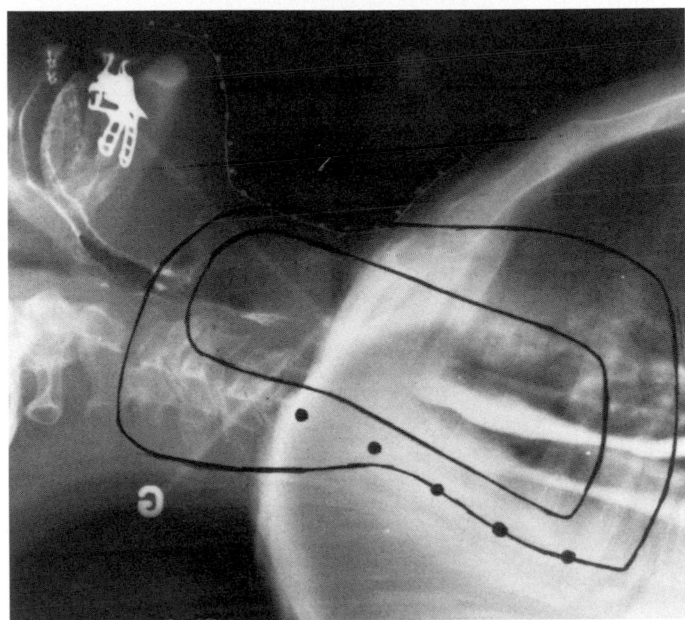

B

C

D

Figure 20.23 **A:** Patient in position for treatment of right lateral portal. Note beeswax bolus, Lipowitz metal blocks (Cerrobend), and foam body mold. The portal is set up by an isocentric method. The beeswax bolus is placed in position after the portal is aligned. The lateral portal should be checked frequently by imaging films. **B:** Lateral and reduced lateral portals for a cancer of the cervical esophagus located at the inlet. A second and final reduction would just cover the gross lesion. The initial lower border is generous because of the inability to evaluate the mediastinal nodes by palpation. The initial lateral portal bows posteriorly on its superior aspect to cover the posterior cervical nodes, and bows anteriorly on its inferior aspect to cover the anterior mediastinal nodes. Note the proximity of the spinal cord to the esophagus. For this patient, it is 2 to 2.5 cm from the posterior wall of the esophagus to the anterior portion of the cervical spinal cord and about 3 cm to the thoracic spinal cord. Black dots mark the posterior aspect of the vertebral bodies. Solder wire with lead shot spaced at 1 cm outlines the midline anterior skin surface. **C,D:** Isodose curves for four-field box technique using 17 MeV x- ray beam: **(C)** section at level of C6 vertebra; **(D)** section at level of T2 vertebra. (From Mendenhall WM, Million RR, Bova FJ. Carcinoma of the cervical esophagus treated with radiation therapy using a four-field technique. *Int J Radiat Oncol Biol Phys* 1982;8: 1435–1439, with permission.)

SURGICAL TECHNIQUES FOR TREATING CARCINOMA OF THE HYPOPHARYNX AND CERVICAL ESOPHAGUS

Roy B. Sessions

Excision of carcinomas of the posterior hypopharyngeal wall is performed through a transhyoid or a lateral pharyngotomy. Tumors of the piriform sinus are excised by a partial pharyngectomy in conjunction with a supraglottic or total laryngectomy. Tumors of the postcricoid region and circumferential tumors of the hypopharynx require a total laryngopharyngectomy with resection of varying portions of the cervical esophagus, trachea or both. In these advanced cases, the preoperative evaluation must be conducted in a systematic manner to determine the resectability of the tumor. Unfortunately, despite the progress made in imaging technology, it is not always possible to determine whether or not a hypopharyngeal tumor invades the prevertebral tissues or how far it extends submucosally into the esophagus. Consequently, it is prudent to carry out such operations in a systematic, step-by-step manner to determine that the tumor can be dissected from the carotid arteries and the prevertebral tissues. Only then, the pharynx and trachea are transected, making the operation irreversible. If the esophagus is to be included in the resection, proper traction using the mobilized pharyngolarynx can aid in the mediastinal dissection (Fig. 20.24).

Following resection of a hypopharyngeal cancer, reconstruction is ideally accomplished in a one-stage procedure, using reliable tissue and it would afford good functional results with the least morbidity. Selection of the reconstructive method is based on the location and the extent of the hypopharyngeal defect created by the resection.

Small posterior pharyngeal defects can be repaired with a skin graft, or by securely suturing the mucosal edges to the prevertebral fascia, allowing remucosalization to cover the defect. Subtotal hypopharyngeal defects in which a posterior strip of mucosa is preserved can be repaired, ideally with a pectoralis major myocutaneous flap, except in obese individuals and in women with large breasts. The main disadvantage to this flap is a tendency for stenosis at the inferior suture line between the flap and the esophagus.

Reconstruction of total pharyngolaryngectomy defects depends on how much of the cervical esophagus was resected. When enough cervical esophagus is left that an anastomosis can be accomplished safely through the neck, three methods of reconstruction are currently used. For details of these methods, the reader is referred to the Chapter 9. The reconstructive options consist of:

1. The radial forearm free flap is relatively easy to harvest, it provides pliable tissue that is easily tubed, the microvascular anastomosis is facilitated by the relatively large caliber of its vessels, and donor site morbidity is minimal.
2. The jejunal free graft can be used to repair long defects from the level of the nasopharynx to the thoracic inlet. Although it is associated with a low incidence of stenosis and fistula, it requires a laparotomy with intestinal anastomosis.
3. The trapezius myocutaneous flap, unlike the pectoralis myocutaneous flap, provides relatively thin skin and subcutaneous tissue that is easy to tube. The length of the pedicle may, however, be insufficient depending on the origin of the transverse cervical artery. Finally, the morbidity associated with the donor site may be significant.

When the amount of cervical esophagus that remains following excision is insufficient to permit a safe anastomosis through the neck, the two methods of reconstruction that can be used are the gastric transposition (Fig. 20.25) and the colon interposition (Fig. 20.26). Both require major abdominal surgery; the gastric transposition also requires dissection of the posterior mediastinum. As a result, operative morbidity and mortality rates are high. The colon interposition is used infrequently as a method for hypopharyngeal reconstruction. The perioperative morbidity is similar to that of the gastric transposition. With this operation, however, it is not necessary to dissect the posterior mediastinum to bring the colon into the neck. When this method of reconstruction is anticipated, a preoperative mesenteric angiogram must be done to ensure that the intended segment of colon is adequately vascularized.

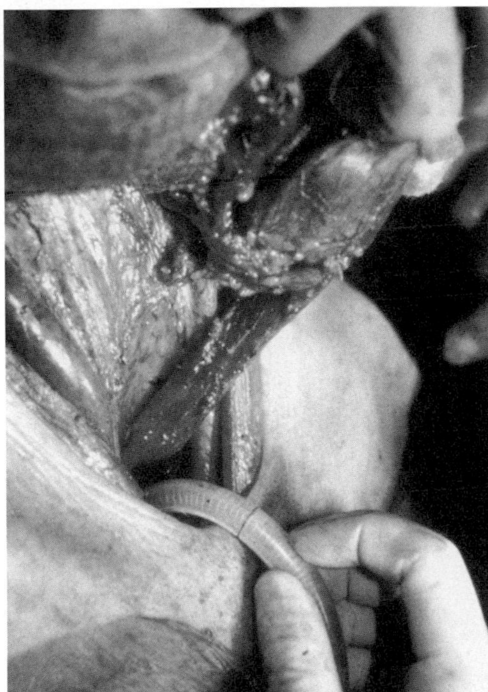

Figure 20.24 Laryngopharynx on left in the grasp of the surgeon. Note the cervical esophagus is still attached and the posterior mediastinum is being dissected and the entire esophageal is being mobilized in preparation for a gastric transposition for creation of a neopharynx. Note endotracheal tube on right of picture.

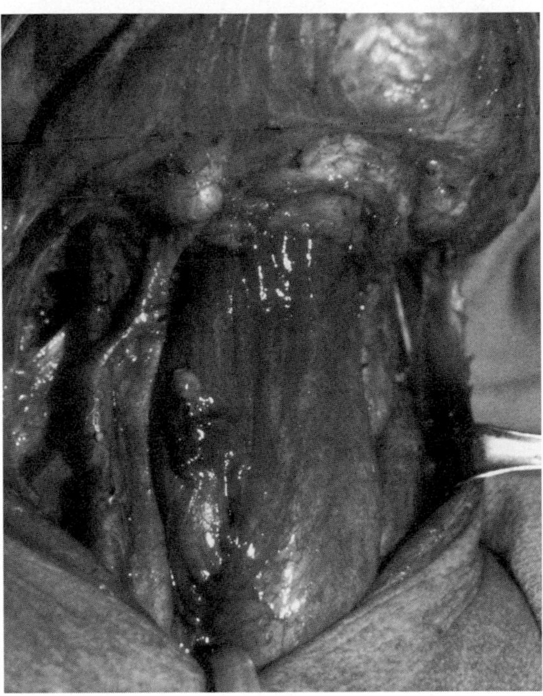

Figure 20.25 Transposed and elevated stomach has been brought up through the posterior mediastinum and is sutured in place in the upper part of the neck; thus, the neopharynx has been reconstituted. Note the endotracheal tube at the bottom of the photograph, prior to creation of a tracheal stoma.

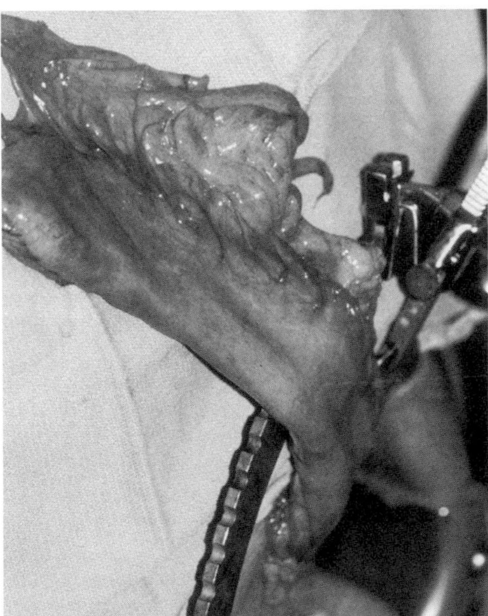

Figure 20.26 A segment of colon ready for movement to the cervical area.

REFERENCES

1. Schechter GL, Kalafsky JT. Cancer of the hypopharynx and cervical esophagus: management concepts. *Oncology* 1988;2:17.
2. Jacobs C. The internist in the management of head and neck cancer. *Ann Intern Med* 1990;113:771.
3. Spitz MR. Epidemiology and risk factors for head and neck cancer. *Semin Oncol* 1994;21:281.
4. Blot WJ. Esophageal cancer trends and risk factors. *Semin Oncol* 1994;21:403.
5. Greene F, Page D, Fleming I, et al. *AJCC cancer staging manual,* 6th ed. New York: Springer-Verlag, 2002.
6. Marks JE, Kurnik B, Powers WE, et al. Carcinoma of the pyriform sinus. An analysis of treatment results and patterns of failure. *Cancer* 1978;41:1008.
7. Vandenbrouck C, Eschwege F, De La Rochefordiere A, et al. Squamous cell carcinoma of the pyriform sinus: retrospective study of 351 cases treated at the Institut Gustave-Roussy. *Head Neck Surg* 1987;10:4.
8. Lefebvre JL. Cancer of the hypopharynx: strategies for larynx preservation. In: Shah JP, Johnson JT, eds. *Proceedings of the 4th International Conference on Head and Neck Cancer.* Madison, WI: Omnipress, 1996:170.
9. Jemal A, Thomas A, Murray T, et al. Cancer statistics, 2002. *CA Cancer J Clin* 2002;52:23.
10. Jacobsson F. Carcinoma of the hypopharynx: A clinical study of 322 cases, treated at Radiumhemmet, from 1939 to 1947. *Acta Radiol* 1951;35:1.
11. Lederman M. Carcinoma of the laryngopharynx: Results of radiotherapy. *J Laryngol Otol* 1962;76:317.
12. Wynder EL, Hultberg S, Jacobsson F, et al. Environmental factors in cancer of the upper alimentary tract. *Cancer* 1957;10:470.
13. Carpenter RJ III, DeSanto LW. Cancer of the hypopharynx. *Surg Clin North Am* 1977;57:723.
14. Jayant K, Balakrishman V Sanghvi LD, et al. Quantification of the role of smoking and chewing tobacco in oral, pharyngeal and esophageal cancers. *Br J Cancer* 1977;35:232.
15. Flanders WD, Rothman KJ. Interaction of alcohol and tobacco in laryngeal cancer. *Am J Epidemiol* 1982;115:371.
16. Slaughter DP, Southwick HW, Smejkal W. "Field cancerization" in oral stratified squamous epithelium: clinical implications of multicentric origin. *Cancer* 1953;6:963.
17. Somers KD, Merrick MA, Lopez ME, et al. Frequent p53 mutations in head and neck cancer. *Cancer Res* 1992;52:5996.
18. Boyle JO, Hakim J, Koch W, et al. The incidence of p53 mutations increases with progression of head and neck cancer. *Cancer Res* 1993;53:4477.
19. Van der Riet P, Nawroz H, Hruban RH, et al. Frequent loss of chromosome 9 p21-22 early in head and neck cancer progression. *Cancer Res* 1994;54:1156.
20. Mineta H, Ogino T, Amano HM, et al. Human papilloma virus (HPV) type 16 and 18 detected in head and neck squamous cell carcinoma. *Anticancer Res* 1998;18(6B):4765.
21. de Villiers EM, Lavergne D, Chang F, et al. An interlaboratory study to determine the presence of human papillomavirus DNA in esophageal carcinoma from China. *Int J Cancer* 1999;81:225.
22. Clayman GL, Stewart MG, Weber RS, et al. Human papillomavirus in laryngeal and hypopharyngeal carcinomas. Relationship to survival. *Arch Otolaryngol Head Neck Surg* 1994;120:743.
23. Andl T, Kahn T, Pfuhl A, et al. Etiological involvement of oncogenic human papillomavirus in tonsillar squamous cell carcinomas lacking retinoblastoma cell cycle control. *Cancer Res* 1998;58:5.
24. Schottenfeld D, ed. *Cancer epidemiology and prevention: current concepts.* Springfield, IL: Charles C. Thomas, 1975:177.
25. Sporn MB, Clamon GH, Dunlop NM, et al. Activity of vitamin A analogues in cell cultures of mouse epidermis and organ cultures of hamster trachea. *Nature* 1975;253:47.
26. Cameron E, Paining L, Leibovitz B. Ascorbic acid and cancer: a review. *Cancer Res* 1979;39:663.
27. Feind CR. The head and neck. In: Haagensen CD, Feind CR, Herter FP, et al., eds. *The lymphatics in cancer.* Philadelphia: WB Saunders, 1972:60.
28. Ballantyne AJ. Significance of retropharyngeal nodes in cancer of the head and neck. *Am J Surg* 1964;108:500.
29. Spiro RH, Lewis JS, Hajdu SI, et al. Mucus gland tumors of the larynx and laryngopharynx. *Ann Otol Rhinol Laryngol* 1976;85:498.
30. Shah JP, Shaha AR, Spiro RH, et al. Carcinoma of the hypopharynx. *Am J Surg* 1976;132:439.
31. Harrison DFN. Role of surgery in the management of postcricoid and cervical esophageal neoplasms. *Ann Otol Rhinol Laryngol* 1972;81:465.
32. Hiroto H. Hypopharyngoesophageal cancer: its surgical treatment. *Kurume Med J* 1963;10:162.
33. Willatt DJ, Jackson SR, McCormick MS, et al. Vocal cord paralysis and tumour length in staging postcricoid cancer. *Eur J Surg Oncol* 1987;13:131.
34. Ballantyne AJ. Principles of surgical management of cancer of the pharyngeal walls. *Cancer* 1967;20:663.
35. Kirchner JA. Pyriform sinus cancer: a clinical and laboratory study. *Ann Otol Rhinol Laryngol* 1975;84:793.
36. Tani M, Amatsu M. Discrepancies between clinical and histopathologic diagnoses in T3 pyriform sinus cancer. *Laryngoscope* 1987;97:93.
37. Guillamondegui OM, Meoz R, Jesse RH. Surgical treatment of squamous cell carcinoma of the pharyngeal walls. *Am J Surg* 1978;136:474.
38. Ballantyne AJ. Methods of repair after surgery for cancer of the pharyngeal wall, postcricoid area, and cervical esophagus. *Am J Surg* 1971;122:482.
39. Hahn SS, Spaulding CA, Kim JA, et al. The prognostic significance of lymph node involvement in pyriform sinus and supraglottic cancers. *Int J Radiat Oncol Biol Phys* 1987;13:1143.
40. Lefebvre JL, Castelain B, De La Torte JD, et al. Lymph node invasion in hypopharynx and lateral epilarynx carcinoma: a prognostic factor. *Head Neck Surg* 1987;10:14.
41. Weber RS, Marvel J, Smith P, et al. Paratracheal lymph node dissection for carcinoma of the larynx, hypopharynx, and cervical esophagus. *Otolaryngol Head Neck Surg* 1993;108:11.
42. Ogura JH, Jurema AA, Watson RK. Partial laryngopharyngectomy and neck dissection for pyriform sinus cancer: conservation surgery with immediate reconstruction. *Laryngoscope* 1960;70:1399.
43. Byers RM, Wolf PF, Ballantyne AJ. Rationale for elective modified neck dissection. *Head Neck Surg* 1988;10:160.
44. Johnson JT, Bacon GW, Myers EN, et al. Medial vs. lateral wall pyriform sinus carcinoma: implications for management of regional lymphatics. *Head Neck* 1994;16:401.
45. Peracchia A. Squamous carcinoma of the esophagus. *Hepatogastroenterology* 1990;37:358.
46. Kelley DJ, Wolf R, Shaha AR, et al. Impact of clinicopathologic parameters on patient survival in carcinoma of the cervical esophagus. *Am J Surg* 1995;170: 427.
47. Kotwall C, Sako K, Razack MS, et al. Metastatic patterns in squamous cell cancer of the head and neck. *Am J Surg* 1987;154:439.
48. Anderson LL, Lad TE. Autopsy findings in squamous-cell carcinoma of the esophagus. *Cancer* 1982;50:1587.
49. Katz AE. Immunobiologic staging of patients with carcinoma of the head and neck. *Laryngoscope* 1983;93:445.
50. O'Neill PA, Romsdahl MM. IgA as a blocking factor in human malignant melanoma. *Immunol Commun* 1974;3:427.
51. Schantz SP, Campbell BH, Guillamondegui OM. Pharyngeal carcinoma and natural killer cell activity. *Am J Surg* 1986;152:467.
52. Schantz SP, Goepfert HG. Multimodality therapy and distant metastases: the impact of natural killer cell activity. *Arch Otolaryngol Head Neck Surg* 1987;113: 1207.
53. Wolf GT, Schmaltz S, Hudson J, et al. Alterations in T–lymphocyte subpopulations in patients with head and neck cancer. *Arch Otolaryngol Head Neck Surg* 1987;113:1200.
54. Schantz SP. Biologic staging of head and neck cancer. *Cancer Bull* 1987;39:103.
55. Santon JB, Cronin MT, MacLeod CL, et al. Effects of epidermal growth factor receptor concentration on tumorigenicity of A431 cells in nude mice. *Cancer Res* 1986;46:4701.
56. Spector JG, Sessions DG, Haughey BH, et al. Delayed regional metastases, distant metastases, and second primary malignancies in squamous cell carcinomas of the larynx and hypopharynx. *Laryngoscope* 2001;111:1079.
57. Bataini P, Brugere J, Bernier J, et al. Results of radical radiotherapeutic treatment of carcinoma of the pyriform sinus: experience of the Institut Curie. *Int J Radiat Oncol Biol Phys* 1982;8:1277.
58. Laccourreye O, Merite-Drancy A, Brasnu D, et al. Supracricoid hemilaryngopharyngectomy in selected pyriform sinus carcinoma staged as T2. *Laryngoscope* 1993;103:1373.
59. French Head and Neck Study Group. Early pharyngolaryngeal carcinomas with palpable nodes. *Am J Surg* 1991;163:377.
60. Dubois JB, Guerrier B, DiRuggiero JM, et al. Cancer of the piriform sinus: treatment by radiation therapy alone and with surgery. *Radiology* 1986;160: 831.
61. Mendenhall WM, Parsons JT, Cassisi NJ, et al. Squamous cell carcinoma of the pyriform sinus treated with radical radiation therapy. *Radiother Oncol* 1987;9:201.
62. Garden AS, Morrison WH, Ang KK, et al. Hyperfractionated radiation in the treatment of squamous cell carcinomas of the head and neck: a comparison of two fractionation schedules. *Int J Radiat Oncol Biol Phys* 1995;31:493.
63. Parsons JT, Mendenhall WM, Stringer SP, et al. Twice-a-day radiotherapy for squamous cell carcinoma of the head and neck: the University of Florida experience. *Head Neck* 1993;15:87.
64. Fein DA, Mendenhall WM, Parsons JT, et al. Pharyngeal wall carcinoma treated with radiotherapy: impact of treatment technique and fractionation. *Int J Radiat Oncol Biol Phys* 1993;26:751.
65. Ogura JH, Biller HF, Wette R. Elective neck dissection for pharyngeal and laryngeal cancers: an evaluation. *Ann Oral Rhinol Laryngol* 1971;8:646.
66. Freeman RB, Marks JE, Ogura JH. Voice preservation in treatment of carcinoma of the pyriform sinus. *Laryngoscope* 1979;89:1855.
67. Goepfert H, Lindberg RD, Jesse RH. Combined laryngeal conservation surgery and irradiation: can we expand the indications for conservation therapy? *Otolaryngol Head Neck Surg* 1981;89:974.
68. Mendenhall WM, Parsons JT, Stringer SP, et al. Radiotherapy in the treatment of squamous cell carcinoma of the hypopharynx and cervical esophagus. In: Shah JP, Johnson JT, eds. *Proceedings of the 4th International Conference on Head and Neck Cancer.* Madison, WI: Omnipress, 1996:175.
69. Sessions DG, Ogura JH. Classification of laryngeal cancer. *Can J Otolaryngol* 1974;3:489.
70. Laccourreye H, Lacau St Guily J, Brasnu D, et al. Supracricoid hemilaryngopharyngectomy: analysis of 240 cases. *Ann Otol Rhinol Laryngol* 1987;96:217.

71. Ho CM, Lam KH, Wei WI, et al. Squamous cell carcinoma of the hypopharynx: analysis of treatment results. *Head Neck* 1993;15:405.
72. Abroad K, Fayos JV. High-dose radiotherapy in carcinoma of the pyriform sinus. *Cancer* 1984;53:2091.
73. Vandenbrouck C, Sancho H, LeFur R, et al. Results of a randomized clinical trial of preoperative irradiation versus postoperative in treatment of tumors of the hypopharynx. *Cancer* 1977;39:1445.
74. Mendenhall WM, Parsons JT, Devine JW, et al. Squamous cell carcinoma of the pyriform sinus treated with surgery and/or radiotherapy. *Head Neck Surg* 1987;10:88.
75. El Badawi SA, Goepfert H, Fletcher GH, et al. Squamous cell carcinoma of the pyriform sinus. *Laryngoscope* 1982;92:357.
76. Wang CC, Blitzer PH, Suit HD. Twice-a-day radiation therapy for cancer of the head and neck. *Cancer* 1985;55[9 Suppl]:2100.
77. Parsons JT, Cassisi NJ, Million RR. Results of twice-a-day irradiation of squamous cell carcinomas of the head and neck. *Int J Radiat Oncol Biol Phys* 1984;10:2041.
78. Tupchong L, Scott CB, Blitzer PH, et al. Randomized study of preoperative versus postoperative radiation therapy in advanced head and neck carcinoma: long-term follow-up of RTOG study 73-03. *Int J Radiat Oncol Biol Phys* 1991;20:21.
79. Head and Neck Contracts Program. Adjuvant chemotherapy for advanced head and neck squamous carcinomas. *Cancer* 1987;60:301
80. Laramore GE, Scott CB, al-Sarraf M, et al. Adjuvant chemotherapy for resectable squamous cell carcinomas of the head and neck: report on Intergroup Study 0034. *Int J Radiat Oncol Biol Phys* 1992;23:705.
81. Paccagnella A, Orlando A, Marchiori C, et al. Phase III trial of initial chemotherapy in stage III or IV head and neck cancers: a study by the gruppo di studio sui tumori della testa a del collo. *J Natl Cancer Inst* 1994; 86:265.
82. Pignon JP, Bourhis J, Domenge C, et al. Chemotherapy added to locoregional treatment for head and neck squamous-cell carcinoma: three meta-analyses of updated individual data. MACH-NC Collaborative Group. Meta-Analysis of Chemotherapy on Head and Neck Cancer. *Lancet* 2000;355:949.
83. El-Sayed S, Nelson N. Adjuvant and adjunctive chemotherapy in the management of squamous cell carcinoma of the head and neck region. A meta-analysis of prospective and randomized trials. *J Clin Oncol* 1996;14:838.
84. Lefebvre J-L, Chevalier D, Luboinski B, et al. Larynx preservation in pyriform sinus cancer: preliminary results of a European Organization for Research and Treatment of Cancer phase III trial. *J Natl Cancer Inst* 1996;88: 890.
85. Koch WM, Lee DJ, Eisele DW, et al. Chemoradiotherapy for organ preservation in oral and pharyngeal carcinoma. *Arch Otolaryngol Head Neck Surg* 1995; 121:974.
86. Hirsch SM, Caldarelli DD, Hutchinson JC Jr, et al. Concomitant chemotherapy and split-course radiation for cure and preservation of speech and swallowing in head and neck cancer. *Laryngoscope* 1991;101:583.
87. Adelstein DJ, Saxton JP, Lavertu P, et al. A phase III randomized trial comparing concurrent chemotherapy and radiotherapy with radiotherapy alone in resectable stage III and IV squamous cell head and neck cancer: preliminary results. *Head Neck* 1997;19:567.
88. Calais G, Alfonsi M, Bardet E, et al. Randomized trial of radiation therapy versus concomitant chemotherapy and radiation therapy for advanced-stage oropharynx carcinoma. *J Natl Cancer Inst* 1999;91:2081.
89. Forastiere AA, Berkey B, Maor M, et al. Phase III Trial to Preserve the Larynx: Induction Chemotherapy and Radiotherapy Versus Concomitant Chemoradiotherapy Versus Radiotherapy Alone, Intergroup Trial R91-11. *Proc Am Soc Clin Oncol* 2001(abst 4).
90. Fu KK, Pajak TF, Trotti A, et al. A Radiation Therapy Oncology Group (RTOG) phase III randomized study to compare hyperfractionation and two variants of accelerated fractionation to standard fractionation radiotherapy for head and neck squamous cell carcinomas: first report of RTOG 9003. *Int J Radiat Oncol Biol Phys* 2000;48:7.
91. Bezjak A, Grilli R, Brownian G. Non-resectability in radiotherapy trials in squamous cell head and neck cancer—implications for generalizability of trial results. *Proc Am Soc Clin Oncol* 1995(abst 296).
92. Vokes EE, Weichselbaum RR. Concomitant chemoradiotherapy: rationale and clinical experience in patients with solid tumors. *J Clin Oncol* 1990;8:911.
93. Forastiere AA. Cisplatin and radiotherapy in the management of locally advanced head and neck cancer. *Int J Radiat Oncol Biol Phys* 1993;27:465.
94. Merlano M, Rosso R, Sertoli MR, et al. Sequential versus alternating chemotherapy and radiotherapy in stage III-IV squamous cell carcinoma of the head and neck: a phase III study. *J Clin Oncol* 1988;6:627.
95. SECOG. A randomized trial of combined multidrug chemotherapy and radiotherapy in advanced squamous cell carcinoma of the head and neck. An interim report from the SECOG participants. *Eur J Surg Oncol* 1986;12: 289.
96. Adelstein DJ, Sharan VM, Earle AS, et al. Simultaneous versus sequential combined technique therapy for squamous cell head and neck cancer. *Cancer* 1990;65:1685.
97. Taylor SG IV, Murthy AK, Vannetzel J-M, et al. Randomized comparison of neoadjuvant cisplatin and fluorouracil infusion followed by radiation versus concomitant treatment in advanced head and neck cancer. *J Clin Oncol* 1994; 12:385.
98. Browman GP, Cripps C, Hodson DI, et al. Placebo-controlled randomized trial of infusional fluorouracil during standard radiotherapy in locally advanced head and neck cancer. *J Clin Oncol* 1994;12:2648.
99. Million RR, Cassisi NJ, Mancuso AA. Management of the neck for squamous cell carcinoma. In: Million RR, Cassisi NJ, eds. *Management of head and neck cancer: a multidisciplinary approach,* 2nd ed. Philadelphia: JB Lippincott Co, 1994:75.
100. Coia LR, Minsky BD, Berkey BA, et al. Outcome of patients receiving radiation for cancer of the esophagus: results of the 1992–1994 Patterns of Care Study. *J Clin Oncol* 2000;18:455.
101. Tai P, Van Dyk J, Yu E, et al. Radiation treatment for cervical esophagus: patterns of practice study in Canada, 1996. *Int J Radiat Oncol Biol Phys* 2000; 47:703.
102. Herskovic A, Martz LK, Al-Sarraf M, et al. Combined chemotherapy and radiotherapy compared with radiotherapy alone in patients with cancer of the esophagus. *N Engl J Med* 1992;326:1593.
103. Spiro RH, Bains MS, Shah JP, et al. Gastric transposition for head and neck cancer: a critical update. *Am J Surg* 1991;162:348.
104. Roka R, Kriwanek S, Roka S. Therapy of cervical esophageal carcinoma. *Recent Results Cancer Res* 2000;155:113.
105. Kelsen DP, Ginsberg R, Pajak TF, et al. Chemotherapy followed by surgery compared with surgery alone for localized esophageal cancer. *N Engl J Med* 1998;339:1979.
106. Mendenhall WM, Sombeck MD, Parsons JT, et al. Management of cervical esophageal carcinoma. *Semin Radiat Oncol* 1994;4:179.
107. Ilson DH, Kelsen DP. Management of esophageal cancer. *Oncology* 1996;10: 1385.
108. Roussel A, Bleiberg H, Dalesio O, et al. Palliative therapy of inoperable oesophageal carcinoma with radiotherapy and methotrexate: final results of a controlled clinical trial. *Int J Radiat Oncol Biol Phys* 1989;16:67.
109. Roussel A, Haegele P, Paillot B, et al. Results of the EORTC-GTCCG phase III trial of irradiation vs irradiation and CDDP in inoperable esophageal cancer. *Proc Am Soc Clin Oncol* 1994(abst 199).
110. Guillamondegui OM, Geoffray B, McKenna RJ. Total reconstruction of the hypopharynx and cervical esophagus. *Am J Surg* 1985;150:422.
111. Rees RS, Ivey GL, Shack RB, et al. Pectoralis major musculocutaneous flaps: long-term follow-up of hypopharyngeal reconstruction. *Plast Reconstr Surg* 1986;77:586.
112. Lau WF, Lam KH, Wei WI. Reconstruction of hypopharyngeal defects in cancer surgery: do we have a choice? *Am J Surg* 1987;154:374.
113. Anthony JP, Singer MF, Mathes SJ. Pharyngoesophageal reconstruction using the tubed free radial forearm flap. *Clin Plast Surg* 1994;21:137.
114. Demergasso F, Piazza MV. Trapezius myocutaneous flap in reconstructive surgery for head and neck cancer: an original technique. *Am J Surg* 1979;138: 533.
115. Coleman JJ, Searles JM, Hester TR, et al. Ten years experience with the free jejunal autograft. *Am J Surg* 1987;154:394.
116. Kato H, Iizuka T, Watanabe H, et al. Reconstruction of the esophagus by microvascular surgery. *Jpn J Clin Oncol* 1984;14:379.
117. Theile DE, Robinson DW, McCafferty GJ. Pharyngolaryngectomy reconstruction by revascularized free jejunal graft. *Aust N Z J Surg* 1986;56:849.
118. Maharaj D, Haffejee AA, Angorn IB, et al. Pharyngolaryngo-oesophagectomy with gastric 'pull-up' for cancer of the hypopharynx and cervical oesophagus. *S Afr J Surg* 1988;26:7.
119. Harrison DFN, Thompson AE. Pharyngolaryngoesophagectomy with pharyngogastric anastomosis for cancer of the hypopharynx: review of 101 operations. *Head Neck Surg* 1986;8:418.
120. Rifai M, Amer F, Abdel-Meguid H, et al. Pharyngeal repair after laryngopharyngectomy: four year experience. *Head Neck Surg* 1987;10:88.
121. Spector JG, Sessions DG, Emami B, et al. Squamous cell carcinoma of the pyriform sinus: a nonrandomized comparison of therapeutic modalities and long-term results. *Laryngoscope* 1995;105(4 Pt 1):397.
122. Ahmad K, Fayos JV. Role of radiation therapy in carcinoma of the hypopharynx. *Acta Radiol Oncol* 1984;23:21.
123. Yu L, Vikram B, Malamud S, et al. Chemotherapy rapidly alternating with twice-a-day accelerated radiation therapy in carcinomas involving the hypopharynx or esophagus: an update. *Cancer Invest* 1995;13:567.
124. Strauss GM. Randomized population trials and screening for lung cancer: breaking the cure barrier. *Cancer* 2000;89[11 Suppl]:2399.
125. Smith TJ, Davidson NE, Schapira DV, et al. American Society of Clinical Oncology 1998 Update of Recommended Breast Cancer Surveillance Guidelines. *J Clin Oncol* 1999;17:1080.
126. Desch CE, Benson III AB, Smith TJ, et al. Recommended Colorectal Cancer Surveillance Guidelines by the American Society of Clinical Oncology. *J Clin Oncol* 1999;17:1312.
127. Hong WK, Lippman SM, Itri LM, et al. Prevention of second primary tumors with isotretinoin in squamous-cell carcinoma of the head and neck. *N Engl J Med* 1990;323:795.
128. Hoffman HT, Karnell LH, Shah JP, et al. Hypopharyngeal cancer patient care evaluation. *Laryngoscope* 1997;107:1005.
129. Eckel HE, Staar S, Volling P, et al. Surgical treatment for hypopharynx carcinoma: feasibility, mortality, and results. *Otolaryngol Head Neck Surg* 2001;124: 561.
130. Wang TD. Preservation of laryngeal function after removal of carcinoma of the pyriform sinus. *Chin Med J (Engl)* 1989;102:825.
131. Amdur RJ, Mendenhall WM, Stringer SP, et al. Organ preservation with

radiotherapy for T1-T2 carcinoma of the pyriform sinus. *Head Neck* 2001;23: 353.
132. Garden AS, Morrison WH, Clayman GL, et al. Early squamous cell carcinoma of the hypopharynx: outcomes of treatment with radiation alone to the primary disease. *Head Neck* 1996;18:317.
133. Wang CC. Carcinoma of the hypopharynx. In: Wang CC, ed. *Radiation therapy for head and neck neoplasms: indications, techniques, and results,* 2nd ed. Chicago: Year Book Medical Publishers, 1990:207.
134. Davidson J, Briant D, Guillane P, et al. The role of surgery following radiotherapy failure for advanced laryngopharyngeal cancer. *Arch Otolaryngol Head Neck Surg* 1994;120:269.
135. Stoeckli SJ, Pawlik AB, Lipp M, et al. Salvage surgery after failure of nonsurgical therapy for carcinoma of the larynx and hypopharynx. *Arch Otolaryngol Head Neck Surg* 2000;126:1473.
136. Jones AS. The management of early hypopharyngeal cancer: primary radiotherapy and salvage surgery. *Clin Otolaryngol* 1992;17:545.
137. Johansen LV, Grau C, Overgaard J. Hypopharyngeal squamous cell carcinoma—treatment results in 138 consecutively admitted patients. *Acta Oncol* 2000;39:529.
138. Frank JL, Garb JL, Kay S, et al. Postoperative radiotherapy improves survival in squamous cell carcinoma of the hypopharynx. *Am J Surg* 1994;168:476.
139. Van den Bogaert W, Ostyn F, van der Schueren E. Hypopharyngeal cancer: results of treatment with radiotherapy alone and combinations of surgery and radiotherapy. *Radiother Oncol* 1985;3:311.
140. Slotman BJ, Kralendonk JH, Snow GB, et al. Surgery and postoperative radiotherapy and radiotherapy alone in T3-T4 cancers of the pyriform sinus. Treatment results and patterns of failure. *Acta Oncol* 1994;33:55.
141. Kraus DH, Zelefsky MJ, Brock HA, et al. Combined surgery and radiation therapy for squamous cell carcinoma of the hypopharynx. *Otolaryngol Head Neck Surg* 1997;116(6 Pt 1):637.
142. Meoz-Mendez RT, Fletcher GH, Guillamondegui OM, et al. Analysis of the results of irradiation in the treatment of squamous cell carcinomas of the pharyngeal walls. *Int J Radiat Oncol Biol Phys* 1978;4:579.
143. Nguyen TD, Malissard L, Eschwege F, et al. [Postoperative radiotherapy in carcinoma of the pyriform sinus. Work of the "Groupe radiotherapie de la Federation national des centres de lutte le cancer"]. *Bull Cancer Radiother* 1995;82:318.
144. Donald PJ, Hayes HR, Dhaliwal R. Combined therapy for pyriform sinus cancer using postoperative irradiation. *Otolaryngol Head Neck Surg* 1980;88: 738.
145. Frank JL, Garb JL, Kay S, et al. Postoperative radiotherapy improves survival in squamous cell carcinoma of the hypopharynx. *Am J Surg* 1994;168:476.
146. Teichgraeber JF, McConnel FM. Treatment of posterior pharyngeal wall carcinoma. *Otolaryngol Head Neck Surg* 1986;94:287.
147. Baker SR, Makuch RW, Wolf GT. Preoperative cisplatin and bleomycin therapy in head and neck squamous carcinoma. Prognostic factors for tumor response. *Arch Otolaryngol* 1981;107:683.
148. Yates A, Crumley RL. Surgical treatment of pyriform sinus cancer: a retrospective study. *Laryngoscope* 1984;94(12 Pt 1):1586.
149. Pingree TF, Davis RK, Reichman O, et al. Treatment of hypopharyngeal carcinoma: a 10-year review of 1,362 cases. *Laryngoscope* 1987;97(8 Pt 1):901.
150. Reece GP, Schusterman MA, Miller MJ, et al. Morbidity and functional outcome of free jejunal transfer reconstruction for circumferential defects of the pharynx and cervical esophagus. *Plast Reconstr Surg* 1995;96:1307.
151. Barrett WL, Gluckman JL, Aron BS. Safety of radiating jejunal interposition grafts in head and neck cancer. *Am J Clin Oncol* 1997;20:609.
152. Cole CJ, Garden AS, Frankenthaler RA, et al. Postoperative radiation of free jejunal autografts in patients with advanced cancer of the head and neck. *Cancer* 1995;75:2356.
153. Pfister DG, Strong E, Harrison L, et al. Larynx preservation in combined chemotherapy and radiation therapy in advanced but resectable head and neck cancer. *J Clin Oncol* 1991;9:850.
154. Forastiere AA. Randomized trials of induction chemotherapy. A critical review. *Hematol Oncol Clin North Am* 1991;5:725.
155. Jacobs C, Makuch R. Efficacy of adjuvant chemotherapy for patients with resectable head and neck cancer: a subset analysis of the head and neck contracts program. *J Clin Oncol* 1990;8:838.
156. Zelefsky MJ, Kraus DH, Pfister DG, et al. Combined chemotherapy and radiotherapy versus surgery and postoperative radiotherapy for advanced hypopharyngeal cancer. *Head Neck* 1996;18:405.
157. Clayman GL, Weber RS, Guillamondegui O, et al. Laryngeal preservation for advanced laryngeal and hypopharyngeal cancers. *Arch Otolaryngol Head Neck Surg* 1995;121:219.
158. Denard F, Chauvel P, Santini J, et al. Response to chemotherapy as justification for modification of the therapeutic strategy for pharyngolaryngeal carcinomas. *Head Neck* 1990;12:225.
159. Fountzilas G, Kosmidis P, Zamboglou N, et al. Does substitution of surgery with induction chemotherapy preserve organ function in inoperable head and neck cancer? A retrospective analysis of 73 cases. *J Chemother* 1994;6:272.
160. Karp DD, Vaughan CW, Carter R, et al. Larynx preservation using induction chemotherapy plus radiation therapy as an alternative to laryngectomy in advanced head and neck cancer. A final report. *Am J Clin Oncol* 1991;14:273.
161. Jacobs C, Goffinet DR, Goffinet L, et al. Chemotherapy as a substitute for surgery in the treatment of advanced resectable head and neck cancer. A report from the Northern California Oncology Group. *Cancer* 1987;60:1178.
162. Pfister DG, Harrison LB, Strong EW, et al. Current status of larynx preservation with multimodality therapy. *Oncology* 1992;6:33.
163. Shirinian MH, Weber RS, Lippman SM, et al. Laryngeal preservation by induction chemotherapy plus radiotherapy in locally advanced head and neck cancer: the M. D. Anderson Cancer Center experience. *Head Neck* 1994; 16:39.
164. Kim KH, Sung MW, Rhee CS, et al. Neoadjuvant chemotherapy and radiotherapy for the treatment of advanced hypopharyngeal carcinoma. *Am J Otolaryngol* 1998;19:40.
165. Kraus DH, Pfister DG, Harrison LB, et al. Salvage laryngectomy for unsuccessful larynx preservation therapy. *Ann Otol Rhinol Laryngol* 1995;104:936.
166. The Department of Veterans Affairs Laryngeal Cancer Study Group. Induction chemotherapy plus radiation compared with surgery plus radiation in patients with advanced laryngeal cancer. *N Engl J Med* 1991;324:1685.
167. Beauvillain C, Mahe M, Bourdin S, et al. Final results of a randomized trial comparing chemotherapy plus radiotherapy with chemotherapy plus surgery plus radiotherapy in locally advanced resectable hypopharyngeal carcinomas. *Laryngoscope* 1997;107:648.
168. Gwozdz JT, Morrison WH, Garden AS, et al. Concomitant boost radiotherapy for squamous carcinoma of the tonsillar fossa. *Int J Radiat Oncol Biol Phys* 1997;39:127.
169. Brizel DM, Albers ME, Fisher SR, et al. Hyperfractionated irradiation with or without concurrent chemotherapy for locally advanced head and neck cancer. *N Engl J Med* 1998;338:1798.
170. Keane TJ, Cummings BJ, O'Sullivan B, et al. A randomized trial of radiation therapy compared to split course radiation therapy combined with mitomycin C and 5 fluorouracil as initial treatment for advanced laryngeal and hypopharyngeal squamous carcinoma. *Int J Radiat Oncol Biol Phys* 1993;25:613.
171. Samant S, Kumar P, Wan J, et al. Concomitant radiation therapy and targeted cisplatin chemotherapy for the treatment of advanced pyriform sinus carcinoma: disease control and preservation of organ function. *Head Neck* 1999;21: 595.
172. Bernier J, Domenge C, Eschwege F, et al. Chemo-radiotherapy, as compared to radiotherapy alone, significantly increases disease-free and overall survival in head and neck cancer in patients after surgery: results of EORTC Phase III trial 22931. *Int J Radiat Oncol Biol Phys* 2001;51(Suppl 1):3 (abst, plenary #1).
173. Cooper JS, Pajak TF, Forastiere AA, et al. Postoperative concurrent radiochemotherapy in high risk SCCA of the head and neck: initial report of RTOG 9501/intergroup phase III trial. *Proc Am Soc Clin Oncol* 2002(abst 903).
174. Merlano M, Vitale V Rosso R, et al. Treatment of advanced squamous cell carcinoma of the head and neck with alternating chemotherapy and radiotherapy. *N Engl J Med* 1992;327:1115.
175. Merlano M, Benasso M, Corvo R, et al. Five-year update of a randomized trial of alternating radiotherapy and chemotherapy compared with radiotherapy alone in treatment of unresectable squamous cell carcinoma of the head and neck. *J Natl Cancer Inst* 1996;88:583.
176. Adelstein DJ, Li Y, Adams GL, et al. An Intergroup phase III comparison of standard radiation therapy and two schedules of concurrent chemoradiotherapy in patients with unresectable squamous cell head and neck cancer. *J Clin Oncol* 2003;21:92.
177. Jacobs C, Lyman G, Velez-Garcia E, et al. A phase III randomized study comparing cisplatin and fluorouracil as single agents and in combination for advanced squamous cell carcinoma of the head and neck. *J Clin Oncol* 1992; 10:257.
178. Forastiere AA, Metch B, Schuller DE, et al. Randomized comparison of cisplatin plus fluorouracil and carboplatin plus fluorouracil versus methotrexate in advanced squamous cell carcinoma of the head and neck: a Southwest Oncology Group Study. *J Clin Oncol* 1992;12:1245.
179. Clavel M, Vermorken JB, Cognetti F, et al. Randomized comparison of cisplatin, methotrexate, bleomycin and vincristine (CABO) versus cisplatin and 5-fluorouracil (CF) versus cisplatin (C) in recurrent or metastatic squamous cell carcinoma of the head and neck. A phase III study of the EORTC Head and Neck Cancer Cooperative Group. *Ann Oncol* 1994;5:521.
180. Browman GP, Cronin L. Standard chemotherapy in squamous cell head and neck cancer: what we have learned from randomized trials. *Semin Oncol* 1994;21:311.
181. Gunnlaugsson GH, Wychulis AR, Roland C, et al. Analysis of the records of 1,657 patients with carcinoma of the esophagus and cardia of the stomach. *Surg Gynecol Obstet* 1970;130:997.
182. Pearson JG. Radiotherapy for esophageal carcinoma. *World J Surg* 1981;5:489.
183. Kakegawa T, Yamana H, Ando N. Analysis of surgical treatment for carcinoma situated in the cervical esophagus. *Surgery* 1985;97:150.
184. Collin CF, Spiro RH. Carcinoma of the cervical esophagus: changing therapeutic trends. *Am J Surg* 1984;148:460.
185. Griffiths JD, Shaw HJ. Cancer of the laryngopharynx and cervical esophagus: radical resection with repair by colon transplant. *Arch Otolaryngol Head Neck Surg* 1973;97:340.
186. Hennessy TP, O'Connell R. Carcinoma of the hypopharynx, esophagus, and cardia. *Surg Gynecol Obstet* 1986;162:243.
187. Clayman GL, Weber RS, O'Malley BB. Cancer of the hypopharynx and cervical esophagus. In: Harrison LB, Sessions RB, Hong WK, eds. *Head and neck cancer: a multidisciplinary approach.* Philadelphia: Lippincott-Raven, 1999:529.
188. Bardini R, Ruol A, Peracchia A. Therapeutic options for cancer of the hypopharynx and cervical oesophagus. *Ann Chir Gynaecol* 1995;84:202.

189. Mendenhall WM, Parsons JT, Vogel SB, et al. Carcinoma of the cervical esophagus treated with radiation therapy. *Laryngoscope* 1988;98:769.
190. Newaishy GA, Read GA, Duncan W, et al. Results of radical radiotherapy of squamous cell carcinoma of the oesophagus. *Clin Radiol* 1982;33:347.
191. Gu XZ. Radiotherapy for carcinoma of the esophagus. In: Kai HGJ, Kai WY, eds. *Carcinoma of the esophagus and gastric cardia.* Berlin: Springer-Verlag, 1984: 257.
192. Gaspar LE, Winter K, Kocha WI, et al. A phase I/II study of external beam radiation, brachytherapy, and concurrent chemotherapy for patients with localized carcinoma of the esophagus (Radiation Therapy Oncology Group Study 9207): final report. *Cancer* 2000;88:988.
193. Cooper JS, Guo MD, Herskovic A, et al. Chemoradiotherapy of locally advanced esophageal cancer: long-term follow-up of a prospective randomized trial (RTOG 85-01). Radiation Therapy Oncology Group. *JAMA* 1999; 281:1623.
194. Burmeister BH, Dickie G, Smithers BM, et al. Thirty-four patients with carcinoma of the cervical esophagus treated with chemoradiation therapy. *Arch Otolaryngol Head Neck Surg* 2000;126:205.
195. Soto Parra H, Valente M, Bidoli, P, et al. Definitive chemoradiotherapy in cervical esophageal carcinoma. *Proc Am Soc Clin Oncol* 1997(abst 262).
196. Santoro A, Bidoli P, Salvini PM, et al. Larynx preservation with combined chemotherapy plus radiotherapy in upper squamous cell carcinoma of the esophagus (SCCE). *Proc Am Soc Clin Oncol* 1993(abst 899).
197. Stuschke M, Stahl M, Wilke H, et al. Induction chemotherapy followed by concurrent chemotherapy and high-dose radiotherapy for locally advanced squamous cell carcinoma of the upper-thoracic and midthoracic esophagus. *Am J Clin Oncol* 2000;23:233.
198. Kelsen DP, Ginsberg R, Pajak TF, et al. Chemotherapy followed by surgery compared with surgery alone for localized esophageal cancer. *N Engl J Med* 1998;339:1979.
199. Bosset JF, Gignoux M, Triboulet JP, et al. Chemoradiotherapy followed by surgery compared with surgery alone in squamous-cell cancer of the esophagus. *N Engl J Med* 1997;337:161.
200. Nygaard K, Hagen S, Hansen HS, et al. Pre-operative radiotherapy prolongs survival in operable esophageal carcinoma: a randomized, multicenter study of pre-operative radiotherapy and chemotherapy. The second Scandinavian trial in esophageal cancer. *World J Surg* 1992;16:1104; discussion 1110.
201. Le Prise E, Etienne PL, Meunier B, et al. A randomized study of chemotherapy, radiation therapy, and surgery versus surgery for localized squamous cell carcinoma of the esophagus. *Cancer* 1994;73:1779.
202. Roth JA, Pass HI, Flanagan MM, et al. Randomized clinical trial of preoperative and postoperative adjuvant chemotherapy with cisplatin, vindesine, and bleomycin for carcinoma of the esophagus. *J Thorac Cardiovasc Surg* 1988;96:242.
203. Walsh TN, Noonan N, Hollywood D, et al. A comparison of multimodal therapy and surgery for esophageal adenocarcinoma. *N Engl J Med* 1996;335:462.
204. Goodner JT. Treatment d survival in cancer of the cervical esophagus. *Am J Surg* 1969;118:673.
205. Forastiere AA, Orringer MB, Perez-Tamayo C, et al. Preoperative chemoradiation followed by transhiatal esophagectomy for carcinoma of the esophagus: final report. *J Clin Oncol* 1993;11:1118.
206. Bleiberg H, Jacob JH, Bedenne L, et al. Randomized phase II trial of 5-fluorouracil (5-FU) and cisplatin (DDP) vs DDP alone in advanced esophageal cancer. *Proc Am Soc Clin Oncol* 1991(abst 447).
207. Ajani J, Ilson D, Daugherty K, et al. Activity of Taxol in patients with squamous cell carcinoma and adenocarcinoma of the esophagus. *J Natl Cancer Inst* 1994;86:1086.
208. Kelsen DP, Ilson D, Wadleigh R, et al. A Phase II multi-center trial of paclitaxel as a weekly one-hour infusion in advanced esophageal cancer. *Proc Am Soc Clin Oncol* 2000(abst 1266).
209. Enzinger PC, Kulke MH, Clark JW, et al. Phase II trial of CPT-11 in previously untreated patients with advanced adenocarcinoma of the esophagus and stomach. *Proc Am Soc Clin Oncol* 2000(abst 1243).
210. Lin L, Hecht JR. A phase II trial of irinotecan in patients with advanced adenocarcinoma of the gastroesophageal (GE) junction. *Proc Am Soc Clin Oncol* 2000(abst 1130).
211. Urba S, Orringer M, Iannettoni M, et al. A phase II trial of preoperative cisplatin, paclitaxel, and radiation therapy (XRT) before trans-hiatal esophagectomy (THE) in patients (PTS) with loco-regional esophageal cancer (CA). *Proc Am Soc Clin Oncol* 2000(abst 960).
212. Wright CD, Wain JC, Lynch TJ, et al. Induction therapy for esophageal cancer with paclitaxel and hyperfractionated radiotherapy: a phase I and II study. *J Thorac Cardiovasc Surg* 1997;114:811.
213. Dropkin MJ, Malgady RG, Scott DW, et al. Scaling of disfigurement and dysfunction in postoperative head and neck patients. *Head Neck Surg* 1983;8:559.
214. Pauloski BR, Logemann JA, Rademaker AW, et al. Speech and swallowing function after oral and oropharyngeal resections: one year follow-up. *Head Neck* 1994;16:313.
215. Coia LR, Soffen EM, Schultheiss TE, et al. Swallowing function in patients with esophageal cancer treated with concurrent radiation and chemotherapy. *Cancer* 1993;71:281.
216. Bradford CR, Esclamado RM, Carroll WR, et al. Analysis of recurrence, complications, and functional results with free jejunal flaps. *Head Neck* 1994;16:149.
217. Kemmler G, Holzner B, Kopp M, et al. Comparison of two quality-of-life instruments for cancer patients: the Functional Assessment of Cancer Therapy-General and the European Organization for Research and Treatment of Cancer Quality of Life Questionnaire-C30. *J Clin Oncol* 1999;17:2932.
218. List MA, D'Antonio LL, Cella DF, et al. Performance Status Scale for Head and Neck Cancer Patients and the Functional Assessment of Cancer Therapy-Head and Neck Scale. A study of utility and validity. *Cancer* 1996;77: 2294.
219. McNeil BJ, Weichselbaum R, Pauker SG. Speech and survival. *N Engl J Med* 1981;305:982.
220. List MA, Strack J, Colangel L, et al. How do head and neck cancer patients prioritize treatment outcomes before initiating treatment? *J Clin Oncol* 2000; 18:877.
221. Mohide EA, Archibald SD, Tew M, et al. Postlaryngectomy quality-of-life dimensions identified by patients and health care professionals. *Am J Surg* 1992;164:619.
222. Van der Donk J, Levendag PC, Kuijpers AJ, et al. Patient participation in clinical decision-making for treatment of T3 laryngeal cancer: a comparison of state and process utilities. *J Clin Oncol* 1995;13:2369.
223. Gralla RJ, Osoba D, Kris MG, et al. Recommendations for the use of antiemetics: evidence-based, clinical practice guidelines. American Society of Clinical Oncology. *J Clin Oncol* 1999;17:2971.
224. *Physicians' desk reference.* Montvale NJ: Medical Economics Pub, 2001.
225. Hartsell WF, Thomas CR, Murthy AK, et al. Pilot study for the evaluation of simultaneous cisplatin/fluorouracil infusion and limited radiation therapy in regionally recurrent head and neck cancer. *Am J Clin Oncol* 1994;17:338.
226. Rodriguez J, Point D, Brunin F, et al. Chirurgie de l'hypopharynx apres radiotherapie. *Bull Cancer Radiother* 1996;83:17.
227. Tavorath RJ, Pfister DG. Chemotherapy for recurrent disease and combined modality therapies for head and neck cancer. *Curr Opin Oncol* 1995;7:242.
228. Earlam R, Cunha-Melo JR. Oesophageal squamous cell carcinoma: I. A critical review of surgery. *Br J Surg* 1980;67:381.
229. Minsky BD. Palliation of esophageal cancer: palliative external beam radiation therapy and combined modality therapy. *Dis Esophag* 1996;9:86.
230. Mehran RJ, Duranceau A. The use of endoprosthesis in the palliation of esophageal carcinoma. *Chest Surg Clin North Am* 1994;4:331.
231. Narayan S, Sivak MV. Palliation of esophageal carcinoma. Laser and photodynamic therapy. *Chest Surg Clin North Am* 1994;4:347.
232. Brennan JA, Mao L, Hruban RH, et al. Molecular assessment of histopathological staging in squamous cell carcinoma of the head and neck. *N Engl J Med* 1995;332:429.
233. Lingen MW. Angiogenesis in the development of head and neck cancer and its inhibition by chemopreventive agents. *Crit Rev Oral Biol Med* 1999;10:153.
234. Albanell J, Codony-Servat J, Rojo F, et al. Activated extracellular signal-regulated kinases: association with epidermal growth factor receptor/transforming growth factor alpha expression in head and neck squamous carcinoma and inhibition by anti-epidermal growth factor receptor treatments. *Cancer Res* 2001;6:6500.
235. Herbst RS, Langer CJ. Epidermal growth factor receptors as a target for cancer treatment: the emerging role of IMC-C225 in the treatment of lung and head and neck cancers. *Semin Oncol* 2002;29[1 Suppl 4]:27.
236. Koch WM, Boyle JO, Mao L, et al. p53 gene mutations as markers of tumor spread in synchronous oral cancers. *Arch Otolaryngol Head Neck Surg* 1994; 120:943.

Radiologic Imaging Concerns

237. Low VH, Rubesin SE. Contrast evaluation of the pharynx and esophagus. [Review]. *Radiol Clin North Am* 1993;31:1265.
238. Wenig BL, Ziffra KL, Mafee MF, et al. MR imaging of squamous cell carcinoma of the larynx and hypopharynx. *Otolaryngol Clin North Am* 1995;28:609.
239. Koch J, Halvorsen RA Jr. Staging of esophageal cancer: computed tomography, magnetic resonance imaging, and endoscopic ultrasound [Review]. *Semin Roentgenol* 1994;29:364.
240. Righi PD, Kelley DJ, Ernst R, et al. Evaluation of prevertebral muscle invasion by squamous cell carcinoma. Can computed tomography replace open neck exploration? *Arch Otolaryngol Head Neck Surg* 1996;122:660.
241. Steinkamp HJ, Heim T, Zwicker C, et al. [The value of nuclear magnetic resonance tomography in tumor staging of laryngeal-/hypopharyngeal cancer]. [German] Wertigkeit der Kernspintomographie im Tumorstaging des Larynx-/Hypopharynxkarzinoms. *HNO* 1992;40:339.
242. Garden AS, Morrison WH, Clayman GL, et al. Early squamous cell carcinoma of the hypopharynx: outcomes of treatment with radiation alone to the primary disease. *Head Neck* 1996;18:317.
243. Amdur RJ, Mendenhall WM, Stringer SP, et al. Organ preservation with radiotherapy for T1-T2 carcinoma of the pyriform sinus. *Head Neck* 2001;23: 353.
244. Lee JH, Sohn JE, Choe DH, et al. Sonographic findings of the neopharynx after total laryngectomy: comparison with CT. *AJNR Am J Neuroradiol* 2000; 21:823.
245. Chak A, Canto MI, Cooper GS, et al. Endosonographic assessment of multimodality therapy predicts survival of esophageal carcinoma patients. *Cancer* 2000;88:1788.
246. Minn H, Lapela M, Klemi PJ, et al. Prediction of survival with fluorine-18-fluoro-deoxyglucose and PET in head and neck cancer. *J Nucl Med* 1997;38: 1907.

247. Reisser C, Haberkorn U, Dimitrakopoulou-Strauss A, et al. Chemotherapeutic management of head and neck malignancies with positron emission tomography. *Arch Otolaryngol Head Neck Surg* 1995;121:272.
248. Parsons JT, Palta JR, Mendenhall WM, et al. Head and neck cancer. In: Levitt SH, Khan FM, Potish RA, et al., eds. *Levitt and Tapley's technological basis of radiation therapy: clinical applications,* 3rd ed. Baltimore: Lippincott Williams & Wilkins, 1999:269.
249. Mendenhall WM, Parsons JT, Mancuso AA, et al. Squamous cell carcinoma of the pharyngeal wall treated with irradiation. *Radiother Oncol* 1988;11:205.
250. Mendenhall WM, Million RR, Bova FJ. Carcinoma of the cervical esophagus treated with radiation therapy using a four-field box technique. *Int J Radiat Oncol Biol Phys* 1982;8:1435.
251. Amdur RJ, Parsons JT, Mendenhall WM, et al. Postoperative irradiation for squamous cell carcinoma of the head and neck: an analysis of treatment results and complications. *Int J Radiat Oncol Biol Phys* 1989;16:25.

CHAPTER 21

Cancer of the Nasal Vestibule, Nasal Cavity, and Paranasal Sinus

Surgical Management

Peter D. Costantino, Mark R. Murphy, and Jason A. Moche

The treatment of nasal and paranasal sinus neoplasms has evolved rapidly over the last three decades. Tumors once thought unresectable are now being treated by a combination of complete surgical resection, primary reconstruction, and focused radiation therapy. New methods of extirpation, particularly at the skull base, have spurred advances in primary reconstruction. Survival rates, along with quality of life, have slowly improved as a result of these combined treatment capabilities. Patients now have the option of an oncologically sound surgical resection coupled with excellent functional and cosmetic reconstruction. This is in direct contrast to the historical standard that consisted of resection without any significant attention to reconstruction. We now have the means to surgically remove these lesions, effectively reconstruct the region, and then use focused radiation therapy to effectively optimize the potential for cure while preserving the patient's appearance and function. This chapter will be limited to the surgical management of nasal cavity, paranasal sinus, and anterior cranial base lesions.

ANATOMY

Nasal Vestibule

Beginning anteriorly, the nasal vestibules represent the bilateral entry points of the nasal cavity. The anterior superstructure of the nasal cavity is bounded by the projecting frontal processes of the maxilla, the paired nasal bones, and the junction of the nasal bones with the frontal bone. In the midsagittal plane the perpendicular plate of the ethmoid bone provides support. The remaining component of the superstructure of the nasal vestibule is the cartilaginous vault, consisting of the upper lateral cartilages and adjacent portion of cartilaginous septum. The lobules of the nose consist of the tip, the lower lateral cartilages, the alae and vestibular regions, and the columella (1). Centrally and inferiorly, the anterior border is bounded by the piriform aperture, whereas the posterior limit is the choanae. The anterior floor is predominantly formed by the palatal

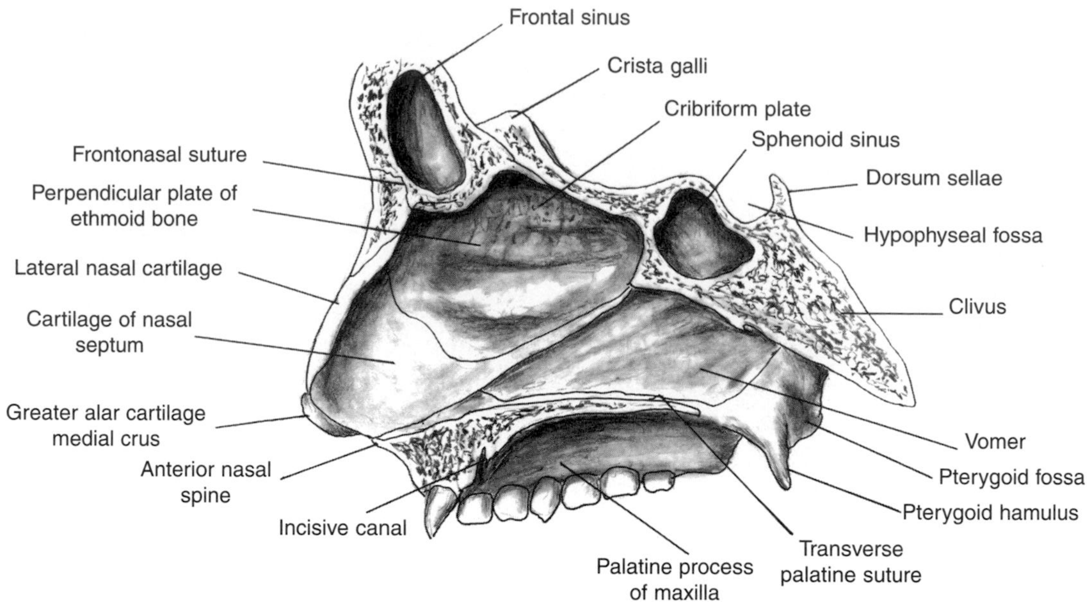

Figure 21.1 Septal anatomy.

process of the maxillary bone, whereas the posterior palate consists of the horizontal process of the palatine bone (Fig. 21.1.).

Posterior to the nasal vestibule is the nasal cavity. The roof of the nasal cavity forms the base of the frontal sinus and cribriform plate. Posteriorly the roof slopes inferiorly to the posterior choanae along the anterior wall of the sphenoid sinus and body of the sphenoid bone. The bony and cartilaginous septum bisects this cavity. The septum consists of the vomer (posteroinferiorly), perpendicular plate of the ethmoid bone (posterosuperiorly), and quadrilateral cartilage (anteriorly). The lateral wall of the cavities is formed by several bony structures: the nasal surface of the maxilla, inferior concha, superior and middle concha of the ethmoid bone, and the perpendicular plate of the palatine bone (Fig. 21.2).

The mucosa of the nasal cavity is psuedostratified, ciliated epithelium containing mucous and serous glands. Olfactory mucosa is found along the roof of the cavity, in communication with the olfactory nerves through the cribriform plate (1). In contrast to the pink respiratory mucosa that lines the majority of the nasal cavity, the olfactory mucosa has a distinct pale tan appearance and is limited to the most superior aspect of the central nasal vault directly above the cribriform plate. The sensory innervation of the nasal cavity emanates primarily from the second division of the trigeminal nerve. Sympathetic innervation is supplied through the branches of the internal and external carotid artery systems. The parasympathetic innervation is through the greater superficial petrosal nerve and branches of the sphenopalatine ganglion.

The rich vascular supply to the nasal cavity is provided through two primary sources: the ethmoid system originating with the ophthalmic artery, and the sphenopalatine vessels, which represent terminal branches off of the external carotid system. The ethmoid arteries are divided into anterior and posterior vessels that both originate from the ophthalmic artery, a branch of the internal carotid. These arteries pierce the medial wall of the orbit at the frontoethmoidal suture. The posterior ethmoidal artery is approximately 0.8 to 1.1 cm anterior to the optic canal, whereas the anterior ethmoidal artery is approximately 2.0 cm anterior to this structure. Both arteries form a horizontal line that generally defines the location of the floor of the anterior fossa at the cribriform plate and fovea ethmoidalis. The sphenopalatine artery represents the terminal branch of the maxillary artery. This vessel runs on the medial surface of the medial pterygoid plate and within the pterygopalatine fossa. Because this vessel is a terminal branch of the external carotid system, it is a "high flow" artery with significant surgical importance. The venous drainage is less defined, but generally follows the arterial supply (1). It should be remembered that venous drainage from the superior nasal cavity, particularly around the orbits, flows into the cavernous sinus system. This is important with respect to the spread of infection, thrombosis, and tumor from these areas of the nasal cavity into the intracranial skull base.

Paranasal Sinuses

There are four named paranasal sinuses: maxillary, sphenoid, frontal, and ethmoid. Each of these sinuses is lined with respiratory mucosa comprised of ciliated, psuedostratified columnar, epithelial cells. Interspersed among these areas are goblet-type mucous cells.

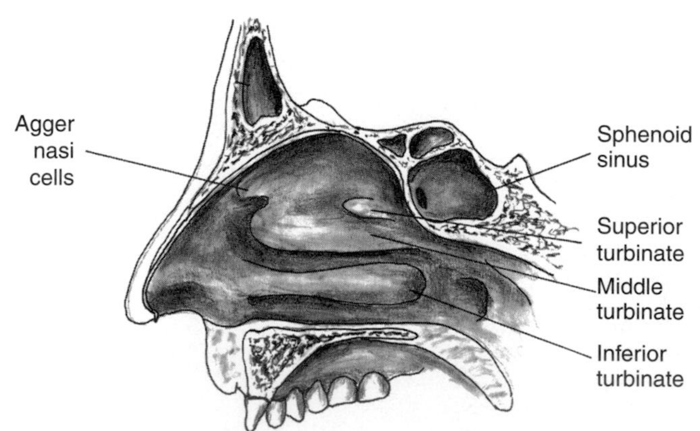

Figure 21.2 Lateral nasal wall anatomy.

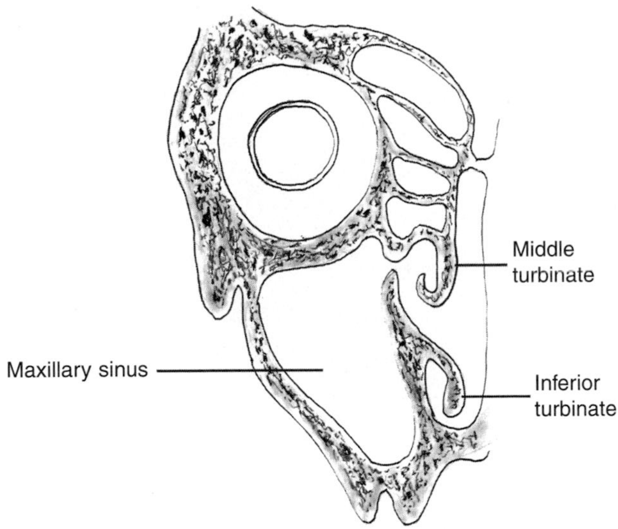

Figure 21.3 Coronal view of paranasal sinus anatomy.

MAXILLARY SINUS

The anterior wall of the maxillary sinus corresponds to the facial surface of the maxilla. The posterior wall corresponds with the infratemporal fossa surface of the sinus. The roof of the maxillary sinus forms the orbital floor, whereas the floor of the sinus is formed by the alveolar process of the maxilla (Fig 21.3). The maxillary sinus derives it blood supply predominately from the maxillary artery with a small contribution from the facial artery. Venous drainage is through the facial vein to the jugular system anteriorly and through tributaries of the maxillary vein posteriorly. A relevant clinical note is the communication between the maxillary vein and pterygoid plexus in the infratemporal fossa. Innervation to the sinus is provided by the maxillary nerve and its branches: the greater palatine, posterolateral nasal, and contributions from the superior alveolar branches of the infraorbital nerve, which emerge from the anterior wall of the maxilla.

ETHMOID SINUSES

The ethmoid sinuses are located directly inferior to the anterior skull base. At their lateral edge lies the lamina papyrcea. The clinical relevance of the lamina papyrcea relates to its permeable nature, which may be penetrated by tumor. The blood supply of the ethmoid sinus is derived through the internal and external carotid systems through the anterior and posterior ethmoid arteries as well as branches off the maxillary artery. The venous drainage is predominantly through two routes; into the nose through the nasal veins or through the ethmoidal veins, which drain into the maxillary system and the cavernous sinus system, respectively. The sinus is innervated by the first and second divisions of the trigeminal system. There are several specific anatomic considerations. The optic nerve lies close to the posterior aspect of the sinus. The anterior cranial fossa may be violated when manipulating the fovea ethmoidalis or the cribriform plate (1).

FRONTAL SINUS

The frontal sinus is extremely variable from patient to patient. Its blood supply is through the supraorbital and supratrochlear arteries, which are branches of the ophthalmic artery from the internal carotid system. An anastomotic network does exist between this supraorbital/supratrochlear system and the superficial temporal artery, also a branch of the external carotid system. Venous drainage is primarily through the superior ophthalmic vein which courses through the superior orbital fissure into the cavernous sinus. Innervation is from the first division of the trigeminal system through the supraorbital and supratrochlear branches (1).

SPHENOID SINUS

The last sinus to be discussed is the sphenoid. Its boundaries are often asymmetric due to the nature of its intersinus septum. The sphenoid sinus derives its blood supply from both the internal and external carotid systems. The maxillary vein and pterygoid plexus are the predominant draining vessels. The mucosa of the sphenoid sinus is innervated by the first and second branch of the trigeminal nerve. This sinus, more so than the others, poses many potential complications. The optic nerve and the pituitary gland lay superiorly, the internal carotid artery and the cavernous sinus laterally. The bone of the lateral wall is usually less than 0.5 mm, and is commonly totally dehiscent (1).

Infratemporal Fossa

The infratemporal fossa lies posterior to the maxillary sinus and has traditionally represented a challenge in terms of tumor clearance in the surgical management of sinus malignancy. The infratemporal fossa is a common site of local tumor spread, but is not addressed by traditional methods of radical maxillectomy. This topic will be addressed later in this chapter. The boundaries of the infratemporal fossa are the mandibular ramus laterally, pterygoid plate medially, maxilla anteriorly, and the greater sphenoid wing superiorly (Fig. 21.4). The maxillary alveolus defines the inferior border with the sphenoid crest defining the superior limit. Vital structures within this space include the foramen ovale, foramen spinosum, and inferior orbital fissure. Also found here is the maxillary artery, muscles of mastication, and third division of the trigeminal nerve. The temporalis muscle inserts on the coronoid process within the fossa, thereby facilitating harvesting it for reconstructive purposes.

Pterygopalatine Fossa

The pterygopalatine fossa is a small space containing branches of the maxillary artery, vidian nerve, foramen rotundum, inferior orbital fissure, second division of the trigeminal nerve, the pterygopalatine and sphenopalatine nerves as well as the

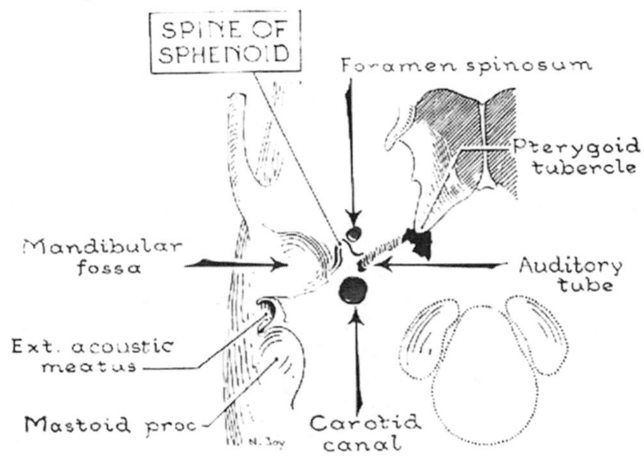

Figure 21.4 Infratemporal fossa anatomy.

greater and lesser palatine nerves and the posterosuperior alveolar nerve. This area serves as a conduit for numerous nerves innervating the teeth, palate, turbinates, sinuses, lacrimal glands, and nasopharynx (2,3).

PATHOLOGY AND ETIOLOGY OF MALIGNANT SINUS TUMORS

Malignant tumors of the sinonasal tract are relatively rare. These neoplasms are predominantly squamous cell carcinomas. Other common malignant lesions include: adenoid cystic carcinoma, adenocarcinoma, neuroectodermal tumors, hemangiopericytoma, lymphoma, melanoma, olfactory neuroblastoma, and sarcomas, with the subsets of angiosarcomas, fibrosarcomas, rhabdomyosarcoma, and chondrosarcoma. Tumors of the salivary gland type constitute 4% to 8% of neoplasms of the sinonasal tract (4,5). After adenoid cystic carcinoma the next most common glandular lesion in the sinonasal tract is intestinal-type sinonasal adenocarcinoma. Malignant melanoma of the sinonasal tract represents 1% of all melanomas (6–8). In children rhabdomyosarcoma stands out as one of the most common tumors, but this is not the case with adults (7).

Even though squamous cell carcinoma is the most common malignancy of the sinonasal tract, it represents only 3% of all malignant tumors of the upper aerodigestive tract (9). The annual incidence is from 0.75 to 1 per 100,000, with the maxillary sinus being the most common location. The ethmoid and sphenoid sinuses are rarely involved. There is a male preponderance with a 2:1 male-to-female ratio (10). These tumors most commonly appear in the sixth decade. Sinonasal squamous cell carcinoma is more frequent among the Japanese, 2.2 to 2.6 per 100,000 in males and 1.2 to 1.4 per 100,000 in females, as well as in particular African populations, 2.5 per 100,000 in males and 1.8 per 100,000 in females (11,12).

Malignancies in the nasal vestibule and paranasal sinuses are rare tumors that pose significant diagnostic and treatment challenges. Lesions arising from these sites often grow unnoticed for extended periods of time secondary to the anatomy. Regional spread is common prior to diagnosis due to the ease of passage within the sinuses. The mode of tumor spread is usually by direct extension (Fig. 21.5). Although the origin of sinus malignancies is the maxillary sinus in 80% of cases, it has been reported that the lesion is confined to this sinus in only 25% of cases (13). This trend continues in the other sinuses as well. Carcinoma arising from the ethmoid sinus is contained within that sinus in less than 25% of patients (13). Primary tumors in the sphenoid and frontal sinuses are extremely rare.

The patterns of proliferation are by direct extension into the orbit or skull base, regionally to lymph nodes, and distant metastasis. Lymphatic spread to regional neck nodes occurs in approximately 15% of cases with distant metastasis in 5% (14). Recurrence is generally an issue of local rather than distant metastases. Distant metastasis of squamous cell carcinoma of the maxillary sinus is approximately 10%, but this is almost always seen in conjunction with local recurrence (15). Secondary primaries are rare but do exist in less than 5% of cases, with the contralateral maxillary sinus the most commonly involved site (16). These lesions are found more commonly in older patients with 95% of maxillary sinus neoplasms occurring in patients older than 40 years (17).

A brief discussion of inverting papillomas is warranted though these are not malignant lesions. There is controversy as to the exact nature of these lesions, which will not be addressed in this chapter. Most inverting papillomas emanate from the lateral wall of the nasal cavity, with subsequent involvement of the maxillary and ethmoid sinuses. These lesions may degenerate into a malignancy in approximately 10% of cases (18). Complete surgical excision is required for cure and radiation therapy is never used as a treatment for inverted papilloma as it can promote malignant degeneration.

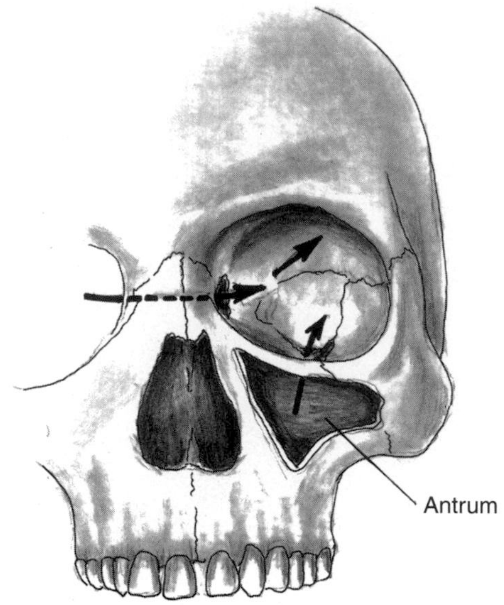

Figure 21.5 Tumor spread to orbit from ethmoid or maxillary antrum malignancies.

The exact etiologic factors contributing to malignant lesions in this region are yet to be fully elucidated. However, numerous factors have been discovered. It has been reported that up to 44% of sinonasal tract malignancies can be traced to occupational exposures. These include nickel, chromium, isopropyl oils, volatile hydrocarbons, and organic fibers found in the wood, shoe, and textile industries (17). Wood dust in particular is associated with a 1,000 times higher incidence of adenocarcinoma of the ethmoid sinuses than found in the general population (19). Infectious agents may also play a role in the pathogenesis of sinonasal carcinoma. Human papilloma virus is associated with inverting papillomas in 24% of cases and in 4% of squamous cell carcinomas (20,21). Evidence linking cigarette smoking as a risk factor is not as clear as it is for other upper aerodigestive tract lesions (22).

CLINICAL PRESENTATION AND DIAGNOSTIC EVALUATION

Tumors emanating from the sinonasal tract are often asymptomatic until they compromise neighboring structures. The symptoms produced by these lesions are dictated by the size and location of the tumor. A unilateral nasal mass must always raise the specter of malignancy especially in older adults. Unilateral nasal congestion, epistaxis, and anosmia are symptoms that require investigation either by telescopic examination, computed tomography, or both.

As stated previously the tumor location has a definitive role in the symptoms produced. Tumors arising from the maxillary antrum most commonly produce proptosis, facial dysesthesias, or asymmetry of the maxillary face secondary to tumor extension (23). Tumors within any of the paranasal sinuses may produce orbital findings, from visual disturbances to orbital displacement, if their growth goes unabated. Intraoral findings are also seen, usually from maxillary lesions, with palatal displacement and loose teeth. Neurologic sequelae are witnessed when the tumor invades the pterygomaxillary space, epidural space, or brain tissue itself. Cranial nerve findings have been stated to be as high as 33% of patients with paranasal carcinoma (24). Cranial nerve deficits commonly include pain, numbness, facial paralysis, and compromised vision.

Patterns of Spread

As one would expect the location of the tumor dictates its pattern of spread. Malignancies of the maxillary sinus often extend posteriorly to the infratemporal fossa and pterygopalatine fossa. These lesions have access to numerous foramina and fissures in the region. They may extend to the orbit through the inferior orbital fissure or the thin bone around the inferior orbital fissure (Fig. 21.5), and intracranially through the foramen rotundum or foramen ovale. They may also traverse the palatine canal or the sphenopalatine foramen to reach the oral cavity. And lastly, they may extend into the petrous portion of the temporal bone through the vidian canal. The major lymphatic drainage pathways for maxillary-based tumors are through the submandibular, parotid, jugulodigastric and retropharyngeal systems. Lymphatic spread of tumors of the nose and paranasal sinuses occurs in 18% to 50% of cases and can be bilateral (25). As a result, the most important step in diagnosis and treatment planning is radiologic imaging as physical examination alone is not adequate to evaluate deep structures that may be involved with tumor. Computed tomography with contrast is one of the most common studies to obtain. The presence of nodal disease and bony invasion are best depicted on these images. Magnetic resonance imaging (MRI) is also a frequently obtained study. Whenever intracranial involvement is a concern an MRI is recommended, as it is superior in detecting dural or cortical involvement. A computed tomography (CT) scan, however, is superior for bony evaluation of disease because MRI is for soft tissue. Angiography is of limited value in evaluating these lesions, but may be useful in assessing feeding vessels and collateral circulation if a large resection is planned, or if the tumor is considered to be an angiofibroma or hemangiopericytoma. Once the clinician is satisfied with the location and extent of tumor, a biopsy is performed. If feasible this may be done in an office setting, however, some of these lesions are vascular and necessitate operating room conditions for safe sampling. After tissue diagnosis is obtained treatment plans may be formulated including surgical options.

STAGING

Lesions of the paranasal sinuses present several difficulties when trying to formulate an adequate staging system. With the numerous vital structures adjacent and frequently involved, assessing the severity of a tumor can often be unclear. As mentioned, these tumors usually have extended beyond their sinus of origin at the time of diagnosis. Sisson et al. (26) proposed a tumor, node, metastases (TNM) staging system in 1963 for antral-based carcinomas. The strengths of their work were in the importance that it placed on the site of extension. Harrison furthered this approach with his 1978 staging system (27). The American Joint Committee on Cancer (AJCC) has also proposed a staging system (28), which is the staging method we recommend.

The AJCC staging system is outlined in Table 21.1. It should be noted that in the 6th edition (28a), which has been recently published, some important updates have been made. These include:

1. A new site has been added. In addition to maxillary sinus, the nasoethmoid complex is described with two regions within that site: nasal cavity and ethmoid sinuses.
2. The nasal cavity region is further divided into four subsites: septum, floor, lateral wall, and vestibule. The ethmoid sinus region is divided into two subsites, right and left.
3. The T staging of ethmoid lesions has been revised to reflect nasoethmoid tumors, and appropriate description of the T staging has been added.
4. For maxillary sinus, T4 lesions have been divided into T4a (resectable) and T4b (unresectable), leading to the division of stage IV into stage IVA, stage IVB, and stage IVC.

MANAGEMENT

Nasal Vestibule Lesions

Lesions within the nasal vestibule are often treated with radiation alone. Patients with selected T3 lesions, and essentially all extensive T4 lesions should undergo surgery combined with radiotherapy for improved cure rates (29). Tumors contained within the nasal vestibule are best addressed through the lateral rhinotomy approach. Fergusson was the first to describe the lateral rhinotomy approach in 1845 (30). The lateral rhinotomy is performed by beginning the incision inferior to the medial aspect of the brow and brought inferiorly roughly halfway between the dorsum and medial canthal attachment (Fig. 21.6A). This incision is performed as a W-plasty to avoid web formation at this site in the postoperative period. The incision continues inferiorly along the alar crease, thereby allowing the nose to be "flipped-open" for access to the anterior nasal cavity.

In the latter half of the 20th century focus was placed on making the approach less disfiguring. There are now several modifications of the technique available to the surgeon, with tumor size and location dictating which incision should be employed (31–33). The incision should be performed in adherence to the aesthetic subunit principle (34) (Fig. 21.6B). Reconstruction of these defects, though often small, are frequently challenging. A variety of flaps are employed, usually rotational and advancement. For larger defects a paramedian forehead flap can be used to avoid prosthesis, or a prosthetic device can be fabricated.

Maxillary Lesions

MAXILLECTOMY: HISTORICAL PERSPECTIVE

Surgical management of the maxillary sinus evolved considerably in the 19th century. Lazars is credited with the precursor of the maxillectomy in 1826. This was soon followed by a successful total maxillectomy with orbital exenteration by Syme in 1828 (35). This approach underwent several modifications throughout the following decades but published results were sparse until the latter half of the 20th century. As supportive measures increased, aggressive surgical management became a viable option in the mid- to latter half of the 20th century. Smith et al. were some of the first to advocate extended maxillectomy in 1954 (36). This movement slowly took hold and in the 1970s acceptable survival rates were published (37). These modifications served as an impetus to expand the type and size of lesions managed by this technique (38). There are a number of different types of maxillectomies, and our preferred method of classifying them is discussed subsequently. The traditional access for maxillectomy consists of a Weber-Furgusson incision which allows complete exposure of the maxillary suprastruc-

TABLE 21.1 2002 American Joint Committee on Cancer Tumor (T) Staging System for Cancers of the Nasal Cavity and Paranasal Sinuses

Primary tumor (T)	
TX	TX: Primary tumor cannot be assessed
T0	T0: No evidence of primary tumor
Tis	Tis: Carcinoma *in situ*
Maxillary sinus	
T1	Tumor limited to maxillary sinus mucosa with no erosion or destruction of bone
T2	Tumor causing bone erosion or destruction including extension into the hard palate or middle nasal meatus, except extension to posterior wall of maxillary sinus and pterygoid plates
T3	Tumor invades any of the following: bone of the posterior wall of maxillary sinus, subcutaneous tissues, floor or medial wall of orbit, pterygoid fossa, ethmoid sinuses
T4a	Tumor invades anterior orbital contents, skin of cheek, pterygoid plates, infratemporal fossa, cribriform plate, sphenoid or frontal sinuses
T4b	Tumor invades any of the following: orbital apex, dura, brain, middle cranial fossa, cranial nerves other than maxillary division of trigeminal nerve (V_2), nasopharynx, or clivus
Nasal cavity and ethmoid sinus	
T1	Tumor restricted to any one subsite, with or without bony invasion
T2	Tumor invading two subsites in a single region or extending to involve an adjacent region within the nasoethmoidal complex, with or without bony invasion
T3	Tumor extends to invade the medial wall or floor of the orbit, maxillary sinus, palate, or cribriform plate
T4a	Tumor invades any of the following: anterior orbital contents, skin of nose or cheek, minimal extension to anterior cranial fossa, pterygoid plates, sphenoid or frontal sinuses
T4b	Tumor invades any of the following: orbital apex, dura, brain, middle cranial fossa, cranial nerves other than (V_2), nasopharynx, or clivus

Stage grouping

Stage 0	Tis	N0	M0
Stage I	T1	N0	M0
Stage II	T2	N0	M0
Stage III	T3	N0	M0
	T1	N1	M0
	T2	N1	M0
	T3	N1	M0
Stage IV	T4a	N0	M0
	T4a	N1	M0
	T1	N2	M0
	T2	N2	M0
	T3	N2	M0
	T4a	N2	M0
Stage IVB	T4b	Any N	M0
	Any T	N3	M0
Stage IVC	Any T	Any N	M1

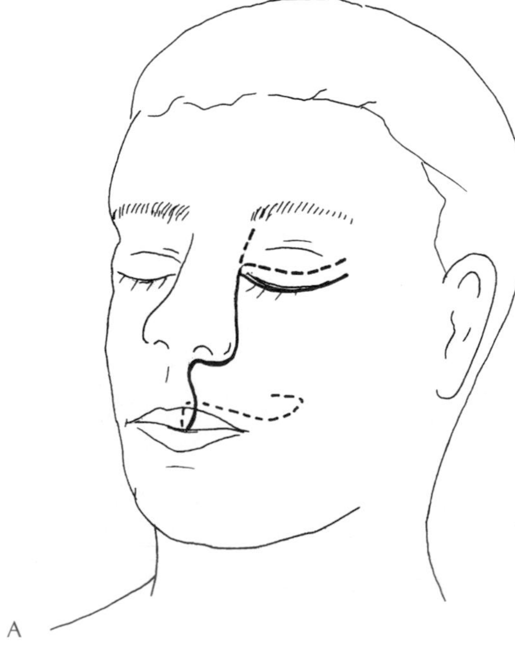

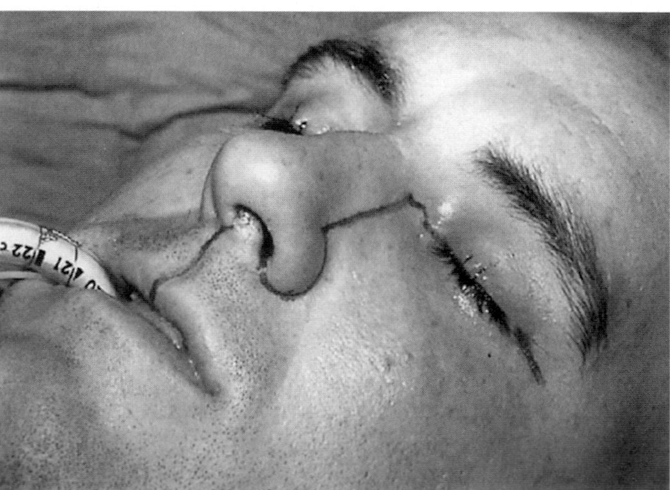

Figure 21.6 **A:** Classic Weber-Fergusson incision includes a lateral rhinotomy coupled with upper lip and lower eyelid extensions. **B:** Modified Weber-Fergusson incision adheres to aesthetic subunits of face.

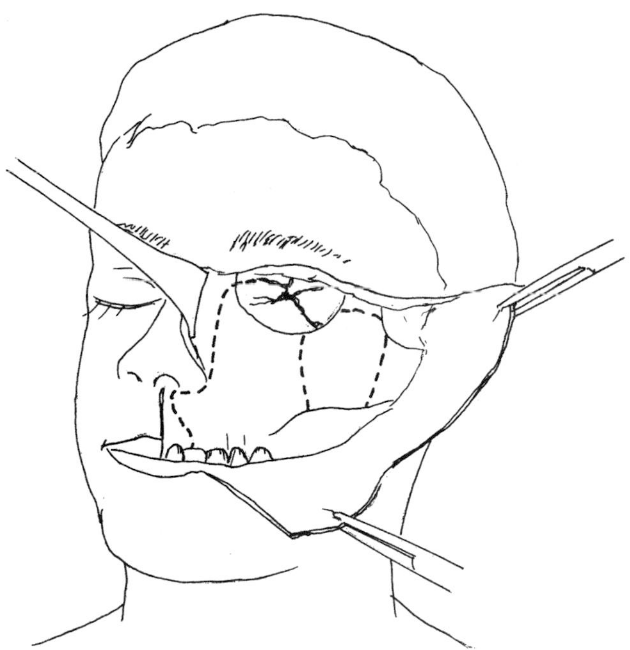

Figure 21.7 Exposure provided by the Weber-Fergusson incision.

ture and infrastructure, and access to the orbit and nasal cavity. This incision follows a line that begins with a subcilliary incision that extends below the medial canthus, along the lateral aspect of the nose and ala, then through the upper lip (Fig. 21.6B). The Weber-Furgusson approach provides wide access to the midface structures for the performance of radical resections for larger tumors (Fig. 21.7).

In contrast to large sinus malignancies, small tumors involving the paranasal sinuses may be treated in a similar fashion to other head and neck tumors, relying on primary radiation for cure. Unfortunately, most tumors have spread to adjacent sinuses and other structures at time of diagnosis and require multimodality therapy. It is our distinct preference that therapy is multimodal, consisting of surgical resection coupled with either preoperative or postoperative radiation therapy. When there is a risk for early orbital involvement by tumor, preoperative radiotherapy has the advantage of potentially sparing the contents of the orbit. If surgical resection is performed first in this setting, either the contents of the orbit will be lost at the time of resection, or the entire orbit will require treatment with radiation in the postoperative phase. When the entire orbit is radiated, visual acuity and globe movement and position can be adversely affected. Preoperative radiation of midface structures does not correlate with a significant increase in postoperative wound healing problems, as compared with other areas of the aerodigestive tract where there is an increase in postsurgical complications following radiation.

Medial Maxillectomy

TRADITIONAL DESCRIPTIONS

Sessions and Larson pioneered the medial maxillectomy (39). Their technique coupled the removal of the medial maxilla and ethmoid sinuses with the lateral rhinotomy incision or modified Weber-Fergusson approach. The indications for medial maxillectomy through this technique include benign and malignant neoplasms exclusively limited to the nasal walls, the medial wall of the maxillary sinus, and the adjacent ethmoid sinuses (32). This is usually achieved by osteotomizing the bone just lateral to the piriform aperture, extending the bone cuts caudally, preserving the lacrimal sac, and achieving a superior line of resection within the ethmoid sinuses (Fig. 21.8). This degree of bone resection is usually associated with an excellent postoperative aesthetic outcome, while achieving an oncologically sound surgical resection. The primary disadvantage of this technique consists of the facial incisions, which can be avoided by the degloving approach, described in the next section. The original technique described by Sessions and Larson has given rise to a number of surgical variants for the purpose of removing skull base tumors, particularly angiofibromas.

FACIAL DEGLOVING APPROACH TO THE MEDIAL MAXILLA

Another approach available to expose the midface for medial maxillectomy is the degloving technique (Fig. 21.9A). The foundations of the degloving approach were established in the early 20th century. Denker and Kahler in 1926 developed an intraoral approach to the nasal cavity through a modification of the Caldwell-Luc incision combined with bony resection. Although this technique did provide acceptable access it was limited with respect to exposure of the superior aspects of the nasal vault (40). Portmann and Retrouvey first described the midfacial degloving approach in 1927. Their approach combined the sublabial and transoral techniques for radical maxillectomy (41). Doyle reported on an extended sublabial incision to approach the maxillary, ethmoid, or sphenoid sinuses in lieu of an extended lateral rhinotomy (42). In 1971 Maniglia presented work coupling the rhinoplastic release of soft tissue with the sublabial technique. The results of 15 years' experience with this technique were reported in 1986 (43). To highlight the cosmetic appeal of this approach one should note that one of the leading papers on this approach was not for oncologic surgery but for reconstructive purposes (44,45). The degloving can be adapted to provide adequate access for a medial maxillectomy, total maxillectomy, and orbital exenteration (46), as well as used in combination with other craniofacial approaches for access to the skull base (47).

Degloving is performed by injecting the nose in a similar fashion for that of a septoplasty. The oral cavity is also injected with local anesthesia containing a vasoconstrictive agent as is done prior to a Caldwell-Luc approach. Mucoperichondrial

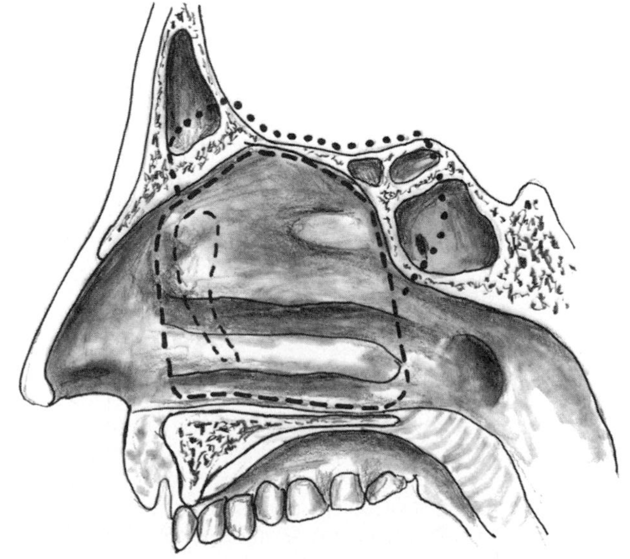

Figure 21.8 Outline of medial maxillectomy.

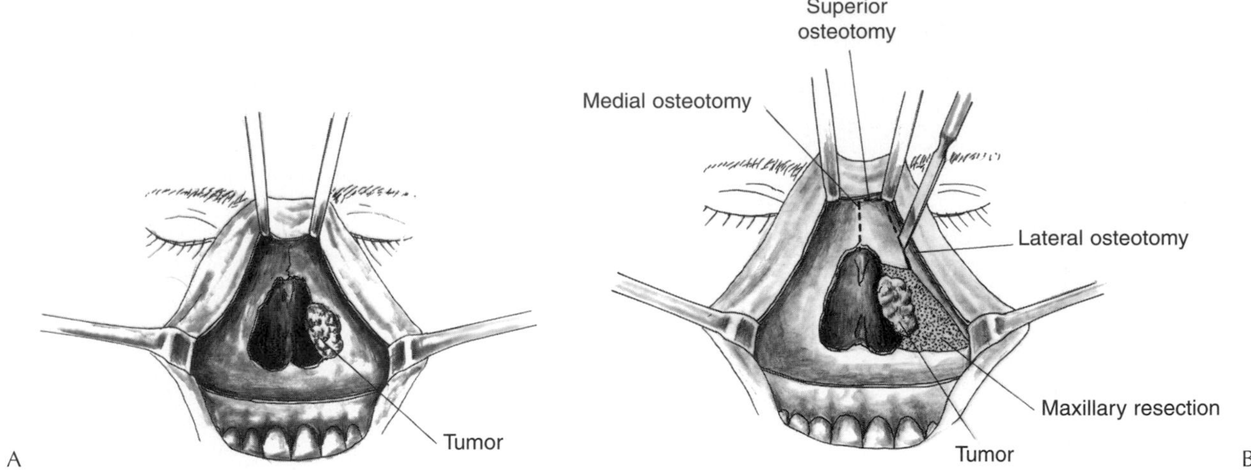

Figure 21.9 **A:** Degloving technique. **B:** Medial maxillectomy through the degloving technique.

flaps are created on both sides of the septum through a complete transfixion incision. The periosteum on the anterior face of the maxilla is elevated, taking care to preserve the infraorbital nerves. This is done through the sublabial approach. The face is then degloved after releasing the remainder of the nasal tissue by performing bilateral intercartilaginous incisions and bilateral piriform aperture releasing incisions. The soft tissues of the face are then retracted to allow direct access to the nasal cavity, nasopharynx, paranasal sinuses, and skull base when coupled with selective osteotomies. Once exposure is attained, the lesion can be excised (Fig. 21.9B). Closure is achieved by securing the septum with transcartilaginous absorbable suture. Packing is inserted and a splint is placed on the dorsum. The intraoral incisions are then closed with a locking running chromic suture (47). The limitation of the facial degloving procedure is an inability to access the most superior aspects of the nasal cavity.

ENDOSCOPIC MEDIAL MAXILLECTOMY

Advancing the concept of cosmetically acceptable surgical approaches is the use of endoscopic equipment. Endoscopic management of sinonasal carcinoma is a controversial field. Over the last decade, a number of surgeons have applied endoscopic techniques to the removal of malignant paranasal sinus tumors (48–50). In this regard, the location, extent, and type of lesion dictate whether an endoscopic approach is appropriate. Though the range of lesions treated by this modality is increasing as surgical experience progresses, it must be remembered that these techniques, by their very nature of a "piecemeal" resection, cannot adhere to time-tested principles of en bloc oncologic surgery. These principles were adopted based on years of experience where non–en bloc techniques demonstrated greater recurrence rates than the complete removal of the tumor as a single specimen. As larger malignant tumors are resected by endoscopic technique, this fact, and previous experience with nonendoscopic "piecemeal" removal, should be considered.

One of the most detailed papers on the subject of endoscopic resection argues that even lesions extending into the orbit, dura, brain, and other structures can be managed endoscopically in trained hands (49). This source describes the endoscopic resection of various carcinomas, melanoma, teratoma, clival chordomas, esthesioneuroblastomas, and leiomyosarcomas in 43 patients. To date the patients have done at least as well as those with external approaches, while attaining excellent functional and overall quality of life (49). It should be noted these authors, and others on the subject, strongly stress a multidisciplinary approach including various combinations of chemotherapy and radiotherapy (49,50). The authors of this chapter do not support these aggressive approaches as controlled randomized trials have not been performed to date, and may not be possible in the United States due to ethical and medicolegal considerations.

For nonmalignant tumors, primarily inverting papilloma, endoscopic approaches enable the surgeon to avoid facial incisions while precisely delineating tumor extent and preserving normal soft tissue structures. Stringent postoperative follow-up is mandatory, as at least an increased theoretical potential for recurrence exists. Currently endoscopic approaches can be the sole method of treatment in a limited number of these patients, usually with nasal, ethmoidal, or limited maxillary disease. More commonly, endoscopic approaches are best combined with external approaches to optimize resection while limiting aesthetic deformity on a patient-to-patient basis (51). Although endoscopy offers great promise, surgeons dealing with these tumors must be adept at the conventional external approaches.

Infrastructure Maxillectomy and Palatectomy

When lesions are limited to the maxillary infrastructure and hard palate, and do not encroach on the orbital floor and into the posterosuperior aspect of the sinus, a palatectomy and partial maxillectomy is often required (Fig. 21.10). These lesions frequently originate in the oral cavity and represent secondary maxillary sinus involvement by direct extension through the hard palate and its overlying mucosa. In this situation, the focus of the procedure is the palate, with those portions of the maxilla that require resection representing secondary components of the surgical procedure. As a result, these lesions can frequently be approached entirely through the oral cavity, avoiding facial incisions. Additionally, the soft palate can frequently be preserved, thereby substantially improving the patient's postoperative function with respect to speech and oral intake.

In the setting of a palatomaxillectomy with preservation of the soft palate, the defect can be left un-reconstructed, relying on the use of a custom obturating denture for oronasal separation. Alternatively, an oral appliance can be permanently avoided by primarily reconstructing the palatal defect with either a temporoparietal vascularized fascial flap or a temporalis muscle flap. The long-term advantage of this approach is obvious, but this type of reconstruction requires an additional incision in the temporal region for flap elevation and rotation.

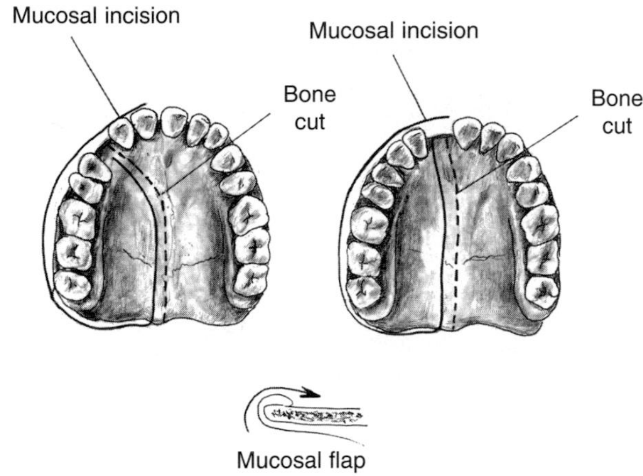

Figure 21.10 Palatectomy incisions.

Further, transfer of a temporalis muscle flap (in contrast to a temporoparietal vascularized fascial flap) leaves a contour deformity of the temporal region that must be reconstructed after flap rotation. This is usually performed at our center with hydroxyapatite cement at the time of resection.

When the soft palate or medial nasal wall is involved with tumor, facial incisions are usually necessary. For lesions that extend posteriorly, clearance of the posterior margin of resection in the proximity of the pterygoid muscles may be necessary. This clearance is enhanced by a second infratemporal fossa exposure if the pterygoid muscles are significantly involved with tumor extension (Fig. 21.11A–D). When the soft palate must be resected, adequate rehabilitation with an obturating denture becomes less satisfactory. Patients frequently have velopalateal insufficiency with the regurgitation of food and liquid into the nasal cavity, along with secondary hygiene problems resulting from this regurgitation. In this setting, primary reconstruction can be considered with either a temporalis muscle flap (smaller defects) (Fig. 21.11E–H) or a radial forearm microvascular transfer (larger defects). It must be remembered that these flaps do nothing to reconstruct the bony dental alveolar arch, and may make denture fabrication and retention more difficult unless the flaps are appropriately tailored and positioned.

For defects where a significant amount of the dental arch is resected, bony reconstruction can be considered with a fibula, iliac crest, or scapula microvascular transfer. It must be remembered that these reconstructions are complex and should only be attempted by teams with significant experience in this type of midface restoration. For younger patients, though, this technical complexity should not be used as an excuse for not informing the patient of the option of primary reconstruction with bone and dental implants, nor understating the long-term dissatisfaction of many patients who use prosthetics for large defect obturation.

Suprastructure Maxillectomy

Isolated suprastructure maxillectomies are rare. In the majority of cases the suprastructure is secondarily involved due to spread from infrastructure components or from tumor involving the medial maxillary wall. Though isolated suprastructure lesions are uncommon, lesions that involve the orbital floor but do not require orbital exenteration are encountered on a regular basis. Our criteria for orbital sparing surgery, without the use of preoperative radiation, require that the fat and muscles of the orbit be free of disease. Involvement of intact periorbita does not require orbital exenteration. In this setting, the periorbita is resected but the orbital contents are preserved. The incision usually consists of a modified Weber-Fergusson, with or without an upper lip-splitting extension. Key considerations include confirming that there is no cranial base involvement in the region of the ethmoids, or involvement of the pterygoid or infratemporal fossa due to posterior tumor extension (Fig. 21.12). If these important areas are compromised, then either a craniofacial resection or an infratemporal fossa approach, respectively, would be required. If there is evidence that the periorbita is overtly breached with involvement of the orbital fat, then preoperative radiation can be considered in an attempt to spare the orbital contents. We do not use this method of orbit sparing, and prefer to recommend orbital exenteration in this setting due to the substantial compromise of eye function and vision following whole-orbital irradiation. We consider eye muscle involvement as an absolute contraindication to any form of orbit-sparing treatment.

In the setting of a resected orbital floor, reconstruction of this area should be considered to prevent predictable and significant posttreatment problems. These problems uniformly consist of varying degrees of extraocular motor dysfunction, globe malposition, visual compromise, and aesthetic deformity. In this setting an isolated orbital floor and orbital rim reconstruction is appropriate. Though "standard" therapy consists of the use of a fascial sling to suspend the orbital contents, we have found this method of reconstruction largely inadequate. Instead, the orbital volume should be reestablished using a rigid material such as titanium mesh. A rigid implant should also be used to re-form an inferior orbital rim and maxillary face when appropriate. This alloplastic reconstruction is then covered with a vascularized flap, consisting of either temporoparietal fascia or temporalis muscle depending on the volume of the defect. Reconstruction of the maxillary suprastructure, orbital floor, and reestablishment of lacrimal system drainage can all be achieved while preserving the opportunity to treat the palatal defect with an obturator. By performing a primary maxillary suprastructure reconstruction coupled with the use of an oral prosthesis, the patient can avoid the problems associated with orbital floor/rim resection without engaging in a complex reconstructive effort, such as a microvascular transfer. We firmly believe that primary maxillary reconstruction will eventually be considered "the standard of care" following the ablation of maxillary sinus cancers.

Maxillectomy with Orbital Involvement

When tumors spread to involve the orbital contents, orbital exenteration is required to achieve clearance of the malignancy. Historically invasion of the periorbita, posterior ethmoid cells, or orbital apex was considered an absolute indication for orbital exenteration (52). Indications for removal of the orbit are now less rigid and we have chosen to preserve the orbital contents even if the periorbita is involved. As previously mentioned, involvement of the intraorbital fat or muscles is an absolute indication for removal of the orbital contents.

The approach for such a resection is exclusively through a classic or modified Weber-Fergusson incision. Though this approach is frequently described as including the removal of the eyelids, we do not agree with this approach. We prefer to preserve the eyelid system unless it is involved with tumor and their resection is required to clear the surgical margins of disease. By preserving the eyelid system, a meaningful orbital reconstruction consisting of an ocular implant and prosthesis remains a possibility. If the eyelid skin is involved with the cancer, then resection of these structures should be performed, narrowing the reconstructive options to a prosthesis or eye patch.

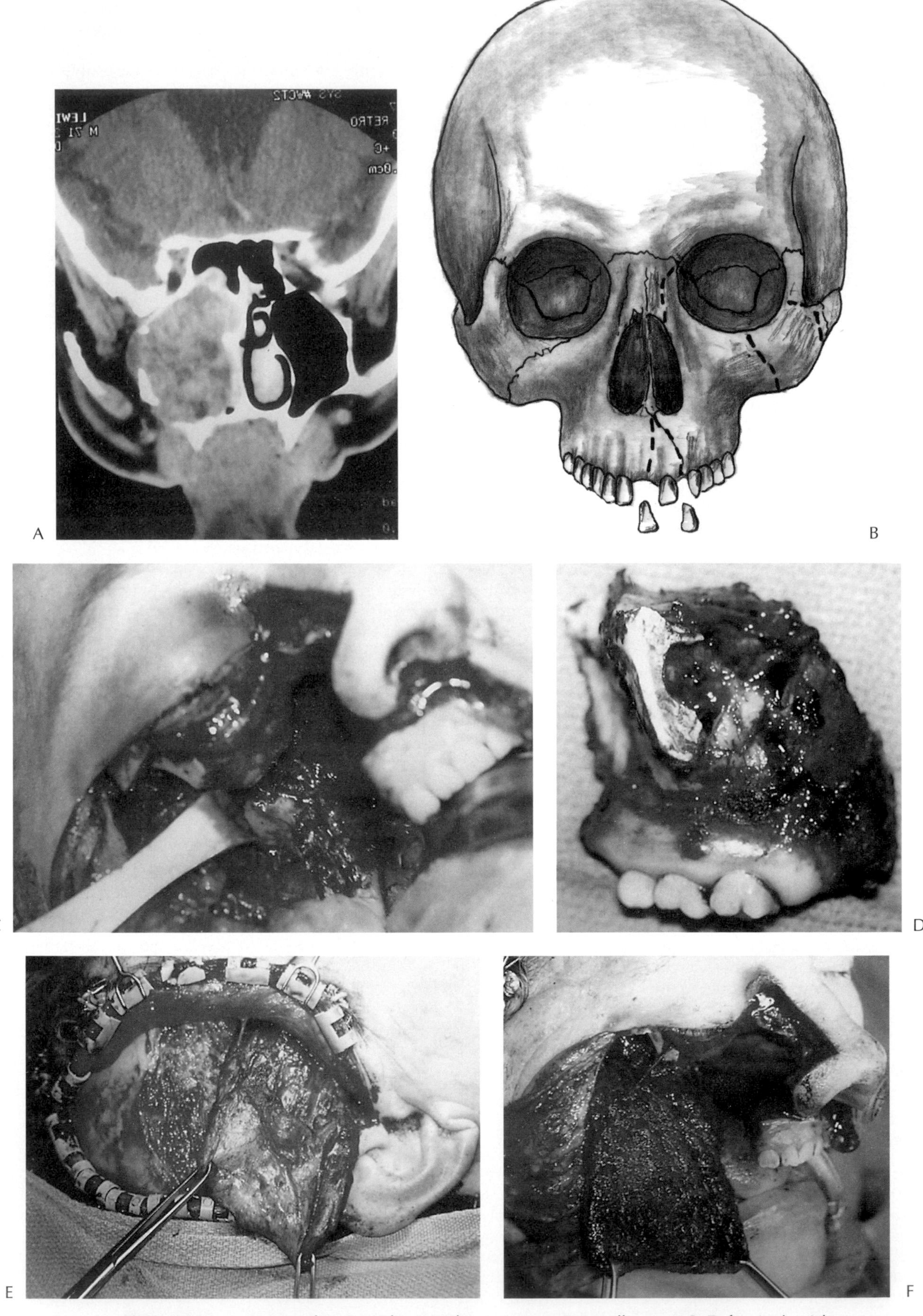

Figure 21.11 **A:** Computed tomography scan showing tumor. **B:** Maxillectomy. **C:** Defect in the right cheek that has been totally resected. **D:** Specimen containing upper jaw and teeth. **E:** Muscle flap from side of head before transfer. **F:** Muscle flap after transfer.

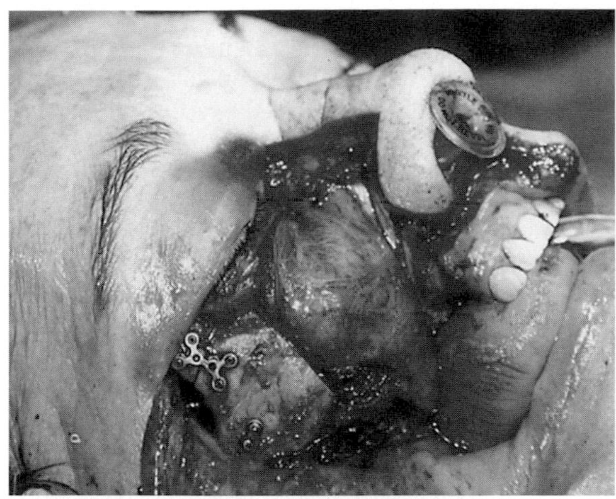

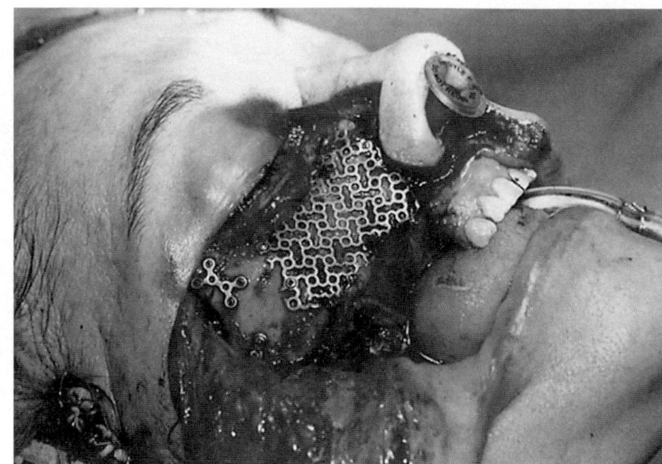

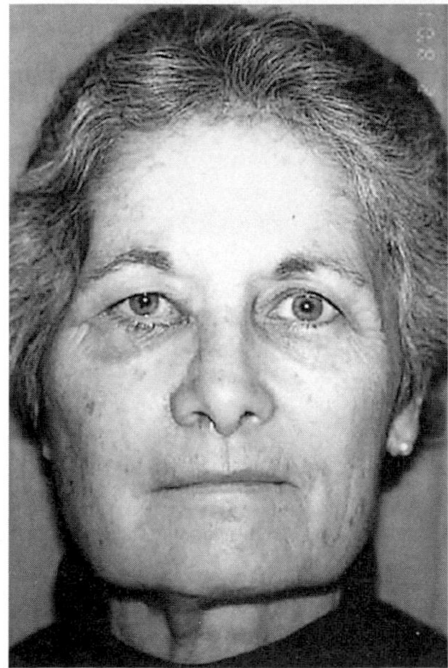

Figure 21.11 *(continued)* **G:** Muscle flap sewn into position. **H:** Titanium mesh to replace lost bone. **I:** Fourteen days after procedure. Note depression in temporal region resulting from flap transfer.

During the process of orbital exenteration, several points should be remembered. First, as the orbital contents are mobilized and increasing traction is placed on the optic nerve, the potential for a vagal response increases. Traction on the optic nerve can result in dramatic drops in both heart rate and blood pressure, and can even precipitate cardiac or cerebral schemia in older adult patients. We do not recommend injection of lidocaine into the optic nerve as is done with carotid body lesions as these injections carry a high risk for direct venous infusion of the lidocaine, or hematoma formation due to puncture of the ophthalmic artery. Instead, gentle traction coupled with adequate osteotomies for specimen mobilization is the preferred method of avoiding this problem. Second, it should be remembered that the ophthalmic artery emanates from the internal carotid artery immediately deep to the optic canal. If significant traction is placed on the optic nerve, or if the resection of the nerve is carried into the optic canal, the internal carotid can be injured in a particularly inaccessible site. The optic nerve stump and the ophthalmic artery that runs within the nerve are best controlled with vascular clips or bipolar cautery prior to transection. During this process care must be taken to avoid injury to the internal carotid which is just deep to the orbital apex.

Following exenteration, a large common cavity consisting of the orbit itself, the maxillary sinus, and the ipsilateral nasal cavity exists. This cavity can be managed in two ways. Either the defect can be skin grafted, depending on the use of an orofacial prosthesis, or vascularized flap reconstruction can be undertaken (53–55). Orofacial prostheses have the advantage of simplicity and afford the practitioner the opportunity to "inspect" the resection cavity for tumor recurrence (56–58). It is our perspective that in the era of high-resolution CT and MRI scanning

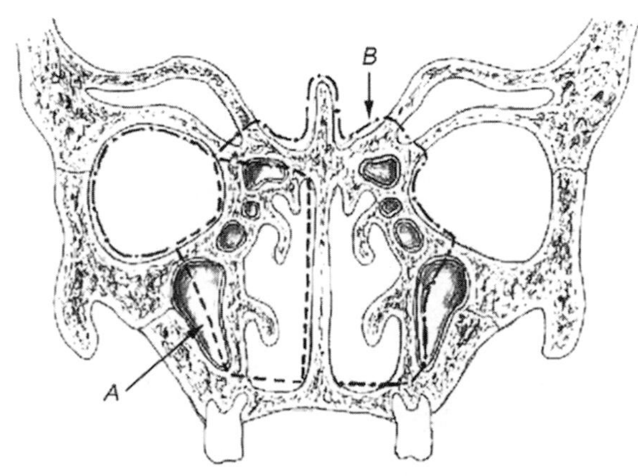

Figure 21.12 Suprastructure maxillectomy. (*A*) Osteotomies if no intracranial involvement; (*B*) if the cranial base is involved with tumor.

that direct cavity inspection is of little management value and does not justify condemning a patient to the use of a prosthesis (59,60). Though these obturators function adequately, the majority of patients with large prostheses complain of a common set of problems relating to difficulty maintaining cavity hygiene, problems with the regurgitation of food into the cavity, and odor emanating from the area.

Unless the patient is elderly or debilitated, it is the strong preference of the authors to engage in flap reconstruction of these defects. In this setting of a combined orbital exenteration and maxillectomy, it is tempting to use local tissue such as a vascularized temporalis muscle flap to fill the defect. Over time this will prove to be an error, as this flap is not of adequate bulk to fully obliterate the resultant cavity. Following atrophy, the temporalis muscle alone achieves little in creating an acceptable reconstruction from either an aesthetic or functional perspective when both the orbit and maxillary sinus require obliteration. Instead, it is our preference to fill this combined cavity with vascularized rectus abdominus muscle/fat or a lateral thigh flap transferred by microvascular technique. The inclusion of substantial amounts of fat serves to minimize muscle atrophy and decrease the risk for secondary soft tissue bulk inadequacy. We have not found an acceptable alternative to this form of flap reconstruction if the implantation of an ocular implant with orbital prosthesis is considered in the setting of a functioning eyelid system. This enhanced volume of vascularized tissue also allows for the reconstruction of the maxillary suprastructure, further enhancing the functional and aesthetic outcome. The situation described assumes an intact palate. Composite defects consisting of the orbit, maxilla, and palate will be discussed in the next section.

Combined Maxillary, Orbital, and Palatal Defects

Tumors that extend to involve the orbit, maxillary sinus, and palate require special comment. These lesions frequently originate in the maxillary sinus, itself, and secondarily involve the palate and orbit. It is rare for ethmoid primaries to extend to involve the palate, and similarly rare for palatal lesions to remain neglected long enough to invade the orbit. Because most of these "three cavity lesions" (oral, sinonasal, orbital) originate in the maxillary sinus, there is a greater chance for tumor extension throughout the posterior wall of the sinus to involve the pterygoid plates and infratemporal fossa. For this reason we approach these lesions with aggressive surgical resection that frequently involves an infratemporal fossa dissection to clear the posterosuperior margin beyond the maxillary sinus. The details of infratemporal fossa dissection are beyond the scope of this chapter. It is strongly recommended that surgeons who choose to care for patients with extensive sinonasal malignancies become familiar with this surgical method of clearing disease from this important area of the skull base.

The resection of a combined maxillary, orbital, and palatal defect leaves a significant defect where vascularized flap should be considered. As long as there is no dural exposure, then flap reconstruction is not mandatory. In the absence of dural exposure, post-resection options include an obturating prosthesis or vascularized flap obliteration of the cavity. Though prostheses are simple and cost-effective, they do little to return patients to their original functional status. These prostheses are difficult to keep clean, leak fluid around their perimeter, and do not adequately support the overlying soft tissues from an aesthetic standpoint. In our opinion, they are most appropriate for older adult patients who would not be capable of undergoing the additional operative time associated with flap reconstruction.

In our experience, the cavity defects are best reconstructed with a microvascular transfer. Flaps that can be used for this purpose include the rectus abdominus, the lateral thigh, the scapula, and the radial forearm. For most defects the rectus flap is more than adequate. Transfer of such a flap in a previously nonoperated patient should add not more than several hours of operative time to the overall procedure, and a success rate of near 100% should be expected. The use of free flaps does have certain advantages. They allow single-stage reconstruction with a generally superior cosmetic result that enhances the patient's quality of life, an often overlooked but vital measure of treatment success.

Ethmoid Lesions

Tumors that extend to, or originate from, the ethmoid sinuses have similar approaches to those lesions that are primary to the nasal cavities. "All unilateral lesions of the anterior ethmoid sinus can be accessed via a curvilinear incision beginning at the inferomedial aspect of the brow and extending inferiorly, midway between the nasal dorsum and medial canthus, along the nasofacial groove" (61). Treatment of ethmoid-based neoplasms has followed a parallel course to that of the nasal cavity, with various modifications of known techniques. For example, Biller et al. report their technique of extending the incision transversely at the level of the nasion for completion of a total rhinotomy as well as a contralateral identical incision, "H"-shaped for bilateral access to the anterior ethmoids (62). As mentioned, endoscopic removal of these lesions is now being performed with some evidence of success.

Ethmoid Lesions with Orbital Involvement

Combined orbital and ethmoid involvement that does not involve either the maxillary sinus or the anterior cranial base is rare. When it occurs, orbital management of ethmoid-based tumors is similar to that of maxillary-based lesions with respect to incision placement. The primary difference is that the resultant cavity is appropriate for obliteration with a vascularized temporalis muscle flap. This flap alone will have adequate volume to fill a combined orbital and ethmoid cavity, and maintain adequate volume following muscle atrophy. This assumes that the orbital floor is intact or has been reconstructed so that the flap does not prolapse into the maxillary sinus. If the maxilla is involved then temporalis muscle alone is usually not adequate. In this situation a microvascular transfer should be considered, particularly if the cranial vault has been breached.

Craniofacial Resection

The evolution of surgical management for nasal and paranasal sinus lesions culminates in the craniofacial resection. In the latter half of the 20th century, skull base surgery teams consisting of an otolaryngologist, neurosurgeon, plastic surgeon and prosthodontist, among other specialists, began to emerge. They sought better treatment options for tumors adjacent to or penetrating the skull base. The aggressive resections performed by such teams reduced local recurrence more than adjuvant therapies such as brachytherapy and chemotherapy did (63). Craniofacial disassembly, largely the result of advances by French plastic surgeon Paul Tessier, began to be seen as a way to access these previously inaccessible lesions (64).

The anterior cranial base floor is formed by the crista galli, cribriform plate, orbital floor, and plenum sphenoidale (Fig. 21.13) Tumor involvement of the anterior cranial base is usually the result of contiguous spread from the ethmoid sinuses, nasal cavity, or nasopharynx. The fundamental surgical goal of cranio-

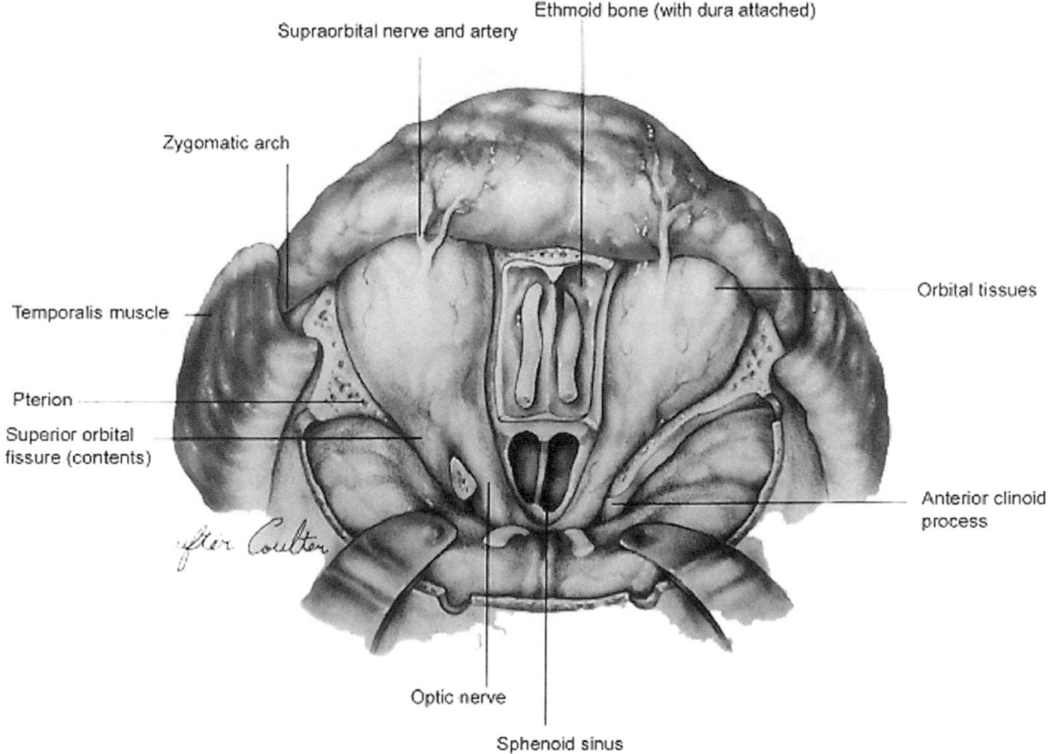

Figure 21.13 Anatomy of anterior cranial base.

facial resection was best stated by Nuss et al. in 1991, "At the cranial base, the surgeon needs to fulfill two disparate sets of therapeutic goals: to protect the brain, the great cerebral vessels, the cranial nerves, the spinal cord, and the organs of special sense; and at the same time, to achieve complete tumor extirpation" (65). There are a variety of approaches available to the cranial base surgeon for access (63,66,67). During the approach the surgeon must be cognizant of the closure at all times, for many of the most serious postoperative complications are directly related to the effectiveness of the reconstruction (i.e., cerebrospinal fluid leaks are due to inadequate repair of the iatrogenic defect).

Our favored approach is through a bicoronal incision. This is made with ample distance from the hairline to preserve an expanse of pericranium for use in the reconstruction. The incision is made being careful to avoid damaging the superficial temporal artery as it extends inferiorly over the temples and anterior to the ears. The forehead tissues are elevated anteriorly to the supraorbital rims in a plane deep to the pericranium. A pericranial flap is meticulously developed ensuring the supratrochlear and supraorbital neurovascular bundles are not transgressed.

Once the cranium is adequately exposed the osteotomies are created. A bifrontal craniotomy can then be performed to expose the dura over the frontal poles. A separate section of bone may be removed between the lateral orbital rims that includes the glabella to the level of the radix and supraorbital rims (Fig. 21.14A) This osteotomy provides direct access to the ethmoid sinuses and maximizes exposure to the subfrontal skull base (Fig. 21.14B) allowing for minimal brain retraction during tumor extirpation (Fig. 21.14C). Postoperative cerebral edema is a well-known complication of these operations secondary to prolonged retraction of the frontal lobes. Therefore the surgeon must plan the osteotomies to minimize this risk. The frontal poles and corresponding dura are then separated from the bony cranial base. If necessary, the olfactory nerves may be transected at this juncture. With this approach, exposure as far posteriorly as the planum sphenoidale and optic chiasma can be attained. If necessary the intracranial portion of the tumor can be circumscribed with osteotomies through the ethmoid air cells.

Additional exposure is often required and can be obtained through facial incisions, degloving, or transpalatal approaches. A lateral rhinotomy is often required to obtain access to the superior limit of the nasal cavity and paranasal sinuses. The lateral rhinotomy can be extended for orbital exenteration if necessary. The facial degloving and transpalatal approaches offer the benefit of avoiding disfiguring incisions but at a cost of limited exposure of the upper vault and ethmoid sinuses (68).

To adequately address some lesions extending into the infratemporal fossa a lateral approach is required, and a variety of infratemporal fossa approaches are available (69). Most of these techniques share several principles. The temporal and infratemporal areas are accessed through a pre- or postauricular incision, which extends onto the cervical region and the scalp in a hemicoronal or bicoronal manner. These incisions allow for exposure of the temporalis muscle, orbitozygomatic complex, parotid gland, and the facial nerve.

The infratemporal fossa is accessed by removing the orbitozygomatic complex (Fig. 21.15) and elevating the temporalis muscle. Extended exposure can be attained by retracting the condylar head and synovial capsule of the temporomandibular joint in an inferior vector. If this maneuver is not sufficient the distraction may be extended. In these circumstances removal of the mandibular neck and condylar head are recommended. Postoperative mandibular dysfunction is limited with removal of the mandibular neck and head when compared with extensive mandibular neck and head distraction and replacement of these structures. The surgeon must be cognizant of the internal maxillary artery and deep temporal vessels when transecting the mandibular neck as these structures lie just medial to the mandibular neck. These vessels are vital to the survival of the temporalis flap which will be employed for reconstruction post-

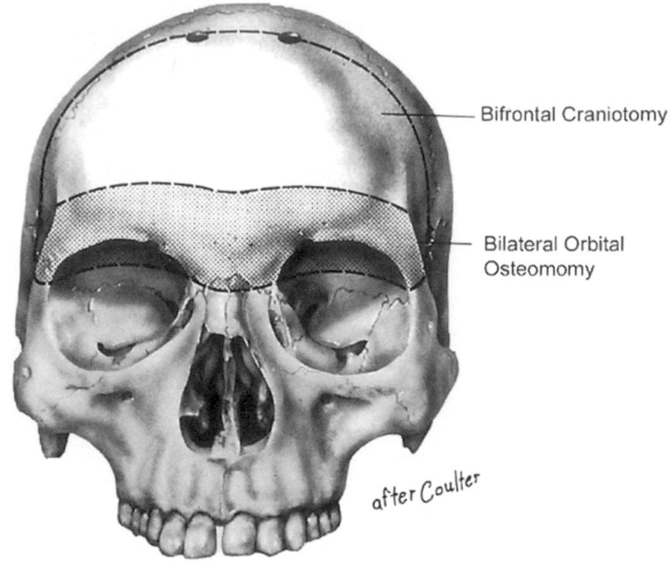

A

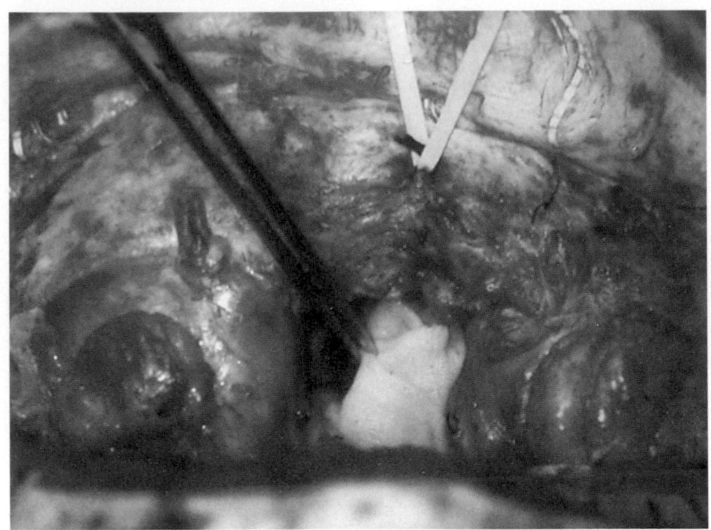

C

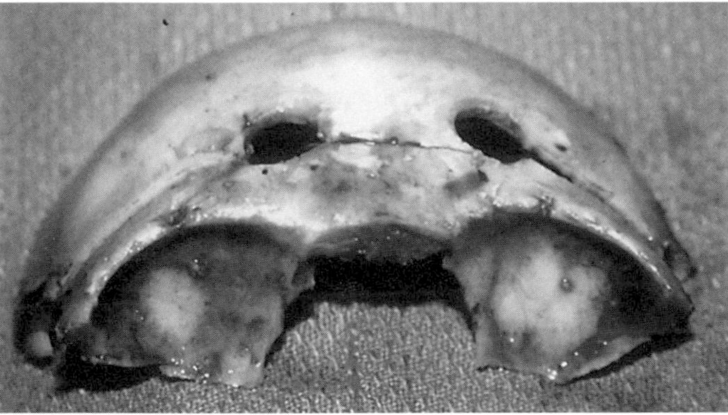

B

Figure 21.14 **A:** Skull illustration demonstrating bilateral bone cuts. **B:** Craniotomy with orbital rims. **C:** Exposure of orbitals.

extirpation. Once transected, the glenoid fossa, spine of the sphenoid, foramen ovale, and spinosum are exposed.

Superior access can be performed at this time through a frontotemporal craniotomy. This exposure allows for brain elevation. The petrous carotid can be isolated by removing the surrounding bone with care. The vessel lies just medial to the osseous eustachian tube as it enters the carotid canal. During the exposure of the carotid the facial nerve and otic capsule must be protected as they lie immediately superior and posterior to the genu of the carotid. Access to the sphenoid is attained between the second and third divisions of the trigeminal nerve.

Craniofacial Defect Reconstruction

The reconstruction has several facets: dural repair, bony reapproximation, and soft tissue defects. The use of the pericranial flap has proven vital in our practice and the literature (70,71). (Fig. 21.16). Pericranium alone is usually adequate, and the use of the galea should be avoided. When raising the galea the vascular supply to the forehead may be compromised, especially if the superficial temporal arteries have been taken. By performing the osteotomies as described, the flap can be placed up to 3 cm further posterior as has been previously described because the flap no longer has to overcome a ridge of bone at the region of the frontal sinus. All dural defects must be addressed prior to reconstructing with the pericranial flap. The scope of materials to repair dural defects continues to expand. We recommend employing autogenous tissue when available. We have also had substantial success with semisynthetic preparations such as acellular dermis. A watertight closure of the dura is vital in preventing postoperative cerebrospinal fluid (CSF) leakage and fibrin tissue sealant can be very useful in this effort. Once this has been achieved the pericranium can be turned intracranially and tacked to the periphery of the resection with sutures.

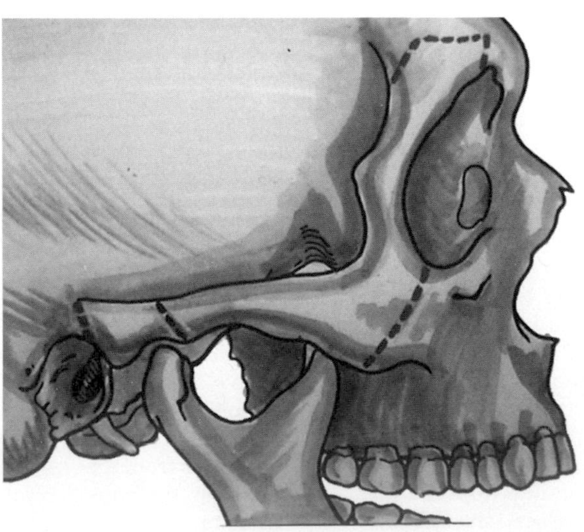

Figure 21.15 Osteotomies for infratemporal fossa approach.

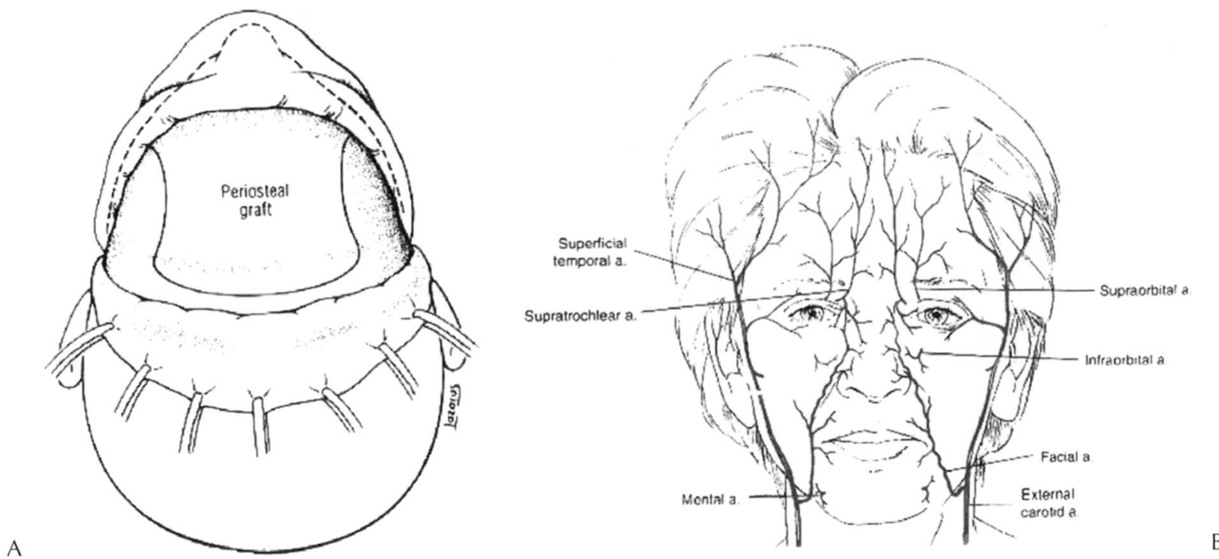

Figure 21.16 **A:** Pericranial flap. **B:** Relevant vasculature for pericranial flap.

The pericranial flap and intact dura often obviate the need for bony grafts to prevent brain herniation into the nasal cavity. If a significant amount of bone is removed from the orbits bone grafting should be considered. Enophthalmos due to posterosuperior retraction of the intraorbital soft tissues can occur if the bony orbital volume is not reestablished. If the surgical defect extends laterally the temporalis muscle or temporoparietal fascial flap can be used in reconstruction. This flap provides vigorous well-vascularized tissue that can be used to successfully separate cranial, oral, and nasal spaces. It can also be employed to obliterate the maxillary cavity postmaxillectomy and orbital cavity postexenteration. Surface defects can also be addressed with this versatile flap (72). In addition, the pericranial flap may be combined with titanium mesh for large anterior skull base defects (73). Skin grafts are rarely needed in the nasal cavity as the pericranial flap is usually mucosalized within several weeks of the procedure.

Free-flap reconstruction of cranial base defects is well reported in the literature (74–77). Reconstruction of cranial base defects now actively employs synthetic materials such as titanium mesh and polyethylene. The use of such materials allows for immediate reconstruction with a low complication rate, 5% with the implants. The etiology of the complication was found to be the patient's soft tissue and not an inherent implant defect. The advantages of synthetic materials are several: availability, easy contouring, stability, tolerance of adjuvant therapy, and overall enhanced cosmetic result which leads to the ultimate goal, improved quality of life for the patient (78).

Frontal Sinus and Sphenoid Lesions

FRONTAL SINUS LESIONS

Frontal sinus tumors are particularly uncommon, with malignant frontal sinus lesions representing reportable events. Though benign frontal sinus-related pathology resulting from chronic infection and inflammation is frequently encountered, actual neoplasms are rare. The frontal sinus, like the sphenoid, is spared from direct exposure to environmental carcinogens. It has been suggested that this relative separation from the "mainstream" nasal cavity may be the reason for this low rate of malignant lesion formation within these two sinuses. When neoplasms do occur in the frontal sinus, they are usually benign primary bone tumors (osteomas) or represent direct extension of more malignant histology from the nasal cavity, ethmoids, or olfactory mucosa.

When addressing lesions involving the frontal sinus a coronal incision provides the maximum exposure. This approach also allows access to neighboring intracranial structures while preserving an acceptable aesthetic outcome (61). This extensive surgical field enables the surgeon to manage a wide variety of lesions, and to easily extend the resection to include neighboring structures, including the anterior fossa. Access to the sinus cavity is usually achieved by removing the anterior table of the sinus, followed by resection of the lesion. This exposure also allows for the management of the subfrontal dura or for the placement of a vascularized pericranial flap into the site for sinus obliteration. If the anterior table is involved with the lesion, it can be replaced with titanium mesh.

Sphenoid Sinus Lesions

Sphenoid tumors usually result from the spread of intracranial tumors through the cranial base into this sinus. These secondary sinus lesions frequently consist of chordomas, chondrosarcomas, pituitary adenomas, and meningiomas. Primary lesions of the sphenoid sinus are even less common than tumors affecting the frontal sinus and represent very specialized care situations from a surgical standpoint.

When secondarily involved by tumor spread through the cranial base, the management of this sinus is intimately related to the method of treatment of the intracranial portion of the lesion, and not specific to the sphenoid sinus itself. As a result, a meaningful discussion of sphenoid sinus tumors is beyond the scope of this chapter. It is recommended that reference sources focused on skull base tumors be consulted for a discussion of this topic. The most logical approach to this sinus for the purpose of achieving a complete tumor resection usually consists of a frontal/subfrontal approach or an infratemporal fossa approach. Other approaches consist of transnasal or transpalatal access, but these approaches result in limited access to the structures deep to the sphenoid sinus itself. The most frequently employed approach in our practice is through the infratemporal fossa. Other approaches have been described, but have yet to become standards of care (79).

RADIOLOGIC IMAGING CONCERNS

Bernard B. O'Malley and Suresh K. Mukherji

The nasal cavity and paranasal sinuses are located centrally in the head, providing structural support for vital functional and cosmetic purposes. The distinction between early and advanced tumors of the nasal cavity and paranasal sinuses is related to the number of subsites and adjacent extraparanasal compartments involved. The concept of the Ohngren plane is applied to the interpretation of modern cross-sectional images. The discussion in this section pertains to small lesions above the Ohngren plane and any lesion below that plane. Lesions of the palate and maxilla are managed in a similar fashion. Unfortunately, patients rarely present to medical care or imaging for the vague symptoms of early paranasal sinus masses. Owing to the frequency of paranasal inflammatory and allergic diseases, in those patients who do eventually undergo scanning, most intrasinus abnormalities that are seen are passed off as incidental. Because paranasal sinus disorders produce vague, nonspecific symptoms, most initial imaging evaluations of the head are designed to examine the brain. Even the scans that do cover the paranasal sinuses are printed at photographic settings to highlight brain structures, obscuring the sinus findings. Consequently, the first imaging procedure performed on patients with unsuspected deep paranasal sinus tumors will not completely define the extent of the tumor.

When a patient finally presents to a referral center with such CT or MRI scans, the imaging workup can usually be completed with a dedicated examination in the alternate modality (MRI or CT) (Figs. 21.17, 21.18). A CT and an MRI generally are considered to provide complementary information (80,81). Although there are some typical features of sinonasal malignancies (82), neither CT nor MRI reveals specific features to render a diagnosis in the majority of neoplasms. Reviewed together they do provide most of the necessary staging information (83). Slow-growing tumors deform more than destroy bone framework. Intermediate grade tumors deform but also cause sclerosis of the involved bone (84). Most epithelial malignancies destroy bone in their path. Only the lymphomas tend to permeate bone more than frankly destroy bone. Position of the tumor suggests the diagnosis in some types. Origin at the uncinate process with a frondlike pattern is typical for inverted papilloma (Fig. 21.19). Origin at the high nasal recess is typical for olfactory neuroblastoma (85), regardless of age (Fig. 21.20). Both CT and MRI can identify skull base invasion. However, CT is superior to MRI for identifying early cortical erosion. This is especially important for evaluating the status of the cribriform plate and orbital walls (86). Magnetic resonance imaging provides exquisite soft-tissue detail and is recommended to evaluate for direct intracranial extension or retrograde perineural extension.

An important complementary role of CT and MR is defining the extent of tumor. The attenuation of most tumors is similar to mucosal thickening making it difficult to distinguish between tumor and adjacent obstructed secretions. This is especially important for tumors that involve the nasal cavity and extend to the frontal recess. It is difficult to determine on CT whether the opacification of the frontal sinus is due to direct tumor extension (requiring a craniofacial approach) or a build up of secretions due to the obstruction of the draining nasofrontal recess. Certain tumors that fall into the latter group may be candidates for endoscopic resection. It has been shown that coronal T2-weighted MR can be very help in differentiating between tumor and obstructed secretions (87). Obstructed secretions tend to be very high brightness on T2-weighted images whereas tumor tends to be lower signal. There is overlap between the signal characteristics between tumor and secretions, but this sequence tends to be very helpful in most cases.

Imaging of paranasal sinus tumors requires a careful analysis of the extent of extraparanasal sinus tumor extension (88,89), particularly in those patients with cranial neuropathies (90). Knowledge of paranasal sinus anatomic variants will prevent mis-staging of tumors before treatment decisions are made (Fig. 21.21). Both CT and MR can be used to detect intraorbital extension. Superior extension requires coronal views of the orbital floor (Fig. 21.22) and cribriform plate or fovea ethmoidalis. Tumors contacting the periorbita or ocular muscle cone have 90% and 100% sensitivity for orbital involvement (91). Careful attention to the second division of the fifth cranial nerve within the infraorbital groove is necessary to exclude retrograde extension to the foramen rotundum. Supplementary sagittal views are helpful for ethmoid tumors (see Fig. 4.14). Axial views are the most useful for retromaxillary extension (Fig. 21.23) and for determining the degree of premaxillary extension. Precontrast T1-weighted views are very useful, given that most of the deep facial space contains natively bright fat signal, which, when involved by tumor, is easily staged and is not affected by artifact. T2-weighted views help to characterize the nature of the lesion and to differentiate between tumor extension and simple (acute or chronic) sinus obstruction (Fig. 21.24) (87).

Preoperative therapeutic embolization of selected hypervascular head and neck tumors should be performed only in experienced hands at referral centers. The risk for operative problems with lesions such as juvenile angiofibroma can be reduced with preoperative embolization. The surgery date should be closely coupled with the embolization (<7 days) to minimize recruitment of collaterals, regardless of the modality available.

Failure at the primary site remains the most important problem in patients with maxillary sinus carcinoma (92). Follow-up imaging of the paranasal sinuses is particularly challenging because of the presence of complex grafts that are typically unique to the individual reconstruction (Fig. 21.25). These layers of tissue are well vascularized and demonstrate intense native contrast enhancement potentially obscuring early local recurrences. A further complicating factor is mucosal reaction due to adjuvant treatment in the remaining sinuses. Because of the attendant increased enhancement of the thickened mucosa and abnormal MRI signal, careful analysis of CT and MRI scans is required by experienced readers before a recurrence is reported (Figs. 21.26 through 21.28). A baseline postoperative scan before discharge probably is not necessary if all margins are reported to be negative (Fig. 21.29). The first postoperative scan can be performed when the operative swelling and induration have resolved appreciably on follow-up. Computed tomography is adequate for this purpose and can reliably be reproduced scan to scan. Magnetic resonance imaging is advantageous for follow-up for high paranasal lesions (93). Metallic miniplates cause artifacts with both CT and MRI. Very thin plates reduce the degree of streak artifact on CT but cause persistent field distortion on MRI and seriously compromise important fat-suppression sequences.

If follow-up imaging reveals a clinically occult abnormality suspicious for recurrence, percutaneous CT-guided needle biopsy procedures can be performed on an ambulatory basis. For patients with suspected recurrences that are deep to well-healed flaps (Fig. 21.30) or that lie in proximity to vital structures, percutaneous needle aspiration or biopsy can provide a minimally invasive route to diagnosis. Subsequent treatment options can then be addressed without the need to compromise the cosmetic success of the reconstruction. Positron emission tomography using fluorodeoxyglucose will eventually be the primary modality to evaluate such patients.

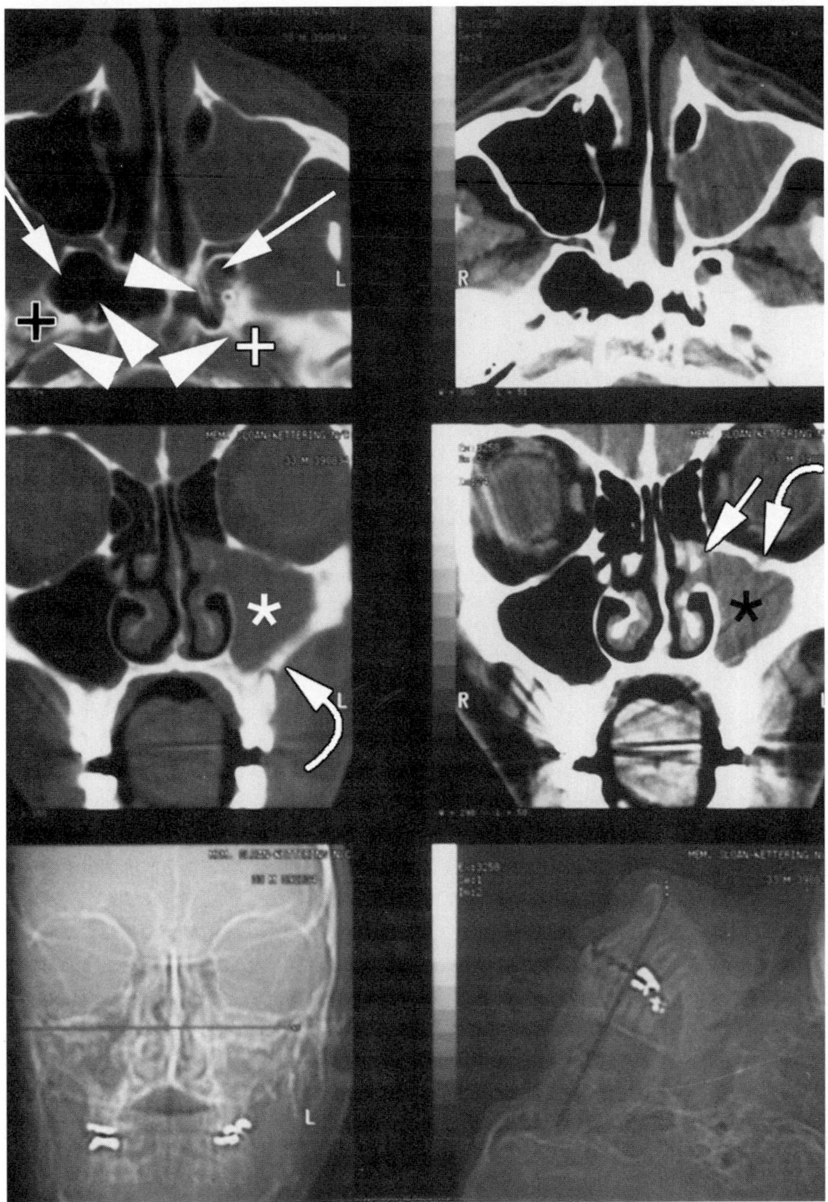

Figure 21.17 Standard paranasal computed tomographic imaging. Top to bottom: Axial and direct coronal views in bone (left) and soft tissue (right) windows, followed by corresponding cross-referenced scout views. A left maxillary mucocele (*asterisk*) is seen filling the infundibulum (*arrow*) of the osteomeatal complex. Bone windows demonstrate thickening of sinus walls (*curved arrows*) due to chronic inflammation. Note the lateral recess of sphenoid sinus (*long arrows*) straddling the vidian canal (*arrowheads*). Foramen ovale (*plus sign*).

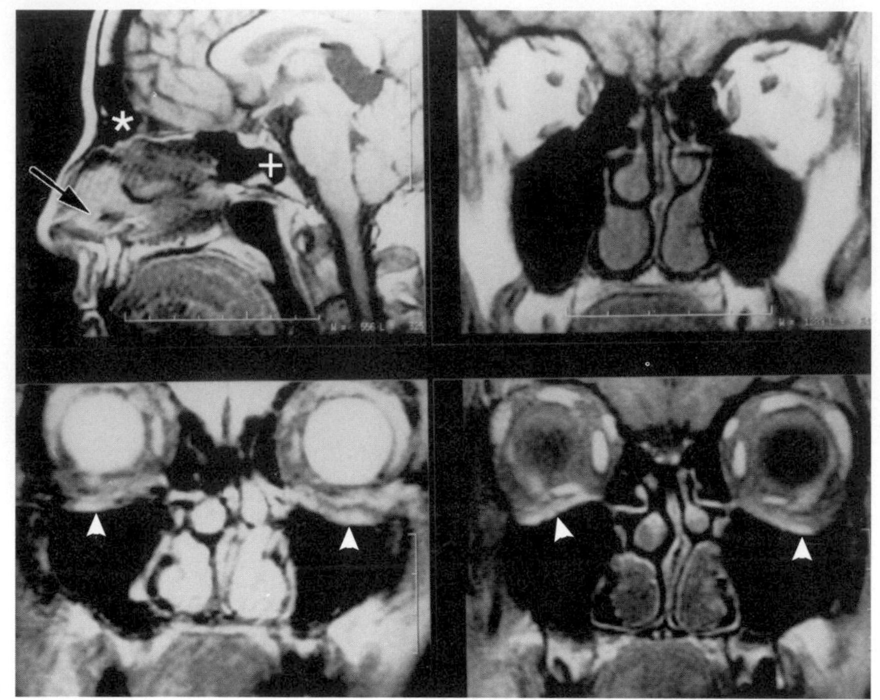

Figure 21.18 **A:** Standard sagittal and direct coronal paranasal magnetic resonance images with **(B)** T1, **(C)** T2, and **(D)** fat-suppressed contrast-enhanced T1 views of normal examination. Midline sagittal view shows septum (*arrow*), anterior skull base, and frontal (*asterisk*) and sphenoid (*plus sign*) sinuses aerating frontal bone and clivus. Coronal views outline normal margin of maxillary sinuses with orbits and ethmoid sinuses with anterior skull base. Bright signal is artifactual, due to magnetic susceptibility at close air–bone–tissue interfaces (*arrowhead*).

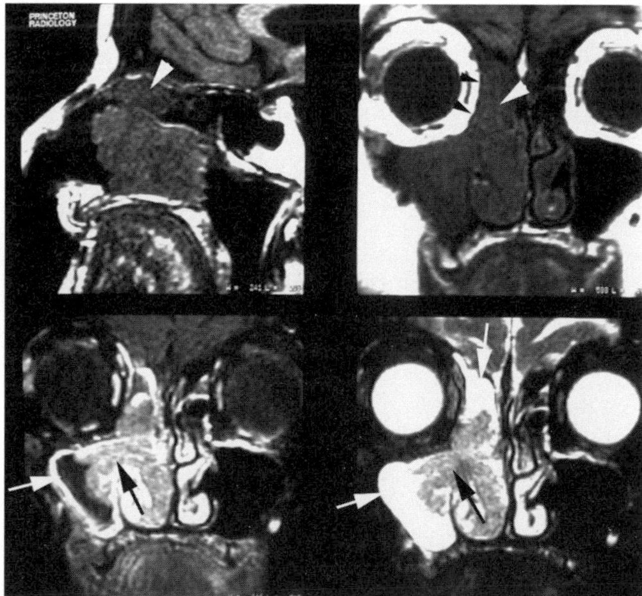

Figure 21.19 Inverting papilloma. Magnetic resonance images (clockwise from top left) include sagittal T1, coronal T1, coronal T2, and enhanced coronal T1. Images show a sinonasal mass straddling the former uncinate process (*black arrow*), limited extension to the ethmoid sinus (*white arrowhead*), causing obstruction of secretions (*white arrows*) but not penetrating the lamina papyracea (*black arrowheads*).

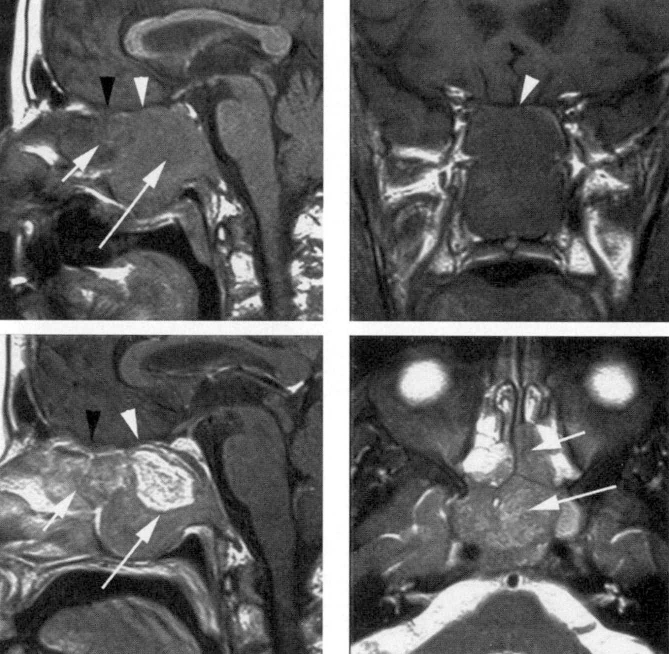

Figure 21.20 Esthesioneuroblastoma. Magnetic resonance images (clockwise from top left) include sagittal T1, coronal T1, axial T2, and enhanced sagittal T1 of a posterior nasal recess mass invading the sphenoid sinus (*long white arrows*), infiltrating the planum sphenoidale (*white arrowheads*) and cribriform plate (*black arrowheads*). No measurable transdural component is present.

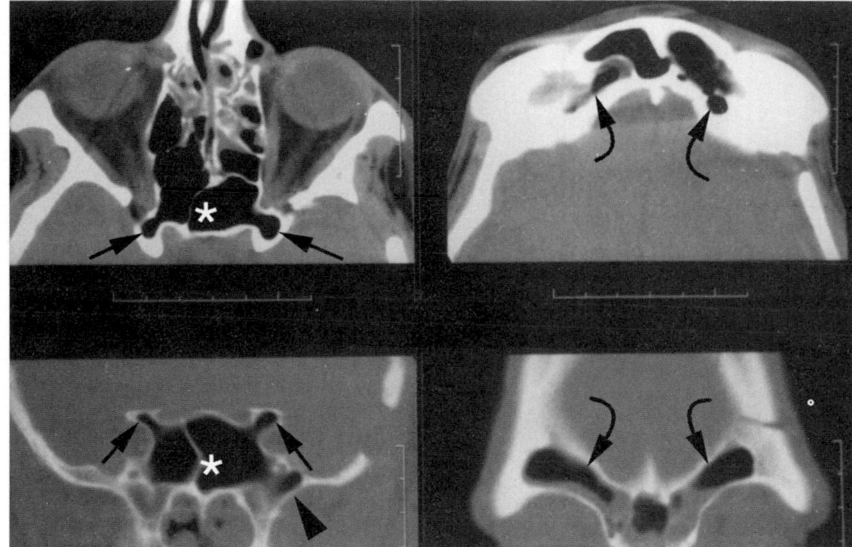

Figure 21.21 Sinus variants. Axial (top) and direct coronal computed tomographic (bottom) bone windows. Aeration of anterior clinoid processes (*arrows*) by well-developed sphenoid sinuses (*asterisk*) (Onodi air cells). Aeration of the orbital roof (*curved arrow*) by lateral extension of right ethmoid sinus. Note the lateral aeration of the sphenoid sinus (*arrowhead*).

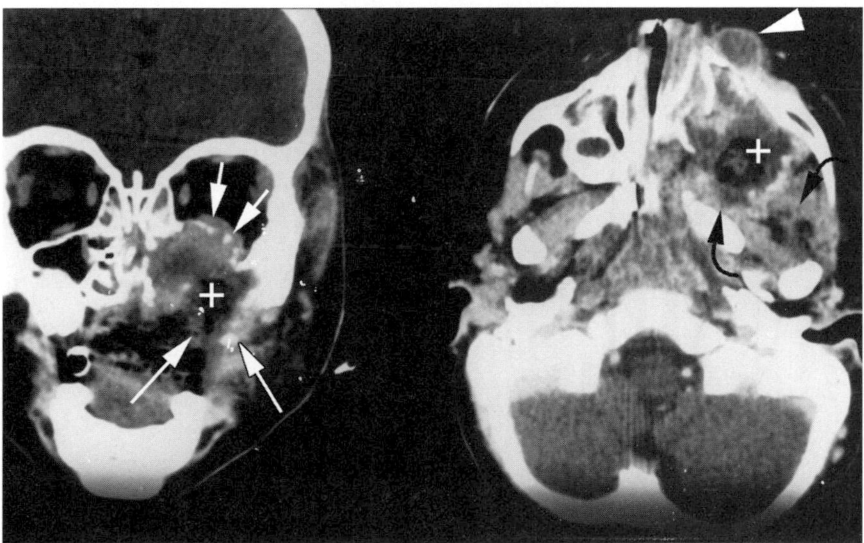

Figure 21.22 Multiplanar computed tomograms of T4 lesions. Large left maxillary mass with central necrosis, orbital invasion (*arrows*), and premaxillary (*arrowhead*) as well as retromaxillary extension (*curved arrows*). The alveolus is destroyed (*long arrows*).

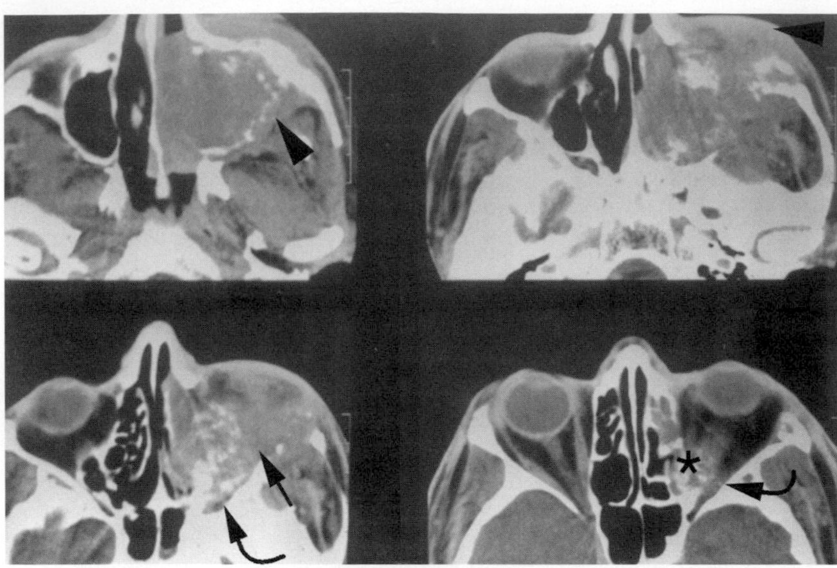
A

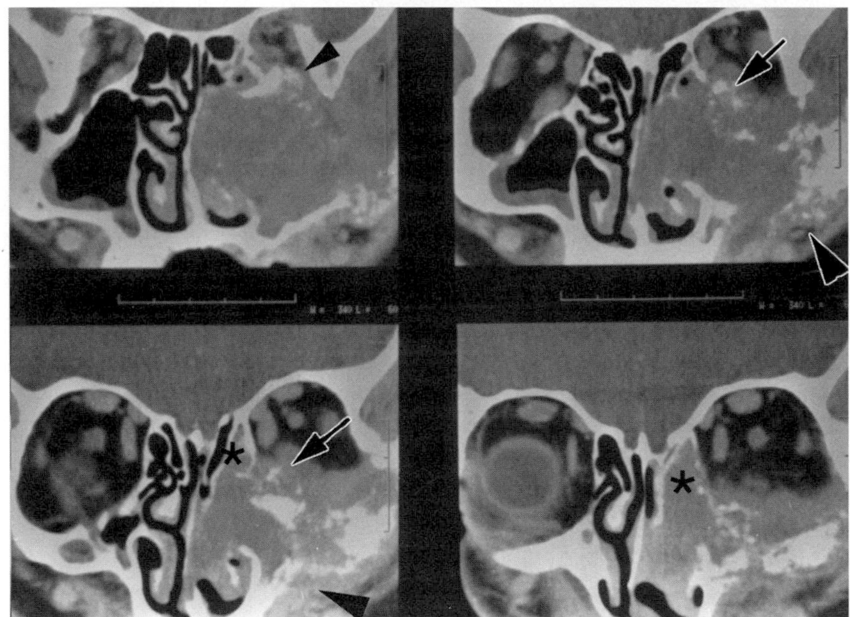
B

Figure 21.23 Multiplanar axial **(A)** and coronal **(B)** contrast computed tomograms of more advanced T4 lesion (more advanced than that shown in Fig. 21.22). Large left maxillary mass with frank orbital invasion (*arrows*) and gross extraparanasal extension (*arrowheads*). The inferior orbital fissure is involved (*curved arrows*) and the ethmoid sinus is infiltrated.

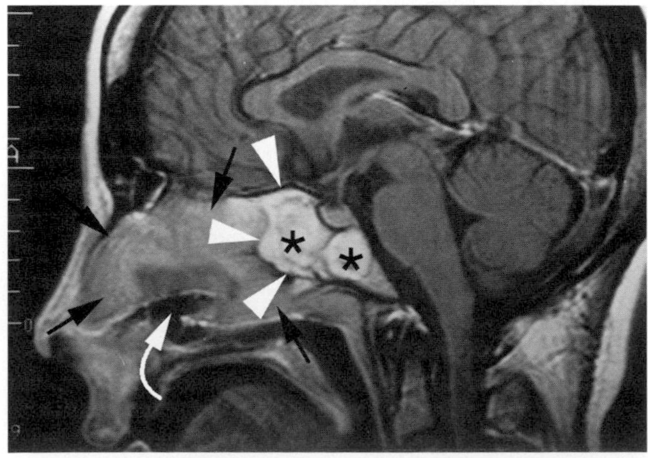
A

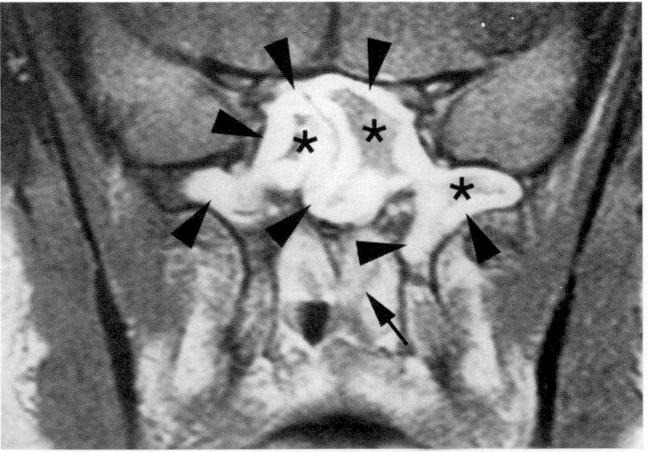
B

Figure 21.24 Obstructed secretions. **A:** Sagittal T1 and **(B)** coronal T2 magnetic resonance images show extensive nasal septal lesion (*arrows*) with central necrosis (*curved arrow*) producing obstructed secretions in the sphenoid sinus, with typical mucosal thickening (*arrowheads*) surrounding the collected secretions (*asterisk*). The secretions usually are bright on T1 but variable on T2 imaging.

A

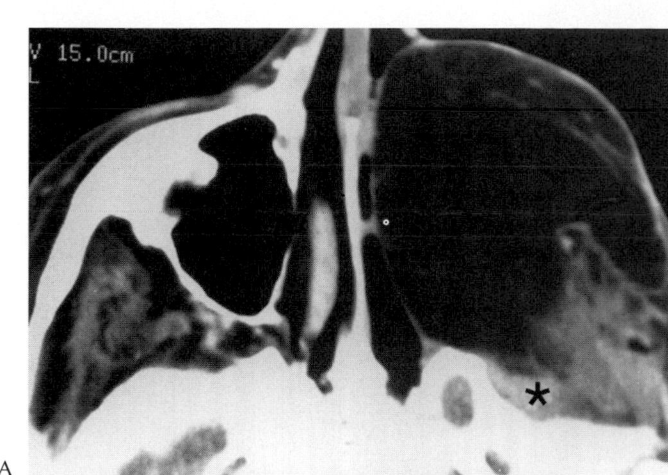

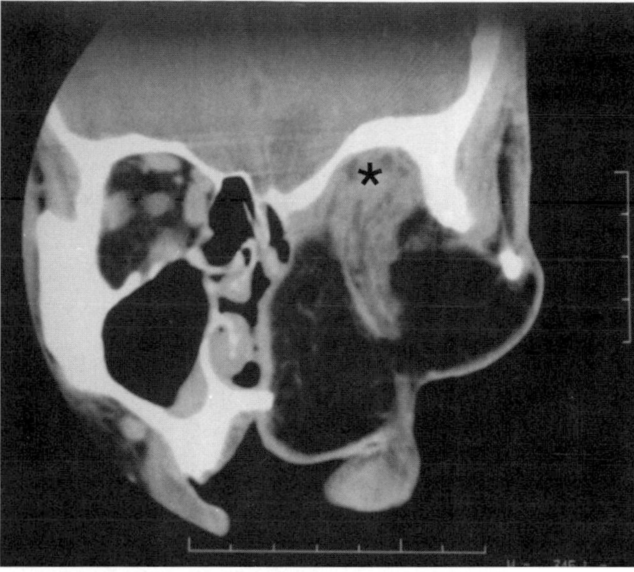

B

Figure 21.25 Appearance after flap reconstruction. Enhanced **(A)** axial and **(B)** direct coronal computed tomograms of facial complex show well-positioned muscular component (*asterisk*) of myocutaneous free flap tucked against the anterior skull base after extended maxillectomy and orbital exenteration. There is no evidence of recurrence.

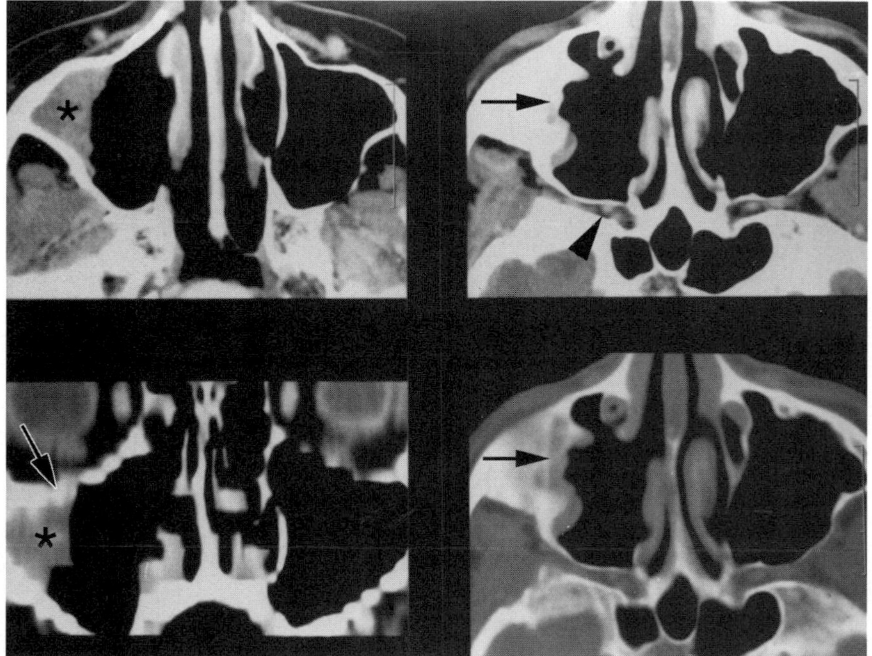

Figure 21.26 Limited local recurrence. Clockwise from top left: Enhanced axial computed tomogram in soft tissue and bone windows and coronal reformatted views of maxillary antra after prior medial maxillectomy show recurrence in the lateral recess (*asterisk*), with equivocal involvement of the infraorbital groove (*arrow*) but no extension to the pterygopalatine fossa (*arrowhead*).

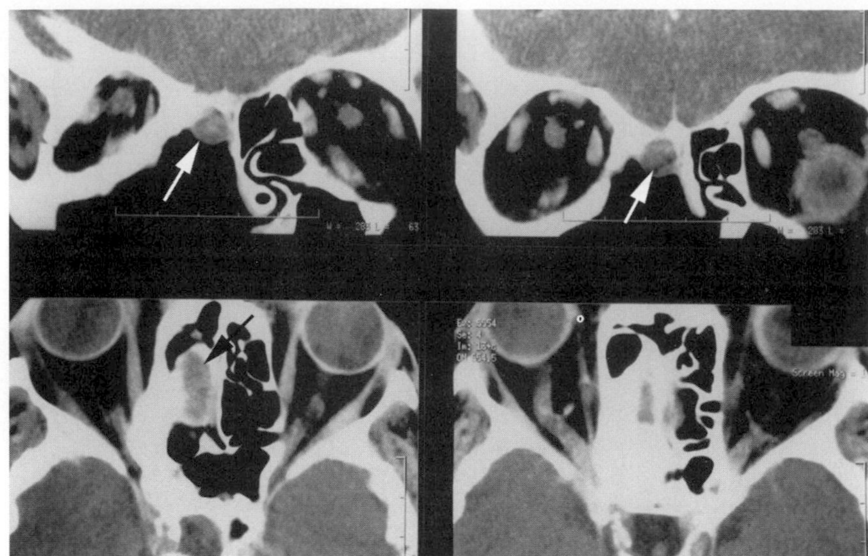

Figure 21.27 Small recurrence of squamous cell cancer. Direct coronal (top) and axial (bottom) contrast computed tomograms show small recurrence at high nasal recess (*arrows*), with minor erosion of cribriform plate.

A

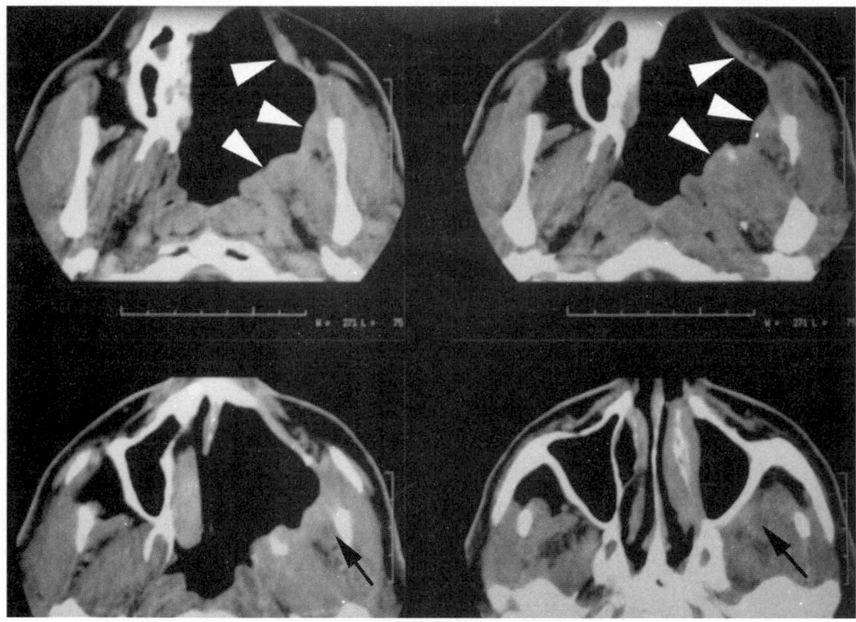

B

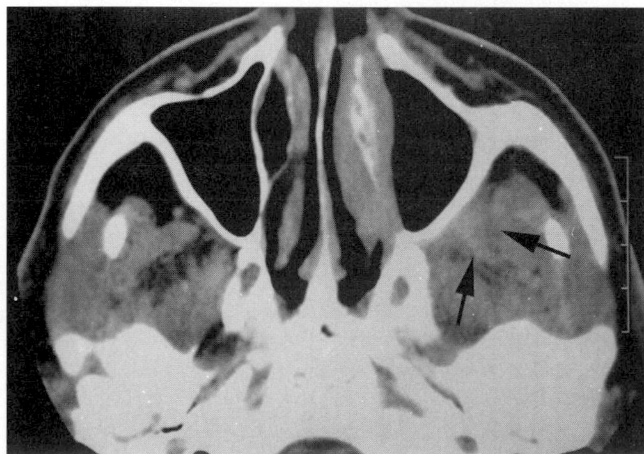

Figure 21.28 Early recurrence. Enhanced **(A)** serial axial and selected **(B)** axial views of early retromaxillary recurrence (*arrows*) hidden behind a well-healed mucosal reconstruction (*arrowheads*).

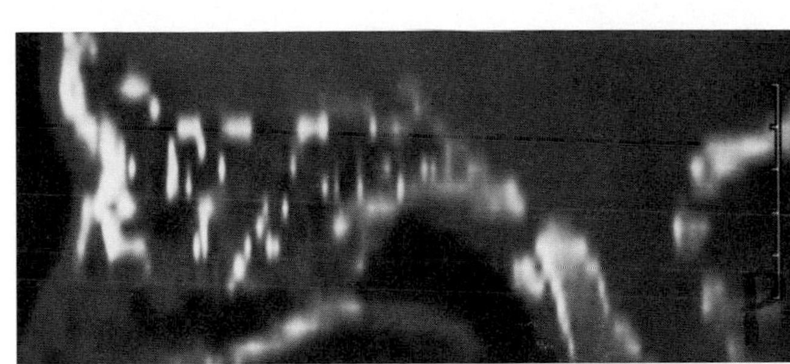
A

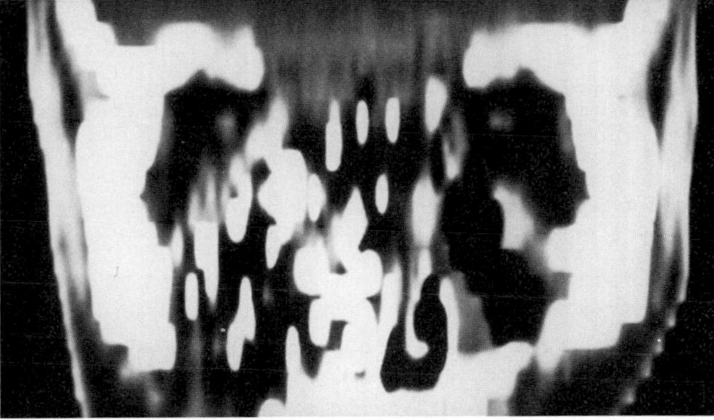
B

Figure 21.29 Immediate follow-up. Reformatted noncontrast **(A)** sagittal bone window and **(B)** coronal soft-tissue window show paranasal sinus wire packing after anterior skull base resection.

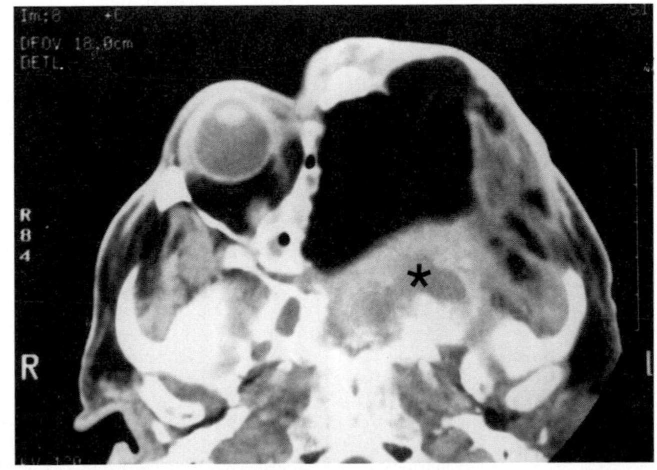
A

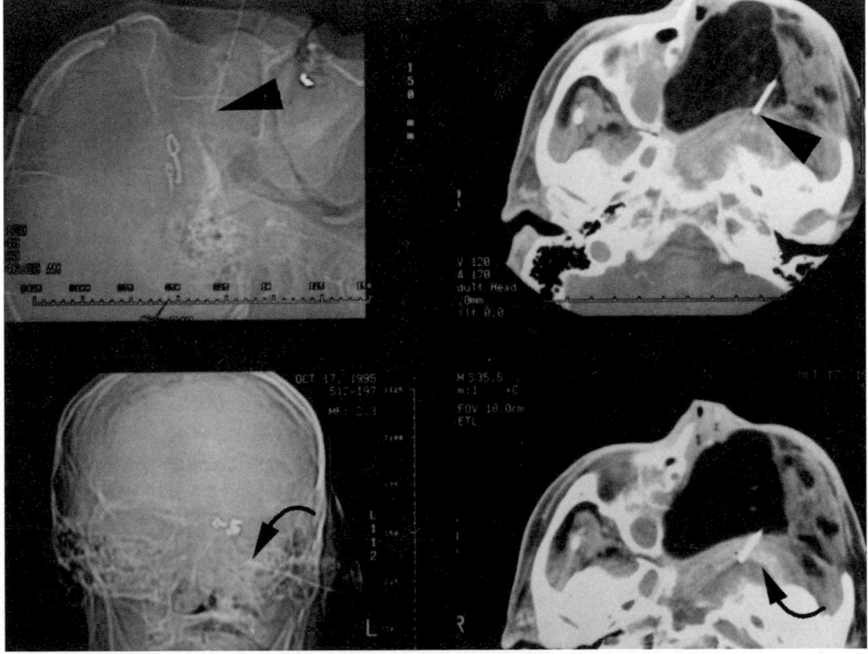
B

Figure 21.30 Follow-up imaging and intervention. **A:** Enhanced axial computed tomogram (CT) shows moderately sized recurrence at the sphenoid bone (*asterisk*) that is not clinically apparent or palpable deep to the well-healed free flap. **B:** Control axial (right) and corresponding "scout radiographic" control images (left), showing CT-guided 20-gauge needle placement into lesion. Note the needle tip at edge of lesion (*arrowhead*) and within lesion (*curved arrows*).

REFERENCES

1. Graney DO, Baker SR. Anatomy. In: Cummings CW, Fredrickson JM, Krause CJ, et al., eds. *Otolaryngology; head and neck surgery*, 3rd ed. St. Louis: Mosby, 1999.
2. Pearson BW, MacKenzie RG, Goodman WS. The anatomical basis of transantral ligation of the maxillary artery in severe epistaxis. *Laryngoscope* 1969;79:969–984.
3. Pearson BW. Surgical anatomy of the nasal cavity and paranasal sinuses. In: Thawley SE, Panje WR, Batsakis JG, et al., eds. *Comprehensive management of head and neck tumors*, 2nd ed. Philadelphia: WB Saunders, 1999.
4. Heffner DK. Sinonasal and laryngeal salivary gland lesions. In: Ellis GL, Auclair PL, Gnepp DR, eds. *Surgical pathology of the salivary glands*. Philadelphia: WB Saunders, 1991.
5. Manning JT, Batsakis JG. Salivary-type neoplasms of the sinonasal tract. *Ann Otol Rhinol Laryngol* 1991;100:691–694.
6. Franquemont DW, Mills SE. Sinonasal malignant melanoma: a clinicopathologic and immunohistochemical study of 14 cases. *Am J Clin Pathol* 1991;96: 689–697.
7. Perez-Ordonez B, Huvos AG. Nonsquamous lesions of the nasal cavity, paranasal sinuses, and nasopharynx. In: Gnepp DR, ed. *Diagnostic surgical pathology of the head and neck*. Philadelphia: WB Saunders, 2001.
8. Schantz SP, Harrison LB, Forastiere AA. Tumors of the nasal cavity and paranasal sinuses, nasopharynx, oral cavity and oropharynx. In: DeVita VT Jr, Hellman S, Rosenberg SA, eds. *Cancer: principles and practice of oncology*, 5th ed. Philadelphia: Lippincott-Raven Publishers, 1997.
9. Pillevuit O, Maire R, Lang FJ. Evaluation of combined neurosurgical and trans-facial excision of extensive rhinosinus tumors infiltrating the anterior skull base. *Ann Oto-Laryngol Chir Cervico-Faciale* 1999;116:270–277.
10. Osguthorpe JD. Sinus neoplasia. *Arch Otolaryngol Head Neck Surg* 1994;120: 19–25.
11. Muir CS, Nectoux J. Descriptive epidemiology of malignant neoplasms of the nose, nasal cavities, middle ear and accessory sinuses. *Clin Otolaryngol* 1980;5: 195–211.
12. Slootweg PJ, Richardson M. Squamous cell carcinoma of the upper aerodigestive system. In: Gnepp DR, ed. *Diagnostic surgical pathology of the head and neck*. Philadelphia: WB Saunders, 2001.
13. Rice DH, Stanley RB. Surgical therapy of the nasal cavity, ethmoid sinus, and maxillary sinus tumors. In: Thawley SE, Panje WR, Batsakis JG, et al., eds. *Comprehensive management of head and neck tumors*, 2nd ed. Philadelphia: WB Saunders, 1999.
14. Robin PE, Powell DJ. Regional node involvement and distant metastases in carcinoma of the nasal cavity and paranasal sinuses. *J Laryngol Otol* 1980;94: 301–309.
15. Lindeman P, Eklund U, Petruson B. Survival after surgical treatment in maxillary neoplasms of epithelial origin. *J Laryngol Otol* 1987;101:546.
16. Miyaguchi M, Sakai S, Takashima H, et al. Lymph node and distant metastases in patients with sinonasal carcinoma. *J Laryngol Otol* 1995;109:304–307.
17. Roush GC. Epidemiology of cancer of the nose and paranasal sinuses: current concepts. *Head Neck Surg* 1979;2:3–11.
18. Delank KW, Alberty J, Schroter D, et al. Diagnosis and treatment modalities in sinonasal inverted papillomas. *Laryngo-Rhino-Otol* 2000;79:226–232.
19. Acheson ED, Cowdell RH, Jolles B. Nasal cancer in the Northamptonshire boot and shoe industry. *BMJ* 1970;1:385–393.
20. Kashima H, Kessis T, Hraban R, et al. Human papilloma virus in sinonasal papillomas and squamous cell carcinoma. *Laryngoscope* 1992;102:973–976.
21. Leung SI, Yuen ST, Chung LP, et al, Epstein-Barr virus is present in a wide histological spectrum of sinonasal carcinomas. *Am J Surg Pathol* 1995;19:994–1001.
22. Zheng W, McLaughlin JK, Chow WH, et al. Risk factors for cancer of the nasal cavity and paranasal sinuses among white men in the United States. *Am J Epidemiol* 1993;138:965–972.
23. Miller RH, Sturgis EM, Sutton CL. Neoplasma of the nose and paranasal sinuses. In: Myers EN, Suen JY, eds. *Cancer of the head and neck*, 2nd ed. Philadelphia: WB Saunders, 1993.
24. Weisberger EC, Dedo HH. Cranial neuropathies in sinus disease. *Laryngoscope* 1977;87:357–363.
25. Dodd GH, Collins LC, Egan RL, et al. The systemic use of tomography in the diagnosis of carcinoma of the paranasal sinuses. *Radiology* 1959;72:379.
26. Sisson GA, Johnson NE, Mir A. Cancer of the maxillary sinus: clinical classification and management. *Ann Otol Rhinol Laryngol* 1963;72:1050.
27. Harrison DF. Critical look at the classification of maxillary sinus carcinomata. *Ann Otol Rhinol Laryngol* 1978;87:3–9.
28. American Joint Committee on Cancer. Maxillary sinus. In: *AJCC cancer staging manual*, 5th ed. Philadelphia: Lippincott-Raven Publishers, 1997.

28a. Greene F, Page D, Fleming I, et al. *AJCC cancer staging manual*, 6th ed. New York: Springer Verlag, 2002.

29. Mendenhall WM, Stringer SP, Cassisi NJ, et al. Squamous cell carcinoma of the nasal vestibule. *Head Neck* 1999;21:385–393.
30. Harrison LB, Pfister DG, Bosl GJ. Chemotherapy as part of the initial treatment for nasopharyngeal cancer. *Oncology* 1991;5:67–70.
31. Noorily AD. A lateral rhinotomy closure technique to avoid alar blunting. *Ear Nose Throat J* 1995;74:403–403.
32. Weisman R. Lateral rhinotomy and medial maxillectomy. *Otolaryngol Clin North Am* 1995;28:1145–1156.
33. Vural E, Hanna E. Extended lateral rhinotomy incision for total maxillectomy. *Otolaryngol Head Neck Surg* 2000;123:512–213.
34. Burget GC, Menick FJ. The subunit principle is nasal reconstruction. *Plast Reconstr Surg* 1985;76:239–247.
35. Pearson BW. Surgical therapy of the nasal cavity and paranasal sinuses. In: Thawley SE, Panje WR, Batsakis JG, et al, eds. *Comprehensive management of head and neck tumors*. Philadelphia: WB Saunders, 1987.
36. Smith RR, Klopp CT, Williams JM. Surgical treatment of cancer of the frontal sinus and adjacent areas. *Cancer* 1954;7:991.
37. Ketchum AS, Chretien PB, Van Buren JM, at al. The ethmoid sinuses: a re-evaluation of surgical resection. *Am J Surg* 1973;126:469–476.
38. Bridger GP. Radical surgery for ethmoid cancer. *Arch Otolaryngol* 1980;106: 630–634.
39. Sessions RB, Larson DL. En bloc ethmoidectomy and medial maxillectomy. *Arch Otolaryngol* 1977;103:195–202.
40. Carrau RL, Snyderman CH. Juvenile nasopharyngeal angiofibroma. In: Myers EN, ed. *Operative otolaryngology head and neck surgery*. Philadelphia: WB Saunders, 1997.
41. Portmann G, Retrouvey. *Le cancer du nez*. Paris: Gaston Doin et Cie, 1927.
42. Doyle PJ, Riding K, Kahn K. Management of nasopharyngeal angiofibroma. *J Otolaryngol* 1977;6:224–232.
43. Maniglia AJ. Indications and techniques of midfacial degloving: a 15-year experience. *Arch Otolaryngol Head Neck Surg* 1986;112:750–752.
44. Casson PR, Bonnano PC, Converse JM. The midfacial degloving procedure. *Plast Reconstr Surg* 1974;53:102–113.
45. Conley J, Price JC. Sublabial approach to the nasal cavity and nasopharyngeal cavity. *Am J Surg* 1979;38:615–618.
46. Price JC, Holliday MJ, Johns ME, et al. The versatile midface degloving approach. *Laryngoscope* 1988;98:291–295.
47. Maniglia AJ, Phillips DA. Midfacial degloving for the management of nasal, sinus, and skull-base neoplasms. *Otolaryngol Clin North Am* 1995;28:1127–1143.
48. Casiano RR, Numa WA, Falquez AM. Endoscopic resection of esthesioneuroblastoma. *Am J Rhinol* 2001;15:271–279.
49. Stammberger H, Anderhuber W, Walch C, et al. Possibilities and limitations of endoscopic management of nasal and paranasal sinus malignancies. *Acta Oto-Rhino-Laryngol Belg* 1999;53:199–205.
50. Tufano RP, Mokadam NA, Montone KT, et al. Malignant tumors of the nose and paranasal sinuses: Hospital of the University of Pennsylvania experience 1990–1997. *Am J Rhinol* 1999;13:117–123.
51. Sham CL, Woo JK, van Hasselt CA. Endoscopic resection of inverted papilloma of the nose and paranasal sinuses. *J Laryngol Otol* 1998;112:758–764.
52. Larson DL, Christ JE, Jesse RH. Preservation of the orbital contents in cancer of the maxillary sinus. *Arch Otolaryngol* 1982;108:370–372.
53. Cordeiro PG, Santamaria E. A classification system and algorithm for reconstruction of maxillectomy and midfacial defects. *Plast Reconstr Surg* 2000;105: 2331–2346.
54. Davison SP, Sherris DA, Meland B. An algorithm for maxillectomy defect reconstruction. *Laryngoscope* 1998;108:215–219.
55. Larson Dl. A classification system and algorithm for reconstruction of maxillectomy and midfacial defects. *Plast Reconstr Surg* 2000;105:2347–2348.
56. Hochman M. Reconstruction of midfacial and anterior skull-base defects. *Otolaryngol Clin North Am* 1995;28:1269–1277.
57. Johnson JT, Aramany MA, Myers EN. Palatal neoplasms: reconstructive considerations. *Otolaryngol Clin North Am* 1983;16:441–456.
58. Schuller DE. Extensive defects of the sino-orbital region. *Arch Otolaygol Head Neck Surg* 1992;118:859–860.
59. Freje JE, Campbell BH, Yousif J, et al. Reconstruction after infrastructure maxillectomy using dual free flaps. *Laryngoscope* 1997;107:694–697.
60. Pollice PA, Frodel JL Jr. Secondary reconstruction of upper midface and orbit after total maxillectomy. *Arch Otolaryngol Head Neck Surg* 1998;124:802–808.
61. Catalano PJ, Sen C. Management of the anterior ethmoid and frontal sinus tumors. *Otolaryngol Clin North Am* 1995;28:1157–1174.
62. Biller HF, Slotnick D, Lawson W, at al. Superior rhinotomy for en bloc resection of bilateral ethmoid sinus tumors. *Arch Otolaryngol Head Neck Surg* 1989; 115:1463–1466.
63. Osguthorpe JD, Patel S. Craniofacial approaches to sinus malignancy. *Otolaryngol Clin North Am* 1995;28:1239–1257.
64. Tessier P, Guiot G, Rougerie J, et al. [Osteotomies cranio-naso-orbito-faciales hypertelorisme]. *Ann Chir Plast* 1967;12:103–118.
65. Nuss DW, Janecka IP, Sekhar LN, at al. Craniofacial disassembly in the management of skull-base tumors. *Otolaryngol Clin North Am* 1991;24:1465–1497.
66. Janecka IP. Surgical approaches to the skull base. *Neuroimag Clin North Am* 1994;4:639–656.
67. McCutcheon IE, Blacklock JB, Weber RS, et al. Anterior transcranial (craniofacial) resection of tumors of the paranasal sinuses: surgical technique and results. *Neurosurgery* 1996;38:471–479.
68. Krause CJ, Baker SR. Extended transantral approach to pterygomaxillary tumors. *Ann Otol* 1982;91:391–398.
69. Fisch U, Pillsbury HS. Infratemporal fossa approach to lesions in the temporal bone and base of skull. *Arch Otolaryngol* 1979;105:99–107.
70. Mustoe TA, Corral CJ. Soft tissue reconstructive choices for craniofacial reconstruction. *Clin Plast Surg* 1995;22:543–554.
71. Scher RL, Cantrell RW. Anterior skull base reconstruction with the pericranial flap after craniofacial resection. *Ear Nose Throat J* 1992;71:210–212, 215–217.
72. Yucel A, Yazar S, Aydin Y, et al. Temporalis muscle flap for craniofacial reconstruction after tumor resection. *J Craniofacial Surg* 2000;11:258–264.
73. Badie B, Preston JK, Hartig GK. Use of titanium mesh for reconstruction of large anterior cranial base defects. *J Neurosurg* 2000;93:711–714.

74. Besteiro JM, Aki FE, Ferreira MC, et al. Free flap reconstruction of tumors involving the cranial base. *Microsurgery* 1994;15:9–13.
75. Izquierdo R, Leonetti JP, Origitano TC, et al. Refinements using free-tissue transfer for complex cranial base reconstruction. *Plast Reconstr Surg* 1993;92:567–574.
76. Shah JP, Kraus DH, Bilsky MH, et al. Craniofacial resection of malignant tumors involving the anterior skull base. Long term results. *Arch Otolaryngol Head Neck Surg* 1997;123:1312–1317.
77. Spinelli HM, Pershing JA, Walser B. Reconstruction of the cranial base. *Clin Plast Surg* 1995;422:555–561.
78. Janecka IP. New reconstructive technologies in skull base surgery: role of titanium mesh and porous polyethylene. *Arch Otolaryngol Head Neck Surg* 2000; 126:396–401.
79. Lalwani AK, Kaplan MJ, Gutin PH. The transphenoethmoid approach to the sphenoid sinus and clivus. *Neurosurgery* 1992;31:1008–1014.

Radiologic Imaging Considerations

80. Hofmann E, Nadjmi M. [Modern neuroradiologic diagnosis and interventional strategies for the ENT physician] [Review] [German]. *HNO* 1995;43:584–589.
81. Kraus DH, Lanzieri CF, Wanamaker JR, et al. Complementary use of computed tomography and magnetic resonance imaging in assessing skull base lesions. *Laryngoscope* 1992;102:623–629.
82. Mafee MF. Preoperative imaging anatomy of nasal-ethmoid complex for functional endoscopic sinus surgery. *Radiol Clin North Am* 1993;31:1–20.
83. Gualdi GF, Melone A, Di Biasi C, et al. [Tumors of the nose, paranasal sinuses and facial bones: the role of computerized tomography and MRI in the assessment of the damage]. *Clin Ter* 1997;148:257–265.
84. Savy L, Lloyd G, Lund VJ, et al. Optimum imaging for inverted papilloma. *J Laryngol Otol* 2000;114:891–893.
85. Pickuth D, Heywang-Kobrunner SH, Spielmann RP. Computed tomography and magnetic resonance imaging features of olfactory neuroblastoma: an analysis of 22 cases. *Clin Otolaryngol* 1999;24:457–461.
86. Maroldi R, Farina D, Battaglia G, et al. [Magnetic resonance and computed tomography compared in the staging of rhinosinusal neoplasms: a cost-effectiveness evaluation] [Italian]. *Radiologica Medica* 1996;91:211–218.
87. Som PM, Shapiro MD, Biller HF, et al. Sinonasal tumors and inflammatory tissues: differentiation with MR imaging. *Radiology* 1988;167:803–808.
88. Allbery SM, Chaljub G, Cho NL, et al. MR imaging of nasal masses [Review]. *Radiographics* 1995;15:1311–1327.
89. Chow JM, Leonetti JP, Mafee MF. Epithelial tumors of the paranasal sinuses and nasal cavity [Review] [32 refs]. *Radiolog Clin North Am* 1993;31:61–73.
90. DeMonte F, Ginsberg LE, Clayman GL. Primary malignant tumors of the sphenoidal sinus. *Neurosurgery* 2000;46:1084–1091; discussion 1091–1082.
91. Eisen MD, Yousem DM, Loevner LA, et al. Preoperative imaging to predict orbital invasion by tumor. *Head Neck* 2000;22:456–462.
92. Paulino AC, Marks JE, Bricker P, et al. Results of treatment of patients with maxillary sinus carcinoma. *Cancer* 1998;83:457–465.
93. Derdeyn CP, Moran CJ, Wippold FJ 2nd, et al. MRI of esthesioneuroblastoma. *J Comput Assist Tomogr* 1994;18:16–21.

CHAPTER 22

Cancer of the Nasal Vestibule, Nasal Cavity, and Paranasal Sinus

Radiation Therapy and Chemotherapy Management

James T. Parsons and Merrill S. Kies

Neoplasms of the paranasal sinuses and nasal cavity account for 3% to 4% of head and neck cancers (1). The male-to-female ratio for all sites and histologies is approximately 3:2 (2,3). Most tumors are advanced at presentation, and the exact site of origin may be uncertain.

Tumors may arise from any of six separate anatomic locations: maxillary sinus, ethmoid sinus, frontal sinus, sphenoid sinus, nasal cavity, or nasal vestibule. Unlike other head and neck sites, in which the vast majority of tumors are squamous cell carcinomas, nonsquamous cell malignant tumors comprise about half of all malignant tumors of these sites (4,5). In addition to squamous cell carcinomas, multiple other histologic subtypes are encountered with some frequency: esthesioneuroblastoma, sinonasal undifferentiated carcinoma (SNUC), small cell carcinoma, adenocarcinoma, adenoid cystic carcinoma, mucoepidermoid carcinoma, inverting papilloma, lethal midline granuloma (nasal natural killer/T-cell CD56-positive lymphoma), malignant melanoma, sarcoma, plasmacytoma, and T-cell or B-cell lymphoma. The majority of these malignancies have dissimilar natural histories. The occasional occurrence of metastatic adenocarcinoma (particularly renal cell, lung, or breast) to this region should also be kept in mind. Anatomic complexity, a high frequency of tumor unresectability, patient refusal to undergo mutilating resection, and tumor proximity to vital structures (brain, brainstem, pituitary, cavernous sinus, and visual apparatus) add further challenge to the management of these tumors. Surgical resections are often piecemeal; even when margins of resection are deemed "negative," local recurrence occurs in more than 50% of patients after surgery alone (4). Management of these tumors often requires a multimodal approach, involving surgery, radiation therapy (RT), and increasingly in recent years, chemotherapy.

From a therapy standpoint, the central issue is usually local control, which for many of these tumors is tantamount to cure. Primary site and histology are important. Local control rates are highest for cancers of the nasal vestibule, followed in order by the nasal cavity, ethmoid sinus, and maxillary sinus; local control rates for sphenoid sinus and frontal sinus lesions are both poor (6). Although there are notable exceptions (e.g., nasal vestibule, esthesioneuroblastoma, adenocarcinoma of the nasal cavity), most patients who experience local failure are not able to be successfully salvaged by secondary treatment, so it is important that the first treatment course maximizes the chance for success. For all sites and histologies combined, the incidence of lymph node metastasis at presentation (about 10%) is low compared with other head and neck mucosal sites. Many authors note poor 5-year survival rates (about 10%) in patients who present with regional lymph node metastasis, considerably lower than the rates achieved in patients with lymph node metastasis from other head and neck primary sites (7). Distant metastasis as the sole site of failure occurs in 10% of patients (6). We organize much of this chapter by anatomic site.

The maxillary sinus is the primary site of approximately 60% of tumors that arise in the paranasal sinuses or nasal cavity. Men are affected twice as often as women. Mean and median ages are both in the early to mid-60s (8–11). Thorotrast, used in the past as a contrast medium for roentgenographic study of the maxillary sinuses, contains the radioactive metal thorium and is a known etiologic agent in maxillary sinus carcinoma.

Cancers of the ethmoid sinus account for 10% to 15% of all nasal cavity/paranasal sinus cancers. Mean and median age are both in the late 50s to early 60s (12–16). The male-to-female ratio is approximately 2.5:1 (13,14); however, in some European series, more than 90% of patients are male (12,16–19), a finding particularly noted in series containing a high proportion of patients with adenocarcinoma or occupational exposure. There is a well-known association between occupational exposure to wood dust and primary ethmoid sinus carcinoma, particularly adenocarcinoma. In a number of series, half or more of patients with ethmoid sinus carcinoma have had such exposure, with exposure times ranging from one to five decades (12,13). Increased risk of nasal and ethmoid sinus carcinoma has also been observed in shoemakers, bakers, flour millers, and workers exposed to nickel, mustard gas, or isopropanol and other chemicals (14,20–22). Cigarette smoking has not been implicated. Series in which a high proportion of patients had such occupational exposure have a preponderance of adenocarcinoma in comparison with squamous cell carcinoma or undifferentiated cancer by a ratio of approximately 2:1 (13,16,17); in series where few patients have such exposure, the proportions of adenocarcinoma to squamous cell carcinoma are generally reversed (14,15).

Primary malignant tumors of the sphenoid sinus represent 1% to 2% of all paranasal sinus tumors. There is a slight male predominance. Mean age is 50 (1).

Frontal sinus carcinoma is extraordinarily rare, accounting for less than 0.3% of paranasal sinus carcinomas (7). Peak incidence is in the fifth and sixth decades with a male-to-female ratio of 5:1 (23,24).

Nasal cavity tumors account for 20% to 25% of tumors of the paranasal sinus/nasal cavity region. Few series report on nasal cavity primaries alone. Most series are reported as part of a larger series of patients with paranasal sinus tumors, and in some series, nasal vestibule cancers are included. The male-to-female ratio is approximately 2:1 (25,26). Median and mean age are both in the late 50s to early 60s (25–27). Nasal cavity adenocarcinomas are linked to occupational exposure to wood dust (furniture industry, saw millers, carpenters); such occupational cancers characteristically arise from the middle turbinate and have a 20:1 male-to-female predominance (28). In addition, nickel refinery workers (29,30) have a 40-fold increased risk of developing squamous cell carcinoma of the nasal cavity; the primary site is also almost invariably the anterior tip of the middle turbinate. Satoh et al. (31) report four cases of squamous cell carcinoma of the nasal cavity among employees at a chromate factory in Japan. Length of industrial exposure was 19 to 32 years. Wegener granulomatosis (32) has also been recently implicated.

Esthesioneuroblastoma has a bimodal age distribution (10–20 years and 50–60 years of age) (33–36), a roughly equal sex distribution, and no racial predilection; it is unusual before the age of 10 or after the age of 70.

Sinonasal undifferentiated carcinoma (SNUC) occurs more often in men than women (37–41). The tumor usually presents in middle age (mean and median ages both approximately 55; range, 20–80).

Malignant melanoma accounts for approximately 5% of malignant tumors of the nasal cavity and paranasal sinuses (42). Sinonasal melanomas present later in life than cutaneous malignant melanomas, mostly in the sixth to ninth decades (43). There is a slight male predilection (42,44). In the Armed Forces Institute of Pathology series, 16% of patients were black (45). Most other series report a lesser percentage (approximately 5%) of blacks (46,47).

Inverting papilloma is a benign sinonasal tumor constituting 0.5% to 4% of all sinonasal tumors (48). Inverting papilloma occurs primarily in the fifth to sixth decades of life, with a male-to-female ratio of 3:1 to 4:1 (49–51). Although rare in childhood and adolescence, inverting papilloma in the young has similar biologic behavior to that observed in older patients, including a high frequency of recurrence and association with malignancy (52,53). The etiology is uncertain although viral infection, chronic sinusitis, and occupational exposure have all been suggested as contributory (54–56). There is no relationship to allergy or nasal polyps (57).

Lethal midline granuloma occurs more frequently in Asia, Mexico, and South America than in European or North American populations (58). The male-to-female ratio is 2:1 (59–61). Mean and median ages are 40 to 45 years. A source of much confusion, the term *lethal midline granuloma* is now being replaced by the more appropriate descriptor, nasal natural killer (NK)/T-cell lymphoma.

Cancer of the nasal vestibule differs from nasal tumors that develop above and behind the limen nasi, the latter being considered part of the nasal cavity proper. The nasal vestibule is lined with skin; squamous cell carcinoma arising from this site has a natural history that is more aggressive than that of skin cancers of the external nose, but less aggressive than nasal cavity or paranasal sinus cancers. Treatment results for vestibule lesions should be separated from those of the posterior nasal cavity. The male-to-female ratio for patients with nasal vestibule cancers is 2:1, with average age of 60 to 65 years (range, approximately 40–80 years). The tumor is rare among blacks.

ANATOMY

Maxillary Sinus

Whole-organ sections through the maxillary antrum are shown in Figures 22.1 and 22.2 (62). The maxillary sinuses are single pyramidal cavities in the bodies of the maxillae with average dimensions of 3.7 cm vertically, 2.5 cm transversely, and 3 cm anteroposteriorly, with a volume of about 15 cm^3 in adults. Each sinus has four walls: nasal (medial), orbital (roof), facial (anterolateral), and infratemporal (posterolateral). The base of each pyramid is formed by the nasal wall (lateral wall of the nasal cavity); the apex extends into the zygomatic process of the maxilla. The roof contains the infraorbital canal. Behind the canine region, the medial (lingual) surface of the alveolar process aligns with the lateral wall of the nose while the lateral (buccal) surface of the alveolar process aligns with the facial surface of the maxilla such that the alveolus itself forms the floor of the antrum. The antral floor is usually about 1.25 cm below the floor of the nasal cavity. The roots of the first and second molar teeth, and occasionally other teeth, may project into the floor of the sinus. The nasal wall has one or more openings that communicate with the middle meatus under the middle turbinate; an accessory ostium is frequently present (Fig. 22.3) (62). These openings are nearer the roof than the floor of the sinus. The sinuses drain by mucociliary action. The junction of the orbital and nasal surfaces of the antrum forms the floor of the ethmoid sinus (antroethmoid septum). The posterolateral wall borders the infratemporal and pterygopalatine fossae. The pterygopalatine fossa lies immediately behind the maxilla and serves as a distribution center of nerves and blood vessels to many areas. Viewed in transverse computed tomographic (CT) sections, the posterior wall describes a lazy "S."

The facial or anterior surface is slightly concave and faces anteriorly and laterally. Most of the surface below the infraorbital foramen is palpable through the gingivobuccal sulcus above the premolar teeth, and the portion above the foramen is easily palpated through the skin.

Before it emerges onto the face, the infraorbital nerve gives off an anterior superior alveolar branch that runs in the facial wall of the maxillary sinus to the incisor and canine teeth. The posterosuperior alveolar nerve arises from the maxillary nerve in the pterygopalatine fossa and runs downward and forward to pierce the infratemporal surface of the maxilla then descends under the mucosa of the maxillary sinus.

Ethmoid Sinus

The ethmoid sinuses each consist of a labyrinth of air cells between the medial wall of the orbit and lateral wall of the nasal cavity (Figs. 22.3–22.6) (62). The air cells vary in number and

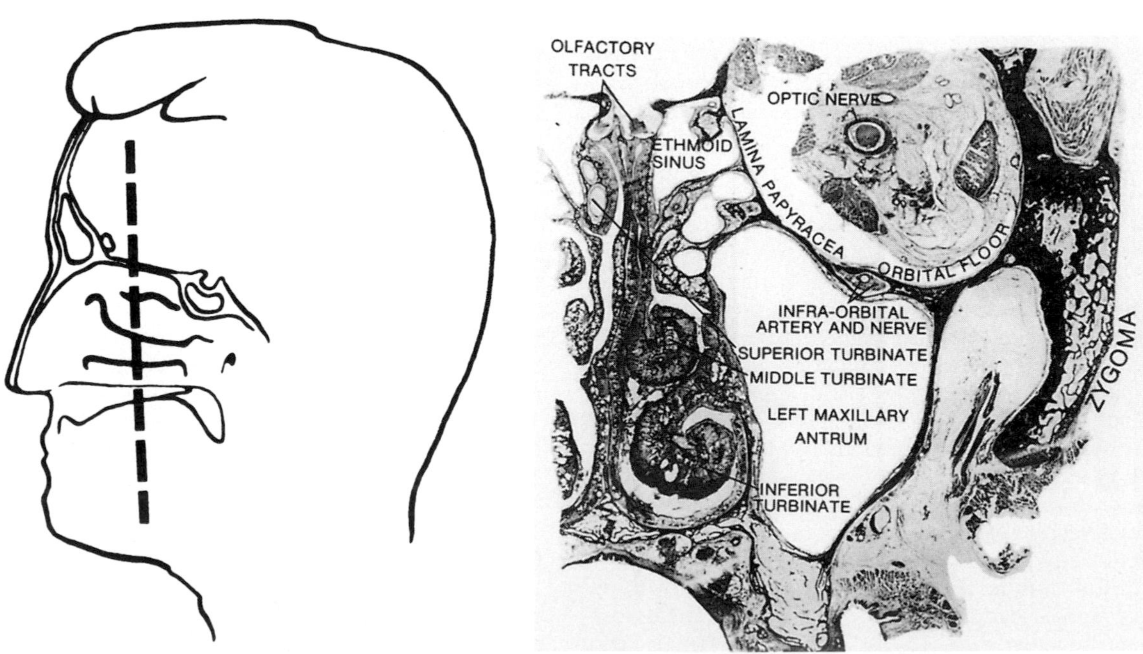

Figure 22.1 Coronal section through the maxillary antrum. Note the thinness of all walls except the hard palate. Lateral to the antrum is the buccinator muscle and fat pad. (Modified from Bridger MWM, van Nostrand AWP. The nose and paranasal sinuses—applied surgical anatomy: a histologic study of whole organ sections in three planes. *J Otolaryngol* 1978;7[Suppl 6]:1–30, with permission.)

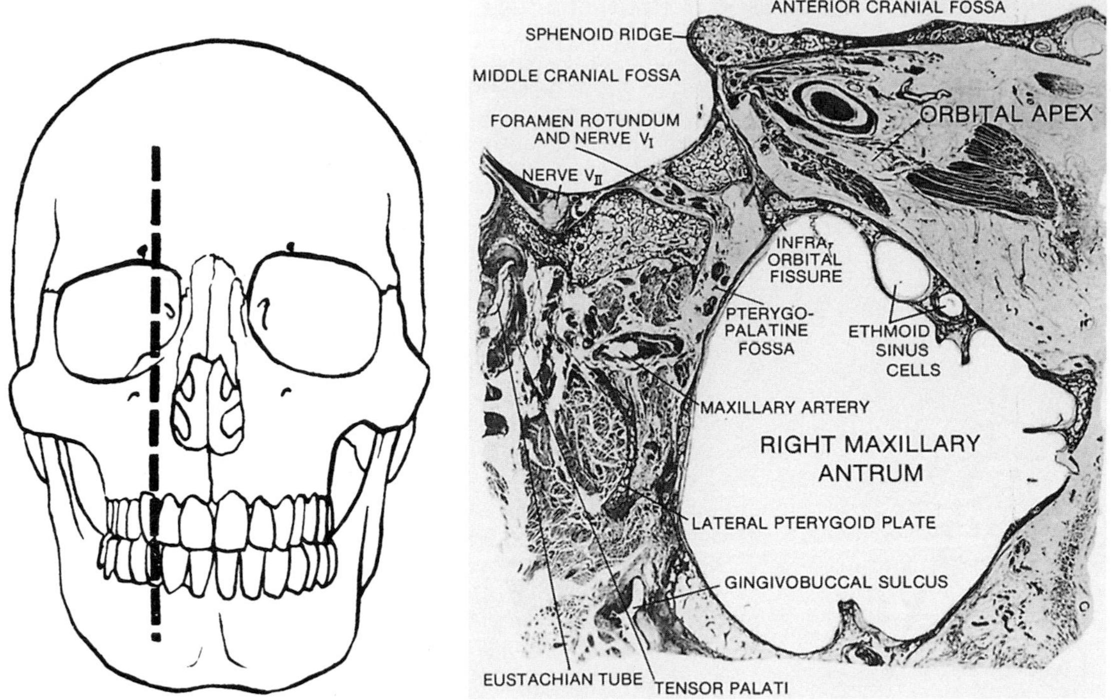

Figure 22.2 Sagittal section through antrum and apex of the orbit. The orbital apex communicates with the pterygopalatine fossa by way of the infraorbital fissure. Extension of antral tumor through the posterior wall provides access to the middle cranial fossa along cranial nerves and vascular foramina. (From Bridger MWM, van Nostrand AWP. The nose and paranasal sinuses—applied surgical anatomy: a histologic study of whole organ sections in three planes. *J Otolaryngol* 1978;7[Suppl 6]:1–30, with permission.)

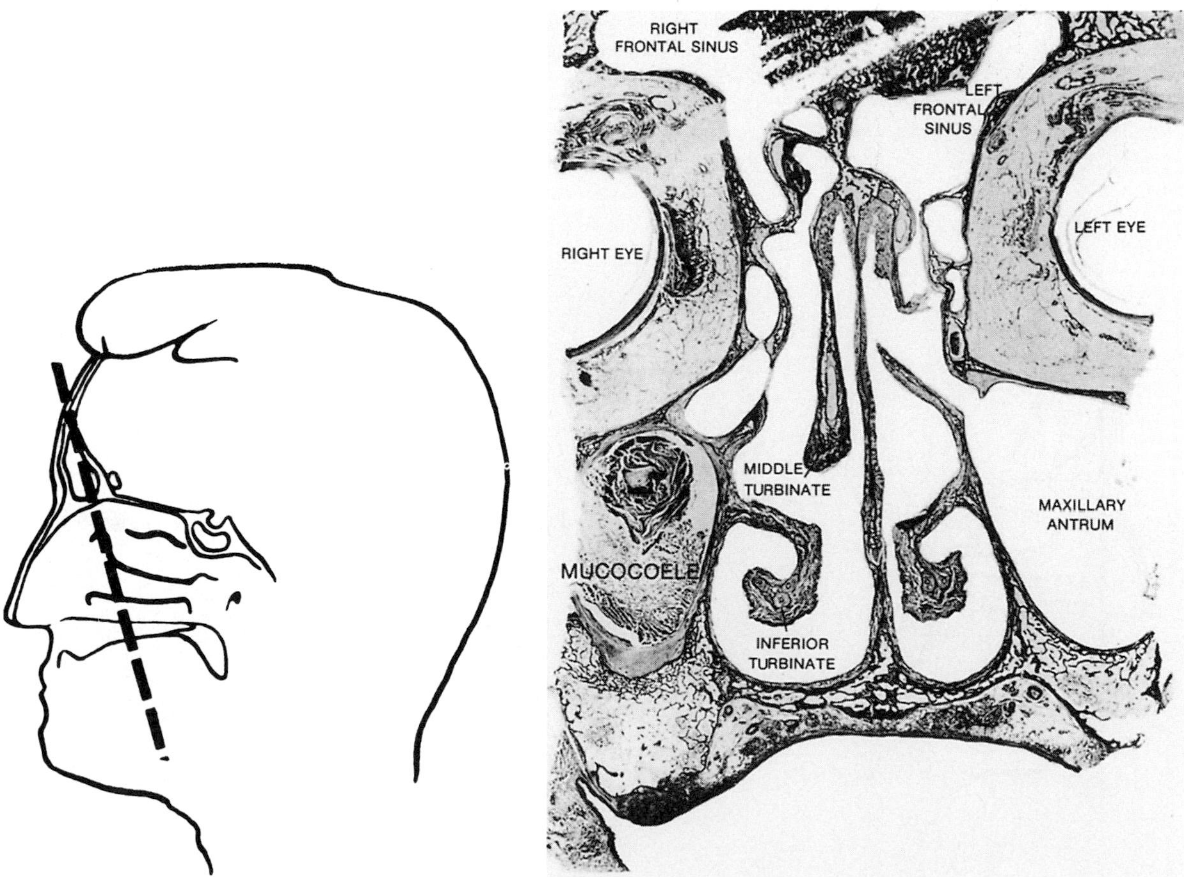

Figure 22.3 Coronal section through frontal sinuses, midnose, and anterior ethmoids. Note left frontonasal duct and ostium of the left maxillary antrum, which open into the middle meatus. The middle turbinate appears to arise from the roof of the nasal cavity near the septum, which is the appearance during physical examination. (From Bridger MWM, van Nostrand AWP. The nose and paranasal sinuses—applied surgical anatomy: a histologic study of whole organ sections in three planes. *J Otolaryngol* 1978; 7[Suppl 6]:1–30, with permission.)

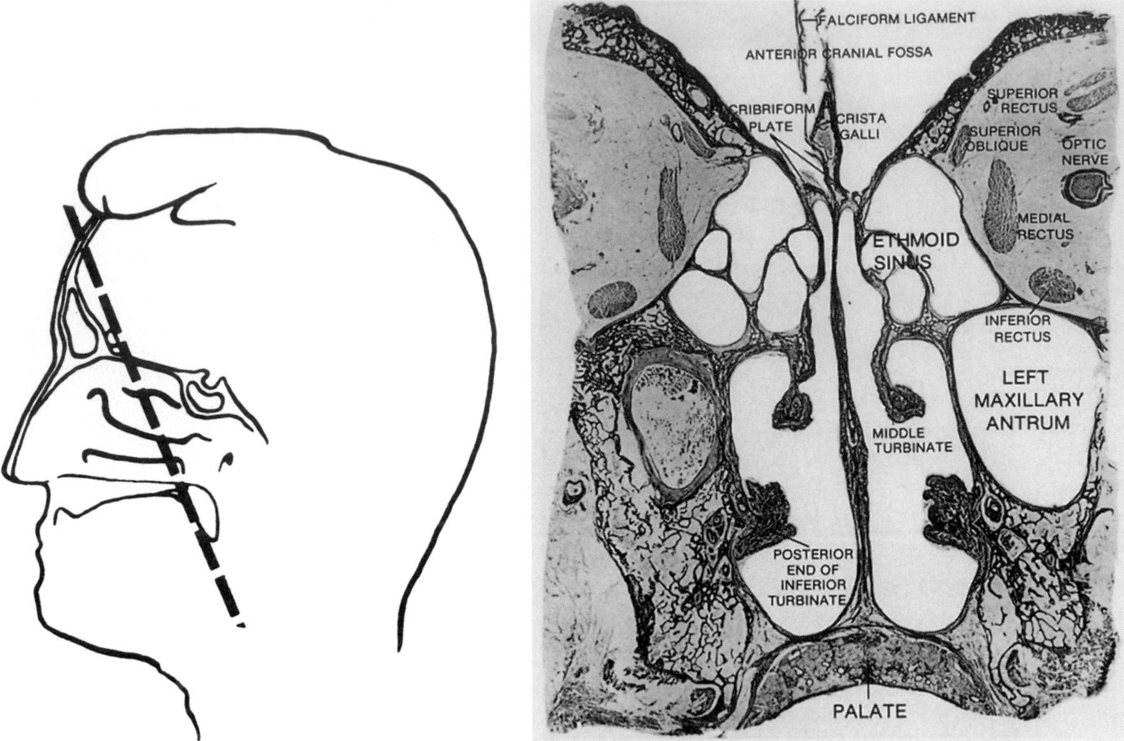

Figure 22.4 Coronal section through the cribriform plate, middle ethmoid sinuses, and posterior inferior turbinates. Note the thinness of the wall separating sinuses from the orbits and nasal cavity. The right and left ethmoid sinuses are completely separated at all levels by the nasal septum and by the narrow superior extension of the nasal cavities. (From Bridger MWM, van Nostrand AWP. The nose and paranasal sinuses—applied surgical anatomy: a histologic study of whole organ sections in three planes. *J Otolaryngol* 1978;7[Suppl 6]:1–30, with permission.)

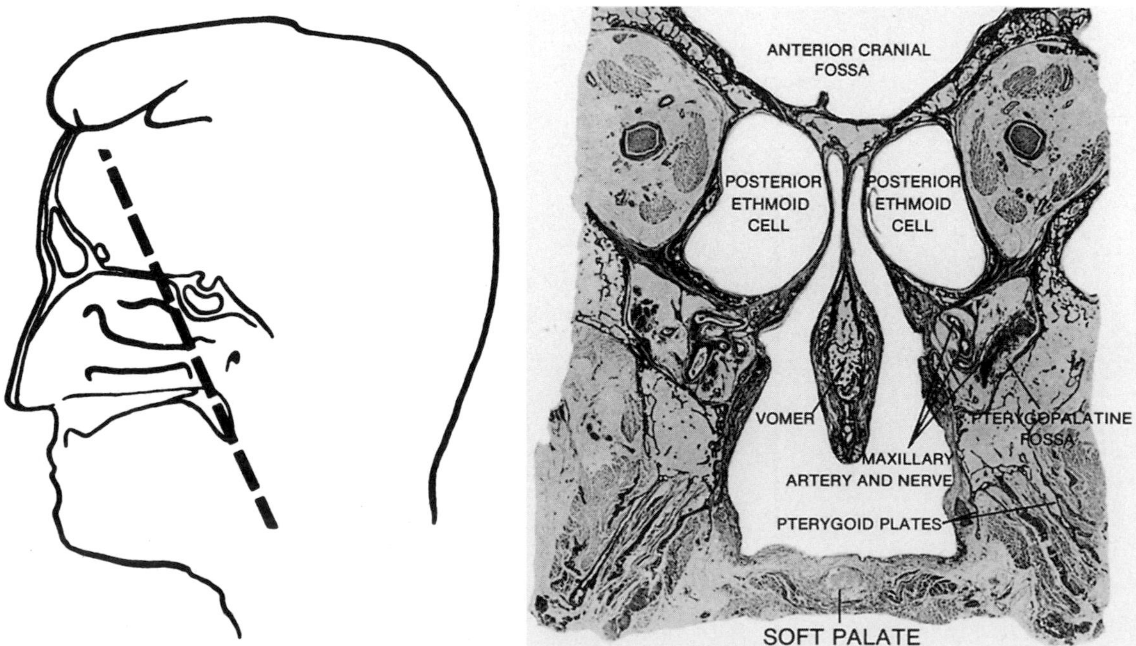

Figure 22.5 Coronal section posterior to the maxillary antrum and anterior to sphenoid sinus and nasopharynx. Note relationships in the pterygopalatine fossa. (Fom Bridger MWM, van Nostrand AWP. The nose and paranasal sinuses in applied surgical anatomy: a histologic study of the whole organ sections in three planes. *J Otolaryngol* 1978;7[Suppl 6]:1–30, with permission.)

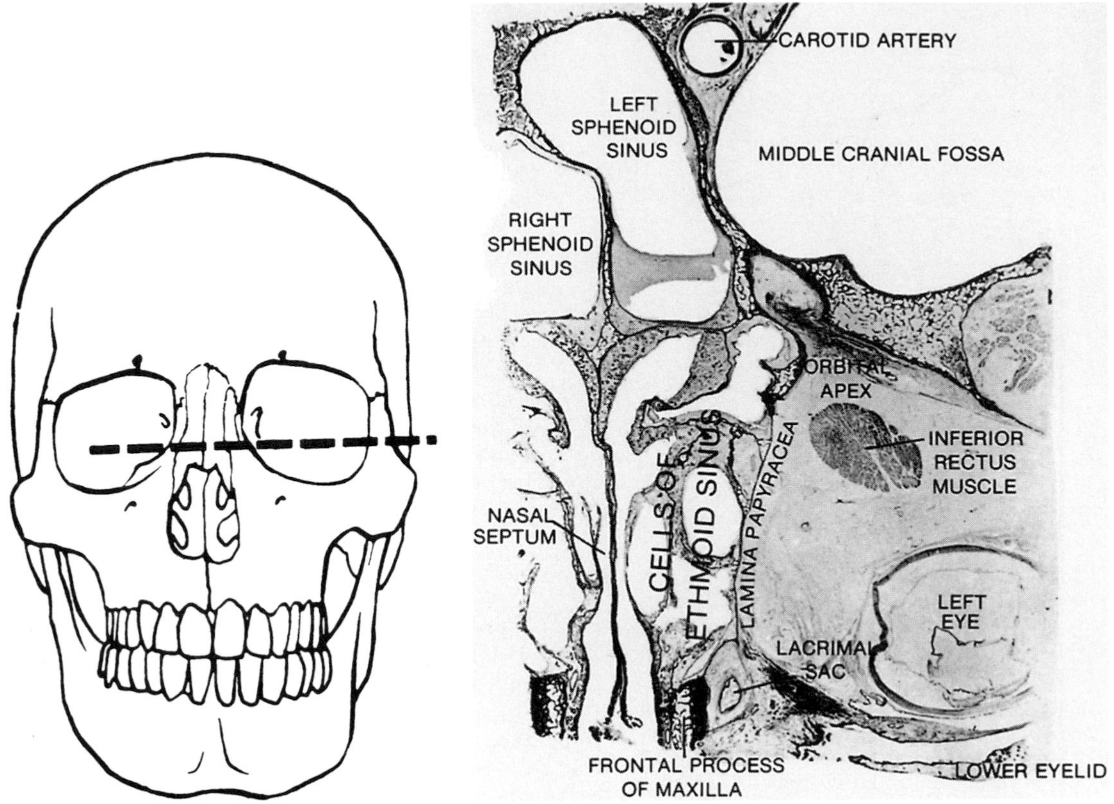

Figure 22.6 Horizontal section through lacrimal sac, orbit, and ethmoid and sphenoid sinuses. The posterior ethmoid cells extend farther laterally than the anterior cells. The sphenoid sinus is in close relationship to the optic nerve and orbital apex. Note the short distance between the anterior ethmoid sinuses and the inner canthus. (From Bridger MWM, van Nostrand AWP. The nose and paranasal sinuses—applied surgical anatomy: a histologic study of whole organ sections in three planes. *J Otolaryngol* 1978; 7[Suppl 6]:1–30, with permission.)

size from 3 large to 18 small sinuses on each side. On each side, they form three groups, anterior, middle, and posterior, which are distinguished from each other on the basis of their sites of communication with the nasal cavity. The sinuses are separated from the orbits by the lamina papyracea, a thin, incomplete porous bone that is easily penetrated by tumor; the orbital periosteum (periorbita) is quite resistant to tumor spread, however (63). The middle ethmoid air cells bulge into the lateral wall of the nasal cavity producing a rounded elevation on the wall of the nasal cavity called the bulla ethmoidalis; the middle ethmoid air cells open anterior and slightly inferior to the bulla via the ethmoid infundibulum and hiatus semilunaris into the middle meatus. The posterior ethmoids are closely related to the optic canal and optic nerve. The ethmoid air cells extend far anteriorly; for this reason, anterior ethmoid lesions may present as a subcutaneous mass in the inner canthus (Fig. 22.6) (62). The anterior cells are covered laterally by the lacrimal bone. The right and left ethmoid sinuses are anatomically separated by the nasal septum (perpendicular plate of the ethmoid) and the narrow cephalic extensions of the nasal cavities themselves. The roof of the ethmoid sinuses relates to the anterior cranial fossa. The portion of frontal bone that comprises the roof of the anterosuperior ethmoid air cells is called the fovea ethmoidalis.

Sphenoid Sinus

The sphenoid sinus is a midline structure in the body of the sphenoid bone. It is in close proximity to the dura, pituitary gland, optic nerves and chiasm, cavernous sinuses, internal carotid arteries, cranial nerves III, IV, V1, V2, and VI, and pterygoid canal and nerve. The clivus and brainstem are posterior. Pneumatization of the sinus varies widely and can extend into all portions of the sphenoid bone. Clival mineralization and fat content also vary considerably. If the sphenoid bone is extensively pneumatized, the sinus may partially surround the optic nerve, carotid artery, and maxillary and vidian nerves. The sinus frequently extends into the roots of the pterygoid processes or even the greater wings of the sphenoid. Although separated by a thin septum, the right and left sides are considered as one in treatment planning; the sides are frequently asymmetric. Occasionally, the bony walls have gaps, and the mucus membrane may lie directly against the dura. The posterior ethmoid air cells may extend into the body of the sphenoid bone and largely replace the sphenoid sinus. Each sinus connects with the nasal cavity in the sphenoethmoid recess via an aperture in the upper part of its anterior wall (Fig. 22.7) (62).

Frontal Sinus

The frontal sinuses are two irregular, usually asymmetric, air cavities separated by a thin, bony septum lying between the outer and inner tables of the frontal bone. They connect to the middle meatus of the nasal cavity by either the frontonasal recess (Fig. 22.3) (62) or ethmoid infundibulum. Frontal sinus air cells may extend far laterally in the orbital process of the frontal bone. They are separated from the anterior ethmoid cells by thin bony walls. The posterior wall, separating the frontal sinus from the anterior cranial fossa, is thick in most patients.

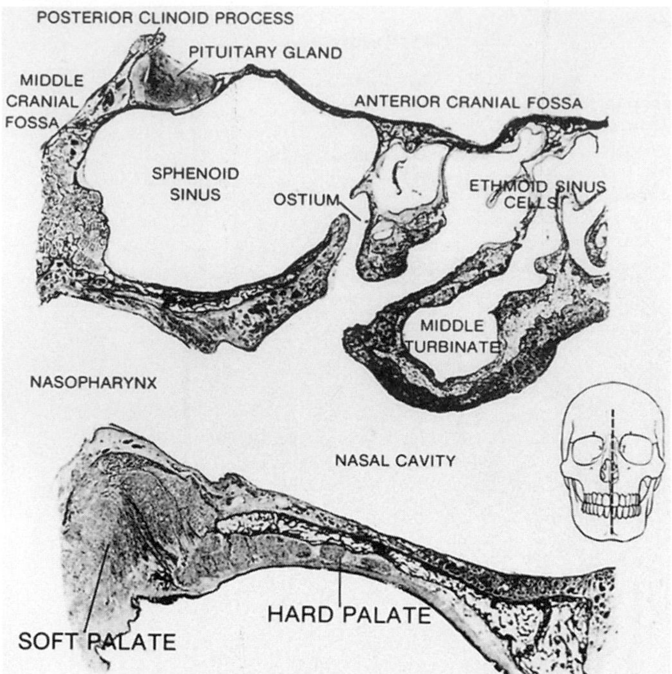

Figure 22.7 Sagittal section through nasopharynx and sphenoid sinus, just left of midline. Note relationship of sphenoid sinus ostium to nasopharynx and posterior nasal cavity. The anterior wall of the sphenoid sinus and the floor of the sella are thin bone. (From Bridger MWM, van Nostrand AWP. The nose and paranasal sinuses—applied surgical anatomy: a histologic study of whole organ sections in three planes. *J Otolaryngol* 1978;7[Suppl 6]:1–30, with permission.)

Nasal Cavity

The nasal cavity begins at the limen nasi (transition from skin to mucosa) and ends at the posterior nasal apertures or choanae, immediately above the posterior border of the hard palate. The choanae are framed laterally by the medial pterygoid plates and superiorly by the base of skull. The posterior choanae communicate directly with the nasopharynx; each aperture is about 2.5 cm high and 1.25 cm wide. The nasal cavity extends from the hard palate inferiorly to the base of skull superiorly and is divided into right and left halves by a midline septum. The composition of the septum and bones and cartilages that compose the roof and sides of the external nose are shown in Figure 22.8 (64). The vomer extends from the undersurface of the body of the sphenoid and forms the lower and posterior septum. The perpendicular plate of the ethmoid forms the upper and anterior septum and is continuous above with the cribriform plate; it is thin and offers little barrier to tumor spread. The septum is often deflected to one side, with deflection most often occurring along the lines joining the vomer with the perpendicular plate of the ethmoid. The septal cartilage forms the majority of the anterior nasal septum.

Whole-organ sections of the nasal cavity and adjacent sinuses are shown in Figures 22.3 through 22.6 (62). Each lateral wall is composed of thin bony folds that project into the nasal cavity. These are the inferior, middle, and superior nasal conchae (turbinates). Each turbinate forms the roof of a passage or meatus which communicates freely with the nasal cavity. The nasolacrimal duct enters the nasal cavity via the inferior meatus. The frontal sinus and anterior and middle ethmoid air cells connect to the nasal cavity via the middle meatus. The superior meatus is short and shallow. It receives the opening of the pos-

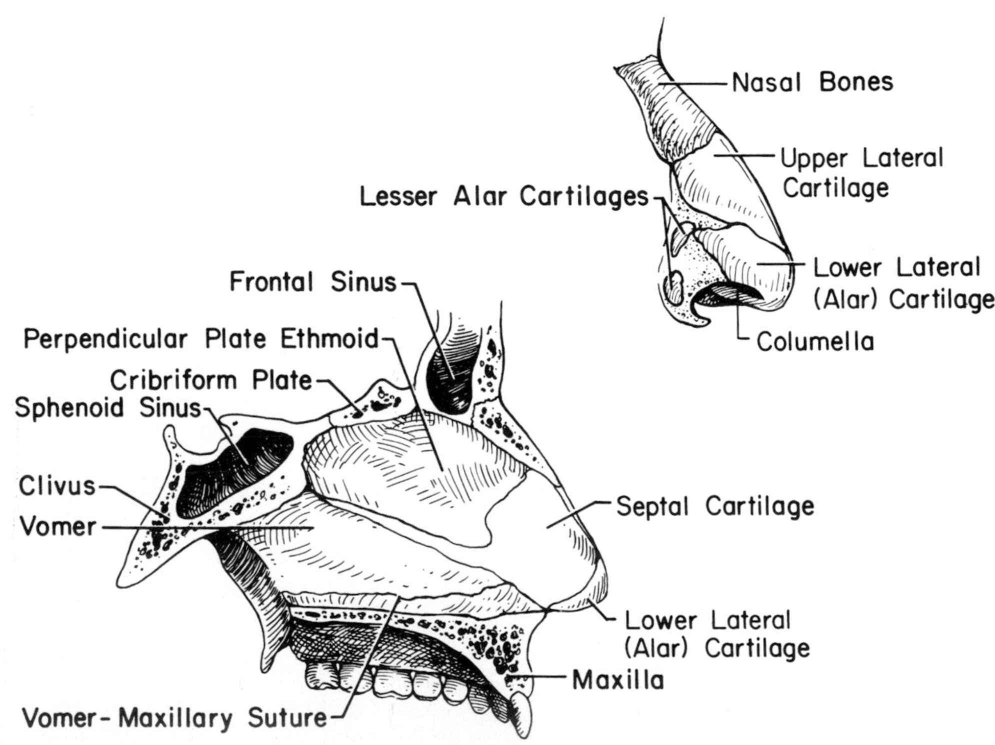

Figure 22.8 Relationship of bones and cartilages of the nose. (From Million RR, Cassisi NJ, Wittes RE. Cancer in the head and neck. In: DeVita VT Jr, Hellman S, Rosenberg SA, eds. *Cancer: principles and practice of oncology*, 2nd ed. Philadelphia: JB Lippincott Co, 1985:407–506, with permission.)

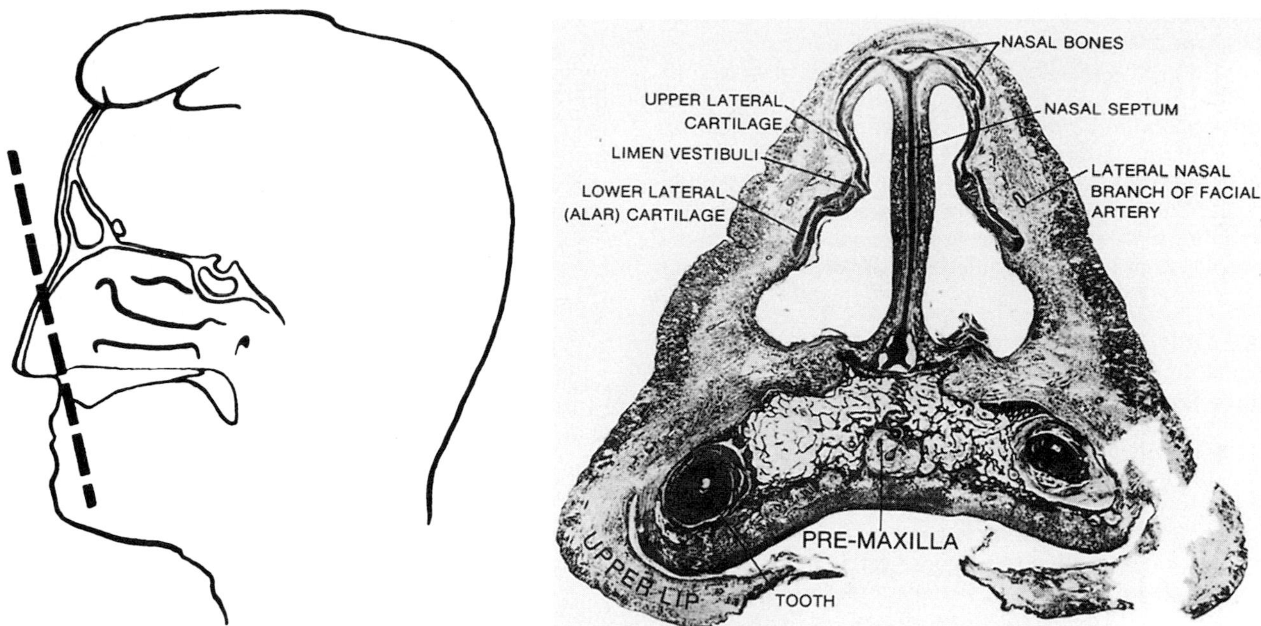

Figure 22.9 Coronal whole-organ section through the vestibule. The upper lateral alar cartilages fuse with the cartilaginous septum. The nasal bones overlap the upper and lower cartilages. The limen vestibuli is the junction of the upper and lower lateral cartilages. (From Bridger MWM, van Nostrand AWP. The nose and paranasal sinuses—applied surgical anatomy: a histologic study of whole organ sections in three planes. *J Otolaryngol* 1978;7[Suppl 6]:1–30, with permission.)

terior ethmoid air cells. Immediately behind the superior meatus, the sphenopalatine foramen (which opens into the pterygopalatine fossa) pierces the lateral wall of the nasal cavity. The pterygopalatine fossa lies just inferior to the inferior orbital fissure, and the infraorbital nerve lies just superior to the fossa as it enters the foramen rotundum. The inferior orbital fissure is immediately contiguous to the superior orbital fissure and middle cranial fossa. The sphenoid sinus opens into the nasal cavity through an opening in the anterior wall of the sinus (Fig. 22.7) (62).

The olfactory nerves enter the nasal cavity through its roof (the cribriform plate of the ethmoid bone) and distribute nerve fibers over the upper third of the septum and superior nasal turbinate. The cribriform plate is slightly caudad to the roof of the ethmoid sinuses; the external landmark for the cribriform plate is the medial canthal ligament. About 20 branches of the olfactory nerve penetrate the cribriform plate, providing an avenue for tumor spread to the anterior cranial fossa (Fig. 22.4) (62). In addition to these foramina, the roof presents a separate foramen, situated anteriorly, for passage of the anterior ethmoid nerves and vessels. More posteriorly, the foramen for the posterior ethmoid artery lies 5 to 7 mm from the optic canal. The olfactory region of the nasal cavity is limited to the superior nasal concha, upper 10 mm of the septum, and nasal roof. The respiratory region comprises the rest of the cavity. The olfactory epithelium is tall, pseudostratified, and columnar with highly specialized cilia. The respiratory epithelium is ciliated columnar. Normally, the mucosal cilia sweep the mucous blanket posteriorly at a rate of 6 to 7 mm per minute into the pharynx; mucociliary clearance rates are markedly reduced after RT (65). Numerous collections of lymphoid tissue and mucous glands exist beneath the epithelium.

Nasal Vestibule

The nasal vestibule is the entrance to the nasal cavity. It is lined by skin having numerous hair follicles and sebaceous and sweat glands. Each vestibule is a three-sided, pear-shaped cavity 1.5 to 2.0 cm in diameter, bounded laterally by the ala nasi and medially by the lower portion of the cartilaginous septum, the membranous septum, and the columella. The vestibule ends posteriorly at the limen nasi, the junction of the lower and upper lateral cartilages (Figs. 22.8, 22.9) (62,64). The floor of the nasal vestibule is approximately 1 cm in length.

ANATOMY: LYMPHATICS

Nasal Cavity and Paranasal Sinuses

The lymphatics of the nasal cavity are separated into olfactory and respiratory groups. According to Rouviere (66), they do not communicate with each other. The lymphatic network of the olfactory region is connected with the subarachnoid space, which allows some absorption of cerebrospinal fluid by the lymphatics. The importance of this connection is uncertain. The lymphatics of the olfactory region run posteriorly to terminate in lymph nodes medial to the carotid artery at the C1-C2 level (i.e., retropharyngeal lymph node). The lymphatics of the respiratory region run posteriorly to terminate a bit lower, either in a junctional, subdigastric, or submandibular lymph node.

Knowledge of the lymphatics of the paranasal sinuses is imperfect (66); the lymphatics are rather sparse. Metastases from carcinoma of the paranasal sinuses are relatively uncommon in comparison with other head and neck mucosal sites, even though lesions are frequently advanced. It is almost unheard of for a patient with an occult paranasal sinus tumor to present with cervical lymphadenopathy.

Nasal Vestibule

The lymphatic trunks run mainly to the submandibular lymph nodes. A small risk for involvement of facial nodes exists, especially those just behind the commissure of the lip in the cheek (buccinator nodes) and those at the crossing of the facial vessels over the mandible (mandibular nodes). The buccinator nodes are located in the thickness of the cheek at the level of, or slightly above, a line drawn from the lip commissure to the base of the auricle. The mandibular nodes are located on the external surface of the mandible in front of the masseter muscle near the crossing of the facial vessels over the mid-body of the mandible. Preauricular lymph nodes are rarely involved. Drainage is ipsilateral but may be bilateral, particularly when the tumor invades the columella, floor of the vestibule, and adjacent upper lip (67).

PATHOLOGY

Maxillary Sinus

Squamous cell carcinoma accounts for 65% to 75% of malignant tumors of the maxillary sinus. The remaining 25% to 35% are minor salivary gland (adenoid cystic, adenocarcinoma, mucoepidermoid, or malignant mixed carcinomas) or undifferentiated carcinoma; adenosquamous carcinoma is rarely reported. Malignant lymphoma, malignant melanoma, and sarcoma are also seen. The maxillary sinus may also be the site of renal cell or other metastases.

Ethmoid Sinus

The common histologies in the ethmoid sinus are squamous cell carcinoma, adenocarcinoma, undifferentiated carcinoma, and adenoid cystic carcinoma. Most adenocarcinomas relate to occupational exposure.

Sphenoid Sinus

Most neoplasms of the sphenoid sinus are malignant. There is a slight predominance of metastatic tumors (usually from breast, kidney, or prostate) over primary lesions. The most common primary malignancies are squamous cell carcinomas, followed by minor salivary gland tumors, lymphoreticular malignancy (lymphoma or plasmacytoma), primary sarcoma (chondrosarcoma being the most common), and very rarely, malignant melanoma (1,68,69).

Frontal Sinus

In the frontal sinus, squamous cell carcinoma outnumbers adenocarcinoma by approximately 20:1 (24).

Nasal Cavity

Approximately 55% to 65% of nasal cavity tumors in the United States are squamous cell carcinoma, 30% are adenocarcinoma or other glandular type, and a few percent each are anaplastic, malignant melanoma, or esthesioneuroblastoma (25,27).

Esthesioneuroblastoma (Olfactory Neuroblastoma)

Esthesioneuroblastoma is a malignant tumor of the superior nasal cavity. It is derived from neuroectodermal cells of the olfactory epithelium and constitutes 3% of all intranasal neoplasms. A neural derivation is indicated ultrastructurally by dense core neurosecretory granules and neuritic processes within tumor cells. Immunohistochemically it is indicated by expression of neurofilament protein, neuron-specific enolase, and S-100 protein. Although morphologically similar to neuroblastoma, the tumor is believed to have more in common with primitive neuroectodermal tumors. Esthesioneuroblastoma has a different clinical presentation than neuroblastoma, rarely occurs in early childhood, rarely is associated with catecholamine secretion, and does not share the N-myc amplification characteristic of neuroblastoma (70). On light microscopy, it may be confused with lymphoma, extramedullary plasmacytoma, undifferentiated carcinoma, malignant melanoma, and rhabdomyosarcoma.

Hyams et al. (71), in a review of cases at the Armed Forces Institute of Pathology, developed a pathologic system classifying esthesioneuroblastomas into four grades. Seventy percent (36 of 51) of patients had low-grade tumors (grade 1–2), and 30% were high-grade (grade 3–4). Reported cure rates exceeded 80% for low-grade tumors compared with 33% for high-grade disease. Few other investigators (37,72–74) have evaluated treatment results according to Hyams grade. Although Levine et al. (72) concluded that the grading system did not correlate with clinical outcome in the University of Virginia series, their data suggest otherwise: of 20 grade 1 to 2 tumors, 7 (35%) relapsed, compared with 4 of 5 (80%) grade 3 tumors (the authors had no grade 4 tumors, preferring instead to group them with sinonasal undifferentiated carcinoma). In the Mayo Clinic series, Foote et al. (73) note that the only significant predictor for 5-year overall survival (81% for low-grade vs. 36% for high-grade, $p < 0.0001$); disease-free survival (61% vs. 25%, $p = 0.0008$); and 5-year local relapse-free survival (73% vs. 38%, $p = 0.0026$) was Hyams grade. Analysis of patients from the University of Cincinnati (37) produced identical findings: 3 of 4 patients (75%) with high-grade tumors died of their disease versus 1 of 7 (14%) with low-grade disease. Eriksen et al. (74) note similar findings: low-grade, 5-year survival and continuous disease-free survival, both 80%; high-grade, 12%, 5-year survival and 17% continuous disease-free survival. Cure is rare in grade 4 tumors (37,71). Of 149 total patients included in the aforementioned series, 103 (69%) had low-grade disease and 46 (31%) had high-grade disease. High-grade tumors were noted to have generally shorter duration of symptoms, higher stage disease at diagnosis, higher rates of all types of failure, shorter disease-free intervals, and more tumor-related deaths than low-grade tumors. Confusion and overlap still exist between Hyams grade 4 tumors and sinonasal undifferentiated carcinomas (37,72).

Sinonasal Undifferentiated Carcinoma

Sinonasal undifferentiated carcinoma (SNUC) is a rare and aggressive malignancy that was first recognized as a separate pathological entity in 1986 (40). The tumor is composed of medium-sized polygonal cells arranged mainly in nests and sheets with oval nuclei showing moderate pleomorphism and large nucleoli, brisk mitotic activity, prominent necrosis, vascular space invasion, frequent perineural involvement, and positive immunocytochemical staining for cytokeratin and epithelial membrane antigen. S-100, leukocyte common antigen and tests for desmin, and antihuman melanoma antibody-45 are negative (75). As therapy differs, it is essential not to confuse SNUC with esthesioneuroblastoma. Esthesioneuroblastoma, unlike SNUC, is typically composed of small cells with sparse cytoplasm and a small round nucleus without a large nucleolus. Immunohistochemical tests further help to differentiate the tumors (75). Nucleoli are prominent and chromatin is coarse in contrast to the more bland-appearing olfactory neuroblastoma (38). Yet another distinct entity, sinonasal neuroendocrine carcinoma (SNEC) has been described and further complicates an already confusing array of disease types (38). Poorly differentiated sinonasal, esthesioneuroblastoma and small cell carcinomas may be difficult to separate histologically.

Inverting Papilloma

The histologic picture of an inverting papilloma is that of a proliferating epithelium inverting into the underlying stroma rather than growing outward from the surface. Rarely the papilloma may be composed almost entirely of cylindrical cells (76). Cylindrical cell papilloma and inverting papilloma have similar biologic behavior, although the former involves paranasal sinuses more often than the latter. Inverting papilloma is a true epithelial neoplasm rather than simply an inflammatory or hyperplastic process (77–80). In approximately 10% (7% at initial diagnosis, and 3% subsequently) of cases, squamous cell carcinoma occurs in association with inverting papilloma (48,57,81,82). The squamous cell carcinoma may be invasive or *in situ*. In patients who develop a metachronous squamous cell carcinoma, the average time to occurrence of the malignancy is approximately 5 years (48,81). The occurrence of metachronous squamous cell carcinoma in these patients is part of the natural history of the disease; there are no data to suggest that the administration of RT increases the risk above the baseline incidence (54,82).

Lethal Midline Granuloma

Lethal midline granuloma is an ambiguous clinical term used to describe a neoplasm leading to progressive destruction of the midface. It is a true neoplasm, with a progressive, disseminated, and fatal course. Other diseases producing a similar clinical picture must be excluded, including infectious diseases, collagen-vascular diseases, Wegner granulomatosis, and other lymphoid and nonlymphoid neoplasms. Polymorphic reticulosis, malignant granuloma, midline malignant reticulosis, lymphomatoid granulomatosis, midline granuloma, nonhealing granuloma, and other terms have been used to describe the same process and are a source of considerable confusion. Recently, it has been generally accepted that most cases of so-called lethal midline granuloma are T-cell lymphomas, and that the tumor cells often express the NK-cell marker CD56. Histologically, the CD56-positive lymphoma cells exhibit a broad morphologic spectrum with frequent angiocentricity (preferential concentration of tumor cells around and within blood vessels, with infiltration and destruction of the blood vessel wall) and necrosis. The tumor has a characteristic immunophenotypic profile (83). The Epstein-Barr viral genome is present in almost all cases. Histologic diagnosis may be difficult because of extensive tissue necrosis, as well as admixtures of reactive inflammatory cells, often requiring multiple deep biopsies (83–85). Nasal NK/T-cell lymphomas are somewhat more common than nasal lymphomas of T-cell or B-cell (usually diffuse, large-cell lymphomas) immunophenotype and are associated with higher relapse rates and lower survival rates (58,60). Although most NK/T-cell CD56-positive lymphomas arise in the nasal cavity, they have also been described outside of the aerodigestive tract in the skin, testis, muscle, gastrointestinal tract, spleen, and liver (84).

Malignant Melanoma

Approximately three fourths of sinonasal malignant melanomas originate in the nasal cavity, followed in order of frequency by the maxillary sinus, ethmoid sinus, and frontal sinus. Primary involvement of the sphenoid sinus is rare (68,69,86). The anterior nasal septum is the most frequent site of origin. Satellitosis and multicentricity are less frequently noted than in cutaneous melanoma (46,87). Preexisting melanosis or pigmented lesions are usually not found. The tumor may be heavily pigmented (brown-black) or achromatic (pink-tan). Histologically, over two thirds of the lesions manifest readily identifiable melanin. In some cases, Fontana and other stains will identify pigment, whereas in other instances, fine-structural study is necessary to demonstrate premelanosomes. When melanin is sparse, diagnostic mistakes may occur. An immunohistochemical profile of positive staining with anti–S-100 protein, HMB-45, and antivimentin confirms the hematoxylin-eosin impression. Mitoses are frequent (42,88).

PATTERNS OF SPREAD

Maxillary Sinus

The pattern of spread is largely dependent on the site of origin within the sinus. Lesions of the anterolateral infrastructure tend to invade the lateral inferior wall and present in the oral cavity, where tumor erodes through the maxillary gingiva or gingivobuccal sulcus. Tumor is at first submucosal, causing elevation of the mucosa, loosening of teeth, or improper fitting of a denture. Ulceration may lead to development of an oral–antral fistula.

Lesions arising on the medial infrastructure readily extend to the nasal cavity. Lesions of the posterior infrastructure erode the posterolateral wall to enter the infratemporal fossa, or invade directly posterior to the pterygopalatine fossa and pterygoid plates. Pterygopalatine fossa involvement greatly reduces the likelihood of cure. Cancer in the fossa has access to the middle cranial fossa through the foramen rotundum; the foramen lacerum through the pterygoid canal; the nasopharynx through the sphenopalatine foramen; the infratemporal fossa through the pterygomaxillary fissure; and the orbital apex through the inferior orbital fissure (Fig. 22.2) (62,89).

Tumor extending to the retroantral fat may involve the pterygoid muscle or the temporalis muscle insertion on the coronoid process. Extension to the orbit may occur through the roof of the maxillary sinus, the ethmoid sinus, or the pterygopalatine fossa and inferior orbital fissure.

Tumors of the suprastructure may grow laterally and invade the malar process of the maxilla and zygomatic bone, producing a mass below the lateral floor of the orbit. The mass may ulcerate, producing an antrocutaneous fistula. The orbit is invaded laterally, displacing the eye inward and upward. The temporal fossa and zygomatic arch are involved in advanced lesions.

Alternatively, suprastructure cancers may grow medially into the nasal cavity, ethmoid sinus, frontal sinus, lacrimal apparatus, and medial inferior orbit. Tumors involving the roof of the antrum may extend perineurally along the infraorbital nerve, through the inferior orbital fissure, across the upper pterygopalatine fossa, and then into the middle cranial fossa through the foramen rotundum.

The incidence of lymph node metastases at diagnosis is 10% to 20% in maxillary sinus squamous cell carcinoma (9,11,90–96) and metastases subsequently may evolve in another 10% to 20%. Lymph node metastases are rare in patients with T1 to T2 disease (96). Patients with lymph node relapse are rarely cured and have a high rate of distant metastasis (96). Lymph node metastasis occurs in 5% of patients with adenoid cystic carcinoma of the antrum. The rate of distant metastasis in all patients with maxillary sinus carcinoma is approximately 15% to 25% (9,91–93,96).

Ethmoid Sinus

Tumor confined to the ethmoid sinus without involvement of surrounding structures is rare (14,15,97). In the M. D. Anderson

Cancer Center series (14), tumor extended to the ipsilateral nasal cavity in 76% of patients; maxillary sinus in 56%; orbit, 53%; sphenoid sinus, 35%; anterior cranial fossa, 32%; frontal sinus, 18%; and nasopharynx, 12%. Surprisingly, involvement of the contralateral ethmoid sinus was rather unusual, reported in only 12% of patients. The relative infrequency of contralateral ethmoid involvement has also been noted by others (18,63,97). Invasion of tumor through the cribriform plate and ethmoid roof is common; in most instances, the dura is compressed but not involved (63). Bony destruction without dural invasion does not carry a particularly poor prognosis, whereas histologically proven dural invasion is a poor prognostic factor (14,97).

The incidence of lymph node metastases in patients with ethmoid sinus carcinoma is substantially less than in maxillary sinus cancer. In the series from M. D. Anderson Cancer Center, only 1 of 34 patients (3%) presented with lymph node metastases (14). In the series from Princess Margaret Hospital, the incidence was 2 of 29 (7%) (15). In a series by Tiwari et al., no patients (out of a total of 50) presented with lymph node metastases (17). Approximately 10% of patients subsequently develop lymph node metastases when the lymph nodes are not electively treated (14).

Distant spread in the absence of locoregional failure is rare (<5%) (14,15).

Sphenoid Sinus

Sphenoid sinus primary malignancies almost always show signs of bone destruction. Cavernous sinus extension and intracranial spread to the anterior or middle cranial fossae are frequent, as are extensions to the ethmoid sinuses (63%), clivus (52%), sella turcica (48%), nasal cavity (48%), nasopharynx (44%), and orbit (22%) (1).

Frontal Sinus

Bony destruction is usually present. Tumor extension into the anterior ethmoids, orbit, subcutaneous tissues of the forehead, and anterior cranial fossa is common.

Nasal Cavity

The routes of spread are essentially the same for the various histologic types with the exception that minor salivary gland tumors have a greater propensity for perineural spread and esthesioneuroblastoma is more inclined to intracranial spread.

Nasal cavity tumors may destroy the septum and may invade through the nasal bone to the skin. Lesions involving the lateral wall of the nasal cavity invade the medial wall of the maxillary sinus, ethmoid sinus, pterygomaxillary fossa, and orbit.

The incidence of regional lymphatic metastases on admission from nasal cavity carcinomas is less than 5%. Another 5% of patients develop lymph node metastases later in the disease course when the neck is not electively treated (25,98,99).

Approximately 10% of patients with nasal cavity carcinomas develop distant metastases. The incidence is higher in patients with malignant melanoma or undifferentiated carcinoma.

ESTHESIONEUROBLASTOMAS

Esthesioneuroblastomas invade the ethmoid sinuses, orbit, anterior cranial fossa, and fairly commonly the frontal lobe of the brain (100–103). Intracranial spread of esthesioneuroblastomas was noted at presentation in 17 (35%) of 49 previously untreated Mayo Clinic patients and occurred at some time during the disease course in 26 patients (53%) (104). Central nervous system (CNS) extension through the olfactory nerves without dural involvement is sometimes noted (34,105). Occasionally patients present with massive intracranial or brain involvement and minimal nasal cavity or paranasal sinus disease, simulating a primary intracranial neoplasm (105). Spread into the cerebrospinal fluid may lead to dissemination of esthesioneuroblastoma throughout the craniospinal axis (106,107).

Clinical evidence of lymph node metastasis is present in 5% to 15% of patients with esthesioneuroblastoma at initial presentation (35,104,108), and as many as 20% to 30% eventually develop cervical lymph node metastasis as a component of disease failure at some time during the disease course (35,73, 109–111). Most lymph node metastases are to the submandibular or jugulodigastric area, but parotid area lymph node metastases have been reported by several authors. Ten percent of patients with clinically negative necks whose primary site remains continuously disease-free after treatment subsequently develop lymph node metastasis (109). Distant metastasis (most commonly to bone and lung) occurs as a solitary event in 10% of patients (36,112,113) and as a component of multi-site recurrence in an additional 15% to 20% of patients.

SINONASAL UNDIFFERENTIATED CARCINOMA

Sinonasal undifferentiated carcinoma (SNUC) demonstrates rapid growth; affected patients typically present with advanced disease. Tumor usually involves the nasal cavity and multiple sinuses. Orbital invasion occurs in two-thirds of patients (39–41, 75) and invasion of the anterior cranial fossa in 40% at diagnosis (39–41,75). In collected series (38–41,75) approximately 20% of patients present with lymph node metastasis. The occurrence of distant metastasis at diagnosis or shortly thereafter is common.

MALIGNANT MELANOMA

Most melanomas arise in the nasal cavity. Those that arise in the paranasal sinuses tend to be relatively advanced at diagnosis. Spread occurs by the same routes as squamous cell carcinoma. The incidence of regional lymph node metastases on admission is approximately 5% to 15% (88); approximately 30% to 40% of patients develop lymph node metastases at some time during the disease course (43,44,87). The submandibular lymph nodes are most commonly involved.

INVERTED PAPILLOMA

Inverted papilloma of the nasal cavity and paranasal sinuses is a relatively rare lesion that usually (96%) (48) arises from the lateral wall of the nasal cavity in the area of the middle meatus and middle turbinate. Approximately 10% to 15% of tumors do not extend beyond the nasal cavity (114). Bone erosion (by pressure) and extension to the paranasal sinuses are common. Spread to the orbit and anterior skull base is less common. Orbital involvement is rare even in recurrent cases; the presence of associated squamous cell carcinoma increases the risk (57, 115). The anatomic distribution in 112 patients who underwent surgical resection at Mt. Sinai Medical Center (48) was as follows: nasal cavity, 100%; ethmoid sinus, 57%; maxillary sinus, 50%; sphenoid sinus, 10%; frontal sinus, 6%; cribriform plate, 5%; nasopharynx, 5%; and intracranial, 2%; no tumors were bilateral. A small percentage of cases arise in the sinuses without nasal cavity involvement (114), and occasionally tumors arise from the nasal septum (48) or occur bilaterally (114,116).

LETHAL MIDLINE GRANULOMA

Twenty percent of patients have disseminated (stage III or IV) disease at diagnosis. Some 10% to 15% of patients present with regional lymphadenopathy (59,61), and another 10% with clinically negative necks develop regional lymph node failure when the lymphatics are not electively treated (61). Twenty-five percent of patients with initially localized disease develop systemic relapse (61), most often involving skin (subcutaneous nodules with or without ulceration), testis, lung, bone, soft tissue, distant lymph nodes, or gastrointestinal tract (59,83).

Nasal Vestibule

Early lesions often present as superficial ulcerations of the membranous septum or columella with physical findings limited to a crust or scab and possibly mild tenderness. More advanced lesions perforate the membranous or cartilaginous septum or invade the alar cartilage and grow through to the skin surface. The upper lip and columella are frequently invaded. Posterior growth into the nasal cavity occurs late or after recurrence. Advanced lesions grow into the gingivolabial sulcus and adhere to or invade the premaxilla. Nasal vestibule carcinomas are often deceptive and more extensive than perceived, an observation confirmed by the numerous patients seen with positive margins or recurrence after attempted local excision.

Lymph node spread from nasal vestibule cancer is usually to a solitary ipsilateral submandibular node, but may be bilateral. The facial nodes are also at risk. The buccinator nodes are best detected by bimanual (simultaneous intraoral and extraoral) palpation of the cheek; the mandibular nodes are located in the subcutaneous tissues in front of the anterior facial vein. Parotid and submental lymph nodes are at low risk of involvement. Lymph node involvement is most likely in patients with extension to the floor of the vestibule, base of the columella or upper lip, and in patients with recurrent local disease. Inflammatory (reddened) changes may signify dermal lymphatic involvement, placing the patient at high risk for lymph node involvement. Lymph node metastases are noted on admission in about 5% of patients (117–119) and subsequently in another 15% when the lymphatic areas have not been electively treated. The incidence is greater in patients with advanced or recurrent tumors. Distant metastasis as the only site of failure is rare, occurring in 2% of patients in the University of Florida series (119,120).

CLINICAL PRESENTATION

Maxillary Sinus

Maxillary sinus cancers produce few symptoms until they extend beyond the sinus. Advanced disease (T3–T4) is found in 75% to 80% of patients at presentation. Orbital invasion is evident in 60% (94). Nasal obstruction, nasal discharge, epistaxis, "sinus pain," and a sense of fullness over the involved antrum are common. Proptosis, diplopia, and chemosis result from orbital invasion. A mass may be present in the cheek or temporal region. Posterior extension produces trismus and headache secondary to invasion of the pterygoid muscles and base of skull. Cranial neuropathy may result from invasion of the skull base or infraorbital nerve in the orbital floor. Inferior tumor extension leads to jaw pain and loosening of upper teeth. Patients frequently consult a dentist, and teeth may be extracted. In edentulous patients, intraoral extension may cause improper fitting of a denture. An oral–antral fistula may be present in the gingivobuccal sulcus or upper gum.

Ethmoid Sinus

The most common symptoms of ethmoid sinus cancer occur as a result of tumor extension to the nasal (74%) or orbital (35%) cavities, producing nasal obstruction, epistaxis, diplopia, proptosis, tearing, or inner canthal mass. The latter may be interpreted as dacryocystitis, leading to inappropriate incision and drainage. Some 15% to 20% of patients complain of frontal headache (14,97).

Sphenoid Sinus

Patients with sphenoid sinus tumors typically present with neurologic rather than rhinologic complaints. Two thirds of patients have severe headaches, which are often most severe in the morning and may awaken the patient (1,68,69). Cranial neuropathy (most commonly involving nerves II–VI) is present in over 50% of patients. Some 50% to 60% of patients have diplopia, and 30% have vision loss due to optic nerve involvement. Facial numbness is present in 25% of patients and 25% have ptosis. Only 5% to 10% have epistaxis or obstructive symptoms. Cerebrospinal fluid rhinorrhea is occasionally noted (1,68). One third of patients have completely normal physical examinations and normal fiberoptic examinations at presentation (1).

Frontal Sinus

Patients with frontal sinus carcinoma present with pain and unilateral or bilateral swelling of the supraorbital ridge or glabella. There is frequently a palpable defect in the frontal bone. Diplopia due to invasion of the extraocular muscles is common. Intracranial extension may lead to confusion and seizures (24).

Nasal Cavity

Nasal cavity tumors usually cause nasal obstruction, blood-tinged mucus, and epistaxis. Headache, local pain, epiphora, diplopia, proptosis, ophthalmoplegia, anesthesia of the maxillary division of the trigeminal nerve, and expansion of the nasal dorsum resulting in ill-fitting eyeglasses may also be present. Patients with small septal tumors usually present with crusting and ulceration.

ESTHESIONEUROBLASTOMA

Esthesioneuroblastomas produce the most unusual array of symptoms of any primary head and neck tumor. In addition to the usual symptoms and signs produced by other nasal tumors, esthesioneuroblastoma may produce isolated symptoms of severe hyponatremia secondary to inappropriate secretion of antidiuretic hormone (ADH) due to production of arginine vasopressin (sometimes in association with hypertension (35, 121–125); Cushing syndrome due to ectopic adrenocorticotropic hormone secretion (126); anosmia; personality change due to frontal lobe invasion (102,127,128); massive epistaxis (either spontaneous or after biopsy) (100); or sudden blindness (128–130) due to nerve compression at the orbital apex/optic canal. Esthesioneuroblastoma may also be associated with atypical back or buttock pain due to leptomeningeal metastasis (so-called drop metastasis) to the lumbar spinal cord or cauda equina, or a tumor-packed bone marrow producing bony pain despite normal plain radiographs and normal bone scan. In the latter circumstance, pancytopenia is common secondary to marrow aplasia.

Although esthesioneuroblastoma cells contain neurosecretory granules, the tumor is not associated with elevated urinary secretion of dopamine, vanillylmandelic acid (VMA), or homovanillic acid (HVA). In patients with inappropriate secretion of ADH or Cushing syndrome, elimination of the tumor leads to resolution of the hormone disturbance.

There is tremendous variability in clinical aggressiveness. Some patients may be symptomatic for years before diagnosis and have indolent courses with multiple local recurrences spanning decades (36,100,102,131,132) without ever developing distant metastases. Other patients rapidly develop metastases and die within months. It seems likely (but remains unproven due to sparse literature on the subject) that such diverse behavior correlates with tumor grade.

SINONASAL UNDIFFERENTIATED CARCINOMA

Patients with SNUC typically present with multiple sinonasal symptoms of short duration (2 to 16 weeks). Ocular complaints (e.g., diplopia or decreased visual acuity) and pain are common.

MALIGNANT MELANOMA

Malignant melanoma typically presents with nasal obstructive symptoms and epistaxis. Many tumors are heavily pigmented, but 10% to 30% are amelanotic and appear as fleshy masses (87, 33,134).

INVERTED PAPILLOMA

The most common presenting symptom of inverted papilloma is unilateral nasal obstruction. A history of allergy is not common. Rhinorrhea, epistaxis, sinus pressure, and headaches are also seen. Some 50% to 60% of patients underwent previous surgical procedures (polypectomy, Caldwell-Luc procedure, or intranasal ethmoidectomy) for other presumed diagnosis by the time they presented for definitive treatment (48,79,114).

LETHAL MIDLINE GRANULOMA

Lethal midline granuloma is characterized by progressive ulceration and destruction of the midface, and is invariably fatal if left untreated. The nasal cavity is the most frequent site of involvement (85%–90%) (58,59,61) followed by the paranasal sinuses (10%) and hard palate (5%). Presenting symptoms are predominantly nasal: obstruction, 82%; nasal purulence or bloody discharge, 67%; midfacial destruction, 47%; cheek or orbital swelling, 45%; fever, night sweats, or weight loss, 30% to 80% (59–61); epistaxis, 21%; pain, 16%; neck lymphadenopathy, 14%; headache, 8%; ocular symptoms, 8%; facial paresthesia, 5%; or other, 16%. Most patients (80%) present with disease confined to the head and neck region (59). Hemophagocytic syndrome characterized by fever, pancytopenia, hemophagocytic histiocytes in the bone marrow, and frequent rapid deterioration in liver function is seen in a small percentage of patients (58).

Nasal Vestibule

Lesions of the nasal vestibule present with few symptoms other than a mass growing in the entrance to the nose, producing crusting, scabbing, and occasional minor bleeding. Pain is usually modest, even with destruction of cartilage or involvement of the lip. Secondary infection is sometimes present, resulting in extreme tenderness of the nose and lip. The lesion may be localized to one area of the vestibule, but frequently it fills the nasal vestibule so that the site of origin cannot be easily determined.

DIAGNOSTIC EVALUATION AND CLINICAL STAGING

Physical Examination

NASAL CAVITY AND PARANASAL SINUSES

The nasal cavity is inspected via nasal speculum and with a 30-degree rigid fiberoptic nasoscope after topical anesthesia and shrinkage of the mucosa. It is usually not feasible to adequately examine the upper nasal cavity with a flexible fiberoptic nasopharyngoscope. The cranial nerves are examined. Evidence of tumor extension into the orbit is sought by simultaneous palpation of the orbits with the index fingers; the tips of the fingers are placed between the bony orbital wall and the eyeball, and findings are compared with the normal side. A 90-degree Hopkins laryngopharyngoscope provides an excellent panoramic view of the nasopharynx and posterior nares. Facial asymmetry should be noted.

In patients with maxillary sinus cancer, examination should independently address anesthesia in each of the following areas because each has specific implications regarding tumor spread: upper lip and lateral nose (infraorbital nerve); buccal side of the posterior alveolus in the area of the premolar and molar teeth (posterior superior alveolar nerve); canine and incisor teeth and adjacent gums (anterior superior alveolar nerve); and hard palate (greater palatine nerve). If the incisor teeth and upper lip are both numb and no mass is palpable in the gingivobuccal sulcus, one can predict involvement of the orbital floor. Numbness of the incisor teeth may be a result of destruction of the anterolateral wall of the antrum or may be a result of a Caldwell-Luc procedure. Hemipalatal anesthesia may result from invasion of the pterygopalatine fossa (in which case tearing may also be absent because of involvement of secretomotor fibers from the sphenopalatine ganglion to the lacrimal gland) or from invasion of the greater palatine nerve, which is in close proximity to the posterior inferior nasal wall of the sinus. Loss of sensation in the posterior alveolus or molar and premolar teeth suggests destruction of the infratemporal wall; unless the maxillary nerve is also involved, sensation of the face remains intact (89). Signs of orbital invasion, cranial neuropathy, and soft tissue extension to the cheek or temporal fossa should be noted. The maxillary teeth, gingivobuccal sulcus, alveolus, and hard palate should be inspected and palpated. The nasal cavity and nasopharynx should be examined with a rigid fiberoptic nasoscope. Submucosal fullness on the posterolateral pharyngeal wall may represent either primary tumor extension or retropharyngeal lymphadenopathy.

An intranasal mass is present in over half of the patients with ethmoid sinus primary tumors. At least 25% will have a palpable medial canthal mass or exophthalmos. Epiphora is present in 5% to 10% of patients. Pathologic diagnosis of ethmoid sinus tumors is usually obtained via biopsy of the intranasal mass, or if no mass is present, external ethmoidectomy or transantral ethmoidectomy (97).

In patients with nasal vestibule cancer, erythema or induration of the upper lip may be subtle. The gingivolabial sulcus is inspected and palpated with the index finger. Tumor that has grown into the sulcus is generally tender and it may not be possible to separate the usually pliable upper lip from the gingiva when tumor involves this site. Advanced lesions infiltrate the entire upper lip, producing a rigid, tender mass that extends from one nasal labial crease to the other and often produces subtle widening, induration, rigidity, and tenderness of the columella and one or both ala or entire external nose. Bone invasion of the premaxilla is noted on physical examination by observing either a tender mass in the region or by noting a spongy softening of the bone at this site. The primary lesion in the vestibule is best visualized by retracting the ala with the wood end of a cotton-tipped applicator stick, because the blades of the nasal speculum obscure adequate visualization. Posterior tumor extension is sought with the fiberoptic telescope. Buccinator and facial nodal regions are palpated bimanually with the index finger of one hand sweeping over the buccal mucosa intraorally while the other hand simultaneously palpates the exterior of the cheek. Special attention is directed to bimanual examination of the submandibular lymph nodes.

DIAGNOSTIC IMAGING

Nasal Cavity and Paranasal Sinuses

Patients should undergo axial and coronal computed tomography (CT) of the neck and magnetic resonance imaging (MRI) of the paranasal sinuses and brain. These are complementary studies (135). A CT scan is better at detecting cervical lymph node metastasis and bone destruction and MRI is superior in assessing extent of intracranial or brain involvement and in distinguishing tumor from retained secretions. An MRI is also better than CT in evaluating retropharyngeal lymph nodes. The ability to distinguish one histologic tumor type from another on imaging studies is limited.

The appearance of esthesioneuroblastoma is relatively nonspecific with both expansile (bowing or molding of sinus walls) and destructive characteristics, usually centered in the superior nasal cavity and ethmoid sinuses, with occasional punctate intratumoral calcifications (105,136) or cystic areas (105,136, 137). Bone scan is performed if the patient has bone pain. Bone marrow biopsy is advised in patients with low blood cell counts (113). Magnetic resonance imaging of the spine is indicated in patients with intracranial disease extension who have symptoms or signs of leptomeningeal spread, although such spread usually occurs late.

CLINICAL STAGING FOR SINUS MALIGNANCIES

The 1997 staging system of the American Joint Committee on Cancer (AJCC) for maxillary sinus and ethmoid sinus cancers is outlined in Table 22.1 (138).

TABLE 22.1 1997 American Joint Committee on Cancer Staging Systems for Maxillary Sinus and Ethmoid Sinus Cancers

Definition of tumor, node, metastasis	
Maxillary sinus primary tumor (T)	
TX	Primary tumor cannot be assessed
T0	No evidence of primary tumor
Tis	Carcinoma *in situ*
T1	Tumor limited to the antral mucosa with no erosion or destruction of bone
T2	Tumor causing bone erosion or destruction, except for posterior antral wall, including extension into the hard palate or the middle nasal meatus
T3	Tumor invades any of the following: bone of the posterior wall of maxillary sinus, subcutaneous tissues, skin of cheek, floor or medial wall of orbit, infratemporal fossa, pterygoid plates, ethmoid sinuses
T4	Tumor invades orbital contents beyond the floor or medial wall including any of the following: the orbital apex, cribriform plate, base of skull, nasopharynx, sphenoid, frontal sinuses
Ethmoid sinus primary tumor (T)	
T1	Tumor confined to the ethmoid with or without bone erosion
T2	Tumor extends into the nasal cavity
T3	Tumor extends to the anterior orbit, or maxillary sinus
T4	Tumor with intracranial extension, orbital extension including apex, involving the sphenoid, or frontal sinus or skin of external nose
Regional lymph nodes (N)	
NX	Regional lymph nodes cannot be assessed
N0	No regional lymph node metastasis
N1	Metastasis in a single ipsilateral lymph node, 3 cm or less in greatest dimension
N2	Metastasis in a single ipsilateral lymph node, more than 3 cm but not more than 6 cm in greatest dimension, or in multiple ipsilateral lymph nodes, none more than 6 cm in greatest dimension, or in bilateral or contralateral lymph nodes, none more than 6 cm in greatest dimension
N2a	Metastasis in a single ipsilateral lymph node more than 3 cm but not more than 6 cm in greatest dimension
N2b	Metastasis in multiple ipsilateral lymph nodes, none more than 6 cm in greatest dimension
N2c	Metastases in bilateral or controlateral lymph nodes
N3	Metastasis in a lymph node more than 6 cm in greatest dimension
Distant metastasis (M)	
MX	Distant metastasis cannot be assessed
M0	No distant metastasis
M1	Distant metastasis

	Stage grouping		
Stage 0	Tis	N0	M0
Stage I	T1	N0	M0
Stage II	T2	N0	M0
Stage III	T3	N0	M0
	T1	N1	M0
	T2	N1	M0
	T3	N1	M0
Stage IVA	T4	N0	M0
	T4	N1	M0
Stage IVB	Any T	N2	M0
	Any T	N3	M0
Stage IVC	Any T	Any N	M1

Source: American Joint Committee on Cancer. *AJCC cancer staging manual,* 5th ed. Philadelphia: Lippincott Williams & Wilkins, 1997:47–50.

The 2002 AJCC staging system for maxillary sinus and nasoethmoid lesions is shown in Table 22.2 (138a). This is the most relevant new information added to the staging system by the AJCC. All other data quoted in this chapter are from the 1997 AJCC staging classification, which is essentially the same, with major exception being noted in Table 22.2.

The staging system used at the University of Florida for cancers of the nasal cavity, sphenoid sinus, and frontal sinus is outlined in Table 22.3.

At least six different staging systems have been proposed by various institutions for esthesioneuroblastoma: Massachusetts General Hospital (the Kadish system) (130); Mt. Sinai Medical

TABLE 22.2 2002 American Joint Committee on Cancer Staging for Maxillary Sinus and the Nasoethmoid Complex

Definition of tumor, node, metastasis

Primary tumor (T)	
TX	Primary tumor cannot be assessed
T0	No evidence of primary tumor
Tis	Carcinoma *in situ*
Maxillary sinus	
T1	Tumor limited to maxillary sinus mucosa with no erosion or destruction of bone
T2	Tumor causing bone erosion or destruction including extension into the hard palate or middle nasal meatus, except extension to posterior wall of maxillary sinus and pterygoid plates
T3	Tumor invades any of the following: bone of the posterior wall of maxillary sinus, subcutaneous tissues, floor or medial wall of orbit, pterygoid fossa, ethmoid sinuses
T4a	Tumor invades anterior orbital contents, skin of cheek, pterygoid plates, infratemporal fossa, cribriform plate, sphenoid or frontal sinuses
T4b	Tumor invades any of the following: orbital apex, dura, brain, middle cranial fossa, cranial nerves other than maxillary division of trigeminal nerve (V_2), nasopharynx, or clivus
Nasal cavity and ethmoid sinus	
T1	Tumor restricted to any one subsite, with or without bony invasion
T2	Tumor invading two subsites in a single region or extending to involve an adjacent region within the nasoethmoidal complex, with or without bony invasion
T3	Tumor extends to invade the medial wall or floor of the orbit, maxillary sinus, palate, or cribriform plate
T4a	Tumor invades any of the following: anterior orbital contents, skin of nose or cheek, minimal extension to anterior cranial fossa, pterygoid plates, sphenoid or frontal sinuses
T4b	Tumor invades any of the following: orbital apex, dura, brain, middle cranial fossa, cranial nerves other than (V_2), nasopharynx, or clivus
Regional lymph nodes (N)	
NX	Regional lymph nodes cannot be assessed
N0	No regional lymph node metastasis
N1	Metastasis in a single ipsilateral lymph node, 3 cm or less in greatest dimension
N2	Metastasis in a single ipsilateral lymph node, more than 3 cm but not more than 6 cm in greatest dimension, or in multiple ipsilateral lymph nodes, none more than 6 cm in greatest dimension, or in bilateral or contralateral lymph nodes, none more than 6 cm in greatest dimension
N2a	Metastasis in a single ipsilateral lymph node, more than 3 cm but not more than 6 cm in greatest dimension
N2b	Metastasis in multiple ipsilateral lymph nodes, none more than 6 cm in greatest dimension
N2c	Metastasis in bilateral or contralateral lymph nodes, none more than 6 cm in greatest dimension
N3	Metastasis in a lymph node, more than 6 cm in greatest dimension
Distant metastasis (M)	
MX	Distant metastasis cannot be assessed
M0	No distant metastasis
M1	Distant metastasis

Stage grouping

Stage 0	Tis	N0	M0
Stage I	T1	N0	M0
Stage II	T2	N0	M0
Stage III	T3	N0	M0
	T1	N1	M0
	T2	N1	M0
	T3	N1	M0
Stage IVA	T4a	N0	M0
	T4a	N1	M0
	T1	N2	M0
	T2	N2	M0
	T3	N2	M0
	T4a	N2	M0
Stage IVB	T4b	Any N	M0
	Any T	N3	M0
Stage IVC	Any T	Any N	M1

Source: Greene F, Page D, Fleming I, et al. *AJCC cancer staging manual,* 6th ed. New York: Springer-Verlag, 2002:59–68.

TABLE 22.3 University of Florida Staging System for Cancers of the Nasal Cavity, Sphenoid Sinus, and Frontal Sinus

Stage I	Limited to site of origin
Stage II	Extension to adjacent sites (e.g., orbit, nasopharynx, paranasal sinuses, skin, pterygomaxillary fossa)
Stage III	Base of skull or pterygoid plate destruction; intracranial extension

Center (139); University of California, Los Angeles (140); Mayo Clinic (73), Institut Gustave-Roussy (141); and Johns Hopkins Hospital (110). Despite deficiencies, the Kadish system is still the most widely used classification. It defines stage A as tumor confined to the nasal cavity; stage B as tumor involving nasal cavity and paranasal sinuses; and stage C as extension beyond the nasal cavity and sinuses. Approximately 20% of patients present with stage A, 30% with stage B, and 50% with stage C (142). Although not all authors have noted good correlation between survival and stage, reasonably good correlation has been noted in most large reviews (33,143). The Kadish system is hampered by heterogeneity within stage C, which includes some patients with relatively favorable prognoses (tumor involving orbit or base of skull), patients with less favorable prognoses (extensive intracranial or brain involvement, lymph node metastases), and patients who have little or no likelihood of cure (distant metastases). It also takes no account of tumor grade.

Nasal Vestibule

Nasal vestibule cancers are staged according to the 1997 AJCC (144) staging system for skin cancer: T1, primary tumor 2 cm or less in maximum diameter; T2, greater than 2 cm but not more than 5 cm in maximum diameter; T3, greater than 5 cm in maximum diameter; and T4, invasion of cartilage, bone, or nerve. Because almost all tumors greater than 5 cm in diameter have cartilage or bone invasion, T3 tumors are rare. T4 tumors can be stratified into favorable lesions, less than 4 cm in diameter with no bone invasion, and unfavorable tumors, ≥4 cm in diameter, with invasion of the premaxilla or, less commonly, the bony septum; most T4 tumors are the more favorable type, with their T4 designation based on cartilage invasion.

SELECTION OF TREATMENT MODALITY

Maxillary Sinus

The mainstay of treatment is surgical resection. Early infrastructure lesions may be cured by surgery alone, but in most cases, RT is given after surgery even if margins are clear. Massive tumor extension to the base of skull, nasopharynx, or sphenoid sinus usually contraindicates surgery. Borderline resectable tumors are treated with neoadjuvant chemotherapy, sometimes followed by preoperative RT, followed by surgery if feasible. If the tumor becomes resectable after chemotherapy alone, some authors prefer to operate before RT is administered. In the era before chemotherapy, RT alone was the only treatment option for patients with locally advanced, unresectable squamous cell carcinoma of the antrum, and 5-year survival rates were low (10%–15%) (Fig. 22.10) (145). The usefulness of neoadjuvant or concurrent chemotherapy is still unknown. As reviewed subsequently, reports on the role of induction chemotherapy (often cisplatin and fluorouracil in the past) are inconclusive. Chemotherapy may have a role in preserving the orbital contents. It is commonly recommended as an adjunct to RT in patients who refuse surgical resection.

SURGICAL TREATMENT

The majority of patients undergo radical maxillectomy, including removal of the entire maxilla and ethmoid sinus. The globe and orbital floor are preserved for inferiorly situated tumors. Orbital exenteration is indicated when tumor has spread through the periorbita. Craniofacial resection (CFR) may be required if the roof of the ethmoids is involved. Reconstructive techniques such as rectus abdominus free-flap repair of maxillary defects and rib reconstruction of the orbital floor have significantly reduced long-term surgical morbidity.

RADIATION TREATMENT

The radiation treatment volume includes the entire maxilla, adjacent nasal cavity, ethmoid sinus, nasopharynx, and pterygopalatine fossa, and at least a portion of the adjacent orbit. The anterior field is usually angled cephalad to parallel the orbital floor to minimize the amount of globe that is irradiated. Three-dimensional conformal therapy, fractionated stereotactic treatment, or intensity modulated RT are all appropriate means of increasing the target dose while reducing the dose to normal dose-limiting tissues, most notably brain and visual apparatus.

ELECTIVE NECK TREATMENT

Jiang et al. (92) report a 0% incidence of lymph node failure among 17 patients who received elective neck RT versus 11 of 50 failures (22%) when elective neck treatment was not administered. The incidence was the same for T2 to T4 disease. The 5-year incidence of distant metastasis was 0% among the 17 who received elective neck treatment versus 31% among 50 patients who did not ($p = 0.03$). The same findings were observed at the University of California San Francisco/Stanford University Medical Center; Le et al. (96) report a 0% incidence of lymph node failure among 26 patients who received elective neck irradiation versus 20% lymph node failure among patients who did not receive elective neck RT. All lymph node failures occurred in patients with T3 and T4 disease. Patients who developed lymph node failure also had a significantly higher rate (81%) of distant metastases on multivariate analysis ($p = 0.006$) than patients without lymph node failure. We recommend elective neck RT in all patients with T2 to T4 or poorly differentiated cancers.

CHEMOTHERAPY

There are several ways in which chemotherapy and RT have been combined:

1. Neoadjuvant chemotherapy followed by radical RT (146)
2. Neoadjuvant chemotherapy, followed by surgery, followed by postoperative RT (147)
3. Neoadjuvant chemotherapy, followed by preoperative RT, followed by surgery (148)
4. Concurrent chemotherapy and RT (149)
5. Superselective intraarterial infusion chemotherapy (150)

Each method is discussed in the following paragraphs.

Kim et al. (146) performed a matched-control study in patients with squamous cell carcinoma of the maxillary sinus comparing standard RT (70 Gy) to the same RT preceded by two or three cycles of neoadjuvant cisplatin and fluorouracil. There were 34 patients in each group. Patients were matched for sex, age, Karnofsky performance status, pathologic grade, tumor location, AJCC stage, and local tumor extension. Most patients had stage IV disease. Six percent of the chemotherapy patients achieved a complete response, and 53% had a partial response.

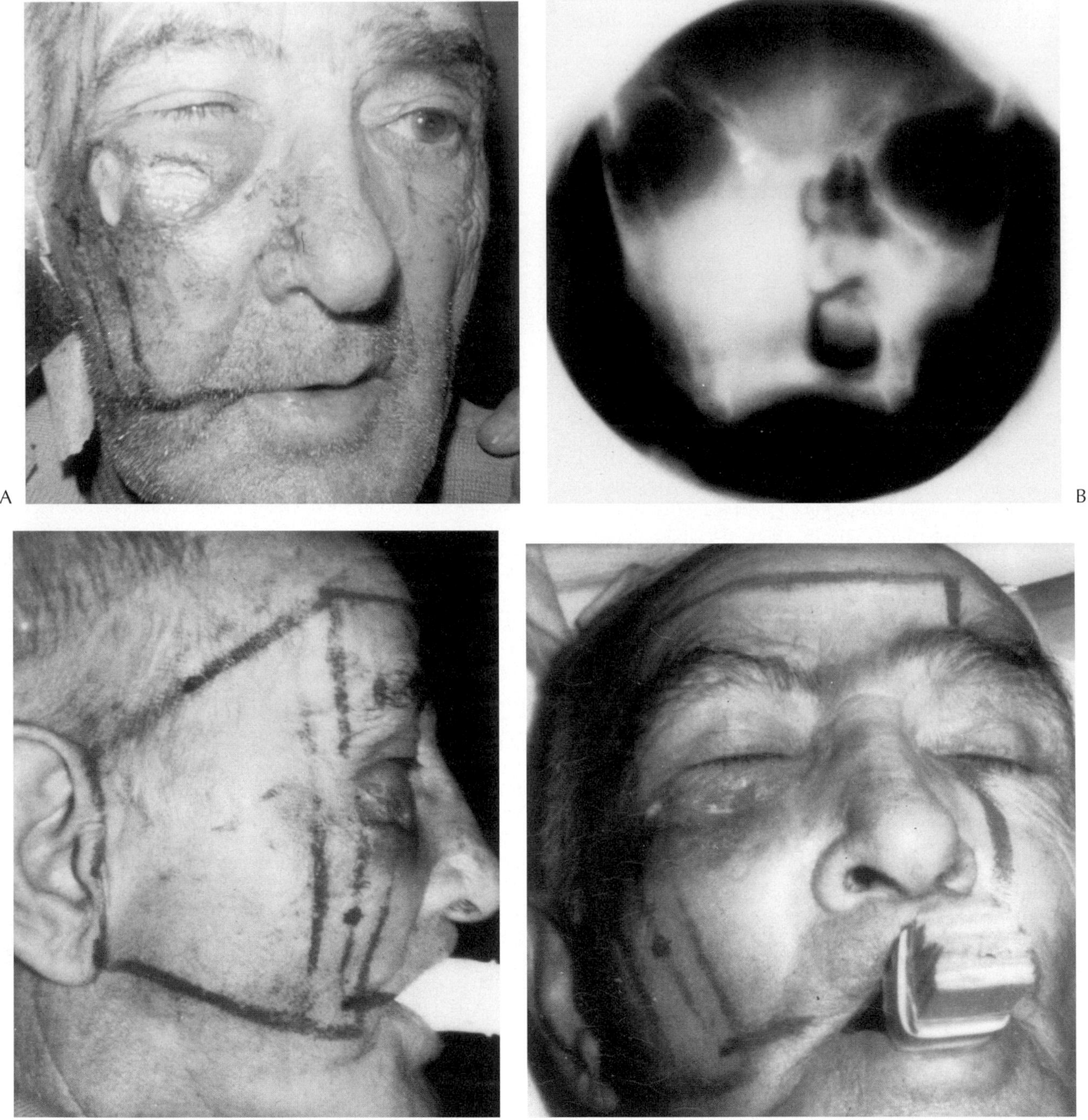

Figure 22.10 A 71-year-old man with a long history of sinusitis, treated by polypectomy and bilateral ethmoidectomies. Two months before admission, he noticed pain in the right cheek and a mass below the right orbit. The mass spontaneously drained through the skin. There was a recent onset of diplopia. **A:** Pus was draining from the right cheek mass, the lids were erythematous and edematous, and there was proptosis of the right eye. The orbit was filled with an indurated mass. The nasal cavity was occluded by tumor, but the nasopharynx was normal (T4 N0). Biopsy revealed squamous cell carcinoma. **B:** Tomography showed opacification of the right maxillary antrum, right ethmoid and sphenoid sinuses, and right nasal cavity with destruction of the medial and inferior orbital walls. There was no intracranial extension. Computed tomography confirmed the above. The patient refused any form of operation and received radiation treatment using ^{60}Co. **C:** The anterior portal. **D:** The right lateral portal. A stack of tongue blades was used to depress the tongue out of irradiation portals. Anterior and lateral portals overlapped on the skin surface.

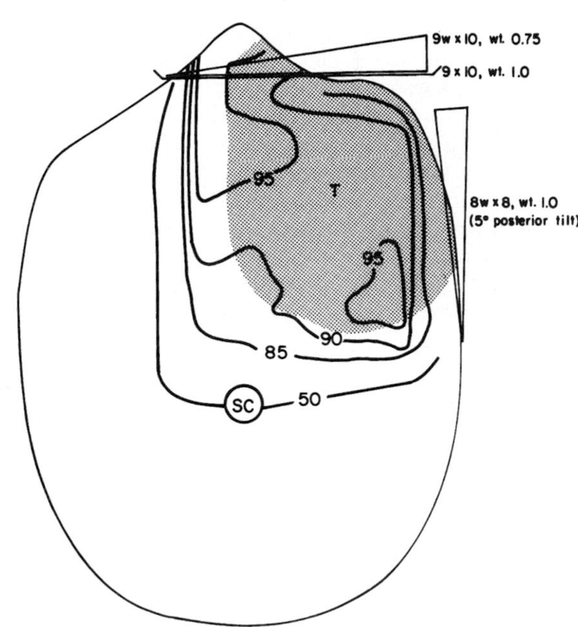

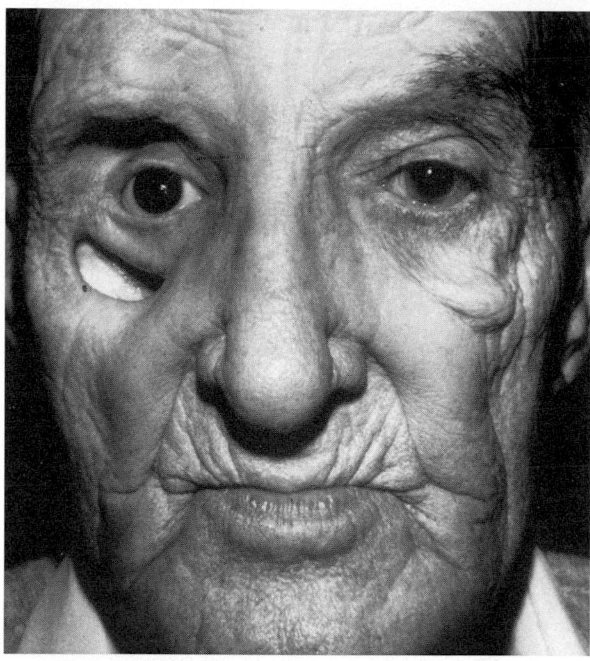

Figure 22.10 ***(continued)*** **E:** The minimum tumor dose was 70 Gy in 40 fractions, specified at 85% of maximum isodose line, administered by continuous-course irradiation. There was complete clinical regression of tumor after 50 Gy. Diplopia disappeared, and vision returned to normal. Pneumatic equalization tubes were inserted for bilateral serous otitis media. Blurry vision developed at 14 months, due to superficial keratitis secondary to dry eye syndrome and a cataract. The right cornea perforated spontaneously at 22 months and was repaired with a corneal transplant. The transplant failed, and the right eye was enucleated. **F:** At 5 years, an artificial eye was inserted, but caused intermittent discomfort. The antrocutaneous fistula persisted, but was asymptomatic and provided a porthole for antrum examination. No evidence of disease existed at 11 years. (**A–D, F** from Parsons JT, Stringer SP, Mancuso AA, et al. Nasal vestibule, nasal cavity, and paranasal sinuses. In: Million RR, Cassisi NJ, eds. *Management of head and neck cancer: a multidisciplinary approach,* 2nd ed. Philadelphia: JB Lippincott Co, 1994:551–598, with permission; **E** from Parsons JT, Million RR. Cancer of the nasal cavity and paranasal sinuses. In: Perez CA, Brady LW, eds. *Principles and practice of radiation oncology.* Philadelphia: JB Lippincott Co, 1997: 41–959, with permission.)

Both groups experienced a 65% rate of local recurrence. The 5-year survival rates after RT alone or neoadjuvant chemotherapy and RT were 32% and 30%, respectively. It was concluded that neoadjuvant chemotherapy failed to demonstrate therapeutic benefit over RT alone.

Lee et al. (147) report on 19 patients with stage III to IV paranasal sinus carcinoma treated with induction chemotherapy at the University of Chicago between 1984 and 1996. Most patients received three cycles of cisplatin and fluorouracil followed by surgical resection, in turn followed by concurrent chemotherapy and RT (hydroxyurea and fluorouracil in a 1-week-on, 1-week-off sequence, with a total RT dose of 60 Gy). Eighty-seven percent of patients treated with induction chemotherapy had a significant (>50%) response and 38% had no tumor in the surgical specimen (pathologic complete response). Five-year overall survival, disease-free survival, and local control rates were high: 73%, 67%, and 76%, respectively.

Björk-Eriksson et al. (148) treated 12 patients with advanced carcinoma of the maxillary sinus or nasal cavity with three cycles of induction cisplatin (100 mg/m^2 on day 1) and fluorouracil (1,000 mg/m^2/24 hours on days 1–5 continuous infusion), followed by 48 Gy preoperative RT, followed by limited resection (without orbital exenteration) 4 weeks after RT. Eight of twelve patients had no residual cancer in the resected specimen and three had minimal microscopic residual disease. Local control was achieved in 11 of 12 patients (92%) at 10 to 50 months follow-up (mean, 27 months; median, 22.5 months).

Harrison et al. (149) report on 12 patients with carcinoma of the paranasal sinuses treated with concurrent chemotherapy and RT at Memorial Sloan-Kettering Cancer Center between 1988 and 1995. All had T4 disease. Radiotherapy was administered by concomitant boost technique (70 Gy in 6 weeks). Most patients received cisplatin 100 mg/m^2 on days 1 and 22 (several patients also received mitomycin C, but the latter was discontinued after observing several deaths related to sepsis). The 3-year local control rate was a remarkable 78%, with 42% 3-year survival.

Lee et al. (150) report on patients who underwent superselective intraarterial and systemic chemotherapy for advanced cancers of the paranasal sinus/nasal cavity region prior to definitive treatment (surgery or RT) at the M. D. Anderson Cancer Center between 1986 and 1988. Neoplasms of the paranasal sinuses are particularly suitable for intraarterial infusion because they are usually encompassed within the territory of the terminal branches of the internal maxillary artery, which can be consistently and repeatedly catheterized in its pterygoid (second) segment. Patients received cisplatin (100 mg/m^2) and bleomycin sulfate (30 U) via intraarterial infusion, followed by intravenous fluorouracil by continuous infusion over 5 days. The procedure was repeated every 3 to 4 weeks for 3 to 4 courses, followed by surgery or RT. Two patients died suddenly and inexplicably within one week of infusion. In another patient, the infusion could not be performed because of arterial spasm. Of 21 evaluable patients, 9 (43%) had complete response and 10 had partial response (48%), for a major response rate of 91%. Two patients who achieved complete response underwent surgical resection; in one no tumor was found, and in the other there was minimal residual tumor. The other seven patients with complete response underwent RT and all remained free of disease. One additional patient had a nonfatal stroke. In an ongoing project at the M. D. Anderson Center, patients with maxillary sinus tumors involving the orbit are treated with neoadjuvant intraarterial cisplatin and systemic paclitaxel and ifosfamide for three cycles (MSK, personal communication). The regimen is highly active with partial or complete responses obtained in 90% of evaluable patients. Decisions then follow with respect to definitive local treatment but an effort is made to preserve the orbit and vision.

Ethmoid Sinus

The preferred treatment for both early and advanced lesions is surgery followed by postoperative RT. Margin status is difficult to determine because of the usual piecemeal manner in which the specimen is removed. Surgery alone without postoperative RT is rarely indicated. Occasional patients with papillary low-grade adenocarcinoma can be successfully treated by limited excision alone (151). The majority of ethmoid tumors are extirpated through medial maxillectomy and *en bloc* ethmoidectomy, including the entire lateral nasal wall, ethmoid labyrinth, lamina papyracea, and inferior and middle turbinates. If tumor involves the fovea ethmoidalis or cribriform plate, then a combined CFR approach is required. Resection may be extended to include the cavernous sinus or sphenoid sinus, but cure rates are dismal when these areas are involved. The operation does not allow adequate *en bloc* resection of tumors involving the orbital apex, nasopharynx, or deeply infiltrating the pterygoid space (145). In U.S. institutions, CFR is the most common procedure for these tumors (14,97). Although some early reports (152) stressed the importance of orbital exenteration as a component of CFR, it is now much less frequently performed (approximately 20% of cases) (14,97); sparing the orbital contents has not been detrimental to tumor control or survival (12,13,17,97). Erosion of the lamina papyracea is common, but the orbital periosteum is relatively resistant to tumor invasion; if the periorbita is not involved, then orbital exenteration is not necessary, even in patients with pretreatment symptoms of orbital invasion (97). When the lesion extends through the bony skull base, the overlying dura should be left attached to the specimen. Rarely, cure of patients with frontal lobe involvement has been reported (97).

If the patient is not a surgical candidate, then RT alone controls 50% to 65% of these tumors (6,13–15,153), but carries with it a higher risk to the visual apparatus and brain than lower dose postoperative RT (15,153). The expectation that surgery will salvage RT failures is not very realistic because few failures are successfully salvaged (14,15).

The current postoperative dose that we recommend is 59.4 Gy at 1.1 Gy twice a day; higher doses are administered if there is known residual disease. Treatment today is often delivered with three-dimensional conformal techniques, frequently with frameless stereotactic repositioning to assure accuracy of setups. The anterior portal is usually angled slightly cephalad to parallel the orbital floor and thus minimize the volume of eyeball irradiated. Careful attention is paid to limiting the dose to the optic nerves.

Neoadjuvant chemotherapy produces high response rates in patients with undifferentiated carcinoma of the ethmoid sinus (14). Some tumors that extensively involve the orbit undergo enough regression after neoadjuvant chemotherapy that sparing of the orbital contents becomes feasible.

Knegt et al. (18) describe a unique 23-year experience of 70 patients with ethmoid sinus adenocarcinoma treated at the University of Rotterdam (The Netherlands) between 1976–1997. Although treatment would be regarded as unconventional by most U.S. practitioners, the results were excellent. Surgical debulking was performed via extended anterior maxillary antrostomy, performing in essence a complete medial maxillectomy and sphenoethmoidectomy. As much tumor as possible was removed, taking care to preserve periorbita and dura. After surgery, areas of tumor involvement were liberally covered with a topical 5% fluorouracil emulsion and the cavity packed with tetracycline-impregnated gauze. Twice weekly, in the outpatient department, packs were removed along with meticulous removal and suction of necrotic material (identified as a painless gray tissue layer) followed by further fluorouracil application. A total of eight such dressing changes and necrotomies were performed. At 12 to 16 weeks, patients were returned to the operating room for repeat extensive biopsies. If no tumor was present, the patient had follow-up. If tumor remained, it was removed, followed by further treatment with topical fluorouracil and external beam radiation therapy (EBRT). Although this approach has never gained acceptance in the United States where CFR is the most widely accepted approach, the results from the Rotterdam series certainly argue for its consideration. Five- and 10-year survival rates of 79% and 64%, respectively, exceed those reported by more conventional exenterative surgery and RT in the United States. Overall, eight patients (12%) developed local recurrence; one developed a lymph node metastasis; and five (8%) developed distant metastases. The orbital contents were preserved and complications were mostly minor.

Sphenoid Sinus

Although some sphenoid sinus tumors are amenable to surgical resection (mostly through transseptal or combined lateral and anterior approaches) (1,69), most are too advanced for surgery and are treated with primary RT with or without chemotherapy. In the series from M. D. Anderson Cancer Center, 50% of all patients with sphenoid sinus primary tumors underwent attempted resection; negative margins were obtained in 43% of that group. *En bloc* resection is impossible. Piecemeal resection via drill curettage is the method used and, because of uncertainty of margins with this approach, postoperative RT is indicated.

Frontal Sinus

Prognosis in patients with frontal sinus carcinoma is poor. The poor prognosis is attributed to the advanced stage of disease at presentation, complex anatomy that makes resection technically difficult, and reluctance of surgeons to aggressively resect these tumors because of serious cosmetic sequelae (23). Cure with surgery alone is unlikely; combined surgery and RT produce a few cures (24).

Nasal Cavity

Based on a report by Ang et al. (25) of 45 patients treated at M. D. Anderson Cancer Center, we make the following treatment recommendations. For small tumors of the lower septum, interstitial implant (approximately 60–65 Gy over 6–7 days) alone produces a high rate of tumor control; alternatively, surgical resection via lateral rhinotomy similarly produces a high rate of tumor control. More extensive lesions of the septum may be treated with either EBRT or surgery plus RT. Lateral nasal wall or nasal floor lesions receive surgery plus RT. We generally favor a combination of surgery and RT over high-dose RT alone to reduce the risk of injury to the visual pathways. If satisfactory excision would require extensive removal of the external nose, RT alone is preferred.

ESTHESIONEUROBLASTOMA

We recommend combined treatment for all stages of disease. The advantages of this approach are twofold: (a) reduction of the rate of locoregional recurrence, which in turn reduces both the ultimate risk of distant metastases as well as development of unresectable local tumor spread to brain or leptomeninges, and (b) reduction of the toxicity of each individual treatment (especially with regard to high-dose RT alone and its potential for producing optic neuropathy, retinopathy, or other CNS injury). As discussed later, there is no convincing evidence that postoperative RT may be safely deleted, even in patients with early stage disease.

For Kadish A and early B lesions, we recommend CFR followed by postoperative RT, usually 59.4 Gy at 1.1 Gy twice a day. No elective neck treatment is recommended.

For advanced Kadish B or C lesions or Hyams grade 3 to 4 tumors that are resectable, we recommend neoadjuvant cisplatin–etoposide chemotherapy; followed by CFR (and neck dissection if clinically positive lymph nodes persist after chemotherapy), followed by 59.4 Gy at 1.1 Gy twice a day.

For unresectable advanced tumors or tumors that extensively invade brain or orbit, we recommend neoadjuvant chemotherapy. Various scenarios may follow. If the tumor becomes resectable after chemotherapy, we recommend CFR followed by postoperative RT (59.4 at 1.1 Gy twice a day). If it remains unresectable after neoadjuvant chemotherapy, then we recommend preoperative RT (59.4 Gy at 1.1 Gy twice a day), followed by resection if feasible. If the tumor remains unresectable at the completion of 59.4, then RT is continued to higher doses, depending on size and location of the tumor. Koka et al. (113) showed that the disease-free interval in patients who received such a multimodal approach was significantly longer than in patients who did not receive chemotherapy ([$p < 0.05$]).

Patients with direct brain extension are treated with curative intent in the appropriate setting (good overall medical condition) because occasional cures are reported (102,154). We are not aware of permanent cures in patients with diffuse leptomeningeal seeding or distant metastases, but aggressive treatment may be warranted with combinations of chemotherapy, RT, with or without autologous bone marrow transplant (in young patients), as long-term remission is sometimes possible.

We recommend bilateral elective neck RT for patients with advanced stage B or C disease or Hyams grade 3 to 4 disease, as failure in the lymphatics occurs in at least 20% of these patients when no elective treatment is administered (109,111,113,155, 156). Koka et al. (113) report no neck failures in 12 patients who received elective neck RT compared with 4 failures in 21 patients (19%) when elective neck RT was not administered. Their data further suggest that chemotherapy may reduce the risk of neck failure (0 of 14 patients who received chemotherapy vs. 7 of 19 [37%] among patients who did not [$p = 0.06$]).

Most authors report low survival rates when lymph node metastases are present (35,113,157). Combined chemotherapy, RT, and surgery will produce some cures (158).

Surgery

Since the mid-1970s, there has been a gradual evolution from lateral rhinotomy to CFR in the treatment of esthesioneuroblastoma. Craniofacial resection is logical because it allows removal of the cribriform plate and direct inspection of dura and brain. Koka et al. (113) report that lateral rhinotomy is associated with a substantially higher rate of local failure than CFR ($p = 0.07$). The same authors also noted that the local failure rate was significantly higher in patients who had no surgical resection of the primary site (80% vs. 44%, $p = 0.02$), and in patients whose tumors responded poorly to chemotherapy (100% failure in nonresponders vs. 33% in patients with complete response, $p = 0.01$).

Radiation Therapy

Esthesioneuroblastoma is relatively radiosensitive. Radiation therapy is generally used before or after surgery rather than as sole modality. If tumor is unresectable, RT is given after neoadjuvant chemotherapy, followed by surgery if possible. Local control is achieved with RT alone in approximately 50% of patients (155,156,159,160), but the required doses are high and potential morbidity is higher than after resection plus lower dose RT. In approximately 10% of patients, no response at all is seen with high-dose RT (132,136,161). Histologic proof (negative pathologic specimens) of radiation responsiveness has been reported by several institutions that use preoperative RT (130). We prefer postoperative over preoperative RT if the lesion is resectable, because one can more safely deliver higher doses in the postoperative setting. We disagree with authors who suggest that RT is unnecessary in completely resected low-grade (Hyams grade 1 and 2) or early stage (Kadish A and B) tumors (139). Paradoxically, these are the patients most likely to benefit from the addition of postoperative RT. Patients with less favorable tumors have such a high rate of developing distant metastases that any benefits in terms of local control are less evident. At the Mayo Clinic, 17 patients with low-grade tumors underwent gross total resection alone. In this group, there was a progressive decline in the local relapse-free survival curve with time: 88% local control at 3 years, 76% at 5 years, and 48% at 8 years (73). Ten other patients with low-grade tumors received postoperative RT and had a 100% 8-year rate of local control. The same phenomenon was observed among patients with low-stage (Kadish A or B) tumors: 5- and 10-year local control rates were 83% and 49%, respectively, after gross total resection alone, compared with no failures in patients who underwent gross total resection and postoperative RT.

Chemotherapy

In the early years, chemotherapy generally consisted of agents known to be active against childhood neuroblastoma, namely cyclophosphamide and vincristine, with or without doxorubicin; these regimens produced major response rates in 30% to 40% of patients (113). In recent years, cisplatin and etoposide have produced higher rates of response, often with complete radiographic or histologic regression even in patients with unresectable disease. Zappia et al. (154) describe two patients from the University of Michigan treated with cisplatin and etoposide for clinically unresectable tumors; both showed complete radiographic response. At Massachusetts General Hospital, Bhattacharyya et al. (162) administered cisplatin and etoposide to nine patients. Eight responded dramatically on radiography; the only patient who failed to respond radiographically underwent resection and no tumor was noted in the resected specimen, leading to an overall radiographic or histologic response rate of 100%. Among patients with unresectable primary tumors, response to chemotherapy significantly predicted survival ($p = 0.02$) and disease-free interval ($p = 0.007$) in the series from the Institut Gustave-Roussy (113). Polin et al. (143) report 34 patients treated at the University of Virginia. In a multivariate regression analysis of potential prognostic factors, 21 patients were identified as having had preoperative RT or neoadjuvant chemotherapy with alkylator-based regimens. Responding patients ($n = 14$) had lower disease-related mortality with 5- and 10-year survival rates of 81% and 55%, respectively. A subsequent review by this group (163) concluded that although the number of reported patients is limited, integration of chemotherapy as a component of primary management in patients with advanced stage disease is warranted.

Sinonasal Undifferentiated Carcinoma

Treatment of this highly aggressive tumor should be initiated promptly. Most authors recommend neoadjuvant chemotherapy (cyclophosphamide, doxorubicin, and vincristine), followed by preoperative RT, then surgical resection, usually CFR (164). In our experience, performing surgery first seldom achieves negative margins and is often followed by rapid recurrence in multiple sites (skin of face, orbit, anterior cranial fossa) before the patient can begin postoperative RT. The frequency of lymph node metastasis suggests that elective neck RT should be administered (38).

Malignant Melanoma

Treatment of malignant melanoma is the same, stage for stage, as squamous cell carcinoma (i.e., surgery and postoperative RT). Kingdom and Kaplan (165) note that the addition of postoperative RT led to improved local control, delay in time to recurrence, and higher survival than surgery alone at the University of California, San Francisco; this was true even in patients whose margins of resection were negative. Improved local control with postoperative RT has also been observed by others (166,167).

It has been the experience of the authors as well as others (42, 43,133,168,169) that mucosal melanoma of the nasal cavity and paranasal sinuses is radiosensitive, more so than cutaneous melanoma. Furthermore, the tumor is sensitive using conventional (1.8–2.0 Gy) fraction sizes. Gaze et al. (133) report complete response in 8 of 13 patients (62%) after RT alone at the University of Edinburgh; disease control was sustained in 5 patients (38%). Gilligan and Slevin (43) treated 28 patients with mucosal melanoma of the nasal cavity and paranasal sinuses with RT alone at the Christie Hospital and Holt Radium Institute and noted initial complete response in 22 (79%); actuarial local control at 3 years was 49%. Stern and Guillamondegui (168) note 5-year local control in 2 of 5 patients (40%) treated with RT alone at the M. D. Anderson Cancer Center. Ghamrawi and Glennie (170) at the Belvedere Hospital in Glasgow radically irradiated five patients, three (60%) of whom had a complete response, and two (40%) of whom had sustained local control. Harwood and Cummings (171) report complete response in 7 of 9 patients (78%) and sustained control in 4 (44%) with mucosal melanoma of the nasal cavity or paranasal sinuses treated with RT alone at the Princess Margaret Hospital. Berthelsen et al. (172) report complete response in 5 of 6 patients (83%) with nasal cavity melanoma after RT alone at the Radium Centres in Arhus, Copenhagen, and Odense, Denmark; 3 of 6 patients (50%) had sustained local control. Summarizing these six series, the complete response rate was 45 of 61 (74%), and the sustained local control rate was 30 of 66 (45%).

Elective neck treatment is not indicated.

Inverted Papilloma

SURGERY

Treatment of inverted papilloma is primarily surgical; local recurrence rates are higher (70%) after transnasal polypectomy or other limited excisions (antrostomy, ethmoidectomy, or turbinectomy) than after more radical procedures (48,49,51, 173–175). Although benign, complete removal is essential for long-term control. Lateral rhinotomy with *en bloc* medial maxillectomy, and removal of the middle and inferior turbinates and all mucosa in the ipsilateral paranasal sinuses is associated with low (5%–10%) recurrence rates and acceptable cosmetic and functional results (48,79,175). More conservative procedures are rarely applicable, but are sometimes used in patients with very localized disease or in patients who refuse *en bloc* resection (48, 176). Anterior skull base erosion calls for CFR (48).

RADIATION THERAPY

Experience with RT for inverted papilloma is limited. It is useful in cases associated with malignancy, multiple recurrent tumors, medically inoperable patients, or unresectable tumors (54,82,177–179). Although some authors express concern that RT may induce malignant transformation of benign inverted papilloma to squamous cell carcinoma (and several examples of such "conversion" have been cited), it must be remembered that metachronous development of squamous cell carcinoma also occurs spontaneously in 3% to 4% (79) of patients after surgery alone; there is no evidence that RT increases this risk.

Lethal Midline Granuloma

When disease is limited to the upper aerodigestive tract, RT is the treatment of choice. The dose is 45 to 50 Gy (59–61,180) and is delivered to the entire nasal cavity, all paranasal sinuses bilaterally, and to the entire hard palate. We generally treat all areas to 39.6 Gy, then boost the site of initial disease to 50.4 Gy at 1.8 Gy per fraction. More limited treatment volumes are associated with a 20% rate of marginal miss (61).

Although chemotherapy is being used with increasing frequency, there is no convincing evidence that it markedly improves outcome for patients with limited disease over RT alone (58–60). When used as primary treatment, chemotherapy produces a lower complete response rate and lower survival rate than primary RT, and in some patients it has been associated with uncontrollable fatal bleeding from the primary site (181). Conventional chemotherapy for relapsed disease is usually not successful. Liang et al. (182) report that two of three patients with relapsed nasal T-/NK-cell lymphoma who received high-dose chemotherapy and autologous bone marrow rescue at Queen Mary Hospital remained in complete remission at 12 and 44 months, respectively.

Nasal Vestibule

Radiation therapy is usually recommended because adequate excision often produces deformity. Early, superficial, well-demarcated lesions of the nasal septum are readily amenable to surgical excision with clear margins and repair by skin graft. Most other lesions are best treated by RT. Tumors involving the alar side of the vestibule often infiltrate the cartilage, and adequate repair of the defect after surgical excision is often less than ideal. Likewise, cancers that involve the floor of the vestibule or columella frequently extend submucosally into the upper lip; resection produces a defect that is difficult to correct. The volume of such cancers may be significant and both EBRT as well as brachytherapy may have to be combined (183). Rhinectomy is generally to be avoided except as a salvage procedure after failed RT.

Although cartilage that has been compromised by tumor invasion, infection, or prior surgery is theoretically more vulnerable to radiation injury, the risk of necrosis is low with properly fractionated EBRT (with or without interstitial implant), even after substantial doses. The probability of tumor control correlates better with tumor volume than with the presence or absence of cartilage invasion (184).

SURGERY

Excision of nasal vestibule tumors often requires removal of cartilage as well as skin. Depending on the site of the lesion, either the columella or alar cartilages may be removed and may be difficult to reconstruct, particularly if surgery is for RT failure. When the alar cartilage is removed, either a composite graft consisting of skin and cartilage from the ear or a nasolabial flap can be used to repair the defect. If the entire external nose is resected, a prosthesis usually is used to cover the defect because examination for recurrent disease is easier and total nasal reconstruction is cosmetically unacceptable.

In the last 10 years, patients with very advanced (≥4 cm) T4 disease with bone invasion of the premaxilla have been treated with full-dose preoperative RT (e.g., 74.4 Gy–76.8 Gy twice a day) followed by surgical resection of the bony component of the tumor and limited soft tissue resection. The rationale is to attempt cure of the soft tissue component with high-dose RT alone so that the scope of resection may be reduced compared with surgery alone. This approach proved successful in providing long-term local control in all four patients in whom it was used; pathologic specimens in three of four patients were negative. Radiotherapy alone produced no cures in three other similarly staged patients despite high doses, which in some patients exceeded 80 Gy (120).

RADIATION THERAPY

Selection of technique depends on extent of disease and experience of the radiation oncologist.

External Beam

Supervoltage beams are theoretically preferable to orthovoltage to reduce the dose to cartilage and adjacent bone. Orthovoltage therapy fractionated over 4 to 6 weeks, however, produces good results. Shorter courses with higher daily fractions may cure the cancer, but long-term cosmetic results may be suboptimal.

For T1 lesions, when EBRT alone is selected, the dose-fractionation schedule should be somewhat more aggressive than that used for skin cancers involving the external nose. Doses of 60 Gy in 25 fractions or 70 Gy over 6 weeks are usually most appropriate (185). The remainder of lesions (e.g., T2 or T3) are best treated with a combination of EBRT and interstitial implantation. Very advanced lesions with invasion of bone (T4) are treated with high-dose EBRT and surgical resection; a full potentially curative dose of RT is applied before surgery with twice daily RT. Patients with smaller T4 lesions (staged T4 on the basis of invasion of adjacent cartilage) are treated as previously described for T2 and T3 disease.

Interstitial Implant

Interstitial implants of the nasal vestibule use after-loading iridium-192 techniques and are highly individualized. The dose varies between 55 Gy to 75 Gy (depending on the size of the lesion) when treatment is by interstitial RT alone. When combined with EBRT (50 Gy), the dose from the implant is 20 to 30 Gy.

Interstitial implants should be used whenever feasible: either alone for early (T1 and selected T2) cancers; or in combination with EBRT for more advanced tumors. Reported local control rates from institutions that use implants exceed 95% (117,186–190). Although there are a few reports of high control rates (119,185) using EBRT alone, many authors report mediocre results (191–193). Poulsen and Turner (193) note local control in only 10 of 16 (63%) T1 to T2 lesions treated at the Queensland Radium Institute with EBRT alone, despite doses (55 Gy in 20 fractions) that would produce a high rate of control for skin cancers at other sites. In Rotterdam, Baris et al. (117) report local control in only 66% of patients with early lesions treated by EBRT alone (vs. 21 of 22 of patients, or 96%, who received interstitial implantation). Mazeron et al. (194) also note local control in only 21 of 33 lesions (64%) treated by EBRT at the Institut Gustave-Roussy. Kagan et al. (195) similarly report local control in only 5 of 7 patients (71%) with early stage disease after 60 to 70 Gy EBRT. Furthermore, in the Kagan series, of 11 patients with early stage disease who underwent surgery and postoperative RT (60 Gy) because of positive margins, only 5 (45%) were cured. These latter patients should be treated the same way as those with *de novo* tumors are treated (i.e., with interstitial RT alone or interstitial plus EBRT); they are given the same total doses as if no surgery had been performed.

A variety of implant techniques have been described (186–188, 196); all require special apparatus, sophisticated dosimetry, and operator experience. Equally good results have been reported with each technique.

TREATMENT OF LYMPHATICS

The neck usually is observed when clinically negative because of the low risk (10%–15%) of subclinical disease.

Elective neck irradiation is used for advanced, recurrent, or poorly differentiated lesions. Patients with multiple postsurgical recurrences may develop in-transit lymphatic metastases. Although electrons may be used to electively irradiate the transit lymphatics (the so-called Fu Manchu technique) (118), the technique is infrequently required.

TREATMENT RESULTS

Maxillary Sinus

SQUAMOUS CELL CARCINOMA

In the past several decades, there have been few fundamental changes in either management or rate of cure of squamous cell carcinoma of the maxillary sinus. The concept of combining surgery and RT was established by Ohngren (197) 70 years ago; in his series, a 5-year survival rate of 38.5% was achieved. Today, combined surgery and RT are almost a routine procedure for patients with resectable tumors. Reported 5-year overall survival rates remain in the 30% to 40% range (8,9,90–94,96, 198–203). Most refinements of surgery and RT techniques over the last 20 years are intended to reduce morbidity and preserve function (e.g., preservation of orbital contents) or improve RT dose distribution (e.g., CT-based treatment planning; multibeam three-dimensional conformal RT to limit the dose to the brainstem, frontal lobes, and visual apparatus; stereotactically administered treatment that allows precise treatment reproducibility and dose delivery; and intensity-modulated RT which allows favorable shaping of isodose distributions), but will probably not substantially impact overall 5-year survival rates.

Le et al. (95) report on 97 patients curatively treated at the University of California, San Francisco (UCSF) or Stanford University Medical Center (SUMC) between 1956 and 1996. Fifty-eight patients had squamous cell carcinoma, 16 had undifferentiated carcinoma, 19 had adenocystic carcinoma, and 4 had adenocarcinoma. Eighty-nine (92%) had T3 or T4 tumors. Sixty-one patients received combined surgery and RT (most commonly administered after surgery) and 36 received RT alone. Histologic subtype had no impact on survival. Overall 5- and

10-year actuarial survival rates were 34% and 31%, respectively. Five-year survival according to the 1997 AJCC staging system is: stage II, 75%; stage III, 37%; and stage IV, 28%. In multivariate analysis, factors that negatively affect survival were older age ($p < 0.001$; T4 (vs. T2 and T3), $p = 0.001$; lymph node involvement at diagnosis ($p = 0.002$); male sex ($p = 0.04$); and treatment with RT alone (vs. combined treatment, $p = 0.009$). Five-year survival was 46% in those who received combined treatment versus 19% after RT alone. A survival advantage for combined treatment was noted for all stages, but not all differences were significant. The 5-year survival rates after combined treatment or RT alone, respectively, according to T stage were as follows: T2, 80% versus 67% ($p = 0.78$); T3, 42% versus 17% ($p = 0.12$); and T4 43% versus 14% ($p = 0.003$). Combined treatment was superior in all age groups. Shorter overall RT treatment time nearly reached statistical significance ($p = 0.06$).

Eighty-six percent of recurrences in the UCSF/SUMC series (56 of 65) occurred within 2 years (6 of the 9 late recurrences were adenocystic carcinoma). The predominant pattern of failure was local. Actuarial 5-year local control in the UCSF/SUMC series was 43% (T2, 62%; T3, 53%; and T4, 36%). Median time to local recurrence was 7 months. The only significant prognostic factor positively affecting local control in multivariate analysis was combined treatment (vs. RT alone, $p < 0.001$). For patients treated with surgery, margin status was the only factor that correlated with local control ($p = 0.007$). For patients treated with RT alone, higher radiation dose (12% local control with doses <65 Gy vs. 29% with doses ≥65 Gy, $p = 0.007$) and shorter overall treatment time ($p = 0.04$) were associated with lower recurrence rates in multivariate analysis.

The 5-year freedom from distant metastasis rate was 66%; on multivariate analysis, freedom from distant metastasis correlated significantly with lymph node status at presentation (N0, 71% vs. N-positive 24%, $p < 0.0001$), T stage ($p = 0.01$), and lymph node recurrence ($p = 0.007$). This incidence of neck node failure among patients who received elective neck RT (26 patients) was 0% versus a 20% rate of nodal failure when elective neck treatment was not administered (96).

Jiang et al. (92) reported on 73 patients with maxillary sinus carcinoma who underwent surgical excision and postoperative RT (50–60 Gy at 2 Gy per fraction) at the M. D. Anderson Cancer Center between 1969 and 1985. Primary disease control was achieved in 57 patients (78%). Salvage surgery was attempted in only 1 of 16 patients with local failure, without success. Of 50 patients without palpable lymphadenopathy who did not receive elective neck RT, 11 (22%) developed nodal relapse (6 before the course of RT was complete and 4 more before 2 years). The incidence of nodal failure was approximately the same for T2, T3, and T4 lesions; tumor grade had no bearing on the incidence of nodal failure. None (0%) of the 17 patients who received elective neck RT developed lymph node failure; these incidences of lymph node metastasis, with or without elective treatment, were almost identical to findings reported by Le et al. (96). Twenty-three percent of patients in the M. D. Anderson series developed distant metastases. The 5-year incidence was 0% among 17 patients who received elective neck RT and 31% among 50 patients who did not receive elective neck RT ($p = 0.03$). The 5-year rates of overall survival, relapse-free survival, and disease-specific survival were 48%, 51%, and 64%, respectively.

Waldron et al. (8) report on 110 patients treated at Princess Margaret Hospital for squamous cell or undifferentiated carcinoma of the maxillary sinus. Seventy-five percent received RT alone with surgery reserved for salvage; the remainder received planned combined RT and surgery. Five-year overall survival was 30%. Five-year cause-specific survival was 43% after RT alone and 55% after combined treatment. Five-year local control was 36% after RT alone and 57% after combined treatment. Of 63 local failures, salvage surgery was performed in 25 patients (40%) and yielded a 5-year cause-specific survival rate of 31% among operated patients (i.e., 12% of all patients with local failure were successfully salvaged).

Kurohara et al. (202) report on 174 patients with squamous cell carcinoma of the maxillary sinus with negative lymph nodes treated at the Roswell Park Memorial Institute between 1925 and 1963. Five-year survival after RT alone was achieved in 13 of 37 patients (35%) with T1 and T2 lesions and 10 of 100 patients (10%) with T3 and T4 disease. Radical surgery plus RT was used in only seven T1 and T2 patients. For T3 and T4 disease, surgery followed by RT produced 5-year survival in 6 of 21 patients (29%).

Lee and Ogura (93) report on 96 patients with maxillary sinus carcinoma who received treatment at Washington University in St. Louis from 1960 to 1976; 74 (77%) had squamous cell carcinoma. After preoperative RT (mostly 50–70 Gy) and surgery, 5-year absolute no-evidence-of-disease survival rates were 60%, 45%, 28%, and 38% in patients with T1, T2, T3, and T4 tumors, respectively. Radiation therapy alone (mostly 60–74 Gy) failed to produce a single 5-year survivor among 23 patients (2 with T2, 6 with T3, and 15 with T4 tumors). Similarly, Cheng and Wang (204) report 22% 5-year survival following RT alone versus 48% after combined therapy at Massachusetts General Hospital.

St-Pierre and Baker (9) report on 66 patients with squamous cell carcinoma of the maxillary sinus treated at the University of Michigan between 1964 and 1975. Eighty-seven percent had T3 or T4 disease. Five-year survival was 16% after RT alone, 20% after surgery alone, and 58% after combined treatment. Five-year survival was 75%, 29%, and 20% for T2, T3, and T4 lesions, respectively. No patient developed lymphatic or distant metastases in the absence of recurrence at the primary site.

Amendola et al. (205) report a 35% 5-year survival rate and a 35% rate of continuous disease control at the primary site (3 years minimum follow-up) in 20 patients (2 with T2 and 18 with T4) with squamous cell carcinoma of the maxillary antrum treated by RT alone. Bataini and Ennuyer (203) report the Curie Foundation results for 27 patients with squamous cell carcinoma of the maxillary antrum treated by supervoltage RT between 1959 and 1965. Only three patients had limited primary disease. The 3- and 5-year disease-free survival rates were 41% (11 of 27 patients) and 32% (6 of 19 patients), respectively.

Frich (201) irradiated 18 patients with T3 or T4 squamous cell carcinoma of the maxillary sinus with curative intent. Six patients (33%) remained continuously free of disease at 5 years after 60 to 70 Gy. Local control was obtained in 6 of 8 suprastructure lesions versus 0 of 7 infrastructure lesions.

In summary, 5-year survival rates of 60% to 70% for T1 and T2 tumors and 30% to 40% for T3 and T4 cancers are observed after resection and postoperative RT. Poor prognostic factors include positive lymph nodes, erosion of the pterygoid plates, pterygopalatine fossa invasion, and orbital invasion (94,206). For advanced unresectable T4 disease, 5-year survival rates are 10% to 15% after high dose RT alone. For T2 and T3 disease, RT alone produces 5-year survival rates that are one-half to two-thirds of the rates achieved with combined surgery and RT. As noted earlier, combined chemotherapy and RT appear promising, but few results have been reported.

MAXILLARY SINUS ADENOID CYSTIC CARCINOMA

Goepfert et al. (207) report on 33 patients with adenoid cystic carcinoma who received treatment with curative intent at M. D. Anderson Hospital between 1951 and 1980. Eight (24%)

remained free of disease 5 or more years after treatment, which usually consisted of surgery and postoperative RT (23 patients). Patients were divided into high-grade and low-grade histologic groups, depending on whether solid areas made up more or less than 30% of the tumor. Eight of 17 patients (47%) with low-grade lesions versus 0 of 16 patients (0%) with high-grade tumors remained free of disease beyond 5 years. Distant metastases occurred in two patients with low-grade disease and in nine patients with high-grade tumors. The finding of poorer prognosis in patients with solid histologic pattern has been confirmed by others (208,209).

Rafla (210) reports on 16 patients from the Royal Marsden Hospital with adenoid cystic carcinoma of the nasal cavity and paranasal sinuses. In 10 patients, tumor arose in the maxillary antrum. Half of the patients received RT alone, and half received surgery plus RT. Three of 13 patients (23%) at risk for 5 years were disease-free.

Leafstedt et al. (211) report the Roswell Park Memorial Institute results for nine patients with adenoid cystic carcinoma of the maxillary sinus treated between 1940 and 1965. Most received surgery alone; there were no cures.

Ethmoid Sinus

Jiang et al. (14) report results on 34 patients with ethmoid sinus carcinoma treated at M. D. Anderson Cancer Center between 1969 and 1993. There were 12 undifferentiated carcinomas, 8 squamous cell carcinomas, 9 adenocarcinomas, 4 adenoid cystic carcinomas, and 1 transitional cell carcinoma. Twenty-one patients received surgery plus RT, and 13 received RT alone; 9 patients received adjuvant chemotherapy. Patients were staged according to the Kadish system for esthesioneuroblastoma (130) (stage T1, 6 patients; T2, 13 patients; and T3, 15 patients).

Five- and 10-year actuarial local control rates were both 71% (T1, 100%; T2, 79%; T3, 53%, at both 5 and 10 years). Surgery plus RT produced a slightly higher rate of local control than RT alone at 10 years (74% vs. 64%, respectively). Surgical salvage was attempted in only one patient and was unsuccessful. Five-year overall, disease-free, and cause-specific survival rates were 55%, 58%, and 58%, respectively. Cervical lymphatic metastases developed in 3 of 31 patients (9%) who did not receive elective neck RT. Four patients (12%) developed distant metastases; in three of the four, lymph node metastasis preceded distant metastasis. Histologically proven dural invasion was associated with poor local control (30% vs. 80% without dural invasion, $p < 0.01$) and survival (40% vs. 83%, $p < 0.02$). A complete response was noted in three patients (all undifferentiated) and partial response in four patients (three undifferentiated and one adenocarcinoma) after induction chemotherapy.

Tiwari et al. (17) at University Hospital V.U. in Amsterdam report treatment results in 50 patients (46 men, 4 women) with carcinoma of the ethmoid sinus who underwent surgery and postoperative RT (usually 65 Gy over 7 weeks). Craniofacial resection was seldom used. Twenty-nine patients had adenocarcinoma, nine had squamous cell carcinoma, five had undifferentiated carcinoma, six had adenoid cystic carcinoma, and one had transitional cell carcinoma. None had lymph node metastases at diagnosis; two patients (4%) developed lymph node metastases after treatment. Twelve (24%) developed distant metastases. The 5-year survival rate was 65%. Local recurrence occurred in 38% of patients. Late local recurrence was a feature of adenocarcinoma.

Other authors have generally reported 5-year overall survival rates between 45% and 65% when surgery and RT were combined (13,212,213) versus approximately 40% overall survival (55% to 60% cause-specific survival) when RT alone was used (14,15). Tumor control and survival rates were similar for the various histologies (13,16).

Sphenoid Sinus

M. D. Anderson Cancer Center reports a 32% 5-year cause-specific survival rate after various combinations of treatment. A significant ($p = 0.05$) reduction in 5-year survival was noted among patients with cranial neuropathies (1). There were no survivors in the Mayo Clinic series beyond 6 years (69).

Nasal Cavity

Ang et al. (25) report results of 45 patients with carcinoma of the nasal cavity (excluding nasal vestibule) who received treatment with curative intent at the M. D. Anderson Cancer Center between 1968 and 1985. Eighteen patients received definitive RT (5 brachytherapy alone and 13 EBRT); 27 patients received surgery and RT. There were 30 squamous cell carcinomas, 9 adenocarcinomas, 5 adenoid cystic carcinomas, and 1 undifferentiated carcinoma. Patients were staged according to the University of Florida staging system (153).

Fourteen patients had nasal septal tumors. All were squamous cell carcinoma. Most (11 of 14, 79%) presented with stage I disease and most (12 of 14, 85%) received definitive RT (including 5 patients treated with brachytherapy alone for tumors of the inferior nasal septum).

In 31 patients tumors arose from the lateral nasal wall or floor. Compared with septal primaries, tumors of the nasal wall and floor tended to be more advanced at presentation (20 of 31, 65%, were stage II and III); half (15 of 31) had nonsquamous histology; and most (25 of 31, 81%) received combined surgery plus RT.

Table 22.4 lists rates of local control; 5- and 10-year overall survival, relapse-free survival, disease-specific survival; and nodal and distant failure according to site of origin within the nasal cavity. Patients with septal primaries had higher initial and ultimate rates of local control, overall survival, and disease-specific survival than patients with lateral wall or nasal floor primaries. All six local recurrences of squamous cell carcinoma were manifest by 2 years, whereas five of the six recurrences of adenocystic carcinoma or adenocarcinoma occurred after 3 years.

Fradis et al. (99) operated (via external rhinotomy, wide excision, and split-skin graft closure) on 16 patients (11 with invasive squamous cell carcinoma, 5 with squamous cell carcinoma *in situ*) with nasal septal carcinoma between 1976 and 1990. All patients with invasive carcinoma received postoperative RT. There were no recurrences; 15 had follow-up more than 2 years, and 10 had more than 5 years of follow-up.

ESTHESIONEUROBLASTOMA

Literature on esthesioneuroblastoma is confusing and fragmented. Most series are small, include patients with short follow-up, and suffer from lack of a consistent treatment approach. For this disease, in which recurrence frequently occurs late, it is probably not worthwhile to report on patients with less than 5 years' follow-up. Furthermore, many reported series did not use conventional methods of end-results reporting, (e.g., 5- and 10-year actuarial survival, relapse-free survival, cause-specific survival, etc.).

Table 22.5 summarizes four series from the pre–CFR era. Patients with less than 5 years' follow-up were excluded. Although 5-year survival rates for each series were 50% to 60%, continuous disease-free rates (≥5 years) were only 5% to 20%. Only the Institut Gustave-Roussy reported 10-year survival: 21%. Local or locoregional recurrence rates ranged from 62% to 74%. Some patients in these series underwent 10 or more oper-

TABLE 22.4 Nasal Cavity Carcinoma: Results According to Primary Tumor Site Within the Nasal Cavity (M. D. Anderson Cancer Center, Houston, 1968–1985)

Endpoint	Nasal septum	Lateral wall or floor	Total
Local control			
Initial	12/14 (86%)	21/31 (68%)	33/45 (73%)
Salvage	2/2	3/10 (30%)	5/12 (42%)
Ultimate	14/14	24/31 (77%)	38/45 (84%)
5-year survival			
Overall	92%	67% ($p = 0.03$)	75%
Relapse free	69%	69%	69%
Disease specific	100%	76%	83%
10-year survival			
Overall	83%	49% ($p = 0.04$)	60%
Relapse free	69%	52%	58%
Disease specific	100%	71%	80%
Neck failure without elective neck treatment	2/8 (25%)	0/28%	2/36 (6%)
Distant metastasis	0/14	4/31 (13%)	4/45 (9%)

Source: Ang KK, Jiang GL, Frankenthaler RA, et al. Carcinomas of the nasal cavity. *Radiother Oncol* 1992;24:163–168.

ations for recurrent disease (36). Brain extension was a component of local failure in 10 of 21 Mayo Clinic patients (48%). Three of the four series reported individual patient data, from which death rates due to tumor were calculated. Unlike other head and neck cancers, there is no apparent decline in the death rate beyond 5 years. In each of the three series, approximately 40% of patients who were evaluable for 5 years died of tumor within 5 years. Of patients who survived 5 years, another 40% died of esthesioneuroblastoma between 5 and 10 years. Furthermore, these series present no convincing evidence that the death rate declines after 10 years. Schwaab et al. (35) report that several patients were alive at 10 years with uncontrolled tumor. This pattern of death is consistent with the observation that some patients have indolent courses punctuated by repeated recurrences, which eventually become unmanageable, leading to death from local extension or metastasis. It is also consistent with the hypothesis that operations in the pre–CFR era were often palliative rather than curative. Approximately 30% to 50% of local failures were successfully salvaged by one or more operations (within the time frame of the analyses).

Table 22.6 shows data on patients with 5-year minimum follow-up from 12 institutions in the CFR era. Just as some patients reported in Table 22.5 underwent CFR, not all patients in Table 22.5 underwent CFR. Five-year survival rates were generally 65% to 75%, and 10-year rates were approximately 60%, representing improvements over results from the pre–CFR era (Table 22.5). Rates of continuous freedom from disease (5-year minimum) also increased (from 5% to 20% in the pre–CFR era to 35% to 40% in the CFR series). Locoregional recurrence remained the most common pattern of failure, occurring in 50% to 60% of all patients and accounting for 75% to 80% of all failures. Although median time to local or locoregional failure is short (6–18 months) (73,74,113), approximately 35% to 40% of local or locoregional failures occurred after 5 years (104,108,109,113). For esthesioneuroblastoma, 5-year survival figures do not portray an entirely accurate picture of treatment efficacy. Many patients who were reported as survivors at 5 years in Table 22.6 were living with uncontrolled disease; had already undergone surgical salvage of locally recurrent disease; or were destined to have their first recurrence beyond 5 years. Some survivors at 10 years also had uncontrolled disease. Approximately two thirds of local or regional failures were suitable for salvage attempts, which were successful in 40% to 45% of patients, leading to successful salvage rates of approximately 25% among all patients with locoregional recurrence (104,108,113). Although treatment results have improved in the CFR era, results are not good enough to allow any indicated component (surgery, RT, or chemotherapy) of therapy to be safely deleted as has been sug-

TABLE 22.5 Esthesioneuroblastoma: Results of Treatment in the Precraniofacial Resection Era

Institution (reference)	Survival: 5 years	Survival: 10 years	Survival: CFD (5-year minimum)	Tumor-related death rate: 0–5 years	Tumor-related death rate: 5–10 years	Tumor-related death rate: Local or locoregional recurrence
Memorial Sloan-Kettering Cancer Center, New York City, 1981 (36)	52%	ND	2/31 (6%)	ND	ND	23/31 (74%)
University of Michigan, Ann Arbor, 1982 (112)	50%	ND	4/21 (19%)	6/16 (38%)	3/10 (30%)	14/21 (67%)
Mayo Clinic, Rochester, MN, 1983 (34)	58%	ND	4/19 (21%)	8/20 (40%)	5/12 (42%)	13/21 (62%)
Institut Gustave-Roussy, Villejuif, France, 1988 (35)	60%	21%	5/31 (16%)	14/34 (41%)	9/20 (45%)	24/36 (67%)

CFD, continuously free of disease; ND, no data.

TABLE 22.6 Esthesioneuroblastoma: Results of Treatment in the Craniofacial Resection Era

Institution (reference)	Years of treatment	Survival: 5 years	Survival: 10 years	CFD (5-year minimum)	Local or locoregional recurrence
University of Virginia, Charlottesville, 1988 (244)	1976–1985	71%[a]	66%[a]	24% (9 yr)	7/12 (58%)
Mt. Sinai Medical Center, New York City, 1990 (139)	1977–1989	ND	ND	4/5 (80%)	1/5 (20%)
Memorial Sloan-Kettering Cancer Center, New York City, 1991 (109)	1975–1985	86%	70%	57% (5 yr) 41% (10 yr)	8/13 (62%)
University of California, Los Angeles, 1992 (140)	1970–1990	74%	60%	8/18 (44%)	9/17 (53%)
Mayo Clinic, Rochester, MN, 1993 (104)	1951–1990	69%	60%	34% (10 yr)	25/49 (51%)[b]
University of Michigan, Ann Arbor, 1993 (154)	1978–1989	9/15 (60%)	ND	5/15 (33%)	9/15 (60%)
Princess Margaret Hospital, Toronto, Ontario, 1997 (245)	1981–1994	5/6 (83%)	ND	3/6 (50%)	3/6 (50%)
Institut Gustave-Roussy, Villejuif, France, 1986 (113)	1980–1995	51%	ND	38% (5 yr)	24/40 (60%)
Martin Luther University, Halle/Saale, Germany, 1999 (246)	1986–1998	10/15 (67%)	ND	5/15 (33%)	9/15 (60%)
University of Cincinnati, Ohio, 2000 (37)	1970–1999	6/11 (54%)	ND	4/10 (40%)	4/10 (40%)
Odense University Hospital, Odense, Denmark, 2000 (74)	1977–1997	45%	30%	17%	ND
Universities of Cologne and Münster, Germany, 2001 (155)	1981–1998	6/13 (46%)	3/9 (33%)	5/13 (38%)	6/17 (35%)

CFD, continuously free of disease; ND, no data.
[a]Cause-specific survival.
[b]Local failure only.

gested by some authors who suggested that CFR alone might suffice. Biller et al. (139) report on five patients with highly select "early" T1 disease with a minimum 5-year follow-up after CFR. Although four of five tumors were locally controlled, we do not believe that this small experience in a tiny subset of favorable patients can be generalized.

Foote et al. (73) reviewed 49 patients with previously untreated esthesioneuroblastoma treated at the Mayo Clinic from 1951 to 1990. Five-year actuarial overall survival was 69%. Twenty-three of 47 evaluable patients (49%) developed local recurrence. The only significant predictor of overall survival, disease-free survival, and local control was Hyams grade. The Mayo Clinic data provide evidence for a benefit of postoperative RT for all grades and stages of disease after gross total excision. The 8-year actuarial local control rate in 22 patients after gross total excision alone was 41% versus 88% in 16 patients after gross total excision plus RT, even though the latter group had less favorable disease characteristics (94% of RT patients had stage C or D disease vs. 45% of surgery-alone cases; 38% of the RT patients had Hyams grade 3 or 4 tumors vs. 15% of the gross total excision-alone patients). Tables 22.7 and 22.8 show local control results by Hyams grade and Mayo Clinic stage according to treatment technique. The data suggest a role for postoperative RT for all patients after gross total resection. High-grade tumors recurred rapidly, whereas low-grade lesions had more indolent courses, a finding that may explain the marked variability in clinical courses observed by many other authors who did not use the Hyams grading system.

SINONASAL UNDIFFERENTIATED CARCINOMA

Inability to achieve local control (often with an intracranial component of failure) remains the biggest problem (39,75). Distant metastasis is also frequent. Reported median survival time is in the range of 10 to 16 months. Five-year survival rates are approximately 15% (37,39). The best results have been reported after neoadjuvant chemotherapy, preoperative RT, and surgical resection (164).

MALIGNANT MELANOMA

Malignant melanomas of the nasal cavity have a higher rate of 5-year survival than those that arise in the paranasal sinuses (87,214). Local recurrence, even in patients with negative surgical margins, is common (46,87,165). At least 50% to 60% of patients develop distant metastases, often preceded by local recurrence (42,43,46,87,215,216). Reported 5-year survival rates are 15% to 25% (43,44,46,87,133,165,214,217,218) and 10-year rates are 0 to 10% (87,218) with no decline in the death rate with time (87,133). Distant metastases may occur as late as 15 to 30 years after treatment (133). Ultimately, cure is rarely achieved.

TABLE 22.7 Esthesioneuroblastoma: 8-Year Local Control According to Treatment Technique (Mayo Clinic, 1951–1990)

Hyams grade	Local control at 8 years: Gross total resection alone (n = 22)	Local control at 8 years: Gross total resection plus RT (n = 16)
1–2	45%	100%
3–4	0%	55%

RT, radiation therapy.
Source: Foote RL, Morita A, Ebersold MJ, et al. Esthesioneuroblastoma: the role of adjuvant radiation therapy. *Int J Radiat Oncol Biol Phys* 1993;27:835–842.

TABLE 22.8 Esthesioneuroblastoma: 8-Year Local Control According to Treatment Technique (Mayo Clinic, 1951–1990)

Mayo Clinic stage	Local control at 8 years	
	Gross total resection alone (n = 22)	Gross total resection plus RT (n = 16)
A–B	47%	100% (1 patient)
C–D	40%	84%

RT, radiation therapy.
Source: Foote RL, Morita A, Ebersold MJ, et al. Esthesioneuroblastoma: the role of adjuvant radiation therapy. *Int J Radiat Oncol Biol Phys* 1993;27:835–842.

INVERTED PAPILLOMA

Recurrence after limited excision usually occurs within 2 years (175); more extensive operations (lateral rhinotomy–medial maxillectomy) are associated with both lower rates of recurrence and longer intervals to recurrence (48). The predominant sites of recurrence after resection are the ethmoid and maxillary sinuses (48).

Lawson et al. (48) operated on 112 patients at Mt. Sinai Medical Center from 1973 to 1993. In 84%, *en bloc* excision through lateral rhinotomy–medial maxillectomy was performed. The recurrence rate in these patients was 13.8%, with an average interval to recurrence of 56 months (range, 15–144 months). Only 4 of 13 recurrences (31%) occurred within 2 years, and 5 (38%) occurred at 7 to 12 years. Conservative removal of tumor (septectomy, intranasal sphenoethmoidectomy, or transantral sphenoethmoidectomy) was performed in 15 patients who demonstrated localization to the septum, inferior turbinate, or middle meatus, with minimal extension to the adjacent ethmoid or maxillary sinuses. There were three recurrences (20%) in the latter group.

Ten patients with advanced or recurrent inverted (eight patients) or cylindrical (two patients) papillomas of the nasal cavity and paranasal sinuses were treated with RT at the University of Florida between 1969 and 1989 (54). Two patients had concomitant invasive squamous cell carcinoma and one had squamous cell carcinoma *in situ*. Nine of the ten patients had experienced one or more local recurrences before RT. Most received 60 to 65 Gy at 1.8 Gy per fraction.

Three patients were treated with RT alone (one medically inoperable, two incompletely resectable). One died of local recurrence (frontal lobe invasion) at 17 months; another developed local recurrence at 12 years and was alive with disease at 15 years; the third patient died of unrelated cause at 7 years with local tumor control. In the latter patient, there was 60% to 70% regression of tumor at the completion of RT and complete disappearance at 6 months.

Six patients received postoperative RT for gross residual (2 patients), microscopic residual (1 patient), questionable margins (2 patients), or associated invasive cancer (1 patient). Five of six patients remained locally controlled at 8.5, 8.5, 9, 9, and 20.5 years. One patient developed local recurrence at 6.5 years and died of local (brain) progression at 7.5 years.

One patient received preoperative RT for poorly resectable inverted papilloma with invasive squamous cell cancer. Tumor regressed by 70% at the completion of RT. Surgery was performed 6 weeks later; there was no tumor in the specimen. Local recurrence (verrucous carcinoma involving the orbit) developed at 13 years. The patient is alive at 16 years with local recurrence after several unsuccessful salvage attempts.

Of the three patients with squamous cell carcinoma or *in situ* cancer at diagnosis, one developed local recurrence (verrucous carcinoma) at 13 years; one recurred with squamous cell carcinoma at 6.5 years and died with brain invasion at 7.5 years; and the third had no evidence of disease at 8.5 years.

No patient developed transformation from benign to malignant tumor which is consistent with other reports (79,82,177, 219). The fact that three of four local recurrences occurred beyond 6 years reinforces the need for long-term follow-up.

Between 1977 and 1990, 25 patients were treated at Massachusetts General Hospital and Massachusetts Eye and Ear Infirmary with RT for inverted papilloma (7 patients) or inverted papilloma associated with squamous cell carcinoma (18 patients) (82). All had advanced or recurrent tumors. After presentation to Massachusetts General Hospital, 16 patients underwent gross total resection followed by RT, 8 had subtotal resection followed by RT, and 1 was unresectable and received RT alone. One-third of the patients had less than 2 years' follow-up. Local control was achieved in 22 of 25 patients (88%). Two patients died of recurrent disease.

Lethal Midline Granuloma (Nasal NK/T-Cell Lymphoma)

Thirty-four patients with polymorphic reticulosis limited to the upper aerodigestive tract and draining lymph nodes were treated with primary RT at the Mayo Clinic between 1936 to 1983 (61). The nasal cavity was involved in 91% of patients. Profound constitutional symptoms were common (62%): weight loss (median, 25 lbs), 44%; fever (usually >103°F), 50%; and night sweats, 21%. Chemotherapy was delivered to seven patients at relapse. Twelve patients relapsed with polymorphic reticulosis and 3 with diffuse histiocytic lymphoma, mostly within 3 years of treatment. Four of the 12 were successfully salvaged with chemotherapy (1 patient) or re-irradiation (3 patients) with 5 to 7 years of follow-up after salvage treatment. Actuarial survivals at 5, 10, and 20 years were 67%, 62%, ad 43%, respectively. Because the series spanned five decades, there was considerable variation of RT technique and dose. Time–dose analysis was performed based on both time–dose fractionation (TDF) scheme (220) and total RT dose. In-field failure rates at 10 years for TDF less than 65 versus ≥65 were 65% and 0%, respectively ($p = 0.0003$). Higher TDFs were also associated with higher survival rates ($p = 0.15$). In-field failure rates after less than 40 Gy versus ≥40 Gy were nearly significantly different ($p = 0.08$). Twenty percent of patients failed in the primary tumor area outside of the initial RT treatment volume (marginal failure). Neither age nor constitutional ("B") symptoms correlated with overall survival. Women had higher survival rates than men ($p = 0.04$).

Chen et al. (59) administered RT to 92 patients with lethal midline granuloma at the National Taiwan University Hospital between 1959 and 1993. Twenty patients also received combination chemotherapy, most commonly cyclophosphamide, doxorubicin, vincristine, and prednisone (CHOP). Eighty percent had disease confined to the head and neck area, whereas 20% had more disseminated disease. Of patients who received chemotherapy, 75% had tumors confined to the head and neck region. Five-, 10-, and 20-year survival rates were 60%, 56%, and 41%, respectively. Survival did not differ between those who did or did not receive adjuvant chemotherapy ($p = 0.63$). Five-, 10-, and 20-year disease-free survival rates were 57%, 53%, and 38%, respectively. Ten patients (11%) developed local recurrence. Fourteen patients (15%) developed systemic relapse; in 5 of the 14, distant relapse was associated with local recurrence. Two of 19 patients who experienced relapse were successfully salvaged at 3.5 to 4.0 years, one by re-irradiation and the other by chemotherapy.

Nasal Vestibule

Local control rates after RT or surgery are similar for comparably staged lesions.

SURGERY

Goepfert et al. (221) report on 10 patients treated surgically for squamous cell carcinoma of the nasal vestibule at the M. D. Anderson Cancer Center; all had 2-year minimum follow-up. Local control was obtained in 9 of 10 patients; 1 patient with local recurrence was successfully salvaged (ultimate local control rate, 100%). Five patients were treated with surgery at the Princess Margaret Hospital; four had early lesions and one patient had an advanced cancer (222). Local control was obtained in all five patients. Of nine patients treated surgically at the University of Leiden for relatively early stage cancers, local control was observed in eight patients (223). Oriba and Snow (224) treated three patients with squamous cell carcinoma 1.5 cm in diameter with Mohs surgery at the University of Wisconsin; disease was locally controlled in all patients at 0.7, 0.8, and 4.3 years, respectively. Seven patients were treated with surgery and postoperative RT at the Queensland Radium Institute for early stage cancer (T1, 4; T2, 1; TX, 2); the local control rate was 66% (193). Four patients with advanced T4 cancers ≥4 cm in size with bone invasion were treated with high-dose preoperative RT and surgery at the University of Florida; local control was obtained in all four patients.

RADIATION THERAPY

Sixty-three patients with squamous cell carcinoma of the nasal vestibule were treated with RT at the Dr. Daniel den Hoed Cancer Center in Rotterdam between 1978 and 1988; all had follow-up ≥46 months (187). Patients received EBRT alone (17 patients), brachytherapy alone (37 patients), or both modalities (9 patients). Local control was observed in 35 of 36 patients (97%) with tumors limited to the nasal vestibule and 20 of 27 patients (74%) with cancers extending to adjacent sites. The overall ultimate local control rate, including patients successfully salvaged after local recurrence was 92% (58 of 63 patients). Five-year absolute and cause-specific survival rates were 65% and 90%, respectively.

McNeese et al. (118) report results of 32 previously untreated patients with squamous cell carcinoma of the nasal vestibule who received RT alone at the M. D. Anderson Cancer Center between 1967 and 1984. None had lymph node metastases at diagnosis. In 11 patients with small, well-demarcated lesions, disease was controlled by interstitial radium or iridium implant. Disease was controlled in 20 of 21 patients treated with EBRT (electrons or electrons plus photons). Fourteen patients received elective neck RT to the upper neck and/or the facial nodes; none developed nodal failure. Four of 18 patients who received no elective nodal irradiation developed neck node recurrences; 2 were successfully salvaged. One significant complication occurred (maxillary osteoradionecrosis).

Between 1970 and 1995, 60 patients were treated with RT alone (56 patients) or RT followed by surgery (4 patients) at the University of Florida. Local control after RT alone was: T1 and T2, 94%; T4, 71%; and overall, 85%. Tumor size and bone invasion significantly influenced the rate of local control.

The neck remained continuously controlled in 88% of patients in whom primary control was achieved when no elective neck treatment was administered. All five neck failures were salvaged. Of eight patients who failed locally, successful surgical salvage was achieved in four. Distant metastases developed in 3 of 60 patients (5%): 1 of 46 (2%) who had continuous locoregional control versus 2 of 14 (14%) who experienced locoregional recurrence. The overall 5-year survival rate was 74%.

TABLE 22.9 Nasal Vestibule Cancer: 5-Year Local Control According to Tumor Size, Extent, and Dose After External Beam Irradiation (Princess Margaret Hospital, 1958–1983)

	Tumor dose	
Tumor size	<50 Gy/5 wk	≥50 Gy/5 wk
<2 cm	11[a] (100%)[b]	22 (95%)
≥2 cm	11 (30%)	11 (82%)
Extension to cartilage, bone, lip, ala, columella		
No	7 (86%)	20 (95%)
Yes	15 (51%)	13 (85%)

[a]Number of patients in category.
[b]Percentage of patients whose tumors were controlled locally at 5 years.
Source: Modified from Wong CS, Cummings BJ, Elhakim T, et al. External irradiation for squamous cell carcinoma of the nasal vestibule. *Int J Radiat Oncol Biol Phys* 1986;12:1943–1946.

Five-year cause-specific survival rates for 56 patients treated with RT alone were as follows: T1 and T2, 94%; T4, 86%; and overall, 91%. All four patients treated with preoperative RT followed by resection for advanced (>4 cm with bone invasion) T4 disease remained alive and disease-free at 27, 33, 33, and 47 months, compared with 0 of 3 patients who received RT alone (120).

Wong et al. (119) report results of 46 patients who underwent EBRT for squamous cell carcinoma of the nasal vestibule at the Princess Margaret Hospital between 1958 and 1983. The 5-year local control rate for 34 patients with tumors less than 2 cm in size was 97% versus 57% for patients with larger tumors. Patients whose tumors extended to cartilage, bone, upper lip, skin of the ala or columella had a lower rate of local control (68%) than those without such extensions (90%). When higher doses were given, the adverse effects of size and tumor extension were partially overcome (Table 22.9). Mak et al. (225) note almost identical effects of dose and lesion size on local control rates in 47 patients who received EBRT at the Rotterdam Radiotherapy Institute.

The highest rates of local control have been obtained after interstitial implant alone: 26 of 27 T1 and T2 lesions treated with iridium at the Institut Gustave-Roussy (189); 9 of 9 cancers treated with radium at the University of Florida; 11 of 11 cancers treated with iridium or radium at the M. D. Anderson Cancer Center (118); 35 of 36 cancers treated by interstitial iridium in Rotterdam (187); and 11 of 11 T1 and T2 tumors treated with iridium at the Norwegian Radium Hospital (186). These high rates of local control (92 of 94, 98%) are partly due to case selection, but also are a result of delivering high-dose (55–75 Gy) RT in a short overall treatment time (5–7 days).

COMPLICATIONS OF RADIATION THERAPY

Nasal Cavity and Paranasal Sinuses

Serious complications of RT consist of osteoradionecrosis of the maxilla; radiation-induced injury to the brain or brainstem; and radiation-induced injury to the visual apparatus. Also at risk is the pituitary–hypothalamic axis which receives incidental RT. The risk of complications is higher in patients who undergo high-dose RT alone than in patients who undergo surgery and lesser dose RT.

BONE

The maxilla is relatively resistant to injury from high-dose RT in comparison with the mandible. Necroses are sometimes precipitated by dental extractions in the post-RT period. Patients in whom extractions must be performed after high-dose RT currently undergo a course of prophylactic hyperbaric oxygen (HBO) therapy (20 preextraction dives, followed by extractions, followed by 10 postextraction dives), which significantly reduces the risk of this complication (226).

BRAIN AND BRAINSTEM

Approximately 10% of patients who receive incidental high-dose RT to the brain develop transient CNS syndrome consisting usually of lethargy, decreased cerebration, vertigo, and headaches. The syndrome typically appears 2 to 3 months after treatment, lasts 2 to 6 weeks, then disappears spontaneously. Patients should be forewarned of this alarming problem because it appears about the time that they have fully recovered from acute effects of RT. The syndrome is believed to result from transient demyelination secondary to incidental brain RT. The latent period corresponds to the turnover time for myelin; the syndrome may be similar in etiology to Lhermitte sign of the spinal cord.

Brain necrosis in a carefully fractionated RT scheme using 1.8 Gy per fraction once a day or 1.1 to 1.2 Gy twice a day is rare. The complication is irreversible, progressive, and sometimes fatal. Signs and symptoms depend on the area and volume of brain irradiated and may simulate an intracranial mass. The essential lesion is demyelination with loss of oligodendrogliocytes and focal or diffuse white matter necrosis. Both small vessel and glial cell damage are responsible. Time to development is 6 months to 2 years, although occasionally injury is seen later. Injury may result in impaired mental function in adults, learning disabilities in children, seizures, dementia, and death. No specific therapy exists. Some necrotic foci act like mass lesions; resection may be life saving in this circumstance. Corticosteroid treatment may relieve surrounding cerebral edema. The differential diagnosis includes recurrent cancer or other CNS disease that produces a similar clinical picture.

Brainstem necrosis is also unusual. Time to onset is usually approximately 1 year, and death usually follows within 1 to 6 months. Common signs and symptoms include nystagmus, cranial nerve palsies, ataxia, paralysis, and anesthesia. Bowden reports the combination of unilateral seventh-nerve palsy and contralateral hemiplegia (227).

PITUITARY

The pituitary and hypothalamus usually receive incidental irradiation. Hypopituitarism resulting from RT was not recognized until the mid-1960s. The problem is much more widely recognized today, using sophisticated radioimmunoassay and stimulation tests that rely on synthetic hypothalamic hormones not available to earlier investigators. The incidence of clinical hypopituitarism in adults treated for paranasal sinus tumors is approximately 3% to 4%. Pretreatment measurements of thyroxine (T_4), thyroid-stimulating hormone (TSH), and morning serum cortisol are performed in all patients. Testosterone levels are obtained in male patients. Follicle-stimulating hormones (FSH) and luteinizing hormones (LH) are checked in postmenopausal female patients. Tests are repeated annually or as indicated.

VISUAL APPARATUS

The largest body of data on time–dose relationships for ocular and optic nerve injury comes from the University of Florida series, which spans almost four decades (228–231).

When results of CFR were first reported in the 1970s, it was suggested (152) that orbital exenteration should be performed whenever the ethmoid sinuses were involved; failure to do so frequently led to orbital recurrence and survival rates were reduced by half. Extrapolating from these data, it became institutional policy at the University of Florida to encompass the majority of the ipsilateral eye within the RT treatment portals when the ethmoid sinuses were involved. Computed tomography and MRI were not available at the time to assess the degree of orbital involvement, so the initial treatment volumes tended to be generous. Furthermore, it was thought in the 1960s and early 1970s that the retina and optic nerve were relatively resistant to the effects of RT. The sparse literature that existed at that time considerably overestimated the tolerance of these areas, suggesting that 68 Gy in 30 fractions at 2.27 Gy per fraction was within retinal tolerance (232).

Following recognition of some cases of radiation retinopathy and optic neuropathy in the early 1970s, all patients at the University of Florida who subsequently received incidental ocular or optic nerve RT underwent baseline ophthalmologic evaluations. All patients were followed by ophthalmologists both during the course of RT and indefinitely after RT, providing over 20 years of prospectively acquired clinical data from approximately 1976 to the present.

Also since the mid-1970s, doses to the optic nerves and retina were calculated prospectively during treatment planning so that accurate dose calculations were available in the majority of patients. This dataset is unlikely to be duplicated in modern times because practice concepts, treatment techniques, imaging abilities, and our understanding of RT injury have all changed.

Several types of RT injury may lead to blindness, some of which are correctable but most are not. A brief summary of the most common scenarios follows.

Lens

If one irradiates the lens, one can reasonably expect development of a cataract, which is often delayed for a number of years. If the dose or RT was not so high as to produce retinal injury, then the cataract can be extracted and vision restored.

Lacrimal Tissue

If all of the orbital contents are radiated, then there is a risk of injury to the major lacrimal gland and accessory lacrimal tissue in the lids. Between 1964 and 1989, 33 patients at the University of Florida with extracranial head and neck tumors received RT to an entire orbit. Most were treated with cobalt-60. The dose to the lacrimal apparatus was calculated at a depth of 1 cm from the anterior skin surface, the approximate depth of the major lacrimal gland. The end point of the study was "severe dry eye syndrome" sufficient to produce visual loss secondary to corneal opacification, ulceration, or vascularization.

The tear film itself is a complex structure consisting of three layers; a lipid outer layer, middle aqueous layer, and inner mucus layer. Loss of any of the three normal constituents of the tear film leads to rapid tear film breakup with resultant dry spots that expose the corneal epithelium to damage. Paradoxically, patients with "dry eye syndrome" may actually complain of excess lacrimation, but the tears are of poor quality and are insufficient to protect the corneal epithelium.

Thirteen patients did not develop severe dry eye complications. Symptoms in those patients were either absent (9 patients) or mild (4 patients who had tearing and sensitivity to wind without reduction in visual acuity).

Three patients with severe dry eye complications that occurred after low doses (32 Gy/16 fractions/22 days; 35.5 Gy/20 fractions/32 days; and 45 Gy/21 fractions/29 days) slowly developed corneal vascularization and opacification over periods of 4, 8, and 11 years, respectively. Seventeen other patients who developed severe dry eye complications received higher doses and had more fulminant courses; the latter patients were usually severely symptomatic within 1 month of completion of RT and were noted to have severe corneal opacification and vascularization by 9 to 10 months. Ultimate visual acuity in the 20 patients with severe dry eye syndrome was "counts fingers" (1 patient), "hand motion" (1 patient), light perception (5 patients), and no light perception (13 patients). Observed corneal reactions included edema, ulceration, bacterial infection, vascularization, opacification, and perforation of the globe. Five patients with corneal ulceration developed iritis in association with the ulceration. Symblepharon was noted in one patient. One patient developed phthisis bulbi. Three globes perforated spontaneously. Conservative measures, including artificial tears, lubricating ointments, topical or systemic antibiotics, steroids, narcotic analgesics, tranquilizers, bandage contact lens, retro-orbital alcohol injections, conjunctival flaps, and tarsorrhaphy were generally unsuccessful in alleviating pain. Twelve patients required enucleation or evisceration because of continued pain or perforation of the globe. The incidence of severe dry eye complications was not affected by patient age. Figure 22.11 (230) summarizes time–dose data from the University of Florida and several other sources. In this sigmoid dose response curve, it is seen that the probability of severe dry eye complications increases steeply above approximately 35 Gy.

Retina

If it is possible to shield enough lacrimal tissue to prevent "severe dry eye syndrome," then at higher doses, one risks radiation retinopathy. Radiation retinopathy usually develops 2 to 3 years

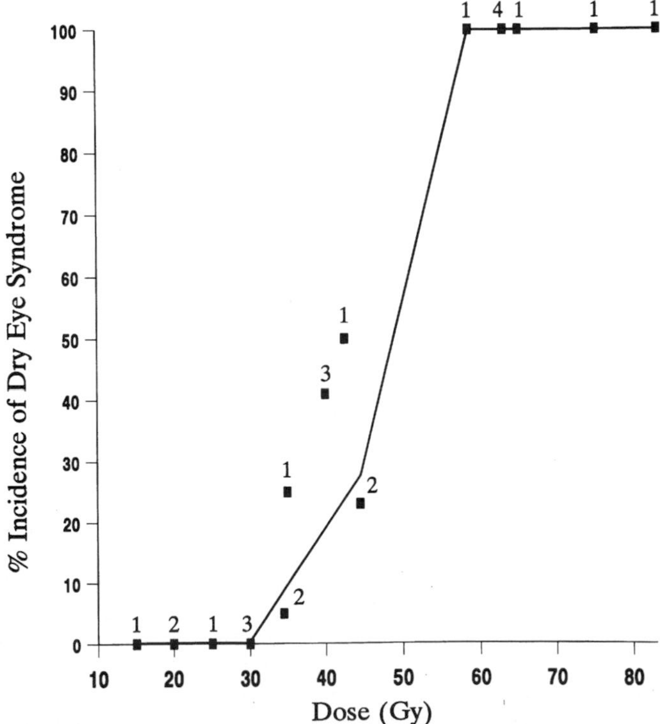

Figure 22.11 Sigmoid dose response curve for production of dry eye complications. Points are numbered to correspond with authors: *1*, Parsons et al. (230); *2*, Bessell et al. (234); *3*, Letschert et al. (235); and *4*, Morita and Kawabe (248). (From Parsons JT, Bova FJ, Fitzgerald CR, et al. Severe dry-eye syndrome following external beam irradiation. *Int J Radiat Oncol Biol Phys* 1994;30:775–780, with permission.)

after RT and has many characteristics of diabetic retinopathy, including retinal neovascularization; retinal hemorrhage; retinal detachment; and neovascularization of the face of the iris (rubeosis iridis), which in turn can lead to neovascular (i.e., "closed-angle") glaucoma, retinal destruction, retinal edema, and blindness. Blindness secondary to retinopathy is usually painless unless glaucoma develops. If severe glaucoma occurs, ocular removal is frequently necessary for pain control because this type of glaucoma often responds poorly to medical management.

At the University of Florida, 68 retinae in 64 patients received EBRT. All patients had a minimum of 3 years' ophthalmologic follow-up (range, 3–26 years; mean, 9 years; median, 8 years). Twenty-seven eyes in 26 patients developed radiation retinopathy resulting in visual acuity of 20/200 or worse, at mean and median times of 2.8 and 2.5 years (range, 1–6.5 years), respectively. Fourteen patients developed rubeosis iridis or neovascular glaucoma.

The earliest symptom of radiation retinopathy was usually diminished vision; in two patients the earliest reported symptoms were neovascular complications (pain due to glaucoma in one and hyphema in the other). Visual acuity and ophthalmoscopic appearance of the fundus remained normal in most patients until symptoms appeared, then rapidly deteriorated over a period of several months, with the onset of retinal hemorrhages, exudates, cotton-wool spots, neovascularization, and areas of capillary nonperfusion on fluorescein angiogram. In three patients, retinal hemorrhages, microaneurysms, cotton-wool spots, or retinal pigment epithelium atrophy preceded the onset of visual deterioration by 1 to 2 years. Four patients considered to be at high risk of developing proliferative retinopathy were treated electively with panretinal laser photocoagulation in an attempt to prevent neovascular complications. In three patients, the laser was applied when retinopathy was first detected (at 16 months, 20 months, and 4 years). In the fourth patient, in whom the retinal dose was 77.6 Gy, prophylactic laser treatment was applied 2 months after RT. None of the four eyes receiving laser treatment developed rubeosis or neovascular glaucoma.

Fourteen of the remaining 23 eyes developed rubeosis iridis or neovascular glaucoma, including the contralateral non-lasered eye in one of the four patients treated with panretinal laser photocoagulation. Rubeosis iridis or glaucoma was first detected 17 months to 5.5 years after RT (mean, 32 months; median, 28 months). Neovascular glaucoma was generally first recognized weeks to months after the onset of visual deterioration due to retinopathy. One of the 14 patients with rubeosis was treated with panretinal laser photocoagulation and direct laser of new vessels on the face of the iris 2 years after RT, when early rubeosis was noted. Fluorescein angiography at that time showed a deficit in the choriocapillaris circulation. Over the next month, severe rubeosis developed with marked increase in intraocular pressure. Another patient who underwent laser treatment of new vessels on the iris showed marked regression of rubeosis and return of intraocular pressure to normal. Six patients required enucleation of blind painful eyes after failure to control glaucoma. In two patients, intraocular pressure was controlled with glaucoma medications which included corticosteroids; in both patients, rubeosis regressed or disappeared.

The occurrence of radiation retinopathy according to total dose and dose per fraction is shown in Table 22.10 (229). Radiation retinopathy was not observed in 33 eyes that received doses less than 45 Gy. For doses between 45 and 54.99 Gy, the incidence was 6 of 12 (50%); between 55 and 64.99, 10 of 12 (83%), and above 65 Gy, 11 of 11 (100%). There was increased risk in patients treated with fraction sizes ≥1.9 Gy; those who received chemotherapy; older patients; and those with diabetes mellitus, although none of these factors reached statistical significance.

TABLE 22.10 Incidence of Vision Loss Due to Radiation Retinopathy According to Dose and Dose per Fraction (68 Eyes in 64 Patients) (University of Florida, 1964–1989)

	Dose (Gy) per fraction		
Dose (Gy)	<1.9	≥1.9	Total
<30	0/5	0/2	0/7
30–39.99	0/10	0/6	0/16
40–44.99	0/8	0/2	0/10
45–49.99	3/6	2/3	5/9
50–54.99	1/3	No data	1/3
55–59.99	1/2	2/2	3/4
60–64.99	4/5	3/3	7/8
65–69.99	2/2	1/1	3/3
70–74.99	4/4	1/1	5/5
≥75	2/2	1/1	3/3

Source: Parsons JT, Bova FJ, Fitzgerald CR, et al. Radiation retinopathy after external-beam irradiation: analysis of time-dose factors. *Int J Radiat Oncol Biol Phys* 1994;30:765–773.

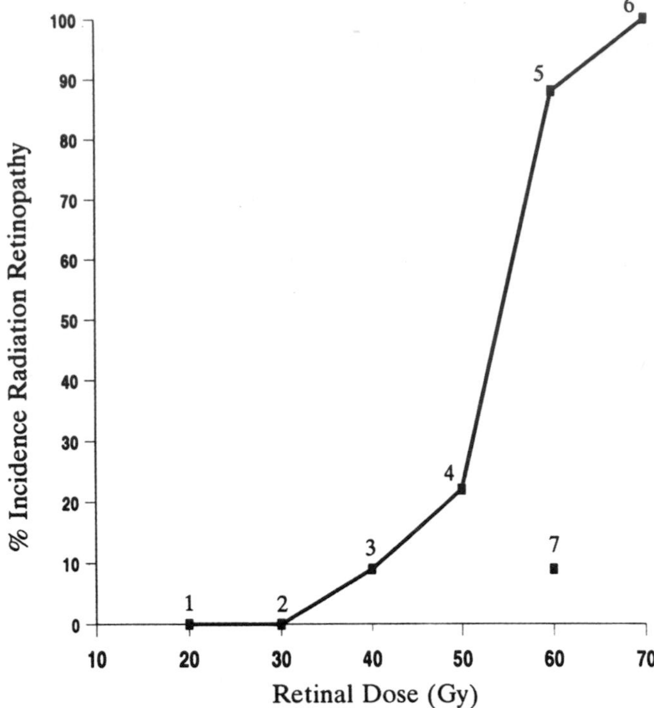

Figure 22.12 Percent incidence of radiation retinopathy for patients whose total doses were administered in fraction sizes of ≤2 Gy. Points are numbered to correspond with authors: *1,* Peterson et al. (233), 20 Gy in 10 fractions, incidence 0 of 242 patients; *2,* Peterson et al. (233), 30 Gy over 15 fractions, incidence 0 of 69 patients; and Bessell et al. (234), 25–30 Gy in 15 fractions, incidence 0 of 10 patients; *3,* Letschert et al. (235) 40 Gy in 20 fractions, incidence 2 of 22 patients (9%); *4,* Parsons et al. (229) 45–55 Gy (≤2.05 Gy/fraction), incidence 2 of 9 patients (22%); *5,* Parsons et al. (229) 57.5–63 Gy (≤2 Gy/fraction), incidence 7 of 8 patients (88%); *6,* Parsons et al. (229) 65–74 Gy (≤2.06 Gy/fraction) incidence 8 of 8 patients (100%); *7,* Chan and Shukovsky (236), 60 Gy in 30 fractions, incidence 2 of 22 patients (9%). (From Parsons JT, Bova FJ, Fitzgerald CR, et al. Radiation retinopathy after external-beam irradiation: Analysis of time-dose factors. *Int J Radiat Oncol Biol Phys* 1994;30: 765–773, with permission.)

Time–dose data from Peterson et al. (233), Bessell et al. (234), Letschert et al. (235), Chan and Shukovsky (236), and Parsons et al. (229) were used to construct the sigmoid dose–response curve in Figure 22.12. The data are for treatments administered with fraction sizes ≤2 Gy per fraction. In the University of Florida data, patients with unusual risk factors (diabetes mellitus, chemotherapy) are excluded. The curve begins to ascend steeply after 45 Gy.

Optic Nerve

If the patient does not experience retinal injury, blindness may still result from optic nerve or optic chiasm injury. Developmentally, the optic nerve is part of the CNS and has approximately the same radiation sensitivity as the spinal cord. Between 1964 and 1989, 215 optic nerves in 113 patients received fractionated EBRT at the University of Florida (minimum ophthalmologic follow-up was 3–21 years). After 1976, all had follow-up prospectively in anticipation of possible injury.

Seventeen nerves developed optic neuropathy, usually at 2 to 3 years (range, 1–14 years) (Table 22.11) (231). No injuries were observed in 106 nerves that received total doses less than 59 Gy. Among nerves that received ≥60 Gy, dose per fraction was more important than total dose (Fig. 22.13) (231). The 15-year actuarial risk of optic neuropathy after ≥60 Gy was 11% with fraction sizes less than 1.9 Gy versus 47% with ≥1.9 Gy per fraction. There was an increased risk with increasing age. Table 22.12 (231) is an analysis of dose compared with patient age for 123 optic nerves that received ≥55 Gy. No patient under 50 years of age developed optic neuropathy. There is no proven effective treatment for optic neuropathy, although hyperbaric oxygen and corticosteroids are worth trying. Retinopathy did not occur in any eyes that developed optic neuropathy.

Two types of optic neuropathy were recognized, anterior ischemic optic neuropathy and retrobulbar optic neuropathy. Anterior ischemic optic neuropathy is believed to be caused by vascular injury to the nerve head. Edema of the disc with flame-shaped hemorrhage in a sectoral pattern may be present. Ischemic neuropathy occurred in five eyes in 4 patients at 2, 2, 2.5, 3, and 4 years (mean, 2.7 years) after doses shown in Table 22.11 (231). Loss of vision was gradual (over several months) and painless. Optic atrophy was noted eventually in all five eyes.

Retrobulbar optic neuropathy is believed to represent more proximal injury to the optic nerve. Disc edema and hemorrhage do not occur. Retrobulbar optic neuropathy developed in 12 nerves in 10 patients (Table 22.11) (231). Latent intervals were 1 to 14 years (mean, 47 months; median, 28 months). Three injuries were detected after 5 years. The initial symptom was a visual field defect in six patients. In three eyes, the patients noted sudden blindness, whereas in the other nine, vision deteriorated over a period of a few days to 2 months. Initial funduscopic examination usually revealed no abnormalities. In one patient, pallor of one sector of the disc was noted at presentation. Eventually optic atrophy occurred in all 12 eyes.

The length of follow-up of uninjured nerves was 3 to 21 years (mean, 8.1 years and median, 7.0 years). Eleven of 17 injuries (65%) were evident by 3 years. The occurrence of optic neuropathy according to total dose, fractionation scheme, and dose per fraction is given in Table 22.13 (231).

Compression of the visual pathways by recurrent neoplasm must be excluded with CT or MRI. There is frequently pathologic enhancement of the radiation-injured segment of the nerve on gadolinium-enhanced MRI.

A dose–response curve at 10 years for patients who received treatment at ≤2 Gy per fraction is shown in Figure 22.14 (231). Data from the University of California, San Francisco (237) are

TABLE 22.11 Time-Dose Parameters in Patients Who Developed Radiation-Induced Ischemic or Retrobulbar Optic Neuropathy (University of Florida, 1964–1989)

Patient number	Dose (Gy)	No. fractions	Overall treatment time (d)	Treatment course	Latent interval (yrs)	Final visual acuity
Ischemic optic neuropathy (5 eyes)						
1	60	30	76	Split	2	NLP
	60	30	76	Split	2	NLP
2	65	32	57	Split	3	NLP
3	67	35	49	Continuous	2.5	20/400
4	63	29	44	Continuous	4	20/400
Retrobulbar optic neuropathy (12 eyes)						
5	75	35	59	Split	14	20/400[a]
6	65	25	36	Continuous	1	NLP
7	68	35	64	Split	2.3	LP
8	70	41	63	Continuous	4	NLP
9	66	40	57	Continuous	6	NLP
	66	40	57	Continuous	8	NLP
10	59	30	43	Continuous	1.2	NLP
	62	30	43	Continuous	1.3	NLP
11	70	41	58	Continuous	2	NLP
12	72	68 (BID)	54	Continuous	2.5	NLP
13	74	39	55	Continuous	1.75	NLP
14	70	40	58	Continuous	3.75	NLP

[a]Altitudinal defect and constricted field.
LP, light perception; NLP, no light perception.
Source: Parsons JT, Bova FJ, Fitzgerald CR, et al. Radiation optic neuropathy after megavoltage external-beam irradiation: analysis of time-dose factors. *Int J Radiat Oncol Biol Phys* 1994;30:755–763.

also included. Dose data from the University of Florida (designated by 1 in Fig. 22.14) (231) are tabulated at 10 years of follow-up for patients whose treatments were administered at ≤2 Gy per fraction. Data are recorded in the middle of each dose range. Doses ranges and incidences of neuropathy were as follows: 25 to 34.99 Gy, 0 of 6 eyes; 35 to 44.99 Gy, 0 of 14 eyes; 45 to 54.99 Gy, 0 of 11 eyes; 55 to 64.99 Gy, 3 (25%) of 12 eyes; and 65 to 74.99 Gy, 9 (35%) of 26 eyes. Data from the University of California, San Francisco (designated by 2 in Fig. 22.14) (231) are recorded as the mean dose (54 Gy) for 49 patients whose follow-up was 1.5 to 18 years (median and mean follow-up approximately 4 and 5 years, respectively); optic neuropathy developed in 1 patient (2%). Almost simultaneous with the University of Florida publication, Jiang et al. (238) published a sigmoid dose–response curve based on the 5-year incidence of optic neuropathy and chiasm injury as a function of radiation dose for

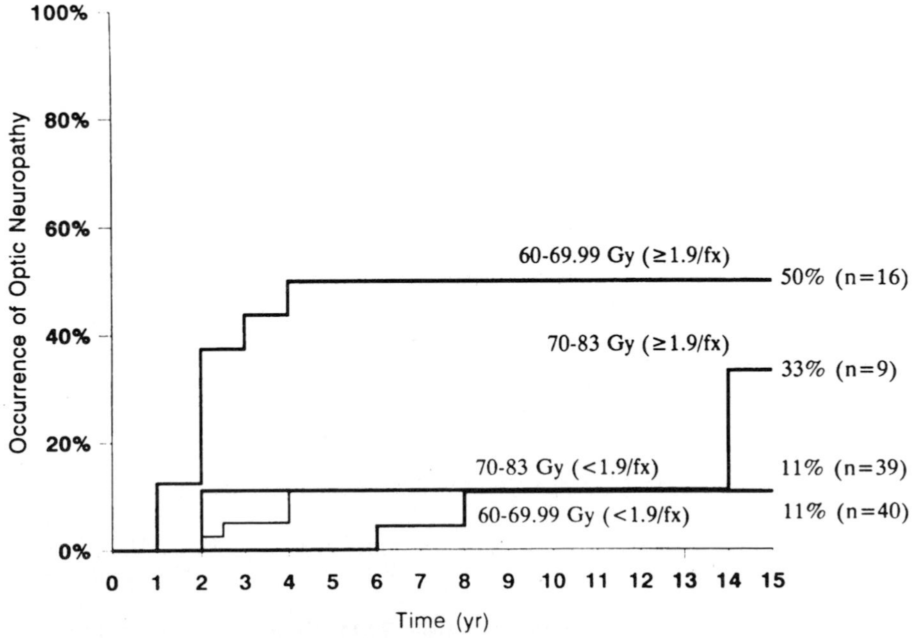

Figure 22.13 Probability of occurrence of optic neuropathy according to total dose and dose per fraction. University of Florida 1964–1989. *fx,* fraction. (From Parsons JT, Bova FJ, Fitzgerald CR, et al. Radiation optic neuropathy after megavoltage external-beam irradiation: analysis of time-dose factors. *Int J Radiat Oncol Biol Phys* 1994;30:755–763, with permission.)

TABLE 22.12 Optic Neuropathy According to Patient Age and Total Dose (University of Florida, 1964–1989)

Dose range (Gy)	Age at time of treatment (yr) <20	20–50	51–70[a]	>70[b]
55–59.99	0/1	0/9	1/6 (17%)	0/3
60–64.99	0/1	0/5	1/9 (11%)	3/4 (75%)
65–69.99	No data	0/14	3/15 (20%)	3/8 (38%)
70–74.99	No data	0/7	2/27 (7%)	3/4 (75%)
≥75	0/2	0/3	1/5 (20%)	No data
Total	0/4	0/38	8/62 (13%)	9/19 (47%)

[a]Optic nerve doses in Gy (fraction size in Gy) in injured patients (51–70 yrs): 59 (1.97); 62 (2.07); 67 (1.91); 68 (1.94); 65 (2.03); 72 (1.06); 70 (1.75); 75 (2.14).
[b]Optic nerve doses in Gy (fraction size in Gy) in injured patients (>70 yrs): 60 (2); 60 (2); 63 (2.17); 66 (1.65); 66 (1.65); 65 (2.6); 70 (1.71); 70 (1.71); 74.25 (1.9).
Source: Parsons JT, Bova FJ, Fitzgerald CR, et al. Radiation optic neuropathy after megavoltage external-beam irradiation: analysis of time-dose factors. *Int J Radiat Oncol Biol Phys* 1994;30:755–763.

patients treated at M. D. Anderson Cancer Center. The shape and inflection points of the curve are almost identical to those in Figure 22.14 (231).

Vision loss is most often unilateral, but bilateral blindness may also occur. The most common scenario leading to bilateral blindness includes ipsilateral radiation retinopathy (which is often "expected" when there is extensive orbital invasion) and contralateral optic neuropathy. Bilateral optic neuropathy or chiasm injury may also occur. The radiation oncologist responsible for treatment planning is advised to pay close attention to time–dose parameters for injury. Three-dimensional conformal and intensity-modulated RT techniques are both useful in limiting the dose to these vital structures. Despite all efforts, optic neuropathy will still occasionally be seen when attempting to control advanced disease with high-dose RT.

Nasal Vestibule

Irradiation of nasal vestibule carcinoma may result in nasal synechiae and occlusion of the nasal passages unless measures are taken to prevent this complication. The patient is instructed to douche the nose with a dilute saline solution and use long cotton-tipped applicator sticks to apply petrolatum jelly and gently lyse any developing adhesions twice daily until healing is complete. The patient is instructed to return to the clinic weekly until healing is complete to receive assistance in breaking down

TABLE 22.13 Optic Neuropathy According to Optic Nerve Dose, Fractionation Scheme, and Dose per Fraction (University of Florida, 1964–1989)

Dose range (Gy)	Once Daily: dose/fraction (Gy) <1.9 Gy[a]	≥1.9 Gy[b]	Twice daily[c] (1.2 Gy/fraction)
<30	0/7	0/3	0/2
30–39.99	0/25	No data	0/1
40–49.99	0/34	0/4	0/4
50–54.99	0/10	0/1	0/1
55–59.99	0/15	1/1	0/3
60–64.99	0/6	4/6	0/7
65–69.99	2/24	4/10	0/3
70–74.99	3/27	1/7	1/4
≥75	0/4	1/2	0/4

Median and mean lengths of follow-up: [a]8 and 7.5 years; [b]13 and 11 years; [c]4 and 4 years.
Source: Parsons JT, Bova FJ, Fitzgerald CR, et al. Radiation optic neuropathy after megavoltage external-beam irradiation: analysis of time-dose factors. *Int J Radiat Oncol Biol Phys* 1994;30:755–763.

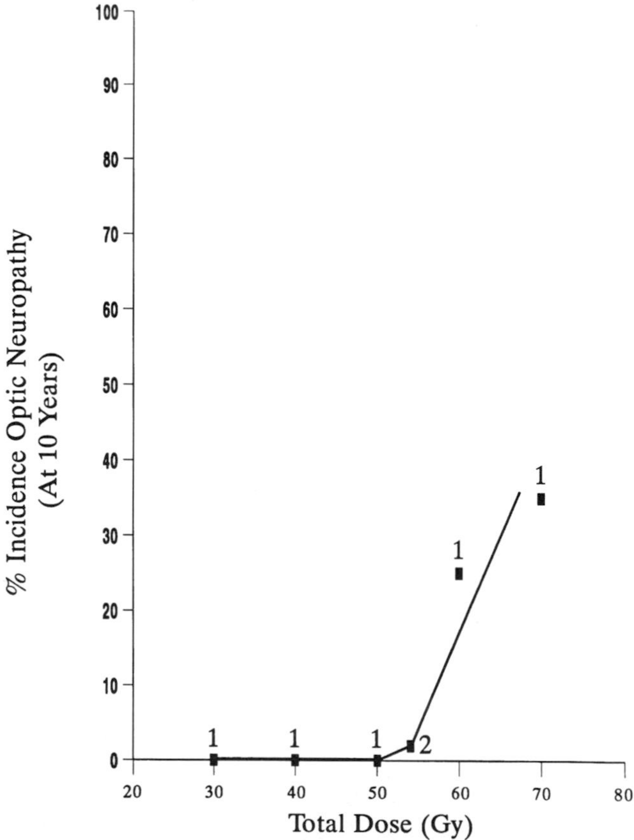

Figure 22.14 Dose–response data from the University of Florida and the University of California, San Francisco (237) for the development of optic neuropathy. *1*, University of Florida data; *2*, University of California, San Francisco data. (From Parsons JT, Bova FJ, Fitzgerald CR, et al. Radiation optic neuropathy after external-beam irradiation: analysis of time-dose factors. *Int J Radiat Oncol Biol Phys* 1994;30:755–763, with permission.)

any developing synechiae. Once mucosal healing is complete, most patients continue to douche the nose to remove crusts. Severe necroses of cartilage, soft tissue, or bone are uncommon. Small, asymptomatic defects in the nasal septum that were produced by tumor extension may persist after RT and do not require surgical repair. Small pits in the nasal dorsum at the sites of implanted radioactive needles may also persist.

In the University of Florida series (120) a total of 19 complications developed in 13 of the 56 patients (23%) treated with RT alone to the primary site. Eleven patients experienced minor, self-limited soft tissue necrosis that healed with conservative management within 6 months. One patient developed necrosis that lasted longer than 6 months. An additional patient with very extensive primary disease developed bilateral cataracts. Two of the four patients treated with high-dose preoperative RT and surgery experienced significant complications (bone exposure, wound breakdown). A third patient underwent resection of tissues thought to be recurrent tumor, but no tumor was noted in the specimen. Cosmesis was good in two patients and poor in the other two.

MANAGEMENT OF RECURRENCE

Nasal Cavity and Paranasal Sinuses

Salvage of primary recurrence generally consists of surgical resection plus postoperative RT if it has not already been administered. Unresectable recurrences are treated initially with chemotherapy or RT in hopes of making them resectable. If surgery cannot be used, high-dose RT with or without chemotherapy will produce some cures. Neck failure is managed by neck dissection RT.

For patients with esthesioneuroblastoma, salvage of neck failure by neck dissection and RT is successful in approximately 50% of patients (104,154). Cervical metastasis significantly predicts development of distant metastasis (113). Death following distant metastasis usually occurs within 2 to 3 years despite aggressive chemotherapy (35,74,104,110); rare long-term survivors are, however, reported (35). Combination chemotherapy in myeloablative doses with autologous bone marrow transplant has been used with occasional success (103).

Nasal Vestibule

Frequent follow-up for 3 years is important because recurrences often are salvaged by second-line treatment. Particular attention is paid to regional lymphatics. Primary recurrences after RT are excised and postsurgical failures are usually treated by RT. Management of recurrence is often successful, but deformity may be significant.

All five patients from the University of Florida who developed lymph node metastases with the primary site continuously controlled were successfully salvaged with neck dissection.

FUTURE DIRECTIONS

Treatment of tumors of the nasal cavity and paranasal sinuses should focus on cure as well as function. The era of super-radical single modality treatment is over. Cure with function is best achieved by combining at least two and sometimes all three modalities: surgery, RT, or chemotherapy. A future challenge will be how to use therapies that best complement each other in different circumstances. Some examples of common scenarios follow.

A patient with an early or moderately advanced resectable tumor of the paranasal sinuses or nasal cavity without orbital or intracranial extension would typically undergo surgery and postoperative RT.

A patient with more advanced, but still resectable, cancer of the paranasal sinuses whose tumor has breached the medial orbital wall and orbital floor with displacement of the globe would be a poor candidate for radical RT because the eye would almost certainly be destroyed. Likewise, preoperative RT would necessarily include a large segment of the ipsilateral globe. Surgery might first be a reasonable alternative if adequate reconstructive skills are available so that the eye can be suspended at its normal (cephalocaudad) level (assuming that tumor did not breach the periorbita and the eye can be preserved). If, however, the eye becomes ptotic after surgery and drops into the maxillary defect, not only will the patient have diplopia, but he or she may later develop blindness because the eye will receive full-dose RT due to its position within the tumor bed. As an alternative to a surgery-first approach, neoadjuvant chemotherapy might be used to produce initial tumor shrinkage; regression of intraorbital tumor would then allow the radiation oncologist to treat the eye to a lesser dose and lesser volume, followed by surgical resection. The same general philosophy applies to patients with intracranial extension.

Although both periorbita and dura are relatively resistant to tumor penetration, such penetrations do occur in a small percent of patients. These patients may have direct extension into the brain or orbital muscular cone. One can either surgically sacrifice these structures, or use neoadjuvant chemotherapy followed by RT with or without concurrent chemotherapy (usually cisplatin). Intraarterial chemotherapy may have a role in these patients, but few centers have any experience and complication rates are significant. In the event of complete response to chemotherapy, one still must choose between high-dose RT, or more moderate-dose RT and surgery. Questions that remain are whether the operation is necessary at all after complete chemotherapy response, and whether the surgery can be of more limited scope than would have been required had surgery been the first treatment. Our current preference would be modest-dose RT followed by a somewhat more limited resection.

Numerous scenarios are possible and there are many opportunities to be creative. Stereotactically aided treatment setups, three-dimensional conformal RT, and intensity-modulated RT will all likely become routine in managing these tumors in the coming decade (239–243). These techniques allow precise patient positioning and field reproducibility; unconventional angles of beam entry; geometric shaping of the radiation beam so that its contour corresponds to the "beam's-eye" view of the target; and geometric shaping of the isodose distribution by altering beam intensity (fluence) thus allowing deliberate inhomogeneity across target and avoidance areas. Although these techniques are of proven value in allowing dose reductions to critical structures in many patients, the techniques have not yet been proven to increase tumor control rates. Further, one can readily envision scenarios in patients with advanced cancers where these techniques will not allow dose reduction to optic nerves or chiasm because these structures may be situated within the tumor.

Another question that remains to be answered is how best to combine chemotherapy and RT. It is important that the treatments be given in such a way that there is an enhancement of tumor sensitization without an increase in late effects on tissues such as the visual pathway and brain. The future holds much promise as novel compounds are under active investigation. We are on the verge of moving to a new phase of molecularly targeted strategies with ultimate goals of providing more directed treatment with increased therapeutic efficacy and diminished associated morbidity.

RADIOLOGIC IMAGING CONCERNS

Bernard B. O'Malley and Suresh K. Mukherji

Advanced lesions of the nasal cavity and paranasal sinuses emphasize the pivotal role of imaging for directing treatment. The number of vital structures at risk and the variety of pathways for perineural and occult deep spread strongly warrant the need for pretreatment imaging. Computed tomography and MR play complementary roles for evaluating the skull base (249–252). Computed tomography is widely available and superior for evaluating the bony structures especially invasion of the periosteum of the lamina papyracea and erosion of the cribriform plate. Magnetic resonance imaging is superior for evaluating for retrograde perineural extension and degree of extension into the soft tissues. An important area that is often neglected is to determine the presence and degree of "intracranial involvement." Magnetic resonance imaging helps differentiate between a tumor that has eroded the cribriform plate but is extradural and a tumor that extends along the dural and a tumor that has invaded brain parenchyma. These various scenarios are all forms of "intracranial involvement" but are treated differently and are associated with different prognoses.

Both CT and MRI should be performed with contrast and should be acquired with a high spatial resolution algorithm, not the standard type used for brain imaging. Planning the MRI scan should also take advantage of matching the imaging planes of a CT protocol. This will allow close correlation between the modalities. Involvement of the orbit and its contents is pivotal and must be evaluated carefully by an experienced reader (253). The CT mages should be obtained in both the axial and the direct coronal plane for all sinonasal neoplasms. These images must be processed in the standard and bone algorithm and printed appropriately. Helical (spiral) CT techniques can produce reformatted views that can be presented in the coronal and sagittal planes and an infinite number of oblique views from the original dataset (see Fig. 4.14). This is especially useful in older adult who may have limited neck flexibility. Properly designed CT imaging protocols can answer most clinical questions, leaving MRI to resolve the remaining issues. Selective catheter angiography can assist in dose escalation by delivering chemotherapy directly to the primary site. In addition, producing higher intratumoral doses, novel combinations of local and systemic treatments have been devised to reduce local and systemic toxicity (253,254).

Magnetic resonance imaging for paranasal disorders can be performed in the standard "head coil," but the sections should be thinner than those used for brain imaging. The standard gap between sections should be minimized or eliminated by using volume acquisitions. The three most important types of "pulse-sequences" for MRI are the T1 and fat-suppressed contrast T1 and fast T2 series. Intravenous contrast is essential and post-contrast T1-weighted images should be performed in all three planes with fat suppression techniques.

Magnetic resonance imaging in this region is often lengthy. These series are performed as matched-image sets in at least two primary planes (Fig. 22.15). Each of these performed in all three primary imaging planes would result in 135 to 180 individual images per scan. This does not allow for additional series, such as magnetic resonance angiography (MRA) or time spent repeating a series because of patient motion.

Because local extraparanasal tumor extension is one of the important prognostic factors (255), each institution must develop standard imaging protocols that allow for proper sequencing of the more important images first. These can be followed by the supplemental projections later. This would, of course, vary slightly depending on the site of origin of the lesion. The simplest and most productive series for the paranasal sinuses are the T1-weighted images, as they have a strong signal and provide an exquisite outline of the extra-paranasal component of tumors against the background of the native fat planes of the deep face. Contrast-enhanced T1-weighted series are necessary to rule out perineural extension and tumor tracking away from the primary site along fascial planes. This series requires that fat suppression provide incremental benefit over CT. The T2-weighted series are vital for determining the extent to which the intrasinus signal abnormality represents tumor, reactive mucosal thickening, or obstructed secretions (256) (see Fig. 21.24). Fat-suppression applied to contrast-enhanced T1-weighted images helps suppress bright signal from surrounding fat, better revealing enhancement related to tumor. These images can be very helpful, however one must be aware of the "susceptibility artifacts" that obscure visualization of foramen rotundum and the nerve of the vidian canal in patients with well-pneumatized sphenoid sinuses. The presence of perineural extension cannot be evaluated in these patients. Fat-suppression is very helpful in post-operative patients, especially those with myocutaneous flaps. However, the presence of metallic clips creates susceptibility artifact in the surrounding tissue and prohibits visualization of the adjacent area.

Magnetic resonance angiography is an important adjunct to the imaging workup. There are several techniques of MRA. Evaluation of the carotid is now routinely being performed using intravenous gadolinium contrast. Noncontrast techniques are most commonly used to evaluate the intracranial circulation. It is important to review not only the reformatted images of the circle of Willis but also the axial "source" images which are used to create the projection images. Unanticipated abnormalities revealed by MRA occasionally determine the unresectable status of a given patient (Fig. 22.16).

The skull base can be divided into three segments from the perspective of extraparanasal tumor extension: the anterior, central, and lateral skull base. The *anterior* skull base is best evaluated in the direct coronal plane with CT or MRI. Computed tomography confirms the integrity of the anterior skull base at the cribriform–fovea complex. Because intracranial extension can occur without obvious bone destruction (Fig. 22.17), contrast-enhanced coronal MRI is required for that site and outperforms CT on that criterion. Furthermore, MRI better characterizes the degree of dural involvement, transdural extension, and brain cortex involvement if present (255) (Figs. 22.18, 22.19). Magnetic resonance imaging can overestimate the degree of dural involvement because of reactive dural thickening, but the thickened membranes should be considered positive until proved otherwise by frozen or permanent section.

The *central* skull base consists of the sphenoid bone, which is oblique to both the conventional axial and coronal imaging planes. Although this would ideally be imaged in a semi-axial plane, such as with nasopharynx primary tumors, most physicians are used to correlating between the axial and coronal views (Fig. 22.20). The coronal view is excellent for evaluation of the foramina lacerum, ovale and rotundum, the pterygoid canal, and the cavernous sinus and orbital fissures (Figs. 22.21, 22.22). Cavernous sinus involvement should be confirmed or excluded by carefully matched precontrast and postcontrast images.

The *lateral* skull base is occasionally involved by retromaxillary extraparanasal extension. This component is readily examined in the familiar axial plane (Fig. 22.23), tracking tumor through the parapharyngeal and carotid spaces and along the lateral pterygoid muscle to the temporal bone (257,258). The degree of distal internal carotid artery involvement is assessed on the spin-echo images and patency of the lumen confirmed with MRA sequences, which may preclude catheter angiography in some instances.

The absolute contraindications for resectability for cure are well known. The *relative* contraindications for resection may have a local variation between institutions. These features must be well known at the time of interpretation of pretreatment images to help with accurate patient selection. Deep involvement of the central skull base or cavernous sinus can occur despite the relatively innocuous clinical appearance of a sinus (259) or nasal cavity lesion (Fig. 22.24).

Follow-up imaging is discussed in Chapter 21. The most important feature of follow-up imaging is absolute consistency of imaging protocols from scan to scan. This is particularly true for cases managed on an "unresectable protocol," wherein treatment response depends heavily on changes in the imaging findings (Fig. 22.25). Biopsy can be avoided when imaging findings are concordant with the clinical pattern. Positron emission tomography scans may prove useful for follow-up in instances of persistent but stable-appearing imaging abnormalities (260) (Fig. 22.26). For deep skull-base involvement and treatment thereof, MRI is more valuable for the early detection of recurrence at the extracranial margin and is more sensitive for intracranial progression (261) (Fig. 22.27).

Percutaneous CT-guided needle biopsy can be performed on an ambulatory basis for diagnostic indications or to rule out recurrence. The percutaneous method is particularly helpful when continued nonsurgical management is desired.

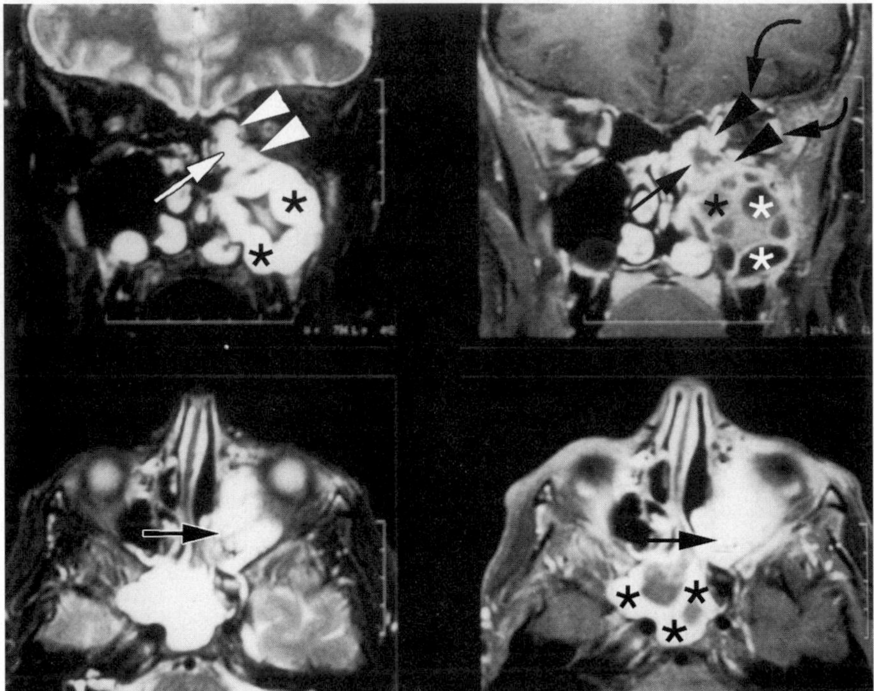

Figure 22.15 Standard magnetic resonance image projections. Matched coronal (top) and axial (bottom) views with fat-suppressed T2 and contrast T1 views of a left ethmoid cancer (*arrows*) without penetration of the periorbita (*arrowheads*). Note the mucosal thickening in the adjacent sinuses (*asterisk*) and the normal intense enhancement of the extraocular muscles (*curved arrows*).

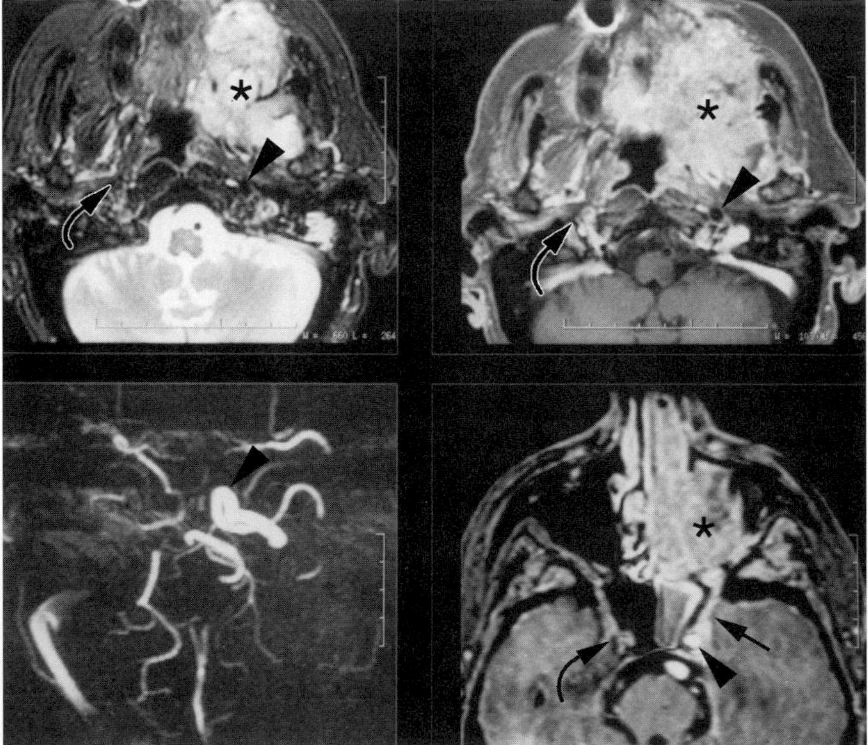

Figure 22.16 Important incidental abnormality. Axial magnetic resonance imaging and phase-contrast magnetic resonance angiography show occluded right internal carotid artery (*curved arrows*) contrasted with normal left internal carotid artery (*arrowheads*), which precluded radical skull-base resection of left cavernous sinus extension (*arrow*) of T4 squamous cell cancer of left maxillary sinus (*asterisk*).

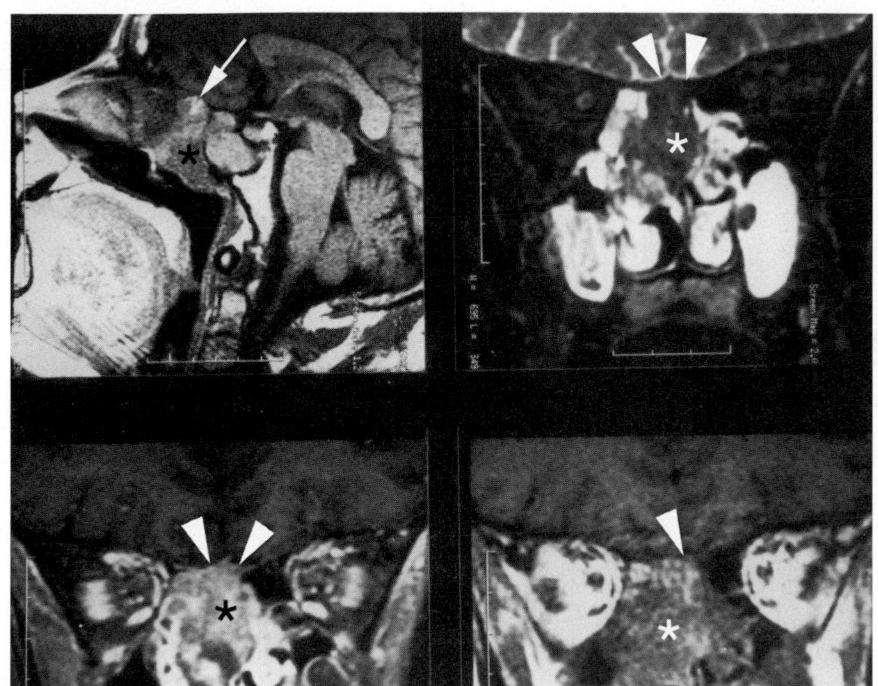

Figure 22.17 Early skull-base penetration. Clockwise from top left: Sagittal T1 and matched coronal T2 (fat-suppressed), coronal T1 and fat-suppressed contrast coronal T1 views show early permeation of the planum sphenoidale (*arrow*), with intracranial disease (*arrowheads*) limited to the extradural space. There is no brain edema. Note the primary lesion in the posterior nasal cavity (*asterisk*).

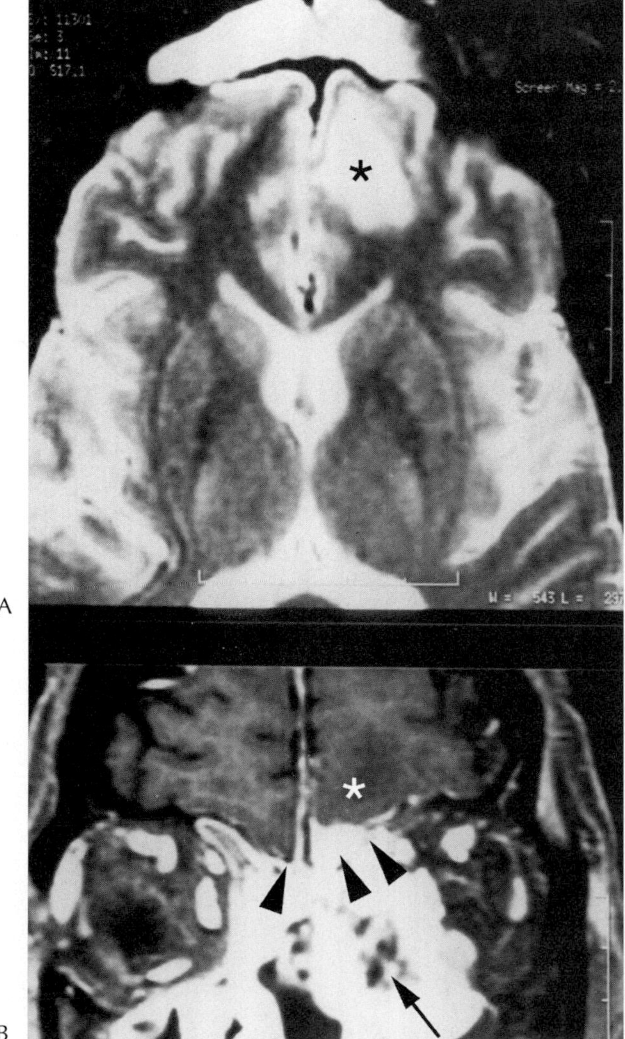

A

B

Figure 22.18 Early brain involvement. Axial T2 **(A)** and fat-suppressed contrast coronal T1 **(B)** views of advanced sinonasal tumor (*arrow*) show left frontal brain edema (*asterisk*) due to penetration of the anterior skull base (*arrowheads*).

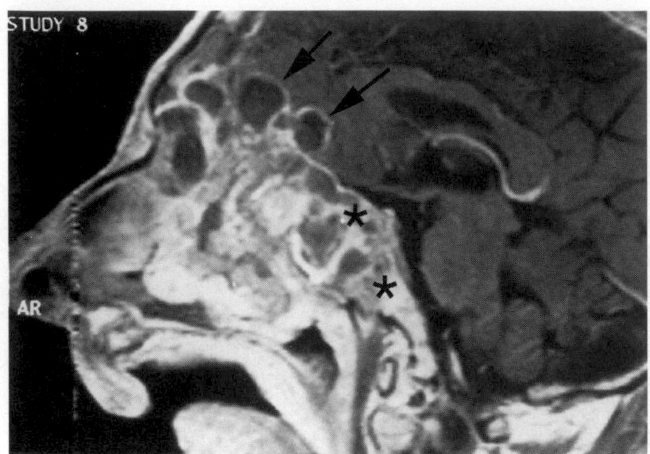

Figure 22.19 Massive sphenoethmoid mass. Sagittal enhanced magnetic resonance imaging view of large, neglected, midline squamous cancer with frank brain invasion at frontal lobe (*arrows*) and sphenoid bone invasion (*asterisk*). (Courtesy of William Donovan, M.D.)

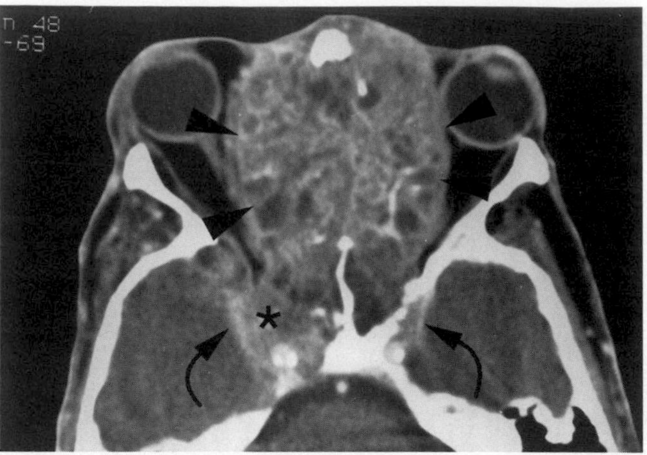

Figure 22.20 Central skull-base involvement. Enhanced axial computed tomographic view of same patient as in Figure 22.19, showing bilateral orbital invasion (*arrowheads*) and bilateral cavernous involvement (*curved arrows*). (Courtesy of William Donovan, M.D.)

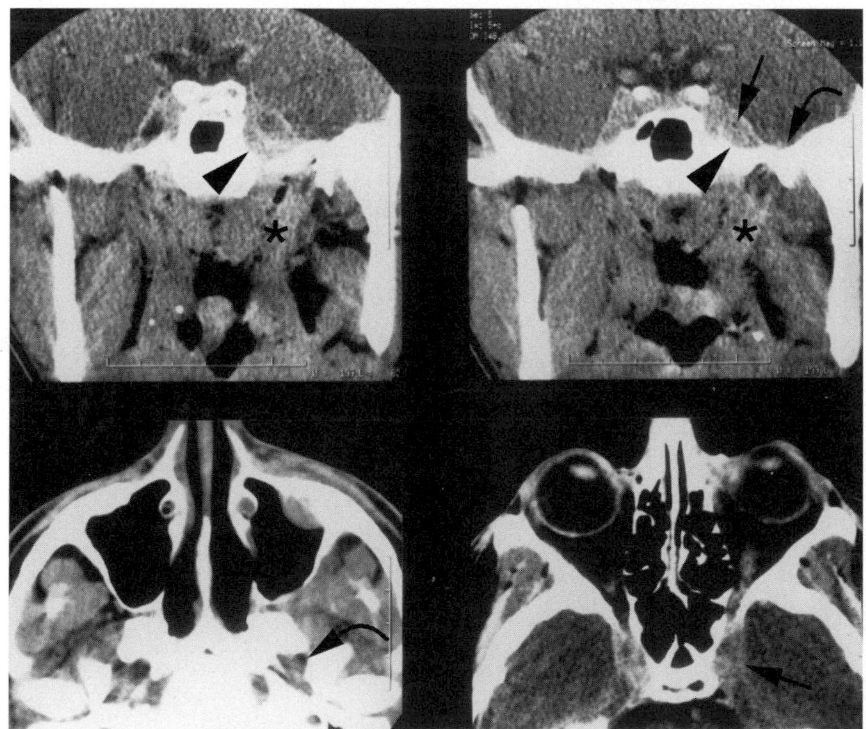

Figure 22.21 Basal foramen penetration. Adjacent enhanced direct coronal (top) and axial (bottom) views of a posterior nasal tumor that tracked through the nasopharynx (*asterisk*) and the foramen lacerum (*arrowheads*) into the cavernous sinus (*arrow*), sparing the foramen ovale (*curved arrow*).

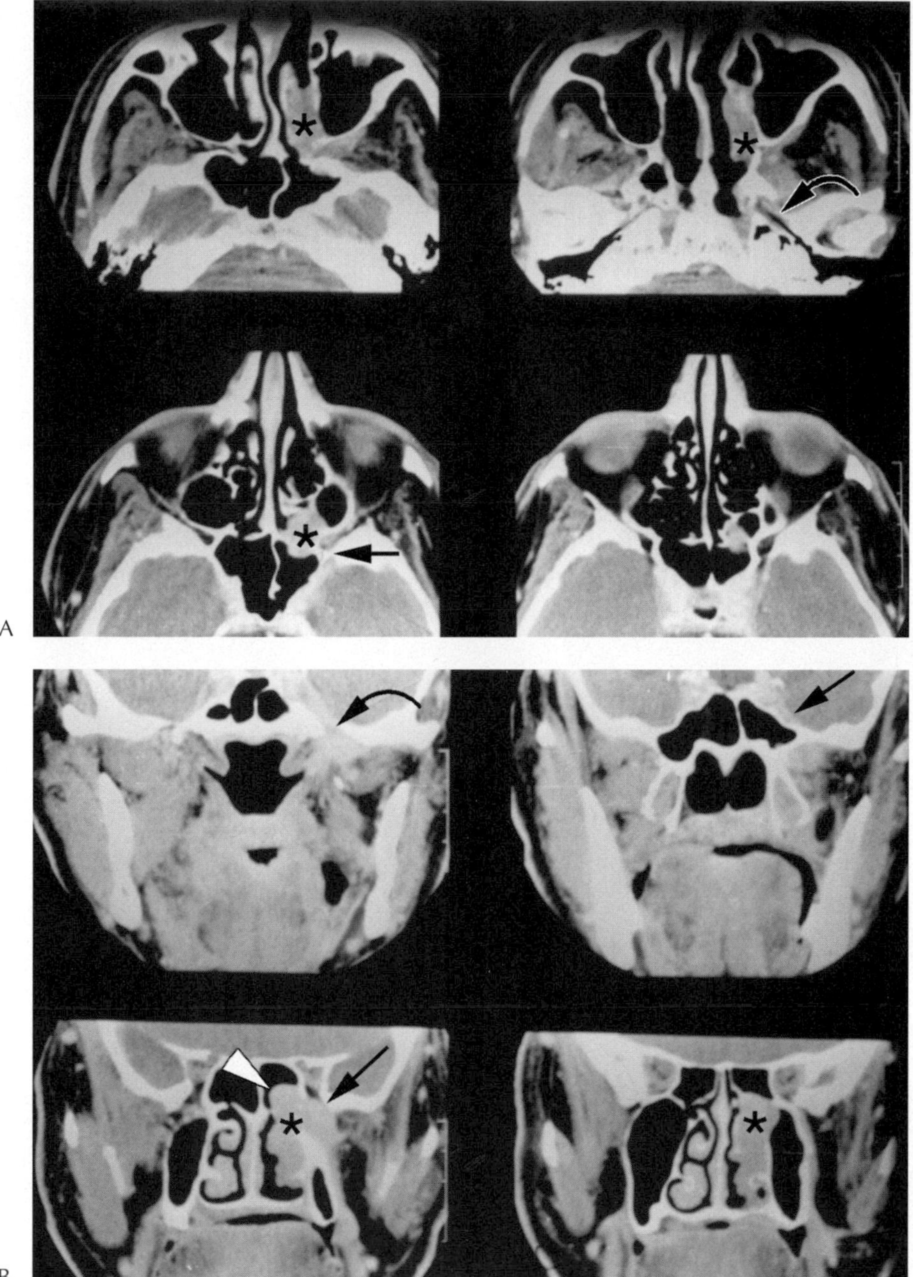

Figure 22.22 Early nasal cancer with deep extension. Contrast axial **(A)** and direct **(B)** coronal sinus computed tomograms show small squamous cell cancer of left posterior nasal cavity (*asterisk*), with contiguous involvement of pterygopalatine fossa and extension to cavernous sinus along both the second (*arrows*) and third (*curved arrows*) divisions of the fifth cranial nerve. The lesion involves the sphenoid sinus (*arrowhead*) and approaches the inferior orbital fissure (*long arrow*).

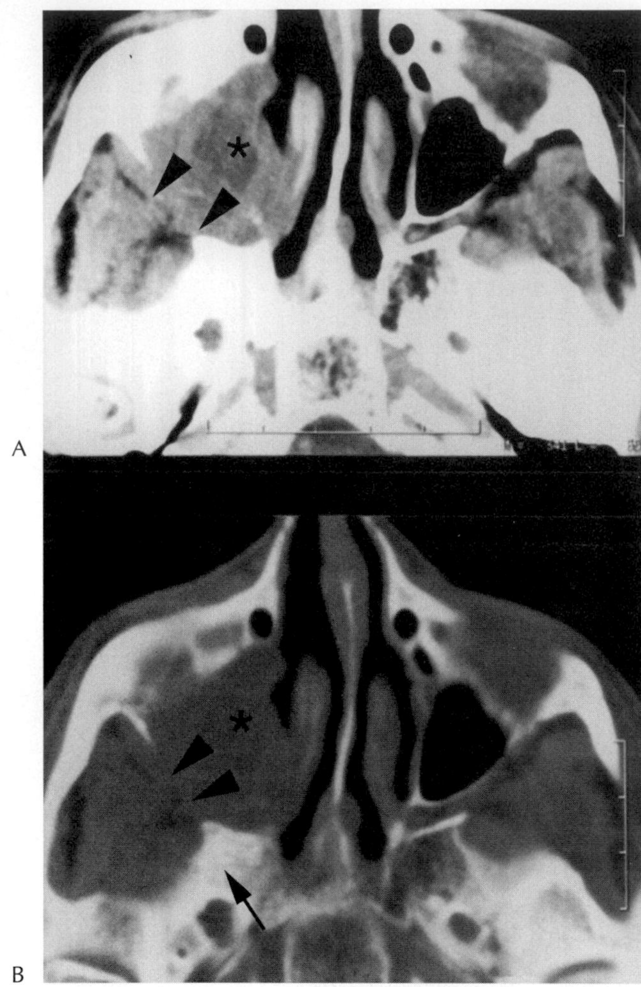

Figure 22.23 Retromaxillary extension. Matched, enhanced, axial computed tomographic **(A)** and corresponding bone-window **(B)** views of T4 squamous cell carcinoma of the right antrum (*asterisk*), with penetration through the posterior wall (*arrowheads*) into the retromaxillary space and early infiltration of the sphenoid bone (*arrow*) showing sclerosis.

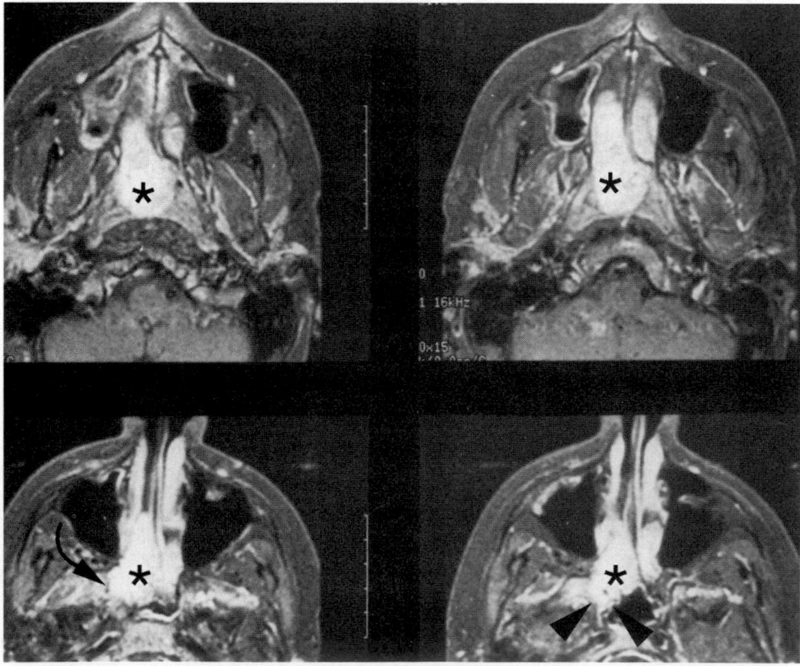

Figure 22.24 Serial enhanced fat-suppressed axial T1-weighted images of the nasal cavity show occult deep involvement. Clinically well-circumscribed lesion of right nasal cavity (*asterisk*) bulging into the choana, invading the lateral recess of the right sphenoid sinus (*curved arrow*), and infiltrating the sphenoid bone (*arrowheads*).

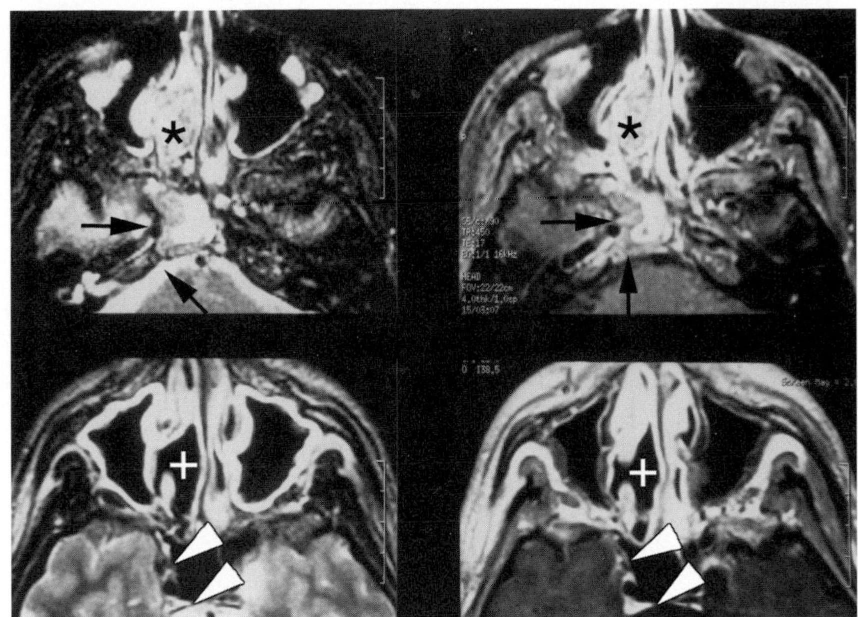

Figure 22.25 Unresectable treatment protocol. Matched pretreatment (top) and posttreatment (bottom) T2 (left) and enhanced T1 (right) magnetic resonance imaging views of an advanced, poorly differentiated squamous cell cancer (*asterisk*) with sphenoid bone involvement (*arrows*) showing complete radiographic clearance of nasal (*plus sign*) and sphenoid components (*arrowheads*) after chemotherapy combined with radiation therapy.

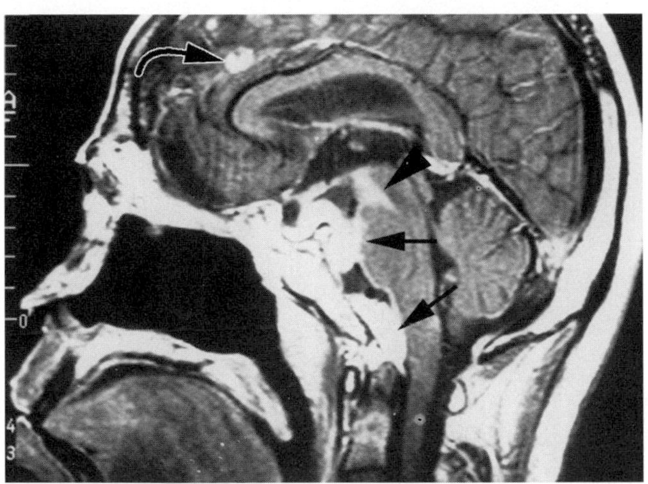

Figure 22.26 Recurrent esthesioneuroblastoma. Enhanced sagittal magnetic resonance image shows widespread progression in subarachnoid spaces despite lack of recurrence within paranasal primary site. Note interhemispheric fissure (*curved arrow*), interpeduncular cistern (*arrowhead*), and prepontine and perimedullary cistern (*arrows*) disease.

RADIATION THERAPY TECHNIQUE*

Louis B. Harrison, Rudolph Woode, and William M. Mendenhall

The usual technique for nasal cavity and paranasal sinus cancers involves a wedged pair. This is typically an anterior field with one or two lateral opposed fields. The anterior field is weighted more heavily, and is contoured to protect as much of the orbital contents as possible. The lateral field(s) is set up to be retro-orbital. We use a central axis block placed just posterior to the orbit, thereby diminishing the divergence into the eye. Sometimes we use a contralateral lateral field only (combined with the anteroposterior field) so as to maximally protect the contralateral eye, but most often we use bilateral lateral fields. These fields are shaped to protect the optic chiasm as much as possible. With this field arrangement, most of the dose to the optic chiasm is exit dose from the anterior field, and is usually no more than 70% to 75% of the prescription dose. Therefore, the total dose to the optic chiasm remains within tolerance. Some radiation oncologists prefer to angle the lateral fields a few degrees posteriorly, which is also an acceptable technique.

A demonstrative case is presented in Figure 22.27.

*Please refer to the Appendix, Imaging Considerations for Radiation Therapy Treatment Planning. This section shows the important radiologic anatomy that allows the radiation oncologist to design the target volumes for treatment planning.

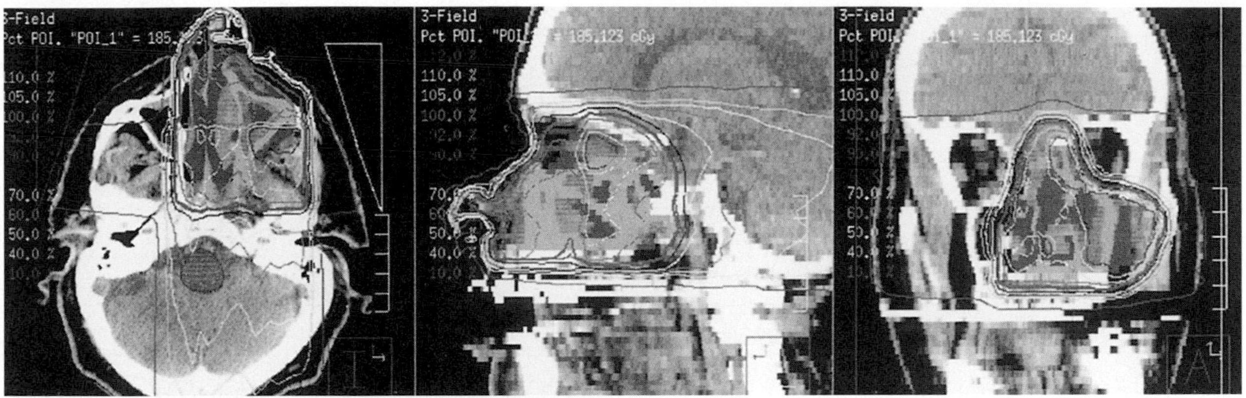

A,B

C

D

Figure 22.27 This patient had a squamous cell cancer involving the left nasal cavity that extended to the ethmoid sinus and was very close to the left optic nerve. He was referred to us after an endoscopic resection. He was not a medical candidate for craniofacial resection. We used three-dimensional conformal radiation therapy. Axial **(A)** and sagittal **(B)** computed tomography (CT) scan cuts show the PTV (*shaded*) and the isodose contours for this patient. The coronal contour **(C)** shows the shape of the anteroposterior field. Two lateral (retro-orbital, with central axis block as described) were also used. **D:** CT cut showing the dose distribution at the level of the ethmoid sinuses, showing relative protection of the right retina, right lens, and right optic nerve. The left retina and left lens are also relatively safe. By virtue of the location of the tumor, a portion of the left optic nerve receives high dose. The optic chiasm (*shaded*) receives between 70% and 75% of dose. With a total dose of 63 Gy in 7 weeks, it should be relatively safe. (***continued on next page***)

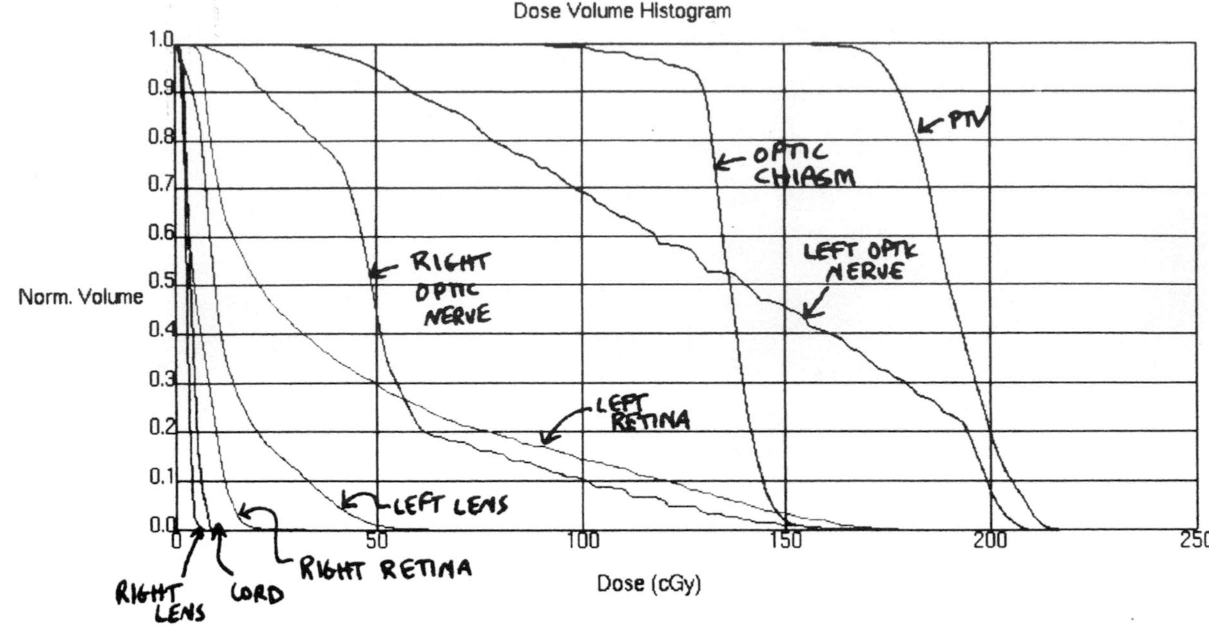

Figure 22.27 (*continued*) E: Dose-volume histogram showing the dose-volume relations for the PTV as well as the important normal structures.

REFERENCES

1. DeMonte F, Ginsberg LE, Clayman GL. Primary malignant tumors of the sphenoidal sinus. *Neurosurgery* 2000;46:1084–1091.
2. Hopkin N, McNicoll W, Dalley VM, et al. Cancer of the paranasal sinuses and nasal cavities. Part I. Clinical features. *J Laryngol Otol* 1984;98:585–595.
3. Lewis JS, Castro EB. Cancer of the nasal cavity and paranasal sinuses. *J Laryngol Otol* 1972;86:255–262.
4. Spiro JD, Soo KC, Spiro RH. Nonsquamous cell malignant neoplasms of the nasal cavities and paranasal sinuses. *Head Neck* 1995;17:114–118.
5. Tufano RP, Mokadam NA, Montone KT, et al. Malignant tumors of the nose and paranasal sinuses: Hospital of the University of Pennsylvania experience 1990–1997. *Am J Rhinol* 1999;13:117–123.
6. Parsons JT, Kimsey FC, Mendenhall WM, et al. Radiation therapy for sinus malignancies. *Otolaryngol Clin North Am* 1995;28:1259–1268.
7. Grau C, Jakobsen MH, Harbo G, et al. Sino-nasal cancer in Denmark 1982–1991—a nationwide survey. *Acta Oncol* 2001;40:19–23.
8. Waldron JN, O'Sullivan B, Gullane P, et al. Carcinoma of the maxillary antrum: a retrospective analysis of 110 cases. *Radiother Oncol* 2000;57: 167–173.
9. St-Pierre S, Baker SR. Squamous cell carcinoma of the maxillary sinus: analysis of 66 cases. *Head Neck Surg* 1983;5:508–513.
10. Shibuya H, Takagi M, Horiuchi J, et al. Clinicopathological study of maxillary sinus carcinoma. *Int J Radiat Oncol Biol Phys* 1985;11:1709–1712.
11. Pezner RD, Moss WT, Tong D, et al. Cervical lymph node metastases in patients with squamous cell carcinoma of the maxillary antrum: the role of elective irradiation of the clinically negative neck. *Int J Radiat Oncol Biol Phys* 1979;5:1977–1980.
12. Brasnu D, Laccourreye O, Bassot V, et al. Cisplatin-based neoadjuvant chemotherapy and combined resection for ethmoid sinus adenocarcinoma reaching and/or invading the skull base. *Arch Otolaryngol Head Neck Surg* 1996;122:765–768.
13. Dilhuydy JM, Lagarde P, Allal AS, et al. Ethmoidal cancers: a retrospective study of 22 cases. *Int J Radiat Oncol Biol Phys* 1993;25:113–116.
14. Jiang GL, Morrison WH, Garden AS, et al. Ethmoid sinus carcinomas: natural history and treatment results. *Radiother Oncol* 1998;49:21–27.
15. Waldron JN, O'Sullivan B, Warde P, et al. Ethmoid sinus cancer: twenty-nine cases managed with primary radiation therapy. *Int J Radiat Oncol Biol Phys* 1998;41:361–369.
16. Karim AB, Kralendonk JH, Njo KH, et al. Ethmoid and upper nasal cavity carcinoma: treatment, results and complications. *Radiother Oncol* 1990;19: 109–120.
17. Tiwari R, Hardillo JA, Tobi H, et al. Carcinoma of the ethmoid: results of treatment with conventional surgery and post-operative radiotherapy. *Eur J Surg Oncol* 1999;25:401–405.
18. Knegt PP, Ah-See KW, vd Velden LA, et al. Adenocarcinoma of the ethmoidal sinus complex: surgical debulking and topical fluorouracil may be the optimal treatment. *Arch Otolaryngol Head Neck Surg* 2001;127:141–146.
19. Roux FX, Brasnu D, Devaux B, et al. Ethmoid sinus carcinomas: results and prognosis after neoadjuvant chemotherapy and combined surgery—a 10-year experience. *Surg Neurol* 1994;42:98–104
20. Acheson ED, Cowdell RH, Hadfield E, et al. Nasal cancer in woodworkers in the furniture industry. *Br Med J* 1968;2:587–596.
21. Acheson ED, Cowdell RH, Jolles B. Nasal cancer in the Northamptonshire boot and shoe industry. *Br Med J* 1970;1:385–393.
22. Acheson ED, Hadfield EH, Macbeth RG. Carcinoma of the nasal cavity and accessory sinuses in woodworkers. *Lancet* 1967;1:311–312.
23. Chowdhury AD, Ijaz T, El-Sayed S. Frontal sinus carcinoma: a case report and review of the literature. *Australas Radiol* 1997;41:380–382.
24. Brownson RJ, Ogura JH. Primary carcinoma of the frontal sinus. *Laryngoscope* 1971;81:71–89.
25. Ang KK, Jiang GL, Frankenthaler RA, et al. Carcinomas of the nasal cavity. *Radiother Oncol* 1992;24:163–168.
26. Bosch A, Vallecillo L, Frias Z. Cancer of the nasal cavity. *Cancer* 1976;37: 1458–1463.
27. Badib AO, Kurohara SS, Webster JH, et al. Treatment of cancer of the nasal cavity. *Am J Roentgenol Radium Ther Nucl Med* 1969;106:824–830.
28. Ironside P, Matthews J. Adenocarcinoma of the nose and paranasal sinuses in woodworkers in the state of Victoria, Australia. *Cancer* 1975;36:1115–1124.
29. Barton RT, Hogetveit AC. Nickel-related cancers of the respiratory tract. *Cancer* 1980;45:3061–3064.
30. Torjussen W, Solberg LA, Hogetveit AC. Histopathologic changes of nasal mucosa in nickel workers: a pilot study. *Cancer* 1979;44:963–974.
31. Satoh N, Fukuda S, Takizawa M, et al. Chromium-induced carcinoma in the nasal region. A report of four cases. *Rhinology* 1994;32:47–50.
32. Stein J, Sridharan ST, Eliachar I, et al. Nasal cavity squamous cell carcinoma in Wegener's granulomatosis. *Arch Otolaryngol Head Neck Surg* 2001;127: 709–713.
33. Elkon D, Hightower SI, Lim ML, et al. Esthesioneuroblastoma. *Cancer* 1979; 44:1087–1094.
34. Olsen KD, DeSanto LW. Olfactory neuroblastoma. Biologic and clinical behavior. *Arch Otolaryngol* 1983;109:797–802.
35. Schwaab G, Micheau C, LeGuillou C, et al. Olfactory esthesioneuroma: a report of 40 cases. *Laryngoscope* 1988;98:872–876.
36. Shah JP, Feghali J. Esthesioneuroblastoma. *Am J Surg* 1981;142:456–458.
37. Miyamoto RC, Gleich LL, Biddinger PW, et al. Esthesioneuroblastoma and sinonasal undifferentiated carcinomas: impact of histological grading and clinical staging on survival and prognosis. *Laryngoscope* 2000;110:1262–1265.
38. Smith SR, Som P, Fahmy A, et al. A clinicopathological study of sinonasal neuroendocrine carcinoma and sinonasal undifferentiated carcinoma. *Laryngoscope* 2000;110:1617–1622.
39. Gallo O, Graziani P, Fini-Storchi O. Undifferentiated carcinoma of the nose and paranasal sinuses. An immunohistochemical and clinical study. *Ear Nose Throat J* 1993;72:588–595.
40. Frierson HF Jr, Mills SE, Fechner RE, et al. Sinonasal undifferentiated carcinoma. An aggressive neoplasm derived from schneiderian epithelium and distinct from olfactory neuroblastoma. *Am J Surg Pathol* 1986;10:771–779.

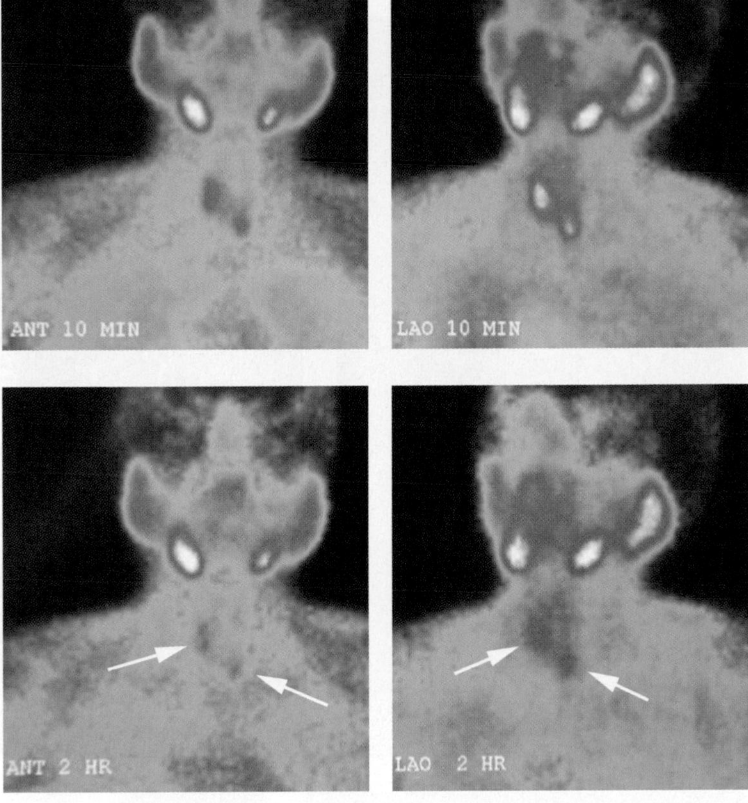

Color Plate 1. Parathyroid imaging. Technetium sestamibi nuclear scans in the early phase (**top**) and delayed phase (**bottom**) show multiple bilateral sites of retained activity in a patient with multifocal parathyroid hyperplasia. *Ant,* anterior; *LAO,* left anterior oblique. (See Fig. 4.27.)

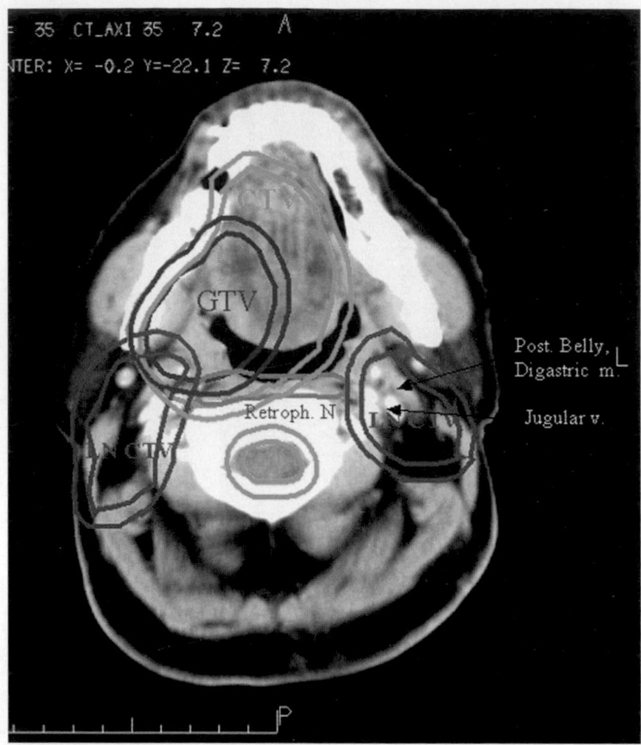

A

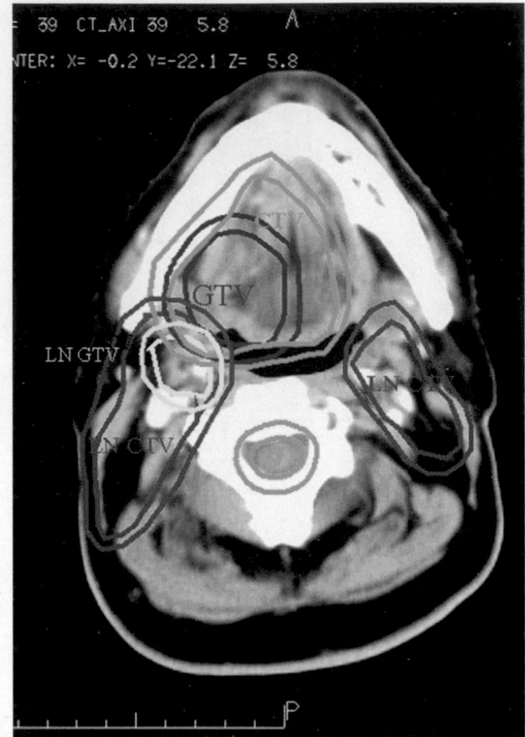

B

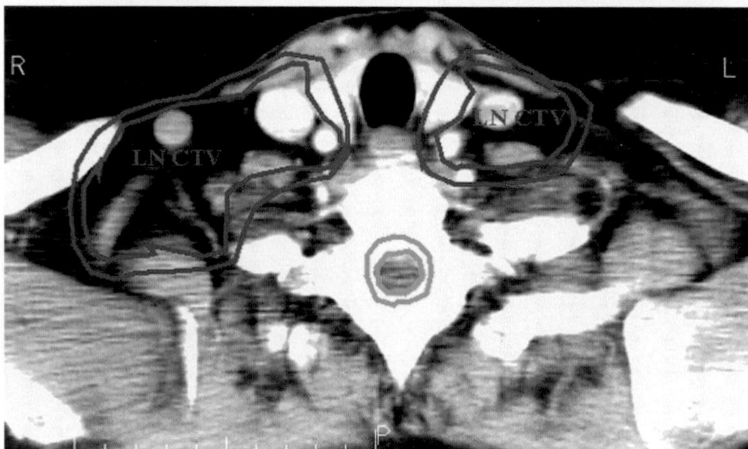

C

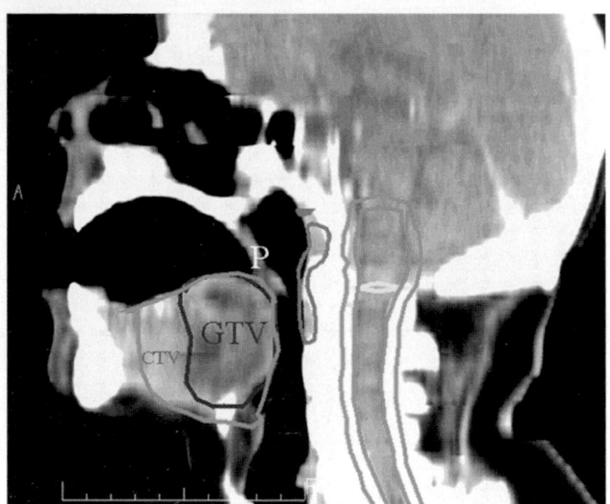

D

Color Plate 2. The targets outlined on planning computed tomography (CT) in a case of stage T2, N1 carcinoma of the right tonsil, involving the lateral base of tongue. The gross target volume (*GTV*), primary tumor clinical target volume (*CTV*), and lymphatic GTV and CTVs are each expanded uniformly by 0.5 cm to yield the corresponding planning tumor volume (*PTV*). **A:** Level II nodal targets in the ipsilateral neck, and the retropharyngeal nodes bilaterally, are outlined through the base of skull. Level II nodes in the contralateral neck are outlined up to the level in which the posterior belly of the digastric muscle crosses the jugular vein. Cephalad to this level, only the ipsilateral level II nodal CTVs and the retropharyngeal nodes are outlined. In cases where the contralateral neck contains clinical or radiologic evidence of metastasis, or in the case of nasopharyngeal cancer, level II is outlined through the base of skull bilaterally. **B:** Nodal metastasis in the LN neck is outlined as a nodal GTV, expanded to yield its PTV. **C:** In the LN lower neck, nodal levels IV and V are included in the CTV. Only level IV is outlined in the contralateral lower neck (the contralateral neck did not have clinical evidence of metastasis). **D:** A sagittal reconstruction of the CT may help in the assessment of the extent of disease. On axial images, it is difficult to distinguish the soft palate from the base of the tongue that contains the targets. The sagittal view facilitates the exclusion of the soft palate (*P*) from the targets. (See Fig. 5.1.)

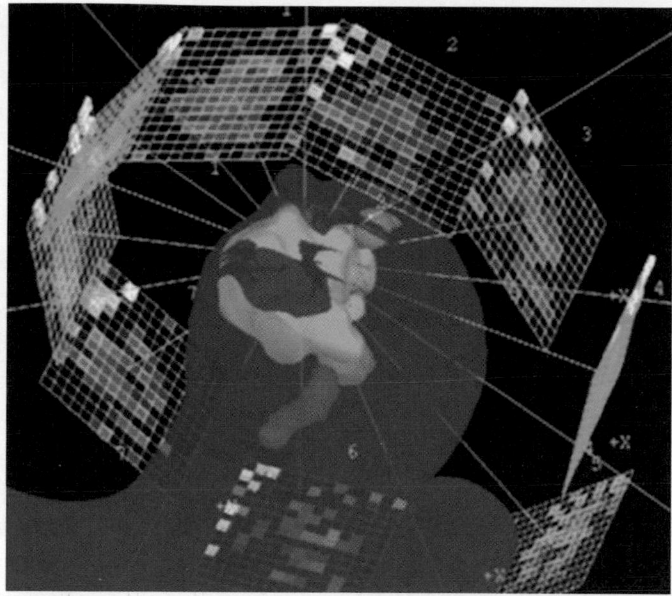

Color Plate 3. Beam arrangement for intensity modulated radiotherapy using a multileaf collimator. Nine coplanar, equidistant beams are used, each containing 1 × 1 cm or 0.5 × 0.5 cm pencil "beamlets." (See Fig. 5.2.)

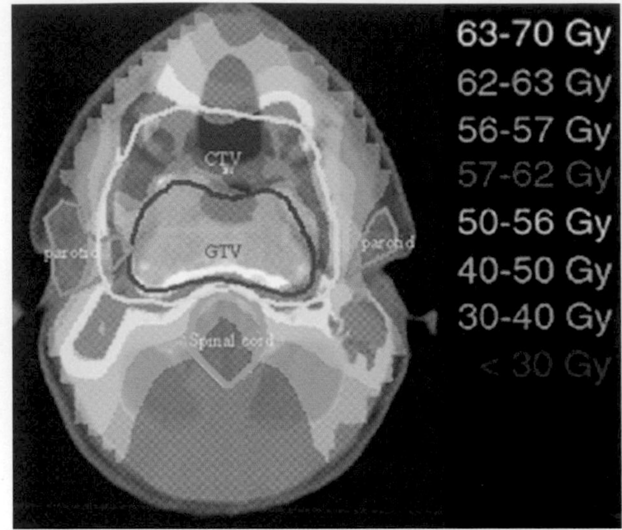

A

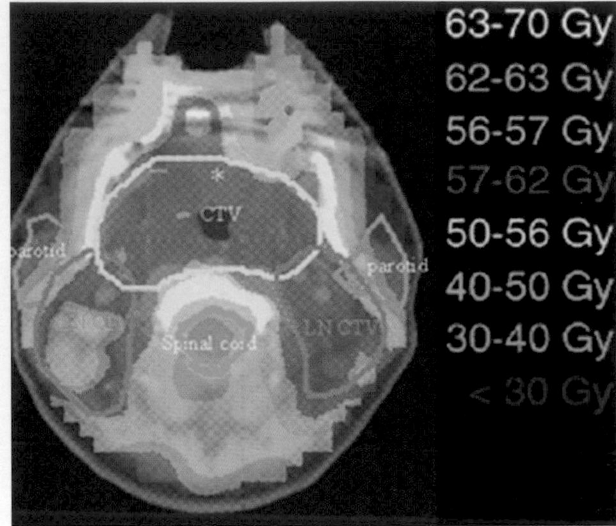

B

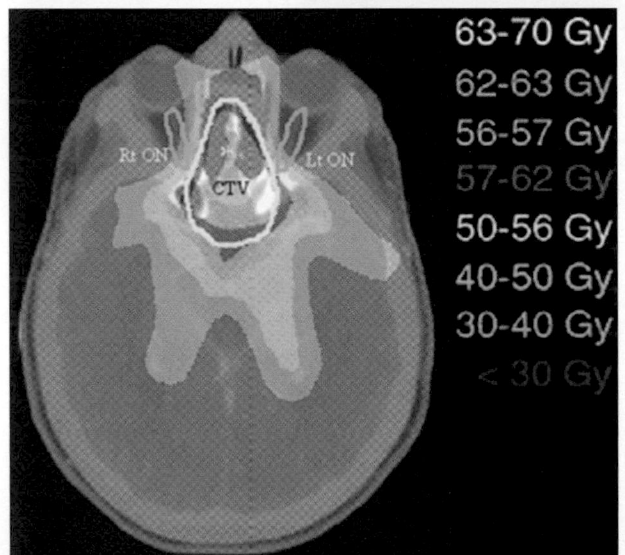

C

Color Plate 4. Targets and doses in intensity modulated radiotherapy of nasopharyngeal cancer. **A:** The gross target volume (*GTV*) was outlined following registration of the planning computed tomography with diagnostic magnetic resonance imaging. The clinical target volume (*CTV*) includes the base of skull, the posterior paranasal sinuses, the clivus, and the parapharyngeal space. **B:** Caudal to the GTV, the CTV contains the parapharyngeal and posterior pharyngeal space through midtonsils. Level II nodal CTVs are outlined through the base of skull bilaterally. **C:** The CTV encompasses the sphenoid and cavernous sinuses in locally advanced cases. Limiting the dose to the optic pathways is an important objective of planning. **D:** Dose-volume histograms of the case described in **A–C**. Both parotid glands are spared while the targets are adequately irradiated. (See Fig. 5.3.)

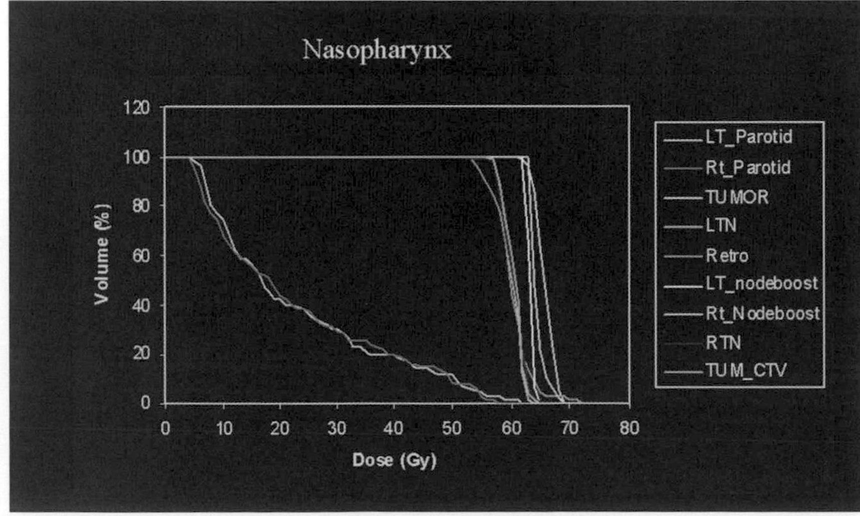

D

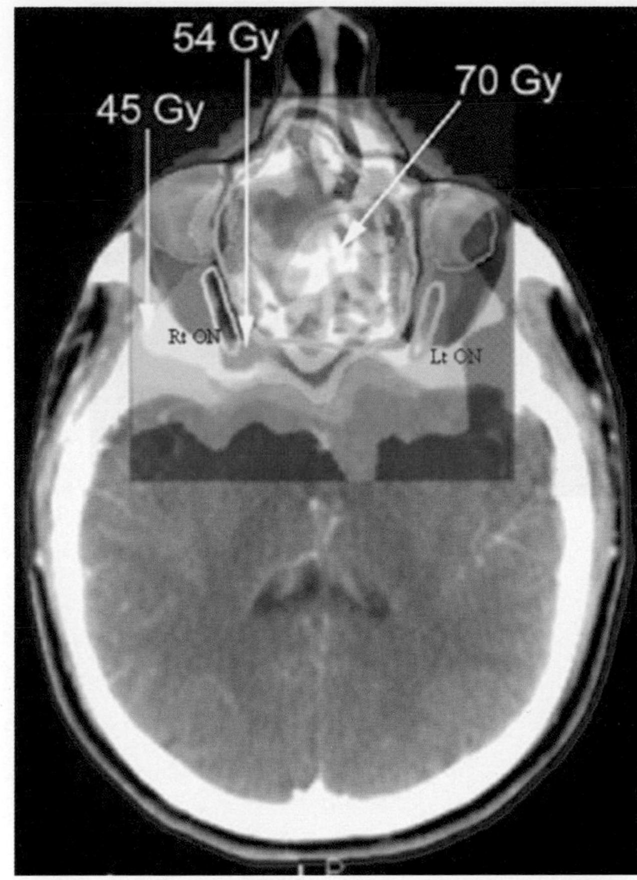

A

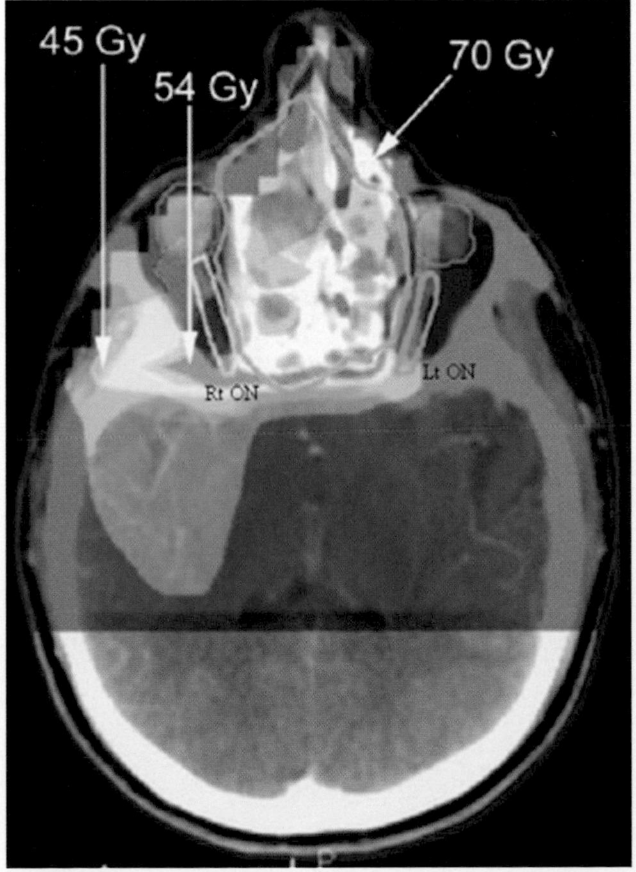

B

Color Plate 5. A,B: Isodoses of intensity modulated radiotherapy for advanced paranasal sinus cancer. Sparing the optic pathways was a major planning objective. (See Fig. 5.4.)

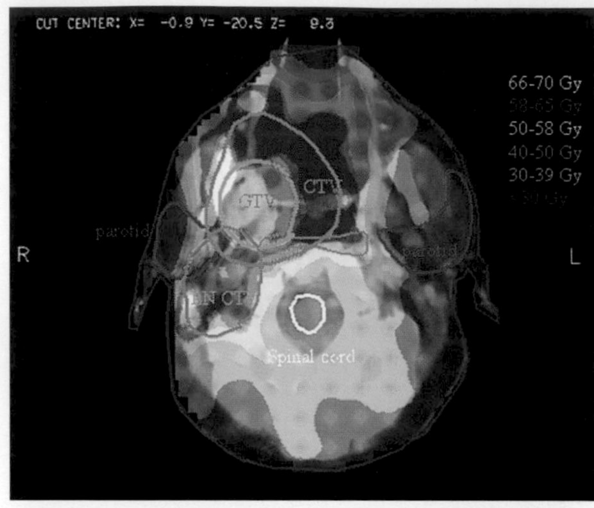

A

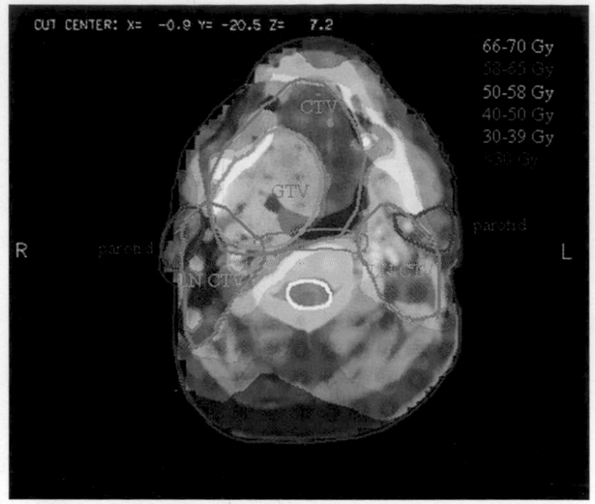

B

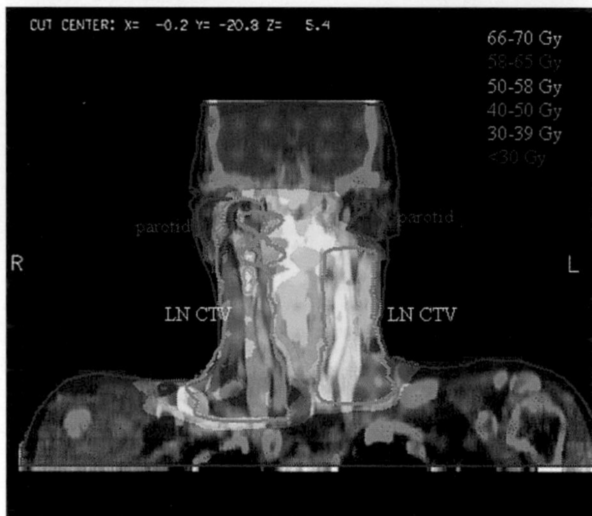

C

Color Plate 6. A–C: Isodoses of intensity modulated radiotherapy for the patient described in Figure 5.1 (see also Color Plate 2). The contralateral parotid gland received a low dose (mean, 17 Gy) and the ipsilateral gland a moderate dose (mean, 32 Gy). CTV, clinical target volume; GTV, gross target volume. (See Fig. 5.5.)

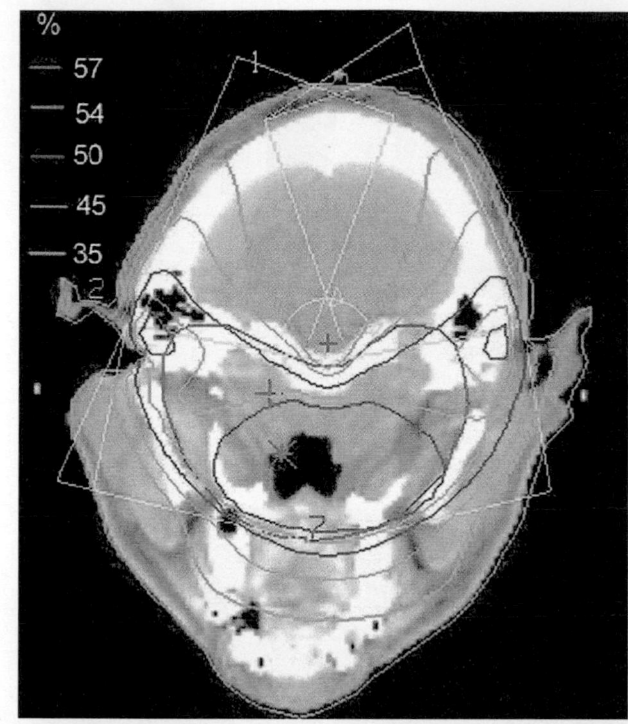

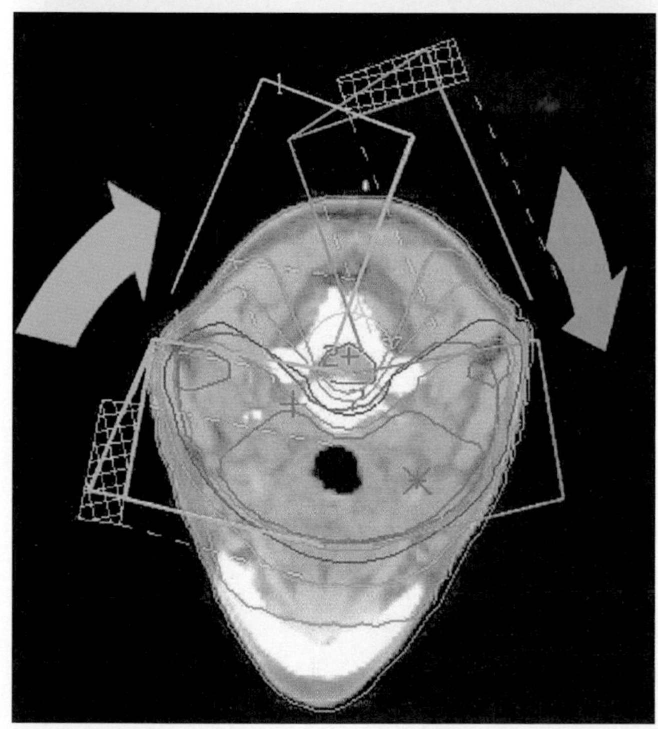

Color Plate 7. "Boomerang"-shaped isodoses achieved by rotating arc fields at the primary tumor **(A)** and upper neck **(B)**. (See Fig. 23.5.)

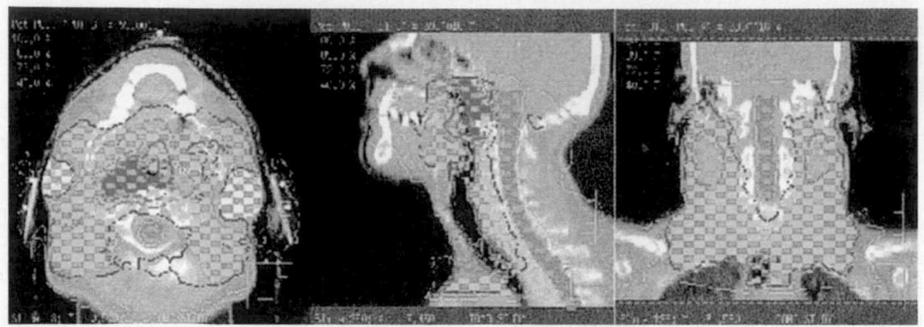

Color Plate 8. Isodose distribution obtained with tomotherapy planning for a patient with advanced nasopharyngeal cancer. The 100%, 80%, 72%, and 40% isodose lines are shown. Bilateral parotid glands and spinal cord are specifically identified for conformal avoidance. (See Fig. 23.6.)

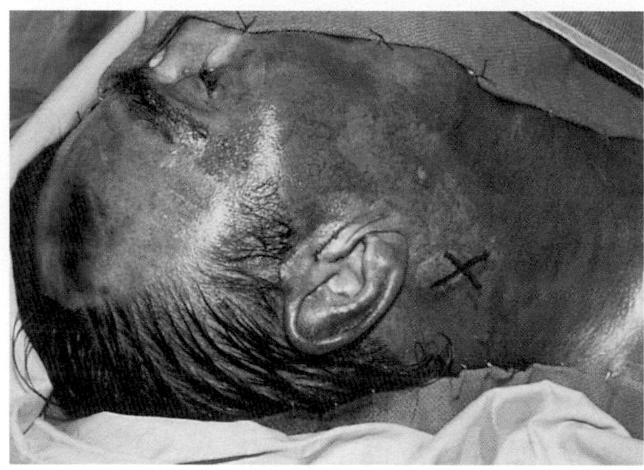

A

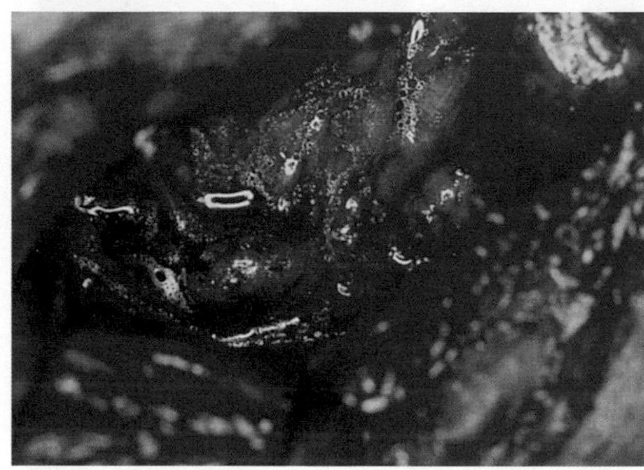

B

Color Plate 9. Intraoperative lymphatic mapping and sentinel lymph node biopsy. **A:** Blue dye has been injected around the primary lesion. **B:** The major draining lymphatic channel and sentinel node are stained with blue dye (See Fig. 25.9B,C).

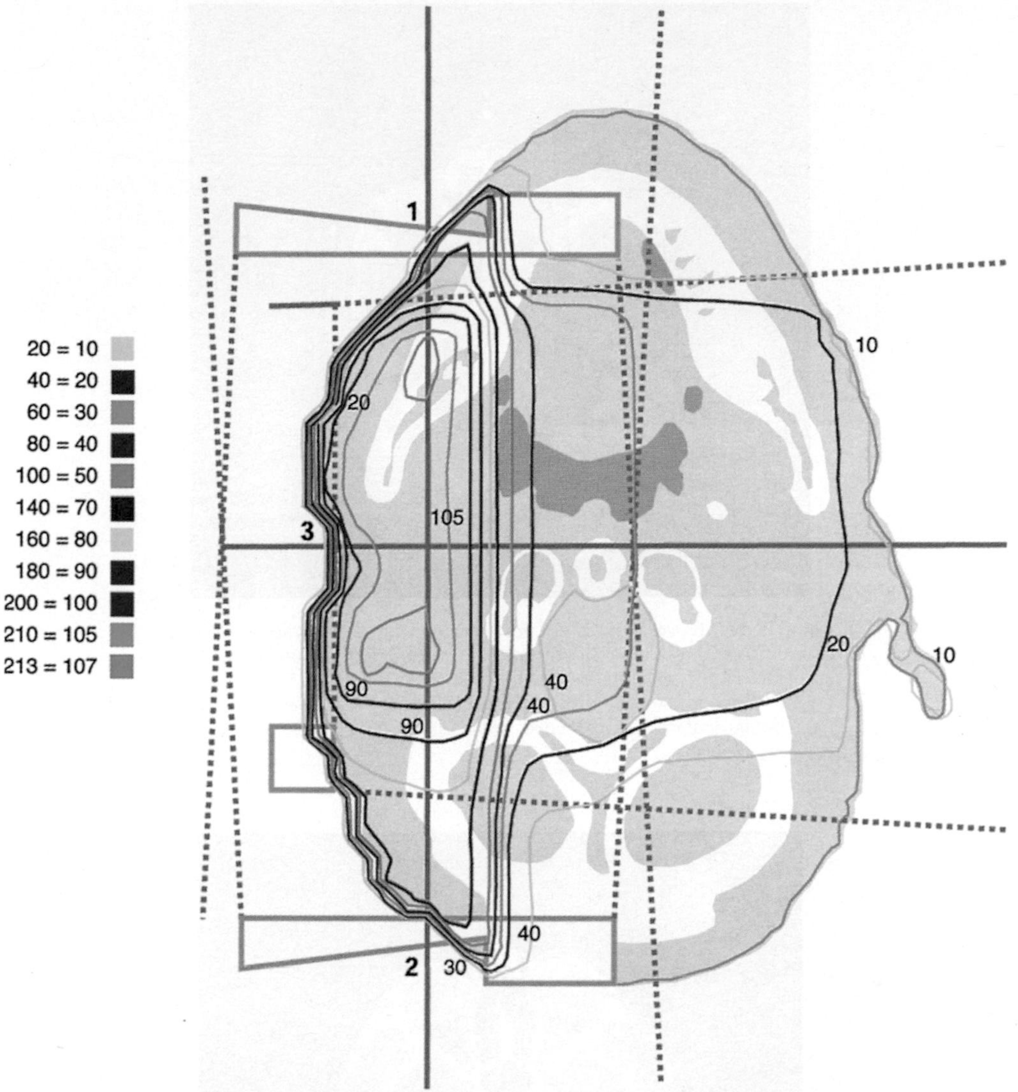

Color Plate 10. Sample radiation therapy treatment plan for parotid malignancy. (See Fig. 26.4.)

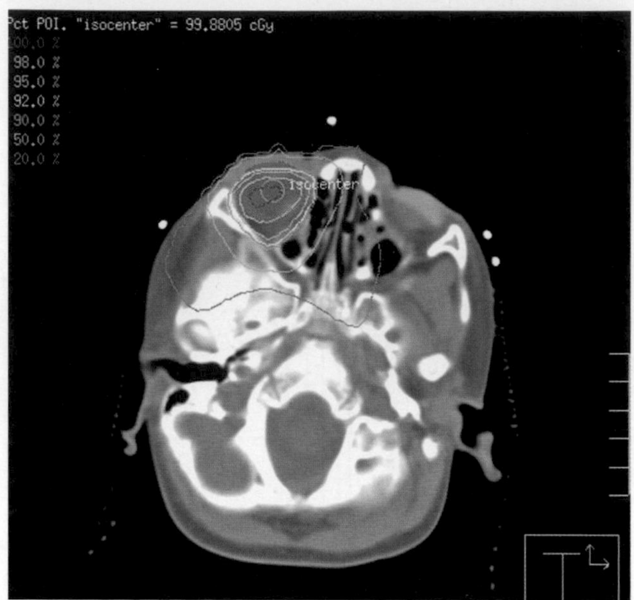

Color Plate 11. Isodose distribution obtained through computed tomographic scan three-dimensional image reconstruction showing four-field arrangement for unilateral retinoblastoma cases. Note the 50% line covers the orbit and the dose drops off fast protecting the chiasm, hypothalamus, pituitary gland, opposite eye, and so forth. (See Fig. 32.8.)

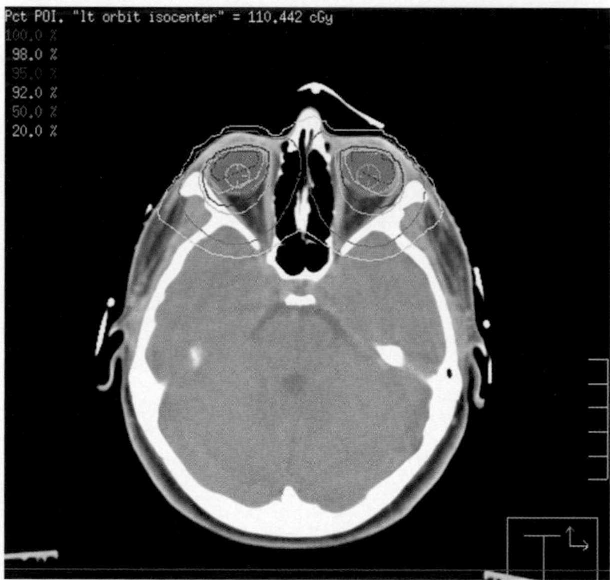

Color Plate 12. Three-dimensional reconstructed image planning for bilateral retinoblastoma using six-field arrangement. Significant sparing effect of different structures close to the eyes and orbits. (See Fig. 32.9.)

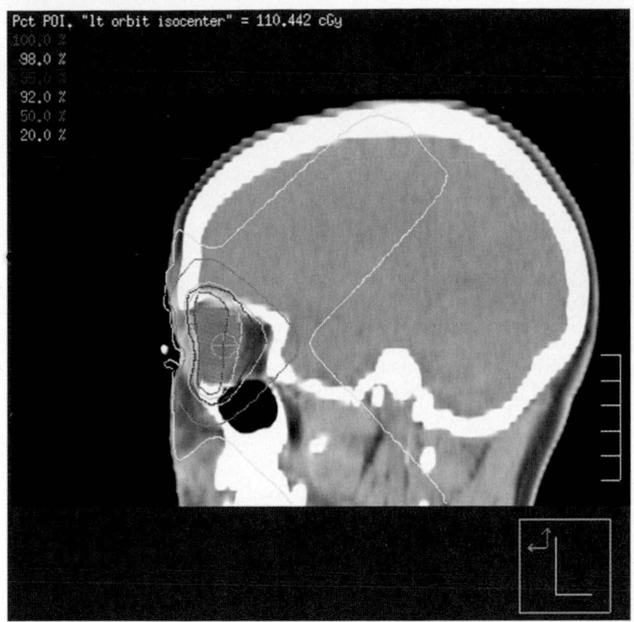

Color Plate 13. Field orientation for anterosuperior oblique and anteroinferior oblique beams used in conjunction with two additional fields: anteromedial oblique and anterolateral oblique beams in unilateral cases. (See Fig. 32.10.)

A

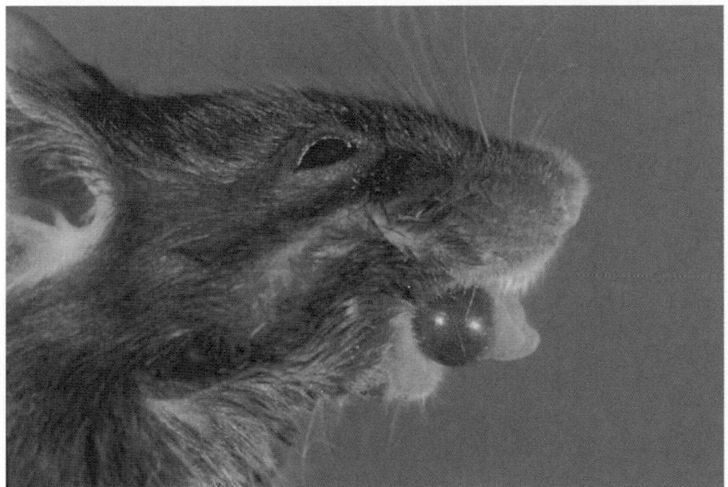

B

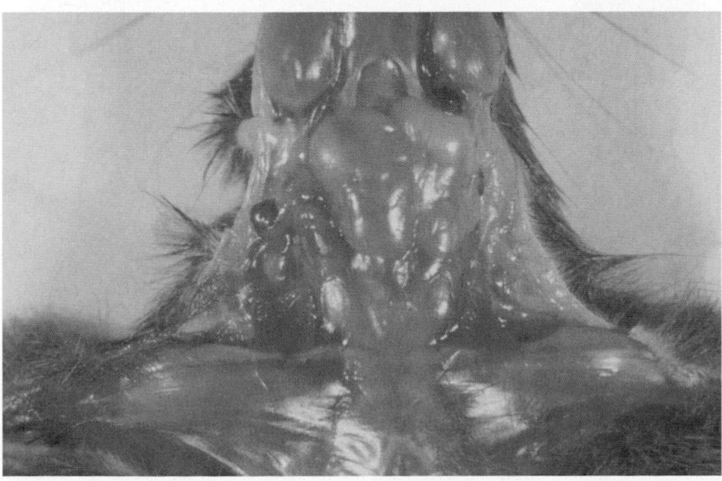

Color Plate 14. The tongues of C57 black mice were inoculated with syngeneic B16/BL6 melanoma cells and mice were killed after 14 days and necropsy performed. An obvious tumor is seen in the tongue. Bilateral metastases are easily identified by melanotic pigmentation within the cervical lymph nodes. (See Fig. 38.11.)

A,B

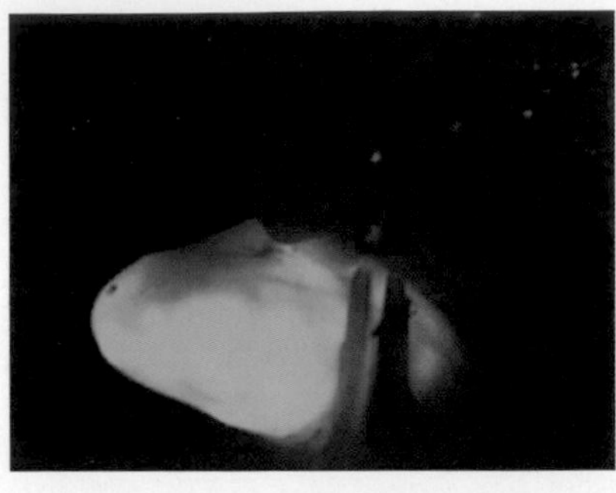

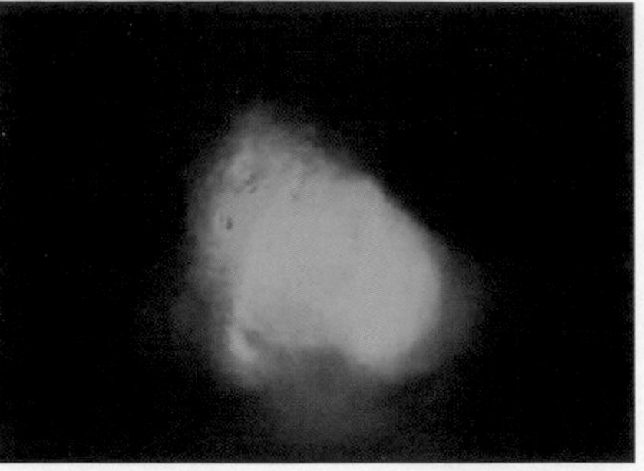

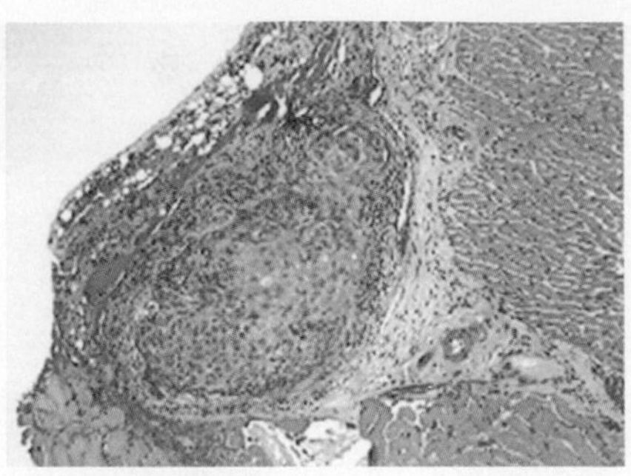

C

Color Plate 15. Photographed under a fluorescent dissecting stereomicroscope, Tu167GFP formed a tumor after injection into the anterior tongue **(A)**, which led to a submandibular metastatic deposit **(B)** that was confirmed by histologic evaluation of the resected fluorescent tissue **(C)**. (See Fig. 38.12.)

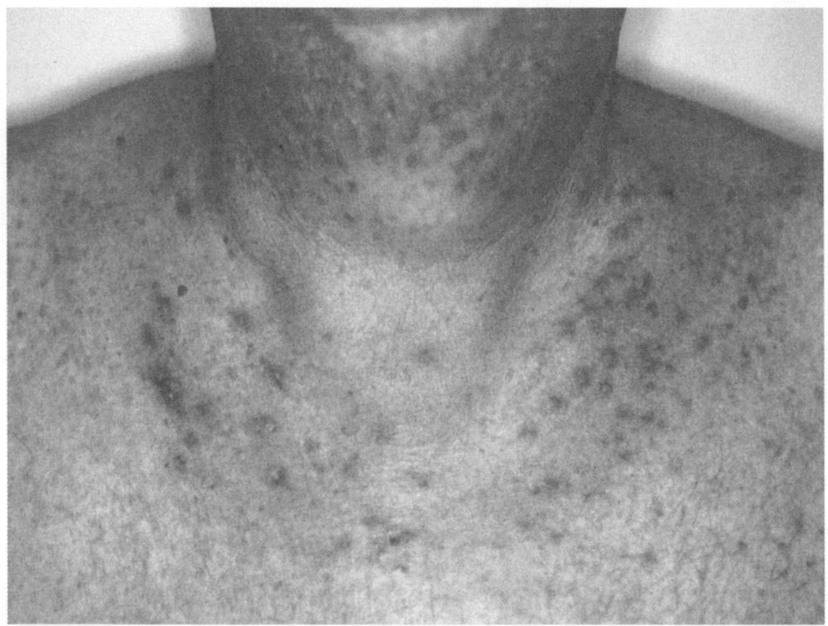

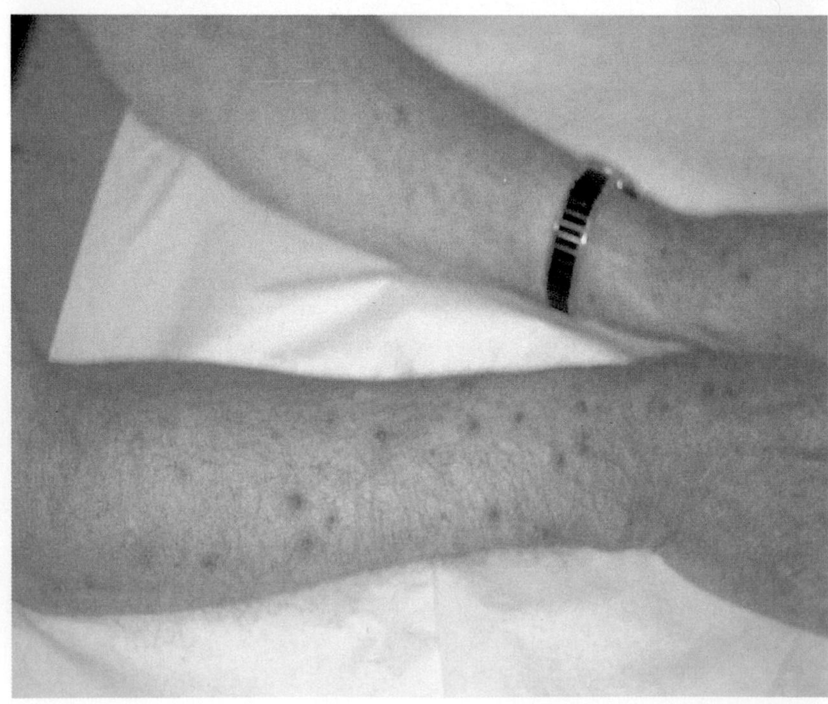

Color Plate 16. Characteristic appearance of folliculitis in a patient receiving weekly C225 during a course of head and neck radiation. This cutaneous reaction commonly manifests across the face, neck, upper torso, and arms, and resolves spontaneously over several weeks or months following completion of therapy. (From Harari PM, Huang S-M. Head and neck cancer as a clinical model for molecular targeting of therapy: combining EGFR blockade with radiation. *Int J Radiat Oncol Biol Phys* 2001;49:427–433, with permission.) (See Fig. 41.14.)

41. Gorelick J, Ross D, Marentette L, et al. Sinonasal undifferentiated carcinoma: case series and review of the literature. *Neurosurgery* 2000;47:750–754.
42. De Meerleer GO, Vermeersch H, van Eijkeren M, et al. Primary sinonasal mucosal melanoma: three different therapeutic approaches to inoperable local disease or recurrence and a review of the literature. *Melanoma Res* 1998; 8:449–457.
43. Gilligan D, Slevin NJ. Radical radiotherapy for 28 cases of mucosal melanoma in the nasal cavity and sinuses. *Br J Radiol* 1991;64:1147–1150.
44. Harrison DF. Malignant melanomata of the nasal cavity. *Proc R Soc Med* 1968; 61:13–18.
45. Holdcraft J, Gallagher JC. Malignant melanomas of the nasal cavity and paranasal sinus mucosa. *Ann Otol Rhinol Laryngol* 1969;78:5–20.
46. Shah JP, Huvos AG, Strong EW. Mucosal melanomas of the head and neck. *Am J Surg* 1977;134:531–535.
47. Ravid JM, Esteves JA. Malignant melanoma of the nose and paranasal sinuses and juvenile melanoma of the nose. *Arch Otolaryngol* 1960;72: 431–444.
48. Lawson W, Ho BT, Shaari CM, et al. Inverted papilloma: a report of 112 cases. *Laryngoscope* 1995;105:282–288.
49. Trible WM, Lekagul S. Inverting papilloma of the nose and paranasal sinuses: Report of 30 cases. *Laryngoscope* 1971;81:663–668.
50. Norris HJ. Papillary lesions of the nasal cavity and paranasal sinuses. Part II. Inverting papillomas. A study of 29 cases. *Laryngoscope* 1963;73:1–17.
51. Suh KW, Facer GW, Devine KD, et al. Inverting papilloma of the nose and paranasal sinuses. *Laryngoscope* 1977;87:35–46.
52. D'Angelo AJ Jr, Marlowe A, Marlowe FI, et al. Inverted papilloma of the nose and paranasal sinuses in children. *Ear Nose Throat J* 1992;71:264–266.
53. Eavey RD. Inverted papilloma of the nose and paranasal sinuses in childhood and adolescence. *Laryngoscope* 1985;95:17–23.
54. Gomez JA, Mendenhall WM, Tannehill SP, et al. Radiation therapy in inverted papillomas of the nasal cavity and paranasal sinuses. *Am J Otolaryngol* 2000;21:174–178.
55. Bernauer HS, Welkoborsky HJ, Tilling A, et al. Inverted papillomas of the paranasal sinuses and the nasal cavity: DNA indices and HPV infection. *Am J Rhinol* 1997;11:155–160.
56. Deitmer T, Wiener C. Is there an occupational etiology of inverted papilloma of the nose and sinuses? *Acta Otolaryngol* 1996;116:762–765.
57. Batsakis JG, Suarez P. Schneiderian papillomas and carcinomas: a review. *Adv Anat Pathol* 2001;8:53–64.
58. Cheung MM, Chan JK, Lau WH, et al. Primary non-Hodgkin's lymphoma of the nose and nasopharynx: clinical features, tumor immunophenotype, and treatment outcome in 113 patients. *J Clin Oncol* 1998;16:70–77.
59. Chen HHW, Fong L, Su IJ, et al. Experience of radiotherapy in lethal midline granuloma with special emphasis on centrofacial T-cell lymphoma: a retrospective analysis covering a 34-year period. *Radiother Oncol* 1996;38:1–6.
60. Sakata K, Hareyama M, Ohuchi A, et al. Treatment of lethal midline granuloma type nasal T-cell lymphoma. *Acta Oncol* 1997;36:307–311.
61. Smalley SR, Cupps RE, Anderson JA, et al. Polymorphic reticulosis limited to the upper aerodigestive tract—natural history and radiotherapeutic considerations. *Int J Radiat Oncol Biol Phys* 1988;15:599–605.
62. Bridger MWM, van Nostrand AWP. The nose and paranasal sinuses—applied surgical anatomy: a histologic study of whole organ sections in three planes. *J Otolaryngol* 1978;7:18–19.
63. Wax MK, Yun KJ, Wetmore SJ, et al. Adenocarcinoma of the ethmoid sinus. *Head Neck* 1995;17:303–311.
64. Million RR, Cassisi NJ, Wittes RE. Cancer of the head and neck. In: DeVita VT Jr, Hellman S, Rosenberg SA, eds. *Cancer: principles and practice of oncology*, 2nd ed. Philadelphia: JB Lippincott Co, 1985:407–506.
65. Stringer SP, Stiles W, Slattery WH, III, et al. Nasal mucociliary clearance after radiation therapy. *Laryngoscope* 1995;105:380–382.
66. Rouviére H. Anatomy of the human lymphatic system. Tobias MJ (translator). Ann Arbor, MI: Edwards Brothers, 1938:1–28, 77–78.
67. Samaha M, Yoskovitch A, Hier MP, et al. Squamous cell carcinoma of the nasal vestibule. *J Otolaryngol* 2000;29:98–101.
68. Lawson W, Reino AJ. Isolated sphenoid sinus disease: an analysis of 132 cases. *Laryngoscope* 1997;107:1590–1595.
69. Cakmak O, Shohet MR, Kern EB. Isolated sphenoid sinus lesions. *Am J Rhinol* 2000;14:13–19.
70. Sorensen PH, Wu JK, Berean KW, et al. Olfactory neuroblastoma is a peripheral primitive neuroectodermal tumor related to Ewing sarcoma. *Proc Natl Acad Sci U S A* 1996;93:1038–1043.
71. Hyams VJ, Batsakis JG, Michaels L. *Atlas of tumor pathology.* Second series. Fascicle 25: tumors of the upper respiratory tract and ear. Washington, DC: Armed Forced Institute of Pathology, 1988:226–257.
72. Levine PA, Gallagher R, Cantrell RW. Esthesioneuroblastoma: reflections of a 21-year experience. *Laryngoscope* 1999;109:1539–1543.
73. Foote RL, Morita A, Ebersold MJ, et al. Esthesioneuroblastoma: the role of adjuvant radiation therapy. *Int J Radiat Oncol Biol Phys* 1993;27:835–842.
74. Eriksen JG, Bastholt L, Krogdahl AS, et al. Esthesioneuroblastoma—what is the optimal treatment? *Acta Oncol* 2000;39:231–235.
75. Righi PD, Francis F, Aron BS, et al. Sinonasal undifferentiated carcinoma: a 10-year experience. *Am J Otolaryngol* 1996;17:167–171.
76. Hyams VJ. Papillomas of the nasal cavity and paranasal sinuses. A clinicopathological study of 315 cases. *Ann Otol Rhinol Laryngol* 1971;80:192–206.
77. Vrabec DP. The inverted Schneiderian papilloma: a 25-year study. *Laryngoscope* 1994;104:582–605.
78. Lawson W, Biller HF, Jacobson A, et al. The role of conservative surgery in the management of inverted papilloma. *Laryngoscope* 1983;93:148–158.
79. Myers EN, Fernau JL, Johnson JT, et al. Management of inverted papilloma. *Laryngoscope* 1990;100:481–490.
80. Vrabec DP. The inverted Schneiderian papilloma: a clinical and pathological study. *Laryngoscope* 1975;85:186–220.
81. Lesperance MM, Esclamado RM. Squamous cell carcinoma arising in inverted papilloma. *Laryngoscope* 1995;105:178–183.
82. Hug EB, Wang CC, Montgomery WW, et al. Management of inverted papilloma of the nasal cavity and paranasal sinuses: importance of radiation therapy. *Int J Radiat Oncol Biol Phys* 1993;26:67–72.
83. Skarin A. Lethal midline granuloma revisited: nasal T/natural-killer cell lymphoma. *J Clin Oncol* 1999;17:1322–1325.
84. Kwong YL, Chan AC, Liang RH. Natural killer cell lymphoma/leukemia: pathology and treatment. *Hematol Oncol* 1997;15:71–79.
85. Harrison DF. Midline destructive granuloma: fact or fiction. *Laryngoscope* 1987;97:1049–1053.
86. Asano K, Sobata E, Yamazaki K, et al. Malignant melanoma arising from the sphenoidal sinus—case report. *Neurol Med Chir (Tokyo)* 2000;40:329–334.
87. Freedman HM, DeSanto LW, Devine KD, et al. Malignant melanoma of the nasal cavity and paranasal sinuses. *Arch Otolaryngol* 1973;97:322–325.
88. Batsakis JG. Thawley SE, Panje WR, et al., eds. Pathology of tumors of the nasal cavity and paranasal sinuses. In: *Comprehensive management of head and neck tumors*, 2nd ed. Philadelphia: WB Saunders, 1999:522–539.
89. Pearson BW. The surgical anatomy of maxillectomy. *Surg Clin North Am* 1977; 57:701–721.
90. Giri SP, Reddy EK, Gemer LS, et al. Management of advanced squamous cell carcinomas of the maxillary sinus. *Cancer* 1992;69:657–661.
91. Ahmad K, Cordoba RB, Fayos JV. Squamous cell carcinoma of the maxillary sinus. *Arch Otolaryngol* 1981;197:48–51.
92. Jiang GL, Ang KK, Peters LJ, et al. Maxillary sinus carcinomas: natural history and results of postoperative radiotherapy. *Radiother Oncol* 1991;21: 193–200.
93. Lee F, Ogura JH. Maxillary sinus carcinoma. *Laryngoscope* 1981;91:133–139.
94. Gullane PJ, Conley J. Carcinoma of the maxillary sinus. A correlation of the clinical course with orbital involvement, pterygoid erosion or pterygopalatine invasion and cervical metatases. *J Otolaryngol* 1983;12:141–145.
95. Le QT, Fu KK, Kaplan M, et al. Treatment of maxillary sinus carcinoma. A comparison of the 1997 and 1977 American Joint Committee on Cancer staging systems. *Cancer* 1999;86:1700–1711.
96. Le QT, Fu KK, Kaplan MJ, et al. Lymph node metastasis in maxillary sinus carcinoma. *Int J Radiat Oncol Biol Phys* 2000;46:541–549.
97. Kraus DH, Sterman BM, Levine HL, et al. Factors influencing survival in ethmoid sinus cancer. *Arch Otolaryngol Head Neck Surg* 1992;118:367–372.
98. Barton RT. Management of carcinoma arising in the lateral nasal wall. *Arch Otolaryngol* 1980;106:685–687.
99. Fradis M, Podoshin L, Gertner R, et al. Squamous cell carcinoma of the nasal septum mucosa. *Ear Nose Throat J* 1993;72:217–221.
100. Obert GJ, Devine KD, McDonald JR. Olfactory neuroblastomas. *Cancer* 1960; 13:205–215.
101. Silcox LE. Olfactory neuroblastoma. *Laryngoscope* 1966;76:665–673.
102. Djalilian M, Zujko RD, Weiland LH, et al. Olfactory neuroblastoma. *Surg Clin North Am* 1977;57:751–762.
103. O'Conor GT, Jr., Drake CR, Johns ME, et al. Treatment of advanced esthesioneuroblastoma with high-dose chemotherapy and autologous bone marrow transplantation. A case report. *Cancer* 1985;55:347–349.
104. Morita A, Ebersold MJ, Olsen KD, et al. Esthesioneuroblastoma: prognosis and management. *Neurosurgery* 1993;32:706–715.
105. Ho HW, Awwad EE, Martin DS, et al. Olfactory neuroblastoma mimicking primary intracranial neoplasm. *Comput Med Imaging Graph* 1991;15:125–127.
106. Riemenschneider PA, Prior JT. Neuroblastoma originating from olfactory epithelium (esthesioneuroblastoma). *AJR Am J Roentgenol* 1958;80:759–765.
107. Louboutin JP, Maugard-Louboutin C, Fumoleau P. Leptomeningeal infiltration is esthesioneuroblastoma: report of two cases with poor prognosis. *Eur Neurol* 1994;34:236–238.
108. Eden BV, Debo RF, Larner JM, et al. Esthesioneuroblastoma. Long-term outcome and patterns of failure—the University of Virginia experience. *Cancer* 1994;73:2556–2562.
109. Beitler JJ, Fass DE, Brenner HA, et al. Esthesioneuroblastoma: is there a role for elective neck treatment? *Head Neck* 1991;13:321–326.
110. Resto VA, Eisele DW, Forastiere A, et al. Esthesioneuroblastoma: the John Hopkins experience. *Head Neck* 2000;22:550–558.
111. Davis RE, Weissler MC. Esthesioneuroblastoma and neck metastasis. *Head Neck* 1992;14:477–482.
112. Appelblatt NH, McClatchey KD. Olfactory neuroblastoma: a retrospective clinicopathologic study. *Head Neck Surg* 1982;5:108–113.
113. Koka VN, Julieron M, Bourhis J, et al. Aesthesioneuroblastoma. *J Laryngol Otol* 1998;112:628–633.
114. Phillips PP, Gustafson RO, Facer GW. The clinical behavior of inverting papilloma of the nose and paranasal sinuses: report of 112 cases and review of the literature. *Laryngoscope* 1990;100:463–469.
115. Elner VM, Burnstine MA, Goodman ML, et al. Inverted papillomas that invade the orbit. *Arch Ophthalmol* 1995;113:1178–1183.
116. Astor FC, Donegan JO, Gluckman JL. Unusual anatomic presentations of inverting papilloma. *Head Neck Surg* 1985;7:243–245.
117. Baris G, Visser AG, Van Andel JG. The treatment of squamous cell carcinoma

of the nasal vestibule with interstitial iridium implantation. *Radiother Oncol* 1985;4:121–125.
118. McNeese MD, Chobe R, Weber RS, et al. Carcinoma of the nasal vestibule: treatment with radiotherapy. *Cancer Bull* 1989;41:84–87.
119. Wong CS, Cummings BJ, Elhakim T, et al. External irradiation for squamous cell carcinoma of the nasal vestibule. *Int J Radiat Oncol Biol Phys* 1986;12: 1943–1946.
120. Mendenhall WM, Stringer SP, Cassisi NJ, et al. Squamous cell carcinoma of the nasal vestibule. *Head Neck* 1999;21:385–393.
121. Singh W, Ramage C, Best P, et al. Nasal neuroblastoma secreting vasopressin. A case report. *Cancer* 1980;45:961–966.
122. Srigley JR, Dayal JR, Gregor RT, et al. Hyponatremia secondary to olfactory neuroblastoma. *Arch Otolaryngol* 1983;109:559–562.
123. Wade PM, Jr., Smith RE, Johns ME. Response of esthesioneuroblastoma to chemotherapy. Report of five cases and review of the literature. *Cancer* 1984; 53:1036–1041.
124. Al Ahwal M, Jha N, Nabholtz JM, et al. Olfactory neuroblastoma: report of a case associated with inappropriate antidiuretic hormone secretion. *J Otolaryngol* 1994;23:437–439.
125. Morris MR, Morris WJ. Esthesioneuroblastoma: an unusual presentation complicating the surgical approach. *Am J Otolaryngol* 1994;15:231–236.
126. Arnesen MA, Scheithauer BW, Freeman S. Cushing's syndrome secondary to olfactory neuroblastoma. *Ultrastruct Pathol* 1994;18:61–68.
127. Mills SE, Frierson HF Jr. Olfactory neuroblastoma. A clinicopathologic study of 21 cases. *Am J Surg Pathol* 1985;9:317–327.
128. Wilson WM, Cullen G. Olfactory groove tumor causing sudden blindness. A case report. *Can J Ophthalmol* 1967;2:133–138.
129. Berman EL, Chu A, Wirtschafter JD, et al. Esthesioneuroblastoma presenting as sudden unilateral blindness. Histopathologic confirmation of optic nerve demyelination. *J Clin Neuro-ophthalmol* 1992;12:31–36.
130. Kadish S, Goodman M, Wang CC. Olfactory neuroblastoma. A clinical analysis of 17 cases. *Cancer* 1976;37:1571–1576.
131. Schenck NL, Ogura JH. Esthesioneuroblastoma. An enigma in diagnosis, a dilemma in treatment. *Arch Otolaryngol* 1972;96:322–324.
132. Oberman HA, Rice DH. Olfactory neuroblastomas. A clinicopathologic study. *Cancer* 1976;38:2494–2502.
133. Gaze MN, Kerr GR, Smyth JF. Mucosal melanomas of the head and neck: the Scottish experience. The Scottish Melanoma Group. *Clin Oncol (R Coll Radiol)* 1990;2:277–283.
134. Blatchford SJ, Koopmann CF Jr, Coulthard SW. Mucosal melanoma of the head and neck. *Laryngoscope* 1986;96:929–934.
135. Girod D, Hanna E, Marentette L. Esthesioneuroblastoma. *Head Neck* 2001;23: 500–505.
136. Vanhoenacke P, Hermans J, Sneyers W, et al. Atypical aesthesioneurblastoma: CT and MRI findings. *Neuroradiology* 1993;35:466–467.
137. Som PM, Lidov M, Brandwein M, et al. Sinonasal esthesioneuroblastoma with intracranial extension: marginal tumor cysts as a diagnostic MR finding. *AJNR Am J Neuroradiol* 1994;15:1259–1262.
138. American Joint Committee on Cancer. *AJCC cancer staging manual,* 5th ed. Philadelphia: Lippincott Williams & Wilkins, 1997:47–50.
138a. Greene F, Page D, Fleming I, et al. *AJCC cancer staging manual,* 6th ed. New York: Springer Verlag, 2002:59–68.
139. Biller HF, Lawson W, Sachdev VP, et al. Esthesioneuroblastoma: surgical treatment without radiation. *Laryngoscope* 1990;100:1199–1201.
140. Dulguerov P, Calcaterra T. Esthesioneuroblastoma: the UCLA experience 1970–1990. *Laryngoscope* 1992;102:843–849.
141. Bourhis J, Fortin A, Dupuis O, et al. Very accelerated radiation therapy: preliminary results in locally unresectable head and neck carcinomas. *Int J Radiat Oncol Biol Phys* 1995;32:747–752.
142. Broich G, Pagliari A, Ottaviani F. Esthesioneuroblastoma: a general review of the cases published since the discovery of the tumour in 1924. *Anticancer Res* 1997;17:2683–2706.
143. Polin RS, Sheehan JP, Chenelle AG, et al. The role of preoperative adjuvant treatment in the management of esthesioneuroblastoma: the University of Virginia experience. *Neurosurgery* 1998;42:1029–1037.
144. American Joint Committee on Cancer. *AJCC cancer staging manual,* 5th ed. Philadelphia: Lippincott Williams & Wilkins, 1997:157–160.
145. Weymuller EA Jr. Cummings CW, Fredrickson JM, et al, eds. Neoplasms. In: *Otolaryngology; head and neck surgery*. St. Louis: Mosby, 1986:923–936.
146. Kim GE, Chang SK, Lee SW, et al. Neoadjuvant chemotherapy and radiation for inoperable carcinoma of the maxillary antrum. A matched-control study. *Am J Clin Oncol* 2000;23:301–308.
147. Lee MM, Vokes EE, Rosen A, et al. Multimodality therapy in advanced paranasal sinus carcinoma: superior long-term results. *Cancer J Sci Am* 1999; 5:219–223.
148. Björk-Eriksson T, Mercke C, Petruson B, et al. Potential impact on tumor control and organ preservation with cisplatin and 5-fluorouracil for patients with advanced tumors of the paranasal sinuses and nasal fossa. A prospective pilot study. *Cancer* 1992;70:2615–2620.
149. Harrison LB, Raben A, Pfister DG, et al. A prospective phase II trial of concomitant chemotherapy and radiotherapy with delayed accelerated fractionation in unresectable tumors of the head and neck. *Head Neck* 1998;20:497–503.
150. Lee YY, Dimery IW, Van Tassel P, et al. Superselective intra-arterial chemotherapy of advanced paranasal sinus tumors. *Arch Otolaryngol Head Neck Surg* 1989;115:503–511.
151. Shah UK, Hybels RL, Dugan J. Endoscopic management of low-grade papillary adenocarcinoma of the ethmoid sinus: case report and review of the literature. *Am J Otolaryngol* 1999;20:190–194.
152. Ketchum AS, Chretien PB, van Buren JM, et al. The ethmoid sinuses: a re-evaluation of surgical resection. *Am J Surg* 1973;126:469–476.
153. Parsons JT, Mendenhall WM, Mancuso AA, et al. Malignant tumors of the nasal cavity and ethmoid and sphenoid sinuses. *Int J Radiat Oncol Biol Phys* 1988;14:11–22.
154. Zappia JJ, Carrol WR, Wolf GT, et al. Olfactory neuroblastoma: the results of modern treatment approaches at the University of Michigan. *Head Neck* 1993; 15:190–196.
155. Eich HT, Staar S, Micke O, et al. Radiotherapy of esthesioneuroblastoma. *Int J Radiat Oncol Biol Phys* 2001;49:155–160.
156. Slevin NJ, Irwin CJ, Banerjee SS, et al. Olfactory neural tumours—the role of external beam radiotherapy. *J Laryngol Otol* 1996;110:1012–1016.
157. Homzie MJ, Elkon D. Olfactory esthesioneuroblastoma—variables predictive of tumor control and recurrence. *Cancer* 1980;46:2509–2513.
158. Lai CH, Wang CH, Tsang NM, et al. Kadish stage C olfactory neuroblastoma successfully treated by chemoradiotherapy: report of two cases. *Changgeng Yi Xue Za Zhi* 1998;21:487–492.
159. Daly NJ, Voigt JJ, Combes PF. Diagnosis and treatment of olfactory neuroblastomas in seven patients. *Int J Radiat Oncol Biol Phys* 1980;6:1735–1738.
160. Guedea F, van Limbergen E, van den Bogaert W. High dose level radiation therapy for local tumour control in esthesioneuroblastoma. *Eur J Cancer* 1994; 30A:1757–1760.
161. Tyler TC, Chandler JR, Wetli C, et al. Olfactory neuroblastoma. *South Med J* 1974;67:640–643.
162. Bhattacharyya N, Thornton AF, Joseph MP, et al. Successful treatment of esthesioneuroblastoma and neuroendocrine carcinoma with combined chemotherapy and proton radiation. Results in 9 cases. *Arch Otolaryngol Head Neck Surg* 1997;123:34–40.
163. Sheehan JM, Sheehan JP, Jane JA, Sr., et al. Chemotherapy for esthesioneuroblastomas. *Neurosurg Clin N Am* 2000;11:693–701.
164. Deutsch BD, Levine PA, Stewart FM, et al. Sinonasal undifferentiated carcinoma: a ray of hope. *Otolaryngol Head Neck Surg* 1993;108:697–700.
165. Kingdom TT, Kaplan MJ. Mucosal melanoma of the nasal cavity and paranasal sinuses. *Head Neck* 1995;17:184–189.
166. Liebross RH, Morrison WH, Garden AS, et al. Mucosal melanoma of the head and neck. *Int J Radiat Oncol Biol Phys* 1997;39:159.
167. Snow GB, van der Esch EP. Mucosal melanomas of the head and neck. *Head Neck Surg* 1978;1:24–30.
168. Stern SJ, Guillamondegui OM. Mucosal melanoma of the head and neck. *Head Neck* 1991;13:22–27.
169. Pergolizzi S, Ascenti G, Settineri N, et al. Primitive sinonasal malignant mucosal melanoma: description of a case treated with radiotherapy (0-7-21 regimen). *Anticancer Res* 1999;19:657–660.
170. Ghamrawi KA, Glennie JM. The value of radiotherapy in the management of malignant melanoma of the nasal cavity. *J Laryngol Otol* 1974;88:71–75.
171. Harwood AR, Cummings BJ. Radiotherapy for mucosal melanomas. *Int J Radiat Oncol Biol Phys* 1982;8:1121–1126.
172. Berthelsen A, Andersen AP, Jensen TS, et al. Melanomas of the mucosa in the oral cavity and the upper respiratory passages. *Cancer* 1984;54:907–912.
173. Calcaterra TC, Thompson JW, Paglia DE. Inverting papillomas of the nose and paranasal sinuses. *Laryngoscope* 1980;90:53–60.
174. Dolgin SR, Zaveri VD, Casiano RR, et al. Different options for treatment of inverting papilloma of the nose and paranasal sinuses: a report of 41 cases. *Laryngoscope* 1992;102:231–236.
175. Segal K, Atar E, Mor C, et al. Inverting papilloma of the nose and paranasal sinuses. *Laryngoscope* 1986;96:394–398.
176. Han JK, Smith TL, Loehrl T, et al. An evolution in the management of sinonasal inverting papilloma. *Laryngoscope* 2001;111:1395–1400.
177. Weissler NC, Montgomery WW, Turner PA, et al. Inverted papilloma. *Ann Otol Rhinol Laryngol* 1986;95:215–221.
178. Guedea F, Mendenhall WM, Parsons JT, et al. The role of radiation therapy in inverted papilloma of the nasal cavity and paranasal sinuses. *Int J Radiat Oncol Biol Phys* 1991;20:777–780.
179. Levendag PC, Annyas AA, Escajadillo JR, et al. Radiotherapy for inverted papilloma: a case report. *Radiother Oncol* 1984;2:13–17.
180. Halperin EC, Dosoretz DE, Goodman M, et al. Radiotherapy of polymorphic reticulosis. *Br J Radiol* 1982;55:645–649.
181. Sobrevilla-Calvo P, Meneses A, Alfaro P, et al. Radiotherapy compared to chemotherapy as initial treatment of angiocentric centrofacial lymphoma (polymorphic reticulosis). *Acta Oncol* 1993;32:69–72.
182. Liang R, Chen F, Lee CK, et al. Autologous bone marrow transplantation for primary nasal T/NK cell lymphoma. *Bone Marrow Transplant* 1997;19:91–93.
183. Goepfert H. The vex and fuss about nasal vestibule cancer. *Head Neck* 1999; 21:383–384.
184. Million RR. The myth regarding bone or cartilage involvement by cancer and the likelihood of cure by radiotherapy. *Head Neck* 1989;11:30–40.
185. Chobe R, McNeese M, Weber R, et al. Radiation therapy for carcinoma of the nasal vestibule. *Otolaryngol Head Neck Surg* 1988;98:67–71.
186. Evensen JF, Jacobsen AB, Tausjo JE. Brachytherapy of squamous cell carcinoma of the nasal vestibule. *Acta Oncol* 1996;35:87–92.
187. Levendag PC, Pomp J. Radiation therapy of squamous cell carcinoma of the nasal vestibule. *Int J Radiat Oncol Biol Phys* 1990;19:1363–1367.
188. Haynes WD, Tapley N. Proceedings: radiation treatment of carcinoma of the nasal vestibule. *Am J Roentgenol Radium Ther Nucl Med* 1974;120:595–602.

189. Chassagne D, Wilson JF. Brachytherapy of carcinomas of the nasal vestibule. *Int J Radiat Oncol Biol Phys* 1984;10:761.
190. McCollough WM, Mendenhall NP, Parsons JT, et al. Radiotherapy alone for squamous cell carcinoma of the nasal vestibule: management of the primary site and regional lymphatics. *Int J Radiat Oncol Biol Phys* 1993;26:73–79.
191. Horsmans JD, Godballe C, Jorgensen KE, et al. Squamous cell carcinoma of the nasal vestibule. *Rhinology* 1999;37:117–121.
192. Fornelli RA, Fedok FG, Wilson EP, et al. Squamous cell carcinoma of the anterior nasal cavity: a dual institution review. *Otolaryngol Head Neck Surg* 2000; 123:207–210.
193. Poulsen M, Turner S. Radiation therapy for squamous cell carcinoma of the nasal vestibule. *Int J Radiat Oncol Biol Phys* 1993;27:267–272.
194. Mazeron JJ, Chassagne D, Crook J, et al. Radiation therapy of carcinomas of the skin of nose and nasal vestibule: a report of 1676 cases by the Groupe Europeen de Curietherapie. *Radiother Oncol* 1988;13:165–173.
195. Kagan AR, Nussbaum H, Rao A, et al. The management of carcinoma of the nasal vestibule. *Head Neck Surg* 1981;4:125–128.
196. Parsons JT, Stringer SP, Mancuso AA, et al. Nasal vestibule, nasal cavity, and paranasal sinuses. In: Million RR, Cassisi NJ, eds. *Management of head and neck cancer: a multidisciplinary approach,* 2nd ed. Philadelphia: JB Lippincott Co, 1994:551–598.
197. Ohngren LG. Malignant tumors of the maxillo-ethmoidal region: a clinical study with special reference to the treatment with electrosurgery and irradiation. *Acta Otolaryngol (Stockh)* 1933;XIX:229–274.
198. Stern SJ, Goepfert H, Clayman G, et al. Squamous cell carcinoma of the maxillary sinus. *Arch Otolaryngol Head Neck Surg* 1993;119:119–964.
199. Zaharia M, Salem LE, Travezan R, et al. Postoperative radiotherapy in the management of cancer of the maxillary sinus. *Int J Radiat Oncol Biol Phys* 1989;17:967–971.
200. Lavertu P, Roberts JK, Kraus DH, et al. Squamous cell carcinoma of the paranasal sinuses: the Cleveland Clinic experience 1977–1986. *Laryngoscope* 1989;99:1130–1136.
201. Frich JC Jr. Treatment of advanced squamous carcinoma of the maxillary sinus by irradiation. *Int J Radiat Oncol Biol Phys* 1982;8:1453–1459.
202. Kurohara SS, Webster JH, Ellis F, et al. Role of radiation therapy and of surgery in the management of localized epidermoid carcinoma of the maxillary sinus. *Am J Roentgenol Radium Ther Nucl Med* 1972;114:35–42.
203. Bataini JP, Ennuyer A. Advanced carcinoma of the maxillary antrum treated by cobalt teletherapy and electron beam irradiation. *Br J Radiol* 1971;44: 590–598.
204. Cheng VS, Wang CC. Carcinomas of the paranasal sinuses: a study of 66 cases. *Cancer* 1977;40:3038–3041.
205. Amendola BE, Eisert D, Hazra TA, et al. Carcinoma of the maxillary antrum: surgery or radiation therapy? *Int J Radiat Oncol Biol Phys* 1981;7:743–746.
206. Som ML. Surgical management of carcinoma of the maxilla. *Arch Otolaryngol* 1974;99:270–273.
207. Goepfert H, Luna MA, Lindberg RD, et al. Malignant salivary gland tumors of the paranasal sinuses and nasal cavity. *Arch Otolaryngol* 1983; 109:662–668.
208. Matsuba HM, Simpson JR, Mauney M, et al. Adenoid cystic salivary gland carcinoma: a clinicopathologic correlation. *Head Neck Surg* 1986;8:200–204.
209. Million RR, Cassisi NJ, Clark JR. Cancer in the head and neck. In: DeVita VT Jr, Hellman S, Rosenberg SA, eds. *Cancer: principles and practice of oncology,* 3rd ed. Philadelphia: JB Lippincott Co, 1989:488–580.
210. Rafla S. Mucous gland tumors of paranasal sinuses. *Cancer* 1969;24:683–691.
211. Leafstedt SW, Gaeta JF, Sako K, et al. Adenoid cystic carcinoma of major and minor salivary glands. *Am J Surg* 1971;122:756–762.
212. Sisson GA Sr, Toriumi DM, Atiyah RA. Paranasal sinus malignancy: a comprehensive update. *Laryngoscope* 1989;99:143–150.
213. Klintenberg C, Olofsson J, Hellquist H, et al. Adenocarcinoma of the ethmoid sinuses. A review of 28 cases with special reference to wood dust exposure. *Cancer* 1984;54:482–488.
214. Loree TR, Mullins AP, Spellman J, et al. Head and neck mucosal melanoma: a 32-year review. *Ear Nose Throat J* 1999;78:372–375.
215. Brandwein MS, Rothstein A, Lawson W, et al. Sinonasal melanoma. A clinicopathologic study of 25 cases and literature meta-analysis. *Arch Otolaryngol Head Neck Surg* 1997;123:290–296.
216. Lee SP, Shimizu KT, Tran LM, et al. Mucosal melanoma of the head and neck: the impact of local control on survival. *Laryngoscope* 1994;104:121–126.
217. Trapp TK, Fu YS, Calcaterra TC. Melanoma of the nasal and paranasal sinus mucosa. *Arch Otolaryngol Head Neck Surg* 1987;113:1086–1089.
218. Hoyt DJ, Jordan T, Fisher SR. Mucosal melanoma of the head and neck. *Arch Otolaryngol Head Neck Surg* 1989;115:1096–1099.
219. Lawson W, Le Benger J, Som P, et al. Inverted papilloma: an analysis of 87 cases. *Laryngoscope* 1989;99:1117–1124.
220. Orton C, Ellis F. A simplification in the use of the NSD concept in practical radiotherapy. *Br J Radiol* 1973;46:529–537.
221. Goepfert H, Guillamondegui OM, Jesse RH, et al. Squamous cell carcinoma of nasal vestibule. *Arch Otolaryngol* 1974;100:8–10.
222. Weinberger JM, Briant TDR, Cummings BJ, et al. The role of surgery in the treatment of squamous cell carcinoma of the nasal vestibule. *J Otolaryngol* 1988;17:372–375.
223. De Jong JMA, Schalekamp W, Hordijk GJ. Squamous carcinoma of the nasal vestibule. *Clin Otolaryngol* 1981;6:205–208.
224. Oriba HA, Snow SN. Tumors of the nasal columella treated by Mohs micrographic surgery. *Laryngoscope* 1997;107:1647–1650.
225. Mak AC, Van Andel JG, van Woerkom-Eijkenboom WMH. Radiation therapy of carcinoma of the nasal vestibule. *Eur J Cancer* 1980;16:81–85.
226. Marx RE, Johnson RP, Kline SN. Prevention of osteoradionecrosis: a randomized prospective clinical trial of hyperbaric oxygen versus penicillin. *J Am Dent Assoc* 1985;111:49–54.
227. Bowden G. Radiation myelitis of the brain-stem. *J Sac Radiol* 1950;2:79–94.
228. Parsons JT, Fitzgerald CR, Hood CI, et al. The effects of irradiation on the eye and optic nerve. *Int J Radiat Oncol Biol Phys* 1983;9:609–622.
229. Parsons JT, Bova FJ, Fitzgerald CR, et al. Radiation retinopathy after external-beam irradiation: analysis of time-dose factors. *Int J Radiat Oncol Biol Phys* 1994;30:765–773.
230. Parsons JT, Bova FJ, Fitzgerald CR, et al. Severe dry-eye syndrome following external beam irradiation. *Int J Radiat Oncol Biol Phys* 1994;30:775–780.
231. Parsons JT, Bova FJ, Fitzgerald CR, et al. Radiation optic neuropathy after megavoltage external-beam irradiation: analysis of time-dose factors. *Int J Radiat Oncol Biol Phys* 1994;30:755–763.
232. Shukovsky LJ, Fletcher GH. Retinal and optic nerve complications in a high dose irradiation technique of ethmoid sinus and nasal cavity. *Radiology* 1972; 104:629–634.
233. Petersen IA, Kriss JP, McDougall IR, et al. Prognostic factors in the radiotherapy of Graves' ophthalmopathy. *Int J Radiat Oncol Biol Phys* 1990;19: 259–264.
234. Bessell EM, Henk JM, Whitelocke RA, et al. Ocular morbidity after radiotherapy of orbital and conjunctival lymphoma. *Eye* 1987;1:90–96.
235. Letschert JG, Gonzalez-Gonzalez D, Oskam J, et al. Results of radiotherapy in patients with stage I orbital non-Hodgkin's lymphoma. *Radiother Oncol* 1991;22:36–44.
236. Chan RC, Shukovsky LJ. Effects of irradiation on the eye. *Radiology* 1976;120: 673–675.
237. Goldsmith BJ, Rosenthal SA, Wara WM, et al. Optic neuropathy after irradiation of meningioma. *Radiology* 1992;185:71–76.
238. Jiang GL, Tucker SL, Guttenberger R, et al. Radiation-induced injury to the visual pathway. *Radiother Oncol* 1994;30:17–25.
239. Brizel DM, Light K, Zhou SM, et al. Conformal radiation therapy treatment planning reduces the dose to the optic structures for patients with tumors of the paranasal sinuses. *Radiother Oncol* 1999;51:215–218.
240. Kuppersmith RB, Teh BS, Donovan DT, et al. The use of intensity modulated radiotherapy for the treatment of extensive and recurrent juvenile angiofibroma. *Int J Pediatr Otorhinolaryngol* 2000;52:261–268.
241. Lohr F, Pirzkall A, Debus J, et al. Conformal three-dimensional photon radiotherapy for paranasal sinus tumors. *Radiother Oncol* 2000;56:227–231.
242. Pommier P, Ginestet C, Sunyach M, et al. Conformal radiotherapy for paranasal sinus and nasal cavity tumors: three-dimensional treatment planning and preliminary results in 40 patients. *Int J Radiat Oncol Biol Phys* 2000; 48:485–493.
243. Leybovich LB, Dogan N, Sethi A, et al. Comparison of IMRT plans for treatment of paranasal sinus and nasopharynx tumors: tomographic technique with and without couch angulation and MLC-based static step-and-shoot technique with coplaner versus non-coplaner beams. *Int J Radiat Oncol Biol Phys* 2001;48:152–153.
244. Spaulding CA, Kranyak MS, Constable WC, et al. Esthesioneuroblastoma: a comparison of two treatment eras. *Int J Radiat Oncol Biol Phys* 1988;15:581–590.
245. Irish J, Dasgupta R, Freeman J, et al. Outcome and analysis of the surgical management of esthesioneuroblastoma. *J Otolaryngol* 1997;26:1–7.
246. Pickuth D, Heywang-Kobrunner SH. Imaging of recurrent esthesioneuroblastoma. *Br J Radiol* 1999;72:1052–1057.
247. Parsons JT, Mendenhall WM, Stringer SP, et al. Nasal cavity and paranasal sinuses. In: Perez CA, Brady LW, eds. *Principles and practice of radiation oncology,* 3rd ed. Philadelphia: Lippincott-Raven Publishers, 1997:941–959.
248. Morita K, Kawabe Y. Late effects on the eye of conformation radiotherapy for carcinoma of the paranasal sinuses and nasal cavity. *Radiology* 1979;130: 227–232.

Radiologic Imaging Concerns

249. Hofmann E, Nadjmi M. [Modern neuroradiologic diagnosis and interventional strategies for the ENT physician]. [Review] [German]. *HNO* 1995;43: 584–589.
250. Kraus DH, Lanzieri CF, Wanamaker JR, et al. Complementary use of computed tomography and magnetic resonance imaging in assessing skull base lesions. *Laryngoscope* 1992;102:623–629.
251. Gualdi GF, Melone A, Di Biasi C, et al. [Tumors of the nose, paranasal sinuses and facial bones: the role of computerized tomography and MRI in the assessment of the damage]. *Clin Ter* 1997;148:257–265.
252. Eisen MD, Yousem DM, Loevner LA, et al. Preoperative imaging to predict orbital invasion by tumor. *Head Neck* 2000;22:456–462.
253. Kerber CW, Wong WH, Howell SB, et al. An organ-preserving selective arterial chemotherapy strategy for head and neck cancer. *AJNR Am J Neuroradiol* 1998;19:935–941.
254. Yokoyama J, Shiga K, Saijo S, et al. [Superselective intra-arterial infusion chemotherapy of high-dose cisplatin for advanced paranasal sinus carcinomas]. *Gan To Kagaku Ryoho* 1999;26:967–973.
255. Dulguerov P, Jacobsen MS, Allal AS, et al. Nasal and paranasal sinus carcinoma: are we making progress? A series of 220 patients and a systematic review. *Cancer* 2001;92:3012–3029.

256. Som PM, Shapiro MD, Biller HF, et al. Sinonasal tumors and inflammatory tissues: differentiation with MR imaging. *Radiology* 1988;167: 803–808.
257. Allbery SM, Chaljub G, Cho NL, et al. MR imaging of nasal masses [Review]. *Radiographics* 1995;15:1311–1327.
258. Chow JM, Leonetti JP, Mafee MF. Epithelial tumors of the paranasal sinuses and nasal cavity [Review]. *Radiolog Clin North Am* 1993;31:61–73.
259. DeMonte F, Ginsberg LE, Clayman GL. Primary malignant tumors of the sphenoidal sinus. *Neurosurgery* 2000;46:1084–1091; discussion 1091–1082.
260. Chaiken L, Rege S, Hoh C, et al. Positron emission tomography with fluorodeoxyglucose to evaluate tumor response and control after radiation therapy. *Int J Radiat Oncol Biol Phys* 1993;27:455–464.
261. Derdeyn CP, Moran CJ, Wippold FJ 2nd, et al. MRI of esthesioneuroblastoma. *J Comp Assist Tomogr* 1994;18:16–21.

CHAPTER 23

Cancer of the Nasopharynx

Lester J. Peters, Danny Rischin, June Corry, and Paul M. Harari

Cancer of the nasopharynx, in the generic sense, includes carcinomas, sarcomas, and lymphomas. Throughout the world, however, "nasopharyngeal cancer" pragmatically refers to a specific category of carcinoma, abbreviated as NPC.

The etiology of NPC is very likely multifactorial: genetic, environmental, and viral. There are at least three major risk factors: (a) a genetically determined predisposition allowing an Epstein–Barr virus (EBV) infection of the type that permits (b) integration of the genome of the virus into the chromosomes of some nasopharyngeal epithelial cells, thereby priming them for (c) neoplastic transformation by some environmental cofactor. Alternatively, the environmental agent(s) may trigger the viral genome in the cells to oncogenic activity.

Although environmental factors appear to be essential, the high frequency in disparate ethnic groups points to different operative agents for each group (1–3). As judged by age-specific incidences, Scandinavians and both blacks and whites in the United States appear to have a different etiologic origin for NPC from that of Chinese Americans or Hong Kong or Singapore Chinese. Among those of Chinese ancestry, the incidence curves rise sharply after the third decade; the curves for non-Chinese individuals show a rise after the fourth or fifth decade. Native Alaskans have a curve pattern similar to that of Chinese individuals, but Tunisians have a bimodal curve, with an early peak in the second decade. In all ethnic groups, the incidence in males is two to three times greater than that in females.

Based on data published in the latest edition of *Cancer Incidence in Five Continents* (4) the world's highest incidence rates of NPC are found in Hong Kong. With its population primarily derived from Guangdong Province in southeastern China, Hong Kong has consistently reported very high rates of NPC of about 25 to 30 per 100,000 in males and 10 to 15 per 100,000 in females. Cantonese Chinese who have migrated to other parts of the world retain a high predisposition to the disease, although at a lesser rate than those living in China (5). Intermediate rates (5–15 per 100,000 in males) are reported in other peoples of Southeast Asia (Malays, Indonesians, Filipinos, Thais, and Vietnamese), Eskimos, and North African Arabs. A relatively low to moderate incidence (1–5 per 100,000) occurs among Northern Chinese, Polynesians, Maltese, and Central Africans. The disease is rare, less than 1 per 100,000 in Caucasians, Japanese, Koreans, and the population of the Indian subcontinent (Table 23.1).

In Europe the populations of the southern countries (Spain, Italy, France, Balkan states) are at a relatively higher risk for NPC than those from northern countries. In the past the increased risk was linked to populations living on the coast of the Mediterranean Sea. Recent data do not seem to confirm this finding. In fact only Malta and Israel (Jews born in Africa or Asia) show higher incidence rates whereas the coastal populations of Spain, Italy, and the Balkan states have a lower incidence than those living in the interior parts of those countries.

TABLE 23.1 Age-Adjusted Incidence Rates by Ethnic Grouping

Incident	Rate	Ethnic grouping
Very high	>25	Indigenous Southern Chinese
High	15–25	Emigrant Southern Chinese (Singapore, US)
Intermediate	5–15	Non-Chinese Southeast Asians, Arabs, Eskimos
Moderate to low	1–5	Northern Chinese, Polynesians, Central Africans, Maltese
Rare	<1	Caucasians, Subcontinent Indian, Japanese, Koreans

Levine et al. (6) have studied demographic patterns for NPC in the United States. These were obtained from the Third National Cancer Survey, the Surveillance Epidemiology and End Results (SEER) Program, and the Connecticut Tumor Registry. Approximately seven out of every eight malignant tumors of the nasopharynx (1,202 patients) were classified as NPC. Although 84% of white patients with cancer of the nasopharynx had NPC, more than 90% of nonwhite patients had NPC. The preponderance of NPC in the case material held for all but the youngest patients; sarcomas were the more frequent among whites under 10 years of age. White patients had the highest frequency of squamous cell carcinomas. Undifferentiated carcinomas were more common in African American and Chinese American patients and were relatively frequent in young patients of all races. Chinese Americans have a greater risk for developing NPC than any other racial/ethnic group in the United States. Whites and blacks have similar risks, except at young ages where there is a minor post-adolescent age peak in NPC risk that is more pronounced for blacks in the United States than for whites (7). A similar young age peak has been observed in other parts of the world such as India, Tunisia, and the Sudan but remains unexplained. The apparent excess risk in the young African American population has been considered to be related to rural residence and low socioeconomic status (8).

The morbidity data from the United States do not show outstanding geographic or temporal variation in NPC risk for whites (6,8). Only the relatively high mortality rate in Alaska stands out as a significant factor in mortality studies of the states and their counties.

EPSTEIN–BARR VIRUS AND BIOLOGIC IMPLICATIONS

The Epstein–Barr virus is ubiquitous in humans and antibodies to polypeptides of the virus are present in over 80% of human serum samples from the United States; even higher percentages are found among Asian and African populations (3,9). Practically no one escapes infection from this herpes-group virus. Primary infections often remain clinically unapparent or not recognized as being due to EBV, particularly in children under the age of 3 to 5 years.

Consequences of EBV infection vary in different populations (i.e., it is associated predominantly with infectious mononucleosis in the Western hemisphere, Burkitt lymphoma in Africa, and NPC in Asia). Occurrence of these three EBV-associated diseases is unusual outside their normally associated populations, which suggests strongly the role of additional factors in the populations at risk. The apparent differences in geographic distribution of the three main EBV-associated diseases have also prompted suggestions that different strains of EBV are prevalent in different areas. This has not been verified and likely is not a factor (3).

Clinically manifest or not, primary EBV infections establish a permanent EBV carrier state in the lymphatic system and also in the major salivary glands (10). This is reflected in the lifelong persistence of EBV-specific antibodies, at almost constant titers, and an intermittent excursion of EBV into the oropharynx (11).

The association between EBV and NPC was initially discovered in 1966 by Old et al. (12) who showed that patients with undifferentiated carcinoma of the nasopharynx had elevated immunoglobulin G (IgG)- and IgA-antibody titers against EBV early and viral capsid antigens. Since then a large number of studies have shown that essentially all cases of undifferentiated carcinoma of nasopharyngeal type throughout the world contain the EBV genome regardless of the local incidence of the tumor or the ethnicity of the patient. Epstein–Barr nuclear antigen 1 (EBNA 1) is expressed in practically all NPCs. Evidence tightening the causal association of EBV with NPC in genetically predisposed groups was provided by a demonstration that showed preinvasive lesions of the nasopharynx contain clonal copies of the EBV genome (using the criterion of terminal repeat reiteration frequency), which indicates that EBV infection is likely to be an early initiating event in the development of NPC (13). Reports on the association between EBV and differentiated [World Health Organization (WHO) type 1] NPC are contradictory. Although some studies have been unable to demonstrate the presence of EBV in squamous cell carcinomas others have shown positive hybridization signals, although expression of viral-encoded transcripts appears to be down-regulated once tumor cells differentiate and produce keratin (14).

Although EBV infection is clearly an important factor in the pathogenesis of NPC its ubiquitous distribution contrasted with the distinct geographic epidemiology of NPC implicates a multistep process. Genetic predisposition is obviously a factor (15). It would also appear that in high-risk groups environmental carcinogens such as salted fish may play a role (16).

GENETICS

Several genetic systems have been investigated in patients with NPC. In southern Chinese populations a strong association with HLA locus A and B antigens is well established (17). Data from other races are inconclusive. Burt et al. (18) investigated associations between NPC and HLA antigens at the HLA-A, B, C, and DQ loci and alleles at the DRB1 locus in a population-based multicenter study in the United States. Data from 82 cases and 140 controls were presented making this the largest study yet performed in Caucasians. An analysis was undertaken to compare their results with previously published findings. This found a significant protective association with A2 antigen in non-Chinese, a protective association with A11 across all races, and increased risk associated with B5 in Caucasians. Associations were found to be more pronounced in younger patients.

Molecular genetic investigations have demonstrated nonrandom and consistent loss of genetic material in defined regions of chromosomes 3p, 9p, 11q, and 14q (19–22). It is well recognized that frequent allelic loss or homozygous deletion within a specific chromosomal region suggests the presence of a tumor suppressor gene. This would indicate the possibility of multiple tumor suppressor genes involved in the pathogenesis of NPC. One of the key molecular genetic events identified in primary NPC is the homozygous deletion as well as aberrant methylation of the *p16* and *p15* genes mapped to chromosome 9p21. These genes are upstream regulators of RB and thus affect critical cellular regulatory pathways that may be pathogenetically linked to NPC development.

GROSS AND MICROSCOPIC ANATOMY

Gross Anatomy

The roof of the nasopharynx begins behind the posterior nasal choanae and slopes downward where it becomes continuous with the posterior wall. The bony roof and posterior wall are formed serially by the basisphenoid, basiocciput, and anterior arch of the atlas. The lateral and posterior walls are, in part, upward extensions of the boundaries of the oropharynx. In the lower part of the lateral wall, the superior constrictor muscle sends its fibers posteriorly to attach to the basisphenoid. Between the upper border of the superior constrictor and the skull base is stretched the pharyngobasilar fascia with the eustachian tube lodged between the medial pterygoid plate and the superior constrictor. The inward bulge of the tubal ampulla creates a slitlike space between it and the posterior wall; the pharyngeal recess or fossa of Rosenmüller is filled, in part, by the levator palati muscle which lies between the pharyngobasilar fascia and the mucous membrane (23).

The nasopharyngeal lymphoid tissue or adenoid is concentrated at the junction of the roof and posterior wall of the postnasal space. There are other lymphoid aggregates about the tubal openings. The sensory nerve supply to the postnasal space is provided by the glossopharyngeal and maxillary nerves. Beneath the mucous membrane of the roof is the vestigial pharyngeal hypophysis. Lying in the midline near the vomerosphenoidal articulation, its presence is a reminder of the embryologic origin of the anterior pituitary from the Rathke pouch. The hypophyseal vestige may be partly or completely surrounded by the basisphenoid. Also in the midline, but dorsal along the roof and separated from the pharyngeal hypophysis by adenoidal tissue, is an epithelial recess. This is sometimes called the pharyngeal bursa and is an occasional locus of inflammation or cyst formation. Believed to be formed by a tethering of pharyngeal endoderm to the tip of the embryonic notochord, the recess has no relationship with the Rathke pouch (23).

Microscopic Anatomy

Batsakis et al. (1) have summarized our current knowledge of the histology of the mucosa of the nasopharynx. It is composed of three basic cell types: pseudostratified columnar (respiratory) cells, squamous cells, and intermediate (pseudostratified) cuboidal cells. All three types are found during fetal development with the respiratory type being the first to evolve. There is an increase in squamous epithelium until, in the adult nasopharynx, the dominance of respiratory over squamous epithelium is reversed. A commensurate increase in the intermediate type of epithelium is not seen, but it persists at junctions between respiratory and squamous epithelia with its greatest density at the junction of the oropharynx and nasopharynx. In the adult, squamous epithelium covers approximately 60% of the entire nasopharyngeal surface. The intermediate epithelium is aptly named because it is intermediate in a topographic as well as cytologic sense. Investigations in nonhuman species have indicated change of some of the intermediate cells to either ciliated respiratory or squamous cells (1). Resembling the intermediate cell layers in both respiratory and squamous epithelia, the greatest density of the intermediate epithelium is in the sites of predilection for NPC. This is also the closest normal histologic homolog of the nonkeratinizing or undifferentiated carcinomas of the nasopharynx (1).

PATHOLOGY

Classification and Histology of Nasopharyngeal Carcinoma

Over the years, diversity of diagnostic nomenclature and an absence of a uniform histologic reporting system have bedeviled correlation with results of therapy and prognosis. Cognizant of this, the World Health Organization (WHO) has divided NPC into three histologic types: squamous cell, nonkeratinizing, and undifferentiated (1,2,24). The categories are distinct and cover the spectrum of NPC micromorphology (Table 23.2).

Microscopically, squamous cell carcinoma of the nasopharynx is like squamous cell carcinomas in other anatomic sites of the upper aerodigestive tracts. The carcinomas manifest obvious and readily identifiable keratin products and their growth pattern is typical of that found in any squamous cell carcinoma In general, the carcinoma is moderately differentiated and is accompanied by a desmoplastic host response. Because it is preponderantly a surface growth, endoscopic examination of the nasopharynx usually identifies the carcinoma. The average age of patients with squamous cell carcinoma of the nasopharynx is somewhat older than that for all NPC patients. It is rarely found in patients younger than 40 years of age (24).

Nonkeratinizing carcinoma of the WHO classification is distinct from both squamous cell and undifferentiated carcinomas. It is a category accommodating carcinomas that are neither keratinizing nor undifferentiated. Like the squamous carcinomas, nonkeratinizing carcinomas exhibit variable degrees of differentiation within the limits of their definition. The cells have a maturation sequence that ends without good light optic evidence of squamous differentiation. Growth may be papillary or

TABLE 23.2 Classification of Nasopharyngeal Carcinoma

	WHO classification	Former terminology
Type 1:	Squamous cell carcinoma	Squamous cell carcinoma
Type 2:	Nonkeratinizing carcinoma without lymphoid stroma	Transitional cell carcinoma intermediate cell carcinoma
	With lymphoid stroma	Lymphoepithelial carcinoma (Regaud)
Type 3:	Undifferential carcinoma without lymphoid stroma	Anaplastic carcinoma: clear cell carcinoma
	With lymphoid stroma	Lymphoepithelial carcinoma (Schmincke)

WHO, World Health Organization.

plexiform. The cells have fairly well-defined cell margins and the neoplastic islands are usually quite well delineated from the adjacent stroma. In some of the carcinomas, there is a pseudostratified arrangement of cells, not unlike that noted for the intermediate epithelium of the nasopharynx. Although histologic differences between squamous cell carcinoma and nonkeratinizing carcinomas are sharp, the differences between nonkeratinizing and undifferentiated carcinomas are sometimes vague and may be arbitrary. The clinical features and the serologic association with EBV suggest that the last two carcinomas are closely related and give support to the notion that there are really only two major subtypes of NPC: squamous cell carcinomas and the less differentiated forms (24,25).

Undifferentiated carcinoma of nasopharyngeal type (UCNT; also known as anaplastic and poorly differentiated NPC) is composed of primitive cells whose most consistent feature is a single, prominent nucleolus and a nucleus with distinct membrane and, in many cases, nuclear vesiculation. In contrast to the other NPC types, the cell margins of this carcinoma are often indistinct and the tumor often has a syncytial appearance. The cellular arrangement, however, is variable with masses, strands, or individual cells lying in a lymphoid stroma. A variety of cytoplasmic forms and growth patterns has given rise to descriptive terms such as *anaplastic, clear cell, spindle cell, simplex,* and *lymphoepithelioma.* Undifferentiated NPC has a striking invasive and metastasizing capability and tissue reactions to the infiltrating tumor are usually limited. Fibrosis or desmoplasia, for example, are never prominent unless there has been prior radiation therapy (24). Usually there is no discernible reaction and the carcinoma maintains an intimate relationship with lymphoid tissues.

The presence or absence of lymphocytes in NPC is not a factor in making the diagnosis. It is now firmly established that the lymphocytes are not neoplastic or integral to the carcinomas. They can be found in all three of the WHO types, but are most often associated with undifferentiated carcinomas. Approximately 98% of undifferentiated, 70% of nonkeratinizing, and 37% of squamous cell carcinomas of the nasopharynx are associated with lymphocytes. The lymphoid "stroma" is not entirely passive. Metastases of undifferentiated NPC to nonlymphoid tissues may also have an accompaniment of lymphoid cells.

Several histologic findings of a host response to NPC merit mention. Some may have as yet unknown prognostic value while others, in the presence of undifferentiated NPC, may mislead the surgical pathologist to a diagnosis of lymphoid neoplasm. A mixture of lymphoid cells, plasma cells, sometimes associated with polymorphonuclear leukocytes, is found in nearly all forms of NPC. A mild to moderate stromal eosinophilia is evident in about one fourth of the carcinomas, most often with the undifferentiated types, where it may be a conspicuous feature. Some authors have also reported an amyloid-like material in the stroma and also sometimes in the cytoplasm of the carcinoma cells (26). The amyloid, unlikely to be of a secondary type, is found most often in association with nonkeratinizing NPC. In the lymphoid tissue immediately adjacent to undifferentiated NPC, there may be a predominance of T lymphocytes. This is a finding of possible significance because of the inherently B-cell nature of the lymphoid tissue of the nasopharynx. T-zone histiocytes (Langerhans cells and precursors) at primary carcinoma sites may also play a role in an immune reaction (27). In lymph nodes with or without metastases from NPC and on occasion, in the nasopharynx itself, tuberculoid granulomas are found. Usually around neoplasm, the epithelioid granulomas may be accompanied by large numbers of eosinophils, fibrosis, and caseous necrosis. Infective granulomas or Hodgkin disease may be simulated.

Despite the variations in histologic appearance of the WHO types, their proposed mode of histogenesis, the lability and maturational tendencies of the nasopharyngeal epithelium, and clinicopathologic findings suggest all three types may be histologically homogeneous. The tendency for an epidermoid differentiation and the light optic findings of a mixed cell or intermediate population in otherwise prototypic histologic classes support this homogeneity, as does ultrastructure. Shanmugaratnam et al. (2) have indicated that features of more than one histologic type were present in 25% of all NPCs studied in a Singapore population. In such instances, classification is based on the predominant type found in the primary lesion.

Carcinomas histologically similar or indistinguishable from NPC types 2 and 3 have been found elsewhere in the epithelium of the Waldeyer ring (28), in the larynx (29), the thymus (30), the major salivary glands (10), and the cervix (31). The role of EBV in some of these carcinomas is strongly suggested by serologic profiles, presence of EBV-associated nuclear antigen in the carcinoma cells, and by high levels of viral genomes in the DNA. A histomorphologic feature common to all is an intimacy of epithelium and lymphoid cells, not unlike that of the nasopharyngeal mucosa. This "lymphoepithelium" is found in the base of the tongue, tonsillar and adenoidal crypts, in association with salivary ducts, laryngeal "tonsil," and obviously in the thymus. These "lymphoepithelial carcinomas" are infrequent (e.g., <5% of base of tongue and tonsil carcinomas), but their biologic behavior and response to treatment qualifies them further as *carcinomas of nasopharyngeal type.*

PATTERNS OF SPREAD AND CLINICAL PRESENTATION

Nasopharyngeal carcinoma, especially of the WHO types 2 and 3, usually arises in the region of the fossa of Rosenmüller. The primary tumor may extend anteriorly into the nasal cavity, superiorly into the floor of the sphenoid sinus or through the foramen lacerum into the cavernous sinus, anterosuperiorly into the posterior ethmoid air cells and orbits, laterally into the parapharyngeal space and sphenopalatine fossa, and inferiorly into the oropharynx (Fig. 23.1). Lymphatic spread most commonly involves the jugular chain of lymphatics and the posterior cervical chain. In addition, retropharyngeal nodes may be involved.

The early symptoms of the disease are neither pathognomonic nor specific. The clinical presentation of NPC in the

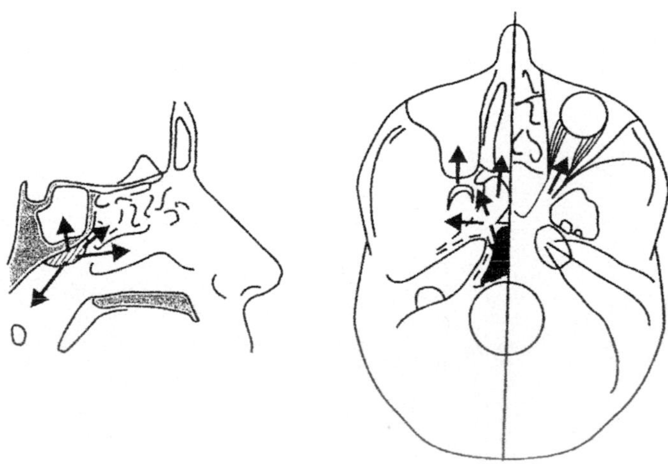

Figure 23.1 Potential routes of spread of primary tumor.

North American population has been documented in a collaborative prospective study (32).

Over a third of patients will notice a mass in the neck as their first symptom and about an equal number will have a sensation of unilateral ear fullness or plugging and hearing loss. Persistent serous otitis media, especially if unilateral in an otherwise healthy adult, should arouse suspicion of a carcinoma of the nasopharynx. A cancer of the nasopharynx will seldom produce choanal or nasal obstruction but initial bleeding or bloody nasal drainage is noticed by about one fifth of patients. The triad of a mass in the neck, a conductive hearing loss, and nasal obstruction with bloody-tinged drainage is frequently present by the time the diagnosis of NPC is made.

The proximity of foramen lacerum and thus the floor of the middle cranial fossa allows for direct tumor extension into the cranium and involvement of adjacent nerves. One fifth of the patients will have symptoms of cranial nerve involvement at the time of diagnosis. Facial pain and paresthesias suggest tumor infiltration of the branches of the trigeminal nerve and diplopia from paralysis of the lateral rectus muscle is a sign of involvement of the abducens nerve. Involvement of cranial nerves III and IV indicates more advanced disease along the cavernous sinus. Tumor extension may occur laterally into the parapharyngeal space and involve cranial nerves IX, X, and XI, thus producing a jugular foramen syndrome. A persistent occipitotemporal headache, especially unilateral, is reported by one of every six patients. Rarely will NPC invade the parotid gland and cause facial nerve paralysis. Proptosis will occur when cancer invades through the posterior portion of the orbit. Trismus is an indication of pterygoid muscle invasion and cancer extension into this space.

At the time of diagnosis, nine of every ten patients will have palpable lymph node metastases with bilateral involvement in half of them. The lymph nodes most frequently involved are in the sub-digastric area and in the chain along the spinal accessory nerve in the posterior triangle. The sentinel lymph node for NPC is located underneath the upper insertion of the sternocleidomastoid muscle. Frequently the neck mass is large and painless and it can enlarge quite rapidly due to necrosis or hemorrhage. Retropharyngeal lymph node metastasis, when extensive, produces a characteristic syndrome of pain referred to the ipsilateral neck, ear, head, forehead, and orbit. It may be associated with a stiff neck or pain when cervical dorsiflexion is attempted.

Physical examination includes inspection of the nasopharynx, either indirectly with a mirror or preferably by direct visualization through a fiberoptic endoscope. The tumor usually appears as an asymmetric mass with telangiectasia on its friable surface and is centered in the fossa of Rosenmüller. Depending on the size of the primary tumor, distortion of the soft palate can occur. Straw-colored serous otitis media is usually unilateral. Evaluation of the cranial nerves may uncover subtle signs of tumor infiltration. The earliest signs are usually extraocular muscle dysfunction, especially lateral rectus palsy, and signs of trigeminal nerve involvement such as hyperesthesia and atrophy of masticatory muscles. The relative frequency of involvement of each cranial nerve is indicated in Table 23.3 (33).

For patients in whom the tumor in the nasopharynx is clinically obvious, biopsy can usually be done under the topical anesthetic by cocaine applications through the nasal cavity. Sometimes however, no primary lesion is evident in the nasopharynx but NPC is suspected on the basis of the presence and location of cervical lymph nodes. In such cases, fine-needle aspiration cytology will usually establish whether the cell type is consistent with NPC. If it is, radiologic assessment of the nasopharynx may indicate a target lesion for biopsy at examination under anesthesia. If not, a core biopsy of an involved node will provide tissue for fluorescent *in situ* hybridization analysis to detect EBV viral genome constituents in the neoplastic cells, which is sufficient to establish the diagnosis of NPC (Fig. 23.2).

TABLE 23.3 Frequency of Individual Cranial Nerve Involvement when Cranial Nerves are Involved in Cancer of the Nasopharynx

Cranial nerves	No. of patients	Frequency (%)
I	1	.05
II	114	4.0
III	236	8.2
IV	207	7.2
V	521	18.1
VI	600	20.9
VII	133	4.6
VIII	49	1.7
IX	264	9.2
X	233	8.1
XI	154	5.4
XII	358	12.5

DIAGNOSTIC EVALUATION AND STAGING

Radiologic evaluation of the nasopharynx, the base of the skull, paranasal sinuses, and the neck is mandatory for appropriate staging and treatment. Computed tomography (CT) allows for the definition of the extent of primary tumor and the amount of invasion and infiltration of surrounding structures. Bone destruction about the floor of the sphenoid sinus, the adjacent middle cranial fossa, the clivus, and the pterygoid plates can be documented as well as the extension of tumor through the foramen lacerum into the middle cranial fossa, laterally into the parapharyngeal space, anteriorly into the nasal cavity, and anterolaterally into the orbit. It is important to demonstrate invasion into the posterior ethmoid cells and adjacent portion of the maxillary antrum. Radiographic documentation of invasion into the base of skull is present in at least one-fourth of patients. Magnetic resonance imaging (MRI) is a valuable complementary study to CT and is recommended whenever possible. An MRI is particularly valuable in discriminating fluid retention from tumor invasion of the sinuses. It also provides a sensitive means of detecting occult invasion of the marrow space of the clivus (Fig. 23.3) and intracranial extension (34).

Both CT and MRI examinations may also reveal metastatic spread to lymph nodes that is undetectable clinically. For example, Figure 23.3 also shows an involved left retropharyngeal lymph node. Such information is vital for radiotherapy treatment planning to avoid the risk for a geographic miss.

The majority of patients with NPC Present with locoregionally advanced disease, and at least one fifth of patients can be deduced to have had occult distant metastases at the time of presentation on the basis of relapse patterns following treatment by radiotherapy alone (35,36). Sites of predilection for metastatic spread are presented in Table 23.4 (37)—the top three sites are bone, lung, and liver. The relative risk for developing metastatic disease as a function of T and N stage at presentation has been analyzed in depth by Lee et al. (38). Appropriate screening for distant metastases is based on the probability of detection versus the cost of screening. We currently recommend that patients with T4 or N+ disease have a metastatic workup including CT of the chest and upper abdomen and a bone scan

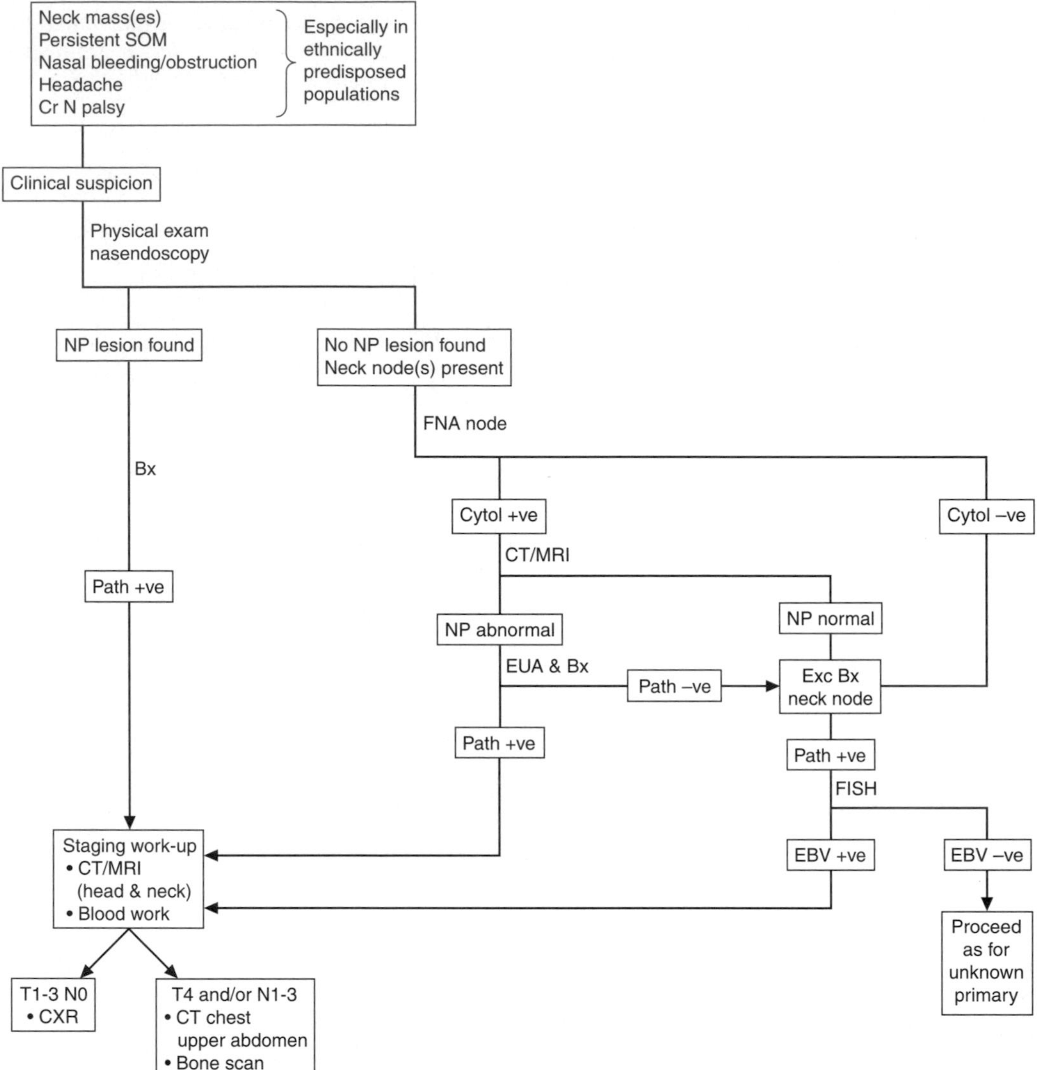

Figure 23.2 Diagnostic algorithm for nasopharyngeal carcinoma. CT, computed tomography; CXR, chest x-ray; EBV, Epstein–Barr virus; EUA, examination under general anaesthetic; FISH, fluorescent *in situ* hybridization; FNA, fine needle aspirate; MRI, magnetic resonance imaging; NP, nasopharyngeal; SOM, serous otitis media; +ve, positive; -ve, negative.

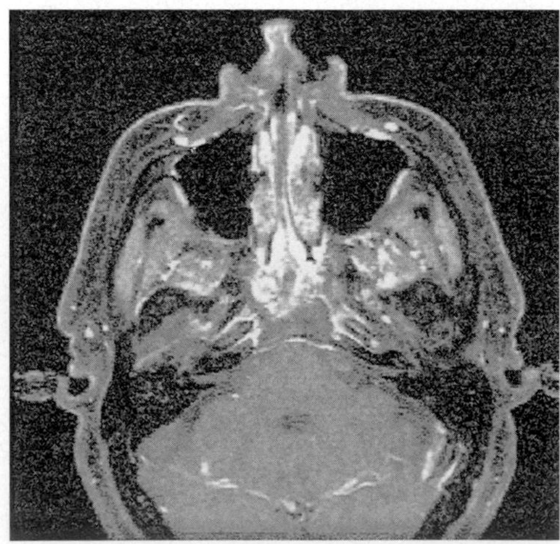

Figure 23.3 Magnetic resonance imaging scan showing subtle invasion of the clivus and a small left retropharyngeal node.

TABLE 23.4 Distant Metastatic Sites of Nasopharyngeal Carcinoma: A Study of 2,637 People

Metastatic site	No. of patients	Frequency (%)
Bones	342	41
Lungs	256	30
Liver	121	1
Distant lymph nodes	101	1
Brain	18	2
Other	3	1
Total:	841	32

Source: Huang SC, Chu GL. Nasopharyngeal cancer: study 11. *Int J Radiat Oncol Biol Phys* 1981;7:713–716.

TABLE 23.5 Unified Tumor (T) and Node (N) Staging System

Primary tumor (T)		Regional lymph nodes (N)	
TX	Primary tumor cannot be assessed	NX	Regional lymph nodes cannot be assessed
T0	No evidence of primary tumor	N0	No regional lymph node metastasis
Tis	Carcinoma *in situ*	N1	Unilateral metastasis in lymph node(s), 6 cm or less in greatest dimension, above the supraclavicular fossa
T1	Tumor confined to the nasopharynx	N2	Bilateral metastasis in lymph node(s), 6 cm or less in greatest dimension, above the supraclavicular fossa
T2	Tumor extends to soft tissues of oropharynx or nasal fossa T2a without parapharyngeal extension T2b with parapharyngeal extension	N3	Metastasis in a lymph node(s) N3a greater than 6 cm in dimension N3b extension to the supraclavicular fossa
T3	Tumor invades body structure or paranasal sinuses		
T4	Tumor with intracranial extension or involvement of cranial nerves, infratemporal fossa, hypopharynx, or orbit		

(alternatively, a whole body positron emission testing scan can substitute for both these tests). For patients with T1 to T3 N0 disease, the yield is too low to justify these tests and the recommended screen is limited to a plain chest film plus routine blood work (Fig. 23.2).

Staging

For many years three separate staging systems have been used for NPC. Among Caucasians the system developed by the American Joint Committee on Cancer (AJCC) was most commonly used in the United States and the similar International Union against Cancer system, or UICC, was used elsewhere in the Western world. By contrast, in Southeast Asia the Ho system (39) was used. One of the major achievements of the past 5 years has been the successful development of a single staging system with international consensus. The new staging system has been ratified by both the UICC in the 5th edition of the *TNM Classification of Malignant Tumours* (40) and the AJCC in its 5th and 6th editions of the *AJCC Cancer Staging Manual* (41,41a). The 6th edition of the AJCC manual maintains the same information for the nasopharynx site as the 5th edition. It embraces many of the features of the Ho system and its derivatives and thus provides a staging system for NPC that is quite different from that of other head and neck cancers. Details of the new unified system are provided in Table 23.5 and the stage groupings are listed in Table 23.6.

Central to the AJCC staging system is use of cross-sectional imaging with CT or MRI to demonstrate the extent of primary tumor and nodal involvement. The principle was adopted that data guiding the staging revision should be based on tumors whose extent was assessed using cross-sectional imaging because outcomes based on previous clinical and radiologic findings would likely be invalid. The main differences between the previous UICC/AJCC staging systems and the new classification are as follows:

T Categories

- T1—Includes all tumors confined to the nasopharynx. The old classification recognized different subsites within the nasopharynx. The lack of validity of these subdivisions in prognosis has been demonstrated by many authors [e.g., Sham et al. (42)].
- T2—Includes involvement of the oropharynx or nasal fossa which under the old system was categorized as T3. Also, recognition of parapharyngeal space extension is provided. This is defined as posterolateral infiltration beyond the pharyngobasilar fascia. A paradoxical situation can arise with the new staging system with respect to patients in whom parapharyngeal space extension is present without involvement of the nasal cavity or oropharynx. Such patients properly belong in the T2 category. This paradox has been rectified in the 6th edition.
- T3—Includes tumors invading the skull base or paranasal sinuses, which were previously categorized as T4.
- T4—This now requires intracranial extension or involvement of cranial nerves or involvement of the infratemporal fossa, hypopharynx, or orbit.

N Categories

The critical prognostic significance of level of lymph node involvement in the neck, as well as size, has been recognized. Multiplicity and clinical fixity of nodes are not criteria for staging (43).

TABLE 23.6 Stage Grouping Nasopharynx

Stage 0	Tis	N0	M0
Stage I	T1	N0	M0
Stage IIA	T2a	N0	M0
IIB	T1	N1	M0
	T2a	N1	M0
	T2b	N0	M0
	T2b	N21	M0
Stage III	T1	N2	M0
	T2a	N2	M0
	T2b	N2	M0
	T2b	N2	M0
	T3	N0	M0
	T3	N1	M0
	T3	N2	M0
Stage IVA	T4	N0	M0
	T4	N3N1	M0
	T4	N2	M0
IVB	Any T	N3	M0
IVC	Any T	Any N	M1

- N1—Unlike other head and neck cancers the N1 category includes one or more nodes up to 6 cm in greatest dimension provided they are unilateral and above the supraclavicular fossa.
- N2—Includes bilateral lymph nodes above the supraclavicular fossa of the neck up to 6 cm in size.
- N3—Presence of nodes greater than 6 cm in diameter or any involvement of or extension to the supraclavicular fossa.

A detailed analysis and comparison of the prognostic significance of the new staging system relative to its predecessors was published by Lee et al. (38).

MANAGEMENT STRATEGIES

Historically, nasopharyngeal cancer has traditionally been treated with radiation therapy alone. However, although good control is achieved in most patients with early stage disease, high rates of both local recurrence and distant metastatic spread have been reported in patients presenting with advanced locoregional disease (44–46). These poor results, with 5-year survival of 15% to 50%, have led to investigation of the benefit of adding chemotherapy either sequentially, concurrently, or both to the primary management strategy for patients with stage III to IV disease. The results of these studies, discussed in detail in late stage disease section, provide the evidence for our current treatment management strategies:

- Stage I and small volume stage II—Radiation therapy alone using three-dimensional (3D) conformal treatment techniques.
- Bulky stage II and stages III to IV—Radiation therapy plus both sequential and concurrent chemotherapy (Fig. 23.4).

Radiotherapy Philosophy and Technique

The propensity of cancer of the nasopharynx to metastasize and to spread locally beyond the confines of the nasopharynx mandates large treatment volumes for all stages of disease. Delineation of the primary target volume is based on the extent of disease determined by clinical and radiologic evaluation. The latter should include both transverse and coronal CT cuts. As in all radiotherapy, the objective of treatment is to deliver a dose to the target volume tailored to the amount of disease present while respecting the tolerance of the normal tissues irradiated. To achieve this objective is technically difficult. Nonetheless, the wide availability of CT-based treatment planning systems and sophisticated treatment delivery systems using customized shielding permits an adequate plan to be devised for virtually all patients except those with extensive intracranial disease or involvement of the sphenoid sinus or posterior orbit with tumor in close proximity to the optic nerves and chiasm. In such patients a compromise has to be struck between the probability of achieving tumor control and the risk for radiation-induced blindness when a dose in excess of 54 Gy is specified.

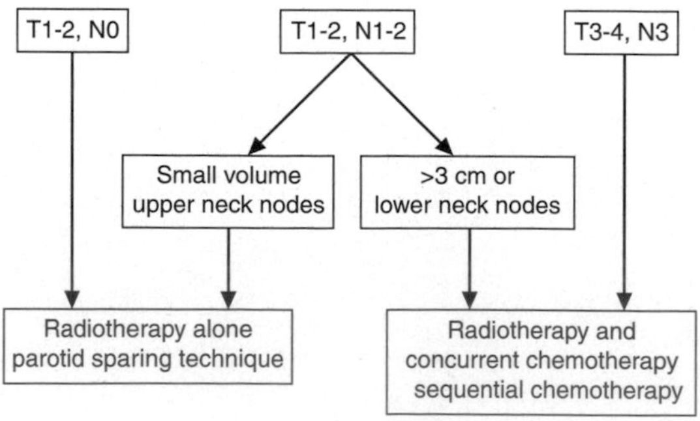

Figure 23.4 Treatment algorithm for nasopharyngeal carcinoma.

Treatment Plan

Although standard treatment planning with parallel opposed fields and an off-cord reduction provides good coverage of the planning target volume (PTV) for early stage disease, it produces unnecessary morbidity associated with irradiation of the major salivary glands and hence has given way to 3D-conformal treatment using parotid sparing techniques. For more advanced disease, especially when there is bilateral posterolateral spread from the primary tumor site, nonstandard plans are essential to achieve adequate coverage. At the Peter MacCallum Cancer Institute (PMCI), we have developed a technique, known as the "boomerang" for treating such cases. This technique, though not strictly 3D-conformal, provides an acceptable alternative for centers where conformational planning technology is not available (Fig. 23.5; see Color Plate 7 following page 524).

The shape of the boomerang isodose curve marries nicely with the extent of disease commonly seen in locally advanced NPC. The posteromedial extent of disease represents a "cold area" with standard techniques, typically receiving almost 30% less dose in the off-cord treatment phase. In the boomerang technique the off-cord component of treatment begins at 36 Gy in 18 fractions. The patient is immobilized in a prone position to obviate treatment through the treatment couch rails. The optimal patient position is one that places the posterior clivus (brainstem) in line with the spinal cord, as seen on the image intensifier. This allows two asymmetric arcs to rotate around the spinal cord/brainstem, typically from 340° to 80° and 280° to 20°. Although we have used this technique to deliver a total dose of 60 Gy (90% of the PTV receives 94% of the dose) it can be used to deliver 70 Gy, keeping within the spinal cord and brainstem dose constraints by using the off-cord arc technique from the outset of treatment. This will then generate a minor parotid-sparing effect; however, the middle ear receives the full prescribed dose.

Three-Dimensional Conformal Treatment

Recent advances in the technology of radiotherapy planning and treatment delivery systems have made it possible to achieve dose distributions that conform closely to any predetermined 3D shape. Such technology offers the prospect of both improving the cure rates of radiotherapy (through dose escalation) and reducing the morbidity of treatment by excluding critical normal structures from the high-dose volume. Planning for 3D-conformal therapy requires definition of the target volume on serial cross-sectional CT images. In the treatment of NPC this involves defining not only gross (imagable) disease at the primary site and in the neck but also potential sites of subclinical spread. In principle it should be possible to define a target volume excluding a substantial part of the major salivary glands thus mitigating xerostomia—one of the most troublesome side effects of conventional treatment. Clearly the risk for defining tighter target volumes is that the probability of a geographic miss of occult disease increases; furthermore the consequences of small errors in reproducing patient setup from day to day are magnified. Extreme precision is needed because of the proximity of the primary tumor to critical normal structures such as the optic pathway and the brainstem and of the retropharyngeal and upper jugular nodes to the parotid glands.

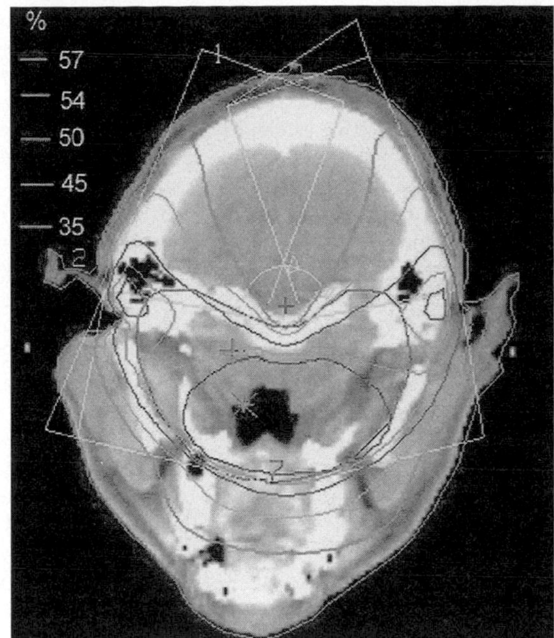

A

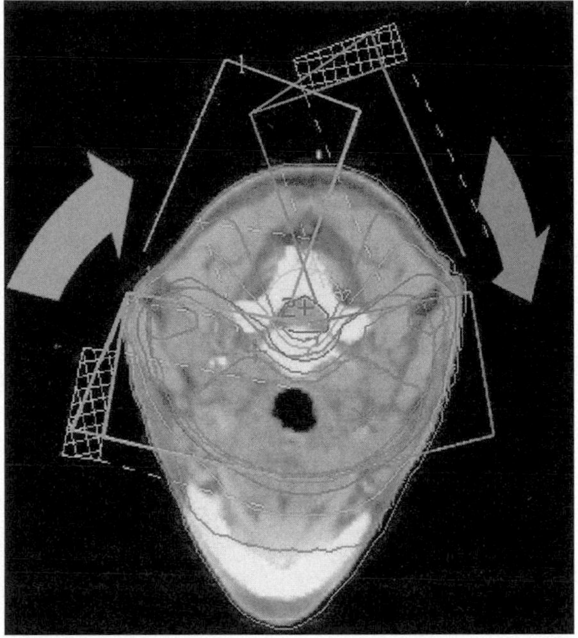
B

Figure 23.5 "Boomerang"-shaped isodoses achieved by rotating arc fields at the primary tumor **(A)** and upper neck **(B).** (See Color Plate 7 following page 524.)

The best conformal plans currently available use intensity modulated radiation therapy (IMRT), which enables virtually any shape of dose distribution to be achieved. However, successful implementation of IMRT requires both sophisticated equipment and a major commitment of time from both the oncologist (to define both PTVs and normal tissues to be spared on cross-sectional imaging) and the physicist to provide proper quality assurance (47). Only a few centers have treated significant series of patients with NPC with IMRT. The largest of these is from the University of California at San Francisco, where Sultanem et al. (48) reported their initial experience on 35 patients treated between April 1995 and March 1998. This series was updated in abstract form in 2001 (49), with outcome data on 67 patients (71% stage III–IV) treated through March 2001. Fifty-one patients received concurrent and adjuvant chemotherapy according to the Intergroup 0099 protocol. With a median follow-up of 28 months, the actuarial 4-year local progression-free survival (PFS), locoregional PFS, and overall survival were 100%, 97%, and 94%, respectively. At 24 months, all evaluable patients had less than grade 2 xerostomia. These excellent results obviously require further follow-up and confirmatory studies but illustrate the potential for a major advance in the therapeutic ratio with IMRT.

As sophisticated as they are, it is likely that currently available IMRT systems may soon be superseded. In the future patients with NPC may be treated with helical tomotherapy, which represents a new generation of technological advancement in the planning and delivery of radiation therapy. Briefly, helical tomotherapy represents the integration of a linear accelerator and a CT scanner within a single unit (50). Although standard radiotherapy is currently delivered using several static fields, helical tomotherapy delivers treatment using a continuously rotating, intensity-modulated fan beam. With the patient steadily translated through a ringlike gantry while the fan beam rotates, the treatment beam forms a helical shape. The beam delivery is similar to that of a CT scanner. The fan beam is shaped or "conformed" to match the shape of the desired tumor/target. The tomographic imaging capacity of the unit (through megavoltage CT) provides a precise verification of both patient setup and delivered dose. Figure 23.6 (see also Color Plate 8 following page 524) shows the extent of conformal avoidance of normal tissues that can be achieved with tomotherapy.

Just as the early generation IMRT studies have shown high promise in their capacity to avoid uninvolved normal tissue structures such as salivary glands, helical tomotherapy should provide even further reduction in these normal tissue doses. The adaptive verification processes of tomotherapy should ensure greater conformity of dose. Specific attention to salivary and auditory toxicities will be paid during the early tomotherapy clinical studies. Although the adverse impact of radiation on salivary gland function is well appreciated, the impact of

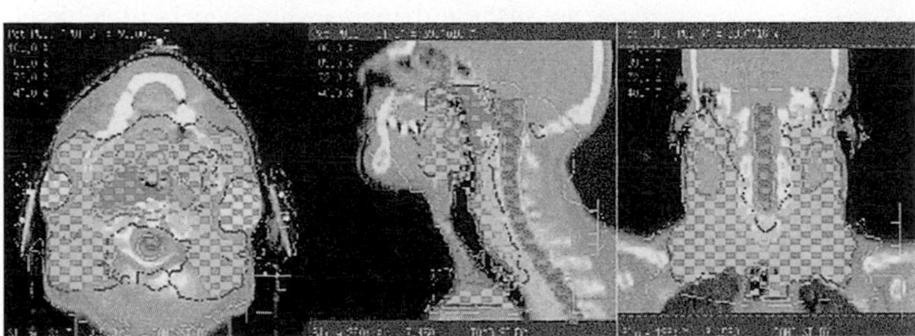

Figure 23.6 Isodose distribution obtained with tomotherapy planning for a patient with advanced nasopharyngeal cancer. The 100%, 80%, 72%, and 40% isodose lines are shown. Bilateral parotid glands and spinal cord are specifically identified for conformal avoidance. (See Color Plate 8 following page 524.)

radiation on auditory function is not broadly recognized. Particularly with increasing trends for the use of ototoxic chemotherapy (namely platinum derivatives) concurrent with radiation for advanced head and neck cancer patients, conformal avoidance of dose delivery to auditory structures will become even more important with regard to ultimate patient quality of life. Paralleling the recent advances in nasopharyngeal irradiation using IMRT, a primary objective for tomotherapy in the treatment of nasopharynx cancer is to maintain the highest possible rate of locoregional disease control while continuing to reduce normal tissue toxicities.

Dose Prescription

The standard radiation dose prescribed to the primary site in nasopharyngeal cancer in most centers is an equivalent of 70 Gy over 7 weeks. Similar doses are given to involved nodes, and clinically uninvolved nodes typically receive 50 Gy in 5 weeks. Surprisingly, there have been no randomized studies specifically addressing the question of radiation dose response in nasopharyngeal cancer, and these recommended doses have largely been derived empirically. Consequently, there remains ongoing controversy regarding optimal radiation dose. Proponents of a dose response above 60 Gy have relied on retrospective data that span treatment periods of 20 to 30 years (51–53). Major changes in radiation technique occurred concurrently, confounding the dose issue (54). Others have noted no difference in local control or survival within the dose range of 60 to 70 Gy (55), particularly if the coverage of the PTV is poor or if treatment includes chemotherapy (56). Wang (57) reports improved locoregional control for a cohort of patients treated after 1979 with accelerated radiotherapy compared with a pre-1979 patient cohort treated with daily radiotherapy. Retrospective comparisons such as these may be compounded by the major advances that have occurred in diagnostic imaging, with subsequent improved tumor volume definition. In addition, although a statistical benefit was found, the historical locoregional control comparison for this study was suboptimal (e.g., 55% local control for T1–T2 lesions). The only randomized study comparing different radiation dose schedules in NPC was terminated prematurely because of unacceptable neurologic toxicity in the high-dose arm. This study did not show improved locoregional control or overall survival in the higher dose arm (58). However, as only half the planned accrual was achieved before the study was terminated, adequate statistical power was lacking.

With the increased availability of IMRT there is an expectation that dose escalation can be safely achieved and should thus be used. It is an opportune time for a randomized trial to establish the optimal radiation dose required in the context of defined WHO histology, UICC 5th edition staging and use of concurrent chemotherapy. It may be that it is the minimum dose to the entire PTV that is more critical for local control than a high(er) median dose.

OUTCOMES AND RESULTS

Early Stage Disease

For the purposes of this discussion, we define early stage disease as T1 to T2 N0 to N1, with the proviso that only N1 cases up to a maximum nodal size of 3 cm are included.

Most reported series of patients with NPC treated by radiotherapy alone show good to excellent local control rates for early stage disease (i.e., T1–T2). In the very large experience of the Queen Elizabeth Hospital in Hong Kong reported by Lee et al. (54), 4,128 patients were treated with radiotherapy alone between 1976 and 1985. Of these patients 1,527 were stage I and 586 were stage II using the Ho staging system, which is similar to the current UICC/AJCC 5th edition. Overall there was a 19% local failure rate for T1 and a 20% rate for T2 with a median follow-up of 4 years. When results obtained pre- and post-1980 were compared, the actuarial 5-year local failure-free survival improved from 77% to 83% for T1 and from 69% to 79% for T2. This coincided with a marked increase in the number of patients staged by CT and a corresponding increase in the relative proportion of stage II versus stage I patients.

The largest experience of Caucasian patients treated by radiotherapy alone is from the University of Texas M. D. Anderson Cancer Center where 378 patients were treated between 1954 and 1992 (55). Of these patients, 55 were staged T1 and 138 were staged T2 using the 4th edition UICC criteria, which made them somewhat less advanced than comparably staged patients in the Hong Kong series. Actuarial 5-year local control rates were 93% for T1 and 79% for T2. The only significant factor predicting for local control other than stage was tumor histology, with lymphoepitheliomas (WHO types II and III) faring significantly better than squamous cell carcinomas (WHO type I).

These results provide a minimum expectation of the local radiocurability of early stage NPC. With modern-day imaging and treatment techniques it is almost certain that these results would be improved and therefore there is no reason to use combined modality treatment on the basis of T stage for the T1 and T2 categories.

With regard to neck nodal disease, the cutoff point for acceptable results with radiotherapy alone is less clear. Regional control of the neck is excellent with radiotherapy regardless of N stage and isolated neck failure is rare (55). However the risk for metastatic disease is highly dependent on the size and location of involved nodes as reflected in the UICC 5th edition/AJCC Cancer Staging Manual, 6th edition staging system. The impact of these factors was specifically examined in the M. D. Anderson series where the 10-year risk for distant metastases increased from 10% for patients with nodes less than 3 cm in size in the upper two thirds of the neck to 65% for those with large nodes in the lower one third (59). Using the current staging system, we would therefore include only the subset of N1 patients having nodes less than 3 cm in size in the early stage category.

Although the results achieved with radiotherapy alone for early stage disease are very good, a recent publication from Taiwan (60) has questioned whether they might be even better with the addition of concurrent and adjuvant chemotherapy. In a series of 32 patients with stage II disease treated with four cycles of cisplatin/5-fluorouracil (5-FU) (two concurrent and two sequential) and followed for a median of 34 months, these authors reported a 3-year actuarial locoregional control rate of 100% and disease-free survival of 97%. In the absence of any randomized studies however, combined modality treatment cannot be recommended as the standard of care for early stage disease.

Late Stage Disease

Late stage disease includes patients with T3 to T4 or N2 to N3 disease plus N1 greater than 3 cm. The available evidence suggests that these patients are best treated with combined modality chemoradiotherapy.

Although nonrandomized trials have reported promising results with the addition of chemotherapy (61,62), randomized trials have yielded mixed results about the possible role of chemotherapy given in conjunction with radiotherapy as part of the primary treatment of locally advanced NPC (Table 23.7). The most influential trial has been the U.S. Intergroup trial, which compared 70 Gy conventionally fractionated radiation and three

TABLE 23.7 Randomized Trials of Radiation Alone Versus Chemoradiation

Trial	No. of patients	Eligibility	Chemotherapy: Induction	Chemotherapy: Concurrent	Chemotherapy: Adjuvant	Median follow-up	Relapse-free survival[a]	Overall survival	Comments[b]
VUMCA I (74)	339	WHO II–III any tumor, node ≥2	Cisplatin, bleomycin, epirubicin	—	—	74 mo	6 yr: 30% vs. 41% ($p < 0.02$)	5 yr: 45% vs. 40% (p = NS[c])	Decreased locoregional and distant failures; 8% treatment-related mortality
Asian-Oceanian (65)		334	WHO II–III, Ho stage III/IV or node ≥3 cm	Cisplatin, epirubicin	—	—30 mo	3 yr: 42% vs. 48% ($p = 0.45$)	3 yr: 71% vs. 78% ($p = 0.57$)	Subgroup with nodes >6 cm—improved local control, RFS and OS
Ma et al. (75)	456	Low neck node or ≥4 cm or base of skull involvement	Cisplatin, bleomycin, 5-FU	—	—	Not available	5 yr: 49% vs. 59% ($p = 0.05$)	5 yr: 56% vs. 63% ($p = 0.11$)	Decreased locoregional failures, no different in distant failures. Only 30% received 3 cycles of chemotherapy
Chan et al. (76)	82	Ho N3 or node ≥4 cm	Cisplatin, 5-FU	—	—	28.5 mo	2 yr: 72% vs. 68% (p = NS)	2 yr: 81% vs. 80% (p = NS)	
U.S. Intergroup (63,64)	147 (193 entered)	Stages III/IV (UICC 92)	—	Cisplatin	Cisplatin, 5-FU	Minimum follow-up 5 yr	5 yr: 29% vs. 58% ($p < 0.001$)	5 yr: 37% vs. 67% ($p = 0.001$)	Decreased locoregional and distant failures
Chan et al. (71)	350	Ho N2/N3 or node ≥4 cm	—	Cisplatin	—	—	2 yr: 67% vs. 77% ($p = 0.077$)		Ho T3 subgroup—significant improvement in PFS
Kwong et al.[d] (72)	157	Ho T3 or N2, N3 or node ≥4 cm	—	UFT	—	34 mo	3 yr: 53% vs. 71% ($p = 0.019$)	3 yr: 76% vs. 84% ($p = 0.29$)	Decreased locoregional and distant failures
			—		Alternating cisplatin, 5-FU/vincristine, bleomycin, methotrexate	34 mo	(NS) 61% vs. 63%	(NS) 78% vs. 82%	
Rossi et al. (73)	229	CR to radiation ± neck dissection	—	—	Vincristine, doxorubicin, cyclophos-phamide	32 mo	4 yr: 56% vs. 58% (p = NS)	4 yr: 67% vs. 59% (p = NS)	Poor compliance with chemotherapy

[a]Results presented as radiation alone vs. chemoradiation.
[b]Refer to chemoradiation arm compared to the radiation alone arm.
[c]NS, not significant
[d]factorial design
5-FU, 5-fluoracil; CR, complete remission; NS, not significant; OS, overall survival; PFS, progression-free survival; RFS, relapse-free survival; UFT, uracil and tegafur; UICC, International Union against Cancer system.

cycles of concurrent cisplatin 100 mg/m^2 followed by three cycles of adjuvant cisplatin 80 mg/m^2 and infusional 5-FU 1,000 mg/m^2 for 4 days to radiation alone (63). Patients with stages 3 and 4 (UICC 4th edition, 1992) were eligible, but 91% were in fact stage 4. The Intergroup trial demonstrated a marked improvement in progression-free and overall survival. The magnitude of the difference detected at the first interim analysis was so large as to precipitate early closure of the study. This is unfortunate since it has meant that the strongest evidence of efficacy of chemotherapy is based on a small trial with significant methodological flaws. Al-Sarraf et al. (64) recently reported the updated results with a minimum 5-year follow-up. The overall survival was 29% in the radiation alone arm and 58% in the chemoradiation arm. In this trial there was a decrease in both locoregional and distant failures. Although the results of this trial altered practice in many centers, many investigators have recommended caution in the interpretation of the results. The high proportion of patients with WHO stages I and II histology (59%) casts doubt on the relevance of the results to populations with predominantly undifferentiated NPCs (65). In particular, 24% had WHO I histology, which has a different natural history and response to treatment from that of undifferentiated NPC. Moreover, the practicality of the Intergroup regimen has been questioned: on the chemoradiation arm only 73% patients completed treatment as planned, with 63% receiving all three cycles of concurrent chemotherapy and 55% receiving the three planned cycles of adjuvant chemotherapy. Of the 193 patients entered only 147 were considered eligible and included in the analysis. The high proportion of ineligible patients was an initial concern, but it has subsequently been explained that 38 patients were deemed to be ineligible based on insufficient documentation, and with the inclusion of these patients in the analysis the survival differences remained significant (66). Another issue that has been raised is the poor survival in the radiation arm compared with results in other randomized trials, and the possibility that chemotherapy compensated for suboptimal radiation (67). The Intergroup trial accrued a small number of patients from many centers, so it is likely that many participating centers had limited experience with the complex radiation treatment planning required for NPC compared with larger centers. However, the poor results could be partly accounted for by the high number of WHO I patients, who had much poorer survival than the WHO II and WHO III patients in this study (64).

The design of the Intergroup trial does not permit one to determine the relative contributions of concurrent versus adjuvant chemotherapy to the improved outcome compared with radiation alone. However, there is increasing evidence that concurrent chemoradiation in a variety of malignancies may improve locoregional control and overall survival (68–70). Furthermore, the role of concurrent chemoradiation in NPC is supported by the preliminary results of two randomized trials in NPC from Hong Kong (71,72). In one trial conducted at the Prince of Wales and Queen Elizabeth hospitals patients were randomized to receive radiation with or without concurrent cisplatin 40 mg/m^2 weekly (71). Three hundred and fifty eligible patients, with 99% having WHO II or III histology, were entered. There was a trend for improved PFS, which was significant in the subgroup with Ho's T3 (UICC 5th edition 1997, T3/T4). Recently, the preliminary results of a randomized trial from the Queen Mary Hospital were presented (72). This trial had a 2 × 2 factorial design testing the addition of concurrent UFT and adjuvant chemotherapy to radiation. As presented at the 2001 ASTRO meeting, accrual was stopped at 157 patients after an interim analysis showed excessive toxicity in the adjuvant chemotherapy arms. Ninety-nine percent of patients had WHO III histology. With a median follow-up of 34 months this trial showed a significant improvement in locoregional control, distant metastases-free survival, and relapse-free survival with concurrent chemoradiation, but no significant improvement in overall survival. No benefit from adjuvant chemotherapy was seen. There has only been one randomized trial that looked solely at the addition of adjuvant chemotherapy to radiation (73). No survival benefit was seen in this trial. In this trial patients were randomized only after they had achieved a complete response to radiotherapy; thus selecting for patients with more radiocurable tumors, a non-cisplatin–containing regimen was used and compliance with the chemotherapy was poor.

The three large trials of induction without concurrent chemotherapy have not demonstrated improved overall survival compared with radiation alone (65,74,75). The International Nasopharynx Cancer Study Group VUMCA I trial demonstrated improved disease-free survival, but not improved overall survival (74). In that trial, which was restricted to patients with N2 or N3 undifferentiated carcinomas and used an induction regimen of three cycles of bleomycin, epirubicin, and cisplatin (BEC), significant toxicity and 8% treatment-related mortality was reported. In the Asian–Oceanian Clinical Oncology Association Trial, which was restricted to patients with Ho's T3 or N2 to N3 or any stage with node size greater than 3 cm and poorly or undifferentiated carcinomas, no difference in relapse-free or overall survival was reported (65). Subset analyses in evaluable patients and in patients with nodes greater than 6 cm favored the chemotherapy arm. The chemotherapy regimen was two to three cycles of epirubicin (110 mg/m^2) and cisplatin (60 mg/m^2). In a recently reported trial, performed in Guangzhou, China, no difference in overall survival was seen, although there was a significant difference in relapse-free survival (75). In this trial the chemotherapy regimen consisted of two to three cycles of cisplatin (100 mg/m^2), bleomycin (10 mg/m^2, days 1 and 5), and 5-FU (800 mg/m^2 continuous infusion, days 1 to 5), with only 32% receiving three cycles and 68% receiving two cycles. The chemotherapy regimens used in these three trials may not have been optimal, with the BEC regimen having unacceptable toxicity, a relatively low dose of cisplatin in the Asian–Oceanian trial, and difficulty in administering the protocol-specified chemotherapy in the Guangzhou trial. The other published randomized trial is the study of Chan et al. (76), which was small and used low doses of chemotherapy. It included only 82 patients, two thirds of whom had upper neck nodes, thus limiting the potential for demonstrating a survival advantage for chemotherapy.

Although these trials of induction chemotherapy without concurrent chemotherapy have not shown any improvement in overall survival they do suggest some impact on local control. In the International Cancer Study Group trial the improved disease-free survival was due to a decrease in both locoregional relapses and distant metastases as sites of first failure (74). In the Asian–Oceanian Clinical Oncology Association Trial, the subgroup analysis in patients with bulky neck nodes showed a significant difference in relapse-free survival that was due to improved local control in the induction chemotherapy arm, without any difference in incidence of distant metastases as the site of first failure (65). Similarly, in the Guangzhou trial there was a significant difference in relapse-free survival that was due to improved local control (75).

A large retrospective series from Hong Kong has been reported demonstrating improved local control in patients who received two cycles of induction chemotherapy compared with patients treated with radiation alone for locally advanced node-positive NPC (55). Multivariate analysis identified administration of chemotherapy as being of independent significance in determining the local failure rate.

It has been generally thought that the addition of concurrent chemotherapy may improve locoregional control and, hence, its major impact would be in patients with advanced T-stage disease (54) and that induction or adjuvant chemotherapy may be most beneficial in patients with advanced N-stage or low neck disease, the group most at risk for distant metastases (59). However, the results of randomized trials are not so straightforward with evidence that induction chemotherapy may also contribute to locoregional control (74,75) and that the use of concurrent chemotherapy may be associated with a decrease in the incidence of distant metastases (72).

Although the available randomized trials have not definitively determined the role or optimal schedule of chemotherapy when given with radiation for NPC, the results of the Intergroup trial taken in conjunction with the emerging results from other trials and a recent meta-analysis (77) would support the use of chemotherapy in patients with locally advanced NPC. Trials of concurrent chemotherapy without sequential (induction or adjuvant) chemotherapy and trials of sequential chemotherapy without concurrent chemotherapy have demonstrated improvements in local control and PFS, but not overall survival. The U.S. Intergroup trial is the only study to show a significant improvement in overall survival (63,64). Despite some of the limitations of this trial, when taken together with the results of the other randomized trials it is reasonable to speculate that both concurrent and sequential chemotherapy are required to achieve a significant improvement in overall survival in patients with locally advanced NPC. Ongoing randomized trials in Hong Kong and Singapore will confirm whether the Intergroup regimen of concurrent and adjuvant chemotherapy is superior to radiation alone in populations with predominantly WHO III NPC.

Although the Intergroup study used adjuvant chemotherapy, there is little other supporting evidence for a role of adjuvant chemotherapy in NPC. One advantage of induction compared with adjuvant chemotherapy is the greater ability to administer full-dose chemotherapy as planned. Another potential advantage of induction over adjuvant chemotherapy is the reduction in tumor bulk juxtaposed to vital dose-limiting structures prior to radiation. Although PTVs should not be reduced on the basis of chemotherapy-induced response, the tumor bulk reduction following induction chemotherapy increases the probability that gross residual disease receives the full radiation dose. This could explain the contribution of induction chemotherapy to local control, which would not be expected with adjuvant chemotherapy. The lack of benefit with induction chemotherapy in other head and neck cancers is most likely due to accelerated repopulation of surviving tumor clonogens which offsets the cytotoxic effect of chemotherapy. However, as accelerated repopulation is a function of tumor differentiation, this is unlikely to limit the effectiveness of induction chemotherapy in an undifferentiated tumor such as WHO II and WHO III NPC (78). In the phase II setting, the approach of induction chemotherapy followed by concurrent chemoradiation has been shown to be feasible and it is associated with excellent compliance and promising results. We have recently reported our results with three cycles of induction chemotherapy with epirubicin 50 mg/m^2 and cisplatin 75 mg/m^2 combined with continuous infusion 5-FU 200 mg/m^2 daily for 9 weeks, followed by concurrent chemoradiation, 60 Gy in 2 Gy fractions with cisplatin 20 mg/m^2 daily for 5 days in weeks 1 and 6 (79). All patients received three cycles of induction chemotherapy, and 97% completed chemoradiation. The estimated 4-year PFS rate was 81% (95% CI: 59%–93%) and the estimated 4-year overall survival rate was 90% (95% CI: 74%–97%). This approach warrants testing in randomized trials.

COMPLICATIONS

Radiotherapy

Because of the location of the nasopharynx and the need for wide field treatment to encompass potential routes of spread, the morbidity associated with radiotherapy of NPC is substantial.

Acute mucositis aggravated by acute changes in salivary volume and texture, progresses to a patchy or confluent grade in the great majority of patients and up to a third may require enteral tube feeding during and immediately after treatment. Scrupulous hygiene, prophylactic antifungal medication, adequate analgesics, and expert dietetic advice are key elements of managing acute mucosal reactions. Skin reactions may also be distressing with around one-fourth of patients developing some degree of moist desquamation. When skin breakdown occurs, we recommend occlusive dressings with Solugel to promote healing. Acute radiation reactions can be exacerbated in patients receiving concurrent chemotherapy, especially regimens containing 5-FU.

Although acute reactions can be distressing, it is the late complications of treatment for NPC that are of greatest concern. Until recently, virtually every patient would lose most of his or her salivary function with consequent comorbidities, especially radiation-related dental caries. Injury to the auditory apparatus is also a frequent though poorly reported late complication of radiotherapy for NPC. Most treatment techniques result in high doses being delivered to the ears and when ototoxic chemotherapy is also used, the risk for symptomatic hearing loss is significant. The forward lobes of the brain can also be injured by radiotherapy. Hong Kong researchers have eloquently documented the frequency of temporal lobe injury (ranging from subtle neurologic changes to frank necrosis) in patients treated with the Ho technique (80). Modern technology now permits selective sparing of the sensitive normal tissues responsible for major late toxicities in the majority of patients. However, even with conventional techniques, many of the complications of radiotherapy for NPC can be prevented or minimized by careful pretreatment assessment, meticulous treatment planning, and assiduous follow-up.

Every patient should have a careful dental evaluation done before treatment. Teeth showing signs of decay or periodontal disease need to be restored or extracted. For patients with advanced disease in whom the pituitary and hypothalamus will be in the primary radiation beam, baseline endocrine assessments of hypophyseal function should be done prior to commencement of radiotherapy. This permits early identification of hormonal deficiencies and the initiation of appropriate replacement therapy (81).

After completion of therapy patients should be examined at regular intervals, every 2 months for the first year after, quarterly for the second and third year, and every 6 months through the fifth year after treatment. A follow-up evaluation is done every year thereafter. During follow-up the disease status is evaluated in search for recurrence at the primary site or the neck nodes and for clinical signs of distant metastases. Attention should be also directed to possible sequelae of treatment and prevention of secondary complications. The external auditory canals will be deficient in normal cerumen production and patients should be instructed in prevention of external otitis. The auditory canal will be dry and the normal migration of the epithelium within the auditory canal is impaired. As a result, debris tends to collect and may impact. Patients should be advised to avoid manipulation of the ear canal and to seek medical advice promptly if irritation develops. Patients with carcinoma of the nasopharynx often present with serous otitis media. After treatment, this may subside but it may persist in a chronic form even after sterilization of the NPC. If this sequela causes bothersome symptoms, it can be managed with indwelling tympanic membrane ventilation tubes.

Dental and oral cavity care should be meticulous and the application of fluoride solutions in the form of stannous fluoride or sodium fluoride by custom-fitted carriers is mandatory. Dental extractions after radiation therapy should be avoided whenever possible. If extractions are unavoidable, extreme precautions are necessary to minimize the risk for osteoradionecrosis (82). Radiation to the temporomandibular joints and masticatory muscles, especially in patients who receive systemic chemotherapy may cause trismus. This usually does not set in before 3 to 6 months after treatment, but is progressive. Patients need to be instructed in its prevention by encouraging active jaw exercises, especially in teenagers and young adults. The effect of irradiation on the mucosa of the sinonasal tract is a metaplastic transformation of the epithelium from ciliary-columnar respiratory epithelium to cuboidal or squamous-stratified epithelium with loss of ciliary function and very often loss of the mucous-secreting elements. In spite of these changes, it is rare that patients experience sinonasal infections. Nevertheless, if they do occur they should be treated promptly and aggressively to avoid undesirable necrosis of soft tissue and osteoradionecrosis of facial bones. Irradiation of all or part of the pituitary hypothalamic axis is unavoidable when there is cancerous bony invasion of the base of the skull. In such patients an annual evaluation of the pituitary function and of the thyroid and pituitary adrenal axis is therefore recommended. Proper replacement therapy should be tailored to deficiencies. Even in patients whose hypothalamus/pituitary is not irradiated, long-term thyroid insufficiency can develop as a direct effect of irradiating the thyroid gland in the neck.

Chemotherapy

Both concurrent and sequential chemotherapy regimens are predominantly cisplatin-based, with 5-FU frequently given with cisplatin in induction or adjuvant regimens. The major acute side effect of cisplatin is nausea and vomiting, which may be immediate or delayed. The use of 5HT3 antagonists together with dexamethasone has led to much higher rates of control of acute emesis (83,84). Although dexamethasone is also beneficial for the control of delayed emesis, this remains a significant toxicity (85). The neurokinin 1 receptor antagonists that are currently in clinical trial have shown preliminary evidence of efficacy in controlling delayed emesis (86). Other toxicities of cisplatin include ototoxicity, peripheral neuropathy, and renal impairment. Regimens that include concurrent and sequential cisplatin may have high cumulative doses of cisplatin with greater risk for ototoxicity and peripheral neuropathy. Cisplatin ototoxicity manifests initially as high-frequency hearing impairment and is generally irreversible (87). Both cisplatin and radiation may contribute to significant ototoxicity in patients with NPC. The peripheral neuropathy is predominantly sensory and generally reversible, but recovery may be slow (88). Renal toxicity can be generally avoided by administration with adequate hydration, and avoidance of the drug in patients with significant renal impairment. With multiple cycles of platinum chemotherapy, anemia may occur. As anemia is associated with poor outcome with radiation, the hemoglobin needs to be monitored during radiation and blood transfusion or erythropoietin may be required.

The more common acute side effects of infusional 5-FU include mucositis and diarrhea. Therapy with 5-FU may be complicated by cardiac toxicity, most commonly manifested as chest pain with electrocardiographic changes consistent with myocardial schemia. In a prospective trial of high-dose infusional 5-FU as commonly used in head and neck cancers including NPC, 7.6% patients experienced a cardiac event related to 5-FU (89). Patients with dihydropyrimidine dehydrogenase deficiency may experience severe toxicity related to 5-FU (90).

MANAGEMENT OF RECURRENT OR METASTATIC DISEASE

Radiotherapy

Locally recurrent NPC, especially if limited to the primary site, without intracranial extension, should be considered for re-treatment with radiotherapy as salvage is possible in a significant proportion of patients. Lee et al. (91) report on a series of 706 patients re-irradiated between 1976 and 1985. Of these patients, 364 had rT1 to rT2 tumors and achieved a 32%, 5-year local failure-free survival. In another Hong Kong series, Chua et al. (92) report a 5-year overall survival of 55% in 33 patients with rT1 to rT2 disease treated by re-irradiation between 1984 and 1995. In a Western series, Pryzant et al. (93) report the results of re-treatment of 53 patients with megavoltage irradiation at the M. D. Anderson Cancer Clinic between 1954 and 1989. Overall 5-year actuarial local control was 35%. Much better results were achieved in a subset of nine patients with recurrent disease confined to the nasopharynx in whom treatment with an intracavitary brachytherapy boost was possible: seven of these patients achieved durable local control. In this series 8 of 53 patients sustained severe complications of re-treatment which were fatal in 5. The most significant factor predicting for severe complications was a total cumulative dose of external beam therapy ≥100 Gy. Similar results were reported by Fu et al. (94) in a series of 74 patients re-treated at the University of California, San Francisco between 1957 and 1995. Overall locoregional PFS was 40%. Significant factors predicting for locoregional control were histologic type (WHO type I worse), time to diagnosis of recurrence (longer than 5 years best), and use of brachytherapy in patients with disease confined to the nasopharynx. Complications were significantly increased in patients who received cumulative doses ≥120 Gy. The definitive study of risk factors for complications of re-treatment is from Hong Kong where Lee et al. (95) report on a series of 654 patients re-treated between 1976 and 1992. Of these patient, 539 received external beam therapy alone. The biologically effective dose (BED) of the initial treatment and to a lesser extent the re-treatment BED were significant determinants of risk; interestingly there was no evidence that the time gap between treatments influenced residual tolerance. In all series there is clearly less morbidity when a component of brachytherapy is used reflecting the smaller volume of tissue receiving a high re-treatment dose. The limitation of brachytherapy in treating disease that extends beyond the nasopharynx can be partially overcome by using modern stereotactic conformal techniques or heavy particle therapy (96–98). No long-term results of re-treatment with conformal photon beam therapy have yet been published. Although it is virtually certain that these techniques will reduce morbidity, there is also a greater risk for geographic miss of tumor, thus limiting overall salvage rates. For example in the series treated with heavy particles, the long-term local control rate was 45%, comparable to that achieved with conventional treatment (98). The use of stereotactic radiosurgery in treating small volume recurrent/residual disease was recently reported by Chua et al. (99). Of 11 patients treated, 9 achieved a complete response, and the estimated 1-year local control rate was 82%.

Radiotherapy also has a role in the palliative treatment of regional or distant metastatic sites in patients with incurable disease. The most common indication is for painful bony or liver metastases.

Surgery

Technical advances in skull base surgery along with better imaging to define the extent of recurrent disease make salvage surgery another option for patients with localized recurrence. A variety of approaches have been described but fall into three main groups: inferior/inferolateral (100–102), lateral (103,104), and anterolateral (105). Long-term control rates averaging 38% have been reported in published series (100–102,105), a figure that compares favorably with re-treatment by radiotherapy. However it is likely that a greater degree of selection is applied to patients being considered for surgical resection than for re-irradiation.

Isolated neck recurrences after treatment of NPC are rare (especially for WHO type II and III). However, for patients who do relapse regionally, and in whom no distant disease can be demonstrated, neck dissection is indicated and can be curative. For example, Wei et al. (106) report on 51 patients who underwent radical neck dissection for persistent or recurrent neck disease following radiotherapy. Actuarial 5-year survival and neck control rates were 38% and 66%, respectively. More recently Yen et al. (107) published outcome data on 31 patients undergoing salvage neck surgery in Taiwan over a 14-year period (emphasizing the rarity of the condition). In this series, overall 5-year survival from neck dissection was 67%.

Chemotherapy

Despite the high incidence of nasopharyngeal cancer in some areas of the world, relatively few trials of chemotherapy in the relapsed or metastatic setting have been conducted. In many Western series, patients with NPC were included in trials investigating chemotherapy in patients with squamous cell carcinomas of the head and neck. Although patients with nasopharyngeal cancer represented a small minority in these trials, they were often among the best responders with the most durable responses. Over recent years there has been increasing acceptance that the mixing of NPC with other sites of head and neck cancer in clinical trials is not appropriate owing to the different biologic behavior and greater chemosensitivity of NPC.

Based on the activity of platinum and 5-FU in head and neck cancer, regimens including a platinum and 5-FU have been studied in phase II trials in patients with NPC, but no phase III trials have been reported. In chemonaive patients these regimens have consistently reported response rates of 50% to 80% with complete response rates of 15% to 20% (108–112). The median time to progression is 8 to 9 months. There are reports of durable responses following chemotherapy for metastatic disease. Investigators from the Institut Gustav-Roussy have reported on 20 long-term survivors who were treated with chemotherapy for metastatic NPC over a period of 18 years at their institution (113). Long-term survival was defined as a disease-free period greater than 36 months after attaining a complete response to chemotherapy. Tumor sites were bone in 15 patients, lung in 4, and biopsy-proven liver involvement in 2 (one patient had disease in two sites). It is of interest that consolidation radiation was given to 13 patients with bone metastases. The authors report that approximately 10% of all patients with metastases treated at their institution since 1985 have achieved long-term survival following treatment with cisplatin-based regimens. However, the authors also reviewed a total of 16 other published reports and identified 31 cases of long-term survivors (3%) among 1,003 patients treated with chemotherapy. Long-term survivors had predominantly bone or lung metastases, and only four patients were known to have been treated with regimens that did not contain platinum. The available data support a potentially curative role for chemotherapy albeit in a very small proportion of patients with metastatic disease.

Other chemotherapeutic agents with demonstrated single-agent activity include mitoxantrone, which had a 25% response rate in a large multicenter trial (114), and paclitaxel, which had a response rate of 22% (115). The combination of carboplatin and paclitaxel yielded response rates of 59% to 75%, which is similar to platinum and 5-FU (116,117). Ifosfamide-containing regimens are active in NPC, including patients previously treated with a platinum and 5-FU regimen based on a small study of ifosfamide and 5-FU (118). More recently, preliminary reports have suggested significant activity of gemcitabine in both previously untreated patients and in patients previously treated with a platinum-containing regimen (119).

Although the impact of chemotherapy on quality of life and palliation of symptoms has not been well studied in patients with recurrent or metastatic nasopharyngeal cancer, there is little controversy about the role of chemotherapy in patients who have not previously received chemotherapy. With the increasing use of chemotherapy as part of first-line treatment, studies assessing the efficacy of re-treatment with platinum-based regimens are required. Furthermore, reports of trials of new drugs for patients with platinum-pretreated NPS should also report response and duration of response to last platinum-based regimen. Identification of novel drugs with activity in platinum-resistant NPC should be a major research priority. There is increasing interest in oncology in the activity of agents that inhibit specific molecular targets [e.g., epidermal growth factor receptor (EGFR) inhibitors and anti-angiogenic agents]. Epidermal growth factor receptor inhibitors have shown promising activity in several malignancies and warrant study in NPC, as EGFR may be up-regulated in NPC by latent membrane I, an EBV-encoded oncogenic protein (120).

SPECIAL ISSUES AND FUTURE DIRECTIONS

Substantial changes in both the strategy and technique of management of NPC have occurred over the past decade. Although important advances have undoubtedly been made, much remains to be done to optimize the management of this disease. The pivotal improvements that have been made in therapeutic efficacy mean that the great majority of patients with NPC can now be cured. The corollary of this fact is that greater attention now needs to be paid to reducing the toxicities (especially long-term sequelae) of treatment. Major unanswered questions that will define the future directions of clinical research on NPC include:

- What is the appropriate staging cutoff for patients to receive concurrent or sequential chemotherapy?
- Can less toxic or more effective chemotherapy combinations be found?
- Might more effective chemotherapy allow a reduction of radiation dose so as to reduce late treatment-related morbidity?
- Might more accurate functional imaging allow a reduction in the volume of the neck treated electively?
- Can sophisticated IMRT treatment techniques be extrapolated to general radiation oncology practice, especially in endemic areas?

- Is there a role for novel targeted agents such as EGFR-signal transduction inhibitors in this disease?
- Can molecular phenotyping predict biologic behavior of tumors or identify patients hypersensitive to chemoradiotherapy?
- What is the role of EBV-DNA in patient monitoring?

CONCLUSIONS

Strong evidence from recent series indicates that the outcome of treatment for NPC is significantly influenced by the quality of medical care rendered. Results have improved dramatically over the past two decades and can confidently be predicted to improve further as a result of revolutions in medical imaging, radiotherapy technical capability, and understanding of the optimal way to combine radiotherapy and chemotherapy. To ensure that patients with NPC receive optimum treatment they should ideally be managed in a major cancer center where the experience and expertise to handle the complexities of the disease are available. Furthermore they should, wherever possible, be enrolled in clinical trials designed to resolve unanswered questions surrounding the disease and its management. As the medical resources available to countries with high endemic rates of NPC increase, opportunities for international collaboration to test new treatment strategies in a timely way should not be lost.

RADIOLOGIC IMAGING CONCERNS

Bernard B. O'Malley and Suresh K. Mukherji

The nasopharynx is reported to be a common site of occult primary squamous cancer. However, in our experience, occult tumors are eventually identified in the tonsil, glossotonsillar sulcus, and piriform sinus. The adenopathy often is usually well out of proportion to the size of the nasopharyngeal primary tumor, and coronal images of the paranasal sinuses and nasopharynx should supplement the axial scans of the neck in that setting (Fig. 23.7).

The widespread availability of the flexible office endoscope allows convenient initial detection and diagnosis of NPC. Imaging plays an essential role in staging of NPC as several of the criteria such as parapharyngeal extension and skull base involvement can only be accurately identified by cross-sectional imaging. The new 6th edition of the AJCC staging manual places even more emphasis of the role of imaging as an essential adjunct for staging (121).

One of the most commonly used planes to image the nasopharynx is a plane that is parallel to the hard palate. This hard palate is a readily identified landmark that can be used for both CT and MRI. Coronal imaging is required for both modalities. Multiple studies have shown the superiority of MRI over all other imaging modalities for the initial staging of NPC (122–124).

Clinical staging of the number of mucosal subsites can be confirmed with cross-sectional imaging. Conventional CT or MRI scans show right- or left-sided involvement (or both) and extension to or through the choana or oropharynx (Fig. 23.8). Computed tomography cannot detect the soft tissue changes as well as MRI, and one study shows it can even overestimate the extent of disease (122). Imaging clearly is necessary to determine the lymph node status of the lateral retropharyngeal and high posterior chain groups. Both CT and MRI are adequate for involvement of these compartments, but MRI better distinguishes between direct infiltration and true lymphatic metastasis (Fig. 23.9). Fluorodeoxyglucose-positron emission tomography (FDG-PET) provides a distinct advantage in staging the neck over cross-sectional imaging (125). The extent of soft tissue involvement must be accurately mapped because both local control (124) and rates of distant metastases and survival (126) correlate with paranasopharyngeal extension. Perineural involvement must be carefully sought because it usually remains asymptomatic (127) until it becomes more difficult to treat at the symptomatic intracranial levels. Computed tomography may not detect central perineural extension until it reaches the cavernous level. Lateral parapharyngeal extension also is occult to the clinical examination and can be accurately staged with imaging (Fig. 23.10). Progression of disease out of the mucosal compartment into the parapharyngeal space and, ultimately, into the masticator space (Fig. 23.11) can be documented with CT or MRI. Careful correlation of the diagnostic imaging with treatment portals has become even more important with the application of IMRT to radiation planning (128). Computed tomography can also be used to guide placement of brachytherapy catheters for more precise positioning (129).

Skull base involvement must be carefully excluded or properly staged when present. Skull base involvement occurs in three main patterns. The most common is the *widening* of the petroclival fissure, indicating the earliest type of skull base involvement (Fig. 23.12). This abnormality is seen well on CT or MRI when performed in the axial or semi-axial plane. The next form of skull base involvement is *direct bone infiltration* (Fig. 23.13). Because there is a survival decline between T3 and T4 tumors related to bone involvement its detection is of utmost importance. Originally CT was responsible for "upstaging" many clinically staged patients (130). Why would a subgroup of T4 patients with minimal bone disease have a more favorable prognosis (131)? Most studies show MRI to be more sensitive than CT for bone infiltration at the skull base (123,132). Because tumor can infiltrate the cancellous layer of bone before frank destruction of the overlying cortical bone occurs, MRI is the better modality at the skull base (Fig. 23.14). This finding is readily seen on noncontrast T1, or fat-suppressed fast T2 or contrast T1, views. Computed tomography can demonstrate cortical bone involvement that is less apparent on MRI. Perhaps cancellous bone involvement is less serious as indicated by the favorable local recurrence rates when bone involvement is shown by MRI alone (133) and more likely to be within the margin of a standard treatment portal. Patients that cannot tolerate MRI should have CT scanning supplemented by nuclear bone scan with single photon emission computed tomography (SPECT) images through the skull base (134) because of the high false-negative rate of CT. With more advanced lesions, the infiltration extends into the retroclival extradural space (Fig. 23.15). The third pathway of skull base involvement is extension through the *preexisting basal foramina.* The most common extensions include foramen ovale, foramen lacerum, and the orbital fissures. Lateral extension through the basipharyngeal fascia allows access to the main trunk of V-3 as it exits the skull base and the tumor tracks proximally into the cavernous sinus (Fig. 23.16). A more infiltrative perivascular pattern along the internal carotid artery results in permeation through the cartilage that covers the foramen lacerum. Larger nasopharyngeal lesions that extend forward and infiltrate the pterygoid processes gain access to the orbital fissures and then to the intracranial compartment. All of these fissures and foramina are covered on the axial neck images in the nasopharyngeal CT protocol. Supplementary direct coronal views can be obtained for advanced lesions.

For the initial staging of nasopharyngeal tumors, MRI holds a distinct advantage over CT (135) that should be employed at initial diagnosis. Because of the greater sensitivity for disturbance of the cancellous bone marrow signal, MRI should be used at that time. In addition to the MRI, because CT is so efficient (132) and reproducible between visits and different laboratories, a CT scan should also be obtained as part of the pretreatment baseline examination (136). Computed tomography is a convenient tool for surveillance and is less expensive than MRI for continued follow-up. Computed tomography is often performed regardless, as many radiation therapy departments now use the CT data obtained from patients in the final treatment position for treatment planning. However, it is *essential* for the radiation oncologist to be aware that MRI is superior to CT for identifying the full extent of disease. As a result, there is a substantial risk for a geographic miss if tumor contours are obtained on only CT, especially if the CT scans are performed with suboptimal imaging technique and without the use of intravenous contrast.

Persistent posttreatment mucosal asymmetries are indeterminate on clinical inspection and on CT. An MRI is more accurate than CT at differentiating treatment change from recurrence (137) (Fig. 23.17). If progressively diminishing T2 signal and T1 contrast enhancement can be shown on MRI, an argument can be made to assume the abnormality is scar tissue, in the absence of changing clinical symptoms. Both modalities, however, have relatively low sensitivity and only moderate specificity for recurrence (137). Computed tomography can actually show reconstitution of bone, which typically has a favorable impact on prognosis for treatment response and local control (138). When treatment-related central nervous system injury is an issue, MRI holds another advantage over CT. The standard nasopharyngeal imaging protocol should include the segments of brain, brainstem, and upper cervical spinal cord in the treatment portal that are at risk (Fig. 23.18). Early white-matter changes are apparent on T2 images and may evolve to enhancing lesions on the contrast T1 series. Ultimately FDG-PET is more useful in determining the likelihood of persistent or recurrent disease than MRI (139) (Fig. 23.19).

A simpler approach to metabolic assessment is the use of a standard nuclear camera with thallium-201 (^{201}Tl) SPECT. The nasopharynx is one subsite where ^{201}Tl has certain advantages over FDG-PET. Unlike glucose, which is used for FDG-PET scans, the normal brain does not use thallium. Thus, tumors involving the skull have the potential to be obscured when imaged with FDG but are more conspicuous when imaged with thallium due to the absence of adjacent brain activity.

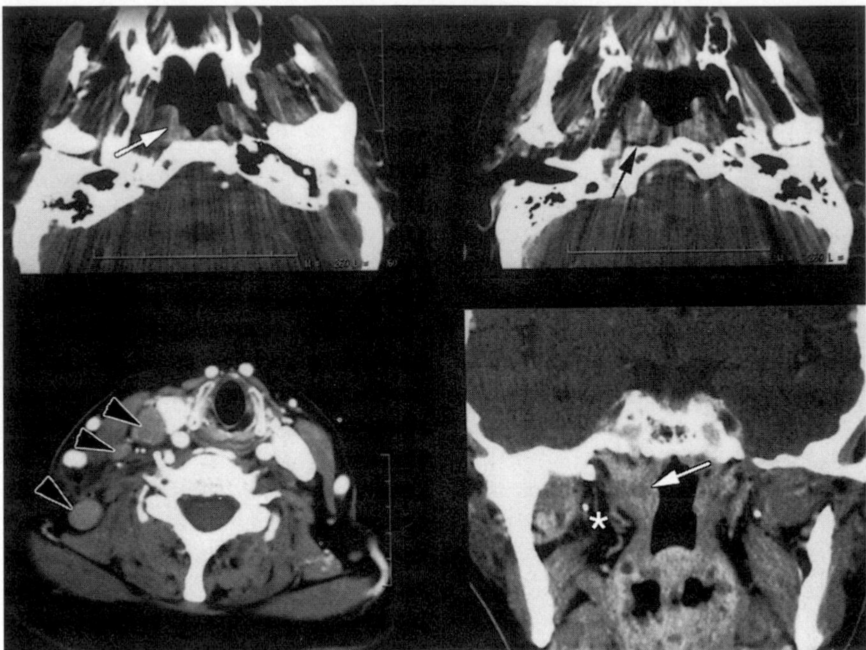

Figure 23.7 Early nasopharyngeal cancer. Enhanced axial computed tomography (top panels and bottom left) and direct coronal view (bottom right) show several pathologic right neck nodes (*arrowheads*) in a patient with squamous cell carcinoma of unknown origin. Axial and coronal views show a T1-stage lesion of the right nasopharynx (*arrows*). The parapharyngeal space is normal (*asterisk*).

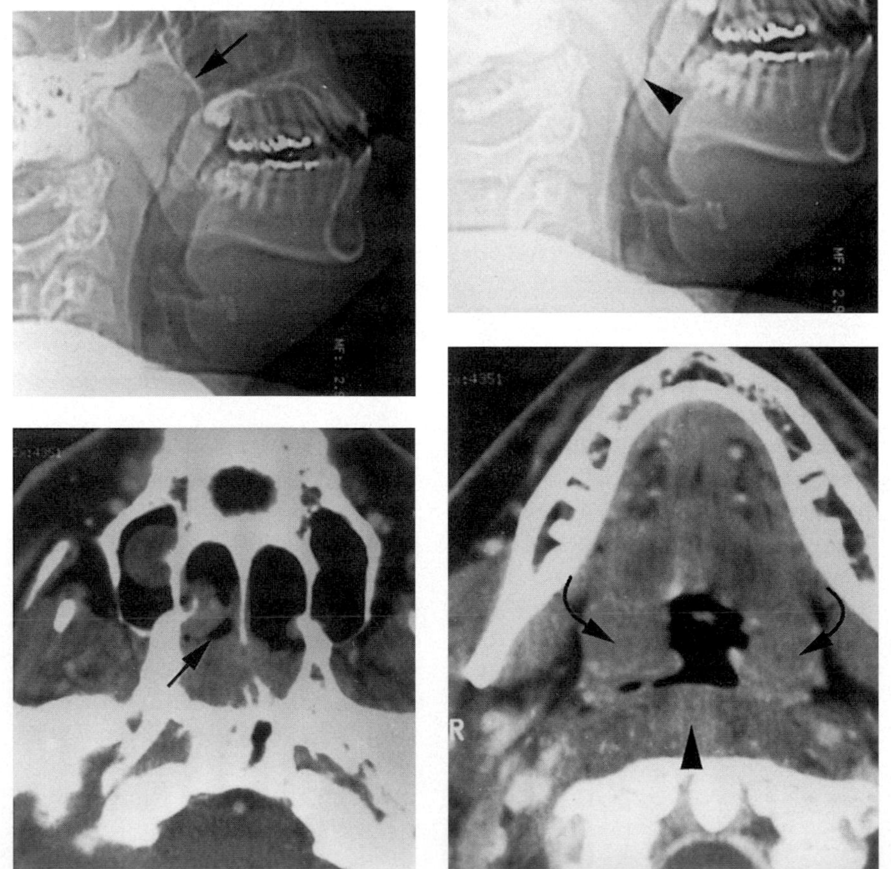

Figure 23.8 Scout lateral and enhanced axial computed tomographic views **(A)** of a large nasopharyngeal mass with anterior choanal involvement (*arrows*) and **(B)** a large nasopharyngeal mass with inferior extension to the level of the oropharynx (*arrowheads*). Note tonsils (*curved arrows*).

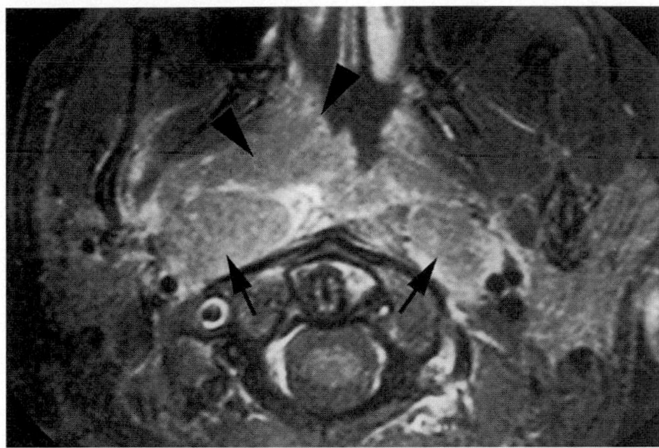

Figure 23.9 Enhanced axial contrast T1 magnetic resonance imaging showing nasopharyngeal mass (*arrowheads*) with bilateral lateral retropharyngeal lymphadenopathy (*arrows*).

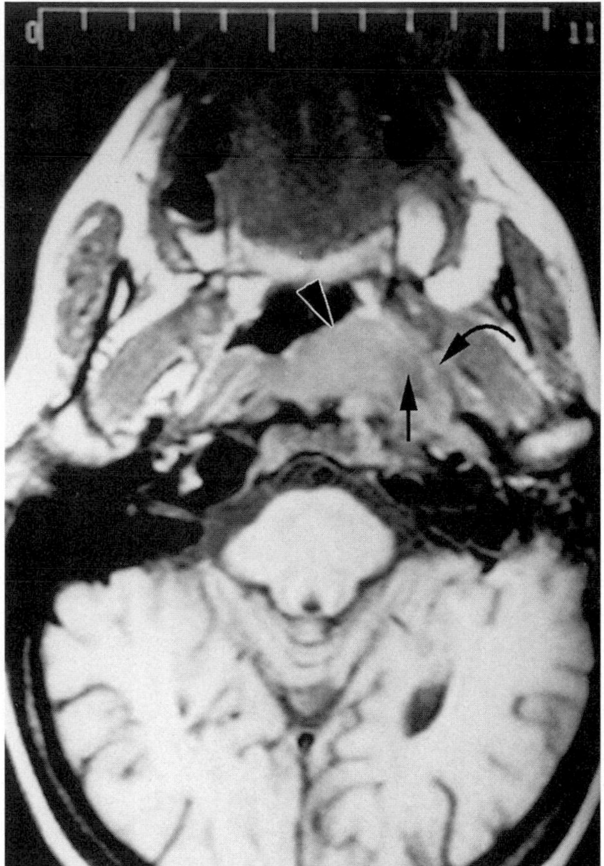

Figure 23.10 Early parapharyngeal space involvement. Semiaxial T1 magnetic resonance imaging shows lateral nasopharyngeal mass (*arrowhead*) with involvement of parapharyngeal space (*arrow*), approaching but not involving the boundary of the masticator space (*curved arrow*).

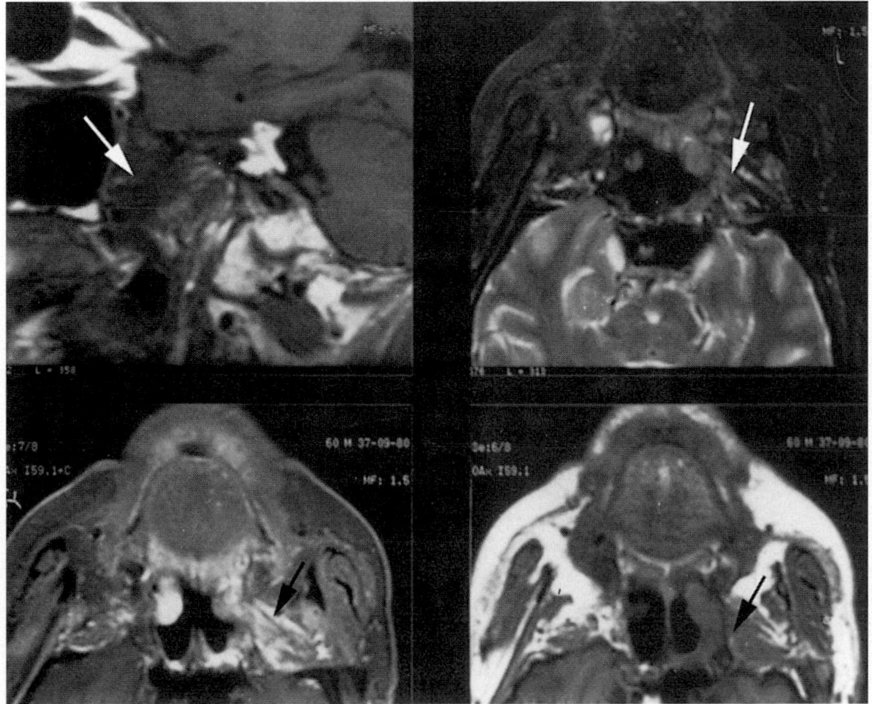

Figure 23.11 Early masticator space involvement. Parasagittal T1 and matched semiaxial T2, T1, and fat-suppressed contrast T1 views of ulcerating lateral nasopharyngeal mass penetrating through the parapharyngeal space and infiltrating the lateral pterygoid muscle (*arrows*).

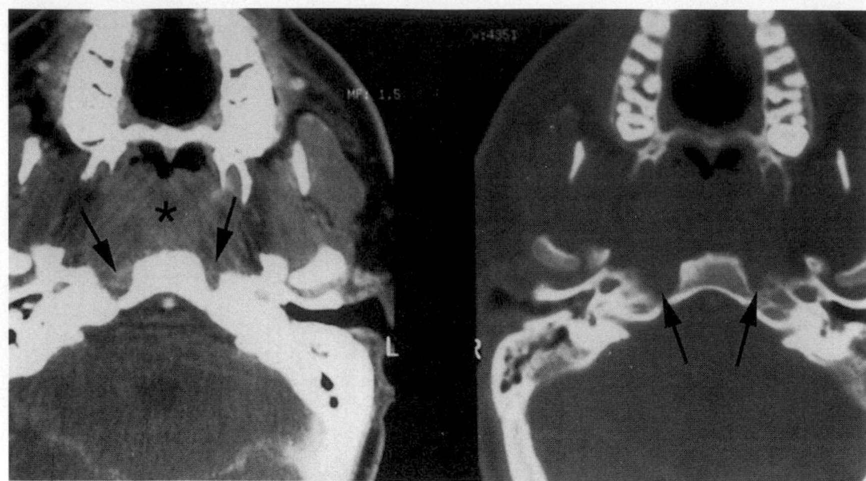

A,B

Figure 23.12 Early skull base involvement. Matched semiaxial soft tissue **(A)** and bone windows **(B).** Computed tomographic views of a large nasopharyngeal mass infiltrating both petroclival fissures (*arrows*), the right more than the left.

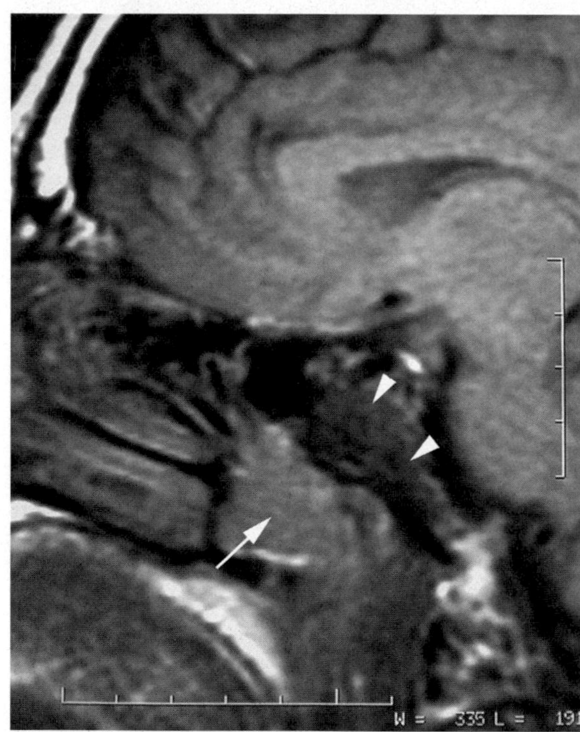

A

Figure 23.13 Direct bone infiltration. **A:** Midsagittal T1-weighted magnetic resonance imaging shows large mass (*arrow*) and abnormal decreased signal in the marrow of the clivus (*arrowheads*). **B:** Direct coronal computed tomography (CT) shows the sclerosis of the cancellous bone of the clivus (*black arrowheads*) due to direct tumor (*white arrows*) infiltration. **C:** Direct coronal CT soft tissue window matches the bone window showing the nasopharyngeal mass (*white arrows*) and intracranial tumor component on the other side of the skull base (*white arrowheads*).

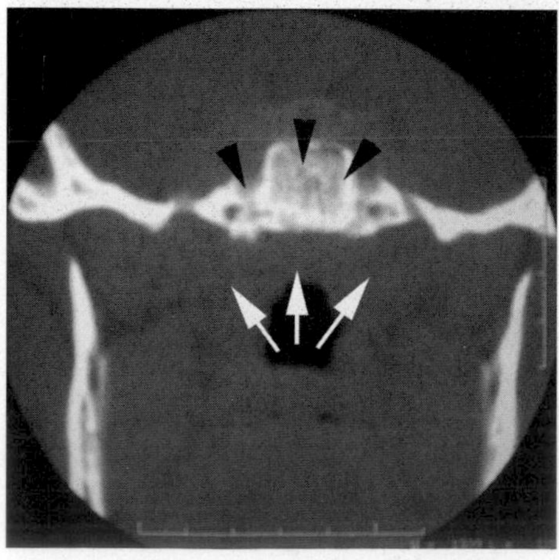

B

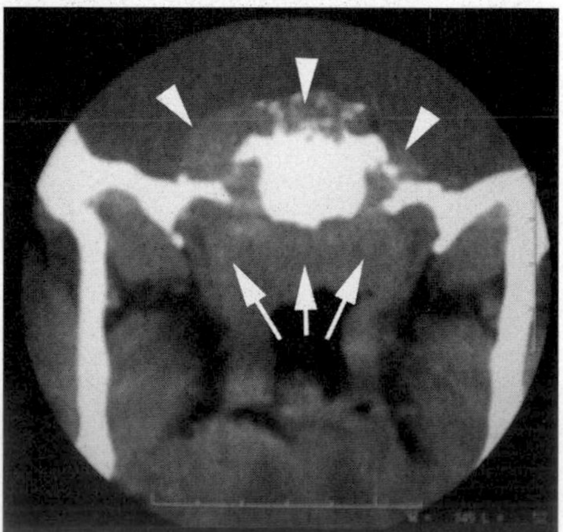

C

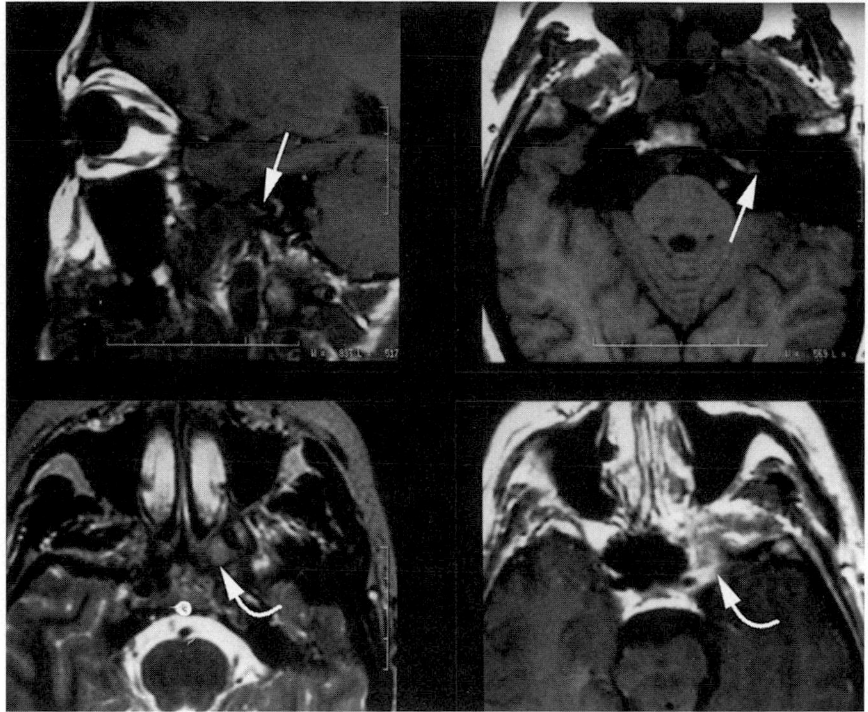

Figure 23.14 Direct skull base infiltration. Sagittal and matched semiaxial T1, T2, and enhanced T1 views of direct invasion of the petrous apex (*arrows*) and sphenoid bone (*curved arrows*).

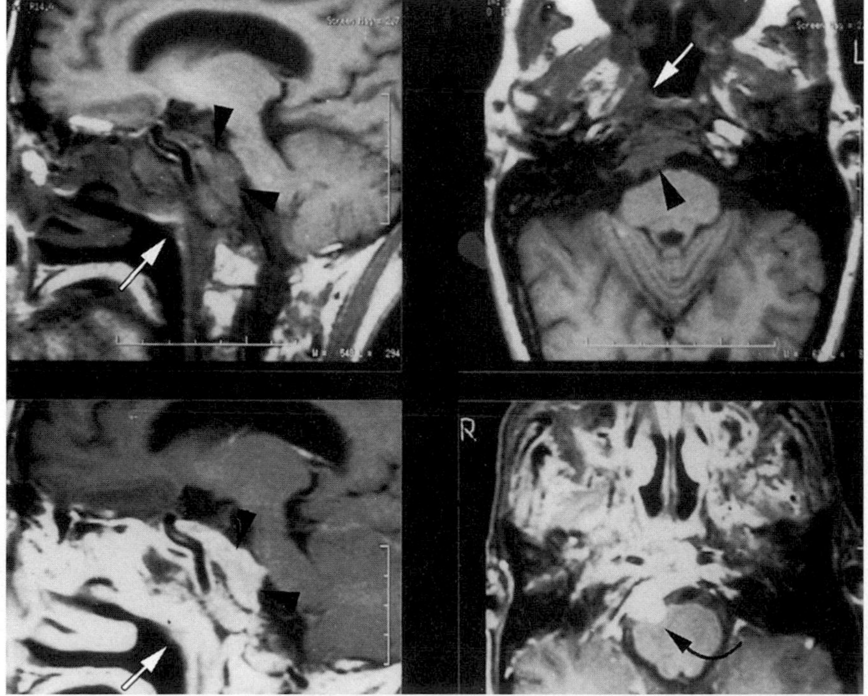

Figure 23.15 Transclival extension. Matched sagittal (left) and semiaxial (right) precontrast and post-contrast views of nasopharyngeal mass responding at the mucosal margin (*arrows*) but progressing through the clivus to the prepontine cistern (*arrowheads*), impinging on the brainstem (*curved arrow*).

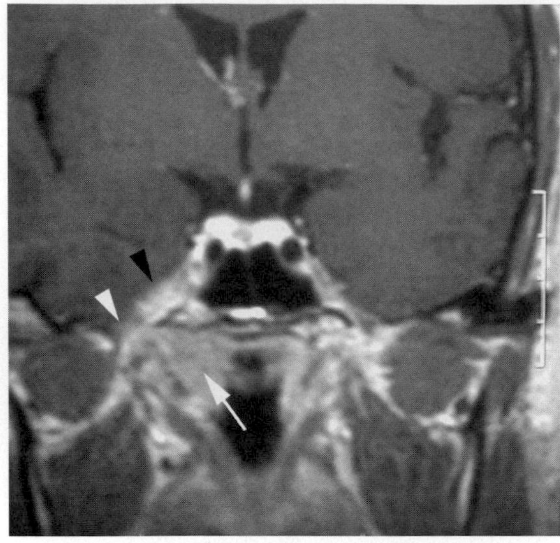

Figure 23.16 Foraminal invasion. Direct coronal T1 magnetic resonance image with contrast shows the cavernous sinus involvement (*black arrowhead*) related to the small nasopharynx tumor (*white arrow*) tracking through the right foramen ovale (*white arrowhead*).

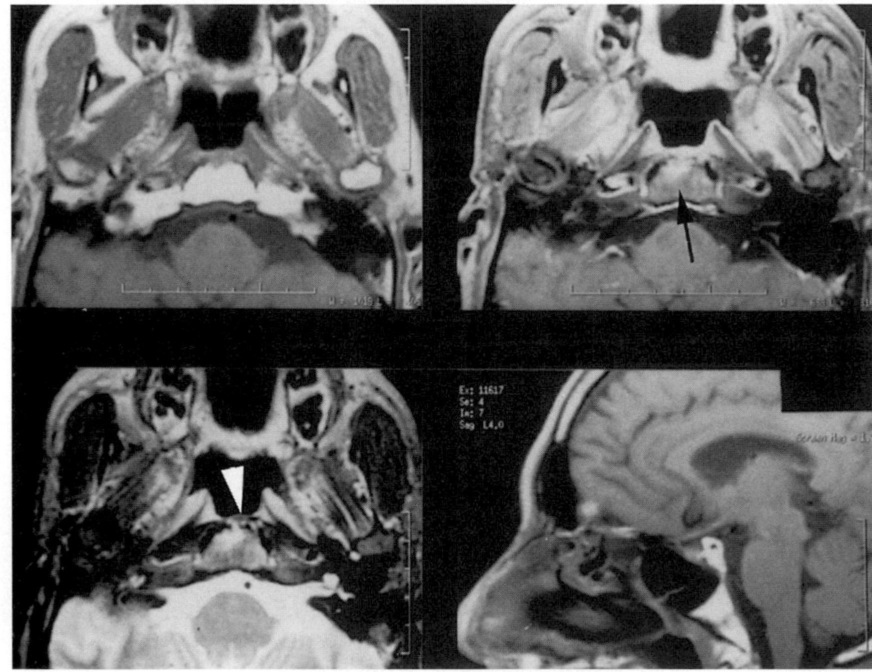

Figure 23.17 Follow-up magnetic resonance imaging. Matched semiaxial T1, contrast T1, T2, and sagittal T1 images show minor residual mucosal irregularity (*arrowhead*) at mucosa and minimal residual abnormal enhancement at the clivus (*arrow*).

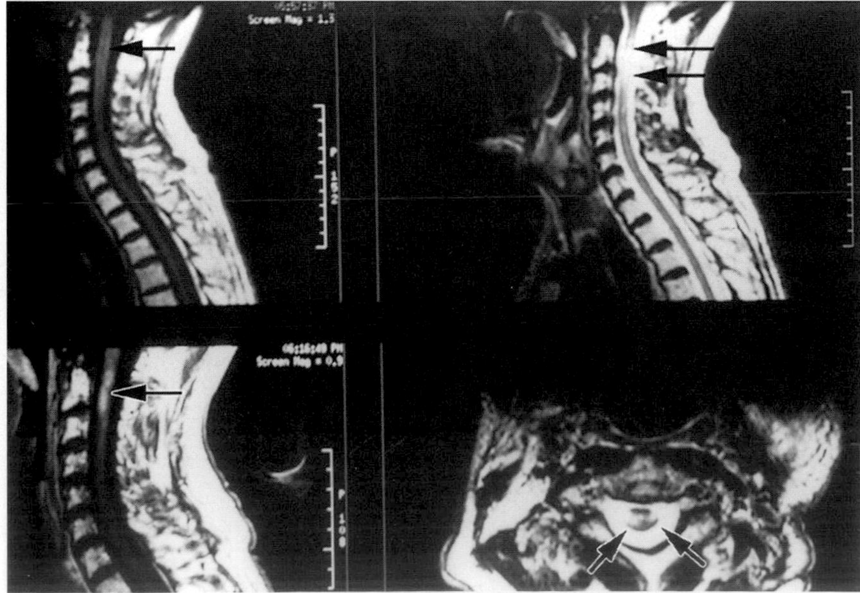

Figure 23.18 Radiation treatment myelitis. Sagittal T1, T2, axial T2, and contrast sagittal T1 magnetic resonance images show segmental intramedullary enhancement (*arrows*) within the portal at the C-2 level. The patient shows no evidence of nasopharyngeal carcinoma.

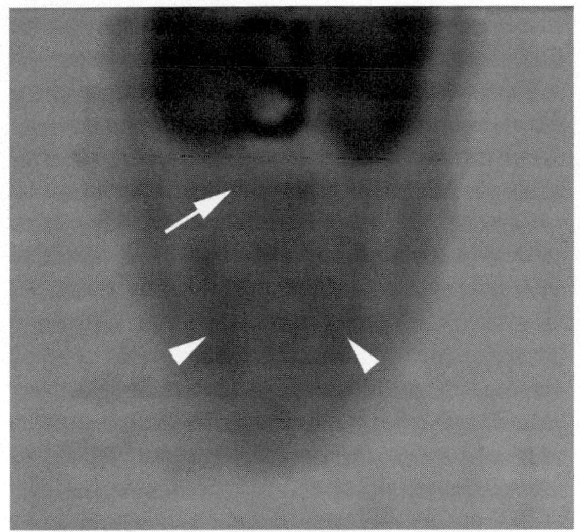

A

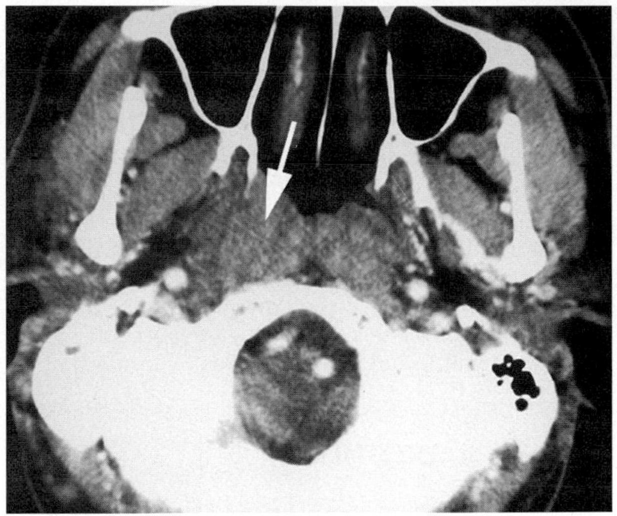

B

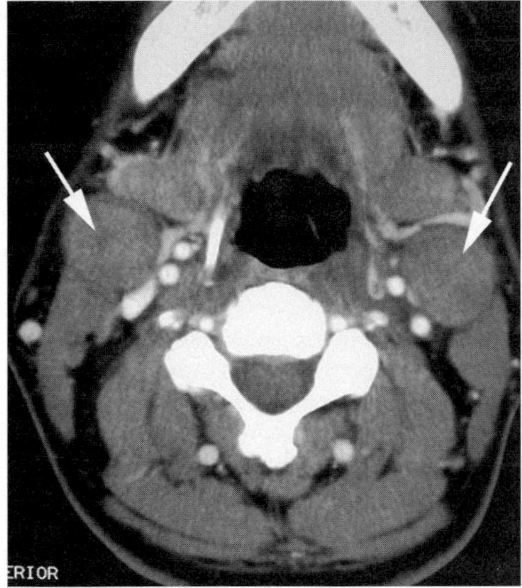

C

Figure 23.19 Fluorodeoxyglucose-positron emission tomography (FDG-PET) follow-up of nasopharynx cancer. **A:** Coronal composite FDG-PET scan image shows absent metabolic activity at primary right nasopharynx site (*white arrow*) after radiation therapy. There is no hypermetabolism related to the treated bilateral lymphadenopathy, only physiologic salivary activity (*white arrowheads*). **B:** Pretreatment computed tomography (CT) shows primary squamous cell carcinoma of the right nasopharynx (*white arrow*). **C:** Pretreatment CT of the neck shows bilateral adenopathy (*white arrows*).

RADIATION THERAPY TECHNIQUE*

Louis B. Harrison, Rudolph Woode, and William M. Mendenhall

Radiation therapy is the primary treatment for nasopharyngeal cancer. It is used either alone or with chemotherapy. Patients are usually treated with conventional external beam radiation therapy, but 3D-conformal techniques have become increasingly favored. A new approach is IMRT, which is reviewed in Chapter 5. This approach is considered too new in order for us to describe a standard of care for this approach. In this section, we will review conventional techniques as well as 3D-conformal techniques.

CONVENTIONAL RADIOTHERAPY

Early stage nasopharyngeal cancers can often be treated by conventional radiation therapy. This involves lateral opposed fields for the primary site and upper neck, with a matching low anterior neck field. The spinal cord is protected after 45 Gy, and the primary site is boosted to 66 to 70 Gy. As long as there is not significant posterior extension or retropharyngeal adenopathy, this technique should be adequate. Care should be taken to include the retropharyngeal lymph node chain in the field. Patients without obvious nodal metastasis receive 54 Gy in 6 weeks to the bilateral upper neck nodes, and 50 Gy to the bilateral low neck field. Patients with involved lymph nodes are considered to have locoregionally advanced disease, and are treated with chemotherapy/radiotherapy. In that situation, the area of involved nodes receives at least 70 Gy with chemotherapy. An additional 5 to 10 Gy electron boost to a bulky lymph node can be considered, depending on the specific circumstances.

The patient should be simulated with head extension and a bite block. The primary fields are designed to treat the entire nasopharynx with adequate margin. Usually, the posterior one third to one half of the nasal cavity is in the field, depending on the exact disease extent. The skull base is included, as well as the adjacent ethmoid sinus and sphenoid sinus. After 45 Gy, the field is reduced. The spinal cord is shielded, and the primary site and upper neck fields are continued. The final boost field is taken to a total dose of 66 to 70 Gy.

After the spinal cord is shielded, the upper posterior neck is treated with electrons. Generally, 6 to 12 MeV are used, depending on the neck thickness. The posterior necks are treated with a dose of 50 to 54 Gy. That completes the elective irradiation. Involved nodes are taken to the same dose as the primary site. Currently, patients with involved lymph nodes are treated with chemotherapy/radiation therapy. In this setting, it is our practice to treat the involved lymph nodes to the same dose as the primary site. The low neck is treated with a single anteroposterior field. Generally, 50 Gy in 5 weeks is delivered. The larynx is blocked, and there is protection to the infraclavicular region, thereby minimizing the dose to the underlying lung tissue.

THREE-DIMENSIONAL CONFORMAL RADIATION THERAPY

Because parapharyngeal extension, or retropharyngeal metastasis, is such an important feature of NPC, the comprehensive irradiation of this region is an important aspect to therapy. Conventional techniques run the risk for underdosing the parapharyngeal region. If there is clear disease extension to this area, then conventional radiation therapy is inadequate. In these situations, more sophisticated treatment planning and delivery is required.

Three-dimensional treatment planning and intensity modulated treatment planning allow for adequate coverage of the parapharyngeal area. Because IMRT is in its infancy, there is no agreed on technique for its use in nasopharyngeal radiation therapy. Chapter 5 discusses IMRT approaches.

The underdosage of the parapharyngeal region is particularly significant once the spinal cord block is added during conventional radiotherapy. Three-dimensional conformal techniques allow for the coverage of these tissues and for the delivery of full therapeutic doses, with proper protection of the spinal cord and brainstem. The usual approach is to begin with conventional radiotherapy that comprehensively encompasses the primary site and upper neck, matched to a low neck field. After approximately 30 Gy, the field arrangement is changed to a 3D-conformal arrangement. This arrangement typically involves a seven-field plan. This includes two lateral fields, two sets of posterior oblique fields, and a single posteroanterior field. The spinal cord and brainstem are protected in all of these fields. However, with the inclusion of the oblique fields and the posteroanterior field, the parapharyngeal region is adequately encompassed by the prescription isodose. The involved lymph nodes in the neck, as well as the primary site, are included in these fields. These fields are treated to the prescription isodose.

The 3D-conformal fields encompass the primary site and parapharyngeal region. These fields are matched to opposed lateral fields that encompass the bilateral upper neck region. Our technique uses a spinal cord block on these fields. In this way, the upper neck is irradiated with lateral opposed fields, and the posterior necks are supplemented with matching electron fields. This technique eliminates any risk for spinal cord overlap. Because there may be field overlap with the mandible, our practice is to feather the junction between the upper neck fields and the 3D fields, usually with a moving junction to avoid overdosing the mandible.

When using this technique, there is a portion of the upper posterior neck that happens to be included in the 3D-conformal plan. The lymph nodes in this area usually receive approximately 50% of the prescription dose. A small electron field can be added to the upper posterior neck, thus bringing these lymph nodes to their daily prescription dose. The remainder of the posterior neck is treated with an appropriate electron field. This field is continuous with upper posterior neck field. In general, the entire field, including the upper posterior neck field is treated for half the dose. At that time, the upper posterior portion is blocked, and the remainder of the posterior neck is continued to the prescription dose. This assures full treatment to the entire posterior cervical chain.

The mid-neck fields are junctioned with a matching anterior neck field. The larynx is blocked in the upper midline of this field, with also serves to protect the spinal cord. This is the same field that is used for low neck treatment in the conventional approach.

Figures 23.20 and 23.21 show specific cases. These cases show all of the treatment fields that have been discussed.

*Please refer to the Appendix, Imaging Considerations for Radiation Therapy Treatment Planning. This section shows the important radiologic anatomy that allows the radiation oncologist to design the target volumes for treatment planning.

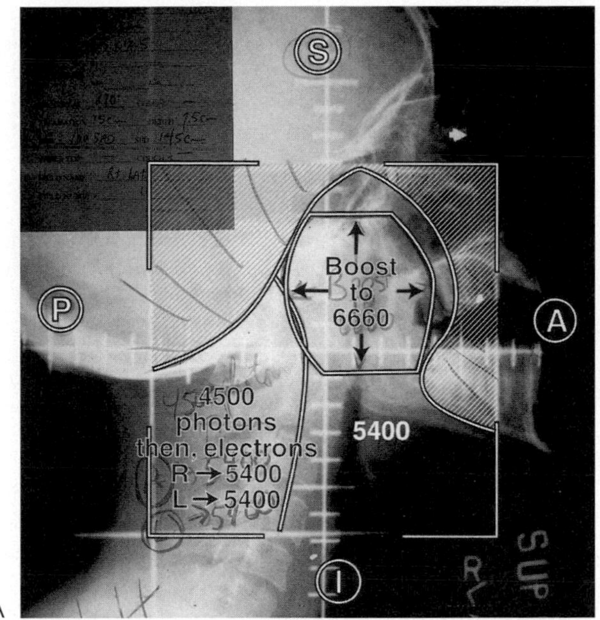

A

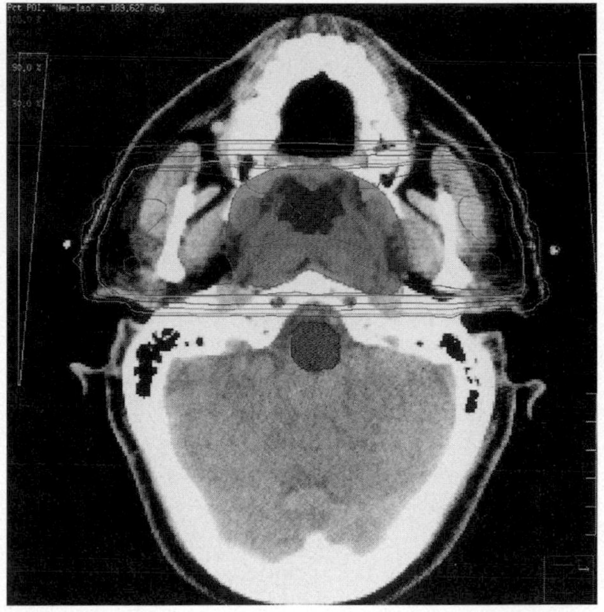

B

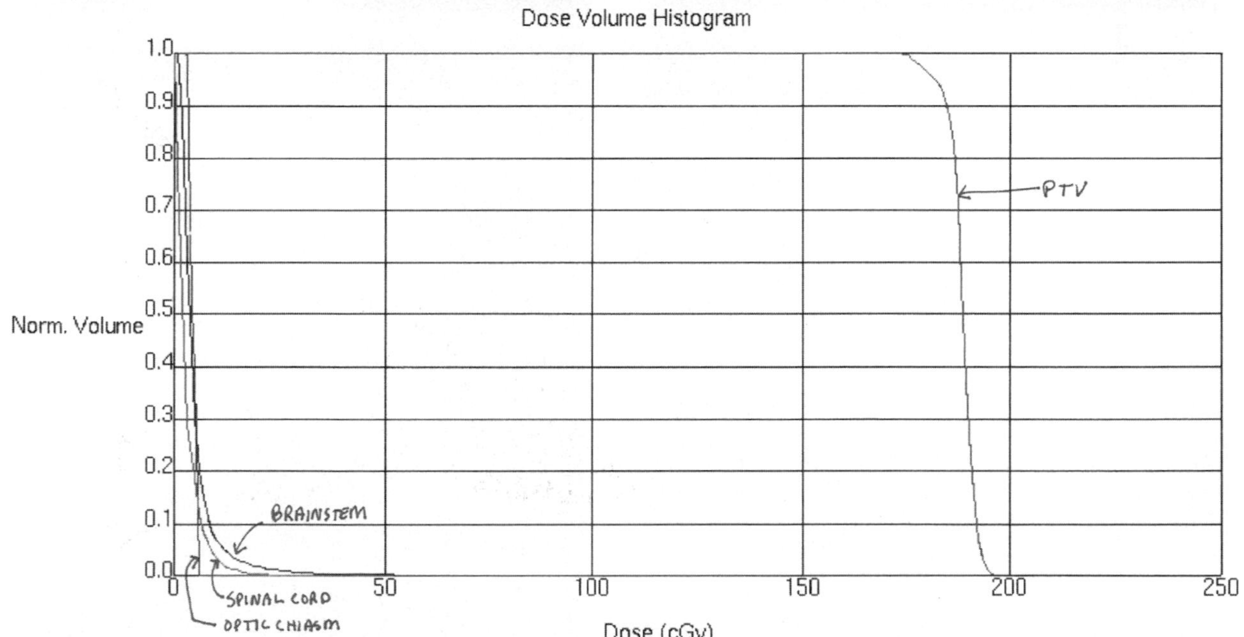

C

Figure 23.20 Nasopharynx—conventional radiotherapy technique. This patient is a 32-year-old man with a T1N0 M0 American Joint Committee on Cancer stage I carcinoma of the nasopharynx. We treated him with conventional radiotherapy alone. **A:** We used lateral opposed fields matched to a low anterior neck field. The initial fields include the upper neck nodes on both sides, the retropharyngeal nodes, and the primary site. Generous margin is used so that the entire floor of the skull base, sphenoid sinus, and posterior aspect of the ethmoid sinuses are in the field. The posterior half of the nasal cavity is in the field. After 4,500 cGy, the spinal cord is protected. The fields are continued to 5,400 cGy. At this point, all areas of microscopic disease should be adequately treated. Electrons are used for the posterior neck, also bringing them to 5,400 cGy. A boost field is created to encompass the nasopharynx proper. This area is treated to a total dose to 6,660 cGy. **B:** An axial dose distribution for the boost field is shown. The primary site is well encompassed. **C:** A dose-volume histogram for the boost field is shown. This clearly reveals that the target is adequately covered, but that structures such as the optic chasm, spinal cord, and brainstem are well protected.

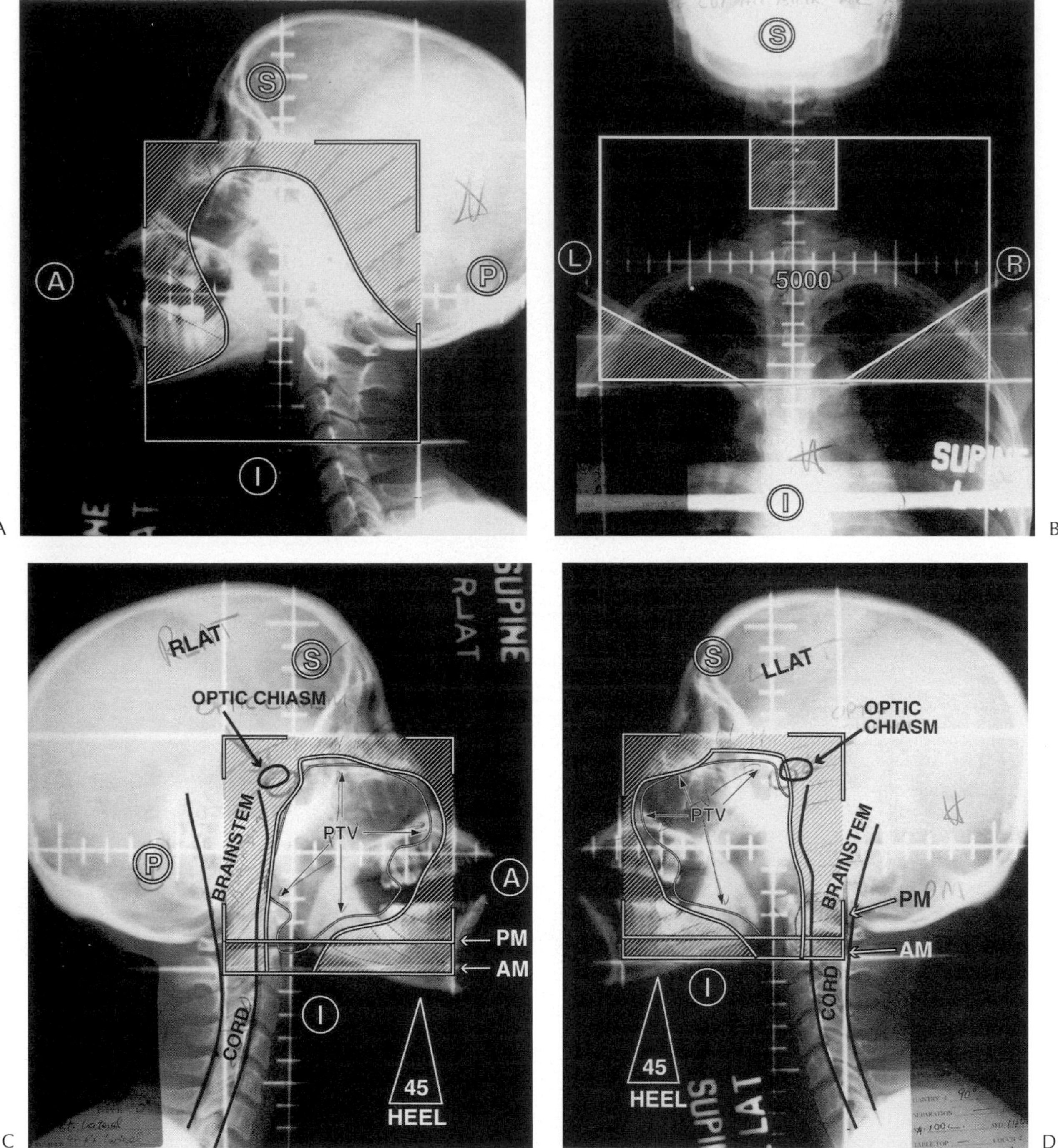

Figure 23.21 Nasopharynx—three-dimensional (3D) conformal radiation therapy technique. This patient is a 35-year-old woman who presented with a T4 N0 M0 American Joint Committee on Cancer stage IV squamous cell carcinoma of the nasopharynx. Her tumor involved the roof of the nasopharynx with bone erosion of the floor of the sphenoid sinus. There were no obvious clinical or radiologic lymph node metastases. She was treated with concomitant chemotherapy and radiotherapy, followed by adjuvant chemotherapy. **A:** The radiation technique begins with opposed lateral fields that includes the primary site and upper neck nodes. This includes the parapharyngeal nodes as well. The initial fields include the nasopharynx, with adequate margin. Included are the entire sphenoid sinus, posterior aspect of the nasal cavity, entire skull base including external auditory canal, and floor of the ethmoid sinus. The blocks are fashioned so as to eliminate the roots of the teeth. The junction with the low neck field **(B)** is above the larynx, so as to protect the larynx. These fields are similar to the conventional fields shown in Figure 23.20. After 3,060 cGy, we changed to a 3D-conformal treatment plan. This is a seven-field plan. It includes two lateral fields **(C,D)**, two sets of posterior oblique fields **(E–H)**, and a single posteroanterior (PA) field **(I)**.

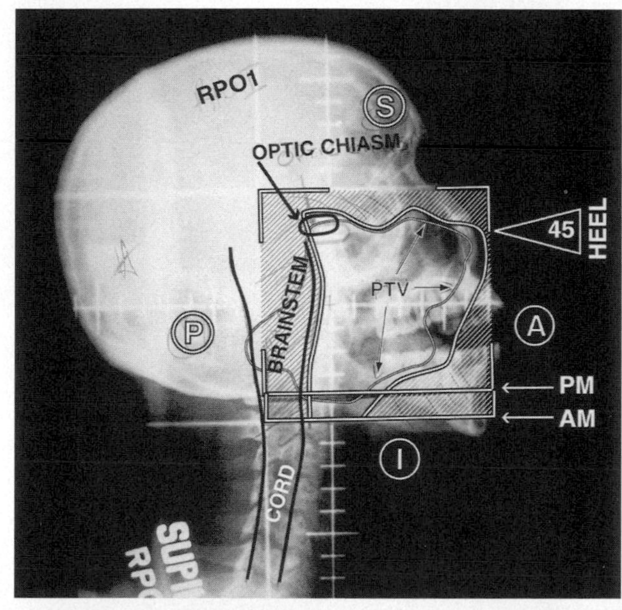

E

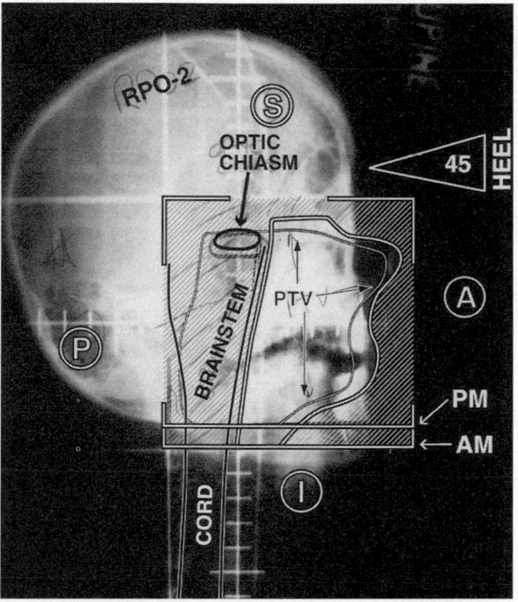

F

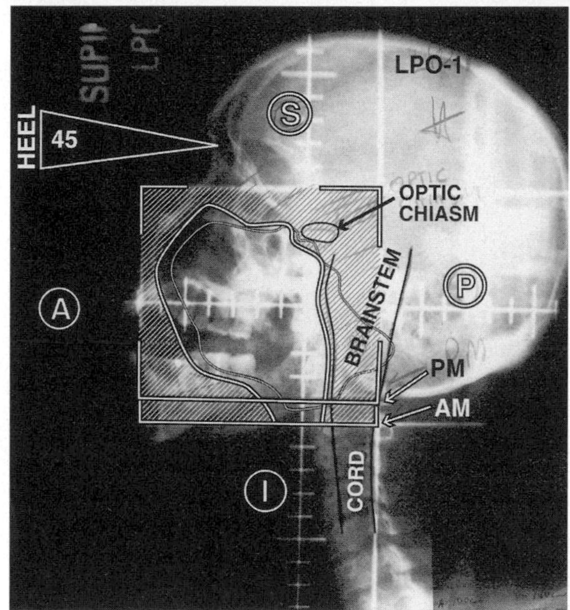

G

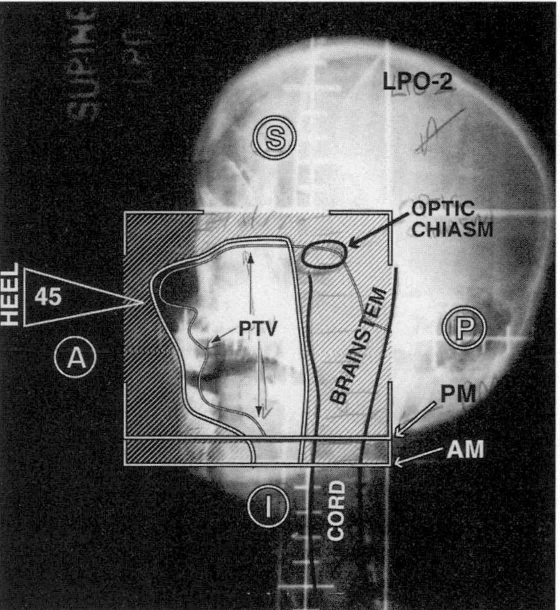

H

Figure 23.21 ***(continued)*** This field design allows for adequate inclusion of the parapharyngeal space, while it also confers adequate protection to the brainstem and upper spinal cord. Obviously, structures such as the optic chiasm are properly protected. This field arrangement gives superb coverage of the target volume, including the parapharyngeal area, without overdosing normal structures. The parapharyngeal regions are included as a result of this field arrangement. The PA field protects the midline structures, but treats both parapharyngeal spaces. The oblique fields adequately encompass the parapharyngeal space on the side of that particular field. With this arrangement, each parapharyngeal space is encompassed by the PA field and both ipsilateral oblique fields. In protecting the spinal cord, it is omitted from each contralateral oblique field. The composite result, however, is a dose distribution that adequately covers the entire region.

(continued on next page)

I

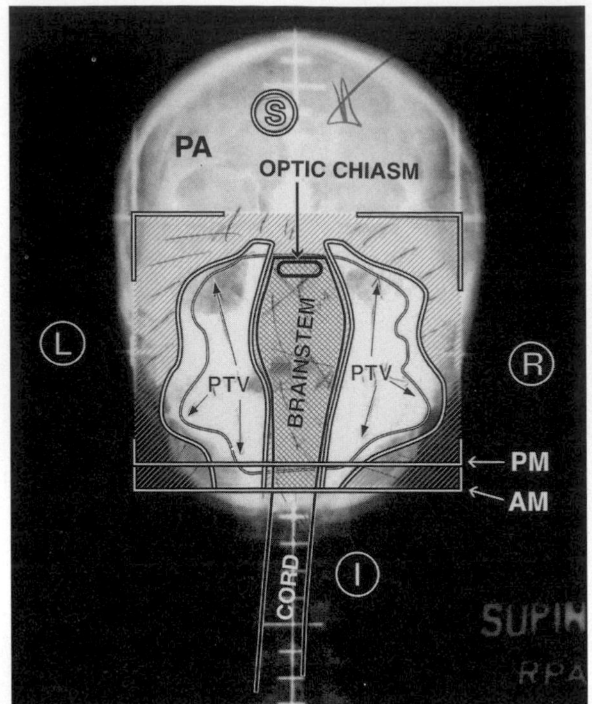

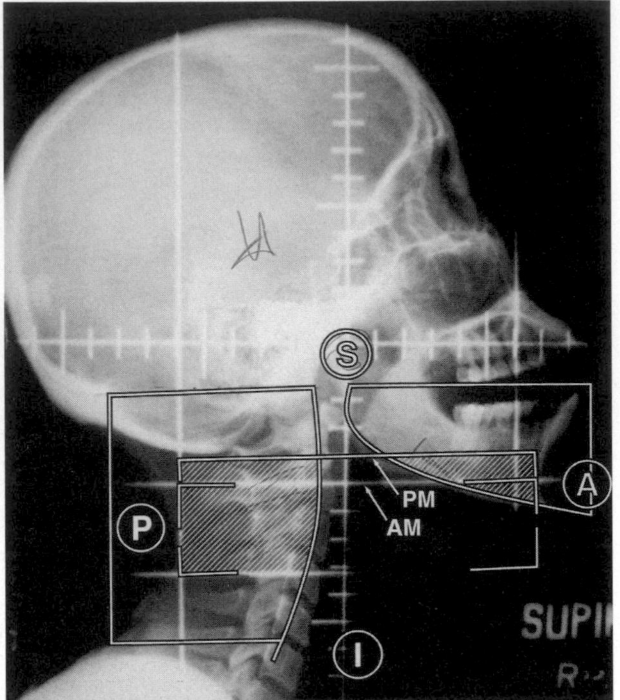

J

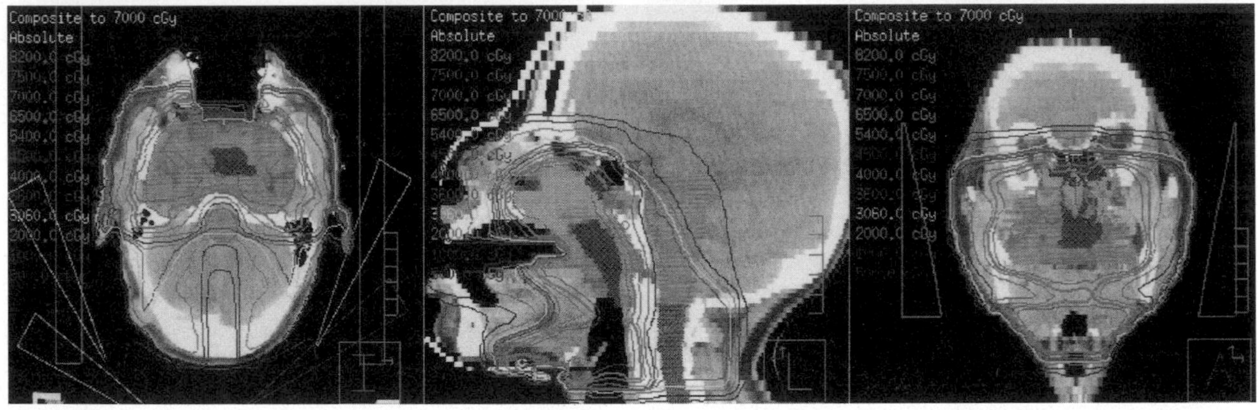

K

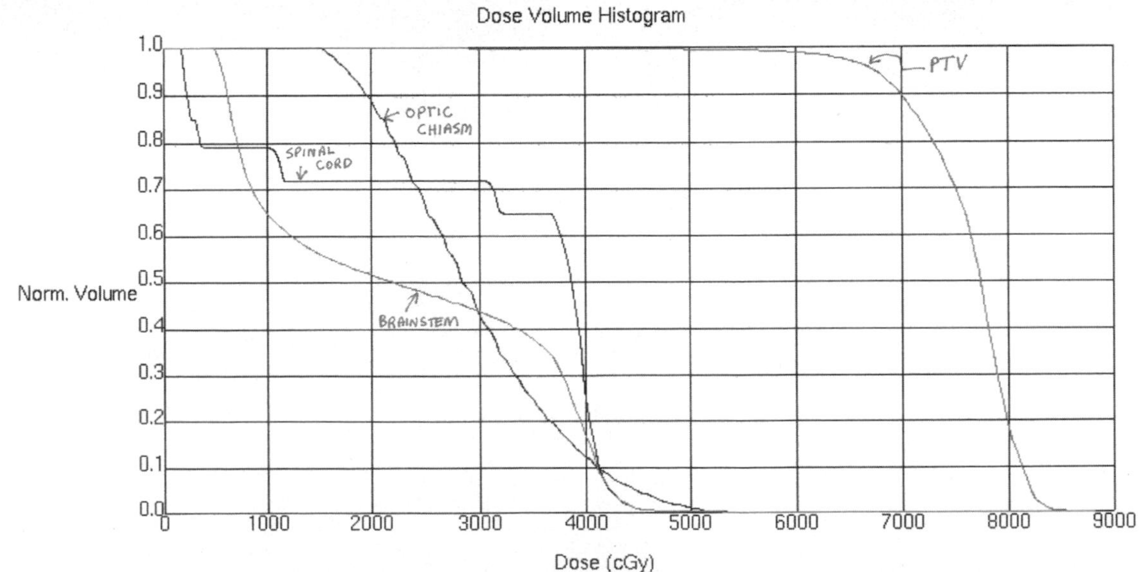

L

Figure 23.21 ***(continued)*** **J:** These mid-neck fields (opposed laterals) are junctioned with the 3D-conformal fields for the primary site (shown previously). The spinal cord is blocked, and the posterior neck is treated with electrons. This eliminates the risk for spinal cord overlap. There is overlap over a small portion of the mandible to prevent complications. This junction is feathered with an AM and PM junction. The AM and PM refer to the fact that these fields are treated with the concomitant boost technique, with an AM and PM fraction. **K:** An axial, sagittal, and coronal dose distribution shows excellent coverage of the target volume. **L:** A composite dose-volume histogram analysis shows excellent coverage of the target volume, and adequate protection of the key normal structures, such as the optic chiasm, spinal cord, and brainstem.

REFERENCES

1. Batsakis JG, Solomon AR, Rice DH. The pathology of head and neck tumors: carcinoma of the nasopharynx, part II. *Head Neck Surg* 1981;3:511–524.
2. Shanmugaratnam K, Chan SH, de-The G, et al. Histopathology of nasopharyngeal carcinoma. Correlations with epidemiology, survival rates and other biological characteristics. *Cancer* 1979;44:1029–1044.
3. Henle W, Henle G. Epidemiologic aspects of Epstein–Barr virus (EBV-associated) diseases. *Ann N Y Acad Sci* 1980;354:326–331.
4. Parkin DM, Whelan SL, Ferley J, et al., eds. Cancer incidence in five continents. *IARC Sci Pub* 1997;143.
5. Lee HP, Duffy SW, Day NE, et al. Recent trends in cancer incidence among Singapore Chinese. *Int J Cancer* 1988;42:159–166.
6. Levine PH, Connelly RR, Easton JM. Demographic patterns for nasopharyngeal carcinoma in the United States. *Int J Cancer* 1980;26:7418.
7. Greene MH, Fraumeni JF, Hoover R. Nasopharyngeal cancer among young people in the United States: racial variations by cell type. *J Natl Cancer Inst* 1977;58:1267–1270.
8. Easton JM, Levine PH, Hyams VJ. Nasopharyngeal carcinoma in the United States. A pathologic study of 177 US and 30 foreign cases. *Arch Otolaryngol* 1980;106:8891.
9. Neel HB. A prospective evaluation of patients with nasopharyngeal carcinoma: an overview. *J Otolaryngol* 1986;15:137–144.
10. Wolf H, Haus M, Wilmes E. Persistence of Epstein–Barr virus in the parotid gland. *J Virol* 1984;51:795–798.
11. Lung ML, So SY, Chan KH, et al. Evidence that respiratory tract is a major reservoir for Epstein–Barr virus. *Lancet* 1985;1:889–892.
12. Old LJ, Boyse EA, Oettgen HE, et al. Precipitating antibodies in human serum to an antigen present in cultured Burkitt's lymphoma cells. *Proc Natl Acad Sci U S A* 1966;56:1699.
13. Pathmanathan R, Prasad U Sadler R, et al. Clonal proliferation of cells infected with Epstein–Barr virus in preneoplastic lesions related to nasopharyngeal carcinoma. *N Engl J Med* 1995;333:693–698.
14. Rajadurai P, Prasad U, Gangatharan C, et al. Undifferentiated, nonkeratinizing and squamous cell carcinoma of the nasopharynx: variants of EBV infected neoplasia. *Am J Pathol* 1995;146:1355.
15. Choi PHK, Suen MWM, Huang DP, et al. Nasopharyngeal carcinoma: genetic changes, Epstein–Barr virus infection, or both. A clinical and molecular study of 36 patients. *Cancer* 1993;72:2873–2878.
16. Ho JHC. An epidemiological and clinical study of nasopharyngeal carcinoma. *Int J Radiat Oncol Biol Phys* 1978;4:182–198.
17. Ren EC, Chan SH. Human leucocyte antigens and nasopharyngeal carcinoma. *Clin Sci* 1996;91:256–258.
18. Burt RD, Vaughan TL, McKnight B, et al. Associations between human leukocyte antigen type and nasopharyngeal carcinoma in Caucasians in the United States. *Cancer Epidemiol Biomark Prevent* 1996;5:879–887.
19. Lo KW, Tsao SW, Leung SF, et al. Detailed deletion on the short arm of chromosome 3 in nasopharyngeal carcinomas. *Int J Oncol* 1994,4:1359.
20. Huang DP, Lo KW, van Hasselt CA, et al. A region of homozygous deletion on chromosome 9p21-22 in primary nasopharyngeal carcinoma. *Cancer Res* 1994;54:4003–4006.
21. Hui ABY, Lo KW, Leung SF, et al. Loss of heterozygosity on the long arm of chromosome 11 in nasopharyngeal carcinoma. *Cancer Res* 1996;56:3225–3229.
22. Cheng RYS, Lo KW, Huang DP, et al. Loss of heterozygosity on chromosome 14 in primary nasopharyngeal carcinoma. *Int J Cancer* 1997 (in press).
23. Watson CRR. The anatomy of the post-nasal space: its significance in local malignant invasion. *Australas Radiol* 1972;16:118–122.
24. Weiland LH, Neel HB, Pearson GR. Nasopharyngeal carcinoma. *Curr Hematol Oncol* 1986;4:379.
25. Krueger GRF, Kottaridis SD, Wolf H, et al. Histological types of nasopharyngeal carcinoma as compared to EBV serology. *Anticancer Res* 1981;1:187–194.
26. Prathap K, Looi LM, Prasad U. Localized amyloidosis in nasopharyngeal carcinoma. *Histopathology* 1984;8:27–34.
27. Nomori H, Watanabe S, Nakajima T, et al. Histiocytes in nasopharyngeal carcinoma in relation to prognosis. *Cancer* 1986;57:100–105.
28. Moller P, Wirbel R, Hofmann W, et al. Lymphoepithelial carcinoma (Schmincke type) as a derivate of the tonsillar crypt epithelium. *Virchows Arch–A. Pathologic Anat Histopathology* 1984;405:83–93.
29. Micheau C, Luboinski B, Schwaab G, et al. Lymphoepitheliomas of the larynx (undifferentiated carcinomas of nasopharyngeal type). *Clin Otolaryngol* 1979;4:43–48.
30. Rosai J. "Lymphoepithelioma-like" thymic carcinoma. Another tumor related to Epstein–Barr virus? *N Engl J Med* 1985;312:1320–1322.
31. Mills SE. Austin MB, Randall ME. Lymphoepithelioma-like carcinoma of the uterine cervix with inflammatory stroma. *Am J Surg Pathol* 1985;9:883–889.
32. Neel HB. Nasopharyngeal carcinoma: clinical presentation, diagnosis, treatment and prognosis. *Otolaryngol Clin North Am* 1985;18:479–490.
33. Sawaki S, Sugano H, Hirayama T. Analytical aspects of symptoms of nasopharyngeal malignancies. In: de-The G, Ito Y, eds. Nasopharyngeal carcinoma: etiology and control. *IARC Sci Pub* 1978;20:147–163.
34. Chong VFH, Fan YF, Khoo JBK. Nasopharyngeal carcinoma with intracranial spread: CT and MRI characteristics. *J Comput Assist Tomogr* 1996;20:563–569.
35. Vikram B, Mishra UB, Strong EW, et al. Patterns of failure in carcinoma of the nasopharynx. Failure at distant sites. *Head Neck Surg* 1986;8:276–279.
36. Geara FB, Sanguineti G, Tucker SL, et al. Carcinoma of the nasopharynx treated by radiotherapy alone: determinants of distant metastasis and survival. *Radiother Oncol* 1997;43:53–61.
37. Huang SC, Chu GL. Nasopharyngeal cancer: Study 11. *Int J Radiat Oncol Biol Phys* 1981;7:713–716.
38. Lee AW, Foo W, Law SC, et al. Staging of nasopharyngeal carcinoma: from Ho's to the new UICC system. *Int J Cancer* 1999;20:179–187.
39. Ho JH. Stage classification of nasopharyngeal carcinoma: a review. *IARC Sci Pub* 1978;20:99–113.
40. International Union Against Cancer. In: Sobin LH, Wittekind CH, eds. *TNM classification of malignant tumours,* 5th ed. New York: Wiley-Liss, 1997.
41. Fleming I, et al., eds. *AJCC cancer staging manual,* 5th ed. Philadelphia: Lippincott-Raven, 1997.

41a. Greene F, Page D, Fleming I, et al. *AJCC cancer staging manual,* 6th ed. New York: Springer-Verlag, 2002.

42. Sham J, Wei W, Nicholls J, et al. Extent of nasopharyngeal carcinoma involvement inside the nasopharynx. *Cancer* 1992;69:854–859.
43. Lee A, Foo W, Poon Y, et al. Staging of nasopharyngeal carcinoma: evaluation of N-staging by Ho and UICC/AJCC systems. *Clin Oncol* 1996;8:146–154.
44. Petrovich Z, Cox J D, Middleton R, et al. Advanced carcinoma of the nasopharynx 2. Pattern of failure in 256 patients. *Radiother Oncol* 1985;4: 15–20.
45. Qin D, Hu Y, Yan J, et al. Analysis of 1379 patients with nasopharyngeal carcinoma treated by radiation. *Cancer* 1988;61:1117–1124.
46. Lee AWM, Poon Y F, Foo W, et al. Retrospective analysis of 5037 patients with nasopharyngeal carcinoma treated during 1976–1985: overall survival and patterns of failure. *Int J Radiat Oncol Biol Phys* 1992;23:261–270.
47. Hunt MA, Zelefsky MJ, Wolden S, et al. Treatment planning and delivery of intensity-modulated radiation therapy for primary nasopharynx cancer. *Int J Radiat Oncol Biol Phys* 2001;49:623–632.
48. Sultanem K, Shu HK, Xia P, et al. Three-dimensional intensity-modulated radiotherapy in the treatment of nasopharyngeal carcinoma: the University of California–San Francisco experience. *Int J Radiat Oncol Biol Phys* 2000;48: 711–722.
49. Lee N, Xia P, Akazawa C, et al. Intensity-modulated radiotherapy in the treatment of nasopharyngeal carcinoma: an update of the UCSF experience. *Int J Radiat Oncol Biol Phys* 2001;51:3[Suppl 1] (abst 145:81–82).
50. Mackie TR, Balog J, Ruchala K, et al. Tomotherapy. *Semin Radiat Oncol* 1999; 9:108–117.
51. Perez A, Devinei VR, Marcial-Vega V, et al. Carcinoma of the nasopharynx: factors affecting prognosis. *Int J Radiat Oncol Biol Phys* 1991;23:271–280.
52. Santos JA, González C, Cuesta P, et al. Impact of changes in the treatment on nasopharyngeal carcinoma: an experience of 30 years. *Radiother Oncol* 1995;36:121–127.
53. Vikram B, Mishra UB, Strong EW, et al. Patterns of failure in carcinoma of the nasopharynx: 1. Failure at the primary site. *Int J Radiat Oncol Biol Phys* 1985; 11:1455–1459.
54. Lee AW, Law SC Foo W, et al. Nasopharyngeal carcinoma: local control by megavoltage irradiation. *Br J Radiol* 1993;66:528–536.
55. Sanguineti G, Geara FB, Garden AS, et al. Carcinoma of the nasopharynx treated by radiotherapy alone: determinants of local and regional control. *Int J Radiat Oncol Biol Phys* 1997;37:985–996.
56. Teo PML, Chan ATC, Lee WY, et al. Enhancement of local control in locally advanced node-positive nasopharyngeal carcinoma by adjunctive chemotherapy. *Int J Radiat Oncol Biol Phys* 1999;43:261–271.
57. Wang CC. Accelerated hyperfractionated radiation therapy for carcinoma of the nasopharynx. *Cancer* 1989;63:2461–2467.
58. Teo PML, Leung SF, Chan ATC, et al. Final report of a randomised trial on altered fractionated radiotherapy in nasopharyngeal carcinoma prematurely terminated by significant increase in neurologic complications. *Int J Radiat Oncol Biol Phys* 2000;48:1311–1322.
59. Geara FB, Sanguineti G, Tucker SL, et al. Carcinoma of the nasopharynx treated by radiotherapy alone: determinants of distant metastasis and survival. *Radiother Oncol* 1997;43:53–61.
60. Cheng SH, Tsai SYC, Yen L, et al. Concomitant radiotherapy and chemotherapy for early-stage nasopharyngeal carcinoma. *J Clin Oncol* 2000;18: 2040–2045.
61. Dimery IW, Peters LJ, Goepfert H, et al. Effectiveness of combined induction chemotherapy and radiotherapy in advanced nasopharyngeal carcinoma. *J Clin Oncol* 1993;11:1919–1928.
62. Bachouchi M, Cvitkovic, Azli N, et al. High complete response in advanced nasopharyngeal carcinoma with bleomycin, epirubicin, and cisplatin before radiotherapy. *J Natl Cancer Inst* 1990;82:616–620.
63. Al-Sarraf M, LeBlanc M, Giri PGS, et al. Chemoradiotherapy versus radiotherapy in patients with advanced nasopharyngeal cancer; Phase III randomised Intergroup study 0099. *J Clin Oncol* 1998;16:1310–1317.
64. Al-Sarraf M, LeBlanc M, Giri P, et al. Superiority of five year survival with chemo-radiotherapy vs radiotherapy in patients with locally advanced nasopharyngeal cancer. Intergroup 0099 Phase III study: final report. *ASCO* 2001;905:227a(abst).
65. Chua DTT, Sham JST, Choy D, et al. Preliminary report of the Asian-Oceanian Clinical Oncology Association randomized trial comparing cisplatin and epirubicin followed by radiotherapy versus radiotherapy alone in the treatment of patients with locoregionally advanced nasopharyngeal carcinoma. *Cancer* 1998;83:2270–2283.
66. Fu KK. Combined radiotherapy and chemotherapy for nasopharyngeal carcinoma. *Semin Radiat Oncol* 1998;8:247–253.

67. Siu LL, Tannock IF. Comments on "Chemotherapy in advanced nasopharyngeal cancer." *Oncology* 2000;14:1237–1241.
68. Brizel DM, Albers ME, Fisher SR, et al. Hyperfractionated irradiation with or without concurrent chemotherapy for locally advanced head and neck cancer. *N Engl J Med* 1998;338:1798–1804.
69. Morris M, Eifel P J, Lu J, et al. Pelvic radiation with concurrent chemotherapy compared with pelvic and para-aortic radiation for high-risk cervical cancer. *N Engl J Med* 1999;340:1137–1143.
70. Schaake-Koning C, Van Den Bogaert W, Dalesio O, et al. Effects of concomitant cisplatin and radiotherapy on inoperable non-small cell lung cancer. *N Engl J Med* 1992;326:524–530.
71. Chan AT, Teo PM, Ngan RK, et al. A phase III randomized trial comparing concurrent chemotherapy-radiotherapy with radiotherapy alone in locoregionally advanced nasopharyngeal carcinoma. *Proc ASCO* 2000;19:1637 (abst).
72. Kwong DL, Sham JS, Au GK. Preliminary report on a randomised controlled trial of concomitant UFT/radiation and adjuvant chemotherapy for locoregionally advanced non-metastatic nasopharyngeal carcinoma. *Int J Radiat Oncol Biol Phys* 2001;51:3[Suppl 1] (abst 71:42).
73. Rossi A, Molinari R, Boracchi P, et al. Adjuvant chemotherapy with vincristine, cyclophosphamide, and doxorubicin after radiotherapy in local regional nasopharyngeal cancer: results of a 4-year multicenter randomised study. *J Clin Oncol* 1988;6:1401–1410.
74. International Nasopharynx Cancer Study Group. Preliminary results of a randomized trial comparing neoadjuvant chemotherapy (cisplatin, epirubicin, bleomycin) plus radiotherapy vs radiotherapy alone in stage IV (> N2, M0) undifferentiated nasopharyngeal carcinoma: a positive effect on progression-free survival. *Int J Radiat Oncol Biol Phys* 1996;35:463–469.
75. Ma J, Mai H-Q, Hong M-H, et al. Results of a prospective randomized trial comparing neoadjuvant chemotherapy plus radiotherapy with radiotherapy alone in patients with locoregionally advanced nasopharyngeal carcinoma. *J Clin Oncol* 2001;19:1350–1357.
76. Chan ATC, Teo PML, et al. A prospective randomized study of chemotherapy adjunctive to definitive radiotherapy in advanced nasopharyngeal carcinoma. *Int J Radiat Oncol Biol Phys* 1995;33:569–577.
77. Huncharek M, Kupelnick B. Combined chemoradiation versus radiation therapy alone in locally advanced nasopharyngeal carcinoma: results of a meta-analysis of 1528 patients from six randomised trials. *Am J Clin Oncol* 2002;25:219–223.
78. Peters L, Rischin D. Chemotherapy for head and neck cancer—different strategies for different cancers. *Lung Cancer* 2001;34:S16.
79. Rischin D, Peters L, Smith J, et al. A phase II trial of epirubicin, cisplatin and infusional 5FU followed by radiotherapy and concurrent cisplatin in patients with locally advanced nasopharyngeal cancer. *ASCO* 2001;904:227a(abst).
80. Lee AWM, Foo W, Chappell R, et al. Effect of time, dose, and fractionation in temporal lobe necrosis following radiotherapy for nasopharyngeal carcinoma. *Int J Radiat Oncol Biol Phys* 1998;40:35–42.
81. Samaan, NA, Vieto R, Schult RN, et al. Hypothalamic, pituitary and thyroid dysfunction after radiotherapy of the head and neck. *Int J Radiat Oncol Biol Phys* 1982;8:1857–1867.
82. Daly T. Dental care in the irradiated patients. In: Fletcher GH, ed. *Textbook of radiotherapy*, 3rd ed. Philadelphia: Lea & Febiger, 1980:229.
83. Marty M, Pouillart P, Scholl S, et al. Comparison of the 5-hydroxytryptamine3 (serotonin) antagonist ondansetron (GR 38032F) with high-dose metoclopramise in the control of cisplatin-induced emesis. *N Engl J Med* 1990;322: 816–821.
84. Roila F, Tonato M, Cognetti F, et al. Prevention of cisplatin-induced emesis: a double-blind multicenter randomized crossover study comparing ondansetron and ondansetron plus dexamethasone. *J Clin Oncol* 1991;9:675–678.
85. Dexamethasone alone or in combination with ondansetron for the prevention of delayed nausea and vomiting induced by chemotherapy. The Italian Group for Antiemetic Research. *N Engl J Med* 2000;342:1554–1559.
86. Campos D, Pereira JR, Reinhardt RR, et al. Prevention of cisplatin-induced emesis by the oral neurokinin-1 antagonist, MK-869, in combination with granisetron and dexamethasone or with dexamethasone alone. *J Clin Oncol* 2001;19:1759–1767.
87. Fleming S, Peppard S, Ratanatharathorn V, et al. Ototoxicity from cis-platinum in patients with stages III and IV previously untreated squamous cell cancer of the head and neck. *Am J Clin Oncol* 1985;8:302–306.
88. Cavaletti G, Marzorati L, Bogliun G, et al. Cisplatin-induced peripheral neurotoxicity is dependent on total-dose intensity and single-dose intensity. *Cancer* 1992;69:203–207.
89. de Forni M, Malet-Martino MC, Jaillais P, et al. Cardiotoxicity of high-dose continuous infusion fluorouracil: a prospective clinical study. *J Clin Oncol* 1992;10:1795–1801.
90. Diasio RB, Beavers TL, Carpenter TJ. Familial deficiency of dihydropyrimidine dehydrogenase. Biochemical basis for familial pyrimidinemia and severe 5-fluorouracil-induced toxicity. *J Clin Invest* 1988;81:47–51.
91. Lee AW, Law SC, Foo W, et al. Retrospective analysis of patients with nasopharyngeal carcinoma treated during 1976–1985: survival after local recurrence. *Int J Radiat Oncol Biol Phys* 1993;26:773–782.
92. Chua DT, Sham JS, Kwong DL, et al. Locally recurrent nasopharyngeal carcinoma: treatment results for patients with computed tomography assessments. *Int J Radiat Oncol Biol Phys* 1998;41:379–386.
93. Pryzant RM, Wendt CD, Delclos L, et al. Re-treatment of nasopharyngeal carcinoma in 53 patients. *Int J Radiat Oncol Biol Phys* 1992;22:941.
94. Fu KK, Hwang JM, Phillips T. Re-irradiation of locally recurrent nasopharyngeal carcinoma. Proceedings of the UICC Workshop on Nasopharyngeal Cancer; February 11–14, 1998; Singapore; pp. 173–187.
95. Lee, AW, Foo W, Law SC, et al. Reirradiation for recurrent nasopharyngeal carcinoma: factors affecting therapeutic ratio and ways for improvement. *Int J Radiat Oncol Biol Phys* 1997;34:43–52.
96. Buatti JM, Friedman WA, Bova FJ, et al. Linac radiosurgery for locally recurrent nasopharyngeal carcinoma: rationale and technique. *Head Neck* 1995;17: 14–19.
97. Cmelak AJ, Cox RS, Adler JR, et al. Radiosurgery for skull base malignancies and nasopharyngeal carcinoma. *Int J Radiat Oncol Biol Phys* 1997;37:99–1003.
98. Feehan PE, Castro JR, Phillips TL, et al. Recurrent locally advanced nasopharyngeal carcinoma treated with heavy charged particle irradiation. *Int J Radiat Oncol Biol Phys* 1992;23:8814.
99. Chua DTT, Sham JST, Hung K-N, et al. Salvage treatment for persistent and recurrent T1-2 nasopharyngeal carcinoma by stereotactic radiosurgery. *Head Neck* 2001;23:791–798.
100. Fee WE, Robertson JR, Goffinet DR. Long-term survival after surgical resection for recurrent nasopharyngeal cancer after radiotherapy failure. *Arch Otolaryngol–Head Neck Surg* 1991;117:123–136.
101. Tu G-Y, Hu Y-H, Xu G-Z, et al. Salvage surgery for nasopharyngeal carcinoma. *Arch Otolaryngol–Head Neck Surg* 1988;114:328–329.
102. Morton RP, Liavaag PG, McLean M, et al. Transcervico-mandibulo-palatal approach for surgical salvage of recurrent nasopharyngeal cancer. *Head Neck* 1996;18:352–358.
103. Panje WR, Gross CE. Treatment of tumours of the nasopharynx: surgical therapy. In: Thawley SE, Panje WR eds. *Comprehensive management of head and neck tumours.* Philadelphia: WB Saunders, 1987;1:662.
104. Fisch U. The infratemporal approach for nasopharyngeal tumours. *Laryngoscope* 1983, 93:36–43.
105. Wei WI, Ho CM, Yuen PW, et al. Maxillary swing approach for resection of tumours in and around the nasopharynx. *Arch Otolaryngol–Head Neck Surg* 1995;121:638–642.
106. Wie WI, Lam KH, Ho CM, et al. Efficacy of radical neck dissection for the control of cervical metastasis after radiotherapy for nasopharyngeal carcinoma. *Am J Surg* 1990;160:439–442.
107. Yen KL, Hsu LP, Sheen TS, et al. Salvage neck dissection for cervical recurrence of nasopharyngeal carcinoma. *Head Neck Surg* 1997;123:725–729.
108. Boussen H, Cvitkovic E, Wendling JL, et al. Chemotherapy of metastatic and/or recurrent undifferentiated nasopharyngeal carcinoma with cisplatin, bleomycin and fluorouracil. *J Clin Oncol* 1991;9:1675–1681.
109. Wang TL, Tan YO. Cisplatin and 5-fluorouracil continuous infusion for metastatic nasopharyngeal carcinoma. *Ann Acad Med* 1991;20:601–603.
110. Au E, Ang PT. A phase II trial of 5-fluorouracil and cisplatinum in recurrent or metastatic nasopharyngeal carcinoma. *Ann Oncol* 1994;5:87–89.
111. Su WC, Chen TY, Kao RH, et al. Chemotherapy with cisplatin and continuous infusion of 5-fluorouracil and bleomycin for recurrent and metastatic nasopharyngeal carcinoma in Taiwan. *Oncology* 1993;50:205–208.
112. Yeo W, Leung TW, Leung SF, et al. Phase II study of the combination of carboplatin and 5-fluorouracil in metastatic nasopharyngeal carcinoma. *Cancer Chemother Pharmacol* 1996;38:466–470.
113. Fandi A, Bachouchi M, Azli N, et al. Long-term disease-free survivors in metastatic undifferentiated carcinoma of nasopharyngeal type. *J Clin Oncol* 2000;18:1324–1330.
114. Dugan M, Choy D, Ngai A, et al. Multicenter phase II trial of mitoxantrone in patients with advanced nasopharyngeal carcinoma in Southeast Asia: an Asian-Oceanian Clinical Oncology Association Group study. *J Clin Oncol* 1993;11:70–76.
115. Au E, Tan EH, Ang PT. Activity of paclitaxel by three-hour infusion in Asian patients with metastatic undifferentiated nasopharyngeal cancer. *Ann Oncol* 1998;9:327–329.
116. Tan EH, Khoo KS, Wee J, et al. Phase II trial of a paclitaxel and carboplatin combination in Asian patients with metastatic nasopharyngeal carcinoma. *Ann Oncol* 1999;10:235–237.
117. Yeo W, Leung TW, Chan AT, et al. A phase II study of combination paclitaxel and carboplatin in advanced nasopharyngeal carcinoma. *Eur J Cancer* 1998; 34:2027–2031.
118. Chua DT, Kwong DL, Sham JS, et al. A phase II study of ifosfamide, 5-fluorouracil and leucovorin patients with recurrent nasopharyngeal carcinoma previously treated with platinum chemotherapy. *Eur J Cancer* 2000;36:736–741.
119. Ngan KC, et al. *Proc ASCO* 2001;234.
120. Sheen TS, Huang YT, Chang YL, et al. Epstein–Barr virus-encoded latent membrane protein 1co-expresses with epidermal growth factor receptor in nasopharyngeal carcinoma. *Jpn J Cancer Res* 1999;90:1285–1292.

Radiologic Imaging Concerns

121. Chong VF, Mukherji SK, Ng SH, et al. Nasopharyngeal carcinoma: review of how imaging affects staging. *J Comput Assist Tomogr* 1999;23:984–993.
122. Curran WJ, Hackney DB, Blitzer PH, et al. The value of magnetic resonance imaging in treatment planning of nasopharyngeal carcinoma. *Int J Radiat Oncol Biol Phys* 1986;12:2189–2196.
123. Ng SH, Chang TC, Ko SF, et al. Nasopharyngeal carcinoma: MRI and CT assessment. *Neuroradiology* 1997;39:741–746.
124. Sakata K, Hareyama M, Tamakawa M. Prognostic factors of nasopharynx

tumors investigated by MR imaging and the value of MR imaging in the newly published TNM staging. *Int J Radiat Oncol Biol Phys* 1999;43:273–278.

125. Kao CH, Hsieh JF, Tsai SC, et al. Comparison of 18-fluoro-2-deoxyglucose positron emission tomography and computed tomography in detection of cervical lymph node metastases of nasopharyngeal carcinoma. *Ann Otol Rhinol Laryngol* 2000;109(12 Pt 1):1130–1134.
126. Teo P, Lee WY, Yu P. The prognostic significance of parapharyngeal tumour involvement in nasopharyngeal carcinoma. *Radiother Oncol* 1996;39:209–221.
127. Su CY, Lui CC. Perineural invasion of the trigeminal nerve in patients with nasopharyngeal carcinoma. Imaging and clinical correlations. *Cancer* 1996; 78:2063–2069.
128. Hunt MA, Zelefsky MJ, Wolden S, et al. Treatment planning and delivery of intensity-modulated radiation therapy for primary nasopharynx cancer. *Int J Radiat Oncol Biol Phys* 2001;49:623–632.
129. Kremer B, Klimek L, Andreopoulos D, et al. A new method for the placement of brachytherapy probes in paranasal sinus and nasopharynx neoplasms. *Int J Radiat Oncol Biol Phys* 1999;43:995–1000.
130. Yamashita S, Kondo M, Hashimoto S. Conversion of T-stages of nasopharyngeal carcinoma by computed tomography. *Int J Radiat Oncol Biol Phys* 1985;11:1017–1021.
131. Altun M, Tenekeci N, Kaytan E, et al. Locally advanced nasopharyngeal carcinoma: computed tomography findings, clinical evaluation, and treatment outcome. *Int J Radiat Oncol Biol Phys* 2000;47:401–404.
132. Chong VF, Fan YF, Khoo JB. Nasopharyngeal carcinoma with intracranial spread: CT and MR characteristics. *J Comput Assist Tomogr* 1996;20:563–569.
133. Nishioka T, Shirato H, Kagei K, et al. Skull-base invasion of nasopharyngeal carcinoma: magnetic resonance imaging findings and therapeutic implications. *Int J Radiat Oncol Biol Phys* 2000;47:395–400.
134. Lee CH, Wang PW, Chen HY, et al. Assessment of skull base involvement in nasopharyngeal carcinoma: comparisons of single-photon emission tomography with planar bone scintigraphy and x-ray computed tomography. *Eur J Nucl Med* 1995;22:514–520.
135. Casselman JW. The value of MRI in the diagnosis and staging of nasopharynx tumors. *J Belge Radiol* 1994;77:67–71.
136. Olmi P, Fallai C, Colagrande S, et al. Staging and follow-up of nasopharyngeal carcinoma: magnetic resonance imaging versus computerized tomography. *Int J Radiat Oncol Biol Phys* 1995;32:795–800.
137. Chong VF, Fan YF. Detection of recurrent nasopharyngeal carcinoma: MR imaging versus CT. *Radiology* 1997;202:463–470.
138. Fang FM, Leung SW, Wang CJ, et al. Computed tomography findings of bony regeneration after radiotherapy for nasopharyngeal carcinoma with skull base destruction: implications for local control. *Int J Radiat Oncol Biol Phys* 1999;44:305–309.
139. Chaiken L, Rege S, Hoh C, et al. Positron emission tomography with fluorodeoxyglucose to evaluate tumor response and control after radiation therapy. *Int J Radiat Oncol Biol Phys* 1993;27:455–464.

CHAPTER 24

Basal and Squamous Cell Skin Cancers of the Skin of the Head and Neck

Randal S. Weber, Geoffrey L. Robb, and Adam S. Garden

Basal and squamous cell skin cancers are the most common malignancies affecting humans (1). In the United States, an estimated 600,000 to 1 million new cases are diagnosed annually (2–4). Although the head and neck region accounts for only 10% of the body surface area, it receives considerably higher actinic exposure compared with the other skin surfaces, a factor that accounts for the higher incidence of skin cancer in that region (5). Basal cell carcinomas predominate over squamous cell carcinomas by a factor of four (5). In addition, men develop this type of skin cancer twice as frequently as do women. In the U.S. population, one in six will develop skin cancer and the age group most commonly afflicted is that of individuals who are between 50 and 75 years old (2).

A cause for concern is the finding that since the early 1960s, squamous cell skin cancer is increasing by an annual rate of 4% to 8% (6). Recent surveys of skin cancer incidence point to a 65% increase since 1980. Although mortality rates for nonmelanoma skin cancer are low, accounting for only 2,000 deaths per year (7), the large number of patients in whom this disease is diagnosed results in medical expenditures in the range of $500 million annually (8).

ULTRAVIOLET CARCINOGENESIS

The principal cause of basal and squamous cell skin cancer is exposure to sunlight (8–11). Recent increases in the incidence of skin cancer are multifactorial but are related to more available leisure time spent in the sun, outdoor occupations, the perception that a tan enhances one's appearance, and potential depletion of the atmospheric ozone (12).

The ozone layer is responsible for reducing the amount of ultraviolet B radiation reaching the earth's surface. It is estimated that for every 1% reduction in atmospheric ozone, a 2% to 4% increase in skin cancer rates will occur (2,13–15). Chlorofluorocarbons (a commonly used refrigerant) deplete stratospheric ozone, which results in a higher intensity of ultraviolet (UV) radiation reaching the earth's surface (16–18). Ozone depletion may be partly responsible for the increased incidence of both melanoma and nonmelanoma skin cancer (19,20).

Another important risk factor for the development of skin cancer is the geographic area of habitation, with individuals living at lower latitudes being at higher risk (21–26). The age-adjusted incidence of nonmelanoma skin cancer in Tucson, Arizona, is more than double that of Rochester, Minnesota (21,27). For every 8- to 10-degree decrement in latitude, the incidence of squamous cell carcinoma of the skin is estimated to double (28,29). In Australia, where the incidence of basal and squamous cell skin cancer is one of the highest reported, the rate is 650 per 100,000 in the temperate south as opposed to 1,560 per 100,000 in the subtropical north (23,26). Finally, such phenotypic characteristics as light skin complexion, hair color, and the ease of sunburning influence the risk for developing skin cancer (30,31). Darker-skinned individuals or those who develop a tan when exposed to the sun have a much lower risk for skin cancer than do those with poorly pigmented or nonpigmented skin (e.g., Celtic and albino) (32).

The UV region of the solar spectrum consists of three principal segments: UVA (320 to 400 nm), UVB (280 to 320 nm), and UVC (200 to 280 nm). The principal carcinogen for the induction of skin cancer is wavelengths in the UVB region (33). Though initially considered noncarcinogenic, UVA has been shown to cause skin cancer in animals when they are exposed to high doses over a long period (34). In addition, due to its deeper level of penetration, UVA is primarily responsible for the sun's aging effects, such as wrinkling and loss of skin elasticity. UVC, a very potent carcinogen, plays a negligible role in the pathogenesis of skin cancers, because it is filtered out by the atmospheric ozone layer.

Induction of skin cancer by exposure to UVB is thought to be due to three mechanisms: direct DNA damage, inadequacy of the genetic DNA repair mechanism, and alteration of the host immune system. Formation of pyrimidine dimers are the signature UV-induced lesion in the genomic DNA. The predominant UV-induced DNA photoproducts are the cyclobutanol-type pyrimidine dimers, resulting in the formation of a ring structure with four members, which reduces the angle between the bases (35). The end result is distortion in the DNA helix. Ultraviolet radiation also produces single-strand breaks in DNA protein cross-links. When fair-skinned individuals (type I) are exposed to UV radiation, a higher amount of pyrimidine dimer formation occurs than in those with sun-insensitive (type IV) skin. The production of cyclobutanol dimers has been shown to cause mutations in human cells (36).

The carcinogenic process usually is a multistep one, involving initiation, promotion, and progression (29). Ultraviolet radiation, either administered as a single large dose or representing an accumulation of several small doses, is sufficient to induce skin cancers in experimental animals; therefore, it is a complete carcinogen. The carcinogenic cascade begins when UVB irradiation damages cellular DNA, producing a series of events that includes DNA repair, mutation, and cellular transformation. Removal of DNA lesions by the repair process is a critical step in the prevention of cellular transformation. Hereditary diseases, such as xeroderma pigmentosum, Fanconi anemia, and ataxia telangiectasia, have been shown to be unusual in their processing of damaged DNA. Patients with xeroderma pigmentosum are hypersensitive to sunlight and are highly prone to the induction of skin cancers, owing to their inability to repair pyrimidine dimers. Analogous to the induction of other solid tumors, the mechanism of UV carcinogenesis involves point mutations, deletions, insertions, and translocations. These genetic alterations of oncogenes serve to produce overexpression of a more potent form of the gene product, leading to the transformed phenotype. Conversely, mutations may downregulate the function of tumor suppressor genes, allowing a relative overexpression of genes that promote cell division and growth. Mutations of the H-*ras* oncogene, a growth control gene involving signal transduction, have been identified in aggressive head and neck skin cancers (37). Ultraviolet radiation–induced mutations of the *p53* tumor suppressor gene have also been identified and detected in squamous cell carcinomas of the skin, supporting the etiologic role of UV radiation in the carcinogenic process. Kanjilal et al. (38) have demonstrated a high-frequency incidence (88%) of *p53* mutations in aggressive nonmelanoma skin cancer of the head and neck.

HISTOPATHOLOGIC CONSIDERATIONS

The term *basal cell carcinoma* is derived from the cellular morphology of this tumor. Its basaloid appearance resembles the basal cell layer of the epithelium. The tumor grows as large islands, cords, and trabeculae in a teardrop, festooning pattern. Peripherally, the nests and lobules of basal cell carcinoma are oriented perpendicular to the basement membrane and have the appearance of a palisading growth pattern. At times, basal cell carcinomas may display polyappendageal differentiation resembling adnexal tumors of the skin.

The most common type of basal cell carcinoma is the nodular growth type that resembles a translucent papule with telangiectatic borders and central ulcer. Neglected nodular basal cell carcinomas may become quite large and exophytic (Fig. 24.1). Nodular basal cell carcinomas are composed of large to small islands encased in the characteristic mucin-rich stroma. Squamous differentiation may occur in the center of the tumor islands, giving rise to the term *basosquamous carcinoma*. Pigmented basal cells may at times be confused clinically with melanoma. Melanin-rich tumors are of the nodular type. The melanocytes, however, have a benign appearance and may actually transfer the melanin pigment through a process of apocapation to the tumor cells. When necrosis occurs, the melanin usually is concentrated in melanophages.

The morphea basal cell carcinoma or the sclerosing type consists of small islands and cords encased in dense fibrosis. The actual parenchymal cords of tumor may comprise only a small percentage of the mass of densely fibrotic skin cancer. At the periphery of these tumors, microscopic extension may occur imperceptibly into the surrounding dermis. The morpheaform tumor usually presents as a flat, indurated, whitish to yellow ill-defined plaque (Fig. 24.2). As these tumors enlarge, they tend to become depressed and resemble a scar.

Another variant, superficial basal cell carcinoma, usually presents as a red, scaly lesion, often on the trunk or extremities. They occasionally occur on the head and neck as well and may become fairly large, forming crusted, scaling erythematous patches resembling a nonspecific dermatitis.

Although the majority of basal cell carcinomas are due to UV radiation, an autosomally transmitted disorder—the basal cell nevus syndrome—is associated with multiple basal cell carci-

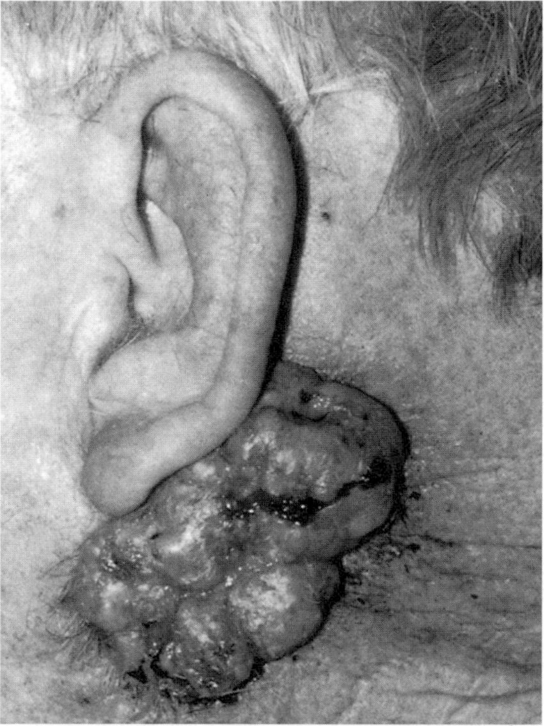

Figure 24.1 An elderly man with a 10-year history of a nodular growth posterior and inferior to the left ear. A biopsy revealed basal cell carcinoma nodular type. (From Weber RS. Surgical principles. In: Weber RS, Miller MJ, Goepfert H, eds. *Basal and squamous cell skin cancers of the head and neck.* Philadelphia: Williams & Wilkins, 1996, with permission.)

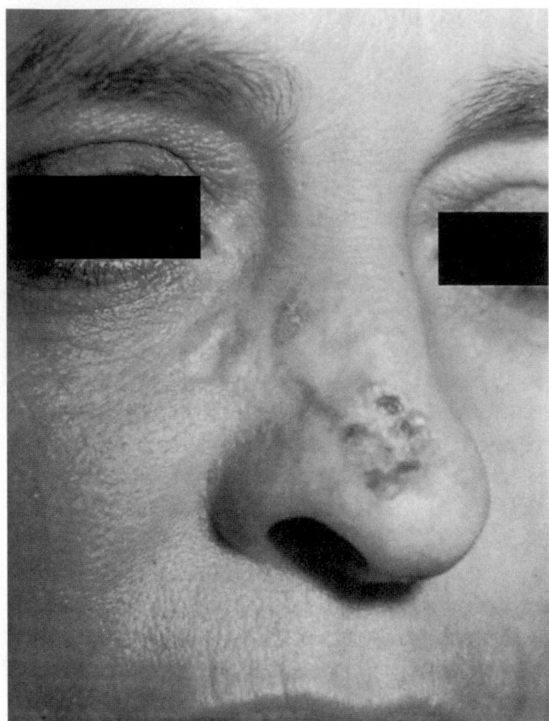

Figure 24.2 A morphea basal cell carcinoma of the nasal tip extending superiorly and laterally toward the medial canthus.

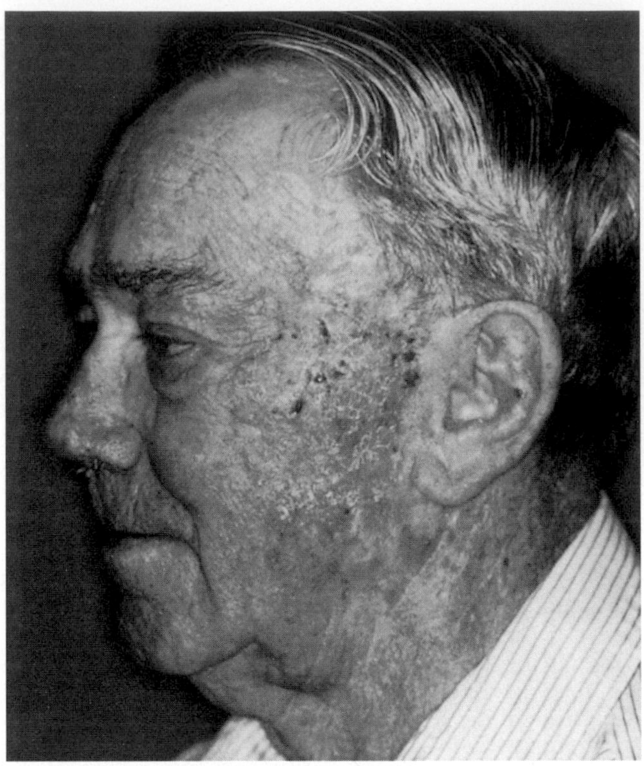

Figure 24.3 A patient with a long history of sun exposure developed a scaling area of the left side of the face. Biopsy revealed Bowen disease (carcinoma *in situ*). (From Weber RS. Clinical assessment and staging. In: Weber RS, Miller MJ, Goepfert H, eds. *Basal and squamous cell skin cancers of the head and neck.* Philadelphia: Williams & Wilkins, 1996, with permission.)

nomas in conjunction with palmar-plantar pits and jaw keratocysts. Among patients afflicted, the first skin cancers appear in childhood or adolescence and usually arise on the eyelids, nose, cheeks, and forehead.

Unlike basal cell carcinoma, which has no precursor lesion, invasive squamous cell carcinoma of the skin may be preceded by actinic keratoses or Bowen disease (squamous cell carcinoma *in situ*). Although UVB radiation is the most common etiologic factor in the development of squamous cell carcinoma, other factors, such as ionizing radiation, genodermatosis, human papilloma virus, exposure to arsenicals and petrochemicals, and chronic ulcerations of the skin, have been associated with the development of skin cancer. Renal transplantation patients or chronically immunosuppressed individuals are prone to develop multiple skin cancers, some of which may behave in an aggressive fashion.

Squamous cell skin cancers arise from a common progenitor cell, the keratinocyte. Common precursor lesions, actinic keratoses are red and scaly and appear on sun-exposed areas of the head and neck, most commonly the forehead, scalp, nose, malar eminence, and the helix of the ear (39). Approximately 8% to 10% of actinic keratosis may progress to invasive squamous carcinomas (39,40). Bowen disease or squamous cell carcinoma *in situ* appears as a single, red, scaling plaque or nodule and is difficult to differentiate from eczema or psoriasis (Figs. 24.3 and 24.4). These lesions may be multifocal and precede the development of invasive skin cancer by many years. Bowen disease is treated by excision or radiotherapy in selected cases (41). Squamous cell carcinoma usually appears as a firm, red nodule with elevated borders and indistinct edges. As these lesions grow, they may ulcerate centrally. Morphologically, there are several distinct types of squamous cell carcinomas of the skin. The most common is typical squamous cell carcinoma, which may be categorized as well, moderately, or poorly differentiated. These designations are based on the amount of keratin present and

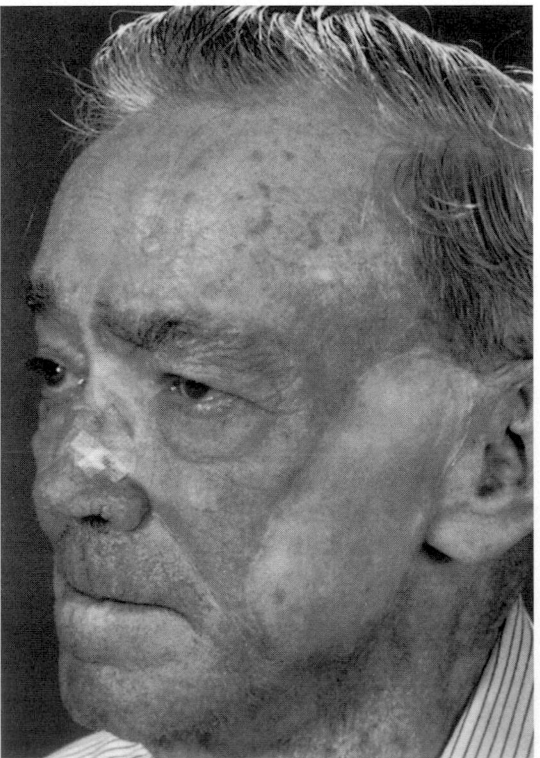

Figure 24.4 The same patient as in Figure 24.3 after wide excision and graft reconstruction.

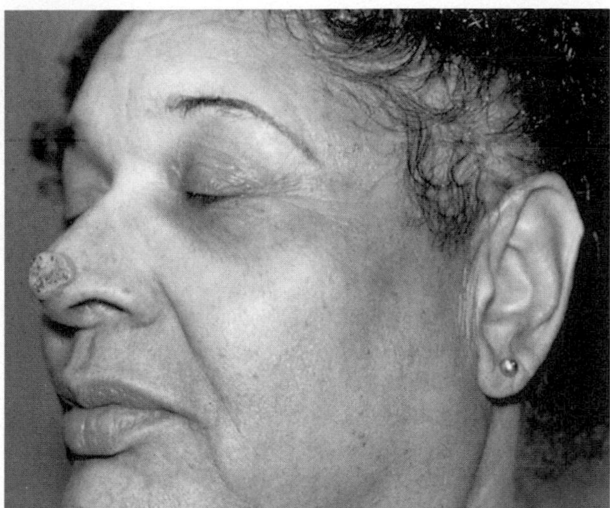

Figure 24.5 A keratoacanthoma arising on the nasal tip. Note the large central keratin plug. (From Weber RS. Clinical assessment and staging. In: Weber RS, Miller MJ, Goepfert H, eds. *Basal and squamous cell skin cancers of the head and neck.* Philadelphia: Williams & Wilkins, 1996, with permission.)

how closely these cells mimic the stratum spinosum of the skin. In the well-differentiated type, keratin pearl formation is common and appears as whorling about a central mass of concentrically arranged keratinocytes with absent nuclei. Poorly differentiated carcinoma is composed of irregular nests and cords with striking nuclear atypia and a high nucleus-to-cytoplasm ratio. Keratin may be scant to absent, whereas necrosis and a high mitotic activity are usually present. In the common type of squamous cell carcinoma of the skin, a dense inflammatory infiltrate may be present. Another interesting variant, clear cell carcinoma of the skin, results from glycogen accumulation. The glycogen is lost during the fixation and staining process, thus giving rise to the so-called clear cell. Spindle-cell carcinoma of the skin often arises in severely sun-damaged areas, in previously irradiated skin, or in an area of a chronic burn scar. The differential diagnosis includes all spindle cell tumors, including malignant melanoma and atypical fibroxanthoma. The diagnosis of squamous cell carcinoma may be contingent on finding epidermal origin, focal squamous differentiation, or immunohistochemical stains that are positive for keratin. Another interesting variant is the acantholytic or pseudoglandular squamous cell carcinoma. The growth pattern of this tumor mimics a glandular neoplasm by the appearance of ducts and glands.

One entity warranting special comment is the so-called keratoacanthoma (Fig. 24.5). This lesion usually appears on sun-exposed skin and displays a period of rapid growth, evolving from a papule to an umbilicated nodule with a central keratinous core. Most keratoacanthomas are 1 to 3 cm in diameter and are reported to regress spontaneously after several weeks. Nevertheless, biopsy demonstrates squamous keratinocytes with cytologic atypia and mitoses. Because keratoacanthomas may behave aggressively and have been associated with metastasis, they should be managed as squamous cell carcinomas, with wide excision and assessment of the margins (42,43).

PHENOTYPICALLY AGGRESSIVE HEAD AND NECK SKIN CANCER

The majority of head and neck skin cancers are localized and readily cured with either complete excision or external-beam radiation therapy. Nevertheless, a subset exists, displaying an aggressive growth pattern; these cancers are difficult to eradicate with radical surgery and radiation therapy. An estimated 2,000 to 3,000 deaths per year in the U.S. are attributable to basal and squamous cell skin cancer (7). Although the mortality is low, the morbidity associated with the treatment of head and neck skin cancer is significant, and the economic and psychosocial impact may be great, especially for advanced disease.

Several factors have been shown to correlate with the risk for local recurrence and regional metastases for basal and squamous cell skin cancer. These include anatomic site of origin, depth of invasion, diameter of the tumor, histologic type, and a history of prior treatment (44,45). Skin cancers arising in the so-called H-zone of the face tend to invade more deeply and are difficult to eradicate (Fig. 24.6) (36). These tumors tend to display vertical growth as opposed to lateral spread in a superficial direction. Areas of concern include the nasolabial sulcus, the alar rims, and the posterolateral nares. In addition, the glabella, the columellolabial junction, and the medial canthus are associated with a higher rate of local recurrence. Periauricular skin cancers, particularly those arising on the helix or anterior to the ear, tend to invade deeply and may spread along cartilage.

The tendency for tumors in these areas to spread deeply has been attributed to the presence of facial embryologic fusion planes. Panje and Ceilley (46) noted tumors of the nasal dorsum, tip, and columella tend to spread in a cephalic-caudad direction. Tumors arising on the columella invade the upper lip and premaxilla, whereas those arising on the nasal ala tend to invade deeply into the nasolabial fold or pyriform aperture, another problem area of great clinical significance.

Basal and squamous cell skin cancers of the medial canthus may display deep invasion, involving the medial canthal tendon, the lacrimal apparatus, the ethmoid sinuses, and the periorbita. Once these neoplasms invade the ethmoid sinuses, extension to the skull base may occur, greatly reducing the possibility of cure. Recurrent or neglected tumors in the medial canthal region frequently require a radical surgical approach and (at times) orbital exenteration.

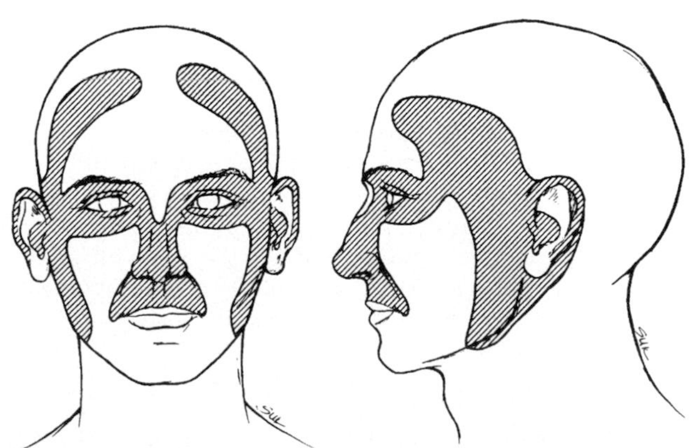

Figure 24.6 The H-zone of the face. The zone includes the nose, nasolabial regions, upper lip and columella, periauricular skin, and the frontozygomatic area. Tumors arising in this location have a propensity for deeper invasion and are associated with higher rates of recurrence. (Reprinted with permission from Weber RS. Clinical assessment and staging. In: Weber RS, Miller MJ, Goepfert H, eds. *Basal and squamous cell skin cancers of the head and neck.* Philadelphia: Williams & Wilkins, 1996, with permission.)

Other authors have attributed the high recurrence rate in the H-zone to other factors such as high nerve density, the proximity of the perichondrium and periosteum to the dermis, and the increased number of sebaceous glands in the midface (47). Insertion of the mimetic muscles directly into the dermis may allow tumors in the H-zone to spread directly into the underlying muscle. Three other factors that the authors posit as predisposing to the higher recurrence rate noted in the midface include the tendency of tumors in this area to invade deeply, underestimation of the tumor thickness, and sensitive cosmetic and functional sequela from surgical resection, leading to less aggressive excision (47).

Diameter and Depth

A direct relationship exists between the diameter of the tumor and the risk for local recurrence. Basal cell carcinomas greater than 6 mm in diameter tend to recur more frequently than those smaller (8). In addition, squamous cell carcinomas of the face equal to or greater than 2 cm in diameter have a higher local recurrence rate than correspondingly smaller tumors (7,28,44). In a series of patients with aggressive basal and squamous cell skin cancers, the local recurrence rate for tumors less than 2 cm in diameter was 7.4%, as opposed to lesions greater than 2 cm, which were associated with a recurrence rate of 15.2% (44). Depth of invasion also correlates with recurrence risk. Rowe et al. (44) noted that lesions less than 4 mm thick or displaying Clark's level I to level III invasion had a local recurrence rate of approximately 5%, whereas those equal to or greater than 4 mm thick or Clark's level IV or V had a local recurrence rate of 17.2%.

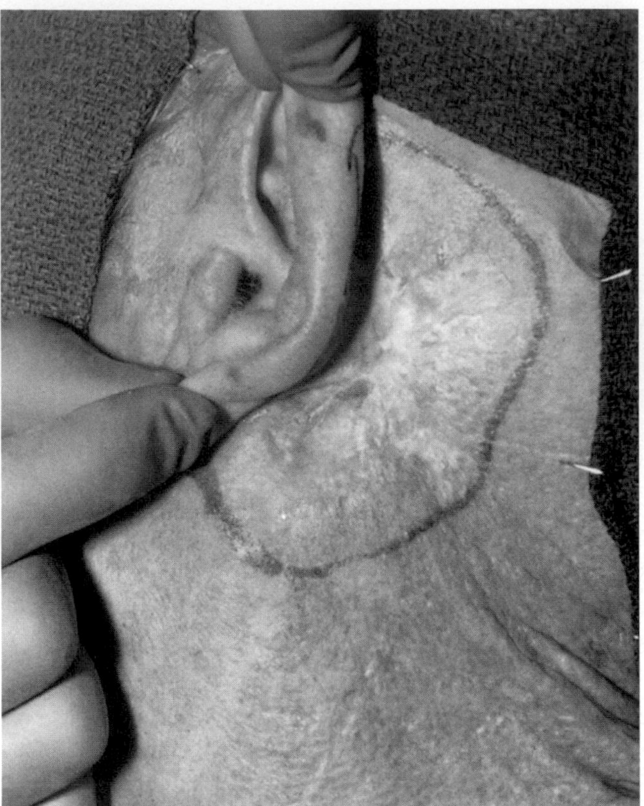

Figure 24.7 A morphea basal cell carcinoma involving the posterior ear and neck region. Note the indistinct borders, which make estimation of the tumor extent difficult. (From Weber RS, Miller MJ. Multidisciplinary management of advanced basal and squamous cell skin cancer of the head and neck. In: Lucent FE, ed. *Highlights of the instructional courses,* vol 7. St. Louis: Mosby-Year Book, 1995, with permission.)

Histology

Tumor morphology, differentiation, and growth pattern may correlate with the risk for tumor recurrence and progression. For example, the nodular basal cell carcinoma remains well circumscribed and has a high cure rate with complete excision. In contrast, the morpheaform basal cell carcinoma seen in approximately 10% of patients displays a more permeative growth pattern and extends peripherally beyond the apparent clinical margin (48). Nests of tumor cells are often separated from the main tumor mass and are surrounded by sclerotic bands of collagen that contribute to difficulty in determining the peripheral extent of the tumor (Figs. 24.7 and 24.8). For these reasons, morpheaform tumors tend to have a higher rate of local recurrence (48).

Poorly differentiated squamous carcinoma (grade III) has a reported local recurrence rate of 28%, as opposed to 13% for well-differentiated tumors (33). The acantholytic or pseudoglandular squamous carcinoma of the skin has a propensity to occur in the periauricular region and is associated with a higher incidence of perineural extension. Spindle-cell carcinomas are recognized as behaving in a more aggressive fashion.

Perineural Invasion

Spread of basal and squamous cell skin cancer along peripheral sensory and motor nerves of the head and neck is well described. Squamous cell cancers demonstrate a much higher propensity for this mode of spread than do basal cell carcinomas. The incidence of perineural invasion in cutaneous squamous cell carcinoma ranges from 2.4% to 14.0% (49,50). Neurotropism may be evident in small peripheral nerve twigs or (in advanced stages) in a major nerve trunk. Skin cancers of the forehead, temporal region, and infraorbital skin may spread along V_1 and V_2, respectively (Figs. 24. 9 through 24.11). Perineural invasion also occurs more frequently in association with tumors arising in the H-zone of the face. The spindle-cell and adenosquamous variants more frequently assume a perineural growth pattern. Perineural spread occurs in fewer than 1% of basal cell carcinomas and, when present, is found in the setting of multiple recurrences after surgery or prior radiation therapy (51,52).

Neurotropism allows tumor to spread along the loose connective tissue of the perineurium. Individual cells may break away from the main tumor mass without surrounding stroma and produce little inflammatory response. The cellular and molecular basis for neurotropic spread remains elusive. Ultrastructural studies have demonstrated a loss of perineural cells and nerve sheath at the advancing front of tumor invasion. The mechanisms of perineural spread include adhesion of tumor cells to the nerve sheath, degradation of the sheath, and motility along the axon. Studies have demonstrated a possible role of nerve cell adhesion molecule for binding of tumor cells to the nerve sheath (53). Furthermore, neurotropic tumors may produce lamin 5, an important constituent of the extracellular matrix that may be important for tumor cell motility (54).

Tumors invading the fifth cranial nerve may spread proximally along the nerve sheath to involve the ganglion and then spread peripherally along another nerve branch or extend along the base of the skull and brain. Most patients (60%) with perineural invasion in the series reported by Goepfert et al. (49) were asymptomatic (51,55). Clinical signs and symptoms of nerve invasion include pain, a burning sensation of the skin, anesthesia, paresthesia, facial paralysis, diplopia or blurred

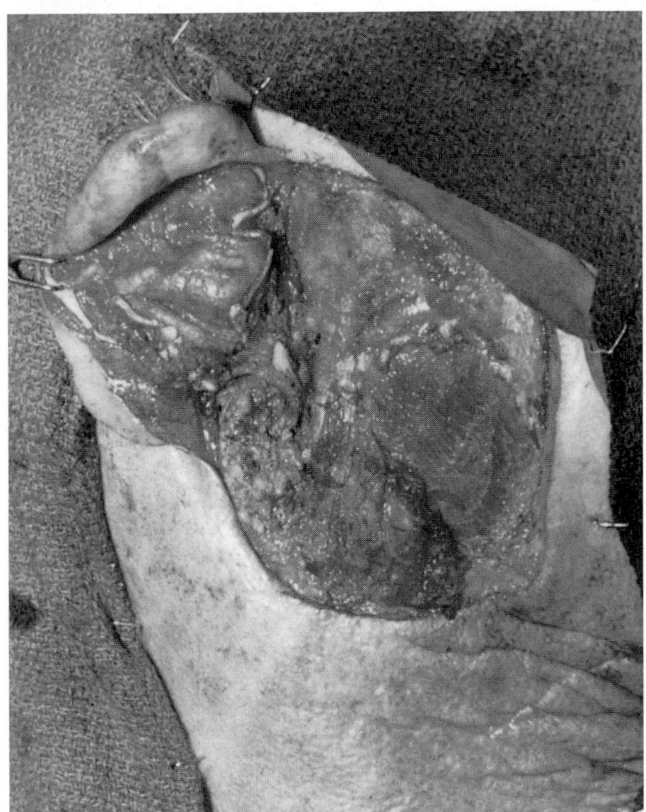

Figure 24.8 Extensive wide local excision of the lesion. Included in the procedure were the postauricular skin, ear cartilage, and upper sternocleidomastoid muscle, to achieve tumor-free margins. (From Weber RS, Miller MJ. Multidisciplinary management of advanced basal and squamous cell skin cancer of the head and neck. In: Lucent FE, ed. *Highlights of the instructional courses*, vol 7. St. Louis: Mosby-Year Book, 1995, with permission.)

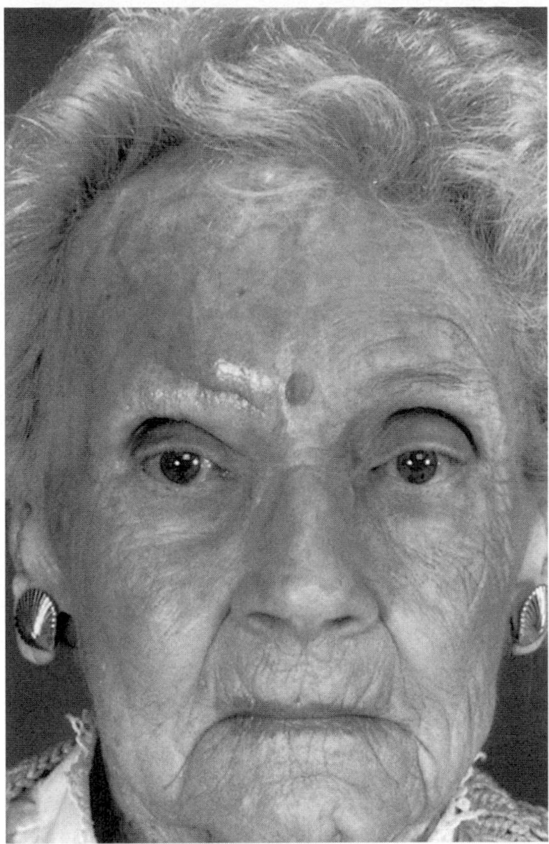

Figure 24.10 The same patient in Figure 24.9 after wide excision of the forehead skin and supraorbital nerve. The supraorbital nerve was positive for squamous cell carcinoma at the superior orbital fissure. The patient received postoperative radiation therapy to the forehead, orbit, and fifth nerve ganglion.

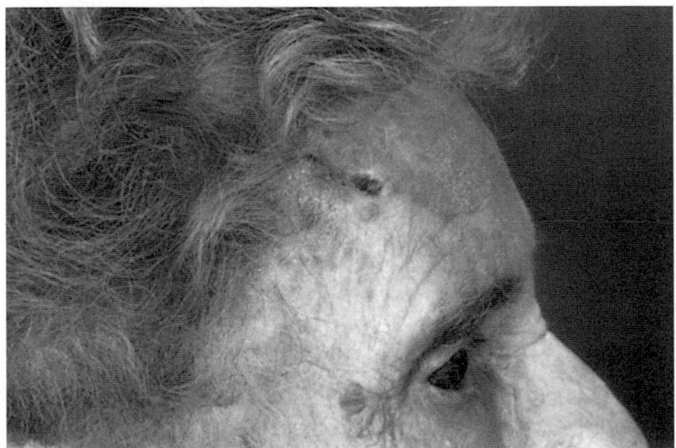

Figure 24.9 An elderly female with a previous history of a cutaneous squamous cell carcinoma arising on the right forehead. One year after excision, this tumor recurred and physical examination revealed decreased sensation of the forehead and a cord of tumor extending from the central ulcer to the supraorbital foramen. (From Weber RS. Clinical assessment and staging. In: Weber RS, Miller MJ, Goepfert H, eds. *Basal and squamous cell skin cancers of the head and neck.* Philadelphia: Williams & Wilkins, 1996, with permission.)

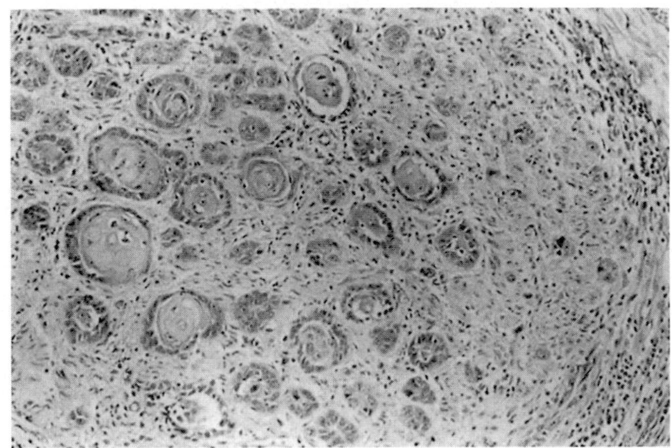

Figure 24.11 Supraorbital nerve seen in cross-section (the same patient as in Figs. 24.9 and 24.10). Note the multiple tumor nests within the nerve sheath.

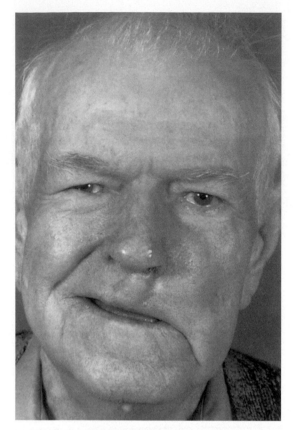

Figure 24.12 Patient previously treated for a squamous cell carcinoma of the upper lip and nasolabial region. Note the flat, white scar just inferior to the nasal ala on the left. One year after treatment, the patient developed significant pain in the left cheek, with paralysis of the midface branches of the facial nerve. (From Weber RS. Clinical assessment and staging. In: Weber RS, Miller MJ, Goepfert H, eds. *Basal and squamous cell skin cancers of the head and neck.* Philadelphia: Williams & Wilkins, 1996, with permission.)

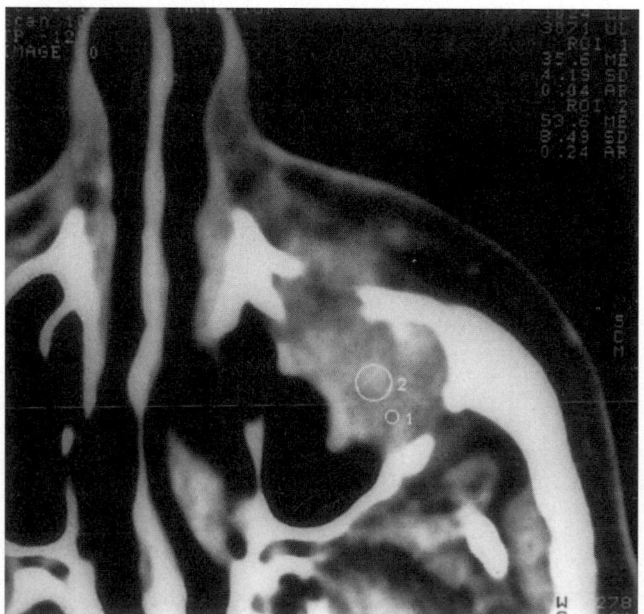

Figure 24.13 Computed tomography scan of the patient in Figure 24.12. Demonstrated are destruction and widening of the infraorbital foramen and tumor infiltrating the maxillary sinus. (From Weber RS. Clinical assessment and staging. In: Weber RS, Miller MJ, Goepfert H, eds. *Basal and squamous cell skin cancers of the head and neck.* Philadelphia: Williams & Wilkins, 1996, with permission.)

TABLE 24.1 Aggressive Nonmelanoma Skin Cancer

Histopathology
Depth of invasion ≥4 mm
Perineural invasion
Lymph node metastasis
Invasion of cartilage, bone, muscle
Morphea basal cell carcinoma
Spindle or acantholytic squamous cell carcinoma
Clinical
Rapid growth
H-zone primary tumors
Scar carcinomas
Immunosuppressed host: transplant patients
Fanconi anemia, chronic lymphocytic leukemia

vision, and jugular foramen syndrome (Figs. 24.12 and 24.13). Major nerve trunk invasion has serious implications for long-term survival. Perineural extension is associated with a higher risk for recurrence, as noted by Goepfert et al. (49), who reported a 47.2% local relapse and a 34.8% incidence of regional metastasis. In that series, less than 30% of patients with this finding were alive at 5 years.

Regional Metastasis

Regional metastasis in cutaneous squamous cell carcinoma is an unusual event occurring in less than 5% of patients (56,57). Metastatic spread may be more common from primary tumors arising on the external ear and in immunocompromised patients (58). The parotid gland is the most common site of metastatic spread, followed in descending order by the lymph nodes in the submandibular triangle and the upper jugular digastric region. Knowledge of the cutaneous lymphatic drainage of the head and neck is important for determining the lymph node groups at risk for harboring metastasis. Tumors of the scalp and forehead arising anterior to a coronal plane through the ear canals spread preferentially to the parotid and upper jugular lymph nodes. Those arising posterior to this line will drain to the suboccipital, the postauricular, and the spinal accessory lymph nodes. In general, the parotid is the watershed for lymphatic drainage and metastasis of the upper face and anterior scalp. Therefore, a parotidectomy is often necessary in the management of regional metastasis from cutaneous malignancies. Table 24.1 lists the clinical and histopathologic factors of cutaneous nonmelanoma skin cancer associated with aggressive behavior.

DIAGNOSTIC IMAGING

Though most skin cancers are well localized and their extent can be determined by physical examination, deeply invasive or recurrent skin cancers may require diagnostic imaging to assess fully the extent of disease. For example, tumors arising in the periauricular region may invade along the cartilaginous canal or extend directly into the parotid gland. Medial canthal basal cell carcinomas fixed to the underlying bone should be imaged to detect osseous invasion or extension into the ethmoid sinuses and orbit. Invasion of the temporal bone may occur when tumors arise in the external ear canal or in those of the external ear that have recurred after unsuccessful treatment. Imaging in these cases is mandatory to determine the extent of disease.

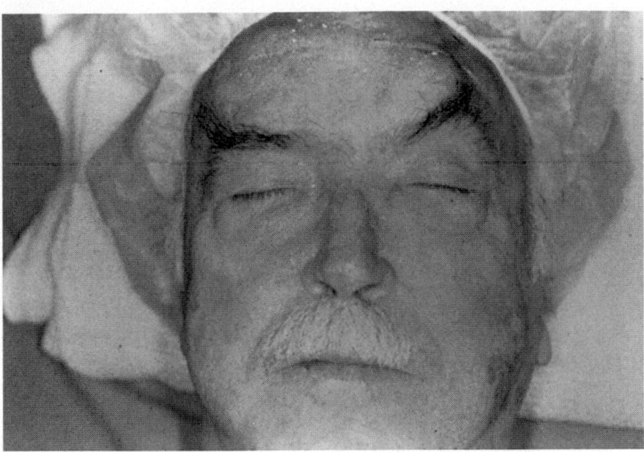

Figure 24.14 Patient with previously treated squamous cell carcinoma of the forehead skin. The patient developed a large subcutaneous recurrence that was fixed to the underlying calvarium. (From Weber RS. Surgical principles. In: Weber RS, Miller MJ, Goepfert H, eds. *Basal and squamous cell skin cancers of the head and neck.* Philadelphia: Williams & Wilkins, 1996, with permission.)

To plan the surgical resection properly and to protect adjacent vital structures, imaging is necessary to delineate areas of involvement. The principal modalities are computed tomography (CT) and magnetic resonance imaging (MRI). A contrast-enhanced CT scan is the modality of choice for determining bone invasion or lymph node metastasis. Axial and coronal images should be obtained with bone settings when evaluating a patient for osseous involvement. Involved lymph nodes of greater than 1.5 cm in diameter appear on CT and demonstrate central hypodensity and peripheral ring enhancement. Loss of adjacent fat or soft tissue planes supports the presence of extranodal extension.

Magnetic resonance imaging, on the other hand, provides superior soft tissue detail, and is the procedure of choice for evaluating intracranial extension, spread within the orbit, or involvement of a major nerve trunk such as the fifth cranial nerve (59). Gadolinium enhancement with fat suppression often demonstrates subtle invasion of a major sensory nerve. Furthermore, extension along the base of the skull or intracranial spread may be better imaged with MRI than CT (Figs. 24.14 and 24.15).

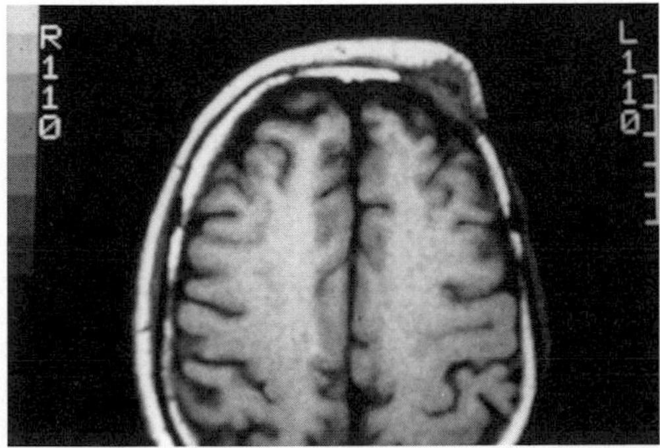

Figure 24.15 Magnetic resonance imaging demonstrating soft tissue extension of the tumor and invasion of the skull. Note that the bright signal of bone marrow is replaced by tumor in the left frontal bone. (From Weber RS. Surgical principles. In Weber RS, Miller MJ, Goepfert H, eds. *Basal and squamous cell skin cancers of the head and neck.* Philadelphia: Williams & Wilkins, 1996, with permission.)

CLINICAL ASSESSMENT

In evaluating a patient with cutaneous basal or squamous cell skin cancer, the initial step is to obtain a complete history and physical examination. Important information includes a history of prior skin cancers and the method of their treatment (60). The patient should be questioned carefully regarding the presence of pain, paresthesias, diplopia, and facial weakness. A history of previous therapeutic radiation therapy to the head and neck should be elicited, as it may preclude further use of this modality. The degree of sun exposure and the patient's current occupation are also useful from a prevention standpoint (60). Family history, especially the patient's ancestral origin, in conjunction with the patient's degree of skin pigmentation and skin type will provide a risk profile and an estimation of the likelihood of developing a second primary skin cancer (61,62).

Pertinent physical findings include the location of the primary tumor and involvement of structures the loss of which would have major cosmetic or functional implications. When surgical excision requires resection of the lacrimal system, eyelids, auditory canal, skull, or dura, immediate reconstruction may be necessary and should be included in the overall treatment plan. Patients with a primary squamous cell carcinoma or recurrent basal cell carcinoma should be examined carefully for signs of facial weakness, ocular dysmotility, or sensory deficits. A neurologic examination should include assessment of extraocular function and facial movement and sensation. The facial skin should be examined for perception of light touch and pinprick. Each side of the face should be compared with the other, and any sensory differences should be noted. In cases when a patient is referred with a prior history of skin cancer and Bell's palsy (or nerve VII paralysis), neurotropic involvement of nerve VII should be strongly considered. Patients may not remember the initial skin cancer excision and should be questioned carefully about prior treatment.

As part of the complete head and neck examination, an assessment of the presence or absence of regional adenopathy is important. Particular lymph node groups requiring careful examination include the parotid, postauricular, upper cervical, and submandibular lymph nodes (63). Enlargement of these lymph nodes may be secondary to an inflammatory process from the skin cancer or from metastatic spread.

STAGING

The clinical and pathologic classifications for staging skin cancer are similar (64,64a). The American Joint Committee on Cancer Staging has been updated in a 6th edition in 2002 (64a). However, the staging criteria for skin cancers are unchanged from the 5th edition (64). The staging system is based on inspection, palpation, tumor dimensions, and a clinical assessment of regional lymph node involvement. Diagnostic imaging may be used as an adjunct to the clinical examination. A T1 tumor is 2 cm or less in greatest dimension, whereas a T2 tumor is greater than 2 cm but not more than 5 cm. T3 cancers are those greater than 5 cm, whereas a T4 tumor is one that invades cartilage, skeletal muscle, or bone. Regional metastasis is designated as N0 (no clinical evidence of spread) or N1 (regional lymph node metastasis present). Pathologic evaluation may be additive from the standpoint of staging. For instance, a T3 squamous carcinoma of the skin found on pathologic examination to invade a major nerve trunk would be designated *pT4*.

MULTIDISCIPLINARY MANAGEMENT OF AGGRESSIVE SKIN CANCER

Aggressive or advanced skin cancers may be arbitrarily defined as tumors that are greater than 2 cm in diameter and invade underlying muscle, cartilage, or bone; extend along peripheral nerves; or have metastasized to regional lymph nodes (7). These tumors not only have a higher recurrence rate but also are associated with a significant degree of cosmetic and functional morbidity (45). In managing these patients, the best oncologic, aesthetic, and functional result will be obtained through multidisciplinary planning and management (65). The multidisciplinary team managing advanced or aggressive skin cancer includes the head and neck oncologic surgeon, Mohs' micrographic surgeon, the plastic surgeon, the radiation oncologist, the medical oncologist, the neurosurgeon, the dental prosthodontist, and the pathologist. Many times, the head and neck surgeon is the first individual to evaluate these patients, is responsible for the initial assessment, and coordinates the treatment team. The radiation oncologist should evaluate the patient before surgery to assess the extent of disease and to plan the postsurgical treatment volume required. Specific indications for postoperative radiation therapy, however, are frequently determined by thorough pathologic evaluation of the resected specimen. The medical oncologist may be called on to manage with systemic therapy those patients who have advanced unresectable tumors or those with distant metastatic spread. Neurosurgical support is obtained when tumor ablation may require a skull-base resection for tumors originating in the paranasal sinuses or periauricular region.

Because these defects are massive, the best management is provided by an ablative surgeon, who focuses on complete tumor removal, and by a second team led by the reconstructive surgeon who can plan the cosmetic and functional restoration with assurance that the margins are reliably free of tumor. In some high-risk patients in whom the adequacy of tumor removal is uncertain or when the risk for tumor recurrence is high, an interim facial prosthesis may be indicated. The dental prosthodontist may need preoperative facial impressions to provide a postsurgical prosthesis. For patients who may require postoperative radiation therapy, the pretreatment dental status is evaluated and any nonrestorable teeth are extracted.

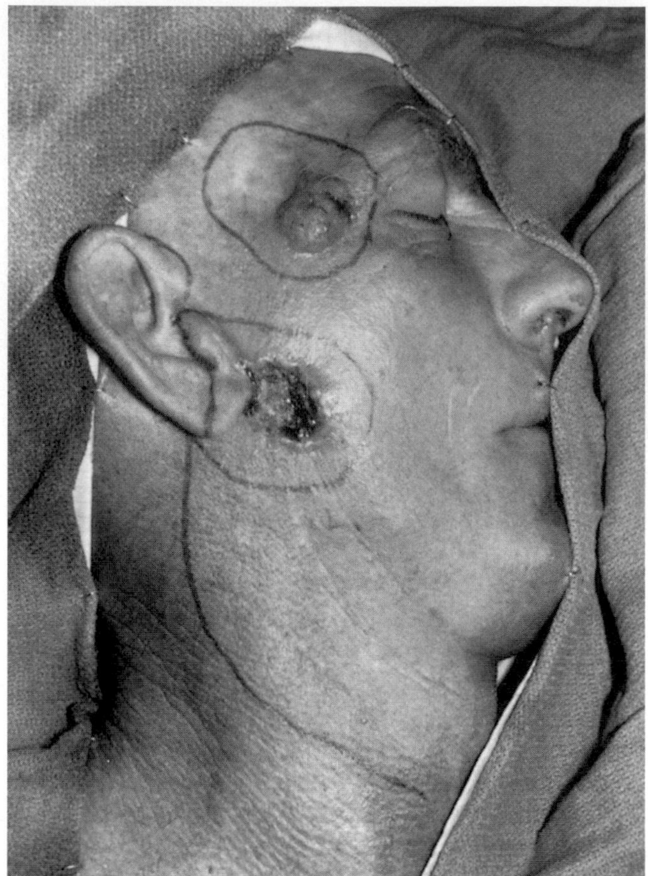

Figure 24.16 Patient with deeply invasive squamous carcinoma of the periauricular region. A secondary cancer is also present in the temporal zygomatic skin. Because of the deeply infiltrative nature of this tumor, a parotidectomy was necessary to ensure an adequate deep margin of resection and protection of the facial nerve.

Surgical Treatment

Before the definitive surgical excision, a biopsy should be obtained to confirm the clinical diagnosis. Tumor histology influences the margin of normal tissue necessary to ensure complete excision. For example, a nodular ulcerative basal cell carcinoma would require a smaller margin than a morphea basal cell, which tends to have indistinct margins. As a general rule, squamous cell carcinomas of the skin require greater margins than basal cell carcinomas of equal size. When clinically evident metastasis is present, a planned regional dissection is indicated, to include the parotid and jugular lymph nodes. Elective lymph node dissection is seldom performed for skin cancer; however, when the parotid gland is directly invaded by tumor, a parotidectomy with regional lymph node dissection is necessary to ensure an adequate deep margin and to protect the facial nerve when this structure is not involved by tumor (Figs. 24.16 through 24.18) (66).

TUMOR EXCISION

The most important tenet of surgical management is complete tumor excision. Cosmetic and functional concerns are secondary and should not compromise treatment. An underestimation of the extent or aggressiveness of a cutaneous malignancy may result in a high risk for local recurrence. Few clinical encounters are more difficult for the patient and clinician than uncontrollable skin cancer in the head and neck region.

Surgical resection is site-dependent. For skin cancers involving the nose, tumors adherent to the underlying cartilage or bone require a partial rhinectomy. Particularly difficult areas in which to ensure complete excision are the medial canthus and the nasal labial fold. In every instance, a close collaboration between the surgeon and pathologist is necessary so that frozen-section margin assessment may be obtained to ensure complete tumor resection. The situation of excising a skin cancer and performing an immediate reconstruction without assurance that the margins are free of tumor should be discouraged. A therapeutic dilemma is created when the tumor has been excised and a complex reconstruction is performed only to find a margin involved by tumor on final pathologic examination. Should the patient be observed, should the cancer be reexcised, or should postoperative radiation be administered? This scenario can be avoided by careful intraoperative frozen-section analysis of the margins.

Periorbital skin cancer has important management implications from the standpoint of functional, cosmetic, and psychological sequelae. Orbital exenteration is rarely necessary in the management of skin cancer in this location. When tumors directly invade the orbital periosteum or the orbital septum or

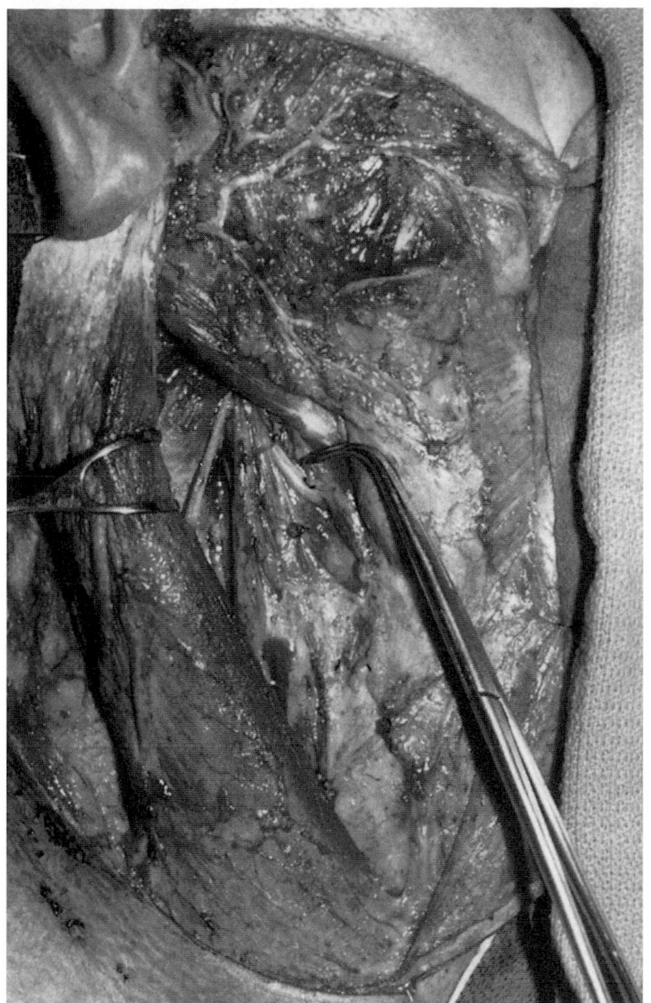

Figure 24.17 Intraoperative photograph after partial auriculectomy, superficial parotidectomy with sparing of the facial nerve, and dissection of lymph nodes in levels II and III.

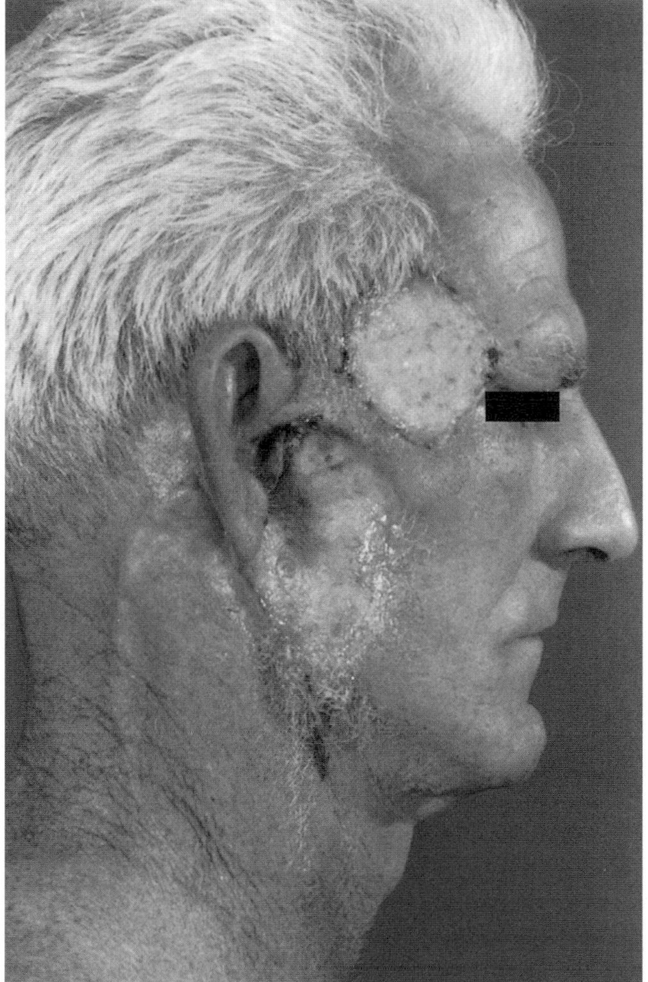

Figure 24.18 Reconstruction with skin grafts to allow for surveillance of tumor recurrence.

when perineural extension results in invasion of the orbital fat, exenteration is necessary. Frequently, this procedure is performed in conjunction with partial maxillectomy, when tumors invade the infraorbital nerve. At the time of exenteration, nerves in the posterior orbit should be examined by frozen section and should be followed in a retrograde fashion until a clear margin is obtained, if feasible. Tumors arising in the medial canthus not only may involve the orbit but also may extend into the ethmoid sinuses. *En bloc* resection of the ethmoid sinuses, a portion of the nose, and the upper maxilla are frequently required to extirpate these tumors.

Periauricular skin cancers require partial or total auriculectomy depending on the extent. Because the skin is thin on the anterior concha, tumors arising in this location may at an early stage invade the auricular cartilage. The skin and underlying cartilage are resected, and a skin graft is placed on the underlying tissue bed. Tumors arising in the conchal bowl or the lateral aspect of the external ear canal may extend into the canal, requiring a sleeve resection. Recurrent tumors fixed to the mastoid or invading the middle ear require a lateral temporal bone or total temporal bone resection, depending on the medial extent. Recurrent cancers of the ear and the preauricular region may invade the parotid, the masseter muscle, and the ascending ramus of the mandible. These extensive lesions require massive *en bloc* resection and immediate reconstruction.

Recurrent, aggressive, and extensive skin cancers require *en bloc* resection analogous to techniques used for upper aerodigestive tract cancer (Figs. 24.19 through 24.21). In these types of tumors, preservation of adjacent skin is not an overriding issue. Wide aggressive resection is necessary to diminish the chance of local recurrence. For basal cell carcinomas, Wolf and Zitelli (67) determined that the maximal subclinical extension ranged from 1 to 6 mm. Furthermore, the authors noted that subclinical invasion was wider when the diameter of the tumor was greater than 2 cm. For basal cell carcinomas less than 2 cm in diameter, a 4-mm margin would totally eradicate 98% of tumors. The authors also recommended greater margins for tumors that were larger than 2 cm. In actual clinical situations, the initial margin is based on inspection, palpation, and imaging studies. For instance, a 2-cm recurrent squamous cell carcinoma of the anterior cheek may require a 1-cm (or greater) margin and a parotidectomy to ensure an adequate deep plane of resection.

For squamous cell carcinoma, Brodland and Zitelli (68) noted that for tumors 1 to 19 mm in diameter, a 4-mm margin of resection would completely remove the tumor in 95% of cases. For tumors 20 mm or greater, a minimum 6-mm margin was required to clear 95% of these cancers. Therefore, the degree of subclinical extension varies directly with the size of the primary. In general, the tendency for tumors to invade into

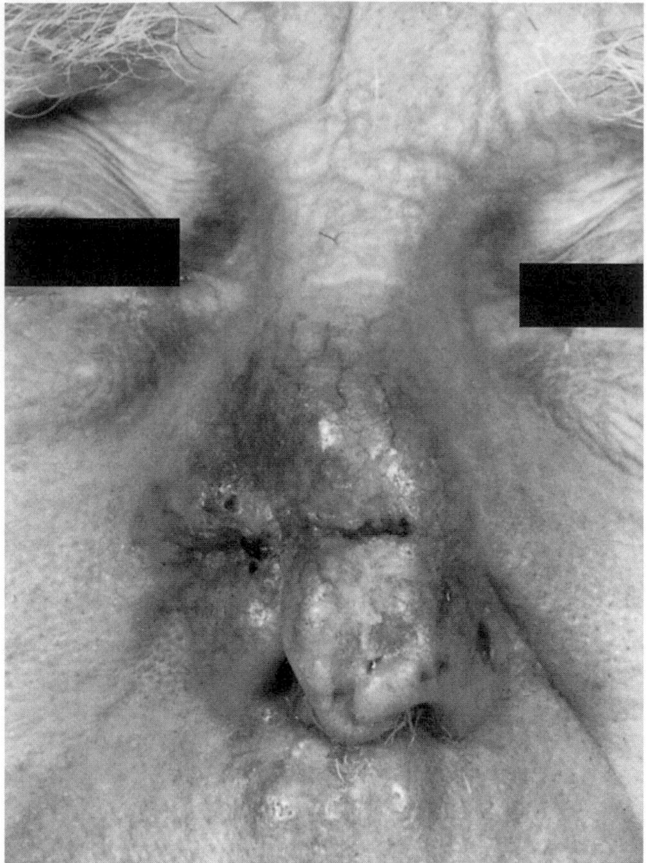

Figure 24.19 Recurrent basosquamous carcinoma of the nose extending into the upper lip. Note the retraction of the right nasal ala and the deep infiltration of the tumor in this location.

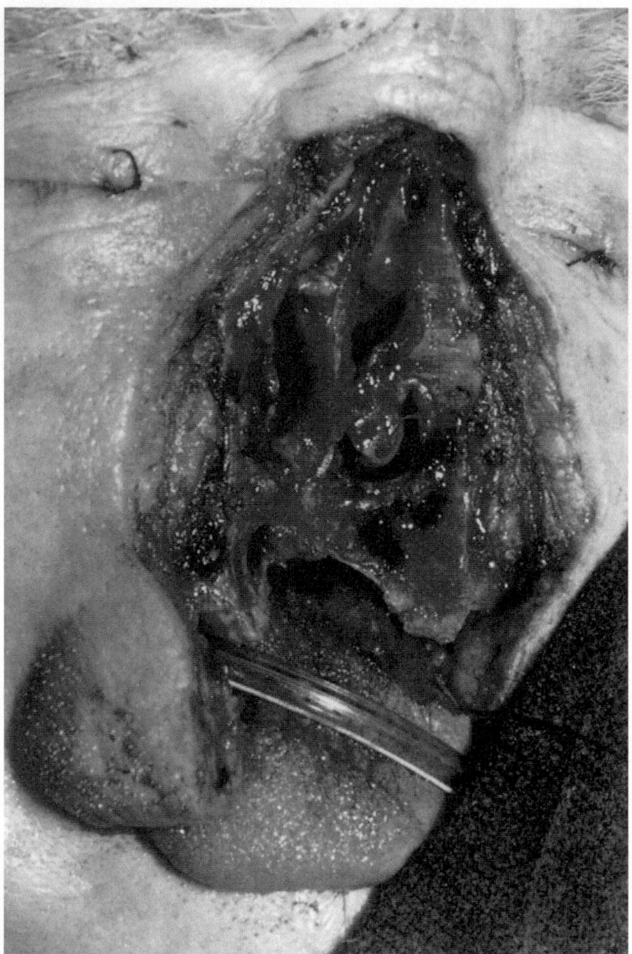

Figure 24.21 Surgical defect after total rhinectomy and resection of the upper lip. The patient's upper lip was reconstructed with bilateral nasolabial advancements, and the nasal defect was rehabilitated with a prosthesis.

the subcutaneous tissue is related to the degree of differentiation and cross-sectional diameter. Poorly differentiated tumors and those greater than 2 cm tend to invade more deeply and require greater margins.

As stated, a close working relationship between surgeon and pathologist is necessary. Once the specimen is removed from the patient, it is taken by the surgeon directly to the pathology suite for frozen-section analysis. Through the use of a suture or hemostat to mark the orientation, the surgeon describes to the pathologist the primary site and the geometric orientation (Fig. 24.22). A specimen map or diagram is then prepared, and all the margins are painted with ink to maintain spatial orientation (Fig. 24.23). For large specimens, *en face* or circumferential margins should be obtained in every instance. The deep margin may be examined with serial sections or *en face,* depending on the size of the specimen. Any areas of tumor involvement are noted on the specimen diagram, which allows the surgeon to locate the exact area of residual disease and to obtain additional margins from the patient. Once the surgeon is assured that the tumor has been completely resected, the defect may be repaired by the reconstructive surgeon using a variety of methods. These range from simple to complex and depend on the risk for recurrence and cosmetic and functional considerations.

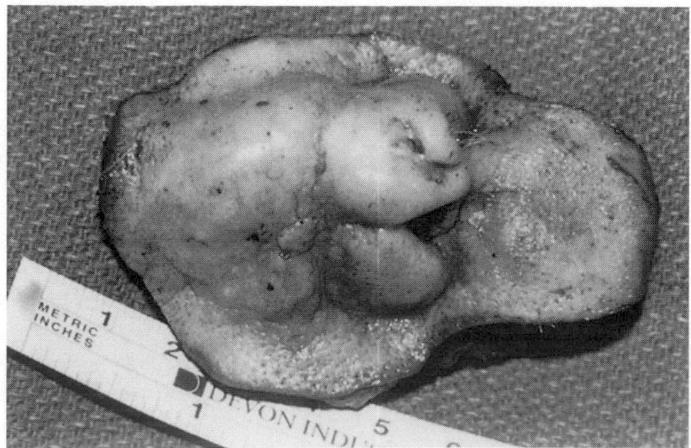

Figure 24.20 Total rhinectomy and upper lip resection *en bloc.*

RECONSTRUCTION

Reconstruction of complex defects in the head and neck after the ablation of advanced skin cancers has advanced through many stages of evolution in the last 50 years. Local skin flaps and waltzing tubed flaps were popular in the early years of reconstruction and were often quite successful in experienced hands. However, the overall lack of adequate local healthy tissue, the frequent necessity of delay of flaps, and poor healing and cosmetic outcomes (especially when radiation therapy was involved) prompted further efforts to enhance reconstruction in the head and neck area.

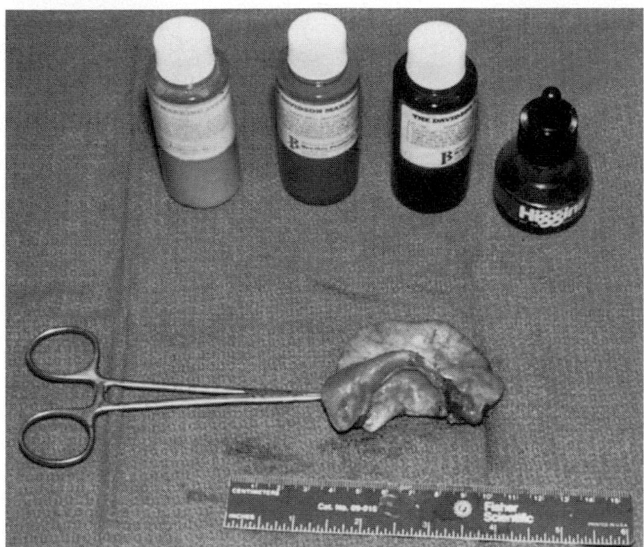

Figure 24.22 Resected specimen in which a hemostat marks the superior origin. Note the various inks used to identify each margin of the specimen and to maintain geometric orientation. (From Yeatman TJ, Weber RS, Balch CM. Malignant diseases of the skin. In: Levine BA, et al., eds. *Current practice of surgery.* New York: Churchill Livingstone, 1993, with permission.)

Numerous types of axial skin and muscle flaps were subsequently developed over the following 20 to 30 years, incorporating regional tissue from the chest and back that could be rotated and advanced into the head and neck defects, with more reliable healing and more predictable successful outcomes. The use of skin flaps such as the deltopectoral flap (69) and thoracoacromial, lateral trapezius, forehead, cervicofacial (70), and cervicothoracic flaps (71) represented a significant advance in reliable skin closure and intraoral coverage. The donor-tissue areas were from outside the radiation zones and brought in additional new blood supply to help in the healing process. However, the need for flap staging and the problem of partial flap necrosis were still frequent constraints that added to patient morbidity and prolonged treatment periods. Adjunctive cancer treatments were also delayed when complications with the flap reconstructions occurred.

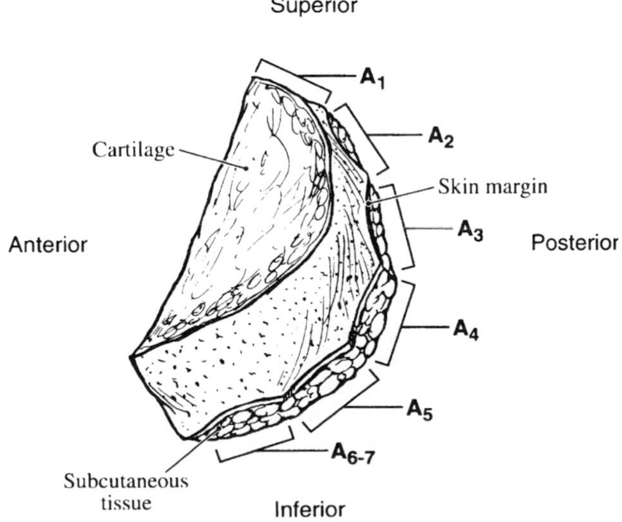

Figure 24.23 Tumor map prepared from the specimen. Map identifies each histologic section. Communication between the pathologist and surgeon allows for identification of any margins involved by tumor and permits the surgeon to resect additional tissue from the precise location of margin positivity. (From Weber RS. Surgical principles. In: Weber RS, Miller MJ, Goepfert H, eds. *Basal and squamous cell skin cancers of the head and neck.* Philadelphia: Williams & Wilkins, 1996, with permission.)

The advent of myocutaneous flaps from the chest and back, such as the pectoralis major (72), latissimus dorsi (73), and trapezius (74), finally added well-vascularized, one-stage flap solutions that represented a quantum leap for the success of head and neck reconstructions. These flaps and their variations, which included bone, became reconstructive workhorses for a number of years, limited in application only by the respective flap's arc of rotation on the vascular pedicle at its origin.

The subsequent development and refinement of microvascular surgical techniques in the 1980s further revolutionized head and neck surgery because it allowed more radical ablative surgery while providing a much broader source of reconstructive tissues, such as bowel, bone, skin, and muscle. These free-tissue transfers are extremely well vascularized and add considerable healing capacity to the typical head and neck compromised or contaminated wound environment. The complexity and compound nature of the defects after the ablation of many advanced head and neck skin cancers are much more formally addressed using distant tissues (without the constraints of an arc of rotation) that are vascularized with the easily accessible high-flow vessels in the neck (75).

Goals of Reconstruction

The primary goal of the multidisciplinary team, composed of the head and neck surgeon, radiation oncologist, medical oncologist, dental oncologist, and plastic surgeon, is the eradication of the head and neck skin cancer. Creation of the head and neck surgical defect must occur as the initial comprehensive event. The aim of reconstructive surgery for the head and neck defect is to provide or maintain as high a quality of life as possible for the patient with regard to the functional and cosmetic outcome.

The reconstructive approach depends on the extent of the ablative defect. An accurate and thorough assessment of the defect should define the subsequent reconstructive needs in terms of function and aesthetics. The scope of solutions for the reconstruction might extend from a simple split-thickness skin graft (76) for a superficial defect to a free bone graft (77) with overlying muscle and skin for a full-thickness cheek and mandible reconstruction after excision of a large or aggressive tumor. Here, it is important for one to think of a reconstructive "elevator" rather than the traditional "stairway," wherein the simplest solution is always the appropriate choice before considering something more complex. The free-tissue transfer may be the most expedient solution to facilitate the patient's reconstructive dilemma and to minimize wound morbidity or to eliminate the need for multiple procedures, especially when adjuvant therapy is necessary.

Thorough knowledge of the basic principles of flaps and grafts facilitates successful processing from the planning stage through completion of the inset of the selected flap. Vigilant prudence should always be exercised in the execution of head and neck reconstructive flaps, with an accent on providing adequate flap vascular supply, to minimize complications and distortion of facial aesthetics. Successful head and neck cancer reconstructions ultimately are measured by the surgeon's ability to cure advanced skin cancer patients and to restore them to a quality of life with satisfactory function and social interaction.

Reliability of Reconstruction

The reconstructive solution for any defect resulting from the excision of an advanced skin cancer should be, of necessity, reliable, expedient, and compatible with satisfactory function and facial aesthetics. Reliability is probably the most critical feature for complex head and neck reconstructions because of its direct relation to uncomplicated primary wound healing (75). This single factor of primary healing can have the domino effect: if the domino falls, it knocks down its neighbors in a well-known cascade effect. In similar fashion, when the primary healing is impaired, the patient can be subject to a cascade of serious (if not life-threatening) complications, such as carotid blowout, aspiration, cavernous sinus thrombosis, or meningitis. Intensive care requirements are extended, more surgical procedures are necessary, hospitalizations are prolonged, timely opportunities for adjuvant therapy are delayed, and quality of life plunges, perhaps permanently.

A reliable reconstruction mandates that the technique of wound closure and the flap tissue used have a high margin of safety for the patient, with a greater degree of predictability of successful outcome for the procedure. Reconstructions must provide the necessary coverage of important neurovascular structures, bone, or brain while also complementing form and function (78). Experimental reconstructive techniques have no place in the treatment armamentarium for patients with head and neck skin cancer. Neither is there a place for a flap that has marginal perfusion in precisely the portion that is necessary for the reconstruction. A poor choice of tissue or an inadequate method of reconstruction that yields ischemic wound margins, especially in a defect with a hostile healing environment, certainly risks sentencing the patient with perhaps an already uncertain prognosis to a morbid and prolonged recovery.

Evaluation of Candidates for Reconstruction

Advanced squamous cell and basal cell carcinoma of the head and neck can very easily involve functionally critical tissues, such as the orbital, nasal, and oral sphincter areas. These tumors can infiltrate multiple tissue layers in sensitive sphincter locations and create intractable facial pain, ectropion and epiphora, dysphonia, nasal obstruction, and facial paralysis. These advanced tumors can present with considerable bulk as well as erosion of the involved tissues, creating significant regional distortion.

Hence the most important aspects of the management of the patient with an advanced skin cancer are the preliminary analysis and diagnosis. Here, the head and neck surgeon and plastic surgeon must accurately assess the tumor and outline the optimal treatment options for the patient. The plastic surgeon needs to counsel the patient as to the size, nature, and location of the ablative defect and must determine the simplest, most effective, and efficient reconstructive solution. However, the reconstructive surgeon must regard the physical as well as the psychological impact of the whole process on the patient. All patients are apprehensive about scarring, facial distortion, and functional loss. Some patients unrealistically expect minimal, if any, alteration in their normal appearance, despite facial deformity that may already exist from the advanced skin cancer. Therefore, patients with advanced skin cancers, in particular, require appropriate preoperative counseling regarding the overall perspective of the tumor excision and reconstruction, to prepare them for early facial edema and distortion, the inevitable surgical scars, and the eventual cosmetic and functional result, which may be less than optimal.

Reconstructive Ladder

A high percentage of advanced primary or recurrent head and neck skin cancers occur in patients who are middle-age or older and who usually have other health problems. Therefore, the reconstructive goal should be to restore the patient to as normal an appearance and function as possible while minimizing the risk for operative morbidity and avoiding the need for prolonged recovery. Primary closure or simple skin grafting are frequently not viable options for many of the more complex defects resulting from advanced skin cancers, unless the patient is not a good candidate for a more aggressive surgical option because of advanced age or concurrent medical conditions. Likewise, secondary healing as a process of gradual wound contraction and epithelialization is rarely used as a primary healing modality, except occasionally on the forehead or scalp (79). The wound morbidity and general inconvenience for the patient, especially over the protracted period necessary for healing, make this approach undesirable for most.

For typical ablative defects seen after excision of advanced skin cancers, the best reconstructive solution is often a local flap, the selection of which depends on the size, depth, and location of the defect (80). The flap can be accomplished on an immediate or delayed basis in relation to the removal of the skin cancer. The excellent blood supply in the head and neck allows for a ready variety of both axial and random flaps of skin and subcutaneous tissue that can be reliably advanced, rotated, or transposed into the local defect. In some circumstances in which there is a high risk for local recurrence, such as total rhinectomy for recurrent squamous cell carcinoma, a period of observation of at least 6 months to a year should precede any consideration of nasal reconstruction so as to inspect for recurrent disease. The patient is fitted for a nasal prosthesis during this period; ultimately, the patient may decide that the prosthesis is a satisfactory solution for the rhinectomy defect, and no further reconstruction is done. Occasionally, initially completed local flaps may have to be staged or revised, such as in lip reconstruction, in which a later procedure can provide a commissure-plasty, for example, and improve the overall symmetry and function of the mouth.

Local Flap Dynamics

The most important features of any external reconstruction in the head and neck, aside from the functional aspect involved, are facial contour, skin color, and skin texture (81). Combining different skin colors and textures in the facial area, such as in skin grafting, contributes to a patchwork-quilt appearance that can certainly detract from an otherwise satisfying reconstruction. The main advantage of local flaps is that they readily provide the best color and texture match to the skin surrounding the defect, as would be expected. In the same way, the local tissues supply tissue similar to that which was excised, providing capacity for functional support, if needed. For example, in lip reconstruction, continuity of the lip orbicularis oris muscle should be restored after full-thickness lip excisions for optimal function. The lip defect can often be closed by rotating and advancing local lip flaps (82) that include innervated orbicularis muscle to reestablish the intact oral muscle sphincter.

In delayed reconstructions, tissue expansion techniques are useful to augment the amount of local tissue available as well as to facilitate closure of the donor area. This expansion approach is common and preferred by some surgeons in nasal reconstructions using the midline forehead flap, which can be expanded before surgery to accommodate larger flaps for nasal reconstructions while allowing an easier donor-site closure. The scalp (83), cheek (84), and neck (84) are also appropriate areas for tissue expansion when extra skin coverage alone for defects is the desired result. Although most advanced skin cancer defects are reconstructed on an immediate basis rather than being delayed, this tissue expansion technique is excellent for secondary facial reconstruction. Extra local composite tissues can be prefabricated with the desired color and texture of the neighboring skin. This technique also allows skin grafts previously used for facial reconstruction and perhaps noncosmetic or functionally problematic to be directly excised and replaced with the normal surrounding skin that is expanded.

Limitations of Local Flaps

Schemia in the local tissue flaps available for reconstruction is unusual because of the excellent blood supply in the head and neck area. However, the converse is true when the defect area has been irradiated and the local irradiated tissue is incorporated into a reconstructive flap. There is a high risk for flap failure in these circumstances because of compromised vascularity and established fibrosis in the tissue. The dermal plexus blood supply of the irradiated flap has been significantly decreased, with a greater degree of fibrosis and stiffness in the epidermis and subcutaneous layer that adversely affects the elasticity and flexibility of the tissue necessary for transfer into the defect. Only local tissues that are nonirradiated should be considered in designing any type of local flap. Other high-risk circumstances for marginal local flap performance include obesity, current smoking history, and large defect size.

Poorly designed local flaps with deficient vascularity can fail, secondarily contribute to a greater degree of locoregional hypertrophic scarring, and ultimately produce an inferior aesthetic result. Local flaps should be designed, if possible, so that the flap orientation takes maximum advantage of skin laxity where it occurs in proximity to the defect, usually in the cheek, around the lips, perinasally, or in the periorbital area. Incisions should preferentially be placed in, or parallel to, the facial creases (Fig. 24.24) (85). This approach takes advantage of the relaxed skin tension naturally present along these lines. Many of the advanced skin lesions occur in older patients, who tend to have greater skin laxity overall that benefits the design of local flaps.

Local Flap Selection

A reasonable perspective of three-dimensional facial geometry and an appreciation of facial and scalp skin dynamics contribute to a successful reconstruction with local flaps (80). Good working knowledge of facial anatomy is important for the appropriate design and safe elevation of head and neck local flaps to optimize blood supply while preserving normal sensation and the natural relationships between such landmarks as the brow, hairline, nasal ala, nasolabial fold, orbital canthi, and the oral commissure.

Most local flaps on the head and neck are of a random pattern, depending on perfusion from unnamed subdermal network vessels. The flaps are designed on the basis of well-known surgical principles of rotation, advancement, and transposition. For defects after the resection of advanced or recurrent facial skin cancers, the local flaps usually used include scalp, galeal, and forehead flaps; cheek flaps; cervicofacial and cervicothoracic flaps; eyelid flaps; and a variety of nasolabial and lip flaps.

Scalp and Forehead Reconstruction

With the excision of most advanced skin cancers involving the scalp or forehead, local flaps are usually sufficient for wound closure. However, incisions in the scalp should be designed to preserve possible flap blood supply for the local flaps, typically based on the supratrochlear, supraorbital, superficial temporal, postauricular, and occipital vessels. Large scalp flaps are very reliable and are usually needed for the reconstruction of advanced or recurrent lesion sites for which primary closure cannot be achieved and skin grafting is not indicated. The most common scalp flaps are designed as large rotation (86), sliding (87), pinwheel (86), or Orticochea-type flaps (88). Larger resections (in excess of 80 cm^2) that leave inadequate scalp for flap design will require free-flap reconstruction with skin-grafted muscle (89).

Most scalp flaps are harvested under the galeal layer, preserving the pericranium on the outer table of the skull. This vascular layer directly adherent to the bone can simply be skin-grafted, if the overlying scalp flap is transposed or rotated away, leaving a defect. Frequently, the geometry of the movement of a scalp flap permits closure of enough of the donor-site defect with another scalp flap such that no skin graft is necessary. Small remaining open areas of the scalp or forehead may be allowed to heal by granulation and contraction, with minimal deformity. This approach is commonly used with local "gull-wing" forehead flaps for larger defect nasal reconstruction in which the forehead defect cannot be completely closed and must heal secondarily. The forehead cosmetic result is very acceptable (79).

For most small to moderate defects of the forehead extending above the brow, the midline forehead flap (especially as an island flap) provides excellent defect repair and simultaneous primary closure of the midline donor. The more difficult lateral forehead area can be repaired with a large temporal scalp rotation flap or with an anteriorly rotated temporalis fascia flap that can then be skin-grafted for a level contour.

All the local scalp flap options contain skin, subcutaneous tissue, and galea in a composite unit. The flaps are ideally based on the previously mentioned primary vasculature of the scalp. Other variations of composite scalp flaps, especially the long, narrow flaps typical of hairline restoration procedures, frequently require one or more delays to ensure flap survival (90). Scalp flaps are usually elevated in the subgaleal plane, which is relatively bloodless. To maximize flap length, galeal release incisions are usually made parallel to the wound margin in series, 1 to 2 cm apart for most of the flap length. Kazanjian and Holmes (91) found that this procedure allows significant stretching of the scalp flap to aid in covering the convex surface area of the skull. The galeal releases should be performed carefully to avoid damaging either the galeal or the subcutaneous blood supply of the flap.

Surprisingly, even small scalp defects can require larger flaps than anticipated for satisfactory closure, because of the inelasticity of the scalp tissue. V-to-Y advancements based on a subcutaneous pedicle, as described by Sakai et al. (92) in 1988, can reliably close some small defects, but surgeons still seem to be more comfortable with larger traditional rotation-type flaps, with pinwheel or double-opposing patterns that are ideal for scalp vertex defects.

For larger defects, a scalp transposition flap or bipedicle flap is a dependable option. The transpositional flap can be used anywhere on the scalp or forehead but may require skin grafting of the donor site. The bipedicle scalp flap can be oriented transversely or axially and then moved over the skull to cover the defect. The donor area usually requires skin grafting, unless the defect is smaller, and the surrounding scalp can be undermined and advanced to the flap without undue tension. Passing flaps over the vertex of the skull requires adequate elasticity inherent in the correct design of the flap pivot points.

Excellent results can also be achieved using the three- or four-flap scalp closure technique described by Orticochea (93), in which the remaining scalp is divided into multiple flaps primarily based on the main scalp vasculature. The flaps usually need galeal releases before being interposed to best advantage for closure of the defect.

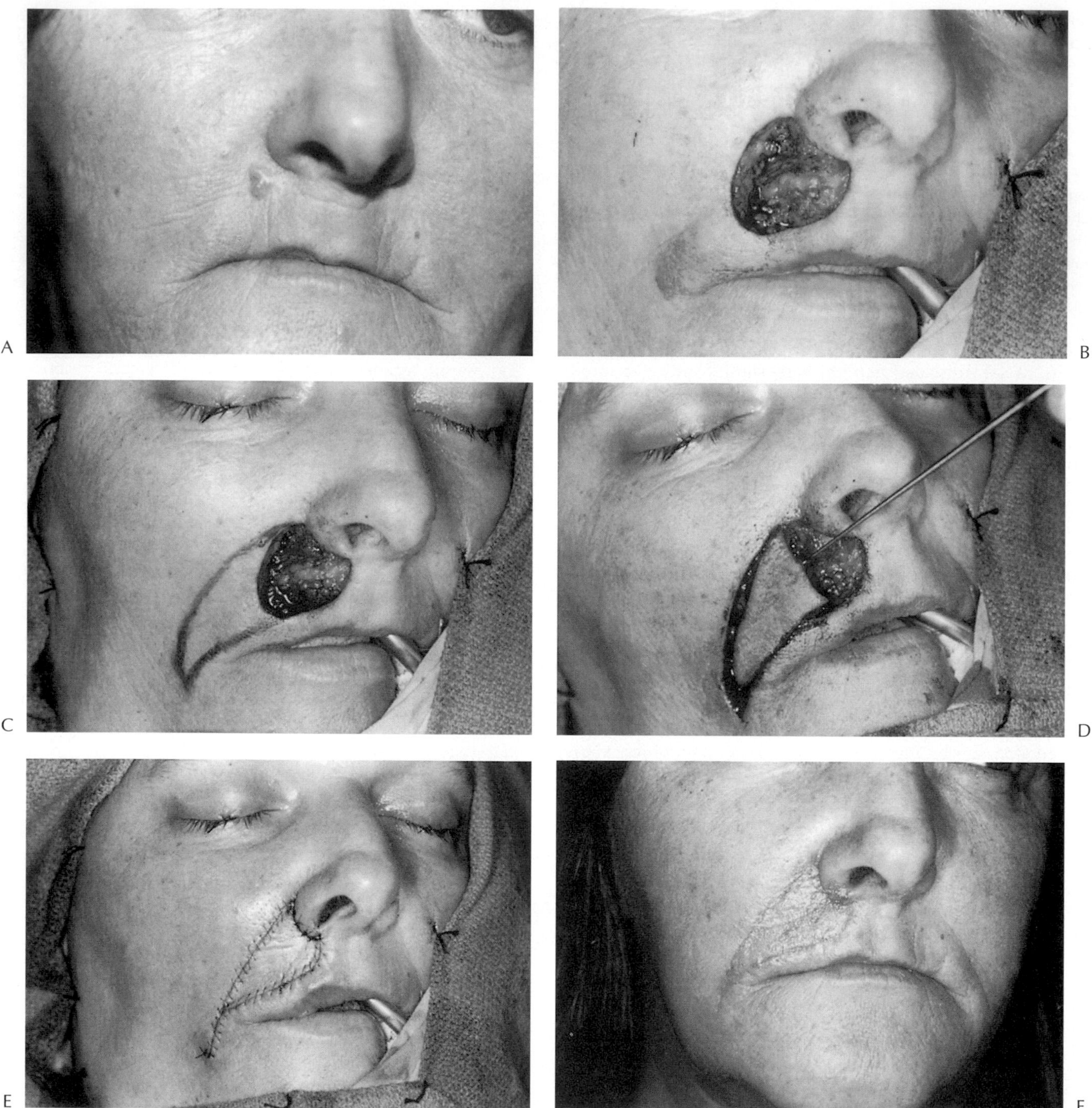

Figure 24.24 Flap reconstruction of basal cell carcinoma of upper lip. **A:** Nodular basal cell carcinoma, right upper lip. **B:** Excision defect at alar base. **C:** V-to-Y advancement flap design using the nasolabial fold. **D:** Advancing the flap to the alar base with minimal tension. **E:** Inset of the advancement flap without lip or nasal distortion. **F:** Early healed flap with normal lip and nasal landmarks.

Cheek Reconstruction

Most cheek defects secondary to advanced skin cancers are extensive and deep, sometimes involving the full thickness of the cheek into the oral cavity, which would require a regional flap or free-tissue transfer for reconstruction. When locally advanced disease erodes the partial thickness of the cheek, it may not be possible to close the defect primarily after adequate excision of the tumor. Any closure under tension can result in distortion of such facial landmarks as the nasal ala, nasolabial fold, commissure, and (especially) the lower eyelid, possibly resulting in an ectropion deformity. The abundant vascularity and general laxity of the cheek soft tissues permit a generous variety of local flap options for cheek reconstruction, with satisfactory camouflage of flap scars in the nasolabial fold or the resting skin tension lines. Properly designed local flaps place vectors of tension primarily into or parallel to the lines of least resistance, minimize the risk for a poor outcome, and maximize the opportunity for healing with minimal scarring and distortion (80).

Local rotation-advancement cheek flaps (94), rhombic flaps (94), bilobed flaps (95), transposition flaps (94), and V-to-Y advancement flaps provide dependable closure methods for most advanced skin cancers, with occasional skin grafting necessary for such donor sites as the preauricular area after the rotation-advancement flap, when it cannot be closed primarily without significant tension or distortion of the tragus.

The most common local flaps for the majority of advanced skin cancers in the cheek are cervicofacial flaps (96). These flaps use the remaining skin of the cheek and take advantage of the preauricular skin laxity. In this way, natural cheek contours are preserved and incisions are placed in existing skin creases. Several variations of the design of the flaps are possible, all medially or inferiorly based, with a postauricular hairline extension for larger flaps (Fig. 24.25). More extensive cheek defects may require extension of the flap design onto the upper chest as a cervicopectoral flap (71), based laterally on the thoracoacromial perforators and rotating the flap anteriorly along the natural facial crease of the nasolabial fold. The flap can also be based medially on the internal mammary perforations and advanced along the lateral face creases, similar to the rotation cheek flap. All these flaps rotate and advance along their arc of rotation and are usually closed primarily by redistribution of the skin tension across the incision.

Nasal Reconstruction

For most patients with advanced skin cancers, local facial flaps usually offer a satisfactory method of reconstruction. However, for advanced disease requiring a rhinectomy, a prosthesis may be the best solution for some patients. Other patients may be dissatisfied with the artificial nose, especially if it cannot be secured well. These patients prefer autogenous reconstruction, which is especially difficult, because many of them have received irradiation to the entire perinasal complex. In these circumstances, a free-tissue transfer, such as a radial forearm flap, may be necessary for reconstruction of the lining, because there is a significant shortage of local tissue for a nasal reconstruction. Typically, a forehead flap (97), expanded or not according to the surgeon's preference, is the primary choice for external cover for the nasal reconstruction because of the color and skin texture match of the forehead skin for the nose.

Lesser reconstructive needs, such as those for partial-thickness nasal defects, can be solved with skin grafts (98), local flaps, and forehead flaps. Skin grafts can be used as an expedient reconstructive solution, especially in questionably complete tumor excisions in which further local observation for recurrence will be necessary over time. A full-thickness graft is a better choice over a split graft, with less contraction and preferred color result (98). If desired, the healed graft can be simply excised later, and a more cosmetic repair can be completed.

Local and regional flaps usually provide the best solution for these defects, again because of the color and texture match obtained. Cheek tissues, usually located superiorly along the nasolabial fold (99), can reliably rotate or advance to close lateral nasal defects. Bilobed flaps (98) offer an excellent closure option for intermediate defects on the lateral or dorsal aspects of the nose. The dorsal nasal flap (100), which advances the redundant glabellar tissue dorsally, allows closure of larger defects, especially at the nasal tip, without sacrificing the forehead flap option, which may be needed for repair at a later time.

Forehead flaps offer the best option for large defects, especially when most or all of the nasal dorsum is involved. The donor forehead site can usually be primarily closed, but occasionally the donor site may require secondary healing, which proceeds with acceptable cosmesis. The flap trochlear blood supply is usually not interrupted until most of the remodeling necessary for the inset of the flap is completed (101).

Full-thickness nasal defects represent a significant challenge to reconstruct lining and external cover and to achieve an aesthetic result. If skeletal support is missing, cartilage or cantilever bone grafts are necessary for the dorsum. Intranasal lining can be provided by turned-in skin flaps, nasolabial flaps, septal cartilage and mucosa flaps, free-skin flaps, and (less often) by skin grafts. The nasal airways should not be obstructed with bulky flap tissue that will tend to protrude into the airway with gravity. Ultimately, multiple revisions may be necessary to shape the alae, sometimes with appropriate cartilage grafts, or to reduce the overall bulk.

Lip Reconstruction

Nowhere in facial reconstruction for advanced skin cancers is function more important than in lip reconstruction. Complete innervated muscle continuity is needed to support the lip level and to prevent drooling, which is the primary complaint of many lip reconstruction patients. It seems prudent that the reconstructed lip be made out of remaining lip, which contains muscle.

For defects of up to one fourth of the upper lip or one third of the lower lip, a layered primary closure is appropriate. For larger defects, the Abbe flap (102), the Estlander flap (103), the Karapandzic flap (82), and the Bernard flap (104) are all local options that incorporate muscle into the repair. Distant flaps have the distinct disadvantage of not including muscle. The Abbe flap is especially helpful for upper lip defects but requires a second stage for vascular pedicle separation for completion. The Estlander flap rotates primarily about the lateral commissure from the upper or lower lip, with the advantage that a second stage is not usually required. The Karapandzic method allows the remaining upper and lower lip segments to be elevated, with preservation of nerve and blood supply, and to be rotated to close large, usually midline, lower lip defects. The procedure can be reversed as an option for a defect of the upper lip.

The modified Bernard flap technique (104) after excision of lateral skin triangles advances intact lateral lip muscle medially with advancement of buccal mucosa to cover the muscle in dealing with large lower lip defects. This approach results in excellent cosmetic and functional restoration in difficult lip reconstructions.

Regional Flaps for Head and Neck Reconstruction

The first regional flap with an axial blood supply developed for head and neck reconstruction was the deltopectoral flap devel-

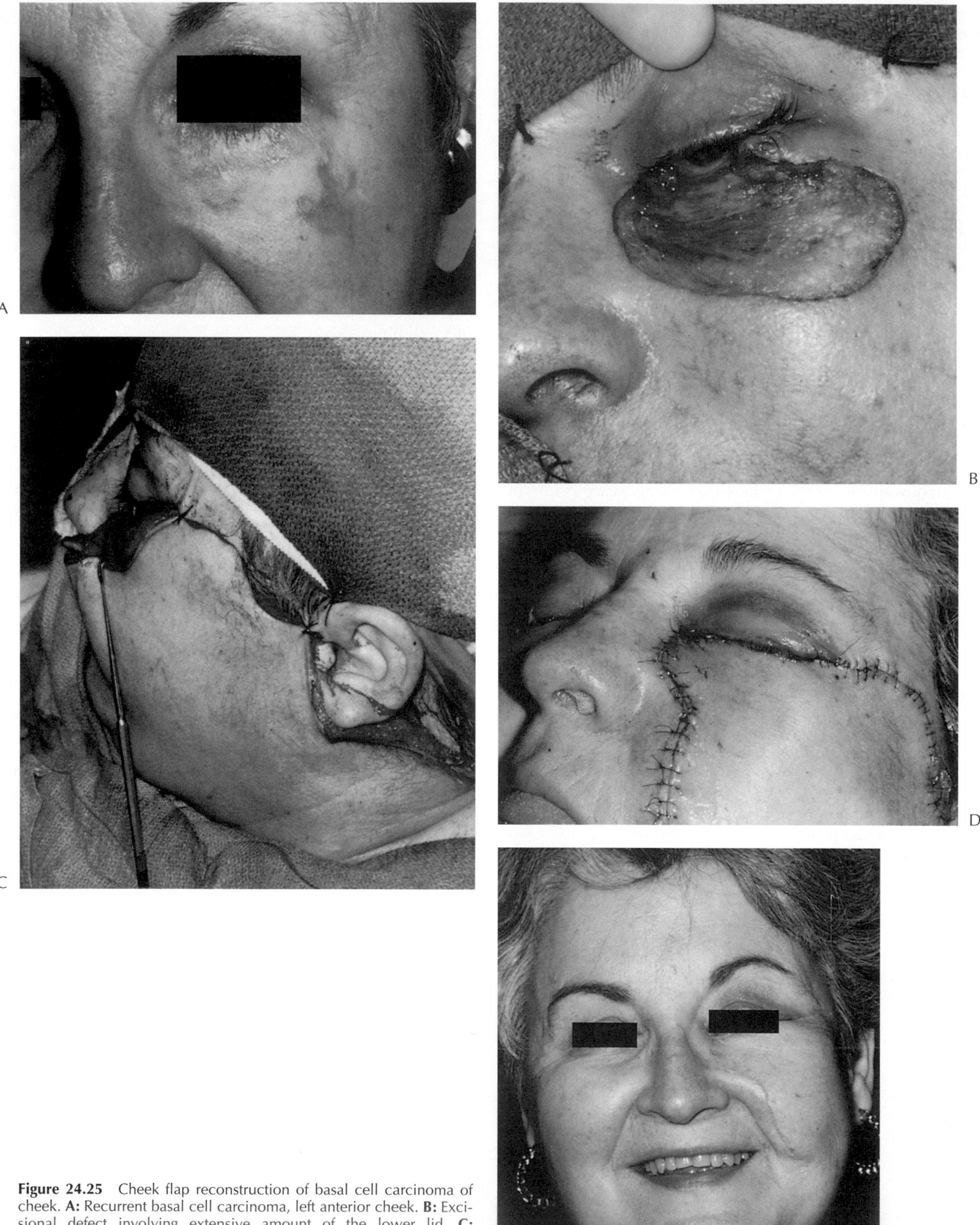

Figure 24.25 Cheek flap reconstruction of basal cell carcinoma of cheek. **A:** Recurrent basal cell carcinoma, left anterior cheek. **B:** Excisional defect involving extensive amount of the lower lid. **C:** Advanced cheek flap with extensive postauricular incision for mobility. **D:** Cheek flap inset over lower lid, nasal cartilage graft. **E:** Healed cheek flap reconstruction.

oped by Bakamjiam (69) in the 1960s. An effective source of new blood supply beyond that possible with skin grafts and local flaps at the time, this flap application was still limited by a short arc of rotation and required a delay for the transfer of the distal end of the flap.

The development of regional myocutaneous flaps that did not require staging advanced the quality of reconstruction possible in the head and neck. The first flap described was the pectoralis major myocutaneous flap by Ariyan (72) in 1979. Once the concept of the more dependable muscle vascular carrier flap with the attached skin island was more universally accepted, other regional muscles, such as the temporalis, trapezius, sternocleidomastoid, and latissimus dorsi, were quickly adopted for use in head and neck defects. Defects from advanced cutaneous cancers could be more reliably reconstructed in one stage using these well-vascularized muscle tissues, with minimal donor-site morbidity. The main limitation for the use of these flaps continues to be the restriction on placement of the flaps within the arc of rotation defined by the location of the primary vascular pedicle of the flap.

The temporalis muscle is a fan-shaped muscle located in the temporal fossa that is very useful for reconstructive applications in the orbit, lateral maxilla, and temporal bone area. In particular, the flap has been used for filling the defects caused by orbital exenteration or soft tissue loss in the forehead or lateral cheek, extending down to the palate. The muscle also has applications for coverage of the frontal dura and separating the dura from the respiratory epithelium of the sinuses or oropharynx. The lateral location of the muscle allows for excellent coverage for bone grafting necessary for the orbit (105).

As an additional reconstructive tool, the temporoparietal fascia (105) overlying the muscle, supplied by the superficial temporal artery, provides a very thin fascial flap to cover the bone of the forehead, orbit, cheek, ear, or temporal bone. The fascia must be carefully skin-grafted, generally without a bolster, to minimize excessive pressure.

The sternocleidomastoid muscle has limited application in head and neck reconstruction (106) because of its segmental blood supply and tendency to unreliability. When successful, the flap can be used to close anterior neck and lateral face defects extending to the palate superiorly. This flap has been replaced for the most part by the pectoralis muscle flap.

The pectoralis myocutaneous flap (72) is one of the most useful regional flaps for head and neck reconstruction, with its thoracoacromial vascular supply present at the base of the neck allowing for a more extensive arc of rotation extending up the lateral face to the zygomatic arch, the orbit, maxilla, oral cavity, lip complex, and neck. Thus, orbital exenterations, temporal bone resections, midface defects, and anterior lower facial defects can be covered effectively (Fig. 24.26). The difficult repair of through-and-through cheek defects can be accomplished reliably with double-paddle pectoralis myocutaneous flaps, which possibly avoids the need for a free-tissue transfer in an elderly patient who may be at a greater morbidity risk in a longer operation.

The trapezius flap (74) is less widely used because it involves a position change and an extended reach for most anterior head and neck applications, unless it is intended for the posterolateral neck, occiput, or lateral temporal areas. For anterior transfer, the muscle should be entirely detached from the scapula, and for more extended anterior coverage, such as the orbit, sacrifice of the spinal accessory nerve may be necessary. However, it is possible with this reach to include bone from the scapula to reconstruct the zygomatic-malar complex or lateral orbit. The main advantage of the vertical trapezius flap is a long flap reach toward the vertex of the posterior scalp, which has a certain incidence of advanced skin cancers. No other regional flap application can reach this high posteriorly. The horizontal trapezius flap, based on the occipital vessels, is a separate muscle or myocutaneous flap that is rarely used today because of the shoulder donor-site morbidity.

The latissimus dorsi flap (73) is yet another versatile myocutaneous flap, most useful for extensive superficial defects that will require well-vascularized tissue, especially if other options, such as the pectoralis major flap, are unavailable or in circumstances where additional bulk and cover are still necessary in conjunction with other flaps. The skin island is quite reliable, even placed distally on the muscle, and the island can be positioned on the muscle to allow for wound coverage as high as the zygoma and as anterior as the chin. The best applications for this flap are the lateral neck and lower face, as the flap is transferred up through the axilla over the clavicle. Positional change in surgery may be necessary, unless the patient can be placed laterally on a bean bag and sterilely draped initially, followed by table rotation so that an anterior approach can still be performed.

Free-Tissue Transfer

The refinement of microvascular techniques has further expanded the utility of muscle, myocutaneous, bone, and fasciocutaneous flaps for reconstruction of advanced skin cancers of the head and neck. Distant tissue sources are now available in a better variety so that improved contouring, function, and cosmesis can be achieved in head and neck reconstruction. The extent of tissue requirements for reconstruction in advanced skin cancers ranges from small and thin to large and thick. Free-tissue transfer offers this same variety in flap choices, with relatively modest donor-site morbidity. This degree of flap flexibility, adaptability, vascularity, and reliability, without the vascular leash restriction of pedicle flaps, has catapulted free-tissue applications to the forefront of head and neck reconstruction, redefining the reconstruction ladder as the *reconstructive elevator.* The flap transfer success has approximated 97% and has allowed faster and more reliable healing in shorter hospital stays for the majority of head and neck patients. Overall, fewer complications are seen with free-tissue transfers performed by experienced microsurgeons, permitting a higher degree of uneventful primary healing, especially important in head and neck patients with prior surgery or radiation therapy (75).

The rectus abdominis muscle or myocutaneous flap (107), the anterolateral thigh flap, the radial forearm fasciocutaneous flap (75), the scapular flap from the back (108), the omentum (109), and the fibular osteocutaneous flap (77) have found extensive application in the reconstruction of defects after the ablation of advanced skin cancers of the head and neck. The rectus flap, as an intermediate-sized muscle, finds excellent utility in the reconstruction of orbital exenterations or maxillectomy defects from aggressive tumors commonly located in these areas. A portion of the muscle may have a skin island to line the oral cavity, palate, or orbital cavity, as necessary. The rectus abdominis, latissimus dorsi, or omentum with a skin graft can be used to cover broad portions of the skull where local flaps are unavailable or extensively irradiated. These healed flaps have an excellent cosmetic appearance.

The transverse rectus abdominis myocutaneous (TRAM) or vertical rectus abdominis myocutaneous (VRAM) flap (depending on the skin island orientation), the anterolateral thigh flap, the radial forearm flap, and the scapular flap all have application to the repair of full-thickness cheek defects. The thinner fasciocutaneous flaps are preferred over the thicker muscle flaps, allowing for better facial symmetry, as the muscle flaps tend to be too bulky for the lower cheek. Any of the flaps mentioned

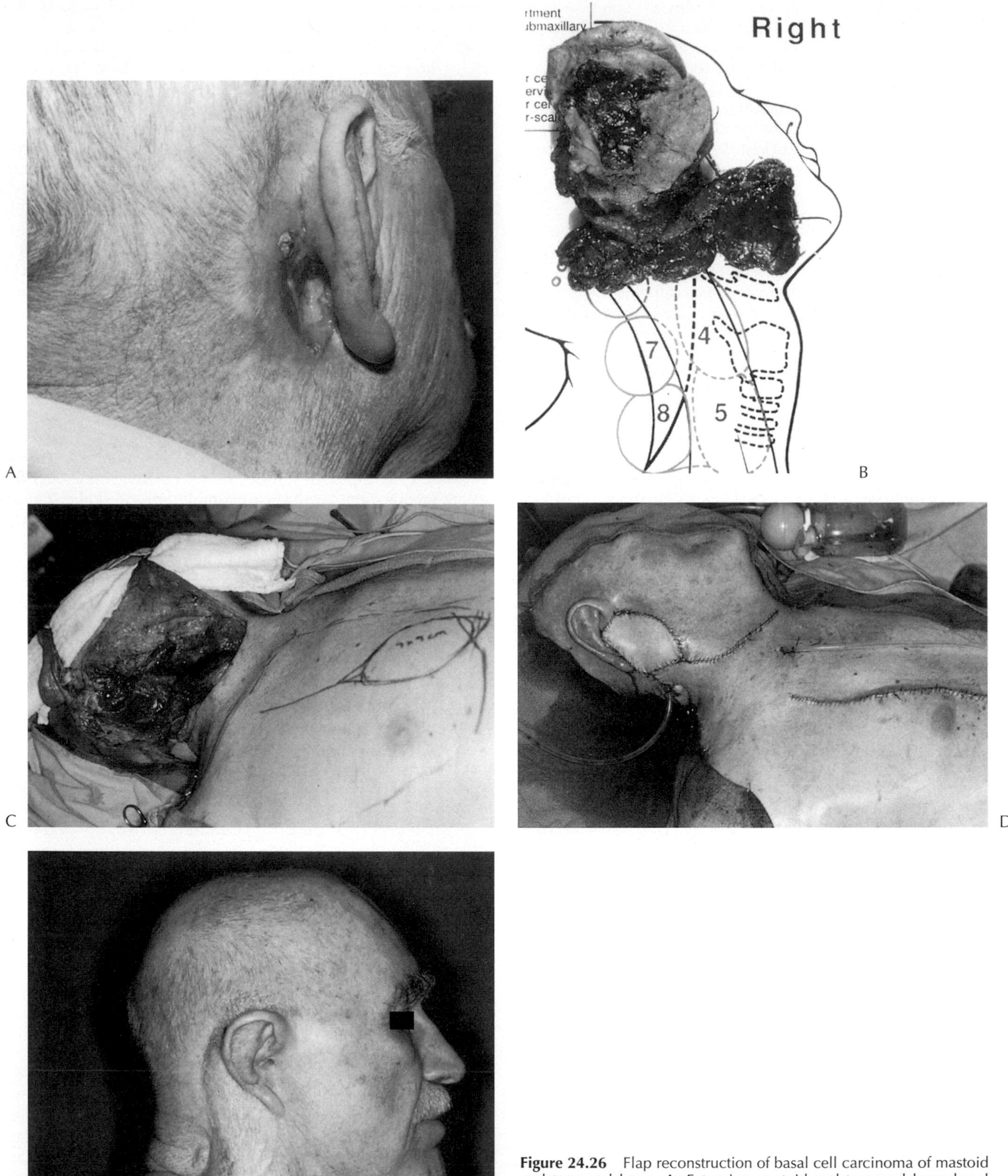

Figure 24.26 Flap reconstruction of basal cell carcinoma of mastoid and temporal bone. **A:** Extensive mastoid and temporal bone basal cell carcinoma. **B:** Pathologic specimen of lesion and neck dissection contents. **C:** Posterolateral facial defect with pectoralis major myocutaneous flap design. **D:** Pectoralis flap inset and donor site closure. **E:** Healed flap with transposition of lobule.

can be effectively used for coverage of temporal bone excisions. Very large tumors requiring essentially hemifacial excisions from the temporal area to the clavicle are addressed with the VRAM or TRAM flaps, which are used more commonly because they are easily accessible from the abdomen without a position change and historically are very reliable, highly vascular flaps (Fig. 24.27). The latissimus dorsi myocutaneous flap is also a good choice for large defects, but the position change is often considered enough of a hindrance to preferentially use the abdominal tissue sources.

Aggressive lip tumors often involve the central or anterolateral portions of the mandible in addition to an extensive area of the local soft tissue of the lip and chin. In these circumstances, the mandible must be reconstructed with bone because of the poor results obtained with reconstruction with soft tissue only in these areas. Often, surgeons will need to use multiple free tissue transfers because of the extended size of the defect of both bone and soft tissue. However, both the fibular and scapular osteocutaneous flaps supply adequate bone and an abundance of skin and soft tissue that can potentially reconstruct the lower lip and chin or cheek all in one stage and in one flap. When the skin flap is turned in intraorally for lining, it may be prudent not to de-epithelialize the flap at the turn and to accept a temporary fistula until the early healing has progressed satisfactorily. The fistula can be easily repaired under local anesthesia some weeks later. Placement of dental implants into these flaps can even be considered at a later time for the fitting of dentures, if desired (110).

Difficult reconstructions after large midface ablations with radiation therapy now focus on the use of bone flaps strategically placed to allow for the placement of implants to facilitate the fitting and stabilization of a cosmetic and functional prosthesis (111). Excellent prostheses are now used routinely in all types of head and neck reconstruction, providing extremely satisfactory results that promote the patient's quality of life and ability to socialize as soon as possible after surgery (112).

Advanced skin cancers of the head and neck are a difficult challenge for all the members of the multidisciplinary team that diagnoses, treats, reconstructs, and rehabilitates these patients. The strategy is to maximize control of the tumor and minimize complications of treatment and reconstruction. The plastic surgeon contributes reconstructive surgical expertise that provides the best local, regional, or free-flap option available to repair the ablative defect, restore form and function for the patient, and facilitate rehabilitation to a satisfactory quality of life.

Radiation Therapy

Success rates of treatment for early-stage skin cancer, often a single modality, are high. The choice of treatment is often based, therefore, not only on the probability of cure that may be equivalent though obtained by different methods but also on the cosmetic and functional outcome. The patient's age, general condition, occupation, and desires are also factored into the decision making.

Most skin cancers of the head, neck, and face are slow growing. They typically have discrete borders, are confined to the skin without invasion into adjacent structures, and have a well-differentiated histologic appearance. Though these lesions are likely to be curable by radiation therapy, most commonly they can be treated as effectively and more efficiently with a variety of surgical techniques. Radiation therapy offers an advantage in several differing scenarios. In particular, irradiation is a useful modality for treating lesions where the surgical deficit may result in an unfavorable functional or cosmetic deficit. Specific sites for which radiation therapy can be used in lieu of surgery include the eyelids, nose, ears, and lips. Radiation therapy is often a good choice for elderly debilitated patients whose surgical procedures might otherwise require a general anesthetic or for those patients in whom even excisions under a local anesthetic are impractical. Radiation therapy also can be potentially advantageous for patients in whom considerable tissue would have to be removed because of concerns of microscopic disease extension beyond the grossly visible lesion or in patients with a field of multiple small lesions that can be encompassed in a radiation portal but would require removing a significant amount of tissue to clear the multiple sites (Fig. 24.28).

Historically, prior to the introduction of linear accelerators as a common modality to administer radiation therapy, skin cancers were treated with superficial or orthovoltage x-rays. Though ideal for treating these superficial tumors, these machines have been largely replaced by higher-energy equipment for the treatment of other malignancies. Many linear accelerators can generate therapeutic low-energy electrons that have depth-dose characteristics suitable for treating most skin cancers, and, if necessary, for deeper-seated tumors, photons can also be applied. The narrow range of electrons allows for the high dose to be delivered to the tumor and for limited doses to be delivered to the underlying tissues. Though limiting doses to underlying tissues is a theoretic advantage, large series (113) using superficial x-rays have reported few complications; if too low an electron energy is selected, unappreciated deeper tumor extension may be missed.

Few series have compared the differing modalities. Sinesi et al. (114) described the M. D. Anderson Cancer Center experience using electron beam for eyelid tumors. The control rate was 89% in 54 patients, and the cosmetic result was judged as good to excellent in more than 80% of the patients. More inferior cosmetic results were felt to be secondary to tumor rather than to treatment effect. Lovett et al. (115) described the experience at the Mallinckrodt Institute using radiation therapy for epithelial cancers. In their retrospective analysis of 112 patients with basal cell carcinomas between 1.1 and 5 cm in size, there was a statistically significant advantage in control rates for patients treated with superficial x-rays rather than with electrons. Additionally, they described a better cosmetic advantage for patients treated with superficial x-rays (97% good cosmesis versus 78% with electrons).

Amdur et al. (116) performed a dosimetric comparison between 250-kVp x-rays and 6- to 8-MeV electrons for a hypothetical 1-cm basal cell carcinoma of the midportion of the lower eyelid. They found that (a) despite internal shielding of the globe when using electrons, the ocular structures obtained a two- to fourfold increased dose compared with the 250 kVp beam; (b) a larger field was needed for electrons, owing to the beam characteristics at the edge of the field; and (c) their monetary charges for equivalent dose-fractionation schedules were 15% less for treatment with superficial x-rays. The theoretic disadvantage of a significantly higher bone absorption of dose with superficial x-rays has not been borne out by clinical experience. In large series reporting the use of radiation therapy for treating skin cancer with x-rays, few cases of bone necroses were noted. The findings from these series suggest that electrons are an effective therapy for skin cancers, are becoming more commonplace, but require greater diligence and technical expertise in their delivery to be as effective as the huge reported clinical experiences with superficial x-rays.

In addition to understanding the physical capabilities of the radiation beam, an understanding of the effects of differing fractionation schedules is critical. Skin cancers, particularly small ones, can often be cured with a few large fractions of irradiation. Fitzpatrick (113) described equivalent 5-year control

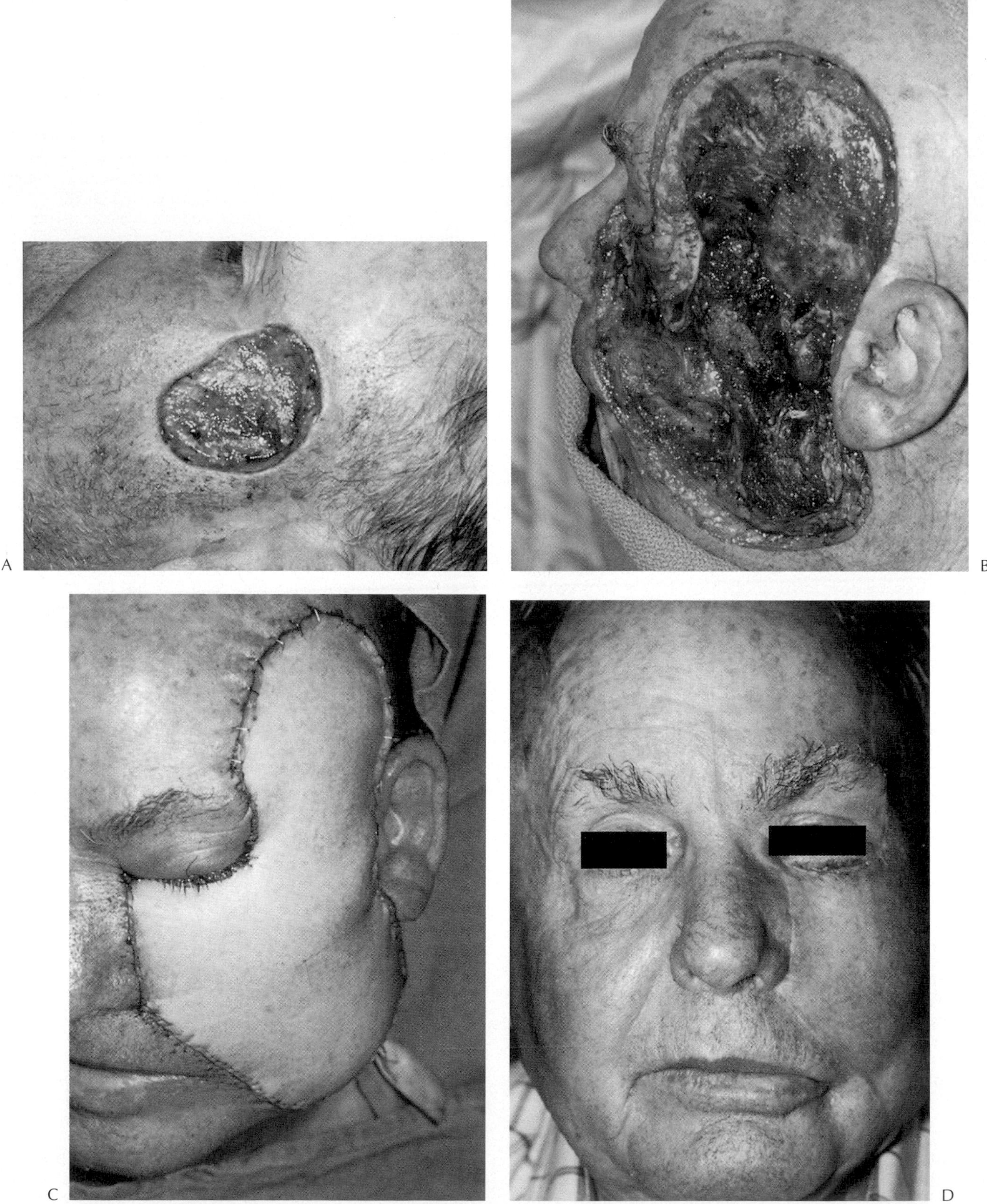

Figure 24.27 Flap reconstruction of recurrent basal cell carcinoma. **A:** Recurrent basal cell carcinoma. **B:** Extensive defect to achieve negative margins with perineural invasion. **C:** Rectus abdominis myocutaneous flap reconstruction of defect. **D:** Healed free rectus abdominis myocutaneous flap.

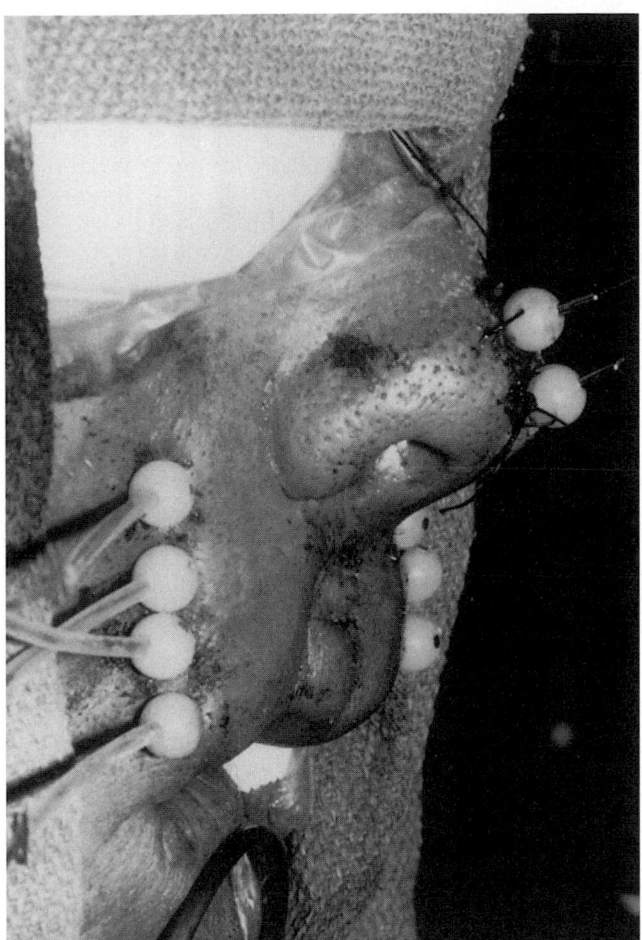

Figure 24.28 Basal cell carcinoma originating in the right nasolabial fold in a 55-year-old man. The lesion recurred repeatedly, despite multiple surgeries that obtained clear margins. The man presented with a recurrent mass involving the columella, nasal septum, and upper lip. He was treated with a combination of external-beam radiation and brachytherapy.

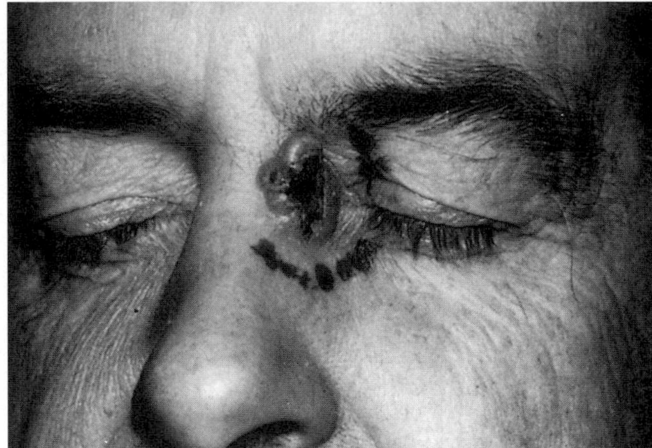

Figure 24.29 Basal cell carcinoma involving the medial canthus of the eye.

rates of 92% and 95%, respectively, in patients treated with one versus multiple fractions of irradiation. In his experience, 20 Gy in one fraction was an effective dose. As the tumor size increases and the irradiation volume increases, multiple fractions are preferred to lessen the likelihood of complications and poorer cosmesis. For larger lesions (greater than 3 cm) schedules ranging from 55 Gy in 4 weeks to 70 Gy in 7 weeks may be more appropriate. Smaller tumors may be treated with schedules as varied as 20 Gy in one fraction (suitable for the elderly debilitated patient for whom transport to a treatment center is extremely difficult and to whom cosmesis is unimportant) to 60 Gy in 6 weeks for small lesions around critical areas where cosmesis and function are critical. A variety of schedules in between these extremes have been described elsewhere.

Skin tumors of the eyelid, particularly those of more than 0.5 cm that would require resecting a significant portion of the eyelid, are ideally suited for treatment with radiation (Fig. 24.29). The radiosensitive ocular structures are protected by gold or tungsten shields, scarring is usually minimal, and, both from a functional and cosmetic standpoint, a good result is obtained. Fitzpatrick et al. (117) described their experience of treating more than 1,000 eyelid skin cancers with radiation therapy. Five-year control rates were greater than 93% and equally good in patients treated primarily and in those treated for recurrent disease after surgery. The complication rate was less than 10% and was most commonly skin atrophy. Ocular damage, mainly keratinization of the cornea, occurred in 3% and was primarily believed to be due to the inability to protect the globe fully for patients with large lesions.

Lesions of the nose, including the alar regions and nasal vestibule, can be treated effectively with radiation therapy and with good cosmetic results. Mazeron et al. (118) reported on a European experience of irradiating more than 1,600 patients with skin cancers of the nose, with control obtained in 93% of the patients and necrosis in only 2%. Control rates with surgery for cancers of the nasal vestibule are approximately 90% but often result in loss of a major portion of the nose. A review of multiple radiation therapy series (119) revealed control rates of 80% for all patients and control rates of 90% for patients with small (2 cm or less) lesions. Early lesions are often amenable to treatment with interstitial therapy. In reviewing multiple series for the results of irradiation, it is important that both dose and technique be evaluated. An insufficient dose or a technique for larger lesions that treats the nose through opposing lateral fields with wax bolus may underdose the floor of the nose and result in inferior outcomes.

Larger skin cancers are uncommon and may require a combination of therapies. Similar to other cancers of the head and neck, cure by radiation therapy depends on multiple factors, including tumor volume. Thus, larger lesions can be cured with radiation therapy, but the success rate is not as high as that achieved for smaller lesions. Lovett et al. (115) analyzed results of radiation therapy treatment of 339 skin cancers. Though they were not tested for statistical significance, there was an obvious trend in the data of higher cure rates for smaller lesions. The crude control rates for lesions of less than 1 cm, of 1.1 to 5 cm, and of more than 5 cm were 96%, 84%, and 71%, respectively. Similarly, Mendenhall et al. (120) reported a 5-year control rate of 54% for irradiation of previously untreated T4 skin cancers, compared with 93% for stage T2 lesions. If radiation alone is unsuccessful, surgical salvage rates are high, and the ultimate control rates of patients with T4 disease is 90% (121).

More commonly, radiation therapy is recognized as an effective postoperative treatment for eliminating suspected microscopic residual disease in patients with unfavorable tumors invading deep contiguous structures. Cancers of the external auditory canal are uncommon, but they are notorious for invading underlying cartilage, and frequently they invade the temporal bone. Austin et al. (122) reviewed the experience in treating such tumors at the M. D. Anderson Cancer Center and concluded that patients who received combination radiation therapy and surgery fared better than those patients treated with either modality alone. Radiation therapy is also advocated in patients with perineural invasion of their skin cancers. McCord et al. (123) reported that control rates in patients treated with surgery and radiation for an incidental microscopic finding of perineural invasion was 78%. When gross clinical perineural invasion was present, the control rate was only 50% (124).

Postoperative radiation therapy is also useful as an adjunctive treatment in the setting of squamous cell skin cancers and (rarely) basal cell cancers that have metastasized to parotid lymph nodes. Spread to parotid lymph nodes is uncommon and is estimated to occur in less than 2% of cases. Spread to cervical lymph nodes is even less common and develops in less than 25% of patients with skin cancer treated with parotidectomy and elective neck dissection (Fig. 24.30). Jackson and Ballantyne (63) reported a local and regional control rate of greater than 70% for patients treated with parotidectomies for metastatic skin cancers. In a selected subgroup of 26 patients treated with planned radiation therapy in addition to surgery, local regional control rates were 88%. Similar results were reported by delCharco et al. (125) from the University of Florida, with a control rate of 89% in 53 patients treated with radiation alone.

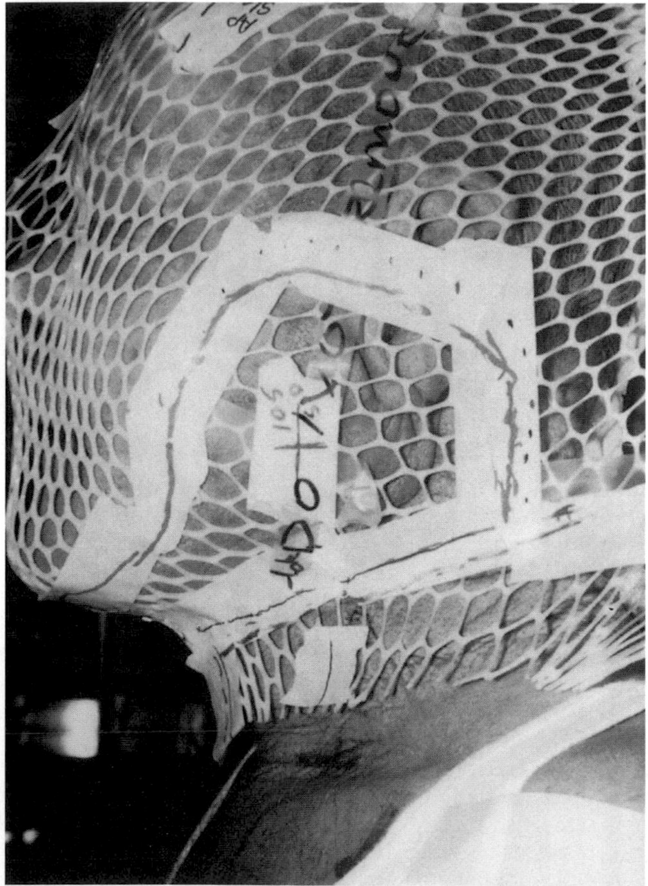

Figure 24.30 Numerous squamous and basal cell cancers of the face and scalp of a 67-year-old man. Patient presented with metachronous right neck and subsequent left neck disease. Each neck region was treated surgically, and multiple nodes were found to contain squamous cell carcinoma. The man received irradiation of 60 Gy to each parotid bed and side of the neck after the dissections. The left upper neck field is shown. The tumor sites remain regionally controlled, though cutaneous lesions of the face and scalp continue.

It is rare for patients presenting with disease metastatic to parotid lymph nodes to have inoperable disease. These patients can be treated with curative radiation therapy. Wang (126) analyzed the results of radiation therapy for treatment of parotid metastases and described a crude control rate of 75% in 24 patients with more than 2 years' follow-up and a survival rate of 57%. delCharco et al. (125) reported a 53% control rate in 15 patients treated with radiation alone (2).

RADIOLOGIC IMAGING CONCERNS

Bernard B. O'Malley and Suresh K. Mukherji

The evaluation of nonmelanoma skin cancer of the scalp, face, and neck is usually performed without cross-sectional imaging. Deeply infiltrating (Fig. 24.31), recurrent, multiple, and critically located lesions require imaging to determine the extent of the primary site and metastatic disease to nodal groups that are primary echelon nodal sites (Figs. 24.32 through 24.34). Imaging also helps to determine the need for preoperative recruitment of plastic-reconstructive surgeons or other members of the interdisciplinary team (Figs. 24.35 through 24.37). Problem areas are the functionally and cosmetically sensitive areas such as the eyelid where basal cell cancer is the most common (129).

The actual superficial cutaneous component of the lesion cannot be outlined as well as the clinical examination, particularly after preceding treatment. Involvement of subcutaneous layer, deep facial planes, and underlying musculoskeletal structures is readily imaged with CT or MRI (Fig. 24.38). The radiologist examining the patient or reviewing a graphic copied from the patient's chart facilitates comprehensive coverage of the lesion. Careful evaluation of the CT bone window images and properly photographed CT soft tissue windows is necessary to avoid underestimation of the depth and extent of the skin lesion.

Perineural extension of skin cancers is difficult to determine based on clinical examination alone (130). Risk factors for perineural extension include sex, size of the lesion, previous therapy (131), and histology. The incidence of perineural invasion with basal cell cancer is greater than previously recognized (132) and more common in the micronodular form (133). Central neurotropic extension is more typical of basal cell or basaloid squamous lesions (Figs. 24.39 and 24.40), which have a greater propensity for local recurrence (134). Imaging can contribute to the proper selection of more aggressive therapy for perineural disease, providing a better disease-free survival (135). Although perineural extension may be detected on CT (136), MRI is clearly the modality of choice (Fig. 24.41) for evaluating the possibility or perineural extension (137,138). When the perineural abnormality is not palpable or develops deep to a well-healed flap, an imaging-guided percutaneous needle biopsy (Fig. 24.42) is instrumental in confirming (or excluding) malignancy. Merkel cell carcinoma is staged locally and regionally with similar imaging for other cutaneous lesions. In addition to risk for nodal disease, these patients are at high risk for local recurrence. Nuclear imaging with ^{123}I MIBG has added useful staging information for this disorder.

Either CT or MRI is useful for lymph node staging for skin cancer. Although CT requires intravenous contrast for lymph node staging, it requires more patient repositioning than is required for MRI. Lymph node metastases are usually a late manifestation of skin cancer, and adenopathy should prompt a search for an alternate primary tumor (139). A noncontrast T1-weighted image is often the most helpful sequence if specifically evaluating for intraparotid lymph nodes.

Follow-up imaging examination is usually reserved for patients who become symptomatic or need surveillance of operative beds because of insensate composite flaps. Careful duplication of imaging protocols is essential for detecting subtle recurrences on the background of evolving treatment changes and ongoing plastic surgery graft revisions. Recurrences are usually local and not completely resectable when perineural invasion developed (140).

An important topic is when to perform CT or MRI for evaluating skin cancers. Imaging for very early superficial lesions is probably not necessary. However, imaging should be strongly considered in the following scenarios:

1. Moderately to advanced scalp lesion to evaluate to bony invasion (CT) and to evaluate for occult parotid lymph node metastases.
2. Tumor situated in areas that have high likelihood of retrograde perineural extension should be imaged with contrast-enhanced MRI. Images should be carried to the cavernous sinus. Such areas include above the eyebrow (V_1) and the infraorbital region (V_2)
3. Neoplasms involving the cheek should be evaluated with CT for deep extension and the possibility for occult parotid or facial lymph node metastases.

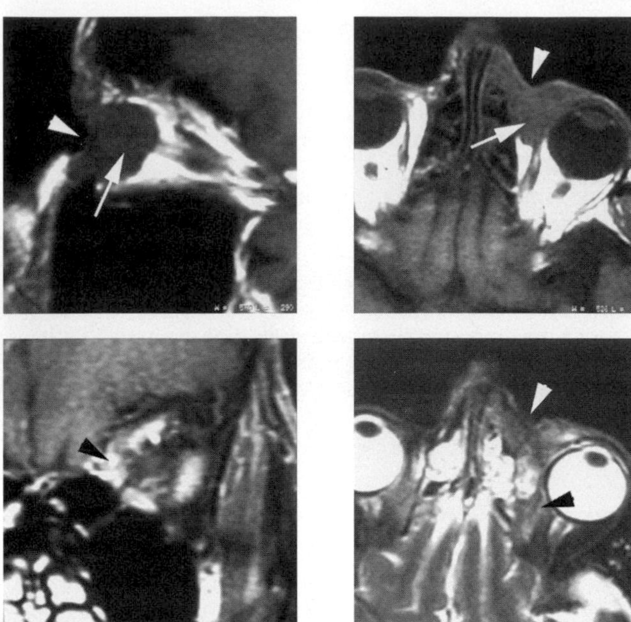

Figure 24.31 Recurrent skin cancer. Clockwise from top left: sagittal T1, axial T1, axial T2, and contrast coronal T1 images show an ulcerated squamous cancer recurrent at the medial canthus of the eye (*white arrowheads*) with deep postseptal extension (*arrows*) and invasion of the extraocular muscles (*black arrowheads*).

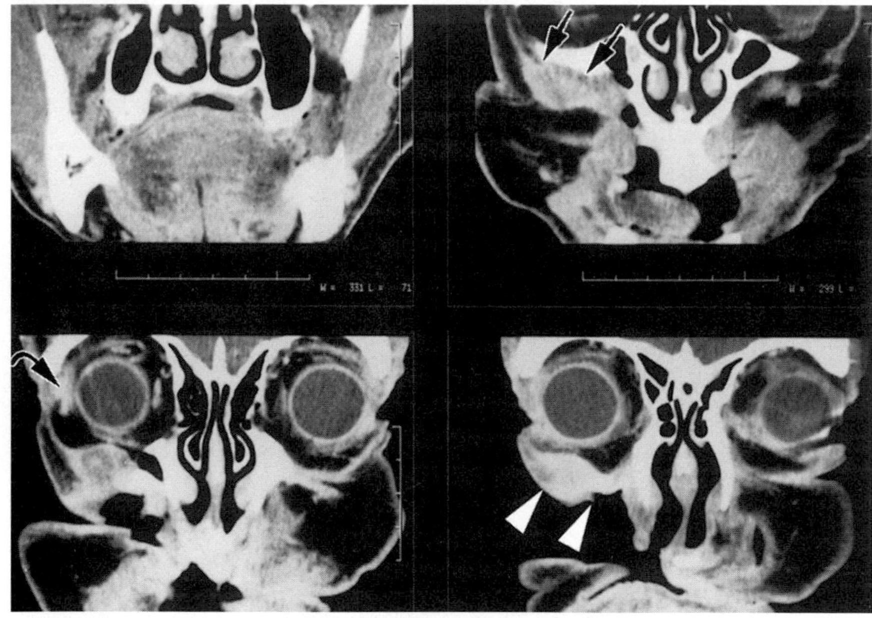

Figure 24.32 Limited orbital involvement. Enhanced direct coronal views through the face show ulcerating skin lesion (*arrowheads*) poorly marginated with the orbital rim (*arrows*), with early invasion of the extraconal compartment of the orbit. Normal lacrimal gland (*curved arrow*).

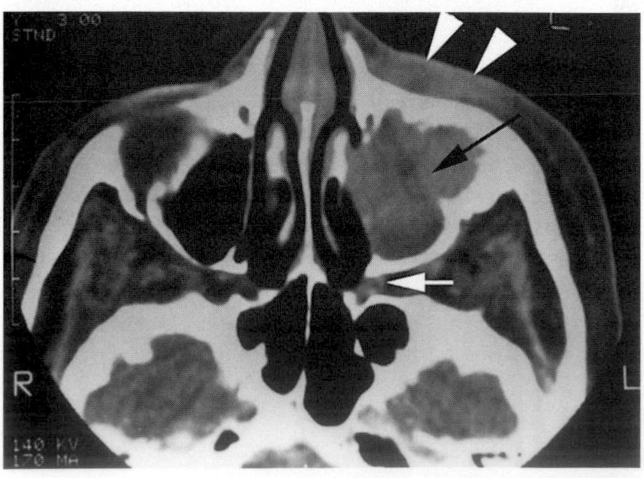

Figure 24.33 Moderate facial invasion. Enhanced axial computed tomography shows moderate extension of skin cancer (*arrowheads*) into the left antrum (*long arrow*), with perineural disease at the pterygopalatine fossa (*arrow*).

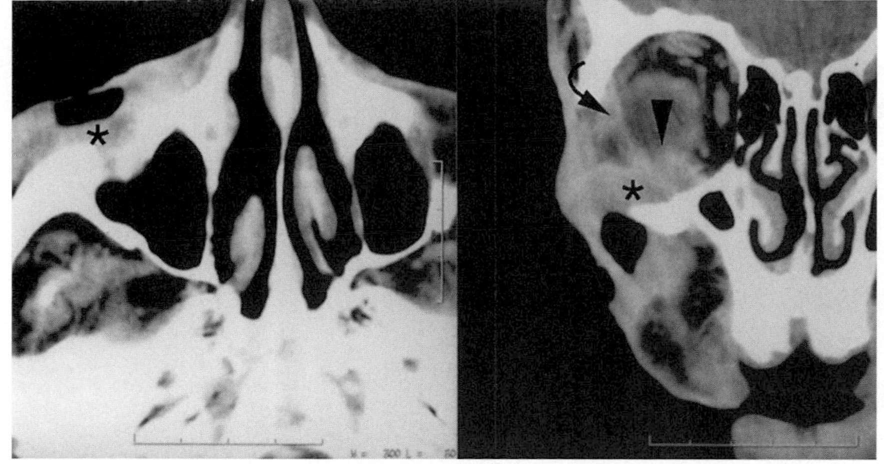

Figure 24.34 Advanced orbital involvement. Locally invasive skin cancer with frank osseous involvement and large orbital component (*asterisk*) infiltrating the globe, muscle cone (*arrowhead*), and lacrimal fossa (*curved arrow*).

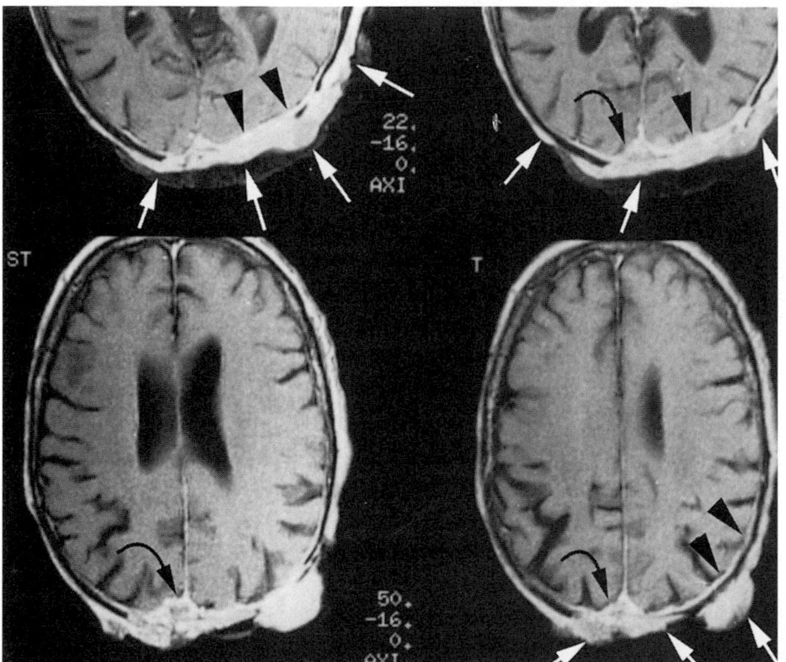

A

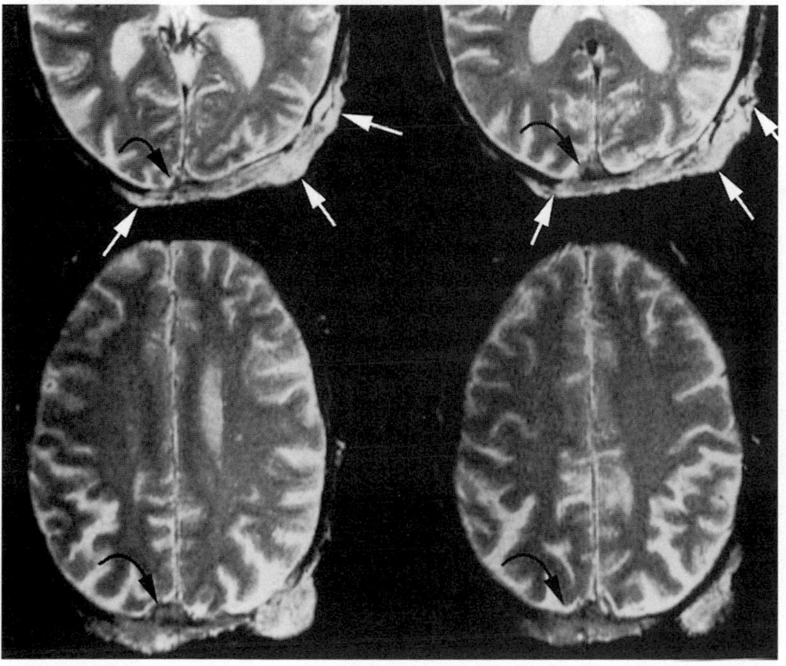

B

Figure 24.35 Extensive scalp cancer. **A:** Serial-enhanced axial T1 magnetic resonance imaging. **B:** T2 magnetic resonance imaging shows extensive scalp lesion (*arrows*) with an intracranial extradural component (*arrowheads*) and direct invasion of the superior sagittal sinus (*curved arrow*). No cortical abnormality to indicate pial involvement.

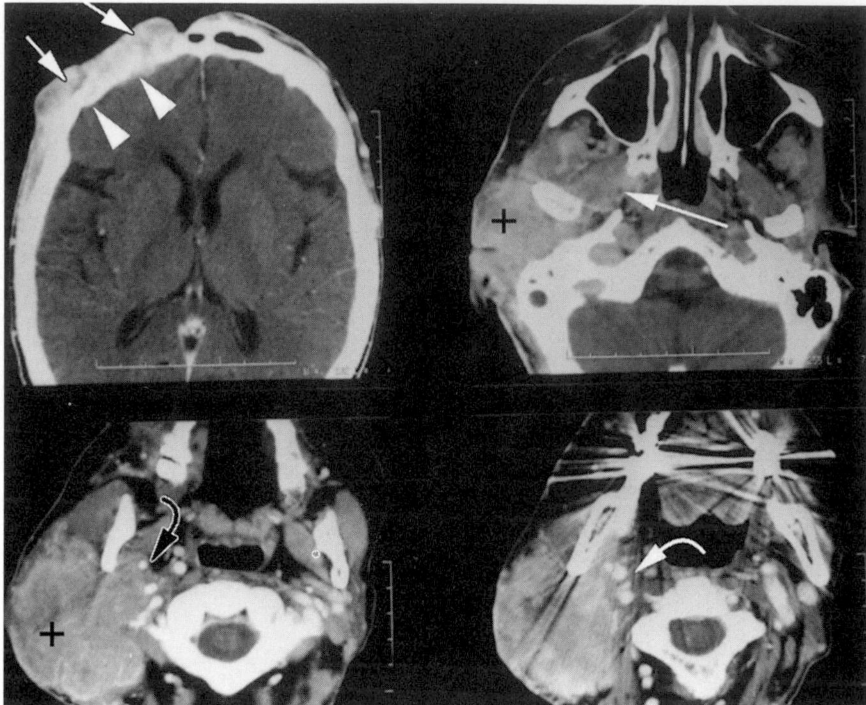

Figure 24.36 Extensive scalp lesion. Enhanced axial computed tomography of head and upper neck shows extensive plaque of tumor of right frontal bone (*arrows*) with permeation of the inner table to epidural space (*arrowheads*) after prior outer table composite resection. Note right cranial nerve V (*long arrow*). Lower images show huge metastasis to right parotid bed (+) invading the parapharyngeal (*curved arrows*) and masticator spaces.

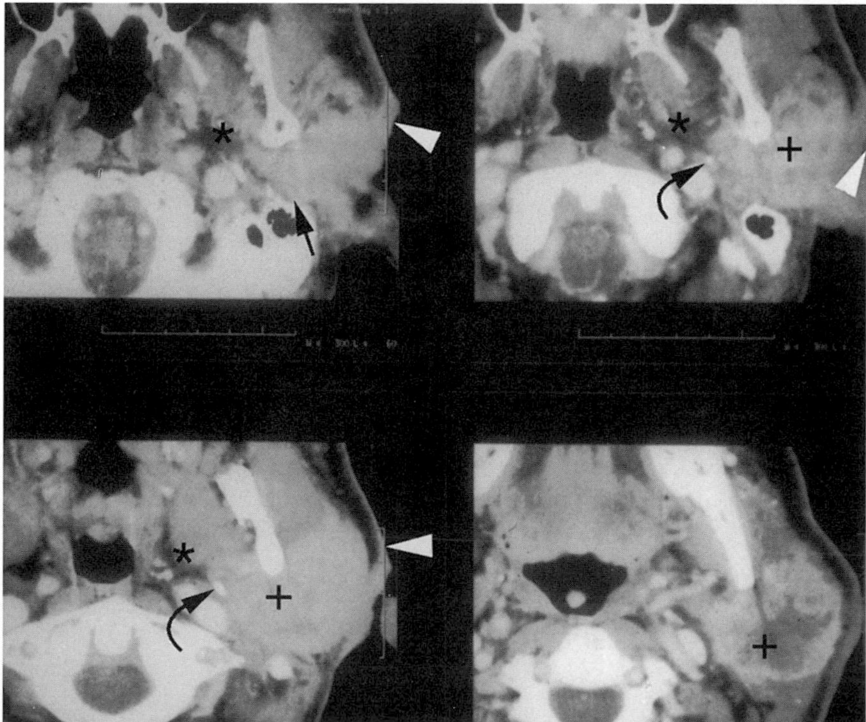

Figure 24.37 Locally invasive skin cancer. Enhanced serial axial computed tomography through left parotid bed shows ulcerating preauricular skin lesion (*arrowheads*) directly infiltrating the parotid space (+), approaching parapharyngeal space (*asterisk*), poorly marginated with the mastoid (*arrow*) and carotid space (*curved arrow*).

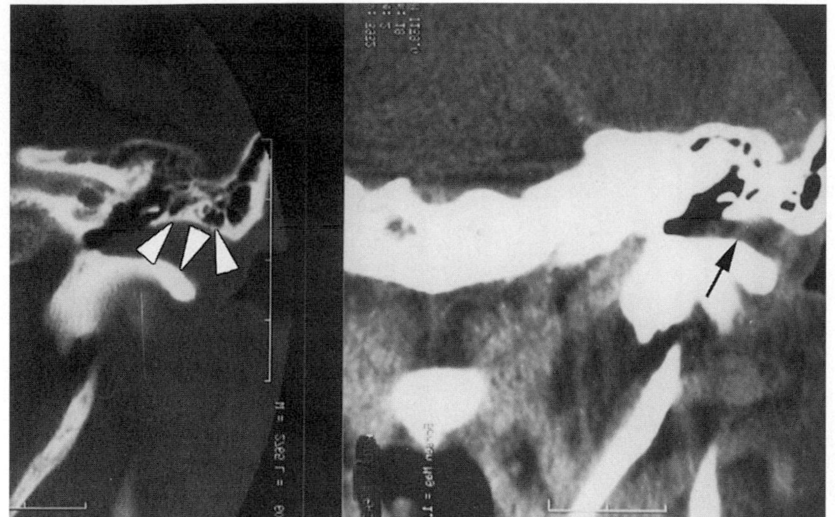

Figure 24.38 Recurrent squamous cancer of external auditory canal. Enhanced coronal computed tomography of recurrent skin cancer filling the right external auditory canal (*arrow*) without bone destruction (*arrowheads*) after prior sleeve resection.

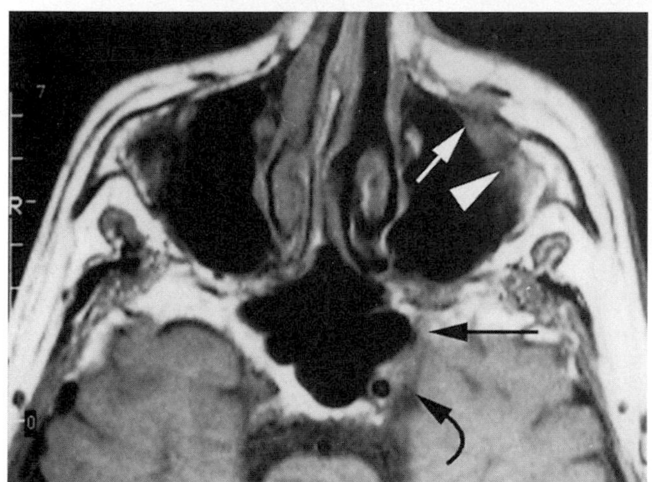

A

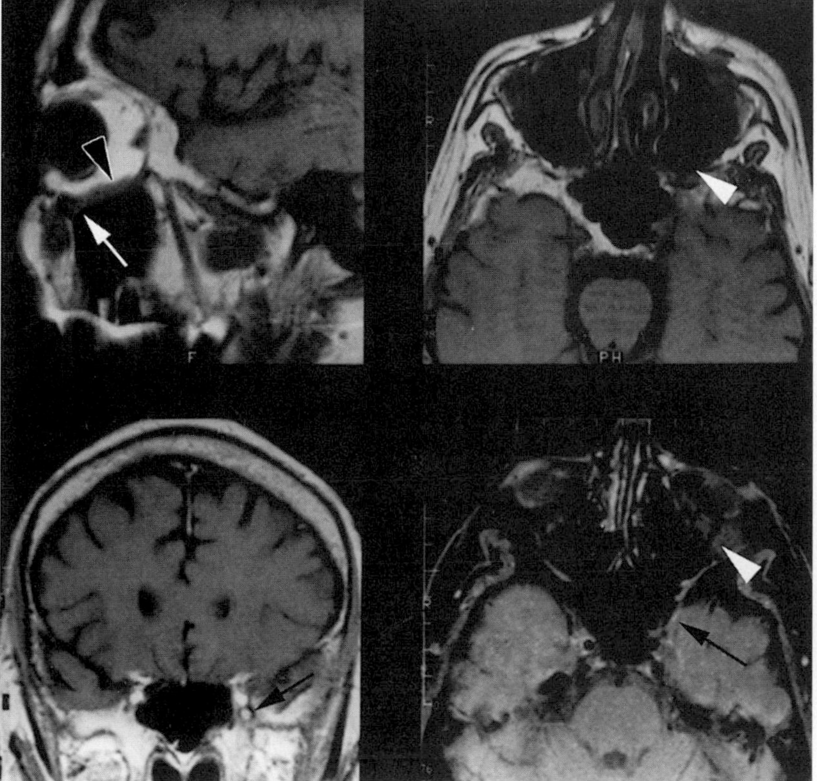

B

Figure 24.39 Neurotropic basal-squamous cancer. Axial T1 magnetic resonance imaging **(A)** and fat-suppressed contrast axial T1 **(B)** views showing proximal neurotropic involvement entering the infraorbital foramen (*arrow*), extending along the inferior orbital groove (*arrowheads*), through the expanded foramen rotundum (*long arrow*), and into the cavernous sinus (*curved arrow*), producing anesthesia of the second division of the fifth nerve despite healed primary nasolabial site.

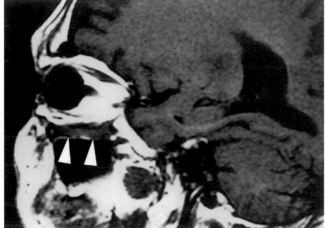

A

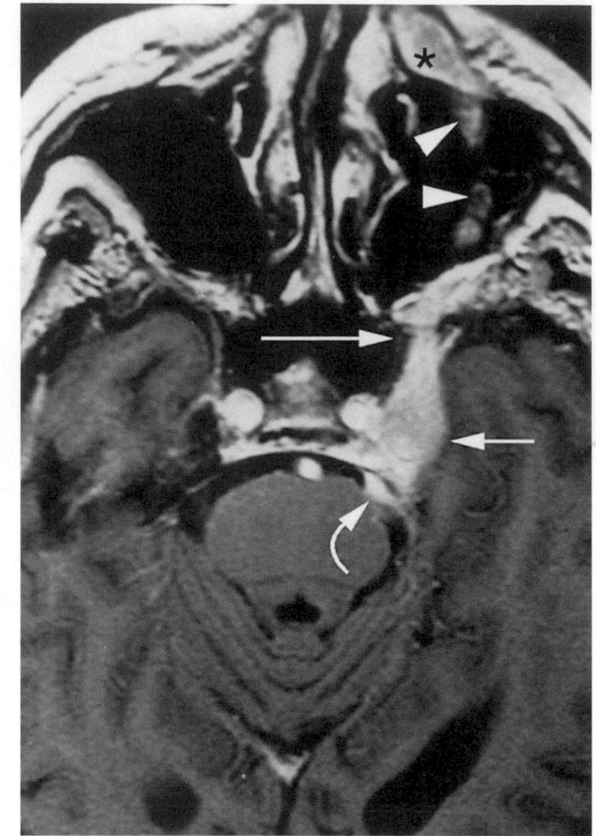

B

Figure 24.40 Progressive neurotropic melanoma. Left parasagittal T1 **(A)** and enhanced axial T1 **(B)** of the face show progressive amelanotic melanoma at left nasolabial site (*asterisk*), growing proximally along the second division of cranial nerve V at the infraorbital groove (*arrowheads*), expanded foramen rotundum (*long arrow*), cavernous sinus (*arrow*), and prepontine cistern (*curved arrow*).

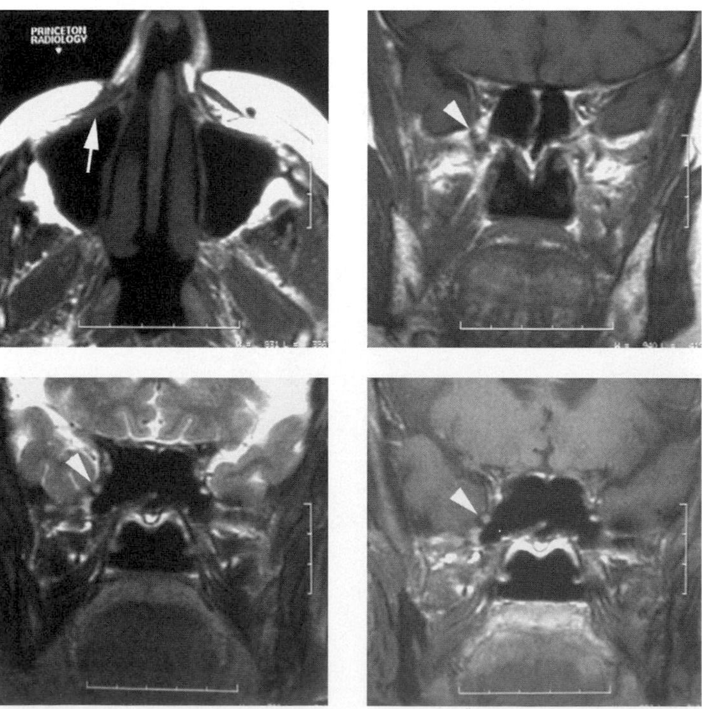

Figure 24.41 Neurotropic extension. Abnormal enhancing signal at right foramen rotundum (*arrowheads*) remote from recurrent right nasolabial lesion (*arrow*) related to perineural extension along the maxillary nerve.

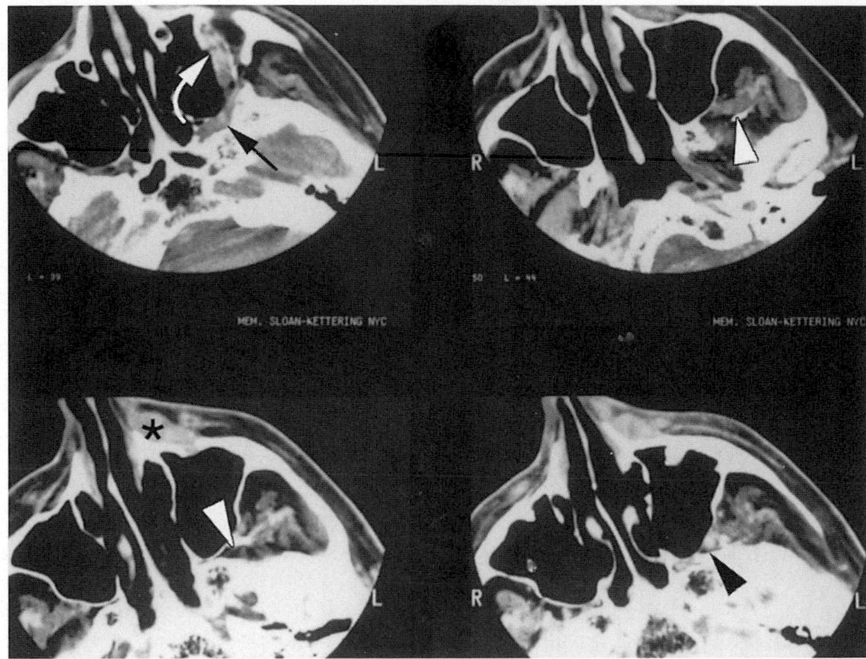

Figure 24.42 Imaging-guided biopsy. Sequential-control computed tomography images of patient in Fig. 24.41 show disease in the left pterygopalatine fossa (*arrow*) and progressive advancement of 20-gauge needle (*arrowheads*) into pterygopalatine fossa.

RADIATION THERAPY TECHNIQUE

William M. Mendenhall

Radiation therapy is most commonly indicated for small lesions around the nose, eye, ear, upper lip, and commissure of the lip; for advanced lesions invading bone and cartilage; after an incomplete excision; for advanced lesions in general; for patients at poor medical risk for a surgical procedure; for multiple adjacent small lesions (e.g., on the nose); and for metastatic spread to regional lymph nodes.

A wide range of techniques is available for the treatment of skin cancer, including orthovoltage and supervoltage x-rays, electrons, and interstitial techniques. The selection of technique is highly individualized and depends on the tumor volume, normal tissues to be protected, available equipment, the experience of the radiation therapist, and patient mobility. Orthovoltage irradiation is associated with a higher probability of local control compared with electron-beam irradiation (141).

Guidelines for selection of the external-beam dose, based on the size of the lesion, the functional or cosmetic result desired, and patient age and mobility, are given in Table 24.2 (142). Short treatment schemes of one to five treatments are curative for small or medium-sizes lesions, but eventually a depressed scar or other complications may result. The late effects of these short schemes have given radiation therapy a bad name in the management of skin cancer, and rightly so, because it usually falls on the surgeon to manage the late complications. These short treatments are particularly undesirable around the eye, nose, and ear. The short regimens are mostly used for the immobile, elderly patient who is able to make only a few visits to the radiation therapy department.

Eyelid

Almost all early lesions of the canthi and lids are treated with orthovoltage techniques. Low-energy electrons might seem advantageous compared with orthovoltage x-rays from a theoretic standpoint, but they require larger portals (~2 cm greater) because of low doses at the beam edges; it is more difficult to protect the eyeball owing to the production of high-energy x-rays in metal eye shields, and they are two to three times more expensive (143). Additionally, Lovett et al. (141) reported a significantly lower rate of local control for basal cell carcinoma 1.1 to 5.0 cm in diameter treated at the Mallinckrodt Institute of Radiology (St. Louis) with electron beam compared with orthovoltage x-rays. A set of eye shields is essential for treatment of these lesions and gives nearly complete protection of the eyeball. Radiation therapy should not be attempted without availability of these shields (Fig. 24.43) (142).

Amdur et al. (143) compared the dose distribution of 250-kVp x-rays and 6- to 20-MeV electron beam using a face phantom constructed out of solid pieces of water-equivalent epoxy to simulate the radiation treatment of an eyelid cancer. The doses that the cornea, lens, and retina would receive beneath the midpoint of the inferior hemisphere of the shield were measured using thermoluminescent and film dosimetry. They noted that for 6- to 8-MeV electrons, the cornea dose was two to four times higher than with 250-kVp x-rays (Table 24.3) (143). Corneal and lens doses rose rapidly with increasing electron-beam energy such that with 10- to 20-MeV electrons, the shield would provide relatively poor ocular protection. An ion chamber and film dosimetry were used to determine the isodose profiles of 250-kVp x-rays and 6-MeV electron beams for a 3-cm diameter field collimated on the surface. With 250-kVp x-rays, the 95% isodose area was 32% wider than with 6-MeV electrons (Fig. 24.44) (143). If electrons are used, therefore, the fields must be enlarged 1.0 to 1.5 cm in all directions and bolus must be applied. Additionally, the dose must be increased 10% to 15% to account for the difference in radiobiologic effectiveness (RBE). They concluded that, because of the ease of eye shielding and the ability to minimize field size, kilovoltage x-rays were the beam of choice for early skin cancer near the eye, as well as for other anatomic sites.

A lead face mask is prepared to sharply limit the radiation field and to reproduce the exact treatment portal each day (144). Because the treatment portals are irregular in outline, each one is calibrated separately. Slight reduction occurs in percentage depth dose at the edge of small orthovoltage beams collimated on the skin, which must be taken into account for treatment planning. These differences in depth dose give a built-in shrinking field technique, and, therefore, field reductions seldom are necessary. Additional layers of lead or lead putty must be added to the lead mask to further eliminate transit irradiation.

The skin of the eyelids is thin and delicate, and fractionation schedules of 3 to 5 weeks that employ relatively small doses per fraction should be adopted for optimal results.

TABLE 24.2 Guidelines for Selection of External-Beam Dose

Orthovoltage dose (Gy)[a]	Examples
65 Gy/7 wk	Large untreated lesion with bone or cartilage invasion, or large recurrent tumor[b]
60 Gy/7 wk	Large untreated lesion with minimal or suspected bone or cartilage invasion[b]
55 Gy/6 wk	Moderate to large inner canthus, eyelid, nasal, or pinna lesions (20–30 cm^2 area)
50 Gy/4 wk	Small, thin lesion (<1.5 cm) around eye, nose, or ear (10 cm^2 area)
45 Gy/3 wk	Moderate-sized lesion of free skin or postoperative cut-through of moderate size on free skin[c]
40 Gy/2 wk or 30 Gy/1 wk	Small lesions (1 cm) or free skin[c]
The following schemes are used when the late cosmetic result is not important and travel for the patient is difficult:	
40 Gy/10 fractions or 30 Gy/5 fractions or 20 Gy/1 fraction	Rapid fractionation schemes produce a high cure rate for small lesions, but the cosmetic result may be less than optimal after 5 years

[a]Add 10% to dose for supervoltage therapy.
[b]All, or a portion, of the therapy given with supervoltage photons or electrons.
[c]*Free* indicates no involvement of ear, nose, eye, or lid.
Source: Mendenhall WM, Million RR, Mancuso AA, et al. Carcinoma of the skin. In: Million RR, Cassisi NJ, eds. *Management of head and neck cancer: a multidisciplinary approach.* Philadelphia: Lippincott, 1994:643–691, with permission.

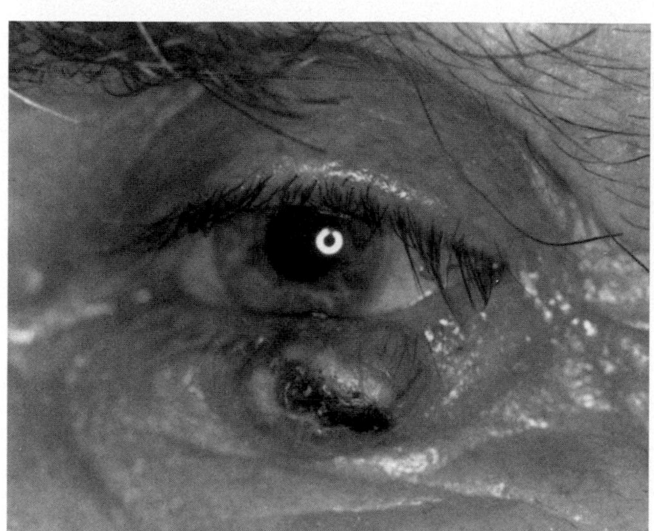
A

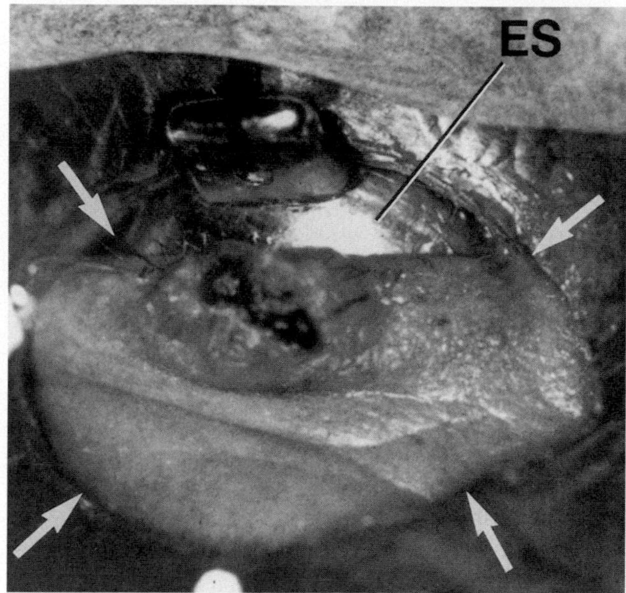

C

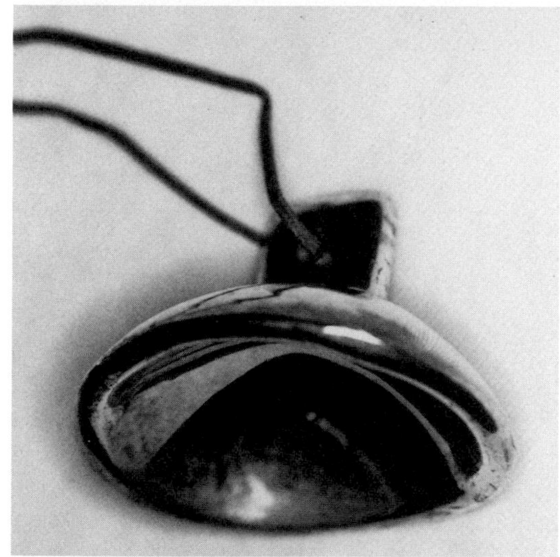
B

Figure 24.43 **A:** 1 × 1cm basal cell carcinoma of the midportion of the lower eyelid. **B:** Eye shield. **C:** The treatment setup that was used to irradiate the patient. ES, eye shield. *Arrows* indicate the field edge. (From Mendenhall WM, Million RR, Mancuso AA, et al. Carcinoma of the skin. In: Million RR, Cassisi NJ, eds. *Management of head and neck cancer: a multidisciplinary approach.* Philadelphia: Lippincott, 1994:643–691, with permission.)

Nose

Techniques for irradiation of nasal lesions vary from simple to highly individualized and complex treatments. We prefer the preparation of a face mask for most *en face* portals for orthovoltage and electron-beam therapy. Lead strips covered with wax may be inserted into the nares to reduce the transit dose to normal tissues when orthovoltage or electrons are used. A combination of photons and electrons may be used in certain situations to reduce depth dose. Supervoltage beams with bolus are useful when bone or cartilage is involved to gain a more homogeneous irradiation and avoid the increased dose in bone and cartilage associated with orthovoltage therapy. When supervoltage or low-energy electrons are used, a bolus is necessary to achieve full surface dose; uninvolved skin areas may not need a bolus. Lesions of the tip of the nose and nasal alar fold are frequently more extensive than judged by palpation, and treatment volumes must be generous.

There may be multiple small foci of cancer scattered over the nose and adjacent cheek with normal intervening skin. It is usually better to encompass all lesions in a single portal rather than to use multiple tiny adjacent portals.

Ear

Small lesions of the pinna may be easily treated with single-portal orthovoltage irradiation. Large lesions, especially those invading cartilage and involving the postauricular sulcus, are frequently treated with supervoltage beam and a wax bolus to

TABLE 24.3 Ocular Protection: Dose Beneath the Eye Shield[a]

Structure	Depth (mm)	250 kVp x-ray (HVL 1.4 mm³)	Electron-beam energy (MeV) 6	8	10	12	14	17	20
Cornea	1	10%	18%	37%	64%	75%	93%	98%	102%
Lens	8	9%	9%	19%	36%	46%	61%	70%	87%
Retina	23	10%	10%	22%	22%	21%	23%	25%	29%

[a]Dose is expressed as a percentage of the dose to depth of maximum dose deposition (D_{max}).
Source: Amdur RJ, Kalbaugh KJ, Ewald LM, et al. Radiation therapy for skin cancer near the eye: kilovoltage x rays versus electrons. *Int J Radiat Oncol Biol Phys* 1992;23:769–779, with permission.

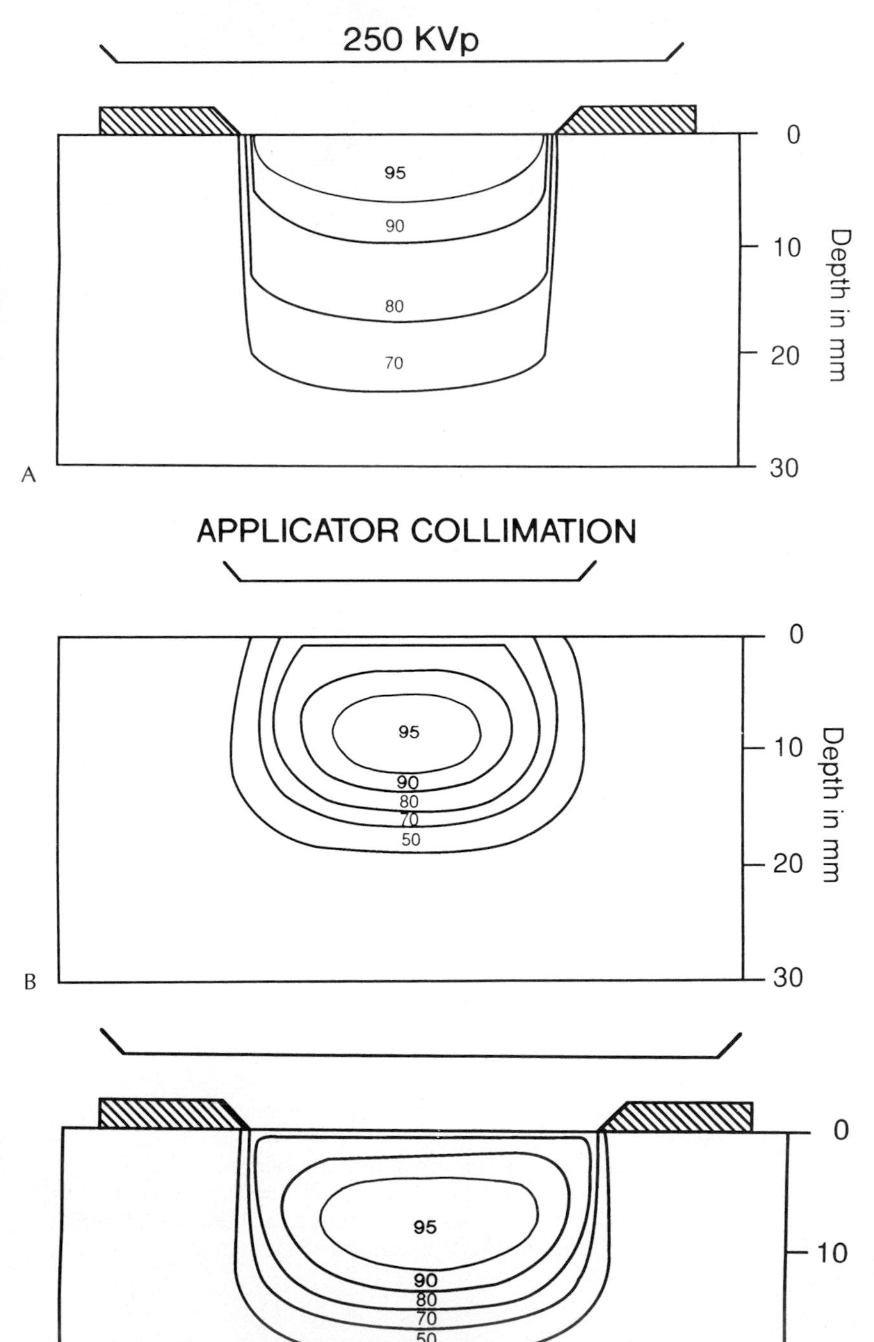

Figure 24.44 Isodose distributions were measured through the center of a 3 × 3 cm square field defined on the surface of a water phantom. Curves are labeled with isodose percentages. **A:** 250-kVp x-rays (half-value layer 1.4 mm³) with secondary collimation on the phantom surface. Source-to-surface distance (SSD) is 50 cm. **B:** 6-MeV electron beam with secondary collimation 5 cm above the phantom surface (at the level of the electron cone). Source-to-collimator distance (SCD) is 95 cm. SSD is 100 cm. **C:** 6-MeV electron beam with tertiary collimation on the phantom surface. SSD equals SCD, which equals 100 cm. (From Amdur RJ, Kalbaugh KJ, Ewald LM, et al. Radiation therapy for skin cancer near the eye: kilovoltage x-rays versus electrons. *Int J Radiat Oncol Biol Phys* 1992;23: 769–779, with permission.)

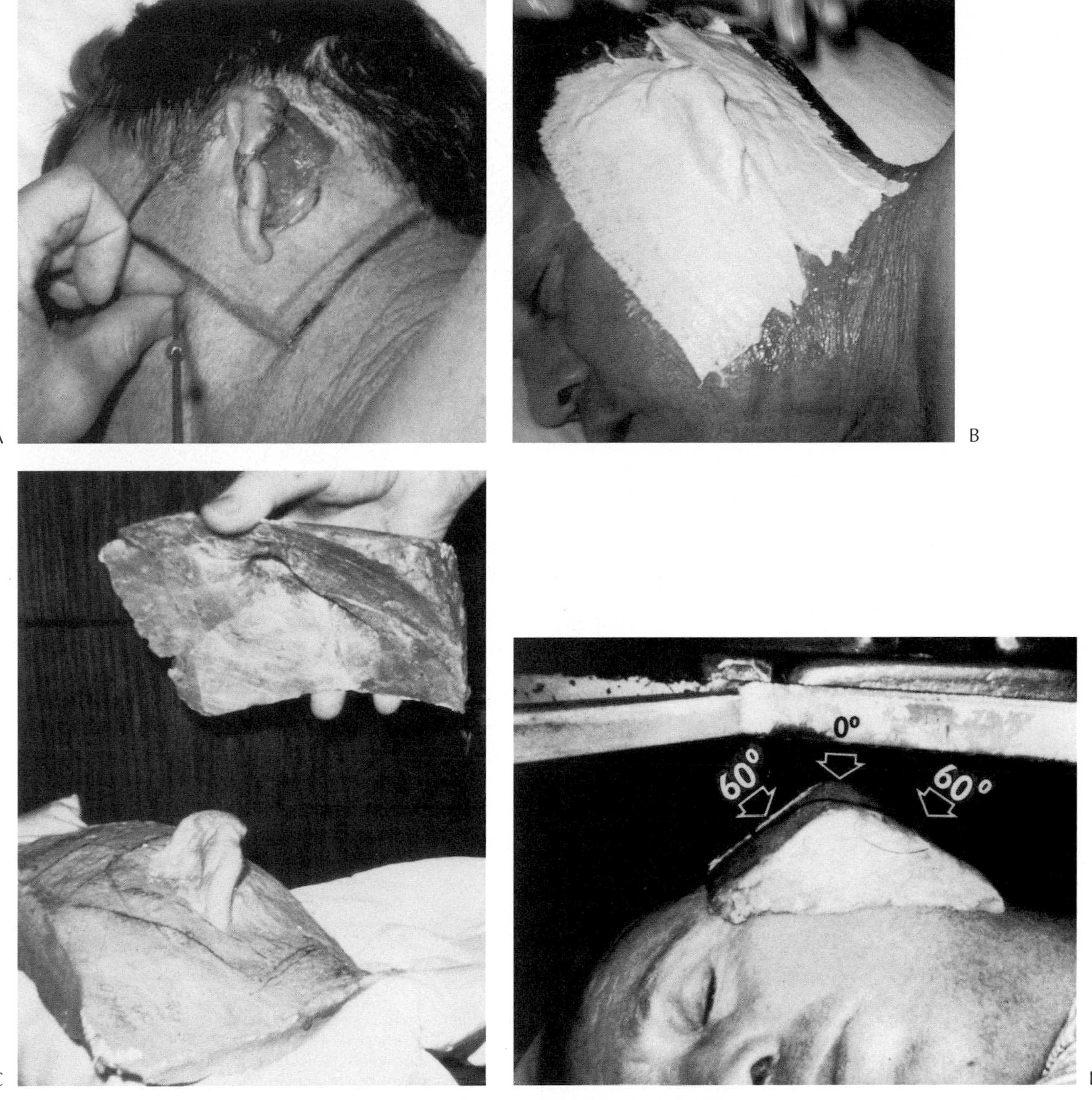

Figure 24.45 **A:** Squamous cell carcinoma of the left ear with cartilage invasion (patient was blind in the right eye). Treatment plan was 65 Gy over 7½ weeks, ^{60}Co, with beeswax bolus, three-field technique: superior and inferior portals angled 60 degrees with wedges, and a straight lateral open field (0 degree). **B:** Preparation of plaster mold. **C:** Plaster cast. **D:** Beeswax bolus in place.

(continued on next page)

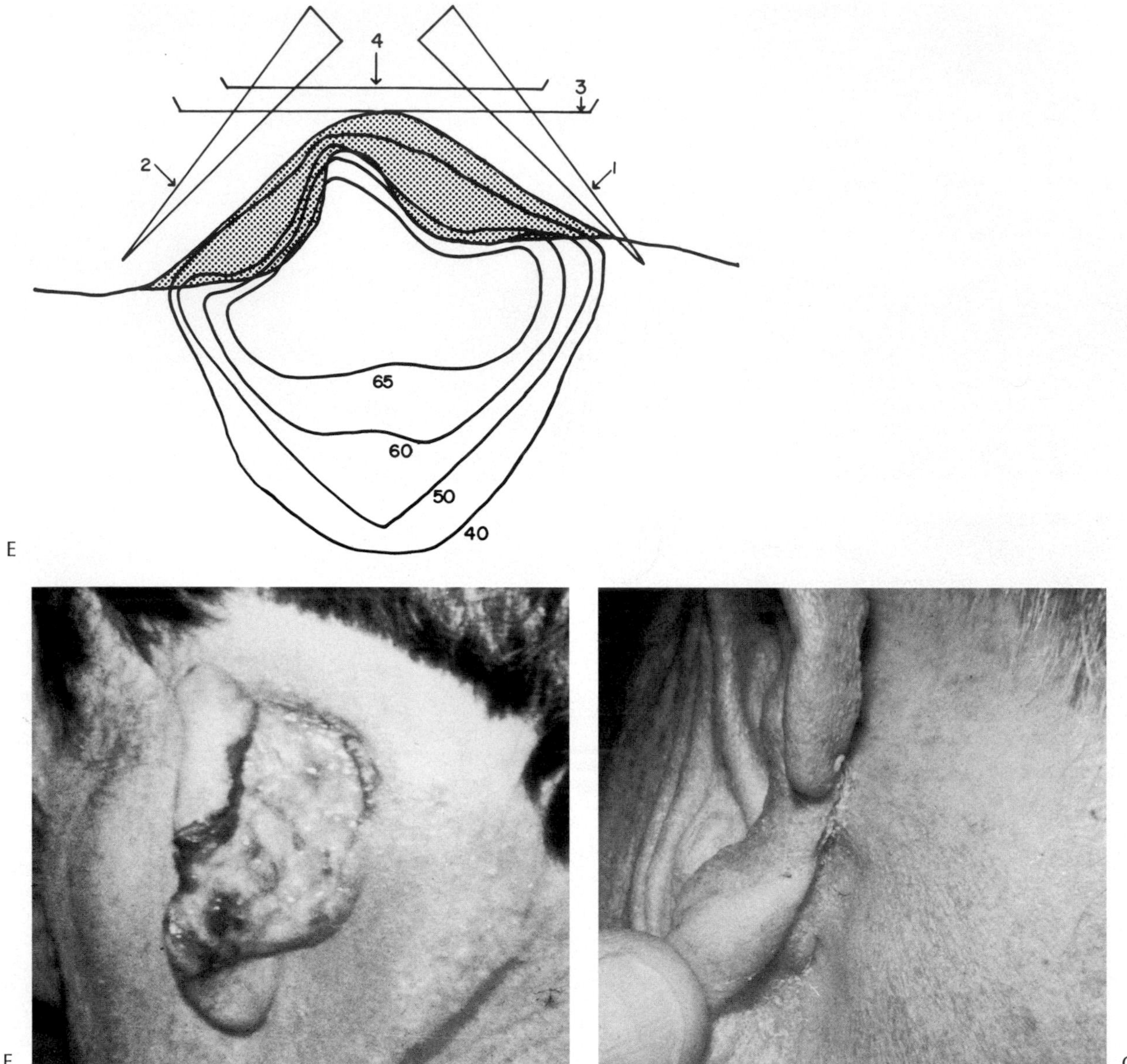

Figure 24.45 ***(continued)*** **E:** Isodose distribution. *Stippled area* represents beeswax compensator. The dose to the midline was approximately 50 Gy over 7½ weeks. **F:** Appearance at 40 Gy. **G:** No evidence of disease was seen at 5½ years. The patient remained alive and disease-free 13½ years after irradiation. (From Mendenhall WM, Million RR, Mancuso AA, et al. Carcinoma of the skin. In: Million RR, Cassisi NJ, eds. *Management of head and neck cancer: a multidisciplinary approach.* Philadelphia: Lippincott, 1994:643–691, with permission.)

ensure homogeneous irradiation and reduce the differential absorption in bone and cartilage. Angled wedge fields, a three-field technique, or mixed beams reduce irradiation to normal structures deep to the ear (Fig. 24.45) (142). Lesions located in the concha and the external auditory canal are more difficult to control and have vague borders; surgical resection with postoperative radiation therapy may be advantageous in the infiltrative, ulcerated lesions.

Upper Lip

Lesions greater than 1 cm often involve the vermilion or the commissure of the lip or extend near the base of the columella or alar cartilages. They may be treated with external-beam irradiation, interstitial implant, or a combination of both. A lead shield is inserted behind the upper lip to reduce transit irradiation when external-beam therapy is used; the shield is coated with wax. A gauze roll is inserted behind the upper lip at the time of the implant to reduce gingival irradiation. The dose to the lens from an upper lip implant is calculated to be 1 to 2 Gy over 6 days when the primary lesion receives 60 Gy at 0.5 cm from a 3 × 1.5 cm single-plane implant.

Scalp

Small scalp lesions are usually managed by excision, but some lesions, although superficial, may involve an extensive area. The latter are usually managed by radiation therapy. Advanced, destructive lesions or multiple invasive lesions usually are treated by radiation therapy; the treatment plans are individualized. Electrons are an advantage, but a variety of photon or electron beams can be mixed for the desired effect. A certain amount of brain irradiation is unavoidable in treatment of massive lesions.

Temple

Small and moderate-sized lesions (2 to 3 cm) are usually managed by excision. Squamous cell carcinomas of the temple area are particularly prone to local and regional recurrence after surgical excision and should be watched closely. If the margins are close or positive, postoperative radiation therapy should be considered rather than reexcision. The larger carcinomas should be considered for radiation therapy. Electrons are advantageous to avoid unnecessary brain irradiation.

Preauricular Area (Cheek)

The majority of the lesions in the preauricular area present early and can be successfully managed by a surgical modality. The advanced lesions require careful staging and treatment planning, however, because they frequently invade the parotid, the pinna, and the external and internal auditory canals; approximate or invade the facial nerve; and invade the zygoma or mandible. Some may be cured by radiation therapy alone in spite of cartilage and bone invasion. If feasible, patients with clinical evidence of nerve invasion should be operated on to remove grossly involved nerves before irradiation.

The radiation treatment plan often is a lateral supervoltage external beam with a wax bolus to provide surface dose. A combination of photons and electrons or electrons alone produce the best distributions. The initial portals should be generous, and the depth-dose specification should be adequate.

REFERENCES

1. Boring CC, Squires TS, Tong T. Cancer statistics, 1991. *CA Cancer J Clin* 1991; 41:19.
2. Scotto J, Fears TR, Fraumeni JF Jr. *Incidence of nonmelanoma skin cancer in the United States.* NIH publication number 83-2433. Washington, DC: Government Printing Office, 1983.
3. Padgett JK, Hendrix JD Jr. Cutaneous malignancies and their management. *Otolaryngol Clin North Am* 2001;34:523.
4. Strom SS, Yamamura Y. Epidemiology of nonmelanoma skin cancer. *Clin Plast Surg* 1997;24:627.
5. Andrade R, Gumport SL, Popkin G, et al. *Cancer of the skin.* Philadelphia: WB Saunders, 1976.
6. Glass AG, Hoover RN. The emerging epidemic of melanoma and squamous cell skin cancer. *JAMA* 1989;262:2097.
7. Weber RS, Lippman SM, McNeese MD. Advanced basal and squamous cell carcinomas of the skin of the head and neck. In: Jacobs C, ed. *Carcinomas of the head and neck: evaluation and management.* Boston: Kluwer Academic, 1990:61.
8. Preston DS, Stern RS. Nonmelanoma cancers of the skin. *N Engl J Med* 1992; 327:1649.
9. Emmett EA. Ultraviolet radiation as a cause of skin tumors. *CRC Crit Rev Toxicol* 1973;2:211.
10. Leffell DJ. The scientific basis of skin cancer. *J Am Acad Dermatol* 2000;42:18.
11. Vitasa BC, Taylor HR, Strickland PT, et al. Association of nonmelanoma skin cancer and actinic keratosis with cumulative solar ultraviolet exposure in Maryland watermen. *Cancer* 1990;65:2811.
12. Czarnecki D, Meehan C, O'Brien T, et al. The changing face of skin cancer in Australia. *Int J Dermatol* 1991;30:715.
13. Henriksen T, Dahlback A, Larsen SH, et al. Ultraviolet radiation and skin cancer: effect of an ozone layer depletion. *Photochem Photobiol* 1990;51:579.
14. Kelfkens G, de Gruijl FR, van der Leon JC. Ozone depletion and increase in annual carcinogenic ultraviolet dose. *Photochem Photobiol* 1990;52:819.
15. Coldiron BM. Ozone depletion update. *Dermatol Surg* 1996;22:296.
16. Madronich S, McKenzie RL, Bjorn LO, et al. Changes in biologically active ultraviolet radiation reaching the Earth's surface. *J Photochem Photobiol B* 1998;46:5.
17. Oikarinen A, Raitio A. Melanoma and other skin cancers in circumpolar areas. *Int J Circumpolar Health* 2000;59:52.
18. Slaper H, Velders GJ, Daniel JS, et al. Estimates of ozone depletion and skin cancer incidence to examine the Vienna Convention achievements. *Nature* 1996;384:256.
19. Diffey BL. Stratospheric ozone depletion and the risk of non-melanoma skin cancer in a British population. *Phys Med Biol* 1992;37;2267.
20. Urbach F. Potential effects of altered solar ultraviolet radiation on human skin cancer. *Photochem Photobiol* 1989;50:507.
21. Scotto J, Kopf AW, Urbach F. Non-melanoma skin cancer among Caucasians in four areas of the United States. *Cancer* 1974;34:1333.
22. Schreiber MM, Shapiro SI, Berry CZ, et al. The incidence of skin cancer in southern Arizona (Tucson). *Arch Dermatol* 1971;104:124.
23. Giles GG, Marks R, Foley P. Incidence of non-melanocytic skin cancer treated in Australia. *BMJ* 1988;296:13.
24. Marks R, Jolley D, Dorevitch AP, et al. The incidence of nonmelanocytic skin cancers in an Australian population: results of a five year prospective study. *Med J Aust* 1989;150:475.
25. Magnus K. The Nordic profile of skin cancer incidence: a comparative epidemiologic study of the three main types of skin cancer. *Int J Cancer* 1991;47:12.
26. Kricker A, English DR, Randell PL, et al. Skin cancer in Geraldton, Western Australia: a survey of incidence and prevalence. *Med J Aust* 1990;152:399.
27. Chuang TY, Popescu A, Su WP, et al. Basal cell carcinoma: a population based incidence study in Rochester, Minnesota. *J Am Acad Dermatol* 1990;22:413.
28. Johnson TM, Rowe DE, Nelson BR, et al. Squamous cell carcinoma of the skin (excluding lip and oral mucosa). *J Am Acad Dermatol* 1992;26:467.
29. Barton IJ, Paltridge GW. The Australian climatology of biologically effective ultraviolet radiation. *Australas J Dermatol* 1979;20:68.
30. Vitaliano PP, Urbach F. The relative importance of risk factors in nonmelanoma carcinoma. *Arch Dermatol* 1980;116:454.
31. Hunter DJ, Colditz GA, Stampfer MJ, et al. Risk factors for basal cell carcinoma in a prospective cohort of women. *Ann Epidemiol* 1990;1:13.
32. Kaidbey KH, Agin PP, Sayre RM, et al. Photoprotection by melanin: a comparison of black and Caucasian skin. *J Am Acad Dermatol* 1979;1:249.
33. Strickland PT, Vitasa BC, West SK, et al. Quantitative carcinogenesis in man: solar ultraviolet B dose dependence of skin cancer in Maryland watermen. *J Natl Cancer Inst* 1989;81:1910.
34. Strickland PT. Photocarcinogenesis by near-ultraviolet (UVA) radiation in Sencar mice. *J Invest Dermatol* 1986;87:272.
35. Friedberg EC. DNA damage and human disease. In: Friedberg EC, ed. *DNA repair.* New York: WH Freeman, 1985:505.
36. Kanjilal S, Pierceall WE, Ananthaswamy HN. Ultraviolet radiation in the pathogenesis of skin cancers: involvement of ras and p53 genes. *Cancer Bull* 1993;45:205.
37. Kanjilal S. Unpublished data, 1995.
38. Kanjilal S, Strom SS, Clayman GL, et al. P53 mutations in nonmelanoma skin cancer of the head and neck: molecular evidence for field cancerization. *Cancer Res* 1995;55:604.
39. Salasche SJ. Epidemiology of actinic keratoses and squamous cell carcinoma. *J Am Acad Dermatol* 2000;42:4.
40. Lober BA, Lober CW, Accola J. Actinic keratosis is squamous cell carcinoma. *J Am Acad Dermatol* 2000;43:881.
41. Dupree MT, Kiteley RA, Weismantle K, et al. Radiation therapy for Bowen's disease: lessons for lesions of the lower extremity. *J Am Acad Dermatol* 2001; 45:401.
42. Schnur PL, Bozzo P. Metastasizing keratoacanthoma: the difficulties in differentiating keratoacanthomas from squamous cell carcinomas. *Plast Reconstr Surg* 1978;62:258.
43. Skidmore RA Jr, Flowers FP. Nonmelanoma skin cancer. *Med Clin North Am* 1998;82:1309.
44. Rowe DE, Carroll RJ, Day CL. Prognostic factors for local recurrence, metastasis, and survival rates in squamous cell carcinoma of the skin, ear, and lip: implications for treatment modality selection. *J Am Acad Dermatol* 1992;26: 976.
45. Lai SY, Weinstein GS, Chalian AA, et al. Parotidectomy in the treatment of aggressive cutaneous malignancies. *Arch Otol Head Neck Surg* 2002;128:521.
46. Panje WR, Ceilley RI. The influence of embryology of the midface on the spread of epithelial malignancies. *Laryngoscope* 1979;89:1914.
47. Wentzell JM, Robinson JK. Embryologic fusion planes and the spread of cutaneous carcinoma: a review and reassessment. *J Dermatol Surg Oncol* 1990;16: 1000.
48. Emmett AJ. Surgical analysis and biological behaviour of 2277 basal cell carcinomas. *Aust NZ J Surg* 1990;60:855.
49. Goepfert H, Dichtel WJ, Medina JE, et al. Perineural invasion of squamous cell skin carcinoma of the head and neck. *Am J Surg* 1984;148:542.
50. Mohs FE. *Chemosurgery: microscopically controlled surgery for skin cancer.* Springfield, IL: Charles C Thomas, 1978.
51. Ballantyne AJ, McCarter AB, Ibanez MI. The extension of cancer of the head and neck through peripheral nerves. *Am J Surg* 1963;106:651.
52. Niazi ZB, Lamberty BG. Perineural infiltration in basal cell carcinomas. *Br J Plast Surg* 1993;46:156.
53. McLaughlin RB Jr, Montone KT, Wall SJ, et al. Nerve cell adhesion molecule expression in squamous cell carcinoma of the head and neck: a predictor of propensity toward perineural spread. *Laryngoscope* 1999;109:821.
54. Anderson TD, Feldman M, Weber RS, et al. Tumor deposition of laminin-5 and the relationship with perineural invasion. *Laryngoscope* 2001;111:2140.
55. Dodd GD, Dolan PA, Ballantyne AJ, et al. The dissemination of tumors of the head and neck via the cranial nerves. *Radiol Clin North Am* 1970;8:445.

56. Dinehart SM, Pollack SV. Metastases from squamous cell carcinoma of the skin and lip: an analysis of twenty-seven cases. *J Am Acad Dermatol* 1989;21: 241.
57. Moller R, Reymann F, Hou-Jensen K. Metastasis in dermatological patients with squamous cell carcinoma. *Arch Dermatol* 1979;115:703.
58. Byers R, Kesler K, Redmon B, et al. Squamous carcinoma of the external ear. *Am J Surg* 1983;146:447.
59. Harms SE. Magnetic resonance imaging of the neoplasms involving the head. *Semin Surg Oncol* 1985;1:188:195.
60. Karagas MR, Stukel TA, Greenberg ER, et al. Risk of subsequent basal cell carcinoma and squamous cell carcinoma of the skin among patients with prior skin cancer. *JAMA* 1992;267:3305.
61. Robinson JK. Risk of developing another basal cell carcinoma: a 5 year prospective study. *Cancer* 1987;60:118.
62. Epstein E. Value of follow-up after treatment of basal cell carcinoma. *Arch Dermatol* 1973;108:798.
63. Jackson GL, Ballantyne AJ. Role of parotidectomy for skin cancer of the head and neck. *Am J Surg* 1981;142:464.
64. American Joint Committee on Cancer. *Manual for staging of cancer.* Philadelphia: Lippincott, 1992.
64a. Greene F, Page D, Fleming I, et al. *AJCC cancer staging manual,* 6th ed. New York: Springer-Verlag, 2002.
65. Weber RS, Miller MJ. Multidisciplinary management of advanced basal and squamous cell skin cancer of the head and neck. In: Lucente FE, ed. *Highlights of the instructional courses,* vol 7. St. Louis: Mosby, 1995:37.
66. Talmi YP, Gal R, Finkelstein Y, et al. Squamous and basal cell cancers directly invading major salivary glands. *Ann Plast Surg* 1991;26:483.
67. Wolf DA, Zitelli JA. Surgical margins for basal cell carcinoma. *Arch Dermatol* 1987;123:340.
68. Brodland DG, Zitelli JA. Surgical margins for excision of cutaneous squamous cell carcinoma. *J Am Acad Dermatol* 1992;27:241.
69. Bakamjiam VY. A two-stage method for pharyngoesophagus reconstruction with a primary pectoral skin flap. *Plast Reconstr Surg* 1965;36:173.
70. Mercer DM. The cervicofacial flap. *Br J Plast Surg* 1988;41:470.
71. Becker DW. A cervicopectoral rotation flap for cheek coverage. *Plast Reconstr Surg* 1978;61:868.
72. Ariyan S. The pectoralis major myocutaneous flap. A versatile flap for reconstruction in the head and neck. *Plast Reconstr Surg* 1979;63:73.
73. Quillen CG. Latissimus dorsi myocutaneous flaps in head and neck reconstruction. *Plast Reconstr Surg* 1979;63:664.
74. Bertotti JA. Trapezius musculocutaneous island flap in the repair of major head and neck cancer. *Plast Reconstr Surg* 1980;65:16.
75. Shestak KC. Microvascular free tissue transfer for reconstruction of head and neck cancer defects. *Oncology* 1992;6:101.
76. Thomas JR. Skin grafts. In: Thomas JR, ed. *Cutaneous facial surgery.* New York: Thieme, 1992:72.
77. Hildago DA. Fibula free flap: a new method of mandible reconstruction. *Plast Reconstr Surg* 1989;84:7.
78. Miyamoto V. Cranial coverage involving scalp, bone, and dura using free epigastric flap. *Br J Plast Surg* 1986;39:483.
79. Burget GC, Menick FJ. Subtotal and total nasal reconstruction. In: Burget GC, Merrick FJ, eds. *Aesthetic reconstruction of the nose.* St. Louis: CV Mosby, 1994: 57.
80. Jackson IT. General considerations. In: Jackson IT, ed. *Local flaps in head and neck reconstruction.* St. Louis: CV Mosby, 1985:1.
81. Thomas JR. Local skin flaps. In: Thomas JR, Roller J, eds. *Cutaneous facial surgery.* New York: Thieme, 1992:77.
82. Karapandzic M. Reconstruction of lip defects by local arterial flaps. *Br J Plast Surg* 1974;27:93.
83. Manders EK. Skin expansion to eliminate large scalp defects. *Ann Plast Surg* 1984;12:305.
84. Hugo N. Basic principles of reconstruction of the lip, oral commissure, and cheek. In: Georgiade GS, ed. *Textbook of plastic, maxillofacial, and reconstructive surgery.* Baltimore: Williams & Wilkins, 1992:527.
85. Sykes JM, Morakami C. Principles of local flaps in head and neck reconstruction. Operative techniques in otolaryngology. *Head Neck Surg* 1993;4:2.
86. Cupp CL, Larrabee WE Reconstruction of the forehead and scalp. Operative techniques in otolaryngology. *Head Neck Surg* 1993;4:11.
87. Kroll SS, Margolis R. Scalp flap closure with primary donor site closure. *Ann Plast Surg* 1993;30:452.
88. Rohrick RJ. Scalp reconstruction. *Sel Read Plast Surg* 1989;5(16):20.
89. McGregor IA, McGregor FM. Scalp, forehead, and cheeks. In: McGregor IA, ed. *Cancer of the face and mouth.* Edinburgh: Churchill Livingstone, 1986:271.
90. Juri J, Juri C. Aesthetic aspects of reconstructive scalp surgery. *Clin Plast Surg* 1981;8:243.
91. Kazanjian VH, Holmes EM. Reconstruction after radical operation for osteomyelitis of the frontal bone: experience in 38 cases. *Surg Gynecol Obstet* 1944;79:397.
92. Sakai S, Soeda S, Terayama 1. Subcutaneous pedicle flaps for scalp defects. *Br J Plast Surg* 1988;41:25.
93. Orticochea M. Four-flap scalp reconstruction technique. *Br J Plast Surg* 1967; 20:159.
94. Jackson IT. Cheek reconstruction. In: Jackson IT, ed. *Local flaps in head and neck reconstruction.* St. Louis: CV Mosby, 1985:189.
95. Murakami CS, Odland PB. Bilobed flap variations. Operative techniques in otolaryngology. *Head Neck Surg* 1993;4:2.
96. Juri J, Juri C. Advancement and rotation of a large cervicofacial flap for cheek defects. *Plast Reconstr Surg* 1979;64:692.
97. Millard DR. Reconstructive rhinoplasty for the lower half of a nose. *Plast Reconstr Surg* 1974;54:133.
98. Antia NH, Daver BM. Reconstructive surgery for nasal defects. *Clin Plast Surg* 1981;8:535.
99. Lawrence WT. The nasolabial rhomboid flap. *Ann Plast Surg* 1992;29:269.
100. Rigg BM. The dorsal nasal flap. *Plast Reconstr Surg* 1973;52:361.
101. Kroll SS, Rosenfield L. Delayed pedicle separation in forehead flap nasal reconstruction. *Ann Plast Surg* 1989;23:327.
102. Abbe RA. A new plastic operation for the relief of deformity due to the double hare lip. *Med Rec* 1898;53:477.
103. Estlander JA. Eine methode aus der einen lippe substanzverluste deranderen zu ertzetzen. *Arch Klin Chir* 1872;14:622.
104. Freeman BS. Myoplastic modification of the Bernard cheiloplasty. *Plast Reconstr Surg* 1958;21:453.
105. Matsoba HM. The temporal fossa in head and neck reconstruction. Twenty-two flaps of scalp, fascia, and full-thickness cranial bone. *Laryngoscope* 1988; 98:444.
106. Larson DL, Goepfert H. Limitations in the sternocleidomastoid musculocutaneous flap in head and neck cancer reconstruction. *Plast Reconstr Surg* 1982; 70:328.
107. Kroll SS. Comparison of the rectus abdominis free flap with the pectoralis major myocutaneous flap for reconstruction in the head and neck. *Am J Surg* 1992;164:615.
108. Swartz WM. The osteocutaneous scapular flap for mandibular and maxillary reconstruction. *Plast Reconstr Surg* 1986;77:530.
109. McLean DH, Burke HJ. Autotransplant of omentum to a large scalp defect with microsurgical vascularization. *Plast Reconstr Surg* 1972;49:268.
110. Robb GL. Free scapular flap reconstruction of the head and neck. *Clin Plast Surg* 1994;21:45–58.
111. Martin JW, Lemon JC. Prosthetic rehabilitation. In: Bailey BJ, ed. *Head and neck surgery–otolaryngology,* 1st ed. Philadelphia: Lippincott, 1993:1431.
112. Robb GL, Marunick MT, Martin JW, et al. Midface reconstruction: surgical reconstruction versus prosthesis. *Head Neck* 200;23(1):48.
113. Fitzpatrick PJ. Radiation therapy of tumors of the skin of the head and neck. In: Thawley S, Panje W, Batsakis J, et al., eds. *Comprehensive management of head and neck tumors.* Philadelphia: WB Saunders, 1987:1208.
114. Sinesi C, McNeese MD, Peters LJ, et al. Electron beam therapy for eyelid carcinomas. *Head Neck Surg* 1987;10:31.
115. Lovett RD, Perez CA, Shapiro SJ, et al. External irradiation of epithelial skin cancer. *Int J Radiat Oncol Biol Phys* 1990;19:235.
116. Amdur RJ, Kalbaugh KJ, Ewald LM, et al. Radiation therapy for skin cancer near the eye: kilovoltage x-rays versus electrons. *Int J Radiat Oncol Biol Phys* 1992;23:769.
117. Fitzpatrick PJ, Thompson GA, Easterbrook EM, et al. Basal and squamous cell carcinoma of the eyelids and their treatment by radiotherapy. *Int J Radiat Oncol Biol Phys* 1984;10:449.
118. Mazeron JJ, Chassagne D, Crook J, et al. Radiation therapy of carcinomas of the skin of nose and nasal vestibule: a report of 1676 cases by the Groupe Europeen de Curietherapie. *Radiother Oncol* 1988;13:165.
119. Wong CS, Cummings BJ, Elhakim T, et al. External irradiation for squamous cell carcinoma of the nasal vestibule. *Int J Radiat Oncol Biol Phys* 1985;12:1943.
120. Mendenhall WM, Parsons IT, Mendenhall NP, et al. T2-T4 carcinoma of the skin of the head and neck treated with radical irradiation. *Int J Radiat Oncol Biol Phys* 1987;13:975.
121. Al-Othman MO, Mendenhall WM, Amdur RJ. Radiotherapy alone for clinical T4 skin carcinoma of the head and neck with surgery reserved for salvage. *Am J Otolaryngol* 1999;22:387.
122. Austin JR, Steward KL, Fawzi N. Squamous cell carcinoma of the external auditory canal. *Arch Otolaryngol Head Neck Surg* 1994;120:1228.
123. McCord MW, Mendenhall WM, Parsons JT, et al. Skin cancer of the head and neck with incidental microscopic perineural invasion. *Int J Radiat Oncol Biol Phys* 1999;43:591.
124. McCord MW, Mendenhall WM, Parsons JT, et al. Skin cancer of the head and neck with clinical perineural invasion. *Int J Radiat Oncol Biol Phys* 2000;47:89.
125. delCharco JO, Mendenhall WM, Parsons JT, et al. Carcinoma of the skin metastatic to the parotid area lymph nodes. *Head Neck* 1998;20:369.
126. Wang CC. The management of parotid lymph node metastases by irradiation. *Cancer* 1982;50:223.
127. Woodruff WW Jr, Yeates AE, McLendon RE. Perineural tumor extension to the cavernous sinus from the superficial carcinoma: CT manifestations. *Radiology* 1986;161:395.

Radiologic Imaging Concerns

128. Catalano PJ, Sen C, Biller HE. Cranial neuropathy secondary to perineural spread of cutaneous malignancies. *Am J Otol* 1995;16:772.
129. Selvin GJ. Basal cell and squamous cell carcinomas. *Optom Clin* 1993;3:17–28.
130. Catalano PJ, Sen C, Biller HF. Cranial neuropathy secondary to perineural spread of cutaneous malignancies. *Am J Otol* 1995;16:772–777.

131. Lawrence N, Cottel WI. Squamous cell carcinoma of skin with perineural invasion. *J Am Acad Dermatol* 1994;31:30–33.
132. Ratner D, Lowe L, Johnson TM, et al. Perineural spread of basal cell carcinomas treated with Mohs micrographic surgery. *Cancer* 2000;88:1605–1613.
133. Hendrix JD Jr, Parlette HL. Micronodular basal cell carcinoma. A deceptive histologic subtype with frequent clinically undetected tumor extension. *Arch Dermatol* 1996;132:295–298.
134. Martin RC 2nd, Edwards MJ, Cawte TG, et al. Basosquamous carcinoma: analysis of prognostic factors influencing recurrence. *Cancer* 2000;88: 1365–1369.
135. Ampil FL, Hardin JC, Peskind SP, et al. Perineural invasion in skin cancer of the head and neck: a review of nine cases. *J Oral Maxillofac Surg* 1995;53:34–38.
136. Woodruff WW Jr, Yeates AE, McLendon RE. Perineural tumor extension to the cavernous sinus from superficial facial carcinoma: CT manifestations. *Radiology* 1986;161:395–399.
137. ten Hove MW, Glaser JS, Schatz NJ. Occult perineural tumor infiltration of the trigeminal nerve. Diagnostic considerations. *J Neuroophthalmol* 1997;17: 170–177.
138. Boerman RH, Maassen EM, Joosten J, et al. Trigeminal neuropathy secondary to perineural invasion of head and neck carcinomas. *Neurology* 1999;53:213–216.
139. Talmi YP, Horowitz Z, Wolf M, et al. Delayed metastases in skin cancer of the head and neck: the case of the "known primary." *Ann Plast Surg* 1999;42: 289–292.
140. McCord MW, Mendenhall WM, Parsons JT, et al. Skin cancer of the head and neck with clinical perineural invasion. *Int J Radiat Oncol Biol Phys* 2000;47:89–93.

Radiation Therapy Technique

141. Lovett R, Perez CA, Shapiro DL, et al. External irradiation of epithelial skin cancer. *Int J Radiat Oncol Biol Phys* 1990;19:235–242.
142. Mendenhall WM, Million RR, Mancuso AA, et al. Carcinoma of the skin. In: Million RR, Cassisi NJ, eds. *Management of head and neck cancer: a multidisciplinary approach,* 2nd ed. Philadelphia: Lippincott, 1994:643–691.
143. Amdur RJ, Kalbaugh KJ, Ewald LM, et al. Radiation therapy for skin cancer near the eye: kilovoltage x-rays versus electrons. *Int J Radiat Oncol Biol Phys* 1992;23:769–779.
144. Bova FJ. Treatment planning for irradiation of head and neck cancer. In: Million RR, Cassisi NJ, eds. *Management of head and neck cancer: a multidisciplinary approach,* 2nd ed. Philadelphia: Lippincott, 1994:291—309.

CHAPTER 25

Melanoma of the Head and Neck

Ann M. Gillenwater and Robert M. Byers

Each year, there are more than 40,000 cases of malignant melanoma diagnosed in the United States. In 1999, more than 9,000 people in this country died from this disease (1). Although these numbers are small compared with those for the more common malignancies of the lung, breast, and colon, the incidence of malignant melanoma in the United States has been increasing by approximately 7% per year. The risk for developing malignant melanoma was estimated to be 1 in 1,500 in 1935; by 1980, it was 1 in 250, and for the year 2001, it is estimated to be 1 in 75 (2). Increases in the incidence of melanoma have been reported from other parts of the world as well (3). The cause of the recent rise in incidence has not been fully elucidated, but may be related to increased sun exposure or to improved detection. In addition, melanoma often strikes the young; the median age at diagnosis in the United States is 53, and 25% of cases are diagnosed in persons younger than 40 years old (4). Melanoma is the sixth most common malignancy diagnosed in adolescents between the ages of 15 and 19 in the United States (5). Approximately 60% of the persons who die from melanoma are younger than 60 years, resulting in a significant loss of potential life years (6).

Malignant melanoma is usually readily curable if detected early. It is therefore increasingly important for physicians to maintain knowledge and skill in the diagnosis and treatment of this malignancy. Since primary lesions occur in the head and neck area approximately 25% to 30% of the time, it is particularly important for otolaryngology–head and neck surgeons to keep abreast of the latest breakthroughs and recommendations for management of melanoma patients (7). This chapter describes the natural history and presentation of head and neck melanoma and makes recommendations for the diagnostic evaluation and treatment of patients with each stage of the disease. Current research efforts and clinical trials aimed at the prevention and treatment of advanced stage and recurrent disease are described.

SKIN ANATOMY

The skin is divided into two layers: the epidermis, which is composed predominately of keratinocytes, and the dermis, which is made up of connective tissue. The basement membrane separates the two layers (Fig. 25.1). The epidermis is a stratified squamous epithelium of varying thicknesses derived from the ectoderm. Keratinocytes located in the basal layer actively divide; as they differentiate and become keratinized, they migrate toward the surface. The dermis is made up of ground substance interspersed with connective tissue fibers (collagen, reticular and elastic fibers) and many cell types, including fibrocytes, macrophages, mast cells, and inflammatory cells. The dermis has two layers also. The papillary layer is located just deep to the basement membrane; the reticular layer contains more intermediate filaments.

Melanocytes are located between the keratinocytes in the basal layer of the epidermis. They produce melanin and supply it to the keratinocytes via cellular processes that interdigitate in intercellular spaces between individual keratinocytes.

NATURAL HISTORY

Epidemiology

The cause of malignant melanoma is multifactorial. Interactions between genetic factors and environmental factors such as ultraviolet light exposure are complex and as yet incompletely understood. Melanoma occurs most often in fair-skinned per-

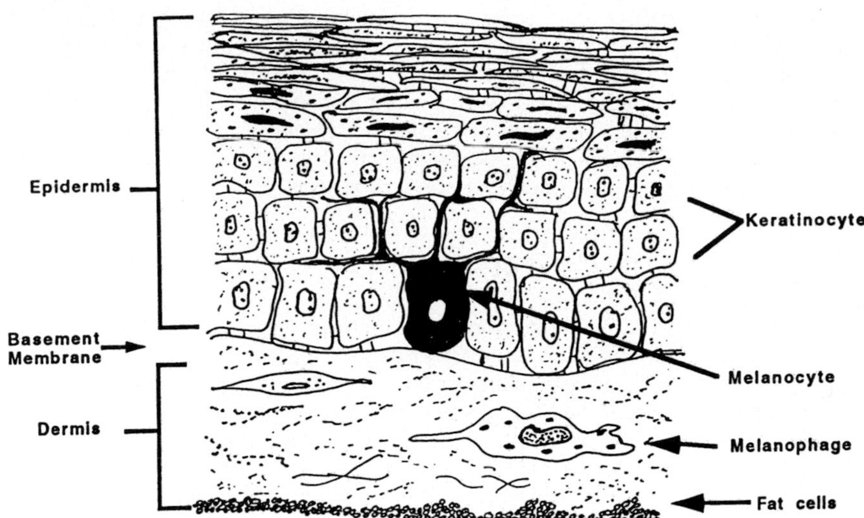

Figure 25.1 The melanocytes are located along the basal layer of the epidermis. Dendritic processes interdigitate between the keratinocytes, supplying them with melanin. (From Wilborn WH, Hyde BM, Montes LF, eds. *Adult skin. Scanning electron microscopy of normal and abnormal human skin.* Deerfield Beach, FL: VCH, 1985, with permission.)

sons of Celtic or Nordic background. Blonde or red hair, blue eyes, tendency toward freckling, and inability to tan are characteristics of people who are most susceptible to melanoma. Geography also plays an important role: prevalence of melanoma by region grows with decreases in latitude. These risk factors have been well established in many epidemiologic surveys and clearly are closely related to the degree of solar exposure.

Melanomas can occur at any cutaneous (or mucosal) site, but there is a predilection for specific sites in different population groups. Jelfs et al. (8) analyzed data on cutaneous malignant melanoma patients from Australia in cancer registries for the year 1989. In this cohort, melanoma was found more commonly on the trunk in males and in the lower limbs in females. Melanoma of the head and neck was more frequent in males than females at a ratio of 1.74. Fifty-two percent of melanomas were thinner than 0.76 mm. Thick lesions were more common in the head and neck region than in other regions of the body.

Although malignant melanoma is predominately a disease of fair-skinned races, it does occur in other ethnic groups. A review of melanoma in African Americans revealed that although its incidence was small, the stage of presentation was more advanced: 77% of patients had a Clark's level IV or higher lesion, and 50% of the lesions were thicker than 3 mm. In 62% of the patients, the melanoma was located on the foot; in 50% it was located in the head and neck region (9).

The occurrence of melanoma in prepubertal children is unusual. A review by Chun et al. (10) of the Puerto Rico Cancer registry revealed only seven cases of melanoma occurring in persons younger than 16 years of age between 1973 and 1990.

Risk Factors

Exposure to ultraviolet radiation is the major cause of cutaneous melanoma. Most epidemiologic studies show an association between sun exposure and development of melanoma. Intermittent exposure to sun appears to be more deleterious than chronic exposure. A history of sunburn, especially at a young age, is associated with increased risk of melanoma (11). The increased incidence of melanoma in people who live close to the equator is also indirect evidence for the role of solar radiation in the development of the disease. Because the development of nevi is thought to be directly related to the degree of sun exposure, the presence of multiple nevi in a person may be a useful biologic marker indicating a susceptibility to develop melanoma.

Several interesting papers have discussed the role of sunscreen use in the development of melanoma. A case-control study performed in Sweden demonstrated that sunscreen use did not protect against the development of malignant melanoma (12). In contrast, there appeared to be an increased risk of melanoma in people who did use sunscreens. A study conducted by the European Organization for Research and Treatment of Cancer (EORTC) Melanoma Cooperative Group produced similar results. Again, sunscreen had no protective effect against melanoma; in fact, an increased risk of melanoma was found with sunscreen use in this study also, especially sunscreen containing psoralens (13). It is suggested that the ability of sunscreens to prevent sunburn may actually encourage longer exposure to ultraviolet (UV) radiation and thus actually increase the risk of melanoma development. Animal studies have supported the epidemiologic findings. Sunscreens applied to mice prior to UV radiation exposure had a protective effect for the development of sunburn but did not alter the incidence of melanoma formation (14).

Another factor complicating this issue is the impact of the wavelength of UV radiation on the pathogenesis of melanoma. Because UVB radiation (at 280- to 320-nm frequency) is the primary cause of most sunburns and is absorbed strongly by DNA, investigators have focused on this region of the UV spectrum as the most likely causative factor for development of melanoma (15). However, evidence is now accumulating that suggests that UVA radiation (320- to 400-nm frequency) may also play an important role in the etiology of melanoma (15–18). If substantiated, the causative role of UVA radiation has substantial implications for the epidemiologic assessment and prevention efforts for melanoma. Sunscreen products were developed to prevent sunburn, and therefore first protected mainly against UVB radiation. Although chemicals to protect against UVA radiation were introduced in sunscreens in 1989, many products only provided partial protection, and the sun protection factor (SPF) only provides an indication of the protection against sunburn, not UVA radiation (15). In addition, most of the tanning lamps in current use emit almost 100% UVA radiation (19). Approximately 25 million people in the United States use sun beds or sunlamps each year (20). Epidemiologic evaluations comparing the use of sun beds and sunlamps to melanoma incidence have produced equivocal results, although several have documented a positive correlation between the use of tanning lamps and the development of melanoma (15,20–22). A population-based, matched case-control study demonstrated a significantly increased odds ratio [1.8; 95% confidence interval (CI), 1.2–2.7] for development of melanoma with repeated use of sun beds (22). In light of these findings, it would be prudent to recommend that persons with fair skin or other potential risk factors for melanoma abstain from using sunlamps until further evidence regarding the possible association with melanoma development is obtained.

Other risk factors that are currently under investigation include genetic susceptibility, dietary composition, and socioeconomic factors. It is estimated that 5% to 12% of people diagnosed with malignant melanoma have a family history of the disease (23,24). Many familial cases are associated with the development of numerous dysplastic nevi in the familial atypical multiple-mole melanoma syndrome (25). Multiple primary lesions are more common in familial cases; 17% of such cases in one series displayed multiple primary lesions (26). The observed familial risk is greater than that which would be expected from similar environmental risks and the hereditary factor of skin coloring.

Because of the observed clustering of cases of melanoma within families, the existence of a major susceptibility gene was hypothesized. The gene that encodes the $p16^{INK4}$ protein [also known as cyclin-dependent kinase inhibitor 2A(CDKN2A)], which is an important cell cycle regulator located on chromosomal region 9p21, has been identified as a possible tumor suppressor gene involved in the initiation or progression of melanoma (27). Mutation or inactivation of $p16^{INK4}$ has been detected in virtually every melanoma cell line, whether derived from familial or sporadic cases. Germline mutations in this gene have been identified in 30% to 50% of families with multiple cases of melanoma (28). In addition, families who carry a $p16^{INK4}$ mutation have a significantly higher risk of developing pancreatic cancer (29–31). Germline mutations have been identified in the gene encoding cyclin-dependent kinase 4 (CDK4) in three melanoma kindreds. Mutation of this gene, which lies on chromosome 12q14, likely occurs in only a very small percentage of families with melanoma (31). Further investigation is required to determine the roles played by these genes and others in melanoma development in the context of other epidemiologic risk factors.

Data on the role of other factors involved in the development of melanoma are limited. Dietary studies have implicated increased consumption of alcohol as a risk factor for melanoma (32). The role of other dietary substances such as polyunsaturated fats, zinc, selenium, ascorbic acid, and vitamins A and D remains uncertain (33). Malignant melanoma is seen more commonly in immunodeficient people; this suggests a role for local immune surveillance defects in the development of this tumor. Experimental studies in mice showing decreased skin immunity after UV irradiation and increased tumor growth in irradiated and immunodeficient skin support this concept (34).

Patterns of Spread

The clinical course of patients who develop melanoma can vary widely. Melanoma arises in the skin, but can spread through the dermal lymphatic channels as well as via blood. Satellite lesions (defined as melanoma lesions that arise within 2 cm of the index primary lesion) and metastases in-transit (cutaneous or dermal nodules within draining lymphatic channels) are not uncommon with this tumor. Metastases to the draining lymph node basins are frequent with more advanced lesions. Cutaneous melanoma of the head and neck does not always progress in an orderly fashion from the primary lesion to the nodule drainage basin and then on to distant sites. Sometimes, melanoma cells travel directly to distant sites and there produce the first manifestation of metastatic spread. The advent of distant visceral metastases carries a grave prognosis.

CLINICAL PRESENTATION

Clinical recognition of the features typical of melanoma in skin lesions is the key to diagnosis of this tumor. A pigmented lesion with an irregular border or surface and variegated coloring should lead the physician to suspect melanoma (Fig. 25.2). Up to 70% of cutaneous malignant melanomas arise in preexisting moles; a recent change in the size, shape, texture, color, or behavior of a mole is characteristic. The development of nodularity, itching, stinging, erythema, bleeding, or ulceration in a preexisting nevus suggests malignant melanoma. Melanomas may be nonpigmented also. Malignant melanoma primary lesions are most often confused with benign nevi. Benign nevi tend to remain smaller and more regular and do not change in appearance. Other items on the differential diagnosis list include pigmented basal cell carcinomas and seborrheic keratoses. The halo nevus, a benign mole surrounded by a ring of hypopigmented tissue, can also be confused with malignant melanoma.

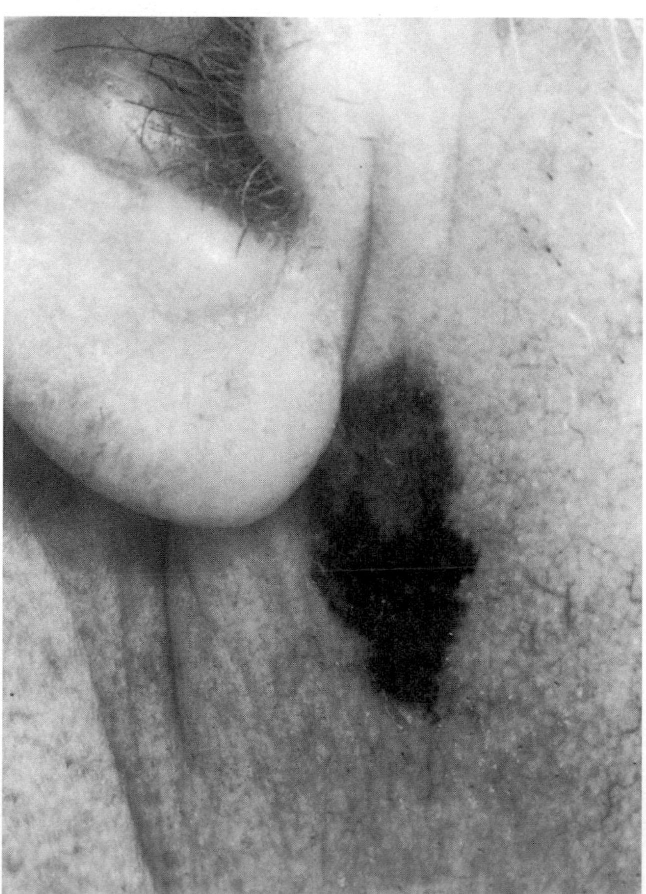

Figure 25.2 Malignant melanoma primary lesion. Note the variegated border.

Diagnostic Staging and Evaluation

The definitive diagnosis of malignant melanoma is based on histologic analysis of the lesion. An excisional biopsy of the suspected primary tumor is the method of choice; it allows accurate identification of the tumor thickness and depth of penetration while avoiding any transgression of tumor boundaries. However, an excisional biopsy may not be feasible if the lesion is too large or located near vital structures such as the eyelid or lip. In this situation, a small incisional or punch biopsy that reaches the full depth of the lesion is indicated. A superficial shave biopsy should not be performed for pigmented lesions, because it makes accurate evaluation of the depth of the lesion impossible. The thickness of a localized primary melanoma is the single most important prognostic factor (35). Thus, because the definitive treatment and overall prognosis of the patient with localized disease depends on the depth of the melanoma primary tumor, a shave biopsy can irreparably interfere with the clinical pathologic evaluation and treatment planning.

STAGING

Once a diagnosis of melanoma is made, the patient requires further evaluation for staging. Staging of the primary tumor is extremely important because of the strong correlation with patient outcome. The melanoma staging system was recently revised by the American Joint Committee on Cancer (AJCC) (36) and is presented in Tables 25.1 and 25.2. Several major changes were introduced. First, although the new staging classification still uses primary tumor thickness to differentiate between T stages, the Breslow microstaging system (37), which uses a quantitative measurement of the vertical height of the melanoma from the granular layer to the point of deepest infiltration, is now the major determinant. The Clark microstaging system (38), which qualitatively categorizes the depth of tumor penetration into distinct histologic layers, is used only to subclassify T1 lesions. The Breslow and Clark microstaging systems are presented in Table 25.3. Second, the presence or absence of ulceration has been introduced as a major criterion for T stage classification. Third, the upper threshold for T1 lesions has been raised from 0.75 mm deep in the 1997 version to 1.0 mm in the current system, and the threshold for T levels is defined as even integers of 1.0, 2.0, and 4.0 mm.

The classification of regional metastases has also changed considerable in the new staging system. Nodal stage is now determined by the number of metastatic nodes, rather than by the size of the nodes. In addition, the nodal groupings are subdivided as micrometastases, which are detected pathologically, or macroscopic metastases, which are clinically evident and confirmed pathologically, or exhibit extracapsular extension of disease. The distant metastases classification has also been altered, to separate lung metastases from other visceral metastases, due to evidence showing increased length of survival with metastatic disease only to the lung. Changes were also introduced in the overall stage groupings. In the most recent system, patients with localized disease are grouped as stage I or II, those with regional metastases are now stage III, and patients with distant metastases are classified as stage IV. The stage groupings also now separate clinical from pathologic staging, and incorporate information obtained from pathologic assessment of resected nodes in the staging system. A description of the new staging system, including a discussion of alterations from the previous system and the rationale for these changes, is presented by Balch et al. (36).

TABLE 25.1 Melanoma TNM Classification

T classification	Thickness	Ulceration status
T1	≤1.0 mm	a: without ulceration and level II/III b: with ulceration or level IV/V
T2	1.01–2.0 mm	a: without ulceration b: with ulceration
T3	2.01–4.0 mm	a: without ulceration b: with ulceration
T4	>4.0 mm	a: without ulceration b: with ulceration
N classification	**No. of metastatic nodes**	**Nodal metastatic mass**
N1	1 node	a: micrometastasis[a] b: macrometastasis[b]
N2	2–3 nodes	a: micrometastasis[a] b: macrometastasis[b] c: in transit met(s) satellite(s) without metastatic nodes
N3	4 or more metastatic nodes, or matted nodes, or in transit met(s)/satellite(s) with metastatic nodes(s)	
M classification	**Site**	**Serum lactate dehydrogenase**
M1	Distant skin, subcutaneous, or nodal mets	Normal
M1b	Lung metastases	Normal
M1c	All other visceral metastases	Normal
	Any distant metastasis	Elevated

[a]Micrometastases are diagnosed after sentinel or elective lymphadenectomy.
[b]Macrometastases are defined as clinically detectable nodal metastases confirmed by therapeutic lymphadenectomy or when nodal metastasis exhibits gross extracapsular extension.

TABLE 25.2 Proposed Stage Groupings for Cutaneous Melanoma

	Clinical staging[a]			Pathologic staging[b]		
	T	N	M	T	N	M
0	Tis	N0	M0	Tis	N0	M0
IA	T1a	N0	M0	T1a	N0	M0
IB	T1b	N0	M0	T1b	N0	M0
	T2a	N0	M0	T2a	N0	M0
IIA	T2b	N0	M0	T2b	N0	M0
	T3a	N0	M0	T3a	N0	M0
IIB	T3b	N0	M0	T3b	N0	M0
	T4a	N0	M0	T4a	N0	M0
IIC	T4b	N0	M0	T4b	N0	M0
III[c]	Any T	N1	M0			
		N2				
		N3				
IIIA				T1-4a	N1a	M0
				T1-4a	N2a	M0
IIIB				T1-4b	N1a	M0
				T1-4b	N2a	M0
				T1-4a	N1b	M0
				T1-4a	N2b	M0
				T1-4a/b	N2c	M0
IIIC				T1-4b	N1b	M0
				T1-4b	N2b	M0
				Any T	N3	M0
IV	Any T	Any N	Any M1	Any T	Any N	Any M1

[a]Clinical staging includes microstaging of the primary melanoma and clinical/radiologic evaluation for metastases. By convention, it should be used after complete excision of the primary melanoma with clinical assessment for regional and distant metastases.
[b]Pathologic staging includes microstaging of the primary melanoma and pathologic information about the regional lymph nodes after partial or complete lymphadenectomy. Pathologic staging 0 or stage IA patients are the exception; they do not require pathologic evaluation of their lymph nodes.
[c]There are no stage III subgroups for clinical staging.
Source: Adapted from Balch CM, Buzaid AC, Soong S-J, et al. Final version of the American Joint Committee on Cancer Staging System for cutaneous melanoma. *J Clin Oncol* 2001;19:3635.

TABLE 25.3 Melanoma Microstaging Systems

Clark's qualitative system	
Level I	*In situ;* all tumor cells are within the epidermis, superficial to the basement membrane
Level II	Tumor involves but does not completely fill the papillary dermis
Level III	Tumor fills the interface between the papillary and reticular dermis
Level IV	Tumor cells invade the reticular dermis
Level V	Tumor involves the subcutaneous tissue
Breslow's quantitative system	
Lesion thickness cutoff values	
≤0.75 mm	
0.76–1.49 mm	
1.50–3.99 mm	
≥0.4 mm	

Source: Clark's qualitative system is adapted from Clark WH Jr, From L, Bernardino EA, et al. The histogenesis and biologic behavior of primary human malignant melanomas of the skin. *Cancer Res* 1989;29:905. Breslow's quantitative system is adapted from Breslow A. Thickness, cross-sectional areas, and depth of invasion in the prognosis of cutaneous melanoma. *Am Surg* 1970;172:902.

EVALUATION

When head and neck cutaneous melanoma is diagnosed, a full-body skin examination should be performed to locate any other melanotic lesions. A complete head and neck examination should be conducted to detect and evaluate satellite lesions or in-transit or nodal metastases. A thorough skin and scalp evaluation is sometimes difficult if the hair is thick; however, shaving the head is not recommended. Recommendations for the diagnostic evaluation for metastatic disease according to stage of disease at presentation are presented in Table 25.2. Full-body computed tomography (CT) scans are not cost-effective because of their very low diagnostic yields in the asymptomatic patient with stage 0 or stage IA disease. If there is any clinical doubt about the presence of a cervical lymphadenopathy in patients with T1b or deeper primary lesions, high-resolution ultrasound or a CT scan of the neck should be performed. The use of lymphoscintigraphy and sentinel lymph node biopsy (SLNB) to determine the status of regional disease is becoming increasingly accepted as standard of care for patients with melanoma. The risks and benefits of this technique are discussed later. For a patient presenting with stage III or IV disease, the staging workup (in the absence of guiding symptoms) should consist of a chest x-ray, screening blood tests including lactate dehydrogenase (LDH), high-resolution ultrasound or CT scan of the head and neck, CT scans of the chest, abdomen, and pelvis, and magnetic resonance imaging (MRI) of the brain (39,40).

Positron emission tomography (PET) with ^{18}F-fluorodeoxyglucose (FDG) is a more recent imaging technique that is being increasingly employed for the assessment of disease burden in cancer patients. The use of FDG-PET for assessment of occult regional and distant metastases has been investigated for patients initially presenting with melanoma (41,42). At this time, however, data are lacking regarding the sensitivity and specificity of PET scans, compared to clinical evaluation and traditional imaging modalities for the detection of occult metastatic disease (43).

Which lymph node groups are most likely to contain microscopic metastatic disease can often be determined by the anatomic location of the primary tumor and the known patterns of lymphatic drainage from the skin of the head and neck (Fig. 25.3). The median plane divides the areas drained by each side of the body; midline lesions can drain to either side or bilaterally. A coronal plane drawn at the level of the external auditory canals separates the anterior and posterior lymphatic drainage beds. Those lesions anterior to the tragus drain to the periauricular and parotid nodes, the facial nodes, the submaxillary and submental nodes, and the jugular nodes. Lesions posterior to the tragus drain to the retroauricular and occipital nodes as well as the spinal accessory and posterior triangle nodal groups. Although it has been suggested that these clinical predictions of the sites of metastatic spread are unreliable (44), others report good results using this approach. A retrospective study of 106 patients who electively underwent neck dissections according to clinically predicted drainage patters revealed only three recurrences of disease outside the dissected field over a 6-year follow-up period (45). In a prospectively documented series of 169 patients, the pathologically positive nodes were found in clinically predicted nodal groups in 92.3% of cases (46), lending further support for the high degree of correlation of clinically predicted patterns of lymphatic spread with pathologic distribution of nodal metastases.

Radionuclide lymphoscintigraphy is a technique being investigated to improve the clinical prediction of the lymphatic drainage basins at risk. For patients with no clinical or radiographic evidence of nodal metastases, a radionuclide can be injected into the dermis at the primary tumor site, and a scan or a cutaneous probe can be used to detect the radiolabeled lymphatic channels and primary echelon nodal groups. Technetium Tc-99m antimony trisulfide colloid or technetium Tc-99m human serum albumin are the agents most frequently used.

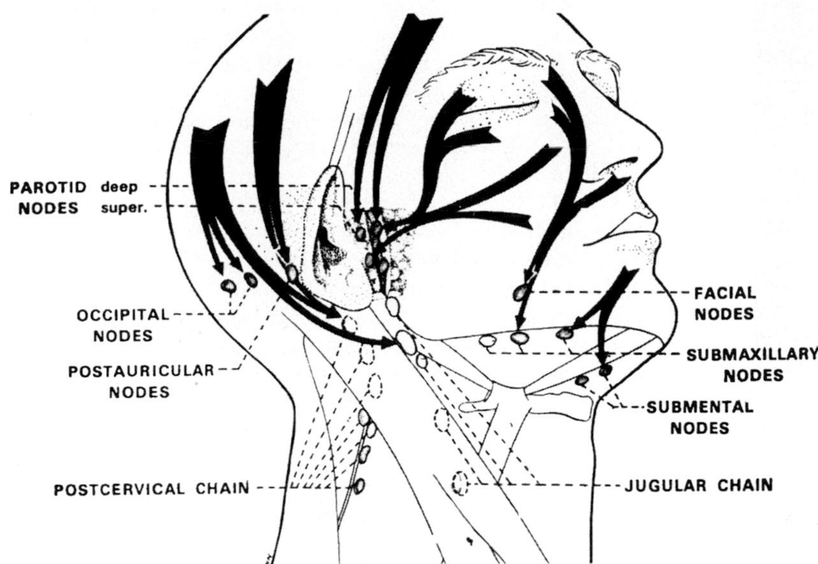

Figure 25.3 Cutaneous lymphatic drainage patterns from the scalp and face. (From Byers RM, Medina JE, Wolf PF. Regional node dissection of the head and neck. In: Balch CM, ed. *Pigment cell. Surgical approaches to cutaneous melanoma*, vol 7. Basel, Switzerland: Karger, 1985, with permission.)

O'Brien et al. (47) identified a sentinel node in 95 of 97 scans using this technique. These authors noted that in 22% of the patients, a sentinel node was identified outside the parotid and major neck nodal regions. In 34% of the patients, the scans identified a sentinel node outside of the clinically predicted nodal drainage basin. However, the clinical importance of these radiographically identified sentinel nodes is undetermined. Even so, this technique may improve our ability to tailor treatment for individual patients. An advantage of performing preoperative lymphoscintigraphy prior to SLNB is that it allows the surgeon to counsel the patient about the likely incision sites and potential complications, such as potential injury to the facial nerve during assessment of a sentinel lymph node (SLN) in the parotid bed. Further study is needed to determine the role of preoperative lymphoscintigraphy in the evaluation of patients with head and neck melanoma in the N0 stage.

Sentinel lymph node biopsy has become an increasingly accepted modality for assessing the status of lymphatics in patients with stage II melanoma outside the head and neck. Several large series documented that SLNB is an efficient way to identify patients who would benefit from a lymph node dissection (48–51). Sentinel node biopsy results can provide prognostic information on patients by revealing microscopic lymph node involvement, while sparing the majority of patients the morbidity of an elective lymph node dissection (ELND).

The rationale for the procedure is based on the concept of an orderly progression of metastatic disease to a primary first-echelon node, the "sentinel node," and from this node to the secondary echelon nodes without skip metastases. If the SLNB is negative for melanoma, theoretically there should be no further metastases within the nodal basin. If the SLNB is positive for melanoma, the patient has a higher risk of additional nodal metastatic disease, and ultimately distant metastases.

CLINICAL MANAGEMENT

The management of malignant melanoma requires the physician to address the primary lesion, the draining lymphatics, and potential distant metastases. The patient's disease stage dictates the extent of the treatment. Complete surgical excision of the primary lesion is mandatory. Table 25.4 outlines the treatment guidelines as practiced at the University of Texas M. D. Anderson Cancer Center.

Surgical Margins and Techniques

The optimal width of the margin of normal tissue to be excised with the primary tumor has been a topic of contention over the years. In the early 1900s, William Sampson Handley (52) described a postmortem examination in a case of metastatic disease from a primary melanoma of the heel. Although Handley was unable to document the extent of the disease around the primary lesion, after his report was published wide excision margins (5 cm or greater) became the standard in the first half of the 20th century. The microstaging systems developed by Clark et al. (38) and Breslow (37) solidified the relationship between tumor thickness and prognosis, and allowed the extent of surgical margins to be decided in a systematic fashion, based on the depth of the lesion.

What constitutes adequate width of surgical margins for primary lesions has been addressed in the reports of several large series of patients with melanoma. In a prospective randomized trial performed by the World Health Organization, wherein 612 patients with primary lesions <2 mm thick were randomly

TABLE 25.4 Treatment Guidelines

Stage	Treatment
I	Wide local excision (WLE) primary

II	WLE primary
	Lymphatics
	  Sentinel node biopsy
	  XRT
	  ELND
	  Observation
	Consider adjuvant systemic therapy for pT4

III	WLE primary Neck dissection Consider postoperative XRT Adjuvant systemic therapy
IV	WLE primary Neck dissection (if not N0) Systemic therapy Site-directed surgery or XRT Supportive care

ELND, elective lymph node dissection; XRT, x-ray therapy.

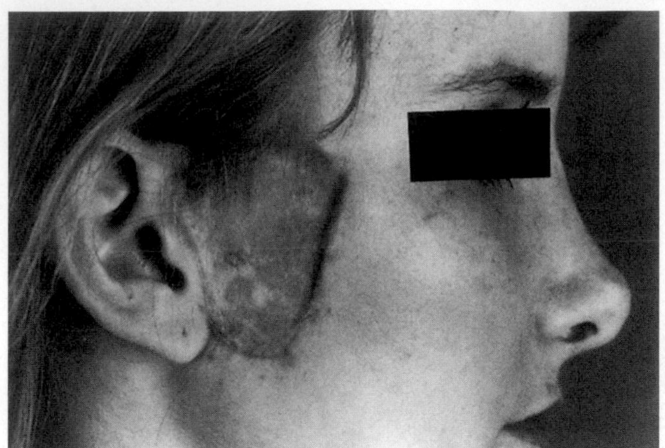

Figure 25.4 This patient had a malignant melanoma primary tumor located just anterior to the tragus. An excessive amount of normal tissue was resected from the cheek, leaving an unnecessarily poor cosmetic result.

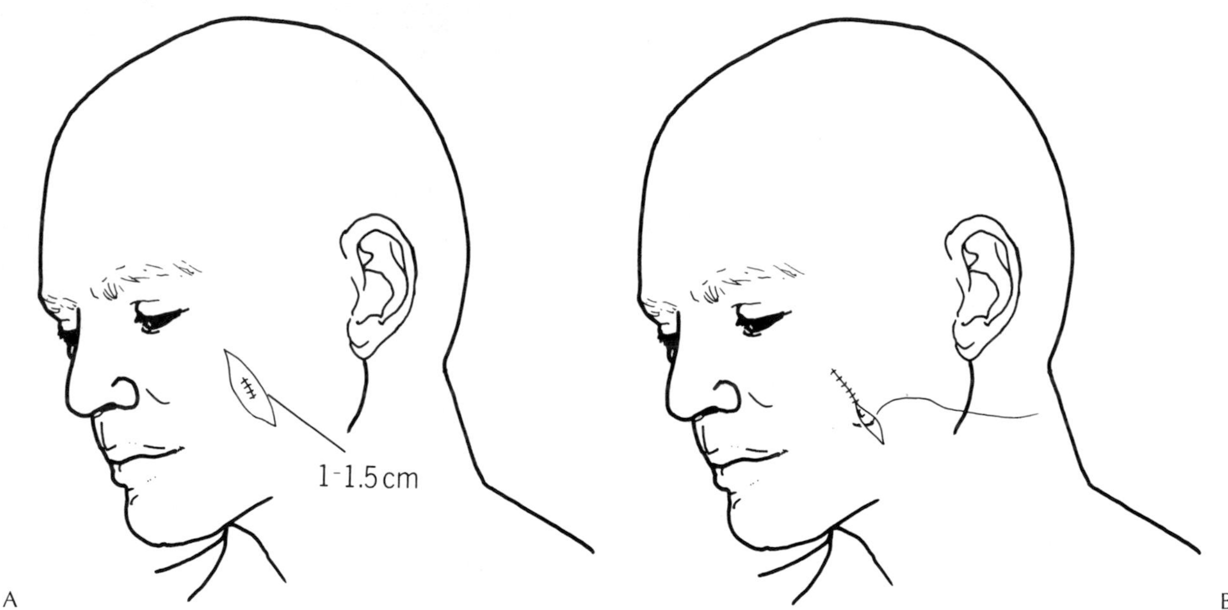

Figure 25.5 **A:** A 1- to 1.5-cm excision suitable for primary closure. **B:** Primary closure. Note proper alignment in relaxed skin tension line, thus minimizing deformity.

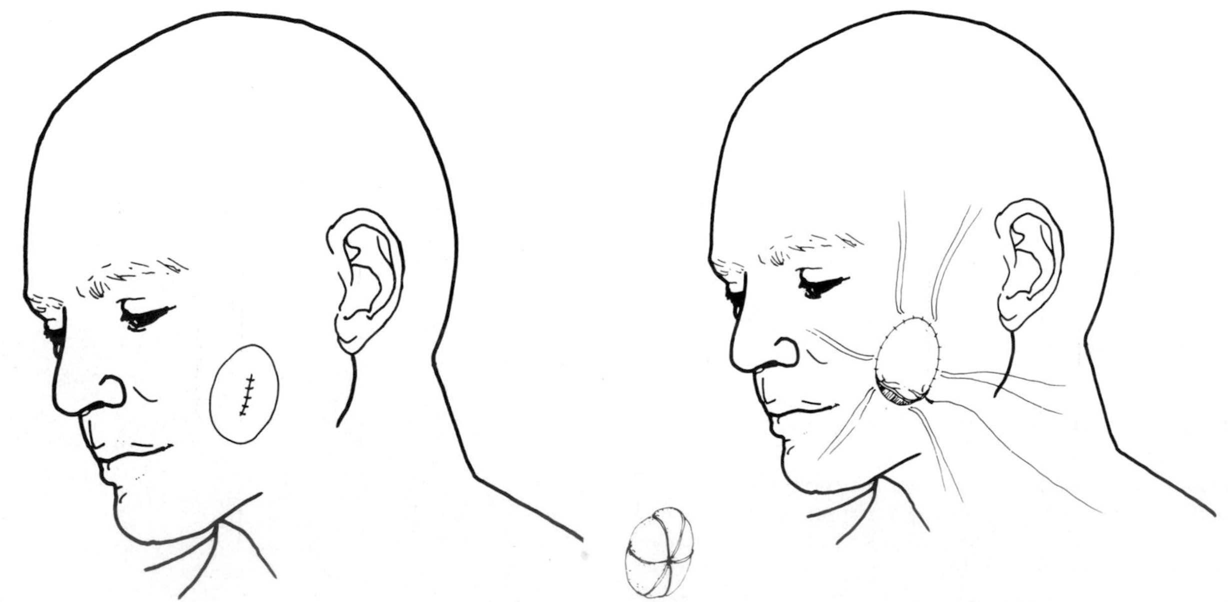

Figure 25.6 **A:** Wide excision that probably would not be suitable for primary closure. More appropriate closure should be local flap reconstruction or skin graft. **B:** Note skin graft placement with gauze bolstered with overtying of sutures.

assigned to undergo primary tumor excision with either 1-cm or 3-cm margins, the survival rates were identical in both groups (53). The authors of this study concluded that for melanoma lesions <2 mm thick (and especially for those <1 mm thick), a surgical excision margin of 1 cm was adequate. A multiinstitution prospective randomized surgical trial reported by Balch et al. (54) compared the excision margins in tumors of intermediate thickness (1 to 4 mm). No significant difference in locoregional recurrence rates, in-transit metastases, or overall 5-year survival rates were found between patients whose lesions were excised with a 2-cm surgical margin and those whose lesions were removed with a 4-cm margin. Patients whose surgery involved 4-cm margins, however, needed more skin grafting and had longer hospital stays than those in the other group. The conclusion reached after this evaluation was that 2-cm margins were adequate for primary melanoma lesions of intermediate thickness (54).

It should be noted that these recommendations were given for melanomas in all body sites; in the head and neck region, anatomic and cosmetic consideration may preclude 2-cm margins or even 1-cm margins. The width of the surgical margins should be uniform. It does not benefit the patient whose closest margin is at the eyelid or ear to take a 2-cm margin from the cheek (Fig. 25.4).

When possible, surgical defects created during wide local excision of a melanoma should be closed primarily (Fig. 25.5). If primary closure is not practical, local flap reconstruction or skin grafting is necessary (Figs. 25.6 and 25.7). Specific solutions for particular lesions are multiple. For example, melanomas of the external ear are usually adequately treated with a partial amputation of the pinna. A small lesion of the helix may be adequately excised with a wedge resection and primary closure (Fig. 25.8). Only when an external ear lesion is extensive, recurrent, or centrally located should the entire pinna be removed. Many melanomas of the nasal skin are adequately removed by excision of the skin and underlying subcutaneous tissues, preserving the underlying perichondrium and/or periosteum. A full-thickness skin graft can then be used to cover the defect. When a large area of nasal skin is affected, it is preferable to excise the skin and subcutaneous tissue of the entire aesthetic unit of the nose and replace it with a full-thickness skin graft. The cosmetic result of this operation is usually good.

In areas such as the scalp or lower neck, a 2-cm margin can be taken around intermediate and deep lesions without causing undue morbidity. In more superficial lesions, a 1-cm margin is usually adequate. In those lesions that do require a wide excision, split-thickness skin grafting provides excellent coverage and reasonable appearance (Fig. 25.7).

If there is any question as to the adequacy of the surgical margin, flap reconstruction should be delayed until permanent pathology reports are obtained. Lentigo maligna and lentigo maligna melanomas often have extensive subclinical horizontal extension of atypical melanocytes. In patients with these pathologic subtypes, strong consideration should be given to skin grafting or delayed reconstruction after excision of the primary.

Management of Regional Lymphatics

Appropriate management of the regional lymphatics with potential to contain occult metastatic disease in patients with malignant melanoma depends on two factors: (a) the location of the lymph nodes at risk to contain microscopic disease, and (b) the risk-to-benefit ratio of each management modality. In clinically N0 patients, management of the regional lymphatics is based on the T stage of the primary, particularly the invasive depth of the primary lesion and the presence or absence of ulceration. Primary melanomas can be separated into three groups: thin—Tis, T1a (≤1.0 mm, no ulceration, and Clark's level <III); intermediate— T1b (≤1.0 mm, with ulceration or Clark's level IV or V); and T2 or T3 (1.01–4 mm), and deep (>4 mm). For patients with thin primary lesions, the risk of regional metastasis is low, and ELNDs or SLNBs are not warranted. After wide excision of the primary tumor, treatment of these patients is limited to observation.

Management of the regional lymphatics in patients with intermediate primary lesions (stage Ib and II disease) remains highly controversial. This subgroup of patients has a comparatively high risk of regional metastasis but a lower risk of distant metastasis (55). Many head and neck surgeons recommend ELND for these patients, reasoning that removal of microscopic disease in the neck will improve regional control and decrease the incidence of distant metastasis, thereby leading to improved overall survival rates. This argument is based on the theory that melanoma progresses in a stepwise fashion from the primary tumor through the draining lymphatics and from there on to distant metastases. However, the efficacy of ELND in improving locoregional disease control and patient survival rates has not been proven. Despite the publication of several retrospective analyses and four prospective studies, the role of ELND for the management of patients with stage I and stage II disease is still unclear (56–63). These large studies have addressed the issue of ELND in melanomas from all body sites; fewer studies have focused on the prognostic benefit of ELND for patients with head and neck melanoma.

One of the largest series of patients with head and neck melanoma was reported by O'Brien et al. (63). In this retrospective analysis, ELNDs were performed in 234 patients (the exact

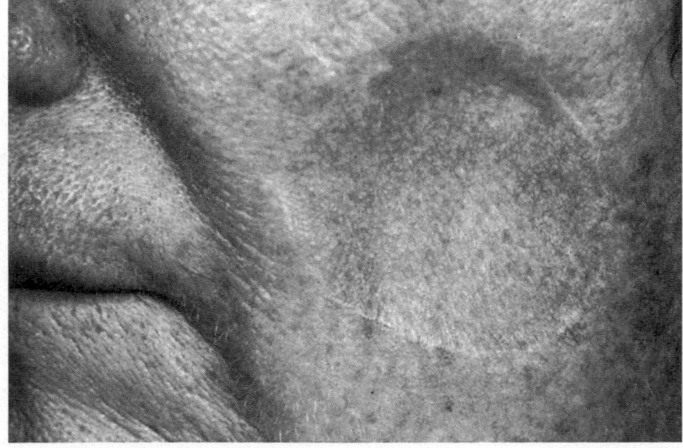
C

Figure 25.6 (***continued***). **C:** Example of long-term result of wide excision site repair by skin graft.

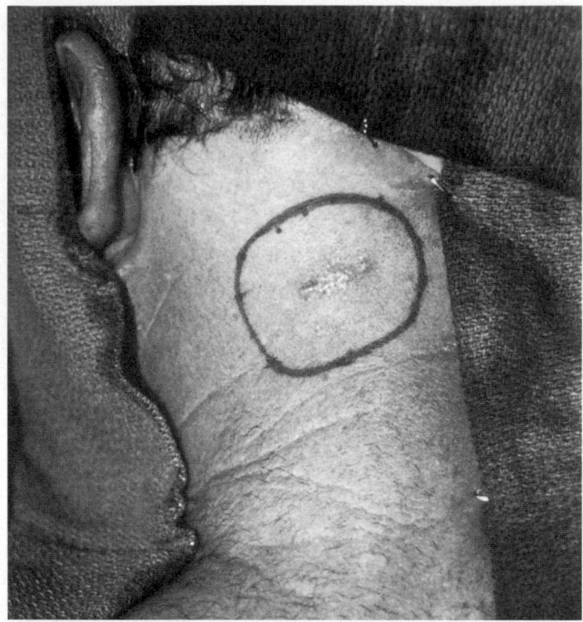

A

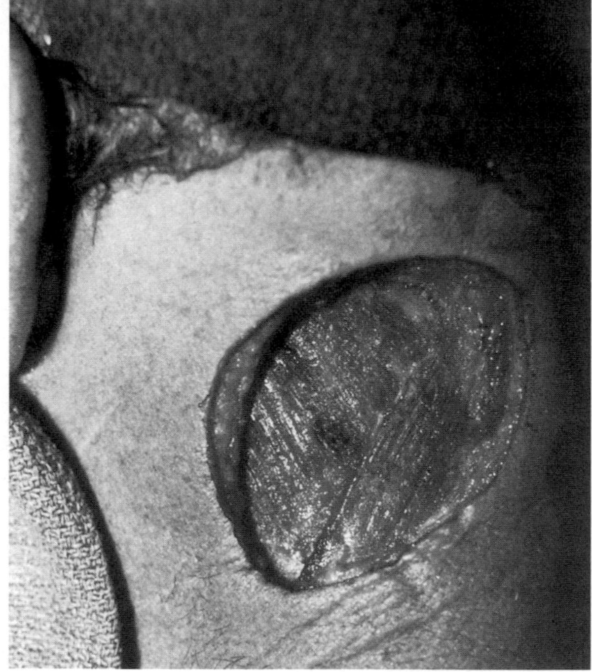

B

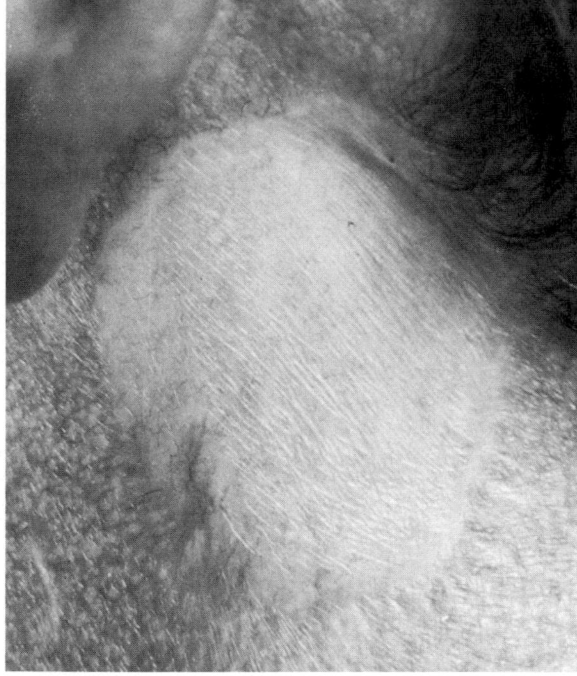

C

Figure 25.7 **A:** Melanoma posterior-lateral neck proposed wide excision. **B:** Wide excision of lesion in **A**. Note depth of excision includes the fascia overlying the underlying neck muscle. **C:** Skin graft repair of lesion shown in **A** and **B**.

thickness of the primary lesions in all of these patients was not clearly delineated). Histologic studies showed that 7% of lymph nodes were positive for disease despite being thought disease-free upon clinical examination. In a univariate analysis of the data, 76% of the patients undergoing ELNDs remained alive at 10 years, whereas only 57% of patients who did not have ELNDs remained alive. However, in a multivariate analysis, ELND was no longer significant in terms of patient survival. Thus, it is still unclear whether ELND in patients with intermediate melanomas of the head and neck provides any improvement in locoregional disease control or survival time as compared with expectant management of the draining lymphatics.

Certainly, ELND is an effective technique to stage the extent of regional metastases and to thereby provide important prognostic information that helps physicians identify patients who might benefit from adjuvant therapy. However, the benefits derived from accurate regional staging must be balanced against the potential morbidity of the procedure.

A more recent but increasingly utilized option for management of the clinically negative neck is intraoperative lymphatic mapping and SLNB. This technique was introduced as an alternative method to detect the presence of occult regional metastases without performing an extensive nodal dissection. This technique offers two major advantages over ELND. First, many patients who undergo lymphatic mapping and SLNB may avoid the potential morbidity and added cost of the more extensive complete lymphadenectomy procedure. Second, identification of sentinel nodes facilitates the detailed analysis of one or

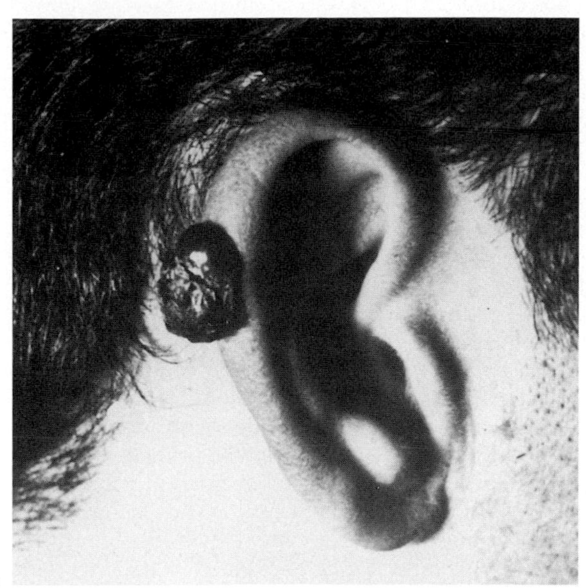
A

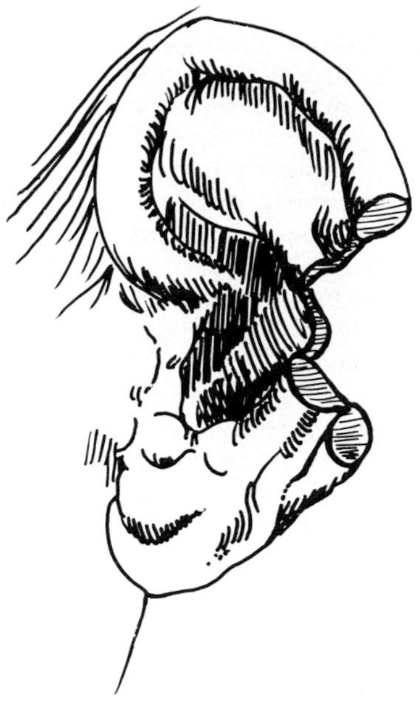

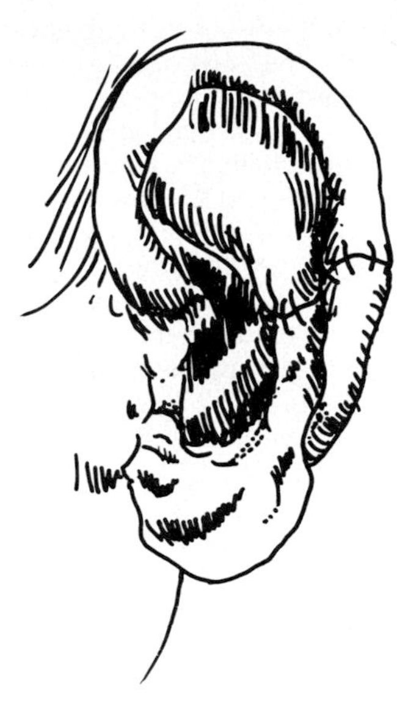
B

Figure 25.8 **A:** Nodular melanoma of external ear, suitable for limited resection. **B:** Wedge resection of lesion similar to that in **A**. Right: Note primary closure of wedge resection.

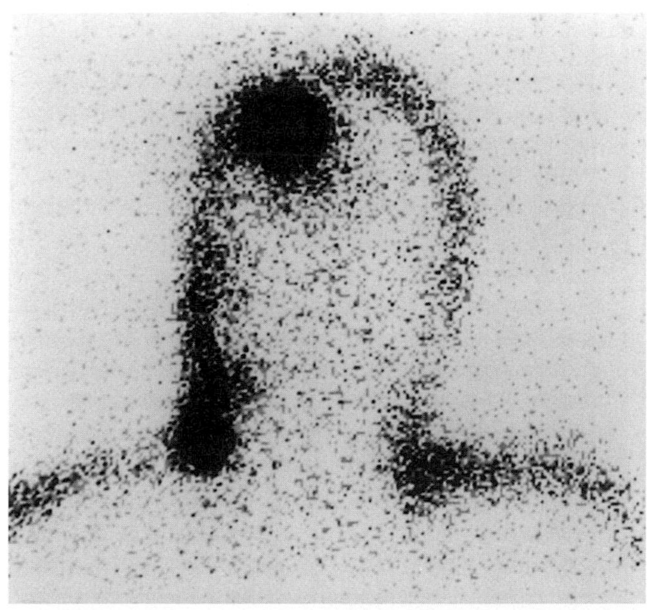
A

Figure 25.9 **A:** Radionuclide lymphoscintigraphy. The primary tumor site on the side of the right forehead was injected with technetium Tc-99m human serum albumin. Note the sentinel lymph node on the upper right side of the neck. **B,C:** Intraoperative lymphatic mapping and sentinel lymph node biopsy. **B:** Blue dye has been injected around the primary lesion. **C:** The major draining lymphatic channel and sentinel node are stained with blue dye. (See Color Plate 9 following page 524.)

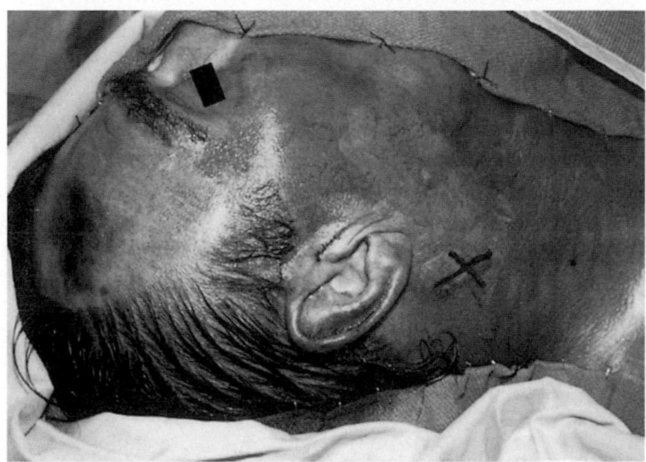
B

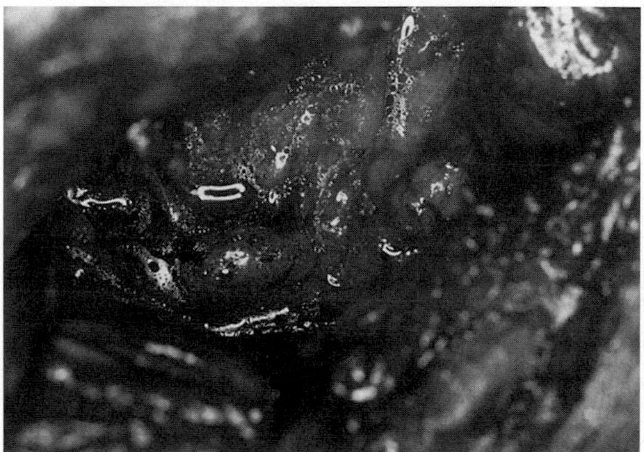
C

a few nodes with the highest potential for metastatic disease, rather than less detailed examination of multiple nodes within the resected specimen. This has potential to improve the accuracy of nodal staging (64).

Intraoperative lymphatic mapping is performed by injection of a radionuclide and/or blue dye into the primary tumor or adjacent to the scar from a previous limited biopsy procedure (Fig. 25.9A). After waiting 1 to 2 hours after radionuclide injection, or several minutes after injection of the blue dye, an incision is made in the skin over the primary lymph node basin, and the lymphatic channel stained with the blue dye is followed to the primary, blue-stained lymph node (Fig. 25.9B). The technical aspects of this procedure have been greatly improved with the addition of preoperative lymphoscintigraphy to identify the proper draining nodal basin and the use of intraoperative gamma probe to identify the site of the sentinel node and to allow a small incision to be made directly over the node.

Lymphatic mapping and SLNB have now been accepted as the standard of care for patients with melanomas located in the trunk and extremities. The efficacy of this technique was verified in several large prospective trials, where the results of the SLNB were confirmed by pathologic analysis of subsequent complete lymphadenectomy (49–51). Thompson et al. (51) performed a preoperative lymphoscintigraphy and intraoperative lymphatic mapping in 118 patients with melanoma for whom ELND was planned as part of their treatment. These physicians were able to localize an SLN in 87% of the patients. They also noted a learning curve, as identification of SLNs improved with increased experience of the surgeon. In 21% of the cases, the SLN contained microscopic metastatic disease; in 17%, this was the only lymph node positive; and in 4%, additional non-SLNs were positive for metastatic disease. Only 2% of non-SLNs had microscopic metastases when the SLN was negative. It should be noted that in 8.5% of the patients, there was a discrepancy noted between the frozen section evaluation and the permanent pathology reading; in each case, the frozen section produced a false negative. The results of this study suggest that the technique of SLNB can reliably predict the presence of microscopic metastatic melanoma in regional lymph nodes (51). Most of these series, however, contained only small numbers of patients with melanoma in the head and neck region.

Because of the complex lymphatic drainage system in the head and neck area, and the close proximity of the primary site to the first-echelon lymph nodes, the technique of lymphatic mapping and SLNB may not be as successful or accurate in patients with head and neck primary lesions. Several studies have investigated the applicability of this technique to head and neck melanoma patients (65–69). One prospective trial verified the accuracy of lymphatic mapping and SLNB in head and neck melanoma patients with pathologic analysis of subsequent elective complete lymphadenectomy (65). In this series, 43 patients underwent preoperative lymphoscintigraphy and intraoperative lymphatic mapping and sentinel node identification, followed by elective node dissection with or without superficial parotidectomy. A total of 155 SLNs in 94 nodal basins were identified in these 43 patients. Nine patients (21%) had metastatic disease in an SLN. Importantly, no patient with a negative SLN had a positive non-SLN; therefore, the false-negative rate was zero. The authors also pointed out some of the technical difficulties associated with performing SLNB in patients with melanoma of the head and neck.

Another series of 72 patients with cutaneous melanoma of the head and neck or of the upper chest and back underwent intraoperative mapping and SLNB (69). Thirty of these patients underwent preoperative lymphoscintigraphy because the primary lymphatic drainage basin was not known. In 71 (90%) of 79 regional basins examined, SLNs were identified. Elective lymph node dissection was performed in 22 patients to evaluate the effectiveness of the technique. Twelve other patients underwent therapeutic procedures because biopsy results showed metastasis within the nodes. Additionally, 15 patients underwent parotidectomy during the SLNB or as part of a lymph node dissection. The authors reported that 15% of the SLNs were positive for micrometastases. Importantly, no non-SLN was found to be positive when the SLN was negative; thus, the false-negative rate was zero. The authors reported only minor complications related to the procedure; retained blue coloration at the injection site and delayed healing of the incision in one patient (69). However, other series of SLNBs in head and neck melanoma patients have found a high rate of regional recurrences after negative SLNBs (47). Because of the complicated anatomy of the head and neck region, one can anticipate difficulties with identification and removal of the SLN, especially when the primary drainage echelon is in the parotid region. Further evaluation will be necessary to fully assess the cost-benefit ratio of this technique in patients with head and neck melanoma. Obviously, lymphatic mapping and SLNB should not be performed in patients with clinically or radiographically evident nodal metastases, as these patients require a formal lymphatic resection.

The method used to pathologically analyze the SLNs is of major importance for accurately detecting microscopic foci of disease. Rather than bivalving the nodes and examining them only with routine hematoxylin and eosin staining, SLNs are serially sectioned and also stained with melanoma specific antibodies. Molecular staging using reverse-transcriptase polymerase chain reaction (RT-PCR) for melanoma specific molecules, such as tyrosinase messenger RNA (mRNA), can also significantly increase the ability to detect extremely low numbers of metastatic cells within lymph nodes (70).

Current practice dictates performing a completion nodal dissection after detection of a positive SLN due to the fact that up to 20% of these patients will have additional positive nodes identified (71). This practice has not been rigorously analyzed to determine whether certain patient groups, such as those with thin melanomas, should be managed differently. The incidence of additional positive nodes has also not been determined specifically for head and neck patients.

Another treatment option for patients with stage II melanoma is adjuvant radiation therapy. In a prospective nonrandomized trial, 79 patients with stage II head and neck melanoma were treated with elective radiation therapy to the primary excision site and draining lymphatics (72). Of the 79 patients, 61% had intermediate lesions, 27% had deep lesions, and the rest had thin lesions but Clark's level IV disease. All patients underwent wide local excision of the primary lesion followed by external beam radiation therapy to the tumor bed and to at least two echelons of the draining lymphatics. The total dose was 30 Gy in 6 Gy per fraction over 2.5 weeks. In this group of patients, the rate of locoregional disease control at 5 years was 85% to 88%. Five patients out of 79 developed locoregional disease recurrence without evidence of disseminated disease. In two of these patients, the recurrence was outside the radiation portal, and so represented a geographic miss. Interestingly, the thickness of the primary lesion had no significant influence on the rate of locoregional disease control, although it did have a significant effect on the ultimate 5-year survival rate. The radiation therapy regimen was well tolerated by patients, producing very limited morbidity (72).

In patients with stage II disease and deep primary tumors, the risk of distant metastasis is high. These patients are more likely to have, and ultimately die of, distant metastases before complications from regional metastases develop. In this situation, observation of the draining lymphatics and performance of therapeutic neck dissections if nodal disease becomes manifest is an accepted treatment strategy. An alternative management plan is to treat those patients with deep lesions with radiation therapy to the draining lymphatics because of the very limited morbidity associated with such adjuvant treatment. However, with the increasing acceptance of lymphatic mapping and SLNB, most adjuvant systemic protocols now require pathologic assessment of the regional lymphatics prior to enrollment. Furthermore, accurate determination of the nodal status allows better characterization of the patient's overall prognosis. For these reasons, consideration should be given to performing SLNB in patients with clinically staged T2 N0 lesions. The role of adjuvant systemic therapy for patients with stage II melanoma is currently being evaluated and is discussed later.

STAGE III DISEASE

In patients with metastatic nodal disease, a therapeutic functional neck dissection is indicated. In addition to adequate excision of the primary tumor, all lymph nodes involved by the tumor as well as those that are at risk to contain microscopic metastases should be removed. It should be remembered that the parotid lymph nodes are often the primary nodal echelon for cutaneous lesions anterior to the coronal plane drawn through the tragus. A superficial parotidectomy with facial nerve sparing should be included in dissections for primary tumors located in this area. When the primary tumor is located posterior to the plane, it is important to dissect the postauricular and suboccipital nodes as well as all level V lymph nodes. The external jugular chain of nodes is also frequently involved in cases of cutaneous primary tumors and should be resected. Important anatomic structures including the spinal accessory nerve and internal jugular vein should be spared unless grossly involved by tumor.

Adjuvant postoperative radiation therapy has improved locoregional control rates after therapeutic neck dissection performed in cases of stage III disease (72,73). A series of 32 patients who received adjuvant radiation therapy combined with limited neck dissections after presenting to their physicians with palpable lymphadenopathy was reported by Ang et al. (72). In the series, 25 patients received 30 Gy in five fractions postoperatively. Seven patients received 24 Gy in four fractions preoperatively to the tumor bed and ipsilateral draining lymphatics. Locoregional disease was controlled in 93% of the patients. This result compares favorably with the 50% incidence of recurrent disease in a group of patients whose similar primary tumors were treated with surgery alone (63,74). It is interesting that the rate of locoregional control in patients receiving adjuvant radiation therapy after neck dissection was not affected by the presence of multiple positive nodes or extracapsular extension of disease. This postoperative regimen of 30 Gy in five fractions (6 Gy per fraction) spread over 2.5 weeks is well tolerated by patients. It should be pointed out that if postoperative radiation therapy is planned, then consideration can be given to performing selective neck dissection rather than a full functional neck dissection. Others argue that there is no indication for postoperative x-ray therapy (XRT) in the absence of extranodal spread, due to the low (14%) incidence of regional recurrence after a comprehensive neck dissection (75). The efficacy of postoperative XRT after neck dissection to control locoregional disease needs to be further evaluated in a prospective randomized trial.

In summary, patients with clinically or radiographically evident nodal metastases require wide local excision of the primary lesion and surgical resection of the draining lymphatics to remove all grossly involved lymph nodes as well as those at risk for occult disease. Postoperative radiation therapy should be considered if multiple positive nodes are found on pathologic examination of the specimen. Because of the high rate (nearly 80%) of distant metastasis in patients who have developed regional metastases, adjuvant systemic therapy should be considered.

Adjuvant Systemic Therapy of Stage IIb and III Disease

Adjuvant systemic therapy is often recommended in patients with deep primary lesions or metastatic regional disease, due to the high rate of developing distant metastases in these patients. Different types of agents, including immunotherapy, chemotherapy, and biochemotherapy, are being investigated for potential efficacy for preventing distant metastases and improving overall survival rates.

Because melanoma is one of the most immunogenic malignancies, the concept of immunotherapy to prevent recurrences or treat metastatic disease is extremely attractive. Various types of immune-modulating agents have been evaluated for adjuvant use in stage II and III melanoma patients. These include biologic response modifiers such as interferons and interleukins, general immunostimulants such as Bacille Calmette-Guérin (BCG) and levamisole, and several types of vaccines.

TABLE 25.5 Studies Evaluating Adjuvant Interferon

Study group	Staging	Agent	Regimen	Results DFS	Results OS
High-dose interferon					
NCCTG 83705	T3/N1	IFN-α2a	20 MU/m^2 i.m. 3×/week × 3 months vs. observation	–	–
ECOG 1684	T4/N1	IFN-α2b	20 MU/m^2 i.v. 5×/week × 1 month, then 10 MU/m^2 s.c. 3×/week for 11 months vs. observation	+	+
ECOG 1690	T4/N2	IFN-α2b	20 MU/m^2 i.v. 5×/week for 1 month, then 10 MU/m^2 s.c. 3×/week for 11 months vs. 3 MU s.c. 3×/week for 2 years vs. observation	+	–
Low-dose interferon					
WHO 16	N1–N2	IFN-α2a	3 MU s.c. 3×/week for 3 years	–	–
Austrian	T3/N0	IFN-α2a	3 MU s.c. 3×/week for 1 year	+	–
French	T3/N0	IFN-α2a	3 MU s.c. 3×/week for 18 months	+	–

DFS, disease-free survival; IFN, interferon; OS, overall survival; WHO, World Health Organization.
Source: Adapted from Whittaker S. Adjuvant therapy in melanoma. *Clin Exp Dermatol* 2000;25:497–502.

Interferon is the best-studied agent for use in melanoma patients in the adjuvant setting; however, the results of several clinical trials are equivocal (summarized in Table 25.5) and the efficacy and cost/benefit ratio of this treatment remains unclear (76,77). In the Eastern Cooperative Oncology Group (ECOG) 1684 trial (78), a randomized control study of interferon-α2b (IFN-α2b) administered as adjuvant therapy for deep primary or regional metastatic melanoma, the drug was given at 20 $MU/m^2/d$ intravenously for 1 month followed by 10 $MU/m^2/d$ subcutaneously three times per week for 3 years (78). Patients who received this therapy had an improved overall survival rate compared with those managed with observation alone. Patients with either clinically or pathologically evident lymph node metastases had the greatest improvement in disease control. Significant toxic effects were reported with this treatment regimen, however; 67% of patients had severe, grade III toxic effects, and life-threatening toxic effects were seen in 9% of the patients during the treatment. The United States Food and Drug Administration approved IFN-α2b for adjuvant treatment in patients with melanoma after the results of this trial were obtained. Subsequent clinical trials have failed to duplicate the improvements in overall survival seen with adjuvant interferon in the ECOG 1684 trial (76). Interestingly, the survival rates for the observation group in the ECOG 1690 trial were substantially improved (54%) when compared to (37%) in the observation group in ECOG 1684 (79). Several factors have been suggested to explain the improved survival rates in both the treatment and control arms in the later trial, including lower numbers of patients with node positive disease, and more aggressive surgical and adjuvant therapy for patients with regional recurrences while in the study. More than 30% of the patients on the observation arm of ECOG 1690 were treated with surgery and adjuvant IFN off-study after developing a recurrence, potentially confounding the comparison of survival rates between the treatment arms (80). When considering whether or not to recommend that patients receive IFN, it is also important to consider the substantial toxicity that can be associated with this treatment (81).

Several types of vaccines have been investigated as adjuvant treatment in patients with resected stage II or stage III melanoma. In small phase II trials, several vaccines have shown promise for improving patient outcome with limited toxicities (82–85); however, no large, randomized study has yet demonstrated a survival advantage for patients treated with any melanoma vaccine (86). A phase III study (ECOG 1694) demonstrated decreased relapse-free and overall survival in the treatment arm with a ganglioside expressed on the surface of most melanoma cells (GM2) conjugate vaccine, compared to the treatment arm with high-dose IFN-α2b (87). Several large randomized phase III trials with melanoma vaccines as adjuvant therapy are currently underway to further evaluate this modality.

STAGE IV DISEASE

Evidence of distant metastasis implies a poor prognosis no matter what type of treatment is initiated. Nevertheless, because of the devastating effects of uncontrolled locoregional tumors,

A

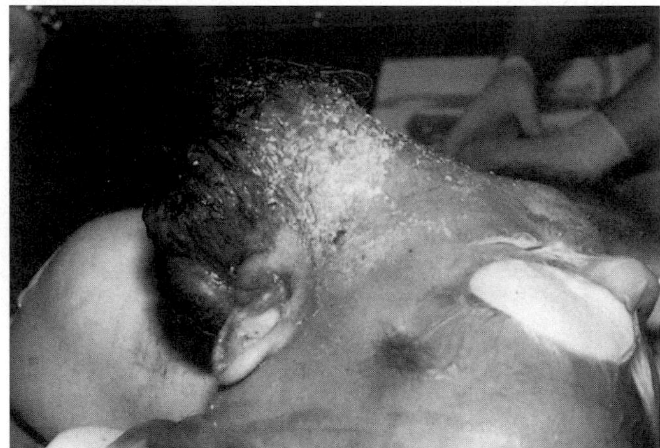

B

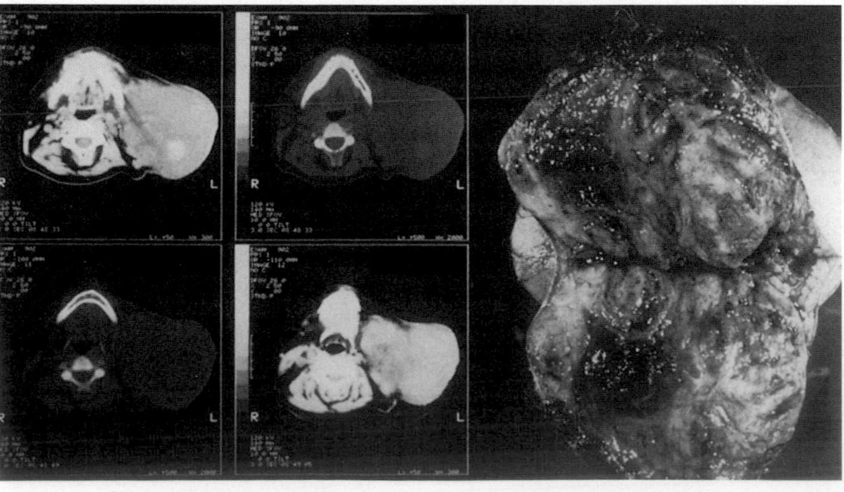

Figure 25.10 Extensive lymphatic metastases of malignant melanoma. The patient was experiencing significant pain and wound problems from uncontrolled regional metastases. **A:** Metastatic melanoma tumor just prior to surgery. **B:** Resected surgical specimen and preoperative computed tomography scan.

aggressive management of locoregional disease is extremely important even when distant metastases are present (Fig. 25.10).

Because results of treatment for stage IV melanoma are poor, no single management strategy can be considered the standard of care. Combinations of local therapy (e.g., surgery and radiotherapy) directed to specific disease sites and systemic therapies such as chemotherapy or biotherapy are often used.

SURGERY FOR DISTANT METASTASIS

Although the development of distant metastasis heralds systemic spread of disease, surgical resection of some metastatic lesions when feasible can offer long-term palliation and in some instances prolong survival. The most common site for initial metastasis is the lung. The relatively improved survival of patients with lung metastases compared to those with metastases to other visceral sites is now reflected in the 2002 staging system. One study documented a 25% 5-year survival rate in patients who underwent thoracotomy for resection of lung metastases from malignant melanoma (88). Because of the considerable variability in the biologic aggressiveness of melanoma, it is difficult to determine which patients would benefit from surgical resection of distant metastasis. Criteria for resection include absence of metastasis at other anatomic sites, control of the primary tumor, and potential for complete resection (89). Consideration should also be given to a trial of systemic therapy prior to surgical resection to evaluate disease response. Radiotherapy is indicated for palliation of large symptomatic lesions.

Systemic Treatment

Chemotherapy

The most active single chemotherapeutic agent for the systemic treatment of melanoma is dacarbazine [dimethyltriazeno-imidazole carboxamide (DTIC)]. The response rates, however, are only about 10% to 20%, and the durations of response are short (median 4 to 6 months) (90,91). Although different treatment schedules and doses have been given, a 1-day treatment of 850 to 1,000 mg/^{2} repeated every 3 to 4 weeks is reasonable. Side effects include nausea, vomiting, suppression of bone marrow function, local pain at injection sites, flu-like symptoms, and malaise. The DTIC analog of this agent demonstrated some activity against metastatic melanoma, but additional clinical trials will be necessary to evaluate its efficacy. The nitrosoureas carmustine [bischloroethylnitrosurea (BCNU)], lomustine [chloroethylcyclohexylnitrosurea (CCNU)], and other agents in this class have also been shown to produce a 10% to 25% response rate in patients with malignant melanoma. Other agents that have shown some response in small clinical trials include vincristine, Taxotere, and a protein kinase C inhibitor, bryostatin-1 (91).

Because of the limited efficacy of single-agent chemotherapy, combination regimens have been evaluated. Most of these combination regimens, however, have not markedly improved response rates but have caused a general increase in toxicity to patients. The combination of DTIC, BCNU, cisplatin, and tamoxifen, however, was reported to generate an overall response rate of 46% and a complete response rate of 11% in a series of 141 patients (91). A randomized study is required to further evaluate the efficacy of this regimen.

Biologic Therapy

The goal of biologic therapy is to mobilize the patient's immunologic defense system to attack malignant cells. Several different methods have been tried, including administration of interleukin-2 (IL-2) and other cytokines, stimulation of the patient's T cells and natural killer cells, and administration of antitumor vaccines. A review of clinical trials using IL-2 has not shown a significant response rate (92).

The strategy behind vaccination for melanoma is to stimulate the patient's immune response against tumor-associated antigens. Investigators are using several different approaches to develop melanoma vaccines (93,94), including antibody response to tumor antigen vaccines, whole-cell vaccines, peptide vaccines, DNA vaccines, dendritic cell vaccines, and others. Several reports of early clinical trial results (82,95–99) have suggested a potential therapeutic role for melanoma vaccines (reviewed in refs. 86 and 100). For example, a trial of 38 patients with resected regional metastases showed an increased time to disease progression in those who received melanoma vaccine compared to placebo (82). However, the authors stressed that the positive results should be interpreted with caution due to the small study size. Indeed, despite the promise hinted at by these small trials and anecdotal reports, melanoma vaccines have not yet been proven to be clinically effective in randomized double-blind trials (101), and this approach remains experimental. Several large multicenter randomized phase III trials are being conducted to address this issue. These trials include (a) GM2 conjugate vaccine versus high-dose IFN by ECOG, (b) melanoma cell lysate vaccine vs. placebo by the Southwest Oncology Group (SWOG), and (c) allogeneic melanoma cell vaccine vs placebo by the John Wayne Cancer Institute (100). The results of these trials should help determine the therapeutic efficacy of this approach to treating melanoma patients.

Biochemotherapy, the combination of cytotoxic chemotherapeutic agents with biologic modifiers such as IL and IFN, improved response rates in several preliminary clinical trials. One combination regimen including DTIC, vincristine, bleomycin, lomustine, and IFN-α produced an overall response rate of 62% and a complete response rate of 13% (101). Yet, a prospective randomized trial that compared sequential combination of CDDP, DTIC, and tamoxifen with IL-2/IFN-α to CDDP, DTIC, and tamoxifen alone showed no significant difference in response rate or median survival time between the two treatment arms (102). The biochemotherapy regimen used at the M. D. Anderson Cancer Center consists of cisplatin, vinblastine, DTIC, IL-2, and IFN-α. This regimen can produce high response rates (up to 60%) but has considerable toxicity (103). Future prospective randomized trials need to be performed to further clarify the cost/benefit ratio of combining cytotoxic chemotherapy with biologic response modifiers for the treatment of metastatic melanoma.

Gene Therapy

An exciting new approach to treatment of systemic melanoma is the use of gene transfer or gene therapy. Extensive *in vitro* and animal experiments have been conducted to devise a strategy for the use of gene therapy against melanoma. Different approaches to gene therapy are being explored (104,105). One technique is to directly transfer a cytokine gene such as *IL-2* into melanoma cells. Theoretically, this would increase the immunogenicity of the melanoma cells and result in inhibition of tumor growth. Another method is to transduce cytokine genes into autologous fibroblasts *in vitro*. The fibroblasts are then mixed with irradiated tumor cells in suspension and reinjected into patients. The aim of this technique is again to elicit a melanoma-specific immune response. A third strategy is the direct transfer of genes into the melanoma *in vivo*. One such gene, *HLA-B7*, is thought to increase the immunogenicity of melanoma. The results of early clinical trials have demonstrated the safety and feasibility of this approach (106). As these clinical trials are all preliminary, the ultimate role of gene therapy in the systemic treatment of metastatic melanoma has not been established (104,105).

Follow-Up

The purpose of routine follow-up of patients after treatment of melanoma is early detection of local disease recurrence, regional and distant metastases, and new primary tumors. A follow-up schedule that was derived by polling eight melanoma experts has been published. Follow-up for patients with melanomas <0.75 mm thick should be every 6 months for the first 2 years and then annually thereafter; for melanomas 0.76 to 1.5 mm thick, every 3 months for years 1 and 2, every 6 months for years 3, 4, and 5, and then annually; for melanomas >1.5 mm thick, every 3 months for years 1, 2, and 3, and every 6 months for years 4 and 5 (107). After 5 years it is recommended that all patients have follow-up annually. The cost-effectiveness of this regimen was not evaluated, however. Brandt et al. (108) evaluated 206 patients with stage I melanomas less than 1.5 mm thick to assess the effectiveness of long-term follow-up. These authors found that disease recurred in only 11 (5.3%) patients, of whom only four (2%) patients were successfully treated. They concluded that aggressive follow-up was not indicated for patients with thin melanomas.

Weiss et al. (109) evaluated the utility and cost-effectiveness of screening tests in follow-up of patients with malignant melanoma. They found that 68% of the patients had disease symptoms that led to the diagnosis of the recurrence. In an additional 26%, recurrent disease was found on routine physical exam. Only 6% of the patients had disease recurrence documented by abnormal chest x-rays, and abnormal laboratory values were never the sole indicator of recurrence. This study suggests that the use of chest x-rays and laboratory values may not be cost-effective in the follow-up of patients with malignant melanoma (110).

Two new technologies, FDG-PET scans and RT-PCR, are under investigation for detection of recurrent or systemic disease in melanoma patients. Data regarding the sensitivity and specificity of a PET scan to detect occult disease is equivocal due to insufficient patient numbers and proper analysis; however, the preliminary studies indicate that it may be more useful for the detection of systemic disease rather than regional disease, and it currently lacks the sensitivity to detect microscopic disease (43,110). With the enhanced sensitivity of RT-PCR, it is theoretically possible to detect and distinguish the rare melanoma tumor cells from the normal cells circulating in the bloodstream. Tyrosinase, an enzyme involved in the synthesis of melanin, is the mRNA marker that has been used most often to detect melanoma. However, investigations have shown marked variability in the sensitivity and reproducibility of this technology (reviewed in ref. 111). A modification of this technique that uses multiple melanoma-associated antigens to improve sensitivity is being investigated (111).

One reasonable approach would be to schedule follow-up exams for patients with intermediate to thick primaries ever 3 or 4 months for the first 2 years, every 6 months for the next 2 years, and annually thereafter, with an annual chest x-ray and liver enzyme tests.

Survival Rates and Prognostic Factors

The efficacy of treatment strategies for patients with stage I and stage II disease can be measured by locoregional disease control, as well as by survival rate. For patients with stage I or stage II disease, both locoregional control and survival rates are affected by the depth of the tumor. In patients with localized primary tumors less than 1.5 mm thick, the prognosis is excellent. In one series, the 15-year cancer-specific survival rate was 92.3% (108). In another series analyzing melanomas from all body sites, the 5-year survival rate for lesions less than 0.75 mm thick was 95%; for those 0.75 mm to 1.49 mm, it was 85% (112). The 5-year survival rates for patients with intermediate and thick primary lesions are approximately 66% and 46%, respectively. Primary tumor thickness is also an important prognostic indicator of time to disease recurrence (113).

Regional and distant metastasis carries a much worse prognosis than localized primary melanoma. In a retrospective analysis of 312 patients with metastatic melanoma, the 5-year survival rate for those with regional metastases was 43.4% and for those with distant metastases, 4.9% (114). These patients were treated with a variety of modalities.

Several prognostic factors are not considered in the current AJCC-UICC staging system, among them the sex of the patient, the location of the primary lesion, and tumor ulceration. In a large review of patients with head and neck melanoma in Sweden, multivariate analysis revealed that the sex of the patient and the anatomic site of the primary tumor were independent prognostic factors akin to tumor thickness (115). Although controversial, many studies have indicated that a primary melanoma on the upper back, posterior arm, neck, or scalp (BANS) carries a worse prognosis than does a lesion in any other location (116). Lesions of the ear (pinna) are also often particularly lethal (117). Primary tumors on the scalp and neck had a worse prognosis than those localized to the face. Furthermore, a lesion on the hair-bearing area of the scalp has a worse prognosis than one on the non–hair-bearing scalp (118). Ulcerated lesions also carry a worse prognosis.

As more information accumulates concerning the natural history of this disease, the importance of other factors for predicting metastasis and survival becomes apparent. For instance, ploidy status has been shown in one study to be predictive of 5-year survival (119). Other factors currently undergoing investigation include *p53* status, chromosomal instability, expression of markers of cell proliferation such as Ki-67, cell cycle regulation such as $p16^{INK4}$, angiogenesis such as vascular endothelial growth factor (VEGF), and apoptosis such as *p53*, Bcl-2, and $p21^{WAF1}$ (120,121).

COMPLICATIONS

The most common complications related to wide local excision of a primary tumor are local wound infection, graft or flap failure, and a poor cosmetic result. The incidence of these complications is reduced by keeping margins of excision to 2 cm or less. The complications of treatment of lymphatic basins are related to the modality of treatment and the anatomic site involved. Potential complications of parotidectomy and anterior neck dissection include facial nerve injury and injury to the spinal accessory nerve. Cervical anesthesia and shoulder weakness can also occur in posterior neck dissections. Experience with intraoperative lymphatic mapping and SLNBs is more limited, and complication rates have not been established; however, complications associated with these procedures include retained blue discoloration at the injection site and injury to the structures at risk during neck dissection and parotidectomy. The major morbidity associated with external beam radiation therapy includes a mild skin reaction and residual fibrosis. A major complication of locoregional treatment is failure to control disease. This can lead to significant pressure and pain difficulties as well as problems with wound care.

Many of the systemic treatment regimens cause severe side effects. Nausea, emesis, fever, malaise, pancytopenia, and neurotoxicity are quite common. The risks and complications related to the new experimental therapies are still being evaluated in phase I and phase II trials.

MANAGEMENT OF DISEASE RECURRENCE

Recurrent disease developing in the skin, subcutaneous tissue, or lymph nodes can be surgically excised when lesions are few and isolated. It is important to try to control these lesions before they become bulky and symptomatic. Other treatment options include radiation therapy, intralesional injection of chemotherapeutic or immunotherapeutic agents, and systemic chemotherapy. Patients with surgically resectable distant metastasis often benefit from metastasectomy.

The development of metastases in the liver and other abdominal visceral organs usually indicates widespread metastatic disease. Patients with liver metastases have poor prognoses and an average life span of only 2 to 4 months. In these patients, consideration should be given to systemic chemotherapy or biologic therapy versus supportive care only. Brain metastasis is not uncommon in patients with metastatic melanoma. Headache and mental deficits are usually the presenting symptoms, and the diagnosis is usually made after MRI or CT imaging. Steroids can help reduce edema surrounding the tumor and improve symptoms. For solitary lesions, surgical excision with postoperative radiation may be indicated. Patients with brain metastases survive only an average of 6 months after surgery, however (89).

SPECIAL ISSUES

Desmoplastic Melanoma

Desmoplastic melanoma is a histologic variant that displays certain distinct clinical features. These lesions are characterized pathologically by malignant spindle-shaped tumor cells in a fibrotic stroma. Many desmoplastic melanomas display neurotropism, and most are amelanotic. The diagnosis may be difficult to establish, but staining with S100 protein may facilitate this process. Desmoplastic melanomas tend to be thicker than nondesmoplastic melanoma lesions at the time of diagnosis, and they have a high potential for local recurrence at the primary site. The tendency for perineural spread also exacerbates the difficulties of obtaining local disease control. Regional nodal metastases are less common in the cases of desmoplastic melanoma than they are in nondesmoplastic primary tumors (122). Because of the propensity for local recurrence, it is important to obtain adequate surgical margins. All margins should be verified by pathologic evaluation and carefully inspected for evidence of perineural spread. Large nerves should be checked at the time of surgery for perineurial involvement by disease. Overall survival rates for patients with desmoplastic melanoma are comparable to those for patients with nondesmoplastic melanoma when adjusted for lesion thickness (123).

Unknown Primary Lesion

There is an unusual subset of patients in whom the primary melanoma is never detected. The prognosis for these patients is not worse than for patients with known primary tumors. Prognosis is dependent on the location and extent of the nodal metastasis. Patients should be treated by surgical dissection tailored to the location and extent of the nodal disease. Adjuvant radiation therapy and systemic therapy should also be considered, just as they would be for other patients with stage III disease.

Mucosal Melanoma

Rarely, melanoma will arise in the mucosal lining of the upper aerodigestive tract, particularly the nasal cavity, paranasal sinuses, and oral cavity. Patients are usually diagnosed with advanced disease, presenting with nasal obstruction, epistaxis, or a symptomatic mass. Those patients who have resectable tumors should undergo surgical removal. Adjuvant radiation therapy may be indicated to control local disease, especially for patients with questionable surgical margins. Elective lymph node dissection is probably not indicated, because distant metastasis many times develops before the appearance of nodal disease. The status of the lymph nodes does not appear to affect overall survival rates, but the development of distant metastasis portends a grave prognosis. The average length of survival after development of distant metastasis is only 6 month. Systemic therapy has not proven effective at increasing survival rates for patients with this variant of melanoma. Five-year survival rates for patients with mucosal melanoma range from 15% in early series (124) to more than 40% in others (125,126).

RADIOLOGIC IMAGING CONCERNS

Bernard B. O'Malley and Suresh K. Mukherji

Management of the neck in the setting of a primary melanoma of the head or neck usually is determined by parametric data regarding primarily the thickness of the specimen (127). Scanning the primary site for deep extension is described in Chapter 24. Imaging of the neck for melanoma usually involves cervical and deep facial lymph node staging scans for skin lesions or imaging of the brain to rule out intracranial metastases. Both sides of the neck should be carefully evaluated, especially for midline lesions and in patients with a previously treated neck. It is important to remember that tumors inherit the lymphatic drainage of the areas that they involve. Melanoma nodal metastases (Fig. 25.11) and hepatic metastases (Fig. 25.12) tend to show early necrosis, simulating squamous metastases. Less commonly there is a solid very intensely enhancing appearance (Fig. 25.13). The diagnostic accuracy of nodal staging with imaging is reduced in patients who have undergone any form of prior treatment (128).

Assessment of nodal involvement serves two main purposes. Most important is the determination of the direction of nodal drainage for synchronous lesions involving multiple sites. Pretreatment nodal evaluation has been shown to be more useful in the head and neck compared to the extremities (129). Another important role is identifying the SLN(s) for excisional biopsy prior to formal therapeutic neck dissection in superficial lesions (130). The SLN staging process has been aided by the use of hand-held gamma probe guided localization (131). Sentinel node results provide prognostic information (132). Lymphoscintigraphy may be unnecessary for cervical skin lesions (133).

Desmoplastic melanomas are most common in the head and neck but less conspicuous because of their amelanotic predominance (134). This form of melanoma has a much higher incidence of neurotropic involvement, which has an adverse effect on prognosis (135) and should influence the extent of local resection (136).

Facial melanomas in the distribution of the fifth cranial nerve are at risk for retrograde perineural extension (137). These facial melanomas are most commonly seen at the second division of the fifth nerve, perhaps because of concern for cosmesis at the nasolabial region at the time of initial resection (Fig. 25.14). Tumors in this location should be evaluated with contrast-enhanced MRI to evaluate for retrograde perineural extension into the cavernous sinus.

Mucosal melanomas of the aerodigestive tract are most common in the oral and sinonasal sites. Survival has not improved despite refinements in treatment (138) or imaging (139). This may be due to the dual lymphatic and hematogenous metastasis pattern and the frequency of distant failure despite local/regional control (140). Melanoma of the various subsites of the aerodigestive tract and orbit are discussed in separate chapters.

Aside from chest x-ray, a survey shows that most patients are followed clinically without imaging (141). This may be due to the pessimism when recurrence is encountered. Early reports suggest that melanoma is markedly hypermetabolic and shows intense activity on FDG-PET scans. However, in our experience, the uptake in melanoma is variable. But PET scanning is better for systemic staging compared with locoregional staging (142).

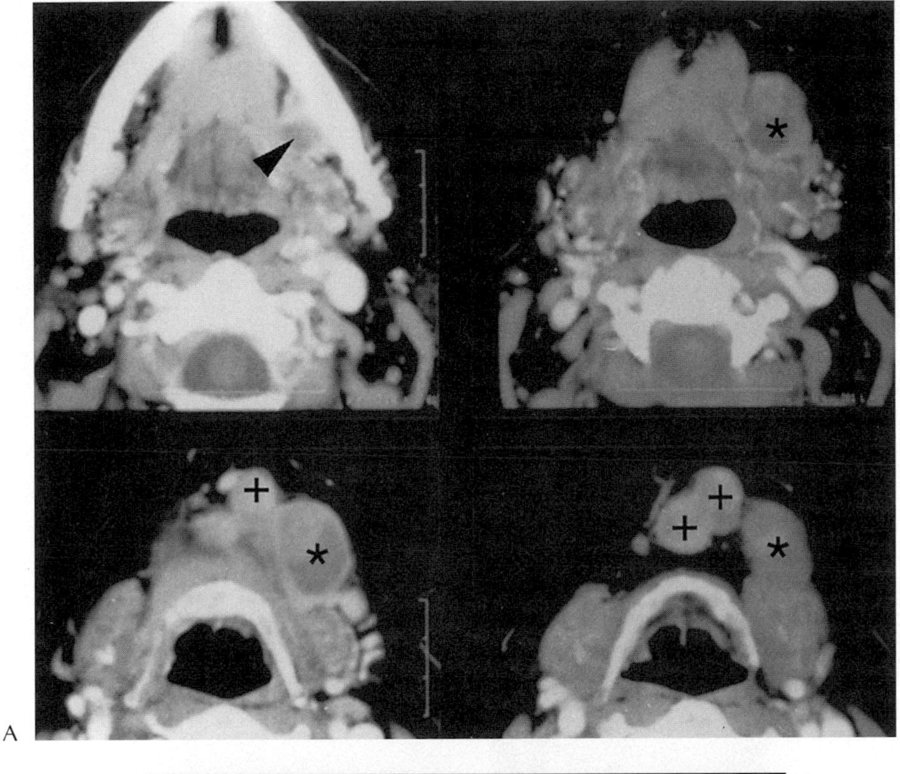

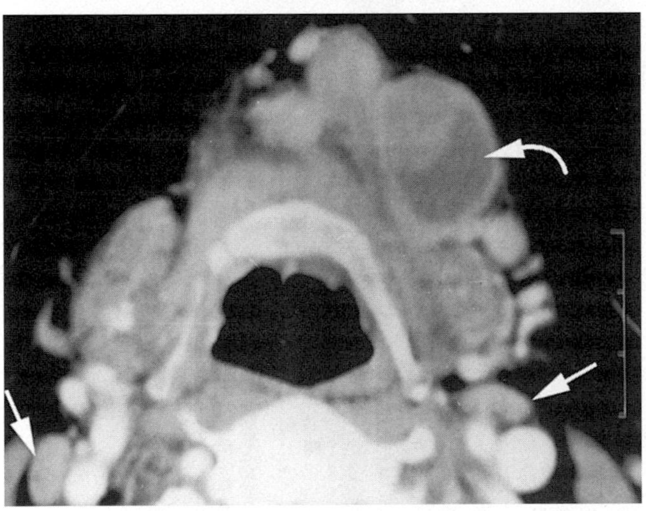

Figure. 25.11 Cervical adenopathy. **A:** Serial enhanced axial computed tomography views of the suprahyoid neck show several pathologic lymph nodes in the submental (+), submandibular (*asterisk*), and sublingual (*arrowhead*) spaces in a patient with a melanoma of the upper lip. **B:** Selected axial views show a mixed pattern of adenopathy: solid enhancement at level II nodes (*arrows*) and necrosis (*curved arrow*) in the larger, level Ib node.

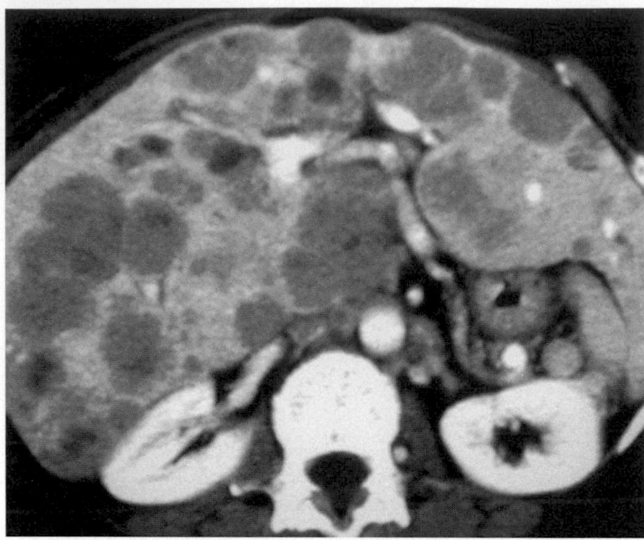

Figure 25.12 Hepatic metastases. Enhanced computed tomographic scan of the liver shows widespread low attenuation metastases indicating necrosis.

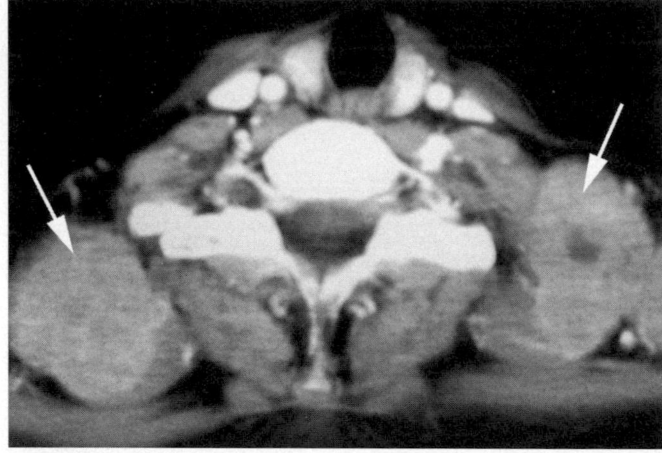

Figure 25.13 Cervical adenopathy. Enhanced computed tomographic scan of the neck shows intensely enhancing masses related to metastatic melanoma (*arrows*).

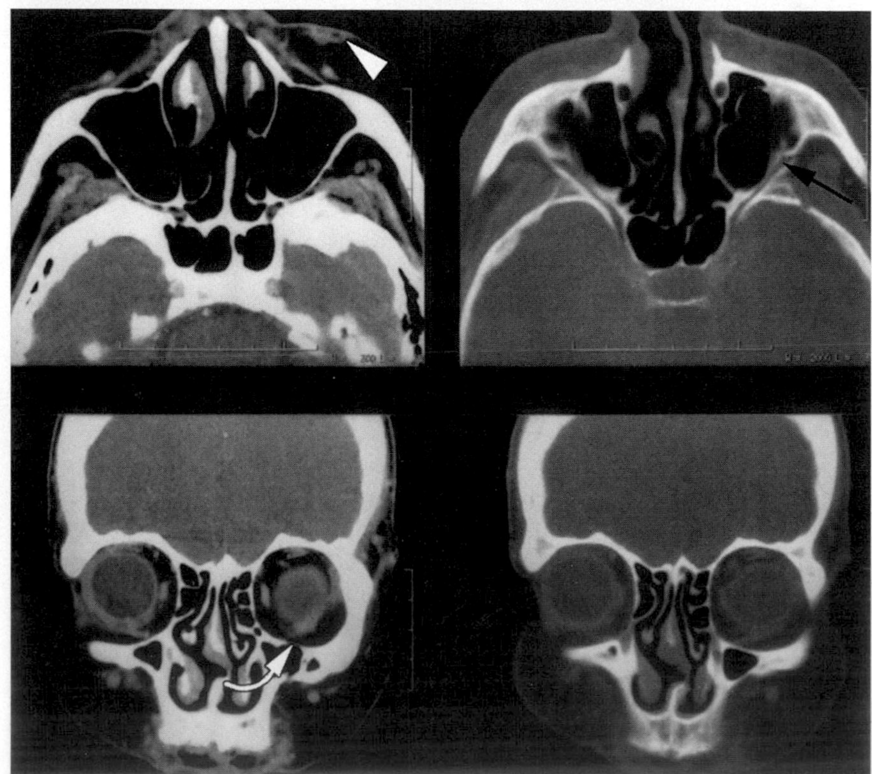

Figure 25.14 Recurrent facial melanoma. Enhanced axial (*top panel*) and direct coronal (*bottom panel*) computed tomographic views in soft tissue (*left*) and bone (*right*) windows show irregular infiltration (*arrowhead*) of the premaxillary subcutaneous plane related to an overlying recurrent melanoma. There is no evidence of involvement of the infraorbital nerve anteriorly near the foramen (*curved arrow*) or as it approaches the pterygomaxillary space (*arrow*).

REFERENCES

1. American Cancer Society. Cancer facts and figures—1999. Atlanta: American Cancer Society, 1999:4.
2. Borzena SH, Fenske NA, Perez IR. Epidemiology of malignant melanoma, worldwide incidence, and etiologic factors. *Semin Surg Oncol* 1993;9:165.
3. Burton RC, Coates MS, Hersey P, et al. An analysis of a melanoma epidemic. *Int J Cancer* 1993;55:765.
4. Edman RL and Wolfe JT. Prevention and early detection of malignant melanoma. *Am Fam Physician* 2000;62:2277.
5. Kim HJ. Photoprotection in adolescents. *Adolesc Med* 2001;12:181.
6. Borden EC. Reducing primary melanoma mortality. *Curr Oncol Rep* 2000;2: 289.
7. Goldsmith HS. Melanoma: an overview. *Cancer* 1979;29:194.
8. Jelfs PL, Giles G, Shugg D, et al. Cutaneous malignant melanoma in Australia, 1989. *Med J Aust* 1994;161:182.
9. Vayer A, Lefor AT. Cutaneous melanoma in African-Americans. *South Med J* 1993;86:181.
10. Chun K., Vazquez M, Sanchez JL. Malignant melanoma in children. *Int J Dermatol* 1993;32:14.
11. Elwood JM. Recent developments in melanoma epidemiology, 1993. *Melanoma Res* 1993;3:149.
12. Westerdahl J, Olsson H, Masback A, et al. Is the use of sunscreens a risk factor for malignant melanoma? *Melanoma Res* 1995;5:377.
13. Autier P, Dore JF, Schifflers E, et al. Melanoma and use of sunscreens: an EORTC case-control study in Germany Belgium, and France. *Int J Cancer* 1995;61:749.
14. Wolf P, Donawho CK, Kripke ML. Effect of sunscreens on UV radiation-induced enhancement of melanoma growth in mice. *J Natl Cancer Inst* 1994; 86:99.
15. Wang SQ, Setlow R, Berwick M, et al. Ultraviolet A and melanoma: a review. *J Am Acad Dermatol* 2001;44:837.
16. Drobetsky EA, Turcotte J, Chateauneuf A. A role for ultraviolet A in solar mutagenesis. *Proc Natl Acad Sci USA* 1995;92:2350.
17. Kvam E, Tyrrell RM. Induction of oxidative DNA base damage in human skin cells by UV and near visible radiation. *Carcinogenesis* 1997;18:2379.
18. Marrot L, Belaidi FP, Meunier JR, et al. The human melanocyte as a particular target for UVA radiation and an endpoint for photoprotection assessment. *Photochem Photobiol* 1999;69:686.
19. Miller SA, Hamilton SL, Wester UG, et al. An analysis of UVA emissions from sunlamps and the potential importance for melanoma. *Photochem Photobiol* 1998;68:63.
20. Swerdlow AJ, Weinstock MA. Do tanning lamps cause melanoma? An epidemiologic assessment. *J Am Acad Dermatol* 1998;38:89.
21. Chen YT, Dubrow R, Zheng T, et al. Sunlamp use and the risk of cutaneous malignant melanoma: a population-base case-control study in Connecticut, USA. *Int J Epidemiol* 1998;27:758.
22. Westerdahl J, Ingvar C, Masback A, et al. Risk of cutaneous malignant melanoma in relation to use of sunbeds: further evidence for UV-A carcinogenicity. *Br J Cancer* 2000;82:1593.
23. Piepkorn MW. Genetic basis of susceptibility to melanoma. *J Am Acad Dermatol* 1994;31:1022.
24. Ostlere LS, Houlston RS, Path MRC, et al. Risk of cancer in relatives of patients with cutaneous melanoma. *Int J Dermatol* 1993;32:719.
25. Schrier PL. Melanoma genetics and cytogenetics. *Clin Dermatol* 1992;10:31.
26. Frank W, Rogers GS. Melanoma update. Second primary melanoma. *Dermatol Surg* 1993;19:427.
27. Reed JA, Loganzo F Jr, Shea CR, et al. Loss of expression of the p16/cyclin-dependent kinase inhibitor 2 tumor suppressor gene in melanocytic lesions correlates with invasive stage tumor progression. *Cancer Res* 1995;55:2713.
28. Aitken J, Welch J, Duffy D, et al. CDKN2A variants in a population-based sample of Queensland families with melanoma. *J Natl Cancer Inst* 1999;92:446.
29. Whelan AJ, Bartsch D, Goodfellow PJ. Brief report: a familial syndrome of pancreatic cancer and melanoma with a mutation in the CKN2 tumor-suppressor gene. *N Engl J Med* 1995;333:975.
30. Goldstein AM, Fraser MC, Struewing JP, et al. Increased risk of pancreatic cancer in melanoma-prone kindreds with p16INK4 mutations. *N Engl J Med* 1995;333:970.
31. Greene MH. The genetics of hereditary melanoma and nevi. 1998 update. *Cancer* 1999;86(suppl 11):2464.
32. Bain C, Green A, Siskind V, et al. Diet and Melanoma. An exploratory case-control study. *Ann Epidemiol* 1993;3:235.
33. Marchand LE. Dietary factors in the etiology of melanoma. *Clin Dermatol* 1992;10:79.
34. Kripke ML. Ultraviolet radiation and immunology: something new under the sun [presidential address]. *Cancer Res* 1994;54:6102.
35. Balch CM, Houghton A, Milton GW, et al., eds. *Cutaneous melanoma,* 2nd ed. Philadelphia: JB Lippincott, 1993:216.
36. Balch CM, Buzaid AC, Soong S-J, et al. Final version of the American Joint Committee on Cancer Staging System for cutaneous melanoma. *J Clin Oncol* 2001;19:3635.
37. Breslow A. Thickness, cross-sectional areas, and depth of invasion in the prognosis of cutaneous melanoma. *Am Surg* 1970;172:902.
38. Clark WH Jr, From L, Bernardino EA, Mihn MC. The histogenesis and biologic behavior of primary human malignant melanomas of the skin. *Cancer Res* 1989;29:705.
39. Buzaid AC, Tinoco L, Ross MI, et al. Role of computed tomography in the staging of patients with local-regional metastases of melanoma. *J Clin Oncol* 1995;13:2104.
40. Lentsch EJ, Myers JN. Melanoma of the head and neck: current concepts in diagnosis and management. *Laryngoscope* 2001;111:1209.
41. Kokoska MS, Olson G, Kelemen PR, et al. The use of lymphoscintigraphy and PET in the management of head and neck melanoma. *Otolaryngol Head Neck Surg* 2001;125:213.
42. Steinert HC, Voellmy DR, Trachsel C, et al. Planar coincidence scintigraphy and PET in staging malignant melanoma. *J Nucl Med* 1998;39:1892.
43. Mijnhout GS, Hoekstra OT, van Tulder MW, et al. Systematic review of the diagnostic accuracy of 18F-fluorodeoxyglucose positron emission tomography in melanoma patients. *Cancer* 2001;91:1530.
44. Wanebo HJ, Harpole D, Teates D. Radionuclide lymphoscintigraphy with technetium 99m antimony trisulfide colloid to identify lymphatic drainage of cutaneous melanoma at ambiguous sites in the head and neck trunk. *Cancer* 1985;55:1403.
45. O'Brien CJ, Peterson-Schaefer K, Ruark D, et al. Radical, modified, and selective neck dissection for cutaneous malignant melanoma. *Head Neck* 1995; 17:232.
46. Pathak I, O'Brien CJ, Petersen-Schaeffer K, et al. Do nodal metastases from cutaneous melanoma of the head and neck follow a clinically predictable pattern? *Head Neck* 2001;23:785.
47. O'Brien CJ, Uren RF, Thompson JF, et al. Prediction of potential metastatic sites in cutaneous head and neck melanoma using lymphoscintigraphy. *Am J Surg* 1995;170:461.
48. Reintgen D, Cruse CW, Wells K, et al. The orderly progression of melanoma nodal metastases. *Ann Surg* 1994;220:759.
49. Morton DL, Wen DR, Wong JH, et al. Technical details of intraoperative lymphatic mapping for early stage melanoma. *Arch Surg* 1992;127:392.
50. Ross MI, Reintgen D, Balch CM. Selective lymphadenectomy: emerging role for lymphatic mapping and sentinel node biopsy in the management of early stage melanoma. *Semin Surg Oncol* 1993;9:219.
51. Thompson JF, McCarthy WH, Bosch CMJ, et al. Sentinel lymph node status as an indicator of the presence of metastatic melanoma in regional lymph nodes. *Melanoma Res* 1995;5:255.
52. Handley WS. The pathology of melanotic growths in relation to their metastases of melanoma. *Lancet* 1907;1:927.
53. Veronesi U, Cascinelli N. Narrow excision (1 cm margin), a safe procedure for thin cutaneous melanoma. *Arch Surg* 1991;126:438.
54. Balch CM, Urist MM, Karakousis CP, et al. Efficacy of 2-cm surgical margins for intermediate-thickness melanomas (1 to 4 mm). Results of a multi-institutional randomized surgical trial. *Ann Surg* 1993;218:262.
55. Balch CM. The role of elective lymph node dissection in melanoma: rationale, results, and controversies. *J Clin Oncol* 1988;6:163.
56. Sim FH, Taylor WF, Pritchard OJ, et al. Lymphadenectomy in the management of stage I malignant melanoma: a prospective, randomized study. *Mayo Clin Proc* 1986;61:697.
57. Verones U, Adamus J, Bandiera DC, et al. Inefficiency of immediate lymph node dissection in stage I melanoma of the limbs. *N Engl J Med* 1977;297:627.
58. Elder DE, Guerry D, Van Horn M, et al. The role of lymph node dissection for clinical stage I malignant melanoma of intermediate thickness (1.51–3.99). *Cancer* 1985;56:413.
59. Balch CM, Soong SJ, Milton GW, et al. A comparison of prognostic factors and surgical results in 1,786 patients with localized (stage I) melanoma treated in Alabama, USA and New South Wales, Australia. *Ann Surg* 1982; 196:677.
60. Milton GW, Shaw HM, McCarthy WH, et al. Prophylactic lymph node dissection in clinical stage I cutaneous malignant melanoma: results of surgical treatment in 1,319 patients. *Br J Surg* 1982;69:108.
61. Sutherland CM, Bather FJ. Prophylactic lymph node dissection for malignant melanoma: what to do while we wait. *J Surg Oncol* 1992;51:1.
62. McCarthy WH, Shaw HM, Cascinelli N, et al. Elective lymph node dissection for melanoma: two perspectives. *World J Surg* 1992;16:203.
63. O'Brien CJ, Coates AS, Peterson-Schaefer K, et al. Experience with 998 cutaneous melanomas of the head and neck over 30 years. *Am J Surg* 1991;162: 310.
64. White RR, Tyler DS. Management of node-positive melanoma in the era of sentinel node biopsy. *Surg Oncol* 2000;9:119.
65. Eicher SA, Clayman GL, Myers JN, et al. A prospective study of intraoperative lymphatic mapping for head and neck cutaneous melanoma. *Arch Otolaryngol Head Neck Surg* 2002;128:241.
66. Carlson GW, Murray DR, Greenlee R, et al. Management of malignant melanoma of the head and neck using dynamic lymphoscintigraphy and gamma probe-guided sentinel lymph node biopsy. *Arch Otolaryngol Head Neck Surg* 2000;126:433.
67. Jansen L, Koops HS, Nieweg OE, et al. Sentinel node biopsy for melanoma in the head and neck region. *Head Neck* 2000;22:27.
68. Patel SG, Coit DG, Shaha AR, et al. Sentinel lymph node biopsy for cutaneous head and neck melanomas. *Arch Otolaryngol Head Neck Surg* 2002;128:285.
69. Morton DL, Wen D-R, Foshag LJ, et al. Intraoperative lymphatic mapping and selective cervical lymphadenectomy for early-stage melanomas of the head and neck. *J Clin Oncol* 1993;11:1751.

70. Shivers S, Weng X, Li W, et al. Molecular staging of malignant melanoma. Correlation with clinical outcome. *JAMA* 1998;280:1410.
71. Gershenwald JE, Thompson W, Mansfield PF, et al. Multi-institutional melanoma lymphatic mapping experience: the prognostic value of sentinel lymph node status in 612 stage I or II melanoma patients. *J Clin Oncol* 1999;17:976.
72. Ang KK, Peters LJ, Weber RS, et al. Postoperative radiotherapy for cutaneous melanoma of the head and neck region. *Int J Radiat Oncol Biol Phys* 1994;30: 795.
73. O'Brien CJ, Petersen-Schaefer K, Stevens GN, et al. Adjuvant radiotherapy following neck dissection and parotidectomy for metastatic malignant melanoma. *Head Neck* 1997;19:589.
74. Byers RM. The role of modified neck dissection in the treatment of cutaneous melanoma of the head and neck. *Arch Surg* 1996;121:1338.
75. Shen P, Wanek LA, Morton DL. Is adjuvant radiotherapy necessary after positive lymph node dissection in head and neck melanomas? *Ann Surg Oncol* 2000;7:554.
76. Lens MB, Dawes M. Interferon alpha therapy for malignant melanoma: a systematic review of randomized controlled trials. *J Clin Oncol* 2002;20:1818.
77. Agarwala SS, Kirkwood JM. Update on the role of adjuvant interferon for high risk melanoma. *FORUM Trends Exp Clin Med* 2000;10:230.
78. Kirkwood JM, Strawderman MH, Ernstoff MS, et al. Interferon alfa-2b adjuvant therapy of high-risk resected cutaneous melanoma: the Eastern Cooperative Oncology Group trial EST 1684. *J Clin Oncol* 1996;14:7.
79. Gray RJ, Pockaj BA, Kirkwood JM. An update on adjuvant interferon for melanoma. *Cancer Control* 2002;9:16.
80. Kirkwood JM, Ibrahim JG, Sondak VK, et al. High- and low-dose interferon alfa-2b in high-risk melanoma: first analysis of Intergroup trial E1690/S9111/C9190. *J Clin Oncol* 2000;18:2444.
81. Spitler LE. Adjuvant therapy of melanoma: at what cost? *J Clin Oncol* 2001; 19:1226.
82. Brystryn JC, Zeleniuch-Jacquotte A, Oratz R, et al. Double-blind trial of a polyvalent, shed antigen, melanoma vaccine. *Clin Cancer Res* 2001;7:1882.
83. Morton DL, Barth A. Vaccine therapy for malignant melanoma. *CA Cancer J Clin* 1996;46:225.
84. Berd D, Maguire HC Jr, Schuchter LM, et al. Autologous hapten-modified melanoma vaccine as postsurgical adjuvant treatment after resection of nodal metastases. *J Clin Oncol* 1997;15:2359.
85. Sosman JA, Unger JM, Liu P-Y, et al. Adjuvant immunotherapy of resected, intermediate-thickness, node-negative melanoma with an allogenic tumor vaccine: impact of HLA Class I antigen expression on outcome. *J Clin Oncol* 2002;20:2067.
86. Livingston P. The unfulfilled promise of melanoma vaccines. *Clin Cancer Res* 2001;7:1837.
87. Kirkwood JM, Ibrahim JG, Sosman JA, et al. High dose interferon α-2b significantly prolongs relapse-free and overall survival compared with GM2-KLH/QS-21 vaccine in patients with resected stage IIB-III melanoma: results of intergroup trial E1694/S9512/C509801. *J Clin Oncol* 2001;19:2370.
88. Gorenstein LA, Putnam JB Jr, Natarajan G, et al. Improved survival after resection of pulmonary metastases from malignant melanoma. *Ann Thorac Surg* 1991;52:204.
89. Mansfield PF, Lee JE, Balch CM. Cutaneous melanoma: current practice and surgical controversies. *Curr Probl Surg* 1994;31:255.
90. Philip AP, Flaherty LE. Biochemotherapy for melanoma. *Curr Oncol Rep* 2000; 2:314.
91. Lee M, Betticher DC, Thatcher N. Melanoma: chemotherapy. *Br Med Bull* 1995;51:609.
92. Kirkwood JM, Agarwala S. Systemic cytotoxic and biologic therapy of melanoma. *Principles Pract Oncol Updates* 1993;7:1.
93. Brinckerhoff LH, Thompson LW, Slingluff CL. Melanoma vaccines. *Curr Opin Oncol* 2000;12:163.
94. Haigh PI, Difronzo LA, Gammon G, et al. Vaccine therapy for patients with melanoma. *Oncology* 1999;13:1561.
95. Chang AE, Aruga A, Cameron MJ, et al. Adaptive immunotherapy with vaccine-primed lymph node cells secondarily activated with anti-co3 and interleukin-z. *J Clin Oncol* 1997;15:796.
96. Adler A, Schachter J, Barenholz Y, et al. Allogenic human liposomal melanoma vaccine with or without IL-2 in metastatic melanoma patients: clinical and immunobiological effects. *Cancer Biotherapy* 1995;10:293.
97. Quan WD Jr, Dean GE, Spears L, et al. Active specific immunotherapy of metastatic melanoma with an antiidiotype vaccine: a phase I/II trial of I-mel-2 plus SAF-m. *J Clin Oncol* 1997;15:2103.
98. Wallack MK, Sivanandham M, Ditaranto K, et al. Increased survival of patients treated with a vaccinia melanoma oncolysate vaccine: second interim analysis of data from a phase III, multi-institutional trial. *Ann Surg* 1997;226:198.
99. Slingluff CL Jr, Yamshchikov G, Neese P, et al. Phase I trial of a melanoma vaccine with gp100 (280–288) peptide and tetanus helper peptide in adjuvant: immunologic and clinical outcomes. *Clin Cancer Res* 2001;7:3012.
100. Pardoll D. Cancer vaccines. *Nat Med* 1998;4(suppl 5):525.
101. Pyrhonen S, Hahka-Kempinen M, Muhonen T. A promising interferon plus 4-drug chemotherapy regimen for metastatic melanoma. *J Clin Oncol* 1993; 10:1919.
102. Rosenberg SA, Yang JC, Schwartzentruber DJ, et al. Prospective randomized trial of the treatment of patients with metastatic melanoma using chemotherapy with cisplatin, dacarbazine, and tamoxifen alone or in combination with interleukin-2 and interferon α-2b. *J Clin Oncol* 1999;17:968.
103. Legha SS, Ring S, Eton O, et al. Development of a biochemotherapy regimen with concurrent administration of cisplatin, vinblastine, dacarbazine, interferon alpha, and interleukin-2 for patients with metastatic melanoma. *J Clin Oncol* 1998;16:1752.
104. Sotomayor MG, Hu H, Antonia S, et al. Advances in gene therapy for malignant melanoma. *Cancer Control* 2002;9:39.
105. Parmiani G, Colombo MP. Somatic gene therapy of human melanoma: preclinical studies and early clinical trials. *Melanoma Res* 1995;5:295.
106. Stopeck AT, Jones A, Hersh EM, et al. Phase II study of direct intralesional gene transfer of allovectin-7, an HLA-B7/beta2-microglobulin DNA-liposome complex, in patients with metastatic melanoma. *Clin Cancer Res* 2001;7: 2285.
107. Romero JB, Stefanato CM, Kopf AW, et al. Follow-up recommendations for patients with stage I malignant melanoma. *Dermatol Surg Oncol* 1994;20:175.
108. Brandt SE, Welvaart K, Hermans J. Long-term follow-up justified after excision of a thin melanoma (<1.5 mm)?: a retrospective analysis of 206 patients. *J Surg* 1990;43:157.
109. Weiss M, Loporinzi CL, Creagan ET, et al. Utility of follow-up tests for detecting recurrent disease in patients with malignant melanomas. *JAMA* 1995;274:1703.
110. Tyler DS, Onaitis M, Kherani A, et al. Positron emission tomography scanning in malignant melanoma. *Cancer* 2000;89:1019.
111. Taback B, Morton DL, O'Day SJ, et al. The clinical utility of multimarker RT-PCR in the detection of occult metastasis in patients with melanoma. *Recent Results Cancer Res* 2001;158:78.
112. Morton DL, Davytan DG, Wanek LA, et al. Multivariate analysis of the relationship between survival and the microstage of primary melanoma by Clark Level and Breslow Thickness. *Cancer* 1993;1971:3737.
113. Schultz S, Kane M, Rosuh R, et al. Time to recurrence varies inversely with thickness in clinical stage I cutaneous melanoma. *J Am Coll Surg* 1990;171:393.
114. Roses DF, Karp NS, Oratz R, et al. Survival with regional and distant metastasis from cutaneous melanoma. *J Am Coll Surg* 1991;172:262.
115. Rangborg U, Afzelius L-E, Lagerlorf B, et al. Cutaneous malignant melanoma of the head and neck. Analysis of treatment results and prognostic factors in 581 patients: a report from the Swedish Melanoma Study Group. *Cancer* 1993;71:751.
116. Bernengo MG, Reali UM, Doveil GC, et al. BANS: discussion of the problem. *Melanoma Res* 1992;2:157.
117. Byers RM, Smith JL, Russell N, et al. Melanoma of the external ear: a review of 102 cases. *Am J Surg* 1980;140:518.
118. Shumate CR, Carlson GW, Giacco GG, et al. Scalp melanoma: location as a prognostic indicator. *Melanoma Lett* 1991;9:3.
119. Kheir SA, Bines SD, Vonroenn JH, et al. Prognostic significance of DNA aneuploidy in stage I cutaneous melanoma. *Ann Surg* 1988;207:455.
120. Reed JA, Albino AP. Update of diagnostic and prognostic markers in cutaneous malignant melanoma. *Clin Lab Med* 2000;20:817.
121. Kashani-Sabet M, Sagebiel RW, Ferreira CMM, et al. Tumor vascularity in the prognostic assessment of primary cutaneous melanoma. *J Clin Oncol* 2002;20: 1826.
122. Beenken S, Byers R, Smith JL, et al. Desmoplastic melanoma. Histologic correlations with behavior and treatment. *Arch Otolaryngol Head Neck Surg* 1989; 115:374.
123. Smithers BM, McLeod GR, Little JH. Desmoplastic melanoma: patterns of recurrence. *World J Surg* 1992;16:186.
124. Conley J, Pack GT. Melanoma of the mucous membranes of the head and neck. *Arch Otolaryngol Head Neck Surg* 1974;99:315.
125. Stern SJ, Guillamondegui OM. Mucosal melanoma of the head and neck. *Arch Otolaryngol Head Neck Surg* 1991;13:22.
126. Patel SG, Prasad ML, Escrig M, et al. Primary mucosal malignant melanoma of the head and neck. *Head Neck* 2002;24:247.

Radiologic Imaging Concerns

127. Wilmes EBJ. Recommendations for therapy of head and neck cutaneous melanoma. *Am J Otolaryngol* 1993;14:267–270.
128. Kelemen PR, Essner R, Foshag LJ, et al. Lymphatic mapping and sentinel lymphadenectomy after wide local excision of primary melanoma. *J Am Coll Surg* 1999;189:247–252.
129. Morris KT, Stevens JS, Pommier RF, et al. Usefulness of preoperative lymphoscintigraphy for the identification of sentinel lymph nodes in melanoma. *Am J Surg* 2001;181:423–426.
130. Wells KE, Rapaport DP, Cruse CW, et al. Sentinel lymph node biopsy in melanoma of the head and neck. *Plast Reconstr Surg* 1997;100:591–594.
131. Alex JC, Krag DN, Harlow SP, et al. Localization of regional lymph nodes in melanomas of the head and neck. *Arch Otolaryngol Head Neck Surg* 1998;124: 135–140.
132. Reintgen D, Cruse CW, Wells K, et al. The orderly progression of melanoma nodal metastases. *Ann Surg* 1994;220:759–767.
133. Leong SP SI, et al. Optimal selective sentinel lymph node dissection in primary malignant melanoma. *Arch Surg* 1997;132:666–672.
134. Carlson JA, Dickersin GR, Sober AJ, et al. Desmoplastic neurotropic melanoma. A clinicopathologic analysis of 28 cases.*Cancer* 1995;75:478–494.
135. Batsakis JG, Raymond AK. Desmoplastic melanoma. *Ann Otol Rhinol Laryngol* 1994;103:77–79.
136. Beenken S, Byers R, Smith JL, et al. Desmoplastic melanoma. Histologic correlation with behavior and treatment. *Arch Otolaryngol Head Neck Surg* 1989; 115:374–379.

137. Majoie CB, Hulsmans FJ, Castelijns JA, et al. Perineural tumor extension of facial malignant melanoma: CT and MRI. *J Comput Assist Tomogr* 1993;17: 973–975.
138. Brandwein MS, Rothstein A, Lawson W, et al. Sinonasal melanoma. A clinicopathologic study of 25 cases and literature meta-analysis. *Arch Otolaryngol Head Neck Surg* 1997;123:290–296.
139. Steinert HC, Huch Boni RA, Buck A, et al. Malignant melanoma: staging with whole-body positron emission tomography and 2-[F-18]-fluoro-2-deoxy-D-glucose. *Radiology* 1995;195:705–709.
140. Manolidis S, Donald PJ. Malignant mucosal melanoma of the head and neck: review of the literature and report of 14 patients. *Cancer* 1997;80:1373–1386.
141. Virgo KS, Chan D, Handler BS, et al. Current practice of patient follow-up after potentially curative resection of cutaneous melanoma. *Plast Reconstr Surg* 2000;106:590–597.
142. Wagner JD, Schauwecker D, Davidson D, et al. Prospective study of fluorodeoxyglucose-positron emission tomography imaging of lymph node basins in melanoma patients undergoing sentinel node biopsy. *J Clin Oncol* 1999;17:1508–1515.

CHAPTER 26

Management of Malignant Salivary Gland Tumors

David W. Eisele and Lawrence R. Kleinberg

Malignant tumors of the salivary glands represent a diverse group of neoplasms with varied biologic behavior. The salivary glands consist of major salivary glands, including the paired parotid, submandibular, and sublingual glands, and the minor salivary glands, which are distributed throughout the upper aerodigestive tract. Salivary gland malignancies are uncommon and occur with an incidence of approximately 1 to 2 per 100,000 population per year. Because of the infrequent occurrence of salivary gland malignancies, single-institution experience with these tumors is usually limited, rendering treatment studies difficult. In addition, the great variety of histopathologic diagnoses associated with salivary gland malignancies and the different biologic behavior of each tumor type result in further difficulty in planning therapy for salivary gland malignancies. An accurate pathologic diagnosis and an understanding of the behavior of each tumor type, therefore, are necessary for the development of an appropriate treatment plan for the individual patient.

The etiologic factors for salivary gland malignancies are poorly understood. Unlike epidermoid carcinoma of the upper aerodigestive tract, tobacco and alcohol use are not considered etiologic factors for salivary gland malignancies. Low-dose radiation therapy or cumulative exposure to irradiation, such as dental radiographs, has been implicated as causal factors for both benign and malignant salivary gland neoplasms (1). Therapeutic, high-dose radiation therapy is not associated with the development of salivary gland neoplasms. Exposure to hardwood dust has been linked to the development of nasal cavity and paranasal sinus minor salivary gland adenocarcinomas (2).

RELEVANT ANATOMY

Parotid Gland

The parotid gland, the largest of the major salivary glands, is a unilobular gland located anteroinferior to the ear. The gland is positioned between the mandibular ramus and mastoid and tympanic portions of the temporal lobe. The gland extends anteriorly over the masseter muscle, superiorly to the zygomatic arch, posteriorly over the sternocleidomastoid muscle, and medially between the mandible and temporal bone. The medial aspect of the gland abuts the lateral parapharyngeal space; therefore, parotid neoplasms may involve this important potential cavity. Superficially, the gland lies in close proximity to the skin and is encased by the superficial layer of the deep

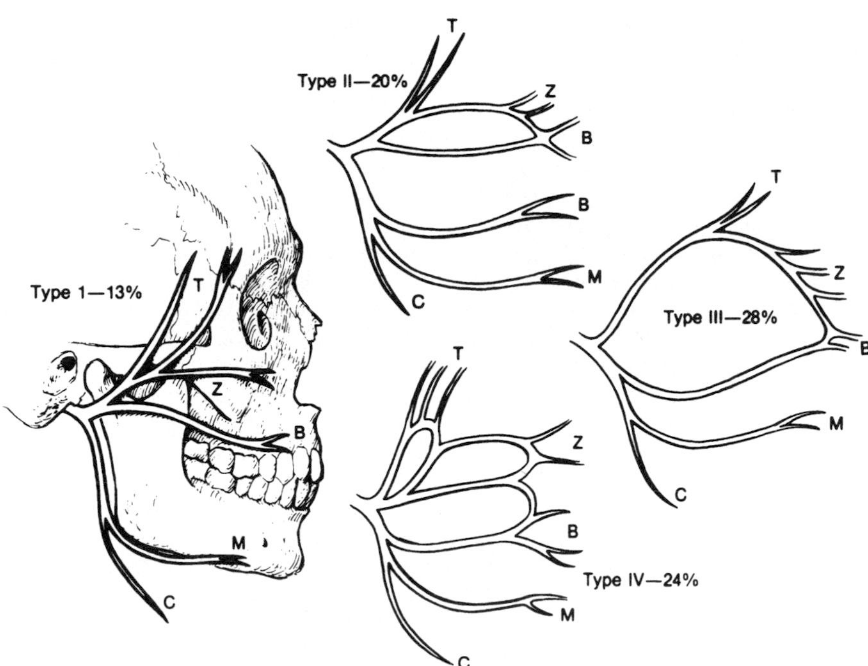

Figure 26.1 Anatomic variations of facial nerve branching. *B,* buccal; *C,* cervical; *M,* marginal mandibular; *T,* temporal; *Z,* zygomatic. (From Johns ME, Kaplan MJ. Malignant neoplasms. In: Cummings CW, Fredrickson JM, Harker LA et al., eds. *Otolaryngology—head and neck surgery,* 2nd ed. St. Louis: Mosby-Year Book, 1993:1048, with permission.)

cervical fascia, subcutaneous tissue, and anteroinferiorly by the platysma muscle.

Although the gland is unilobular, the portion of the gland lateral to the facial nerve is termed the *superficial lobe* and that medial to the nerve the *deep lobe* of the gland. These two lobes are actually contiguous and are not distinct anatomic structures. Rather, they are the consequence of surgical dissection.

Multiple projections of the gland can exist and are variable. The presence of these processes renders total removal of all parotid tissue difficult during total parotidectomy.

Stensen's duct, or the parotid duct, drains the parotid gland. It courses anteriorly over the masseter muscle from the anterior aspect of the gland and then courses medially through the buccinator muscle and buccal fat pad, entering the oral cavity opposite the second upper molar. Accessory parotid tissue separate from the parotid gland can occur adjacent to Stensen's duct and is present in approximately 20% of patients (3).

The facial nerve exits the temporal bone via the stylomastoid foramen and enters the parotid gland. Within the gland, the nerve divides at the pes anserinus into temporofacial and cervicofacial trunks. The nerve then divides in a variable pattern into five branches: frontal, zygomatic, buccal, mandibular, and cervical (Fig. 26.1) (4). Variable patterns of anastomosis exist between the upper branches. The distal branches of the facial nerve innervate the ipsilateral facial muscles.

Landmarks for identification of the facial nerve during parotidectomy are shown in Table 26.1. Wide surgical exposure is necessary for adequate landmark visualization. The surgeon should be prepared to use any of the anatomic landmarks for nerve identification.

TABLE 26.1 Anatomic Landmarks for Facial Nerve Identification

Targal pointer (nerve approximately 1 cm medial and anteroinferior to tip of pointer)
Tympanomastoid structure (nerve approximately 6–8 mm medial to suture)
Diagastric muscle attachment to diagastric groove (nerve just superior and on same plane as muscle attachment)
Nerve within mastoid bone
Retrograde dissection from distal nerve branch

The parotid gland receives parasympathetic secretomotor innervation. Preganglionic parasympathetic fibers originate in the inferior salivary nucleus of the brainstem and travel in the glossopharyngeal nerve. Fibers then course in the tympanic branch of the glossopharyngeal nerve to the tympanic plexus and then in the lesser superficial petrosal nerve to the otic ganglion. Postganglionic parasympathetic fibers from the otic ganglion reach the parotid gland via the auriculotemporal nerve. The parotid gland receives sensory innervation from the trigeminal nerve.

The arterial supply to the parotid gland consists of the superficial temporal and internal maxillary arteries. The gland's veins drain via the superficial temporal vein and maxillary vein, which join to form the retromandibular vein.

The parotid gland lymphatics drain to intraglandular lymph nodes, which are entrapped within the gland during embryologic development, and to extraglandular periparotid nodes. Cervical lymphatics drain to submandibular and deep upper jugular nodes.

Submandibular Gland

The submandibular gland is located within the submandibular triangle. Anteriorly, a portion of the gland lies superior to the mylohyoid muscle. Wharton's duct, the submandibular duct, lies in proximity to this anterior, superior portion of the gland and courses superior to the mylohyoid muscle and lateral to the hyoglossus muscle. The duct enters the oral cavity as an elevated papilla just lateral to the lingual frenulum. Posteriorly, the submandibular gland is near the parotid gland and is separated from it by the stylomandibular ligament. Medially, the gland is adjacent to the hyoglossus muscle. Laterally, the upper portion of the gland is adjacent to the mandible. Inferiorly, the gland is adjacent to the digastric sling and extends lateral to the anterior and posterior bellies of the digastric muscle. With age, the gland may become ptotic and occupy a lower position in the neck.

Three nerves of importance lie close to the submandibular gland. The marginal mandibular branch of the facial nerve courses superficial to the fascia overlying the gland and deep to the platysma muscle. The hypoglossal nerve courses between the gland and the hyoglossus muscle. The lingual nerve lies superior to the gland. Postganglionic parasympathetic innervation originating in the superior salivary nucleus reaches the submandibular ganglion via the facial nerve and chorda tympani. Postganglionic parasympathetic fibers course from the submandibular ganglion to the submandibular gland. The vascular supply to the submandibular gland is the facial artery, which is close to the medial aspect of the gland. The gland's veins drain via the lingual vein. The submandibular gland's lymphatics drain to submandibular nodes and deep jugular nodes.

Sublingual Gland

The sublingual gland, the smallest of the major salivary glands, is located proximal to the submandibular duct, superior to the mylohyoid muscle. Laterally, it is close to the mandible, and medially it lies adjacent to the hyoglossus muscle posteriorly and the genioglossus muscle anteriorly. The gland is located just deep to the oral mucosa in the floor of the mouth. Saliva from the sublingual gland enters the oral cavity via multiple small sublingual ducts. These ducts may unite to form a larger duct, Bartholin's duct, which joins the submandibular duct. Postganglionic parasympathetic nerve fibers from the submandibular ganglion supply the sublingual gland. The arterial supply to the sublingual gland is the sublingual branch of the lingual artery and the submental branch of the facial artery. The sublingual gland's lymphatics drain to the submandibular and deep jugular nodes.

Minor Salivary Glands

The minor salivary glands, of which there are approximately 750 to 1,000, are distributed throughout the upper aerodigestive tract and are concentrated primarily in the oral cavity and oropharynx. Minor salivary glands also are located in the nose and nasal cavity, paranasal sinuses, nasopharynx, larynx, and trachea. The lymphatic drainage of the minor salivary glands is site-specific and approximates the recognized lymphatic drainage of the site. Rarely, ectopic salivary gland tissue, such as that found in the mandible, undergoes neoplastic transformation (5).

CLINICAL PRESENTATION

Parotid Gland Malignancies

On presentation, patients with malignant tumors of the parotid gland are approximately a decade older than patients with benign parotid neoplasms, with an average age at presentation of approximately 55 to 60 years (6–8). Malignant parotid tumors are distributed evenly between the sexes (6), with a slight male predominance reported in several series (7,9).

Most patients (65% to 80%) present with an asymptomatic parotid mass (7,8,10). A significant proportion of malignant parotid tumors are clinically indistinguishable from a benign neoplasm. The duration of symptoms before presentation averages approximately 4 to 8 months (6,8). Approximately 10% of patients, however, have a history of a long-standing mass (6). In one study, palpable cervical lymph nodes, facial nerve palsy, deep tumor fixation, and rapid tumor enlargement were statistically significant symptoms and signs suggestive of malignancy by multivariate analysis (11).

Pleomorphic adenoma of the parotid can undergo malignant degeneration (carcinoma ex pleomorphic adenoma) at a rate of approximately 5% (12,13). This is most likely to occur in patients with a long-standing pleomorphic adenoma (14). A rapid change in the size of a chronic parotid mass and development of new symptoms related to the mass in a previously asymptomatic patient should raise suspicion of the possibility of malignant transformation. Rapid increase in size of a benign parotid neoplasm, however, can also occur.

Approximately 10% to 15% of patients with malignant parotid neoplasms present with pain. Pain is not a reliable indicator for malignancy, however, as it occurs in approximately 5% of patients with benign parotid tumors (15). Pain associated with a malignant neoplasm is associated with a worse prognosis, as compared with an asymptomatic parotid malignancy (10,16).

Facial nerve paralysis, either generalized or partial, occurs in 10% to 20% of patients with malignant parotid tumors (9,17–19). Other symptoms on presentation can include sensory loss (10%) and trismus (4%) (9).

The superficial lobe of the gland is the primary site of parotid cancers in approximately 90% of patients (9). Malignant parotid neoplasms may present as parapharyngeal space masses (20). Approximately 5% of parotid malignancies have clinically apparent parapharyngeal space extension at the time of presentation (8,9). The accessory parotid gland is involved primarily by parotid malignancies 2% of the time (10).

Clinically apparent cervical lymph node metastases are found at presentation in approximately 10% to 15% of patients (9,19), and periparotid nodes are evident in 6% of patients (9).

Submandibular Gland Malignancies

The average patient age at presentation with submandibular gland malignancies is similar to that of patients with parotid malignancies (55 to 60 years old) (21). There is a slight male predominance, with a male-female ratio of 1.2:0 (21).

Submandibular gland malignant neoplasms present as an asymptomatic mass in most patients (21,22). Pain is present in 6% to 7% of patients (21,22). Duration of symptoms before presentation averages some 6 months (21). Tumors that are present for more than 5 years are usually low-grade mucoepidermoid carcinomas or malignant mixed tumors (22).

Skin attachment or deep tumor fixation was noted in 28% of patients in one study (22). Local tumor invasion involving the marginal mandibular nerve, the lingual nerve, or the hypoglossal nerve can infrequently occur. Cervical lymph node metastases are clinically apparent in 14% to 16% of patients at presentation (21,22).

Sublingual Gland Malignancies

Most patients (45%) with malignant neoplasms of the sublingual gland present with asymptomatic floor-of-mouth swelling (23,24). Some tumors (20%) are identified incidentally by dental practitioners (23). At presentation, approximately 15% of patients already are experiencing pain (23). Other presenting symptoms include impaired denture retention and tongue sensory loss (23).

Minor Salivary Gland Malignancies

The clinical presentation of minor salivary gland malignancies depends on tumor site of origin, histopathologic type, and size. Most malignant tumors of minor salivary glands involve the oral cavity, with the hard palate being the most common site (25). Most patients present with a painless submucosal mass (26). Pain is uncommon and ulceration is unusual (26,27). Except for those that arise in the hard palate, most are mobile

(26). The average duration of symptoms is approximately 6 months, but 30% of patients have symptoms present for greater than 1 year before diagnosis (27).

Malignant tumors of the nasal cavity and paranasal sinuses present most commonly with epistaxis, nasal obstruction, or chronic sinusitis (28). Tumors arising in the maxillary sinus are associated with facial pain and swelling (26). Tumors that invade the orbit may present with decreased visual acuity, diplopia, epiphora, or proptosis (28). Neoplasms arising from the nasopharynx may present with hearing loss due to eustachian tube dysfunction or nasal obstruction.

Laryngeal minor salivary gland malignancies most commonly involve the supraglottic larynx and present with throat pain, hoarseness, and dysphagia (26). Those arising in the subglottic larynx usually present with airway obstruction (26). Primary tracheal malignancies commonly present with hoarseness, dyspnea, and cough (26).

Ectopic salivary gland tumors of the mandible may present clinically and radiographically similar to odontogenic tumors. Pain, jaw swelling, and trismus are the most frequent complaints (5).

DIAGNOSTIC EVALUATION AND STAGING

Fine-Needle Aspiration Biopsy

Fine-needle aspiration biopsy (FNAB), a simple and well-tolerated procedure, is a highly accurate method for the diagnosis of salivary gland neoplasms. We use FNAB in the initial assessment of most patients with suspected major salivary gland neoplasms. Some suspected neoplasms are determined by FNAB to be nonneoplastic, inflammatory processes or cysts, and thus surgery may be avoided (29,30). In other patients, the scope of the surgery may be modified. For example, if lymphoma of the parotid is diagnosed by FNAB, incisional biopsy of the mass (rather than formal parotidectomy) is sufficient for lymphoma classification.

The routine use of FNAB for the assessment of parotid neoplasms is controversial (31). Opponents of its routine use argue that it infrequently alters the standard approach—parotidectomy—which provides a definitive diagnosis for, and cures the majority of, parotid neoplasms. One benefit of FNAB for parotid masses is its ability to diagnose malignancy before surgery. This allows the surgeon to plan for prompt therapy, obtain appropriate imaging studies, and obtain preoperative consultations with radiation oncologists and dentists, if necessary. The patient can be counseled regarding the scope of the surgery and treatment plan. If a metastatic malignancy to the parotid is suspected, a search for the primary neoplasm can be undertaken. Most of the time, however, a benign neoplasm is diagnosed, and the patient can be immediately reassured regarding the suspected diagnosis.

Fine-needle aspiration biopsy for salivary gland masses is very accurate; however, the accuracy of FNAB depends on the skill of the cytopathologist. Sensitivities of greater than 90% and specificities of greater than 95% have been reported (32–37). Lower rates of sensitivity (approximately 60% to 95%) and specificity (approximately 70% to 90%) for FNAB are obtained for malignant tumors (30). False-negative results for malignancy occur 10% to 25% of the time, which is more frequent than for benign tumors (35,37). False-positive results for malignancy, however, are unusual, and, in general, treatment planning appropriate for malignancy can be undertaken based on the FNAB results if malignancy is diagnosed by FNAB. It should be noted that the accuracy of FNAB for specific malignant tumor classification is limited.

Masses evaluated by FNAB that yield inadequate cellular material should be reevaluated by FNAB. We have found that immediate on-site procurement and evaluation of the FNAB specimen provides a higher yield of adequate specimens, compared with biopsies taken without immediate evaluation (38). Fine-needle aspiration biopsy is performed with or by the cytopathologist, and this approach facilitates clinicopathologic correlation. Suspected neoplasms with repeatedly unsatisfactory or suspicious cytopathologic results require surgery for definitive diagnosis.

Fine-needle aspiration biopsy can also be useful for the assessment of accessible minor salivary gland malignancies (e.g., those involving the oral cavity). Parapharyngeal tumors can be evaluated by needle biopsy transorally or with computed tomographic (CT) guidance. Nonpalpable suspicious nodes can be subjected to biopsy under ultrasound guidance.

Diagnostic Imaging

Radiographic evaluation of the aforementioned neoplasms is discussed later. For parotid and submandibular neoplasms, in most instances, CT scans and magnetic resonance imaging (MRI) do not differentiate benign from malignant tumors and are not routinely obtained for the assessment of small mobile, circumscribed tumors. If malignancy is diagnosed before surgery by FNAB, CT scan or MRI may be of value to assess further the local extent of disease and to assess the neck for nonpalpable lymph nodes. Large tumors and neoplasms that are fixed, recurrent, or involve the deep lobe or parapharyngeal space are evaluated by either CT or MRI. Of MRI findings, poorly defined tumor margins appears to be the characteristic finding best predictive of malignancy (39).

At the present time, positron emission tomography (PET) scans appear to have no advantage over CT or MRI in the evaluation of parotid tumors (40). Radionuclide imaging and sialography are no longer used for the evaluation of parotid neoplasms. Imaging is routinely obtained for the assessment of minor salivary gland malignancies involving the nose and paranasal sinuses. Both MRI and CT scans with direct coronal cuts give valuable information regarding extent of disease. Computed tomography is superior to MRI in bone definition, and MRI is sometimes useful in differentiating paranasal sinus obstructive, inflammatory disease from the neoplasm, and therefore is often complementary to CT scan. Minor salivary gland malignancies involving the oral cavity are imaged by CT scan if there is suspected deep invasion (e.g., hard-palate bone involvement). Minor salivary gland malignancies of the pharynx, larynx, and trachea are imaged by either CT or MRI, but MRI has the advantage of multiplanar imaging, which can be especially helpful in the assessment of laryngeal and tracheal tumors.

Staging

The American Joint Committee on Cancer (AJCC) staging system for major salivary gland malignancies is shown in Table 26.2 (41). Recent AJCC changes have been made in T3 and T4 lesions. In addition to tumors having extraparenchymal extension, all tumors larger than 4 cm are considered T3. T4 lesions have been divided into T4a (resectable) and T4b (unresectable), leading to a division of stage IV into IVA, IVB, and IVC. These changes are reflected in the 6th edition of the AJCC Cancer Staging Manual (41a). This system, which is the same system endorsed by the International Union Against Cancer (UICC), is designed for the staging of malignancies of the major salivary glands, including the parotid, submandibular, and sublingual glands but not for minor salivary gland malignancies. The T

TABLE 26.2 Staging System for Major Salivary Gland Malignancies

Primary tumor (T)

TX	Primary tumor cannot be assessed
T0	No evidence of primary tumor
T1	Tumor 2 cm or less in greatest dimension without extraparenchymal extension[a]
T2	Tumor more than 2 cm but not more than 4 cm in greatest dimension without extraparenchymal extension[a]
T3	Tumor more than 4 cm and/or tumor having extraparenchymal extension[a]
T4a	Tumor invades skin, mandible, ear canal, and/or facial nerve
T4b	Tumor invades skull base and/or pterygoid plates and/or encases carotid artery

Regional lymph nodes (N)

NX	Regional lymph nodes cannot be assessed
N0	No regional lymph node metastasis
N1	Metastasis in a single ipsilateral lymph node, 3 cm or less in greatest dimension
N2	Metastasis in a single ipsilateral lymph node, more than 3 cm but not more than 6 cm in greatest dimension; or in multiple ipsilateral lymph nodes, none more than 6 cm in greatest dimension; or in bilateral or contralateral lymph nodes, none more than 6 cm in greatest dimension
N2a	Metastasis in a single ipsilateral lymph node more than 3 cm but not more than 6 cm in greatest dimension
N2b	Metastasis in multiple ipsilateral lymph nodes, none more than 6 cm in greatest dimension
N2c	Metastasis in bilateral or contralateral lymph nodes, none more than 6 cm in greatest dimension
N3	Metastasis in a lymph node more than 6 cm in greatest dimension

Distant metastasis (M)

MX	Distant metastasis cannot be assessed
M0	No distant metastasis
M1	Distant metastasis

Stage grouping

I	T1	N0	M0
II	T2	N0	M0
III	T3	N0	M0
	T1	N1	M0
	T2	N1	M0
	T3	N1	M0
IVA	T4a	N0	M0
	T4a	N1	M0
	T1	N2	M0
	T2	N2	M0
	T3	N2	M0
	T4a	N2	M0
IVB	T4b	Any N	M0
	Any T	N3	M0
IVC	Any T	Any N	M1

[a]Extraparenchymal extension is clinical or macroscopic evidence of invasion of soft tissues. Microscopic evidence alone does not constitute extraparenchymal extension for classification purposes.
Source: American Joint Committee on Cancer. *AJCC cancer staging manual,* 6th ed. New York: Springer, 2002:69–75, with permission.

classification for assessment of the primary tumor is based on size, extraparenchymal extension, facial nerve involvement, and base of skull invasion. The recent changes in AJCC staging have not been made in the UICC system.

The N classification indicates regional lymph node involvement by tumor. The regional lymph nodes for the parotid gland are the intraparotid, infraauricular, and preauricular nodes. For the submandibular gland, the nodes are the submandibular, upper cervical, and submental-internal (upper deep) jugular nodes. Other lymph node metastases are considered distant metastases. The M staging refers to the presence or absence of distant metastases.

The present staging system describes the anatomic extent of tumor spread but does not account for the clinical biologic behavior of the malignancy (42). Tumor grading, based on cellular and molecular factors, in the future may be important in the staging of salivary gland neoplasms (42).

MANAGEMENT

Surgery is the treatment of choice for almost all malignant salivary gland tumors. Radiation therapy is beneficial as adjunctive therapy for certain malignant tumors. Conventional radiation therapy or fast neutron radiation therapy are used for unresectable lesions, but irradiation alone is rarely used for early lesions. Chemotherapy may be useful in select patients for palliation of unresectable or recurrent disease. The following subsections discuss in detail the treatment of site-specific salivary gland malignancies. An algorithm for the management of salivary gland malignancies is shown in Figure 26.2.

Therapy for Major Salivary Gland Malignancies

Surgical resection is a standard component of treatment of all major salivary gland malignancies. Postoperative radiation therapy is given, depending on the stage and pathologic features of the tumor. The principles of treatment of parotid and submandibular malignancies are summarized in Table 26.3. Unresectable salivary lesions are treated with radiation therapy alone, using conventional techniques or neutron radiation therapy.

SURGICAL THERAPY FOR PAROTID MALIGNANCIES

Most parotid neoplasms, both benign and malignant, are located in the superficial lobe of the gland. Parotidectomy with an adequate margin of resection around the tumor cures most neoplasms, including small low-grade malignancies without local extension (T1, T2). If malignancy is diagnosed before surgery by FNAB or intraoperatively by frozen-section evaluation, parotidectomy with complete tumor resection is recommended. The amount of resection is dictated by the degree of tumor extension. Skin, muscles, nerves, mandible, and temporal bone are resected if invaded. Tumors involving the deep lobe are resected after superficial parotidectomy and facial nerve dissection. An algorithm for parotid malignancy management is shown in Figure 26.3.

Parotidectomy Technique

The face and neck are prepared and draped with a transparent adhesive drape to allow visualization of the face during the procedure. A preauricular incision is made, extending inferiorly along the line of attachment of the ear lobule and curving gently into an upper-neck crease. An anterior skin flap is elevated superficial to the parotid fascia to the posterior border of the masseter, avoiding the peripheral branches of the facial nerve anteriorly. The tail of the parotid is dissected from the sternocleidomastoid muscle. The posterior branch of the greater auricular nerve is preserved if possible.

The digastric muscle, exposed as the tail of the parotid gland is elevated, serves as an important landmark for the facial nerve. A second plane of dissection is developed in the pretragal space. This space is opened with blunt dissection parallel to the course

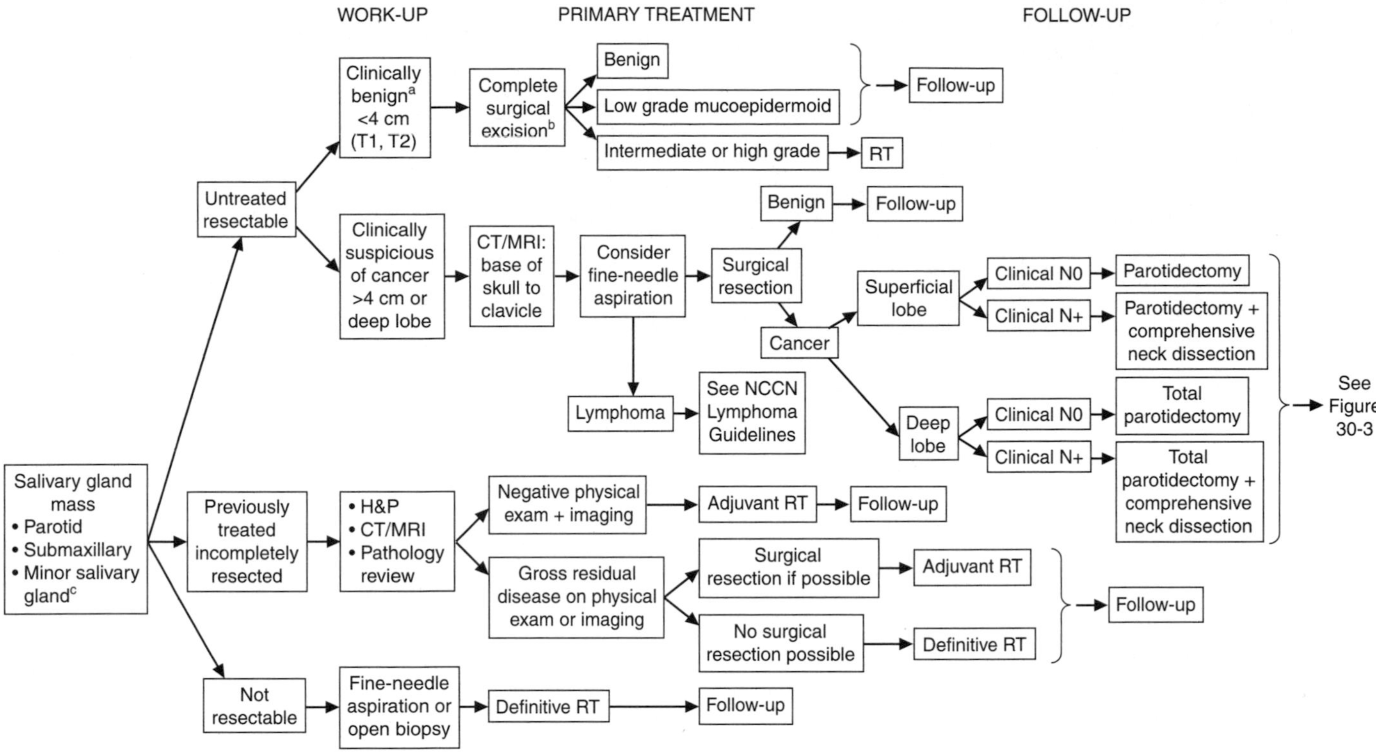

Figure 26.2 National Comprehensive Cancer Network (NCCN) salivary gland mass evaluation and management algorithm. Evaluation, treatment, and follow-up. [a]Characteristics of benign tumor includes superficial lobe, slow growth, painless, VII intact, no neck nodes. [b]Surgical excision of clinically benign tumor: no enucleation of lateral lobe, intraoperative communication with pathologist if indicated. [c]Site and stage determine therapeutic approaches. (From Forastiere AA, Ang K, Brockstein B, et al. *NCCN practice guidelines for head and neck careers.* NCCN, 2000, with permission.)

of the facial nerve. This dissection exposes the tragal pointer and opens a plane from the zygoma superiorly to just above the styloid process inferiorly. With the tail of the parotid gland and the pretragal portion of the parotid gland mobilized, parotid gland fascial attachments to the mastoid remain and are incised. The facial nerve is identified next by anatomic landmarks (see Table 26.1). After the main branch of the facial nerve is identified, the individual branches of the facial nerve are followed peripherally, and the gland is sharply separated from the nerve branches.

Total parotidectomy involves removal of parotid gland tissue, both medial and lateral to the facial nerve. For tumor involving the deep lobe of the gland, superficial parotidectomy and facial

TABLE 26.3 Principles of Treatment for Major Salivary Gland Malignancies

	Stage			
Primary tumor site	**T1 and T2, low grade[a]**	**T1 and T2, high grade[b]**	**T3**	**T4**
Parotid gland	Complete resection by parotidectomy[c]	Complete resection by parotidectomy[c] Neck dissection for N+ neck Postoperative radiation therapy	Complete resection by parotidectomy[c] Neck dissection for N+ neck Postoperative radiation therapy	Complete resection by parotidectomy[c] Resection of skin, mandible, muscles, and temporal bone as necessary to obtain free surgical margins Neck dissection for N+ neck
Submandibular gland	Submandibular gland excision	Wide excision of submandibular triangle Preserve nerves unless involved by tumor Postoperative radiation therapy	Wide excision with neck dissection (including involved nerves) Postoperative radiation therapy	Surgery to fit extent of disease Postoperative radiation therapy

CN, cranial nerve; N+, node positive clinically or radiographically.
[a]Low-grade mucoepidermoid carcinoma and acinic cell carcinoma.
[b]Intermediate and high-grade mucoepidermoid carcinoma, adenocarcinoma, adenoid cystic carcinoma, malignant mixed tumor, undifferentiated carcinoma, and squamous cell carcinoma.
[c]Facial nerve is preserved if functioning preoperatively and surgical plane of dissection between nerve and tumor is present.
Source: Adapted from Eisele DW, Johns ME. Malignant tumors of the salivary glands. In: Niederhuber JE, ed. *Current therapy in oncology.* St. Louis: Mosby-Year Book, 1993:151.

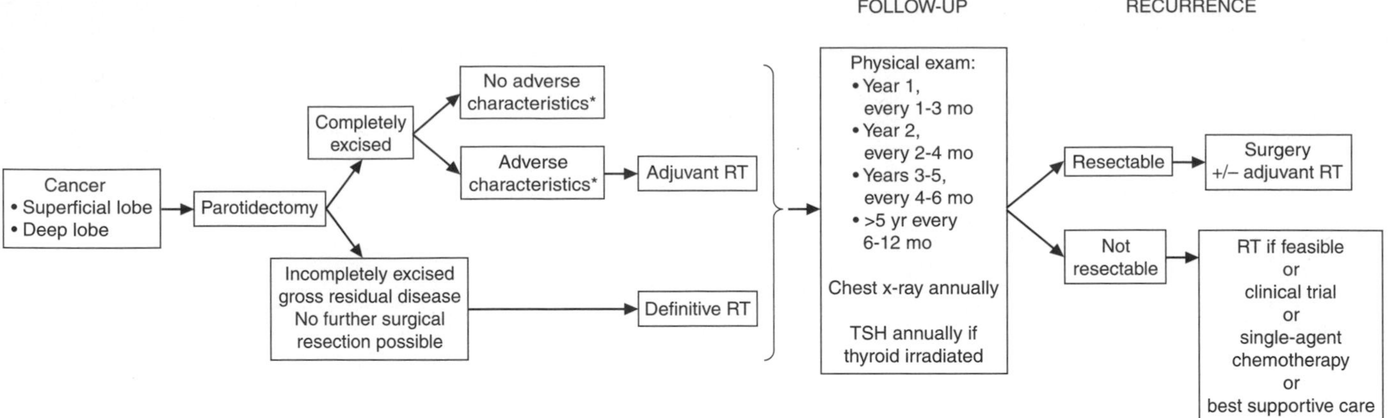

Figure 26.3 National Comprehensive Cancer Network (NCCN) parotid cancer management algorithm. Treatment, follow-up, and recurrence management following parotidectomy. *Asterisk,* Size τ 2 cm, close or positive margins, neural/perineural invasion, lymph node metastasis; consider radiotherapy if lymphatic/vascular invasion, extracapsular spread, or high grade. (From Forastiere AA, Ang K, Brockstein B, et al. *NCCN practice guidelines for head and neck cancers.* NCCN, 2000, with permission.)

nerve dissection are performed first. The deep lobe of the parotid gland is then removed using dissection beneath the nerve.

Extent of Parotidectomy for Malignant Neoplasms

Parotid carcinomas have variable infiltration into adjacent tissues. The surgeon should strive to achieve clear margins of resection, as multiple retrospective studies have shown an increased risk for recurrence (43–45) and decreased survival (46–48) with positive surgical margins of tumor excision. The extent of parotidectomy (partial vs. total) does not appear to impact on local control rates (43) or survival (49). Thus, the dogma that total parotidectomy is the necessary extent of surgery at the primary for parotid malignancies is not supported by the literature. Rather, the extent of surgery for parotid malignancies should be individualized on the basis of clinical findings, imaging studies, and intraoperative findings.

Occasionally, the diagnosis of malignancy is made on evaluation of the permanent pathology after superficial parotidectomy. The need for additional surgery is established after pathologic review of the specimen. If the surgical margins are negative, additional surgery is probably not beneficial to the patient. Positive surgical margins, however, are an indication for additional resection to ensure total tumor removal. Because parotid wound reexploration can be performed safely, oncologic concerns should be paramount in the decision to reoperate (50). The decision for postoperative adjuvant radiation therapy is made on the basis of tumor histopathology and tumor staging. Most patients with malignant tumors—except the low-grade malignancies (low-grade mucoepidermoid carcinoma and acinic cell carcinoma)—that are staged T1 or T2 are candidates for postoperative radiation therapy.

Extent of Surgery for Adenoid Cystic Carcinoma

Controversy has existed over the extent of surgery that is appropriate for adenoid cystic carcinoma because of the proclivity of this malignancy to spread locally, particularly by perineural invasion. This carcinoma also exhibits a tendency for distant metastases, especially to the lungs, yet a relatively low propensity for regional lymphatic metastases.

Radical surgical resection evolved historically as a consequence of the failure of conservative local resection of adenoid cystic carcinoma. Radical surgery, however, carries with it potential serious morbidity, significant functional sequelae, and cosmetic disfigurement. In addition, radical surgery for adenoid cystic carcinoma does not provide significant improvement in survival rates over less radical surgical resection with postoperative radiation therapy.

In addition to perineural spread, adenoid cystic carcinoma typically extend microscopically well beyond the palpable tumor mass (51). The extent of surgical resection should be undertaken with these characteristics in mind. Thus, resection with a wide surgical margin encompassing the tumor, individualized for the specific patient, is recommended. Surrounding structures are inspected for invasion and are resected if involved. Complete resection of the tumor with resection of involved surrounding structures is the surgical goal to attain as the presence of tumor at the surgical margin significantly influences the development of local recurrences (52,53). Thus, surgical judgment must be exercised to be aggressive enough to obtain clear surgical margins, yet not overly radical when all gross disease has been resected (53). Nerves, particularly sensory nerves, should be carefully inspected for thickening, a sign of perineural invasion. Invaded nerves should be resected until clear margins are obtained by frozen section evaluation. A normally functioning facial nerve is preserved unless it is determined to be invaded by tumor or if a plane of dissection between the tumor and nerve cannot be achieved.

Frozen-Section Evaluation

An experienced pathologist and clinical correlation are required for the use of frozen-section evaluation of salivary gland neoplasms. Frozen-section evaluation of parotid masses can be helpful in differentiating neoplastic from nonneoplastic disease as well as in distinguishing malignant from benign disease. Like FNBA, the specific classification of malignant neoplasms can be difficult with frozen section. Also, the complete morphology of a tumor and focal areas of tumor invasion may not be appreciated on frozen-section evaluation (54). Frozen-section evaluations agree with the final histopathologic diagnosis 80% to 90% of the time (55). Malignant tumors are incorrectly called benign tumors 10% to 30% of the time (56–58). On the other hand, false-positive diagnoses for malignancy are unusual.

If frozen-section evaluation provides a definitive diagnosis of malignancy, the surgical procedure appropriate for the

TABLE 26.4 Parotid Mass-Frozen-Section Indications

1. Confirm neoplasm
2. Characterize neoplasm (benign vs. malignant)
3. Ensure specimen distribution for additional studies
4. Guide completeness of surgical resection
5. Assess lymph node for metastasis

malignancy is performed. If, however, a definite diagnosis of malignancy cannot be made by frozen-section assessment, parotidectomy is performed, and further surgery (e.g., facial nerve sacrifice) is deferred until a final histopathologic diagnosis is rendered. Frozen-section evaluations are helpful in assessing surgical margins intraoperatively, and thus are helpful to guide the extent of surgery to ensure complete tumor resection. Enlarged or suspicious periparotid or cervical lymph nodes are evaluated by frozen section, and the decision to perform a neck dissection can be made based on whether metastatic nodes are present. The surgeon should be aware of the limitations of frozen-section evaluation of parotid neoplasms, and, therefore, should keep the request for frozen-section within acceptable indications. Table 26.4 lists reasonable indications for frozen-section evaluation.

In some instances, a definitive histopathologic diagnosis of minor salivary gland malignancies is made by biopsy before surgery. For minor salivary gland malignancies, frozen sections are useful primarily in guiding complete surgical resection.

Facial Nerve Management

Before surgery, a clear understanding of the functional status of the facial nerve by physical examination is necessary as partial or total facial paralysis may be present as a result of tumor invasion. This information is important in guiding the surgeon in intraoperative decision making regarding management of the facial nerve.

Facial nerve branches or the main trunk of the facial nerve invaded by tumor are resected if facial paralysis is present before surgery. If there is no preoperative dysfunction of the facial nerve, however, the facial nerve can be preserved in most cases. Nussbaum and Bortikner (59) reported the need to resect the facial nerve, totally or partially, in 29% of parotidectomies performed for malignancy. They noted a high rate of tumor recurrence in cases with clinical facial nerve paralysis. Importantly, they demonstrated the feasibility of surgical preservation of the facial nerve in the majority of cases of parotid carcinoma (71%) with a low (14%) rate of tumor recurrence. Criteria for nerve preservation included the absence of clinical nerve involvement and the presence of a surgical plane of resection between the tumor and facial nerve.

The surgeon must exercise judgment intraoperatively with regard to management of the facial nerve. Efforts to preserve the nerve should be made if the nerve is normal before surgery, and nerve preservation is feasible without compromising complete tumor resection. Facial nerve branches or the main trunk of the nerve are resected if nerve invasion is noted intraoperatively or tumor encasement precludes complete dissection of the tumor from the nerve. The margins of nerve resection should be checked by frozen-section analysis, and additional resection performed as necessary to ensure negative margins of resection. Proximal facial nerve resection may necessitate mastoidectomy for exposure of the facial nerve within the temporal bone. After facial nerve resection, immediate nerve reconstruction is undertaken with either the sural or greater auricular nerve serving as a graft. Some malignancies, especially adenoid cystic carcinoma, may exhibit perineural skip lesions, and therefore frozen-section margins may not accurately reflect the completeness of tumor resection.

Planned postoperative radiation therapy is not a contraindication to facial nerve grafting (60). Facial nerve function following nerve resection and grafting results in a functional facial nerve in approximately 75% of patients (60). Generally, however, most patients achieve only moderate success, grade III to IV by the House-Brackmann facial grading system (60). For this reason and because of length of time for functional recovery following nerve grafting, simultaneous performance of rehabilitative procedures for facial reanimation is recommended. These include gold-weight upper eyelid implants, lower lid tightening, and static facial slings (61–63).

SURGICAL MANAGEMENT OF THE NECK

For all types of malignant salivary gland tumors, a neck dissection is performed for clinically positive nodes. Even though the type of dissection is dictated by the operative findings, a modified radical neck dissection with preservation of the spinal accessory nerve, jugular vein, and sternocleidomastoid muscle is generally preferred over the classic radical neck dissection. This technique is favored in the absence of extracapsular lymph node extension because of cosmetic superiority and decreased morbidity. If extracapsular extension of tumor is present in the neck, structures invaded are resected to achieve complete tumor removal. Invasion of the carotid artery and deep cervical fascia are ominous intraoperative findings.

For the clinically negative neck, the first-echelon lymph nodes are inspected during parotidectomy or submandibular gland excision. Enlarged or suspicious nodes are removed and examined by frozen-section analysis. A neck dissection is performed if the presence of metastatic disease is determined by frozen section.

Several studies using multivariate analysis have shown that certain factors are associated with a high risk for occult metastases for major salivary gland carcinomas. Armstrong et al. (64) noted a 20% risk for occult metastases for tumors greater than 4 cm and a 49% risk for high-grade tumors. Frankenthaler et al. (65) found a 33% risk for occult metastases for parotid malignancies associated with facial nerve paralysis and an 18% risk for high-grade tumors in general. Regis de Brito Santos et al. (66) noted that T stage, desmoplasia, and histopathologic type were independent predictors of nodal metastases by multivariate analysis. They showed a greater than 50% risk for metastases for the following neoplasms: adenocarcinoma, undifferentiated carcinomas, high-grade mucoepidermoid carcinoma, squamous cell carcinoma, and salivary duct carcinoma.

Because of the increased risk for occult nodal metastases with large (T3, T4) tumors, tumors invading the facial nerve, high-grade tumors, and high-risk histopathologic tumor types, a modified radical neck dissection should be considered for these primary tumor characteristics. Neck dissection can be performed with low morbidity, and it provides additional prognostic pathologic information. At the present time, however, there are no compelling data to support the benefit of elective neck dissection for the clinically negative neck for malignant salivary gland tumors. Adjuvant radiation therapy to the neck is recommended for those patients at high risk for occult cervical metastases.

Surgical Management of Parapharyngeal Space Salivary Gland Neoplasms

The parapharyngeal space can be involved by primary salivary gland neoplasms or by parotid neoplasms that extend from the deep lobe into the parapharyngeal space. Parotid neoplasms extend to the parapharyngeal space by two possible routes. Round tumors extend into the parapharyngeal space posterior to the stylomandibular ligament. Dumbbell tumors penetrate between the mandible and the stylomandibular ligament with a waist-like constriction, to involve the parapharyngeal space. Primary parapharyngeal space neoplasms can be differentiated from deep-lobe parotid tumors radiographically. Most parapharyngeal space salivary gland neoplasms are benign.

The approach for surgical resection of malignant parapharyngeal space neoplasms salivary is dependent on the site of tumor origin. Primary parapharyngeal salivary neoplasms are removed by a transcervical, submandibular approach. Deep-lobe parotid tumors involving the parapharyngeal space are removed by superficial parotidectomy with facial nerve identification followed by resection of deep lobe and parapharyngeal space tumor. Division of the stylomandibular ligament and anterior mandibular dislocation improves access to the parapharyngeal space and facilitates resection. Most parapharyngeal space neoplasms can be bluntly finger-dissected from the space. Mandibulotomy is rarely necessary for access to parapharyngeal space neoplasms. Anterior mandibulotomy and mandibular swing, however, may be necessary to access massive or recurrent benign neoplasms as well as invasive malignant neoplasms. Lateral mandibulotomy is not favored because of attendant inferior alveolar nerve division with resultant sensory loss. Select malignant tumors with local invasion involving the parapharyngeal space may require partial mandibulectomy for resection. In such cases, the parapharyngeal space is exposed via the mandibulectomy site. Occasionally a parapharyngeal space neoplasm presents after inappropriate transoral incisional biopsy. In this case, a combined transcervical-transoral approach may be necessary to ensure complete tumor resection. In all cases, tumor spillage should be carefully avoided so as to minimize the possibility of recurrent tumor.

Recurrent Pleomorphic Adenoma

Although recurrent pleomorphic adenoma (RPA) is not a malignant neoplasm, it is characterized by local invasion and recalcitrance to local control. For these reasons and the therapeutic challenge it poses, RPA is discussed here. Histopathologic features of pleomorphic adenoma include incomplete encapsulation and transcapsular growth with pseudopod extensions. These features account for most recurrences after tumor enucleation because residual tumor is frequently left *in situ* following this procedure. These features also account for the propensity for these neoplasms to rupture during enucleation because surgical dissection is close to the pseudocapsule of the tumor. Surgical violation or tumor spillage is another mechanism for the development of RPA, as pleomorphic adenoma is a highly implantable tumor. Formal parotidectomy decreases the possibility of tumor rupture and spillage compared with lesser surgical procedures. Formal parotidectomy results in a low incidence of RPA of usually less than 2%. There appears to be an increased risk for RPA for variants of pleomorphic adenoma. These include large tumors, deep lobe tumors, tumors approximating the facial nerve, and recurrent tumors (67). Recurrent pleomorphic adenoma is also more common in young patients for unclear reasons (68,69).

A patient with RPA typically presents with a painless mass in or near the previous operative site (70). Demographics reveal a predominance of female patients. The average age of patients with RPA is between 30 and 40 years old (70,71). As stated above, RPA occurs more frequently in patients who develop a primary tumor at an earlier age (68,69). A thorough history is important, and the details of previous surgical management should be understood. Following initial treatment of pleomorphic adenoma, there is usually a long interval before recurrent disease. The mean interval to the time of first recurrence is approximately one decade (71). This length of time stresses the importance of long-term follow-up to assess initial treatment results. Recurrent pleomorphic adenoma typically occurs earlier following tumor enucleation than following formal parotidectomy (72). Fine-needle aspiration biopsy of a suspected RPA is a highly accurate method to confirm the diagnosis and to rule out malignant transformation or a metachronous neoplasm. Frequently the extent of disease in RPA is underestimated. Most (60% to 70%) recurrences are multifocal (71). Imaging studies such as MRI help to provide information providing the number, size, and location of recurrences. Two thirds of RPA involve the superficial lobe and one quarter involve the deep lobe (71). Following diagnosis of RPA, the previous pathology should be reviewed to rule out misdiagnosis of the original tumor. In retrospect, some tumors that were previously diagnosed as benign tumors prove to be malignant. In addition, concern regarding the possibility of malignant transformation of pleomorphic adenoma, or carcinoma ex pleomorphic adenoma, should be raised. Malignant degeneration of pleomorphic adenoma can occur in 5% of cases and occurs more frequently in long-standing recurrent tumors (71).

The treatment of RPA must be individualized (71). Factors that influence the management of RPA include the type of prior surgery, the extent and location of recurrence or recurrences, facial nerve function, the patient's general health status, and the patient's needs. The patient should be informed of all of the risks of a particular treatment and should be an active participant in treatment decision making. Observation alone of RPA in elderly or ill patients may be appropriate (70). Because most recurrences are multifocal, complete resection of the remaining parotid (total parotidectomy) with facial nerve preservation, whenever possible, is the best surgical therapy for RPA in the setting of prior enucleation, tumor spill, or for patients who have previously undergone less than an adequate previous parotidectomy. If total parotidectomy had been previously performed, or in select situations of apparent isolated recurrence, resection of the recurrent tumor mass alone by careful dissection around the capsule of the recurrence may be appropriate (72,73). Although the management of confluent RPA encasing the facial nerve is controversial, facial nerve resection and immediate nerve grafting is optimal for this difficult situation (74).

Significant scarring related to prior surgery can be expected. Meticulous surgical technique with magnification is recommended (72). Identification of the peripheral branch of the facial nerve with retrograde dissection or identification of the facial nerve in the mastoid may be necessary to identify and protect the facial nerve. The use of electrophysiologic monitoring of the facial nerve appears to assist in early nerve identification and to decrease facial nerve trauma (75). The risk for temporary and permanent facial nerve injury increases with each surgery performed for RPA (68). Adjuvant postoperative radiation therapy has shown benefit in decreasing further recurrences following resection of RPA. The presence of gross residual tumor following resection, however, results in a statistically significant increase in the risk for local failure compared with microscopic residual disease (68,76,77).

SURGICAL THERAPY FOR SUBMANDIBULAR GLAND TUMORS

Malignant neoplasms of the submandibular gland are usually confined to that structure. Resection alone is adequate surgery for small low-grade malignancies confined to the gland, but, for all other malignancies, removal of the contents of the submandibular triangle in addition to the gland is recommended. Included in this procedure are the submandibular nodes. For locally invasive tumors, the surgical resection is extended to include the involved structures with an appropriate tumor-free margin. The involved structures may include the skin, the marginal mandibular branch of the facial nerve, the hypoglossal nerve and lingual nerves, the floor of the mouth, or the extrinsic and intrinsic tongue muscles. Nerves invaded by tumor should be resected until tumor-free margins are obtained by frozen section.

After appropriate preparation and draping, submandibular gland excision technique requires that an incision be made in a skin crease several centimeters below the inferior border of the mandible. The incision is extended down through the platysma muscle, and a subplatysmal flap is elevated (with care taken not to injure the marginal mandibular branch of the facial nerve). The superficial layer of the deep cervical fascia is divided, and the anterior facial vein is divided and ligated. Elevation of the fascia exposes the submandibular gland. The dissection is performed superiorly, and the facial artery is divided and ligated. The mylohyoid muscle is retracted anteriorly, and the gland is retracted posteroinferiorly, exposing the lingual nerve and Wharton's duct. The submandibular ganglion is divided, thus freeing the lingual nerve. Wharton's duct is divided and ligated. The hypoglossal nerve is preserved as the inferior border of the submandibular gland is dissected free, and the facial artery is divided again inferiorly and ligated. The wound is then closed in layers over a drain.

POSTOPERATIVE RADIATION THERAPY FOR MAJOR SALIVARY GLAND MALIGNANCIES

There is substantial evidence that postoperative radiation therapy can improve local control when given after surgery to appropriately selected patients with malignant major salivary gland tumors. Numerous series have documented improved local control when postoperative radiation therapy is given (78–82). In general, postoperative radiation therapy is indicated in all situations except low-grade, stage I tumors.

Armstrong et al. (83) used a matched-pair analysis comparing groups of 46 patients treated with and without postoperative radiation therapy to determine which subsets of patients benefit from this approach. Local control was significantly improved for node-positive patients given postoperative radiation therapy (69% vs. 40%). Local control was excellent for stage I and stage II malignancies, regardless of whether they were treated with surgery alone or with surgery and postoperative radiation therapy (91% vs. 79%). Local control by T and N stage after treatment with resection and postoperative radiation therapy was reported by Harrison et al. (81) and is summarized in Table 26.5.

TABLE 26.5 Local Control of Major Salivary Gland Malignancies with Postoperative Radiation Therapy

	Actuarial local control, 5-year
T1	100%
T2	83%
T3	80%
T4	43%
	Actuarial locoregional control, 5-year
N0	83%
N+	58%

Source: Adapted from Harrison LB, Armstrong JG, Spiro RH, et al. Postoperative radiation therapy for major salivary gland malignancies. *J Surg Oncol* 1990;45:52.

Postoperative radiation therapy is routinely recommended for high-grade tumors and stage III and stage IV tumors. Close or positive surgical margins, perineural or perilymphatic invasion, intraparotid or regional nodal metastases, and recurrent disease are also indications for postoperative radiation therapy.

Radiation therapy portals for major salivary gland tumors should include the entire preoperative extent of the gland and tumor with a 2-cm margin. For parotid tumors, the superior margin is generally at the zygomatic arch, the inferior border at the hyoid bone, the posterior border at the mastoid process, and the anterior border at the second molar to include Stensen's duct. Multiple field techniques are used to minimize the radiation therapy dose to the contralateral parotid gland. Common arrangements included three fields (anteroposterior, posteroanterior, and lateral) or anteroposterior and posterior oblique or anterior and posterior oblique wedge pairs. A sample treatment plan is shown in Figure 26.2. Mixed unilateral electron and photon beams are used less commonly. In using these techniques, care must be taken to treat the deep lobe, which extends to the parapharyngeal space, and to limit the dose to the contralateral parotid gland so as to spare its function. In addition, posterior oblique fields must not exit through the orbit. Similar techniques can be used for the treatment of submandibular and sublingual gland malignancies, although opposed lateral fields can be used when the treatment volume extends to the midline and a significant portion of parotid tissue is excluded.

Numerous studies have documented improved local control for adenoid cystic carcinoma of both major and minor salivary glands when postoperative radiation therapy is given. These series demonstrate local control improved from the range of approximately 25% to 40% without postoperative radiology to 75% to 80% with postoperative radiation therapy, although late failures may continue to occur (53,78,81,84,85).

Garden et al. (53) reported a 10-year actuarial local control of 70% if a named nerve was involved and there was a positive margin, 83% when either was involved, and 91% when neither was involved. When the analysis was confined to patients receiving radiation doses in excess of 56 Gy (which would be standard for high-risk patients in the current approach to radiotherapy), local control was actually 88% if there was a positive margin and 89% if a named nerve was involved. For adenoid cystic carcinoma, the radiation therapy portal is generally modified to follow named nerve roots to the base of the skull because of this tumor's propensity for perineural space spread along nerve roots. However, the analysis by Garden and colleagues of the patterns of failure for 198 adenoid cystic tumors treated with surgery and postoperative radiation therapy demonstrated that base-of-skull failure is rare with or without elective treatment of the base of the skull. The authors concluded that it may be justified to eliminate coverage of nerve roots in the absence of significant invasion of named nerves, especially in situations where treatment would involve a substantial modification of radiation therapy portals and increased risk for morbidity. Because base-of-skull failure can lead to significant morbidity and is difficult to treat, we continue to recommend treatment portals for adenoid cystic carcinoma that follow the nerve roots to the base of the skull. Elective neck irradiation is not used for adenoid cystic carcinoma, as the risk for occult nodal metastasis is low.

Tumors of the submandibular gland are less common than parotid tumors, but some series address the outcome with surgery and postoperative radiotherapy. These data suggest that management of submandibular tumors should be based on the same principles that guide therapy of parotid tumors. Sykes et al. (86) reported 5- and 10-year local control of 85% and 73%, respectively, in a group of 30 patients. All relapses after 5 years occurred in patients with adenoid cystic carcinoma. Results have been reported for 83 patients treated after surgery at M. D. Anderson Cancer Center for high-risk features of perineural invasion, positive margins, extraglandular spreads, positive lymph nodes, locally recurrent disease, named nerve involvement, or high-grade histology. Ten-year actuarial local control was 88%. Important adverse prognostic factors identified in multivariate analysis were adenocarcinoma (41% vs. 94% local control), high-grade tumor (69% vs. 95%), positive margin (79% vs. 92%), and radiotherapy prior to 1985 (80% vs. 98%) (87).

RADIATION THERAPY MANAGEMENT OF THE NECK

Elective neck dissection is rarely indicated; however, with the exception of adenoid cystic carcinoma, elective neck irradiation is indicated in most situations in which postoperative radiation therapy to the primary site is used. Unilateral elective neck fields should be added for high-grade and T3 and T4 tumors. Armstrong et al. (64) analyzed the results of elective neck dissection and clinical failure patterns in a series of 474 newly diagnosed major salivary gland tumors. Patients with high-grade tumors and tumors larger than 4 cm were at high risk for subclinical nodal spread, with incidence rates of at least 49% and 21%, respectively. In contrast, T1 and T2 tumors with low- or intermediate-grade histology had a risk for only 7%. Rodriguez-Cuevas et al. (88) confirmed these results in another large group of patients. Postoperative neck irradiation after neck dissection is given for solitary metastatic nodes greater than 1 cm, multiple metastatic nodes, or extracapsular nodal extension.

Therapy for Minor Salivary Gland Malignancies

SURGICAL RESECTION

Like major salivary gland malignancies, adequate surgical resection is also standard therapy for minor salivary gland tumors. Improved disease-specific survival is demonstrated for patients undergoing surgical resection with or without radiation therapy compared with nonsurgical management (89). Postoperative radiation therapy is recommended for select tumors. Conventional or fast neutron radiation therapy is used for unresectable lesions. Primary radiation therapy has been advocated by some as a management alternative for early lesions in cases in which resection would lead to substantial morbidity, but this recommendation is controversial.

Surgery for minor salivary gland malignancies depends on tumor location and extent of disease. Complete surgical resection with tumor-free margins is essential to success. Malignancies involving the paranasal sinuses and nasal cavity may require partial or total maxillectomy. This can be accomplished with a midfacial degloving approach or an external approach. Tumors involving the ethmoid sinuses and extending to or beyond the cribriform plate usually require craniofacial resection. Tumors invading the orbit can sometimes be removed adequately without orbital exenteration if the invasion is limited to the periorbita. More extensive invasion usually necessitates orbital exenteration.

Malignancies involving the oral cavity and oropharynx can usually be removed transorally. Tumors involving the hard palate may require partial maxillectomy. Extensive tumors of the oropharynx may require a combined transoral and external approach with or without mandibulotomy to provide adequate removal.

Minor salivary gland carcinomas involving the larynx are removed using conservation laryngeal surgery. Supraglottic laryngectomy tailored to the disease is recommended for tumors confined to the supraglottic larynx. On the other hand, massive, destructive laryngeal minor salivary gland carcinomas, those with subglottic extension, or those arising in the subglottic larynx require total laryngectomy.

Tracheal malignancies are removed by partial or segmental tracheal resection. End-to-end tracheal anastomosis is the preferred method of reconstruction after resection if feasible. Surgical resection by partial mandibulectomy is recommended for salivary gland carcinomas of the mandible (5).

There is no benefit to elective treatment of the clinically negative neck in patients with minor salivary gland malignancies due to the low (<10%) incidence of neck recurrence for the untreated N0 neck (89,90).

POSTOPERATIVE RADIATION THERAPY FOR MINOR SALIVARY GLAND TUMORS

Although fewer data support the role of postoperative radiation therapy for minor salivary gland than support major salivary gland malignancies, the strategy of using adjuvant radiation therapy for high-risk patients has been successful and leads to local control in the range of 75% (79,91–93) in comparison with local control rates of approximately 50% (25,79,93) without radiation therapy. Indications for adjuvant radiation therapy include positive or close surgical margins; deep infiltration of bone, cartilage, or muscle; lymph node metastasis; large tumor size; and high-grade histology. The application of this strategy has led to a local failure rate of 22% at the M. D. Anderson Cancer Center (91), 26% at the University of Florida (92), and 12% at Stanford (94). Stage of tumor and positive margins may be important predictors of local control (92,94), although even with microscopically positive margins, local failure has been observed to be only 17% (94). In contrast, the local failure rate was 47% in one series, in which 90% of the patients were treated with surgery alone (25).

The treatment fields for the primary site vary with tumor location. In general, the treatment fields and doses used should be similar to the fields that are used for similar squamous cell carcinoma at the same site. As with adenoid cystic carcinoma of the major salivary glands, it is standard to extend the field to follow the named regional nerve roots to the base of the skull for adenoid cystic carcinoma arising in the minor salivary glands.

Elective neck radiation therapy for minor salivary gland malignancies is generally not recommended, although it is used at some centers for tumors located in the tongue, floor of mouth, pharynx, or larynx (90–92). Our policy is to treat only the first-echelon nodes, which are included in the primary treatment volume. Garden et al. (91) found a 2% neck recurrence rate with elective neck radiation therapy and a 5% recurrence rate without neck radiation therapy. Although it is controversial, Garden et al. recommend elective neck radiation therapy for tumors of the floor of the mouth or the tongue or when the neck is entered during resection of the primary tumor. Parsons et al. (92) found similar low-neck failure rates with or without radiation therapy, but considered laryngeal and pharyngeal sites to be at increased risk for nodal metastases requiring treatment. Postoperative radiation therapy after neck dissection should be given to all patients with nodal metastases except solitary metastasis of less than 1 cm without extracapsular extension.

Radiation Therapy Alone for Unresectable Major and Minor Salivary Gland Malignancies

Conventional radiation therapy alone for unresectable salivary gland tumors has not been a successful strategy. Laramore (95) reviewed the literature and found a 26% local control rate.

Neutron radiation therapy, available at a few specialized centers around the world, has led to a superior outcome and has been tested on a large number of patients. A review of the literature has revealed a 67% local control rate for 309 patients treated with neutrons but only 26% for those treated with conventional photon radiotherapy (95). Neutrons appear to have a higher relative biologic effectiveness for salivary gland tumors that leads to a higher tumor killing effect relative to toxic effects on normal tissue than is the case with conventional photon radiation therapy. Neutron radiotherapy deposits more energy while transversing a cell than does photon radiotherapy, which may result in a higher rate of DNA damage from direct "hits" rather than indirect injury from free radicals generated by the radiotherapy. This phenomenon may be especially important in slowly cycling tumors as direct DNA injury may be less amenable to repair and is less dependent on cell cycle distribution. In addition, as direct radiation injury is not dependent on the generation of free radicals, hypoxic areas of tumor are not as resistant to neutron radiotherapy as they are to photon therapy.

A small randomized trial performed by the Radiation Therapy Oncology Group in the United States and the Medical Research Council in Great Britain demonstrated the 10-year actuarial local control to be 56% with neutron therapy, compared with 17% with photon therapy (96). Pooled European data has demonstrated a 65% local control for patients treated with gross residual disease with neutrons and 28% for conventional photons (97). For 120 patients treated at the University of Washington for gross residual tumor of the major salivary gland, local control was 59% (98). For tumors 4 cm or less in size, local control and cause-specific survival were 80% and 73%, respectively, but only 35% and 22%, respectively, for those with larger tumors. The data also suggested that surgical debulking may contribute to improved outcome.

The results for a large group of patients with unresectable or gross residual adenoid cystic carcinoma treated with fast neutron therapy at the University of Washington have been reported (99). Overall 5-year actuarial local control is 57% with a 5-year survival of 72%. Patients with the favorable prognostic factors of surgical debulking and absence of base of skull invasion had local control of 80% at 5 years. Patients with base of skull involvement had 5-year local control of only 23%. Eight patients with microscopic residual disease had 100% 5-year local control. A review of patients with gross residual adenoid cystic carcinoma treated at the University of Heidelberg demonstrated 5-year local control of 75% for those treated with neutron therapy, whereas it was 32% for those receiving conventional photon radiotherapy alone or mixed photon and neutron radiotherapy (100). These findings demonstrate the efficacy of neutron therapy in improving local control in patients with gross residual adenoid cystic carcinoma, although these studies have not suggested a significant survival benefit. Nevertheless, even in the absence of survival benefit, there may be great value in preventing the substantial and potentially prolonged morbidity of local recurrence in a disease that generally has indolent progression of systemic metastasis.

These data suggest that referral to a neutron facility should be considered for patients with gross residual tumor. Complications, however, including tissue necrosis, may be increased compared with conventional photon therapy. It may be the case that if the photon dose was escalated to a point where similar complications would result, then outcome of photons would approach the outcome achieved with neutron irradiation. Wang and Goodman (101) reported that use of hyperfractionated radiation therapy—1.6 Gy twice daily to a dose of 60 to 78.9 Gy—achieved a 5-year local control of 100% for nine parotid malignancies and a 78% 5-year local control for a group of 15 minor salivary gland malignancies, but these results still require confirmation in a larger group of patients with longer follow-up. At the present time, neutron radiotherapy should be considered a standard option. When conventional radiation therapy alone is used, doses to at least 70 Gy should be used to maximize the chances of tumor control.

Radiation Therapy Alone for Early Salivary Gland Malignancies

Although appropriate under limited circumstances, radiation therapy alone is not generally used as an alternative to surgery for early-stage lesions. Neutron radiation therapy has achieved a promising local control of approximately 75% for tumors of less than 4 to 5 cm (102,103). Results do not appear to vary with histology or site of tumor origin for either major or minor salivary glands (102). We recommend consideration of referral to a neutron center when radiation therapy alone is to be used.

Although radiation therapy alone is controversial, Parsons et al. (92) recommended using conventional irradiation for the treatment of salivary gland malignancies under some circumstances. Using conventional radiation therapy, these authors found that seven of nine early adenoid cystic carcinomas and five of five early mucoepidermoid carcinomas and adenoid cystic carcinomas were controlled. Based on these results, they recommended consideration of this approach for early-stage mucoepidermoid carcinoma and adenoid cystic carcinoma. They also recommended that radiation therapy be considered as primary therapy, with the understanding that local control may be reduced.

OUTCOMES AND RESULTS

Survival results for salivary gland malignancies should be interpreted cautiously because these data are generally collected from a heterogeneous group of patients. Information about the prognostic factors of stage, histopathology, and tumor site are of great importance in interpreting survival outcomes. Moreover, the strategy developed in recent years of using adjuvant radiation therapy for all high-risk patients improves outcomes. In most available series, not all patients received adjuvant radiation therapy, and the standard indications for adjuvant treatments were not always defined.

Major Salivary Gland Tumors

Spiro et al. (104) reported benchmark survival results in 474 patients with major salivary gland tumors treated at the Memorial Sloan-Kettering Cancer Center from 1944 to 1982. The 5-, 10-, and 15-year survivals were 54%, 43%, and 34%, respectively, with determinate survivals of 63%, 47%, and 42%, respectively. Multivariate analysis showed that advanced stage, higher histologic grade, and submandibular location were prognostic for a poorer outcome. In addition, treatment after 1966 was found to be an important prognostic factor and was thought to relate to both a higher proportion of low-grade tumors and an increased use of postoperative radiation therapy beginning during this latter period. Although analysis did not reveal a survival benefit with the use of adjuvant radiation therapy, Armstrong et al. (83) performed a matched-pair analysis using patients from this data set and revealed a significantly improved 5-year determinate survival (51% vs. 10%) in stage III and stage IV patients treated with postoperative radiation therapy. An improvement in determinant survival was also observed with adjuvant radiation therapy in node-positive patients (49% vs. 19%). There was no benefit seen in the comparison of stage I and stage II malignancies, with 5-year determinate survivals of 82% with radiation therapy and 92% without radiation therapy. A series of 62 parotid malignancies treated with surgery and postoperative radiation therapy at the Massachusetts General Hospital revealed similar survival rates (105). North et al. (80) also demonstrated a significant survival benefit of postoperative radiation therapy in a multivariate analysis of patients treated at Johns Hopkins Hospital.

Aside from treatment, numerous other prognostic factors have been identified. The most important are stage and tumor histopathology. Prognostic factors are discussed in the following subsections.

TUMOR STAGE

In a Japanese study of 1,683 patients with parotid carcinoma, the validity of the 1997 TNM staging system (Table 26.2) for predicting survival was demonstrated by Numata et al. (106). The 10-year survival rates for stage I, II, III, and IV tumors were 82%, 64%, 50%, and 33%, respectively. There were no significant differences between stage II and III survival curves and stage III and IV survival curves. Thus, additional studies are needed to further refine the present TNM staging system in terms of stage stratification.

TUMOR HISTOPATHOLOGY

Tumor histopathology is a dominant prognostic factor for salivary gland malignancies. Evaluation of tumor behavior based on histopathology has allowed the classification of low-grade tumors, including acinic cell carcinoma and low-grade mucoepidermoid carcinoma, and high-grade tumors, including adenocarcinoma, adenoid cystic carcinoma, carcinoma ex pleomorphic adenoma, squamous cell carcinoma, high-grade mucoepidermoid carcinoma, and undifferentiated carcinoma (Fig. 26.3). Survival rates continue to decrease after 5 years for all tumor types except for the low-grade malignancies, acinic cell carcinoma, low-grade mucoepidermoid carcinoma, and squamous cell carcinoma.

REGIONAL LYMPHATIC METASTASES

Disease with regional lymph node metastases has a poorer prognosis than that without metastasis. High-grade mucoepidermoid carcinoma, squamous cell carcinoma, and adenocarcinoma are the malignant tumors with the highest propensity for cervical metastases. Acinic cell carcinoma and adenoid cystic carcinoma have relatively low rates of lymph node metastases.

Large tumor size is associated with a higher rate of regional lymph node metastases as is associated facial nerve paralysis (10,78,106).

DISTANT METASTASES

Distant metastases, which predict a poor prognosis, occur in approximately 20% of parotid malignancies, and they occur most frequently in adenoid cystic carcinoma and undifferentiated carcinoma. The incidence of distant metastases increases with increased T and N classifications (106). The most common sites for distant metastases (in decreasing order of occurrence) are lung, bone, and brain.

The length of survival for patients with distant metastases depends on tumor type. For example, the median survival for malignant mixed tumors was less than 2 years in one series (107); however, survival of more than 10 years has been reported for adenoid cystic carcinoma with distant metastases (107,108). As adenoid cystic carcinoma patients have a median survival of more than 4 years after the identification of distant metastasis (109), aggressive local treatment of the primary site including complete surgical resection and postoperative radiation therapy is warranted.

LOCATION

There appears to be no difference in survival based on the location of a malignancy within the parotid gland, although parapharyngeal space extension seems to be associated with a poor prognosis (110). In general, parotid malignancies have a better prognosis than do salivary carcinomas arising in other locations. Submandibular gland neoplasms behave more aggressively than parotid gland tumors, but this may be related to local anatomy of the area rather than to biologic differences between tumors.

RECURRENCE

The recurrence rate of parotid carcinoma is substantial for high-grade malignancies. Survival rates are diminished for patients with recurrent malignancies according to some investigators but, using multivariate analysis, North et al. (80) showed no difference in 5-year survival rates between previously untreated disease and recurrent tumors.

PAIN

Pain associated with known malignancy is an ominous symptom. Pain occurs in approximately 6.5% of malignant tumors (15). Spiro et al. (10) reported a 5-year survival of 35% for patients with malignancies associated with pain but a 5-year survival of 68% for patients without pain.

FACIAL NERVE PARALYSIS

Facial nerve paralysis associated with malignant tumor is associated with high incidences of regional and distant metastases and indicates a poor prognosis (80,111). The histologic diagnoses most frequently encountered in patients with facial nerve paralysis are undifferentiated carcinoma, squamous cell carcinoma, adenocarcinoma, and adenoid cystic carcinoma (111).

SKIN INVOLVEMENT

Invasion of skin and other surrounding tissues is associated with decreased survival (80). Skin involvement indicates advanced malignancy and requires excision of the involved structures.

SEX

Sex has been correlated with survival for salivary gland malignancies. Men have poorer outcomes than do women, but the reason for this difference is unknown (80).

Minor Salivary Gland Malignancies

Spiro et al. (25) have reported survival outcome for a large series of minor salivary gland patients. For 492 patients treated at the Memorial Sloan-Kettering Cancer Center, 5-, 10-, and 15-year cause-specific survivals were 75%, 62%, and 57%, respectively, with overall survivals of 73%, 56%, and 46%, respectively. The role of adjuvant radiation therapy could not be adequately assessed for these patients. Series reported from the University of Florida (92) and from the M. D. Anderson Cancer Center (53) have shown similar survivals despite improved local control resulting from the use of postoperative radiation therapy. There are important prognostic factors for minor salivary gland malignancies that are discussed later.

TUMOR HISTOPATHOLOGY

As is the case with major salivary gland malignancies, tumor histopathology is a dominant prognostic factor for minor salivary gland malignancies. Survival data for minor salivary gland malignancies by tumor histopathology are shown in Figure 26.4 (see also Color Plate 10 following page 524). The importance of tumor grade and the long natural history of adenoid cystic carcinomas should again be noted. Spiro et al. (25) found that higher-grade histology, increased extent of disease, and subsite were important prognostic factors.

EXTENT OF DISEASE

Evaluation of the impact of extent of disease has been hampered by the lack of a formal staging system for minor salivary gland malignancies. Spiro et al. (25), however, found extent of disease to be highly predictive of outcome when the TNM staging systems for squamous cell carcinomas of each subsite were applied to the minor salivary gland tumors. For stages I to IV, 10-year overall survivals were 83%, 53%, 35%, and 24%, respectively. The influence of stage according to grade is shown in Figure 26.4 (see also Color Plate 10 following page 524).

Vander Poorten et al. (89) evaluated 55 patients with minor salivary gland carcinoma and staged the tumors using staging guidelines for squamous cell carcinoma of the same region involved. Patients demonstrated 5-year survival rates of 84%, 73%, 60%, and 29% for stages I, II, III, and IV, respectively.

SITE

Minor salivary gland malignancies of the oral cavity have a more favorable prognosis, compared with those arising in the paranasal sinuses (25,89). When minor salivary gland malignancies are staged using the TNM system for squamous cell carcinoma at similar subsites, site is no longer prognostic, although stage was highly predictive of survival outcome (25). Parsons et al. (92) also found that subsite was a significant factor in predicting outcome in univariate analysis but did not predict outcome in a multivariate analysis that accounted for the effect of extent of disease.

DISTANT METASTASES

The presence of distant metastases predicts poor prognosis for minor salivary gland carcinoma. In one series, no patient who presented with distant metastases survived for 5 years, whereas 70% of M0 patients survived 5 years (89).

Results of Neutron Radiation Therapy for Major and Minor Salivary Malignancies

The reported results using neutron radiation therapy for salivary gland malignancies generally combine groups of patients with major and minor gland malignancies. The largest reported series includes 118 patients treated at Fermilab (102). Five-year, disease-free survival rates were 32% for major salivary gland tumors and 36% for minor salivary gland lesions. Of note, local control was 74% for tumors of 5 cm or less, whereas local control was only 30% for malignancies greater than 5 cm. Histology

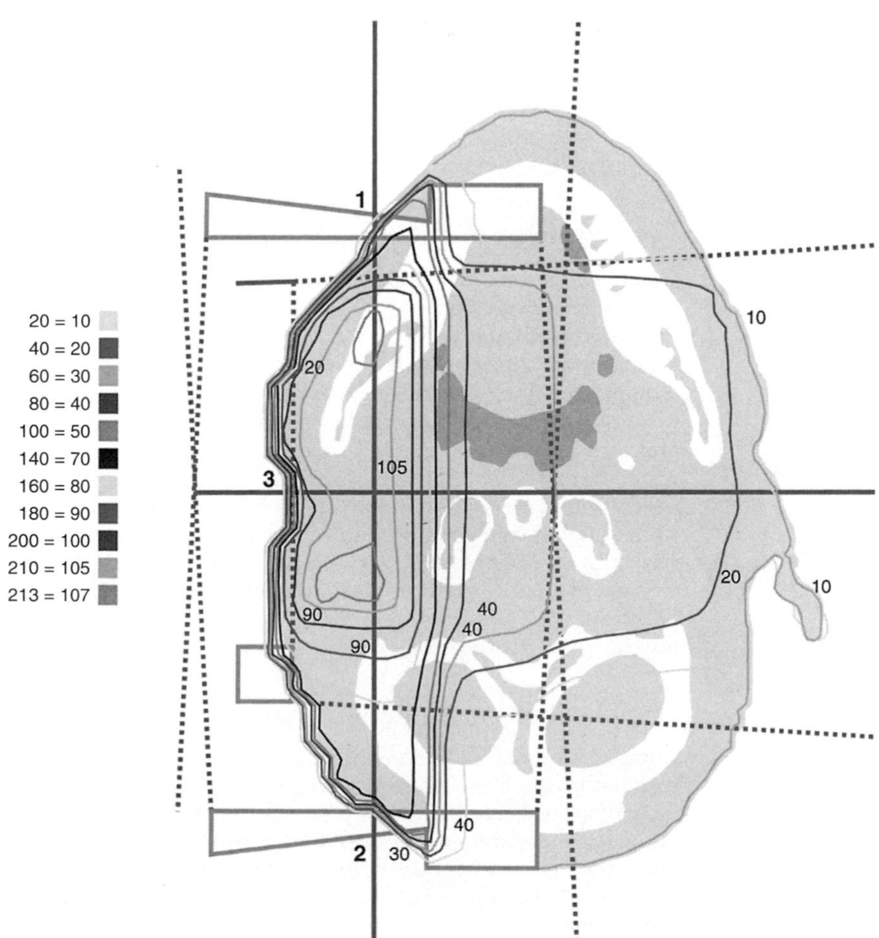

Figure 26.4 Sample radiation therapy treatment plan for parotid malignancy. (See Color Plate 10 following page 524.)

did not affect local control. Similar results have been achieved at the University of Washington (103).

COMPLICATIONS

Complications of Parotidectomy

There are both early and late complications of parotidectomy (Table 26.6) (112). Partial or complete paralysis involving some or all of the branches of the facial nerve can occur as an early complication. Temporary facial nerve paralysis involving all or just one or two branches of the facial nerve occurs in 10% to 30% of cases. Permanent facial nerve paralysis has occurred in less than 3% of the patients undergoing superficial parotidectomy. The incidence of facial nerve paralysis is higher with total parotidectomy than with superficial parotidectomy. This may be related to stretch injury or the result of surgical interference of the vasa nervorum. Temporary paresis usually resolves from weeks to months after surgery. Facial nerve paralysis is also more common after reoperation for recurrent tumors. The branch of the facial nerve most at risk for injury during parotidectomy is the marginal mandibular branch. Nerve transection can occur during surgery and, in this situation, immediate nerve repair should be performed.

Hemorrhage or hematoma after parotidectomy is uncommon and is usually related to inadequate hemostasis at the time of the surgical procedure. Treatment consists of evacuation of the hematoma and control of bleeding vessels.

Infection is rare after parotidectomy, a fact that is probably related to the rich vascular supply of the region. Treatment consists of abscess drainage (if necessary), local care, and antibiotics.

Skin flap necrosis is most commonly located in the distal tip of the postauricular skin flap, and care must be taken in designing the incision to avoid this complication. Smoking may contribute to this complication, and patients should be instructed to avoid smoking before surgery.

Trismus may be related to inflammation and fibrosis of the masseter or other muscles of mastication. This complication is usually mild and transient and usually improves with jaw exercises.

Salivary fistula or sialocele is a relatively common complication after parotidectomy. This occurs if the cut edge of the remaining salivary gland leaks saliva and drains through the wound or collects beneath the flap. Fistula is usually a self-limited problem and is treated with local care and a pressure dressing to overcome the secretory pressure of the salivary tissue. A sialocele may require repeated needle aspiration and the application of a pressure dressing. Chronic salivary fistula is rare.

TABLE 26.6 Complications of Parotidectomy

Early complications
Facial nerve paralysis
Hemorrhage or hematoma
Infection
Salivary fistula or sialocele
Seroma
Long-term complications
Frey syndrome
Recurrent tumor
Hypertrophic scar or keloid
Neuroma of the greater auricular nerve

Wound seroma is an uncommon complication that can usually be managed with aspiration of the accumulated fluid.

Frey syndrome, or gustatory sweating, is a relatively common long-term complication of parotidectomy. This phenomenon is thought to be related to aberrant regeneration of nerve fibers from the postganglionic secretomotor parasympathetic innervation of the parotid gland to the severed postganglionic sympathetic fibers that supply the sweat glands of the skin of the face and the auriculotemporal region. As a result, sweating or dermal flush occur during salivary stimulation. Frey syndrome has been reported for 30% to 60% of patients undergoing parotidectomy. Only some 10% of patients, however, have symptomatic Frey syndrome. This complication may be prevented with the use of a thick skin flap at the time of parotidectomy. Postoperative radiation therapy significantly diminishes the incidence of Frey syndrome. Most patients with Frey syndrome do not seek therapy. Medical treatment of symptomatic Frey syndrome includes topical anticholinergics, such as 1% glycopyrrolate, or botulinum toxin injection.

Hypoesthesia of the greater auricular nerve is an expected sequela of parotidectomy in most cases. Occasionally, this nerve or a branch of the nerve courses posteriorly and can be left intact during parotidectomy. In most cases, however, division of the greater auricular nerve is required, producing long-term sensory loss in the region of the pinna and parotid area. Patients must be cautioned to avoid injury to this area because of the sensory loss. An amputation neuroma of the greater auricular nerve can occur and must be differentiated from cervical lymphadenopathy. Treatment is simple excision.

Significant cosmetic deformity after superficial parotidectomy is uncommon. Most patients have a minor soft tissue deficit in the region of resection. The deficit is usually more pronounced after total parotidectomy. Local muscle flaps, such as a sternocleidomastoid muscle flap, have been recommended to improve the contour after parotidectomy.

Cosmetic complications of parotidectomy include hypertrophic scar and keloid. Scar revision with steroid injections may be necessary.

Complications of Submandibular Gland Excision

Complications of submandibular gland excision are uncommon (112). Hemorrhage, particularly from the facial artery, results in vigorous bleeding if encountered intraoperatively or may cause a hematoma after surgery. Hematoma management requires wound reexploration and control of hemorrhage. Infection is uncommon after submandibular gland excision. Injury to the marginal mandibular branch of the facial nerve can occur and results in loss of lip depressor function. Permanent injury to this nerve is unusual. Temporary paresis of this nerve can occur from a stretch injury acquired during retraction. Other nerves at risk during submandibular gland excision include the hypoglossal and lingual nerves, resulting in ipsilateral tongue paralysis and anesthesia of the anterior two thirds of the tongue, respectively. These nerve injuries are uncommon.

Complications of Radiation Therapy

Complications of radiation therapy for major salivary gland malignancies can include mucositis, xerostomia, hair loss, skin ulceration, osteoradionecrosis of the mandible, fibrosis, injury of the optic apparatus, and brainstem necrosis. Unilateral radiation therapy portals are sufficient for most major salivary gland malignancies, and because this spares the contralateral parotid gland and most of the mucosa of the pharynx, xerostomia is uncommon.

Complications of radiation therapy for minor salivary gland malignancies depend on the site treated. For sites in the oral cavity, xerostomia and osteoradionecrosis of the mandible can occur. A dental consultation before radiation therapy can avert irradiation-related dental complications. Irradiation of the sinonasal region can be complicated by irradiation injury of the eye, optic nerve, brainstem, and pharynx. Facial nerve grafts do not appear to be damaged by postoperative radiation therapy (113).

Neutron radiation therapy has been associated with a high risk for severe complications and necrosis in the early experience, but improved techniques and an increased understanding of normal tissue tolerance have reduced the incidence of severe long-term complications (96,98,99,102,103,114) close to levels seen with external-beam radiation therapy alone for unresectable head and neck tumors. The particular complications are related to the site treated and generally include necrosis or tissue injury, which may be expressed as soft tissue ulceration, osteoradionecrosis, nerve injury, temporal lobe necrosis, eye injury, etc. It should be noted that in some instances these complications were expected based on the extent and difficult anatomy of tumors that may be referred for neutron therapy.

MANAGEMENT OF RECURRENCE

Locally recurrent disease should be managed similarly to disease at initial presentation. Complete surgical resection should be performed, if possible. If prior radiation therapy has not been given, postoperative radiation therapy should be given for all but small, low-grade malignancies resected without positive or close margins. Armstrong et al. (115) found 5- and 10-year survivals of 83% and 58%, respectively, for completely resected low- and intermediate-grade lesions with clinically negative nodes. Local control among these patients was significantly better when the recurrent tumor was less than 3 cm (80% vs. 62% at 5 years and 73% vs. 25% at 10 years). For high-grade malignancies, determinant survivals were 40% and 29% at 5 and 10 years, respectively, with local control rates at 5 and 10 years of 49% and 35%, respectively. Based on these findings, Armstrong et al. (116) recommended postoperative radiation therapy for all but small low- and intermediate-grade malignancies. In most instances, external-beam radiation therapy cannot be given to patients treated previously with this therapy. Brachytherapy can be used in high-risk patients when prior external-beam radiation therapy has been administered (116).

If surgical resection is not feasible, high-dose radiation therapy should be administered for recurrent disease. If no prior radiation therapy has been given, referral to a neutron treatment facility should be considered. Under some circumstances, neutron radiation therapy can be used for retreatment after prior external-beam radiation therapy and should be considered. At the Fermilab, 7 of 10 tumors treated with neutron radiation therapy for recurrent disease after prior external-beam radiation therapy were controlled (102). Brachytherapy can also be used to treat gross disease after prior external-beam radiation therapy (116).

CHEMOTHERAPY

At present, there is no proved benefit of adjuvant chemotherapy in improving locoregional tumor control or survival for malignant salivary gland tumor patients. The primary role of chemotherapy in the management of these malignancies is palliation of symptomatic unresectable recurrent disease. Patients who have advanced unresectable disease and achieve a clinical response to chemotherapy often note significant pain control. Complete or partial responses to chemotherapy are achieved in up to 40% to 50% of patients (117–119). Median response durations reported for palliation with chemotherapy range from 5 to 8 months (120,121).

Multiinstitutional, prospective studies are necessary to evaluate further the role of chemotherapy as adjuvant therapy for salivary gland malignancies. Studies have shown the combinations of paclitaxel and carboplatin (122) and vinorelbine and cisplatin (123) to have moderate activity for salivary gland carcinomas.

SPECIAL ISSUES AND FUTURE DIRECTIONS

The future holds great promise for better understanding of the behavior of the diverse malignancies that affect the salivary glands. Further studies of the molecular biology of various salivary gland malignancies will provide refined understanding of the behavior of variants of the same histopathologic tumor type. Such molecular information may further improve the diagnostic accuracy of FNAB in terms of specific diagnosis of a given malignant neoplasm. Furthermore, such tumor biology information will allow for refinement of the staging system for salivary gland malignancies.

Diagnostic imaging, including PET scans, will continue to evolve and will provide improved diagnostic information regarding the extent of local disease and the presence of regional and distant metastases. The potential for imaging studies to detect early local and regional recurrences will improve.

Treatment modalities including radiation therapy and chemotherapy will improve. Biologic predictors of radiation therapy and chemotherapy responses will help guide patient selection for these treatment modalities. At the present time, no radiation therapy fractionation schedule has been shown to be optimal for salivary gland malignancies. In the future, optimal altered fractionation schemas will be defined. In addition, new intensity-modulated radiation therapy and intraoperative radiation therapy approaches may prove to be effective for salivary gland malignancies. Such approaches may improve tumor control with diminished patient morbidity. Better radiosensitizing and radioprotective agents will be identified to be used in concert with radiation therapy.

Chemotherapeutic agents more active against salivary gland malignancies will be identified and the role of these agents used concurrently with radiation therapy will be defined. Additional potential future treatment modalities for salivary gland malignancies include targeted chemotherapy and radiation therapy, gene therapy, and immunotherapy.

Outcome analyses will provide more information regarding treatment results. For example, studies with longer follow-up intervals will provide data regarding survival following surgery and neutron beam radiation therapy for adenoid cystic carcinoma. Furthermore, outcome studies will give valuable information regarding quality-of-life parameters following different treatment regimens.

RADIOLOGIC IMAGING CONCERNS

Bernard B. O'Malley and Suresh K. Mukherji

Many salivary gland tumors are managed without any preoperative imaging (124). Patients with deep-lobe parotid neoplasms, neurologically symptomatic neoplasms, or recurrent or otherwise large neoplasms of major salivary gland origin warrant pretreatment imaging. Imaging cannot predict the tissue type of any salivary neoplasm. Moreover, the benign or malignant nature cannot confidently be predicted (125). Imaging can suggest benign features allowing a simple approach to excision. Pretreatment imaging can also predict the safest, most appropriate approach to biopsy. At the very least, fine-needle aspiration (FNA) should be performed because of the possibility of discovering lymphoma or metastasis from a regional skin or scalp lesion, which would prompt a different type of workup and prevent a cosmetically sensitive biopsy procedure. Axial views with CT or MRI outline the components of the superficial and deep lobes of the parotid gland and the margin with the mandibular ramus and cortical mastoid. This view also confirms the integrity of the distal internal carotid artery. When cranial nerve VII is involved, the coronal (or sagittal) view is necessary to trace the vertical segment of the nerve trunk above the stylomastoid foramen. This view is easily achieved with MRI (Fig. 26.5) but requires some effort with positioning for CT (Fig. 26.6), particularly if the neck has previously been dissected. Many malignant (Fig. 26.7) as well as benign (Figs. 26.8 and 26.9) salivary neoplasms appear well circumscribed on CT and MRI (126). The true infiltrating extent of some lesions can be underestimated by contrast CT (Figs. 26.10 and 26.11). More accurate characterization of salivary neoplasms can be achieved simply by re-scanning the gland after a brief delay in the equilibrium phase of intravenous contrast (127). Although MRI is more sensitive for soft tissue infiltration (Fig. 26.12), the high signal intensity of the normal adult gland can obscure the true tumor margin on the T2 image. Tumors of the major salivary glands are well depicted on noncontrast T1-weighted images. When malignant tumor is present, enhanced MRI can aid in ruling out proximal neurotropic extension (128). Fat-suppression techniques must be applied to the fast T2 and contrast T1 series (Figs. 26.13 and 26.14). Surface coil techniques applied to the immediate region of interest allow very high resolution of the parotid bed (Fig. 26.15). Sonography is useful tool if needed for guidance of submandibular or superficial lobe parotid gland biopsy (129). It is not comprehensive enough for staging the deep lobe of parotid or parapharyngeal space (Fig. 26.16).

Imaging of the posttreatment gland is challenging because of the hyperintensity present on T2 MRI and the enhancement present on CT and MRI related to scarring (Fig. 26.17). Tumor contrast enhancement occurs early during dynamic scanning and enhancement related to scarring occurs later and persists longer. Either modality is useful only if a discrete lesion is revealed in or near the operative bed (Figs. 26.18 and 26.19). Because of the cosmetic significance of a well-healed incision and the increased risk for nerve VII injury in the treated gland, imaging-guided percutaneous biopsy is a useful adjunct when recurrence is suspected. This is particularly helpful when the lesion is not palpable or exists in the deep lobe. Fluorodeoxyglucose (FDG)-PET requires an appreciable degree of cellular turnover to provide an adequate sensitivity for detection of tumor (Fig. 26.20). Given the variability of tumor grade among salivary neoplasms, PET is less reliable than in other neoplasms.

Submandibular gland lesions are rarely imaged, as they present early and are easily palpated (Figs. 26.21 and 26.22). It should be noted that because large parotid lesions can push down into the submandibular space, the parotid bed should be covered by any examination of the submandibular gland (Fig. 26.23). Obstructing calculi of Wharton duct occasionally result in firm enlargement of the submandibular gland (Fig. 26.24). Enlarged upper cervical lymph nodes can displace and irritate the submandibular gland, causing a pseudomass of the gland.

Lesions of minor salivary gland origin require carefully planned scans if imaging is to be of any benefit to the patient. As these lesions are predominantly malignant, they have a higher risk for deep, unanticipated central neurotropic extension that must be carefully excluded, regardless of the clinically reported duration of the abnormality. Examples of these lesions are demonstrated in other chapters (see Figs. 16.37 and 19.41).

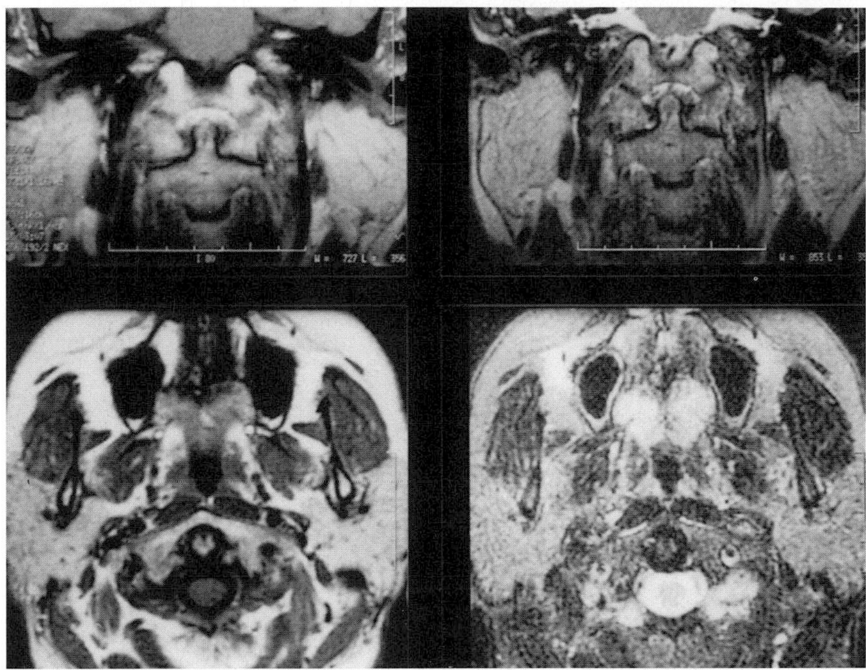

Figure 26.5 Normal variant. Noncontrast magnetic resonance imaging. Clockwise from top left: Coronal T1, coronal T2, axial T2, and axial T1 views showing prominent but normal signal parotid glands.

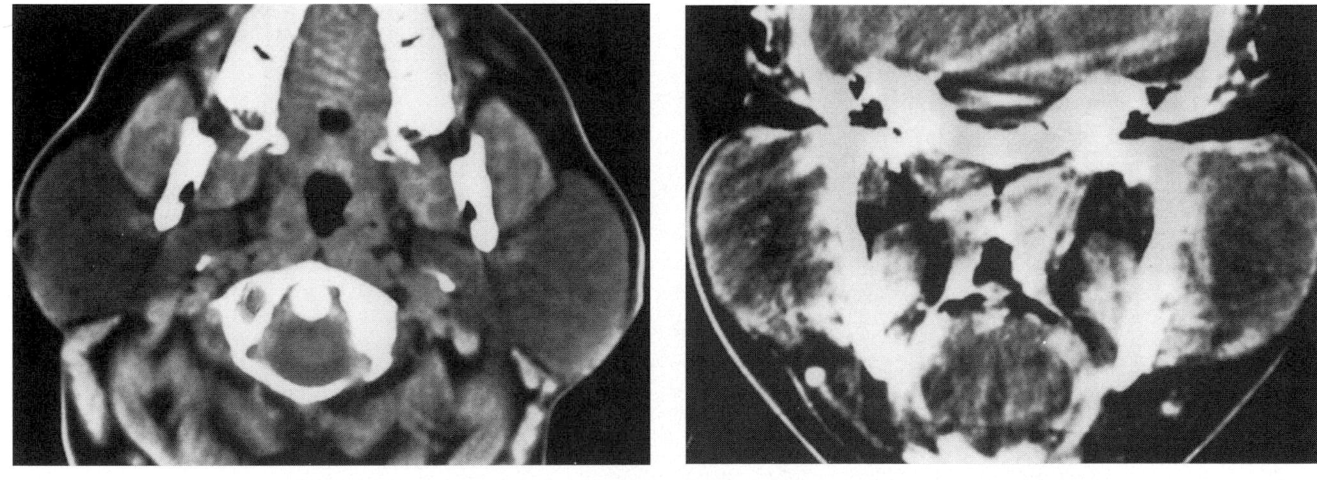

A B

Figure 26.6 Normal variant. Noncontrast computed tomographic axial **(A)** and direct coronal **(B)** views, showing very prominent but normal texture parotid glands.

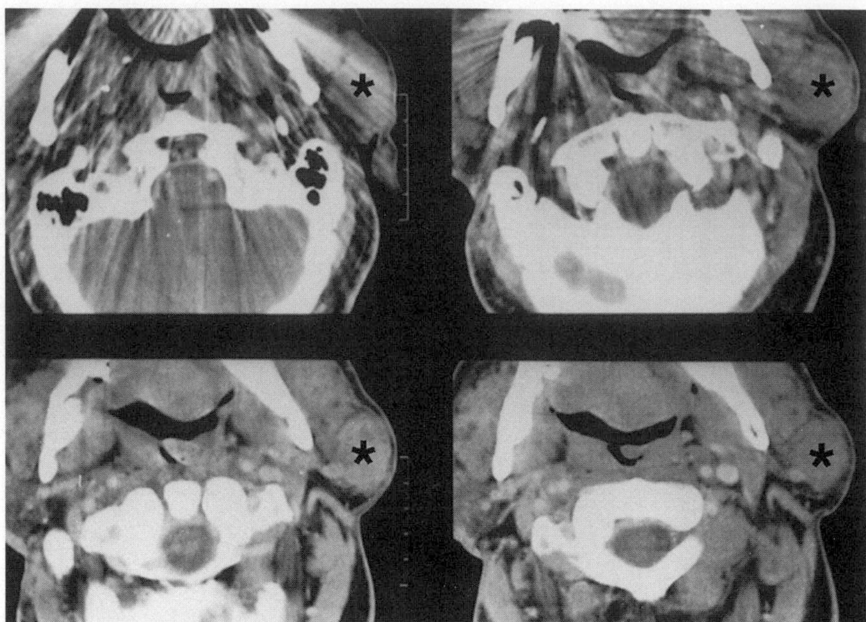

Figure 26.7 Primary parotid lesion. Serial enhanced axial views of a well-defined mass in the superficial lobe of the left parotid gland (*asterisk*).

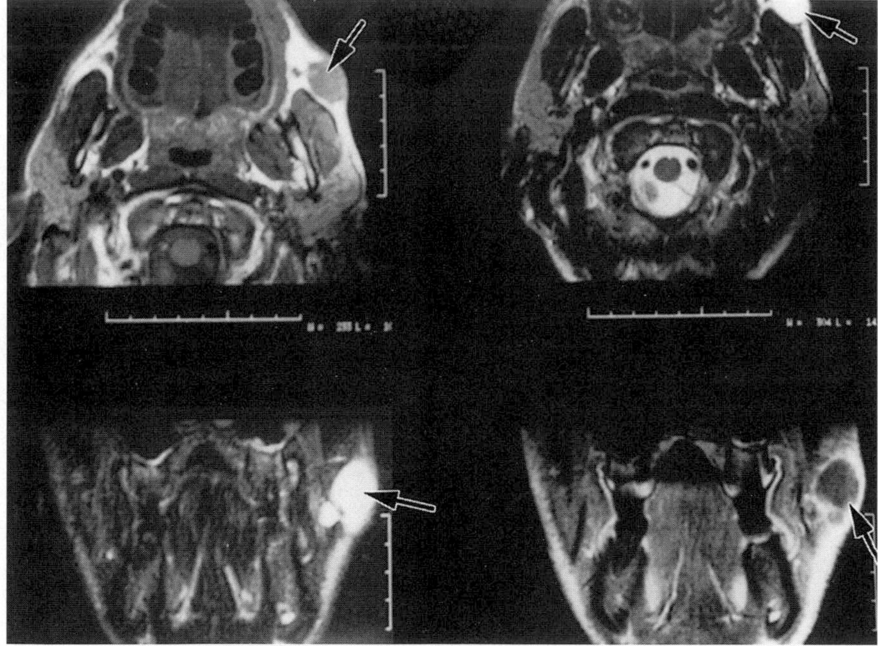

Figure 26.8 Accessory parotid lesion. Multiplanar magnetic resonance imaging. Clockwise from top left: Axial T1, axial T2, contrast coronal T1, and coronal T2 views. Shown is a well-circumscribed lesion (*arrow*) at accessory parotid tissue along Stensen duct, which proved to be a pleomorphic adenoma.

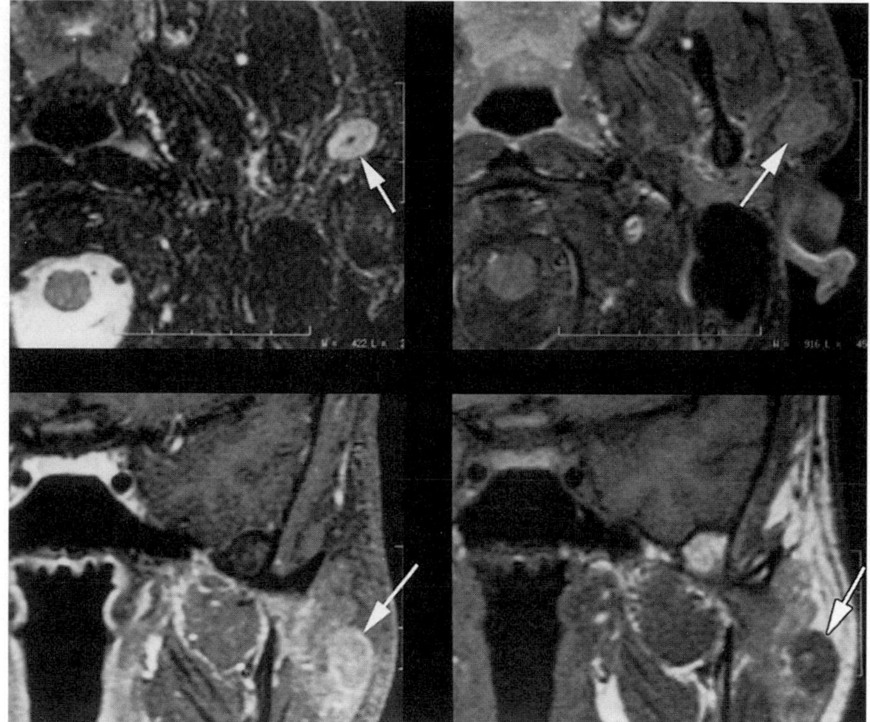

Figure 26.9 Intraparotid lymph node. Contrast magnetic resonance imaging. Clockwise from top left: Axial T2, axial fat-suppressed T1, coronal T1, and coronal fat-suppressed T1 views of a lesion in the superficial lobe (*arrows*). Excisional biopsy revealed hyperplastic lymph node.

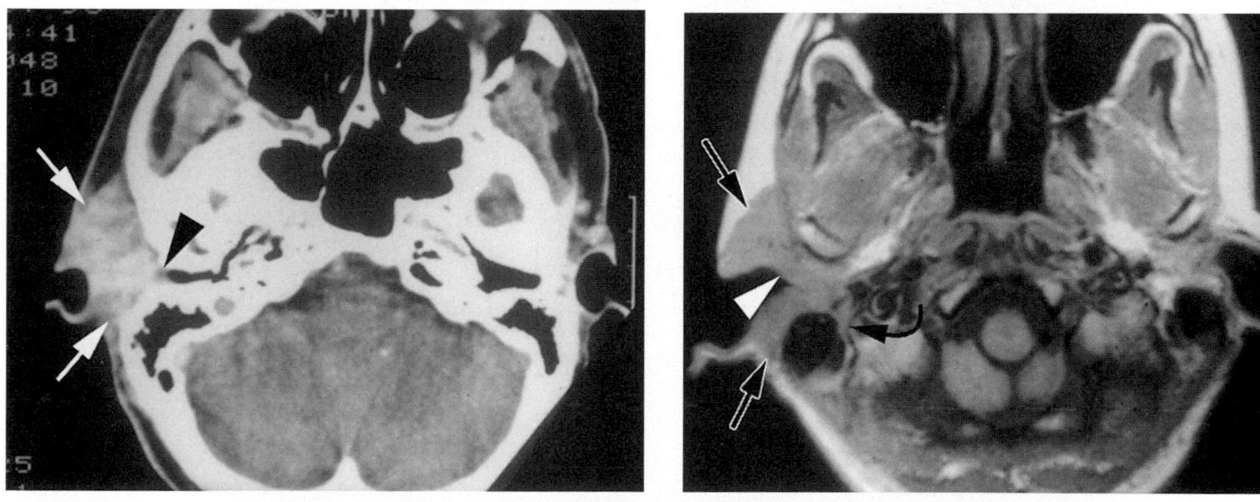

Figure 26.10 Primary parotid lesion. Enhanced axial computed tomography **(A)** and magnetic resonance imaging **(B)** show an infiltrating lesion arising in the superficial lobe of the right parotid gland (*arrows*) surrounding the external auditory canal (*arrowheads*) and infiltrating the stylomastoid foramen (*curved arrow*).

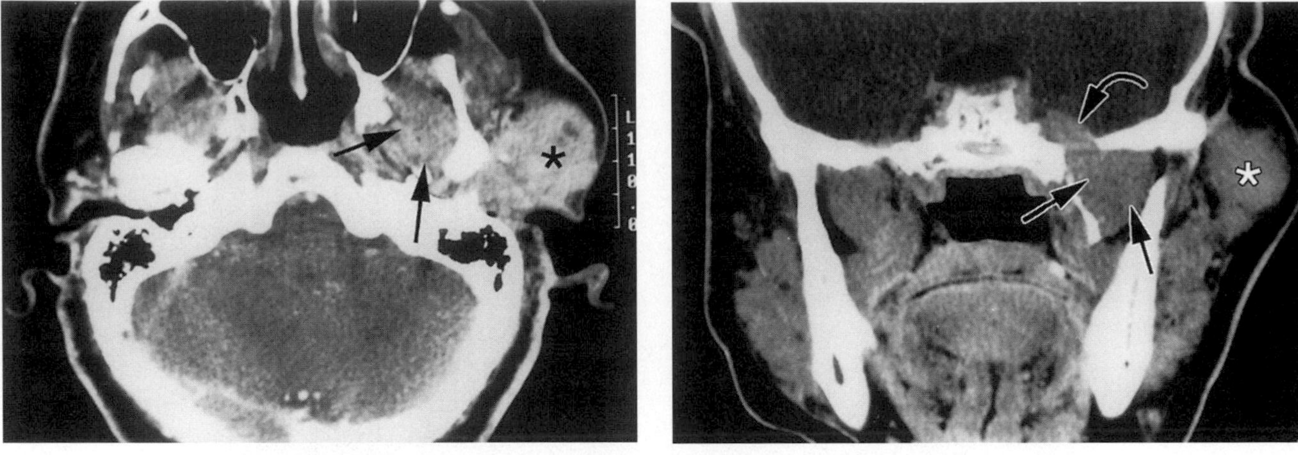

Figure 26.11 Deeply infiltrating lesion. Enhanced axial (A) and direct coronal (B) computed tomographic views of apparently well-circumscribed and palpable lesion in the superficial lobe (*asterisk*). Closer inspection shows contiguous extension from the deep lobe through the masticator space (*arrows*) into the foramen ovale and Meckel cave (*curved arrow*).

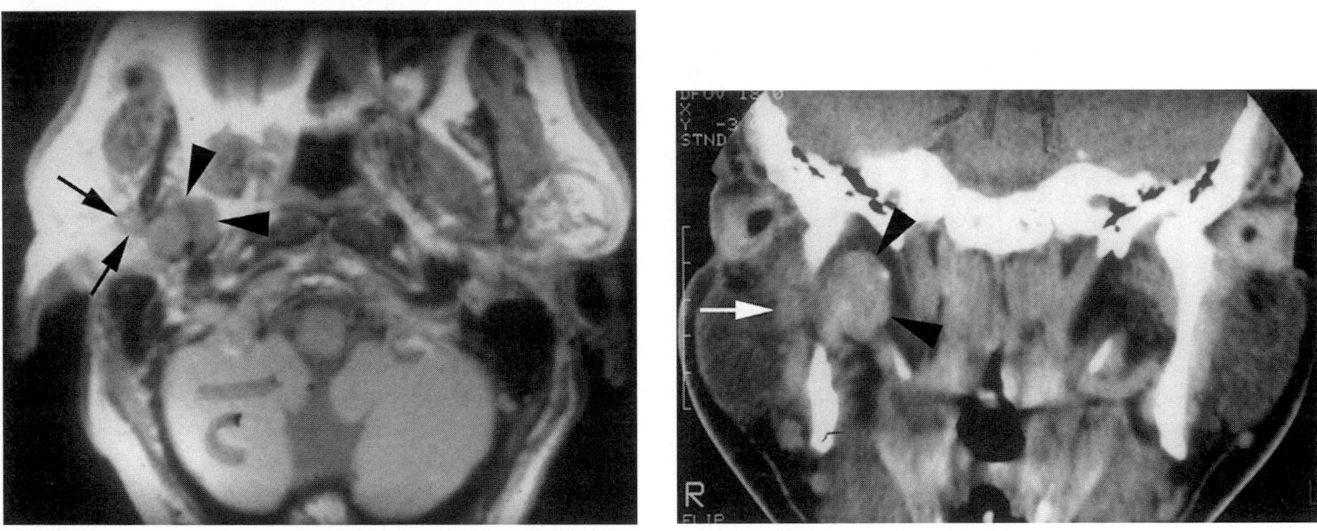

Figure 26.12 Carcinoma expleomorphic adenoma. Both enhanced axial T1 magnetic resonance imaging (A) and direct coronal computed tomography (B) show well-defined medial margins (*arrowheads*) typical of a benign lesion. The stellate-appearing irregular lateral margin (*arrows*) was the site of the carcinoma that produced the facial palsy.

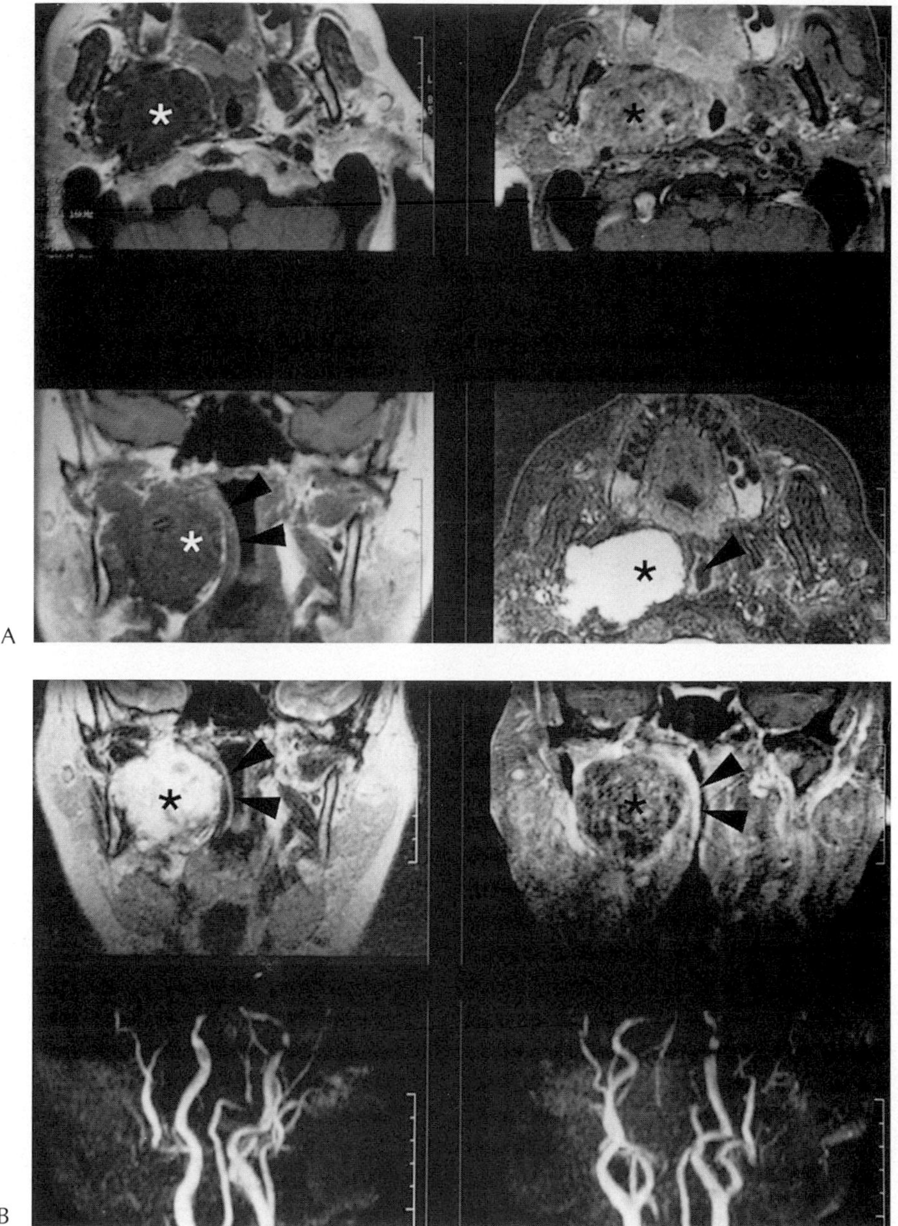

Figure 26.13 Large, deep-lobe mass. **A:** Multiplanar magnetic resonance imaging. Clockwise from top left: Axial T1, contrast T1, T2, and coronal T1 views showing well-defined mass in parapharyngeal space (*asterisk*) with ill-defined connection to the superficial lobe. **B:** Multiplanar magnetic resonance imaging and magnetic resonance angiography show large mass (*asterisk*) in parapharyngeal space, deforming nasopharyngeal airway (*arrowheads*), with no infiltration of the skull base. Magnetic resonance angiography shows displacement of the right internal carotid artery, with no stenosis or occlusion.

A

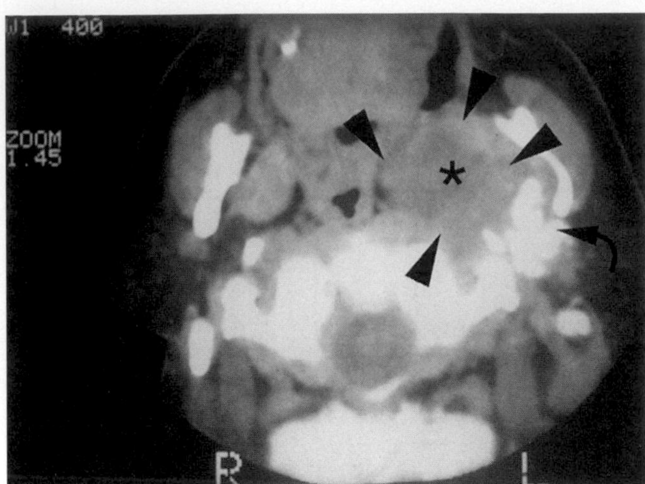

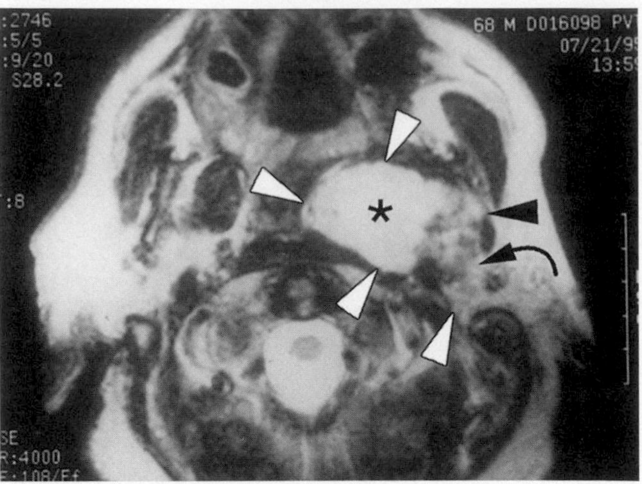

B

Figure 26.14 Untreated pleomorphic adenoma. **A:** Noncontrast axial computed tomography. **B:** T2 magnetic resonance imaging. Shown is a large, very heterogeneous, well-circumscribed mass (*arrowheads*) arising within the deep lobe. The ossified components are dense on computed tomography and produce only a low signal on magnetic resonance imaging (*curved arrows*), secondary to cartilage formation. The larger component bulges medially into the parapharyngeal space (*asterisk*).

A

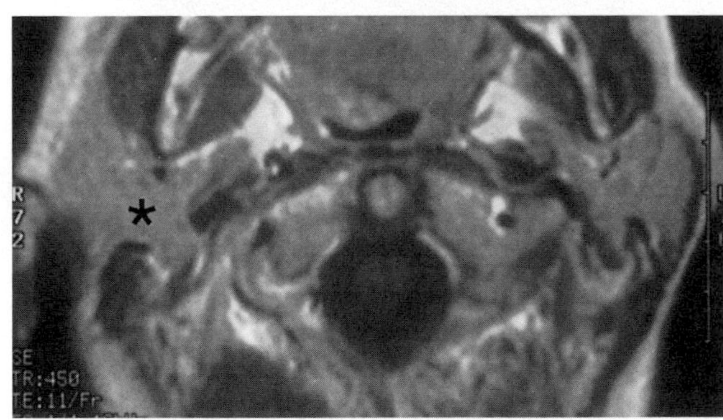

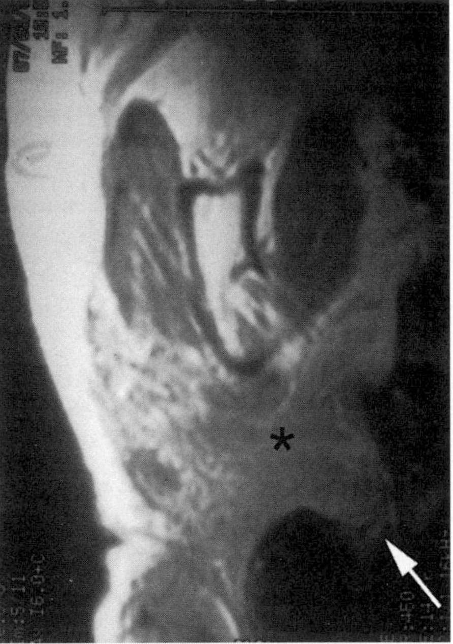

B

Figure 26.15 Surface coil technique. Conventional **(A)** and high-resolution surface coil **(B)** T1 images show infiltrating carcinoma of the entire right parotid gland (*asterisk*), with better resolution of the region with surface receiver coil. Note nerve VII at the stylomastoid foramen (*arrow*).

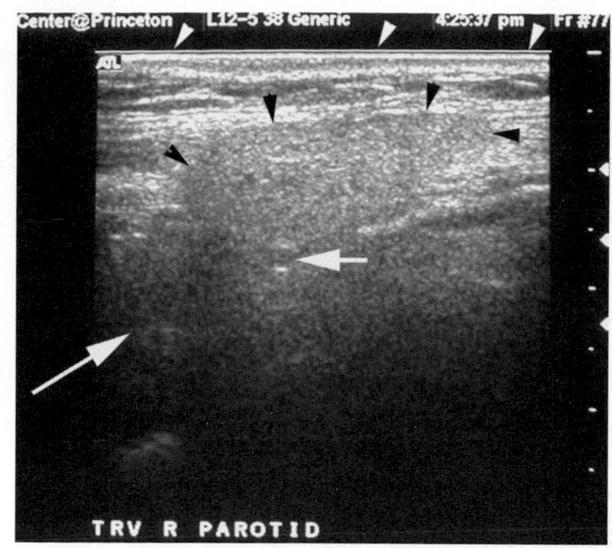

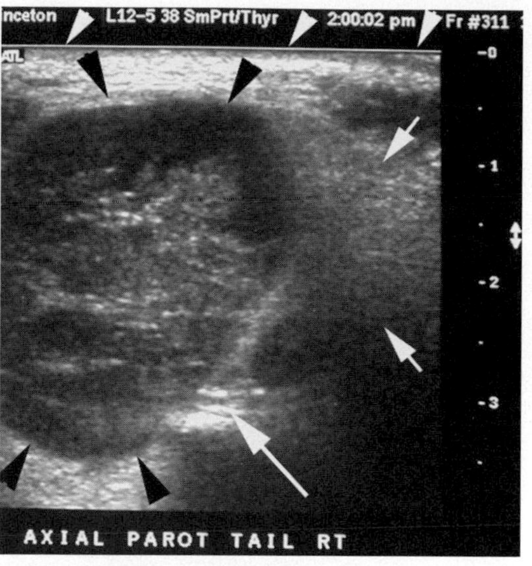

Figure 26.16 Sonography of parotid gland. **A:** Transverse (axial) sonogram of normal parotid gland shows good resolution of superficial structures including skin surface (*white arrowheads*), superficial lobe (*black arrowheads*), and retromandibular vein (*short white arrow*). There is poor definition of deeper landmarks such as the stylomastoid foramen (*long white arrow*) and the capsule of the deep lobe is not outlined. **B:** Large tail of parotid mass shows skin surface (*white arrowheads*), superficial lobe (*white arrows*), mass (*black arrowheads*), and retromandibular vein (*long white arrow*).

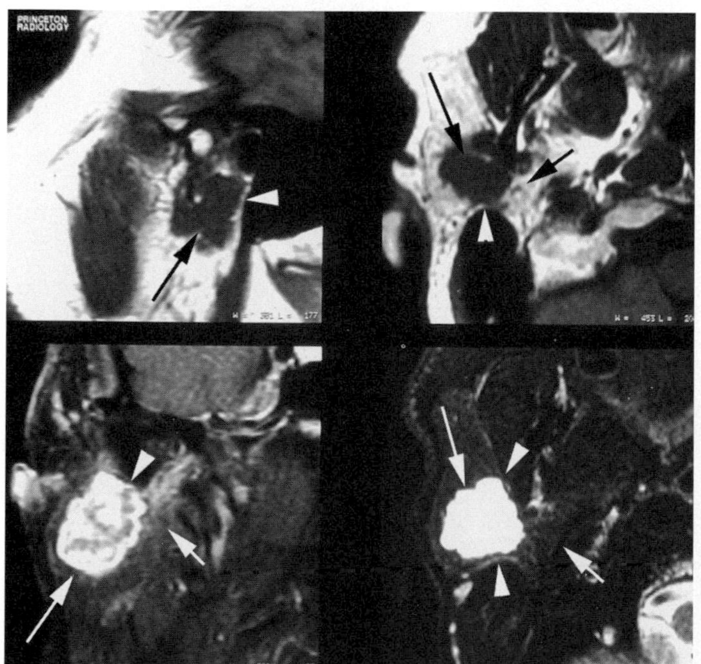

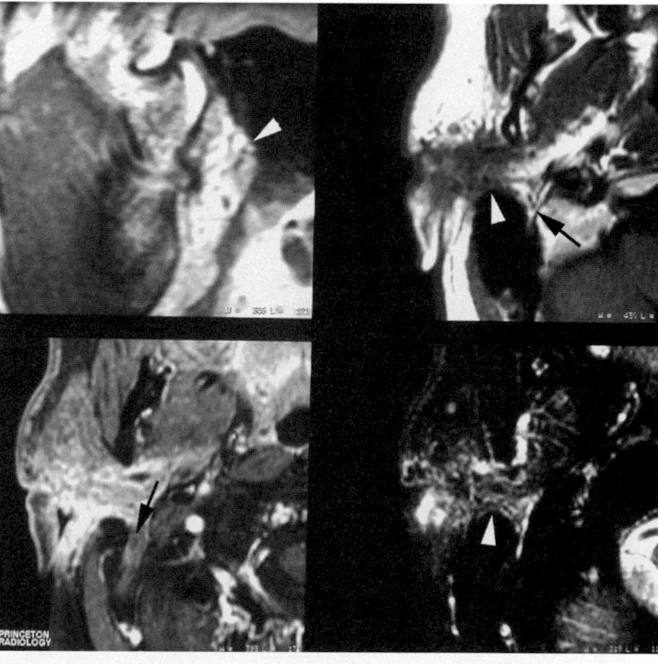

Figure 26.17 Follow-up total parotidectomy. Magnetic resonance imaging, clockwise from upper left: sagittal T1, axial T1, axial T2, and fat-suppressed axial contrast T1 series. **A:** Well-circumscribed malignancy (*long black arrows*) has close margin with cortical mastoid (*white arrowheads*) but does not involve the deep lobe (*short white arrows*). **B:** Postoperative collage shows preservation of the cortical mastoid (*white arrowheads*) and no involvement of the stylomastoid foramen (*black arrow*).

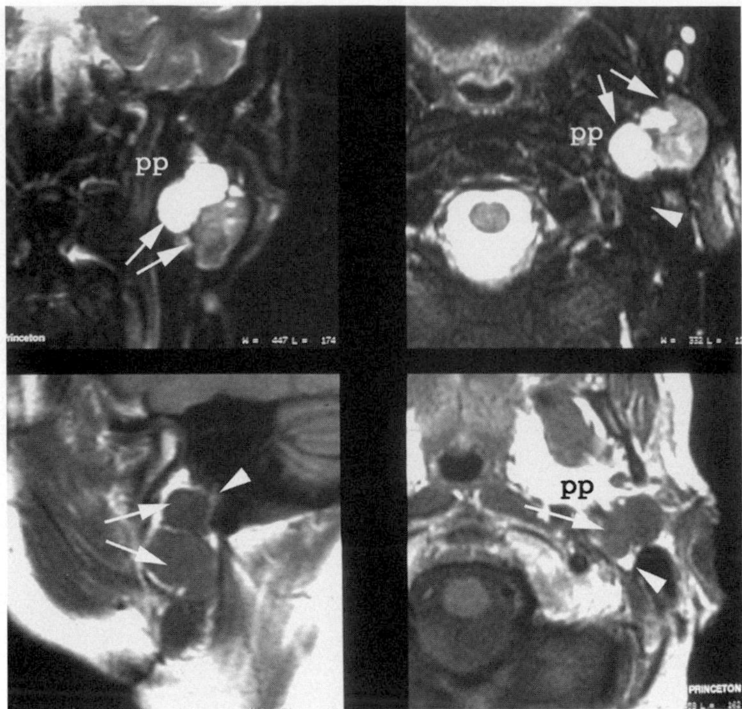

Figure 26.18 Recurrent pleomorphic adenoma, deep lobe recurrence. Magnetic resonance imaging collage, clockwise from top left: coronal T2, axial T2, axial T1, and sagittal T1 images show the deep lobe recurrence (*white arrows*) involving the parapharyngeal space (*pp*), approaching but not infiltrating the stylomastoid foramen (*white arrowhead*).

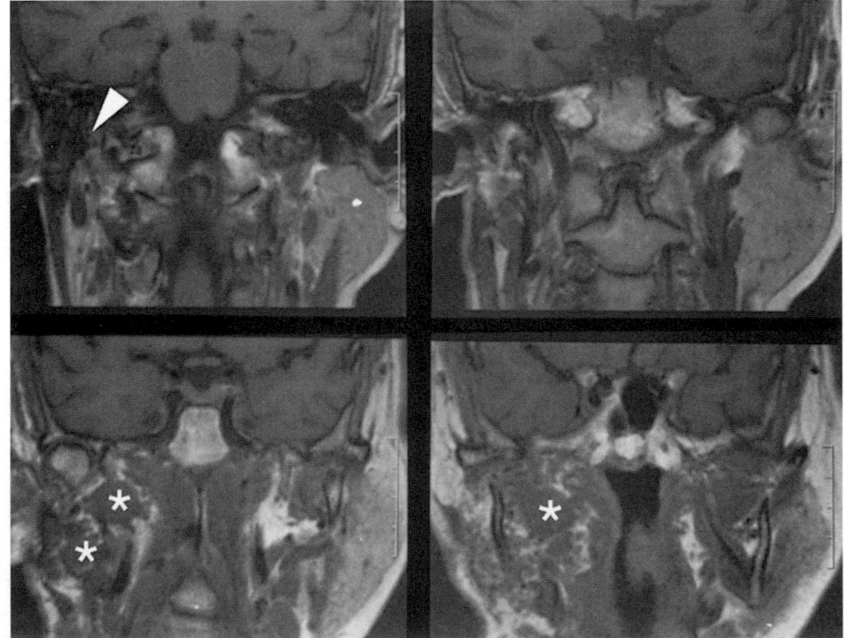

A

Figure 26.19 Deep recurrence of pleomorphic adenoma. Serial coronal T1 **(A)**, axial T2 **(B)**, and fat-suppressed contrast T1 **(C)** magnetic resonance imaging views of the skull base. Shown is multilobular deep-lobe recurrence (*asterisk*) approaching the soft palate (*arrow*) and stylomastoid foramen (*arrowhead*). Mastoid signal (*curved arrow*) is due to dysfunction of the eustachian tube.

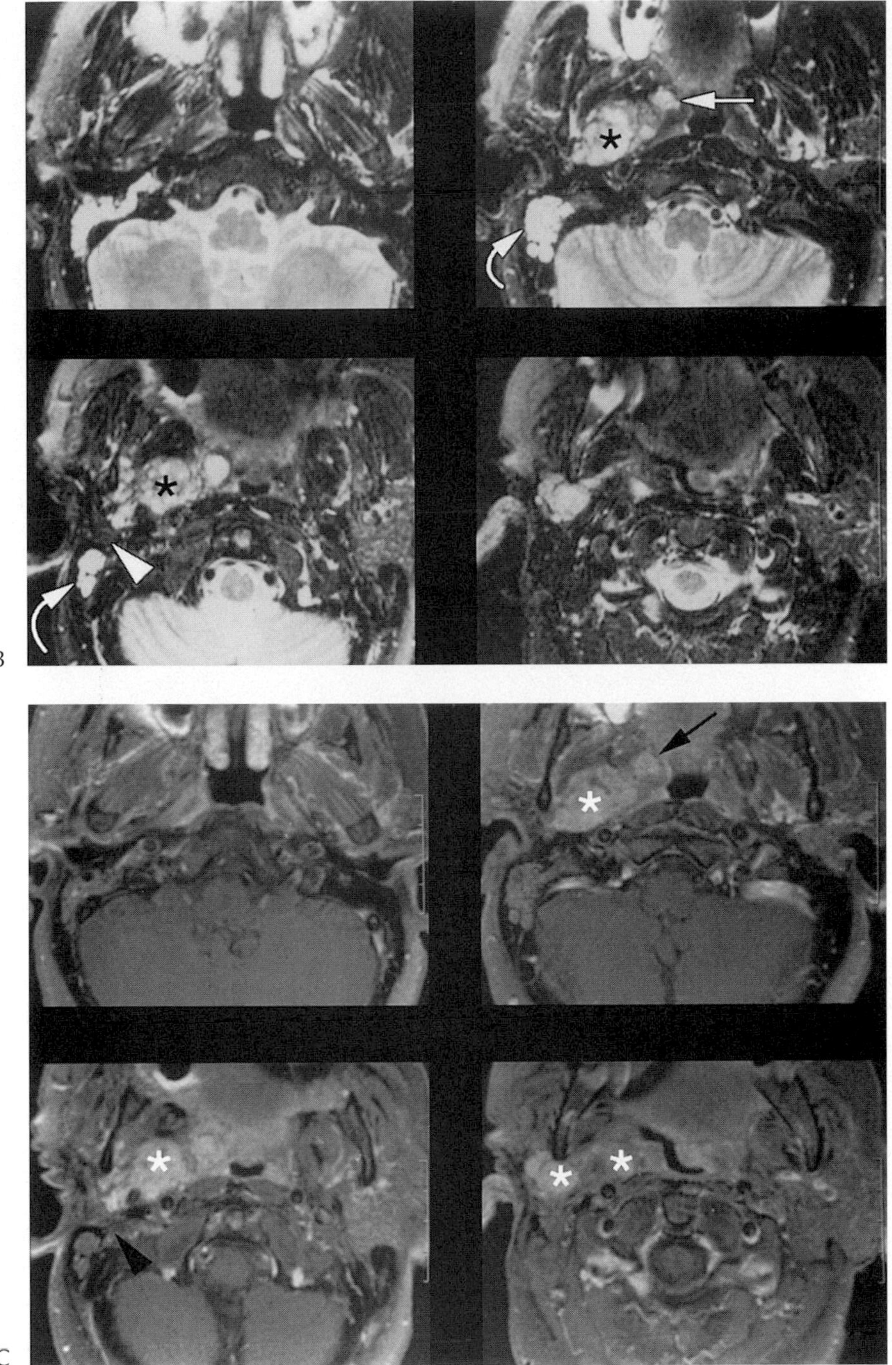

Figure 26.19 *continued.*

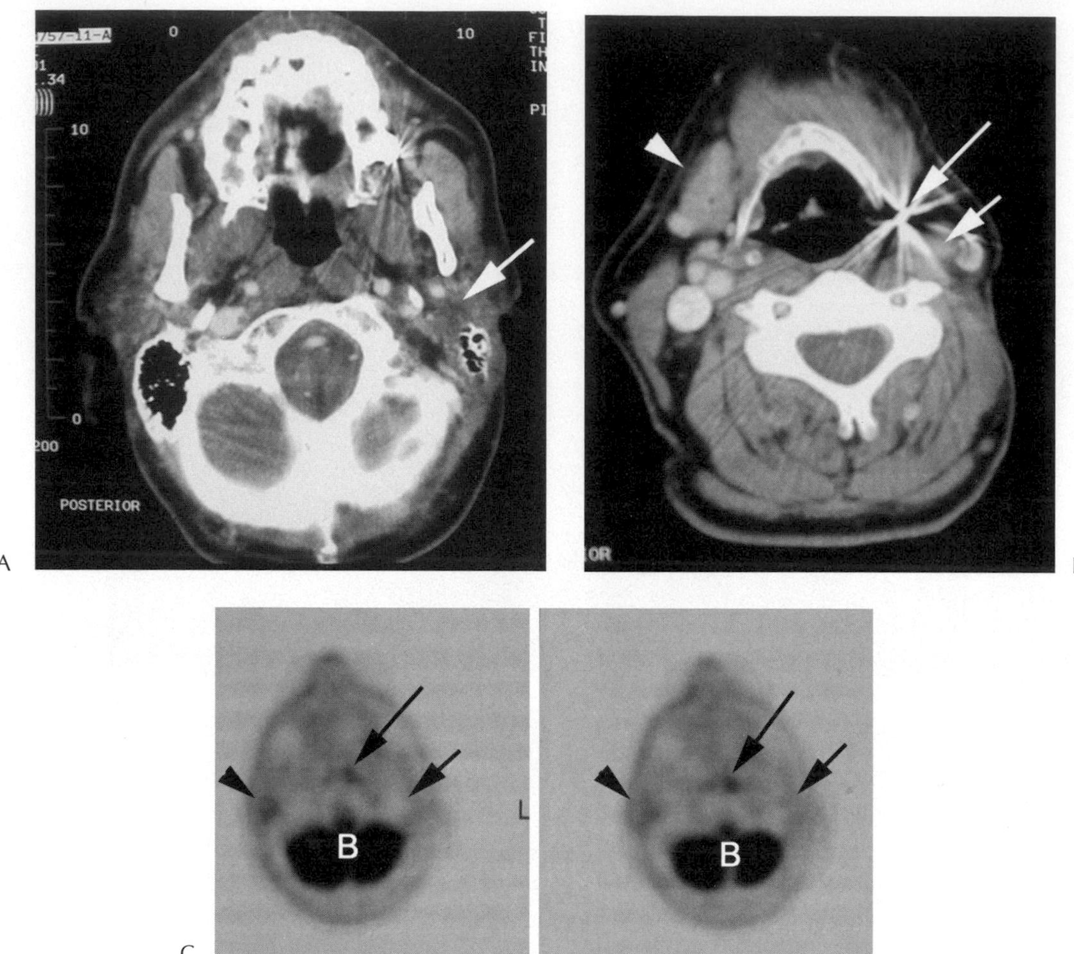

Figure 26.20 Fluorodeoxyglucose–positron emission tomography (FDG-PET) salivary follow-up. Enhanced axial computed tomographic images through **(A)** parotid bed show operative changes status post enucleation left parotid mass (*white arrow*) and **(B)** level II of the neck show poor visualization of the left neck dissection (*short arrow*) due to artifact from operative clip (*long arrow*). Normal submandibular gland (*arrowhead*). **C:** Axial FDG-PET images through the parotid beds show absent metabolic activity in operative bed (*short arrows*), physiologic activity in remaining right parotid bed (*arrowhead*), and asymmetric muscle activity (*long arrow*).

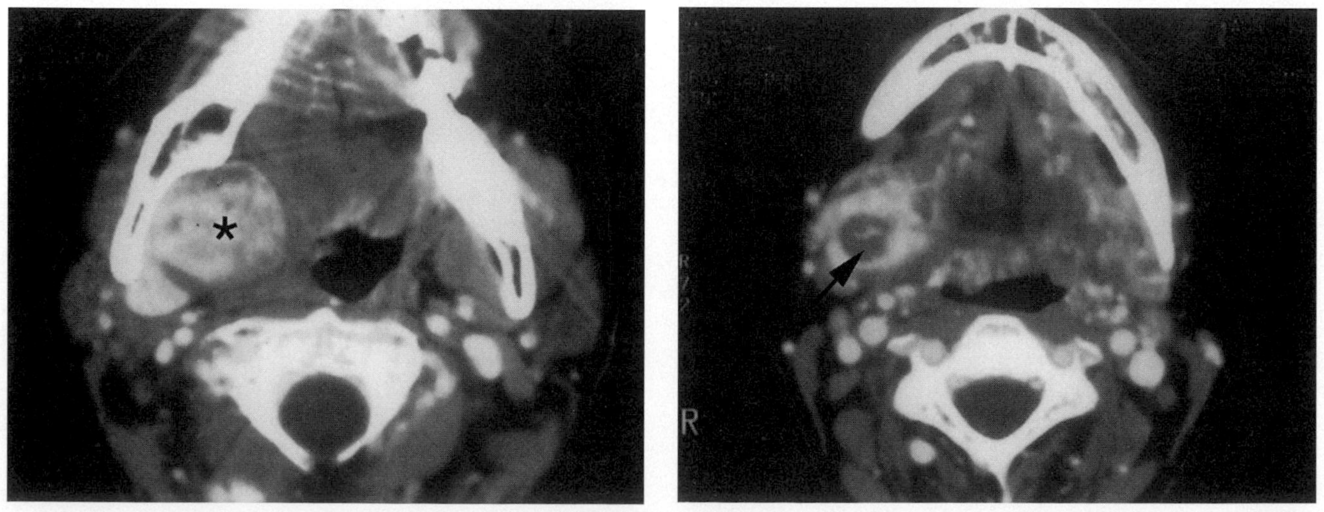

Figure 26.21 Submandibular mass. **A:** Enhanced axial computed tomography reveals enhancing mass within the hilum of the right submandibular gland (*asterisk*). **B:** Lower section shows low attenuation of lower segment of gland reflecting necrosis or obstructed gland (*arrow*).

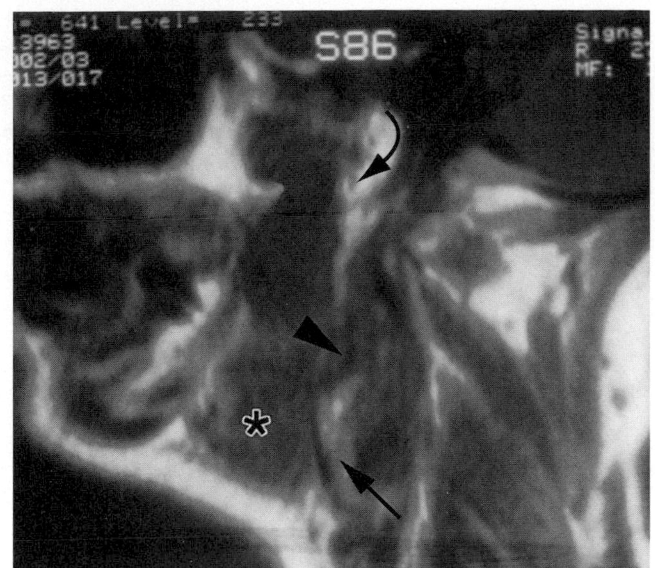

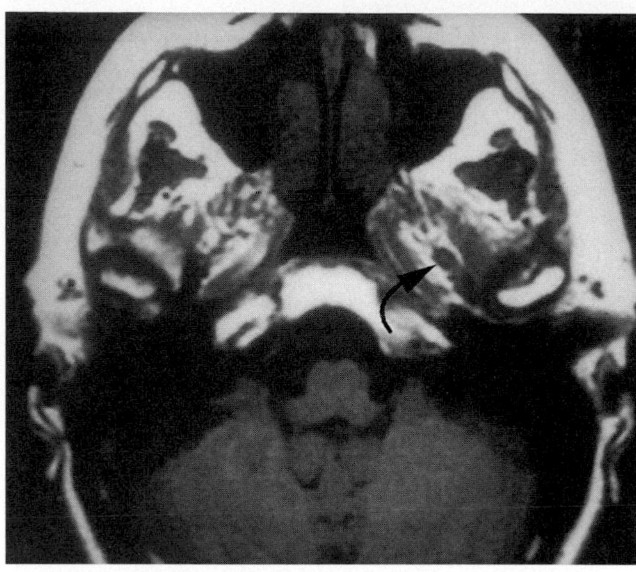

A B

Figure 26.22 Submandibular cancer. **A:** Sagittal T1 view shows submandibular mass (*asterisk*) with poor margin with carotid sheath (*arrowhead*), which appears thickened (*arrow*). **B:** Axial view shows thickening of ipsilateral nerve V approaching the skull base (*curved arrows*).

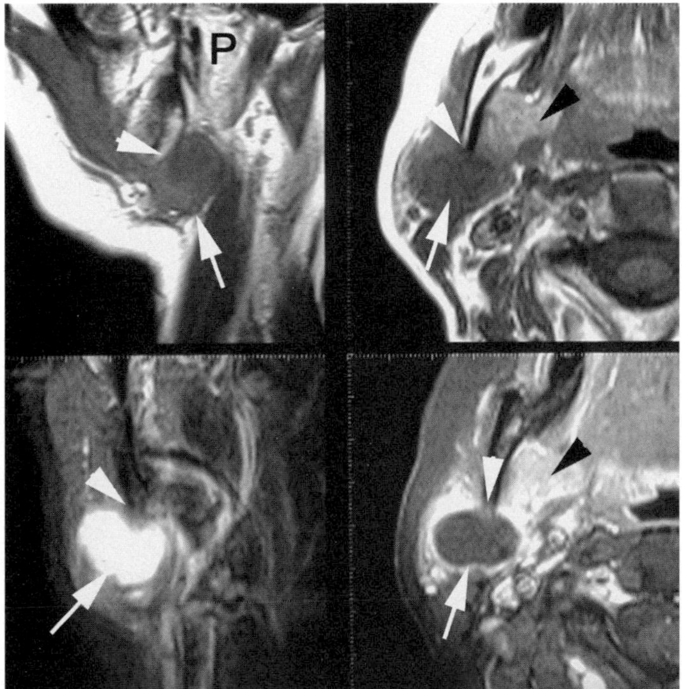

Figure 26.23 Tale of the tail. Magnetic resonance imaging collage, from top left, includes sagittal T1, axial T1, contrast axial T1, and coronal T2. The tail of parotid mass (*white arrows*) appears remote from the parotid gland (*P*) and pushes down against the submandibular gland (*black arrowhead*) contacting the edge of the mandibular ramus (*white arrowheads*).

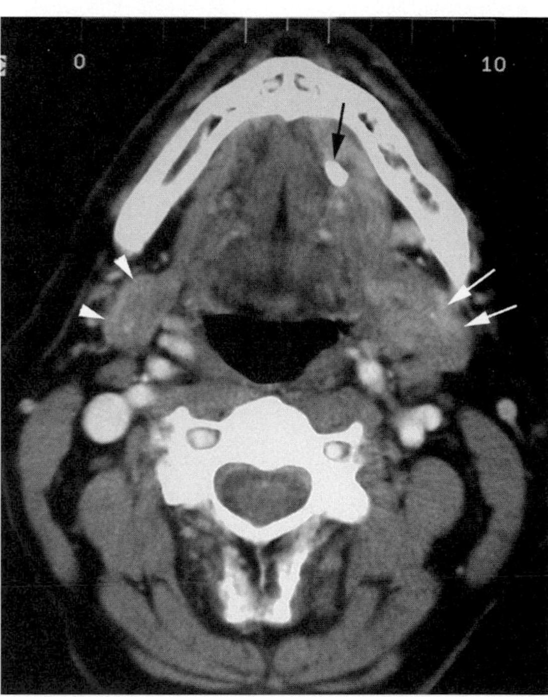

Figure 26.24 Pseudomass of the neck. The left submandibular gland (*white arrows*) is swollen compared with the right (*white arrowheads*) due to an obstructing calculus (*black arrow*) within the left Wharton duct.

RADIATION THERAPY TECHNIQUE

Louis B. Harrison, Rudolph Woode, and William M. Mendenhall

Parotid Gland

Parotid tumors are usually treated either with a wedged pair or a mixed beam technique. It has been our preference to use a wedged pair technique. This allows comprehensive irradiation of the parotid bed, as well as the cervical lymph nodes. The theoretical concern about the influence of the mandible on the electron beam dosimetry is completely avoided by using the wedged pair technique.

Figure 26.25 shows a patient who had a carcinoma ex pleomorphic adenoma. Her treatment included postoperative radiation to the parotid bed as well elective irradiation to the ipsilateral neck. The wedged pair technique is shown, as well as the dose volume histogram analysis. It is usually not a problem to include the entire target volume within the prescription isodose, and keep the spinal cord within tolerance. The contralateral parotid gland should receive less than 10% of the prescription dose. The ipsilateral technique also spares the contralateral minor salivary gland tissues. Therefore, these patients should not have a major problem with xerostomia.

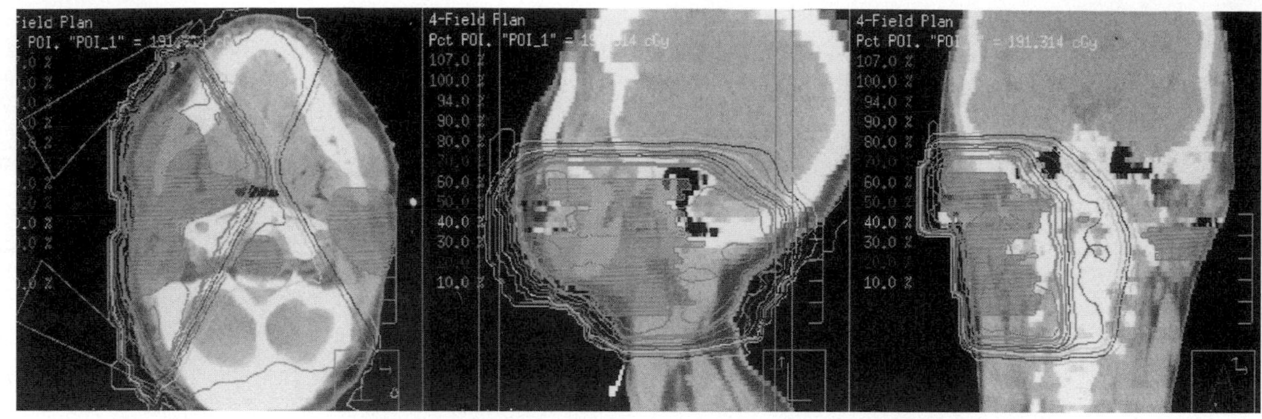

A,B C

Figure 26.25 Parotid gland—wedged pair. This 30-year-old woman underwent a resection for a 2-cm mass in the right parotid. Final pathology showed a carcinoma expleomorphic adenoma. The carcinomatous elements were high grade, and the margin was close. Given this pathology report, we treated the patient with postoperative radiation therapy to the parotid with elective irradiation to the ipsilateral neck. The entire parotid bed was contoured, including the region of the deep lobe. This includes the region where the deep lobe abuts the parapharyngeal space. Also contoured were the ipsilateral neck nodes. The patient was treated using an ipsilateral wedge pair technique for the primary site and upper neck, matched to an ipsilateral low neck field. The wedged pair fields are shown, revealing the PTV. Axial **(A)**, sagittal **(B)**, and coronal **(C)** dose distribution showing the contours as well as the isodose curves. This plan provides excellent coverage of the target volume, with less than 10% of the dose going to the contralateral parotid, which is also outlined.

REFERENCES

1. Preston-Martin S, Thomas DC, White SC, et al. Prior exposure to medical and dental x-rays related to tumors of the parotid gland. *J Natl Cancer Inst* 1988; 80:943.
2. Klintenberg C, Olofsson J, Hellquist M, et al. Adenocarcinoma of the ethmoid sinuses: a review of 28 cases with special reference to wood dust exposure. *Cancer* 1984;54:482.
3. Frommer J. The human accessory parotid gland: its incidence, nature, and significance. *Oral Surg* 1977;43:671.
4. McCormack LJ, Cauldwell EW, Anson BJ. The surgical anatomy of the facial nerve with special reference to the parotid gland. *Surg Gynecol Obstet* 1945; 80:620.
5. Martinez-Madrigal F, Pineda-Daboin K, Casiraghi O, et al. Salivary gland tumors of the mandible. *Ann Diagn Pathol* 2000;4:347–353.
6. Skolnick EM, Freidman M, Becker S, et al. Tumors of the major salivary glands. *Laryngoscope* 1977;87:843.
7. Theriault C, Fitzpatrick PJ. Malignant parotid tumors—prognostic factors and optimum treatment. *Am J Clin Oncol* 1986;9:510.
8. Kane WJ, McCaffrey TV, Olsen KD, et al. Primary parotid malignancies—a clinical and pathologic review. *Arch Otolaryngol Head Neck Surg* 1991;117:307.
9. Frankenthaler RA, Luna MA, Lee SS, et al. Prognostic variables in parotid gland cancer. *Arch Otolaryngol Head Neck Surg* 1991;117:1251.
10. Spiro RH, Huvos AG, Strong EW. Cancer of the parotid gland—a clinicopathological study of 288 primary cases. *Am J Surg* 1975;130:452.
11. Wong DSY. Signs and symptoms of malignant parotid tumors: an objective assessment. *J R Coll Surg Edinb* 2001;46:91–95.
12. Duck SW, McConnell FMS. Malignant degeneration of pleomorphic adenoma-clinical implications. *Am J Otolaryngol* 1993;14:175.
13. Lewis JE, Olsen KD, Sebo TJ. Carcinoma expleomorphic adenoma: pathologic analysis of 73 cases. *Hum Pathol* 2001;32:596–604.
14. Batsakis JG. Tumors of the major salivary glands. In: Batsakis JG, ed. *Tumors of the head and neck. Clinical and pathological considerations,* 2nd ed. Baltimore: Williams & Wilkins, 1979:1.
15. Eneroth CM. Histological and clinical aspects of parotid tumors. *Acta Otolaryngol* 1964;191:1.
16. Mustard RA, Anderson W. Malignant tumors of the parotid. *Ann Surg* 1964; 159:291.
17. Pedersen D, Overgaard J, Sogaard H, et al. Malignant parotid tumors in 110 consecutive patients: treatment results and prognosis. *Laryngoscope* 1992;102: 1064.
18. Dunn EJ, Kent T, Hines J, et al. Parotid neoplasms: a report of 250 cases and review of the literature. *Ann Surg* 1976;184:500.
19. Sullivan MJ, Breslin K, McClatchey KD, et al. Malignant parotid tumors: a retrospective study. *Otolaryngol Head Neck Surg* 1987;97:529.
20. Berdal P, Hall JG. Parapharyngeal growth of parotid tumors. *Acta Otolaryngol* 1970;263:164.
21. Bissett RJ, Fitzpatrick PJ. Malignant submandibular gland tumors. *Am J Clin Oncol* 1988;11:46.
22. Spiro RH, Hajdu SI, Strong EW. Tumors of the submaxillary gland. *Am J Surg* 1976;132:463.
23. Spiro RH. Treating tumors of the sublingual glands, including a useful technique for repair of the floor of mouth after resection. *Am J Surg* 1995;170:457.
24. Rankow RM, Mignogna F. Cancer of the sublingual salivary gland. *Am J Surg* 1969;118:790.
25. Spiro RH, Thaler HT, Hicks WF, et al. The importance of clinical staging of minor salivary gland carcinoma. *Am J Surg* 1991;162:330.
26. Batsakis JG. Neoplasms of the minor and lesser major salivary glands. In: Batsakis JG, ed. *Tumors of the head and neck. Clinical and pathological considerations,* 2nd ed. Baltimore: Williams & Wilkins, 1979:76.
27. Andersen LJ, Therkildsen MH, Ockelmann HH, et al. Malignant epithelial tumors in the minor salivary glands, the submandibular gland and the sublingual gland. Prognostic factors and treatment results. *Cancer* 1991;68:2431.
28. Tran L, Sidrys J, Horton D, et al. Malignant salivary gland tumors of the paranasal sinuses and nasal cavity. *Am J Clin Oncol* 1989;12:387.
29. Qizilbash AH, Sianos J, Young JEM, et al. Fine needle aspiration biopsy cytology of major salivary glands. *Acta Cytol* 1985;29:503.
30. Heller KS, Dubner S, Chess Q, et al. Value of fine needle aspiration biopsy of salivary gland masses in clinical decision-making. *Am J Surg* 1992;164:667.
31. Batsakis JG, Sneige N, El-Naggar AK. Fine needle aspiration of salivary glands: its utility and tissue effects. *Am Otol Rhinol Laryngol* 1992;101:185.
32. Stewart CJR, MacKenzie K, McGarry GW, et al. Fine-needle aspiration cytology of salivary gland: a review of 341 cases. *Diagn Cytopathol* 2000;22:139–146.
33. Frable MAS, Frable WJ. Fine needle aspiration biopsy of salivary glands. *Laryngoscope* 1991;101:245.
34. Roland NJ, Caslin AW, Smith PA, et al. Fine needle aspiration cytology of salivary gland lesions reported immediately in a head and neck clinic. *J Laryngol Otol* 1993;107:1025.
35. Zurrida S, Alasio L, Tradati N, et al. Fine needle aspiration of parotid masses. *Cancer* 1993;72:2306.
36. Layfield JL, Tan P, Glasgow BJ. Fine needle aspiration of salivary gland lesions. *Arch Pathol Lab Med* 1987;111:346.
37. Jayaram G, Verma AK, Sood N, et al. Fine needle aspiration cytology of salivary gland lesions. *J Oral Pathol Med* 1994;23:256.
38. Eisele DW Sherman ME, Koch WM, et al. Utility of immediate on-site cytopathological procurement and evaluation in fine needle biopsy of head and neck masses. *Laryngoscope* 1992;102:1328.
39. Takashima S, Wang J, Takayama F, et al. Parotid masses: prediction of malignancy using magnetization transfer and MR imaging findings. *AJR* 2001;176: 1577–1584.
40. McGuirt WF, Keyes JW, Greven KM, et al. Preoperative identification of benign versus malignant parotid masses: a comparative study including position emission tomography. *Laryngoscope* 1995;105:579.
41. American Joint Committee on Cancer. *AJCC cancer staging manual,* 5th ed. Philadelphia: Lippincott-Raven, 1997:54.

41a. Greene F, Page D, Fleming I, et al. *AJCC cancer staging manual,* 6th ed. New York: Springer-Verlag, 2002.

42. Batsakis JG. Staging of salivary gland neoplasms: role of histopathologic and molecular factors. *Am J Surg* 1994;168:386.
43. Tran L, Sadeghi A, Hanson D, et al. Major salivary gland tumors: treatment results and prognostic factors. *Laryngoscope* 1986;96:1139–1144.
44. Vander Poorten VL, Balm AJM, Hilgers FJM, et al. The development of a prognostic score for patients with parotid carcinoma. *Cancer* 1999;85: 2057–2067.
45. Timon CI, Dardick I, Panzarella T, et al. Clinico-pathological predictors of recurrence for acinic cell carcinoma. *Clin Otolaryngol* 1995;20:396–401.
46. O'Brien CJ, Soong SJ, Herrera GA, et al. Malignant salivary tumors—analysis of prognostic factors and survival. *Head Neck* 1986;9:82–92.
47. Malata CM, Camilleri IG, McLean MR, et al. Malignant tumors of the parotid gland: a 12-year review. *Br J Plast Surg* 1997;50:600–608.
48. Tullio A, Marchetti C, Sessena E, et al. Treatment of carcinoma of the parotid gland: the results of a multicenter study. *J Oral Maxillofac Surg* 2001;59: 263–270.
49. Magnano M, Gervasio CF, Cravero L, et al. Treatment of malignant neoplasms of the parotid gland. *Otolaryngol Head Neck Surg* 1999;121:627–632.
50. Chaffoo RA, Fee WE Jr. Early reexploration of the parotid wound following parotidectomy. *Am J Otolaryngol* 1989;10:38–41.
51. Perzin KH, Gullane P, Clairmont AC. Adenoid cystic carcinoma in the salivary glands: a correlation of histologic features and clinical course. *Cancer* 1978;42:265–282.
52. Namazie A, Alavi S, Abemayor E, et al. Adenoid cystic carcinoma of the base of tongue. *Ann Otol Laryngol* 2001;110:248–253.
53. Garden AS, Weber RS, Morrison WH, et al. The influence of positive margins and nerve invasion in adenoid cystic carcinoma of the head and neck treated with surgery and radiation. *Int J Radiat Oncol Biol Phys* 1995;32:619.
54. Westra WH. The surgical pathology of salivary gland neoplasms. *Otolaryngol Clin North Am* 1999;32:919–943.
55. Heller KS, Attie JW, Dubner S. Accuracy of frozen section in the evaluation of salivary tumors. *Am J Surg* 1993;166:424.
56. Miller RH, Calcaterra TC, Paglia DE. Accuracy of frozen section diagnosis of parotid lesions. *Ann Otol Rhinol Laryngol* 1979;88:573.
57. Hillel AD, Fee WE. Evaluation of frozen section in parotid gland surgery. *Arch Otolaryngol* 1983;109:230.
58. Wheelis RF, Yarington CT. Tumors of the salivary glands, comparison of frozen-section diagnosis with final pathological diagnosis. *Arch Otolaryngol* 1984;110:76.
59. Nussbaum M, Bortikner D. Facial nerve presentation in parotid carcinoma. *Bull NY Acad Med* 1986;62:862–865.
60. Brown PD, Eshleman JS, Foote RL, et al. An analysis of facial nerve function in irradiated and unirradiated facial nerve grafts. *Int J Radiat Oncol Biol Phys* 2000;48:737–743.
61. Frodel JL. Primary facial rehabilitation in facial paralysis. *Arch Facial Plast Surg* 2000;2:249–251.
62. Shindo M. Management of facial nerve paralysis. *Otolaryngol Clin North Am* 1999;32:945–964.
63. Fisher E, Frodel JL. Facial suspension with acellular human dermal allograft. *Arch Facial Plast Surg* 1999;1:195–199.
64. Armstrong JG, Harrison LB, Thaler HT, et al. The indications for elective treatment of the neck in cancer of the major salivary glands. *Cancer* 1992;69:615.
65. Frankenthaler RA, Byers RM, Luna MA, et al. Predicting occult lymph node metastasis in parotid cancer. *Arch Otolaryngol Head Neck Surg* 1993;119:517.
66. Regis de Brito Santos I, Kowalski LP, Cavalcante de Araujo V, et al. Multivariate analysis of risk factors for neck metastases in surgically treated parotid carcinomas. *Arch Otolaryngol Head Neck Surg* 2001;127:56–60.
67. Donovan DT, Conley J. Capsular significance in parotid tumor surgery: reality and myths of lateral lobectomy. *Laryngoscope* 1984;94:324–329.
68. Liu FF, Rotstein L, Davison AJ. Benign parotid adenomas: a review of the Princess Margaret Hospital experience. *Head Neck* 1995;17:177–183.
69. McGregor AD, Burgoyne M, Tan KC. Recurrent pleomorphic salivary adenoma—the relevance of age at first presentation. *Br J Plast Surg* 1988;41: 177–181.
70. Myssiorek D, Ruah CB, Hybels RL. Recurrent pleomorphic adenomas of the parotid gland. *Head Neck* 1990;12:332–336.
71. Phillips PP, Olsen KD. Recurrent pleomorphic adenoma of the parotid gland: report of 126 cases and a review of the literature. *Ann Otol Rhinol Laryngol* 1995;104:100–104.
72. Conley J. Problems with reoperation of the parotid gland and facial nerve. *Otolaryngol Head Neck Surg* 1988;99:480–488.

73. Fee, WE, Goffinet DR, Calcaterra TC. Recurrent mixed tumors of the parotid gland—results of surgical therapy. *Laryngoscope* 1978;88:265–273.
74. Niparko JK, Beauchamp ML, Krause CJ, et al. Surgical treatment of recurrent pleomorphic adenoma of the parotid gland. *Arch Otolaryngol Head Neck Surg* 1986;112:1180–1184.
75. Olsen KD, Daube JR. Intraoperative monitoring of the facial nerve: an aid in the management of parotid gland recurrent pleomorphic adenoma. *Laryngoscope* 1994;104:229–232.
76. Samson MJ, Metson R, Wang CC, Montgomery WW. Preservation of the facial nerve in the management of recurrent pleomorphic adenoma. *Laryngoscope* 1991;101:1060–1062.
77. Maran AGD, Mackenzie IJ, Stanley RE. Recurrent pleomorphic adenomas of the parotid gland. *Arch Otolaryngol* 1984;110:167–171.
78. Fu KK, Leibel SA, Levin ML, et al. Carcinoma of the major and minor salivary glands. Analysis of treatment results and sites and causes of failures. *Cancer* 1977;40:2882.
79. Eapen LJ, Gerig LH, Catton GE, et al. Impact of local radiation in the management of salivary gland carcinomas. *Head Neck Surg* 1988;10:239.
80. North CA, Lee DJ, Piantadosi S, et al. Carcinoma of the major salivary glands treated by surgery or surgery plus postoperative radiotherapy. *Int J Radiat Oncol Biol Phys* 1990;18:1319.
81. Harrison LB, Armstrong JG, Spiro RH, et al. Postoperative radiation therapy for major salivary gland malignancies. *J Surg Oncol* 1990;45:52.
82. Fitzpatrick PJ, Theriault C. Malignant salivary gland tumors. *Int J Radiat Oncol Biol Phys* 1986;12:1743.
83. Armstrong JG, Harrison LB, Spiro RH, et al. Malignant tumors of major salivary gland orgin. *Arch Otolaryngol Head Neck Surg* 1990;116:290.
84. Vikram, B, Strong EW, Shah, JP, et al. Radiation therapy kin adenoid cystic carcinoma. *Int J Radiat Oncol Biol Phys* 1984;10:221.
85. Miglianico L, Eschwege F, Marandas P, et al. Cervico-facial adenoid cystic carcinoma: study of 102 cases. Influence of radiation therapy. *Int J Radiat Oncol Biol Phys* 1987;13:673.
86. Sykes AJ, Slevin NJ, Birzgalis AR, et al. Submandibular gland carcinoma; an audit of local control and survival following adjuvant radiotherapy. *Oral Oncol* 1999;35:187–190.
87. Storey MR, Garden AS, Morrison WH, et al. Postoperative radiotherapy for malignant tumors of the submandibular gland. *Int J Radiat Oncol Biol Phys* 2001;51:952–958.
88. Rodriguez-Cuevas S, Labastida D, Baena L, et al. Risk of nodal metastases from malignant salivary gland tumors related to tumor size and grade of malignancy. *Eur Arch Otorhinalaryngol* 1995;252:139.
89. Vander Poorten VLM, Balm AJM, Hilgers FJM, et al. Stage as major long term outcome predictor in minor salivary gland carcinoma. *Cancer* 2000;89: 1195–1204.
90. Jenkins DW, Spaulding CA, Constable WC, et al. Minor salivary gland tumors: the role of radiotherapy. *Am J Otolaryngol* 1989;10:250–256.
91. Garden AS, Weber RS, Ang KK, et al. Postoperative radiation therapy for malignant tumors of minor salivary glands. Outcome and patterns of failure. *Cancer* 1994;73:2563.
92. Parsons IT, Mendenhall WM, Strenger SP, et al. Management of minor salivary gland carcinomas. *Int J Radiat Oncol Biol Phys* 1996;35:443.
93. Sadeghi A, Tran LM, Mark R, et al. Minor salivary gland tumors of the head and neck: treatment strategies and prognosis. *Am J Clin Oncol* 1993;16:3.
94. Le QT, Birdwell S, Terris DJ, et al. Postoperative irradiation of minor salivary gland malignancies of the head and neck. *Radiother Oncol* 1999;52:165–171.
95. Laramore GE. Fast neutron radiotherapy for inoperable salivary gland tumors: is it the treatment of choice? *Int J Radiat Oncol Biol Phys* 1987;13:1421.
96. Laramore GE, Krall, JM Griffin TW, et al. Neutron versus photon irradiation for unresectable salivary gland tumors: final report of an RTOG-MRC randomized clinical trial. Radiation Therapy Oncology Group. *Int J Radiat Oncol Biol Phys* 1993;30:235.
97. Krull A, Schwarz R, Brackrock S, et al. Neutron therapy in malignant salivary tumors: results at European centers. *Recent Results Cancer Res* 1998;150:88–99.
98. Douglas JG, Lee S, Laramore GE, et al. Neutron radiotherapy for the treatment of locally advanced major salivary gland tumors. *Head Neck* 1999; 21:255–263.
99. Douglas JG, Laramore GE, Austin-Seymour M, et al. Treatment of locally advanced adenoid cystic carcinoma of the head and neck with neutron radiotherapy. *Int J Radiat Oncol Biol Phys* 2000;46:551–557.
100. Huber PE, Debus J, Latz D, et al. Radiotherapy for advanced adenoid cystic carcinoma: neutrons, photons, or mixed beam? *Radiother Oncol* 2001;59: 1621–1627.
101. Wang CC, Goodman M. Photon irradiation of unresectable carcinomas of salivary glands. *Int J Radiat Oncol Biol Phys* 1991;21:569.
102. Saroja KR, Mansell J, Hendrikson FR. An update on malignant salivary tumors treated with neutrons at Fermilab. *Int J Radiol Oncol Biol Phys* 1987; 13:1319.
103. Buchholz TA, Laramore GE, Griffin BR, et al. The role of fast neutron radiation therapy in the management of advanced salivary gland malignant neoplasms. *Cancer* 1992;69:2779.
104. Spiro RH, Armstrong J, Harrison L, et al. Carcinoma of major salivary glands. *Arch Otolaryngol Head Neck Surg* 1989;115:316.
105. Spiro IJ, Wang CC, Montgomery WW, et al. Carcinoma of the parotid gland. Analysis of treatment results and patterns of failure after combined surgery and radiation therapy. *Cancer* 1997;71:2699.
106. Numata T, Muto H, Shiba K, et al. Evaluation of the validity of the 1997 International Union Against Cancer TNM classification of major salivary gland carcinoma. *Cancer* 2000;89:1664–1669.
107. Jackson GL, Luna MS, Byers RM. Results of surgery alone and surgery combined with postoperative radiotherapy in the treatment of cancer of the parotid gland. *Am J Surg* 1983;146:497.
108. Tannock IF, Sutherland DJ. Chemotherapy for adenoid cystic carcinoma. *Cancer* 1980;46:452.
109. Matsuba HM, Spector GJ, Thawley SE, et al. Adenoid cystic salivary gland carcinoma. A histopathologic review of treatment failure patterns. *Cancer* 1986;57:519.
110. Nigro MF, Spiro RH. Deep lobe parotid tumors. *Am J Surg* 1977;134:523–527.
111. Conley J, Hamaker RC. Prognosis of malignant tumors of the parotid gland with facial paralysis. *Arch Otolaryngol* 1975;101:39.
112. Eisele DW, Johns ME. Complications of surgery of the salivary glands. In: Eisele DW ed. *Complications in head and neck surgery.* St. Louis: Mosby-Year Book, 1993:183.
113. Gullane PJ, Havas TJ. Facial nerve grafts: effects of postoperative irradiation. *J Otolaryngol* 1987;16:11.
114. Griffin TW. Optimal treatment for salivary gland tumors. *Int J Radiat Oncol Biol Phys* 1991;21:857–858.
115. Armstrong JG, Harrison LB, Sprio RH, et al. Observation on the natural history and treatment of recurrent major salivary gland cancer. *J Surg Oncol* 1990;44:138.
116. Armstrong JG, Harrison LB, Spiro RH, et al. Brachytherapy for malignant tumors of salivary gland origin. *Endocuriether Hyperthermia Oncol* 1990;6:19.
117. Dreyfuss AI, Clark JR, Fallon BG, et al. Cyclophosphamide, doxorubicin, cisplatin combination chemotherapy for advanced carcinomas of salivary gland origin. *Cancer* 1987;60:2869.
118. Kaplan MJ, Johns ME, Cantrell RW. Chemotherapy for salivary gland cancer. *Otolaryngol Head Neck Surg* 1966;95:165.
119. Dimery IW, Legha SS, Shirinian M, et al. Fluorouracil, doxorubicin, cyclophosphamide, and cisplatin combination chemotherapy in advanced or recurrent salivary gland carcinoma. *J Clin Oncol* 1990;8:1056.
120. Licitra L, Marchini S, Spinazze S, et al. Cisplatin in advanced salivary gland carcinoma. *Cancer* 1991;68:1874.
121. Creagan ET, Woods JE, Rubin J, et al. Cisplatin-based chemotherapy for neoplasms arising from salivary glands and contiguous structures in the head and neck. *Cancer* 1988;62:2313.
122. Airoldi M, Fornari G, Pedani F, et al. Paclitaxel and carboplatin for recurrent salivary gland malignancies. *Anticancer Res* 2000;20:3781–3783.
123. Airoldi M, Pedani F, Succo G, et al. Phase II randomized trial comparing vinorelbine verses vinorelbine plus cisplatin in patients with recurrent salivary gland malignancies. *Cancer* 2001;91:541–554.

Radiologic Imaging Concerns

124. Spiro RH. Changing trends in the management of salivary tumors [Review]. *Semin Surg Oncol* 1995;11:240–245.
125. Freling NJ, Molenaar WM, Vermey A, et al. Malignant parotid tumors: clinical use of MR imaging and histologic correlation. *Radiology* 1992;185:691–696.
126. Freling NJ. Imaging of salivary gland disease. *Semin Roentgenol* 2000;35: 12–20.
127. Choi DS, Na DG, Byun HS, et al. Salivary gland tumors: evaluation with two-phase helical CT. *Radiology* 2000;214:231–236.
128. Yousem DM, Kraut MA, Chalian AA. Major salivary gland imaging. *Radiology* 2000;216:19–29.
129. Gritzmann N. Sonography of the salivary glands. *AJR* 1989;153:161–166.

CHAPTER 27

Cancers Involving the Skull Base and Temporal Bone

Ivo P. Janecka, Silloo Kapadia, Anthony A. Mancuso, Sanjay Prasad, David A. Moffat, and Julian J. Pribaz

Temporal bone is a complex structure of the skull base that houses important sensory and neurovascular anatomy with proximity to many vital structures (1). Cancer of the temporal bone is a rare but aggressive disease. The age-adjusted incidence for a squamous cell carcinoma (SCC) is 1 per 1 million women and 0.8 per 1 million men annually (2). The clinical presentation is often nonspecific, with symptoms and signs of chronic ear infection. In our review (3), reports of otorrhea (or an increase in its volume) were present in 28%, pain in 25.6%, or bleeding in 16.3%, followed closely by facial palsy (11.6%) as the predominant clinical features. In another study by Pensak et al. (4), the symptomatology of patients ranged from ear pain (74%) through hearing loss (62%) and bleeding (28%) to facial numbness (12%) and vertigo (10%). The clinical signs included ear canal lesion (88%), aural discharge (84%), preauricular swelling (25%), facial paralysis (18%), and abnormal neck nodes (8%) (4). Once diagnosed by a biopsy, temporal bone cancer does present a therapeutic challenge. Except for small ear canal tumors, it may not be possible to establish the precise site of tumor origin because, in most cases, both the ear canal and the middle ear are involved (5). Regional lymphatic spread is uncommon (6). Full assessment of tumor perimeter with imaging and specific histologic cell identification is needed before formulation of a therapeutic plan. The first treatment should be the most comprehensive one, as it often correlates directly with a patient's eventual outcome.

Previously, treatment modalities included local excision, variations of mastoidectomy, and temporal bone resection (TBR). Radiation therapy (RT) often was used alone or after surgery. The limitation of direct bone penetration by radiation and the frequent presence of chronic infection with temporal bone cancers are compounding factors that diminish the effectiveness of RT as a primary therapeutic modality.

This chapter discusses the current understanding of pathology, imaging, surgery, and outcomes as they relate to the diagnosis and treatment of cancer of the temporal bone.

PATHOLOGY

Malignant tumors involving the temporal bone include SCC, basal cell carcinoma (BCC), adenocarcinoma, sarcoma, and secondary neoplasms that may involve the temporal bone either by metastases from distant sites or by direct invasion from adja-

This chapter was adapted from Prasad S, Janecka IP. Efficacy of surgical treatments for squamous cell carcinoma of the temporal bone: a literature review. *Otolaryngol Head Neck Surg* 1994;110:270–280; and Sekhar LN, Pomeranz S, Janecka IP, et al. Temporal bone neoplasms: a report on 20 surgically treated cases. *J Neurosurg* 1992;76:578–587, with permission.

cent structures (7–10). Squamous cell carcinoma is the most commonly seen primary malignant tumor of the ear and temporal bone (3,6,10–15). It may originate in the skin of the auricle, the external auditory canal (EAC), or the middle ear cleft. Squamous cell carcinoma of the auricle is second in frequency only to BCC. In advanced cases, when both the EAC and temporal bone are involved, the exact site of origin may be difficult to determine. Spector (15) reported a mean age of 72.6 years (range, 56 to 98 years) for patients with SCC of the temporal bone, with a 2:1 male predominance. Most patients with external ear SCC are elderly white men, with a median age of 60. There is a male predominance of more than 95%, and exposure to actinic rays or frostbite is common (15). In one study, the median age for patients with middle ear SCC was 68 years, with no sex predominance (6).

Squamous cell carcinoma of the auricle presents as an ulcerating bleeding lesion that may be painful. Squamous cell carcinoma of the EAC may present as a polyp, ulcer, or subcutaneous mass, with pain and drainage. Chronic otitis media and otorrhea are common manifestations of SCC of the EAC and middle ear. Hearing loss and facial paralysis may be present.

Histologically, conventional SCC of the external and middle ear may be well differentiated by the presence of keratin formation and intercellular bridges, or it may be moderately to poorly differentiated. Verrucous carcinoma, a well-differentiated variant of SCC with prominent surface keratinization, absent dysplastic features, and a pushing rather than infiltrating advancing edge, may occasionally involve the temporal bone (8,13). The differential diagnosis includes chronic otitis media, actinic keratosis, pseudoepitheliomatous hyperplasia, squamous papilloma, and BCC. Squamous cell carcinoma of the temporal bone shows a capacity to spread via anatomic pathways, along nerves and vascular or fascial planes, and by direct bone erosion. The incidence of metastasis varies from 12% to 16% (15).

Basal cell carcinoma is the most common primary skin cancer. Basal cell carcinoma of the temporal bone arises from the skin of the auricle or EAC (7–9,16,17). Basal cell carcinoma of the external ear accounts for 21% of all neoplasms of the ear and temporal bone (8). In the auricle, BCCs account for 90% of carcinomas and 10% are SCCs, whereas in the EAC, 80% of tumors are SCCs and 20% are BCCs, mainly in its lateral portion (8). There is a 2:1 male predominance. The mean age of patients is in the sixth decade, although any age group may be involved. Most BCCs occur in whites; blacks rarely are affected. The main etiology is exposure to actinic rays.

Histologically, BCC may be of the solid or nodular type, the sclerosing or morphea type, the multicentric or superficial type, or the metatypical or basosquamous type (16). The tumor cells resemble the basal cells of the epidermis. They have hyperchromatic, basophilic, round to oval nuclei, and scant cytoplasm. A characteristic feature is the presence of tumor cell nests in the upper dermis, showing a peripheral radiating or palisading arrangement of tumor cell nuclei. Focal squamous differentiation may be present. The histologic differential diagnosis of BCC mainly includes variants of SCC. Combined surgery and postoperative RT is the preferred treatment of conventional SCC and BCC involving the temporal bone (15). Tumors that initially involve lymph nodes carry a poor prognosis.

Primary adenocarcinomas arising from the region of the middle ear are rare (8,18–26). These neoplasms often belong to the category of low-grade papillary adenocarcinoma (8–25) or, rarely, high-grade adenocarcinoma or adenoid cystic carcinoma (18,26).

Papillary adenocarcinomas of middle ear origin occur in patients with a mean age of 41 years (range, 15 to 71 years) (23). There is no sex predilection. Symptoms include progressive unilateral hearing loss, which is sometimes longstanding (8,18). Tinnitus and vertigo may be present, as may pain and cranial nerve paralysis. Computed tomographic (CT) scans show a lytic lesion with prominent extension into the posterior cranial cavity. Microscopically, these are well-differentiated, low-grade epithelial neoplasms with a papillary-cystic glandular appearance (18,20,23–25). Intracystic papillae and glands are lined by a uniform single layer of cuboidal or columnar epithelial cells. The cells have a vacuolated or clear cytoplasm and round, hyperchromatic nuclei. Mitotic activity is not a feature (23). The papillary projections and colloid-like secretions may superficially resemble papillary thyroid carcinoma.

Low-grade primary adenocarcinomas should be distinguished from the more common adenomas of the middle ear (8,18,23). Bony erosion and facial nerve involvement are more likely to be present in the former. These tumors grow slowly and follow a locally destructive clinical course. Heffner (23) has suggested that papillary low-grade adenocarcinomas of the middle ear probably arise from the endolymphatic sac located in the posteromedial plate of the petrous bone.

Primary high-grade adenocarcinomas and adenoid cystic carcinomas of the middle ear are very rare. Histologically, high-grade adenocarcinomas demonstrate poorly formed glands or sheets of tumor cells displaying hyperchromatic, pleomorphic nuclear features and mitoses. Middle ear adenocarcinomas should be distinguished from malignant tumors arising from ceruminous glands of the external auditory meatus, adenoid cystic carcinomas that spread to the temporal bone from the adjacent parotid area, and metastatic adenocarcinoma. These have a more rapid, destructive clinical course with regional and distant metastasis. Low-grade papillary adenocarcinomas are treated with surgical resection. High-grade adenocarcinoma or adenoid cystic carcinoma may require surgery and postoperative RT.

Sarcomas of the temporal bone are rare. Rhabdomyosarcoma (RMS), a soft tissue sarcoma characterized by skeletal myogenic differentiation, is the most common soft tissue sarcoma in children and the most common sarcoma of the head and neck (27–29). In the head and neck, the orbit is more commonly involved by RMS, followed by the nasopharynx, middle ear–mastoid region, and sinonasal tract. Rhabdomyosarcoma in these nonorbital sites, collectively referred to as *parameningeal sites,* has a propensity to spread to the skull base, and therefore carries a poorer prognosis than orbital RMS (27–29).

Rhabdomyosarcoma of the ear and temporal bone is a rare, highly aggressive neoplasm of infants and children (30–36). When the EAC and middle ear are both involved at onset, the exact site of origin may be difficult to determine. In addition, the temporal bone may be invaded by RMS from adjacent sites, such as the infratemporal fossa and nasopharynx (31). Wiatrak and Pensak (31) studied 12 patients with RMS involving the temporal bone; the RMS arose within the middle ear–mastoid region in 7 cases and the EAC in 2 cases, and invaded the temporal bone from adjacent structures in 3 cases (31). These patients ranged in age from 18 months to 13 years (mean age, 5 years). Early symptoms, such as hearing loss, otalgia, aural discharge, or a polyp in the EAC with penetration of the tympanic membrane, are often mistaken for chronic otitis media and may lead to delay in diagnosis (31). Other prominent but advanced findings include preauricular swelling and skull-base involvement with cranial nerve dysfunction.

Histologically, RMS is classified into embryonal RMS (ERMS), the botryoid variant of ERMS, and alveolar or pleomorphic types, depending on its growth pattern, degree of differentiation, and configuration of the neoplastic cells (27). Most cases of head and neck RMS (approximately 80% to 85%) are of the ERMS type or its botryoid variant, and 10% to 15% are alveolar. Pleomorphic RMS is uncommon. In one study, 11 of 12 cases of temporal bone RMS were of the embryonal type, and one was botryoid (31). In ERMS, varying numbers of rhabdomyoblasts with cytoplasmic cross-striations are found, depending on the tumor's degree of differentiation. Hypercellular areas may alternate with less cellular fibromyxoid areas. Short and spindled rhabdomyoblasts are seen, which feature a central, elongated nucleus and tapered ends. Round cells with darkly staining, hyperchromatic nuclei and scant eosinophilic cytoplasm may also be present with mitoses. The botryoid variant is characterized by a grapelike configuration and distinctive histologic features, including a prominent myxoid stroma displaying a paucity of tumor cells alternating with more cellular areas, and a subepithelial condensation of tumor cells, the cambium layer. In the EAC, botryoid RMS may be mistaken for granulation tissue; however, the presence of spindle-shaped or round rhabdomyoblasts should suggest the diagnosis. Alveolar RMS is composed of noncohesive cells arranged in an alveolar pattern. Tumor cells are attached peripherally to fibrous septa and have hyperchromatic, round, or spindled nuclei with inconspicuous nucleoli and acidophilic cytoplasm.

Rhabdomyosarcoma should be distinguished from Ewing's sarcoma, lymphoma, undifferentiated carcinoma, and melanoma by its skeletal features. The diagnosis may be confirmed by immunostaining for desmin (positive in more than 90% of cases), muscle-specific actin, and sarcomeric actin (37). Although myoglobin is a more specific striated muscle marker, it is much less sensitive. On occasion, RMS may be cytokeratin- or S-100 protein-positive.

Rhabdomyoblastic differentiation can be confirmed ultrastructurally by the demonstration of actin and myosin filaments with Z bands and intermediate filaments. A consistent chromosomal rearrangement—t(2;13)(q35;ql4)—has been found in alveolar RMS (38).

The Intergroup RMS Study clinical staging classification (groups I to IV; Table 27.1) is based primarily on the surgical resectability of the grossly detectable tumor (28,29). Computed tomography scanning and magnetic resonance imaging (MRI) show a soft tissue mass with bone destruction, especially at the skull base, and delineate precisely the extent of tumor. Rhabdomyosarcoma of the ear and temporal bone is an aggressive, locally destructive tumor. The path of spread is usually by invasion of the fallopian canal and facial nerve; from there, tumor extends to the internal auditory canal and leptomeninges of the posterior fossa (35). In approximately 12% of cases, there is regional nodal involvement, and in 15%, distant metastases are seen at diagnosis (31).

TABLE 27.1 Definition of Rhabdomyosarcoma Clinical Groups

Group I	Localized disease, completely resected (regional nodes involved) a. Confined to muscle or organ of origin b. Contiguous involvement, infiltration outside the muscle or organ of origin
Group II	Localized disease with microscopic residual disease or regional disease with no residual or with microscopic residual disease a. Grossly resected tumor with microscopic residual disease(nodes negative) b. Regional disease, completely resected (nodes positive or negative) c. Regional disease with involved nodes, grossly resected, but with evidence of microscopic residual disease
Group III	Incomplete resection or biopsy with gross residual disease
Group IV	Metastatic disease present at onset

Source: Data derived from Maurer HM, Beltangady M, Gehan EA, et al. The Intergroup Rhabdomyosarcoma Study–I: a final report. *Cancer* 1988;61:209–220.

Rhabdomyosarcoma is treated with combined therapy including surgery, RT, and chemotherapy. The selection of a primary therapeutic modality depends on tumor extent and the age of the patient. Most RMSs in children are treated with primary chemotherapy, with surgery and RT being reserved for salvage. Owing to the low occurrence of regional metastasis of RMS, treatment of the neck should be limited to those patients with clinically positive nodes. Adverse prognostic features include parameningeal sites, such as the middle ear and nasopharynx, which are associated with a less favorable prognosis than is the orbit; alveolar histologic type (as compared with embryonal RMS and its botryoid variant); and advanced clinical stage (28,29). According to the Intergroup RMS Study, the overall 5-year survival in RMS patients in group I was 83%; in group II, 70%; in group 111, 52%; and in group IV, 20% (28). Because most patients with RMS of the ear and temporal bone present with advanced disease and develop meningeal extension, the prognosis is poor. Wiatrak and Pensak (31) reported a mean survival of 2.8 years (range, 3 months to 19 years) in patients with RMS of the temporal bone.

Secondary malignant tumors of the temporal bone are relatively uncommon and arise by metastatic hematogenous spread from a distant site, by direct invasion from adjacent structures, or by diffuse leptomeningeal spread (39–43). In a review of 212 reported cases of metastatic temporal bone tumors, Imamura and Mukakamki (42) found that the more common sites of origin were the breast (38 cases), lung (23 cases), kidney (12 cases), prostate (10 cases), salivary gland (10 cases), pharynx or nasopharynx (15 cases), and gastrointestinal tract (17 cases). In 37 cases, the site of origin was undetermined; the remaining cases involved miscellaneous sites, including the leptomeninges, genitourinary tract, other head and neck sites, thyroid, and soft tissue. Direct invasion from adjacent structures occurs from sites such as the pharynx, nasopharynx, parotid, meninges, or metastatic tumor of cervical lymph nodes. Such spread occurs either along natural passages or along planes of least resistance.

In most cases, secondary malignant tumors of the temporal bone present late in the clinical course, although occasionally they may be the initial manifestation. All age groups may be affected. There is no sex predilection. The involvement may be bilateral (39). Secondary disease may be asymptomatic, or the otologic symptoms (hearing loss) may be overshadowed by other lesions. Manifestations might include facial paralysis, otalgia, and periauricular swelling.

The histologic type in hematogenous metastases from distant sites is usually a carcinoma—namely, adenocarcinoma—followed by SCC or, rarely, small-cell carcinoma, malignant lymphoma, melanoma, and sarcoma, which also may disseminate to the temporal bone but are less common (39–43). Secondary malignant tumors originating in adjacent structures include SCC of the pharynx, nasopharyngeal carcinomas, salivary gland tumors [adenoid cystic carcinoma, adenocarcinoma (not otherwise specified), or, rarely, mucoepidermoid carcinoma], and sarcoma of the meninges.

DIAGNOSTIC IMAGING

Diagnostic imaging is critical to planning therapy of malignancies arising in the temporal bone. Computed tomography scanning is normally the first study because the assessment of bone detail is critical to the treatment planned; MRI also is used frequently as a complementary study, to assess cancer spread outside the temporal bone. Especially the infratemporal fossa, cranial nerve, and central nervous system proximate to the temporal bone must be evaluated. The facial nerve and the trigeminal nerve often are affected by temporal bone cancer and provide an avenue for perineural tumor spread intracranially or extracranially (or both). In advanced and deeply infiltrating lesions, CT or MRI may prove adequate for evaluating the status of the sigmoid and transverse venous sinuses and the carotid artery. Conventional angiography is necessary in occasional cases or when a balloon occlusion test of the carotid artery is planned before an anticipated internal carotid artery (ICA) sacrifice during tumor resection. If modern imaging is available, conventional tomography has no role and plain films have little place in the evaluation of these patients. Ultrasonography also plays little or no role in evaluating temporal bone malignancies. Ultrasonography is used occasionally to guide a needle biopsy of a nonpalpable, CT suspicious node; however, it is not used routinely to search for nodal metastases (44).

Radionuclide studies play a limited adjunctive role in the evaluation of patients with cancer affecting the temporal bone. Occasionally, inflammatory disease mimics recurrent cancer. A combination of bone and gallium single photon emission computed tomography (SPECT) can help distinguish between these conditions or follow the progress of a therapeutic trial for infection or tissue necrosis. Also, SPECT or positron emission tomography (PET) may be used with fluorodeoxyglucose (FDG) to help determine whether a mass or signs of recurrent disease are due to a tissue necrosis or recurrent tumor; these studies currently are at the investigational stage of development.

Technique of Examination

The images presented in this chapter are examples of how images should appear. Scans should always be optimized for spatial resolution (i.e., performed with thin slices and a small field of view). Tiny pictures of the anatomic region of interest surrounded by large zones of black are not acceptable for the type of decision making required for treating malignancies of the temporal bone.

For general evaluation of the head and neck region, CT sections should be contiguous and no more than 3 mm thick in the main areas of interest. Contiguous 1- to 2-mm sections are used routinely in the study of the temporal bone and 1-mm thickness is almost always the most appropriate choice. The field of view must be kept as small as possible (e.g., 14 to 16 cm in the neck and 9 to 10 cm in the temporal bone) to ensure the best possible spatial resolution. Image data should be processed at bone and soft tissue algorithms to ensure the best contrast resolution. Images should be photographed and presented in a manner that enhances the conspicuity of any abnormality.

Intravenous contrast is used with CT studies to assess the soft tissue extent of a tumor, the status of the cavernous sinus, and other intracranial spread, and to detect regional metastatic adenopathy. If the study is being done solely for bone detail, intravenous contrast is not necessary.

An MRI should be performed with 3- to 4-mm slice thickness and a field of view from 16 to 18 cm if a 1.0 to 1.5 tesla instrument is being used. Low-field and midfield units may require thicker sections and a larger field of view if imaging time is to be held within acceptable limits; a thicker section or larger field of view limits spatial resolution. An MRI study should always be focused on the precise area of interest. When necessary, a small, localized receiver coil or a phased array set of high-resolution receiver coils may be used. A general type of head MRI protocol is virtually never acceptable for evaluating the local extent of malignant tumors at the skull base.

Intravenous contrast is used with MRI for the same basic reasons as are listed for CT studies. Detection of perineural spread is an additional indication. T1-weighted images *must* be obtained before and after contrast administration, as enhancement can cause lesions to become isointense and, therefore, less visible within fatty marrow or other areas of adjacent fat. Fat saturation techniques may be rendered nondiagnostic owing to field distortion artifacts; however, if used with care and if the pitfalls just mentioned are borne in mind, postcontrast T1-weighted, fat-suppressed images can be used as a substitute for T1-weighted images before and after contrast infusion.

An imaging-directed needle biopsy can be used to sample disease in areas not approachable by other means. Computed tomography usually is used for guidance, although ultrasonography may be used in some cases. An MRI-directed biopsy currently is available at very few institutions.

Limitations of Imaging in Evaluating Tumor Extent

Neither CT nor MRI can distinguish among edema due to the presence of tumor cells scattered in surrounding tissue; tumor emboli in lymphatics; or edema due to peritumoral inflammation, a biopsy, or the like. Areas of swelling must be presumed to be involved with a tumor on imaging studies unless some plausible alternative explanation is available (e.g., a recent biopsy).

A tumor adjacent to bone cannot be distinguished from tumor involving the periosteum. If no cortical erosion or periosteal reaction is visible, the periosteum can likely be taken as a margin; however, this radiographic impression may require intraoperative confirmation. In slower-growing lesions, bone may be thinned to the point of not being visible (dehiscence) and the periosteum may still be intact; these changes of regressive remodeling (i.e., saucerization or "expansion" of bone) usually are associated with smooth rather than irregularly eroded bone at the interface between tumor and bone. In this situation, invasion or adherence to periosteum probably is more likely than in cases in which the bone adjacent to a tumor is completely normal (i.e., not remodeled). Irregular erosion of cortical bone at its interface with a tumor is an unmistakable sign of invasion. Magnetic resonance imaging is better than CT for showing spread of a tumor to the marrow spaces of the skull base and calvarium, but a combination of MRI and CT usually is necessary to understand fully the extent of disease within these bones. However, MRI *cannot* be used under any circumstances to *exclude* bone erosion when tumor lies adjacent to bone.

Tumor invading the skull may displace dura and produce a reactive enhancement. In such cases, the tumor may have invaded or only be adherent to the dura. Irregular dural thickening suggests invasion, and adjacent leptomeningeal or brain invasion confirms transdural spread. In many cases, the surgeon merely is alerted to a probable area of dural involvement, and intraoperative confirmation of suspicious imaging findings is required to ensure the best approach to resection and closure of the area of skull and dural involvement.

Perineural spread is best detected by MRI; however, normal perineural vascular plexus enhancement is present along the exit foramina of the trigeminal nerve, the facial nerve, and within the cavernous sinus. A skilled MRI study interpreter must understand the difference between these normal variants and the signs of perineural tumor spread. An MRI can demonstrate enlargement and enhancement of inflamed nerves that mimic tumoral involvement. Perineural spread *cannot* be excluded on the basis of normal imaging studies because microscopic disease is always a possibility.

Lymph nodes are better evaluated by CT than MRI because metastatic deposits within the nodes can be seen with greater clarity on CT (45). In the absence of such visible metastatic deposits, MRI and CT depend on size criteria for the detection of nodal metastatic disease. Size criteria produce obligatory false-positive (owing to normal size variations and reactive adenopathy) and false-negative (owing to microscopic disease) results. The facial, parotid, and neck nodes are included on the CT studies in most cases of temporal bone malignancies and especially when the primary lesion is a skin cancer. Unfortunately, an MRI study of the neck adds considerable time and cost while offering limited benefit.

Specific Indications for Imaging

DIFFERENTIAL DIAGNOSIS

Lesions of the EAC are normally accessible for a biopsy. A submucosal or subcutaneous mass should be studied with CT or MRI (or both) in almost all cases, before a biopsy is performed. Questionable lesions (e.g., noncholesteatomatous masses) medial to the tympanic membrane are best studied before a biopsy is performed, as this can prevent unnecessary exploration or hemorrhagic complications (e.g., in the case of middle ear extension of a glomus jugulare tumor) or other rare complications (e.g., the inadvertent biopsy of a carotid artery or meningoencephalocele). Occasionally, imaging can help to differentiate among an aggressive infiltrating nonmalignant process (e.g., necrotizing otitis extrema, Langerhans histiocytosis), temporal bone malignancy, or a more generalized malignant tumor such as lymphoma. Imaging might also establish that a "temporal bone tumor" actually is arising elsewhere, such as in the parotid gland or masticator space (e.g., RMS in children) (Fig. 27.1). A prominent spread pattern along the facial or auriculotemporal nerve (and perhaps more proximally to the mandibular nerve) suggests an adenoid cystic carcinoma; however, this pattern can occur in other carcinomas and in benign nerve sheath tumors. Occasionally, slow-growing adenoid cystic carcinoma or adenocarcinoma of the EAC produces a smooth remodeling of adjacent bone. Differentiation of such slow-growing submucosal cancer from a rare adenoma proves difficult on the basis of the imaging findings. A tumor centered along the posterior aspect of the temporal bone in the vicinity of the upper jugular fossa or vestibular aqueduct may be an adenocarcinoma arising from the endolymphatic sac, although some believe the tumor arises from the mastoid air cells in this region.

Metastases to the temporal bone are rare. If a destructive, highly vascular tumor is seen, then a renal cell carcinoma must be considered. Metastases usually are recognized by their highly erosive appearance and atypical site of origin. For instance, sometimes a lesion of the lower clivus is mistaken for a paraganglioma until its center is localized correctly as being outside the jugular fossa. Chordomas and chondrosarcomas have a fairly typical imaging morphology and site of origin, so they should not be mistaken for metastases if good-quality MRI and CT studies are available. When metastases are a reasonable diagnostic concern, a radionuclide bone scan should be performed to look for other sites of skeletal involvement.

LOCAL EXTENT OF THE TUMOR

Computed tomography is used to detect bone erosion (Figs. 27.2 and 27.3). Critical regions of interest for assessing medial tumor spread include the bony and cartilaginous portions of the eustachian tube, the carotid canal, and the carotid artery. Posterior spread involves the jugular fossa and sigmoid plate and sinus. Computed tomography evidence of superior spread to the roof of the mastoid, middle ear, or external canal heralds intracranial invasion, and detailed T1- and T2-weighted coronal MRI studies are mandatory (Figs. 27.4 and 27.5). On MRI with paramagnetic contrast, it may be difficult to distinguish reactive

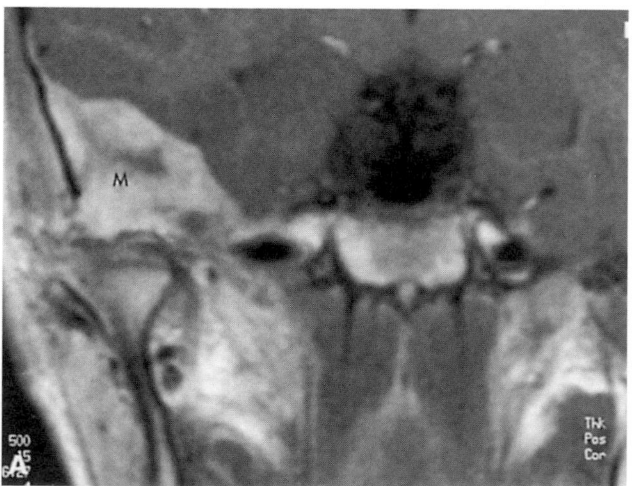

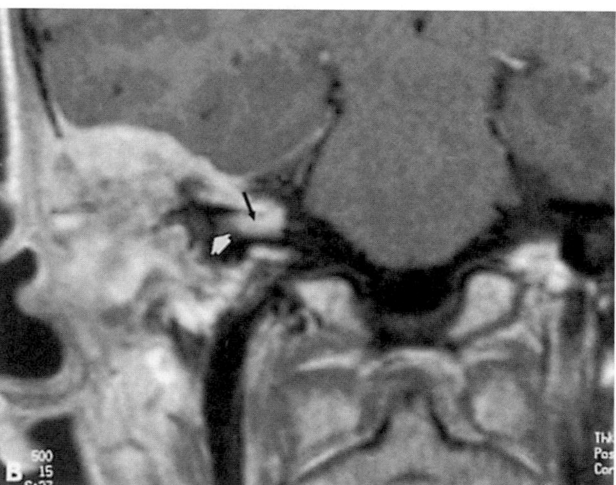

Figure 27.1 A 3-year-old girl presented with a mass in the periauricular region, which subsequently proved to be a temporal bone rhabdomyosarcoma of mastoid origin. **A:** Coronal, T1-weighted, contrast-enhanced magnetic resonance imaging (MRI) shows a partially necrotic mass (*M*) involving the mastoid portion of the temporal bone and extending intracranially, although it remains extradural. This is a good example of bulky parameningeal disease. **B:** Coronal MRI section posterior to that in **A** shows tumor spreading within the internal auditory canal (*black arrow*), probably reaching it through the facial canal. Note the sparing of the bony labyrinth (*white arrow*). This patient is at high risk for central nervous system dissemination because of this spread to the internal auditory canal. (From Million RR, Cassisi NJ, eds. *Management of head and neck cancer: a multidisciplinary approach,* 2nd ed. Philadelphia: Lippincott, 1994:815, with permission.)

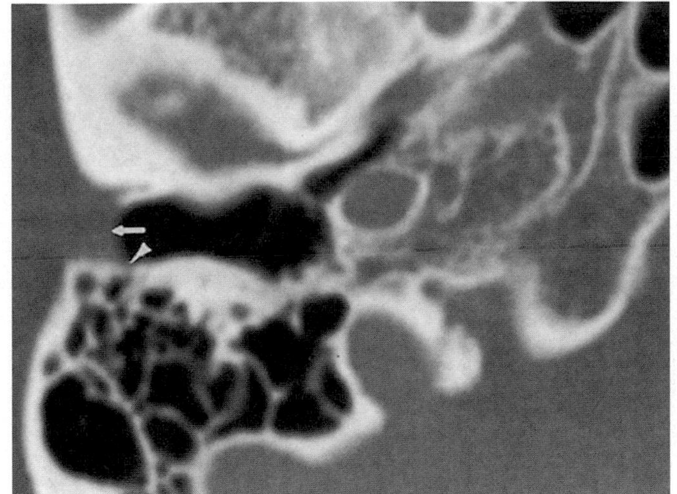

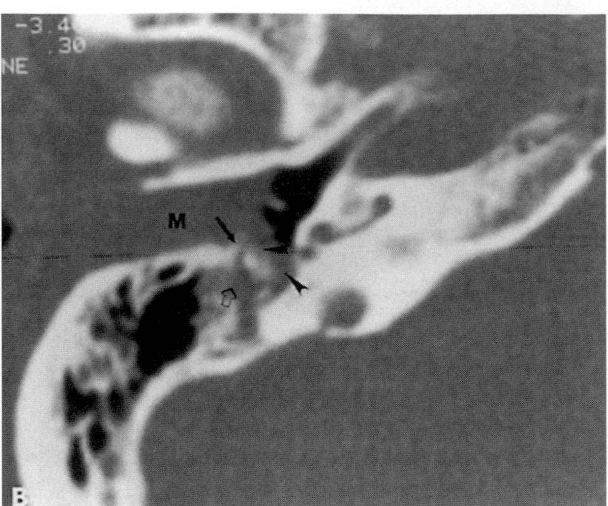

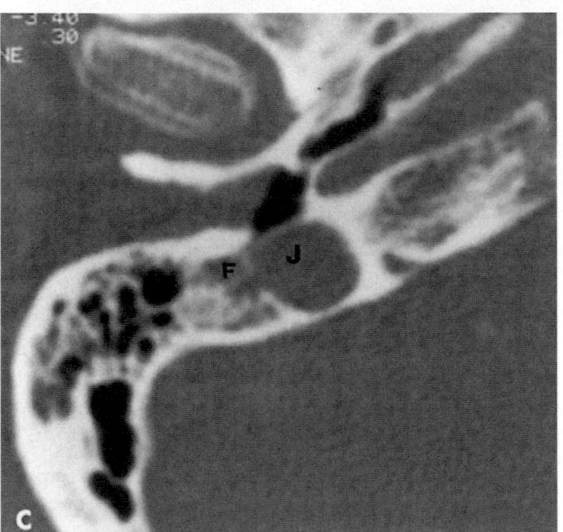

Figure 27.2 Two different patients with masses of the external auditory canal (EAC). Biopsies revealed squamous cell carcinoma. Computed tomography was performed to evaluate the medial extent of tumor and to look for bone destruction. **A:** The first patient's tumor was limited to the junction of the bony and cartilaginous portions of the EAC. Soft tissue filled the canal at its opening (*arrow*). No definite bone erosion is seen; small dehiscences (*arrowhead*) such as that seen here are common, normal anatomic variants and cannot be distinguished from early cortical erosion. **B,C:** The second patient also had a mass in the EAC that totally occluded the external auditory meatus. **B:** The mass (*M*) is seen filling the EAC to the tympanic annulus level. The tumor invades the posterior canal wall (*arrow*), grows into the sinus tympani and lower facial recess (*arrowheads*), and infiltrates the descending facial canal (*open arrow*). **C:** The bone between the enlarged, eroded facial canal (*F*) and the high jugular bulb (*J*) is eroded. (From Million RR, Cassisi NJ, eds. *Management of head and neck cancer: a multidisciplinary approach,* 2nd ed. Philadelphia: Lippincott, 1994:758, with permission.)

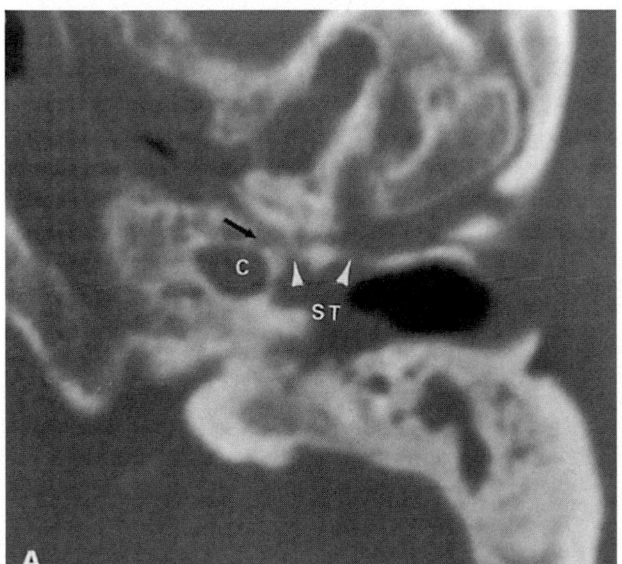

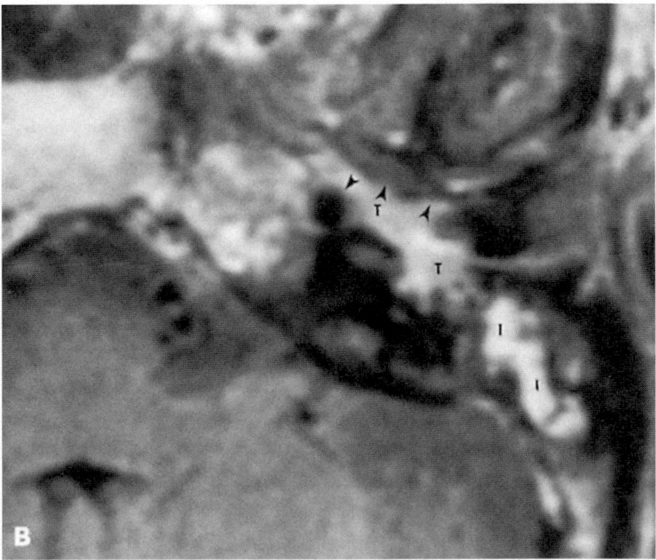

Figure 27.3 A patient with a history of chronic middle ear disease and increasing ear pain. Exploratory tympanotomy and biopsy revealed squamous cell carcinoma of the middle ear. **A:** Axial computed tomographic (CT) scan shows the middle ear filled with soft tissue (*ST*), which is a nonspecific finding. The bone surrounding the middle ear is markedly sclerotic and focally eroded (*arrowheads*); note the focal erosion (*arrow*) between the bony eustachian tube and carotid canal (*C*). **B:** A T1-weighted, contrast-enhanced axial magnetic resonance image at the same level as the CT scan seen in **A**. Tumor (*T*) in the middle ear and mastoid was enhanced less than the inflammatory changes (*I*) in the mastoid. Note the proximity of the tumor to areas of focal bone erosion seen in **A** (*arrowheads*). (From Million RR, Cassisi NJ, eds. *Management of head and neck cancer: a multidisciplinary approach,* 2nd ed. Philadelphia: Lippincott, 1994:759, with permission.)

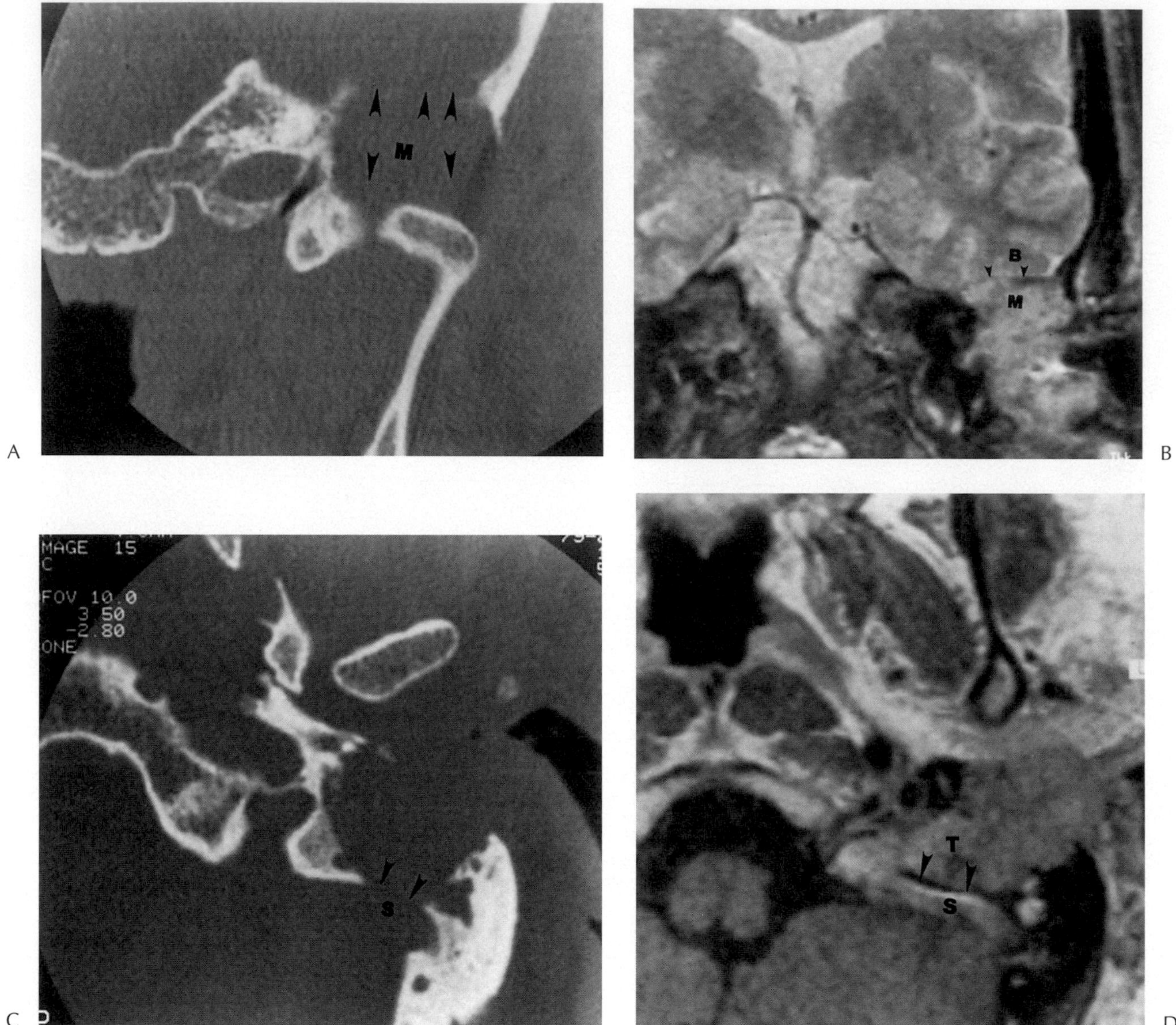

Figure 27.4 A patient with a carcinoma of the external auditory canal (EAC) presenting as a predominantly submucosal mass. **A:** Coronal computed tomographic (CT) section viewed at bone windows shows the mass (*M*) eroding the roof and floor of the EAC (*arrowheads*). **B:** Coronal T2-weighted magnetic resonance image (MRI) at the same position as the CT scan in **A** shows the dura or periosteum (*arrowheads*) continuing to separate the tumor mass (*M*) from the brain **(B)**. **C:** Axial CT scan viewed at bone windows shows the tumor invading the mastoid and eroding the sigmoid plate (*arrowheads*) adjacent to the sigmoid sinus (*S*). **D:** Axial T1-weighted contrast-enhanced MRI at the same level as the CT scan in **C** showing the tumor (*T*) respecting the periosteal-dural margin (*arrowheads*) and not invading the sigmoid sinus (*S*).

dural changes from dural invasion. Any enhancement of dura should be considered as highly suspicious for invasion, and actual confirmation of invasion in subtle cases remains an intraoperative task. Transdural spread to the brain is best confirmed with coronal MRI for the temporal lobes and axial images for the cerebellum.

LOCAL SPREAD PATTERNS OF SKIN CANCER OF THE PINNA AND PERIAURICULAR REGION

Study of the local extent of a tumor almost always begins with CT, because evaluation of the bone is of critical interest. An MRI is added whenever the extent of soft tissue, perineural spread, or intracranial disease is in question after CT scanning in cases of advanced skin cancer.

The deep extent of soft tissue invasion in this location can be difficult to evaluate clinically. Magnetic resonance imaging is particularly good for demonstrating the extent of direct invasion of the masseter, sternocleidomastoid, and posterior belly of the digastric muscles. Spread around the temporomandibular joint (TMJ) capsule and into the deeper masticator or parapharyngeal spaces may be shown by MRI or CT; often both studies are required to evaluate this particularly insidious spread pattern through the petrotympanic fissure and around the periarticular soft tissues of the TMJ (see Figs. 27.3 and 27.4).

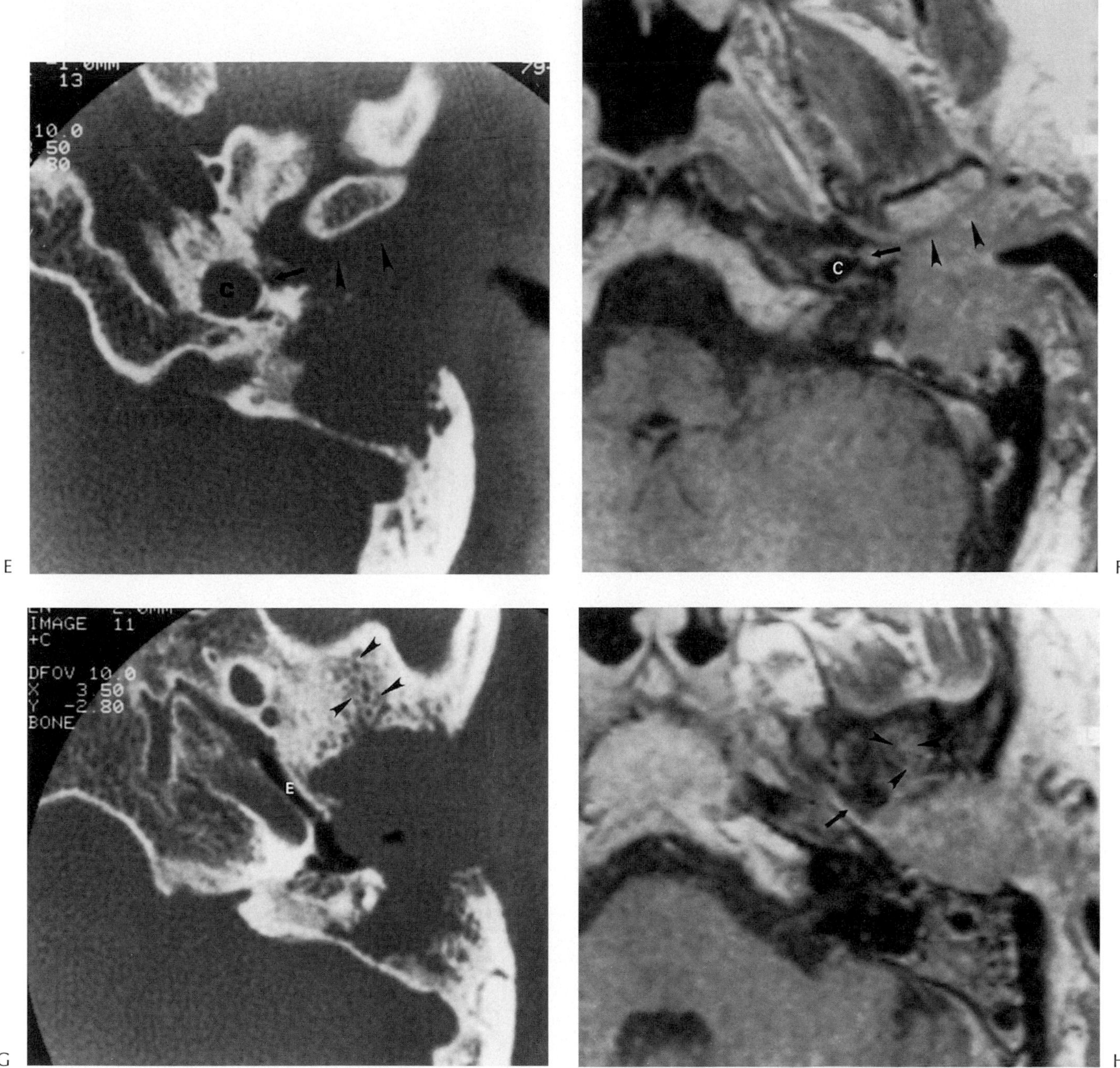

Figure 27.4 ***(continued)*** **E:** Axial CT study viewed for bone detail shows destruction of the anterior wall of the EAC and likely spread to the periarticular tissues of the temporomandibular joint (TMJ; *arrowheads*). Tumor is eroding the bone (*arrow*) adjacent to the carotid canal (*C*). **F:** Axial contrast-enhanced T1-weighted MRI at the same level as the CT scan in **E** confirms tumor in the periarticular tissues of the TMJ and likely invading the joint capsule (*arrowheads*). The tumor in bone (*arrow*) adjacent to the carotid canal (*C*) also is confirmed. **G:** Axial CT scan viewed for bone detail shows tumor infiltrating the marrow space of the zygomatic portion of the temporal bone (*arrowheads*) as well as tumor adjacent to the bony portion of the eustachian tube **E**. **H:** T1-weighted contrast-enhanced MRI at the same position as the CT scan in **G** confirms tumor in the marrow space (*arrowheads*) but cannot distinguish tumor from mucosal thickening in the bony eustachian tube (*arrow*).

Deeply invasive tumors may encase or destroy the zygomatic arch, perhaps by growth along the masseter to its attachment on this bone. The mandible is involved infrequently. It is not unusual for a tumor to grow around the posterior aspect of the TMJ into the uppermost aspect of the poststyloid parapharyngeal space near the point at which the ICA enters the vertical portion of the carotid canal. Before high-resolution sectional imaging, spread to this area could not have been anticipated before surgery. Tumor growing along the temporalis muscle may involve the coronoid process of the mandible.

Tumors of the external ear frequently grow medially to involve the bony-cartilaginous junction of the EAC; early bone invasion here may be difficult to detect without careful com-

A

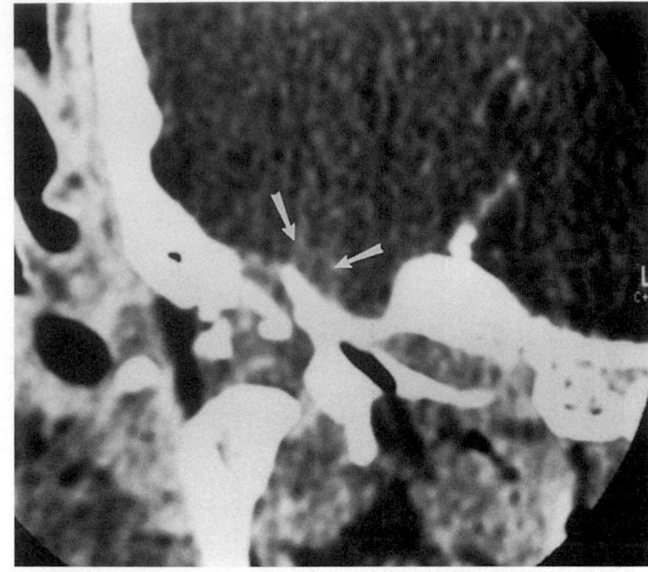

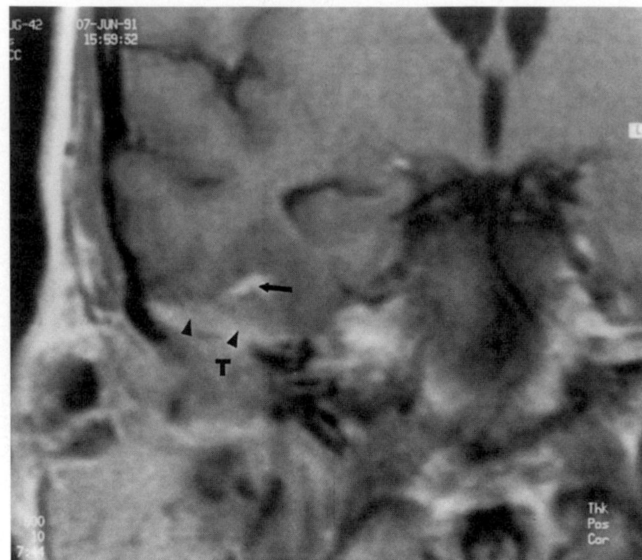

B

C

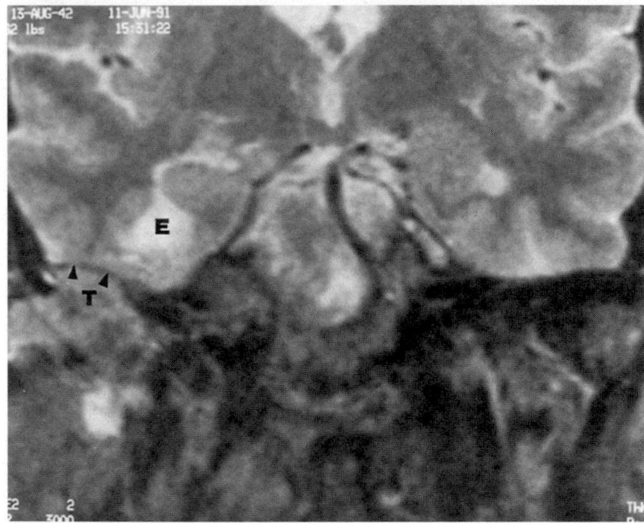

Figure 27.5 A patient with a large, submucosal, poorly differentiated carcinoma of the external auditory canal (EAC). **A:** Contrast-enhanced computed tomographic (CT) scan viewed for brain detail suggests dural and, possibly, brain invasion (*arrows*). **B:** Coronal, contrast-enhanced T1-weighted magnetic resonance image (MRI) at the same position as the CT scan in **A** shows the tumor (*T*) extending transdurally (*arrowheads*) to invade the brain (*arrow*). **C:** T2-weighted MRI matching the MRI seen in **B** shows that although the periosteal–dural interface remains partially intact (*arrowhead*), the inferior temporal lobe is edematous (*E*) and clearly invaded by tumor (*T*). The route of tumor spread could be through leptomeningeal or venous routes.

parison to the opposite side, as the bone at the junction is normally slightly irregular in appearance (Fig. 27.2). Tumors that grow adjacent to the calvarium or mastoid may invade these structures directly. Tumors growing along the posterior belly of the digastric or sternocleidomastoid muscle may invade the skull at the digastric groove and mastoid tip or adjacent skull base. Continued medial growth from areas of mastoid bone involvement may take the tumor margin as far medially as the petrous apex. The favored pathways for spread to the petrous apex are along existing mastoid air cell tracts and along the tympanic bone to the petrotympanic fissure and on to the carotid canal and bony eustachian tube. Spread through the mastoid and petrous bone may lead to invasion of the transverse, sigmoid, and petrosal sinuses.

The predominant nerve at risk is the facial nerve. Proximal spread along the facial nerve can lead to involvement of the geniculate ganglion and greater superficial petrosal nerve. Spread into the inner ear and along cranial nerve VIII may occur in very advanced lesions (Fig. 27.1). The auriculotemporal nerve may be involved in lesions that spread to the facial nerve, upper parotid gland, and perimandibular region. Spread from the auriculotemporal nerve to the mandibular division of the trigeminal nerve or middle meningeal artery can lead to involvement of the skull base at the foramen ovale or spinosum, respectively. Proximal spread along this pathway can lead to cavernous involvement. Spread along any of these cranial nerves (V, VII, or VIII) can lead eventually to brainstem invasion or leptomeningeal spread of tumor.

STAGING OF TEMPORAL BONE CANCERS

There is no uniformly accepted stating system for temporal bone cancers. The structure proposed by the University of Pittsburgh temporal bone cancer staging system has proven to be useful to the authors, and studies indicate that it correlates well with surgical findings. The system closely correlates with patient outcome and is more sensitive than preoperative radiographic staging alone. This staging system is presented in Table 27.2.

TABLE 27.2 University of Pittsburgh Staging System for Squamous Cell Carcinoma of the Temporal Bone

T status
- T1: Tumor limited to the external auditory canal without bony erosion or evidence of soft tissue extension
- T2: Tumor with limited external auditory canal bony erosion (not full thickness) or radiographic finding consistent with limited (<0.5 cm) soft tissue involvement
- T3: Tumor eroding the osseous external auditory canal (full thickness) with limited (<0.5 cm) soft tissue involvement, or tumor involving middle ear and/or mastoid, or patients presenting with facial paralysis
- T4: Tumor eroding the cochlea, petrous apex, medial wall of the middle ear, carotid canal, jugular foramen or dura, or with extensive (>0.5 cm) soft tissue involvement

N status
- Lymph node involvement is a poor prognostic sign and places the patient in an advanced stage, i.e., T1N1 (stage III) and T2, T3, T4, N1 (stage IV)

M status
- M1 disease is stage IV and is considered a very poor prognostic sign

Source: Arriaga M, Curtin H, Takahashi H, et al. Staging proposal for external auditory meatus carcinoma based on preoperative clinical examination and computed tomography findings. *Ann Otol Rhinol Laryngol* 1990;99:714–721, with permission.

EVALUATION OF THE CAROTID ARTERY AND DURAL VENOUS SINUSES

The proximity of tumor to the carotid artery and dural venous sinuses or their invasion by tumor is determined best by a combination of CT and MRI (Figs. 27.3 and 27.4). Magnetic resonance angiography (MRA), static MRI, and contrast-enhanced CT can determine the dominance and patency of major dural sinuses; angiography is usually not necessary for this purpose if the imaging studies are performed with care and the most current techniques. Tumor and thrombus in a major dural venous sinus may be indistinguishable. The jugular vein or a major dural sinus may appear to be completely occluded when it is merely compressed; conventional angiography can be used in the occasional circumstance when differentiation of these two conditions is mandatory for surgical planning. Slow flow in a major vascular structure can be mistaken for complete occlusion even on the best MRA study.

Carotid arteriography with test balloon occlusion may be necessary if carotid sacrifice is anticipated. The artery can then be occluded before surgery with endovascular techniques, if desired. Imaging with CT and MRI determines the proximity of tumor to the carotid artery. Carotid arteriography does not normally provide any additional information about the likelihood of carotid (encasement versus adhesion) involvement with the tumor. Several things should be remembered when carotid angiography is considered. The procedure of performing angiography carries with it an intrinsic risk for complication. Because angiography is only useful in determining cerebrovascular sufficiency via temporary balloon occlusion of the ICA, it should be done only if resection and replacement of the vessel is contemplated. Angiography is not superior to standard imaging (MRI and CT) in visualizing the cerebral vascular supply and venous drainage, and should not be used when noninvasive scanning techniques provide adequate information on the status of these important structures. If carotid replacement is considered, several additional facts should be considered. There is at least a 2% risk for complication from test balloon occlusion, such as femoral hematoma, dissection of the ICA, or transient or permanent stroke. As a result, this test should not be obtained without clear indications. Even if test balloon occlusion indicates adequate cerebral sufficiency, the risk for permanent neurologic deficit following either carotid ligation or replacement is at lease 7%. The complexity added to a temporal bone resection by carotid resection and replacement is substantial, and should only be undertaken by a surgical team highly experienced in this type of procedure.

DETECTION OF RECURRENT DISEASE

Recurrent malignancy of the temporal bone frequently extends much deeper than can be appreciated on physical examination. Whenever the physical examination is inconclusive, MRI or CT (or both) should be performed. In this setting, the rate of detection of bone invasion as well as clinically occult perineural spread and adenopathy will increase as compared with that in an untreated case. If salvage therapy is an option after an initial attempt at cure, one should consider obtaining a baseline imaging study approximately 3 to 4 months after the completion of therapy. The baseline study helps in differentiating early signs of recurrence from posttreatment alterations of the local anatomy. Radionuclide tumor imaging agents may also be used for detecting or confirming recurrence; thallium and FDG are currently being investigated with regard to their accuracy in detecting recurrence. Preliminary data suggest that a negative radionuclide study excludes tumor with a high degree of confidence, but a positive study may be due to tumor, reactive changes, or superimposed infection.

The facial lymph nodes probably are less familiar to surgical and radiation oncologists than are nodes in other head and neck locations. The position of the facial nodes, their relationship to the parotid nodes, and examples of metastatic disease are reported elsewhere (46). Facial nodes can be the source of palpable subcutaneous recurrent disease or occult metastatic disease. Cancer, especially carcinomas of the pinna and periauricular region, also may involve periauricular, retromastoid, and occipital nodes, which are infrequent sites of nodal metastases in noncutaneous head and neck malignancies; these nodes should be included on CT or MRI studies whenever the primary site places them at risk.

OPERATIVE TECHNIQUE

Historical Perspectives

In 1954, Parsons and Lewis (47) pioneered *en bloc* TBR for tumors. In 1975, Lewis (48) reviewed 100 cases of limited *en bloc* petrous bone resection for cancer. He reported a 5% perioperative mortality and a 27% 5-year cure rate. Subsequent clinical series were reported by Conley and Schuller (49), Lewis (50), Ariyan (51), Graham et al. (52), and Schramm (53).

Anesthesia, Monitoring, and Position

General endotracheal anesthesia aims to achieve brain relaxation and to allow monitoring of cranial nerves. A lumbar subarachnoid drain and sequential compression stockings are used. The potential for extensive blood loss must be considered. Neurophysiologic monitoring may include an electroencephalogram, somatosensory evoked responses, and brainstem evoked responses from the contralateral ear. Cranial nerve monitoring is used when preservation of the cranial nerves is a goal. The patient is placed in a supine position on a Mayfield headrest, with the head rotated 60 degrees contralaterally. Sur-

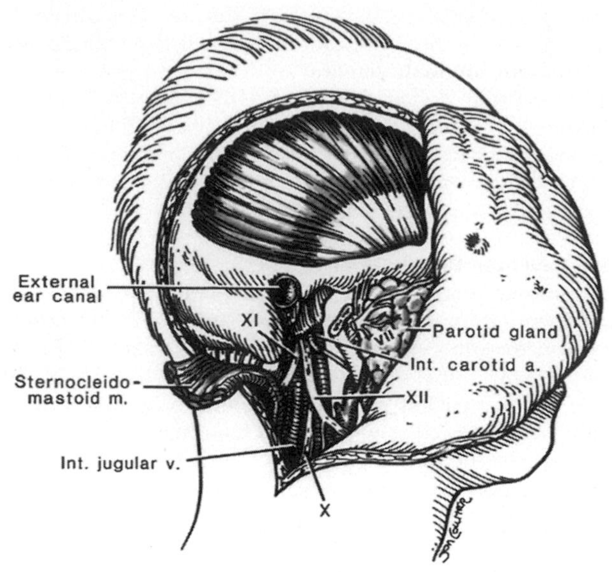

Figure 27.6 Wide exposure of temporal bone and surrounding structures before temporal bone resection. The extracranial facial nerve and the temporomandibular joint have been transected; lower cranial nerves have been exposed in the neck. *Int.*, internal; *m.*, muscle; *v.*, vein.

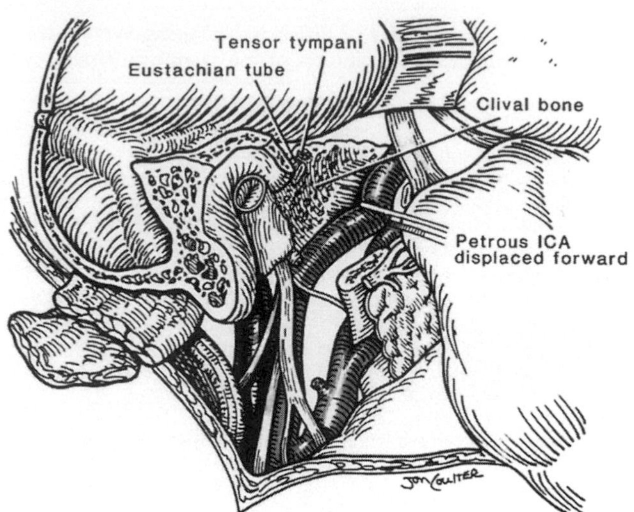

Figure 27.8 The petrous internal carotid artery (*ICA*) has been mobilized anteriorly.

gical exposure is related to the planned extent of surgical resection, based on preoperative imaging studies of the tumor perimeter. The goals include tumor-free excisional margins and preservation or reconstruction of uninvolved critical anatomic structures. Surgical safety and facilitation of the best possible postoperative quality of life are emphasized.

Temporal Bone Resection

A C-shaped retroauricular incision is made, and the external ear canal is transected and sutured. The skin flap is reflected forward. When the external ear is involved with tumor, modification of exposure incisions focuses on surgical tumor margins and viability of elevated soft tissue. Among the options is basing the external ear on a superior or posterior scalp pedicle. The ICA, jugular vein, and regional cranial nerves are isolated in the neck. The extracranial facial nerve is exposed also. An appropriate regional lymph node group, if involved, is dissected (neck, parotid gland, etc.). The temporalis muscle is elevated and reflected anteroinferiorly. A zygomatic osteotomy is performed. The TMJ is opened, and the ipsilateral condyle and neck of the mandible are excised (Fig. 27.6). A temporo-occipital craniotomy is performed (Fig. 27.7). Then an extradural middle-fossa dissection is performed, and the petrous ICA is unroofed, allowing anterior mobilization (Fig. 27.8). The anterior end of the transected eustachian tube is sutured shut to prevent cerebrospinal

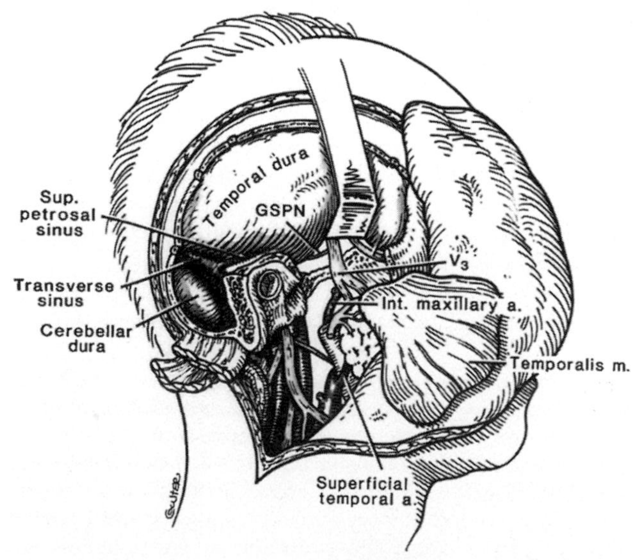

Figure 27.7 Temporal and suboccipital craniotomies with zygomatic osteotomies have been performed. The trigeminal nerve ($V_{2,3}$) has been exposed. GSPN, greater petrosal superficial nerve; *Int.*, interior; *m.*, muscle; *sup.*, superior.

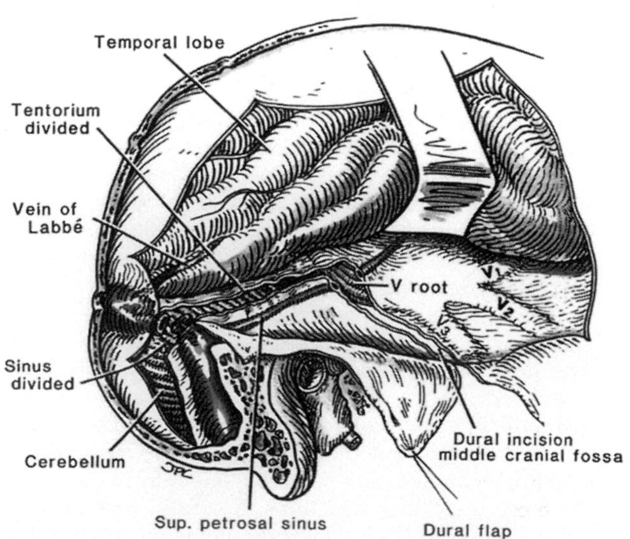

Figure 27.9 The temporal and the retrosigmoid dura and the tentorium have been opened. The lateral sinus has been ligated distally to the vein of Labbé. *Sup.*, superior.

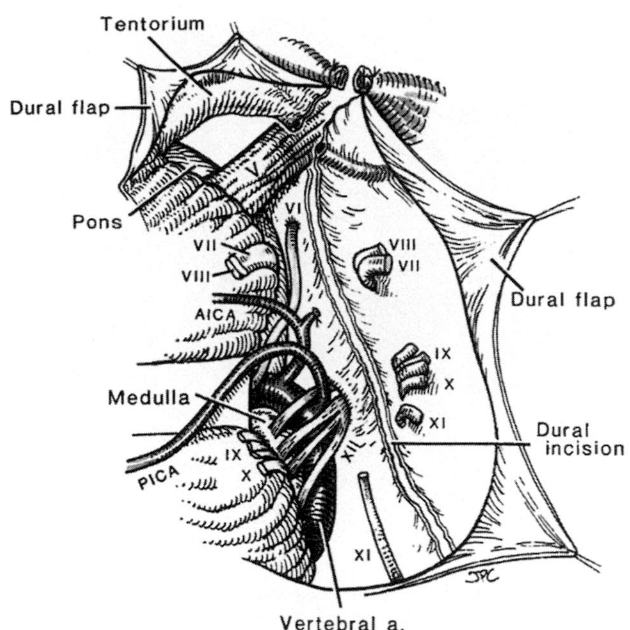

Figure 27.10 Cranial nerves VI through XI have been transected, and the posterior dura (medial face of the temporal bone) is incised. *PICA*, posterior inferior cerebellar artery.

fluid (CSF) leakage. The transverse or sigmoid sinus and the internal jugular vein are ligated only if they are nondominant and communicate with the other side (assessed from preoperative studies) (Fig. 27.9). An intraoperative test occlusion using a temporary clip can be performed. Brain is observed for possible secondary swelling. After anterior displacement of the petrous ICA, the petroclival bone is drilled away to disconnect the temporal bone medially. The dura around the temporal bone is transected, as are the cranial nerves and petrosal sinuses. *En bloc* tumor resection includes the seventh and eighth cranial nerves and the lower cranial nerves (Fig. 27.10). The petrous bone is disconnected from the occipital bone and the clivus by use of a drill or rongeur. Venous bleeding from the basilar and petrosal sinuses may be profuse and require packing with oxidized cellulose. Progressively greater degrees of temporal bone resection are presented in Figure 27.11. The degree of temporal bone resection is determined by the tumor extent.

Neurovascular Reconstruction

Petrous ICA reconstruction may be performed with a saphenous vein interposition graft. The seventh, ninth, eleventh, and twelfth cranial nerves also can be reconstructed using nerve grafts (Fig. 27.12). A hypoglossal-facial nerve neurorrhaphy usually is not performed because loss of 12th cranial nerve function would worsen the condition of the swallowing mechanism, which is already affected by the loss of the ninth and tenth cranial nerves. The dural defect is reconstructed with autologous pericranium or fascia lata. Achievement of water-

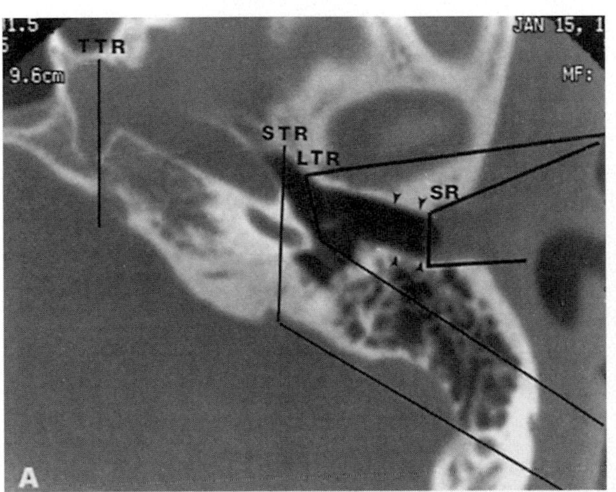

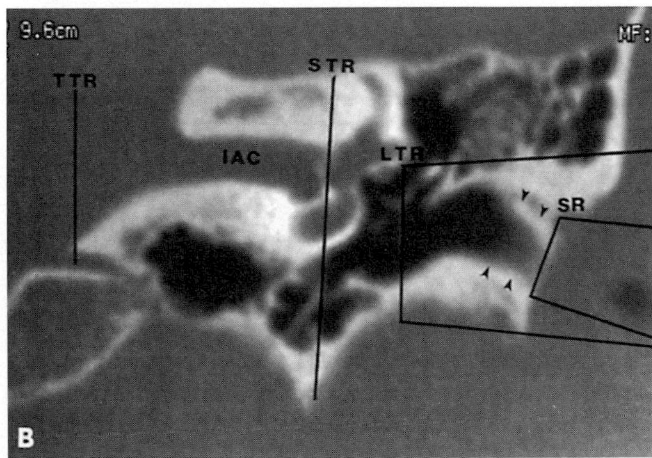

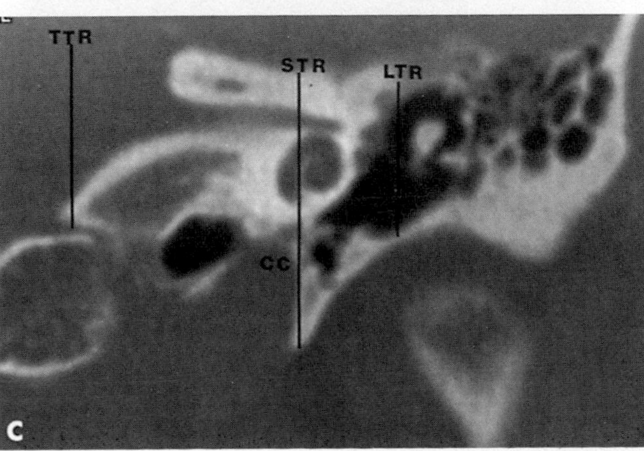

Figure 27.11 Three sections from a temporal bone computed tomographic (CT) scan marked to show the basic limits of various temporal bone resections. *Black lines* represent the medial limits of each procedure including (from lateral to medial): sleeve resection (*SR*), lateral temporal bone resection (*LTR*), subtotal temporal bone resection (*STR*), and total temporal bone resection (*TTR*). **A:** Axial CT scan through the external auditory canal, hypotympanum, basal turn of cochlea, and horizontal carotid canal. *Arrowheads* show optional medial extension of sleeve resection to include part of the bony external ear canal. **B:** Coronal CT scan through the external ear canal and internal auditory canal (*IAC*). *Arrowheads* show optional medial extension of sleeve resection to include part of the bony external ear canal. **C:** Coronal CT scan obtained more anterior than that in **B** to show medial margins of resection relative to the carotid canal (*CC*) and petrous apex. (From Million RR, Cassisi NJ, eds. *Management of head and neck cancer: a multidisciplinary approach,* 2nd ed. Philadelphia: JB Lippincott, 1994:759, with permission.)

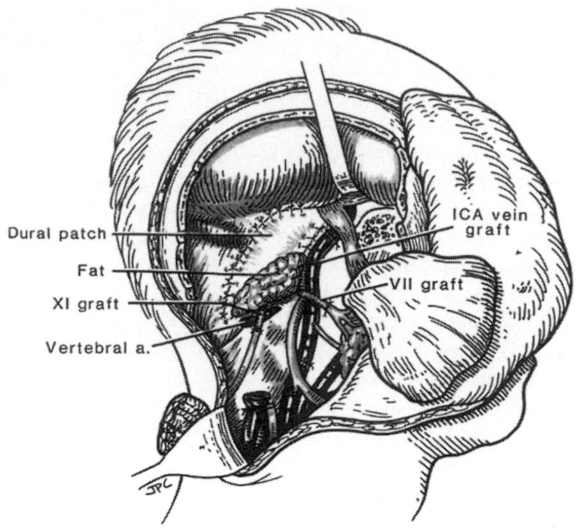

Figure 27.12 Reconstruction of the petrous internal carotid artery (*ICA*) with a saphenous vein graft. Facial nerve and accessory nerve grafts are completed. *a.*, artery.

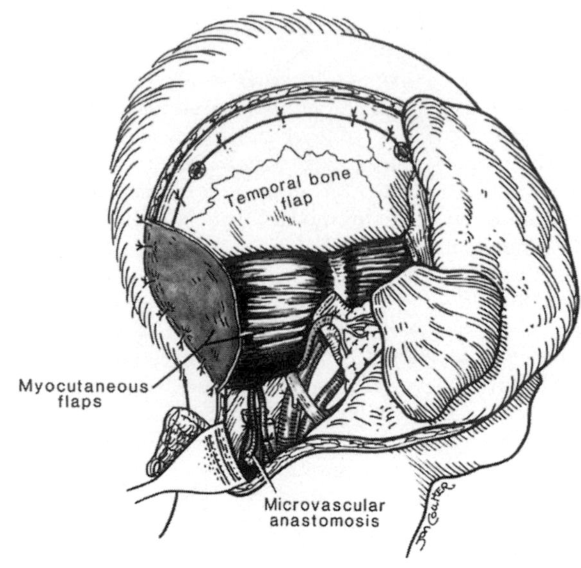

Figure 27.14 Surgical defect is filled with a transferred microvascular rectus abdominis myocutaneous flap anastomosed to the external carotid system.

tight closure is difficult. The temporalis muscle, if usable, can be rotated posteriorly and sutured to the periphery of the surgical defect, providing the initial layer of soft tissue reconstruction (Fig. 27.13). If temporalis muscle is not available, a microvascular flap is used (Fig. 27.14). A closed-system drain is left under the skin flap for 2 to 4 days as a gravity-activated drain (Fig. 27.15).

Auxiliary Operations

Because of the deficits of the seventh, ninth, and tenth cranial nerves, a tarsorrhaphy, tracheostomy, and gastrostomy may be performed at the time of or subsequent to the TBR. Vocal cord augmentation may also be needed at a later time to facilitate swallowing. In our own cases, 10 of the 20 patients had temporary tracheostomies, 8 received vocal cord augmentation, and 8 underwent temporary gastrostomies (3). Twelve had tarsorrhaphies, one a cricopharyngeal myotomy, and one a ventriculoperitoneal shunt placement.

Partial Temporal Bone Resections

Temporal bone resection can be scaled down from the extent of total extirpation. This is done on the basis of limited tumor extent and may vary from canal resection to lateral and subtotal TBR. The most medial extent of resection is the tympanic membrane for the former and the middle ear promontory for the latter. In both procedures, the facial nerve as well as the lower cranial nerves are preserved. The defect usually is reconstructed with rotation of the temporalis muscle.

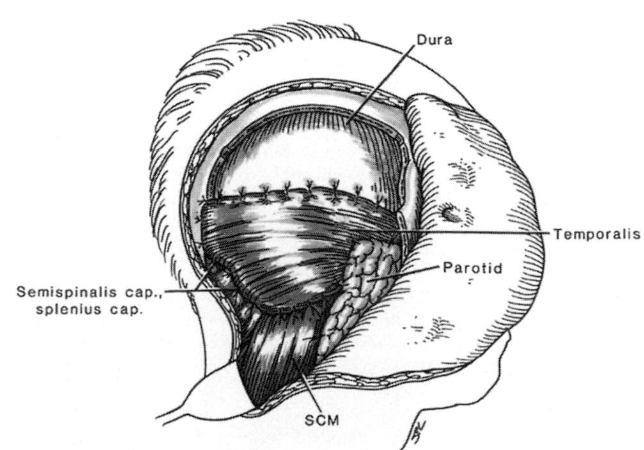

Figure 27.13 Temporalis muscle is rotated over the defect. *cap.*, capitis; *SCM*, sternocleidomastoid muscle.

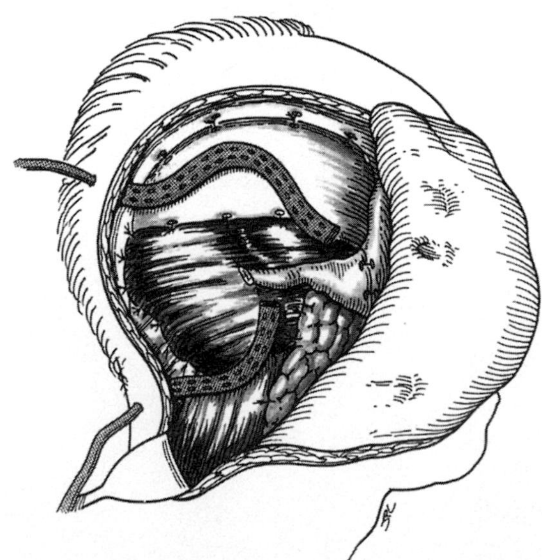

Figure 27.15 Replacement of zygoma over transferred muscle flap and placement of suction drains.

POSTOPERATIVE CARE

After surgery, the patient is observed in an intensive care unit until both the neurologic and pulmonary status are stable. Lumbar CSF drainage via a spinal drain [intermittent (e.g., 50 mL every 8 hours)] is required. Sequential compression stockings are used until the patient is fully ambulatory to lessen the chances for deep vein thrombosis. Tracheostomy care is provided. When gastrostomy has been performed, its removal requires the demonstration, by a modified barium swallow, of adequate swallowing without aspiration. Vocal cord mobilization assists better swallowing and speech. Recovery of facial nerve function to grade III or IV (54) is expected to occur 12 to 18 months after nerve graft reconstruction.

A CT scan usually is obtained on the day after surgery (to look for intracranial air, blood, etc.) or as indicated by the patient's clinical status. Angiographic studies are carried out if the ICA was repaired or grafted or if possible intraoperative damage to the vessel is suspected. After the patient's discharge, clinical follow-up examinations are accompanied by CT or MRI studies at 3 months (a baseline study) and then at 6 to 12 months, to look for possible tumor recurrence.

Adjuvant Treatment

Adjuvant treatment might include intraoperative brachytherapy (afterloading), external-beam RT, radiosurgery, or chemotherapy. Over the past decade stereotactic radiosurgery as a method of treating skull base tumors has gain acceptance and is now much more commonly available. Temporal bone cancers certainly fall into the category of lesions that could benefit from radiosurgery following tumor resection. This modality of treatment substantially limits the need for brachytherapy as a means of delivering high-dose radiation to the skull base while sparing important nearby structures and the skin. The oldest and most accurate form of radiosurgery is delivered by gamma knife systems. With this form of radiosurgery the patient's head is placed in a fixed frame, which then guides targeted beams of gamma radiation that emanate from a helmet-like cobalt source into which the patient's head is placed. This form of stereotactic radiation is very accurate, but limited in that it cannot treat lesions that extend any significant distance below the skull base. In contrast, newer forms of stereotactic radiosurgery utilize beams of gamma energy originating from a Linac machine that are targeted on the tumor site by computer, much as a tomography would visualize a specific site in the body. As a result, they are much more flexible in treating other areas of the body, beyond the brain and skull base. Cervical structures can be radiated, and this radiation can be combined with standard external beam sources of radiotherapy. Though not as accurate as gamma knife, Linac-based systems are much less expensive and have expanded the use of radiosurgery to more types of lesions in an expanded population of patients. The utility of radiosurgery in achieving high dosage levels to skull base sites cannot be overstated. Virtually all patients with malignancies that involve the skull base and temporal bone should be considered for radiosurgery, subject to the details of their unique clinical situation (55).

Complications

A TBR is a major invasive procedure. Critical neurovascular structures are manipulated, and some may even require resection (portion of a brain, cranial nerves, ICA, sigmoid and petrosal sinuses, jugular vein, labyrinth). Blood loss may be significant. This produces an immediate intraoperative challenge to a patient's homeostasis (brain edema, coagulopathy, schemia, etc.). After surgery, the challenge continues with additional requirements for a patient's spontaneous respiration, deglutition, vocalization, ambulation, social contact, and so forth. Preservation of key uninvolved anatomic structures (aided by intraoperative monitoring) or immediate reconstruction assists the patient in overall rehabilitation.

In our series of 20 patients (3), we encountered no perioperative deaths. Intraoperatively, one 65-year-old patient had transient profound brachycardia and hypotension, which may have occurred due to trigeminal nerve stimulation. This patient made a slow postoperative recovery. One patient developed an intraoperative coagulopathy. After surgery, two patients developed a flap hematoma that necessitated evacuation. One pseudomeningocele spontaneously subsided. One patient developed sepsis, five developed pneumonia, and one had a urinary tract infection. Two patients had inappropriate antidiuretic hormone secretion with prolonged hyponatremia. Three patients had dysphagia and confusion that resolved within 5 weeks (one following resection of the vein of Labbé of the dominant hemisphere). Three patients had a single seizure, despite appropriate anticonvulsive prophylaxis. One patient experienced massive pulmonary emboli 2 days after surgery and required resuscitation, and another had minor myocardial schemia. One patient had hepatitis, and one had prolonged TMJ pain.

RECONSTRUCTION OF THE LATERAL SKULL BASE

Tumor resection of the lateral skull base often includes scalp, auricle, adjacent parotid gland, and the facial nerve. The underlying temporal bone, middle and inner ears, ascending ramus of the mandible, and TMJ may be resected as well. More invasive tumors extending to the middle and posterior cranial base may involve bone, dura, cranial nerves as they exit the skull, the ICA, and the internal jugular vein. Such resections may expose the underlying brain. More extensive tumors may extend anteriorly to involve the zygoma, maxilla, maxillary antrum, and pharynx, thereby exposing the skull base and brain additionally to the aerodigestive tract. Preoperative imaging provides preliminary information about the type of defect resulting from radical resection. However, the actual extent of the defect, especially in the soft tissues, often is not known until frozen sections of the margins have been analyzed and tumor excision has been completed.

Planning

Once the resection has been completed, a careful appraisal must be made of the defect, its surrounding tissues, and the requirements for reconstruction. Dural defects are considered first. The neurosurgeon often uses a fascia lata graft to obtain a watertight closure. Once the dura is reconstructed, attention can be directed toward the remainder of the defect. Here, careful planning is required. An assessment is made of both the area of skin needed to resurface the cutaneous defect and the volume of tissue required to fill the potential dead space and restore the contour. The viability of surrounding tissues, the scars, and the presence of radiation damage must be appreciated. The missing bone generally is not replaced; the soft tissue deficit is reconstructed with soft tissue. With more extensive defects, the need to separate the sinuses and aerodigestive tract from the cranial base necessitates the use of flaps with separate cutaneous paddles (56–61).

The continuity and functional potential of the facial nerve must be assessed. A segmental defect of the nerve, with an adequate nerve stump and peripheral plexus, may simply be grafted. More extensive lesions growing into the substance of the cheek may be reconstructed using a functional muscle transfer. Ancillary procedures to address lagophthalmos, including a lateral canthopexy or static facial sling, may be appropriate at this time. The insertion of gold weights into the upper eyelid typically is performed during a secondary operation.

Attention then is directed toward the actual wound closure. Several types of flaps are available to the reconstructive surgeon challenged with complex temporal bone defects. The best flap will depend on the exact location and size of the defect, the volume of tissue required, and any special functional needs for the reconstruction. Local and regional flaps are used for smaller defects, whereas free-tissue transfers are employed for larger, deeper, and more complex reconstruction.

Local and Regional Flaps

Several local and regional flaps are available to reconstruct lateral skull-base defects. However, some areas may not be candidates for tissue transfer because of previous irradiation or scarring from previous operations. For instance, the temporalis muscle and temporoparietal fascial flaps, which commonly are used in reconstruction of the anterolateral skull base, may be compromised during resection of a lateral skull-based tumor (53,62). Compromise of the temporalis muscle flap, a very useful local pedicled muscle flap in the reconstruction of temporal bone defects, occurs if the blood supply to this muscle is involved by tumor in the preauricular region or infratemporal fossa. This muscle is supplied by the deep temporal artery, which emanates from the internal maxillary system. It therefore can be compromised by involvement of the deep temporal artery, which runs deep to the neck of the mandible, or due to loss of the external carotid system from disease or surgery involving the ipsilateral neck. If the glenoid fossa and head/neck of the mandible are involved by tumor spread, it is very likely that the temporalis flap will not be useful. From a practical standpoint, this muscle flap should be elevated as if it could be used for reconstruction, and the pedicle may prove to be involved as the operation progresses. If involved, the muscle should then be amputated and another form of reconstruction should be employed. This situation requires that alternate forms of reconstruction should be anticipated before surgery and incorporated in the patient's operative preparation.

In contrast to the temporalis muscle flap, the temporoparietal fascial flap is rarely compromised by either temporal bone cancers or by the ablative surgery itself. The value of this flap in preventing CSF fistula cannot be overstated, and it has been largely unreported for this application in the treatment of temporal bone malignancies. The blood supply for this flap is the superficial temporal artery, which emanates from the external carotid system. As a result, it is usually spared from tumor spread to the infratemporal fossa. This flap should be used in conjunction with other reconstructive tissues, as it does not contain the bulk necessary to fully fill the void resulting from large resection. It is, though, very useful in covering exposed dura to prevent a CSF leak.

In addition to the temporalis muscle flap and the temporoparietal fascial flap, scalp flaps, cervical flaps, or deltopectoral flaps (63–68) can also be employed. However, these flaps do not have sufficient bulk to fill deeper wounds, where restoration of the contour and obliteration of potential dead space is required. For small, deeper defects, especially in the lower temporal area, the sternomastoid musculocutaneous flap is a good candidate (68–72). The size and reach of the flap are limited by its segmental blood supply; only the upper half of the muscle and its overlying skin can be safely used when the flap is based superiorly (Fig. 27.16).

The pectoralis major (73–76) and the trapezius myocutaneous (77–80) pedicled flaps have been used widely because they provide more tissue to reconstruct larger defects. The pectoralis major musculocutaneous flap, based on the thoracoacromial vessels, is rotated at the midclavicular level. Though this flap provides excellent coverage of the neck, the tissues used to reconstruct the actual temporal defect tend to be in the randomly vascularized, distal portion of the flap. Here, tissue viability is less reliable, and the muscle itself lacks the bulk with which to fill a complex defect. The resulting donor defect on the anterior chest wall can be especially deforming in women.

The trapezius musculocutaneous flap can be oriented either laterally or vertically to close temporal defects. Based on the descending deep branch of the transverse cervical artery, this flap pivots in the posterior triangle of the neck and therefore is able to reach more superiorly in the temporal region. Paravertebral skin forms the cutaneous portion of the flap. Unfortunately, harvesting of the flap necessitates a repositioning of the patient intraoperatively. The donor defect for this may be acceptable if a small flap is taken. However, if a large flap is harvested, the donor site must be skin-grafted, which produces a significant deformity with possible delayed healing of the skin graft. It is possible to raise this flap and maintain the innervation to the anterolateral portion of the trapezius muscle, thereby maintaining its function of shoulder elevation (Fig. 27.17).

Free-Tissue Transfer

COVERAGE AND VOLUME REPLACEMENT

Larger, deeper, and more complex defects, especially in the upper temporal region, are best closed with a free-tissue transfer. Free-tissue transfer has developed into the most reliable form of reconstruction because the best-perfused portion of the flap can be tailored to fill the most difficult portion of the reconstruction (81–91). Most authors report a greater than 96% success rate and a lower complication rate than with pedicled flaps (86).

Because of the plethora of available flaps, reconstructive surgeons now can tailor the flap to meet their reconstructive requirements. For large shallow defects, a fasciocutaneous flap from either the scapular or parascapular area may be a satisfactory solution. However, harvesting tissues from the back requires repositioning the patient once extirpative surgery has been completed. If the patient cannot be repositioned intraoperatively, then a fasciocutaneous or musculocutaneous flap may instead be harvested from the anterolateral thigh. Based on the descending branch of the lateral femoral circumflex vessels, the anterolateral thigh flap (91) has a long vascular pedicle that can easily reach recipient vessels in the neck (Fig. 27.18).

Fasciocutaneous flaps can also come from the volar forearm and lateral arm. Because they are thinner than anterolateral thigh flaps, these forearm and arm flaps have typically been used for intraoral lining and reconstruction of the central third of the face. Smaller, more superficial temporal defects also are good recipient sites for these flaps.

Larger, deeper, and more complex defects having a large potential dead space are best reconstructed with musculocutaneous flaps. The rectus abdominis musculocutaneous flap is the most commonly used of these tissues. This flap is popular

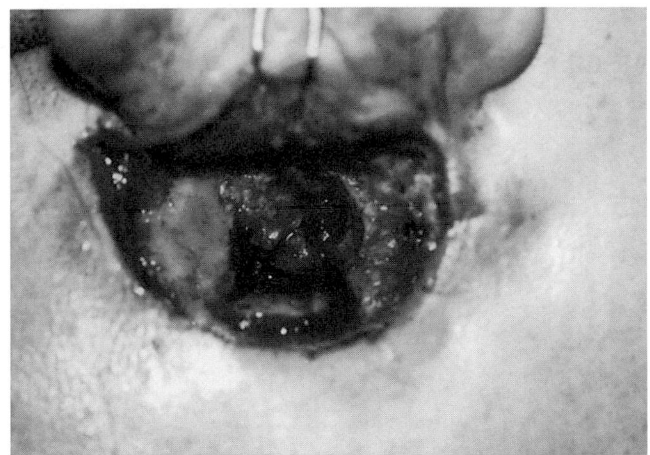
A

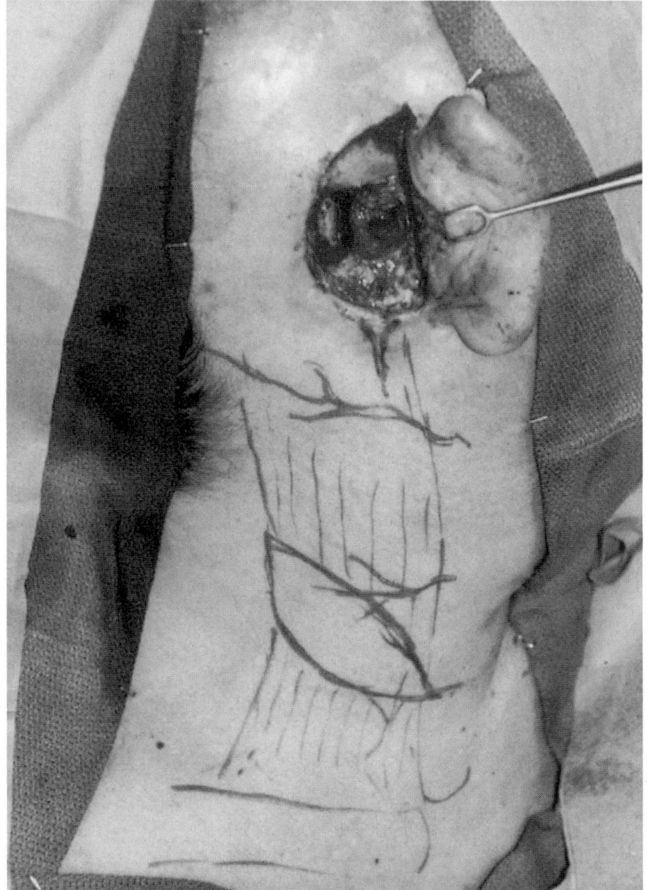
B

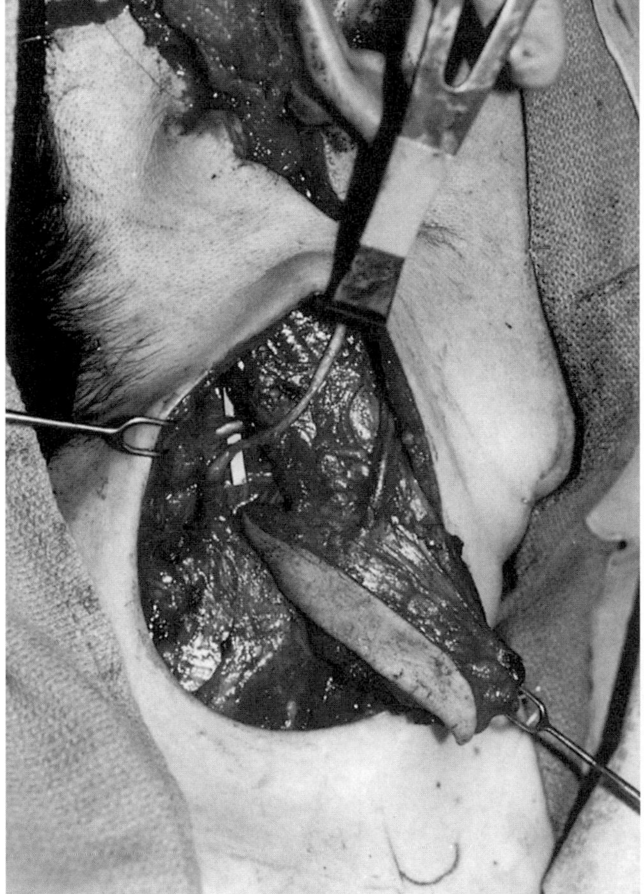
C

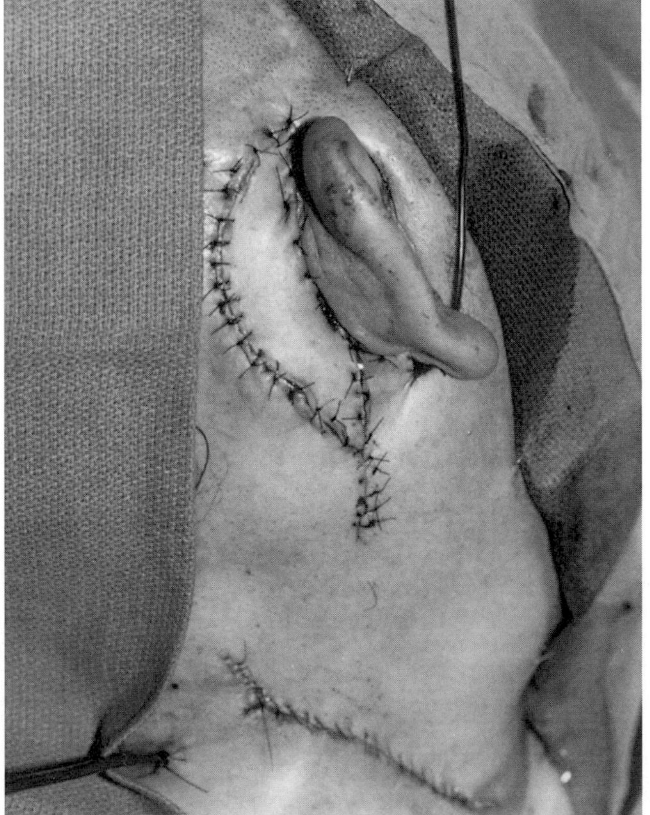
D

Figure 27.16 A 36-year-old woman presented with a long history of drainage from the right ear due to a temporal bone cholesteatoma and temporal lobe abscess. **A:** The patient underwent radical excision of the chronic abscess cavity, including the middle ear and temporal bone. **B:** Outline of reconstruction with a superiorly based sternomastoid musculocutaneous flap. **C:** Intraoperative view of the sternomastoid musculocutaneous flap. **D:** The completed closure.

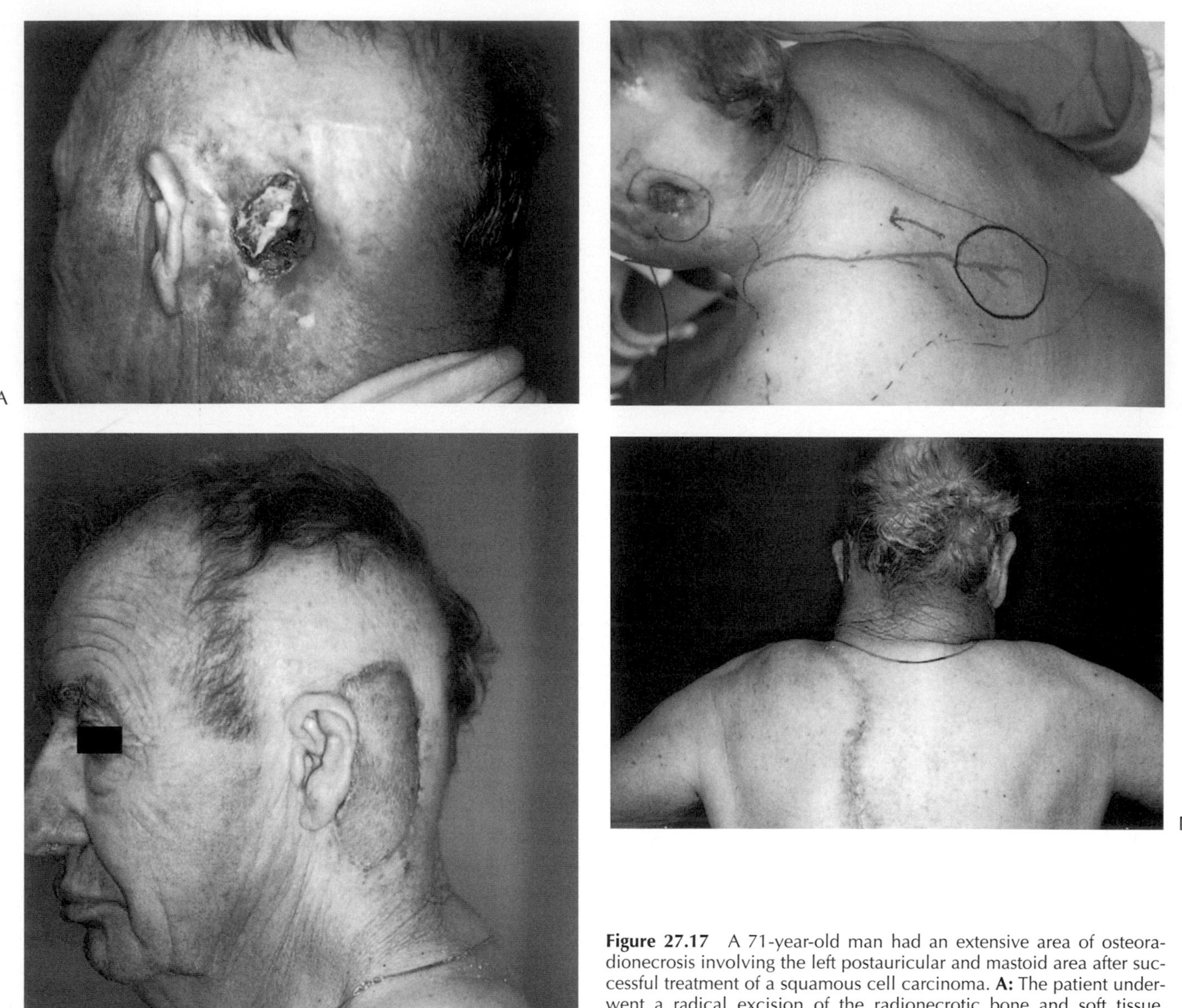

Figure 27.17 A 71-year-old man had an extensive area of osteoradionecrosis involving the left postauricular and mastoid area after successful treatment of a squamous cell carcinoma. **A:** The patient underwent a radical excision of the radionecrotic bone and soft tissue, preserving the middle ear and facial nerve. The 8 × 7 cm defect was reconstructed with a pedicled trapezius myocutaneous flap. **B:** An outline of a reconstructive flap. The trapezius muscle filled the potential dead space, and the cutaneous paddle replaced lost skin. The flap reached the defect through a subcutaneous tunnel. **C:** Healed lateral skull-base defect. **D:** Donor site scar. The patient retained trapezius muscle function because of preservation of the spinal accessory nerve and superolateral portion of the muscle.

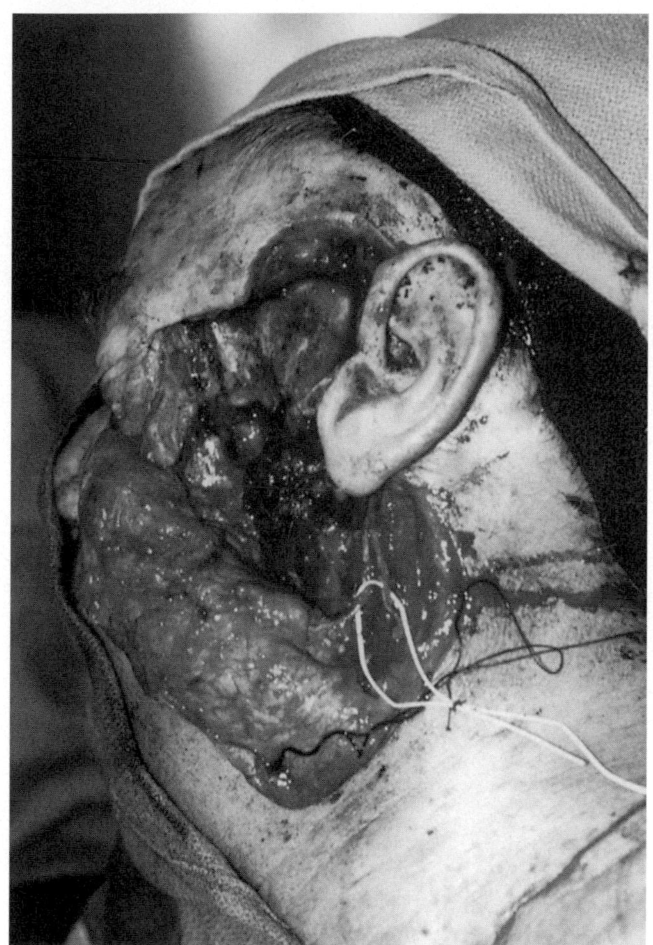

A

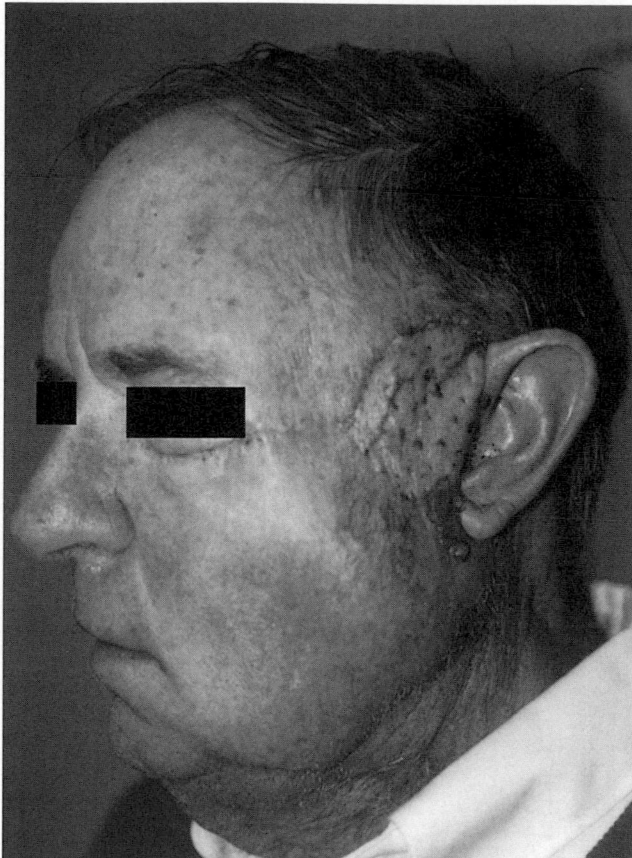

C

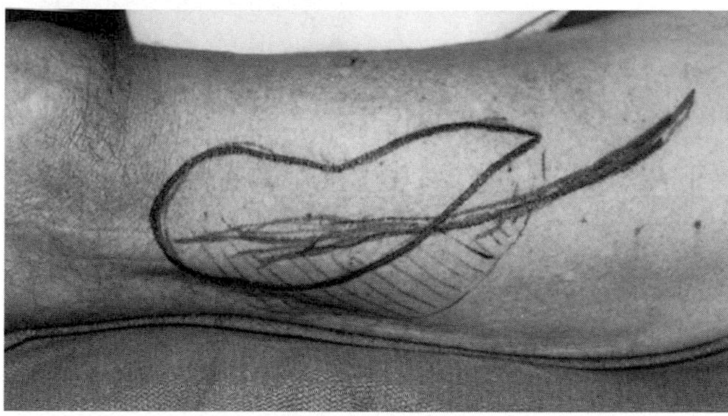

B

Figure 27.18 A 72-year-old man presented with a recurrent melanoma in the left temporal fossa 4 years after resection of a melanoma of the left buccal mucosa and buccal space. **A:** Resection of the recurrence required removal of the temporalis muscle, zygomatic arch, temporomandibular joint, ascending rami of the mandible, and the tissues of the pterygopalatine fossa. The upper three branches of the facial nerve were resected. Here, the vessel loop lies around the lower intact branches of the facial nerve. **B:** This complex defect was reconstructed with an anterolateral thigh free musculofascial flap. A portion of vastus lateralis muscle was included to help to fill the depths of the defect. Skin from the flap donor site was applied over the muscle as a full-thickness graft. The nerve to the vastus lateralis was used as a graft to replace the partially resected facial nerve. **C:** Four months after surgery, the patient's wounds have healed. He awaits facial nerve recovery.

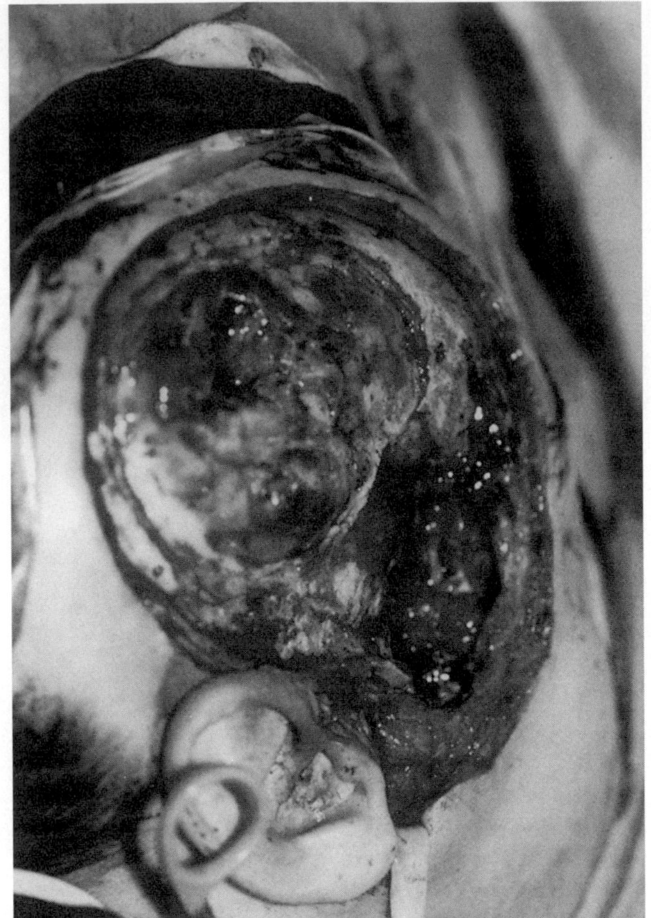

A

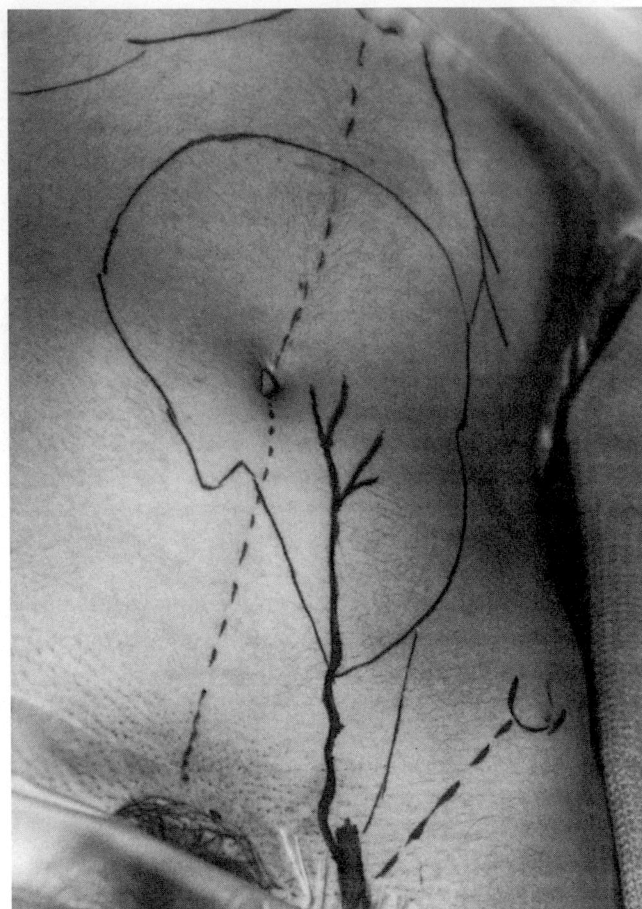

B

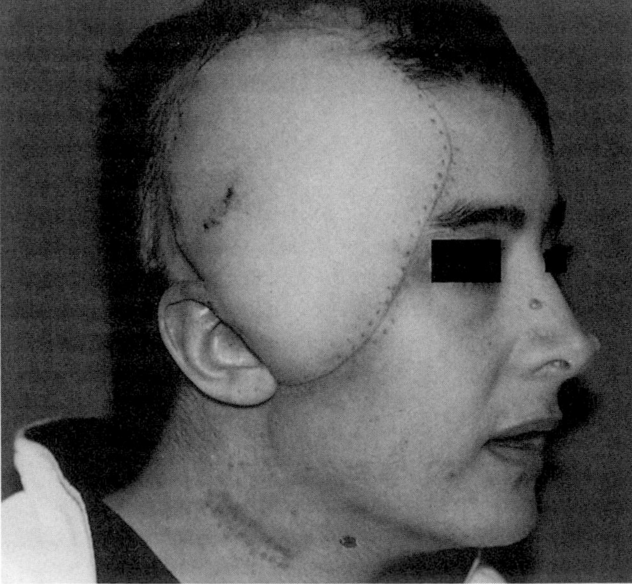

C

Figure 27.19 A 27-year-old woman presented with a recurrent glioblastoma of the temporoparietal region, initially treated with radiation therapy and excision. **A:** This recurrence was radically excised, creating a defect extending from the zygomatic arch into the temporal fossa and pterygoid region. Brain is exposed at the base of the wound. **B:** The closure used a rectus abdominis myocutaneous free flap. The anterior rectus fascia reconstructed the dural defect. The flap pedicle was anastomosed to the facial artery and internal jugular vein. **C:** Postoperative result at 6 weeks.

because it provides substantial tissue, does not require repositioning of the patient, and leaves an acceptable donor-site scar. Based on the deep inferior epigastric vessels, the flap has a long, safe vascular pedicle (Fig. 27.19).

FUNCTIONAL RECONSTRUCTION

If the facial nerve must be reconstructed, suitable nerve grafts may be harvested in concert with the harvesting of the muscle flap; thus, the motor nerve that normally innervates the donor muscle may now serve as a free interpositional nerve graft. Usually, it is not necessary to harvest a sural nerve graft when a free muscle or musculocutaneous flap is needed to reconstruct the defect. Free transfer of a functional muscle is desirable where the resection includes the parotid gland and other soft tissues in the cheek and where a simple facial nerve grafting is insufficient. The planning of a functional muscle flap adds complexity, because the flap must be designed so that the muscle runs obliquely from the lateral aspect of the oral commissure to the zygomatic region. The muscle then will pull the corner of the mouth upward to produce a smile. The motor nerve to the muscle flap is anastomosed to the stump of the facial nerve. Feasible donor muscles include the rectus abdominis (Fig. 27.20), vastus lateralis (Fig. 27.18), and latissimus dorsi.

If a muscle flap is needed both to fill a potential dead space and to animate the face, the best donor site is the combination of the latissimus dorsi and the serratus anterior muscles. The two muscles are both based on the thoracodorsal vascular pedicle. Therefore, both muscles can be vascularized simultaneously

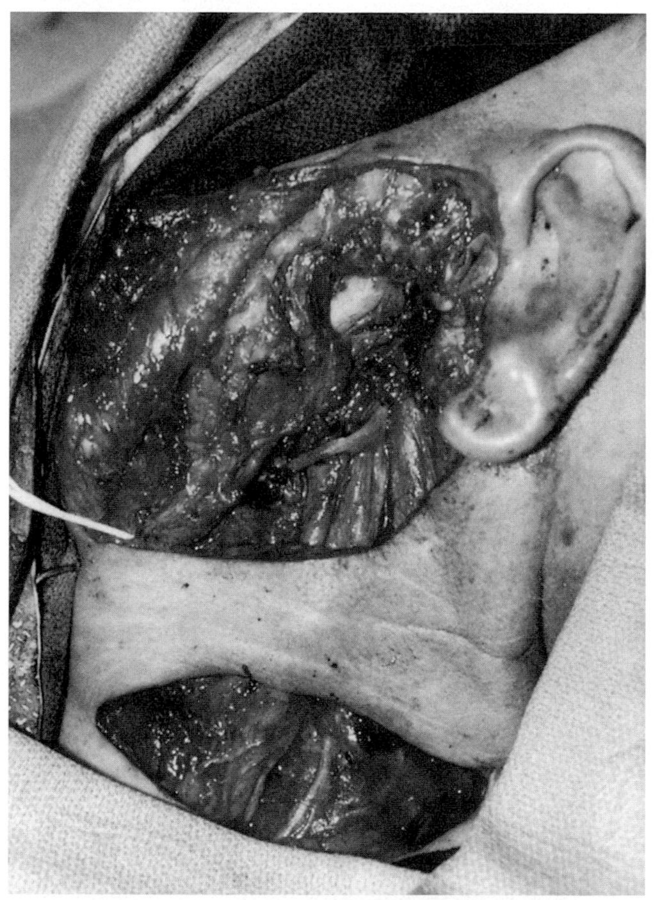

A

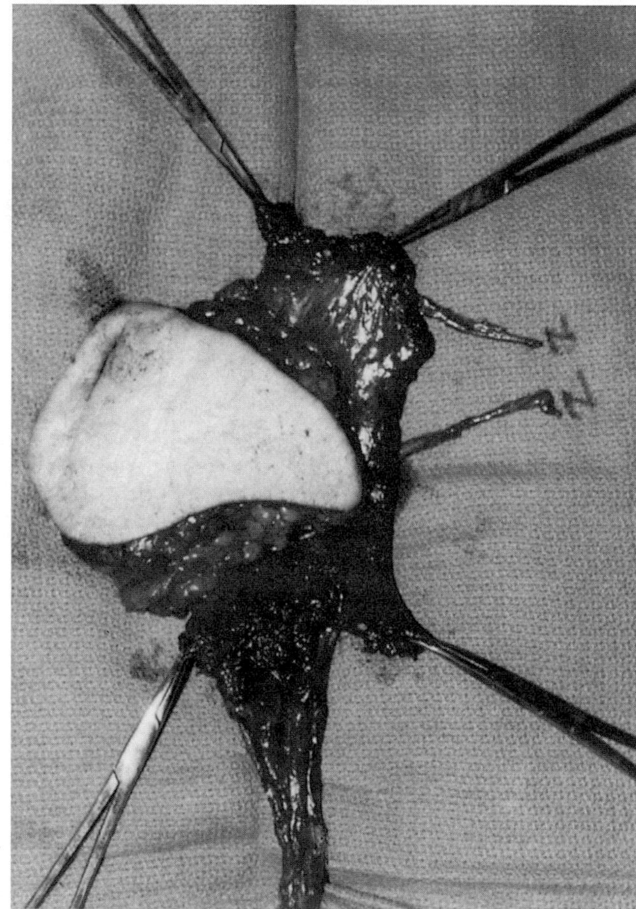

C

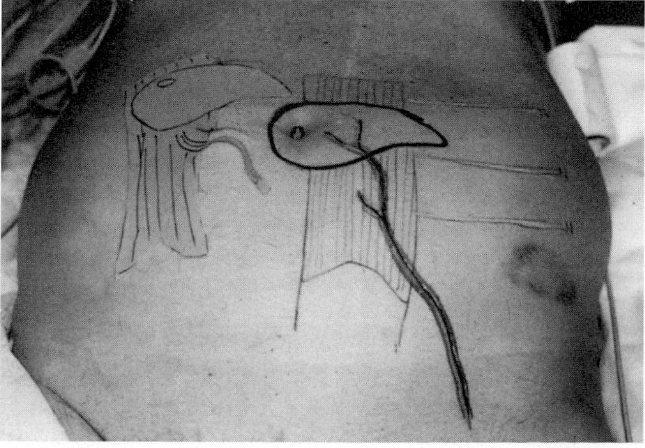

B

Figure 27.20 A 78-year-old man had a recurrent adenocarcinoma of the left parotid gland and infratemporal fossa. **A:** Preauricular and infratemporal fossa tissues, including facial nerve, were radically excised. Radioactive beads were placed in the defect. **B:** A pattern was made of the defect and then drawn on the abdomen. **C:** A functional rectus abdominis myocutaneous flap, here with two intercostal motor nerves exposed, helped to reconstruct the defect.

(Continued on next page)

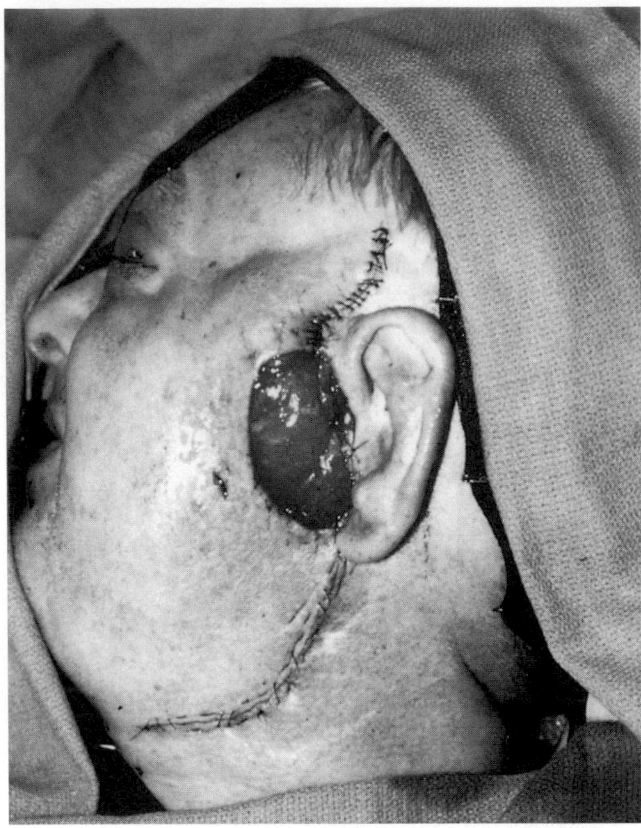
D

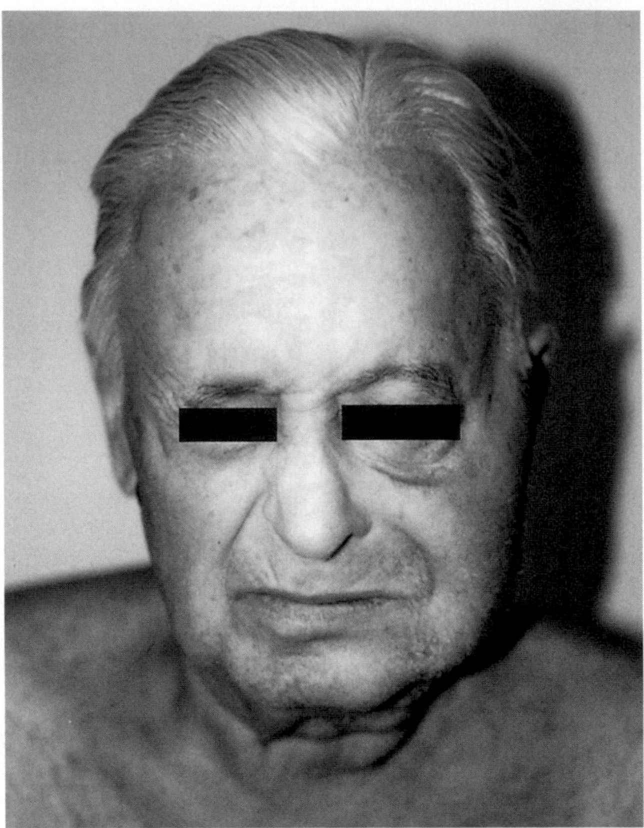
E

Figure 27.20 *(continued)* **D:** A segment of rectus muscle, designed to provide facial animation, was positioned from the corner of the mouth and nasolabial fold to the temporal region. It was innervated by the ipsilateral facial nerve via the two intercostal nerves. The skin paddle was removed, defatted, and reapplied as a full-thickness graft. The anterior belly of the digastric was reoriented to augment the function of the depressor angularis at the corner of the mouth. Blood supply to the flap came from the superior thyroid vessels and anterior jugular vein. Lagophthalmos was treated with a lateral tarsorrhaphy. **E:** Six months after surgery, the lagophthalmos has resolved, and the patient is capable of a grimace.

with a single set of arterial and venous anastomoses, shortening operative time. The lower two or three digitations of the innervated serratus anterior muscle can be used for facial reanimation, whereas the latissimus dorsi muscle can fill the potential dead space created by the extirpative operation.

Radical resections in the temporal area create complex defects that often require innovative reconstructions. Small defects can be managed by local flaps or regional musculocutaneous flaps, whereas larger deficits require free-tissue transfers. The reconstructive surgeon has a plethora of wound closure techniques from which to choose. Reconstruction requires a careful assessment of the missing tissues; the treatment that best closes the wound and restores function should be selected. Therapy must be individualized to each patient's particular needs to obtain the optimum reconstructive result.

RESULTS: CURRENT STATUS

The major impediment in assessing survival and outcome of temporal bone cancer has been the rarity of the lesions encountered. No single institution has sufficient data to allow analysis of results. Previously, we reviewed all publications dealing with surgical treatment for SCC of the temporal bone (92). No randomized or nonrandomized control studies were identified. All studies were case series without control subjects. This review sought answers to the following questions:

1. What is the survival rate of patients with lesions confined to the EAC and treated by surgical resection, and what type of operation should be performed in this instance?
2. Once the disease enters the middle ear, what is the operation that provides optimal survival?
3. Is total TBR ever indicated?
4. How does prognosis change as structures such as the dura mater, brain, and ICA become involved? Is there a role for surgery in these instances?
5. Does the addition of preoperative or postoperative RT enhance survival?

A Medline search was performed to identify all publications in the English language dating back to 1966 that dealt with the treatment of SCC of the temporal bone. Manuscripts dating back to 1915 were identified by searching the *Cumulative Index Medicus* and by reviewing references quoted in recent articles. Ninety-six publications (3,6,7,9,14,15,43,47–50,52,93–176) were encountered, of which 26 articles (6,47,153–176) containing information on 144 patients were analyzed extensively. Among the reasons for exclusion of a study was the lack of information describing the extent of disease (as determined by clinical examination and preoperative imaging), type of treatment, and follow-up for each patient.

Terms used were defined as follows:

- *Mastoidectomy:* includes all types of modified radical and radical mastoidectomy

- *Temporal bone resection, lateral:* removal of the osseous and cartilaginous EAC, malleus, and incus
- *Temporal bone resection, subtotal:* removal of the otic capsule in addition to removal of the osseous and cartilaginous EAC, malleus, and incus
- *Temporal bone resection, total:* removal of the petrous apex in addition to all that is removed in subtotal resection

To simplify analysis, several assumptions had to be made: Because of the lack of adequate preoperative imaging in studies performed until 1975, surgical findings were used to stage the extent of disease. Reference to *middle ear involvement* included tumors that extended from the external canal to involve either the lateral compartment or both the lateral and medial compartments of the middle ear. Most authors did not make a distinction between these two levels of involvement.

All patient records were entered into dBASE III Plus software (SYBEX Corp., Alameda, CA) on an IBM-compatible personal computer (176). Twenty-eight fields were opened and labeled as follows: author, year of publication, patient number, age, sex, histology, extent of disease, presence of regional metastases, presence of distant metastases, preoperative radiation, type of preoperative radiation, preoperative chemotherapy, previous surgery, type of previous surgery, type of operation performed, ICA involvement, resection of ICA, dural invasion, resection of dura, brain invasion, resection of brain tissue, postoperative radiation, type of postoperative radiation, postoperative chemotherapy, survival, follow-up (years), failure to control disease, and site of failure. Each record was given a numeric value under each field, denoting a specific characteristic of the patient. Data retrieval was performed using commands stated in the software manual (176).

For the purpose of analysis, all patients who were reported as *alive with disease* were considered statistically *dead of disease* (DOD) because it was presumed that their survival would be short. All patients who died of other causes and who had no evidence of disease within 1 year after treatment were excluded from the analysis because of inadequate follow-up. Those who died during surgery were considered DOD and were included in the analysis. Patients who were dead of other causes beyond 1 year after treatment were considered disease-free up to that time. Chi-square analysis was used to determine the statistical significance between compared groups. A p value less than 0.05 was considered significant.

General Findings Regarding Publications Analyzed

The quality of the studies was evaluated using the five levels of evidence posited by Cowart (176). No prospective randomized trial (level I or II) was identified. Nonrandomized concurrent cohort comparison studies (level III) also were not found. A nonrandomized historical cohort comparison study (level IV) was found. All remaining studies were case series without control subjects (level V).

Of the 96 publications identified, 26 articles contained sufficient information on 144 patients with regard to extent of disease, type of treatment rendered, and follow-up. Seventy publications were excluded from the analysis for one or more of the following reasons: Eight articles combined multiple histologic types in their report of overall survival. Adequate information on extent of disease, type of treatment, and follow-up was lacking in 8, 4, and 14 articles, respectively. Forty-five articles failed to report all three parameters for each individual patient.

Overall Survival

No statistically significant difference in survival was found between mastoidectomy (5 of 10, or 50% 5-year survival), lateral TBR (17 of 35, or 48.6% 5-year survival), or subtotal TBR (1 of 2, or 50% 5-year survival) when disease was confined to the external canal. There were three perioperative deaths in the group that underwent lateral TBR and one in the group that underwent subtotal TBR.

When disease extended into the middle ear, patients who had subtotal TBR had a 41.7% 5-year survival (5 of 12), and those who had lateral TBR had a 28.6% 5-year survival (2 of 7); the difference was not statistically significant. There was a trend toward lower survival for patients who had a mastoidectomy (6 of 35, or 17.1% 5-year survival) than for those who had subtotal TBR ($\chi^2 = 3.17$; $0.05 < p < 0.10$). The observed difference in survival between patients who underwent lateral TBR and those who underwent mastoidectomy was not statistically significant. The four patients who underwent total TBR had a 0% 1-year survival. There were two perioperative deaths in the subtotal TBR group and one in the total TBR group. Carcinoma that invaded the petrous apex was seen in one patient treated with subtotal TBR (who was DOD at 1 year) and in four patients treated with total TBR (2 of 4, or 50% 1-year survival, and 0 of 4, or 0% 2-year survival). The small numbers precluded statistical analysis.

In a very large single center study comprising 33 patients treated for temporal bone carcinoma, the findings largely agreed with the previous data. This study assessed the outcome for patients with SCC who were treated by mastoidectomy and postoperative radiotherapy. The authors concluded that the results of mastoidectomy with removal of all gross tumor, combined with planned perioperative radiotherapy, makes it a useful approach for the treatment of these SCC lesions. They believe that this method of treatment gives at least as good, and possibly better, 5-year cure rates than traditional temporal bone resection. They found the mastoidectomy procedure to cause less operative morbidity and mortality than more aggressive forms of resection. Though the authors find these data useful, a complete gross resection remains the standard of care and should be attempted even if more aggressive surgery is required. It is clear, though, that the inclusion of postoperative radiotherapy is mandatory in the overall treatment plan for any temporal bone malignancy (177).

Value of Radiation Therapy

The value of preoperative or postoperative RT was analyzed. All patients with disease confined to the external canal who were treated with mastoidectomy or subtotal or total TBR received RT, precluding analysis of these groups. No statistically significant difference in survival was seen between patients treated with lateral TBR and RT (12 of 25, or 48.0% 5-year survival) or lateral TBR alone (4 of 9, or 44.4% 5-year survival). Improvements in RT, from the use of radium and cobalt to the use of electron-beam teletherapy and brachytherapy, and their impact on survival could not be studied adequately.

Patients with carcinoma extending into the middle ear who were treated with mastoidectomy and RT (6 of 30, or 20% 5-year survival) survived longer than did those treated with mastoidectomy alone (0 of 4, or 0% 2-year survival). All patients treated with lateral or total TBR received preoperative or postoperative RT, precluding analysis of the value of RT. The 10 patients treated with subtotal TBR and RT had a 30% 5-year survival (3 of 10), whereas the 3 patients treated with subtotal TBR alone had a 100% 5-year survival (3 of 3). This difference was statistically significant ($\chi^2 = 4.61$; $0.01 < p < 0.05$). All patients with extension of cancer into the petrous apex had either preoperative or postoperative RT, and the value of RT could not be determined.

Dural Invasion

Patients who had carcinomatous involvement of the dura mater had an 11.1% 5-year survival (1 of 9), and treatment by resection of the dura did not change survival rates (Fig. 27.6). Margins of resection, however, were not stated by the authors.

Internal Carotid Artery Involvement

Four patients had extension of disease to involve the ICA. Of the 2 patients treated with total TBR and ICA sacrifice, 1 died from postoperative cerebral schemia and the other was DOD at 14 months with failure at regional and distant sites. Another patient was treated with total TBR alone and was DOD at 8 months, with local persistence. The remaining patient was treated with preoperative RT and lateral TBR and was DOD at 21 days, with local persistence.

Brain Invasion

In two patients, local invasion of carcinoma into the temporal lobe was treated with mastoidectomy and preoperative or postoperative RT. One patient was DOD at 1 month, with local persistence, and the other, who was treated with mastoidectomy, brachytherapy, and teletherapy, also was DOD at 5 months, with local persistence. No patient was treated with resection of involved cerebral or cerebellar tissue.

Site of Failure

Of 77 patients who died of their disease, site of failure was reported by the authors in 54 patients: 45 patients experienced local failure, 5 had locoregional failure, 3 had regional failure alone, and 1 had regional and distant failure. Several inferences were suggested by the available evidence:

1. Patients with carcinoma that is confined to the EAC experience similar survival, regardless of whether mastoidectomy, lateral TBR, or subtotal TBR is performed (50%, 48.6%, and 50% 5-year survival, respectively). Our preference for lateral TBR, which allows *en bloc* resection of tumor for these lesions, remains unchanged. The addition of RT to lateral TBR does not appear to improve survival.
2. When disease extends into the middle ear, survival of patients treated with subtotal TBR (41.7% 5-year survival) appeared to be improved over those treated with lateral TBR (28.6% 5-year survival) or mastoidectomy (17.1% 5-year survival). It appears that more extensive surgery than lateral TBR can prolong survival, though it remains uncertain whether the addition of RT to mastoidectomy improves survival.
3. The value of surgical resection when carcinoma extends to involve the petrous apex remains unclear (0% 1-year survival after subtotal TBR and 50% 1-year survival and 0% 2-year survival after total TBR).
4. Resection of involved dura mater does not appear to improve survival. However, incomplete data regarding margins of resection were reported.
5. Determination of the value of resection of involved brain parenchyma or ICA requires further study.

Some inferences regarding the value of preoperative or postoperative RT for SCC of the temporal bone also are suggested by the review. For tumors confined to the external canal, the addition of RT to lateral TBR appeared to have no survival advantage. The morbidity of RT may possibly be avoided in these patients. For tumors extending into the middle ear, RT appeared to improve survival in patients treated with mastoidectomy. Survival for patients treated with subtotal TBR with or without RT was paradoxical. Patients treated without RT fared better than those with RT. Perhaps the small sample size and patient selection factors in the former group contributed to the discrepancy.

Carcinomatous invasion of the dura mater or brain implies aggressive biologic behavior of the tumor. The role for surgical resection of these structures remains unclear. In our study (91), resection of involved dura did not appear to improve overall survival. However, margins of resection could not be studied adequately. Experience with lesions that extend to involve cerebral tissue has been limited. The two patients in our study who were treated with mastoidectomy and RT were both DOD at 1 month and 5 months, respectively. It is unclear what the survival advantage of surgical removal of resectable brain parenchyma would be, because we were unable to identify any patients who had such treatment.

Experience with carcinomatous involvement and resection of the ICA has also been limited. Of the four patients who had such involvement, two were DOD at 8 months and 21 days, with local persistence, respectively (91). Of the remaining two patients who had resection of the ICA, one patient died from cerebral schemia and the other was DOD at 14 months with regional and distant failure. The recent addition of improved preoperative carotid artery testing, such as the balloon occlusion test of the ICA with ^{100}Xe CT, may better identify those patients with adequate, marginal, or minimal contralateral cerebral blood flow, enabling better selection of patients for ICA sacrifice. Determination of the value of ICA resection—especially as it relates to survival—requires further study.

Several other aspects of this disease could not be studied because of the lack of information provided by the authors. The histologic differentiation of the tumor and its relationship to overall survival is an example. The method of temporal bone removal—whether by *en bloc* resection, piecemeal resection, or a drill-out—and its relationship to survival also require further study. Although the information may be intuitively obvious, a formal study evaluating the relationship between margins of resection in this disease and overall survival is lacking.

Moffat et al. (179) examined the surgical records of their 15 patients who underwent salvage surgery for extensive T3 or T4 temporal bone cancer (recurrent SCC in a radical mastoid cavity after previous treatment by mastoidectomy and RT). The salvage surgery consisted of an extended TBR with supraomohyoid neck dissection. Histologic evidence of local lymph node involvement in the supraomohyoid neck dissection was present in 13% of cases. These authors found histologic evidence also of involvement of the periarterial neural plexus in some cases, but direct involvement of the arterial wall was not seen in this series. There was no sacrifice of the intrapetrous carotid artery, and the tip of the petrous bone was removed using a high-speed air drill as a secondary procedure. Involved dura was excised with as wide a margin as possible. Involved temporal lobe also was excised with a margin when possible. All patients had been followed up for at least 5 years (range, 5 to 12 years). Those patients who succumbed did so in the first postoperative year. All those with poorly differentiated tumors died. The survivors had well- or moderately differentiated tumors. Radical surgery yielded a 47% 5-year survival. Twenty-nine percent of the survivors had temporal lobe involvement that necessitated a partial excision of the temporal lobe of the brain. Three of the survivors experienced dural involvement.

Both patients with well-differentiated SCCs survived, but all four patients with poorly differentiated tumors died (178). The postoperative complications included disequilibrium (21.7%);

palsies of the ninth, tenth, and 11th cranial nerves (each at 17.4%); dysphagia (13%); meningitis (8.7%); and occipital (8.7%) and trigeminal (4.3%) neuralgia.

In another study, Pensak et al. (4) reported on their 10-year experience with 46 patients with temporal bone cancer. Thirty-nine patients were treated with surgery and postoperative RT. Surgery included sleeve resection (one patient; no postoperative RT), lateral TBR (16 of 39), modified lateral TBR (13 of 39), and total TBR (9 of 39; ICA was preserved). Their results showed a tumor-free status at 3 years of 72% (28 of 39) and at 5 years of 51% (20 of 39).

CONCLUSION

Cancer of the temporal bone is treatable, and surgery can achieve beneficial results in selected cases. The key to substantial improvement in control of this serious disease is early diagnosis (high index of suspicion), precise CT and MRI evaluation, and three-dimensional oncologic resection. Immediate reconstruction of involved cranial nerves and soft tissue positively affects a patient's quality of life. Technical capabilities, however, must be balanced with tumor biology and the potential for functional reconstruction. The achievable quality of life, not just life's prolongation, must be assessed before the selection of the treatment of temporal bone cancer.

REFERENCES

1. Tiedemann K. Anatomy. In: Janecka IP, Tiedeman K, eds. *Skull base surgery: anatomy, biology and technology.* Philadelphia: Lippincott-Raven, 1996.
2. Morton RP, Stell PM, Derrick PPO. Epidemiology of cancer of the middle ear cleft. *Cancer* 1984;53:1612–1617.
3. Sekhar LN, Pomeranz S, Janecka L, et al. Temporal bone neoplasms: report on 20 surgically treated cases. *J Neurosurg* 1992;76:578–587.
4. Pensak ML, Gleich LL, Gluckman JL, et al. Temporal bone carcinoma: contemporary perspectives in the skull base surgical era. *Laryngoscope* 1996;106: 1234–1237.
5. Shaheen OH. The management of tumours of the middle ear. *J Laryngol Otol* 1983;97:313–317.
6. Michaels L, Wells M. Squamous cell carcinoma of the middle ear. *Clin Otolaryngol* 1980;5:235–248.
7. Goodwin WJ, Jesse RH. Malignant neoplasms of the external auditory canal and temporal bone. *Arch Otolaryngol* 1980;106:675–679.
8. Hyams VJ, Batsakis JG, Michaels L. Tumors of the upper respiratory tract and ear. In: *Atlas of tumor pathology,* 2nd series, fascicle 25. Washington, DC: Armed Forces Institute of Pathology, 1988.
9. Greer JA, Code TR, Weiland LH. Neoplasms of the temporal bone. *J Otolaryngol* 1976;5:391–398.
10. Nager GT. Squamous cell carcinomas. In: *Pathology of the ear and temporal bone.* Baltimore: Williams & Wilkins, 1993.
11. Arriaga M, Curtin HD, Takahashi H, et al. The role of preoperative CT scans in staging external auditory meatus carcinoma radiologic-pathologic correlation study. *Otolaryngol Head Neck Surg* 1991;105:6–11.
12. Austin JR, Stewart KL, Fawzi N. Squamous cell carcinoma of the external auditory canal. Therapeutic prognosis based on a proposed staging system. *Arch Otolaryngol Head Neck Surg* 1994;120:1228–1232.
13. Edelstein DR, Smouha E, Sacks SH, et al. Verrucous carcinoma of the temporal bone. *Ann Otol Rhinol Laryngol* 1986;95:447–453.
14. Kenyon GS, Marks PV, Scholtz CL, et al. Squamous cell carcinoma of the middle ear: a 25 year retrospective study. *Ann Otol Rhinol Laryngol* 1985;94: 273–277.
15. Spector JG. Management of temporal bone carcinomas: a therapeutic analysis of two groups of patients and long-term follow-up. *Otolaryngol Head Neck Surg* 1991;104:58–66.
16. Nager GT. Basal cell carcinoma. In: *Pathology of the ear and temporal bone.* Baltimore: Williams & Wilkins, 1993.
17. Jacobs GH, Rippey JJ, Altini M. Prediction of aggressive behavior in basal cell carcinoma. *Cancer* 1982;49:533–537.
18. Nager GT. Adenocarcinoma of the middle ear. In: *Pathology of the ear and temporal bone.* Baltimore: Williams & Wilkins, 1993.
19. Glasscock ME, McKennan KX, Levine SC, et al. Primary adenocarcinoma of the middle ear and temporal bone. *Arch Otolaryngol Head Neck Surg* 1987;3: 822–824.
20. Carroll WR, Niparko JK, Zappia JJ, et al. Primary adenocarcinoma of the temporal bone. A case with 40-year follow-up. *Arch Otolaryngol Head Neck Surg* 1991;117:439–441.
21. Schuller DE, Conley JJ, Goodman JH, et al. Primary adenocarcinoma of the middle ear. *Otolaryngol Head Neck Surg* 1983;91:280–283.
22. Gulya AJ, Glasscock ME, Pensak ML. Primary adenocarcinoma of the temporal bone with posterior fossa extension: case report. *Laryngoscope* 1986;96: 675–677.
23. Heffner DE. Low grade adenocarcinoma of probable endolymphatic sac. A clinicopathologic study of 20 cases. *Cancer* 1989;64:2292–2302.
24. Batsakis JG, el-Naggar AK. Papillary neoplasms (Heffner's tumors) of the endolymphatic sac. *Ann Otol Rhinol Laryngol* 1993;102:648–651.
25. Lo WW, Applegate LJ, Carberry JN, et al. Endolymphatic sac tumors: radiologic appearance. *Radiology* 1993;189:199–204.
26. Cannon CR, McLean WC. Adenoid cystic carcinoma of the middle ear and temporal bone. *Otolaryngol Head Neck Surg* 1983;91:96–99.
27. Enzinger FM, Weiss SW, eds. Rhabdomyosarcoma. In: *Soft tissue tumors,* 3rd ed. St. Louis: Mosby, 1995:539–577.
28. Maurer HM, Beltangady M, Gehan EA, et al. The Intergroup Rhabdomyosarcoma Study—I: a final report. *Cancer* 1988;61:209–220.
29. Maurer HM, Gehan EA, Beltangady M, et al. The Intergroup Rhabdomyosarcoma Study—II. *Cancer* 1993;71:1904–1922.
30. Raney RB, Lawrence W Jr, Maurer HM, et al. Rhabdomyosarcoma of the ear in childhood. A report from the Intergroup Rhabdomyosarcoma Study—I. *Cancer* 1983;51:2356.
31. Wiatrak BJ, Pensak ML. Rhabdomyosarcoma of the ear and temporal bone. *Laryngoscope* 1989;99:1188–1192.
32. Jaffe BF, Fox JE, Batsakis JG. Rhabdomyosarcoma of the middle ear and mastoid. *Cancer* 1971;27:29.
33. Naufal PM. Primary sarcomas of the temporal bone. *Arch Otolaryngol* 1973; 98:44.
34. Chasin WD. Rhabdomyosarcoma of the temporal bone. *Ann Otol Rhinol Laryngol Suppl* 1984;112:71–73.
35. Myers EW, Stool S, Wettschew A. Rhabdomyosarcoma of the middle ear. *Arch Otolaryngol* 1968;77:949–956.
36. Goepfert H, Cangir A, Lindberg R, et al. Rhabdomyosarcoma of the temporal bone: is surgical resection necessary? *Arch Otolaryngol* 1979;105:310–313.
37. Parham DM, Webber B, Holt H, et al. Immunohistochemical study of childhood rhabdomyosarcoma and related neoplasms. Results of an Intergroup Rhabdomyosarcoma Study Project. *Cancer* 1991;167:3072–3080.
38. Douglass EC, Shapiro DN, Valentine M, et al. Alveolar rhabdomyosarcoma with the t(2-13): cytogenetic findings and clinicopathologic correlations. *Med Pediatr Oncol* 1993;21:83–87.
39. Nager GT. Metastasis to the temporal bone and cerebellopontine angle. In: *Pathology of the ear and temporal bone.* Baltimore: Williams & Wilkins, 1993: 833–857.
40. Nelson EG, Hinojosa R. Histopathology of metastatic temporal bone tumors. *Arch Otolaryngol Head Neck Surg* 1991;7:189–193.
41. Horowitz SW, Leonetti JP, Azar-Kia B, et al. CT and MR of temporal bone malignancies primary and secondary to parotid carcinoma. *AJNR* 1994;15: 755–762.
42. Imamura S, Mukakamki Y. Secondary malignant tumors of the temporal bone. A histopathologic study and review of the world literature. *Nippon Jibiinkoka Gakkai Kaiho* 1991;94:924–937.
43. Schuknecht HF, Allam AF, Murakami Y. Pathology of secondary malignant tumors of the temporal bone. *Ann Otol Rhinol Laryngol* 1968;77:5–22.
44. Van den Brekel MW, Castelijns JA, Stel HV, et al. Occult metastatic neck disease: detection with US and US-guided fine-needle aspiration cytology. *Radiology* 1991;2:457.
45. Yousem DM, Som PM, Hackney DB, et al. Central nodal necrosis and extracapsular neoplastic spread in cervical lymph nodes: MR imaging versus CT. *Radiology* 1992;3:753–759.
46. Tart RP, Mukherji SK, Avino AJ, et al. Facial lymph nodes: normal and abnormal CT appearance. *Radiology* 1993;188:695–700.
47. Parsons H, Lewis JS. Subtotal resection of the temporal bone for cancer of the ear. *Cancer* 1954;7:995–1001.
48. Lewis JS. Temporal bone resection. Review of 100 cases. *Arch Otolaryngol* 1975;101:23–25.
49. Conley J, Schuller DE. Malignancies of the ear. *Laryngoscope* 1976;86: 1147–1163.
50. Lewis JS. Surgical management of tumors of the middle ear and mastoid. *J Laryngol Otol* 1983;97:299–311.
51. Ariyan S. Tumor surgery of the temporal bone. *Laryngoscope* 1974;84: 645–670.
52. Graham MD Staloff RT, Kemink JL, et al. Total en bloc resection of the temporal bone and carotid artery for malignant tumors of the ear and temporal bone. *Laryngoscope* 1984;94:528–533.
53. Schramm VL Jr. Temporal bone resection. In: Sekhar LN, Scharmm VL Jr, eds. *Tumors of the cranial base: diagnosis and treatment.* Mt. Kisco, NY: Futura, 1987:683–698.
54. House JW. Facial nerve grading systems. *Laryngoscope* 1983;93:1056–1068.
55. Feigenberg SJ, Mendenhall WM, Hinerman RW, et al. Radiosurgery for paraganglioma of the temporal bone. *Head Neck* 2002;24:384–389.
56. Conley JJ, Schuller DE. Reconstruction following temporal bone resection. *Arch Otolaryngol Head Neck Surg* 1977;103:34–37.
57. Schusterman NM, Kroll SS. Reconstruction strategy for temporal bone and external facial defects. *Ann Plast Surg* 1991;26:233–242.

58. Neligan PC, Boyd JB. Reconstruction of the cranial base defect. *Clin Plast Surg* 1995;22:71–77.
59. Mustoe TA, Corral CJ. Soft tissue reconstructive choices for craniofacial reconstruction. *Clin Plast Surg* 1995;22:543–554.
60. Spinelli FFM, Persing JA, Walser B. Reconstruction of the cranial base. *Clin Plast Surg* 1995;22:555.
61. Pribaz JJ, Morris DD, Mulliken JB. Three dimensional free flap reconstruction of complex facial defect using intra operative modeling. *Plast Reconstr Surg* 1994;93:285–293.
62. Horowitz JH, Persing JA, Nichter LS, et al. Galeal-pericranial flaps in head and neck reconstruction. *Am J Surg* 1984;148:489–497.
63. McGregor IA, Jackson IT. The extended role of the deltopectoral flap. *Br J Plast Surg* 1970;23:173.
64. Bakamjian VY, Long M, Rigg B. Experience with the medially based deltopectoral flap in reconstructive surgery of the head and neck. *Br J Plast Surg* 1971;24:174.
65. Stark RB, Kaplan JM. Rotation flaps, neck to cheek. *Plast Reconstr Surg* 1972; 50:230–233.
66. Crow ML, Crow FJ. Resurfacing large cheek defect with rotation flaps from the neck. *Plast Reconstr Surg* 1976;58:196–200.
67. Kaplan L, Goldwyn RM. The versatility of the laterally based cervicofacial flap for cheek repairs. *Plast Reconstr Surg* 1978;61:390.
68. Becker DW. A cervicopectoral rotation flap for cheek coverage. *Plast Reconstr Surg* 1978;61:868–870.
69. Jabalay ME, Heckler FR, Wallace WH, et al. Sternomastoid regional flaps: a new look at an old concept. *Br J Plast Surg* 1979:32:106–113.
70. McCraw JB, Magee WP, Kalwaic H. Uses of the trapezius and sternomastoid myocutaneous flaps in head and neck reconstruction. *Plast Reconstr Surg* 1979;63:49.
71. Conley JJ. The sternomastoid muscle flap. *Head Neck Surg* 1980;2:308–311.
72. Larson DL, Goepfert H. Limitations of the sternomastoid musculocutaneous flap in head and neck cancer reconstruction. *Plast Reconstr Surg* 1982;70:328.
73. Ariyan S. The pectoralis major myocutaneous flap. A versatile flap for reconstruction of the head and neck. *Plast Reconstr Surg* 1979;63:73.
74. Ariyan S, Cuono CB. Use of pectoralis major myocutaneous flap for reconstruction of large cervical, facial or cranial defects. *Am J Surg* 1980;140: 503–506.
75. Sasaki CT, Gardiner LJ, Carlson RD, et al. The extended pectoralis major flap in head and neck reconstruction. *Otolaryngol Head Neck Surg* 1986;94: 274–278.
76. Russell RC, Feller AM, Elliott LF, et al. The extended pectoralis major myocutaneous flap: uses and complications. *Plast Reconstr Surg* 1991;88:814–823.
77. Demergasso F, Plazza MV. Trapezius myocutaneous flap in reconstructive surgery for head and neck cancer. *Am J Surg* 1978;138:533–536.
78. Rosen HM. The extended trapezium musculocutaneous flap for cranioorbital facial reconstruction. *Plast Reconstr Surg* 1985;75:318–324.
79. Mathes SJ, Stevenson TR. Reconstruction of the posterior neck and skull with vertical trapezium musculocutaneous flap. *Am J Surg* 1988;156:248–251.
80. Hagan KF, Mathes SJ. Trapezius muscle and musculocutaneous flaps. In: Strauch B, Vasconez LO, Hall-Findlay EJ, eds. *Grabbs' encyclopedia of flaps.* Boston: Little, Brown, 1990:496–503.
81. Jones NF, Schramm VL, Sekhar LN. Reconstruction of the cranial base following tumor resection. *Br J Plast Surg* 1987;40:155.
82. Fisher J, Jackson IT. Microvascular surgery as an adjunct to craniomaxillofacial reconstruction. *Br J Plast Surg* 1989;42:146.
83. Jones NF, Hardesty RA, Swartz WM, et al. Extensive and complex defect of the scalp, middle third of the face, and palate: the role of microsurgical reconstruction. *Plast Reconstr Surg* 1990;82:937–950.
84. Jones TF, Jones NF. Advances in reconstruction of the upper aerodigestive tract and cranial base with free tissue transfer. *Clin Plast Surg* 1992;19:819.
85. Thompson JG, Restifo RJ. Microsurgery for cranial base tumors. *Clin Plast Surg* 1995;22:563–572.
86. Kroll SS, Reece GP, Miller MJ, et al. Comparison of the rectus abdominis free flap with the pectoralis major myocutaneous flap for reconstruction of the head and neck. *Am J Surg* 1992;164:615.
87. Schusterman MA, Homdeski G. Analysis of morbidity associated with immediate microvascular reconstruction in head and neck cancer patients. *Head Neck* 1992;14:14.
88. Jones NF, Sekhar LN, Schramm VL. Free rectus abdominis muscle flap reconstruction of the middle and posterior cranial base. *Plast Reconstr Surg* 1986;78:471.
89. Urken ML, Turk JB, Weinberg H, et al. The rectus abdominis free flap in head and neck reconstruction. *Arch Otolaryngol Head Neck Surg* 1991;117:85–87.
90. Shestak KC, Jones NF. Microsurgical free tissue transfer in the elderly patient. *Plast Reconstr Surg* 1993;88:259.
91. Pribaz JJ, Orgill DP, Epstein MD, et al. Anterolateral thigh free flap. *Ann Plast Surg* 1995;34:585–592.
92. Prasad S, Janecka L. Efficacy of surgical treatment for squamous cell carcinoma of the temporal bone: literature review. *Otolaryngol Head Neck Surg* 1994;110:270–280.
93. Johns ME, Headington JT. Squamous cell carcinoma of the external auditory canal: a clinicopathologic study of 20 cases. *Arch Otolaryngol* 1974;100:45–49.
94. Campbell E, Volk BM, Burkland CW. Total resection of the temporal bone for malignancy of the middle ear. *Ann Surg* 1951;134:397–404.
95. Coleman CC, Khuri A. A rational treatment for advanced cancer of the external ear and temporal bone. *Va Med Monthly* 1959;86:21–24.
96. Hutcheon JR. Experiences with aural carcinoma over the past six years. *Med J Aust* 1966;2:406–407.
97. Figi FA, Weisman PA. Cancer and chemodectoma in the middle ear and mastoid. *JAMA* 1954;156:1157–1162.
98. Wang CC. Radiation therapy in the management of carcinoma of the external auditory canal, middle ear or mastoid. *Ther Radiol* 1975;116:713–715.
99. Sinha PP, Aziz HI. Treatment of carcinoma of the middle ear. *Ther Radiol* 1978;126:485–487.
100. Boland J. The management of carcinomas of the middle ear. *Radiology* 1963; 80:285.
101. Holmes KS. The treatment of carcinoma of the middle ear by the 4MV linear accelerator. *Proc R Soc Med* 1960;53:242–244.
102. Yamada S, Schuh FD, Marvin JS, et al. En bloc subtotal temporal bone resection for cancer of the external ear. *J Neurosurg* 1973;39:370–379.
103. Hahn SS, Kim JA, Goodchild N, et al. Carcinoma of the middle ear and external auditory canal. *Int J Radiat Oncol Biol Phys* 1983;9:1003–1007.
104. Sorenson H. Cancer of the middle ear and mastoid. *Acta Radiol* 1960;54:4 60–468.
105. Frazer JS. Malignant disease of the external acoustic meatus and middle ear. *Proc R Soc Med* 1930;23:1235–1244.
106. Barnes EB. Carcinoma of the ear. *Proc R Soc Med* 1930;23:1231–1234.
107. Conley JJ. Cancer of the middle ear and temporal bone. *N Y State J Med* 1974;74:1575–1579.
108. Kinney SE, Wood BG. Malignancies of the external ear canal and temporal bone: surgical techniques and results. *Laryngoscope* 1987;97:158–164.
109. Kinney SE. Squamous cell carcinoma of the external auditory canal. *Am J Otol* 1989;10:111–116.
110. Clark LJ, Narula AA, Morgan DAL, et al. Squamous carcinoma of the temporal bone: a revised staging. *J Laryngol Otol* 1991;105:346–348.
111. Corey JP, Nelson E, Crawford M, et al. Metastatic vaginal carcinoma to the temporal bone. *Am J Otol* 1991;12:128–131.
112. Hiraide F, Inouye T, Ishii T. Primary squamous cell carcinoma of the middle ear invading the cochlea: a histopathologic case report. *Ann Otol Rhinol Laryngol* 1983;92:290–294.
113. Schusterman MA, Kroll SS. Reconstruction strategy for temporal bone and lateral facial defects. *Ann Plast Surg* 1983;26:233–294.
114. Haughey BH, Gates GA, Skerhut BE, et al. Cerebral shift after lateral craniofacial resection and flap reconstruction. *Otolaryngol Head Neck Surg* 1989;101: 79–86.
115. Bergetedt HF, Lind MG. Temporal bone scintigraphy. *Acta Otolaryngol* 1980; 89:465–473.
116. Jahn AF, Farkashidy J, Berman JM. Metastatic tumors in the temporal bone-a pathophysiologic study. *J Otolaryngol* 1979;18:85–95.
117. Ruben RJ, Thaler SU, Holzer N. Radiation induced carcinoma of the temporal bone. *Laryngoscope* 1977;87:1613–1621.
118. Katsarkas A, Seemayer TA. Bilateral temporal bone metastases of the uterine cervix carcinoma. *J Otolaryngol* 1976;5:315–318.
119. Ramsden RT, Bulman CH, Lorigan BP. Osteoradionecrosis of the temporal bone. *J Laryngol Otol* 1975;89:941–955.
120. Vize G. Laryngeal metastasis to the temporal bone causing facial paralysis. *J Laryngol Otol* 1974;88:175–177.
121. Arriaga M, Curtin H, Takahashi H, et al. Staging proposal for external auditory meatus carcinoma based on preoperative clinical examination and computed tomography findings. *Ann Otol Rhinol Laryngol* 1990;99:714–721.
122. Adams WS, Morrison R. On primary carcinoma of the middle ear and mastoid. *J Laryngol Otol* 1955;69:115–131.
123. Gacek RR. Management of temporal bone carcinoma. *Trans Penn Acad Otolaryngol Ophthalmol* 1979;32:67–71.
124. Goodman ML. Middle ear and mastoid neoplasms. *Ann Otol Rhinol Laryngol* 1971;80:419–424.
125. Arena S, Keen M. Carcinoma of the middle and temporal bone. *Am J Otol* 1988;9:351–356.
126. Hilding DA, Selker R. Total resection of the temporal bone for carcinoma. *Arch Otolaryngol* 1969;89:98–107.
127. Cundy RL, Sando L, Hemenway WG. Middle ear extension of nasopharyngeal carcinoma via the eustachian tube. *Arch Otolaryngol* 1973;98:131–133.
128. Lewis JS. Squamous carcinoma of the ear. *Arch Otolaryngol* 1973;97:41–42.
129. Lessor RW, Sector GJ, Divinens VR. Malignant tumors of the middle ear and external auditory canal: a 20 year review. *Otolaryngol Head Neck Surg* 1987;96:43–47.
130. Arthur K. Radiotherapy in carcinoma of the middle ear and auditory canal. *J Laryngol Otol* 1976;90:753–762.
131. Tuckre VN. Cancer of the middle ear. *Cancer* 1965;16:642–650.
132. Conley JJ, Novack AJ. The surgical treatment of malignant tumors of the ear and temporal bone. *Arch Otolaryngol* 1960;71:635–652.
133. Conley JJ, Novack AJ. Surgical treatment of cancer of the ear and temporal bone. *Trans Am Acad Ophthalmol Otolaryngol* 1960;71:83–92.
134. Wagenfield DJH, Keane T, Norstrand AWP, et al. Primary carcinoma involving the temporal bone: analysis of 25 cases. *Laryngoscope* 1980;90:912–919.
135. Lewis JS, Parsons H. Surgery for advanced ear cancer. *Ann Otol Rhinol Laryngol* 1958;67:364–399.
136. Lewis JS, Page R. Radical surgery for malignant tumors of the ear. *Arch Otolaryngol* 1966;83:56–61.
137. Lederman M. Malignant tumors of the ear. *J Laryngol Otol* 1965;79:85–119.
138. Frew L, Finney R. Neoplasms of the middle ear. *J Laryngol Otol* 1963;77: 415–421.

139. Lindahl JWS. Carcinoma of the middle ear and meatus. *J Laryngol Otol* 1955;69:457–467.
140. Bradley WH, Maxwell JH. Neoplasms of the middle ear and mastoid: report of 54 cases. *Laryngoscope* 1954;54:533–556.
141. Miller D. Cancer of the external auditory meatus. *Laryngoscope* 1955;65:448–461.
142. Colledge L. Two cases of malignant disease of the temporal bone. *J Laryngol Otol* 1943;58:251–254.
143. Peele JC, Hauser GH. Primary carcinoma of the external auditory canal and middle ear. *Arch Otolaryngol* 1941;34:254–266.
144. Gamett-Passe ER. Primary carcinoma of the eustachian tube. *J Laryngol Otol* 1948;62:314–315.
145. Spencer FR. Malignant disease of the ear. *Arch Otolaryngol* 1938;28:916–940.
146. Means RG, Gersten J. Primary carcinoma of the mastoid process. *Ann Otol Rhinol Laryngol* 1953;62:93–100.
147. Ariyan S, Sasaki CT, Spencer D. Radical en-bloc resection of the temporal bone. *Am J Surg* 1981;142:443–447.
148. Arena S. Tumor surgery of the temporal bone. *Laryngoscope* 1974;84:645–670.
149. Brooker GB. Bilateral middle ear carcinomas associated with Waldenstrom's macroglobulinemia. *Ann Otol Rhinol Laryngol* 1982;91:299–303.
150. Towson CE, Shofstall WH. Carcinoma of the ear. *Arch Otolaryngol* 1950; 51:724–738.
151. Robinson GA. Malignant tumors of the ear. *Laryngoscope* 1931;41:467–473.
152. Buckmann LT, Baffe W. Carcinoma of the middle ear and mastoid. *Ann Otol Rhinol Laryngol* 1943;52:194–201.
153. Liebeskind MM. Primary carcinoma of the external auditory canal, middle ear, and mastoid. *Laryngoscope* 1951;61:1173–1187.
154. Stokes HB. Primary malignant tumors of the temporal bone. *Arch Otolaryngol* 1990;32:1023–1030.
155. Rosenwasser H. Neoplasms involving the middle ear. *Arch Otolaryngol* 1940;32:38–53.
156. Grossman AA, Donnelly WA, Smithman ME. Carcinoma of the middle ear and mastoid process. *Ann Otol Rhinol Laryngol* 1947;56:709–721.
157. Mattick WL, Mattick JW. Some experience in management of cancer of the middle ear and mastoid. *Arch Otolaryngol* 1951;53:610–621.
158. Wahl JW, Gromet MT. Carcinoma of the middle ear and mastoid. *Arch Otolaryngol* 1953;58:121–126.
159. Crabtree JA, Britton BH, Pierce MK. Carcinoma of the external auditory canal. *Laryngoscope* 1976;86:405–415.
160. Hanna DC Richardson GS, Gaisford JC. A suggested technique for resection of the temporal bone. *Am J Surg* 1967;114:553–558.
161. Adams GI, Paparella MM, Fiky FM. Primary and metastatic tumors of the temporal bone. *Laryngoscope* 1971;81:1273–1285.
162. Staloff RT, Myers DL, Lowery LD, et al. Total temporal bone resection for squamous cell carcinoma. *Otolaryngol Head Neck Surg* 1987;96:4–14.
163. Nadol JB Schuknecht HE. Obliteration of the mastoid in the treatment of tumors of the temporal bone. *Ann Otol Rhinol Laryngol* 1984;93:6–12.
164. Arriaga M, Hirsch BE, Kamerer DB, et al. Squamous cell carcinoma of the external auditory meatus (canal). *Otolaryngol Head Neck Surg* 1989;101: 330–337.
165. McCrea RS. Radical surgery for carcinoma of the middle ear. *Laryngoscope* 1972;82:1514–1523.
166. Gacek RR, Goodman M. Management of malignancy of the temporal bone. *Laryngoscope* 1977;87:1622–1634.
167. Scholl LA. Neoplasms involving the middle ear. *Arch Otolaryngol* 1935;22:548–553.
168. Clairmont AA, Conley JJ. Primary carcinoma of the mastoid bone. *Ann Otol Rhinol Laryngol* 1977;86:306–309.
169. Beal DD, Lindsay JR, Ward PH. Radiation-induced carcinoma of the mastoid. *Arch Otolaryngol* 1965;81:9–16.
170. Coleman CC. Removal of the temporal bone for cancer. *Am J Surg* 1966;112: 583–590.
171. Miller D, Silverstein H, Gacek RR. Cryosurgical treatment of carcinoma of the ear. *Trans Am Acad Ophthalmol Otolaryngol* 1972;76:1363–1367.
172. Tabb HG, Komet H McLaurin JW. Cancer of the external auditory canal: treatment with radical mastoidectomy and irradiation. *Laryngoscope* 1964;74: 634–643.
173. Lodge WO, Jones HM, Smith MEN. Malignant tumors of the temporal bone. *Arch Otolaryngol* 1955;61:535–541.
174. Ward GE Loch WE, Lawrence W. Radical operation for carcinoma of the external auditory canal and middle ear. *Am J Surg* 1951;82:169–178.
175. Newhart H. Primary carcinoma of the middle ear: report of a case. *Laryngoscope* 1917;27:543–555.
176. Cowart R. *The ABCs of dBASE III PLUS*. Alameda, CA: SYBEX, 1986:1–265.
177. Zhang B, Tu G, Xu G, et al. Squamous cell carcinoma of the temporal bone: reported on 33 patients. *Head Neck* 1999;21:461–466.
178. Cook DJ, Guyatt GH, Laupacis A, et al. Rules of evidence and clinical recommendations on the use of antithrombotic agents. *Chest* 1992;102: 3055–311S.
179. Moffat DA, Grey P, Ballagh RH, et al. Extended temporal bone resection for squamous cell carcinoma. *Otolaryngol Head Neck Surg* 1997;116:617–623.

CHAPTER 28

Paragangliomas of the Head and Neck

Mark S. Persky, Kenneth S. Hu, and Alejandro Berenstein

Paragangliomas represent highly vascular neoplasms embryologically arising from the paraganglia of neural crest origin and most commonly occurring in the head and neck region. These tumors are closely associated with either blood vessels (carotid artery, jugular bulb) or nerves (vagus, tympanic plexus), and their clinical presentation may involve a wide spectrum of signs and symptoms. A slowly enlarging neck mass and/or findings consistent with cranial nerve (CN) dysfunction are the hallmarks of presentation. A familial history of these tumors may be present, and there is a significant incidence of multicentric tumors, both in familial and sporadic cases. Malignant paragangliomas are uncommon, and their diagnosis can be confirmed only by the presence of metastatic disease, usually within regional lymph nodes. There are no strict histologic criteria within the primary tumor that can differentiate between benign and malignant paragangliomas.

Computerized tomography (CT) and magnetic resonance imaging (MRI) usually establish the diagnosis. Angiography defines the vascular supply and may visualize vessel involvement (invasion), and paves the way for preoperative embolization, if surgery is contemplated.

Paragangliomas are highly vascular, and they characteristically have early blood vessel and neural involvement, in addition to skull base and potential intracranial extension. These factors all contribute to the challenging nature of effectively treating these tumors. Traditionally, surgery has been the preferred method of treatment, especially with the evolution of more sophisticated skull base approaches, safer embolization protocols, and advanced vascular bypass procedures (1). Postoperative CN dysfunction is anticipated in patients with larger tumors and skull base involvement; therefore, a focus on rehabilitation efforts is necessary.

Radiation therapy was traditionally relied on for treating unresectable paragangliomas or tumors in elderly or debilitated patients. Advances in radiation oncology and increasing experience in treating head and neck paragangliomas have translated into improved long-term tumor response with acceptable complications from radiation treatment.

ANATOMY AND PHYSIOLOGY OF PARAGANGLIA

Paraganglia are part of the diffuse neuroendocrine system (DNES), previously known as the amine precursor uptake decarboxylate (APUD) system. These structures are widely dispersed aggregates of specialized (neuroendocrine) tissue that contain cells with the potential to secrete neuropeptides and catecholamines, which function as neurotransmitters, neurohormones, hormones, and parahormones (2,3). Paraganglia, like other members of the DNES, are composed of two predominant cell types: chief cells and sustentacular cells. Neuropeptides and catecholamines are produced and stored in the cytoplasmic granules of chief cells. The sequence of catecholamine production and metabolism is shown in Figure 28.1 (4). Tyrosine is ultimately converted to dopamine, norepinephrine, or epinephrine. The enzyme methyltransferase, necessary for the conversion of norepinephrine to epinephrine, is present only in the adrenal medulla, heart, and brain (5). Therefore, only norepinephrine may accumulate in the chief cells of

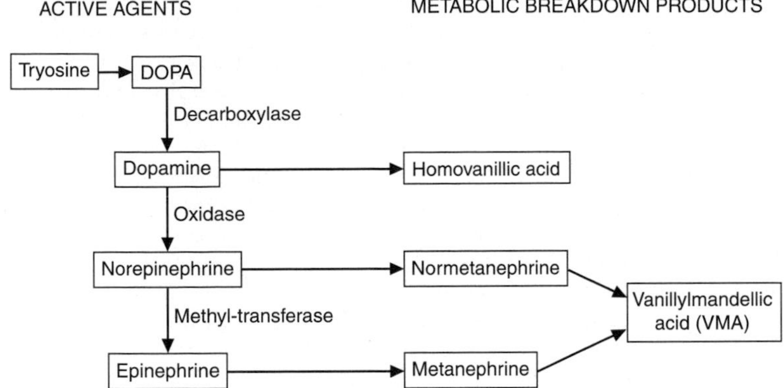

Figure 28.1 Catecholamine metabolism.

extraadrenal paraganglia. Tumors of the adrenal (pheochromocytomas) and extraadrenal (paragangliomas) paraganglionic system have the potential capacity to secrete epinephrine and norepinephrine, respectively. Elevated urinary levels of metanephrines (metanephrine or normetanephrine), and vanillylmandelic acid (VMA), the ultimate breakdown product of catecholamine metabolism, may be found in patients with pheochromocytomas or paragangliomas. Laboratory testing to determine urinary metanephrines and VMA is important in the evaluation of patients with suspected paragangliomas, particularly in the presence of hypertension.

Paraganglia arise from neural crest progenitor cells, whereas other components of the DNES, including the pancreatic islets, pulmonary neuroepithelial bodies, and dispersed neuroendocrine cells of the gastrointestinal tract and lungs, arise from closely related neuroectoderm (Fig. 28.2) (6). Glenner and Grimley (7) developed a classification of paraganglia based on embryology, location, and histology, and divided them into two major groups: the adrenal medulla and the extraadrenal paraganglion system. The latter group is subdivided into branchiomeric (migrating along a branchiomeric distribution), intravagal, aorticosympathetic and viscero-autonomic paraganglia. The carotid bodies, jugulotympanic, laryngeal, and orbital paraganglia are the head and neck paraganglia belonging to the branchiomeric group and are closely associated with CNs and arteries. The jugulotympanic paraganglia and the carotid body arise from the second and third pharyngeal pouches, respectively. In contrast to the other major paraganglia of the head and neck, vagal paraganglia are not closely associated with arteries and do not migrate along a branchiomeric distribution. Accordingly, they have been classified into a separate group of extraadrenal paraganglia by Glenner and Grimley (7).

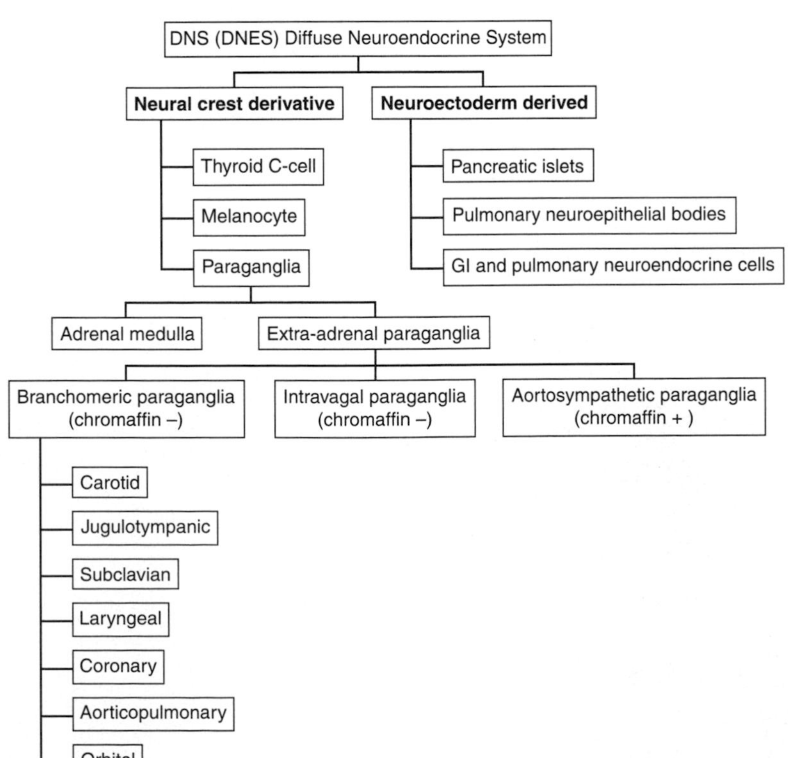

Figure 28.2 Diffuse neuroendocrine system.

Paraganglia are dispersed throughout the head and neck region. Neoplastic transformation (i.e., paragangliomas) most commonly occurs in the carotid body, jugulotympanic, and vagal paraganglia, although paragangliomas have also been reported in the larynx (8), orbit (9), thyroid (10), tongue (11), nasal cavity (12), paranasal sinuses (12,13), external auditory canal (14), and in supratentorial locations (15,16).

Carotid Body

The carotid body is a discrete, ovoid structure arising most commonly from the posteromedial wall of the common carotid bifurcation either within or outside its adventitial layer (Fig. 28.3). The carotid body is affixed to the artery by a band of fibrous tissue known as the ligament of Mayer (17). The major innervation of the carotid body is sensory via the glossopharyngeal nerve. Afferent nerve branches from the carotid body join those from the carotid sinus to form the carotid sinus nerve, also known as the nerve of Hering (18). The carotid body receives its blood supply from glomic arteries, small vessels arising from the carotid bifurcation that course through the ligament of Mayer (19). The carotid body is in close proximity to the baroreceptive carotid sinus and shares a common afferent neural pathway. This relationship becomes of great importance in the surgical management of carotid body tumors.

Reported normal dimensions of the carotid body vary with the greatest diameter, ranging from 3 to 7 mm (17), and the maximum weight is 15 mg (20). A single body is found at each bifurcation in 83% to 95% of cases at necropsy (21,22). Reported variations include double carotid bodies on one side in up to 7% of cases and bilobed carotid bodies in 9% (22).

The carotid body functions as a chemoreceptor and plays a critical role in a ventilation and perfusion homeostasis. The carotid body is intensely vascular, with a perfusion rate greater than that of the heart and brain (17). This richly vascular environment supports its chemoreceptor function. Detected changes in arterial partial pressures of oxygen and carbon dioxide, pH, and temperature trigger a reflex response initiated by the carotid body that results in compensatory changes in cardiovascular and respiratory activity. The carotid body, along with the cardioaortic bodies, are the only paraganglia with demonstrated chemoreceptive function.

Jugulotympanic Paraganglia

Temporal bone paraganglia are derived from neural crest tissue of the second branchial arch and are associated with either the tympanic branch of the glossopharyngeal nerve (Jacobson's nerve) or the auricular branch of the vagus nerve (Arnold's nerve) (23,24). Typically, each ear contains three small discrete paraganglia, measuring 0.1 to 1.5 mm in diameter (24,25). More than 50% of these paraganglia occur in the region of the jugular fossa. Over 20% are found in the inferior tympanic canaliculus, which transmits Jacobson's nerve (24), and another 10% are located in the mucosa of the promontory (24). Although the paraganglia of this region are morphologically and embryolog-

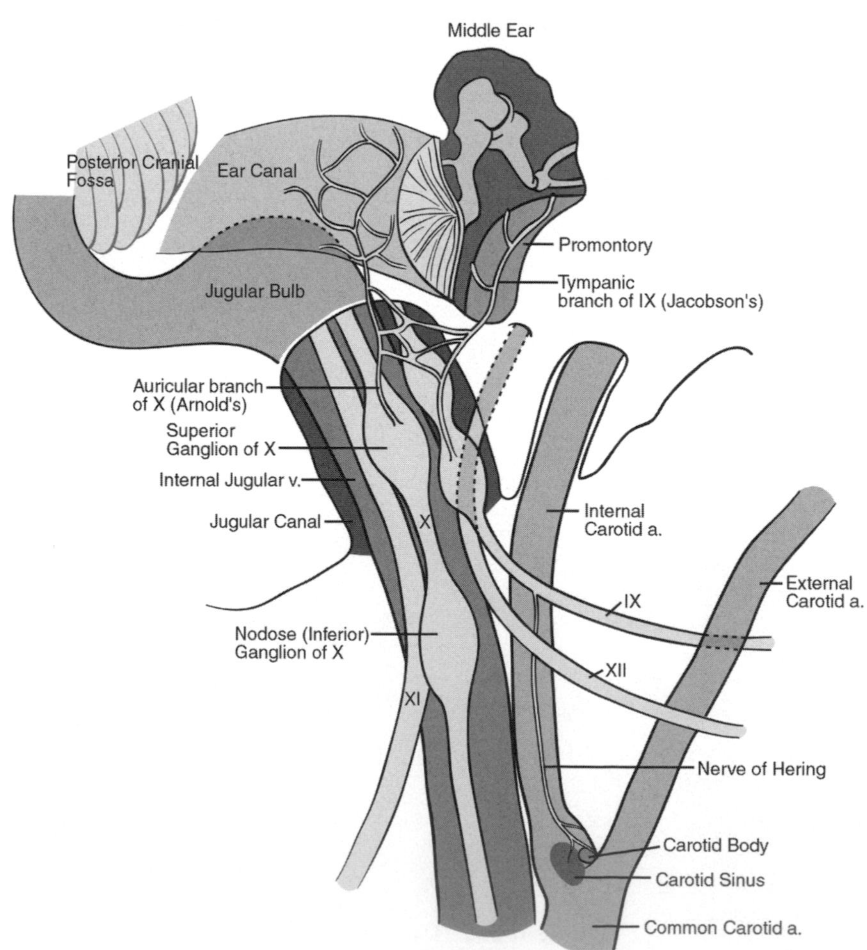

Figure 28.3 Anatomy of common sites of head and neck paraganglia.

ically identical, the neoplasms that arise from them, namely jugular paragangliomas and tympanic paragangliomas, each exhibit distinct clinical behavior that has important diagnostic and therapeutic implications.

Jugulotympanic paraganglia located along Jacobson's nerve arise from the glossopharyngeal nerve, whereas those located along Arnold's nerve are related to the vagus nerve or the glossopharyngeal nerve via anastomoses with the vagus nerve (24). The inferior tympanic branch of the ascending pharyngeal artery serves as the major blood supply to all paraganglia of the jugulotympanic region (24).

Vagal Paraganglia

In contrast to the carotid body, vagal paraganglia are not organized into discrete bodies, but rather are small cell groups dispersed within the perineurium, below the nerve sheath or between nerve fiber fascicles (7). Although they may occur anywhere along the course of the vagus nerve, they are most often located within or just below the nodose (inferior) ganglion and less often within the middle and jugular (superior) ganglion. The jugular ganglion lies within the jugular foramen, with the middle ganglion lying just below the jugular ganglion. The nodose ganglion is the largest, measuring approximately 2.5 cm in length, and is located high in the neck, below the jugular foramen and posterior to the internal carotid artery (ICA) (26) (Fig. 28.3). The vagal paraganglia are adjacent to the CN IX to XII, the sympathetic trunk, jugular vein, and ICA at or just below the skull base. This anatomic relation has important implications in the presentation and management of vagal paragangliomas.

Microscopic Anatomy

The typical microscopic appearance of paraganglia is characterized by organized clusters (zellballen) of chief (type I) cells surrounded by sustentacular (type II) cells embedded in a web of small vessels (24). The chief cells have large round or oval nuclei and abundant, finely granular cytoplasm containing neurosecretory granules that store catecholamines. Two forms of chief cells have been described: the more abundant "light" cell containing clear cytoplasm and uniform spherical granules, and "dark" cells with a dense cytoplasm and irregular granules (7). The sustentacular cells are elongated, have dense ovoid nuclei, have no neurosecretory granules, and are structurally related to the satellite cells of the autonomic ganglia (27). They give off thin cytoplasmic processes that surround aggregates of chief cells, resulting in an organoid appearance (28), and, closely resembling a Schwann cell, the sustentacular cells ensheathe nerve axons (19).

PARAGANGLIOMAS

Evolution of Terms

Our present knowledge of head and neck paragangliomas has evolved over the last century, prompted by advances in science and medicine. Although technologic advances in molecular biology, immunohistology, medical imaging, and the development of the electron microscope have greatly contributed to our understanding of these tumors, this has also led to a confusing array of terms, occasionally resulting in further misunderstanding of these complex lesions.

The carotid body was discovered over 200 years ago and was thought to be a ganglion due to its relationship with the intercarotid nervous plexus (29). Determining that the carotid body was histologically distinct from a ganglion, Kohn in 1900 coined the term "paraganglion" (30,31). In the 1930s, "nonchromaffin paraganglioma" was introduced by Watzka to distinguish the extraadrenal paraganglia from the chromaffin-reacting tissue related to catecholamine production of the adrenal medulla. This has since proved to be nonspecific and inaccurate because the granules within the chief cells of paragangliomas do contain catecholamines. The terms *glomus body* and *glomus jugularis* were introduced by Guild (25) in 1941 when describing a vascular mass in the dome of the jugular bulb and the promontory of the middle ear. Rosenwasser (32), in 1945, was the first to realize that certain vascular middle ear tumors resembling carotid body-like tumors were neoplasms of Guild's glomus jugulare. Mulligan (33) proposed the term *chemodectoma* in 1950, emphasizing the chemoreceptor function of paraganglia. In 1974, Glenner and Grimley proposed a classification system for paraganglia and the tumors that arise from them (Fig. 28.2). Although this classification is the basis for the current nomenclature (e.g., jugular paraganglioma, tympanic paraganglioma, vagal paraganglioma), the term *carotid body tumor* remains popular.

Microscopic Pathology

Paragangliomas are highly vascular tumors and typically retain the general organoid appearance of normal paraganglia with clusters (zellballen) of chief (type I) cells (7,27) and peripheral sustentacular cells (type II) surrounded by a fibrovascular stroma. Chief cells predominate and, when compared with nonneoplastic chief cells, they reveal cytologic pleomorphism with ovoid to polyhedral cells. The nuclei appear vesicular to hyperchromatic and may be round to ovoid in shape (7). Mitotic figures are rare. Electron microscopy identification of neurosecretory cytoplasm granules is similar to those in normal chief cells and is characteristic of paragangliomas (27). Immunohistochemical techniques aid in the pathologic identification of paragangliomas. Chromogranin, synaptophysin, and neuron-specific enolase (NSE) identify chief cells, and S-100 is picked up by sustentacular cells.

Jyung et al. (34) recently reported the expression of angiogenic growth factors in paragangliomas including vascular endothelial growth factor (VEGF) and platelet-derived endothelial cell growth factor (PD-ECGF). These growth factors appear to be important signals in tumor angiogenesis and in part may be responsible for the marked vascularity of head and neck paragangliomas.

The histologic criteria for the diagnosis of a malignant paragangliomas are nonspecific and are frequently identified in benign paragangliomas. These features include increased mitotic activity, central necrosis of the cell nest, and vascular space invasion (35). S-100 staining is often diminished in malignant paragangliomas, indicating a loss of sustentacular cells (6,17,27). Abnormal DNA content is common in paragangliomas and is not indicative of malignancy (17). There is no definite relationship between mitotic activity, perineural or vascular invasion, and the potential for malignant behavior (7,17,36).

Although local invasion is sometimes considered a manifestation of aggressive disease, most pathologists believe malignancy should be diagnosed only by the presence of metastases to regional lymph nodes or distant sites (23,37). Histologically "benign" paragangliomas may locally invade vital structures, including the skull base and adjacent neural and vascular structures, and result in significant nerve dysfunction (37).

Incidence

Paragangliomas of the head and neck are rare tumors, accounting for only 0.012% of tumors reviewed by the surgical pathol-

TABLE 28.1 Distribution of Paragangliomas

Paraganglioma	Number
Carotid body tumor	28
Jugular paraganglioma	14
Vagal paraganglioma	5
Tympanic paraganglioma	3
Other (laryngeal, sphenoid, C-spine)	3
Total	53

ogy department of Memorial Sloan-Kettering from 1938 to 1975 (38). Reports of the relative distribution of paragangliomas in the head and neck are conflicting, which may be due to the variation in nomenclature. Investigators often categorize jugular and tympanic paragangliomas as a single entity (27,31,38). Other reports are from institutions that may have a biased referred patient population (38). The carotid body is the most common site of paragangliomas in the head and neck. Carotid body tumors (CBTs), jugular paragangliomas, and tympanic paragangliomas account for 80% of all head and neck paragangliomas (27), and vagal paragangliomas, another 5% (23). Nasal, orbital, laryngeal, and other paragangliomas occur much less frequently. Our review of 47 patients with 53 paragangliomas treated over a 10-year period (1990–2000) is consistent with the relative incidence of specific paragangliomas as reported by others (Table 28.1) (39).

HIGH-ALTITUDE POPULATION

There is a marked increased incidence of carotid body hypertrophy (40) and CBTs in populations living at high altitudes (41,42), most likely related to chronic hypoxemia (43). Compared with populations living at sea level, there is a ninefold increased incidence of CBTs in those dwelling between 2,000 and 3,000 m above sea level and a 12-fold increase incidence in those living between 3,000 and 4,500 m above sea level (41). Rodriguez-Cuevas et al. (41) reported a retrospective analysis of 120 cases of CBTs occurring in inhabitants living at high altitude (>2,200 m above sea level). As compared with cases occurring in populations living below 1,500 m above sea level, they noted a higher female predominance (8.3:1 vs. 2:1), a lower rate of bilaterality (5% vs. 10–20%), and a less frequent familial history (1% vs. 7–25%). A higher incidence of carotid body hypertrophy (43) and CBTs has also been noted in patients with chronic obstructive pulmonary disease, perhaps related to chronically low pO_2 levels (44).

FAMILIAL OCCURRENCE

There is a well-documented familial occurrence of paragangliomas. The genetic transmission of familial paragangliomas is autosomal dominant with highly variable expressivity and reduced penetrance (45). There is a form of genomic imprinting whereby, regardless of the clinical status of the mother or father, only the paternally transmitted gene leads to symptoms, and the maternally transmitted gene results in carriership without developing tumors (45–47). A detailed family history is essential both for proper patient management and for investigation of family members to identify occult paragangliomas (48). Advances in genetic mapping have linked hereditary paragangliomas to at least two gene loci: 11q23 (47) and 11q13 loci (49).

The known patterns of inheritance and genomic imprinting allows genetic counseling to become more accurate when considering the parent of origin, sex of the patient, and the DNA linkage diagnosis (45). The use of genetic counseling and the subsequent MRI scanning of at-risk individuals has resulted in the detection of small, asymptomatic tumors. The discovery of an early-stage paraganglioma poses a dilemma in management in light of its natural history of slow growth. Some paragangliomas, especially very small ones, have been shown not to be progressive, and a "wait and scan" management may be advisable (50).

Familial or hereditary paragangliomas have been previously reported to account for 5% to 10% (51,52) of all cases of head and neck paragangliomas, but it appears that these estimates were low due to the complex mode of inheritance and variable phenotypic expression (45). It may in actually account for up to 25% to 50% of cases (46,48). Most (90%) cases of hereditary paragangliomas involve the carotid body (36). If a familial history is present, there is a 78% to 87% possibility of multiple paragangliomas (52,53). Bilateral carotid body paragangliomas occur more frequently with familial cases (31.8%) than nonfamilial cases (4.4%) (51). Conversely, data suggest that younger patients who have paraganglia that are multifocal should be evaluated for possible genetic etiology (48).

MULTICENTRIC PARAGANGLIOMAS

Multiple paragangliomas may be present in up to 22% of patients (51,53,54). Approximately 10% of nonfamilial paragangliomas are multicentric (31). The most common multicentric combination is two CBTs (51), which occurs in approximately 20% of patients with CBTs (31). In our series, 5 of 47 patients (11%) with paragangliomas presented with multiple tumors, most commonly another CBT.

The potential to develop multicentric tumors has important clinical implications. The presence of bilateral carotid body paragangliomas presents a difficult challenge in management due to the loss of baroreceptive function and subsequent refractory hypertension following CBT surgery. Multiple tumors, including vagal or jugular paragangliomas, present problems concerning significant morbidity of multiple lower CN dysfunction, perhaps bilaterally, either by direct tumor involvement or resulting from surgical resection. Because multicentric tumors may be metachronous, routine follow-up MRI imaging is indicated.

MALIGNANT VARIANT

Malignant paragangliomas are uncommon. As previously mentioned, the most important criterion of malignancy is documented lymph node or distant metastatic tumor because the histologic examination of the primary tumor is unreliable for establishing a malignant diagnosis. The prevalence of malignancy depends on the site of the primary tumor, and there has been considerable variability in the reported frequency. Malignant CBT has been reported in up to 20% of patients, but most reports indicate a rate of 3% to 6% of cases (55). The metastatic rate to the regional lymph nodes is unknown (56). The most common sites of distant CBT metastases are the bones, lungs, and liver (57). Malignancy is less common in familial paragangliomas compared with sporadic cases. Grufferman et al. (51), in a literature review of CBTs, found a malignancy rate of 12% in nonfamilial tumor compared with a 2% rate in familial tumors. The jugulotympanic paraganglioma malignancy rate ranges widely from less than 1% to 25%, but is most often reported as about 5% (58). The most common sites of metastases, in decreasing incidence, are the lungs, lymph nodes, liver, vertebrae, ribs, and spleen (59). Although the reported rate of malignancy of vagal paragangliomas is as high as 19% (60), a 10% frequency is accepted, with the regional lymph nodes and lungs as the most common sites of metastases (61). Vagal paragangliomas probably represent the highest rate of malignancy of the more common types of head and neck paraganglioma. Primary orbital and laryngeal tumors demonstrate the highest malignant rate of head and neck paragangliomas in 20% to 25% of cases (31).

Pacheco-Ojeda et al. (56), in a review of 43 cases of malignant CBTs, found that locoregional control requires primary tumor resection and neck dissection followed by radiation therapy. There may be a long time interval between primary resection and the appearance of a metastatic lesion, ranging from 20 months to 20 years. The growth rate of metastases is slow with a doubling time of 2,000 days. Disseminated disease is relatively unresponsive to chemotherapy.

Growth Rate

Paragangliomas are slow-growing tumors with a mean growth rate of 1.0 mm/year and a median doubling time of 4.2 years. Jansen et al. (50) reported no significant growth (>20% increase in volume) in 40% of head and neck paragangliomas followed by serial MRI or CT scan for a mean follow-up period of approximately 4.5 years. They also report less growth in very small and very large paragangliomas compared with intermediate-size tumors, suggesting a biphasic growth pattern (50).

FUNCTIONING PARAGANGLIOMAS

Although all paragangliomas have the potential of releasing vasoactive substances such as catecholamines and dopamine (4,61), only 1% to 3% of paragangliomas produce associated clinical findings (4,62). A four- to fivefold elevation of serum norepinephrine is necessary to produce symptoms (28), suggestive of increased catecholamine levels including excessive sweating, hypertension, tachycardia, nervousness, and weight loss (4). Urinary laboratory screening tests, including 24-hour urinary metanephrine (normal <1.3 mg) and VMA levels (normal value is 1.8 to 7.0 mg), are frequently elevated 10 to 15 times normal in patients with actively secreting tumors (4). Serum catecholamine levels, including serum norepinephrine and epinephrine, are also of value in the evaluation of patient. Because head and neck paragangliomas do not have the ability to secrete epinephrine, an elevated serum epinephrine level is suggestive of a concurrent pheochromocytoma (4). There have been several reports of association between pheochromocytoma and both familial and nonfamilial paragangliomas (63–65). Paragangliomas may occur in patients with familial multiple endocrine neoplasia (MEN), both type IIA (pheochromocytoma, medullary thyroid carcinoma, and parathyroid hyperplasia), and type IIB (also includes mucosal neuromas) (66).

Clinical Presentation—Signs, Symptoms, and Patterns of Spread

CAROTID BODY TUMOR

The carotid body is located in the adventitia of the posterior medial aspect of the common carotid artery bifurcation. On gross examination, CBTs are dark tan to purple in color and usually well circumscribed. As the paraganglioma grows, it tends to splay the carotid bifurcation and progressively involve the carotid adventitia (Fig. 28.4). Classically, the ICA is displaced posteriorly and laterally (67). With continued growth, the tumor extends superiorly along the internal carotid to the skull base and may affect adjacent CNs, most commonly the vagal and hypoglossal nerves. Occasionally the sympathetic chain is involved. The intense vascularity of the tumor effects adjacent structures with a suffusion of dilated blood vessels, including the epineurium of nerves.

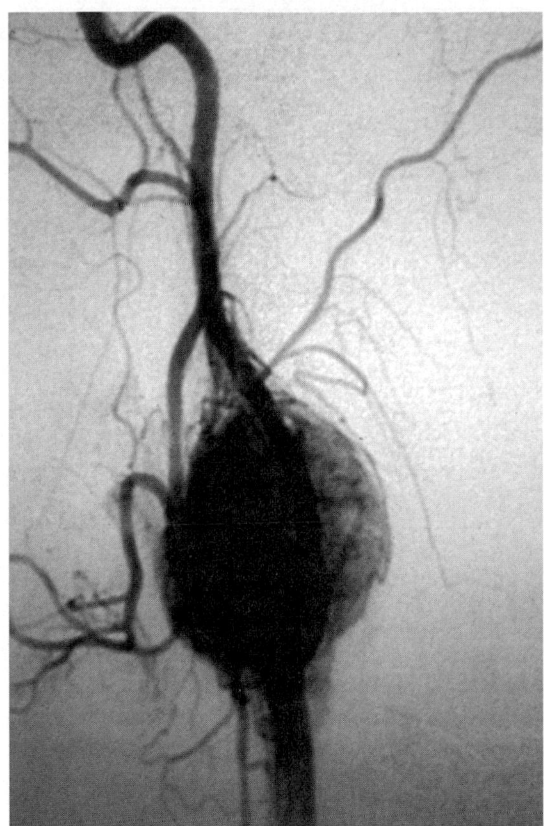

Figure 28.4 Subtracted carotid angiogram demonstrating carotid body tumor splaying the carotid bifurcation.

The median age at presentation is 45 to 54 years, with a range of 12 to 78 years, and most series report a female predominance of approximately 2:1 (68–70).

Carotid body tumors almost always present as a palpable anterolateral neck mass, located at or superior to the carotid bifurcation and deep to the sternomastoid muscle (67,68). In our series, 68% of patients noted an enlarging neck mass and 79% had an evident mass on physical examination (Tables 28.2 and 28.3). Carotid body tumors are slow growing and often are present for months to years before the patient seeks medical attention. On palpation, they are typically vertically fixed and later-

TABLE 28.2 Paraganglioma Symptom

	CBT (n = 28)	JP (n = 14)	VP (n = 5)	TP (n = 3)
Neck mass	19	—	2	—
Tinnitus	—	11	—	3
Pulsatile	—	7	—	2
Dysphagia	—	5	2	—
Hearing loss	—	7	—	—
Hoarseness	—	4	2	—
Pain	3	2	—	1
Vertigo	—	5	—	—
Otorrhea	—	3	—	1
Facial weakness	—	4	—	—

CBT, carotid body tumor; JP, jugular paraganglia; TP, tympanic paraganglioma; VP, vagal paraganglioma.

TABLE 28.3 Paragangliomas: Physical Findings

	CBT (n=28)	JP (n=14)	VP (n=5)	TP (n=3)
Neck mass	22	1	2	—
Nonpulsatile	12	—	2	—
Pulsatile	10	1	—	—
Cranial nerve deficit				
V	—	2	—	—
VII	—	2	—	—
VIII	—	8	—	—
IX	—	3	1	—
X	—	4	1	—
XI	—	—	1	—
XII	—	8	—	—
Ear mass	—	5	—	3
Parapharyngeal mass	2	—	2	—

CBT, carotid body tumor; JP, jugular paraganglia; TP, tympanic paraganglioma; VP, vagal paraganglioma.

ally mobile due to its fixation to the carotid artery (67,70,71) and may be pulsatile (67). Bruits have been reported in 10% to 16% of cases (69,70,72). Pain is present in slightly more than a quarter of the cases (68,69). Medial extension into the parapharyngeal space is reported in 20% of cases and may cause submucosal bulging of the lateral oropharynx (69,73). Cranial nerve neuropathies are present in approximately 10% to 30% of cases at presentation (69,74,75), In some large CBTs, continued growth results in extension to the skull base with bony erosion.

Patients may occasionally present with a history of having undergone an open incisional biopsy, after unsuspecting surgeons assumed they were operating on an enlarged cervical lymph node. Open biopsy should be avoided due to the risk for hemorrhage (76). Brisk bleeding of the mass fixed to the carotid results in an incisional biopsy, which leads to increased hemorrhage and subsequent fibrosis at the operative site. If the diagnosis of CBT is suspected, incisional biopsy is contraindicated. Fine-needle aspiration biopsy may be safely performed with minimal risk for bleeding from this highly vascular tumor.

Grouping of CBTs according to size and vessel involvement has not been consistent in the literature, although the Shamblin (55) classification is based on surgical findings related to carotid artery involvement (Table 28.4).

JUGULAR AND TYMPANIC PARAGANGLIOMAS

Although jugular and tympanic paragangliomas have often been reported as a single entity (i.e., temporal bone paragangliomas), their distinction has important clinical and therapeutic implications. In recognizing the importance of this distinction, as well as to ensure uniformity of nomenclature and comparison of treatment outcome, various classification systems have developed over the years that have been revised as more advanced imaging and surgical techniques have been introduced. In 1962, Alford and Guilford (77) coined the term "glomus tympanicum" to describe those tumors originating from paraganglia within the middle ear and confined to the middle space, as opposed to the "glomus jugulare" of the temporal bone that develop from the jugular bulb and extend to the middle ear cleft and skull base. Fisch (78) subsequently modified a classification system based on tumor extension (Table 28.5). The Glasscock-Jackson classification, based on both the site of origin and extent of tumor involvement, was introduced in 1982 (Table 28.6) (79). These latter two classification systems are most often used today and provide a staging system for comparison of treatment results.

TABLE 28.4 Shamblin's Surgical Classification of Carotid Body Tumors

Group I	Tumors are relatively small with minimal attachment to the carotid vessels
Group II	Tumors are larger with moderate arterial attachment and can be resected with precise surgical dissection
Group III	Larger tumors encasing the carotid arteries and can be resected only with arterial sacrifice

TABLE 28.5 Classification of Temporal Bone Paragangliomas

Class A	Tumors arising along the tympanic plexus on the middle ear promontory
Class B	Tumors arising from the inferior tympanic canal of the hypotympanum; may invade the middle ear and mastoid; cortical bone over jugular bulb is intact; carotid canal is intact
Class C	Tumors arising in dome of jugular bulb and involving the overlying cortical bone
C1	Tumors eroding the carotid canal, but not involving the carotid artery
C2	Tumors involving the vertical carotid canal
C3	Tumors involving the horizontal carotid canal; foramen lacerum free tumor
C4	Tumors involving the foramen lacerum and the cavernous sinus
Class D	Tumors with intracranial extension of posterior fossa
De1	Extradural tumor of less than 2 cm medial dural displacement
De2	Extradural tumor of more than 2 cm medial dural displacement
Di1	Intradural tumor less than 2 cm
Di2	Intradural tumors more than 2 cm
Di3	Neurosurgically unresectable tumors

Source: Modified from Fisch V, Mattox D. *Microsurgery of the skull base.* New York: Thieme, 1988:149–153.

TABLE 28.6 Glasscock-Jackson Classification of Glomus Tumors

Glomus tympanicum	
Type 1	Small mass limited to the promontory
Type II	Tumor completely filling the middle ear space
Type III	Tumor filling the middle ear and extending into the mastoid
Type IV	Tumor filling the middle ear, extending into the mastoid or through the tympanic membrane to fill the external auditory canal; may also extend anterior to the internal carotid artery
Glomus jugulare	
Type I	Small tumor involving the jugular bulb, middle ear, and mastoid
Type II	Tumor extending under the internal auditory canal; may have intracranial extension
Type III	Tumor extending into petrous apex; may have intracranial extension
Type IV	Tumor extending beyond the petrous apex into the clivus or infratemporal fossa; may have intracranial extension

Routes of Spread

Tympanic paragangliomas arise from the paraganglia associated with Jacobson's or Arnold's nerves. They may fill the middle ear cavity and extend posteriorly into the mastoid air cells or inferiorly to the jugular bulb. Within the middle ear, continued growth results in ossicular involvement and a resulting conductive hearing loss. Otorrhea and polyp formation may occur, especially with extension through the tympanic membrane. Continued growth with vestibular involvement produces a sensorineural hearing loss, vertigo, and occasionally pain from the associated inflammatory response.

Jugular paragangliomas tend to spread along the paths of least resistance in multiple directions and gain access to various portions of the temporal bone and base of skull neurovascular foramina. With progressive extensive temporal involvement, additional growth leads to posterior cranial fossa involvement. Intracranial extension can occur via several pathways: posteriorly, directly through the petrous bone, extension into and through the internal auditory canal, or infralabyrinthine extension (80,81). There is early intraluminal jugular extension into the sigmoid sinus and internal jugular vein with possible growth into the inferior petrosal sinus. Tumor can invade into the middle ear cleft, the petrous apex, or into the mastoid and retrofacial air cells with a resulting facial nerve paralysis. Inferiorly, jugular paragangliomas may extend into the infratemporal fossa and post-styloid parapharyngeal space into the neck (Fig. 28.5).

Signs and Symptoms

As with other paragangliomas of the head and neck, jugular and tympanic paragangliomas are slow growing and are occasionally present for many years before diagnosis. Symptoms are typically present for 2 to 3 years (82). The progression of symptoms depends on the location and size of the paraganglioma and the direction of spread.

Tympanic paragangliomas occur most commonly during the sixth decade of life, have a marked female preponderance, and usually present with a conductive hearing loss, pulsatile tinnitus, and a mass behind the tympanic membrane (82) (Table 28.2). On otoscopic examination, a red-blue middle ear mass that blanches on positive pneumatoscopic pressure (Brown's sign) may be present (Table 28.3). Perforation of tumor through the tympanic membrane may occur, producing a vascular "polyp" that may bleed spontaneously. With vestibular invasion, sensorineural hearing loss and vertigo develop. Jugular paragangliomas that invade the middle ear result in signs and symptoms similar to those of a tympanic paraganglioma, but a CT scan evaluation usually can distinguish the two by the presence or absence of erosion of the bony plate at the lateral aspect of the jugular fossa.

Jugular paragangliomas most commonly occur in the fifth and sixth decades of life (83) and demonstrate a female to male ratio of 4:1 to 6:1 (28,77,82). They often demonstrate early skull base involvement, with extension into the middle ear and internal jugular vein. Superior extension into the middle ear results in symptoms similar to tympanic paragangliomas and may result in a conductive or sensorineural hearing loss, depending on the extent of vestibular involvement (1,39). Hearing loss (55–58%) and tinnitus (56–66%) are the most common presenting symptoms (82,84,85) (Table 28.2). Symptoms related to lower CN deficits (VII–XII) are also common. Persky et al. (39) report that in their series all patients with jugular or vagal paragangliomas had dysfunction of at least one CN (Table 28.3). Ogura et al. (84) report that 27 of 72 (38%) patients with jugular paragangliomas had a least one CN palsy at presentation. Gardner et al. (85), in their series of 36 patients, report 58% of

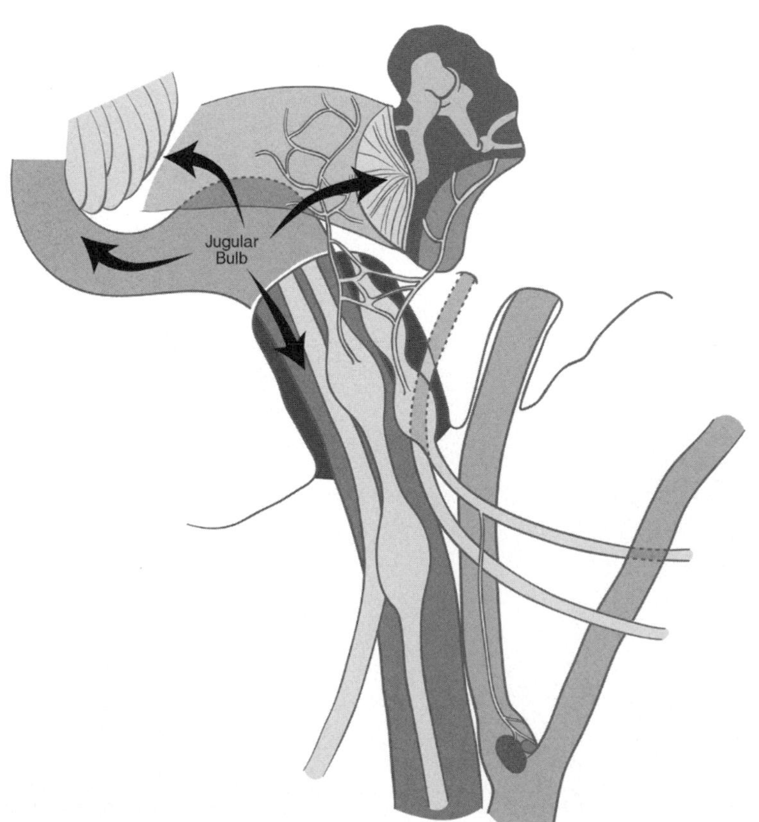

Figure 28.5 Patterns of spread of jugular paragangliomas.

patients with jugular paragangliomas exhibited at least one CN dysfunction before surgery, with 28% having VIII nerve dysfunction alone. Tumors of the skull base without extensive middle ear extension may present with isolated tongue weakness, hoarseness, dysphagia, or shoulder drop, or with symptoms of multiple CN dysfunction. The jugular foramen syndrome (CN IX, X, XI palsy or Vernet syndrome) is occasionally encountered, and CN IX to XII palsy (Collet-Sicard syndrome) occurs in approximately 10% of jugular paragangliomas (82).

VAGAL PARAGANGLIOMAS

Vagal paragangliomas (VPs) are uncommon and account for up to 5% of all head and neck paragangliomas (36,53). Although they most commonly arise from the nodose (inferior) ganglion, VPs may also originate from the middle and superior ganglion and less frequently anywhere along the course of the vagus nerve. Compared with the discrete carotid body, vagal paraganglia are distributed more diffusely within the nerve or perineurium. Vagus nerve fibers fan out or "splay over" the surface of the VP, or early in their development enter the substance of the tumor, and therefore preservation of the vagus nerve is usually not possible with complete tumor resection (53,86,87).

Vagal paragangliomas are ovoid or spindle-shaped tumors and most commonly present as an asymptomatic mass of the upper neck, typically more cephalad than CBTs. Vagal paragangliomas have three basic patterns of spread (53) (Fig. 28.6). Because most VPs originate at the inferior (nodose) ganglion, the tumor tends to spread inferiorly into the post-styloid parapharyngeal area. Extension superiorly toward the skull base in the area of the jugular foramen results in early involvement of the internal jugular vein, adjacent CNs (IX, XI, XII), and ICA, manifesting the typical anterior displacement of this artery (Fig. 28.7). Paragangliomas presumably arising from the middle ganglion, termed "paraganglioma juxtavagale," typically extend into the jugular foramen. Vagal paragangliomas originating from the superior ganglion have a greater chance of assuming a "dumbbell" form with posterior cranial fossa tumor in addition to parapharyngeal extension inferiorly. Parapharyngeal extension may cause a bulge of the lateral oropharyngeal wall and medial displacement of the tonsils. It may not be possible to determine the site of origin with larger tumors.

Vagal paragangliomas are slow growing with a female to male preponderance of 2:1 to 3:1 and a mean duration of symptoms of 2 to 3 years before presentation (36,53,82,88). The most common symptom is a slowly growing, asymptomatic upper neck mass. As the tumor enlarges, it encroaches on the lower CNs and the adjacent sympathetic chain. Various authors report that 33% to 50% of patients have CN neuropathy at presentation (39,82,86,87), involving, in decreasing frequency, the vagal (20–47%), hypoglossal, spinal accessory, and sympathetic plexus nerves (Table 28.3). Signs and symptoms include unilateral vocal cord paralysis, hoarseness, dysphagia, nasal regurgitation, atrophy of the hemitongue, shoulder weakness, and Horner syndrome. Hearing loss and pulsatile tinnitus implies temporal bone extension. The progression of symptoms is often helpful in differentiating VPs from other head and neck paragangliomas. Leonetti et al. (73) reported on five cases of VPs with vocal cord paralysis and hearing loss or tinnitus. In all cases, vocal cord symptoms preceded otologic symptoms by 2 to 2½ years. The initial presence of vocal cord paralysis with or without hoarseness helps differentiate VPs from CBTs (87).

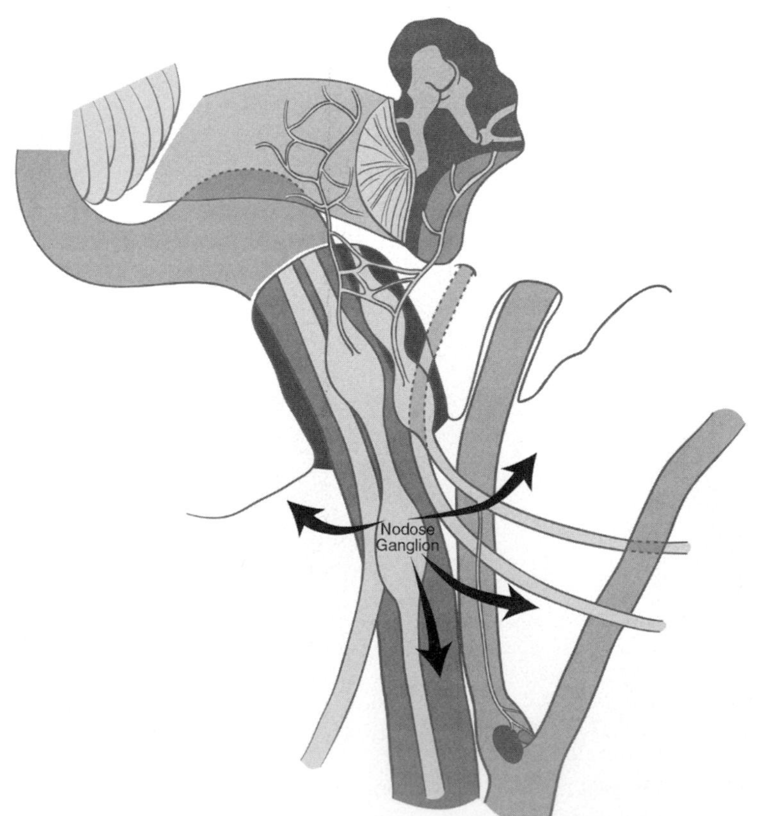

Figure 28.6 Patterns of spread of vagal paragangliomas with nodose ganglion origin.

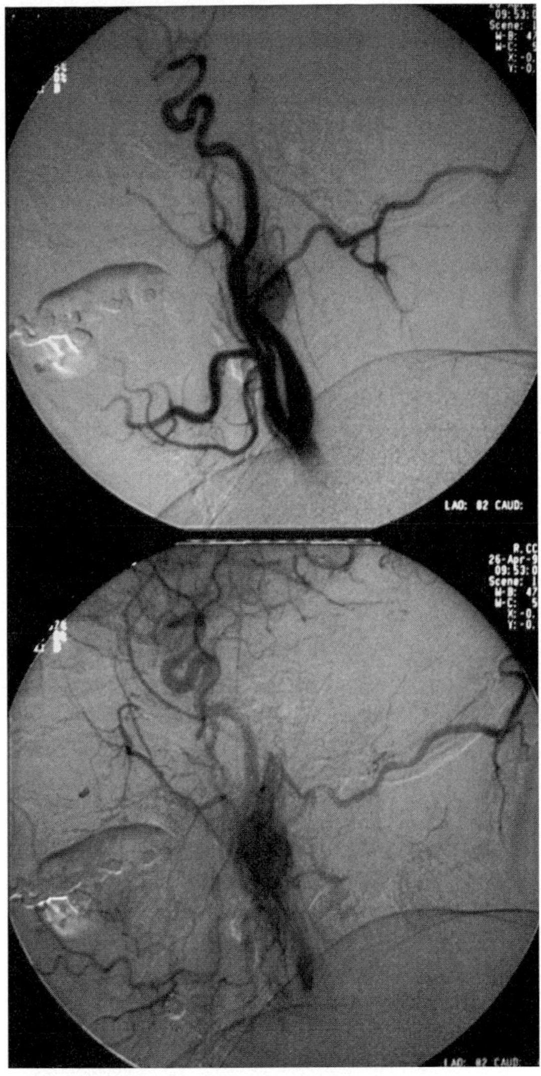

Figure 28.7 Subtracted lateral view of carotid angiogram demonstrating anterior displacement of the internal carotid artery by a vagal paraganglioma (note the vascular tumor blush).

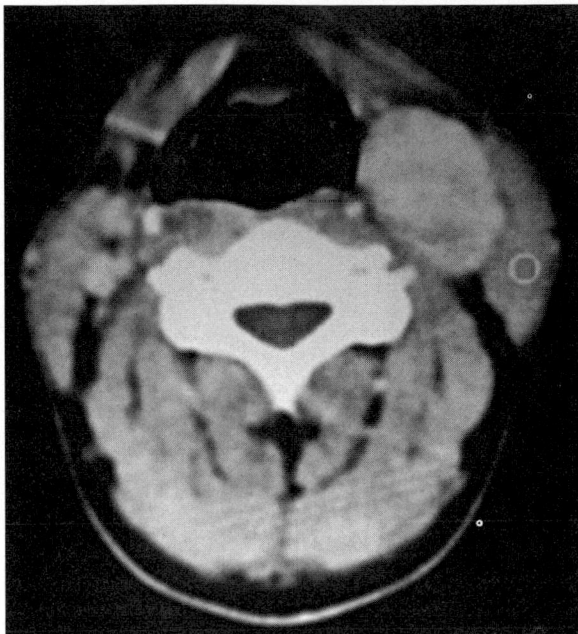

Figure 28.8 Axial computed tomography with contrast revealing a markedly enhancing carotid body tumor.

Diagnostic Evaluation

COMPUTED TOMOGRAPHY

Computed tomography is an excellent imaging technique to identify paragangliomas and to document the extent of tumor with precise evaluation of bone invasion. The classic CT findings of paragangliomas include a homogeneous mass with intense enhancement following intravenous contrast administration (Fig. 28.8). Although this appearance is typical of paragangliomas, it may be seen with other vascular tumors. Tumor location, displacement of major vessels, and patterns of involvement or invasion of surrounding structures aid in the differential diagnosis, which may include neurolemmoma and meningioma (1).

Carotid body tumors typically appear as a well-defined enhancing mass that splays the common carotid bifurcation with posterolateral displacement of the ICA (23). Less often, larger tumors may reveal heterogeneous contrast enhancement secondary to areas of focal thrombi and hemorrhage (89). Vagal paragangliomas may be differentiated from CBTs with CT because they tend to displace both the internal and external carotid arteries anteriorly. Skull base extension of VPs is associated with erosion and widening of the jugular foramen, which is well visualized on CT imaging.

Jugular paragangliomas have similar imaging qualities to other paragangliomas, but early involvement of the skull base and subsequent intracranial extension results in characteristic findings. Thin CT sections (1–3 mm) are necessary to adequately evaluate the intricate anatomy of the temporal bone. Early findings include enlargement of the jugular foramen with irregularity of the bony margins. With tumor enlargement there is the typical "moth-eaten" appearance of the jugular foramen and destruction of adjacent bone, including the caroticojugular spine (23). Erosion of this bony spine is helpful in differentiating jugular paragangliomas that have invaded the middle ear from tympanic paragangliomas originating in the mesotympanum (90). As the tumor continues to grow, it tends to follow the path of least resistance by extending superiorly into the middle ear (23) (Fig. 28.9) Ossicular chain destruction is common. Tumor extension inferiorly results in involvement of the internal jugular vein and infratemporal fossa (23). Intraluminal involvement of the internal jugular vein may extend inferiorly into the neck and superiorly into the sigmoid and transverse sinuses (Fig. 28.10). Lateral extension results in the invasion of the facial nerve canal and infiltration of the nerve (80). Intracranial extension into the posterior fossa occurs by three main routes spread: posteriorly, directly through the petrous bone (80,81); medially, via the intrameatal route into the cerebellopontine angle; and into the cerebellomedullary angle via the infralabyrinthine-inframeatal route (81).

Computed tomographic findings in tympanic paragangliomas usually define a small discrete mass arising from the cochlear promontory and confined to the tympanic cavity (80,81). Ossicular destruction is not typical. Although large lesions may encase the ossicles, ossicular destruction is unusual (80). The presence of air and/or bone between a tympanic cavity mass and the jugular bulb characterizes the tumor as a tympanic paraganglioma rather than a jugular paraganglioma (1).

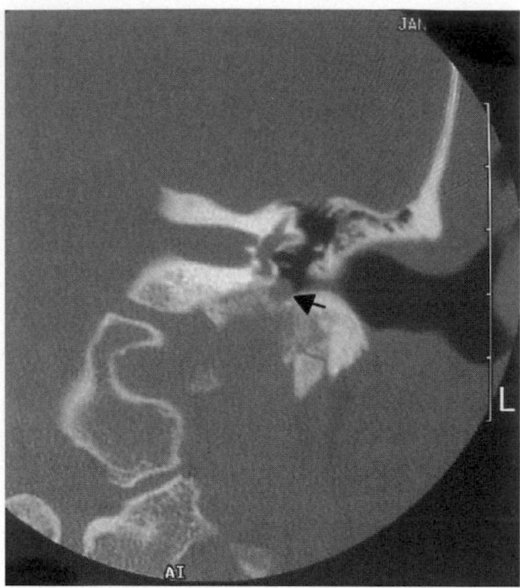

Figure 28.9 Coronal computed tomography of the temporal demonstrating a jugular paraganglioma extending into the hypotympanum (*arrow*). Note the "moth-eaten" appearance of the bony jugular bulb.

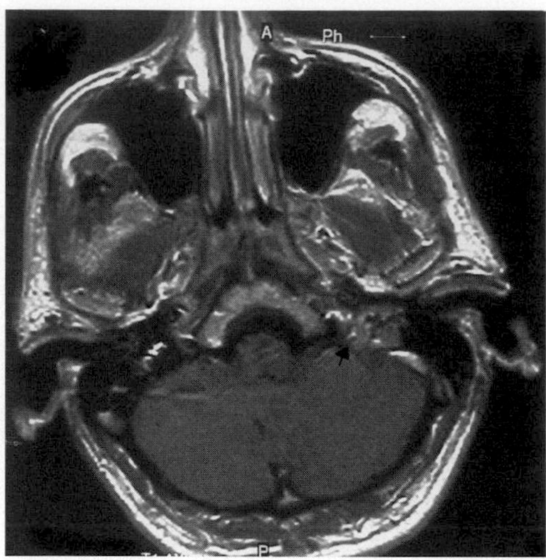

Figure 28.11 Axial magnetic resonance imaging demonstrating petrous bone involvement with a jugular paraganglioma and extension into the posterior cranial fossa (*arrow*).

Posterior extension into the mastoid air cells and anterior extension into the eustachian canal and nasopharynx is uncommon (91).

MAGNETIC RESONANCE IMAGING

Although CT is the study of choice to evaluate bone involvement, MRI provides meticulous soft tissue detail and defines skull base, intracranial, dural, and neural involvement, especially with gadolinium enhancement (39) (Fig. 28.11). Augmented by its ability to image in multiple plans, MRI is superior to CT in defining paragangliomas' relation to adjacent vascular and skull base structures. Carotid body tumors can readily be seen splaying the common carotid bifurcation and displacing the ICA posteriorly and laterally, differentiating it from VPs, which bow the ICA anteriorly (39).

Magnetic resonance imaging studies of paragangliomas demonstrate a background tumor matrix of intermediate-intensity signal on T1-weighted and proton density–weighted images and moderately high-intensity signal on T2-weighted images along with scattered areas of focal signal voids, reflecting high-flow blood vessels (92). Intense homogeneous contrast enhancement is seen (92). On T2-weighted images, the classical

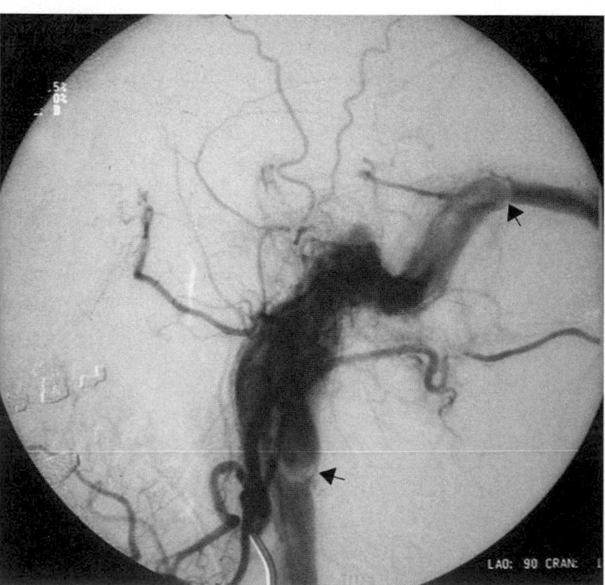

Figure 28.10 Subtracted lateral view of late (venous) phase carotid angiogram demonstrating an extensive intraluminal jugular paraganglioma extending from the transverse sinus superiorly to the internal jugular vein inferiorly (*arrows*).

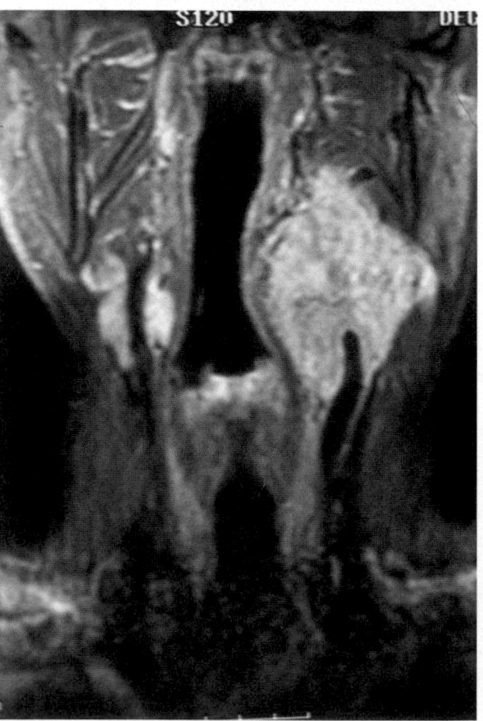

Figure 28.12 Magnetic resonance imaging, T2-weighted study with gadolinium, coronal view demonstrates bilateral carotid body tumors and the "salt and pepper" appearance so common to paragangliomas. Note parapharyngeal extension with bulging of the adjacent oropharyngeal wall.

MRI "salt and pepper" appearance, originally described by Olsen et al. (93) and present in most lesions greater than 1.5 cm in size, reflects signal voids intermixed with regions of focally high signal intensity, the latter of which are probably due to slow flow within the image plane (92) (Fig. 28.12). These findings, however, are not specific for paragangliomas, and may be seen with other hypervascular lesions (e.g., metastatic renal cell carcinoma and thyroid carcinoma). The paragangliomas' typically smooth contour, signal characteristics, and location, coupled with a detailed clinical history and physical findings, should result in an accurate diagnosis.

Magnetic resonance imaging is more effective than CT in identifying small synchronous paragangliomas, especially those tumors smaller than 5 mm. But CT is most effective in demonstrating lesions greater than 8 mm (94).

Magnetic resonance angiography (MRA) provides excellent visualization of the major head and neck vasculature and can demonstrate vessel displacement (Fig. 28.13), gross tumor involvement, and possible compromised blood flow. As previously stated, variations in vessel displacement can differentiate between paragangliomas (e.g., CBT vs. vagal paraganglioma). Magnetic resonance angiography may be useful in defining flow-related enhancement of lesions larger than 1.5 cm (23). Although three-dimension time-of-flight (3D TOF) angiography appears to be superior to other MRA techniques in identifying some tumor feeders, its sensitivity does not appear to be high enough to demonstrate detailed tumor vascular supply, which is best defined by digital subtraction superselective angiography (DSA) (95).

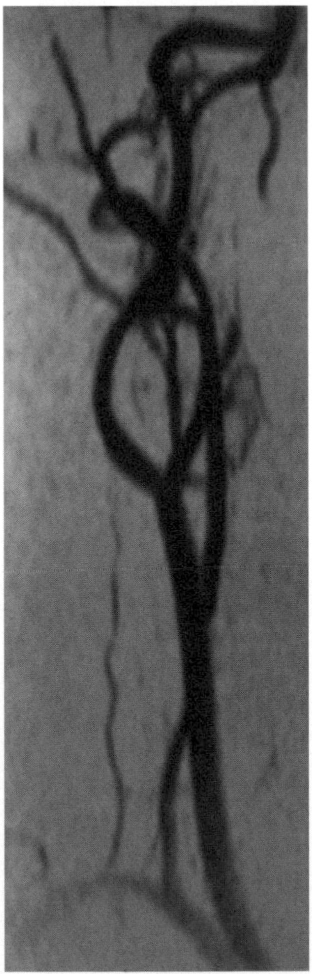

Figure 28.13 Magnetic resonance angiogram of a right carotid body tumor with splaying of the carotid bifurcation and posterior displacement of the internal carotid artery.

RADIOISOTOPE IMAGING

Paragangliomas, like other neuroendocrine tumors, have been found to have a high density of somatostatin type 2 receptors on their cell surface. Octreotide is a somatostatin analog that, when coupled to the radioisotope indium 111, creates a scintigraphic image of tumors expressing somatostatin type 2 receptors. Telischi et al. (96), in a study of 21 patients with presumed head and neck paragangliomas undergoing indium 111–octreotide scintigraphy, demonstrated an accuracy of 90%, a sensitivity of 94%, and a specificity of 75% in tumor detection. Radioisotope scintigraphy provides a noninvasive imaging modality that is particularly useful as a screening method for patients with a family history of paragangliomas. In addition, it is useful in detecting synchronous, metachronous, and metastatic tumors.

ANGIOGRAPHIC EVALUATION

Angiography plays an important role in the evaluation of paragangliomas if surgery is contemplated for definitive treatment. Preoperative evaluation requires a thorough investigation of the tumor blood supply (and possible anastomoses), displacement of vessels, potential vessel compromise by tumor invasion, and adequacy of intracranial circulation if ICA sacrifice is necessary. Superselective angiography also allows safe preoperative embolization of the tumor vasculature, hopefully avoiding proximal vessel occlusion and unexpected migration of embolization material into the cerebral or systemic circulation. Additionally, angiography is very accurate in detecting previously undiagnosed synchronous paragangliomas (97).

Although the clinical presentation is often strongly suggestive of the diagnosis of a paraganglioma, CT and MRI examinations are necessary in ruling out tumors that may mimic paragangliomas (e.g., neurogenic tumors, meningiomas) and in delineating the extent of large masses (Fig. 28.14). Angiography provides exquisite detail of the vascular anatomy and supplies diagnostic information as well. As previously described, CBTs reveal the diagnostic finding of splaying of the internal and external carotid arteries at the carotid bifurcation. The ICA is displaced posteriorly and laterally. Vagal paragangliomas also displace the carotid vessels, but the ICA is bowed anteriorly and medially by these tumors (Fig. 28.15).

We have found that angiography, through percutaneous femoral artery catheterization, also provides important information to the surgeon, aside from providing endovascular access for possible tumor embolization (69). Superselective angiography provides an arterial "map" and identifies the blood supply and flow dynamics to the tumor. This affords the surgeon an advantage of locating displaced vessels and also provides an enhanced view of identifying and ligating feeding vessels. More unpredictable and less accessible feeding vessels from the internal carotid supply would be identified and appropriately managed. Tumor venous outflow is visualized during later phases of the arteriogram. This allows the surgeon to preserve the known venous drainage until the final stages of tumor mobilization, thereby decreasing blood loss. Additionally, the extent of intraluminal venous involvement of jugular paragangliomas within the internal jugular vein inferiorly, and the sigmoid sinus superiorly, can be accurately assessed, thereby allowing adequate resection (98) (Fig. 28.10). Internal carotid angiography may reveal findings that are associated with a higher incidence of intraoperative disruption of the ICA such as irregularity of the arterial wall, significant narrowing of the lumen, and CBT larger than 5 to 6 cm (52,99).

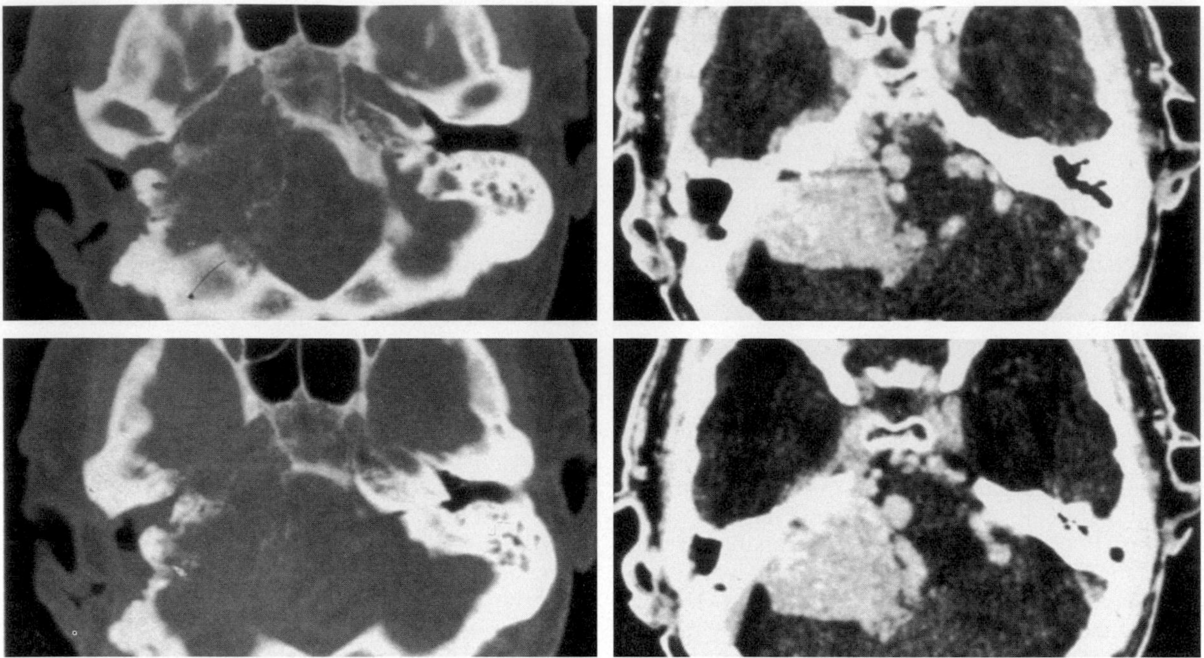

Figure 28.14 A 56-year-old man with a recurrent jugular paraganglioma presenting with cranial nerve VII to XII palsies and brainstem compression findings. Computed tomography demonstrates petrous bone destruction and dilated intracranial venous drainage.

Angiography of the intracranial circulation evaluates patency of the circle of Willis for determining adequate cerebral perfusion if carotid blood flow is interrupted for temporary control or for permanent ligation and sacrifice (Fig. 28.16). Many methods of determining tolerance to occluding carotid circulation have been described, including xenon CT scanning (100), electroencephalogram monitoring, and measurement of distal carotid stump pressures. Our method of internal carotid balloon occlusion under local anesthesia with monitoring of mental functions for 20 minutes seems to be reliable in predict-

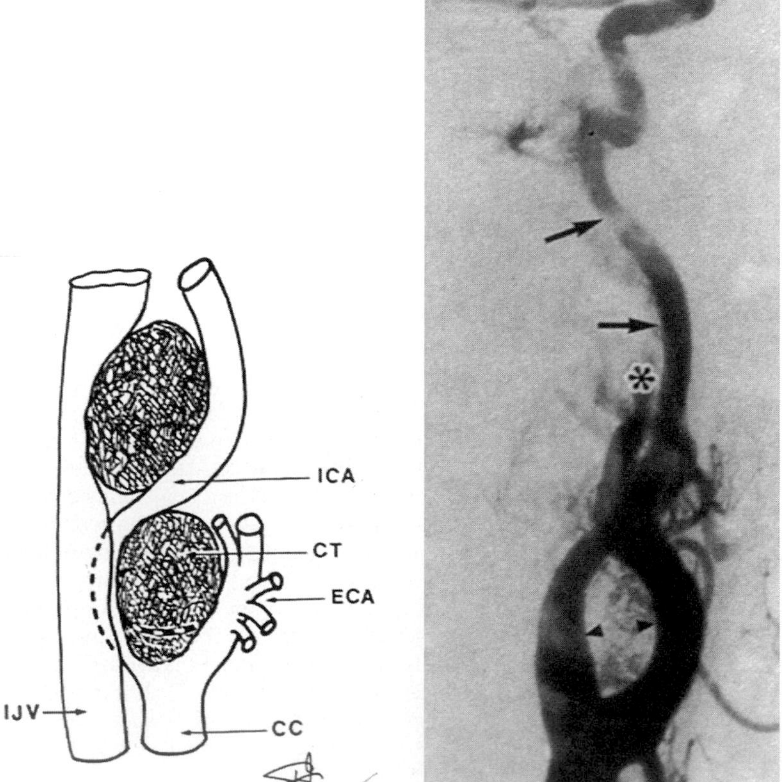

Figure 28.15 **A:** Diagrammatic illustration of the relationship between a carotid body tumor (*CT*) and vagal paraganglioma with the large vessels of the neck. *CC*, common carotid artery; *ECA*, external carotid artery; *ICA*, internal carotid artery; *IJV*, internal jugular vein. **B:** Carotid angiogram in a 50-year-old woman with a vagal paraganglioma and carotid body tumor following embolization of the external carotid branches (*asterisk*). Note the displacement of the vessels related to the vagal (*arrows*) and carotid (*arrowheads*) tumors.

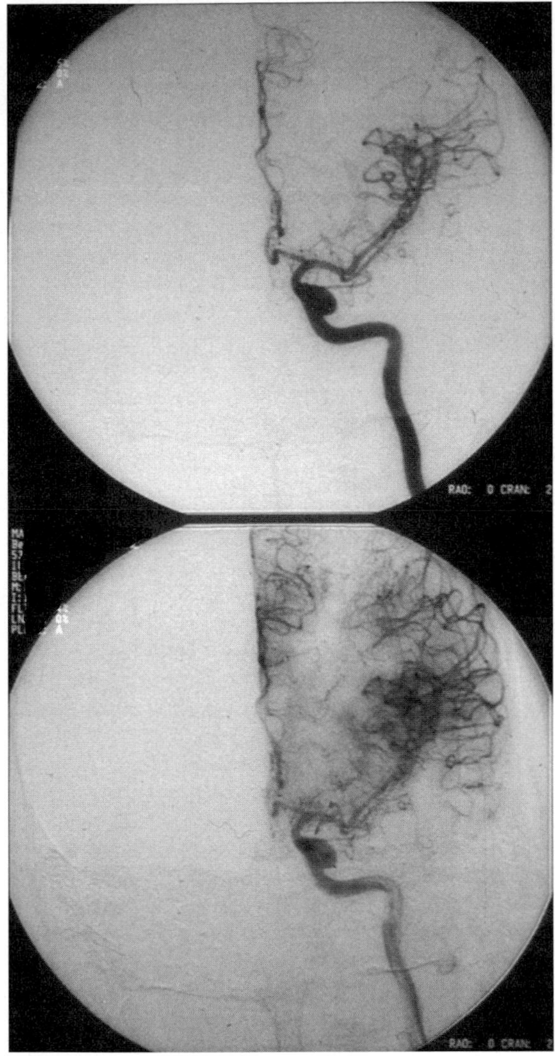

Figure 28.16 Left internal carotid angiogram demonstrating a nonpatent circle of Willis with absence of contralateral cerebral circulation.

ing a patient's tolerance to interruption of carotid blood flow. More recently we rely on angiographic evidence of adequate contralateral cerebral blood without performing elective internal carotid balloon occlusion (Fig. 28.17). In our study of 28 patients undergoing cerebral angiography, 26 patients (93%) demonstrated angiographic or carotid balloon occlusion, testing evidence of tolerance to possible carotid sacrifice (39). With this preoperative information, surgical decisions concerning carotid bypass options can be made. Even with preparation for ICA grafting, a review of multiple series reports a 9.7% rate of strokes and a 2.4% incidence of mortality (99).

Angiography is also a sensitive diagnostic study to evaluate for the presence of a previously undiagnosed synchronous paragangliomas, especially in patients with family histories (54,66,67,69,98). Computed tomography, MRI, and octreotide scans are relatively effective screening tests for occult tumors, but angiography has a higher resolution to identify these highly vascular tumors. In our series, 4 of 47 patients had previously undiagnosed paragangliomas that were discovered on angiography (three CBTs, one VP). For these reasons, bilateral carotid angiography is an important part of the protocol in our comprehensive evaluation of the patient who is to undergo surgery (39).

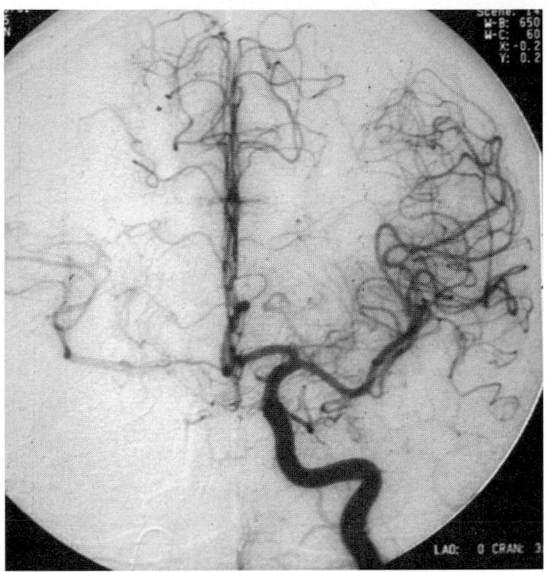

Figure 28.17 Left internal carotid angiogram showing a patent circle of Willis with circulation to contralateral cerebral vessels.

Management Options

Traditionally, surgical resection has represented the mainstay of treatment for these tumors, but the outcome is dependent on many factors that may influence the ideal result of total tumor removal while minimizing postoperative complications. Relative contraindications to surgery include extensive skull base or cranial involvement, advanced age of the patient, medical comorbidities, and bilateral or multiple paragangliomas that may result in unacceptable postoperative morbidity with resultant bilateral lower CN palsies.

If surgery is the chosen treatment course, preoperative embolization is performed. Embolization of paragangliomas has been an extremely useful adjunct in our treatment protocol. Although not uniformly accepted (73,75,86,101,102), there are major advantages in using combined endovascular embolization and subsequent surgery, assuming that certain criteria are fulfilled prior to performing embolization (66,84,103–106). An experienced vascular radiology team must be thoroughly familiar with the complexities and possible variations in head and neck vascular anatomy. Many anastomoses exist between the external and internal carotid system, and without this knowledge, disastrous neurologic consequences may result (107). The safe performance of this procedure by interventional vascular radiology has to be established and documented with an acceptable rate of morbidity and mortality (105,108).

PREOPERATIVE EMBOLIZATION

The main objective is directing the embolism material to selectively permeate only the vascularity of the paraganglioma without proximal occlusion of the feeding artery, and certainly avoiding distal migration of emboli into the general systemic circulation, which would result in possible central nervous system and pulmonary complications. Postembolization angiography should document absence of tumor "blush," with continued patency of the external carotid system (Figs. 28.18 and 28.19. Avoiding proximal vessel occlusion with embolization maintains adequate blood flow to normal tissue, avoids recruitment of internal carotid bloody supply to the tumor, and provides future endovascular access for possible tumor recurrence.

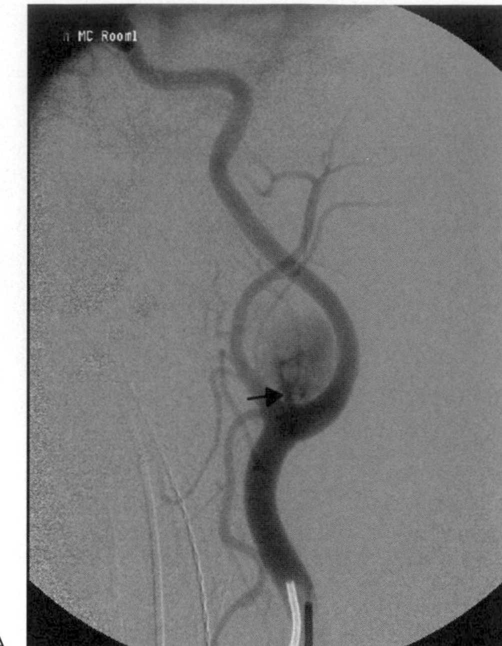

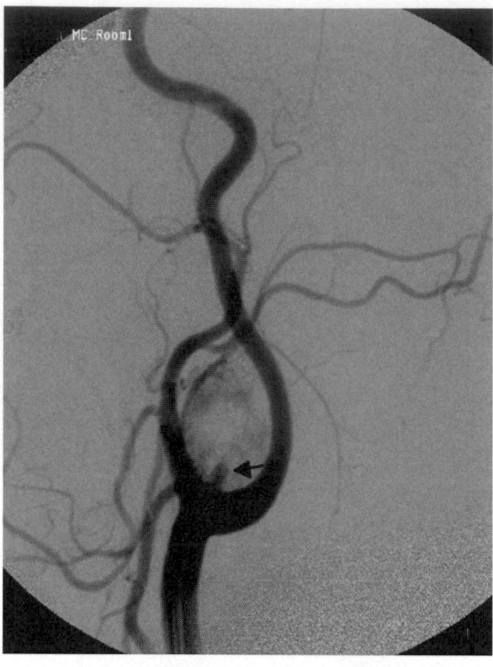

A B

Figure 28.18 A: Common carotid angiogram demonstrating splaying of the internal and external carotid arteries by a carotid body tumor (CBT). Well visualized is the carotid body artery (*arrow*) originating from the carotid bifurcation and supplying the tumor. **B:** Common carotid angiogram postembolization for a CBT. Note the absence of tumor vascularity with preservation of normal carotid artery anatomy. The stump of the carotid body artery is also intact (*arrow*).

The potential invasiveness of embolization must be justified by providing advantages during surgery, which results in improved tumor resection directly related to decreased tumor vascularity. Postembolization paragangliomas often manifest a reduction in tumor size as much as 25% as a result of diminished tumoral blood flow. Clinically, there is a decrease in the pulsatile nature of the tumor with elimination of bruits and pulsatile tinnitus. Reduction in tumor size results in less manipulation of surrounding structures required for exposure during surgery. Embolization of tumor vasculature also provides a major advantage in less blood loss during dissection of the neoplasm (54,67,108,109). This obviously improves exposure, better defines the planes of dissection, and ultimately reduces the need for transfusion (71,105,106). Studies support embolizing only larger tumors (105,110–112). The risk for potential complications from embolization must always be weighed against the advantages of improved surgical exposure, resection, and morbidity.

Not all paragangliomas should be embolized. This decision should depend on the location and extent of the tumor and the

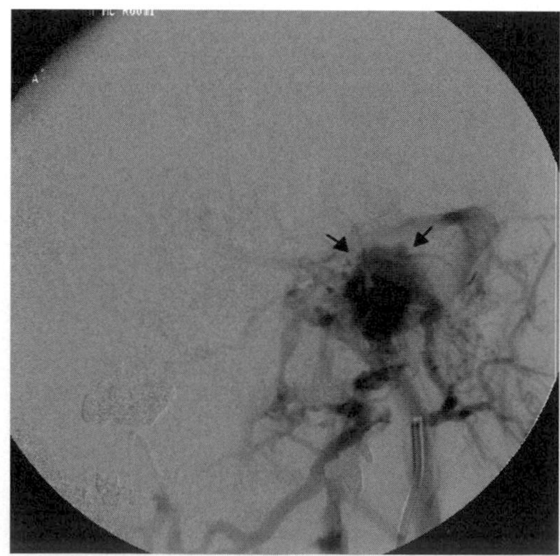

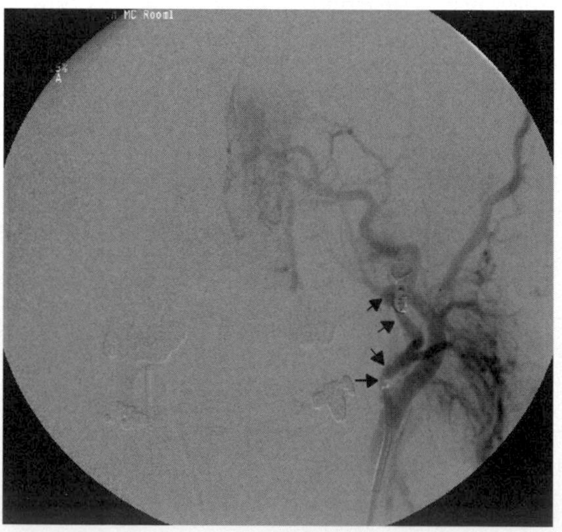

A B

Figure 28.19. A: Posterior auricular angiogram demonstrating tumor vascular "blush" of jugular paraganglioma (*arrows*). **B:** Postembolization posterior auricular angiogram with absence of jugular paraganglioma vascularity and preservation of the artery (*arrows*).

experience of the surgeon and the interventional radiologist. Tympanic paragangliomas confined to the middle ear cavity do not require preoperative embolization if the patient is being treated by an experienced otologic surgeon. In our experience, other types of paragangliomas are routinely treated with preoperative embolization. In our study, the postembolization intraoperative one-unit mean blood loss translates into the infrequent need for transfusions (39). With large CBTs, the paraganglioma may surround the ICA and dissection must proceed through the tumor to gain exposure of the arterial wall as the first step in dissecting and preserving the ICA. Without prior embolization, significant blood loss would result.

More recently, the concept of compartmentalization of the blood supply of paragangliomas has been discussed. Radiologists studying the vascular anatomy of paragangliomas with angiography have concluded that segments of the tumor are supplied by different feeding vessels, and these "compartments" can be put together like a jigsaw puzzle to reveal the entire tumor vasculature (113,114). Superselective angiography to define each feeding vessel assumes even more significance, with eventual identification of the entire arterial supply and embolization of the total tumor mass. The surgeon must also address the marked hypertrophy and hyperplasia of blood vessels involving normal tissues adjacent to intermediate-sized and large paragangliomas. In patients with CBTs there is a marked thickening and hypervascularity of the vasa nervosa of the adjacent vagus nerve and sympathetic plexus. Larger CBTs have extension of this process to the hypoglossal nerve. Embolization of CBTs results in less shunting of blood flow through these adjacent epineural vessels, thereby providing a more distinct plane of dissection for neural preservation and less blood loss. Although elective intraoperative external carotid artery (ECA) ligation for hemostasis has been reported, we believe that this procedure is to be avoided (84,86,109). Paragangliomas have multiple major arterial feeding vessels and proximal ECA ligation does not prevent retrograde flow through the external carotid vessels providing tumor circulation. Proximal ligation, therefore, has little effect on tumor blood flow and complicates the possibility of future endovascular access to this area. In these circumstances, recurrent tumor may require direct tumor puncture for future embolization, although there have been excellent results with primary tumor devascularization before surgery using this technique (115,116). External carotid ligation also results in recruitment of ICA blood supply, especially with recurrent skull base tumors. Embolization of these tumors then becomes extremely hazardous, if not impossible.

SURGERY

Surgery is performed within 2 days of angiography and embolization to avoid recruitment of collateral tumor blood supply and prior to the onset of significant postinflammatory effect (39). Short-term steroids are administered if there is concern about tumor edema that may compromise tumor dissection. The anesthesiologist must be prepared to counteract the α- and β-adrenergic catecholamine cardiovascular effect when dealing with "secreting" tumors.

Carotid Body Tumors

Carotid body tumors are exposed through a transverse incision or oblique incision along the anterior sternomastoid muscle for larger tumors. Proximal and distal control is obtained of the common, internal, and external carotid arteries with vessel loops (Fig. 28.20). The surgeon should be prepared for carotid bypass precautions in case of ICA injury that is unable to be easily repaired, especially with larger tumors. The results of preoperative cerebral angiography are important in determining the need for bypass. Adequate tumor removal requires a subadventitial dissection of the carotid artery. Mobilization of the ICA is the initial step of the tumor dissection, and this vessel is typically displaced over the posterior, lateral aspect of carotid artery tumors. Occasionally, the tumor must be dissected through and "split" to remove the ICA from its encasement. Once the ICA is free, any tumor that extends inferior to the bifurcation should be dissected off the common carotid artery. The ECA and its branches may then be dissected, although difficulty with this part of the procedure may warrant sacrifice of the ECA, if necessary, for adequate tumor excision. The last step is freeing the tumor from the carotid bifurcation, where there is most intimate involvement of the artery because the tumor originates in the carotid body located at this site (Fig. 28.21).

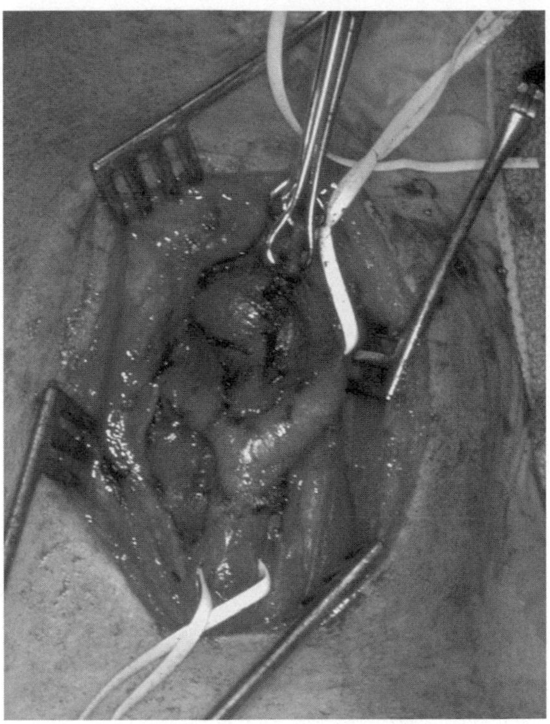

Figure 28.20 Mobilization of a carotid body tumor (in clamp) with vessel loops around the common and internal carotid arteries.

Nerves adherent to, but not infiltrated by, CBTs can usually be mobilized in an intact fashion, and these include the vagus, hypoglossal, and, occasionally, glossopharyngeal nerves. The sympathetic chain and the superior laryngeal nerve are often adherent to tumor, especially those with medial extension into the parapharyngeal space.

Jugulotympanic Paragangliomas

Tympanic paragangliomas confined to the middle ear (Glasscock-Jackson type I, Fisch class A) can be approached through a transcanal approach (117). These small tumors do not require preoperative embolization. If the margins of the tumor are not easily discernible, but the bone over the jugular bulb and the carotid canal is intact (Glasscock-Jackson types II–III, Fisch class B), a postauricular, transmastoid extended facial recess approach provides excellent exposure for tumor resection (117). A tympanoplasty can be performed at that time, if necessary.

Involvement of the jugular bulb requires a combined transmastoid and transcervical approach (118). If there is limited involvement of the jugular bulb without carotid artery involve-

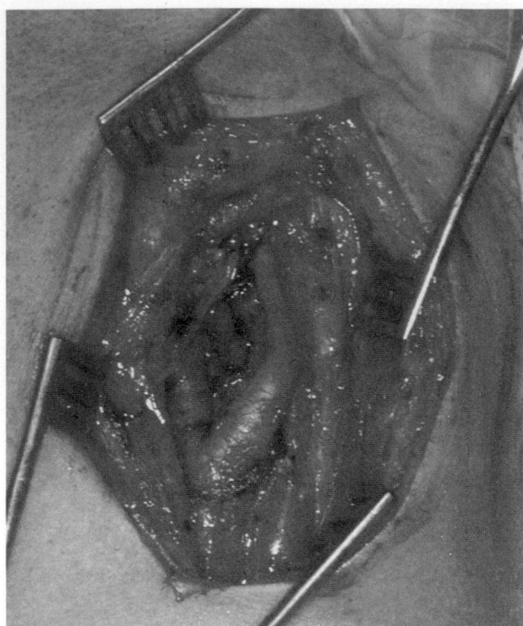

Figure 28.21 Splayed appearance of the carotid bifurcation after excision of a carotid body tumor. The internal and external carotid arteries have been preserved.

ment, a complete mastoidectomy and extended facial recess approach is performed. The sigmoid sinus is exposed and traced to the jugular bulb. Isolation and control of the internal jugular vein and ICA is performed and CNs IX through XII are dissected to the skull base. The internal jugular vein is ligated. Mobilization of the distal facial nerve at the second genu with the stylomastoid periosteum provides excellent exposure of the jugular bulb area. The superior sigmoid sinus is occluded by packing with oxidized cellulose, and the inferior sigmoid sinus is opened with mobilization of the tumor. Bleeding from the inferior petrosal sinus is controlled with careful packing of oxidized cellulose. Careless trauma in this area risks damage to CNs IX through XII in their course through the jugular canal medial to the jugular vein.

More extensive involvement of the jugular bulb or involvement of the intrapetrous ICA requires an infratemporal fossa approach as developed by Fisch (119). A wide mastoidectomy approach is performed with removal of the posterior bony external canal, canal wall skin, tympanic membrane, malleus, and incus. The facial nerve is mobilized from the geniculate ganglion to the stylomastoid foramen with anterior translocation of the nerve. The ICA, internal jugular vein, and CNs IX through XII are dissected to the skull base with ligation of the internal jugular vein and vessel loop control of the ICA. The mandibular condyle is retracted anteriorly. The ICA is followed through its intrapetrous course with resection of the eustachian tube. The sigmoid sinus, jugular bulb, and internal jugular vein are resected with the tumor. Dissection of tumor is meticulously performed off the ICA. The exiting CNs are preserved if they can be adequately separated from the tumor. Additional exposure into the infratemporal fossa can be accomplished with resection of the mandibular condyle and zygomatic arch. Through this approach there is access to the posterior, middle, and anterior cranial fossa, and if necessary, continued tumor resection is accomplished through a neurosurgical, intracranial approach. A pedicled temporalis, temporal-parietal, or sternomastoid flap is used for reconstruction and obliteration of the defect. The external auditory canal is closed at the meatus. Spinal drainage catheters are used after surgery for significant cerebrospinal fluid leaks.

Vagal Paragangliomas

Vagal paragangliomas may vary on the extent of skull base or intracranial involvement. Most VPs originate in the nodose (inferior) ganglion, approximately 2 cm below the jugular foramen. When these tumors grow, they extend to the skull base as well as involve the post-styloid parapharyngeal space. Vagal paragangliomas arising in the middle or superior vagal ganglia have early skull base involvement with intracranial extension. As with all paragangliomas, complete radiographic evaluation with contrast-enhanced MRI and CT studies defines the extent of involvement. A combined cervical-mastoid approach to the skull base is best for safe and wide exposure.

A wide curving postauricular incision is carried into the neck below the level of the hyoid bone. The sternomastoid muscle is retracted posteriorly and the carotid sheath structures and CNs IX to XII are dissected up to the skull base with careful dissection of the ICA off the VP. The posterior belly of the digastric muscle is resected and the styloid process is transected at its attachment to the inferior petrous bone. Vessel loops are placed around the ICA for control of possible vessel disruption. Paragangliomas without skull base involvement can be safely resected with this approach. If tumor extends into the jugular canal, then a mastoidectomy with facial nerve mobilization and transposition allows exposure of the jugular bulb. The sigmoid sinus can be packed off or ligated with subsequent removal of the sigmoid, jugular bulb, and internal jugular vein complex. The carotid canal is dissected superiorly and the ICA is carefully separated off the tumor. The tumor can then be excised, which almost always involves sacrifice of the vagus nerve and additional CNs according to the tumor size and local involvement (53). The surgical approach involves closure by obliterating the mastoid cavity with a fat graft. More extensive defects, or those involving cerebrospinal fluid leakage, require a temporoparietal fascia flap (120) or a sternomastoid muscle flap.

Complications

Complications resulting from head and paraganglioma surgery can be grouped into three main categories: CN injuries, vascular injury, and injury to the carotid body/carotid sinus complex.

CRANIAL NERVE INJURY

Lower CN dysfunction is a common complication of surgical resection of head and neck paragangliomas and often requires postoperative rehabilitation (53). Indeed, larger tumors involving the temporal bone can infiltrate between the fascicles of the CNs, even with normal nerve function. These involved nerves should be sacrificed to effect a total tumor resection (121). Our experience with postoperative CN dysfunction reflects a combination of total paralysis, due to nerve sacrifice, and paresis with ultimate recovery of function due to nerve traction. The frequency of affected nerves is related to tumor type and size and the surgical approach (Table 28.7) (39). Although isolated injury to one of the lower CNs (IX–XII) often results in temporary minor difficulties in swallowing, aspiration, phonation, or tongue motion, multiple CN injury may result in significant morbidity (98). Multiple CN deficits are particularly poorly tolerated in elderly patients. Bilateral lower CN palsies most often represent a severe, potentially life-threatening situation.

Although temporary CN deficits have been reported in up to half of the cases of CBT resection (67,73), many resolve over time. Reports of permanent postoperative CN deficits range widely from 13% to 40% (52,67,70,71,99,122). Large tumor size

TABLE 28.7 Paraganglioma: Postoperative Cranial Nerves

	None	V_3	VII	VIII	IX	X	XI	XII	Sympathetic
CBT (*n* = 28)	14	1(P)			9(P)	2(S), 3(P)	1(P)	1(S)	6(S)
JP (*n* = 14)	4		1(S),5(P)	1(S)	4(S)	3(S)	3(S)	2(S)	
VP (*n* = 5)		1(P)		1(S)	4(S)	1(S)	3(S)		
TP (*n* = 3)		2(P)							

P, paresis; S, sacrificed.

(>5 cm) appears to contribute to the incidence of postoperative CN injury (123,124). Vagus nerve injury is most common with a resulting paretic or paralyzed vocal cord due to either vagal nerve retraction or sacrifice (39). An isolated superior laryngeal nerve paralysis may also result because this nerve is in close proximity to the medial surface of the carotid arteries. In addition, the internal branch of the superior laryngeal nerve provides supraglottic sensory innervation, and immediate postoperative aspiration problems may result. Other commonly injured nerves include the hypoglossal nerve, which can be carefully dissected off the tumor, and the glossopharyngeal nerve, which is at risk with resection of larger, superiorly extending tumors. The accessory nerve frequently approximates the posterior aspect of the tumor, but postoperative dysfunction is uncommon.

Excision of VPs almost always requires the sacrifice of the vagus nerve, usually at the level of the nodose ganglion (39,53,87) (Table 28.7). Resection of the vagus nerve immediately below the skull base results in additional morbidity, besides the expected vocal cord paralysis. Paralysis of the soft palate results in hypernasal voice quality and nasal regurgitation of fluids. There is also superior laryngeal nerve dysfunction with the consequences previously described. Resection of additional CNs (IX–XII) (30–50% of cases) (53,87) and the sympathetic chain (25%) is often necessary (53). Facial nerve damage may result during a transtemporal approach as the nerve is transposed (53). Netterville et al. (53) described a postoperative syndrome in 9 of their 40 patients undergoing VP resection that is characterized by severe pain in the parotid region associated with eating. This pain, which is most severe with first bite of each meal and diminishes over the next several bites, is most prominent in the early postoperative period and gradually improves over time. They termed this syndrome "the first-bite syndrome." The symptoms are thought to be due to spasm of parotid gland myoepithelial cells resulting from denervation supersensitivity of sympathetic receptors after damage or removal of the cervical sympathetics and loss of sympathetic innervation. On oral intake and release of the parasympathetic neurotransmitter, there is cross-stimulation of the sympathetic receptors, resulting in a supramaximal response of the myoepithelial cells. Eight of nine patients with this syndrome had undergone sympathetic nerve resection while the ninth had postoperative Horner syndrome. This syndrome may result in decrease oral intake during the postoperative period, and a bland diet is helpful during this period

Jugular paragangliomas are intimately involved with CNs IX to XII, and therefore few (28%) undergoing surgery have intact postoperative CN function (Table 28.7) (39). Jackson et al. (79), in their series of large glomus tumors, report that although postoperative permanent CN deficiencies were common, almost all were of a single nerve and included CNs IX (18%), X (27%), XI (9%), and XII (9%). Postoperative facial nerve dysfunction is common from manipulation of the nerve during tumor resection (79,85).

Postoperative Rehabilitation

Paraganglioma surgeons should anticipate postoperative nerve dysfunction, and familiarity with rehabilitation techniques is necessary for proper patient care. If tumor resection results in nerve transection, then primary anastomosis, if possible, results in acceptable function. This is especially true of the facial, accessory, and hypoglossal nerves. Cable grafts using greater auricular or sural nerve are also an option, especially with the facial and accessory nerves. Rehabilitation for patients with postoperative nerve dysfunction is dependent on the functional deficit. The following represents the appropriate management of specific nerve dysfunction:

Facial nerve. Intraoperative facial nerve monitoring increases the probability of preserved facial nerve function after surgery. Facial nerve resection with reanastomosis or cable graft reconstruction requires 6 to 12 months for reinnervation. Transposition of the facial nerve may also result in facial weakness that requires 2 to 6 months for improvement. It is most important to provide eye (corneal) protection with facial nerve paralysis. Immediately after surgery, ophthalmic drops of artificial tears and eye ointment protection at night prevent corneal drying and ulceration. Upper lid gold weight implants are effective for long-term rehabilitation (82). If necessary, a tarsorrhaphy can be performed for additional eye protection. If there has been facial nerve resection without reconstruction or there are no signs of returning facial nerve function after 6 months, then temporalis and masseter muscle/fascial slings or adynamic fascial or allograft slings are effective. Prior experience with cross-facial grafting has also been gratifying.

Glossopharyngeal nerve. The resulting oropharyngeal hypesthesia is best managed with swallowing therapy, especially with attempts at directing the food bolus to the contralateral side.

Vagus nerve. The result of vagal dysfunction is quite variable and the debility is frequently related to the age and general medical condition of the patient. Vagus paralysis results in supraglottic hypesthesia and vocal cord paralysis. Early swallowing therapy after surgery helps control aspiration. A cricopharyngeal myotomy may also improve swallowing. If the vagus nerve has not been sacrificed but is not functioning due to neuropraxia, then Gelfoam injection of the vocal cord for medialization is indicated, potentiating swallowing and improving voice quality. If vagus sacrifice was necessary for tumor resection or if there is no return of vagal function after 4 to 6 months, then more permanent vocal cord medialization is necessary. This may be accomplished with fat or bovine collagen injection. Silastic implant medialization is also very effective, and occasionally an arytenoid adduction procedure is also necessary. If there are continuing problems with oral intake and handling secretions, a tracheostomy and gastrostomy may be appropriate for proper care.

In the case of a high vagal nerve dysfunction, there are additional considerations. The vocal cord assumes a more lateral position due to superior laryngeal nerve paralysis, and there is less effective compensation by the contralateral vocal cord. Additionally, there is paralysis of the hemipalate, causing hypernasal voice quality and nasal regurgitation. Transoral hemipalatal adhesion addresses this problem (125).

Accessory nerve. Physical rehabilitation with active and passive range of motion exercises will improve shoulder function with paralysis of the sternomastoid and trapezius muscles.

Hypoglossal nerve. Speech and swallowing therapy will rehabilitate the ipsilateral tongue paralysis. If there is an associated vagal and/or glossopharyngeal nerve dysfunction, intensive swallowing therapy assumes an important role in preventing life-threatening aspiration.

Vascular Injury

The incidence of intraoperative or postoperative stroke has dropped dramatically as surgical and anesthetic techniques have improved. This improvement has been attributed to multiple factors, including detailed preoperative imaging and angiographic evaluation to determine vessel involvement by tumor, carotid occlusion testing, correlation of bilateral cerebral angiography findings with postocclusion cerebral function, and advancements in surgical arterial revascularization techniques. Several series report a 0% to 2% rate of major stroke rate as a complication of CBT resection (67,68,70,71,75,99,122). Earlier series reported a rate of 10% to 20% (71,126). Although the absolute necessity for vessel replacement during CBT surgery cannot be definitely determined before surgery, vessel stenosis and wall irregularity, as well as extreme widening of the carotid bifurcation are among the factors that best predict the need for replacement (41,69,99,127,128). Carotid body tumors larger than 5 (52) to 6 cm (128) are also more likely to require vascular replacement.

Compared with carotid body paragangliomas, VPs are usually not as intimately associated with the great vessels, making vascular injury less likely (87). Netterville et al. (53) reported carotid artery encasement in 5 of 46 patients with VPs. One was treated with radiation, another underwent carotid artery sacrifice, a third underwent carotid artery replacement, and two had carotid artery laceration.

With the infratemporal fossa approach for large glomus tumors of the skull base, the carotid artery can be exposed from the bifurcation to the cavernous sinus, and meticulous tumor dissection can more often preserve the ICA (79). Certainly, large jugular paragangliomas commonly involve the ICA, especially if there is erosion of the bony partition between the internal jugular vein and the ICA. Internal carotid artery damage occurred in only 1% of patients with large paragangliomas of the skull base (129).

Carotid Body/Carotid Sinus Complex

Resection of bilateral CBTs or a CBT and contralateral jugular (and occasionally vagal) paraganglioma can result in baroreceptive dysfunction due to bilateral denervation of the carotid sinus. This dysfunction manifests as sustained hypertension and tachycardia. Netterville et al. (52) reported that 10 of 11 patients undergoing bilateral carotid sinus denervation demonstrated severe labile hypertension/hypotension, headache, diaphoresis, and emotional instability. As the parasympathetic response is lost, unopposed sympathetic stimuli result in the cardiovascular morbidity, which is usually successfully managed medically in the postoperative period with α-adrenergic antagonists. Sodium nitroprusside is used in the early postoperative period to prevent hypertension. The long-term cardiovascular effects are controlled with clonidine or phenoxybenzamine.

RADIATION THERAPY IN THE MANAGEMENT OF PARAGANGLIOMAS

Radiotherapy has traditionally been relegated to the treatment of unresectable paragangliomas (e.g., extensive skull base involvement or intracranial extension) or those tumors involving the medically infirm and elderly. Some have advocated surgery as the only curative option based on the assumption that paragangliomas are radioresistant and ultimately progress following radiotherapy. However, the risk for perioperative morbidity and long-term postoperative complications, including CN dysfunction, can be considerable. Certainly, surgery may be the preferred treatment of paragangliomas in which complete resection entails acceptable morbidity. With technical advances in preoperative embolization, skull base surgery, and reconstruction, a greater proportion of cases can presently be effectively resected. However, if surgery results in significant debility requiring long-term rehabilitation, other effective options should be considered (130,131). Observation of these slow-growing tumors may be considered in patients with small and moderate-sized asymptomatic paragangliomas who can be closely monitored. Alternatively, radiotherapy has been proven for the past several decades to be an effective therapeutic option and should be considered as a form of primary treatment. Therapeutic options always must be judiciously weighed and are dependent on the physician's experience, clinical findings, patient preference, and risks of morbidity.

Radiotherapy has been used primarily to treat jugular paragangliomas of the temporal bone and significantly less frequently for treatment of CBTs or VPs. Both conventionally fractionated radiotherapy and, more recently, stereotactic radiosurgery have been utilized. When primary radiotherapy is considered, the diagnosis should be confirmed either pathologically (e.g., fine-needle aspiration biopsy) or by characteristic CT and MRI criteria. Successful treatment of paragangliomas with radiotherapy must be defined because there is rarely total resolution of the tumor after treatment. Thus, "local control" usually means stability (or regression) of tumor size and nonprogression (or improvement) in neurologic symptoms.

Past Results

LOCAL CONTROL

The first major review demonstrating the efficacy of radiation was reported by Alford and Guilford (132) in 1962 on 106 cases of paragangliomas collected from the literature. Although more advanced lesions were treated with radiotherapy, local control was comparable to surgery, 72% versus 78%, respectively. Unfortunately, follow-up was relatively short for a disease with a long natural history. Since then, numerous reports with follow-up as long as 35 years have demonstrated the effectiveness of radiation in control of head and neck paragangliomas (Tables 28.8 and 28.9). The accumulated data represent a wide variety of dose levels (30 to 70 Gy), radiation techniques (electrons,

TABLE 28.8 Radiotherapy (RT) for Head and Neck Paragangliomas

Institution	No. of patients	Median follow-up	RT dose (range)	Local control	Disease-specific survival	Overall survival	Time to local failure
UF: Hinerman, 2001	71 (80 tumors)	11.1 yr (7 mo–32 yr)	45 Gy (22–60 Gy)	94% (75/80)	98%	NS	3, 5, 8, and 19 yr
UF: Evenson, 1998	15 (23 tumors)	5 yr	45 Gy (35–70 Gy)	96%	89%	NS	5 yr
WF: Mumber, 1995	15	11 yr	50 Gy (45–60 Gy)	100%	NS	NS	NS
Geisenger: Cole, 1994	38	10 yr	(35–45 Gy)	87%	89%	59%	2, 3, 5 yr, and 2 after 10 yr
UVMC: Larner, 1992	29	16.2 yr (5–31 yr)	<30 to >60 Gy	86%	93%		8, 8, 12, and 17 yr
Mayo: Schild, 1992	10	7.5 yr	46 Gy (16–52 Gy)	100%	100%	100%	NS
RMH: Powell, 1992	46	9 yr (1–32)	(35–66 Gy)	85%	NS	NS	NS
Netherlands Cancer Institute: Verniers, 1992	22 (44 tumors)	10 yr (mean)	50 Gy (50–60 Gy)	88% (10 yr)	NS	NS	2 and 9 yr
Krakow: Skolyszewski, 1991	24	7 yr	60 Gy (30–60 Gy)	96%	100%	92%	NS
University of Arizona: Boyle, 1990	10	2–9 yr	45–54 Gy	100%	100%	80%	NS
Hoogenhout, 1990	31	11 yr	40–50 Gy	97%			
Methodist and CTRC: Pryzant, 1989	20	11 yr	45 Gy	94%	NS	NS	8 yr
Iowa: ML Wang, 1988	19	5–35 yr	58 Gy (29–68 Gy)	84%	NS	71% (10 yr)	NS
UF: Friedland, 1988	26	2–18 yr	45 Gy (40–50 Gy)	96%	NS	NS	NS
Copenhagen: Hansen, 1988	39	7 yr	40–60 Gy	92%	95%	82%	Both failed at 1.5 yr
Washington University: Konefal, 1987	26	Minimum 4 yr	24 to >60 Gy	86%	73%	NS	NS
Royal Victory Hospital: Dawes, 1987	55 (58 tumors)		50 Gy/20	83%	95%; DFS, 77%	94% (20 yr)	NS
Johns Hopkins: Zinreich, 1986	15	2 to 10 yr	45 Gy/5 wk	100%	NS	NS	NS
Wessex Regional: Mitchell, 1985	12	6–7 yr (1.5–15 yr)	34.5–60 Gy	92%	92%	83%	Persistent after treatment
St. Bartholomew's: Sharma, 1984	42	11 yr (0–35 yr)	50–65 Gy	83%	93%; DFS, 77%	NS	NS
Rotterdamsch RT I: Lybeert, 1984	28	1.5–18 yr	40–60 Gy	100%	NS	NS	NS
PMH: Cummings, 1984	45	10 yr (3–23 yr)	35 Gy/3 wk	93%	100%	76%	1, 7, and 16 yr
University of Kansas: Reddy, 1983	11	>10 yr	22–56 Gy	100%	100%	NS	NS
UF: Dickens, 1982	14	8 yr (3–12 yr)	47 Gy (38–56 Gy)	100%	100%	100%	NS
UVA: Kim, 1980	40	5–30 yr	12–60 Gy	83%	NS	NS	NS
MGH: CC Wang	45	1–26 yr	NS	96%	NS	93%	6 and 11 yr
University Hospital of Wales: Gibbin, 1978	14	8.7 yr (mean) (1 to 16 yr)	45 Gy (42–50 Gy)	86%	86%	86%	Both within 2 yr after RT
Washington University/ Swedish/Virginia Mason: Simko, 1978	14	7.7 yr (mean) (1.3–17 yr)	28–65 Gy	86%	92%	92%	NS
Queen Elizabeth: Arthur, 1977	20	13 yr	45–50 Gy	95%	100%	75%	3 yr
Washington University: Spector, 1975	20	8 yr (2–27 yr)	46–60 Gy	65%	NS	NS	NS
MDAC: Tidwell, 1975	17	4–18 yr	42–50 Gy	100%	100%	94%	NS
UCSF: Newman, 1973	14		46–55 Gy	93%	93%	93%	Persistent
University of Minnesota and UK: Marayuma, 1972	14	NS	45 Gy (30–60 Gy)	93%	65% (10 yr)	100%	NS
MGH: Hatfield, 1972	23	5 yr (min)	>40 Gy (30–45 Gy)	74%	NS	NS	1 to 18 yr
Mayo: Fuller, 1966	69	10–15 yr (1–32 yr)		88%	95%	88%	NS
University of Michigan: Grubb, 1964	14	4 yr (0 to 10 yr)	40 Gy (22–50 Gy)	86%	100% DFS, 86%	79%	NS
Total	967 (1,009 tumors)			90% (907/ 1,009)			

CTRC, Cancer Therapy and Research Center; DFS, disease-free survival; MDAC, M. D. Anderson Cancer Center; MGH, Massachusetts General Hospital; NS, not stated; PMH, Princess Margaret Hospital; RMH, Royal Marsden Hospital; UCSF, University of California, San Francisco; UF, University of Florida; UK, University of Kentucky; UVA, University of Virginia; UVMC, University of Virginia Medical Center; WF, Wake Forest.

TABLE 28.9 Local Control after Radiotherapy for Carotid Body Tumors and Vagal Paragangliomas

Institution	No. of patients	Median follow-up	Median dose	Local control
Centro Oncologico (Valdagni)	7 (13 tumors)	2.5 yr (1–19 yr)	50 Gy (46–60 Gy)	100%
Rotterdamsch RT I (Lybeert)	9 (11 tumors)	1.5–18 yr	40–60 Gy	100%
Wessex Regional (Mitchell and Clyne)	6	6	37–55 Gy	83%
RMH (Powell)	4	9 yr		100%
UF (Mendenhall)	4 (6 tumors)	3 yr (2–4.5 yr)	45 Gy (41–49 Gy)	100%
UF (Hinerman)	18 (25 tumors)	9 yr (mean)	45 Gy (35–70 Gy)	96%
Total	48 (63 tumors)			97% (61/63)

photons, radium implant), and beam energies (superficial, cobalt, 4–6 megavoltage). Overall, local control rates range from 65% to 100% with an average of 90% based on over 1,000 tumors from 36 series (907/1,009) (Table 28.8) (130,131,133–166). No obvious difference in local control is detectable between those primarily involving the temporal bone versus the CBTs and VPs [local control 97% (61/63)] (Table 28.9) (133,139,151, 153,167,168). Mean or median follow-up was at least 10 years (133,135–137,140,143,144,152,154,161,165) in multiple series with a maximum follow-up over 30 years in some (133,137,139, 145,152,165). Kim et al. (157) reported a local control of 90% on 225 temporal bone tumors from 11 radiotherapy series published from 1965 to 1980. Schild et al. (138) updated the analysis by including studies published from 1965 to 1992. Local control was obtained in 91% (337/370) after radiotherapy. In their report, Kim et al. (157) demonstrated a dose-response relation between local control and total radiotherapy delivered. The optimal dose appeared to be greater than 40 Gy. Local failure was 1% versus 25% if patients received >40 Gy (n = 142) versus ≤ 40 Gy (n = 83), respectively.

In general, a dose of 45 Gy/5 weeks is recommended; however, a Canadian schedule of 35 Gy/3 weeks has also shown to be effective (154). The high rates of local control after radiotherapy led Rosenwasser (169) to conclude that "radiation failures occur, but perhaps they are not so much failures in the sense that irradiation is not effective but that irradiation may not have reached the tumor in its entirety." Paralleling such high rates of control are disease-specific survivals ranging from 65% to 100%, with the majority of series reporting rates between 90% to 100% as well as high rates of overall survival of 65% to 100% (Table 28.8).

NEUROLOGIC RESULTS

There are limited data reported for improvement of symptoms after radiotherapy. The most frequent symptoms associated with temporal bone paragangliomas are hearing loss and tinnitus, presenting in 55% to 58% and 56% to 66% of patients, respectively (135,139,142,144,151,154). After radiotherapy, tinnitus commonly improves or resolves in up to 88% of cases (139,154). Among temporal bone tumors treated with radiation with a median follow-up of 10 years, Cummings et al. (154) demonstrated complete relief of tinnitus in 79% of 38 reported cases and stable or partial relief in 21%. Of the 40 patients with initial hearing impairment, 5% reported a return to normal hearing, 30% reported some improvement, and 62% were unchanged. Others have also reported an 8% to 85% incidence of hearing impairment as a presenting symptom (135,139,142, 144), but do not detail a response to radiotherapy.

The incidence of other lower cranial neuropathy at presentation is usually about 40% for temporal bone tumors but may range from 8% to 60% (135,137–140,144,151). Often, the presenting CN symptoms are long-standing with only a modest possibility of improving after radiotherapy. The probability of improvement is most likely inversely related to the duration of cranial neuropathy (139,153). The reported rates of improvement vary from 0% to 83% with an average of 35% for all series that document response (Table 28.10) (135,138,139,142,144,146,149,151,153,154,156). Complete restoration of CN function can occur in about 10% (range 8–20%); however, the majority show no change. Of particular interest, only about 1% of cranial neuropathies worsen after radiotherapy. Postradiation cranial neuropathy is rare and only four such cases have been reported: two cases of CN VII palsy, one CN VIII dysfunction occurring after high dose of radiotherapy (64–66 Gy) (139,153), and one case of CN VI palsy that the authors stated had an "unclear etiology" (149).

Radiation Effects

RADIOGRAPHIC CHANGES

The majority of lesions remain stable in size or show modest tumor regression on radiographic evaluation after radiotherapy (144,157,170). Mukherji et al. (171) reported the University of Florida experience of 17 patients with 18 paragangliomas treated with definitive radiation who underwent pre- and posttreatment imaging using CT or MRI. Sixty-one percent showed a decrease in tumor size, with an average reduction of 23% (range 8–45%) at a median follow-up of 2½ years. All tumors persisted, but none showed an increase in size. Postradiation MRI findings included reduction in flow voids, decreased het-

TABLE 28.10 Cranial Neuropathy Response after Definitive Radiotherapy

Author	Improved	Complete resolution	Worse
Friedland (146)	33% (19/57)	9% (5/57)	4% (2/57)
Cummings (154)	100% (26/26)[a]	8% (2/26)	0%
Dawes (149)	28% (16/57)	NR	0%
Boyle (142)	50% (2/4)	NR	0%
Mumber (135)	50% (3/6)	NR	0%
Lybert (153)	17% (1/6)	0%	0%
Dickens (156)	47% (14/30)	20% (6/30)	0%
Mitchell (151)	66% (2/3)	NR	0%
Pryzant (144)	0% (0/9)	0%	0%
Powell (139)	19% (5/26)	NR	NR
Schild (138)	83% (5/6)	NR	0%
	33% (67/204)	10% (13/128)	1% (2/204)

Three cases of new cranial neuropathy [2 CN VII after radiotherapy (64–66 Gy) (Powell), and one reported a CN VI with unclear cause (Dawes)].
NR, not reported.
[a]Cranial neuropathy stable or improved, excluded from total analysis of those improved.

TABLE 28.11 McCabe/Fletcher Staging (Temporal Bone Tumors)

Group I (tympanic tumors)
- Absence of bone destruction on radiographic examination
- Intact VII and VIII
- Intact jugular foramen

Group II (tympanomastoid tumors)
- Bone destruction confined to the mastoid
- Facial nerve normal or paretic, jugular foramen nerves intact
- Superior bulb of the jugular vein involved by retrograde jugulography

Group III (petrosal and extrapetrosal tumors)
- Carotid arteriogram evidence of destruction of petrous or occipital bones and jugular fossa
- Jugular foramen syndrome
- Positive retrograde jugulography
- Presence of metastases

erogeneous enhancement, and reduced T2 signal. Computed tomography detected improvement in skull base erosion in rare cases (1 in 8 patients) (144,157). Other smaller studies demonstrate regression in 57% to 73% of patients followed by CT (138,140). Angiographic follow-up may not show significant change in patients with no evidence of clinical progression. Maruyama (164) reported the results of three paragangliomas followed by serial angiography over several years, and though tumors were clinically controlled, only minimal reductions in vascularity were detected angiographically. Thus, paragangliomas show modest radiographic change or stable tumor in the majority of cases.

HISTOPATHOLOGIC CHANGES

The basis by which radiation prevents tumor growth and reduces symptoms is not completely understood because the chief cells can be present long after radiation (131,172–174). Few studies report the radiation effect on paragangliomas (131,172, 173). Gardner et al. (174) studied six irradiated tumor specimens resected 4 to 6 weeks postradiation. The distinctive finding was of vascular endarteritis with mural thrombi when compared with nonirradiated specimens. One of six specimens showed a necrotic infarct, whereas two cases showed changes in tumor cells consistent with pyknotic cellular death. No significant difference in fibrosis was noted between the irradiated and nonirradiated specimens. However, at 6 months after irradiation, Rosenwasser (175) and others (131,176,177) have noted a dramatic increase in stromal fibrous connective tissue with wide separation of tumor nests and diminished vascularity. Chief cells are present but may develop nuclear pleomorphism with coarse chromatin clumping and irregular nuclear outlines. Others have described similar histopathologic findings in irradiated specimens (174,176).

Based on these findings, it seems that radiation induces an obliterative endarteritis with resultant fibrosis, which possibly prevents regrowth in addition to promoting partial tumor involution (131,178). Whether radiation exerts a primary effect on chief cells is difficult to determine because morphologically intact but persistent cells may lose reproductive ability (179).

Local Control—Radiotherapy/Surgery

Extraction of meaningful data from retrospective studies is inherently fraught with difficulty. Single-institution retrospective series often report conflicting results based on small patient numbers and selection bias. For example, Ogura et al. (84) reported a cure rate of 80% (39/49) after surgery alone for jugular paragangliomas versus 25% (3/12) after radiotherapy alone and 64% (7/11) with combined surgery and radiation. In this series and those from Glasscock et al. (180), surgery was recommended as the treatment of choice for resectable tumors and radiotherapy was proposed for large, inoperable tumors. Moore et al. (88) reported successful control in 88% (7/8) of tympanic paragangliomas treated with surgery alone and 25% (1/4) of petrosal/extrapetrosal tumors treated by surgery alone versus 100% (5/5) of similar tumors treated with radiotherapy alone and 88% of tumors treated with surgery followed by radiotherapy. Other series have demonstrated no obvious differences between surgery and radiotherapy (178). Carrasco and Rosenman (181) reported a large series showing similar local recurrence rates after surgery versus radiotherapy occurring in 7% versus 8% (19/283 vs. 24/299), respectively. The mortality rate from progressive disease was low after treatment with either modality, 2.5% (7/283) with surgery versus 6% (18/299) with radiation. Due to the retrospective nature of the data, the impact of selection bias on such an analysis cannot be determined.

In an effort to extract meaningful data, one may compare outcomes based on a common staging system. Few studies report their results based on a staging system that can be used for cross-modality and interinstitutional comparison. However, several series report results based on the McCabe/Fletcher staging system, which categorizes temporal bone paragangliomas into the tympanic, tympanomastoid, and petrosal/extrapetrosal categories (Tables 28.11 and 28.12) (133,137,144,145,157). Although this staging system is based on the use of outdated radiographic examinations, such as plain x-ray films and retrograde jugulography, it is similar in principle to the Fisch and Glasscock/Jackson systems, which are currently preferred. A combined analysis

TABLE 28.12 Local Control after Primary Radiation Therapy vs. Surgery vs. Surgery and Postoperative Radiation in Temporal Bone Paragangliomas[a]

McCabe/Fletcher stage	RT	Sx	Sx + RT[b]	All patients
I	93% (14/15)	87% (27/31)	78% (7/9)	87% (48/55)
II	100% (18/18)	88% (7/8)	70% (7/10)	89% (32/36)
III	92% (56/61)	17% (1/6)	95% (19/20)	87% (76/87)
Total	93% (88/94)	78% (35/45)	85% (33/39)	87% (156/178)

[a]RT, radiation therapy; Sx, surgery.
Based on pooled analysis of five series that reported results by a common staging system (Wang, Larner, Pryzant, Kim, Hinerman).
[b]Note the majority received radiotherapy in conjunction with surgery as upfront definite treatment rather than as salvage.

of five studies reporting the results of surgical or radiotherapeutic treatment of temporal bone tumors staged according to the McCabe/Fletcher system is presented in Table 28.12 (133,137,144,145,157). Patients were treated with radiotherapy alone ($n = 94$), surgery alone ($n = 45$), or surgery and radiation ($n = 39$). Patients in the last cohort received radiation, usually in the postoperative setting, for gross residual disease. Median follow-up ranged from 11 to 16 years. The average local control was 93%, 78%, and 85% for patients treated with radiotherapy, surgery, or combined surgery and radiation, respectively. Despite a selection bias against the radiotherapy group (65% were group III paragangliomas) compared with the surgery alone (13% were group III) or combined surgery and radiation (51% were group III), local control appeared at least as good after radiotherapy alone compared with the other two treatment groups. Local control for group III tumors was better after definitive radiotherapy (92%) or combined modality treatment (95%) versus surgery alone (17%). Patients with early or intermediate group tumors did well regardless of treatment approach. Although McCabe and Fletcher recommended surgery alone for tympanic tumors, combined treatment for tympanomastoid tumors, and radiotherapy alone for petrosal or extrapetrosal tumors (152), the combined analysis suggests that surgery or radiotherapy are equally effective alternatives for group I and II tumors of temporal bone paragangliomas (local control 87% and 88% vs. 93% and 100% after surgery and radiation therapy for group I and II tumors, respectively), and radiotherapy is the preferred treatment option for advanced tumors (local control 92% for group III tumors) (Table 28.12). Moreover, a combined approach does not appear to improve local control compared with radiotherapy alone. Kim et al. (157) also emphasized that there is no obvious benefit of a debulking subtotal resection in conjunction with definitive radiotherapy. The pooled analysis is based on retrospective data on 174 patients and is subject to selection/reporting bias; nevertheless, it represents a comparison based on a common staging system with reasonably long-term follow-up. Unfortunately, the respective morbidities of the different treatment groups were not detailed in these studies.

Salvage Therapy

Late recurrences have been reported up to 19 years after radiotherapy (133) with the majority recurring within 10 years after radiotherapy (Table 28.8), highlighting the need for continued long-term surveillance. If local failure occurs after definitive radiotherapy or surgery, Carrasco and Rosenman (181) concluded that salvage rates are high based on a review of 24 series from 1964 to 1987 comprising 582 patients treated with surgery and/or radiation. Four percent (25/582) died of disease [2.5% (7/283) of surgery patients and 6% of radiation patients (18/299)], and salvage was obtained in 88% in patients failing initial treatment with either surgery or radiotherapy. Of 62 patients recurring after initial resection, 95% (56/59) were salvaged with definitive radiation and 100% (3/3) with additional surgery, for an overall salvage rate of 95% (59/62). Salvage of radiotherapy failures with surgery or additional radiotherapy was successful in 95% (19/20) and 71% (25/35), respectively, for an overall rate of 80% (44/55). Thus, the use of either surgery or radiotherapy as initial treatment does not preclude the success of salvage surgery or radiation for tumor recurrence.

Malignant Paragangliomas

Metastatic disease is often indolent and asymptomatic. The standard treatment of malignant paragangliomas is resection of the primary and regional node dissection followed by postoperative radiation. Data regarding outcome of malignant paraganglioma after definitive radiation is rare. Hinerman et al. (133) reported on three patients with malignant CBTs and neck metastases who underwent definitive radiation (64.8 to 70 Gy) and who were without evidence of disease at 15 months, 4 years, and 6 years.

Toxicity of Fractionated Radiotherapy

Severe complications after radiotherapy have been reported in 30 series involving 795 patients, and are summarized in Table 28.13 (130,133–142,144–146,148,149,151–156,158–163,165,166). This review involves 37 years of literature (1964–2001) with a wide variation in techniques and doses. The incidence of severe complications is 6% (49/795), and treatment related mortality 0.6% (5/795). Four of the five reported deaths resulted from brain complications including necrosis and abscess. Several of these deaths resulted from overdosage of radiation with external beam radiation (66–70 Gy), radium implant, or large-volume brain irradiation. Severe morbidity consisted primarily of osteoradionecrosis [$n = 12$ (1.5%)], chronic otitis [$n = 8$ (1%)], brain necrosis [$n = 6$ (0.8%)], radiation related cranial neuropathy [$n = 4$ (0.5%)], radiation-induced sarcoma [$n = 3$ (0.4%)], external auditory canal stenosis [$n = 2$ (0.3%)], and trismus [$n = 2$ (0.3%)]. The majority of such complications were related to treatment using excessive doses, outdated treatment techniques (orthovoltage, which is preferentially absorbed in the bone or radium implant), or reirradiation. For example, of the four cranial neuropathies related to radiotherapy, three occurred after 64 to 66 Gy. Cole and Beiler (136) reported that all severe complications in their series occurred in the orthovoltage-treated patients and none in those treated with megavoltage. Of importance is the low incidence [0.4% (3/795)] of radiation-induced secondary malignancy, including two fibrosarcomas occurring 15 and 25 years posttreatment and one osteosarcoma occurring 5 years later. One fibrosarcoma developed after a radium implant; the other two malignancies occurred after treatment with 50 and 62 Gy (Table 28.13).

With modern treatment planning and appropriate dosing, definitive radiotherapy for paragangliomas should be well tolerated. In the acute setting, patients may experience dermatitis, alopecia, mucositis, epilation, and alterations in taste and saliva, along with either otitis externa or media. The potential complications vary according to the radiation technique and treatment site. At standard doses of 45 Gy/25 fractions, most of these side effects are transient, and treatment-related mortality is exceedingly rare. Chronic toxicities such as osteoradionecrosis and brain complications should also be negligible. Care must be taken to minimize dose inhomogeneity and volume of treated normal tissues, especially brain (Fig. 28.22).

Stereotactic Radiosurgery

Stereotactic radiosurgery (SRS) has been explored in the primary treatment of paragangliomas. The major advantage of stereotactic radiation is that one large dose of tightly shaped (conformal) radiation may be delivered to the tumor, thereby sparing surrounding tissue. Two methods of delivering stereotactic radiation are (a) the use of radioactive cobalt sources (gamma knife) and (b) the generation of radiation from a linear accelerator (Linac). Typically, all imaging (e.g., CT scan or MRI), planning, and treatment are completed in a one-time treatment session, and the radiation is delivered with the highest precision of all current radiation delivery

TABLE 28.13 Severe Complications after Radiotherapy for Paraganglioma

Author	No. of patients	Severe chronic complications
Hinerman	71	1 transient CNS syndrome preirradiation
		1 transient CN7 palsy 10 months after RT—resolved spontaneously
		1 otitis media requiring myringostomy
		1 severe dental caries
		1 external otitis
Evenson	15	1 transient CNS lethargy
Mumber	15	1 osteosarcoma of occipital bone 5 yr p pt received 62 Gy
Cole	38	3 osteoradionecrosis (all treated with orthovoltage)
		1 recurrent tumor hemorrhage (treated with orthovoltage)
		No serious complications in megavoltage treated patients
Larner	29	None reported
Schild	10	None reported
Powell	46	2 facial nerve palsy p 64–66 Gy
Verniers	22	1 perforation due to otitis media
Skolysweski	23	1 brain cortical atrophy
Boyle	9	None reported
Pryzant	20	None reported
ML Wang	19	EAC stenosis p 67 Gy
		1 encephalopathic death p 66 Gy
Friedland	15	1 revision sequestrectomy for cholesteatoma
		1 revision mastoidectomy and sequestrectomy for bony sequestrum 10 yr p RT
		1 trismus
Konefal	26	1 osteoradionecrosis after 54 Gy to the right ear and bilateral mixed beam treatment
Dawes	55	1 encephalopathy
		2 labyrinthitis
Mitchell	12	1 mastoid sequestrectomy for persistent ear crusting 16 yr p RT
Sharma	42	4 cases of osteoradionecrosis (3 after reirradiation to doses of 80–88 Gy in 2 cases and 1 radium implant)
Lybert	28	1 possible CN8 palsy p 65 Gy
Cummings	45	4 chronic otitis externa
		1 chronic otitis media
		1 EAC stenosis
		1 fatal brain necrosis p 70 Gy accidentally delivered
		1 osteoradionecrosis 10 yr p 58 Gy using electrons
Reddy	11	None reported
Dickens	14	2 choleststeatoma
		1 bony sequestrum
		1 trismus
Wang	45	2 pts with osteoradionecrosis
Gibbin	14	None reported
Simko	14	1 temporal bone necrosis p 57 Gy
Arthur	20	None reported
Tidwell	17	1 fatal + C45 brain necrosis p 50 Gy to large volume (hot spot 63 Gy in brain)
Newman	14	1 lethal fibrosarcoma 15 yr after 50 Gy
Hatfield	23	1 brain abscess
Fuller	69	1 fibrosarcoma 25 yr p radium implant
		1 death from abscess due to necrotic mastoid process p radium implant
Grubb	14	None reported
Total	795	49

EAC, external auditory canal.

techniques. Patients receive one large fraction of radiation (usually 12 to 18 Gy) to a precisely defined area using a localizing stereotactic head frame. The radiobiologic rationale of delivering one large dose is to effectively treat tumors that may be radioresistant while minimizing the amount of normal tissue in the treatment field. A small number of series have reported success using this approach to treat jugular paragangliomas with no reported local failures except in one series (Table 28.14) (170,182–186). Treatments appear to be well tolerated, with no reported severe chronic toxicities. Although initial results appear promising, follow-up is short (median follow-up 20–38 months), and more experience is needed to define its role vis-à-vis conventionally fractionated radiotherapy and surgery. Limitations of SRS include eligibility restrictions lesion size and location as well as a greater risk for geographic miss due to the sharp dose gradient (182). Tumors may be no greater than 4 cm to achieve tight dose conformality. Only lesions located above the stereotactic frame may be treated due to treatment planning constraints. Therefore, primarily skull-based lesions can be treated, but lesions originating from or extending into the upper neck may not be adequately covered.

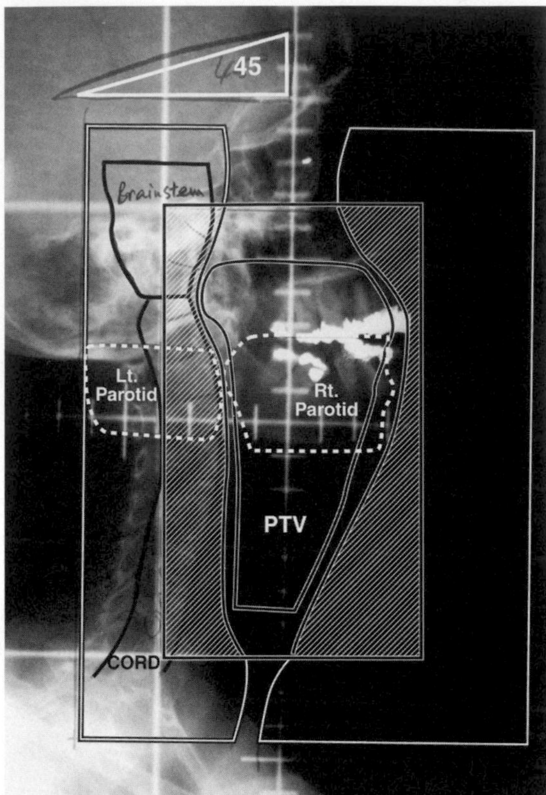

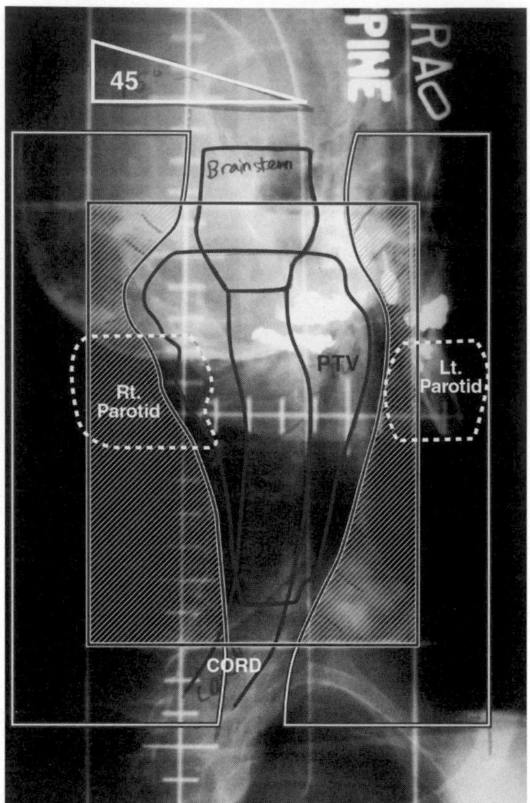

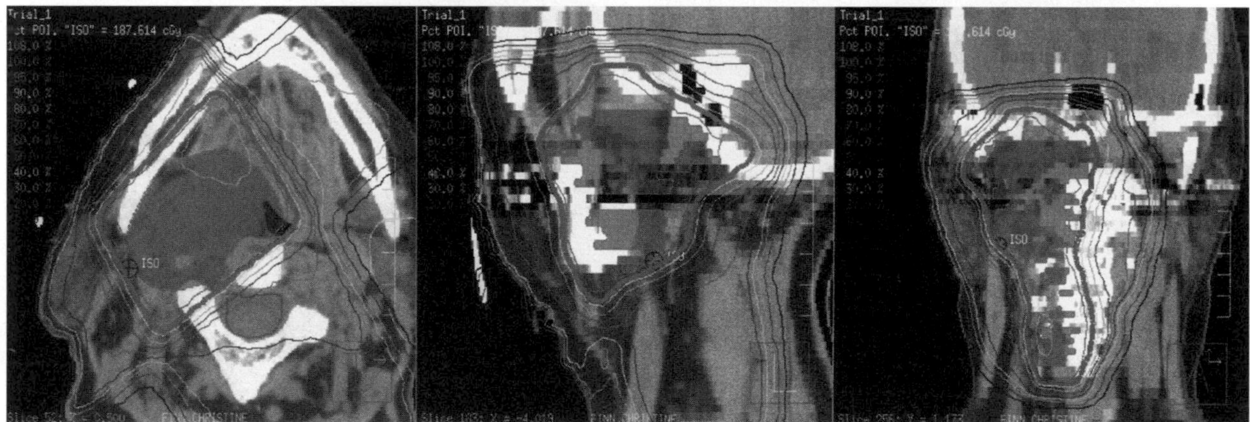

Figure 28.22 Three-dimensional treatment plan of a 69-year-old woman treated with radiation for a vagal paraganglioma. She received a dose of 45 Gy in 5 weeks. Particular effort was made to minimize dose to the contralateral parotid, brainstem, and spinal cord. PTV, planning target volume.

TABLE 28.14 Experience with Stereotactic Radiosurgery

Institution	No. of patients	Median follow-up	RT dose: mean peripheral dose	Local control	Complications
Liscak	14	20 mo	19.4 Gy (10–25 Gy)	100%	Acute: headache and nausea in 2 patients Chronic: hearing decreased in 3 patients
Austria (Eustacchio)	10	38 mo	13.5 Gy	100%	
Mayo (Foote)	9	20 mo	15 Gy (12–18 Gy)	100%	No reported chronic or acute toxicities
University of Texas, Southwestern (Jordan)	8	27 mo	16 Gy (12–20 Gy)	88%	Chronic: intractable vertigo requiring cane resolved—1 patient

TREATMENT STRATEGIES

Patients presenting with signs and symptoms of a paraganglioma should undergo a thorough history and physical examination to evaluate neural function. A positive family history may be strongly indicative of multiple tumors, which should be considered even in the sporadic cases. Computed tomography scanning and MRI will evaluate the extent of tumor, especially skull base or intracranial involvement. These studies usually identify the presence of unsuspected multiple paragangliomas or the possibility of malignant metastatic regional disease. If necessary, fine-needle aspiration biopsy is a diagnostic and safely performed procedure. If surgery is contemplated, angiography is indicated to identify tumor blood supply, to visualize possible vessel invasion, and to evaluate bilateral cerebral blood supply.

The ideal scenario is a patient who is cured of the tumor with minimal morbidity from the treatment. The concept of "cure" must be defined and accepted by the treating physician and, of course, the patient. Certainly, the surgical definition of cure is total tumor resection and long-term confirmation of no tumor recurrence. The radiation therapy literature has defined the criteria of cure, in the paraganglioma patient, as nonprogression of tumor as documented by appropriate long-term follow-up, which is so important in these slow-growing neoplasms. Only infrequently is there appreciable tumor regression, as is often seen in the successful treatment of malignant neoplasms of the head and neck (136). Therefore, the concept of cure in a paraganglioma patient should be modified to include stabilization or nonprogression of tumor growth. With this in mind, the comparison of paraganglioma treatment results between surgery and radiation therapy should focus on the justifiably different definition of cure. If the cure rate of one mode of treatment is statistically convincing, then that form of treatment should be administered. Because surgery and radiation therapy demonstrate equal cure rates (133), as indicated by the previous sections, then the focus should be on the associated morbidity and mortality of each treatment.

Primary surgery should be considered for patients with small to moderate-size CBTs and tympanic paragangliomas without CN dysfunction. These tumors can usually be totally excised without significant morbidity. Primary surgery is also indicated for patients with jugular or vagal paragangliomas in the presence of lower CN dysfunction (CNs VII, IX–XII), whereby resection of the tumor would not result in additional significant functional deficits, especially in younger and middle-aged patients without coexisting medical problems. If a diagnosis of a malignant paraganglioma is established, tumor resection with a neck dissection is indicated, assuming there is no evidence of systemic disease. Primary radiation therapy is presently the accepted treatment of the elderly, poor-risk patients with multiple or severe medical conditions, and patients with extensive skull base or intracranial involvement. Radiation therapy is also indicated in patients with jugular or vagal paragangliomas and no evidence of lower CN dysfunction and in patients with multiple or bilateral tumors with the potential for severe postoperative debility from CN dysfunction (52,54,66,85,87,184,187). Observation without treatment is also an option for older patients who can be closely followed in the setting of these slowly growing tumors (188).

Refinements in surgery, interventional radiology, and medical care have resulted in acceptable surgical mortality rates for even extensive tumors. However, surgical treatment of paragangliomas, especially those with a natural history of early skull base involvement (e.g., jugular paragangliomas) and early CN involvement (e.g., vagal paragangliomas), results in a higher incidence of CN dysfunction as compared with radiation therapy. Indeed, there is even evidence of occasional improved CN function in paragangliomas treated by radiation therapy. Certainly, lower CN dysfunction (CNs VII, IX–XII) represents a potentially significant debility, especially if multiple CNs are affected. Although rehabilitation techniques can improve the patients' ability to cope with these problems, it is still better to avoid these debilities if cure can be obtained. Radiation therapy has the advantage of avoiding the increased morbidity of surgery while offering an equal possibility of cure (133–135). Of course, the morbidity of radiation therapy must be considered, but proper treatment planning with appropriate dosing (4,500 cGy/5 weeks for fractional therapy) results in minimal side reactions. Salvage therapy, either surgery for previously radiated patients or radiation therapy for patients having undergone prior resection, has also been proven effective in controlling local disease. The treatment algorithms are shown in Figures 28.23 and 28.24.

If a diagnosis of a malignant paraganglioma is established (clinical evidence of involved lymph nodes or metastatic disease), tumor resection with a neck dissection and postoperative radiation is indicated, assuming there is no evidence of systemic disease.

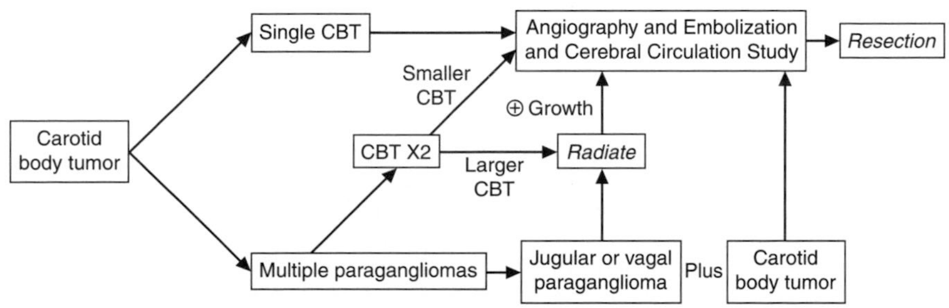

Figure 28.23 Treatment of carotid body tumor (CBT) ± multiple paragangliomas.

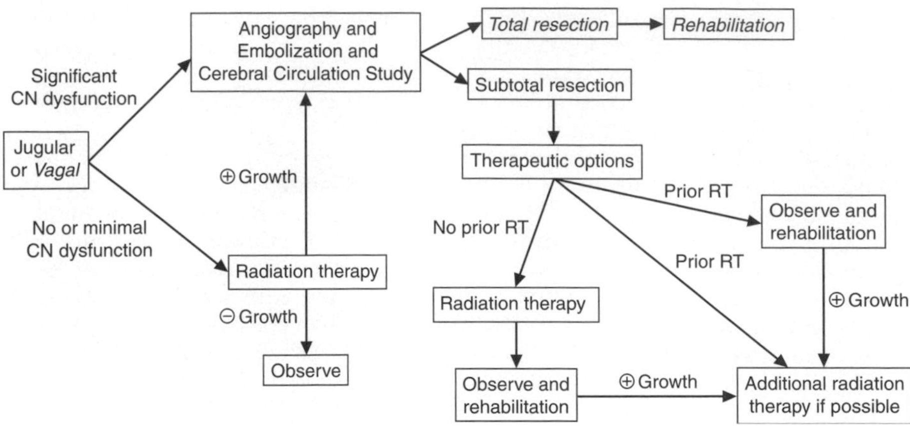

Figure 28.24 Treatment of jugular and vagal paragangliomas. RT, radiation therapy.

RADIOLOGIC IMAGING CONCERNS

Bernard B. O'Malley

Paragangliomas develop in predictable locations with fairly typical imaging features (189) and clinical syndromes (Fig. 28.25). Depending on location, however, they can present clinically at early or very advanced stages. Several modalities can be used for detection and staging of solitary or multiple lesions in the head and neck region (190,191).

Because of the vascular nature of these lesions, contrast CT with proper bolus parameters can detect and stage paragangliomas (Fig. 28.26). In the neck, the degree of vascular encasement can be estimated with either CT or MRI; MRI and MRA can supplant the role of CT, which requires iodinated contrast. The pattern on MRI is different from the homogeneous enhancement of the mass on CT. The typical MRI pattern is low signal (voids) against a background of heterogeneous signal or contrast enhancement (Fig. 28.27). Magnetic resonance angiography can show the position and condition of the lumen of the carotid artery (Fig. 28.27), but prediction of adventitial involvement requires correlation with thin axial sections. Ultimately, the advanced lesions may require catheter angiography for full characterization of the vascular supply (Fig. 28.28). Test carotid balloon occlusion can be performed if there is a risk for needing intraoperative bypass, vascular graft, or sacrifice.

In the skull base, petrous bone, and jugular foramen, CT and MRI are complementary. Lesions of the jugular system (jugulare and nodose) can be obscured by the native enhancement of the vein (and adjacent carotid); MRI and MRA can resolve this issue even on noncontrast series (Fig. 28.29) (192,193). The heterogeneous signal of paragangliomas is detectable against the background of either the high signal of slow (venous) flow or low signal of rapid arterial or venous flow (194). Infiltration of the skull base is observed with MRI, which can differentiate between infiltrated or obstructed mastoid air cells (Fig. 28.30). Computed tomography can demonstrate the degree of mastoid bone destruction and permeation and can outline the course of jugular and carotid canals. It can demonstrate better than MRI the status of the middle ear and ossicles. Both MRI and CT can evaluate involvement of the posterior fossa. Catheter angiography with embolization can be performed to aid in reducing the operative hemorrhage (195) in this critical location.

Follow-up in the neck is challenging because of the vascular nature of scarring, which renders detection of an enhancing lesion difficult. There is a characteristic enhancement profile (196), however, that allows one to differentiate among paraganglioma, solid tumor, and scar (Fig. 28.31). For nonsurgical cases, follow-up imaging shows minor change in overall lesion size in more than half the cases treated (197). There should be a decrease in the characteristic flow-void pattern in the mass, however (197).

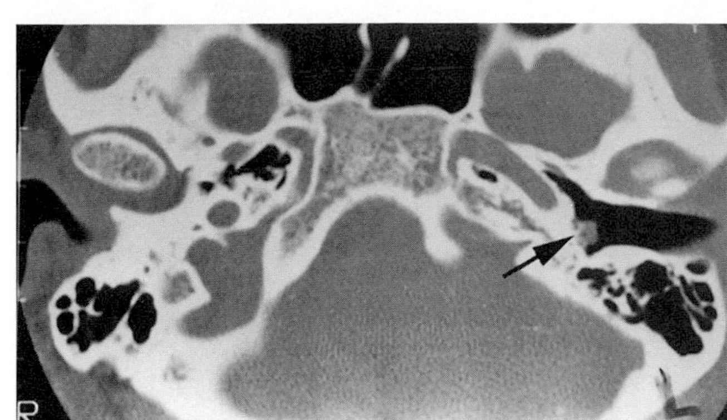

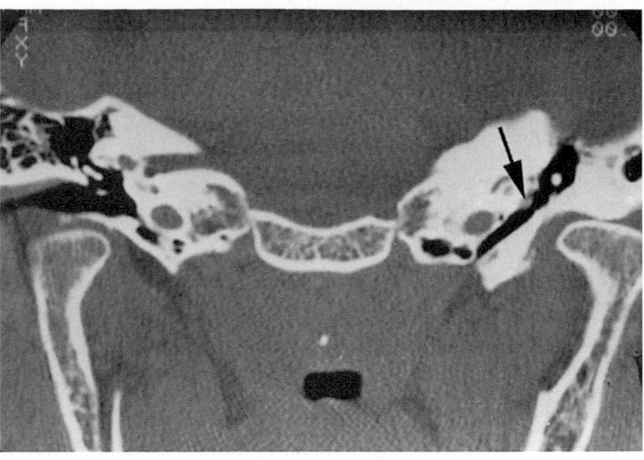

Figure 28.25 Glomus tympanicum. Axial **(A)** and direct coronal **(B)** computed tomography views show a tiny lesion at the cochlear promontory (*arrows*) in a patient with pulsatile tinnitus. Note the grainy pattern of the background soft tissues as a result of processing the images for high spatial (bone) resolution.

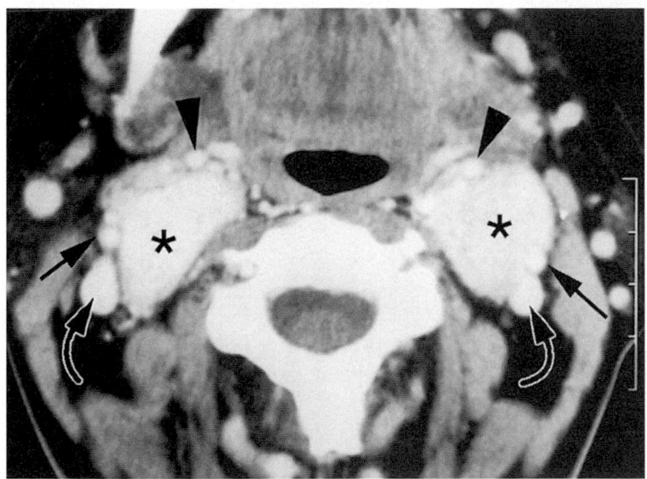

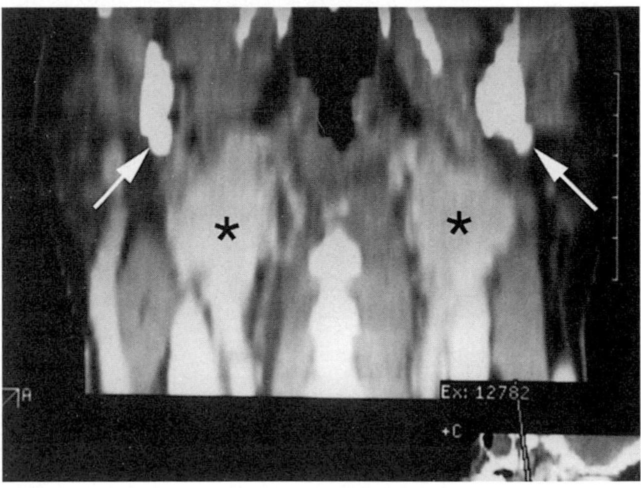

Figure 28.26 Bilateral carotid body tumors. **A:** Enhanced axial computed tomography image of upper neck. Shown are intense homogeneously enhancing masses (*asterisk*) arising in both bifurcations, with displacement of the internal carotid (*arrows*) from the external carotid branches (*arrowheads*). Jugular veins (*curved arrows*). **B:** Coronal reformatted views show bilateral masses (*asterisk*) and angles of mandible (*arrows*).

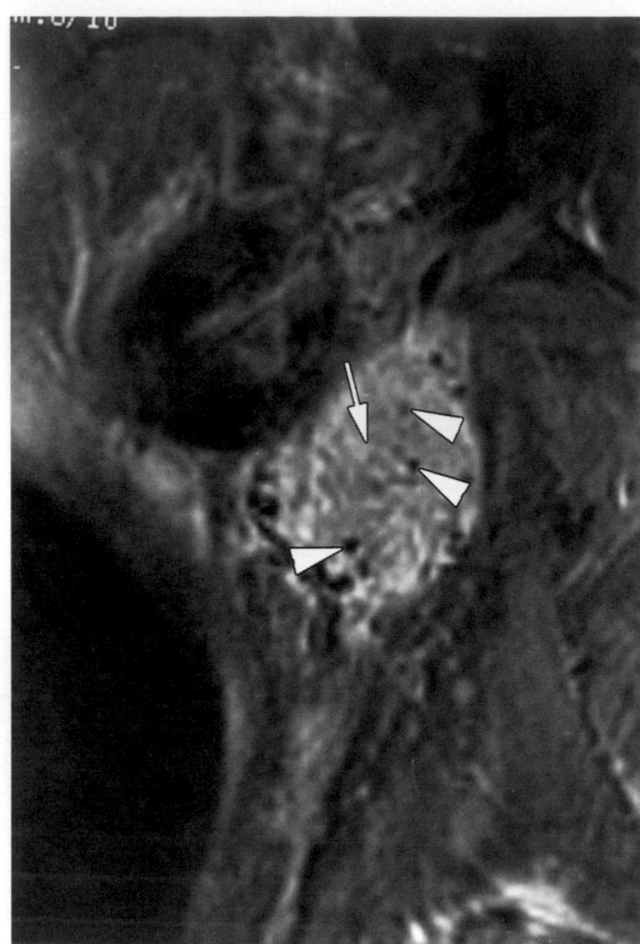

A

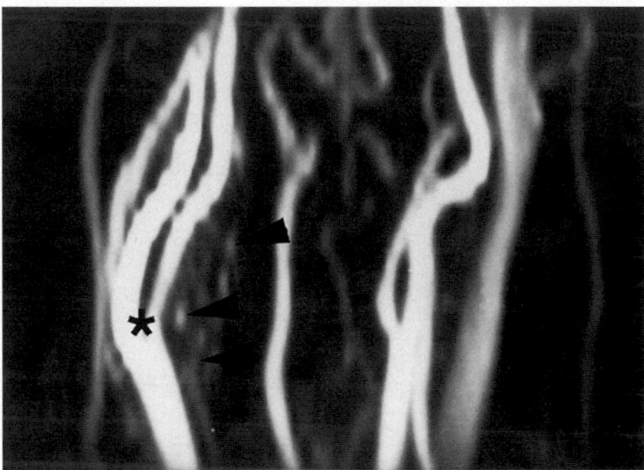

B

Figure 28.27 Unilateral carotid body tumor. **A:** Parasagittal fat-suppressed contrast T1-magnetic resonance imaging shows heterogeneous mass at the left carotid bifurcation, with typical pattern of low-signal voids (*arrowheads*) against a background of heterogeneous signal (*arrow*). **B:** Magnetic resonance angiogram of midneck shows faint linear segments of enhancement (*arrowheads*) related to the mass displacing the carotid bifurcation (*asterisk*) laterally.

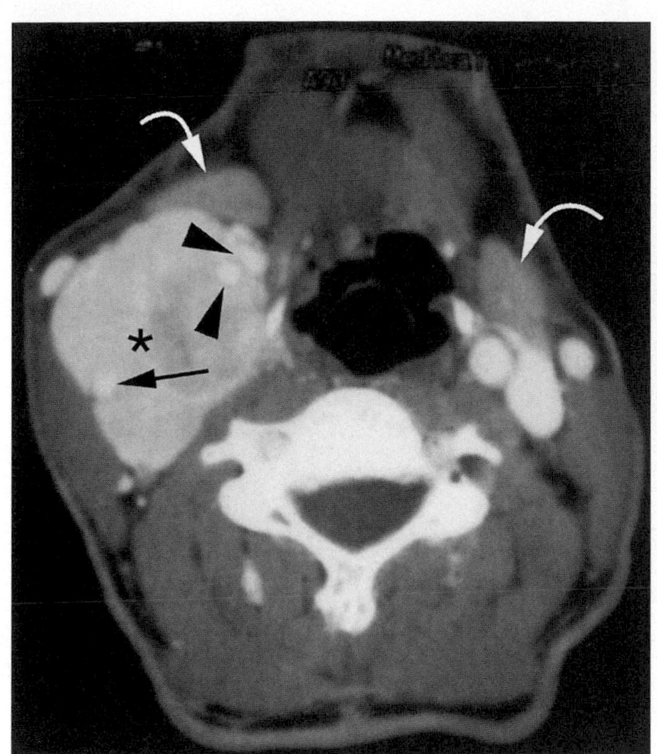
A

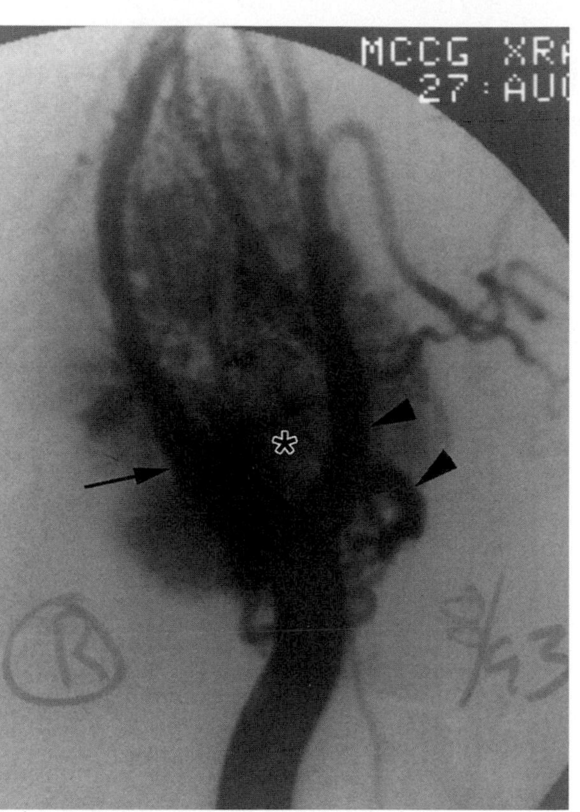

B

Figure 28.28 Huge carotid body tumor. **A:** Enhanced axial computed tomography. **B:** Right common carotid angiogram. Both show huge homogeneously enhancing mass (*asterisk*) splaying the carotid bifurcation. The mass surrounds the internal carotid artery (*arrows*) and branches of the external carotid artery (*arrowheads*). Note the submandibular glands (*curved arrows*).

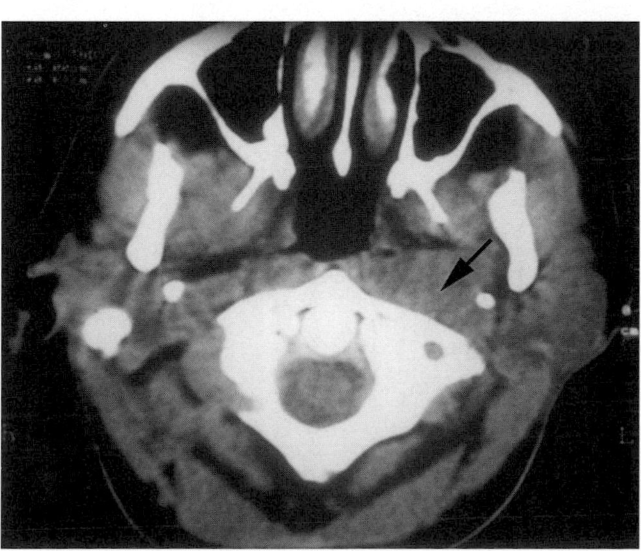
A

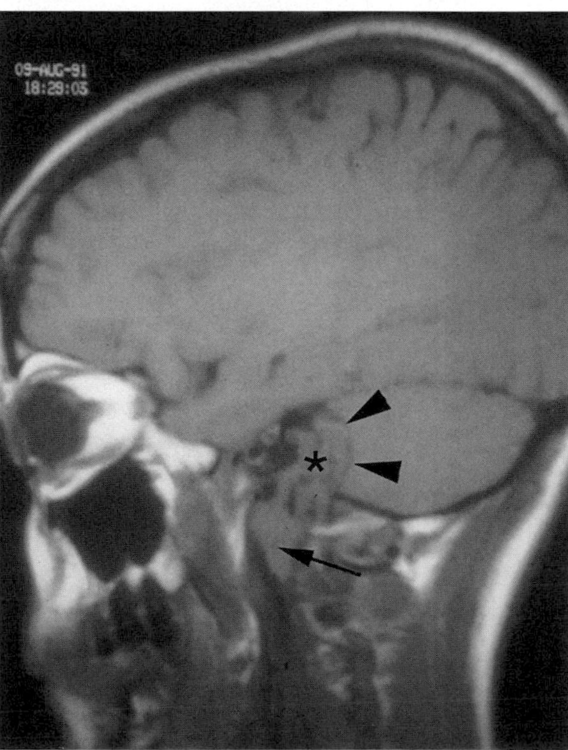

B

Figure 28.29 Glomus jugulare. Noncontrast axial computed tomographic scan **(A)** and noncontrast parasagittal magnetic resonance imaging **(B)** show a heterogeneous mass (*asterisk*) expanding out of the jugular foramen below skull base (*arrows*) and into the (extradural) posterior fossa (*arrowheads*).

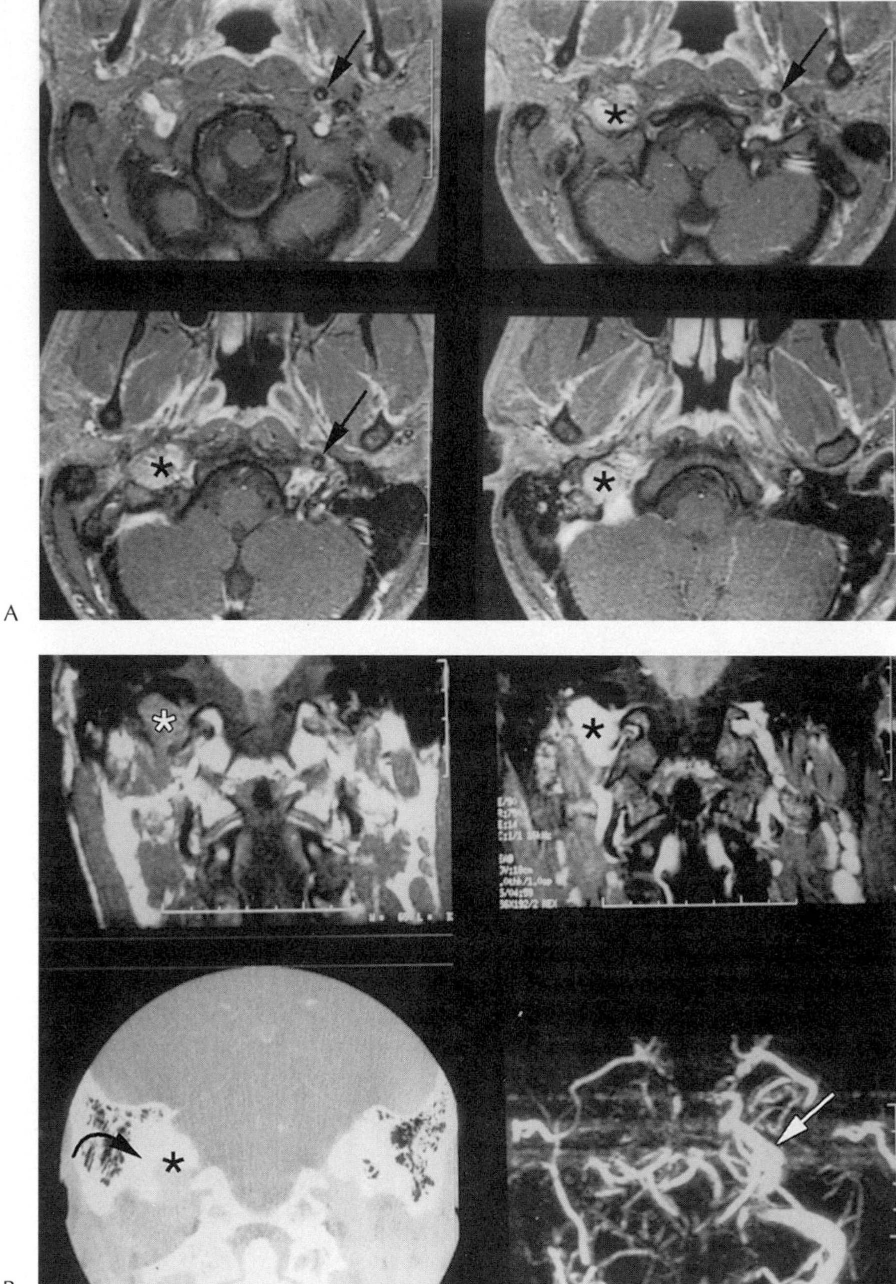

Figure 28.30 Glomus jugulare. **A:** Serial-enhanced, fat-suppressed, axial T1 magnetic resonance imaging views show intense homogeneously enhancing mass within the right jugular fossa (*asterisk*). Note conspicuous absence of right internal carotid artery flow void at skull base, compared with normal left flow (*arrow*). The right carotid artery was sacrificed in the remote past during resection of a huge paraganglioma of the innominate artery. **B:** Matched precontrast (*left*) and postcontrast (*right*) coronal T1-weighted magnetic resonance imaging views of skull base and (*lower panel*) contrast coronal computed tomography and magnetic resonance imaging (*right*) of skull base show same findings. Note sclerotic reaction of mastoid bone about jugular fossa. *Curved arrow* indicates jugular fossa.

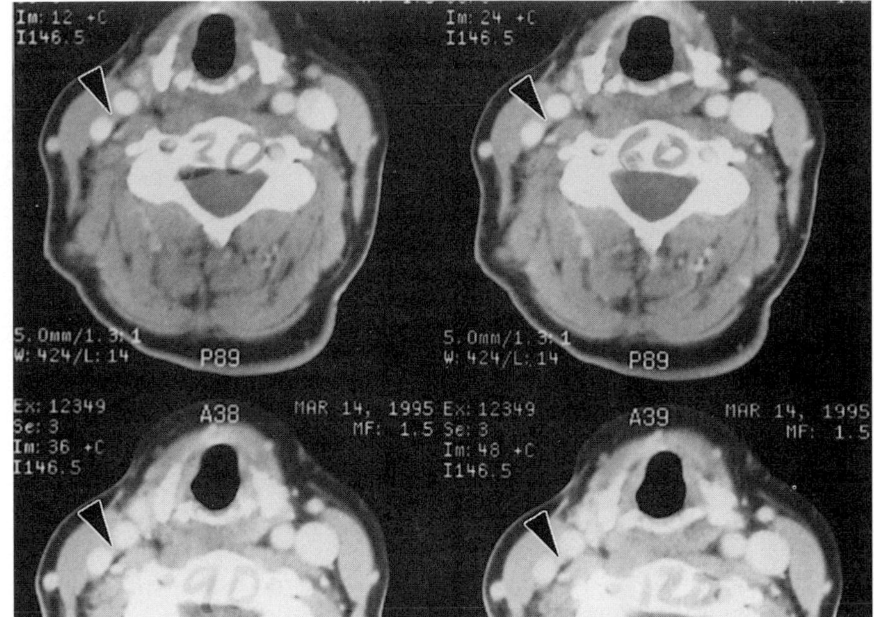

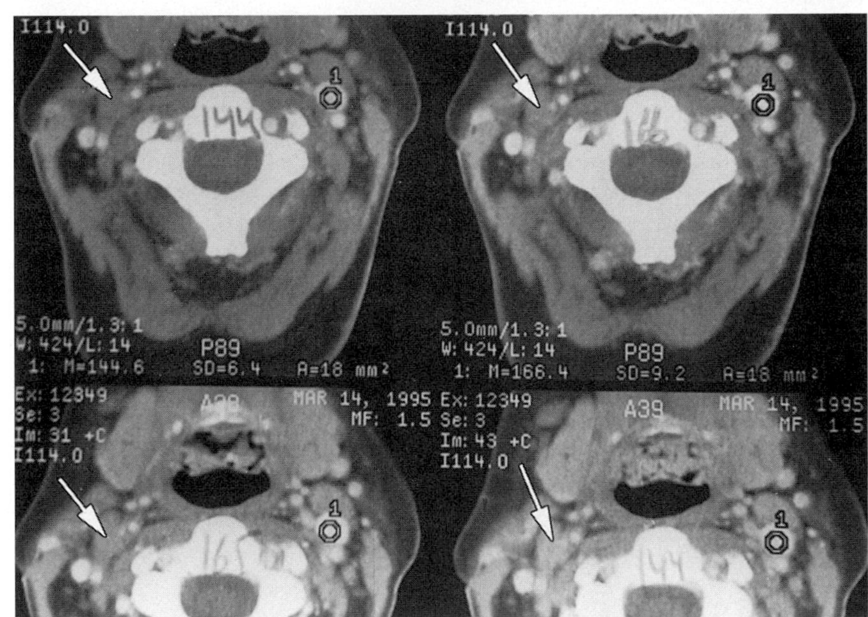

Figure 28.31 Follow-up surveillance. **A:** Timed sequential axial images at 30, 60, 90, and 120 seconds at level of right carotid bifurcation (*arrowhead*). **B:** Timed images above carotid bifurcation show that scarring at the right jugulodigastric level (*arrow*) (interpreted as recurrence on prior magnetic resonance imaging) has little, if any, enhancement. Region of interest measures at left common carotid artery provide reference arterial type curve of Hounsfield units.

RADIATION THERAPY TECHNIQUE

William M. Mendenhall

The treatment technique depends on the location of the tumor, the number of lesions (1 or ≥ 2), and whether the tumor is malignant. The vast majority of tumors are single and benign.

Temporal bone tumors may be treated with stereotactic radiosurgery or fractionated radiation therapy. Stereotactic radiosurgery is performed with either a linear accelerator–based system or a gamma knife; the results with either technique are equivalent (198).

Fractionated radiation therapy may be delivered with stereotactic radiation therapy, intensity-modulated radiation therapy (IMRT), or a wedge pair technique using three-dimensional conformal treatment planning (Fig. 28.32) (199). The lesion is treated with a 1-cm margin of normal tissue to a dose of 45 Gy in 25 fractions over 5 weeks. The disadvantage of the wedge pair technique is that a larger volume of normal tissue is treated. However, even very large tumors can be treated with an ipsilateral technique that will result in a very low dose to the contralateral parotid gland and minimize the risk for xerostomia.

Glomus vagale and carotid tumors are not suitable for stereotactic radiosurgery and are better treated with IMRT or three-dimensional treatment planning using a wedge pair technique.

The technique used for patients with multiple tumors is variable and depends on the location and extent of the lesions. Very large bilateral tumors may require parallel-opposed fields. Alternatively, resection of one lesion and irradiation of the contralateral tumor may minimize the long-term morbidity of treatment if one of the lesions can be resected with acceptable morbidity.

There is little information pertaining to radiation therapy for malignant paragangliomas. The diagnosis of malignancy is based on the presence of metastatic disease. Our philosophy has been to resect lesions that can be resected with acceptable morbidity and to add postoperative irradiation depending on the pathologic findings. In practice, most patients who are operated on for malignant paragangliomas receive adjuvant postoperative irradiation at our institution. The dose fractionation schedules are similar to those employed for other malignancies. Because (by definition) the regional lymph nodes are involved, the ipsilateral lymph nodes must be included in the target volume.

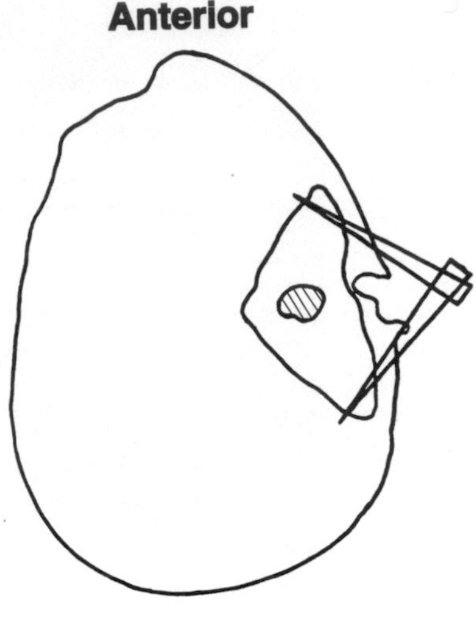

Figure 28.32 Axial contour of skull through the temporal bone depicting the dose distribution for the wedge pair technique. This consists of oblique 6-MV x-ray fields with wedge compensating filters. The fields enter anteroinferiorly and posterosuperiorly so that the beams enter and exit below the eyes. The 93% isodose line encompasses the temporal bone chemodectoma (*hatched area*). (From Mendenhall WM, Friedman WA, Parsons JT, et al. Radiation therapy and stereotactic radiosurgery for temporal bone tumors. *Oper Tech Otolaryngol Head Neck Surg* 1996;7:208–218, with permission.)

REFERENCES

1. Jackson G. Diagnosis for treatment planning and treatment options. *Laryngoscope* 1993;103:17–22.
2. Pearse A. The cytochemistry and ultrastructure of the polypeptide hormone-producing cells of the APUD series and the embryonic, physiologic and pathologic implications of the concept. *J Histochem Cytochem* 1969;17:303–313.
3. Pearse A. The diffuse neuroendocrine system: historical review. *Front Horm Res* 1984;12:1–7.
4. Schwaber M, et al. Diagnosis and management of Catecholamine secreting Glomus Tumors. *Laryngoscope* 1984;94:1008–1015.
5. Matsuguchi H, et al. Noradrenalin-secreting glomus tumor with cyclic change of blood pressure. *Arch Intern Med* 1975;135:1110–1113.
6. Kliewer K, Cochran A. A review of the histology, ultrastructure, Immunohistology, and molecular biology of extra-adrenal paragangliomas. *Arch Pathol Lab Med* 1989;113:1209–1218.
7. Glenner G, Grimley P. Tumors of the extra-adrenal paraganglion system (including chemoreceptors). In: *Atlas of tumor pathology*. Washington, DC: Armed Forces Institute of Pathology, 1974:1–90.
8. Thirlwall AS, et al. Laryngeal paraganglioma in a five-year-old child—the youngest case ever recorded. *J Laryngol Otol* 1999;113:62–64.
9. Venkataramana N, et al. Paraganglioma of the orbit with extension to the middle cranial fossa: a case report. *Neurosurgery* 1989;24:762–764.
10. Kronz J, et al. Paraganglioma of the thyroid: two cases that clarify and expand the clinical spectrum. *Head Neck* 2000;22:621–625.
11. Nielsen TO, Sejean G, Onerheim RM. Paraganglioma of the tongue. *Arch Pathol Lab Med* 2000;124:877–879.
12. Welkoborsky HJ, et al. Biologic characteristics of paragangliomas of the nasal cavity and paranasal sinuses. *Am J Rhinol* 2000;14:419–426.
13. Sharma HS, et al. Malignant paraganglioma of frontoethmoidal region. *Auris Nasus Larynx* 1999;26:487–493.
14. Skinner LJ, et al. Paraganglioma of the external auditory canal: an unusual case. *J Laryngol Otol* 2000;114:370–372.
15. Sambaziotis D, et al. Intrasellar paraganglioma presenting as nonfunctioning pituitary adenoma. *Arch Pathol Lab Med* 1999;123:429–432.
16. Yamauchi T, et al. Paraganglioma in the frontal skull base—case report. *Neurol Med Chir* 1999;39:308–312.
17. Barnes L, Taylor S. Carotid body paragangliomas: a clinicopathologic and DNA analysis of 13 tumors. *Arch Otolaryngol Head Neck Surg* 1990;116: 447–453.
18. Adams W. The comparative morphology of the carotid body and carotid sinus. Springfield, IL: Charles C. Thomas, 1958:272.
19. Heath D. The Human Carotid Body in Health and Disease. *J Pathol* 1991;16:1–8.
20. Heath D, Smith P. The pathology of the carotid body and sinus, vol 17. Baltimore: Edward Arnold, 1985.
21. Smith P, Jago R, Heath D. Anatomical variations and quantitative histology of the normal and enlarged carotid body. *J Pathol* 1982;187:287–304.
22. Khan Q, Heath D, Smith P. Anatomical variations in human carotid bodies. *J Clin Pathol* 1988;41:1196–1199.
23. Rao AB, Koeller KK, Adair CF. From the archives of the AFIP. Paragangliomas of the head and neck: radiologic-pathologic correlation. Armed Forces Institute of Pathology. *Radiographics* 1999;19:1605–1632.
24. Guild S. Glomus jugulare in man, a nonchromaffin paraganglioma, in man. *Ann Otol Rhinol Laryngol* 1953;62:1045–1071.
25. Guild S. A hitherto unrecognized structure, the glomus jugulares in man. *Anat Rec* 1941;79(suppl 2):28.
26. Katsuta T, Rhoton AL, Matsushima T. The jugular foramen: microsurgical anatomy and operative approaches. *Neurosurgery* 1997;41:149–202.
27. Kliewer K, et al. Paragangliomas: assessment of prognosis by histologic, immunohistochemical, and ultrastructural techniques. *Hum Pathol* 1989;20: 29–39.
28. Gulya A. Glomus tumors and its biology. *Laryngoscope* 1993;103:7–15.
29. Lawson W. The neuroendocrine nature of the glomus cells: an experimental, ultrastructural, and histochemical tissue culture study. *Laryngoscope* 1980;90: 120–144.
30. Kohn A. Die paraganglien. *Arch Mikr Anat* 1903;62:263.
31. Sykes J, Ossoff R. Paragangliomas of the head and neck. *Otolaryngol Clin North Am* 1986;19:755–767.
32. Rosenwasser H. Carotid body like tumor involving the middle ear and mastoid bone. *Arch Otolaryngol* 1945;41:64–67.
33. Mulligan R. Chemodectoma in the dog. *Am J Pathol* 1950;26:680–681.
34. Jyung RW, et al. Expression of angiogenic growth factors in paragangliomas. *Laryngoscope* 2000;110:161–167.
35. Lack E, Cubilla A, Woodruff J. Paragangliomas of the head and neck region. A pathologic study of tumors from 71 patients. *Hum Pathol* 1979;10:191–218.
36. Lawson W. Glomus bodies and tumors. *NY State J Med* 1980;80:1567–1575.
37. Wenig B. Pathology of head and neck cancer, part III. In: Harrison L, Sessions R, Hong W, eds. *Head and neck cancer*. Philadelphia: Lippincott-Raven, 1999.
38. Lack E, et al. Paragangliomas of the head and neck region: a clinical study of 69 patients. *Cancer* 1977;39:397–409.
39. Persky MS, Setton A, Niimi Y, et al. Combined endovascular and surgical treatment of head and neck paragangliomas—a team approach. *Head Neck* 2002;24:423–431.
40. Arias-Stella J. Human carotid body at high altitudes. *Am J Pathol* 1969;55:82a.
41. Rodriguez-Cuevas S, Lopez-Garza J, Labastida-Almendaro S. Carotid body tumors in inhabitants of altitudes higher than 2000 meters above sea level. *Head Neck* 1998;20:374–378.
42. Saldana M, Salem L, Travezan R. High altitude hypoxia and chemodectomas. *Hum Pathol* 1973;4:251–263.
43. Edwards C, Heath D, Harris P. The carotid body in emphysema and left ventricular hypertrophy. *J Pathol* 1971;104:1–13.
44. Chedid A, Jao W. Hereditary tumors of the carotid bodies and chronic obstructive pulmonary disease. *Cancer* 1974;33:1635–1641.
45. Oosterwijk J, et al. First experience with genetic counselling based on predictive DNA diagnosis in hereditary glomus tumors (paragangliomas). *J Med Genet* 1996;33:379–383.
46. van der Mey AG, Maaswinkel-Mooy PD, Cornelisse CJ, et al. Genetic imprinting in hereditary glomus tumours: evidence for a new genetic theory. *Lancet* 1989;2:1291–1294.
47. Heutink P, et al. A gene subject to genomic imprinting and responsible for hereditary paragangliomas maps to chromosome 11q23–qter. *Hum Mol Genet* 1992;1:7–10.
48. Drovdlic C, et al. Proportion of heritable paraganglioma cases and associated clinical characteristics. *Laryngoscope* 2001;111:1822–1827.
49. Mariman E, et al. Fine mapping of a putatively imprinted gene for familial nonchromaffin paragangliomas to chromosome 11q13.1: evidence for genetic heterogeneity. *Hum Genet* 1995;95:56–62.
50. Jansen JC, et al. Estimation of growth rate in patients with head and neck paragangliomas influences the treatment proposal. *Cancer* 2000;88:2 811–2816.
51. Grufferman S, et al. Familial carotid body tumors: Case report and epidemiologic review. *Cancer* 1980;46:2116–2122.
52. Netterville JL, et al. Carotid body tumors: a review of 30 patients with 46 tumors. *Laryngoscope* 1995;105:115–126.
53. Netterville JL, et al. Vagal paraganglioma: a review of 46 patients treated during a 20-year period. *Arch Otolaryngol Head Neck Surg* 1998;124:1133–1140.
54. Gardner P, et al. Carotid body tumors, inheritance, and a high incidence of associated cervical paragangliomas. *Am J Surg* 1996;172:196–199.
55. Shamblin W, et al. Carotid body tumor (chemodectoma): clinicopathologic analysis of ninety cases. *Am Surg* 1971;122:732–739.
56. Pacheco-Ojeda L. Malignant carotid body tumors: report of three cases. *Ann Otol Rhinol Laryngol* 2001;110:36–40.
57. Zbaren, Lehman W. Carotid body paragangliomawith metastasis. *Laryngoscope* 1985;95:450–454.
58. Manolidis S, et al. Malignant glomus tumors. *Laryngoscope* 1999;109:30–34.
59. El Finky F, Paparella M. A metastatic glomus jugulare tumor. A temporal bone report. *Am J Otol* 1984;5:197–200.
60. Druck N, et al. Malignant Glomus vagale: report of a case and review of the literature. *Arch Otolaryngol* 1976;102:534–536.
61. Batsakis J. Paragangliomas of the head and neck. In: *Tumors of the head and neck: clinical and pathological consideration*. Baltimore: Williams & Wilkins, 1979:369–380.
62. Zak F, et al. *The paraganglionic chemoreceptor system*. New York: Springer-Verlag, 1982.
63. Irons G, Weiland L, Brown W. Paragangliomas of the neck: clinical and pathologic analysis of 116 cases. *Surg Clin North Am* 1977;57:575–583.
64. Parkin J. Familial multiple glomus tumors and pheochromocytomas. *Ann Otol Rhinol Laryngol* 1981;90:60–63.
65. Revak C, Morris S, Alexander G. Pheochromocytoma and recurrent chemodectomas over a twenty-five year period. *Radiology* 1971;100:53–54.
66. Maier W, Marangos N, Laszig R. Paraganglioma as a systemic syndrome: pitfalls and strategies. *J Laryngol Otol* 1999;113:978–982.
67. Wax M, Briant T. Carotid body tumors: A review. *J Otolaryngol* 1992;21:277–285.
68. Williams M, et al. Carotid body tumor. *Arch Surg* 1992;127:963–968.
69. Gaylis H, Davidge-Pitts K, Pantanowitz D. Carotid body tumours. A review of 52 cases. *S Afr J Surg* 1987;72:493–496.
70. Dickinson P, et al. Carotid body tumour: 30 years experience. *Br J Surg* 1986;73:14–16.
71. Muhm M, et al. Diagnostic and therapeutic approaches to carotid body tumors. Review of 24 patients. *Arch Surg* 1997;132:279–284.
72. Lees C, et al. Tumors of the carotid body: experience with 41 operative cases. *Am J Surg* 1981;142:362–365.
73. Leonetti JP, et al. Perioperative strategies in the management of carotid body tumors. *Otolaryngol Head Neck Surg* 1997;117:111–115.
74. Shedd D, Arias J, Glunk R. Familial occurrence of carotid body tumors. *Head Neck* 1990;12:496–499.
75. Matticari S, et al. Diagnosis and surgical treatment of the carotid body tumors. *J Cardiovasc Surg* 1995;36:233–239.
76. Sakurai H, et al. Chemodectoma of the carotid body treated with radiation therapy: a case report. *Radiat Med* 1995;13:191–194.
77. Alford B, Guilford F. A comprehensive study of tumors of the glomus jugulare. *Laryngoscope* 1962;72:765–787.
78. Fisch U. Infratemporal fossa approach for extensive tumors of the temporal bone and base of the skull. *J Laryngol Otol* 1978;92:949.
79. Jackson C, Glasscock ML, Harris P. Glomus tumors: diagnosis, classification and management of large lesions. *Arch Otolaryngol* 1982;108:401–406.
80. Swartz J, Harnsberger R, Mukherji S. The temporal bone. *Radiol Clin North Am* 1998;36:819–853.

81. Valavanis A, Schubiger O, Oguz M. High-resolution CT investigation of nonchromaffin paragangliomas of the temporal bone. *AJNR* 1983;4:516–519.
82. Jackson CG, et al. Diagnosis and management of paragangliomas of the skull base. *Am J Surg* 1990;159:389–393.
83. Bishop GB Jr, et al. Paragangliomas of the neck. *Arch Surg* 1992;127: 1441–1445.
84. Ogura J, Spector G, Gado M. Glomus jugulare and vagale. *Ann Otol* 1978;87(5 pt 1):622–629.
85. Gardner G, Cocke E, Robertson J. Skull base surgery for glomus jugulare tumors. *Am J Otol* 1985;126–134.
86. Biller H, et al. Glomus vagale tumors. *Ann Otol Rhinol Laryngol* 1989;98(1 pt 1):21–26.
87. Urquhart AC, et al. Glomus vagale: paraganglioma of the vagus nerve. *Laryngoscope* 1994;104:440–445.
88. Moore G, Yarington CT Jr, Mangham CA Jr. Vagal body tumors: diagnosis and treatment. *Laryngoscope* 1986;96:533–536.
89. Som P, et al. Parapharyngeal space masses: an updated protocol based on 104 cases. *Radiology* 1984;153:149–156.
90. Cheng A, Niparko JK. Imaging quiz case 2. Glomus tympanicum tumor of the temporal bone. *Arch Otolaryngol Head Neck Surg* 1997;123:549,551–552.
91. Chakeres D, LaMasters D. Paragangliomas of the temporal bone: high resolution CT studies. *Radiology* 1984;150:749–753.
92. Som P, et al. Tumors of the parapharyngeal space and upper neck: MR imaging characteristics. *Radiology* 1987;164:823–829.
93. Olsen W, et al. MR imaging of paragangliomas. *AJR* 1987;148:201–204.
94. van Gils AP, et al. MRI screening of kindred at risk of developing paragangliomas: support for genomic imprinting in hereditary glomus tumours. *Br J Cancer* 1992;65:903–907.
95. van den Berg R, et al. Vascularization of head and neck paragangliomas: comparison of three MR angiographic techniques with digital subtraction angiography. *AJNR* 2000;21:162–170.
96. Telischi FF, et al. Octreotide scintigraphy for the detection of paragangliomas. *Otolaryngol Head Neck Surg* 2000;122:358–362.
97. Lasjaunias P, Berenstein A. *Surgical neuro-angiography; endovascular treatment of craniofacial lesions,* vol 2. New York: Springer-Verlag, 1987.
98. Jackson C. Skull Base Surgery. *Am J Otol* 1981;3:161–171.
99. Anand VK, Alemar GO, Sanders TS. Management of the internal carotid artery during carotid body tumor surgery. *Laryngoscope* 1995;105(3 pt 1):231–235.
100. Steed D, et al. Clinical observations of the effect of carotid artery occlusion on cerebral blood flow mapped by Xenon computed tomography and its correlation with carotid artery back pressure. *J Vasc Surg* 1990;11:38–44.
101. Brackman D, Kinney S, Fu K. Glomus tumor: diagnosis and management. *Head Neck Surg* 1987;9:306–311.
102. Litle VR, Reilly LM, Ramos TK. Preoperative embolization of carotid body tumors: when is it appropriate? *Ann Vasc Surg* 1996;10:464–468.
103. Merland J, et al. Diagnostic and therapeutic angiography in the evaluation and treatment of glomus jugulare tumors. Apropos of 32 cases (French). *Neuro-Chirurgie* 1985;31:358–366.
104. Smith R, Shetty P, Reddy D. Surgical treatment of carotid paragangliomas presenting unusual technical difficulties. The value of preoperative embolization. *J Vasc Surg* 1988;7:631–637.
105. LaMuraglia, G, et al. The current surgical management of carotid body paragangliomas. *J Vasc Surg* 1992;15:1038–1044; discussion 1044–1045.
106. Ward P, et al. Embolization: an adjunctive measure for removal of carotid body tumors. *Laryngoscope* 1988;98:1287–1291.
107. Lasjaunias P. Nasopharyngeal angiofibromas: hazards of embolization. *Radiology* 1980;136:119–123.
108. Murphy T, Brackmann D. Effects of preoperative embolization on glomus jugulare tumors. *Laryngoscope* 1989;99:1244–1247.
109. Robison JG, et al. A multidisciplinary approach to reducing morbidity and operative blood loss during resection of carotid body tumor. *Surg Gynecol Obstet* 1989;168:166–170.
110. Borges L, Heros R, DeBrun G. Carotid body tumors managed with preoperative embolization. Report of two cases. *J Neurosurg* 1983;59:867–870.
111. Valavanis A. Preoperative embolization of the head and neck: indications, patient selection, goals, and precautions. *AJNR* 1986;7:943–952.
112. Wang SJ, et al. Surgical management of carotid body tumors. *Otolaryngol Head Neck Surg* 2000;123:202–206.
113. Moret J, et al. Interet de l'arteriographie therapeutique dans le traitment des glomus tympano-jugulaires. *Ann Otolaryngol (Paris)* 1977;94:491–498.
114. Moret J, Delvert G, Lasjaunias P. Vascular Architecture of tympanojugular glomus tumors. Its application regarding therapeutic angiography. *J Neuroradiol* 1982;9:237–260.
115. Casasco A, et al. Devascularization of craniofacial tumors by percutaneous tumor puncture. *AJNR* 1994;15:1233–1239.
116. Chaloupka J, et al. Evolving experience with direct puncture therapeutic embolization for adjunctive and palliative management of head and neck hypervascular neoplasms. *Laryngoscope* 1999;109:1864–1872.
117. House W, Glasscock M. Glomus tympanicum tumors. *Arch Otolaryngol* 1968; 87:550.
118. Brackmann D, Arriaga M. Surgery for glomus tumors. In: Brackmann D, Shelton C, Arriaga M, eds. *Otologic surgery.* Philadelphia: WB Saunders, 1994.
119. Fisch V, Mattox D. Microsurgery of the skull base. New York: Thieme, 1988: 149–153.
120. Netterville J, Civantos F. Defect reconstruction following neuro-otologic skull base surgery. *Laryngoscope* 1993;103:55–63.
121. Sen C, et al. Jugular foramen: microscopic anatomic features and implications for neural preservation with reference to glomus tumors involving the temporal bone. *Neurosurgery* 2001;48:838–848.
122. Hallett JW Jr, et al. Trends in neurovascular complications of surgical management for carotid body and cervical paragangliomas: a fifty-year experience with 153 tumors. *J Vasc Surg* 1988;7:284–291.
123. McCaffrey TV, et al. Familial paragangliomas of the head and neck. *Arch Otolaryngol Head Neck Surg* 1994;120:1211–1216.
124. Meyer FB, Sundt TM Jr, Pearson BW. Carotid body tumors: a subject review and suggested surgical approach. *J Neurosurg* 1986;64:377–385.
125. Netterville J, Vrabec J. Unilateral palatal adhesion for paralysis after high vagal injury. *Arch Otolaryngol Head Neck Surg* 1994;120:218–221.
126. Monro R. The natural history of carotid body tumours and their diagnosis and treatment. *Br J Surg* 1950;37:4445–4453.
127. Rosen I, et al. Vascular problems associated with carotid body tumors. *Am J Surg* 1981;142:459–463.
128. Pantanowitz D, Pitts-Davidge K, Demetriades D. The significance of the carotid bifurcation angle in carotid body tumors. *S Afr Med J* 1991;80:318–321.
129. Woods CI, Srasnick B, Jackson CG. Surgery for glomus tumors: the Otology Group experience. *Laryngoscopy* 1993;103:65–70.
130. Hatfield PM, James AE, Schulz MD. Chemodectomas of the glomus jugulare. *Cancer* 1972;30:1164–1168.
131. Spector GJ, et al. Glomus jugulare tumors: effects of radiotherapy. *Cancer* 1975;35:1316–1321.
132. Alford BR, Guilford FR. A comprehensive study of tumours of the glomus jugulare. *Laryngoscope* 1962;72:765–787.
133. Hinerman RW, et al. Definitive radiotherapy in the management of chemodectomas arising in the temporal bone, carotid body, and glomus vagale. *Head Neck* 2001;23:363–371.
134. Evenson L, et al. Radiotherapy in the management of chemodectomas of the carotid body and glomus vagale. *Head Neck* 1998;20:609–613.
135. Mumber M, Greven K. Control of advanced chemodectomas of the head and neck with irradiation. *Am J Clin Oncol* 1995;18:389–391.
136. Cole J, Beiler D. Long-term results of treatment for glomus jugulare and glomus vagale tumors with radiotherapy. *Laryngoscope* 1994;104:1461–1465.
137. Larner JM, et al. Glomus jugulare tumors. Long-term control by radiation therapy. *Cancer* 1992;69:1813–1817.
138. Schild SE, et al. Results of radiotherapy for chemodectomas. *Mayo Clin Proc* 1992;67:537–540.
139. Powell S, Peters N, Harmer C. Chemodectoma of the head and neck: results of treatment in 84 patients. *Int J Radiat Oncol Biol Phys* 1992;22:919–924.
140. Verniers DA, et al. Radiation therapy, an important mode of treatment for head and neck chemodectomas. *Eur J Cancer* 1992;28A(6–7):1028–1033.
141. Skolyszewski J, Korzeniowski S, Pszon J. Results of radiotherapy in chemodectoma of the temporal bone. *Acta Oncol* 1991;30:847–849.
142. Boyle JO, Shimm DS, Coulthard SW. Radiation therapy for paragangliomas of the temporal bone. *Laryngoscope* 1990;100:896–901.
143. Hoogenhout J, et al. Surgery and radiotherapy in the management of glomus body tumors. *Proc ESTRO* 1990:67.
144. Pryzant RM, Chou JL, Easley JD. Twenty year experience with radiation therapy for temporal bone chemodectomas. *Int J Radiat Oncol Biol Phys* 1989;17: 1303–1307.
145. Wang ML, et al. Chemodectoma of the temporal bone: a comparison of surgical and radiotherapeutic results. *Int J Radiat Oncol Biol Phys* 1988;14: 643–648.
146. Friedland JL, et al. Chemodectomas arising in temporal bone structures. *Head Neck Surg* 1988;10:S53–S55.
147. Hansen HS, Thomsen KA. Radiotherapy in glomus tumours (paragangliomas). A 25 year-review. *Acta Otolaryngol Suppl* 1988;449:151–154.
148. Konefal JB, et al. Radiation therapy in the treatment of chemodectomas. *Laryngoscope* 1987;97:1331–1335.
149. Dawes PJ, et al. The management of glomus jugulare tumours. *Clin Otolaryngol* 1987;12:15–24.
150. Zinreich ES, Lee DJ. Radiotherapy for the treatment of paragangliomas in the temporal bone. *Ear Nose Throat J* 1986;65:181–184.
151. Mitchell DC, Clyne CA. Chemodectomas of the neck: the response to radiotherapy. *Br J Surg* 1985;72:903–905.
152. Sharma PD, Johnson AP, Whitton AC. Radiotherapy for jugulo-tympanic paragangliomas (glomus jugulare tumours). *J Laryngol Otol* 1984;98:621–629.
153. Lybeert ML, et al. Radiotherapy of paragangliomas. *Clin Otolaryngol* 1984;9: 105–109.
154. Cummings BJ, et al. The treatment of glomus tumors in the temporal bone by megavoltage radiation. *Cancer* 1984;53:2635–2640.
155. Reddy EK, Mansfield CM, Hartman GV. Chemodectoma of glomus jugulare. *Cancer* 1983;52:337–340.
156. Dickens WJ, et al. Chemodectomas arising in temporal bone structures. *Laryngoscope* 1982;92:188–191.
157. Kim JA, et al. Optimum dose of radiotherapy for chemodectomas of the middle ear. *Int J Radiat Oncol Biol Phys* 1980;6:815–819.
158. Wang CC. Paraganglioma of the head and neck. In: Wang CC, ed. *Radiation therapy for head and neck neoplasms.* Chicago: Year Book Medical Publishers, 1990:371–377.
159. Gibbin KP, Henk JM. Glomus jugulare tumours in South Wales—a twenty-year review. *Clin Radiol* 1978;29:607–609.
160. Simko TG, et al. The role of radiation therapy in the treatment of glomus jugulare tumors. *Cancer* 1978;42:104–106.

161. Arthur K. Radiotherapy in chemodectoma of the glomus jugulare. *Clin Radiol* 1977;28:415–417.
162. Tidwell TJ, Montague ED. Chemodectomas involving the temporal bone. *Radiology* 1975;116:147–149.
163. Newman H, Rowe JF Jr, Phillips TL. Radiation therapy of the glomus jugulare tumor. *AJR Radium Ther Nucl Med* 1973;118:663–669.
164. Maruyama Y. Radiotherapy of tympanojugular chemodectomas. *Radiology* 1972;105:659–663.
165. Fuller AM, et al. Chemodectomas of the glomus jugulare tumors. *Laryngoscope* 1967;77:218–238.
166. Grubb WB, Lampe I. The role of radiation therapy in the treatment of chemodectomas of the glomus jugulare. *Laryngoscope* 1964;75:1861–1871.
167. Valdagni R, Amichetti M. Radiation therapy of carotid body tumors. *Am J Clin Oncol* 1990;13:45–48.
168. Mendenhall WM, et al. Chemodectoma of the carotid body and ganglion nodosum treated with radiation therapy. *Int J Radiat Oncol Biol Phys* 1986;12: 2175–2178.
169. Rosenwasser H. Long term results of therapy of glomus jugulare tumours. *Arch Otolaryngol* 1973;97:49–54.
170. Jordan JA, et al. Stereotactic radiosurgery for glomus jugulare tumors. *Laryngoscope* 2000;110:35–38.
171. Mukherji SK, et al. Irradiated paragangliomas of the head and neck: CT and MR appearance. *AJNR* 1994;15:357–363.
172. Glasscock ME, et al. The surgical management of glomus tumors. *Laryngoscope* 1979;89:1640–1651.
173. Myers EN, et al. Glomus jugulare tumor: A radiographic-histologic correlation. *Laryngoscope* 1971;81:1838–1851.
174. Gardner G, et al. Combined approach surgery for removal of glomus jugulare tumors. *Laryngoscope* 1977;87:665–688.
175. Rosenwasser H. Glomus jugulare tumors. I. Historical background. *Arch Otolaryngol* 1968;88:1–40.
176. Brackmann DE, et al. Glomus jugulare tumors: effect of irradiation. *Trans Am Acad Ophthalmol Otolaryngol* 1972;76:1423–1431.
177. Rosenwasser H. Current management glomus jugulare tumors. *Ann Otol Rhinol Laryngol* 1967;76:603–610.
178. Van Miert PJ. The treatment of chemodectomas by radiotherapy. *Proc R Soc Med* 1964;57:946–951.
179. Suit HD, Gallager HS. Intact tumor cells in irradiated tissue. *Arch Pathol* 1964; 78:648.
180. Glasscock ME, Harris PF, Newsome G. Glomus tumours: diagnosis and treatment. *Laryngoscope* 1974;84:2006–2032.
181. Carrasco V, Rosenman J. Radiation therapy of glomus jugulare tumors. *Laryngoscope* 1993;103(11 pt 2 suppl 60):23–27.
182. Feigenberg SJ, et al. Radiosurgery for paraganglioma of the temporal bone. *Head Neck* 2002;24:384–389.
183. Liscak R, et al. Leksell gamma knife radiosurgery of the tumor glomus jugulare and tympanicum. *Stereotactic Funct Neurosurg* 1998;70(suppl 1):152–160.
184. Eustacchio S, et al. Gamma knife radiosurgery for glomus jugulare tumours. *Acta Neurochirurg* 1999;8:811–818.
185. Foote RL, et al. Stereotactic radiosurgery for glomus jugulare tumors: a preliminary report. *Int J Radiat Oncol Biol Phys* 1997;38:491–495.
186. Foote RL, et al. Glomus jugulare tumor: tumor control and complications after stereotactic radiosurgery. *Head Neck* 2002;24:332–339.
187. Sillars HA, Fagan PA. The management of multiple paraganglioma of the head and neck. *J Laryngol Otol* 1993;107:538–542.
188. Glasscock A. The history of glomus tumors: A personal perspective. *Laryngoscope* 1993;103:3–6.
189. Leverstein H, Castelijns JA, Snow GB. The value of magnetic resonance imaging in the differential diagnosis of Parapharyngeal space tumours. *Clin Otolaryngol* 1995;20:428–433.
190. Kwekkeboom DJ, van Urk H, Now BK, et al. Octreotide scintigraphy for the detection of paragangliomas. *J Nucl Med* 1993;34:873–878.
191. Macfarlane DJ, Shulkin BL, Murphy K, et al. FDG PET imaging of paragangliomas of the neck: comparison with MIBG SPECT. *Eur J Nucl Med* 1995;22:1347–1350.
192. Vogl TJ, Juergens M, Balzer JO, et al. Glomus tumors of the skull base: combined use of MR angiography and spin-echo imaging. *Radiology* 1994;192: 103–110.
193. Held P. MRI of orofacial tumors and paragangliomas with 2D GE sequences: indications and optimal sequence parameters. *Eur J Radiol* 1994;18:38–44.
194. van Gils AP, van den Berg R, Falke TH, et al. MR diagnosis of paraganglioma of the head and neck: value of contrast enhancement. *AJR* 1994;162: 147–153.
195. Tikkakoski T, Luotonen J, Leinonen S, et al. Preoperative embolization in the management of neck paragangliomas. *Laryngoscope* 1997;107:821–826.
196. Som PM, Lanzieri CF, Sucher M, et al. Extracranial tumor vascularity: determination by dynamic CT scanning. Part 11: the unit approach. *Radiology* 1985;154:407–412.
197. Mukherji SK, Kasper ME, Tart RP, et al. Irradiated paragangliomas of the head and neck: CT and MR appearance. *AJNR* 1994;15:357–363.

Radiation Therapy Technique

198. Hinerman RW, Mendenhall WM, Amdur RJ, et al. Definitive radiotherapy in the management of chemodectomas arising in the temporal bone, carotid body, and glomus vagale. *Head Neck* 2001;23:363–371.
199. Mendenhall WM, Friedman WA, Parsons JT, et al. Radiation therapy and stereotactic radiosurgery for temporal bone tumors. *Oper Tech Otolaryngol Head Neck Surg* 1996;7:208–218.

CHAPTER 29

Cancer of the Thyroid Gland

Roy B. Sessions and Kenneth D. Burman

During recent years, we have witnessed a dramatic growth in the literature relating to thyroid cancer, and, as a result, the diagnosis, approach, and treatment is now based on a more scientific understanding. Recent research in molecular genetics and immunology can now be directly applied to improve patient care. Nonetheless, many controversies remain and important differences of opinion still exist among experienced clinicians.

The focus of this chapter is on the diagnosis and treatment of thyroid nodularity and cancer.

HISTORY

Wharton introduced the name *glandular thyroideae* (thyroid glands) to the literature in 1656 (1). Before that time, the thyroid was thought to be made of two separate structures called the *laryngeal glands.* During the 18th century, however, the thyroid was recognized as one entity (1). The word *thyroid* was derived from the gland's adjacency to the thyroid cartilage, and, as such, was a more specific adaptation of the previously used name, *laryngeal glands.* The Greeks were the first to allude to thyroid gland enlargements, referring to them as *bronchoceles* or *hernias of the windpipe* (2). These enlargements were later named from the Latin, *tumid guttur,* a term that eventually became *goitre* when adapted to the French and (even later) *goiter* when Anglicized (3). Having initially been assigned a role as an aesthetic space filler in the anterior neck, the thyroid gland later was thought to be a vascular filtration device related to cerebral circulation (4). The earliest work linking the thyroid gland to body functions occurred in the first quarter of the 19th century (3) and, from that period on, understanding steadily progressed. Hyperthyroidism had been described much earlier by Parry (in 1825), and then by Graves (5) and by Von Basedow (6). According to Halsted (7), myxedema was first described in 1850 by Curling. Reverdin (4) and Kocher (8) made important observations on myxedema and thyroidectomy. Low thyroid function was first treated with thyroid extract by Murray in 1890 (7). Kendall isolated the thyroid hormone in 1914, but it was not synthesized until 1927 (9).

Although it is unknown who performed the first thyroidectomy, Kocher (8) was the predominant innovator in thyroid surgery, performing at least 4,000 thyroid operations with a remarkably low complication rate despite adverse metabolic circumstances. He made significant observations on total and subtotal thyroidectomy, as well as established the relation of both to postoperative metabolic changes. Halsted (7) learned thyroid surgery from Kocher, who had won the Nobel Prize for medicine in 1909 for his work on the thyroid gland.

EPIDEMIOLOGY OF THYROID CANCER

There are approximately 18,000 new cases of thyroid cancer diagnosed yearly in the United States, and it is one of the few cancers that is increasing in frequency. The reason(s) for this fact are unknown, but there are more cases of thyroid cancer diagnosed yearly than multiple myeloma, brain tumors, or lymphoma (10–12). Thyroid cancer accounts for 0.6% of male and 1.6% of female malignancies. The prevalence of thyroid cancer is much more pervasive due to the fact that most patients who have the disease are followed for a long period of time. Accordingly, in the United States approximately 40 persons per 1 million population have thyroid cancer (13,14). The disease causes a low percentage of deaths, with approximately 10% of afflicted patients succumbing over a 20- to 30-year period. In general, the prognosis of thyroid cancer is good, although morbidity may approach 20% to 30% over 20 to 30 years. There are no absolute histologic or clinical criteria that portend a much worse prognosis, although cervical or distant metastases, vascular and lymphatic invasion, and extension beyond the confines of the thyroid gland locally each indicate a worse prognosis. Despite these facts, at present it is impossible to accurately predict which tumors will display a particular aggressive nature and which will be more indolent. Generally speaking, anaplastic and medullary thyroid cancer are more aggressive than follicular and papillary.

Thyroid cancer is less common in children than in adults but still accounts for 1.4% of childhood malignancies (15). The incidence of thyroid cancer in children younger than 15 years is approximately 0.5 per million per year, with a rapid rise occurring after the age of 5. Children with thyroid cancer tend to have more frequent pulmonary metastases, and our knowledge concerning the optimal approach to these patients and the long-term follow-up is still evolving.

In reality, because of the fact that many thyroid cancers never become clinically apparent and as such are never diagnosed, the true incidence is not known. For example, repeated studies have shown that a number of unsuspected nodules are found at autopsy, and a certain percentage of these are invariably malignant (16–21). In addition, when one considers the so-called occult papillary thyroid carcinomas, which rarely become clinically apparent (22–28), it is impossible to know just how many thyroid cancers actually exist in the general population. Autopsy data acquired from deaths of individuals previously unsuspected of having thyroid cancer support this notion. Fukunaga and Yatani (23) reported data from multiple countries in which there was an 11% overall incidence of occult papillary thyroid carcinoma in such autopsies. Other country-specific data addressing this issue have revealed 28% in Japan (Hiroshima and Nagasaki excluded), 6% in Canada, 9% in Poland, 6% in Colombia, and from 6% to 13% in the United States (23,27,28). Undoubtedly, if the number of thyroid cancers that exist in the overall population was really known, it would have a substantial impact on incidence statistics. Nonetheless, most clinicians consider small (less than several millimeter) single focuses of thyroid cancer to be indolent and not of clinical significance, most of the time. These small focuses are considered distinct, from a clinical viewpoint, from incidentally discovered thyroid nodules that are 1 cm or larger in size, which require appropriate attention.

The inexact nature of these statistics is further complicated by the fact that during the last several decades, the incidence of thyroid carcinoma seems to be increasing, particularly among women. It should be noted, however, that because of earlier detection, improved treatment methods, and perhaps an overall decrease in follicular cancer, the overall mortality rate of thyroid cancer has decreased in both sexes (10). The magnitude of the increasing incidence of thyroid cancer in the United States is somewhat unclear and may be due in part to the improvement of diagnostic technology, although this is debated. In addition to the more sophisticated diagnostic methods, the increasing numbers likely correspond somewhat to previous exposure of the neck area of children to ionizing radiation (29). Data from other countries, however, where childhood head, neck, and mediastinal radiation treatment was never widely used, suggest that other factors may be important as well (29–32). In addition, the worldwide trend somewhat contradicts that seen in the United States; some countries have witnessed a leveling of the incidence of thyroid cancer (10,33,34). During the 1970s, the U.S. incidence of both papillary and follicular cancer increased. Recent data, however, suggest a marked decrease in the incidence of follicular carcinoma (35). This decrement may be related to the increase in dietary iodine in the United States, although certainly other factors may be playing a role.

Overall, thyroid nodules are clinically palpable in 6.4% of women and 1.5% of men in the 30- to 60-year age group (19). These numbers, of course, depend on the experience and assiduousness of the examiner. At the time of autopsy, palpable nodules are noted in some 20% of the adult cases, and, on histologic examination, perhaps 50% of these adults have discrete nodules (20,21). Children have a much lower prevalence of thyroid nodules (0.05% to 1.8%) (36,37). The female-male ratio is between 2:1 and 4:1 (19,38). In adults, only 2% to 10% of palpable nodules are found to be cancer at the time of surgery (39,40). Women are affected with thyroid carcinoma more commonly than are men (10,41); furthermore, differentiated thyroid cancer occurs more frequently in women as in men. These sex ratios are similar in whites and blacks; however, in the United States, blacks of both sexes seem to be more commonly affected than whites (42). In patients with medullary and anaplastic cancer, men and women are affected in equal proportions (43–45). Even though the overall incidence of differentiated thyroid carcinoma is higher in women than in men (46) and the overall incidence of thyroid nodules is substantially higher in women than in men, suggesting that a nodule in a man is more likely to be malignant (19).

Other factors have an impact on the discussion of epidemiology. For instance, there are definite age patterns for individual cancers of the thyroid. Only a small percentage of thyroid cancers occur in the young, and, when they do, they usually are papillary carcinoma (47,48). Even though thyroid cancer is less common in children than in adults, it still accounts for 1.4% of childhood malignancies (15). In children, thyroid nodularity is

TABLE 29.1 Relative Incidence of Types of Thyroid Cancer

	Incidence (%)	
Type of carcinoma	MSKCC (n = 1,083) (1930–1960)	Mayo Clinic (n = 1,181) (1926–1960)
Papillary	67	62
Follicular	15	18
Medullary	6	6
Anaplastic	7	14
Other	5	

Statistics show relative incidence of different thyroid malignancies from two large series: Memorial Sloan-Kettering Cancer Center (MSKCC) and the Mayo Clinic. Note the similarity of distribution and time frame.
Source: Sessions R, Diehl W. Thyroid cancer and related nodularity. In: *Cancer of the head and neck,* 2nd ed. New York: Churchill Livingstone, 1989:738, with permission.

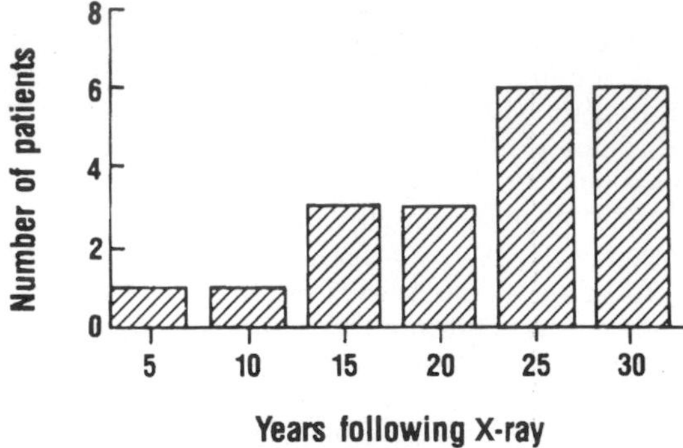

Figure 29.1 Incidence and timing of papillary thyroid carcinoma in patients exposed to ionizing irradiation during childhood. (Adapted from DeGroot M, Sternberg T. *The thyroid and its diseases,* 5th ed. New York: Churchill Livingstone, 1984.)

much more frequently malignant than in adults, and in some studies as many as 50% of thyroid nodules in the pediatric age group are malignant (49). A study by Farahati et al. (48) suggested that papillary thyroid cancer in girls is influenced by sex hormones during puberty. Apparently, such is not the case in boys (48), although the influence of various hormones on the development and progression of thyroid cancer needs further study.

In general, the incidence of papillary carcinoma peaks in early adult life and then gradually decreases in frequency, whereas the incidence of follicular carcinoma tends to peak somewhat later. Anaplastic cancer occurs later in life than differentiated cancer (26), typically occurring in patients over age 40. In both papillary and follicular cancer, the male population has a less pronounced peak incidence than the female population. Overall, papillary carcinoma is more common than follicular. Next in frequency is medullary thyroid cancer, which is more common than anaplastic (50). In some series, anaplastic carcinoma constitutes approximately 10% of all thyroid cancers (51), but this seemingly high figure is undoubtedly influenced by institutional bias (Table 29.1), and most studies suggest that anaplastic thyroid cancer accounts for about 1% to 3% of all thyroid malignancies.

ETIOLOGY OF THYROID CANCER

Exposure to ionizing external radiation is the only proven thyroid carcinogen (29). This relationship was first recognized by Duffy and Fitzgerald (52) in 1950 and has since been substantiated (53,54). Ron et al. (55) demonstrated a strong linear dose relationship between irradiation and thyroid carcinoma in children but not in adults.

It has been noted that after childhood irradiation exposure, the incidence of thyroid cancer increases in a linear manner until the third decade of life (Fig. 29.1). A 10- to 25-year postirradiation latency period has also been previously reported for the development of thyroid abnormalities. Remarkably, this delay has not been noted, however, in the pediatric thyroid cancer cases that have resulted from the Chernobyl nuclear disaster in the Ukraine in 1986, where there has been a dramatic increase in such cancers starting as early as 1989 (56–58). In general, thyroid gland exposure seems to increase the risk for developing nodules; furthermore, the nodules that develop under these circumstances are more likely to be malignant. More than one third of the patients who were exposed to irradiation and went on to have thyroidectomies had carcinoma (59).

According to Schneider and Ron (60), there may be important clinical distinctions between the initiating factors and those that act as promoters of thyroid cancer. Irradiation initiates the carcinoma, but additional factors (e.g., elevated thyroid-stimulating hormone, TSH) probably are required before it becomes clinically evident (60–62). Thyroid-stimulating hormone hypersecretion, though not being sufficient to cause thyroid carcinoma, may stimulate its growth in humans once it is present (61,62). In addition, because irradiation is a mutagen, certain genetic alterations that may be involved in irradiation carcinogenesis are found in some thyroid carcinomas (63).

In contrast to external irradiation, there is no compelling evidence to suggest that internal irradiation from ^{131}I used for therapeutic or diagnostic medical purposes causes thyroid carcinoma in humans (64–67).

The fact that differentiated thyroid cancer is significantly more common in women, the fact that this disparity between the sexes is at its highest at the time of puberty (44), and, finally, the suggestion in some studies that parity may increase the risk for thyroid carcinoma (68–72) suggest that hormonal factors are involved in the pathogenesis of certain thyroid carcinomas (61), although further study in this area is warranted.

Some data suggest a relationship among iodine deficiency, prolonged TSH stimulation, and thyroid carcinomas (30,62,73). Other risk factors may include genetic syndromes, such as Gardner syndrome, Cowden disease, and Carney disease, all autosomal-dominant disorders (74,75). The clear and predictable genetic association with medullary thyroid cancer is discussed at some length later in this chapter. A number of molecular abnormalities have been described in thyroid tissue of patients with papillary and follicular thyroid carcinoma; however, at this time this information is only investigational (76).

Anaplastic thyroid cancer is extremely aggressive and almost invariably fatal. LiVolsi and Merino (77) have stated that 80% of patients with anaplastic carcinoma note a history of antecedent goiter. Anaplastic carcinoma may arise as a result of dedifferentiation from more differentiated disease (78–83). Even though it has been suggested that there is an association between ionizing irradiation and anaplastic transformation of differentiated cancer (82,84), there is no compelling evidence that such is the case (83,85–89). *p53* mutations may play a role in the process of dedifferentiation of carcinoma (90).

EMBRYOLOGY OF THE THYROID AND PARATHYROID GLANDS

The thyroid gland is bipartite in origin, the main body coming from endodermal anlage of the primitive gastrointestinal tract (91,92), and the parafollicular or C cells from the ectodermal neural crest. The gland normally descends from the pharyngeal floor down the midline of the anterior neck, comes into close central proximity to the hyoid cartilage (93), and, when fully developed (by gestational week 7), comes to lie in an anterolateral relationship with the cricoid cartilage and cervical trachea, intimately wrapping around both. Because the medial component of the thyroid is closely associated with the developing heart, the thyroid is essentially directed to its position near the base of the neck as a consequence of the continuing descent of the heart during these early stages of thyroid formation. Full embryonic thyroid gland development occurs by the third month of pregnancy, but the adult weight of 15 to 25 g is attained slowly during the developmental years. From a physiologic standpoint, however, the embryonic gland, even though appropriately small, is functional by the 11th gestational week and is able to concentrate radiolabeled iodine and to synthesize iodothyronines. This period corresponds to the final stages of follicular lumen formation, when colloid is detectable extracellularly (94,95).

Knowledge of the embryonic migration of the thyroid gland is essential in dealing with a variety of midline embryologic ontogeny, such as foramen cecum of the tongue, thyroid ectopia, thyroglossal duct cysts, and neoplasms of the pyramidal lobe. Although less common than afflictions of the gland itself, aberrations of this normal embryonic pathway can occur. As the descending thyroid gland loses its connection with the tongue, the thyroglossal duct usually consists of a tube lined with ciliated pseudostratified epithelium that becomes replaced by constricted fibrous tissue. The distal portion of the duct differentiates to a varying extent, forming the pyramidal lobe or lobes. The lingual part of the duct frequently remains identifiable until late fetal life and may branch to give rise to miniature salivary glands (91). The remaining portion may be represented by a strip of fibrous or muscular tissue called the *levator glandulae thyroideae* (93).

Variations in thyroid development and the presence of aberrant thyroid tissue occur frequently. Though not proved, there have been suggestions of hereditary predisposition to such aberrations (94). Thyroid ectopia is a product of incomplete reabsorption, and it can occur anywhere along the pathway of the median primordium or even along the route of the ultimo branchial components of the thyroid lateral lobes. Ectopic locations of thyroid tissue in the mediastinum (95), cervical lymph nodes (96), heart (97), liver (98), esophagus, larynx, and trachea (99,100) are well documented. Deposits of thyroid tissue in the lateral part of the neck have traditionally clinically been regarded as metastatic differentiated carcinoma, but there is ample explanation embryologically for such an occurrence in the absence of cancer (101–105). Nonetheless, from a clinical viewpoint, the presence of thyroid tissue in the lateral neck must be considered to represent metastatic thyroid cancer, unless it has been proven to the contrary. A common site of thyroid ectopic tissue is the tongue base, and autopsy studies have shown an incidence as high as 10% of children possessing thyroid remnants in this area (106,107). The lingual thyroid can occasionally represent the entire complement of thyroid tissue.

The ectodermally derived component of the thyroid gland is the parafollicular or C cells that migrate from the neural crests to the ultimobranchial bodies of the fourth and fifth branchial pouches and eventually fuse with the follicular cells; hence the name *parafollicular* (108). These calcitonin-producing cells have been shown to be the only mature thyroid cells to originate from this presumptive thyroid primordium. They belong to a vastly more complex system known as the *diffuse neuroendocrine system* (109). The interest in and knowledge of this neuroendocrine system has increased substantially in recent years. Tumors derived from the parafollicular cells are part of a growing number of recognized neuroendocrine neoplasms and as such are not limited to the thyroid gland, (e.g., carcinoid tumors). In the final analysis, however, these tumors present as thyroid problems and are managed as such.

The follicular cells of the thyroid gland are derived from the median endodermal downgrowth of the first and second pharyngeal pouches. By the fifth week of gestation, these cells are separated from the pouches and ultimately fuse with the parafollicular cells.

PHYSIOLOGY OF THE THYROID

Certain aspects of the chemical function of the thyroid gland have a bearing on the etiology, pathogenesis, and natural history of thyroid nodularity in general and thyroid cancer in particular. The follicle is the basic functional unit of the gland, and the follicular sacs within the gland are lined by follicular cells that secrete two active hormones: thyroxine (T_4) (3,5,3′5′-tetraiodothyronine) and 3,5,3′-triiodothyronine (T_3). The follicles are filled with thyroglobulin, a colloid that is the storage form of thyroid hormone. This macromolecular glycoprotein provides a matrix for the synthesis of the thyroid hormones and a vehicle for their subsequent storage. It is also the most abundant of thyroid proteins, comprising the bulk of the follicular colloid as well as a substantial part of the gland's intracellular material. Iodide is extracted from the blood, oxidized, and then coupled with tyrosine radicals to form thyroglobulin, which is actually a mixture that contains T_3 and T_4 (as well as biologically inactive analogues). Release of active hormones into the blood circulation involves intracellular proteolysis and reverse pinocytosis of intrafollicular colloid. In the plasma, T_3 and T_4 are bound to specific binding globulin (e.g., thyroxine-binding globulin, TBG), prealbumin, and albumin. T_3 is more active than T_4 and is the principal intracellular hormone that has widespread effects on cellular metabolism, oxygen consumption, heat production, and growth and development (110). Indeed, present tenets suggest T_4 is mainly a prohormone.

The control of thyroid hormone secretion is an elaborate system of intrinsic autoregulation that in the normal physiologic state involves a continuous automatic feedback control through the pituitary gland and hypothalamus. This mechanism maintains a steady supply of hormones by storage and release. Essentially, TSH secreted from the pituitary gland stimulates the process leading to the synthesis and release of thyroid hormone. The secretion of TSH in turn is regulated by the concentration of unbound thyroid hormone in the blood, which occurs through a feedback message to the pituitary gland, specifically the T_3 receptor. The TSH secretion is also regulated by thyrotropin-releasing hormone from the hypothalamus. Thyroid hormone reciprocally influences TSH secretion. The hypothalamus probably determines the set point of the TSH feedback threshold (Fig. 29.2). It is relevant to the concept of "suppression therapy" that TSH is also the major regulator of the morphologic and functional states of the thyroid gland. Without TSH stimulation the thyroid gland atrophies, and hormone synthesis and secretion decrease.

Thyroglobulin serum measurements are used clinically as a tumor marker for residual or persistent thyroid tissue in

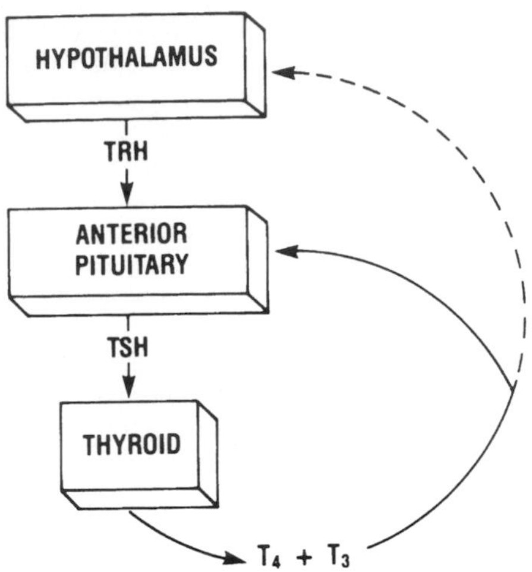

Figure 29.2 Autoregulatory feedback system for thyroid activity. Note ultimate central control. *TRH*, thyrotropin-releasing hormone; *TSH*, thyroid-stimulating hormone.

patients with thyroid cancer. Although this macromolecule is the principal iodoprotein or storage form of thyroid hormone and as such is a major component of the thyroid gland itself, it is also present in normal serum at a given concentration. In effect, this serum concentration reflects thyroid secretion of thyroglobulin. Certain thyroid tumors, thyroiditis, and other disorders are associated with an increased level of thyroglobulin in the blood. Thyroglobulin is increased in both benign and malignant thyroid tumors and is of no value before surgery in distinguishing between the two. After total thyroidectomy in cancer patients (and following ^{131}I therapy) thyroglobulin levels fall to undetectable levels, provided, of course, that metastatic disease is not present. In this context, when measured over time, thyroglobulin serves as a useful marker for tumor persistence or recurrence, the latter of which is usually heralded by a return of the thyroglobulin to a detectable concentration (111,112). Parenthetically, thyroglobulin measurement is complex, and clinical value must be interpreted cautiously, especially in the presence of thyroglobulin antibodies.

Medullary thyroid cancer also secretes calcitonin, and its measurement can also be utilized as a tumor marker in patients especially following a thyroidectomy. Foster et al. (113) postulated that calcitonin emanated from the parafollicular cells. Pearse (114) named them *C cells* to associate synthesis, storage, and secretion of calcitonin. In 1965, Williams (115) suggested that medullary thyroid carcinoma originated in the parafollicular cells, and, in 1968, an association between increased serum calcitonin and this cancer was described (116). Serum calcitonin is normally present at measurable levels, and therefore its elevation in patients with medullary cancer makes it a valuable, although somewhat nonspecific, marker in the management of this tumor. Another product of the pathophysiology of medullary cancer that provides a marker for follow-up is the carcinoembryonic antigen (CEA). Though not specific for medullary carcinoma, this antigen may prove useful in identifying subgroups with a poor prognosis (117,118).

HISTOMORPHOLOGY OF THE THYROID GLAND

The thyroid gland is encapsulated by a delicate but continuous sheet of connective tissue that also encases the small blood vessels entering and leaving its parenchyma. This is the gland's true capsule, and it adheres intimately as it dips as septa in between the glandular lobules, creating a series of compartments. Each lobule consists of 20 to 40 follicles and is supplied with its own artery. The follicle is the functional unit of the thyroid, and each follicle is surrounded by epithelial cells that are cuboidal in the euthyroid state, squamous in the state of decreased glandular function, and columnar after prolonged stimulation by TSH. The follicles are filled with colloid, the density of which depends on the functional activity of the gland.

C cells are located between and around the more numerous follicular cells (119); as the host ages, there seems to be a tendency for C-cell hyperplasia. Unknown is whether this increase in the number of C cells is precursory to the formation of medullary carcinoma, but it does tend to parallel the increasing incidence of this cancer with increasing age (120,121). The distribution of C cells in the thyroid is not homogeneous (122). C cells are more numerous in the central portions of the thyroid gland (i.e., at the junction of the middle and upper third of the thyroid lobes) (121–124).

Oxyphil cells, also known as *Hürthle cells,* are altered follicular cells (125,126) that are commonly found in Graves' disease, autoimmune thyroiditis, thyroids damaged by irradiation, neoplasms, and some adenomatoid nodules (127).

SURGICAL ANATOMY OF THE THYROID GLAND AND ADJACENT AREA

The thyroid gland is a bilobed, horizontally oriented structure that consists of a right and left lobe, a central isthmus between the two, and (in a third of the glands) a pyramidal lobe that extends cephalically for a variable distance. Average gland size varies somewhat but in adults it is usually between 15 and 25 g. The thyroid gland is enclosed between the layers of the deep cervical fascia in the anterior neck. Its surgical capsule is external to the true capsule and is only prominent posteriorly, where it condenses to connect the lobes of the gland to the cricoid cartilage and the first two tracheal rings. This suspensory ligament of Berry is a reflection of the middle layer of the deep cervical fascia.

The bilobed gland drapes around the anterior and lateral aspects of the airway, usually covering the cricoid cartilage and the adjacent trachea. The location of the lower border of the thyroid isthmus varies, depending on the habitus of the person. In certain individuals, the isthmus can actually lie beneath the sternal notch. The lateral lobes lie between the great vessels of the neck and the tracheoesophageal structures. These lobes are confined by their capsule and the vessels within it; once the lateral capsular veins are transected, the lobes can be rotated anteriorly with relative ease. The more medial parts of the thyroid lobes, however, are firmly attached to the underlying airway by the densely adherent ligament of Berry.

The supply and drainage of blood to and from the thyroid gland involves two pairs of arteries, three pairs of veins, and a dense network of connecting vessels that mesh throughout the capsule of the gland. Because of the complexity of capsular vascularity, the vessels can be especially troublesome if not managed meticulously during surgery. The inferior thyroid arteries branch directly from the thyrocervical trunks, which lie lateral to the great vessels of the neck. This bilateral artery is fairly consistent between left and right sides of the neck, extending from lateral to medial, crossing in a slightly upward direction behind (deep to) the common carotid arteries but anterior or superficial to the sympathetic trunk. In the lower neck, the inferior thyroid artery is the only structure that crosses the long axis of the common carotid artery deep to that vessel, and this relationship lends itself to easy identification as it emerges from under the medial edge of the common carotid artery. The inferior thyroid artery enters the thyroid bed at a level above the inferior pole of the gland and then angles inferomedially to enter the gland at its midsection. In the true sense of the word, an inferior thyroid pole artery that corresponds to the veins of the inferior pole does not exist. The artery usually gives off one or two branches, one directed cephalically to the superior parathyroid gland and one directed inferiorly to the inferior parathyroid. Because this blood supply to the delicate parathyroid glands is critical to their function, ligation of the inferior thyroid artery ideally should take place beyond these take-off sites. In many cases of uncomplicated thyroid surgery in which the parathyroid glands seem grossly undisturbed, but in which the calcium level decrease after surgery, the likely explanation is that parathyroid metabolism was altered by schemia or venous congestion, rather than by direct glandular injury.

Even though the relationship of the inferior thyroid arteries to the recurrent laryngeal nerves is variable, the artery provides an efficient means of locating the nerve that lies posterior (deep) to it approximately 70% of the time (Fig. 29.3).

The superior thyroid artery begins as the first branch of the external carotid artery in 80% of individuals and from the common carotid artery in the remainder (128). This vessel usually arises just above the thyroid cartilage and runs inferiorly, deep to the superior belly of the omohyoid muscle and superficial to or on the surface of the superior constrictor muscle. The superior thyroid artery goes to the superior pole of the gland, where it divides to lie on the anterior gland surface and posteriorly on the back surface of the lobe. Here it anastomoses with branches of the inferior thyroid artery that come from below. These posterior branches of the superior thyroid artery occasionally supply the superior parathyroid glands. The superior thyroid artery usually lies posterolaterally and parallel to the external branch of the superior laryngeal nerve (Fig. 29.4B). It is surgi-

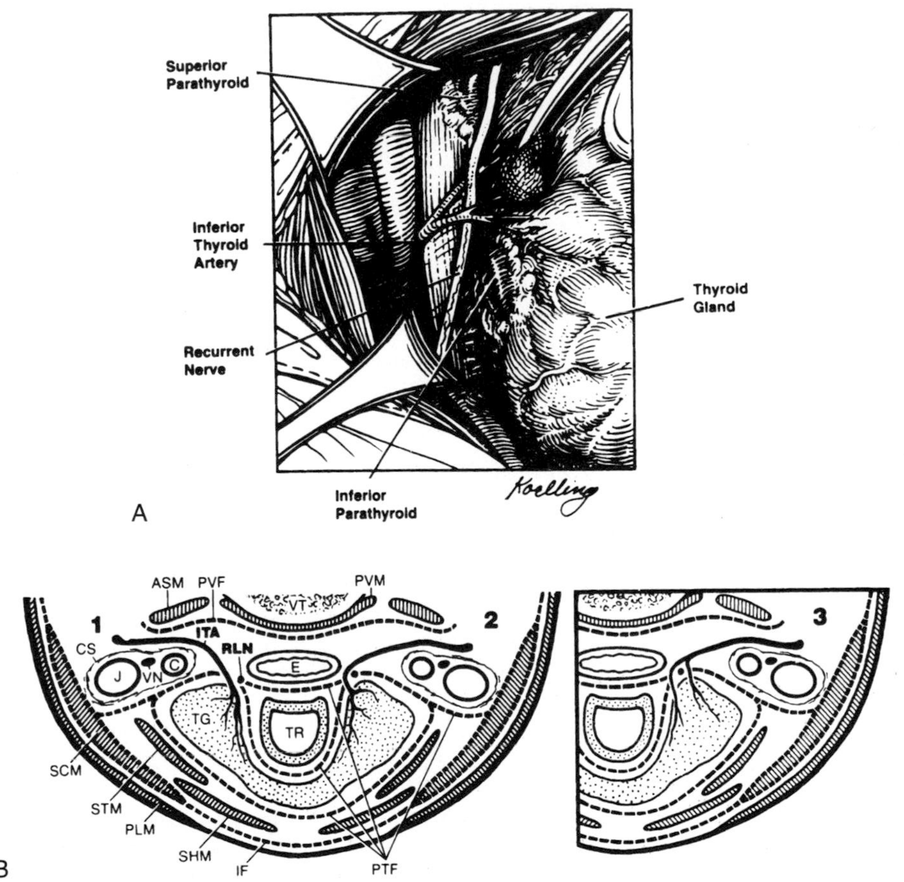

Figure 29.3 The various relationships of the inferior thyroid artery to the recurrent laryngeal nerve. **A:** View of the right side of neck, with thyroid lobe retracted medially. Note artery division with one branch deep and one superficial, thereby straddling the nerve. **B:** Cross-section of neck at thyroid level, showing the anteroposterior relationship of the recurrent laryngeal nerve and the inferior thyroid artery. Note difference between left and right sides of neck (depicted as such for illustration of possible levels of two structures). The inferior thyroid artery can variously be found passing lateral to nerve, as is shown on the left side of drawing 1. This relationship occurs in approximately 70% of necks. Less commonly, the artery passes deep to the nerve, as is depicted on the right side of drawing 2. The least common configuration occurs when the artery straddles the nerve, as illustrated in the drawing 3. Axial diagram (frontal diagram in **A**). *ASM*, anterior scalene muscle; *C*, carotid artery; *CS*, carotid sheath; *E*, esophagus; *IF*, investing layer of deep cervical fascia; *ITA*, interior thyroid artery; *J*, jugular vein; *PLM*, platysma; *PTF*, pretracheal fascia; *PVF*, prevertebral fascia; *PVM*, prevertebral muscle; *RLN*, recurrent laryngeal nerve; *SCM*, sternocleidomastoid muscle; *SHM*, sternohyoid muscle; *STM*, sternothyroid muscle; *TG*, thyroid gland; *TR*, trachea; *VN*, vagus nerve; *VT*, vertebra.

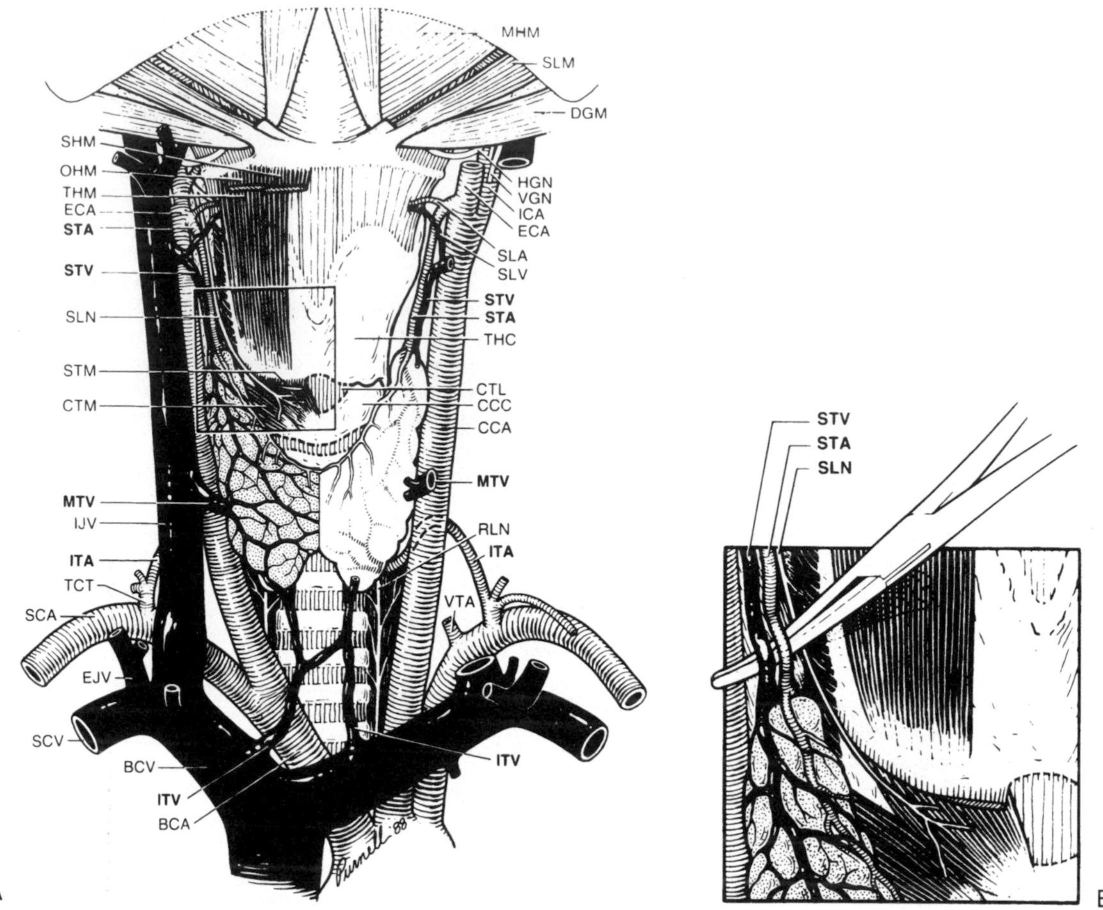

Figure 29.4 **A:** Venous drainage of the thyroid gland (dark vessels). Note that two major venous channels, superior and middle, eventually flow into the internal jugular vein, whereas the inferior veins flow into the brachiocephalic veins. **B:** Artist's depiction of the relationship of the external branch of the superior laryngeal nerve to the superior thyroid vessels. Variations occur; the nerve can be as shown, can loop over or under the vessels, or can be intertwined with them. *BCA*, brachiocephalic artery; *BCV*, brachiocephalic vein; *CCA*, common carotid artery; *CCC*, cricoid cartilage; *CTL*, cricothyroid ligament; *CTM*, cricothyroid muscle; *DGM*, digastric muscle; *ECA*, external carotid artery; *EJV*, external jugular vein; *HGN*, hypoglossal nerve; *ICA*, internal carotid artery; *IJV*, internal jugular vein; *ITA*, inferior thyroid artery; *ITV*, inferior thyroid vein; *MHM*, mylohyoid muscle; *MTV*, middle thyroid vein *OHM*, omohyoid muscle; *RLN*, recurrent laryngeal nerve; *SCA*, subclavian artery; *SCV*, subclavian vein; *SHM*, sternohyoid muscle; *SLA*, superior laryngeal artery; *SLM*, stylohyoid muscle; *SLN*, superior laryngeal nerve (external branch); *SLV*, superior laryngeal vein; *STA*, superior thyroid artery; *STM*, sternothyroid muscle; *STV*, superior thyroid vein; *TCT*, thyrocervical trunk; *THC*, thyroid cartilage; *THM*, thyrohyoid muscle; *VGN*, vagus nerve; *VTA*, vertebral artery.

cally significant that there is perhaps 1 cm of superior thyroid artery between the gland surface and the anterior take-off of the external branch of the superior laryngeal nerve. This space allows safe clamping of the vessel. Whenever possible, the surgeon should dissect the individual branches of the distal artery and ligate them with the nerve in view. To ligate the vessel higher is to invite nerve damage. This is especially important in the approximately 15% of cases in which the superior laryngeal nerve runs between the terminal branches of the superior thyroid artery (129). From its point of adjacency to the superior thyroid artery, the nerve runs medially to pierce the fascia that overlies the surface of the cricothyroid muscle. At surgery, these delicate distal nerve branches are often visible through the thin fascia and, at this location, they are particularly vulnerable to trauma.

Sizable capsular veins drape over the gland within the fibrous capsule and connect directly with the smaller vessels that drain the parenchyma. These capsule vessels drain into the superior, middle, and inferior thyroid veins. All three of these pathways eventually drain into the internal jugular or innominate veins, either directly or indirectly (Fig. 29.4A). The middle thyroid vein is especially important because its transection allows the rotation of the thyroid lobe, which is a maneuver helpful in the identification of the recurrent laryngeal nerve and the parathyroid glands. There is variability in the presence and position of the middle thyroid vein; in some necks, it is absent.

The lymphatic drainage of the thyroid gland is both intraglandular and extraglandular. There is an abundance of the former, and these capillaries readily anastomose with the profuse intraglandular venous capillaries (130). Considering this rich lymphatic-venous network, it is no wonder that multifocal lesions are the norm rather than the exception in certain carcinomas. The incidence of intraglandular metastasis varies considerably from one study to another; this is probably related to the differences in primary tumor size. In effect, larger tumors are associated with a higher incidence of multifocal tumor sites than smaller tumors. There is some disagreement among anatomists, however, over the validity of lymphatic channel-mapping techniques that have been performed by injection studies (131–133). Skeptics suggest that the pressures generated by injection in such studies are nonphysiologic and result in artificial patency of delicate endothelial linings between venous and lymphatic structures. It has been suggested that these multiple intraglandular sites might represent true multicentric and *de novo* foci of tumor rather than intrathyroidal lymphatic dissemination (134); however, the intraglandular metastatic explanation seems more likely.

In any event, the chief efferent lymphatic pathways are superior, inferior, and lateral; they follow the superior blood vessels, the inferior thyroid arteries, and the inferior and middle thyroid veins. In general, the thyroid isthmus drains upward into the prelaryngeal (Delphian) nodes and downward into the mediastinal nodes. The central and lower parts of each lateral thyroid lobe drain down into the tracheoesophageal nodes along the course of the recurrent nerve. The superior pole of the gland drains into the nodes accompanying the superior thyroid vessels (135). The so-called central compartment nodes are the primary sites of drainage, whereas the nodes of the lateral neck (internal jugular, posterior triangle) constitute a zone of secondary drainage (Fig. 29.5). This fact has a significant bearing on the tailored modifications of neck surgery generally used in treating thyroid cancer (135–142). In a significant number of people, there are lymphatics that drain the posterior and superior aspect of the thyroid gland to lymphatics in the retropharyngeal area (143). Metastasis to this space sets the stage for both mediastinal and base-of-skull metastasis (Fig. 29.6). That this pattern occasionally occurs is readily explained by Rouviere's (143) observation that this precise lymphatic drainage pathway existed in more than 20% of his dissection. In point of fact, parapharyngeal space metastasis from thyroid cancer was first reported in 1985 by Robbins and Woodson (144) and has been seen by one of the chapter authors (R.B.S.) in two patients.

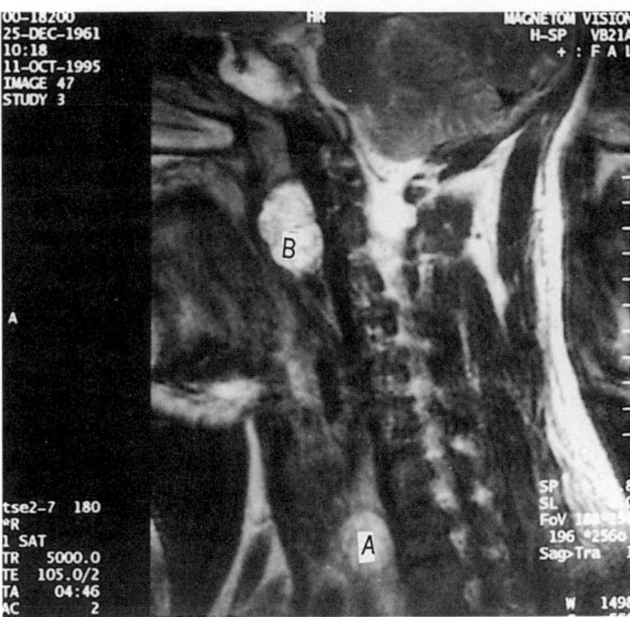

Figure 29.6 Magnetic resonance imaging (left sagittal T2-weighted view). Retropharyngeal (retrovisceral) space adenopathy that represents metastatic papillary thyroid carcinoma in a 30-year-old man (*A*). Metastatic papillary carcinoma to an RP node (*B*).

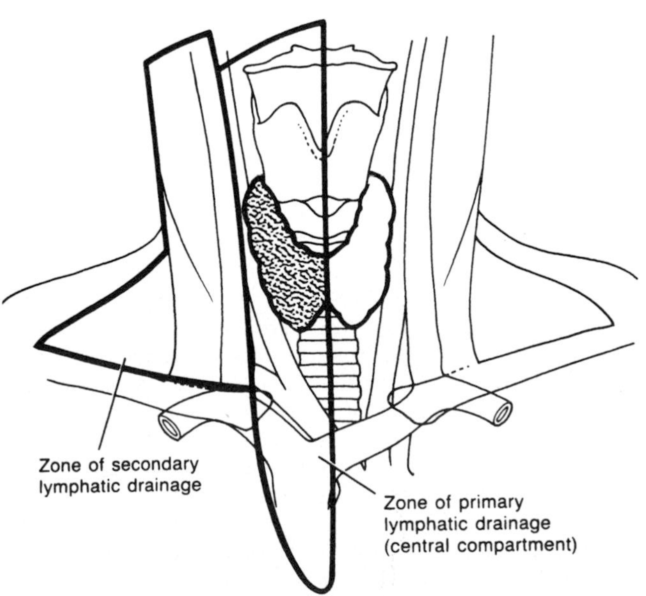

Figure 29.5 Primary and secondary cervical lymphatic drainage zones from the thyroid gland.

Certain clinical studies have concluded that metastasis of papillary thyroid carcinoma occurs first in the paratracheal nodes, regardless of the location of the primary tumor. That is, there may be little or no relationship between the site of the primary tumor and the direction of metastasis. In the earlier stages, metastases are more frequent to the lower part of the neck. It is postulated that the metastases to the upper and submandibular nodes occur in later stages because of lymphatic obstruction that occurs with increasing primary tumor size and also when the pretracheal and paratracheal nodes have become obstructed by metastasis (139). All these facts would tend to justify the skepticism of those who doubt the accuracy of lymphatic mapping techniques that have been done by injection studies.

The reader should remember that many studies on lymphatic drainage and the clinical implications of the patterns observed are developed with a surgical bias; as such, their results depend on the thoroughness of the surgeon's dissection.

SPECIFIC ANATOMIC RELATIONSHIPS

The thyroid's location in a tightly compacted area lends itself to a sometimes intimate relationship with a number of important structures. To dissect in this area in a cavalier manner is to invite injury to one or more of the delicate structures that are constantly in the operative field. Patience, delicate tissue handling, and meticulous hemostasis all play a role in safely performed surgical procedures. Despite ideal circumstances, however, there is still a low but expected percentage of injuries to the superior laryngeal and recurrent laryngeal nerves and to the parathyroid glands. By and large, the frequency of injury to one or more of these structures varies with the extent of the primary pathology and with both the skill and experience of the surgeon. Contemporary techniques that emphasize surgical minimalism in differentiated thyroid cancer, however, are associated with a lessened likelihood for injury than are the more radical procedures.

The thyroid surgeon must have a thorough knowledge of the recurrent laryngeal nerve, its variations, and the areas especially vulnerable to trauma. This nerve ascends on either side of the neck to terminate as one or two branches that enter the larynx deep to the articulation between the cricoid and thyroid cartilages. The recurrent laryngeal nerve provides a motor supply to the larynx but does have some sensory function in the upper trachea and subglottic area and may even divide into sensory and motor terminal branches, which then penetrate the adherent zone of the ligament of Berry (Fig. 29.7) (145). Short of using intraoperative nerve monitoring or nerve electrostimulation, surgeons are unable to differentiate between motor and sensory branches; therefore, all nerves should be preserved unless tumor invades them. The motor functions of the recurrent nerve are far more important, providing stimuli to both abductor and adductor muscles of the larynx. Recurrent laryngeal nerve fibers are incorporated within the vagus nerve trunk, although the fibers are actually from cranial nerve XI in the brainstem (146). The right recurrent nerve leaves the vagus at the base of the neck, loops around the subclavian artery, and then extends into the thyroid bed some 2 cm lateral to the trachea. Normally, the right nerve extends in a superior-medial direction to enter the larynx between the arch of the cricoid cartilage and the inferior cornu of the thyroid cartilage. Rarely, and only on the right side of the neck, a "nonrecurrent" nerve comes off the vagus in the neck and enters the larynx directly from lateral to medial. In this circumstance, there is usually an associated retroesophageal subclavian artery. The left recurrent laryngeal nerve has a somewhat different course than the right; it leaves the vagus nerve at the level of the aortic arch and passes inferior and posterior to the arch, lateral to the ductus arteriosus. It then passes posterior to the carotid sheath and into the thyroid bed, where it is generally closer to and parallel to the tracheoesophageal groove than its counterpart on the right side of the neck.

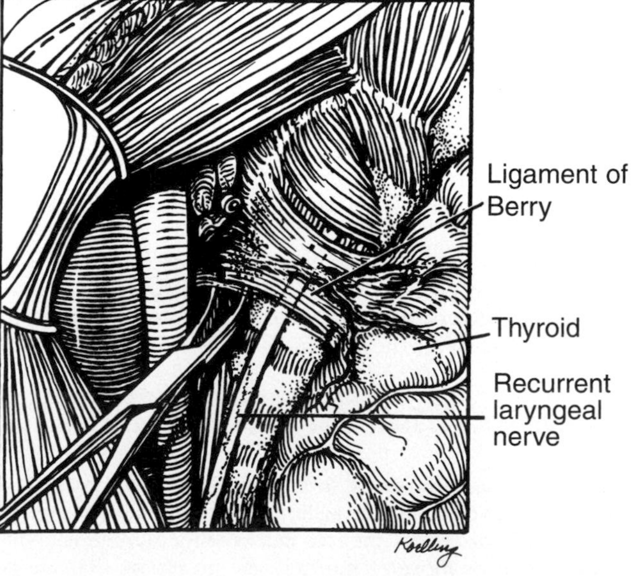

Figure 29.7 Recurrent laryngeal nerve and its relationship to the ligament of Berry (right side of neck). Thyroid gland has been retracted medially.

In both the left and right sides of the neck, as it ascends upward and across the thyroid bed, the recurrent nerve comes into proximity with the inferior thyroid artery—deep to the artery 70% of the time, superficial to or intermingled with it in the remainder. The recurrent laryngeal nerve often branches before it enters the larynx, and these branches are closely associated with the inferior thyroid artery (Fig. 29.3). The nerve generally does not branch below the level of the inferior thyroid artery; therefore, it is safer to identify it inferior to the point where it crosses the artery.

The recurrent laryngeal nerve is especially vulnerable to injury in several specific sites during thyroidectomy. In a substantial percentage of individuals, the nerve lies anterior to the inferior thyroid artery as it traverses the thyroid bed on its pathway to the larynx; under these circumstances, the nerve is especially susceptible to stretching when the thyroid lobe is retracted anteriorly. The second vulnerable area is at the point at which the nerve enters the larynx. Here, there is virtually no laxity along its axis. In this area, the ligament of Berry is especially protective of retraction forces as surgical exposure is sought; however, as this ligamentous tissue is transected, the nerve trunk assumes an increasing proportion of the force of retraction. The distal nerve either enters the larynx just posterior to the edge of the ligament of Berry or penetrates those same ligamentous fibers. Added caution must be employed, therefore, during the final separation of the gland from the posterior area of the cricoid cartilage, lest the delicate nerve fibers are damaged at their entry point. In the area where the recurrent laryngeal nerve traverses the thyroid bed, it is often obscured by fat and areolar tissues. Though it is reassuring for the surgeon to expose the nerve in this area, a vigorous search can lead to injury, either by microvascular compromise or by bruising of the trunk. Though dissection and identification are encouraged, under occasional circumstances it is better left alone, concentrating instead on what is not transected as the gland is removed. The area of the thyroid at which the nerve enters the larynx is particularly susceptible to bleeding from veins, and attempts to control bleeding here must be made with precision, especially avoiding the use of unipolar thermal methods. In general, bipolar electrode thermocoagulation is encouraged once the thyroid has been rotated medially.

The proper management of the parathyroid glands during thyroid surgery is essential because of the significant metabolic alterations and difficulties that can follow their manipulation. The head and neck surgeon should be thoroughly familiar with the physiology, usual locations, variations, and the different appearances of these glands. Autopsy studies report different numbers of glands; in addition, there is considerable variability between these individual studies. This variation has to be interpreted with the realization that the numbers are predicated on the capability of the prosector. Undoubtedly, there are patients with only three parathyroid glands, but some reports of this unusual occurrence probably reflect the inability of the dissector to locate all the glands. Considering this possibility, it is difficult to discern the exact incidence of a three-gland configuration. It seems safe to say, however, that at least 80% of necks have four glands, and probably at least 10% have more than four. Eight glands have been reported, but more than five occur only rarely (105,147–149). On two separate occasions, one of the chapter authors (R.B.S.) has observed six parathyroid glands.

These caramel-colored structures weigh from 30 to 70 mg and usually can be distinguished from adjacent fatty tissue by appearing more tan than yellow. This color difference is somewhat unreliable, however, depending both on the color of the surrounding fat and the amount of fat that is attached to the individual parathyroid glands. Importantly, when traumatized, parathyroid glands turn a distinct mahogany color. Such is not the case with lymph nodes or fat tissue. The shape of parathyroid glands varies but is most often beanlike. Less frequently, when they lie beneath the capsule of the thyroid gland, they can be thin and waferlike or, on other occasions, oblong and tubular.

The locations of the parathyroids vary somewhat but are predictable in most cases. The superior glands are usually located on the undersurface of the thyroid gland at the level of the cricoid cartilage (150). One study (147) found that in about 80% of patients, the parathyroids were located within a circumscribed area of 2 cm^2 in diameter, some 1 cm above the intersection of the recurrent laryngeal nerve and the inferior thyroid artery. The glands tend to lie posterior and medial to the recurrent laryngeal nerve. Unusual locations include positions posterior to the lower pharynx or esophagus, within the wall of the esophagus, and cephalic to the superior pole of the thyroid, adjacent to the superior pole vessels. Frequently, an upper gland is deep to the thyroid capsule, but only rarely are the superior parathyroids found entirely within the thyroid gland (150). One of the chapter authors (R.B.S.) has removed a thyroid gland in which three parathyroids were located. Significantly, in approximately 80% of patients, the position of the glands on one side is similar to its respective counterpart on the opposite side of the neck. For example, when a gland is located, the search for its counterpart on the opposite side should initially be directed to the corresponding area.

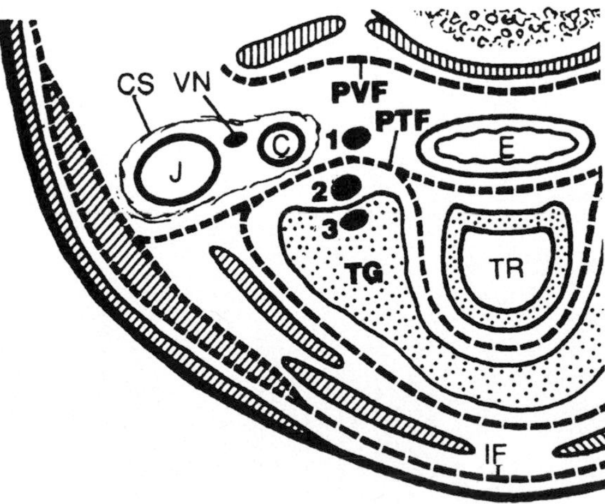

Figure 29.8 Variations in location of inferior parathyroid glands. These glands can be located (*1*) in the tissue between the pretracheal and the prevertebral fascia, (*2*) between the pretracheal fascia and the capsule of the thyroid gland, and (*3*) deep to the capsule of the thyroid gland. Note these various locations depicted by *black dots* representing the parathyroid glands. *C*, carotid artery; *CS*, carotid sheath; *E*, esophagus; *IF*, investing layer of deep cervical fascia; *J*, jugular vein; *PTF*, pretracheal fascia; *PVF*, prevertebral fascia; *TG*, thyroid gland; *TR*, trachea; *VN*, vagus nerve.

The inferior glands are more variable in location than are the superior. In almost 50% of necks, they are located on either the lateral surface of the lower pole of the thyroid gland or just posterior to the pole (149,150). These parathyroids usually lie in the tissue between the pretracheal and the prevertebral fascia or between the pretracheal fascia and the capsule of the thyroid gland caudal to the inferior thyroid artery. Uncommonly, the inferior gland is found beneath the thyroid capsule but not actually within its parenchyma, which is a circumstance occurring only rarely (Fig. 29.8). Perhaps 40% of inferior parathyroid glands lie in the thymic tissue but, even so, only a very small percentage of parathyroid glands are inaccessible from a cervical incision.

PATHOLOGY, PATHOGENESIS, AND NATURAL HISTORY OF THYROID CANCER

Though a variety of staging systems for thyroid cancer have been developed (e.g., Ames, Ages, Macis, Ohio State, and University of Chicago), we believe that the common value for all should be the identification of important prognostic variables and risk factors that ultimately influence clinical decisions. Of equal importance, however, is the fact that interinstitutional comparison of data depends on a common lexicon; hence, the importance of consistent staging methods. For the sake of standardization, we recommend the TNM (tumor, node, metastasis) system developed by the Union International Contre le Cancer and American Joint Committee on Cancer (Table 29.2).

The incidence of metastasis to the thyroid is substantially less than primary occurrence of cancer in that gland. This is somewhat surprising, considering the substantial blood flow through this organ. Direct extension and lymphatic spread from adjacent aerodigestive carcinomas, such as larynx and hypopharynx, occur with a low but consistent rate, and removal of part or all of the thyroid gland is an essential part of treatment in some of these aerodigestive cancers. When blood-borne, however, metastasis to the thyroid gland usually comes from distant organ sites, most frequently kidney and breast.

Most thyroid neoplasms present as nodules and, because of this, glandular nodularity must be part of any meaningful discussion of thyroid cancer. The term *goiter* refers to any generalized enlargement of the gland and, as such, can be either malignant or benign. The word, therefore, is nonspecific and is of little value, even though its use is perpetuated.

Most malignant neoplasms of the thyroid gland come from either the follicular epithelium or the parafollicular C cells. Lymphomas arise from nonepithelial elements.

Primary cancers of the thyroid gland are classified as differentiated (papillary and follicular carcinomas), medullary, undifferentiated or anaplastic, insular carcinomas, squamous cell carcinomas, lymphomas, and sarcomas. There is some variance of incidence among different clinical series, but all agree that papillary carcinoma is the most common histologic type of thyroid cancer, making up 60% to 75% of all malignancies of that gland (142–145). Differentiated cancers (e.g., papillary and follicular) accounts for more than 80% of all thyroid cancers. Follicular carcinoma is thought to occur in 10% to 20% of patients with thyroid cancer; however, data suggest a decreasing incidence of this malignancy (146). Anaplastic carcinoma is uncommon, accounting for less than 5% thyroid cancers (50). Medullary carcinoma is also unusual, making up 5% to 10% of all thyroid cancers (50). Insular thyroid carcinoma is extremely uncommon, and probably should be con-

TABLE 29.2 TNM Staging of Differentiated (Papillary/Follicular) Thyroid Cancer

Primary tumor (T)		
TX	Primary tumor cannot be assessed	
T0	No evidence of primary tumor	
T1	Tumor 1 cm or less in greatest dimension, limited to the thyroid	
T2	Tumor more than 1 cm but not more than 4 cm in greatest dimension, limited to the thyroid	
T3	Tumor more than 4 cm in greatest dimension, limited to the thyroid	
T4	Tumor of any size extending beyond the thyroid capsule	
Regional lymph nodes (N) (i.e., the cervical and upper mediastinal lymph nodes)		
NX	Regional lymph nodes cannot be assessed	
N0	No regional lymph node metastasis	
N1	Regional lymph node metastasis	
N1a	Metastasis in ipsilateral cervical lymph node	
N1b	Metastasis in bilateral, midline, or contralateral cervical or mediastinal lymph node	
Distant metastasis (M)		
MX	Distant metastasis cannot be assessed	
M0	No distant metastasis	
M1	Distant metastasis	
Stage grouping: separate stage groupings recommended for medullary or undifferentiated (anaplastic) carcinomas		
	<45 yr	≥45 yr
Papillary or follicular		
Stage I	Any T, any N, M0	T1, N0, M0
Stage II	Any T, any N, M1	T2, N0, M0
	T3, N0, M0	
Stage III		T4, N0, M0
	Any T, N1, M0	
Stage IV		Any T, any N, M1
Medullary		
Stage I	T1, N0	M0
Stage II	T2, N0	M0
	T3, N0	M0
	T4, N0	M0
Stage III	Any T, N1	M0
Stage IV	Any T, any N	M1
Undifferentiated (anaplastic)[a]		
Stage IV	Any T, any N	Any M

[a]All cases are stage IV.
Source: American Joint Committee on Cancer. *AJCC cancer staging manual,* 5th ed. Philadelphia: Lippincott-Raven, 1997.

sidered a variant of follicular cancer. The exact incidence of primary thyroid lymphoma is uncertain but is thought to be perhaps 2% to 4% of all thyroid tumors (147). Primary squamous cell carcinoma of the thyroid gland accounts for approximately 1% of thyroid cancers (148).

Age plays a role in relative incidence; in people younger than 40, papillary carcinomas are more common, whereas in the population 40 or older the relative incidence of other types of cancer increases (Fig. 29.9). The median age of patients with undifferentiated thyroid carcinoma is 60 years (147). Primary thyroid lymphoma tends to occur in individuals older than age 40, especially in those with a history of long-standing Hashimoto's thyroiditis.

Papillary Thyroid Carcinoma

It is difficult to know the true incidence of papillary carcinoma in the overall population because a substantial number of people have asymptomatic and inconsequential microtumors (occult carcinomas) that are discovered only accidentally, either at autopsy or at the time of surgery for a different problem (149). The mere concept of dormant cancer that is accidentally discovered and that may never have required treatment is nearly unique in the cancer experience. In fact, this intriguing phenomenon serves to call attention to the broad behavioral spectrum of papillary carcinoma in general. There is, for example, evidence that small microscopic foci of thyroid cancer (<1 cm) may develop and remain dormant for the duration of a person's life, whereas metastatic sites of the same tumor continue to grow (22,28,149). Sampson (18) showed that a substantial percentage of occult primary tumors are associated with micrometastases in cervical lymph nodes. This fact should be assigned a low order of therapeutic importance, however, as it appears to be of little clinical consequence, although this issue needs to be analyzed using modern analytic techniques. Sampson further observed that 517 of 518 persons with occult papillary carcinoma of the thyroid gland reached the end of life without any awareness of the presence of these tumors. Data from an extensive series by Woolner et al. (151) showed that no patient with papillary carcinoma died from this cancer when the primary lesion was less than 1.5 cm in diameter. However, it has now been recognized that a family history of microscopic

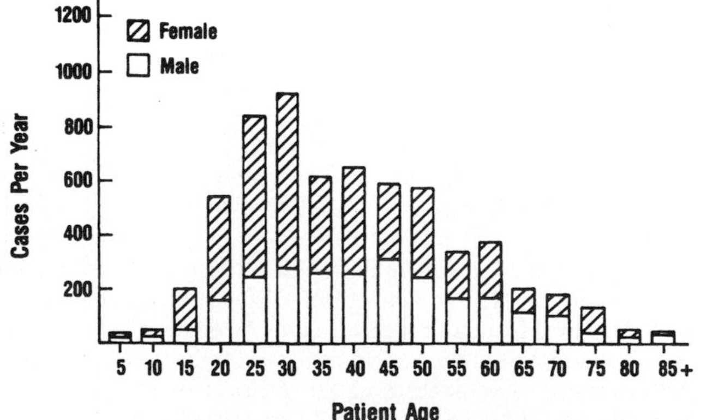

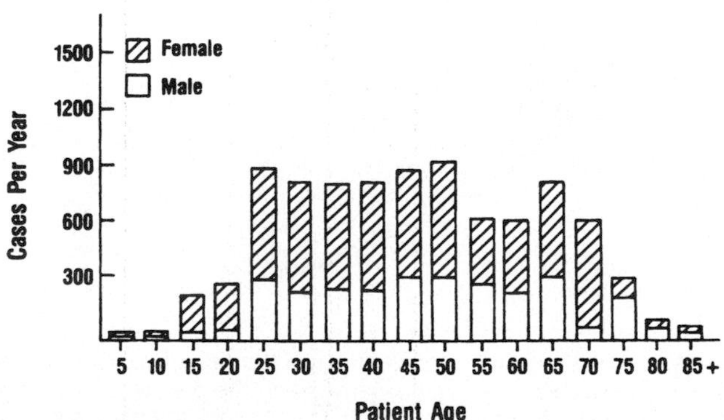

Figure 29.9 **A:** Relative incidence of papillary carcinoma by age. Note the consistent predominance in female subjects (sample taken from period between 1973 and 1977). **B:** Relative incidence of follicular carcinoma by age from 1973 to 1977. (Adapted from Brennan M, McDonald J. Cancer of the endocrine system. In: DeVita V, Hellman S, Rosenberg S, eds. *Cancer: principles and practice of oncology,* 2nd ed. Philadelphia: Lippincott, 1985.)

TABLE 29.3 Extent of Various Papillary Carcinoma at Mayo Clinic (1926–1960)

Category	No.	Cases (%)
Occult	244	35
Intrathyroidal	354	50
Extrathyroidal	68	10
Biopsy only[a]	38	5
Total	704	100

[a]Inoperable.
Source: Adapted from Hutter R, Tollefsen H, DeCosse J, et al. Spindle and giant cell metaplasia in papillary carcinoma of the thyroid. *Am J Surg* 1965;110:660, with permission.

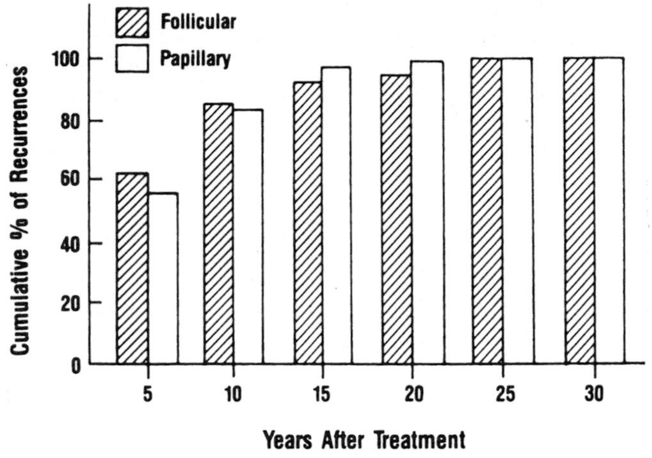

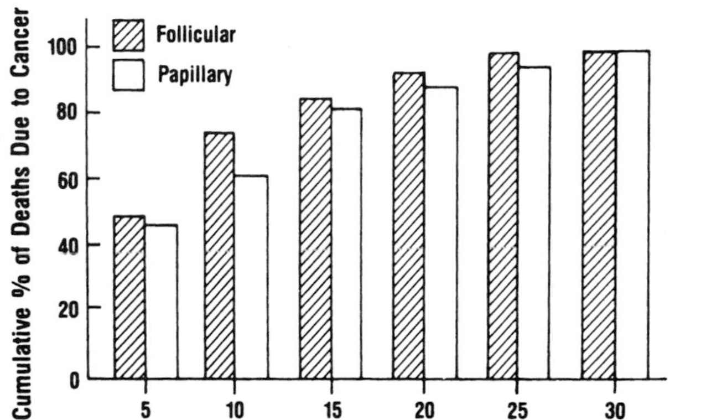

Figure 29.10 **A:** Recurrence of differentiated thyroid carcinoma. Note prolonged natural history. **B:** Death from differentiated thyroid carcinoma. Note prolonged natural history. (Adapted from Cady B. Changing clinical, pathologic, therapeutic and survival pattern in differentiated thyroid carcinoma. *Ann Surg* 1976;184:541.)

papillary thyroid cancer may be associated with a poorer prognosis in a patient discovered to have a microscopic focus of papillary thyroid cancer (152).

One could argue that the differences between occult and clinically obvious papillary carcinoma are only a reflection of the passage of time. After all, don't all tumors begin at a microscopic level? Perhaps some or all of the so-called occult tumors discovered at autopsy would have eventually evolved in size, had the patient lived long enough. On the other hand, perhaps this is a matter of host immune fluctuation, and that a circumstance in which those tumors remain dormant represents a biologic victory of host over tumor.

Papillary carcinoma can be classified as occult (<1.0 cm in greatest diameter), intrathyroidal (>1.0 cm but confined within the gland), and extrathyroidal (extending beyond the capsule to involve surrounding viscera). The relative incidence of the various types is noted in Table 29.3. At the time of clinical presentation, up to 80% to 90% of primary lesions are confined to the gland (i.e., only a limited percentage have extended to the surrounding cervical tissues) (153). Extrathyroidal disease extension seems to be associated with both a substantial morbidity and a survival compromise (154,155). Of course, a pathologist's ability to diagnose thyroid cancer as well as its associated findings depend on his/her experience, the material submitted by the surgeon, as well as the assiduousness of examining the tissue and its blocks.

Usually, papillary carcinoma is indolent. Only half of all recurrences are obvious by 5 years, and, of those patients who ultimately die from the disease, less than 50% do so within this time frame. Actually, both tumor recurrences and death from papillary cancer can occur for two to three decades after discovery (Fig. 29.10). This prolonged natural history substantially complicates the analysis of data, and, unlike with many other head and neck cancers, to discuss thyroid survival in the usual 3- to 5-year survival timetable invites inaccuracies.

The most characteristic histologic feature of papillary carcinoma is the presence of papillary fronds. Most lesions contain follicular elements to a varying extent; few are purely papillary. Though this mixture does not seem to have any impact on biologic behavior or ultimate prognosis and though these mixed tumors demonstrate a papillary behavior pattern, there are those who believe that mixed tumors are more likely to respond to radioactive iodine than are the pure papillary type (156). Whatever the case, from a morphologic standpoint, these tumors may be called *mixed* but, as a practical matter, they are classified as *papillary carcinoma* (157). A version of papillary carcinoma known as a *follicular variant* has a follicular morphology but is thought to behave like, and has the prognosis of, typical papillary carcinoma (158–161). Follicular variant of papillary cancer has become an extremely common diagnosis, and, in some institutions, represents the majority of papillary thyroid cancers. It is believed that this diagnosis represents an authentic change in the presentation of papillary thyroid cancer rather than a modification of nomenclature or classification. Although it is believed that follicular variant of papillary thyroid cancer acts similarly to classic papillary thyroid cancer, this issue needs to be studied (161). An even more unusual variant of papillary carcinoma is the so-called tall cell variant, which features characteristic individual cellular differences, such as the presence of oxyphilic cells. Diagnostically, 30% of the thyrocytes must have basal nuclei and the cells must be twice as tall as wide (162). There obviously is a subjective nature to this diagnosis, and, in fact, the consistency of this diagnosis has not been studied between different pathologists or institutions. Nonetheless, tall cell thyroid cancer is thought to have a more aggressive clinical behavior than typical papillary carcinoma. In fact, even a tall cell lesion less than 1 cm in diameter can behave aggressively.

Most papillary lesions are quite firm and are not encapsulated. Perhaps 10%, however, do have a well-defined capsule, and this finding is generally believed to be a favorable sign (163,164). On cut section, they often grossly appear circumscribed but, even then, can appear to blend into the surrounding gland. In the larger lesions, there is often degeneration that has resulted from hemorrhage and necrosis. Foci of calcium and sclerosis may be present, and laminated products of calcification (psammoma bodies) are almost always found. This finding is of diagnostic significance because it is highly suggestive of this particular cancer (26,66,77), but psammoma bodies have been observed in primary ovarian and lung cancers of the papillary type (165) and in kidney lesions. Of all these lesions, only thyroid carcinoma stains positive for thyroglobulin. When coincidentally found in cervical lymph nodes, the presence of psammoma bodies is highly suspicious for metastatic papillary carcinoma, even in the absence of a primary tumor in the thyroid itself. In some instances, psammoma bodies are found extensively in a thyroid gland that has other sites of proven papillary thyroid cancer. It is controversial whether this constellation of psammoma bodies represents a separate focus of papillary thyroid cancer. However, whether within the gland or within the cervical lymph nodes, whether multiple or singular, the presence of a psammoma body is of no prognostic consequence (166).

Multifocal disease is the rule rather than the exception in papillary thyroid carcinoma, being reported as high as 80% in some series (153,156,167–170). It has been suggested that this finding represents *de novo* multicentric tumor formation, especially in thyroid glands previously exposed to ionizing irradiation (171). On the other hand, other studies suggest that the multifocal nature of the disease actually represents intraglandular metastasis (156,172). Whatever the case, the fact that this occurs in such a high percentage of glands lends compelling logic to the argument for the removal of more, rather than less, thyroid gland in the surgical management of papillary thyroid cancer. One study points out that in patients who have initially had a subtotal procedure and then a completion thyroidectomy, up to 30% have one or more microfoci of carcinoma in the clinically normal lobe (173–176). Some investigators have cited 5% to 20% local recurrence rates in patients with partial thyroidectomy (168,177,178), and, in addition, a higher rate of pulmonary and nodal metastasis in that same group. In analyzing the importance of multifocal disease, Mazzaferri and Jhiang (177) reported a 30-year recurrence rate of 40% among patients who had undergone subtotal thyroidectomy, compared with 26% among patients who had undergone total or near-total thyroidectomy. In contrast, there are those clinical investigators who feel that, regardless of partial or total gland resection, the presence of multifocal disease has no bearing on survival (i.e., local recurrence does not necessarily translate into survival compromise) (179,180), and these investigators recommend a more conservative gland resection in smaller tumors. Regardless of this controversy about mortality, it does appear that multifocal papillary thyroid cancer recurs more frequently than the presence of a single focus, and we believe that prevention of morbidity is an important goal.

Generally, invasive tumors are biologically more aggressive, and the resulting compromise in survival applies to both papillary and follicular cancers (46,48,155,181). The study by Woolner and colleagues (26) of 1,181 thyroid cancer patients showed that no patient died of papillary cancer if the lesion was less than 1.5 cm in diameter and only 3% died when the lesion, although substantially larger, remained intrathyroidal; however, 16% died when the disease was extrathyroidal. According to Woolner et al., long-term comparisons of these classes of papillary carcinoma have been made to normal life expectancy, and only extrathyroidal cancer causes a marked divergence from expected cures (Fig. 29.11). The majority of later studies (177–181), including that of Mazzaferri and Jhiang (177), as well

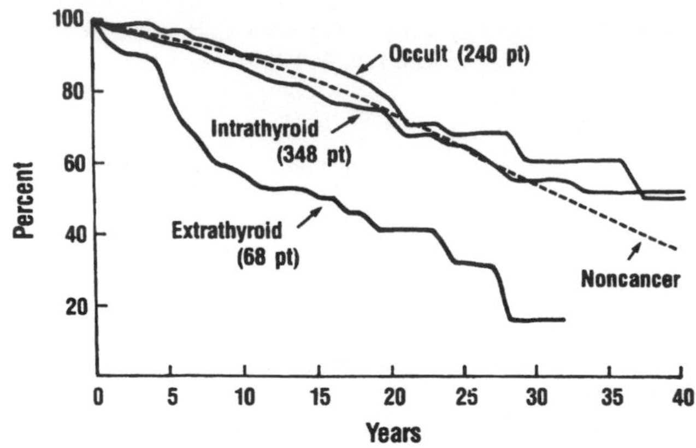

Figure 29.11 Survival of patients with papillary thyroid cancer by degree of local extension relative to noncancer group. Note significant survival compromise with extrathyroidal extension. (Adapted from Woolner L, Beahrs O, et al. Thyroid carcinoma: general considerations and follow-up data on 1,181 cases. In: Young S, Inman D, eds. Thyroid neoplasia. *Proceedings of the second imperial cancer research fund symposium*. London: Academic Press, 1968.)

as our own, suggest that risk factors for both recurrence and mortality include size of the tumor (>4.5 cm), sex (more aggressive in male patients), capsular, lymphatic and/or vascular invasion, multicentricity, and the presence of cervical lymph nodes.

The 10% to 20% of differentiated thyroid tumors that are locally invasive tend to grow into the laryngeal and tracheal framework, the recurrent laryngeal nerves, the pharynx and esophagus, and (most commonly) the overlying strap muscles. Other structures within the area that lie in proximity to the thyroid gland are less commonly subject to invasion (152). Encroachment into adjacent structures can involve any degree from microscopic to gross invasion (173,177), and, on occasion, metastatic nodes filled with tumor can demonstrate extracapsular extension directly into surrounding tissue. Though tumors that invade the strap muscles seem clinically to do better than those that involve the deep neck structures, the former are probably just as biologically aggressive as the latter. The more favorable behavior that is reported probably reflects the fact that these muscles are easily and safely resectable, and such reports probably reflect a more aggressive surgical management. In those cancers that invade the airway, it is our experience that papillary lesions more often involve only the framework (thyroid cartilage and tracheal rings), whereas follicular carcinomas seem to transgress the tracheal wall and appear intraluminally more frequently. This impression is not shared by all, however, and some do not make a distinction between the two types of cancers.

Woolner's (45) data showed that most of the patients demonstrating extrathyroidal disease were older than 40 years. Mazzaferri and Jhiang's (177) studies as well as multicenter cooperative analyses indicate that local invasion is associated with enhanced recurrence rates and decreased survival (178–182).

In papillary carcinoma specifically and in differentiated thyroid cancer in general, older age groups have a somewhat worse survival (46,182–184). Age of the patient at the time of diagnosis is an important prognostic variable. Thyroid cancer recurs more frequently when a patient is diagnosed after age 40 to 50, and the mortality of the disease is increased (177,182,184) (Fig. 29.12).

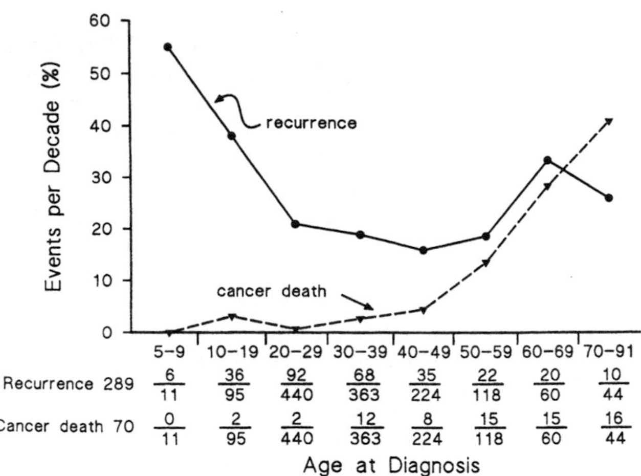

Figure 29.12 Effect of patient age at the time of diagnosis of tumor recurrence and death from differentiated thyroid carcinoma. The numerators are the number of events during the previous interval, and the denominators are the number of patients at the end of the interval. (Adapted from Mazzaferri E, Jhiang S. Long-term impact of initial surgical and medical therapy on papillary and follicular thyroid cancer. *Am J Med* 1994; 97:418.)

A dramatic shift comes at age 50 in women, as contrasted to a linear relationship between age and mortality in men. Some have speculated that this difference between men and women is related to the hormonal changes that occur in menopausal women (185). This explanation is overly simplistic for many reasons, as one would expect those women who first developed cancer in the premenopausal years to experience an acceleration of disease as they pass into and through menopause. In fact, this is not the case; female patients whose disease starts during younger life generally do not have a conversion to a more lethal cancer as they age (186). It would seem that the hormonal or other regulatory factors present in the early development of the cancer are programmed from the tumor's inception for a different biologic behavior pattern.

Other investigators believe that the tumor stage and histologic differentiation are as important as the patient's age in determining prognosis and management (177,187,188). Some question the use of age as an important risk factor, specifically taking issue with the statement that papillary thyroid cancer is more aggressive and associated with a higher mortality rate when found after the age of 40. They contend that the phenomenon probably is due to the fact that the tumor has been present for 10 to 20 years at the time of diagnosis and has therefore gained momentum and aggressiveness. We take issue with the latter of these two views and believe that increasing age is very important in virtually all aspects of these cancers. Indeed, the most commonly used staging system (TNM) takes age into account.

Men younger than age 40 have a prognosis comparable to that of women of the same age. Overall, however, men have a worse survival prognosis, although the difference is believed by some to be small (46,137,179,183,189). The Mazzaferri and Jhiang (177) study, on the other hand, showed that the risk of death from differentiated thyroid cancer was perhaps twice as great in men as in women. There seems to be an increasing incidence of men with differentiated thyroid cancer, and this may ultimately lower the overall survival statistics of the disease. In the last 40 years, the ratio of men to women having papillary thyroid carcinoma has decreased from 1:4 to 1:2 (184).

An association between Graves' hyperthyroidism and thyroid carcinoma has been suggested. In fact, one study reported that this malignancy was found in a higher-than-expected percentage of nodules in patients with Graves' disease (190). It has been suggested that thyroid receptor antibodies may promote tumor growth in these patients (191–193). However, this issue is controversial.

The propensity for papillary cancer to spread in lymphatics within and outside the thyroid gland is striking, and it has become evident that such invasion is associated with an increased risk for recurrence (177). In those papillary cancer patients who are older than 40, anywhere from 40% to 75% have gross evidence of regional nodal metastasis at presentation (47,184,194). In addition, if one considers those patients with only histologic (i.e., subclinical) metastasis, the overall incidence undoubtedly is higher. In Mazzaferri and Jhiang's (177) exhaustive review, the 36% incidence of nodal metastasis in adult papillary carcinoma patients represents a somewhat less impressive but still formidable figure.

Although earlier studies suggested that the presence of nodal metastases was not associated with enhanced recurrence, it is now clear from several analyses that the presence of lymph nodes is associated with increased recurrence and mortality (46,168,170,179,184,195–197). The presence of metastasis of papillary cancer to lymph nodes is detrimental at any age and under most circumstances (181,198). Furthermore, such metastases constitute a risk factor for recurrence and cancer-specific mortality, especially if bilateral cervical or mediastinal lymph node metastases were present (199–204). Clark (184) has made the important point that patients with or without obvious lymph nodes do not necessarily represent two clearly separable groups, because a remarkable percentage of those without palpable disease turn out to have histologically positive nodes when the nodes are empirically sampled surgically. Indeed, the application of molecular techniques to this issue has shown that nodal metastases may exist as demonstrated by the presence of messenger RNA for thyroglobulin without visual light microscopic evidence of cellular evidence of disease (205).

Children with a significantly higher overall rate of nodal metastasis have a better prognosis than do adults (206). The incidence of metastasis in children is remarkable (207,208). Hayles et al. (49) reported that of patients younger than 15 and afflicted with papillary carcinoma, 90% showed cervical metastasis at some time during the course of their disease. Further studies need to be performed assessing the effect of nodal and pulmonary metastases on children with differentiated thyroid cancer.

Long-term studies of patients who developed papillary cancer in adolescence have found that such patients rarely die of thyroid cancer, even though many demonstrate a large overall tumor burden (207,209,210). On the other hand, there have been other studies that suggested a more ominous natural history in those children in whom differentiated thyroid cancer develops (207,209,211). In addition, information suggests that the sex hormones expressed during puberty have a noticeably different impact on these cancers in girls than in boys (48). Welch et al. (211a) have analyzed a large cohort of children and adolescents with thyroid cancer, and it appears that their survival for several decades is not markedly influenced; however, such studies must have extremely long follow-up data before a definitive statement regarding this issue can be made.

In the thyroid literature, the definition of regional metastasis as it pertains to the natural history of papillary carcinoma is somewhat inconsistent. Because the mediastinal lymphatic drainage channels are part of the primary system—the central compartment—to which thyroid cancer drains (Fig. 29.5), some believe that nodes in the thymic and mediastinal areas should be thought of in the same context as cervical nodes, rather than as distant disease. In one Mazzaferri (159) study, data show that papillary carcinoma patients with cervical or mediastinal lymph node metastases had significantly higher 30-year cancer-specific mortality rates than those without metastases, but in this analysis, Mazzaferri makes the point that the most unfavorable carcinomas are those that are locally aggressive, that are associated with cervical as well as mediastinal lymph node metastases, and that exist in patients who are older than age 45. This study, therefore, groups most of the risk factors for ominous clinical behavior (159).

A unique regional nodal presentation that defies classification with routine lymphatic metastases is that circumstance in which papillary carcinoma metastasizes to nodes in the retrovisceral space. In this circumstance, there is ready access to mediastinum and to skull base. We have seen several patients who presented with either retrolaryngeal or parapharyngeal space adenopathy. One such patient was found to have a large lymph node deep to the recurrent laryngeal nerve in the retrovisceral space and in addition a parapharyngeal space node that simulated a deep lobe parotid tumor (Fig. 29.6). Our experience would support a generally conservative attitude toward cervical metastasis in papillary carcinoma, and we stress a continued level of optimism in dealing with this common occurrence. Most important, we are cautious not to overreact to the presence of cervical nodal disease with radical surgical procedures. The suggestion by some that cervical metastasis of papillary carcinoma is insignificant serves to undermine the sanctity of traditional cancer thinking, and undoubtedly frustrates the student of thyroid neoplasia. It should be emphasized, however, that because of a wide spectrum of behavior and substantial differences between notable clinical investigators, there must be a certain tolerance for divergence of treatment strategies for this disease. For example, both the endocrine and surgical management of thyroid tumors vary somewhat between institutions and communities as with no other malignancy. Both the thyroidologist and surgical oncologist, therefore, must demonstrate flexibility in managing this family of tumors.

Clinical performance after distant metastasis depends on a variety of factors. The ability of the tumor to concentrate radioactive iodine, the age of the patient, the site of the metastasis, and (importantly) the actual volume of tumor at the metastatic site affect performance (212,213). Overall, 10% of patients with papillary carcinoma develop distant metastasis at some point in the course of their disease (214). Most commonly, this involves the lungs and occasionally the bones and central nervous system. It is important to note that when distant macrometastasis of papillary carcinoma does occur in adults, death from disease occurs within 1 year after discovery in almost 50% of patients (215). Data from the Memorial Sloan-Kettering Cancer Center between 1982 and 1984 revealed that of the 25 patients who had this disease and had distant metastasis during that time frame, nine deaths occurred. In those who had cancer-related deaths, seven were older than age 40 (50).

Clearly, the general clinical performance of this cancer in children is different, and even distant metastasis is less lethal. It has been reported that up to 20% of children with papillary thyroid cancer have obvious pulmonary metastasis at presentation (205), but this circumstance often seems to have little impact on life or death. In this age group, pulmonary metastases can persist for many years, and the patient may have no clinical symptoms. Such a diagnosis in a child invariably stimulates a strenuous emotional reaction on the part of both family and physician. In this emotionally charged atmosphere, the stage is set for an excessive treatment strategy.

The prognosis of distant metastasis seems to be volume-related. For example, survival is longest with diffuse pulmonary metastasis that is seen only on radioactive iodine scans but not on chest radiographs. Prognosis seems to be worse in those patients whose chest radiographs demonstrate large (as opposed to smaller) lung masses (212,213). In more favorable conditions, chest computed tomography (CT) examinations (generally without the administration of radiocontrast) show small tumors less than 1 cm, whereas larger tumors, perhaps with mediastinal involvement, have a worse prognosis. Distant metastases to bone and the central nervous system also seem to be associated with a more serious prognosis than do those to lungs (215).

The natural history and prognosis of the tall cell variant of papillary carcinoma seem to differ from the standard variety. Various studies suggest a worse overall behavior pattern for this relatively unusual tumor. In an extensive review of the subject, Prendiville et al. (216) originally challenged this simplification, concluding that the tall cell variant has a worse prognosis only in patients older than age 50. It is our view that tall cell cancer indeed does tend to metastasize and recur locally more frequently than non–tall cell papillary cancer. Importantly, there should be more stringent and consistent pathologic criteria between pathologists concerning the diagnosis of tall cell variant papillary thyroid cancer (216).

Follicular Thyroid Carcinoma

Follicular thyroid cancer is less common than papillary cancer. Overall, it is the second most common thyroid cancer, making up some 15% of all malignancies of this gland. In fact, follicular cancer seems to be decreasing in frequency recently. When follicular and papillary cancer are critically compared with each other, it is not entirely clear that they are different; some investigators believe that when matched by age, sex, and stage at the time of diagnosis, these two tumor groups demonstrate the same behavior (217). It has been suggested that the poorer prognosis often alluded to in follicular carcinoma is related to an older mean patient age and a more advanced tumor stage at the time of presentation rather than to a different biology (177,217). Data from Mazzaferri and Jhiang (177) indicate that patients with tumors of comparable stage have similar 30-year recurrence and cancer-specific mortality rates, regardless of papillary or follicular histology of the tumor. Other investigators believe, however, that follicular carcinoma has a less favorable prognosis than papillary, reporting a crude survival rate of approximately 70% at 5 years and 43% at 10 years for follicular cancer as opposed to 90% and 80%, respectively, for papillary cancer (218). Both tumors have an excellent prognosis when confined to the thyroid and demonstrate minimal invasion beyond their tumor boundaries (177,218). Conversely, both papillary and follicular carcinoma have a poor prognosis if they demonstrate significant invasion or if they have metastasized to distant sites (219,220). Particularly worrisome features include size and the presence of vascular invasion.

Invasion must be clearly defined in this cancer. In our view, the term *minimal invasion* refers to that histologic state in which there is cellular invasion into, but not penetrating through, the capsule of the tumor. Frank invasion demonstrates tumor transgression through the capsule. The presence of vascular invasion places this tumor into a separate, more ominous category, and it is incongruent to note that there is "minimal invasion" in the presence of vascular invasion. Such tumors should be considered follicular carcinoma and treated as appropriate. Of course, the presence of invasion only into, but not through, the capsule can be a very subjective diagnosis that depends on the assiduousness of the pathologist and the number of sections taken. Few patients with true minimal invasion have distant metastasis or die of their disease (173,177,221,222). Silverman (223) states that this group consists of neoplasms that closely resemble adenomas, and these lesions are almost always cured by conservative surgical procedures. He states that with such an approach, the recurrence rate is approximately 1%. We believe it is difficult to make a definitive statement regarding the long-term prognosis of minimally invasive follicular carcinoma partly because of these technical factors just noted and also because of the lack of long-term studies. In this situation, we tend to treat minimally invasive follicular carcinoma similarly to frank follicular carcinoma. A discussion with the patient regarding these controversies is always beneficial. Lesions that demonstrate invasion have a poorer prognosis (142). This ominous behavioral characteristic seems to apply to young as well as older patients (184). Furthermore, lesions that demonstrate both capsule and vascular invasion have a worse prognosis than those that have capsular invasion alone (224). We believe that vascular invasion to any degree is an ominous finding and is associated with a poor prognosis.

In those patients who demonstrate moderate to marked parenchymal invasion at the primary site, the survival rate decreases significantly: 34% at 10 years and 16% at 20 years, according to Woolner et al.'s data (142) (Fig. 29.13). The mean survival time in this latter group is 6 years (142). A study by Peake (225) emphasizes the difference in survival between the noninvasive and the invasive tumors by showing that, despite therapy, most patients in the invasive group succumb over 10 to 20 years. In this analysis, it is this group of invasive tumors that account for most differentiated thyroid cancer–related mortality.

Specific definition of the word *invasion* is (again) important in discussion of these cancers; that is to say, tumor capsular invasion, no matter how severe, is not the same as local visceral invasion into trachea, muscle, and other structures. Tumors that demonstrate this regional tendency are probably biologically more aggressive, whether follicular or papillary, and have a worse prognosis (45,155,181).

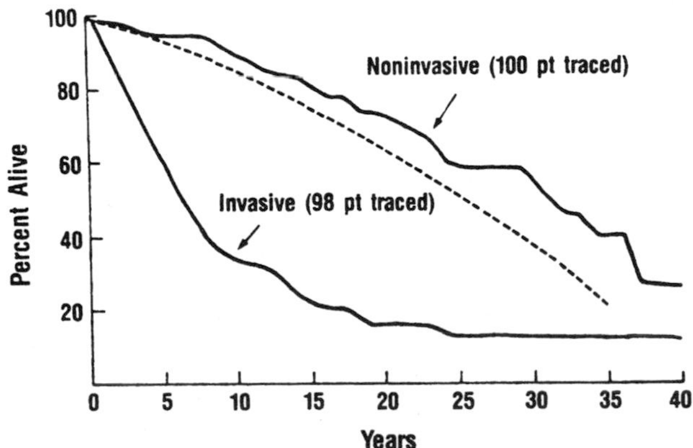

Figure 29.13 Follicular thyroid carcinoma survival relative to invasion. Note significant compromise in survival with extrathyroidal extension. (Adapted from Woolner L, Beahrs O, et al. Thyroid carcinoma: general considerations and follow-up data on 1,181 cases. In: Young S, Inman D, eds. *Thyroid neoplasia. Proceedings of the second imperial cancer research fund symposium.* London: Academic Press, 1968:51.)

In contrast to papillary carcinoma, intrathyroidal multifocal disease rarely occurs in follicular cancers. Instead, these lesions are usually solitary and encapsulated and have a microfollicular histologic pattern that is indistinguishable from their benign counterpart, the follicular adenoma. In follicular carcinoma, those findings that constitute malignancy are not cytologic but instead are histologic (e.g., transcapsular invasion and microvascular invasion of the vessels along the tumor capsule). Thus, there exists an insoluble diagnostic dilemma in distinguishing benign from malignant follicular thyroid lesions by fine-needle aspiration (FNA) techniques in which the cytologist samples only cells from within a given lesion (160,226,227). In this situation, individual cellular characteristics may not reflect the diagnostic features necessary to impose the label of follicular carcinoma. Essentially, the distinction between benign and malignant follicular lesions requires evaluation of multiple sections from the interface of the tumor capsule and the surrounding thyroid gland (77), and the cytopathologist and surgeon must have a realistic discussion regarding this limitation. An analogous problem exists with the analysis of follicular lesions by frozen sections taken at the time of surgery; as many as 5% of the encapsulated lesions called *benign* will eventually prove to be malignant when examined with multiple permanent sections of the capsule. We do not, therefore, recommend obtaining a frozen-section analysis of follicular lesions.

Women with follicular cancer tend to fare better than men in terms of survival, and patients younger than age 40 are more frequently cured than those who are older. Follicular cancer does not commonly involve lymph nodes. When nodes are positive in follicular carcinoma, there usually is significant local disease and (more importantly) significant local visceral invasion (184,227,228).

Regarding distant metastasis, follicular cancers are more likely to spread to bone than are papillary cancers; in fact, bone involvement is often the first presentation of this disease. A pathologic fracture in a person with a thyroid mass therefore should be managed with this in mind. Most patients with bone metastasis do poorly (155,178). Various authors have reported 10- and 15-year survivals to be only 29% and 11%, respectively, in this group (50,181,184). In addition to bone metastasis, follicular carcinoma may produce lung, liver, and cerebral metastases. It is especially important to assess for cerebral metastases because they are potentially lethal and may require adjunctive treatment with external radiation therapy, surgery, or corticosteroids.

Hürthle Cell Follicular Variant Carcinoma (Oxyphilic Cell)

According to the World Health Organization classification, Hürthle cell cancers are probably a type of follicular carcinoma (229); the criteria required to make the distinction between carcinomas and adenomas are the same as in the follicular lesions. Recent studies have questioned whether Hürthle cell cancer is more similar to follicular or papillary thyroid cancer in origin. Some investigators consider them to be more aggressive and to be associated with a mortality rate higher than that of follicular cancer (230,231). Other authors, on the other hand, believe that the behavior patterns are similar (229,232). Two series reported pulmonary metastases of 25% and 35%, respectively (279,233).

It has been (231a) reported that 30% to 50% of Hürthle cell carcinomas are associated with lymph node metastases, compared with 5% to 10% of follicular carcinomas (211). The studies suggested a much worse prognosis for Hürthle cell cancer as compared with follicular cancer. This issue is controversial and recent analysis suggests that it is slightly more aggressive than follicular cancer. Further, the frequency with which Hürthle cell tumors concentrate radioactive iodine has also been reanalyzed, although it appears that many such tumors do have this ability. Practically speaking, we strongly believe that patients with Hürthle cell carcinoma should be considered for radioactive iodine therapy after compulsive preparation including a low-iodine diet (234).

Insular Thyroid Carcinoma

In 1984, this tumor was so named because the clusters of cells within it contain small follicles that resemble the pancreatic islet cells (235). These thyroid cells stain positive with thyroglobulin antibodies but not with calcitonin antibodies. Insular thyroid cancer is a very uncommon malignancy that is either independent within a given gland or can be seen to a variable extent within typical papillary or follicular thyroid cancer. At the time of diagnosis, there usually is vascular and capsular invasion. Generally, this cancer has been perceived to behave less favorably than do both papillary and follicular carcinoma (235).

Burman et al. (149) published an overview of a fragmented literature and have brought clarity to the facts that pertain to this tumor. They concluded that insular thyroid cancer is a very aggressive malignancy and that when compared with both papillary and follicular carcinoma, there appears to be a higher recurrence rate as well as a higher mortality when the insular lesion is not mixed with papillary or follicular lesions. When insular cancer is located within follicular or papillary thyroid cancer, however, the clinical outcome of the well-differentiated component does not seem to be adversely influenced. Finally, many insular thyroid cancers concentrate radiolabeled iodine.

Squamous Cell Carcinoma of the Thyroid Gland

Even though the presence of squamous cells within the thyroid gland is controversial, it is known that squamous metaplasia of thyroid follicular epithelium does occur. It follows, therefore, that the malignant transformation of benign metaplastic squamous cells is probably the histologic basis for squamous cell carcinoma of this gland (149). This tumor is rarely encountered, accounting for approximately 1% of thyroid cancers (148), and it seems to occur most frequently in older patients with a history of thyroid gland enlargement. Squamous cell carcinoma usually progresses rapidly and demonstrates a predilection for local invasion and metastasis. Probably because of cytokine production, squamous carcinoma of the thyroid can present with systemic symptoms of hypercalcemia, fever, and leukocytosis (236). Exclusion of metastasis to the thyroid from another site, such as lung or upper respiratory tract, is important during the workup of patients with this cancer. Early detection and extensive surgery represent the best chance for palliation and cure. The role of radiation therapy has not been clarified, but presumably, as with aggressive squamous cell carcinomas of the aerodigestive tract that also demonstrate a propensity for regional lymphatic metastasis, postoperative therapy is probably important to disease management. Squamous cell carcinoma may be associated with systemic extrathyroidal findings such as fever, hypercalcemia, and leukocytosis, perhaps related to ectopic production of cytokines.

Lymphoma of the Thyroid Gland

Cancers of the thyroid that are of lymphoid origin consist of primary non-Hodgkin lymphoma, Hodgkin lymphoma, and plasmacytoma. The reported frequencies of the various thyroid lymphomas vary, but all agree that the occurrence is unusual; primary lymphomas of the gland constitute approximately 2% of extranodal lymphomas and less than 5% of all malignant thyroid tumors (237–240). The fact that at least 15% of patients with systemic lymphomas demonstrate thyroid gland involvement at autopsy (241,242) confuses this issue, however. This phenomenon of thyroid involvement with systemic disease occurs almost exclusively in non-Hodgkin lymphoma (237), and as this is by far the most common form of primary lymphoma, the impact on overall thyroid data is significant (240). In fact, the vast majority of primary thyroid lymphomas are non-Hodgkin. Hodgkin lymphomas are extremely uncommon, and plasmacytomas are the rarest of the three (243–246). Apparently, lymphomas arise from local lymphoid cells (247,248), and it should be pointed out that the literature of previous years was confused by the inaccuracies of diagnosing small cell anaplastic carcinoma in tumors that are now almost always considered primary lymphomas (83,235,249–251).

The unusual nature of lymphoma as a primary tumor in the thyroid gland serves to emphasize the importance of the diagnostic alertness of the clinician; that is to say, when one makes the diagnosis of primary thyroid lymphoma, it should be done with the reasonable certainty that there is no lymphoma elsewhere. The thyroid surgeon, therefore, should think of lymphoma as a systemic disease, until it is proved otherwise. For example, the association of thyroid gland lymphomas and metastatic Burkitt-like lymphoma from the gastrointestinal tract (252,253) renders a gastrointestinal workup necessary as part of the routine for those patients receiving a diagnosis of primary thyroid lymphoma. Thoracic, abdominal, and pelvic CT or magnetic resonance imaging (MRI) scanning are important in this workup, and positron emission tomography (PET) scans seem particularly useful in diagnosing systemic sites of lymphoma (253).

Lymphoma is commonly observed in a background of autoimmune thyroiditis. In some series, every patient studied had histologic evidence of Hashimoto thyroiditis in the peritumoral tissue (237,251,253–255). Patients with Hashimoto thyroiditis have approximately a 60-fold relative risk for developing non-Hodgkin lymphoma compared with a normal thyroid population (256). It is postulated that chronic autoimmune stimulation is responsible for lymphoma development. This same phenomenon has been described in salivary glands involved in the Sjögren syndrome (257). There does not seem to be an association of primary thyroid lymphoma with either prior irradiation to the area or with human immunodeficiency virus infection (237).

Some 20% of patients with primary thyroid lymphoma have a long-standing nodule or nodules (144,188,258). Hypothyroidism has been reported in up to 40% of lymphoma cases, and this is thought to be secondary to coexisting chronic autoimmune thyroiditis as well as replacement of normal thyroid tissue by the tumor.

Clinically, typical primary lymphomas are painless enlargements that most commonly occur in older people (237). There seems to be about a 3:1 female preponderance. These tumors are often associated with hoarseness, even in the presence of normally working vocal cords (243). Presumably, this is related to generalized edema in the larynx. In our experience, paralysis of the recurrent laryngeal nerve is rarely seen in this disease, even in circumstances in which the entire area of the nerve is

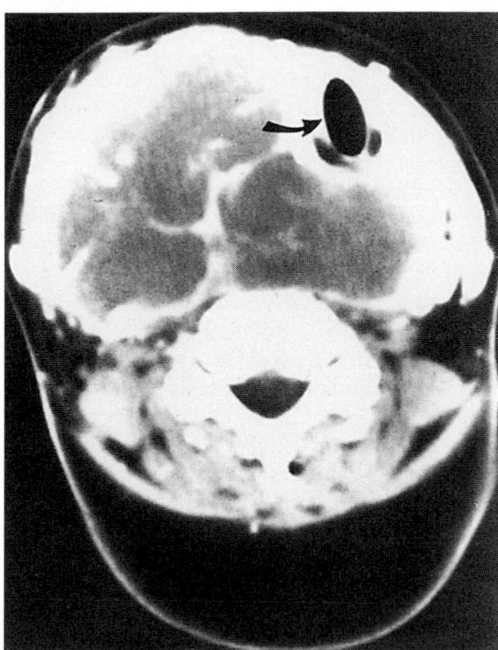

Figure 29.14 Computed tomographic scan (axial view) of extensive thyroid lymphoma. Note lobulated but organized appearance of mass that compresses but does not invade the airway (*arrow*). Note encasement of recurrent nerve area. Nerve function was normal at the time of this scan.

engulfed with tumor. The radiographic image of such a tumor is that of a lobulated but organized mass (Fig. 29.14). When substantial enlargement occurs in the neck, diagnosis is usually forthcoming; however, when the lymphoma develops in the mediastinum, the first symptom can be airway compromise.

Diagnosis of primary thyroid lymphoma is made by history, examination, MRI, and finally by FNA or biopsy. A high percentage of lymphomas are accurately diagnosed by FNA with appropriate immunotyping for monoclonality (237). In cases in which a diagnosis cannot be obtained by this technology, open incisional biopsy may be required to establish a diagnosis. Some surgeons prefer to do a thyroidectomy rather than an open incision and biopsy alone, as this removes a significant mass of tissue that may not respond to chemotherapy. The patient is already receiving general anesthesia and the pathologist then has adequate tissue to examine.

Anaplastic Carcinoma of the Thyroid Gland

Anaplastic carcinoma of the thyroid is a devastating disease that usually overcomes the host in a matter of months, sometimes even weeks. These uncommon cancers represent less than 5% of malignancies of this gland (50,77,88,89,259), and most commonly they occur in elderly women. The natural history of anaplastic thyroid cancer is characterized by rapid and massive locoregional growth, dysphagia, superior vena cava syndrome, and (finally) asphyxiation or exsanguination (82,83,260). Jugular lymph node involvement occurs early and is present in most patients at the time of diagnosis; at that time, more than half of the patients have systemic metastasis, most commonly in the lungs (249). Even in those studies in which achievement of improved locoregional control by multimodal methods has been reported, most patients died of distant metastasis (261,262).

Anaplastic thyroid cancer seems frequently to be associated with antecedent thyroid disease. LiVolsi and Merino (77) reported that 80% of patients note a prolonged history of goiter of some sort. Although there is disagreement, it is possible that some cases of anaplastic carcinoma are associated with the transformation of differentiated cancer (81–83); that is to say, these particular tumors probably represent the terminal stage in the dedifferentiation of a follicular or papillary carcinoma. It should be noted, however, that anaplastic cells do not seem to produce thyroglobulin or to be able to transport iodine, and that thyrotropin receptors are not found in their cell membranes (264). In almost all cases of anaplastic thyroid cancer, some form of differentiated cancer, either papillary, follicular, or Hürthle cell cancer, is seen (43,243) Even a small focus of anaplastic carcinoma in a patient with differentiated thyroid cancer should be considered an ominous sign.

The anaplastic component of these tumors is typically composed of varying proportions of spindle, polygonal, and giant cells (265). Certain papillary carcinomas also demonstrate spindle and giant cell metaplasia; even though they retain their classification as papillary cancer, the natural history of such tumors appears to be more aggressive and is associated with a poorer prognosis than papillary cancer lacking these features (85,266). This aggressive behavior pattern as well as the histomorphologic appearance adds credibility to this theory of tumor evolution and dedifferentiation. The lethality of anaplastic cancer should not be underestimated, even when minimal in size amid a background of predominantly differentiated cancer.

Although there are repeated suggestions in the literature of an association between ionizing irradiation and anaplastic transformation of papillary thyroid cancer (83,85–87), the bulk of the evidence would suggest otherwise. Many anaplastic tumors develop in patients who have not received irradiation for a well-differentiated thyroid carcinoma. In a compilation of data from six series that reported a total of 115 anaplastic thyroid carcinomas, Kapp et al. (82) reported that only 30% had a history of having received ionizing irradiation prior to the development of anaplastic carcinoma. Other studies involving almost 700 cases of differentiated thyroid cancer treated with external-beam radiation therapy (EBRT) and 352 patients with differentiated thyroid carcinoma treated with ^{131}I together yielded only three cases of anaplastic transformation (267–269). Even if most anaplastic thyroid carcinomas are derived from preexisting differentiated thyroid cancers, only a small number of differentiated thyroid carcinomas actually turn into anaplastic cancer. That slight possibility, therefore, should not be allowed to influence significantly the treatment of differentiated thyroid cancer. The employment of radioactive iodine or even EBRT should not be avoided because of the theoretic concern for tumor dedifferentiation.

Medullary Thyroid Carcinoma

Medullary carcinoma is unique among thyroid tumors (270, 271). These malignancies are derived from the nonepithelial parafollicular or C cell, which is a designation that associates the ability of these cells to synthesize and secrete calcitonin. This family of cells possesses the capacity for the ectopic production of peptide hormones and also the predisposition to familial neoplasia, sometimes in multiple organ systems (272). These parafollicular cells are derived from the neural crest and are therefore of neuroectodermal origin. By embryologic definition, they are unrelated to the thyroid follicular cells. The parafollicular cells are part of what was formally known as the *amine precursor uptake and decarboxylation cell system* (273), now more correctly called the *diffuse neuroendocrine system* (109). The new terminology acknowledges that the primary products of these cells—neuropeptides and catecholamines—may serve as neurotransmitters, neurohormones, hormones, and parahormones (169). Those tumors originating in this system generally share certain histochemical and functional similarities. Medullary tumors, for example, have histologic and cytologic features typical of other neuroendocrine tumors, such as carcinoid tumors, pancreatic islet-cell tumors, and pheochromocytomas (26,169).

Medullary thyroid carcinoma occurs in two basic forms, sporadic and familial. Each variety occurs with equal relative frequency in men and women (43). The sporadic tumors make up perhaps 70% to 90% of the total and 10% to 30% of the familial (120,274). Patients with the familial version have inherited medullary carcinoma as an autosomal-dominant trait in one of three distinct clinical syndromes: isolated familial medullary thyroid carcinoma (FMTC), multiple endocrine neoplasia type IIA (MEN-IIA), and multiple endocrine neoplasia type IIB (MEN-IIB). Even though the type I MEN syndromes do not involve the thyroid gland, they are listed in Table 29.4 with the entire group of syndromes.

All three thyroid-associated syndromes are related to specific mutations of the *ret* oncogene located on chromosome 10. Usually, there is a specific point mutation in exons 10 to 15 in MEN-IIA and familial medullary cancer and in exon 16 in MEN-IIB. Exons 10 to 15 code for the extracellular or transmembrane portions of the receptor, and exon 16 codes for the intracellular domain. Tyrosine kinase activation is mediated by each of the mutations (275). The actual incidence of each is somewhat difficult to ascertain because studies may be influenced by the aggressiveness of the family-screening policy at the reporting institution. If the family of each familial tumor patient is properly screened, for instance, a higher relative percentage of familial tumors would be discovered. Even with this consideration, the sporadic version of medullary cancer is almost certainly much more common than the familial. Depending on the particular series quoted, medullary thyroid carcinoma accounts for 3% to 10% of all thyroid cancers (237,276). The fact that any medullary cancer can possibly be part of a syndrome has a considerable impact on the approach to these tumors. In any patient with a medullary tumor, for example, the presence of a pheochromocytoma must be excluded before thyroidectomy.

If one classifies medullary carcinoma in the spectrum of lethality, it tends to have a more favorable prognosis than anaplastic cancer but is less favorable than either papillary or follicular carcinoma. The overall 5-year survival for patients with medullary thyroid cancer ranges from 25% to 75% (277), with a mean survival of near 50% (24,26,278). The survival at 10 years is substantially less than that at 5 years (274). If there is no nodal metastasis, the 5-year survival is 85% or more (274,275,279); however, it drops markedly when cervical or mediastinal nodes become positive. In fact, the 5-year survival of patients who have medullary cancer and positive nodes is 50% at best (275). Because of a remarkable predilection for early regional nodal metastasis, even in microdimensional primary tumors (280,281), prompt detection, classification, and aggressive surgical treatment are essential. Overall, 50% of medullary thyroid cancers demonstrate metastasis at the time of diagnosis (282).

Medullary tumors are usually circumscribed and encapsulated, but this local organization is often deceiving. Although lymphatic spread is its main mode of metastasis, distant hematogenous spread to the lungs, liver, adrenal glands, skin, and other parts can be seen (283). Lymphatic spread is most commonly to the nodes of the central and paratracheal regions and to the jugular chains (284–287). The degree of aggressiveness of medullary cancer varies greatly (288), with some tumors recurring locally or regionally after many years of quiescence, and others following a rapidly fatal course with widespread metastases. Although it is difficult to predict biologic potential from histologic appearances, most clinically aggressive tumors show necrosis, considerable pleomorphism, and many mitoses (284,289,290).

Medullary thyroid cancers typically produce amyloid depositions (291). Such deposits probably are derived from polymerized calcitonin and tend to occur in both primary and metastatic sites (166). Amyloid, however, is present in only 60% to 80% of medullary carcinomas; its absence, therefore, does not rule out this malignancy (292). Calcitonin immunohistochemistry, on the other hand, is probably the most useful adjunct to routine histology, and the homogeneity of the staining of this hormone may even reflect tumor differentiation and ultimate prognosis (281). Familial medullary thyroid cancer or MEN-IIA/B have a tendency to occur at the junction of the upper one third and lower two thirds of the thyroid gland, the location where there is a predominance of C cells. Furthermore, in these syndromes there usually is found multiple smaller sites of medullary thyroid cancer and C-cell hyperplasia.

There are no apparent histologic differences between sporadic and familial medullary tumors, but the two groups do demonstrate different behavioral characteristics. The sporadic tumors are usually located unilaterally within the gland, although they can occasionally be bilateral (293,294). On the other hand, almost all familial tumors are either bilateral or multifocal (294). This relates to the diffuse C-cell (parafollicular) hyperplasia that precedes the development of multiple foci of carcinoma in the familial tumors. This cellular hyperplasia is thought to be premalignant, and invasion through the follicular basement membrane by these cells is the pathologic marker for conversion to malignancy. Histologically, medullary cancer is characterized by areas of C-cell hyperplasia found adjacent to areas of malignancy and by deposits within the thyroid of calcitonin-derived amyloid. Both hyperplasia and medullary carcinoma may lead to a rise in baseline calcitonin production or an abnormal pentagastrin stimulation test of calcitonin. Apparently all thyroid C cells have the potential for hyperplasia in inherited medullary carcinoma (281). It is likely that there is a predilection for specific locations within the gland. The fact that C cells are normally concentrated in the upper two thirds of the

TABLE 29.4 Outline of Multiple Endocrine Neoplasia (MEN) Syndromes

- MEN-I (Wermer syndrome)
  - Parathyroid hyperplasia
  - Pituitary adenomas
  - Pancreatic adenomas
- MEN-IIA (Sipple syndrome)
  - Medullary thyroid carcinoma
  - Parathyroid hyperplasia
  - Pheochromocytoma
- MEN-IIB
  - Medullary thyroid carcinoma
  - Pheochromocytoma
  - Ganglioneuromatosis
  - Marfanoid habitus

thyroid lobes would support the logic of such a tendency (275,294,295).

Functionally, medullary carcinomas secrete a variety of chemicals that can serve as tumor markers (274,296–305), but the most consistent and reliable are the CEA and the peptide hormone calcitonin. Because serum calcitonin levels relate directly to the number of C cells present throughout the body, the measurement of this hormone provides the basis for a sensitive and specific diagnostic test (173). It is not clear, however, whether this represents the combination of C-cell hyperplasia and the tumor.

Inherited medullary carcinoma exists as one of three distinct clinical groups: There is FMTC, an inherited form of medullary thyroid cancer. There are those medullary cancers that are part of syndromes (i.e., MEN). Type IIA and type IIB MENs both involve thyroid and adrenal tissue with medullary carcinoma and pheochromocytoma. In addition, MEN-IIA patients demonstrate parathyroid hyperplasia, and MEN-IIB patients have a typical phenotype consisting of a marfanoid body habitus as well as mucosal neuromas.

Multiple endocrine neoplasias are inherited in an autosomal-dominant trait, and penetrance is reported to be up to 100% (277,306–309). Expression is variable, however, with different features appearing with varying frequency among families or individuals. The many sporadic occurrences of MEN appear to represent *de novo* germline (and thus heritable) mutations. Up to 50% of MEN cases are reported to be *de novo* mutations, and all occurrences are mutations of the paternally derived chromosome (310,311). The gene responsible for both MEN-II and FMTC is the *ret* proto-oncogene located on the long arm of chromosome 10. Therefore, FMTC is genetically related to MEN-II (i.e., it is a heritable form of medullary thyroid cancer that happens to be unassociated with any other inherited neuroendocrine pathology). Of the roughly 25% of all medullary cancers that are identifiable familial variants, some 16% are MEN-IIA, perhaps 3% are MEN-IIB, and approximately 5% are FMTC. For this reason, all medullary thyroid carcinoma patients and their families should be screened for MEN and FMTC. Thirty percent of MEN-II index cases die of medullary thyroid carcinomas or pheochromocytoma (277).

Penetrance of medullary thyroid carcinoma approaches 100% in MEN-II gene carriers (277,306,307,309,312–314). In contrast to the sporadic form, heritable medullary thyroid carcinoma is generally multicentric and bilateral and is histologically found in association with C-cell hyperplasia. MEN-IIB–associated medullary cancer tends to be more aggressive than any of the other types, including the sporadic type. In addition, at the time of serologic detection, this malignancy tends to be more advanced than the sporadic form. The age of persons affected also differs for sporadic versus heritable medullary cancer; the mean age at diagnosis in the sporadic medullary carcinomas is 50 to 60 years, whereas the average age of patients with MEN-II is 16 years. Medullary carcinoma has been diagnosed in MEN-IIB patients as young as age 7 months (315). An earlier onset of this malignancy in female gene carriers has also been described (312). Table 29.5 compares the features of heritable versus sporadic medullary thyroid carcinoma.

The ability to test peripheral white cell DNA for the presence of *ret* oncogene mutations can be efficiently and rapidly performed clinically. This test is mandatory for any patient diagnosed with medullary thyroid cancer, and if a mutation is found, first-degree family members must be tested as well. Extreme care should be taken to ensure that different samples are not confused due to similarities in patient names. If a first-degree family member has the identical mutation as the proband, then serious consideration should be given to evaluating for pheochromocytoma, hypercalcemia, and medullary thyroid cancer in the newly identified patient or relative. In fact, consideration of a "prophylactic" thyroidectomy to prevent the development and progression of medullary thyroid cancer is indicated. Broad, candid discussions with the patient and family as well as with medical authorities from a variety of disciplines, e.g., genetics, endocrine, pediatrics, and surgery, is required.

TABLE 29.5 Comparison of Features of Heritable and Sporadic Medullary Thyroid Carcinoma

MEN-II or FMTCs	Sporadic MTC
Multifocal	Unifocal
Bilateral	Unilateral
More aggressive	Less aggressive
Age onset: second or third decade	Age onset: sixth or seventh decade
Earlier onset in women	Onset age similar for men and women

The features noted represent general comments, and specific exceptions may occur.
FMTC, familial medullary thyroid carcinoma; MEN, multiple endocrine neoplasia; MTC, medullary thyroid carcinoma.

If, however, the *ret* oncogene is normal in the proband or in a family from a proband who has a mutation, the specific follow-up evaluation for the newly identified "normal" family member is controversial (272). Present techniques detect *ret* oncogene mutations in about 95% to 97% of patients with familial disease, meaning that about 3% to 5% of these individuals will not have identifiable mutations. Perhaps these are related to as-yet-unidentified *ret* mutations causing abnormalities, to mutations in genes other than the *ret* oncogene, or to technical or administrative errors. In any case, experts emphasize that a patient with medullary thyroid cancer with a normal *ret* oncogene or a family member (the family has a known mutation) who has a normal *ret* oncogene should have the *ret* oncogene measurement repeated at a later date to ensure its accuracy. The clinical and laboratory follow-up of a negative *ret* oncogene in these circumstances is also debatable, but some endocrinologists suggest the periodic performance of clinical examinations as well as radiologic and chemical studies over time.

Metastasis to the Thyroid Gland

Metastasis of other cancers to the thyroid gland is unusual as a presenting finding; however, because of the extreme vascularity of the gland, micrometastases are commonly found at autopsies of patients with remote malignancies in kidney, lung, breast, or skin (melanoma). Actually, almost any carcinoma has the capacity to spread to the thyroid gland. In patients who die of disseminated carcinomas, up to 24% are reported to have metastatic foci within the thyroid gland at autopsy (316,317). It is essential, therefore, that a patient who has a known carcinoma elsewhere and presents with a thyroid mass be viewed with suspicion for metastatic carcinoma. Such lesions should initially be evaluated by FNA and, if the cytology demonstrates metastasis, the management of the thyroid should involve the more complex paradigm for the overall treatment plan of the primary tumor (318). It should be noted that the thyroid mass may not appear until years after the original cancer diagnosis; furthermore, it may be the only presenting sign of distant metastasis.

Even though one must impose strictly limited indications for any surgery in the setting of disseminated metastatic disease, thyroidectomy in patients with slowly growing metastasis from elsewhere (particularly renal cell carcinoma) can be considered (243) if the palliation gained may benefit the quality of life.

DIAGNOSIS AND CLINICAL PRESENTATION OF THYROID CANCER

To operate on every nodular thyroid would be excessive, and to do so would subject a large number of patients to unnecessary surgery. This point is substantiated by the facts: approximately 7% of women and 2% of men have an enlarged thyroid; a nodule can be palpated in 3% to 4% of U.S. citizens; and the absolute prevalence of cancer in solitary and multinodular glands is 10% to 15% (319). Thus, identifying those persons with thyroid masses that are more likely to be malignant is the critical first step in their management. Certain generalizations about risk factors can be helpful in formulating strategies; age, sex, family history, and exposure to ionizing irradiation are all considerations in the decision process. We consider thorough evaluation of all thyroid nodules that are 1 cm or larger, regardless of whether they are identified by palpation or radiologic techniques. In addition, multinodular goiters should also be evaluated in a similar manner if there are nodules larger than 1 cm. These clinical guidelines may be modified in special circumstances.

Risk Factors

AGE

The probability that a thyroid nodule is malignant changes with age. Even though children are less likely to have thyroid nodules than adults, cancer has been reported to be present in 15% to 60% of nodules present in the young (320–322). This wide divergence of probability confuses the fact that in children who had thyroid nodularity and did not receive neck irradiation, a twofold increased risk for thyroid cancer is present in comparison to adults (323). Persons older than age 60 have a higher chance of malignancy in thyroid nodules (324,325). Although these two extremes of age are comparable in incidence, the natural history is different between the two groups; prognosis for thyroid cancer is significantly worse in the elderly than it is in children and younger adults (326).

SEX

Thyroid nodules are approximately eight times more common in females than in males (326). In striking contrast, the likelihood that a given nodule is malignant is two to three times greater in men than in women (325,327). Thyroid cancer in the pediatric population also occurs more commonly in girls (328).

IRRADIATION EXPOSURE

Exposure of the head and neck to ionizing increases the chance of developing both benign and malignant thyroid nodules. Furthermore, the association of irradiation to the thyroid gland and subsequent malignant transformation within that gland is incontrovertible. Between 1920 and 1950, radiation therapy to the head and neck was administered to more than 1 million Americans for such benign conditions as enlarged tonsils, adenoids, and thymus, tinea capitis, impetigo, sinusitis, keloids, eosinophilic granuloma, and acne (329,330). A possible association between irradiation for hyperthyroidism and the subsequent development of carcinomas was reported in 1949, and by the early 1950s this relationship was well established (331). Radiation therapy has subsequently been banned as the treatment of benign pediatric conditions. In one study, thyroid nodules were noted in 38% of those children exposed to such irradiation (332). Patients who have nodules and a history of irradiation during childhood have an approximately 35% likelihood of malignancy in the nodule (333–335). Children and adolescents, it would seem, are more sensitive to the mutagenic effects of low levels of ionizing irradiation. Among the approximately 15,000 survivors of the atomic bombings of Hiroshima and Nagasaki, young people seemed to be at greatest risk for the development of thyroid abnormalities, and data that have been compiled since have shown the same pattern (336). For instance, of those young persons who had Hodgkin disease and received radiation therapy to the chest, 30% are reported to have thyroid nodules and are at increased risk for developing thyroid cancer (337). Thyroid nodules have been noted in 33% of the Marshall Islands natives (338). The general population (especially children) exposed during the Chernobyl nuclear accident has been noted to have an increased rates of thyroid cancer (339,340). In contrast to our previous understanding and observations, children exposed to the Chernobyl nuclear accident have a particularly aggressive type of papillary thyroid cancer that histologically appears to contain sclerosis (340). Further, these patients have had thyroid cancer observed within several years of the accident, whereas pervious types of radiation exposure were associated with the development of thyroid cancer many years subsequently (340).

The risk for cancer development is directly proportional to exposure doses that range from 7 to 1,000 cGy (332,341). The amount of irradiation exposure seems to be the single most important risk factor in thyroid nodule development. The risk relationship continues until at least 1,500 rad. At levels of 3,000 rad or higher, the pathologic changes usually take the form of hypothyroidism, thyroiditis, or diffuse cellular atypia. Furthermore, it would seem that the risks are inversely proportional to age of exposure (342). Cancers can be seen as early as 3 years after exposure (with a peak occurrence at 15 to 30 years) and then decline over time. Risks remain elevated for at least 45 years after irradiation (343–345). The latency period between exposure and cancer development varies, with the average of 8.5 years. This latency has not been seen, however, in the group exposed during the Chernobyl incident. In this circumstance, carcinogenesis inexplicably seems to be greatly accelerated. Since the Chernobyl accident, discussion has been vigorous regarding the ability of potassium iodine administration to prevent the subsequent development of thyroid nodules and cancer in a population that may be exposed to excessive doses of radioiodine (345).

In contrast to data for external irradiation, little evidence suggests that internal irradiation from therapeutic or diagnostic doses of ^{131}I causes thyroid carcinoma in humans (64–67). There have been suggestions in the European literature of an increased number of gastrointestinal and bladder malignancies in individuals who have been treated with ^{131}I (346–352).

FAMILY HISTORY

Familial inheritance of papillary thyroid carcinoma is very uncommon (353,354), and the pathophysiology of such a familial disorder is unknown. Race contributes to the rate of thyroid cancer: Chinese, Hawaiian, and Filipino groups are at higher risk (355). How much influence dietary factors has on these data is unclear.

In a patient with a thyroid mass, family history of thyroid cancer should raise the consideration of medullary thyroid cancer, which presents as FMTC or as part of MEN. Family or personal history of hyperparathyroidism, urinary stones, and symptoms of such pheochromocytomas as hypertension, sweats, palpitations, and headaches should alert one to this diagnosis.

Gardner syndrome, a familial disorder involving colonic polyps and other benign tumors, is associated with increased thyroid nodules and papillary thyroid carcinoma (356). There has been discussion about whether colon polyps and cancer occur more frequently in patients with differentiated thyroid cancer, although further investigations are needed to assess this possible association. Cowden syndrome is a rare autosomal-dominant disorder associated with hamartomas, breast lesions, gastrointestinal polyps, ovarian cysts, uterine fibroids, and thyroid neoplasms (75). The specific defect in this disorder has been found to be a mutation in the *pTEN* suppressor oncogene.

Clinical Symptoms and Signs

The variety of factors and findings that enter into the decision about whether to operate include the examination, the age and sex of the patient, the family history, and a history of exposure to ionizing irradiation. Various diagnostic aids, such as ultrasonography, radioisotopic scans, FNA, MRI, CT, and routine radiographs, can provide information that helps in assessing whether a mass is benign or malignant. Calcitonin measurement in patients with medullary cancers are required to assess for recurrence or progression of disease, in conjunction with physical examination, history, and radiologic studies. Free T_4 (or less desirably a total T_4), total T_3, and TSH are required in patients with hyperthyroidism. Serial measurement of thyroglobulin levels is required in the evaluation of patients with known differentiated thyroid cancer, in association with appropriate nuclear medicine and radiologic studies (357). It is controversial whether measurement of serum calcitonin is useful in patients with thyroid nodules prior to thyroidectomy, in patients without a known personal or family history of medullary thyroid cancer. Similarly, measurement of serum thyroglobulin prior to thyroidectomy in a patient with a thyroid nodule is probably not useful.

Thyroid cancer most commonly presents as a single neck mass noted incidentally by the patient, physician, family, or friends. In women, previously unsuspected masses are often discovered during routine examinations done by the gynecologist. Persons with thyroid cancer are usually clinically euthyroid. Local symptoms are unusual; pain can occur after spontaneous hemorrhage within a nodule, but this is nonspecific and is just as likely in benign as in malignant lesions. Rarely, dysphagia or hoarseness can occur.

A clinician is often able to establish an early level of suspicion with the basic tools of the history and physical examination. A thyroid mass in a child, no matter its size or consistency, is highly suspicious for malignancy. Regardless of sex, a thyroid mass in elderly patients is more likely to be malignant. Even though more women than men develop thyroid cancer, any given nodule in a man is more likely to be cancer. Regardless of age of presentation of a mass, any patient who was exposed to low-dose irradiation in childhood is at a substantially higher-than-normal risk for thyroid cancer. Medullary carcinoma may be associated with systemic symptoms, such as chronic diarrhea, and, of course, as part of MEN-II the patient may have hypertension, headache, palpitations, and diarrhea associated with a pheochromocytoma, and hypercalcemia, renal stones, and fractures as a result of the primary hyperparathyroidism.

The most consistent sign suggesting malignancy in a thyroid mass is probably the presence of associated significant cervical adenopathy. The primary mass itself, however, can offer valuable clues as to its nature. Although such words as *hard with fixation* can apply to a mass associated with thyroiditis, these characteristics must be viewed with suspicion for malignancy. The opposite must not be assumed, however; soft masses with no fixation to surrounding tissues are not necessarily benign. Rapid enlargement can be deceptive because of the tendency for intralesional hemorrhage. On the other hand, relentless and rapid growth can be seen in a fulminating anaplastic carcinoma.

Cystic masses are likely benign, but cystic carcinomas do occur. Whether a particular mass is solid, cystic, or mixed is probably of some importance in the assessment of potential malignancy, as the reported incidence of malignancy is higher in the solid masses and lower in the cystic masses. However, extreme caution must be used applying this information as only authentic pure cysts have a lower likelihood of harboring cancer. A true cyst is defined as having no internal echoes on thyroid sonogram and showing enhanced echogenicity posterior to the cyst due to enhanced signal through transmission through the cystic mass. Data derived by Ashcraft and VanHerle (319) from an exhaustive compilation of multiple studies of operated lesions that had previously been studied by ultrasonography showed that solid lesions had a 21% incidence of malignancy, cystic lesions had a 7% incidence, and mixed lesions a 12% incidence. These data must be interpreted with consideration of the sample bias of a group that was selected for surgery. In such a sample, one would expect the incidence of cancer to be higher in all three subgroups. The incidence of malignancy in cystic thyroid masses is reported at 2% to 9% overall (358). Although most thyroid cysts are obvious by palpation, some mixed masses feel more solid than cystic, and one must make that clinical judgment with caution. Also, cysts can be deceivingly firm as a result of an abundance of fluid. Approximately 5% to 15% of cysts contain thyroid cancer when the cysts actually having combined solid and cystic components (359).

Clinical judgment of solitary versus multiple nodules must be tempered by the inaccuracy inherent to palpation. For instance, glands that are operated for a solitary nodule have been reported to be multinodular 30% to 75% of the time (319). Undoubtedly, this level of inaccuracy would improve if all thyroids with any nodularity were imaged. Controversy exists, however, as to whether thyroid cancer occurs at a lower rate in solitary nodules as compared with multinodular goiters (326,360–362). Overall, the survey data suggest some 5% to 10% of the multiple nodules and 10% to 20% of the solitary nodules are malignant (363). Though these data are useful for both doctor and patient in achieving a broad-based understanding of the problem, FNA and cytology have simplified these issues greatly. Furthermore, the entire thyroid gland must be considered, and if there is a dominant larger nodule in the setting of multiple smaller nodules, we would consider this to nodule have an equivalent chance of harboring malignancy as does a solitary nodule.

Regarding the issue of vocal cord function relative to thyroid abnormalities, vocal cord weakness or paralysis can be secondary to either benign or malignant growths that are impinging on the recurrent laryngeal nerve. Vocal cord paralysis can be caused by a variety of benign thyroid diseases (167,360,361), although its presence and specifically its new or recent onset is considered an important clinical suggestion of malignancy. Motion changes are often associated with voice change, but such may not be the case if the involvement has been gradual and laryngeal compensation has occurred. Furthermore, the diagnostician must be wary of that circumstance in which a paralyzed vocal cord does not appear to be of recent onset. This is often characterized by a midline or compensated cordal position, which may not be associated with any noticeable voice

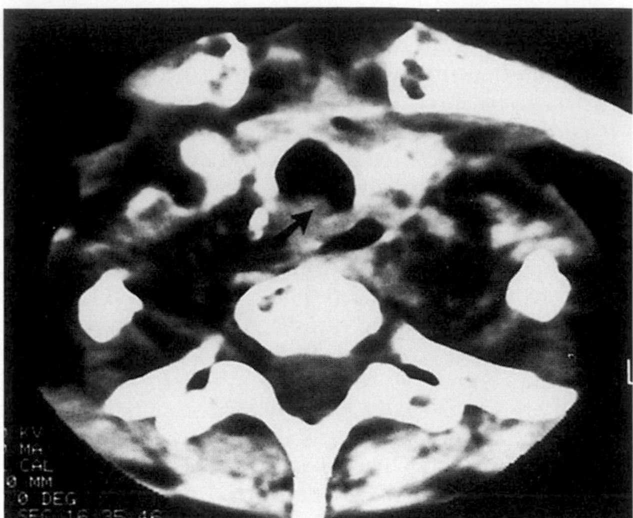

Figure 29.15 Computed tomographic scan of laryngeal level (axial projection). Note posterior invasion into lumen of air column. This luminal encroachment by tumor was visible on laryngeal examination.

change, and may reflect a problem totally unrelated to the thyroid gland, such as previous viral illnesses, diabetes mellitus, and a variety of other afflictions. This is not to suggest that in the setting of a thyroid mass, a paralyzed vocal cord is to be viewed casually; on the contrary, generally it is an ominous sign. The finding, however, should be combined with other parameters of measurement. It is important that any patient with hoarseness in this context be evaluated thoroughly.

Horner syndrome associated with a thyroid mass usually represents a malignant circumstance; however, we have seen several patients with classic eyelid and pupil findings in whom a large benign multinodular thyroid gland was apparently affecting the function of the sympathetic trunk. In one of these patients, on removal of the gland, the Horner syndrome abated.

Large multinodular goiters with or without substernal extension can cause tracheal shift or compression and alteration of the airway (364).

Differentiation must be made between tracheal deviation and significant lumen compression. Pulmonary assessment is helpful with associated flow loops. Tracheal deviation is most commonly caused by benign lesions, and significant compression is more likely associated with a malignant lesion, although these are simply clinical guidelines. Intraluminal tumor extension, however, almost always represents aggressive malignant behavior (Fig. 29.15). The optimal preoperative evaluation for true tracheal invasion with luminal extension is by endoscopy.

In the unusual case in which a thyroid mass is accompanied by the physical examination features of MEN-IIB (mucosal neuromas and marfanoid body habitus) or MEN-IIA (localized cutaneous lichen amyloidosis), medullary carcinoma is suggested (277).

Laboratory Evaluation

Thyroid function tests (e.g., free T_4 and TSH) are typically normal in patients with thyroid malignancy. The vast majority of patients with thyroid cancer are clinically euthyroid. Hyperthyroidism is rarely caused by a malignant toxic nodule (365,366). Thyroid antibodies similarly lack utility in distinguishing malignant from benign nodules (367). It should be remembered, however, that antimicrosomal antibodies are present in almost all patients with Hashimoto disease, and as there is an association between autoimmune thyroiditis and lymphoma, any thyroidal mass in a patient with a high antibody titer should be viewed as a potential lymphoma (368), especially if there has been rapid growth of the thyroid gland.

Thyroglobulin is present in normal human serum in concentrations of 20 to 40 ng per mL, but elevation above this offers no specific information. Thyroiditis and even hyperthyroidism can be responsible for an abnormally high thyroglobulin (369). It should be noted, however, that even though diagnostic sensitivity has not been described, a thyroglobulin level of more than 10 times the upper limit of normal is suggestive of thyroid cancer (370). We believe that the actual discriminating value of this marker is limited in the preoperative patient.

Of all blood products, the plasma calcitonin has the most direct diagnostic value in determining the nature of a thyroid mass. This polypeptide is normally produced exclusively by the C cells, and significant elevation suggests the presence of thyroidal C-cell hyperplasia or medullary cancer (371). Calcitonin levels are elevated in almost all patients with medullary thyroid cancer (372). However, in those patients who do have normal baseline values, detection of microlesions or C-cell hyperplasia associated with MEN-IIA or MEN-IIB can be accomplished with a pentagastrin or calcium stimulation of calcitonin (309). Rarely, calcitonin can be secreted ectopically by such other tumors as small cell lung cancers, pheochromocytomas, and carcinoid tumors. Elevations in serum calcitonin levels can occur in other thyroidal condition, such as Hashimoto thyroiditis, hyperthyroidism, and goiter, and therefore this test has low specificity in the diagnosis of thyroid cancer (372). Benign conditions, in general, are associated with milder elevations than are some thyroid cancers, but small medullary thyroid cancers and C-cell hyperplasia can result in serum elevations that are indistinguishable from other benign thyroid conditions.

Genetic testing is mandatory for first-degree family members (of a propositus with a demonstrated *ret* mutation) at risk for developing medullary cancer. The *ret* proto-oncogene encodes a protein receptor: tyrosine kinase. Mutations of *ret* are highly associated in 95% of hereditary medullary thyroid cancer, MEN-IIA and MEN-IIB, and FMTC (311,373). In contrast to familial forms of medullary thyroid cancer, only a very small percentage of patients with sporadic medullary thyroid cancer have a germline mutation in the *ret* oncogene (311,374), and this circumstance is usually associated with a poor prognosis (375). The germline mutation in the *ret* proto-oncogene is an alteration of cysteine residues in exon 10 or 11 in the case of MEN-IIA and a substitution of a methionine for a threonine in exon 16 in the case of MEN-IIB (375). Persons with MEN-IIA are also at risk for having hyperparathyroidism and pheochromocytoma; therefore, a history of either disorder or even the presence of hypercalcemia or hypertension should be viewed with suspicion. Those with MEN-IIB are at risk for associated pheochromocytoma and neuromas; similarly, they should be screened for all aspects of this endocrine complex.

Imaging

Overall, standard radiographs provide limited information in the evaluation of a thyroid mass and, with the exception of identifying metastatic lung disease, generally provide no specific information about the nature of the primary tumor (376). The chest radiograph should include the lower neck such that the position of the trachea can be visualized. This film can also suggest substernal extension of a large goiter. When calcifications are seen in the gland, and especially if they are bilateral, bulky, and near the junction of the upper one third and lower two thirds of the gland, medullary cancer is suggested. Approximately 40% of patients with this tumor demonstrate such calcifications in the upper and lateral part of the gland, the very areas of greatest concentration of C cells. Such calcifications can also be seen in metastatic medullary cancer that is present in cervical lymph nodes (377). The interpretation of calcification on any image should be made with caution, however, as other types of thyroid cancer and even benign goiters also can demonstrate this finding (378).

Computed tomography and MRI can offer valuable information about the overall three-dimensional relations of gland, tumor, and adjacent viscera. Local invasion seen on any of these images suggests malignancy, although this finding often is obvious on careful physical examination (Fig. 29.15). Finally, the presence of metastatic cervical or mediastinal adenopathy usually is obvious on CT scanning and MRI. The relative values of these two elaborate techniques are debated and may vary between institutions and clinicians. Of course, the use of radiologic studies depends on many factors, but, in general, thyroid sonograms or neck CT (or MRI) examinations may be useful before surgery in the evaluation of a goiter or a nodule for information regarding tracheal deviation or compression or the presence of cervical adenopathy. Once the diagnosis of thyroid cancer is made and the patient has had a thyroidectomy and is being monitored for the presence of recurrent or persistent disease periodic neck, chest and abdominal radiographic studies (e.g., CT or MRI) are very useful. Bone scans can help detect the presence of osseous metastases when appropriate (378). The use of iodine contrast in CT technology can significantly hamper the use of postoperative diagnostic radionuclide imaging, and the casual employment of CT without consideration for the overall strategy can compromise management of a thyroid cancer patient. Of course, the avoidance of CT dyes applies only to patients with differentiated thyroid cancer when radioiodine possibly may be used diagnostically or therapeutically in the near future. The MRI dye (gadolinium) does not interfere with subsequent radioiodine studies. During preoperative assessment, MRI (or CT) may be beneficial in the assessment of tumors that are known to be malignant, for the large gland that is thought to be partially substernal, or for those lesions believed to involve the air column (181). Under such circumstances, the surgeon is best forewarned about the perimeters of the tumor

Positron emission tomography scanning has emerged as extremely helpful in selected patients with thyroid cancer (379). Largely due to cost considerations, it should not be used before surgery in the routine patient with a thyroid nodule or goiter. However, it is interesting that there are now multiple instances in which a PET scan was performed for a different reason and "incidental" thyroid nodule was discovered. In this circumstance, further evaluation of these nodules has suggested that the chance of such a nodule harboring thyroid cancer is at least 90%, assuming the PET showed distinct and unequivocal activity in the thyroid. Indeed, we have seen such a patient who had a previously undiscovered papillary thyroid cancer that at surgery was found to be about 6 to 7 mm in size. The best-documented use of PET scans in patients with differentiated thyroid cancer relates to its capacity to detect cervical or distant disease in patients with negative or poor uptake on radioiodine scans but who have an elevated serum thyroglobulin or small lesions seen in the neck or chest by CT or MRI. Positron emission tomography scans may be useful as well in detecting or monitoring disease in any patient with differentiated thyroid cancer. In general, the less avid the radioiodine uptake by lesions, the greater the uptake of fluorodeoxyglucose on PET scan. Further studies need to be performed to determine whether avidity of fluorodeoxyglucose uptake by a lesion(s) correlates with the aggressiveness of the tumor and ultimately with progression and mortality. Positron emission tomography scanning is also useful in detecting and monitoring disease in patients with other forms of thyroid malignancy such as anaplastic and medullary thyroid cancer.

Ultrasonography defines the size, location, and consistency of a thyroid nodule but provides little discriminating information in the evaluation for malignancy. Whether a lesion is cystic or solid is relatively important because the probability of malignancy seems to be higher in solid lesions (380,381). In contrast, it has been shown that approximately 25% of thyroid cancers present on ultrasonography as partially cystic nodules (382,383). The value of this method for distinguishing malignant from benign lesions is therefore limited. Ultrasonography, however, is important for (a) following change of size of a thyroid nodule, (b) repeated examination of patients with a history of radiation exposure to the thyroid gland, (c) examining calcification within thyroid nodules (181), (d) guiding FNA techniques, (e) evaluating changes in a multinodular gland over time, (f) following thyroid abnormalities during pregnancy, and (g) preoperatively assessing bilateral disease in a thyroid gland in which only a unilateral mass is palpated and in which a lobe or isthmus resection is being considered. In sum, thyroid sonography is extremely important in allowing an accurate determination of whether a nodule or goiter has changed over time, and it has supplanted less accurate or quantitative measurements such as clinical palpation alone.

Radionuclide imaging has been used under a variety of diagnostic circumstances. The underlying premise is that the thyroid gland preferentially traps and disperses certain radioisotopes and, in so doing, visually isolates certain abnormalities within its substance. In fact, radionuclide images, whether obtained with radiolabeled iodine, technetium (Tc)-99m, or technetium-sestamibi, provide little actual information in the routine evaluation of a thyroid nodule (384). Essentially, either cold or warm images can be seen in both benign and malignant lesions, and therefore they have a low specificity (319).

An intrathyroid area that has a higher uptake than its surrounding thyroid tissue is referred to as hot or warm and traditionally is considered less likely to be malignant; the area that fails to concentrate the isotope is referred to as a cold nodule and traditionally has been considered more likely to be malignant. This oversimplification involves a variety of factors that alter the diagnostic value of radionuclide tests. For example, a nodule that functions differently from surrounding gland can be disguised by the overlying tissue; thus, a striking difference in contrast is camouflaged by averaging. A so-called warm nodule may, in reality, be a nonfunctioning nodule, in which the apparent tracer uptake is secondary to overlying normal thyroid tissue. Furthermore, nonfunctional thyroid tissue can represent a variety of nonneoplastic abnormalities such as a cyst, thyroiditis, or hemorrhage into an adenoma. Actually, approximately 80% of cold nodules are benign (181). Hypofunctional nodules can be malignant, even though the probability is relatively low (319). In a series of proved thyroid carcinomas that had been radioactively scanned, Beahrs and Kubista (385) showed that 61% of scans revealed cold nodules, 29% were normal scans, and, importantly, 10% showed hot spots at or near the site of the malignant lesion. Finally, important studies have shown that in all thyroid nodules, whether benign or malignant, 50% to 84% are hypofunctioning or cold, 10% are normal or warm, and 6% are hyperfunctional (50,319). A true hyperfunctional autonomous nodule rarely is associated with thyroid cancer, if the term *autonomous* is restricted to nodules with an undetectable TSH and complete suppression of extranodal tissue on scan.

Other isotopes such as Tc-99m and ^{201}Tl are of limited use in the evaluation of thyroid nodules. Technetium 99m has been shown to be trapped in some thyroid cancer cases, presenting a hot image. Thallium 201 has been shown to be taken up in malignant tissue and has a positive predictive value of 90%, even if the area has failed to image by radiolabeled iodine or technetium (386–388).

Many multinodular thyroid glands contain both functional and nonfunctional nodules and, in that circumstance, the interpretation of a radioisotopic scan is somewhat complicated. Although useful information can be gained from radioisotopic scanning, these techniques are not diagnostic and, because they do not reliably distinguish between benign and malignant lesions, they should not be the determining criteria for lesion removal. In laboriously compiled data, Ashcraft and VanHerle (319) showed that of all patients referred to surgery because of a cold thyroid nodule, only one of six had a malignant tumor. In the usual patient, if a thyroid nodule warrants removal on the basis of clinical, laboratory, radiologic, or cytologic findings, a radioisotopic study need not be done.

Fine-Needle Aspiration and Cytologic Evaluation

Fine-needle aspiration should not be confused with needle biopsies, which require a Tru-cut or Vim-Silverman needle and yield tissue segments for histologic rather than cytologic evaluation (389). Compared with FNA, large-needle biopsy of thyroid nodules is less sensitive for cancer diagnosis and, furthermore, is associated with a higher complication rate (390). Of all diagnostic methods, FNA and cytologic evaluation are the most accurate for diagnosing the character of thyroid nodule. The FNA should be one of the first steps in the decision regarding whether to operate. Follow-up of patients with benign or indeterminate cytologic has yielded an accuracy rate of greater than 90% (391). The false-negative rate is nearly 5%, and false positivity is substantially lower, usually less than 1% to 3%. In most large series, the false-positive diagnoses have occurred early in the series, and distortion of the data often is attributable to the inexperience of the cytopathologist. Lesion size also can cause variation in the false-negative rate of thyroid FNA, with larger nodules have a higher false-negative rate. It is very important that adequate cytologic samples be obtained and that they be analyzed by an experienced cytologist. It is also important that the cytologist and clinician have a mutual understanding of the meaning of the written report to decrease misunderstanding. In some circumstances, second opinions should be requested of another experienced cytologist.

Indications for FNA of the thyroid gland include the evaluation of a single thyroid nodule, a prominent nodule in a multinodular goiter, or the reclassification of a growing nodule that has been previously aspirated. Indeed, a thyroid FNA is indicated in any circumstance in which a thyroid nodule or the thyroid gland itself might be harboring a thyroid malignancy. A thyroid FNA is also indicated when it is important to make a specific thyroid diagnosis that cannot be made clinical or with supporting laboratory data.

It is clear that FNA has reached such a state of refinement and usefulness that to deny its preeminence in evaluating the thyroid mass is to deny an abundance of literature and, more importantly, to invite unwarranted surgery. Since the development of this technique, the number of patients requiring surgery has decreased by 35% to 75%, depending on the series reported (392–395). The yield of malignancy at the time of surgery has almost tripled in these preselected patients (396–398), and it has been estimated that the cost in managing patients with thyroid nodules has been reduced by more than 25% (337,399).

Interpretation of thyroid nodule cytology is generally categorized into four groups: benign, suspicious for malignancy, malignant, or insufficient for diagnosis. Approximately 65% to 70% of aspirates are interpreted as benign, and these consist mostly of adenomatoid (i.e., colloid) nodules, Hashimoto or lymphocytic thyroiditis, and cysts. The false-negative rate in this group is less than 5% when surgery is performed subsequently (214). Approximately 4% of thyroid nodules are interpreted as malignant, and these consist of papillary, medullary, and anaplastic carcinomas and lymphomas. The false-positive rate in this group is less than 5%. Approximately 10% of thyroid nodules are read as suspicious for malignancy, and 15% to 20% of all aspirations are insufficient for diagnosis (400,401). Insufficient specimen may be attributed to a number of factors: the inexperience of the operator or cytologist, nodular vascularity, presence of cystic fluid, and the imposition of very strict criteria to judge adequacy (402–404). Repeat aspiration yields sufficient data in approximately 50% of these cases (405). In lesions that are difficult to palpate, ultrasound guidance with FNA can be helpful (406). The greater the experience of the aspirator and the cytologist, the less the likelihood of obtaining insufficient aspirates. It is very important that an aspirate have sufficient cellularity to render a proper diagnosis, and if there is insufficient cellularity, the aspirate must be repeated, or performed by a more experienced person, until a diagnosis can be made. In our experience, we estimate that less than 1% to 2% of thyroid aspirates have insufficient cellularity for a diagnosis, even after performing repeat aspirations as needed. It has been helpful to have a cytologist on site and immediately review an aspirate for adequacy to ensure maximal efficiency.

The uncertain group includes follicular neoplasms (which could represent follicular carcinoma or follicular variant of papillary cancer), a diagnosis that includes both adenomas and carcinomas. The diagnosis of follicular carcinoma is not made cytologically but instead requires histologic evaluation of the lesion and its interface with the adjacent thyroid gland. Microvascular invasion along the lesion capsule and cellular invasion through the capsule into the surrounding normal thyroid gland are the findings that constitute malignancy. In FNA, the needle samples cells within an encapsulated lesion, and neither the microinvasion nor the tumor encroachment into the capsule is captured by this method. Of those nodules read as follicular neoplasms on FNA, approximately 20% ultimately are found to be thyroid cancer (either follicular neoplasm or follicular variant of papillary cancer), with the remaining 80% being benign adenomas or Hashimoto thyroiditis (407). Additional studies are warranted to better define the percentage of aspirates that are labeled as follicular neoplasm that on histologic examination are in reality follicular cancer or follicular variant of papillary cancer. A similar diagnostic difficulty exists for oxyphilic or Hürthle cell neoplasms, 15% of which turn out to be carcinomas (408). Hürthle cell infiltration can occur in many benign conditions, including Hashimoto thyroiditis and multinodular goiters, especially in older subjects. It frequently is difficult to differentiate significant Hürthle cell infiltration (i.e., neoplasm) from the scattered Hürthle cell infiltration seen in these other benign conditions. Lastly, the presence of lymphocytic infiltration in any aspiration may make it difficult to assess the likelihood of a lesion harboring papillary cancer, because atypical cells may be observed in both situations (409).

When either small lesions or multinodular glands are sampled by FNA, reliability may be somewhat compromised. In the former, the difficulty of precise localization may decrease the yield of tumor tissue, although sonographic localization at the time of the aspiration may be useful. In the latter circumstance, one or even multiple nodules may not represent completely the entire histologic profile of the gland. The judgment of the diagnostician must be more shrewdly employed in making decisions in each of these circumstances. Ultrasonography also enhances needle localization in approaching multinodular goiters. We generally try to aspirate the largest nodules in a multinodular goiter, especially those that are larger than about 1 cm in diameter.

When positive for cancer, FNA offers valuable preoperative planning information that helps the surgeon in preoperative patient counseling. With a positive FNA, the likelihood of error is so low that surgery should be undertaken even though other risk factors or suggestive physical findings are absent. Fine-needle aspiration is reliable in the preoperative diagnosis of papillary thyroid cancer, and it may be helpful in suggesting medullary cancer, in which case specific calcitonin staining of the tissue and measurement of serum calcitonin may be helpful. If medullary cancer is suspected, preoperative evaluation of hypercalcemia and pheochromocytoma must be performed, in conjunction with a thorough family history.

On the other hand, if the FNA is negative, continued skepticism is in order. If other findings and risk factors suggest malignancy, surgical exploration often is warranted, despite a negative FNA. There are few strict guidelines regarding indications for surgery in the context of a negative aspiration. Specific examples include, for example, growth, compression on the esophagus or trachea, voice change related to impingement of the recurrent laryngeal nerve, cervical adenopathy that might represent local metastases, the entire clinical context, and the patient's desires. The size of the lesion also is relevant. In general, if a thyroid nodule is larger than approximately 3 to 4 cm, it is thought that serious consideration for surgery should be entertained because of the chance of the nodule harboring cancer as well as the increased possibility of a false-negative aspiration. In any case, whenever a thyroid nodule is being followed, we believe it is important to utilize clinical and radiologic assessment (e.g., sonograms), and we also think it useful to repeat the FNA periodically. Repeat aspirations decrease the likelihood of a false-negative aspiration.

The use of thyroid hormone suppression to help discern malignant from benign lesions has fallen into disfavor. It is rarely used at the present time because (a) both benign and malignant lesions can increase or decrease with thyroid hormone suppression; (b) suppression mandates that the serum TSH be decreased, and this predisposes a patient for an increased risk for atrial fibrillation and bone loss, especially in elderly women; and (c) size increase in a thyroid nodule is thought to be a poor reflection of the presence of malignancy, especially when a previous aspiration has been benign (480).

Keen diagnostic judgment is required also when a cyst is encountered by FNA. First, adequate cytologic sampling is more difficult in cysts. Except for rare intraglandular thyroglossal duct cysts, true cysts of the thyroid are unusual. The cystic lesions commonly observed are most frequently the result of degeneration of adenomatoid nodules and follicular adenomas; however, papillary and follicular carcinomas also undergo cystic changes (383,389). The overall incidence of carcinoma in all thyroid cysts is less than 9%; the incidence is much higher in those cysts that exceed 4 cm in diameter and less in smaller cysts (319). A negative reading in very large cysts or in cysts that reform soon after aspiration should be viewed with suspicion. The viscosity and color of the fluid of the fluid are nonpredictive (410). Clear, colorless, and watery fluid is highly suggestive of a parathyroid cyst (411,412), and this should be confirmed by measuring parathyroid hormone (PTH) in the fluid obtained. Malignancies metastatic to the thyroid gland from other sites are unusual, but FNA can be useful in identifying their origin (413). Metastases of renal cell carcinoma, lung, breast, colon, and uterine carcinomas all have been cytologically identified within the thyroid gland (414). The ability to identify metastases to the thyroid is an important reason why a thyroid aspiration is recommended prior to surgery in essentially all patients with a thyroid nodule.

Immunostaining for markers of thyroid cancer have not been highly discriminating in cytologic specimens. The presence of thyroglobulin in a cervical lymph node aspirate confirms thyroid cancer and can help differentiate follicular neoplasms from medullary thyroid cancer or metastatic disease from distant sites. These tumors can be suggested or even diagnosed by FNA. Thyroid malignancies have been noted to have lower levels of thyroid peroxidase (415), lower levels of epithelial membrane antigen and Leu-7 antigen (416), and higher levels of epidermal growth factor (417). In addition, cell-surface proteoglycans and glycoproteins of the CD44 family are altered in a number of thyroid cancers. This alteration of intercellular adhesion characteristics may prove to be a valuable marker of malignancy (418).

A number of novel genes have been identified in thyroid cancer cells that, in the future, may assist in identifying malignant thyroid lesions. Markers of malignant transformation of thyroid epithelium are galectin-1 (419) and galectin-3 (420). The *RET/PTC* oncogene activation occurs in 20% of thyroid cancers as detected by combined immunohistochemical and reverse-transcriptase polymerase chain reaction (421). Rearrangement of the *NRRK1* gene, encoding one of the receptors for the nerve growth factor, frequently is detected in thyroid cancers (422). Also noted with increased frequency in thyroid neoplasms is the protein kinase C α-mutant gene expression (423). Mutations of Gs-α and *ras* genes may play important roles in tumorigenesis.

DEVELOPMENT OF A TREATMENT STRATEGY

The intelligent and thoughtful appraisal of a nodular thyroid is best achieved with the use of a variety of technical aids as well as a thorough understanding by both surgeon and endocrinologist of the behavior of the various tumors. An awareness of the various risk factors for thyroid cancer helps one to decide when to operate. The simplest approach, in terms of decision making, would be to remove all masses, but this would subject the majority of patients to unnecessary surgery with its attendant risks.

A number of practical and efficient schemas have been suggested for managing a thyroid nodule (226,424,425). In the setting of a normal pituitary gland, if the TSH level (and T_4 and T_3) indicates hyperthyroidism, the workup should address the differential diagnosis of thyrotoxicosis, and a radioisotopic scan is indicated. In most patients with a thyroid nodule, the TSH level is normal, however, and the next step in the evaluation should be an FNA. If the cytologic material suggests that the nodule is benign, observation of the patient commonly is recommended. Although thyroid hormone suppression has been used in the

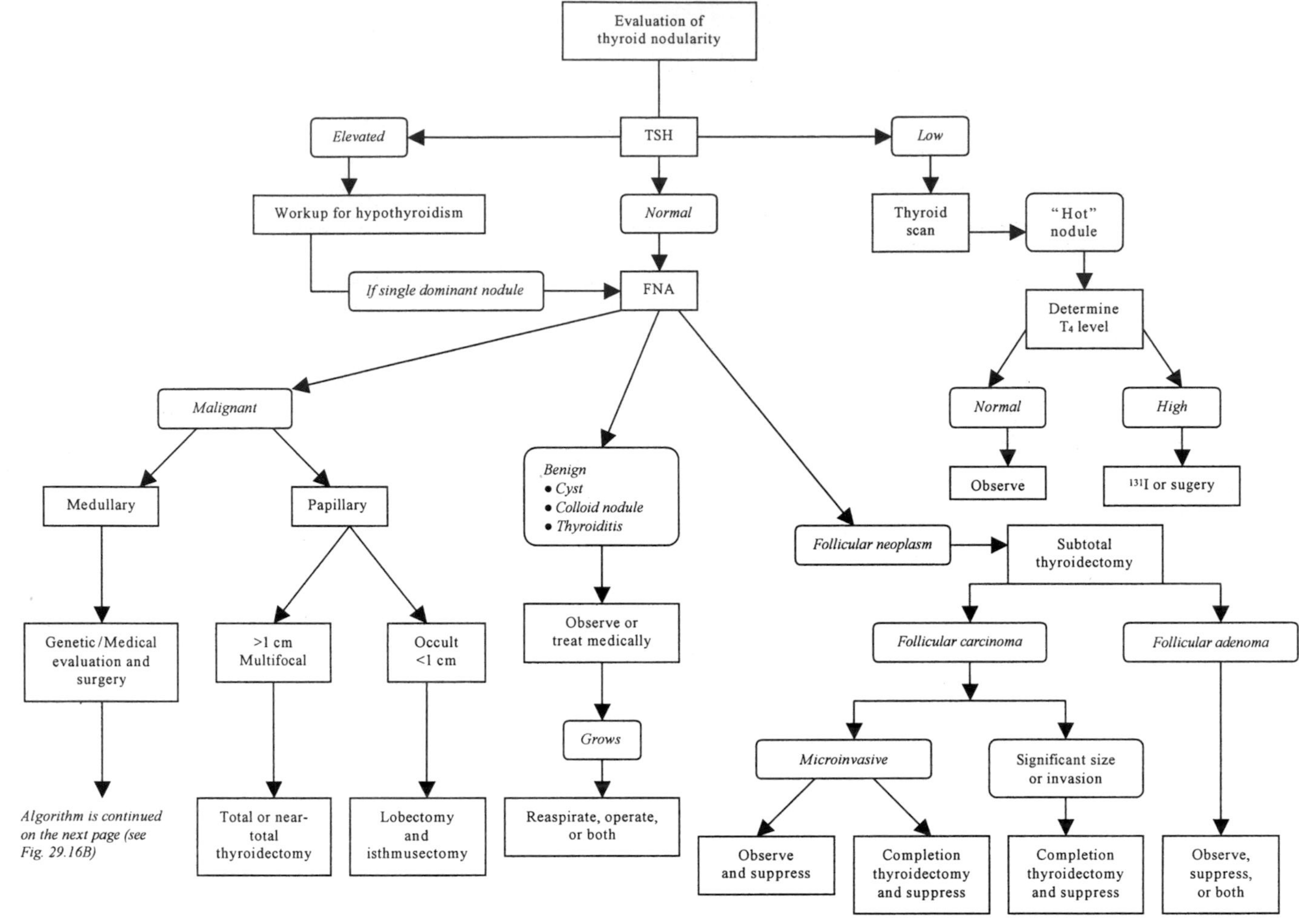

Figure 29.16 **A:** An algorithm for evaluation of thyroid mass. Note: If fine-needle aspiration (FNA) suggests medullary cancer diagnosis, a different pathway of diagnosis and therapeutic workup is followed.

past, especially prior to accurate FNAs, its use has fallen into disfavor (vide supra) (426–433).

There are risks associated with thyroid hormone suppression therapy. Accelerated bone loss and osteopenia (especially in postmenopausal and aged women), the induction of tachycardia, elevated systolic blood pressure, enlargement of cardiac muscle mass, and atrial dysrhythmias can result (434–436). Elderly patients with cardiac arrhythmias are especially vulnerable to these difficulties.

If the cytology from the nodule is highly suspicious for thyroid cancer, surgery is recommended. If the lesion is interpreted as a follicular neoplasm, surgery is required to define the difference between adenoma and carcinoma. When the cytologic evaluation is worrisome but not diagnostic, a practical analysis of risk factors for cancer assists in determining the need for surgery. If a nonsurgical approach is chosen, close ultrasonographic monitoring in conjunction with periodic history and physical examination and a repeat aspiration help to determine which patients will require surgery. Cystic lesions that re-form after two or three aspirations probably should be managed with surgery, despite continued negative cytology (437). If the FNA suggests medullary cancer, appropriate genetic studies are performed in addition to serum calcitonin and urinary screening for MENs and pheochromocytoma [e.g., with urine vanillylmandelic acid (VMA), metanephrines, and catecholamines]. The suggested algorithms for developing a management strategy for this family of diseases is presented in Fig. 29.16.

There is considerable organizational effort currently being devoted to the development of practice guidelines for the diagnosis and management of various cancers. In addition to the algorithm suggested in Fig. 29.16, we have included practice guidelines for medullary carcinoma that have been developed and proposed jointly by the American Society of Head and Neck Surgery and the Society for Head and Neck Surgeons (see "Practice Guidelines for Medullary Thyroid Cancer: Suggested").

In general, there is no standard approach to a thyroid mass. Risk factors, the patient's wishes, and the entire clinical context as well as the knowledge and experience of the clinicians help determine the approach to a given patient. The FNA is the cornerstone of the approach to virtually all thyroid masses. When cervical adenopathy is present and the FNA of that tissue is worrisome for cancer, we recommend thyroid surgery, regardless of patient sex or age. If there is another cancer present that might have metastasized to the thyroid, we first perform an FNA, perhaps with specific staining. Of all the risk factors, we consider advanced age, radiation exposure, and male sex most important for predicting cancer and for judging natural history.

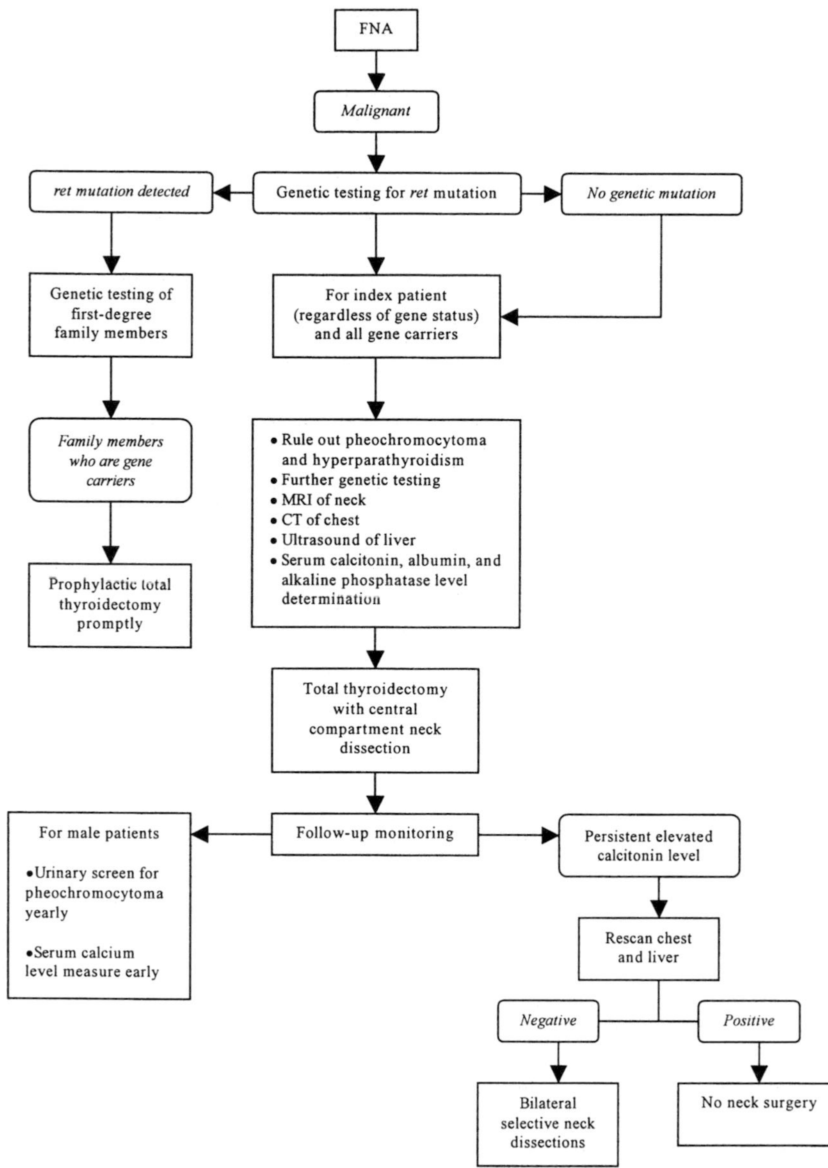

Figure 29.16 *(continued)* **B:** The medullary pathway is shown. *CT*, computed tomography; *MRI*, magnetic resonance imaging; T_4, thyroxine; *TSH*, thyroid-stimulating hormone.

We tend to alter the general approach accordingly, being more likely to intervene surgically in the higher-risk groups. A relative appraisal of the various risk factors is outlined in Table 29.6. Practical algorithms (scheme) for diagnosis and treatment of thyroid masses are outlined in Figs. 29.16 and 29.17. Depending on circumstances, this algorithm can vary considerably depending on the cytology that is discovered.

Selection of an Operation for the Primary Tumor

With the exception of some anaplastic carcinomas and most lymphomas, cancer of the thyroid gland should initially be managed surgically. The different operations that have been described merely represent variations of the amount of gland resected. The partial thyroidectomy can be as limited as a lumpectomy or as extensive as a near-total procedure, which is an operation that includes all but a thin posterior portion of the contralateral deep surface. Between these extremes, the procedure can be a lobectomy, an isthmusectomy, a lobe and isthmus removal, or any variation of these. The total thyroidectomy usually represents the removal of all of the gland that is within the surgical capsule. The actual removal is not always as complete as thought, however, a fact that is demonstrated by studies showing 2% to 5% residual deposits on radioactive iodine scans after presumed "total" thyroidectomy (363).

A considerable body of literature exists that addresses the issue of which operation to perform under particular circumstances. For a variety of reasons, investigators of noted reputation and comparable status directly contradict one another regarding the degree of radical surgery indicated (438–440). Even more remarkably, many of the same disagreements have been perpetuated for decades, much to the frustration of the less experienced thyroidologists and surgeons. As is true in much of therapeutic medicine, however, when there is such diversity between thoughtful investigators, the appropriate approach is probably somewhere between the two extremes. In addition, in matters perpetually in question, surgical trends tend to be cyclic, and attitudes that reflect contemporary thinking serve to influence those cycles. Our approach is to recommend a total or near-total thyroidectomy for all patients with a preoperative FNA that shows papillary thyroid cancer. The exception to this might be in those lesions that are unilateral and are less than 1 cm in diameter, in which a less gener-

TABLE 29.6 Relative Significance for Various Risk Factors in Thyroid Mass

	Low risk		→		High risk
	1	2	3	4	5
Age					
Elderly				X	
Child				X	
Sex					
Male				X	
Female		X			
Low-dose radiation in childhood					X
Family history		X			
Cystic mass[a]		X			
Solid mass				X	
Multiple masses		X			
Solitary mass			X		
Growing mass					X
Stable mass			X		
Hot scan	X				
Cold scan			X		
Warm scan		X			
Fine-needle aspiration (–)		X			
Fine-needle aspiration (+)					X
Associated cervical adenopathy					X
Complete resolution to thyroid suppression	X				
Partial resolution to thyroid suppression			X		
No response to suppression				X	

The characteristics noted and their presumed likelihood of harboring malignancy are subjective. Most reliance should be placed on the history and physical examination and radiologic studies, in conjunction with an adequate thyroid aspiration interpreted by an experienced cytologist.

[a]Most cysts have mixed solid and cystic components. A pure cyst that has no internal echoes on sonogram and has enhanced through transmission may have relatively low frequency of thyroid cancer, but cysts with mixed solid and cystic components likely have a higher chance of malignancy.

ous operation is acceptable. If a preoperative FNA is suspicious for malignancy or suggests a follicular neoplasm, either a lobectomy or a near-total thyroidectomy can be performed. The decision as to which operation to perform depends on the clinician's experience, the clinical context, and the patient's desires. We believe that a preoperative thyroid sonogram can be useful; if it shows a definite contralateral nodule(s), a thyroid ultrasound-guided aspiration can be performed. Even if an aspiration is not performed, the presence of abnormalities on the contralateral side can be helpful. If a lobectomy alone is performed and the final diagnosis shows thyroid cancer, then a completion thyroidectomy must be performed within 2 weeks of the initial surgery. The chance of a follicular nodule containing thyroid cancer is about 10% to 20%, meaning that in the majority of cases the nodule will be benign and no further surgery is needed. If, however, a sonogram showed a contralateral abnormality, then these areas need to be followed to ensure they are benign.

Many clinicians believe that a patient who has only a lobectomy will not require subsequent thyroid hormone replacement; we take issue with this. An increasing percentage of such patients will have an elevated TSH when followed over time, and thyroid hormone suppression will have to be given to perhaps as many as 25% to 50% of these patients when followed for decades. If a near-total thyroidectomy is performed when the preoperative aspiration is suspicious, a completion thyroidectomy would not be needed, and, in addition, the diagnosis of contralateral metastases would be made. However, the risk for hypocalcemia and recurrent laryngeal nerve injury is somewhat higher with a near-total thyroidectomy. Given these considerations, the decision as to which surgery should be performed is a made jointly by the attending physicians and the patient. Surgeons should be cognizant of these facts and should only perform a surgical procedure that they are competent and confident in performing. In some circumstances, consultations and assistance may be helpful. Ablative radioactive iodine can help eradicating residual thyroid tissue after a near-total thyroidectomy, but ^{131}I therapy cannot usually be used to eradicate an entire remaining lobe (210).

In contrast, the case to be made for a liberal employment of total thyroidectomy is compelling; Mazzaferri et al.'s (46) extensive 10-year follow-up study reported the recurrence rate was lowest in patients who had undergone a total thyroidectomy. Other studies by Massin et al. (178), Schlumberger et al. (441), and DeGroot et al. (187) also support such a philosophy. Other advantages also apply to total thyroidectomy, such as increased reliability of serum thyroglobulin levels, the enhanced diagnostic and therapeutic facility of radiolabeled iodine employment, and elimination of the potential for derangement of residual microfoci of papillary carcinoma into undifferentiated cancer.

In general, surgical morbidity is greatest with a total thyroidectomy and least with a lobectomy. All morbidity data, however, must be critically analyzed with knowledge of the skills of the surgeons participating in the study. Occasional thyroid surgeons are expected to be more problem-prone, and the standards for these surgeons should be based on a more conservative rather than a more radical surgical approach. In sophisticated and experienced surgical hands, the operative complications of total thyroidectomy are almost identical to those associated with the partial operation.

The surgical procedures recommended for papillary carcinoma are slightly different from those for follicular carcinoma. Traditionally, in the latter, those lesions that are more than microinvasive require a more aggressive approach. Some investigators, however, believe that the smaller, noninvasive follicular cancers can be treated just as conservatively as papillary

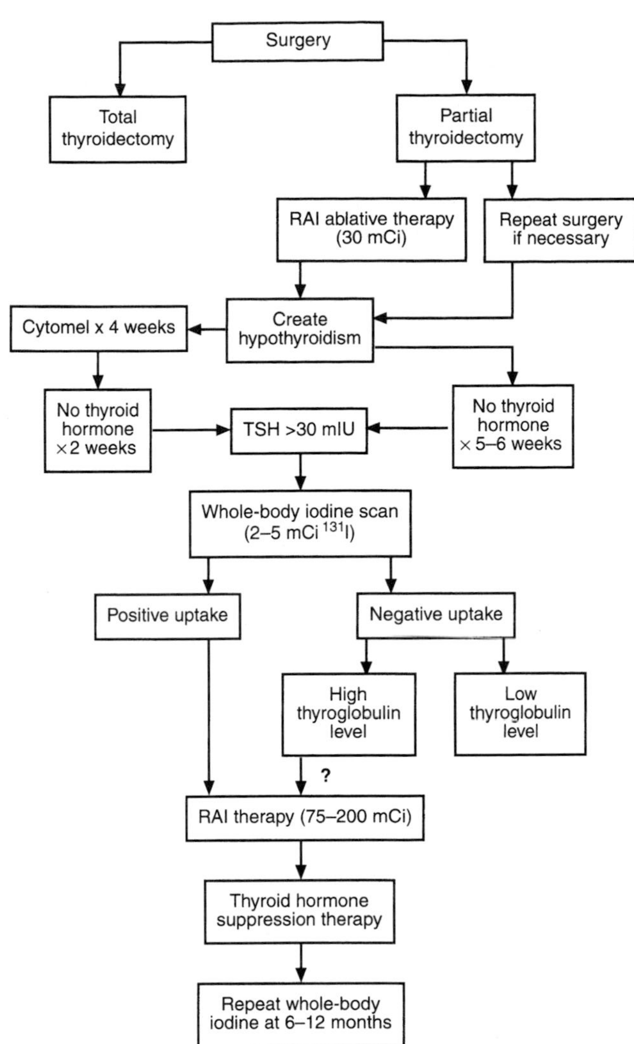

Figure 29.17 Schema showing a practical algorithm for employment of radioactive iodine (RAI) in the evaluation and treatment strategy. *TSH*, thyroid-stimulating hormone.

lesions. Nonetheless, we prefer a near-total thyroidectomy for all patients with follicular cancer, whether microinvasive or extensively invasive. Overall, the somewhat poorer prognosis of follicular over papillary carcinoma may be related to more advanced patient age and more advanced tumor stage at the time of diagnosis than to the actual histology. Furthermore, data show that the survival rates of patients with papillary or follicular carcinoma are similar in patients of comparable age and stage (187). We concur with these conclusions. Hürthle cell and medullary carcinomas are more ominous lesions and, as such, require a more extensive local operation; that is, total rather than partial thyroidectomy should be done routinely.

When a single micropapillary carcinoma (i.e., well encapsulated and <1.0 cm) is covered coincidentally in the pathologic specimens retrieved by surgery for other problems such as adenomas, thyroiditis, or the hemithyroidectomy undertaken with laryngectomy, further surgery usually is not needed. In this circumstance, the impact on life expectancy is thought to be minimal (442). We do recommend periodic assessment (e.g., thyroid sonogram, serum thyroglobulin levels) in individual circumstances, as appropriate.

For larger or multifocal papillary cancers, most surgeons recommend a total thyroidectomy. Because of an unacceptable local recurrence rate, lumpectomy is not advised for any malignant lesion. In papillary carcinomas, total thyroidectomy probably yields a lower recurrence rate in this group of patients and may lower the mortality rate. Overall, in papillary carcinoma, the incidence of multifocal disease is significant, and the local recurrence rate is doubled in those patients who underwent a subtotal rather than a total thyroidectomy (443). Patients who have been treated with lobectomy experience a 5% to 10% local recurrence (444,445). The ability to identify microfoci of papillary thyroid cancer depends on the assiduousness of the examining pathologist and the number of sections analyzed. It is generally believed that three or more microscopic foci, especially if they involve both lobes, should be treated with a near-total thyroidectomy.

In most instances of patient with thyroid cancer, as noted above, a near-total thyroidectomy is the most appropriate procedure. To a great extent, such an operation protects one recurrent laryngeal nerve, minimizes the surgical danger to the parathyroid glands, lessens the likelihood of local recurrence, provides less interference with future diagnostic or therapeutic use of radioactive iodine, and diminishes the possibility that well-differentiated carcinoma will degenerate into anaplastic carcinoma (446).

In circumstances in which papillary carcinoma is suspected in both lobes, total thyroidectomy appears to be indicated. If an isthmus lesion contains papillary thyroid cancer, a total thyroidectomy usually is recommended. If the cancer to be removed is associated with a multinodular gland, a near-total or total thyroidectomy should be performed. In any cancer, it is important to remove all gross disease, as cutting through tumor increases the chance of tumor recurrence and shortens survival (46).

In follicular carcinoma, there is a direct correlation between the degree of vascular invasion and death. When vascular invasion is minimal, 3% die from the tumor; when invasion is moderate to severe, 52% die (142). This finding perhaps should be a major factor in deciding how much surgery should be done—that is, those lesions that demonstrate substantial invasiveness should be managed with a total thyroidectomy. A partial thyroidectomy, consisting of either a lobe and isthmus or a near-total procedure, is recommended by some for lesions characterized by minimal invasiveness, although we prefer that a near-total thyroidectomy be performed as this will allow more reliable follow-up evaluations. Whether the employment of more extensive thyroidectomy directly correlates with a reduction in death rates is somewhat uncertain, however. A preoperative FNA result that is interpreted as follicular neoplasm requires further action. Assuming it represents an adequate sample read by an experienced cytologist, it is customary to recommend surgery. The likelihood of this lesion showing cancer (usually follicular cancer or follicular variant of papillary cancer) on final histologic examination after surgery is approximately 15% to 30%. The type of surgery to recommend with a preoperative diagnosis of follicular neoplasm depends on many factors, including the experience of the surgeon and the wishes of the patient. On the one hand, if a lobectomy and isthmusectomy is performed, and the final histologic diagnosis is cancer, then a completion thyroidectomy is required within 7 to 10 days. On the other hand, if an initial near-total thyroidectomy is performed, the potential risk for hypocalcemia and hoarseness is somewhat higher than if a lobectomy/isthmusectomy is performed initially. Also, as noted, the chance of the lesion harboring cancer is relatively low. There is no single correct answer to this dilemma, except that a mutual decision should be made between the health care team and the patient. In the customary case, we tend to prefer an initial near-total thyroidectomy. This approach also simplifies the longer-term issue as to whether the patient should be taking exogenous L-thyroxine and decreases the likelihood that any remaining tissue will regrow and represent a potential problem in the future.

PRACTICE GUIDELINES FOR MEDULLARY THYROID CANCER: SUGGESTED DIAGNOSTIC EVALUATION

Clinical Evaluation

COMPLETE HISTORY AND PHYSICAL EXAMINATION

The history should document the presence or absence and duration of symptoms referable to hypercalcitonemia (diarrhea and flushing), pheochromocytoma (headache, palpitations/tachycardia, hypertension, diaphoresis, nausea/vomiting, tremulousness/ anxiety), or hyperparathyroidism (renal stones, bone abnormalities), as well as the presence or absence of hoarseness, dysphagia, and stridor. The history should also indicate if there is a family history of non-MEN medullary carcinoma (FMTC), MEN-IIA or -IIB. History of previous or current mucosal neuromata of the oral cavity or gastrointestinal tract should be noted.

COMPLETE HEAD AND NECK EXAMINATION

A complete head and neck examination consists of inspection and palpation of the head and neck; the presence or absence of neuromata of the tongue, thickened lips, or marfanoid facies should be documented. Attention should focus on the characteristics of the palpable thyroid mass, such as the size, consistency, number, and fixation to trachea or larynx. Extrathyroidal extension to involve soft tissues in the central compartment of the neck or the skin should also be documented. The larynx should be visualized and vocal cord function documented.

If enlarged nodes are present, their location (group or level I to VI), number, size, mobility, relationship to adjacent structures, and staging should be documented.

Imaging Studies

CHEST RADIOGRAPH

A chest radiograph should be done to evaluate for metastatic disease.

COMPUTED TOMOGRAPHY SCAN WITH CONTRAST OR MAGNETIC RESONANCE IMAGING

Computed tomography scan of the neck with contrast or MRI is indicated when there is suspicion of tumor extending into the larynx or trachea or into the mediastinum. Magnetic resonance imaging is preferable if well-differentiated thyroid neoplasm remains in the differential at this point (the iodine contrast used for CT scanning may delay postoperative radioactive iodine therapy). An MRI scan is particularly helpful for retrosternal tumors and to evaluate for enlarged mediastinal lymph nodes. If there is evidence of cervical lymph nodes containing medullary thyroid cancer, chest and abdominal CT (or MRI) are useful to help stage this disease and to identify pulmonary and hepatic lesions. A bone scan may also be useful and is especially indicated if there are known metastases outside the thyroid area. A PET scan is also very helpful and should be used for staging the disease and assessing progression in cases where there are known extrathyroidal metastases. Additional radiologic studies such as octreotide scans may be helpful in selected circumstances.

Laboratory Tests

Laboratory tests should include the assessment of the following:

- Serum calcitonin and CEA levels
- Serum calcium (if elevated, obtain PTH level)
- CBC and comprehensive metabolic profile, including liver function tests and alkaline phosphatase levels
- TSH
- 24-hour urine catecholamine (especially if there are symptoms suspicious for pheochromocytoma or if there is known FMTC); some clinicians will also measure plasma metanephrine/normetanephrine

Preoperative laboratory tests should also be performed as indicated by personal experience and institutional guidelines.

Consultations Recommended Before Surgery

- Endocrinology consult
- Anesthesia (if pheochromocytoma previously resected or present workup equivocal)
- General surgery (if pheochromocytoma present)
- Otolaryngology consultation, especially if there are vocal cord issues
- Internal medicine if there are additional complicating medical problems

BIOPSY

If sporadic medullary thyroid carcinoma (MTC) is suspected from elevated calcitonin levels alone, a thyroid FNA is still important, depending on clinical presentation (increased calcitonin levels are present occasionally in other malignancies, bone disorders, renal failure, hemorrhagic disorders, or thyroiditis). Recent studies indicate that calcitonin elevations can occur in a wide variety of benign thyroid conditions, and, furthermore, that an FNA is more accurate in suggesting medullary thyroid cancer than is a serum calcitonin. An FNA of the thyroid is not necessary when there is a known familial *ret* gene mutation.

TREATMENT

Primary Tumor

Treatment of primary tumors include surgery (total thyroidectomy recommended in all cases). Radiation and chemotherapy are not indicated as primary treatment.

Neck

- Surgery
- N0: Medial compartment neck dissection should be performed in all cases; it includes lymph nodes from the level of the hyoid bone to the innominate vein and from one carotid sheath to the other. In addition, all cases merit intraoperative palpation of the jugular nodes and neck dissection if palpable nodes are present.
- N+: In cases with clinical or radiologic suspicion of nodal metastases, a neck dissection should be performed that includes levels II to V and may preserve uninvolved structures (e.g., spinal accessory nerve). It should be recognized during the course of neck treatment that no effective adjunctive treatment has been established for medullary carcinoma.
- Chemotherapy may be employed in selected circumstances when there is known metastatic disease that is progressive.
- External radiation therapy may be useful in the control of focal metastatic lesions (e.g., osseous) and may be used following surgery in selected patients with extensive cervical disease remaining after surgery.

Other

Multiple endocrine neoplasia (MEN-IIA) parathyroid hyperplasia occurs in approximately 30%, and subtotal parathyroidectomy or total parathyroidectomy and autotransplantation should be considered at the time of the primary operation to avoid the potential risk for recurrent laryngeal nerve injury in reoperation of the central compartment. Cryopreservation of one or more removed parathyroid glands may be considered for later reimplantation should hypoparathyroidism result from the initial surgery. The goal of surgery is to avoid impinging any of the parathyroid glands, and autotransplantation or cryopreservation should be used only as needed.

ADJUVANT TREATMENT

Before Surgery

Pheochromocytoma discovered during preoperative workup should be resected before treatment of MTC.

After Surgery

Extracapsular extension of tumor has been associated with poor prognosis in MTC. There is information in the literature suggesting that radiation therapy may be beneficial in patients with multiple, large nodal metastases with extracapsular extension. It may also be beneficial when there is gross or microscopic residual tumor. The usual dose range is 50 to 70 Gy in 1.8- to 2.0-Gy fractions given in 5 to 8 weeks, supplemented by a brachytherapy boost if indicated by pathologic findings.

FOLLOW-UP

The follow-up schedule depends on the patient's clinical course and individual risk for recurrence. In general it is as follows: every 3 to 6 months for 3 years, thereafter every 6 to 12 months for up to 10 years, and then once a year for life. These guidelines are arbitrary and should be modified as needed with an individual case, and they assume that there is no evidence of recurrent or persistent disease. As noted previously, it is mandatory that a *ret* oncogene be measured in all patients with medullary thyroid cancer.

Follow-up evaluations should include the following:

- Examination of the head and neck area in conjunction with a thorough history and physical examination
- Chest CT every 6 to 12 months
- Neck sonogram (or CT/MRI) every 6 to 12 months
- Serum calcitonin and CEA levels every 6 to 12 months
- Yearly determination of serum calcium levels and urine catecholamine, VMA, and metanephrine levels in patients with familial MTC
- Periodic bone scan and octreotide scan and PET scan as appropriate

FAMILY SCREENING

A sporadic case of MTC may represent the index case of a familial MTC kindred. In fact, about 10% to 15% of the time a patient without a family history of medullary thyroid cancer is the index case for such an entity, and a *ret* oncogene mutation is identified. Bilateral tumors or evidence of C-cell hyperplasia may indicate such a situation. Family history of thyroid surgery, a poorly differentiated carcinoma, or sudden death may also indicate a familial MTC, because of inaccurate diagnoses or the use of older histologic criteria. Available members of familial MTC kindreds should be screened for MTC. For FMTC, MEN-IIA and -IIB assessment of peripheral blood for evidence of *ret* gene mutation should be performed.

In Hürthle cell adenomas, a lobe and isthmus resection seems to be adequate for cure; however, in Hürthle cell carcinomas, a completion thyroidectomy should always be undertaken, no matter how harmless the histologic appearance of the lesion. Many investigators believe this follicular variant is more aggressive than standard follicular carcinoma, and, furthermore, Hürthle cell cancers tend to pick up radioactive iodine less actively than do follicular cancers.

The treatment of thyroid lymphoma is controversial but, as with all lymphomas, any strategy must be preceded by a specific diagnosis, typing, and staging of the disease. It should be pointed out, however, that while the development of a treatment strategy is an admirable goal, many of these patients are elderly, exhibit a poor performance status, or may require urgent therapy to relieve symptoms. Generally, the treatment consists of a combination of external radiation and adjuvant chemotherapy in patients with disseminated (stage III and IV) disease, as well as a surgical procedure in selected circumstances. In localized disease (stage I or II), surgical removal can be considered, but debulking techniques rarely are indicated; instead, radiation and chemotherapy usually are recommended. Patients with bulky local disease generally do not do well with chemotherapy alone. The 5-year survival rate for thyroid lymphoma is 75% or higher when the disease is limited to the thyroid gland, 35% to 40% in patients with extrathyroidal extension, and, impressively, 5% with disseminated disease (237,253).

Selection of the Appropriate Operation for Cervical Metastasis

A substantial percentage of patients with papillary thyroid carcinoma have microscopic metastatic regional adenopathy. In many cases, this component of the tumor is treated effectively by radioactive iodine and thus is never clinically apparent (46,155). The exact incidence of metastasis (both clinically apparent and occult) in papillary cancer, therefore, is unknown. It is known that the overall incidence of cervical metastasis is substantially higher with papillary than with follicular cancers. Cervical metastasis occurs frequently in papillary cancer, but is rarely in follicular. In each variety of differentiated thyroid cancer, the underlying theme of surgical neck management is conservatism. In those patients in whom there is no palpable adenopathy, waiting to remove nodes only after they become palpable does not seem to compromise survival (194,447). The clinically negative neck, therefore, provides the surgeon with several options.

Because occult cervical metastasis is unusual in follicular carcinoma, elective neck dissection of any sort is usually unwarranted. However, this issue is not so clear with papillary cancer, which is characterized by frequent metastasis. Some investigators recommend a prophylactic central compartment clean-out in all patients with papillary lesions (448), whereas others claim that elective neck dissections in this disease have not been shown to be more effective than observation and therapeutic dissection when necessary (194,447). We recommend a compromise between the two extremes, performing a regional dissection to retrieve those nodes at highest risk if the primary tumor is larger than 2 cm in diameter or if it is extrathyroidal. Anatomists disagree about the pattern of early thyroid cancer metastasis, but most surgeons consider the medial compartment nodes to be the primary drainage pathway, separate from the deep jugular nodes, which are part of a secondary drainage system. With larger and less favorable primary lesions, therefore, we recommend a dissection that extends from the hyoid bone to the mediastinum and from one jugular vein to the other. Particular attention is paid to those nodal channels that are embedded within the fatty tissue in the tracheoesophageal groove. Despite a paucity of data demonstrating survival enhancement with this approach, we believe the risks of such a dissection are low and the procedure is appropriate. In smaller and more favorable papillary lesions, we do not recommend an elective neck dissection of any sort. In a small percentage of patients in whom there are matted nodes or extranodal extension of disease, a more extensive neck dissection is necessary to remove cervical metastasis.

In all differentiated thyroid cancer in which there is palpable neck disease, a selective neck dissection, designed to remove the regional nodes involved and those otherwise at risk, is performed. If the metastatic disease is in the anterior or thymic area, a central compartment clean-out should include the tissue from the hyoid bone to the mediastinum and from one internal jugular vein to the other. In this setting, the lateral deep jugular area should be carefully inspected by palpation; however, in the absence of obvious adenopathy, we do not recommend dissecting the deep jugular nodes of levels II, III, IV, or V. If there is palpable disease laterally, a lymphadenectomy should be performed that includes these three levels. In this setting, attention should be paid to those nodes that accompany the inferior thyroid artery into the posterior triangle of the neck, and, when there is palpable disease in that area, the dissection should include level V. The submandibular triangle usually is not included in the dissection, as thyroid cancer rarely metastasizes to this area (154). We have treated two patients with papillary carcinoma in whom there was metastasis to the parapharyngeal space nodes (Fig. 29.6), a presentation that has been reported on one other occasion (144). Because of this, we believe that in the presence of cervical nodal metastasis and in patients with noticeably aggressive disease, imaging (either nuclear or magnetic resonance) should be used to visualize the neck in general, including the base-of-skull area. None of the standard neck operations allows the surgeon to approach this remote area and, if significant adenopathy is visualized here, appropriate techniques for its removal should be employed in addition to standard methods for the remainder of the cervical area.

The description of selective neck dissections should be recorded in the standard nomenclature, which has been jointly developed by the American Society of Head and Neck Surgery and the Society of Head and Neck Surgeons (449). Classifying and reporting in this manner promotes interinstitutional standardization of outcomes research.

In patients with medullary thyroid cancer, regardless of the size of the tumor, the general surgical approach to the neck is more aggressive than in differentiated cancer. This philosophy has evolved largely because the uptake of iodine by medullary cancer is negligible, and radioactive ablation does not play a useful role in the treatment of this disease (294). In addition, medullary carcinoma generally is considered somewhat resistant to conventional radiation therapy and, even though there is some interest in the employment of adjuvant EBRT, most studies fail to show improvement in the survival of patients treated in this fashion (294,450). Postoperative radiation therapy may have value in controlling locoregional disease, but this also remains unproved. With medullary cancer, regardless of size or location and even in circumstances in which the neck is clinically negative, most surgeons recommend an extensive central compartment clean-out. If disease is uncovered in any of the areas dissected, the operation is converted to include levels II through V bilaterally. In most cases, the internal jugular veins, the sternocleidomastoid muscles, and the 11th cranial nerves are spared. The value of nodal dissection in medullary thyroid carcinoma has not been analyzed by designed clinical trials, but retrospective analysis of data on clinically negative necks shows a 10-year survival rate of 67% in those patients treated with neck dissections and 43% in those who were not (363). It is unclear whether survival would be enhanced by more than selective neck dissections, but most surgeons believe that in the clinically negative neck, the more conservative approach probably is as effective as the radical or the modified radical neck dissection (451).

If the neck is clinically positive, on the other hand, a more extensive dissection appears to be indicated. The extent of the operation varies depending on the amount and location of disease, but a modified radical neck dissection is employed in many circumstances. Radical neck dissection is employed when strategically placed bulky disease requires a more extensive extirpation. In medullary carcinoma, adequacy of surgical extirpation is so important that the surgeon should take extraordinary measures to remove gross tumor. A reasonable clean-out of the upper mediastinal nodal groups can usually be achieved by means of a standard cervical approach, but the surgeon should be prepared to use a sternotomy to gain access for mediastinal nodal dissection. In light of the uncertainty of the radiosensitivity of this disorder, such extension of surgery seems indicated. Sternotomy and mediastinal nodal clean-out might be justified in all medullary carcinomas in which there is associated cervical nodal metastasis.

Extended Surgery for Extraordinary Circumstances

In both differentiated and medullary carcinoma, a vigorous attempt should be made to remove all gross tumor. The thoroughness of the removal is undoubtedly less important in differentiated cancer, as that disease generally is less lethal and often radioresponsive.

Fixation to the thyroid cartilage or trachea (or both) can require partial- or full-thickness removal of those skeletal structures. Removal of one thyroid cartilage lamina does not create major morbidity, especially if the internal thyroid perichondrium is left intact. The trachea can be partially resected and repaired as part of the *en bloc* tissue removal, or it can be shaved, leaving the internal mucosa intact. When mucosa is left intact, the overlying skeletal defect is reinforced by moving adjacent soft tissues. Isolated full-thickness tracheal wall defects can be repaired with a composite mucosal-cartilage composite graft harvested from the nasal septum. With more extensive tracheal involvement, a segment of up to four rings can be removed and closed with primary anastomosis (452). In those patients with skeletal invasion in whom partial laryngectomy techniques are employed, a significant percentage demonstrate survival benefit (152,453–455).

In differentiated cancer management, rarely is it necessary to sacrifice the recurrent laryngeal nerve. If engulfed or involved with tumor, this important structure should be dissected free whenever possible. Leaving gross disease on the nerve is acceptable in differentiated thyroid cancer. This is not true, however, with medullary cancer, in which the surgeon should consider sacrificing the nerve, especially if doing so is necessary to achieve gross tumor removal. Obviously, the decision must be reevaluated if the tumor left on the nerve is but one of several areas where gross tumor remains. In this situation, to remove a nerve probably is ill-advised.

With differentiated thyroid cancer, total laryngectomy should be used only in the most extreme circumstances of extensive intraluminal invasion (152,456). Most often, some form of partial laryngectomy is possible (457,458). When it is not, we recommend partial tumor removal followed by postoperative EBRT or radioactive iodine (459–461). If this approach fails, one usually can remove the larynx later. With medullary cancer, the uncertainty of radioresponsiveness dictates a more aggressive surgical posture—that is, the indications for laryngectomy are more liberal.

Local invasion of thyroid cancer into the pharyngeal or esophageal wall usually is managed by resection of the immediate area and generally does not require major organ removal. However, segments of the esophagus can be removed and repaired by means of free jejunal transfer.

Surgical Management of Residual Disease in Medullary Thyroid Cancer

Serum calcitonin provides a reliable marker for medullary thyroid carcinoma, and the presence of residual disease can often be judged after surgery. Normalization of the calcitonin value is the standard for documenting complete eradication of this cancer, along with absence of disease using radiologic techniques. In patients with a calcitonin level of less than 10 pg/mL there seems to be a high cure rate. On the other hand, if the calcitonin is 10 pg/mL residual disease is likely. Overall, the rate of persistent hypercalcitoninemia is nearly 50% for patients with nonpalpable microscopic disease and greater than 80% for patients presenting with a palpable tumor (462). This high frequency of persistent hypercalcemia often is due to micrometastasis in regional lymph nodes, and many of these patients fail to demonstrate abnormalities on either imaging or physical examination. Other sites of tumor persistence cause hypercalcitonemia. Liver, lung, and hilar and mediastinal nodes are all sites of potential involvement. In the absence of clinical disease, persistent hypercalcemia presents a troublesome dilemma to the diagnostician. The value of surgical reexploration in the absence of obvious disease is somewhat unclear, but several noted investigators have reported data that would seem to justify a thorough surgical clean-out of the neck or mediastinum. Tisell et al. (463) advocate a "microdissection" technique in patients with residual calcitonin elevation after primary surgery and have been successful in normalizing their levels in 10% to 20% of patients. Moley et al. (464) have reported similar results with reexploration and clean-out of the cervical tissues. There is some controversy regarding this methodology, as others have failed to justify reoperation to normalize calcitonin levels (282). Considerable study that includes long-term follow-up is necessary before the exact value of this prophylactic surgical approach is defined. Until then, our philosophy remains as follows: If a total thyroid removal was accomplished and a thorough central compartment clean-out failed to reveal histologic medullary cancer in cervical nodes, we see little benefit to reoperating on the neck, despite persistence of abnormal calcitonin levels. This assumes, of course, that a thorough radiologic examination was performed (e.g., neck sonogram or MRI, chest CT, perhaps PET scan and octreotide scan) and no specific evidence of disease was identified. On the other hand, if only a thyroidectomy was performed, persistent elevation of calcitonin might well be secondary to histologic neck disease. In this setting, the neck should be dissected to include levels II through V. Before reoperation for medullary carcinoma, a search should be made for possible widespread metastasis to lung or abdomen (liver). Such images as chest and abdominal CT and MRI of the neck (and possibly PET scan) might well reveal disease that would alter the surgical approach.

Treatment Strategy for Anaplastic Carcinoma

Treatment results for anaplastic carcinoma are discouraging. Despite the employment of various aggressive treatment strategies that consist of surgery, radiation therapy, chemotherapy, or combinations of the three, almost all patients with this disease die a cancer-related death. Pathologically, even a single focus of poorly differentiated or undifferentiated thyroid cancer in a background of well-differentiated cancer is believed to carry a prognosis similar to that of anaplastic cancer. The median survival of anaplastic thyroid cancer is 2 to 6 months, and only a few patients have survived for more than 12 months (88,89,189). Clinical investigations and medical trials (Taxol) for this malignancy continue, but to date have not shown sufficiently promising results that they are employed in routine clinical care.

Regarding specific strategies, various combinations of drugs, radiation, and surgery seem to affect local and distant disease somewhat differently, though inevitably with similar outcomes. The most effective single cytotoxic drug is doxorubicin, and, in some patients, this in combination with cisplatin has yielded a favorable response (465). A combination of doxorubicin and hyperfractionated radiation therapy also has been reported (262), and other trials have employed this approach with surgery added (466). Other investigators have employed a combination of doxorubicin, cisplatin, and radiation therapy (264). Multimodal strategies consisting of hyperfractionated radiation therapy, bleomycin, cyclophosphamide, 5-fluorouracilamide, and surgery have yielded variable responses, although accompanied by substantial toxicity (467). Finally, a Swedish trial has shown that certain radiation therapy fractionation alterations have yielded encouraging responses when combined with doxorubicin and surgery (466).

This generally discouraging picture should dictate a practical approach that recognizes that many strategies yield some responsiveness at the primary site, but virtually none do so distantly. Treatment of this disease should be started, therefore, as soon as possible, before distant metastases appear. Even a small histologic focus of anaplastic cancer in a larger tumor should still be approached as anaplastic cancer. If the larger tumor is a differentiated thyroid cancer, the clinician can decide whether ^{131}I therapy may be useful, although attention to the differentiated thyroid cancer (e.g., ^{131}I scan and treatment) should not delay expeditious treatment for the anaplastic cancer. In anaplastic cancer, an inexorable and relentless course toward death is impressive in most cases and, even when distant metastases are obvious, treatment approaches must take into consideration the quality of death to be expected with a massive and invasive cancer that engulfs and encroaches on the airway. When and how to establish a palliative airway, the employment of debulking surgery, and even the deliverance of radiation therapeutic or chemotherapeutic plans all become issues of judgment that should be developed by a thoughtful dialogue between the various oncologic disciplines, as well as with the patient and family.

Treatment Strategy for Thyroid Cancer in Children

Over the last 30 years, the incidence of radiation-associated thyroid carcinoma in childhood has decreased because indiscriminate radiation therapy for benign conditions in infancy and early childhood has ceased. Actually, less than 10% of differentiated thyroid carcinomas occur in patients younger than 20 years (468). Even though children and adolescents commonly present with more advanced disease than do their older counterparts, the prognosis in the young group is generally surprisingly good. With appropriate treatment, the 15- to 20-year survival rate in children and adolescents with papillary carcinoma approaches 90% (469). Even with distant metastases, children respond well to therapy. Actually, the incidence of metastasis at the time of presentation is significant. In one study, 84% had lymph node metastases and 12% had pulmonary metastases (470), and in another study the incidence was 88% and 19%, respectively (471).

Primary management of thyroid cancer in children is surgical, with a near-total or total thyroidectomy being recommended (472). Following surgery, assuming there is a papillary thyroid cancer greater than 1 cm, three or more foci less than 1 cm, follicular cancer or evidence of disease outside the thyroid gland, ^{131}I therapy is usually given. The dose in children has not been studied extensively, but some thyroidologists typically give approximately 100 mCi ^{131}I. If, however, there was relatively minimal disease of papillary thyroid cancer confined to the thyroid gland, we would consider an ablative dose of 29 mCi ^{131}I. In any case, it is important to perform periodic ^{131}I scans to ensure there is no residual activity, in conjunction with periodic serum free T_4, TSH, and thyroglobulin measurements and radiologic studies, such as thyroid sonograms (206,207,220,473,474). After surgery, routine suppression of TSH below the low-normal range should be accomplished (470,475), although this has the possibility of enhancing bone loss. The goal of TSH varies but depends to a large extent on the aggressiveness of the disease and the length of time since surgery. Sufficient L-thyroxine to suppress TSH to less than 0.01 μU/mL is the goal with active or aggressive disease, whereas a goal TSH of 0.1 μU/mL can be used if the disease is less aggressive or if several years have passed since treatment without evidence of disease. The clinician should work closely with the pediatrician and the family to enhance optimal care of the patient's thyroid condition as well as to monitor normal growth and development. Interaction with the family and child is extremely important as numerous issues should be discussed over time, including future fertility, risks of treatment modalities, and the prognosis of the thyroid cancer. This treatment strategy appears to yield excellent results (475,476).

Treatment Strategies for Thyroid Nodularity During Pregnancy

Maternal thyroid gland alteration is significant during pregnancy, with glandular volume increasing even with maternal iodine-sufficient diets. With even a mildly iodine-deficient diet (which has been found to be common in pregnant U.S. women), however, the thyroid gland enlarges substantially, presumably in response to serum thyrotropin elevation. The ability of TSH and, presumably, other thyroid stimulators to promote thyroid growth is potentiated by iodine deficiency. Any palpable thyroid enlargement is considered abnormal for a normal pregnant woman, and if a discrete nodule is present, an FNA and cytologic evaluation should be performed. Should these studies suggest malignancy, the decision to operate should be individualized according to the type of tumor, the growth pattern of the mass, and the timing of the expected birth. To operate during the early stages of a pregnancy is to assume responsibility for the health and well-being of the fetus during a very vulnerable developmental period. The impact of anesthetic agents and other medications on the fetus is never to be underrated, and the earlier the fetal age, the greater is the potential adverse impact. The timing of surgical intervention is a provocative issue that tests to the fullest the capacity for interdisciplinary dialogue and concert among surgeon, endocrinologist, obstetrician, and pediatrician, and fundamental ethical responsibilities to the unborn child must form the matrix among these specialties. Within this context, our general guidelines follow. If the thyroid FNA shows papillary thyroid cancer, we would recommend that a thyroidectomy be performed in the middle trimester of pregnancy. Whether a near-total thyroidectomy should be performed or whether a lobectomy should first be performed, with a completion thyroidectomy being performed after delivery, is a decision that must be made by the patient and the health care team. Serum thyroglobulin, if markedly elevated, as well a thyroid sonogram to identify the size of the nodule and the possibility of bilateral disease (which could be aspirated under ultrasound guidance if needed) and the entire clinical context form the basis for deciding which surgical procedure should be performed. Significant postoperative hypocalcemia requiring large doses of calcium and vitamin D should be avoided in pregnant women, because of the potential effects on the fetus. If the papillary thyroid cancer is identified in the last trimester of pregnancy, it might be preferable to delay surgery until after delivery, although all of the associated information must be considered.

More difficult is the situation in which the FNA is suspicious, but not diagnostic, for follicular neoplasm (or follicular variant of papillary thyroid cancer). Again, consideration of the entire context including a thyroid sonogram is important, as is interaction of the health care team and the patient and her family. It is difficult to even give general guidelines without knowing the information relating to each case as well as the experience of the surgeon. However, if the thyroid nodule is relatively large (>3 to 4 cm) and the aspiration has been read by one, or better yet two, experienced cytologists, then consideration of a lobectomy and isthmusectomy during the second trimester can be entertained. If the lesion is smaller than 3 to 4 cm, it still may be a follicular carcinoma (or follicular variant of papillary cancer) about 10% to 20% of the time, and it would be desirable to extirpate this lesion as soon as possible, and consideration would be given for also performing a lobectomy and isthmusectomy during the second trimester of pregnancy. If the final histology is positive, a decision can be made whether to perform the completion thyroidectomy during or after the pregnancy. If the decision was made to follow a thyroid nodule during pregnancy (e.g., benign aspiration, cooperative decision by patient and physicians to follow a nodule with a suspicious aspiration), then it is important to palpate the nodule and perform a thyroid sonogram periodically to ensure the nodule is not changing its character or growing. Parenthetically, a patient who is taking L-thyroxine during pregnancy for hypothyroidism frequently has marked changes in thyroid hormone metabolism and, therefore, dose requirements throughout pregnancy. Exogenous L-thyroxine should be taken in the morning by itself and not with other mediations, especially iron or calcium that are known to inhibit L-thyroxine absorption. Further, serum T_4, total T_3, and TSH should be measured frequently in a patient taking exogenous L-thyroxine for hypothyroidism, perhaps as often as monthly, with adjustment of the L-thyroxine dose as needed and with consideration of the increasing requirements in many patients as the pregnancy progresses.

Thyroid Hormone Suppression Therapy

Thyroid hormone is necessary to replace the function of the thyroid gland that is lost as a result of surgery or radioactive iodine use and also to suppress TSH levels. The notion that TSH stimulates the growth of thyroid carcinoma forms the basis for the manipulation of this hormone (477,478). Like normal thyroid tissue, most differentiated thyroid carcinomas contain functional TSH receptors, which are more abundant in follicular than in papillary carcinoma (479). TSH has been shown to stimulate thyroid cancer cell growth *in vitro*, to stimulate radioactive iodine uptake into tumor cells *in vivo*, and to enhance thyroglobulin secretion by tumor cells (197,480). Patients with papillary carcinoma who receive suppressive doses of T_4 seem to experience a lower recurrence rate and improved survival (155,197,471). In patients with follicular cancer, the benefits of suppression of thyroid hormone are more controversial, but the evidence seems to demonstrate significant decreases in recurrence and mortality in the suppressed group (481,482).

Levothyroxine, the synthetic form of T_4, provides stable levels of T_4 as well as T_3, which is the product of peripheral conversion of T_4. The therapeutic goal is to achieve high-normal levels of T_4 and to suppress TSH to below-normal levels. Essentially, this creates a state of subclinical thyrotoxicosis. In a small percentage of these patients, an increase in myocardial mass with subsequent diastolic dysfunction can result from this hypermetabolic state (483). One other consequence of these metabolic alterations may be osteoporosis, which may even occur in children (484). However, the main risk for osteoporosis resulting from this treatment is in high-risk groups such as postmenopausal women (477,483). All patients undergoing TSH suppression require regular monitoring of their thyroid hormone and TSH levels to ensure proper dosing, and that monitoring should be more intense in the patients at higher risk for cardiovascular problems and osteoporosis. Changes in estrogen level, liver function, and a number of medications may require thyroid hormone dose adjustment. L-thyroxine should be taken by itself and no other medication should be taken within at least 2 hours, if possible. Calcium, iron, sucralfate and cholestyramine each inhibit L-thyroxine absorption. The addition of estrogen therapy to women already taking L-thyroxine will also alter the L-thyroxine dose requirements.

RADIOLABELED IODINE IN THE MANAGEMENT OF THYROID CANCER

Body Scanning

Whole-body scans using ^{131}I help stage the cancer and determine the need and potential usefulness of radioactive iodine therapy. Iodine is transported actively into thyroid cells via mainly the now characterized sodium-iodide symporter, and the unused or unrecycled iodine is excreted by the kidneys. Its uptake by thyroid cells provides a means of staging functional cancer and targeted therapy. Because of equilibration, the 24-hour urine iodide excretion (or a single spot sample expressed as microgram per day) provides a reasonable estimate of the iodine intake or exposure. Even when functional, however, malignant thyroid cells are significantly less active than normal thyroid tissue, taking up 0.04% to 0.6% of the dose per gram of tumor tissue (485). Therefore, the volume of thyroid tissue competing for the iodine is critical to the ability of the tumor cells to incorporate the isotope.

An elevated TSH level is essential to enhance the uptake of the isotope into thyroid cancer cells. This hormone is the anterior pituitary product that stimulates thyroid hormone synthesis and secretion. In addition, it is the primary regulator of iodine uptake into thyroid tissue. A TSH level of 30 mIU/mL or greater is considered optimal to stimulate adequately radioactive iodine absorption into malignant thyroid cells (486). It is unknown if a higher TSH level of perhaps 100 μU/mL is associated with greater tissue radioiodine uptake than a TSH level of, for example, 30 μU/mL. To stimulate endogenous TSH, circulating thyroid hormone levels must decrease. After total or near-total thyroidectomy, the TSH level usually rises to a maximum level in 4 to 6 weeks (487). In those who have been on thyroid hormone suppression therapy, 6 weeks off of T_4 usually is required to achieve the appropriate level of TSH. The symptoms and signs of prolonged hypothyroidism can be very unpleasant and, in an effort to minimize the impact of thyroid hormone withdrawal, Cytomel (T_3), which has a shorter half-life than T_4 (about 24 hours for T_3 as compared with 7 days for T_4), can be given to the patient during the first 4 weeks of abstinence from thyroxine, and then the Cytomel is stopped about 2 weeks prior to the scan. The duration of the period of TSH elevation should be minimized owing to possible stimulation of residual cancer growth, and because of the symptoms of hypothyroidism the patient develops. On the other hand, the TSH must be sufficiently high to perform an optimal scan. This compromise is generally met with the schedule noted above. Two to three days prior to the isotope scan, we insist on measuring serum TSH, thyroglobulin, the complete blood count (CBC), and comprehensive metabolic profile, as well as β–human chorionic gonadotropin (β-hCG) for all female patients who are capable of becoming pregnant.

Hypothyroidism, especially in elderly or medical ill patients, may result in a variety of abnormalities, including hyponatremia; we also like an assessment of the CBC as an abnormal result may change our treatment plan with ^{131}I. It is extremely important to take an appropriate history and to document a negative β-hCG immediately prior to administering isotope to a woman of child-bearing potential. The use of isotopes and the relevant medical implication should be discussed with the patient as soon as it is clear she will be receiving isotopes in the future. We also routinely place our patients on a low-iodine diet for the last 2 weeks prior to a scan and then measure urine iodine (either 24-hour urine or spot sample) directly before the isotope scan. It is important to take an adequate history to determine if a patient has been exposed to radiopaque dyes that could interfere with the isotope scan and treatment, but, in addition, we believe it is important to actually document relative iodine deficiency in the patient prior to the isotope scan and treatment. The precise iodine concentration needed is not known, but a goal value is less than 200 to 300 μg/day or μg/L, and if the value is greater than 700 to 1000 μg/day or μg/L, consideration is given to delaying the scan and the treatment. In theory, the higher the urine iodine, the greater the iodine stores in the patient and the less effective the administered radioiodine would be.

Considerable effort has been devoted to shortening or eliminating the prolonged postthyroidectomy time spent waiting for the TSH level to rise. Exogenous administration of bovine TSH had been tried, but it stimulates an immunologic response and antibody formation (488). Furthermore, bovine TSH is less effective than endogenous human TSH in stimulating cancer cells to incorporate radioactive iodine (489).

Within the last several years, recombinant human TSH (rhTSH) has been available. Published studies indicate that the use of rhTSH to stimulate TSH uptake and effect an optimal scan is almost equivalent to a scan performed with the customary L-thyroxine withdrawal method detailed above. In fact, when a patient is subjected to a withdrawal scan and measurement of serum thyroglobulin level and these results are compared in the same patient to a scan and thyroglobulin level performed following rhTSH, the ability to detect residual uptake or disease is almost equal. Since its approval by the Food and Drug Administration (FDA), rhTSH has been used widely and its major advantage is that patients can continue their L-thyroxine therapy and avoid the consequences of hypothyroidism. rhTSH is presently approved only for the performance of diagnostic scans, not for treatment. We routinely place the patient on a low-iodine diet for 2 weeks prior to the test. We perform the tests as follows: On Monday, labs are drawn for CBC, comprehensive metabolic profile, TSH, β-hCG (in women of childbearing potential), and thyroglobulin level. Once it is clear the β-hCG is negative, then they receive an intramuscular injection of 0.9 mg rhTSH. On Tuesday, 0.9 mg rhTSH is administered. On Wednesday, the serum TSH is measured, and 4 mCi ^{131}I given orally. On Friday, serum thyroglobulin is measured and the patient undergoes an isotope scan. The rhTSH-stimulated thyroglobulin level should remain less than 1 ng/mL in a patient without evidence of recurrent or persistent disease. If the serum thyroglobulin level rises to greater than 2 ng/mL or if the isotope scan shows uptake, then the patient is considered to have possible remnant tissue or disease, and typically a withdrawal scan is then performed (at least 6 weeks later) and treatment with ^{131}I can be accomplished immediately after that, if required.

Consideration of when to perform an rhTSH scan as compared with a more standard withdrawal scan has been the subject of considerable discussion. Because rhTSH is not approved for use in conjunction with ^{131}I treatment, we have generally been performing standard withdrawal scans in patients who are having their first scan after surgery as well as in patients who were treated a year previously and are undergoing their first post-treatment scan. The reason for the latter category is that we would like to compare the same scan technique and equivalent thyroglobulin levels to ensure there is no evidence or recurrent or residual disease. In addition, if any patient with differentiated thyroid cancer is likely to have residual or recurrent disease or has had aggressive thyroid cancer, we tend to perform a standard withdrawal scan. On the other hand, in patients who have had a negative withdrawal scan 1 year after treatment and have a low likelihood of disease remaining, we tend to perform an rhTSH-stimulated scan. We have been impressed that withdrawal from thyroid hormones can be quite debilitating for many elderly patients or those with significant medical illnesses, and we would prefer to perform an rhTSH-stimulated scan to avoid hypothyroidism if possible. If it is likely a patient will require treatment with ^{131}I, we still perform a withdrawal scan. We believe these guidelines will change over time as more experience with rhTSH scans is obtained. There are several clinical protocols being performed that are assessing the utility of rhTSH in the treatment of patients with ^{131}I, although, as noted, the FDA has not approved this use to date.

The issue of "stunning" should also be discussed. "Stunning" refers to decreased radioisotope trapping, and presumably effectiveness in destroying tissue, if a patient had been recently exposed to a so-called scanning dose of ^{131}I. That is, a scanning dose of 2 to 10 mCi ^{131}I not only may allow scanning and visualization of tissue, but also may actually destroy the tissue to some extent, and perhaps decrease the ability of the cells to trap a subsequent therapeutic dose of ^{131}I, rendering it less effective. The issue of stunning and its clinical importance is hotly debated, and we believe that if it exists it plays a minor clinical role. If stunning has clinical significance, it seems most relevant with higher scanning doses (e.g., 10 mCi vs. 2 mCi ^{131}I) and when the timing between the diagnostic scan and the treatment is delayed for several weeks or months. In practice, most endocrinologists perform a diagnostic scan and then treat with ^{131}I within a week, decreasing the possible importance of stunning as a relevant phenomenon.

If an rhTSH-stimulated scan is performed and then it is noted that a withdrawal scan and treatment must proceed, this time interval is at least 6 weeks, and theoretically stunning could be more relevant. Some clinics are now assessing the utility of ^{123}I for scans rather than ^{131}I because the radiation damage of ^{123}I is negligible and it could not cause stunning. It is not yet known if scans obtained with ^{123}I are as effective in detecting residual tissue as scans performed with ^{131}I, and further work in this area is warranted.

Thus far, no major side effects have been encountered from multiple injections of this genetically engineered product (490,491), but some patients note malaise for several hours after the injection. To date, no patient has developed TSH antibodies, which would be a major problem as it would make measurement of serum TSH problematic. A TSH elevation related to a withdrawal scan or the administration of rhTSH might cause metastatic lesions to enlarge and cause local problems. The presence of cerebral metastases in particular might enlarge with TSH elevation and this can cause neurologic signs and symptoms. Neurologic consultation and perhaps consideration of external radiation and steroids may decrease this likelihood. Similarly, osseous metastases that are impinging on the spinal canal can increase after TSH elevations. It is unknown if rhTSH or withdrawal scans are associated with a greater chance of lesional change.

Using a standard withdrawal technique, a whole-body scan can be performed once the patient's TSH level is elevated to more than 30 μU/mL (492), and the total-body iodine pool should be as low as possible (493). Radioactive iodine uptake at the time of scan or therapy is enhanced by a low-iodine diet prior to administration of the isotope (494–496). A dose of 2 to 10 mCi of ^{131}I is administered and, 48 to 72 hours later, scans of the patient are obtained to determine the level of uptake in the neck, chest, and other regions of the body. If there is a need for ^{131}I treatment, those patients who have significant residual normal thyroid tissue after surgery require either completion thyroidectomy or ^{131}I ablation therapy. Radioisotope scans can have false-positive as well as false-negative results, and scan results must be considered in the entire clinical context and in conjunction with relevant radiologic studies. False-positive uptake commonly can occur in the salivary glands or sinuses as well as in the thymus. Rarer causes include ascites, pulmonary effusion, bronchial duplication cysts, and even artificial eyeballs. Isotope contamination of clothes and residual isotope in the bladder or bowel must be excluded. In many instances, repeating the scan in 1 to 2 days helps to rule out some of these causes, whereas other sources of false-positive studies still may be present. Healthy skepticism must be maintained when examining an isotope scan, especially if the existing clinical, laboratory, and radiologic data are not consonant.

Routine remnant thyroid gland radio ablation is questioned by some investigators (497,498), but is used widely and has considerable appeal (499,500). The dose for ablation varies according to the volume of residual tissue present, but up to 87% of patients can be successfully ablated with ^{131}I after subtotal thyroidectomy (497). Whether achieved by surgery or by radioisotope, elimination of residual thyroid gland confers the advantages of possibly treating multifocal lesions, allowing visualization of distant or local metastatic disease on follow-up scans (501), allowing the rise in TSH (502), and improving the specificity of monitored serum thyroglobulin as a means of detecting cancer growth (503,504). Whether ^{131}I that is administered for ablation of the thyroid remnant actually lowers recurrence rates and improves survival is somewhat controversial; some studies have found that it does, whereas others have failed to corroborate such findings (187,479,505). Whether ^{131}I ablation should be performed with 29 mCi or a larger dose in the range of 150 mCi also is somewhat controversial and depends on the individual case. In general, we prefer to treat with 100 to 150 mCi ^{131}I as this reliably ablates any subsequent uptake on scan in patients with remaining thyroid remnants and there is no evidence that this dose is more harmful than a lower dose of 29 mCi ^{131}I. But 29 mCi ablates the remaining residual tissue only 30% to 50% of the time, and when the patient is scanned a year later there frequently is neck bed uptake with a mildly elevated thyroglobulin level.

We strongly encourage performing an isotope scan prior to treatment even in patients who are going to receive a therapeutic ^{131}I dose, for instance, patients who had a recent thyroidectomy for differentiated thyroid cancer and are going to receive ^{131}I therapy. Our rationale for performing a scan prior to treatment includes the following factors: (a) A diagnostic scan gives a strong indication that there is not exogenous iodine contamination (we also measure urine iodine). A patient may have received radiopaque dyes or may be taking health food supplements (e.g., kelp) and may have failed to mention it to the physician. If such a patient were treated, there would be no uptake after receiving ^{131}I therapy, and the treatment would, in effect, expose the patient to isotope needlessly. (b) A diagnostic scan can be compared with future diagnostic scans to assess progression of disease. It is not possible to accurately compare a posttherapy scan (which we always obtain about 7 days following therapy) to any future diagnostic scans because of the amount of isotope received and the greater number of lesions detected by the larger dose. (c) A diagnostic scan might show disease activity that would require further evaluation prior to receiving ^{131}I therapy. For example, a diagnostic scan may show unanticipated uptake in the chest, bones, or brain. If this were noted, further analysis with radiologic studies (e.g., MRI) and perhaps biopsy might be needed. ^{131}I therapy can cause edema and expansion of metastatic lesions. An osseous lesion in the cervical spine, for example, would require attention prior to ^{131}I therapy, as would a cerebral metastases, which might also require steroid administration at the time of ^{131}I therapy. Taken together, these explanations support the utility of a pretreatment diagnostic isotope scan even if a patient is definitely going to receive a therapeutic dose.

Treatment

Radiolabeled ^{131}I is a highly effective, targeted method of treating differentiated thyroid cancer. It has been used for more than 50 years, both to ablate residual normal thyroid tissue and to treat the cancer. This isotope is transported actively into normal and differentiated thyroid cancer cells, thus creating subsequent destruction with little radiation exposure to adjacent tissues. The beta particles emitted by ^{131}I penetrate and destroy tissue within a 2-mm zone (506). The destructive effect of the isotope depends on the tumor's capacity to concentrate iodine. Even after meticulous preparation, a number of thyroid cancers fail to concentrate radioactive iodine in amounts sufficient for therapy. In the differentiated cancer group, nonfunction is still rare but appears more common in patients older than 40 years and in those with Hürthle cell tumors. Medullary carcinomas and anaplastic cancers do not concentrate radioactive iodine (507). At present, clinically, there are no techniques available to enhance iodine uptake other than ensuring the urine iodine is low and the patient has a sufficiently elevated TSH level.

Isotopes have gained wide utility because differentiated tumors can be infiltrative, locally invasive, and associated with occult regional lymph node metastases. Specifically, the use of ^{131}I has been shown to improve survival, decrease recurrences, and prolong disease-free survival in persons with certain types and stages of thyroid cancer (232,508). Despite extensive efforts toward isolating identifying features of those patients who will benefit from radioactive iodine therapy, the debate over the exact indications for its use continues (509). In general, most authors agree that radiolabeled iodine therapy should be advised for patients with differentiated thyroid cancer except for the relatively small number of subjects considered to be in the low-risk group. As regards papillary cancer, the low-risk group generally is defined as young patients who have tumors smaller than 1 cm that are confined to the thyroid and are well encapsulated (179). This diagnosis assumes that a thorough examination of the thyroid gland was made by the pathologist and that sufficiently frequent histologic sections were made. Low-risk patients may not benefit from radioactive iodine (177,510), although some investigators have advocated its use in those low-risk patients in whom a positive postoperative scan is obtained (232). In all other patients with papillary cancer and in all patients with follicular thyroid cancer, the benefits of radioactive iodine are unquestioned. In this latter group, both tumor recurrence and cancer deaths after thyroid surgery were reduced by half in patients treated with radioactive iodine as compared with those receiving only thyroid hormone therapy or EBRT (177,511). Benefits of radioactive iodine may, in part, relate to the high rate of multifocal papillary carcinoma within the thyroid (512,513). Overall, ^{131}I is concentrated by 60% to 90% of papillary and follicular cancers but by only 36% of Hürthle cell carcinomas (232,496). Of metastatic lesions in either the lungs or bones, only about 50% will concentrate ^{131}I (441), although this number may be higher with adherence to a low-iodine diet and use of more modern nuclear medicine techniques. Inability to concentrate iodine may be due to the small size of lesions and the inherent decreased capacity to identify them by use of nuclear medicine techniques rather than by their decreased ability to actually trap iodine. In these patients, although they may not be detected by scanning procedures, the isotope may still be effective in destroying the tissue. Nonetheless, there certainly exist other lesions that are large and do not trap or respond to radioiodine therapy. Adjunctive use of MRI/CT (without contrast) and sonograms can help identify if lesions are present but not concentrating radioiodine.

The actual impact of ^{131}I on recurrence and survival in patients with macroscopic residual or recurrent disease is disputed. Some investigators deny benefit (514), whereas others extol the effectiveness of the method (459). Despite some disagreement among investigators, considerably more evidence exists to support usage of ^{131}I therapy in those tumors that concentrate the isotope.

Some researchers believe that the presence of cervical lymph node metastasis in papillary carcinoma patients may not affect life expectancy (19,179,515), whereas others believe that its presence is associated with increased disease recurrence rate and death (177). Administration of radioactive iodine to patients with positive lymph nodes has been shown to reduce both recurrence and death rates (155,232).

Those cancers that are locally invasive and unresectable have a high recurrence rate and a mortality rate of 44% at 2 years. If uptake is proved, however, radioactive iodine therapy is useful in reducing these numbers (179,516). Cures and remissions attributable to radioactive iodine in persons with metastatic disease approach 36% (208,517). In patients with lung metastases, survival is significantly better in those with radioactive iodine uptake (232), and the use of radioactive iodine therapy for all patients with lung metastases significantly improves overall survival (178). Complete remission has been demonstrated in 65% of patients with metastatic differentiated lung metastases using cumulative doses of approximately 680 mCi of radioactive iodine (518).

Persons with highly invasive follicular carcinoma have improved survival after ^{131}I therapy (94). In those with less aggressive lesions, the benefit of therapy is more controversial (482). Most institutions routinely prescribe radioactive iodine treatment of follicular thyroid cancer, given the possible benefits seen in various studies and the ability to follow those patients with whole-body radioactive iodine scans. The benefit of ^{131}I therapy in persons with Hürthle cell carcinoma and the tall cell variant of papillary carcinoma is less dramatic than in other patients with differentiated thyroid cancer, but it should still be employed within the confines of the clinical context. It should be remembered that pretherapy diagnostic scans may be negative, but posttherapy scans might indeed show uptake. Of course, ^{131}I therapy should not be used to treat patients with medullary thyroid cancer or anaplastic cancer unless there is an associated differentiated thyroid cancer and the advantages of such therapy outweigh the disadvantages (519). It is still controversial whether to treat a patient with differentiated thyroid cancer and an elevated serum thyroglobulin level and a negative diagnostic radioiodine scan, assuming the patient was prepared properly for the scan and the urine iodine is sufficiently low. The use of associated radiologic studies to assess for disease present is important and the present algorithm assumes as well that these studies are negative. Thus, the clinician is left with no evidence of residual disease except an elevated thyroglobulin level. No definitive guidelines can be issued whether to treat such a patient with ^{131}I until further studies are performed. However, we tend to treat such patients with ^{131}I on one occasion because it is impossible to know ahead of time whether the posttherapy scan will detect disease and it is equally impossible to know if there is a small amount of disease below the threshold sensitivity of scanning techniques that may also be effectively treated with ^{131}I. On the other hand, we do not consider continuing to repeatedly treat such patients unless there is some evidence of effectiveness.

Measurement of serum thyroglobulin is crucial to our assessment of all patients with differentiated thyroid cancer. Using modern assays, a level of serum thyroglobulin greater than 1 ng/mL (assuming a near-total thyroidectomy followed by ^{131}I therapy) suggests the presence of recurrent or residual disease. The serum thyroglobulin level is a more sensitive indicator of disease when the patient is having a withdrawal scan with a concomitantly elevated TSH. Different physicians have various threshold levels at which they would treat with ^{131}I, but this depends as well on the histologic findings of the original tumor, the demonstrated aggressiveness of the tumor, and the results of additional radiologic studies. The threshold thyroglobulin level for the presence of residual or recurrent disease during withdrawal used to be considered 10 ng/mL, although with present assays a value greater than 1 ng/mL bespeaks the presence of tumor cells, but the difficult question is at what level should further treatment with ^{131}I be effected. As noted, this depends on numerous other factors, and no specific guidelines can be formulated.

Thyroglobulin levels are critical to the assessment of any patient with differentiated thyroid cancer, but unfortunately about 20% of thyroid cancer patients have serum thyroglobulin levels that preclude the accurate determination of serum thyroglobulin. Although there are commercial assays touting that they can accurately assess serum thyroglobulin in this circumstance, from a clinical standpoint all measurements of thyroglobulin in the presence of antibodies are problematic. However, over time in some patients the thyroglobulin antibodies dissipate, allowing thyroglobulin measurement; in fact, the decreased titer or disappearance of thyroglobulin antibodies is an indication that the thyroid tissue (and its antigens) are decreasing in mass. Because thyroglobulin titers vary over time, periodic assessment of thyroglobulin levels and antibody may be useful even in patients initially thought to have high titer thyroglobulin antibodies. The issue is more complex because antibodies detected in one assay may not be detected in another, because the thyroglobulin molecule is enormous and different techniques identify different epitopes. To date, there is no sophisticated thyroglobulin assay that identifies one specific known epitope that corresponds to an antibody test that identifies the same epitope.

Patients with high titer thyroglobulin antibodies require the aggressive use of clinical examination and radiologic techniques to identify disease presence, because the utility of serum thyroglobulin levels is abrogated. Lastly, recent advances have suggested that the measurement of serum messenger RNA for thyroglobulin may be a reliable and accurate means to assess the presence of residual thyroid tissue or disease, even in patients with the presence of thyroglobulin antibodies.

The appropriate dose of radioactive iodine can be determined by a quantitative dosimetric approach or by an empiric, standardized dose method. The standardized method is time- and cost-efficient, yet dosimetry may be a better method for calculating doses for those patients with distant metastases or with a prior history of significant cumulative doses. One standard approach (without dosimetric analysis) recommends 100 to 150 mCi for patients with only thyroid bed uptake on radioactive iodine scan, 150 mCi for uptake in cervical nodes, and 175 to 200 mCi for patients with distant metastases (86,219). Doses higher than 200 mCi have not been shown to be more effective in most cases (515). The use of dosimetry requires the administration of a scanning dose of ^{131}I with subsequent measurement of urine and serum isotope levels in conjunction with repeated assessment of whole-body retention. Using a computer formula and with the assistance of an experienced radiation physicist, an analysis can be made of the appropriate ^{131}I dose that should be administered and taken up by tumor tissue but minimizes the dose to the whole body, bone marrow, and lungs. Dosimetric analysis of this kind requires extensive time, equipment and personnel, but it theoretically is better than simply administering a standard ^{131}I dose with no consideration of tissue uptake and the presence of metastatic disease.

Dosimetric analysis can support the use of larger doses of ^{131}I with hopes that the tumor will be more effectively treated and ablated. However, there are no long-term comparison studies assessing the utility and possible side effects of dosimetry versus a routine dose. In fact, such studies are extremely difficult to perform and we don't expect such information to be forthcoming. Therefore, whether to use a routine standard ^{131}I dose or whether to use dosimetry will not be scientifically answered in the near future. Therefore, to summarize our method, for most patients we use a standard ^{131}I dose as detailed above. For a minority of patients, especially those with disseminated disease with osseous or pulmonary metastases or extensive cervical disease, and in patients who have already received several doses of ^{131}I therapy, we consider dosimetry. We use our judgment regarding the dose administered. For example, even if dosimetric analysis indicates that we could give over 300 to 400 mCi ^{131}I in a single dose, we have shied away from this extremely high dose and typically do not give a single dose higher than 300 to 400 mCi, and we use this dose only in unusual circumstances and with the full understanding of the patient. We perform a posttherapeutic scan and measure CBC with white blood cell count every 2 weeks for 3 months following a dosimetrically calculated ^{131}I dose. It is impossible at present to know if such a dose is more effective than a standard ^{131}I dose, but to date we have not seen significant side effects and we have performed this technique in probably several hundred patients over the last two decades and in probably 50 to 75 patients in the last 2 to 3 years. From a purely theoretical standpoint, it makes sense to calculate a dose in this manner as it should administer the maximal dose to the tumor tissue while sparing excessive radiation exposure to the lung, bones, and whole body. Indeed, in some circumstances, such calculations suggest that even a standard dose of 100 to 150 mCi ^{131}I might be excessive. Furthermore, based on theory, if a tumoricidal dose is calculated to be, for example, 300 mCi, does it make more sense to keep treating with separate doses of 100 mCi, given perhaps every year for 3 years, or to give a single tumoricidal dose of 300 mCi? Unfortunately, these questions are unanswerable based on present knowledge.

Means other than dietary alteration and manipulation of the TSH level exist for enhancing the impact of ^{131}I on both normal thyroid and on cancers. For example, lithium reduces the release of iodine from normal thyroid and tumor tissue, and therefore may enhance the retention of the isotope (520). Pending further studies demonstrating the efficacy of this drug, however, we do not advocate its use in routine circumstances. Various radioactive iodine sensitizers such as doxorubicin (Adriamycin) currently are under investigation in the treatment strategy for thyroid cancer patients (521). Recently, 13-*cis*-retinoic acid has been shown to increase radioactive iodine uptake (522–524), although none of the techniques noted has sufficient literature confirmation for us to recommend its use at this time.

Complications from ^{131}I therapy include immediate nausea in a high percentage of patients, thyroiditis in 10% to 20% (525), occasional sialoadenitis (usually temporary or permanent) (526), and, rarely, radiation sickness (527). The parathyroid glands are relatively radioresistant to high-dose ^{131}I therapy (528). Although transient testicular/ovarian failure has been reported, ^{131}I therapy has not been shown to alter fertility in women or to increase abortions or fetal complications when pregnancy is delayed for a year after therapy (529–531). However, these studies are extremely limited in size and scope and must not be considered definitive. In men, associated endocrine changes might occur, but no actual alteration of testosterone levels has been described (531). A reduction in sperm motility has been noted in men treated with ^{131}I, but infertility does not appear to be higher than in the general population. Further study is necessary to solidify confidence regarding these very important reproductive issues. Until such study is accomplished, long-term storage of semen should be offered to selected male patients who are scheduled to receive large doses of radioactive iodine or to those with metastases close to the testes (531). Women should be advised not to get pregnant for at least 6 months, and preferable 12 months, following ^{131}I therapy. The general clinical context should be considered as well, because pregnant women can have only limited diagnostic studies to assess the presence or progression of disease. Men should also be advised not to consider impregnation until at least 6 months after ^{131}I therapy.

Temporary bone marrow suppression can be seen 1 to 6 months after therapy (532). Those patients receiving a mean whole-blood radiation dose of 2.67 Gy from ^{131}I may experience more serious bone marrow suppression (533). A low incidence of leukemia has been reported in patients who have received large cumulative doses of radioactive iodine to the 1-Ci level (66,534,535). Bladder cancer has been described and is seen after repeated high-dose radioactive iodine therapy (486). Pulmonary fibrosis is a concern when pulmonary metastases are present and in circumstances in which doses above 250 mCi are administered (486,536). Concerns regarding increased numbers of gastrointestinal cancers in the higher-dose group have prompted the use of laxatives to accelerate the transit time of the radioisotope through the gastrointestinal tract. Sialagogues likewise are encouraged for flushing the salivary gland tissue. Every patient given a therapeutic dose of ^{131}I is recommended to drink several liters of water or fluids and to suck on lemon drops or similar sialogogues for the first day after ^{131}I therapy. Patients are also advised to wake up 3 a.m. the night following ^{131}I therapy to urinate, drink fluids, and suck on more lemon drops. Laxatives are routinely administered for the first day as well. Antiemetics (e.g., Zofran) are given if a patient has nausea or vomiting following the dose or if the patient or physician expects this to occur. In rare instances, amifostine administration can be considered to prevent ^{131}I uptake by the salivary glands. Although a preliminary study suggests this may be beneficial, it has not yet been proven that amifostine does not alter the effectiveness of ^{131}I on treating tumor tissue. The patient's family and social situation should be considered, and specific advice regarding decreasing radiation exposure of possible contacts should be given. Lastly, these patients are hypothyroid and they should be advised not to make important personal or business decisions or even to drive or operate heavy machinery when hypothyroid.

A practical algorithm for radioactive iodine ablation, scan, and therapy is depicted in Figure 29.17. Within the endocrine and nuclear medicine community, diversity regarding the various alternatives in the use of isotopes is considerable. This algorithm is merely a guideline to a general plan.

External-Beam Radiation Therapy and Chemotherapy Strategies

Probably because of the effectiveness of surgical and radioactive iodine management of the majority of thyroid cancers, experience with both EBRT and chemotherapy in treating this family of neoplasms is limited. Furthermore, the outcome data that have evolved from conventional radiation therapy and chemotherapy strategies are unclear; the actual value of these treatment modalities has not been established by randomized and prospective studies. However, EBRT appears definitely to enhance local control of differentiated thyroid cancer. This is especially true in those patients in whom gross disease remains after surgery. Some of the best responses have been noted when EBRT is used in combination with doxorubicin (189,471, 537–542). The impact of EBRT on survival is unclear (537,543, 544). In anaplastic thyroid cancer, EBRT has been used with extremely limited success to treat locally recurrent disease, and there is some indication that responses are improved by a combination of radiation and doxorubicin. Patients with distant metastases from differentiated cancer, especially to bone, often are older and tend to concentrate iodine poorly in the metastatic sites. In this group, palliation by EBRT directed at these specific lesions seems beneficial (189,541,545).

External radiation therapy to the cervical area does seem beneficial in decreasing recurrences in patients with medullary thyroid carcinoma who have residual neck disease. For patients with metastatic medullary carcinoma, the results of treatment with EBRT or with chemotherapy are somewhat unclear. Some believe that EBRT after surgery does not lower local recurrence rates. On the other hand, investigators from the University of Texas M. D. Anderson Cancer Center and others point out that whereas EBRT is not curative in medullary cancer, its use helps to prevent local recurrence (538–540,546–548). We share this latter view and do employ postoperative irradiation of the neck and mediastinum in those medullary lesions that demonstrate regional nodal metastases. Various drug strategies, including doxorubicin, dacarbazine, streptozotocin, and 5-fluorouracil, have been used for medullary cancers, but generally response rates to both single-agent and combination plans are poor.

With anaplastic carcinoma, EBRT used after surgery may enhance palliation and, because these tumors proliferate rapidly, the use of accelerated fractionation schemes may be useful (261,541). The overall response rate, however, is poor. Given the generally very poor prognosis for anaplastic carcinoma, chemotherapy may be a useful component of the treatment strategy. Under the best of circumstances, the mortality from this disease is approximately 90% (88,89,549,550), and realistic goals must be focused on the palliative benefits of achieving local control to protect the airway. The combination of EBRT and doxorubicin (261–264,531,551–553), often given in combination with cisplatin (554), seems to offer the most reasonable treatment strategy for most of these rapidly growing tumors. When local tumor circumstances permit, thyroid gland removal is desirable for helping to achieve local control. The occasional cure that is achieved usually entails a multimodality approach. However, regardless of the therapy employed, anaplastic thyroid cancer has an extremely grave prognosis.

FOLLOW-UP MONITORING AND SUBSEQUENT THERAPY

Thyroid cancer that is in presumed remission can recur many years after the initial treatment; hence, these patients require lifelong monitoring. For at least two decades after presentation (and possibly even longer), patients with thyroid cancer should undergo routine physical examinations, thyroid blood tests, serum tumor marker level determinations (i.e., thyroglobulin or calcitonin), radioactive iodine scans, and periodic radiologic studies, such as sonogram/MRI of the neck, chest CT (without contrast in patients with differentiated cancer), and perhaps PET scan. The frequency of periodic evaluation is difficult to define as a general policy, as it depends on the clinical context, evidence of recurrent disease, results of measurements of markers, and radiologic studies. Examination of the neck should be performed regularly. Thyroid hormone and TSH levels are monitored to ensure proper dosages and adequate suppression. The serum TSH should be suppressed in patients with differentiated thyroid cancer, although after several years or decades of no evidence of recurrence, the TSH goal can be raised. Markers for cancer are monitored with the caveats noted previously, considering the problems concerning the assessment of serum thyroglobulin levels.

After total thyroidectomy has been performed for differentiated cancer, the thyroglobulin level is predictive of the presence of thyroid tissue. Thyroglobulin, a thyroid-specific glycoprotein, is the prohormone in thyroid hormone synthesis. A rising serum thyroglobulin level suggests recurrent cancer in those patients who have received ablative or therapeutic doses of radioactive iodine or in those who are fully suppressed on thyroid hormone therapy (555). Elevation of serum thyroglobulin is highly sensitive (97%) and specific (100%) for thyroid cancer recurrence. The test has a higher sensitivity than does a radioactive iodine scan (57%), but the specificities of these two tests are similar (556). An elevated thyroglobulin level may warrant follow-up radioactive iodine scan and therapy. An undetectable thyroglobulin level in a patient who is on thyroid hormone therapy may not accurately predict the absence of papillary carcinoma but has been shown to have a low false-negative rate in detecting follicular cancers (557,558), although it has now been recognized that a baseline serum thyroglobulin level can be present even in the presence of cervical disease.

Thyroglobulin is being used in some studies to identify proper suppressive doses of thyroid hormone in patients with thyroid cancer (476). Thyroglobulin measurements are unreliable if thyroglobulin autoantibodies are present (559), and these antibodies have been noted to occur at a higher rate (15% to 30%) in persons with thyroid cancer as compared with persons with normal thyroid glands (560). A worrisome thyroglobulin level in most assays is a detectable level greater than 1 ng/mL, in a patient who has had a near-total thyroidectomy followed by ^{131}I therapy. The normal range on laboratory slips does not apply and is misleading, because normal individuals with functioning thyroid glands have serum levels between about 20 and 60 ng/dL. This range is irrelevant for assessing patients with thyroid cancer following treatment. Recent efforts to have laboratories denote a more appropriate normal range have been successful to some degree. In any case, the physician should be alert to the individual context and what is considered appropriate or elevated. Special care must be taken in patients with thyroglobulin antibodies, in whom the levels are less reliable. In these patients, adjunctive radiologic studies are especially important. It is hoped that serum measurement of messenger RNA for thyroglobulin may be beneficial in assessing for residual thyroid tissue even in the presence of thyroglobulin antibodies.

Treatment controversy arises in the special case in which the thyroglobulin level is elevated and the radioactive iodine uptake is nil. Explanations for this discordance include the presence of small metastases that cannot be visualized with radioactive iodine, high levels of cold iodine (such as that administered with contrast dyes) competing with the radioactive form, excess normal thyroid tissue that obscures metastatic imaging, and false-positive levels of thyroglobulin related to autoantibodies (561,562). Several studies have documented disease activity on scan after radioactive iodine therapy in patients with a false-negative scan and an elevated thyroglobulin level (93,563). As noted, it is important to ensure the urine iodine is appropriately low in these patients and to use radiologic studies to search for evidence of disease activity. Each case must be considered individually, whether treatment with ^{131}I therapy may be warranted in this circumstance. Continued hypercalcitoninemia after surgical management of medullary thyroid cancer indicates persistent disease. Reports claim that 5% to 15% of medullary patients will have abnormal basal or stimulated calcitonin levels after surgery (564). Presumably, this finding indicates either residual local disease or distant metastases. In the face of persistently elevated calcitonin levels, further dissection of the central and lateral neck and upper mediastinum has been promoted. In one study, normalization of serum calcitonin was reported in up to 25% of patients (464). Serologic testing should consist principally of an annual assessment of calcitonin; however, further testing is required to exclude MEN-associated disease or FMTC.

As stressed previously, all patients with medullary thyroid cancer require assessment of their *ret* oncogene to determine if there are mutations identified. If the test is positive, further tests should exclude the presence of hypercalcemia and pheochromocytoma. Calcitonin stimulation tests also should be mentioned. In the past, calcium and/or pentagastrin to stimulate calcitonin were widely employed. However, these tests are time consuming and entail added costs to the patient. In addition, pentagastrin is no longer available commercially. However, serum calcitonin assays have markedly improved and the lower limit of detectability is as low as 1 pg/mL. There are no modern studies directly comparing the ability to detect disease by use of a stimulated calcitonin and by use of unstimulated values in the present assays. Nonetheless, for the reasons mentioned, most frequently at the present time an unstimulated calcitonin in a sensitive assay is used to monitor for the presence of disease.

COMPLICATIONS OF SURGERY

Because informed consent documentation includes explanations of anatomic and physiologic details that often are beyond the patient's comprehension, it is important to emphasize to the patient that, compared with other major surgical undertakings, thyroid operations are actually very safe. The complication rate of thyroid operations is probably among the lowest of what are broadly classified as major head and neck procedures, and, when one considers the anatomic complexity of the area, this extraordinary fact reflects favorably on contemporary surgical training and expertise. On the other hand, the complexity of critical parts in this relatively small area can present substantial difficulties to the inadequately trained or inexperienced surgeon.

Overall safety is illustrated by examination of present and past reports of complication rates associated with thyroid surgery. Though in part a reflection of improved training and sophistication of modern surgery, the improvement of contemporary over historical data undoubtedly also represents more precise scrutiny. For example, historical reporting reflects heterogeneous experiences retrospectively compiled from lengthy studies that included multiple generations of surgeons in multiple institutions. One would expect the complication rate to be lower with a consistent surgical team and prospective analysis of complications.

Postoperative Infection

Postoperative infection is very unusual in thyroid surgery, largely because of the abundant blood supply to the area. On this basis, and because the surgical field is not normally connected with the aerodigestive tract, the routine use of perioperative antibiotics seems unwarranted. In circumstances in which a wound seroma or hematoma forms that requires secondary drainage, the use of antibiotics to combat skin flora is recommended. In addition, many surgeons routinely employ perioperative antibiotics in those cases in which a drain is left in place at the completion of surgery. Postoperative hematomas or seromas can be of sufficient size to cause tracheal compression, and typically this complication is identified within the first day after surgery.

Hemorrhage

Hemorrhage after thyroid surgery occasionally is encountered. Hallmarks of sophisticated thyroid and parathyroid surgery are meticulous hemostasis and compulsive attention to the technical details necessary to "operate dry." Despite the best efforts of skillful surgeons, however, postoperative bleeding still occurs sometimes. Because of the abundant blood supply in the area, thyroid surgical patients might be susceptible to intraoperative oozing. Surgical preparation should include screening for bleeding disorders, a thorough history of bruising or bleeding tendencies, and assurance that the patient is avoiding medications that might interfere with the normal clotting mechanism. Even in those patients who bleed more than usual during surgery, placement of drains in the wound usually offsets the potential problem. The usual cause for significant postoperative hemorrhage leading to wound hematoma is the uncoupling of a ligature or staple that was placed on a vein or artery during the procedure. When such a technical mishap occurs with the superior pole vessels, the middle or inferior thyroid veins, or the inferior thyroid artery, a rapidly enlarging hematoma can develop into life-threatening airway compression in the early postoperative period. The most likely time for such an occurrence is in the recovery room, often after a stormy awakening from anesthesia during which the patient coughs and strains on the endotracheal tube. The anesthesiologist must attend to the importance of a peaceful extubation and postoperative recovery period. When neck swelling and airway compression occur rapidly, the immediate treatment is to open the wound and evacuate collected blood. Under such circumstances, to attempt reintubation before hematoma evacuation invites accentuation of the difficulty. Once the immediate threat of airway compression is allayed, an orderly return to the operating room for reintubation, general anesthesia, reexploration, vascular control, and appropriate irrigation can be accomplished.

During thyroidectomy, bleeding often is encountered just anterior to the point at which the recurrent laryngeal nerve enters the larynx. A troublesome vein is usually found here that must be transected. Caution must be exercised at this point of the surgery because of the vulnerability of the nerve that lies just deep to this vein. Bipolar rather than unipolar electrocoagulation should be employed to minimize the chance for thermal injury to the adjacent nerve. A substantial proportion of recurrent laryngeal nerve injuries occur while the surgeon is attempting to control troublesome bleeding in the thyroid bed.

The recurrent nerve, as it is being stretched during the dissection of Berry's ligament, becomes increasingly vulnerable to injury. This resilient fascial layer provides a source of protection to the nerve at its laryngeal entry point by absorbing the energy imposed by retraction of the thyroid gland. As the ligament is dissected, therefore, retraction of the thyroid gland itself must be applied carefully and with restraint, lest the nerve be stretched.

Pneumothorax and Chylous Fistulae

Pneumothorax and chylous fistulae have been reported only rarely after thyroidectomy and, when encountered, usually result from an extended thyroid or neck procedure for cancer. The treatment for pneumothorax depends on the magnitude of the problem, but when the pneumothorax is substantial, a chest tube is required. Chylous leaks occur more often on the left side and are usually self-limiting if adequate wound drainage is employed.

Wound Seroma

A wound seroma is encountered periodically after thyroidectomy, especially when a large goiter has been removed. After the removal of the standard drain, a transudative fluid can fill the space created by the large gland. Left undrained, this body of fluid can lead to infection. Even large seromas can be effectively treated by simple needle aspiration. Occasionally, repeated aspirations of 10 to 20 mL of straw-colored fluid are required on sequential days to resolve the problem. Only rarely is it necessary to reopen the wound.

Scars

Unsightly scars result from several problems: widening, hypertrophy, and keloid formation. Improper placement and tethering of the central part of the scar to the underlying tissue also create an aesthetically undesirable appearance in the very visible anterior neck. When properly planned and with normal healing, the thyroid incision is aesthetically very acceptable. In those individuals with existing skin creases, every attempt should be made to place the incision within the normal fold, thus ensuring maximal camouflage. In those individuals in whom there are no existing lines, the surgeon should make an attempt to estimate the folds with bimanual pulling of the cervical skin from side to side. This maneuver is best accomplished with the patient in the sitting position, and a mark should be made on the skin to ensure the duplication of localization once the patient is asleep and supine. If the incision curve is too accentuated, or if it is made in a straight rather than a semilunar fashion, the resulting scar appearance is substandard. A common error made in incision design is in placing the incision too low on the neck. The skin over the sternal notch is under considerable tension and, in general, does not heal as inconspicuously as skin elsewhere on the neck. In women with pendulous breasts, or in anyone with a heavy anterior chest wall, the incision should be placed higher. People prone to keloid scar formation are especially susceptible to keloid formation if the incision is placed too low on the neck. Finally, women should be instructed to wear an athletic support bra for approximately 1 month after surgery in an attempt to lessen the downward pull and tension on the horizontally oriented incision.

Nerve Injury

Injury of the important nerve structures that regulate voice production and, to some extent, swallowing, can result from thyroid or parathyroid surgery.

Superior Laryngeal Nerve Injury

The superior laryngeal nerve is especially vulnerable because it often is not seen by the surgeon, is located at the periphery of the operation, and is in proximity to the large superior thyroid pole vessels, which generally are ligated. In fact, the main trunk of the external branch of the superior laryngeal nerve is adjacent to these vessels, and the relation between the two varies somewhat (565). In addition, the delicate terminal nerve fibers that actually penetrate the external surface of the cricothyroid muscle run under the investing fascia. The muscle itself lies deep to the medial edge of the superior pole of the thyroid, and therefore, even with precise dissection of the superior pole vessels, these delicate terminal branches are vulnerable to thermal and instrumental trauma during dissection of that part of the thyroid gland.

Because the visual manifestations of superior nerve paralysis are not readily apparent, the actual incidence of this complication is unknown. Injury to the superior laryngeal nerve might be more common than injury to the recurrent nerve. Furthermore, the result of injury to either nerve often might be temporary and therefore might remain unrecognized (566).

Injury to the superior nerve results in a voice change rather than a compromise of the airway. Any significant injury to the superior nerve denervates the cricothyroid muscle to some extent. The contraction of this muscle normally serves to lengthen (i.e., tense) the vocal cord. Relaxation of the cricothyroid muscle therefore shortens the corresponding vocal cord, which results in difficulty with pitch variation. The ability to achieve upper-register phonation is especially encumbered by superior laryngeal nerve paresis or paralysis. Throughout this process, the voice is not what is commonly known as *hoarse* but rather is restricted in vocal range. Despite these symptoms, physical findings are subtle and generally are not obvious to the less sophisticated laryngeal examiner. Classic electromyographic injury patterns are seen when the cricothyroid muscle is tested; essentially, such findings are diagnostic.

The delicate terminal nerve fibers under the cricothyroid muscle fascia, once injured, cannot be repaired, and whatever regeneration ultimately occurs is beyond the control of the surgeon. The vocal effect of injury to this nerve can be significant, especially in the performing artist or public speaker. Voice therapy offers limited help but can be useful in preventing the vocal ill effects of unsupervised laryngeal compensation.

INFERIOR (RECURRENT) LARYNGEAL INJURY

Even though the true incidence of superior laryngeal nerve(s) injury is unknown, we believe it to be a more common occurrence than injury to the recurrent nerve(s). Despite this, the recurrent nerve(s) injury has historically received far more attention and publicity. The incidence of permanent recurrent nerve paralysis is reported to be from less than 1% to 1.5% for total thyroidectomy and approximately one-half of that for subtotal procedures (155,567,568). The incidence of temporary unilateral vocal cord paresis or paralysis after thyroidectomy is between 2.5% and 5% (565). Our own cases have yielded a paresis or paralysis rate considerably lower than these numbers. We believe that results similar to ours are corroborated by other surgeons. A higher incidence of recurrent nerve injury has been reported in thyroidectomy that is performed in combination with neck dissection (567), but that may reflect a more advanced stage of disease encountered in those patients. One would expect the nerve injury rate to increase with advanced primary disease. We routinely examine the larynx before and after all thyroidectomy and parathyroidectomy procedures, documenting the motion of the patient's cords.

The incidence of bilateral recurrent nerve paralysis is very low. However, when it does occur, the resultant difficulties can be prompt and severe. In completion thyroidectomy (performed in those patients who have undergone a partial thyroidectomy but who, after pathologic study, require a second operation to complete the thyroidectomy), the incidence of nerve injury is the same as one would expect with the initial partial procedure. Others dispute this claim and report a higher incidence of injury in completion thyroidectomy (567). The incidence of nerve injury is undoubtedly higher in patients who have undergone a thyroidectomy and in whom the surgeon must reoperate on a previously dissected site in which there is scar tissue (145). This should not be true, however, if the surgeon is removing the previously unoperated side of the gland. Cancer operations, compared with thyroid surgery for benign disease, probably increase the injury rate (568).

The management of unilateral vocal cord paralysis secondary to recurrent laryngeal nerve injury usually is supportive. If the nerve has been clearly visualized and is believed to be intact, we do not favor reexploration, even when vocal cord paralysis is noted immediately after surgery.

If the nerve has been transected during thyroidectomy, we favor microsurgical repair, even though the resulting vocal cord motion will not duplicate the normal preinjury state (569). The value of this primary repair technique may be in reducing the extent of vocal cord atrophy. Crumley's extensive laboratory experiments, however, suggest that the relinking of the two severed ends of the recurrent nerve is not the ideal method (570,571). Crumley has shown that undesirable laryngeal synkinesis and actual vocal cord hyperadduction can follow reanastomosis. Instead of primary reanastomosis, he believes the better way to reinnervate the denervated larynx is to anastomose branches of the ansa hypoglossal nerve to the distal end of the severed recurrent nerve. Resulting restoration of tone plus the normal adaptation of the contralateral vocal cord appear to minimize the ill effects of recurrent nerve injury (570,571). Despite this provocative work, we favor primary anastomosis.

The immediate voice changes that follow recurrent nerve injury are distinct. A noticeable breathiness and volume limitation occur. After the initial adductive activity associated with acute injury has subsided, the vocal cord drifts to a paramedian position that is slightly off midline. If the ipsilateral superior laryngeal nerve has also been injured, the cord assumes a more lateral (intermediate) position, and the voice is proportionately worse (572). Unilateral vocal cord paralysis only rarely is associated with aspiration, and when this does occur the superior nerve has usually been concomitantly injured. In the face of this combination injury, significant lateralization of the vocal cord invariably is associated with more glottic incompetence, a state that can be followed by vocal deterioration and a tendency to aspirate secretions and other liquids. Undoubtedly, the tendency to aspiration is also a result of sensory deficit that accompanies such injuries.

With an isolated recurrent laryngeal nerve injury, however, the vocal cord remains paramedian rather than in the more lateral position. If the superior nerve is intact, the functional cricothyroid muscle has a slight adductive effect; thus, the vocal cord gradually drifts toward the midline. The time required for this scenario varies from weeks to months. This midline drift may also result from gradual partial reinnervation. During this period of adjustment, the opposite and normally innervated vocal cord can actually hyperadduct, compensating for the glottic incompetence created by the paralyzed cord. Skillful voice therapy during this time can be invaluable. Forced adduction exercises under the supervision of a voice therapist probably have no impact on nerve healing but can hasten the return of glottic competence and relatively normal voice. In addition, the patient is provided real psychological value from this rehabilitative effort. In those patients left with permanent air leak and vocal incompetence despite the best efforts of the voice pathologist and the passage of adequate time for healing, treatment is directed to medialization procedures such as thyroplasty and arytenoid medialization. These procedures have virtually replaced Teflon cord injection (573–576).

The actual voice changes that follow an acute recurrent laryngeal nerve injury during thyroidectomy, though distinct, often are so subtle and short-lived that the patient may not even realize that there was a change. Because the symptoms of unilateral nerve injury during thyroidectomy are elusive, it is essential that all patients undergo a preoperative laryngeal examination by a physician competent in evaluating the subtleties of vocal cord motion. Not uncommonly, a previously unrecognized and asymptomatic unilateral vocal cord paralysis caused by viral or other previous insults is found in the normal population. If such an abnormality has not been documented before surgery, its relation to the thyroidectomy may be misinterpreted.

Bilateral vocal cord paralysis is much more problematic than unilateral paralysis. Major clinical problems develop during two separate phases—immediately after surgery and years after the injury. These fairly consistent changes can be explained on a physiologic basis. When bilateral recurrent laryngeal nerve injuries are acute and isolated, the vocal cords initially have a short period (hours) during which the unopposed adductive laryngeal forces generate a spastic adductive vocal cord contraction (572). This is followed by a period of relaxation, during which the normal elastic forces of the larynx draw each vocal cord laterally but, because of the continuing adductive efforts of the respective left and right cricothyroid muscles, only the paramedian position ultimately is reached bilaterally. Here the paralyzed vocal cords reside indefinitely. Over time (sometimes years), the continued adductive activity of the cricothyroid muscles gradually pulls the cords back to the midline. Immediately after extubation, during the spastic adductive phase that follows bilateral recurrent nerve injury, the airway is obstructed to a variable degree; thus, stridor is produced. This critical phase often occurs in the recovery room, and proper interpretation of the events is vital to appropriate management. The stridor usually passes when the phase of vocal cord abduction begins; thus, reintubation rather than tracheostomy is the strategy of choice during the obstructive phase. On the other hand, successful extubation may not be possible, in which case a tracheostomy becomes necessary. If one is able to support the patient through this spastic phase, extubation often is followed by a breathy and inadequate voice. Aspiration of liquids can result from the bilateral abducted position of the vocal cords. The patient should be denied thin liquids by mouth until adaptation is achieved. Occasionally, aspiration is such a problem that placement of a feeding tube or even a percutaneous gastrostomy becomes necessary.

During the abduction period, the voice often is very weak; however, as the vocal cords begin to return to the midline, the voice improves, but at the expense of the airway. Eventually, the voice may be almost normal, but because of the bilateral midline position of the vocal cords, the airway is compromised substantially. These circumstances may not come to the attention of a physician for years after thyroid surgery; in fact, the patient may not even associate the gradually worsening airway status with the previous thyroidectomy. On questioning, however, the scenario becomes obvious; immediately after thyroidectomy, the patient experienced an initially poor voice but adequate airway followed by gradual return of voice but inadequate airway. Not uncommonly, such patients have received misdiagnoses for years and have been treated unsuccessfully for such conditions as bronchial asthma, chronic obstructive pulmonary disease, or other causes of dyspnea, only to learn that the inexorable bilateral medialization of the vocal cords gradually has compromised the airway.

The various techniques for treating bilateral vocal cord medialization are designed to provide more airway while not sacrificing the voice completely. However, an improvement in airway is, to some extent, always achieved at the expense of vocal strength. Such surgical procedures as arytenoidectomy (577) and transverse cordotomy (578) serve to widen the airway while preserving a usable voice. These procedures are irreversible, however, and should not be performed until adequate time has been allowed for nerve recovery, which can take as long as 12 months. If the injury is secondary to nerve stretching or swelling, the return of function usually occurs within several months. Laryngeal electromyography may be useful in judging the prognosis for recovery in patients with bilateral nerve injuries (579,580). Acoustic evidence suggests that the transverse cordotomy procedure leads to a superior vocal result compared with either the arytenoidectomy or arytenoid lateralization procedures (581). Finally, a significant research effort has been made in recent years to reinnervate the larynx; however, none of this work has yet produced a practical method (569,582–587).

In those circumstances in which both recurrent laryngeal nerves and both superior laryngeal nerves sustain injuries during thyroidectomy, the vocal cords do not move medially over time because the counterforces of the cricothyroid muscles are absent. Therefore, the voice does not improve greatly after the initial insult. On the contrary, patients often demonstrate problems resulting from glottic incompetence rather than an inadequate airway. This circumstance leads to aspiration probably because of a combination of denervation and because of the inability of the larynx to seal at the vocal cord level; essentially, the most phylogenetically primitive and important of laryngeal functions—glottic closure—is lost. Furthermore, this inability of the vocal aperture to seal, with the resulting loss of ability to increase subglottic pressure, is compounded further by subtle cricopharyngeal and upper esophageal malfunction and some loss of sensory sensation to the upper tracheal lumen, all of which results from loss of recurrent laryngeal nerve function.

Metabolic Complications

The metabolic complications of thyroid tumor surgery occur as a result of reequilibration and redistribution of vital biochemical elements after surgical trauma (or removal) of parathyroid glands. It is not within the scope of this chapter to discuss thyroid surgery performed for Graves disease.

A transient drop in the serum calcium level after thyroid tumor surgery is common and can occur even in those circumstances in which the surgeon has performed only a lobectomy, an operation in which there should be minimal disturbance of the environment around the parathyroid glands. The hypocalcemia associated with this circumstance probably does not result from hypoparathyroidism but instead may be due to fluctuations in serum protein binding and a resulting postoperative alteration of acid–base status, albumin concentration, and hemodilution (588). Such fluctuations in serum protein binding, and the ensuing physiologic changes, can result in a decrease in the protein-bound form of serum calcium and generally should not cause symptoms (214). Transient symptomatic hypocalcemia after total thyroidectomy is reported to occur in approximately 7% to 25% of cases, whereas permanent hypocalcemia is less common, occurring in 0.4% to 13.8% of patients (214,589,590). In subtotal thyroidectomy, the incidence of permanent hypocalcemia is reported to be between 0.2% and 1.9% (590). There is, however, no consensus on the appropriate identification or treatment of patients with postthyroidectomy hypocalcemia. In fact, many patients who experience a decrease in serum calcium are asymptomatic, and the decrement of calcium necessary to produce symptoms is variable. For example, numerous patients undergo a decrease from a preoperative normal calcium level to levels such as 8.5 to 9.0 mg/dL. In the absence of symptoms, this decrease is less meaningful.

Measurement of serum ionized calcium (the unbound portion) may be useful, as total calcium can be more influenced by alterations in calcium binding proteins. It is difficult to give specific guidelines, but as a general comment it is preferable to err on the side of treating low calcium levels whenever the low calcium may be significant or contributing to a possible metabolic complication, e.g., cardiac abnormalities. It is also important to measure serum magnesium in such circumstances, as hypomagnesemia may contribute to hypocalcemia. With regard to serum calcium, our approach is to consider giving calcium supplementation to patients with a serum calcium lower than 8.0 mg/dL even in the absence of symptoms such as tetany or paresthesias. It is possible that this calcium level, especially if it decreases rapidly even further, may cause significant cardiac or neurologic problems without prior advance warning or premonitory signs or symptoms. In general, it is important that patients with hypocalcemia have cardiac monitoring with frequent clinical assessment and measurement of electrolytes, calcium, and magnesium. Early aggressive attention to possible hypocalcemia will decrease the chance of significant problems and will shorten the hospital length of stay. Following discharge at an appropriate time, the supplemental calcium and vitamin D administration can be gradually tapered.

Both thyroid and parathyroid surgery should be performed by thyroid surgeons in concert with medical colleagues who are schooled in the endocrine aspects of this subject. The thyroid surgeon, however, must be independently knowledgeable of the pathogenesis, recognition, and, most important, treatment of postoperative hypoparathyroidism. In circumstances in which the calcium decrease results from actual hypoparathyroidism, the rapidity of the drop seems to affect symptoms (i.e., a rapid drop of blood calcium seems more often to be associated with symptoms). The symptoms of digital paresthesia, circumoral numbness, and a generalized sense of cutaneous sensitivity and irritability can result from moderate reductions in ionized calcium. In cases in which the blood calcium is dramatically lowered, enhanced reflexes, muscle contractility and spasm, tetany, seizures, cardiac dysrhythmias, and even death can ensue.

Treatment is tailored to respond to the severity of the problem. Many believe that among those patients who have enough residual parathyroid tissue ultimately to sustain normal blood levels, it is best to treat only those who are experiencing significant symptoms. In these patients, it is argued, the normal glandular tissue will function more readily if calcium supplement is not given during the early stage of the problem. It is argued further that premature administration of calcium tends to suppress the restitution of normal activity in the balance of the parathyroid tissue. Anyone who contemplates adopting this nihilistic philosophy should take into consideration, however, the morbidity of the symptom complex associated with hypocalcemia. We argue strongly against this nihilistic approach. Hypocalcemic patients often complain bitterly of the extreme sense of anxiety and cutaneous sensitivity. When symptoms are severe or life-threatening findings are involved, prompt attention must be given to enhancing the blood calcium level. A lowered ionized calcium level is not to be viewed casually and, whether accompanying symptoms exist or not, we believe treatment is advisable.

The most commonly cited etiology for postthyroidectomy hypocalcemia is parathyroid insufficiency, which has been caused by devascularization, injury, or excision of the very delicate parathyroid glands. Permanent hypocalcemia is fairly uniformly related to these factors. Although risk to the parathyroid glands is reported to be inversely proportional to the experience of the surgeon, transient hypocalcemia may occur despite meticulous identification and preservation of all four (or more) glands by the most skillful surgeon.

The ideal situation in thyroid surgery is for the surgeon to identify the four parathyroid glands in the perithyroid fibrofatty tissue (i.e., independent of and unattached to the thyroid gland). The most common form of injury probably involves the vessels to and from the parathyroids. Subtle vascular compromise often is unrecognized during surgery. Generalized change in the color of a parathyroid gland suggests venous congestion and can herald impending hypofunction. Partial discoloration with a demarcated line of color change across a gland, on the other hand, usually suggests arterial insufficiency. Not infrequently, the surgeon identifies one or more of the parathyroid glands after the thyroid gland is out, and, in this circumstance, the parathyroid glands may have been disrupted and dislocated. If this occurs, the surgeon should prepare the parathyroid tissue properly and reimplant it into a regional muscle. This technique, although followed by a transient loss of PTH secretion from the transplanted glands, is frequently successful in restoring parathyroid function (591).

Although less likely, transient hypocalcemia may also be encountered after hemithyroidectomy in which one thyroid lobe and at least two parathyroid glands are preserved. Other possible etiologies of postthyroidectomy hypocalcemia include an increased uptake of calcium by bone secondary to thyrotoxic osteodystrophy (hungry bone syndrome) (592), prolonged parathyroid suppression in patients with preoperative thyrotoxicosis (592), transient hemodilution with increased renal excretion of calcium (593), and increased calcitonin release secondary to thyroid manipulation in surgery (594). Medications can induce hypocalcemia in the perioperative period. Propylthiouracil and propranolol, both of which are used in Graves disease patients for perisurgical prophylaxis against thyroid storm, have been associated with hypocalcemia (595). A wide variety of medications, including phosphate enemas and azidothymidine, exhibit similar associations.

Finally, Falk (596) has introduced two additional possible etiologies for transient hypocalcemia after thyroidectomy: hypothermia and excessive release of endothelia-1. Hypothermia of the parathyroid glands that results from intraoperative irrigation of the wound can cause transient schemia. Endothelia-1, a vasoconstricting peptide, is present in high concentrations in both the parathyroid and thyroid glands. Intraoperative manipulation of the thyroid or parathyroid gland can induce release of endothelia-1 and cause transient schemia of the remaining parathyroid tissue and subsequent hypocalcemia.

The secretion of each parathyroid gland seems to contribute in a cumulative way to the entire hormone level; therefore, decrease of hormone production as a result of surgical trauma is a proportionate rather than an all-or-none phenomenon.

On rare occasions, the anatomic location of the parathyroid glands is extraordinary and befuddles the surgeon. The ultimate example of this is the situation in which one or more of the parathyroid glands actually lies deep to the capsule of the thyroid gland. This anatomic variation sometimes is recognized only after the thyroid has been removed, and unfortunately the discovery is often made by the pathologist examining the specimen. A more detailed description of the parathyroid anatomy and location was provided in the anatomy and technical sections of this chapter.

Postoperative hypocalcemia can be categorized as symptomatic or asymptomatic. Symptomatic hypocalcemia is either emergent or nonemergent. The signs and symptoms of hypocalcemia are manifold and include Chvostek sign, Trousseau sign, perioral paresthesias, carpopedal spasm, generalized muscle cramps, laryngospasm, arrhythmias, tetany, and seizures. Perioral and upper-extremity paresthesias are the most common symptoms of hypocalcemia.

Symptomatic hypocalcemia requires immediate calcium supplementation. The decision to administer calcium intravenously rather than orally depends on the severity of the symptoms and the extent of the hypocalcemia. Some recommend treating symptomatic hypocalcemia in conjunction with an ionized calcium level of less than 4.0 mg/dL (which roughly corresponds to a total serum calcium of 7.8 mg/dL or an ionized calcium level of 1.0 mmol/L) with a calcium gluconate infusion (1 mg/kg/h) (597). It also is recommended that these patients start oral calcium (1,000 mg of elemental calcium twice daily) and 1,25(OH)$_2$-vitamin D_3 (0.25 to 0.50 μg twice daily). For this treatment regimen, the intravenous calcium is stopped when the level of ionized calcium reaches 4.4 mg/dL (roughly 1.2 mmol/L) or higher. Specific attention by the treating physicians must be paid to the type of calcium preparation employed and the percentage calcium in each preparation. It is very easy to get confused, as calcium contained in a given preparation can be reported as available ionized calcium or as total calcium in, for example, calcium gluconate. We prefer to calculate all calcium given as ionized or free calcium and to record carefully all sources given. Very close monitoring of serum calcium is mandatory in any patient administered calcium, especially in a patient receiving intravenous calcium. In most instances, intensive care unit monitoring with constant cardiac monitoring is required for patients receiving intravenous calcium in this circumstance (598,599).

Our preference is to preoperatively check serum ionized calcium, magnesium, and phosphorus levels in all patients undergoing thyroid surgery. Magnesium levels are particularly important in the hypocalcemic patient, as hypomagnesemia tends to impair PTH secretion in addition to inducing end-organ resistance to PTH (600). It should be noted that the initial effect of hypomagnesemia is a rise in PTH secretion, followed by a more prolonged decrease in this hormonal secretion. Consideration must be given to the fact that a normal PTH level does not rule out hypoparathyroidism. The PTH level should be interpreted in the context of the serum calcium level; a PTH level in the normal range may be inappropriately low in association with a low serum calcium. Measurement of total serum calcium with serum albumin (approximately 50% of serum calcium is bound by proteins such as albumin) is acceptable if ionized calcium is unavailable. Ionized calcium represents unbound serum calcium, and so that level is considered a more accurate test. These studies can be repeated 12 and 24 hours after surgery. The rationale for waiting 12 hours after surgery to obtain these values is to allow serum calcium to stabilize. If a rising or stable trend is noted from 12 to 24 hours and the patient is asymptomatic, the calcium test can be repeated in 1 week. However, these guidelines should be modified based on individual circumstances, and it is preferable to err on the side of more, rather than less, measurements if there is any question or possibility of a problem.

For postthyroidectomy patients, we favor maintaining an ionized calcium level greater than 2.0 mg/dL or a total serum calcium greater than 8.0 mg/dL. Although most hypocalcemic patients present initially with paresthesias, the first sign of hypocalcemia could be arrhythmia, tetany, or seizures. A serum ionized calcium level of less than 2.0 mg/dL or signs and symptoms of hypocalcemia require that the patient receive oral calcium with 1,25$(OH)_2$-vitamin D_3. The dose for oral supplementation is 1.5 mg of elemental calcium per kilogram per day. Calcium carbonate contains 40% elemental calcium; therefore, a 79-kg hypocalcemic patient would require approximately 1 g of elemental calcium per day in addition to normal dietary intake. This corresponds to roughly 650 mg calcium carbonate four times daily. Another form of supplement available is calcium gluconate. Calcium citrate has the advantage of not requiring an acidic environment for absorption. Malabsorption, therefore, occurs less with achlorhydric patients or those taking H_2-blockers.

In stable patients with no intercurrent issues, the serum ionized calcium level should be checked 1 week after surgery. If the value has increased significantly, calcium supplementation can be tapered over the next week in those patients who were discharged on such medication. Those patients who fail to show a rebound in their calcium levels should continue calcium supplementation and return for serum ionized calcium levels weekly.

In emergent situations such as seizures, cardiac arrhythmias, or a very low ionized calcium level, 10 to 30 mL intravenous calcium gluconate can be given over 10 minutes (roughly 93 to 279 mg of elemental calcium). Generally, it is much more desirable to infuse slowly over 3 to 4 hours. The effects of a bolus of intravenous calcium diminishes within 2 hours, and continuous infusion sometimes is necessary. Intravenous infusion can be started at 0.5 mg elemental calcium per kg per hour for symptomatic hypocalcemia of moderate degree, increasing to 1.0 to 1.5 mg/kg/h for more severe cases (601). The ideal target for correcting hypocalcemia is 10 to 15 mg/kg of elemental calcium, to be given over a period of 8 to 24 hours. Maintenance of infusion rates depends on serial serum calcium levels, obtained every 4 hours. Oral calcium supplementation can be started at this time (15 mg/kg/d elemental calcium with 0.25 to 0.50 mg 1,25$(OH)_2$-vitamin D_3). Serum electrolytes, albumin, and magnesium should be monitored in a similar fashion. To prevent precipitation in solution, bicarbonate or phosphate should not be administered via the same intravenous line. The calcium infusion can be discontinued when the ionized calcium level is equal to or exceeds 1.12 mmol/L. Electrocardiographic monitoring during administration is recommended for a symptomatic patient with an ionized calcium level of less than 1.12 mmol/L (4.0 mg/dL). Though there should always be a flexible treatment strategy employed in this dynamic condition, a general guide for management of postthyroidectomy hypocalcemia is outlined in Table 29.7.

TABLE 29.7 Practical Overview and Set of Guidelines for the Management of Postoperative Hypocalcemia

	Definition	Treatment	Monitoring	Length of treatment
Symptomatic emergent hypocalcemia	1. Arrhythmia, seizures, tetany 2. Ca_I level variable, usually <1.0 mmol/L	1. 10–30 mL 10% gluconate can be infused over 10 min–3 hr[a] 2. IV infusion of calcium gluconate from 0.5 to 1.5 mg elemental calcium/kg/hr, for a total of 10–15 mg/kg over 8–24 hours 3. Oral calcium + vitamin D_3 (as below)	1. Continuous cardiac calcium monitoring 2. Ca_I, Mg, P every 2–4 hours	1. Discontinue infusion when Ca_I, >1.12 mmol/L; start oral calcium + vitamin D_3 (as below) 2. Discharge home on oral calcium + vitamin D_3 (as below) 3. Weekly Ca_I, Mg, P 4. Taper calcium supplements based on Ca_I levels
Symptomatic nonemergent hypocalcemia	1. Perioral and upper-extremity paresthesias or signs and symptoms of hypocalcemia, excluding arrhythmia, seizures, or tetany 2. Ca_I level variable	15 mg/kg/d elemental calcium (650 mg $CaCo_3$ PO q.i.d. for 70-kg person) + 0.25–0.5 μg 1,25$(OH)_2$-vitamin D_3 PO daily	1. Ca_I, Mg, P levels every 12 hours until asymptomatic 2. Cardiac monitoring preferred	1. Weekly Ca_I, Mg, P levels 2. Taper calcium supplements based on Ca_I levels
Asymptomatic nonemergent hypocalcemia	Ca_I <1.12 mmol/L (4.0 mg/dL), or serum calcium <4.24 mmol/L (8.0 mg/dL)	15 mg/kg/d elemental calcium (650 mg $CaCo_3$ PO q.i.d. for 70-kg person) + 0.25–0.50 μg 1,25$(OH)_2$-vitamin D_3 PO daily	Ca_I, Mg, P levels at 12 and 24 hours postoperatively	1. Weekly Ca_I, Mg, P levels 2. Taper calcium supplements based on Ca_I levels

This evaluation and treatment should involve considerable flexibility and clinical judgment on the part of the treating physician. In addition, the treating physician must be familiar with the condition and the medications used. It is extremely important to check the actual calcium vials given to ensure the total and elemental calcium given is correct. Frequent confusion occurs in communication regarding total or elemental calcium doses. Many physicians in the acute management of hypocalcemia prefer to obtain both a total and an ionized calcium to better assess the actual serum concentrations of calcium available at the tissue level.
Ca_I, serum-ionized calcium; Mg, magnesium; P, phosphorus.
[a]Slower rate of infusion preferable.

CONCLUSION

This lengthy discussion of thyroid cancer and related issues represents but a small portion of knowledge derived from an extensive literature. Many of the issues that have been debated and discussed for decades persist without closure. It is fortunate, therefore, that because of the long natural history of most thyroid malignancies, failure to answer many questions seems more tolerable. Nonetheless, thyroid cancer can be a devastating disease and, when the cancer is of the less differentiated variety, any inclination to minimize its potential should be avoided. It is also preferable that patients with thyroid cancer be managed by an interdisciplinary health care team whose members have the same philosophy regarding approach and treatment of patients with thyroid cancer. In addition, the importance of including the patient in the management team cannot be over emphasized.

RADIOLOGIC IMAGING CONCERNS

Bernard B. O'Malley and Suresh K. Mukherji

Comprehensive staging of the neck and upper mediastinum for thyroid and related malignancies usually comes about after the diagnosis of cancer has been made by FNA or, less commonly, thyroid lobectomy. Ultrasound of the thyroid is widely performed and provides a good screening test for thyroid masses (Fig. 29.18). Most sonograms of the thyroid gland are performed to establish the size, number, and distribution of nodular masses in the thyroid gland. Most of these patients are followed clinically for small nodules. Patients with hyperparathyroidism generally do not undergo sonography. The sonogram can be helpful for guided FNA (602) but otherwise cannot confirm cancer or determine what type when present. Sonography, in experienced hands, can also be used for regional lymph node staging but cannot be considered comprehensive because of its inability to penetrate the mediastinum.

Nuclear imaging of nodular glands is usually not necessary in metabolically asymptomatic patients. The FNA should not be delayed by the performance or results of radionuclide scans when nodules of 1.0 cm or greater are encountered. These nuclear scans should be interpreted with careful clinical and cross-sectional imaging correlation (Fig. 29.19). Only when multiple nodules are present does a radionuclide scan aid in determining which would be most productive for biopsy. Cold nodules are three times more likely than other nodules to be cancerous. Nuclear imaging with radioactive iodine agents is used widely for papillary and follicular cancer. Not all cell lines are or remain iodine-avid, however. Thallium 201 has been employed as a general tumor marker for thyroid cancers. More recently, with the development of whole-body scanners, PET imaging is being used for regional and systemic scanning (Fig. 29.20). This method, which entails the use of fluorodeoxyglucose, is very sensitive but not as specific as are the radioactive iodine agents for thyroid cell lines. Octreotide nuclear scanning is useful for detecting and staging medullary thyroid cancer (603).

Tumors of the thyroid bed include thyroid cancer (Fig. 29.21), medullary thyroid cancer, and parathyroid disorders (604). Lymphoma (Fig. 29.22 and 29.23) and metastases (Fig. 29.24) rarely involve the thyroid. Magnetic resonance imaging and CT scans allow a global yet detailed staging of the mediastinum and the neck. But CT is limited because iodinated contrast hinders subsequent postoperative nuclear scanning and ablation in patients who are potential candidates for radioiodine therapy. Ultrasonography has a more limited role outside the immediate thyroid bed but can be very useful for image-guided FNA. We use graphical worksheets to help coordinate information between imaging and clinical follow-up (Fig. 29.25). Sonography often is requested for evaluation of the thyroid gland when a nodule is discovered incidentally (602). This may not add any useful information if exploration of the opposite lobe is performed routinely at lobectomy. The best single modality for staging is probably MRI, because of excellent tissue discrimination, for which contrast is not necessary. Regional extension of disease to the mediastinum is easily staged in the coronal and sagittal planes (Fig. 29.26).

Anaplastic tumors (Fig. 29.27) can be well evaluated with contrast CT without iodine considerations. Because of the low position of the thyroid gland in the central compartment and the frequent penetration to the upper mediastinum, CT scans of the thyroid bed often are degraded by artifact. The neck and superior mediastinum are best evaluated by 3- to 5-mm-section CT images (Fig. 29.28) obtained while the patient's arms are positioned along his or her sides. Because of artifact from the shoulder, section thickness in broader patients must be extended to 8 to 10 mm. Another maneuver in attempting to reduce shoulder artifact is to draw the shoulders down passively or actively by having patients reach for their toes.

Our thyroid CT protocol includes a precontrast survey of the thyroid bed to take advantage of the native iodine concentration within the gland (Fig. 29.29). Well-planned contrast CT scans can be reformatted in the coronal or sagittal planes to outline the cephalad (Fig. 29.30) or caudal (Fig. 29.31) extent of disease. Although no single imaging modality can be used to screen, diagnose, and stage thyroid cancer, most thyroid cancers that are detected early require no cross-sectional imaging in the absence of established thyroid cancer risk factors. Most of the attention of thyroid imaging tends to be focused on evaluation of the cervical and paratracheal lymph nodes. However, one must keep in mind that the retropharyngeal lymph nodes are at risk following any form of treatment. These nodes are clinically occult, and we have seen several cases of isolated retropharyngeal nodal involvement without associated nodal involvement of the jugular or paratracheal nodal groups.

Follow-up surveillance imaging of thyroid cancer is performed primarily by the nuclear medicine service with ^{131}I scans. Cross-sectional imaging can be performed with MRI (Fig. 29.32) or noncontrast CT scans to stage the neck and mediastinum and confirm the nuclear findings. Contrast-enhanced CT is acceptable when the residual or recurrent disease is no longer iodine-avid (Fig. 29.33). Computed tomography and nuclear images can be co-registered to improve the overall accuracy of the combined modalities (605). Access to an agent that does not require withdrawal of thyroid hormone replacement for follow-up surveillance scanning would be convenient. Positron emission tomography or the less expensive ^{201}Tl single photon emission computed tomography scans may fulfill that role (606). Fluorodeoxyglucose (FDG) PET has been shown to have a sensitivity of 60% to 71% (607,608). Furthermore, the volume of disease detected by PET can risk stratify patients when correlated with cross-sectional scans (609).

Medullary carcinoma of the thyroid gland requires very careful follow-up imaging (Fig. 29.34), particularly in the familial population. Scans often are requested for rising CEA levels. ^{111}In octreotide scans can locate more disease than cross-sectional scans (603,610,611).

Parathyroid lesions usually are manifest symptomatically via metabolic disturbances or are detected incidentally on biochemical screening. These conditions usually are due to adenomas (Fig.

29.35) or hyperplastic glands (Fig. 29.36). Because of their benign nature, most patients undergo neck exploration with exposure of all parathyroid glands. Not all surgeons obtain preoperative localization scans in the virgin neck. The reported success rate for experienced thyroid surgeons approaches 95% cure of hyperparathyroidism (612). Thallium–Tc-99m subtraction scan was the method used until sestamibi proved simpler to perform and interpret. Some would argue that sestamibi scans are not cost effective (613). Cross-sectional imaging (Fig. 29.37) as an adjunct to sestamibi scanning is most useful in the setting of persistent symptomatology after neck exploration. Preoperative localization (612) and intraoperative gamma-probe guided surgery with sestamibi (614) also approach 95% success rate in cure of persistent/recurrent hyperparathyroidism in the reoperated population. If the occult adenoma is not revealed on imaging of the neck and entire mediastinum, catheter angiography may be necessary to locate or ablate the adenoma(s).

Parathyroid cancer (Fig. 29.38) may be suspected before surgery by excessively high PTH levels or relatively large or invasive-appearing masses in the (posterior) thyroid bed. Despite the preponderance of benign parathyroid lesions, these lesions must be staged carefully, with particular attention paid to the recurrent laryngeal nerves and the tracheoesophageal margin.

Benign disorders of the thyroid gland can cause advanced local organ dysfunction (Fig. 29.39). Large goiters may require resection or debulking because of continued growth despite medical therapy. Either MRI or CT scanning can outline the mass accurately relative to the vital structures of the central compartment. Imaging must outline fully the mediastinal component, particularly in reference to the vascular plane. Most masses remain prevascular, bulging forward between the innominate and left common carotid arteries. Retrosternal extension should be reported promptly to the surgeon because of the compressive effects within the thoracic inlet, especially given the tendency of goiter to undergo spontaneous hemorrhage (615). Radiologists must be aware that goiters assume different configurations in the supine and erect positions. Further, the degree of mediastinal penetration often changes under anesthesia. Involvement of the posterior mediastinum is rare in benign disease. Rarely, a dominant nodule or adenoma enlarges rapidly due to intralesional hemorrhage (Fig. 29.40).

Locally aggressive thyroid cancer puts the recurrent laryngeal nerves at risk primarily and at neck dissection. Occasionally, the venous system is invaded, resulting in tumor thrombus. Careful attention to contrast parameters is necessary with CT (Fig. 29.41) to identify this feature. On various sequences, MRI can readily outline the thrombus relative to the vena cava (Fig. 29.32).

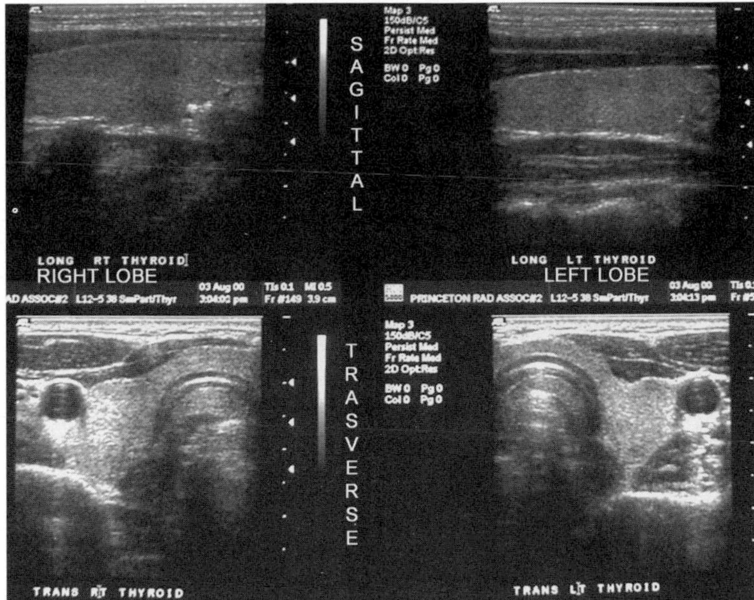

Figure 29.18 Normal thyroid sonogram. Upper and lower panels show sagittal and transverse views of the right and left lobes as labeled demonstrate normal size and homogeneous echotexture of the glands.

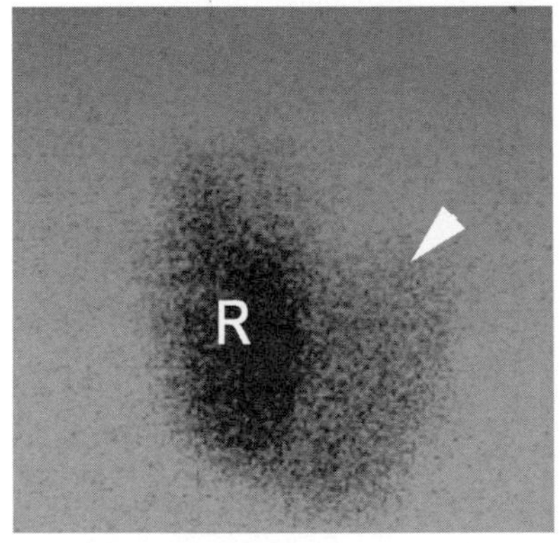

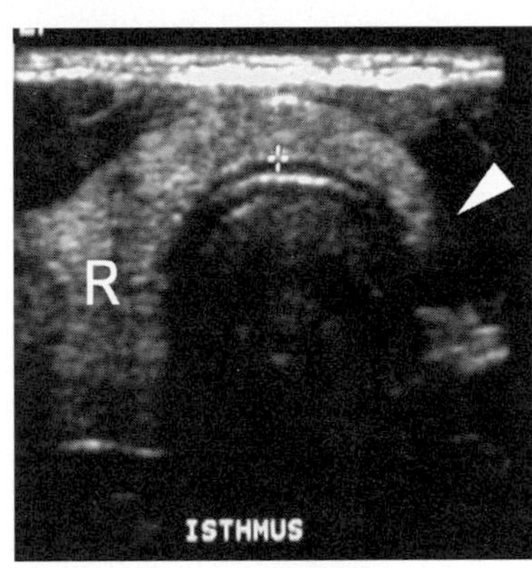

A,B

Figure 29.19 Pseudotumor of thyroid. **A:** Nuclear radioiodine scan shows apparent dominant thyroid mass in a patient with clinical right thyroid prominence (*R*). **B:** Thyroid sonogram shows that the clinical and nuclear scan impressions are related to congenital absence of the left lobe (*arrowhead*).

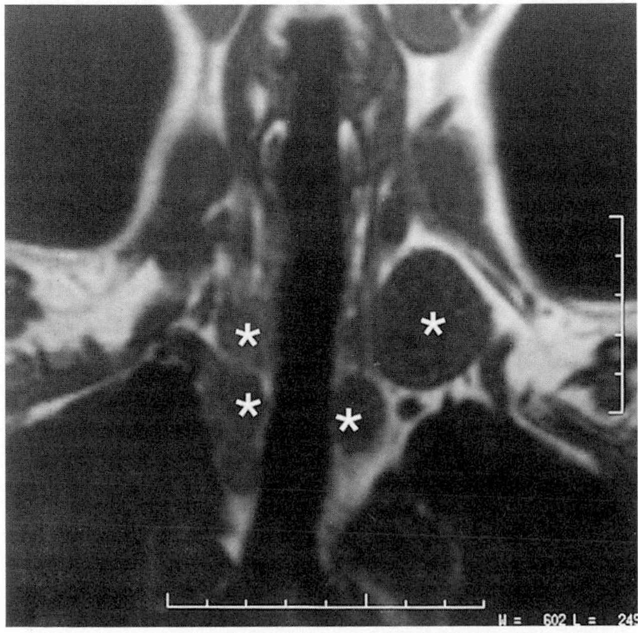

A

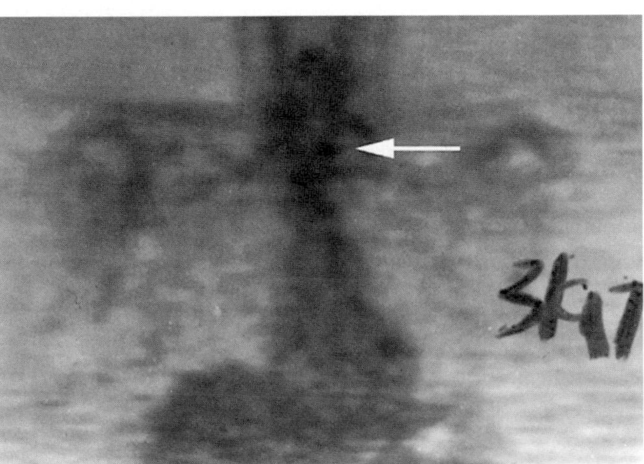

B

Figure 29.20 Follow-up of differentiated thyroid cancer. **A:** Coronal T1-weighted magnetic resonance imaging covering the neck and mediastinum, showing persistent bilateral adenopathy (*asterisk*) despite absence of corresponding abnormality on ^{131}I scan. **B:** Coronal fluorodeoxyglucose-positron emission tomography view, obtained because of the discrepancy, shows one small focus of increased activity (*arrow*), confirming sterilized tumor in the lymph nodes.

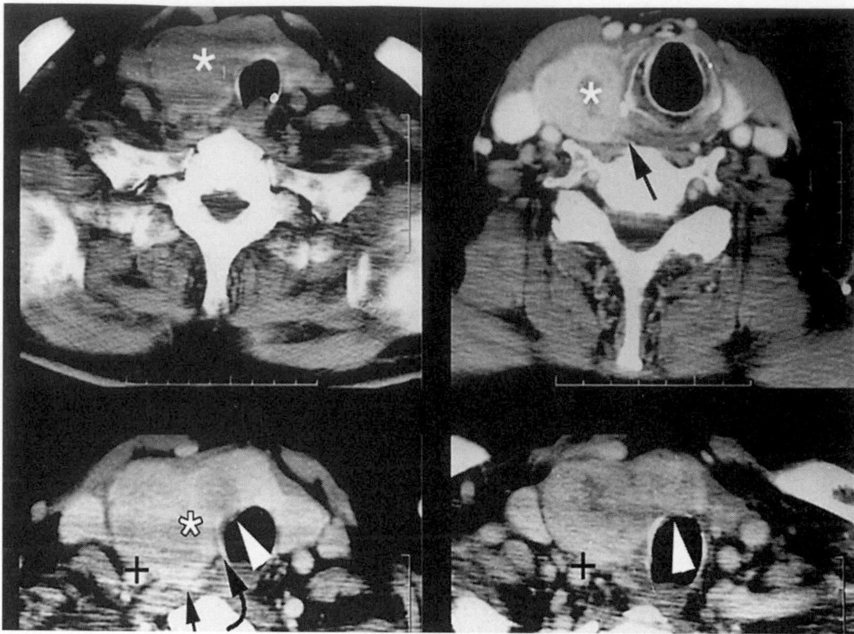

Figure 29.21 Large thyroid cancer. Precontrast (*upper left*) axial computed tomography shows heterogeneous mass expanding the right lobe and isthmus (*asterisk*). Serial postcontrast axial views (beginning with the *upper right panel*) reveal overall size of the mass (*asterisk*), early tracheal invasion (*arrowheads*), infiltration of the tracheoesophageal groove (*curved arrow*), and poor margin with the prevertebral fascia (*arrow*) and internal carotid artery (+).

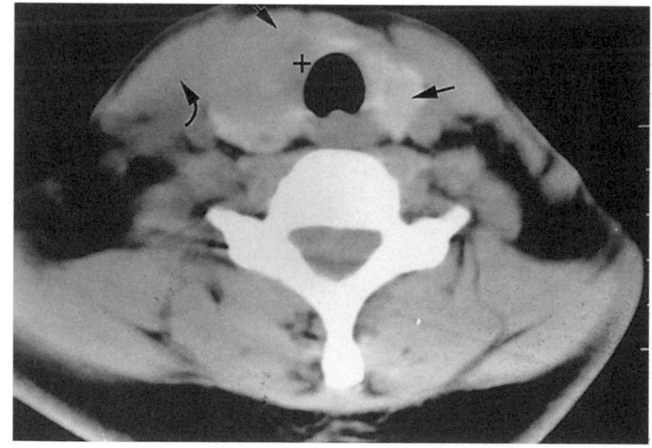

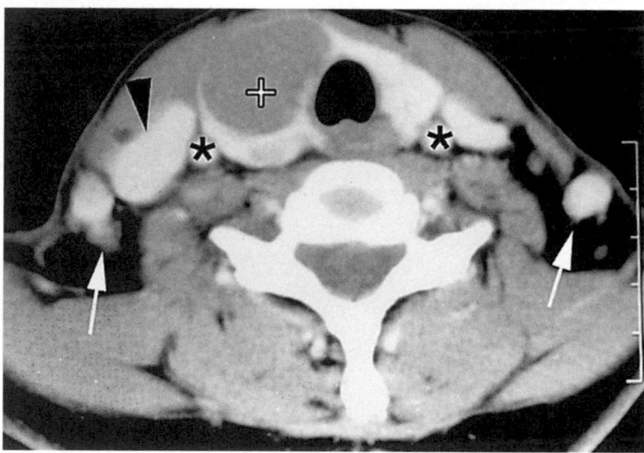

Figure 29.22 Thyroid lymphoma. Matched precontrast **(A)** and postcontrast **(B)** axial computed tomography of low-attenuation lesion expanding the right lobe (+) with less apparent lesions on the precontrast series (*arrows*). Note common carotid artery (*asterisk*), internal jugular vein (*arrowhead*), sternocleidomastoid (*curved arrow*), and external jugular vein (*long arrow*).

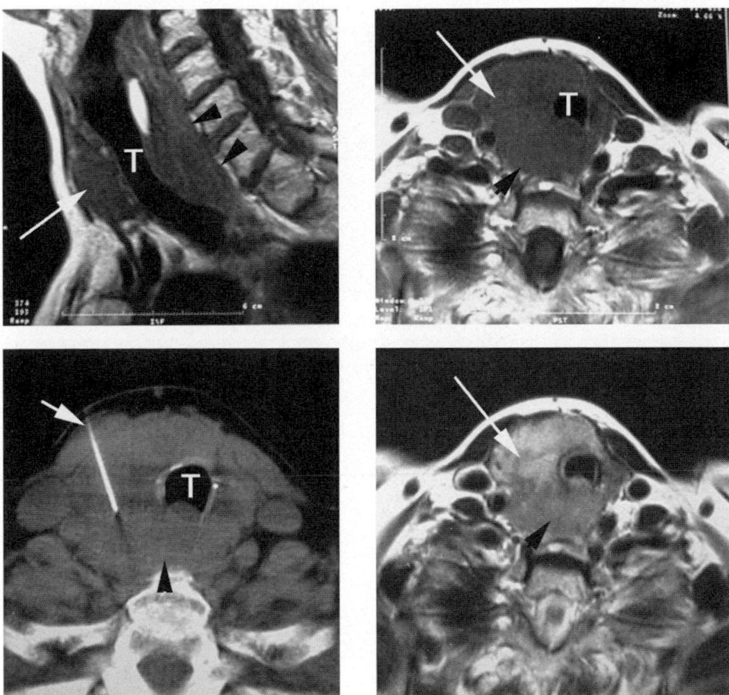

Figure 29.23 Thyroid lymphoma. Magnetic resonance imaging collage from upper left includes sagittal T1, axial T1, axial T2, and axial CT images showing large infiltrating mass (*long arrows*) expanding the gland invading the prevertebral space (*arrowheads*) displacing the trachea (*T*). The computed tomography image without contrast shows core biopsy of mass (*short arrow*).

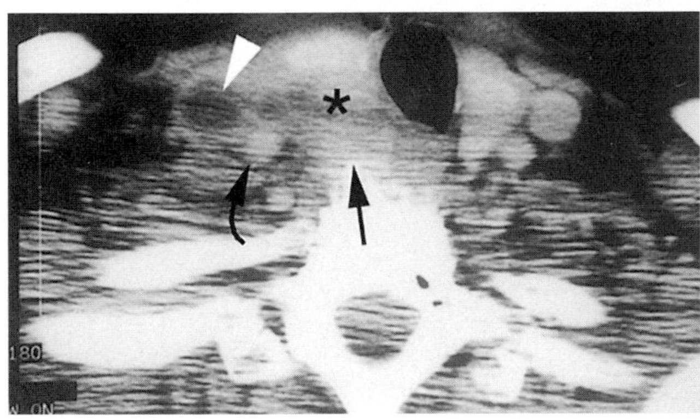

Figure 29.24 Metastatic disease. Enhanced axial computed tomography at thyroid bed (*asterisk*) infiltrating the prevertebral plane (*arrow*). Note common carotid artery (*curved arrow*) and tumor thrombus in the internal jugular vein (*arrowhead*).

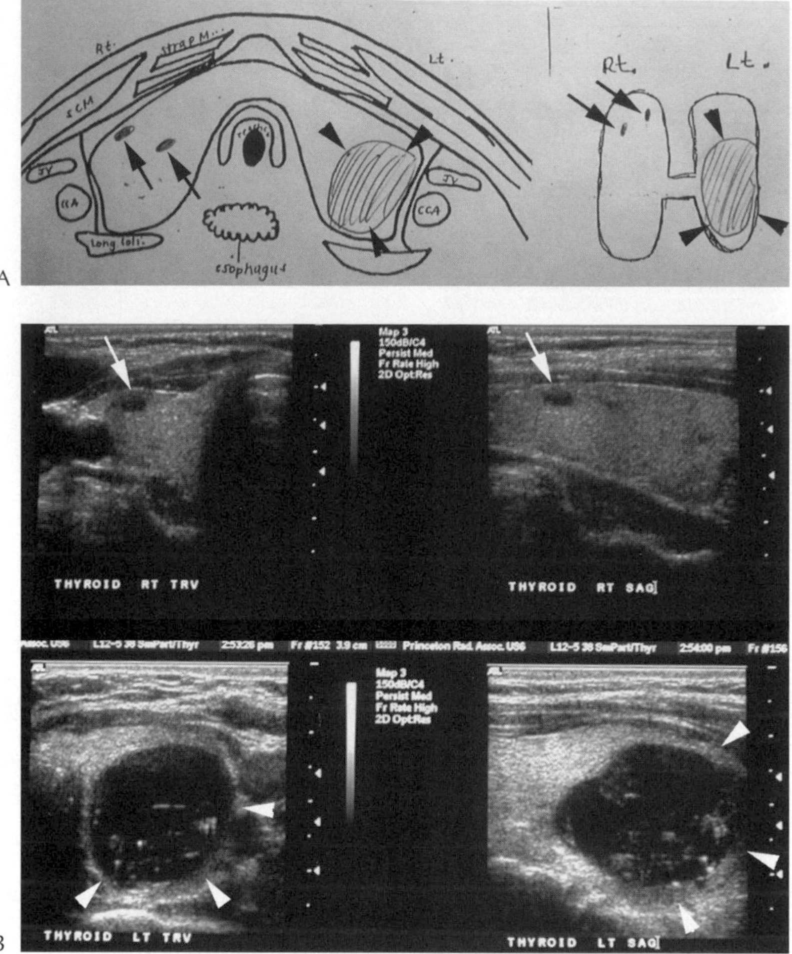

Figure 29.25 Imaging worksheet. **A:** Graphical worksheet outlines the position of the important findings in a reproducible manner showing transverse view on left and coronal view on right. Dominant left lobe mass (*arrowheads*) and smaller right lobe nodules (*arrows*). **B:** Ultrasound collage of thyroid gland with right lobe upper panels and left lobe in lower panels shows small right upper pole nodules (*arrows*) and dominant mass arising in lower pole of left lobe (*arrowheads*).

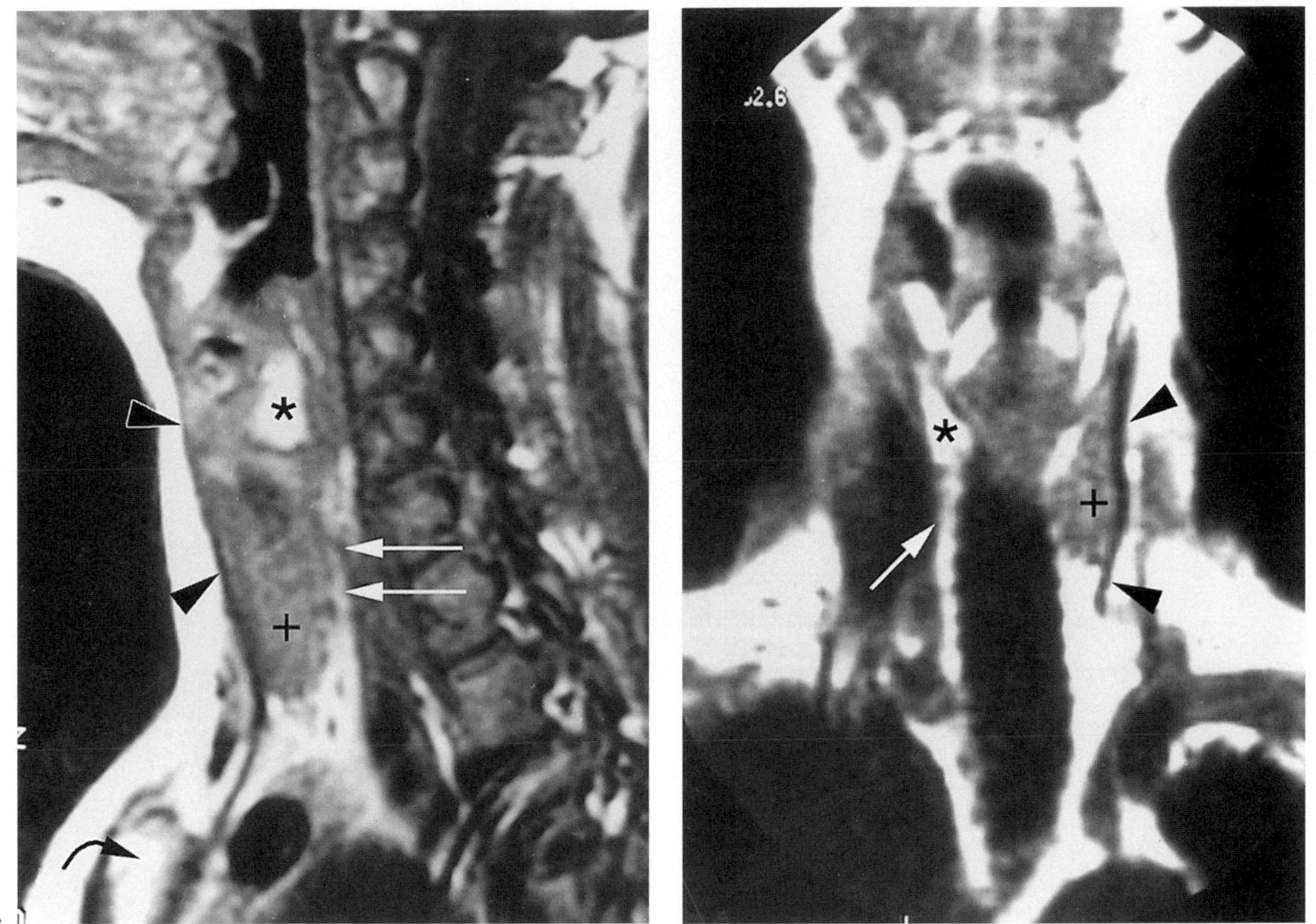

Figure 29.26 Role of magnetic resonance imaging. In addition to axial views, magnetic resonance imaging can project sagittal **(A)** and coronal **(B)** views for disorders that often penetrate the inlet. Note normal thyroid lobe (+), tracheoesophageal groove (*arrows*) after right lobectomy, outer investing fascia (*arrowheads*), cricoid cartilage (*asterisk*), and manubrium (*curved arrow*).

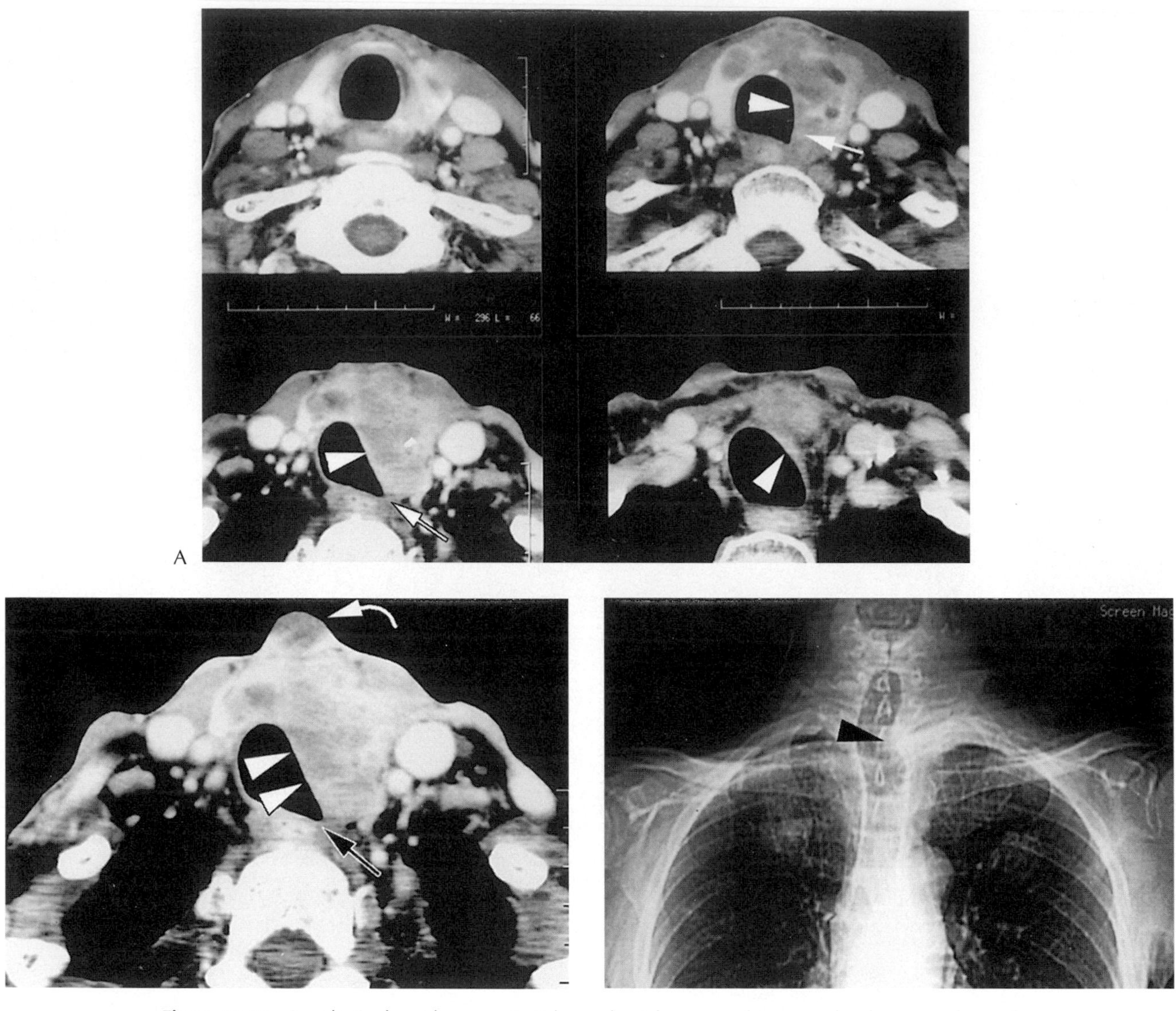

Figure 29.27 Anaplastic thyroid cancer. **A:** Enhanced axial computed tomography shows rapid growth of thyroid mass after initial response to combined therapy. **B:** Note tracheal invasion (*arrowheads*) and tracheoesophageal groove invasion (*arrows*) with penetration of skin (*curved arrow*). **C:** Scout view also shows tracheal compromise (*arrowhead*).

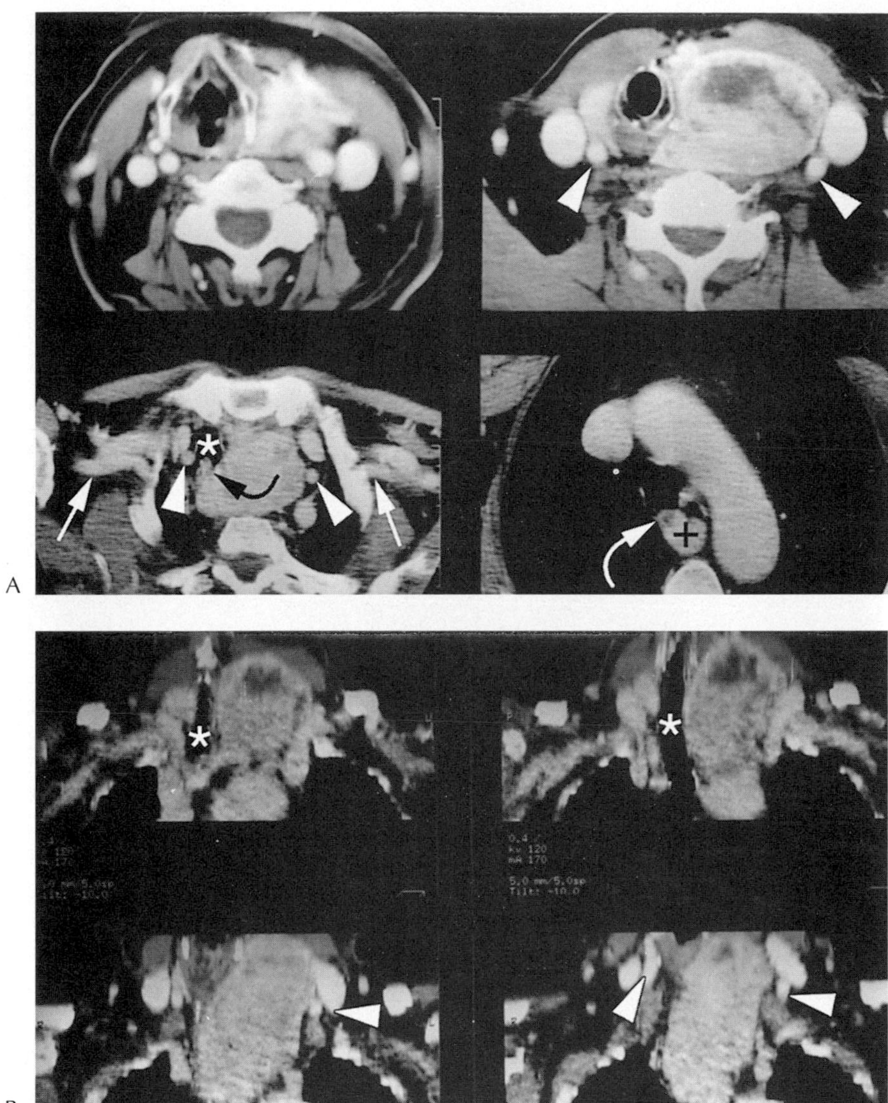

Figure 29.28 Tracking large thyroid masses. **A:** Serial enhanced axial computed tomographic images at the low neck show large mass expanding the left lobe, penetrating the inlet to the posterior mediastinum (+). Bolus technique gives high contrast in the neck without streak artifact at the important inlet landmarks. **B:** Coronal reformatted images lay out the cephalocaudal position of the mass relative to mediastinal structures. Note trachea (*asterisk*), esophagus (*curved arrow*), subclavian arteries (*arrows*), and carotid arteries (*arrowheads*).

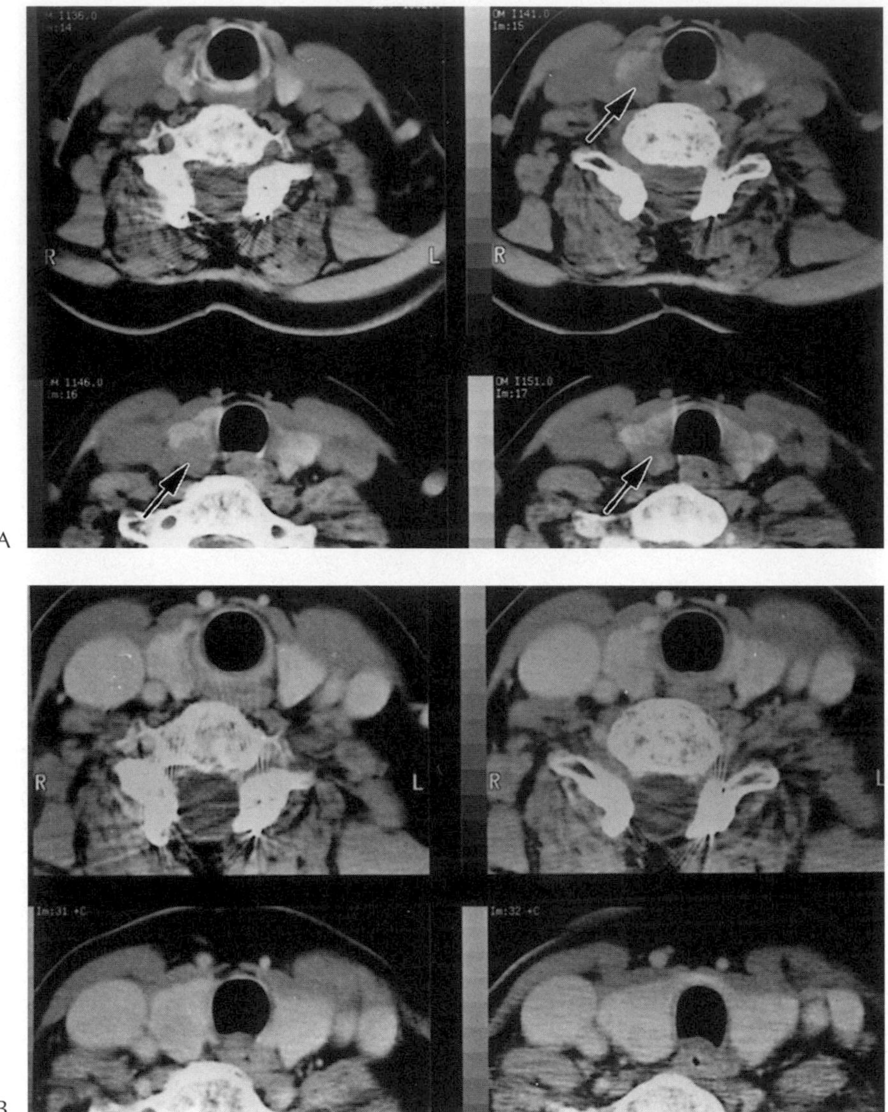

Figure 29.29 Value of precontrast images. **A:** Serial axial computed tomographic images through thyroid bed reveal a focal lesion (*arrows*) within the right lobe against a background of high attenuation related to native iodine accumulation in normal thyroid tissue. **B:** Postcontrast axial computed tomographic images matched to precontrast shows how postcontrast-only imaging can obscure lesions, revealing only the less important cystic or colloid abnormalities.

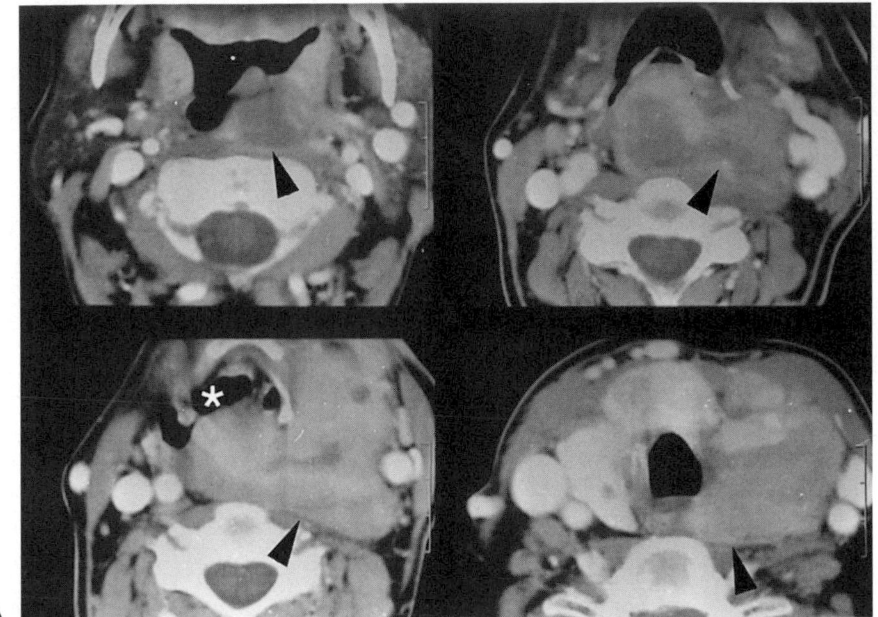

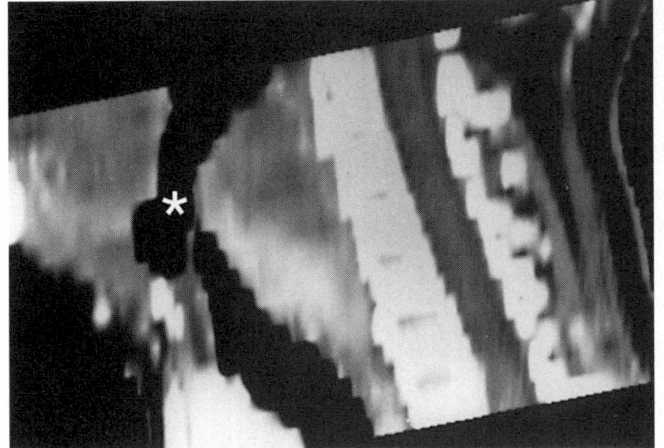

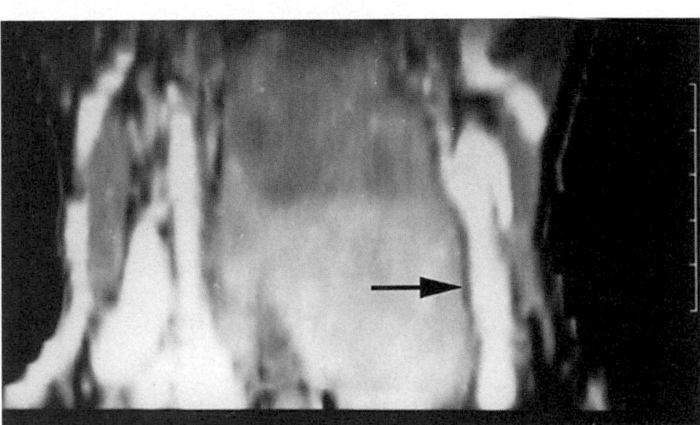

Figure 29.30 Large goiter. **A:** Serial enhanced axial computed tomography of retropharyngeal extension of enlarged left lobe in addition to isthmus. The airway is moderately compromised (*asterisk*), and the prevertebral plane is preserved (*arrowheads*). **B:** Sagittal reformatted view shows extrinsic partial supraglottic airway compromise (*asterisk*). **C:** Coronal reformatted view shows lateral displacement of the left common carotid artery (*arrow*).

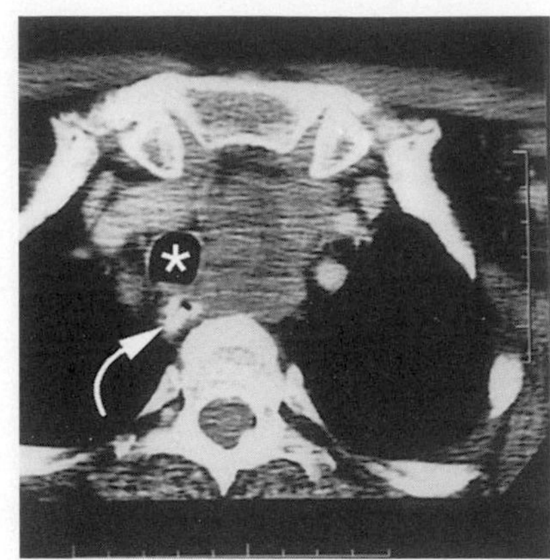

A

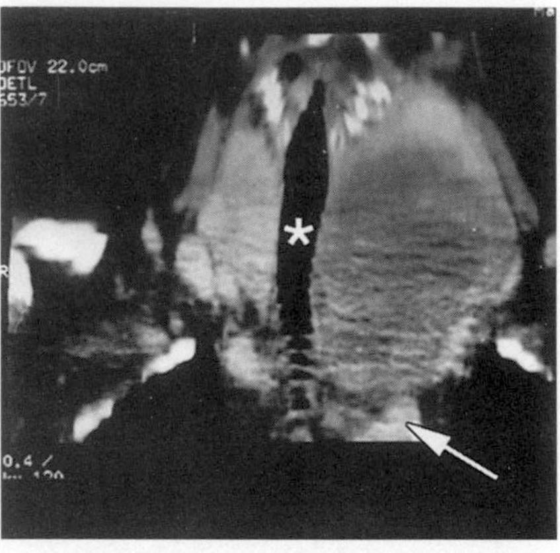

B

Figure 29.31 Limited mediastinal penetration. Enhanced axial computed tomographic view **(A)** and reformatted coronal view **(B)** of bulky left-lobe mass with limited mediastinal penetration. Note trachea (*asterisk*) and oral contrast paste in esophagus (*curved arrow*). Note aortic arch (*long arrow*).

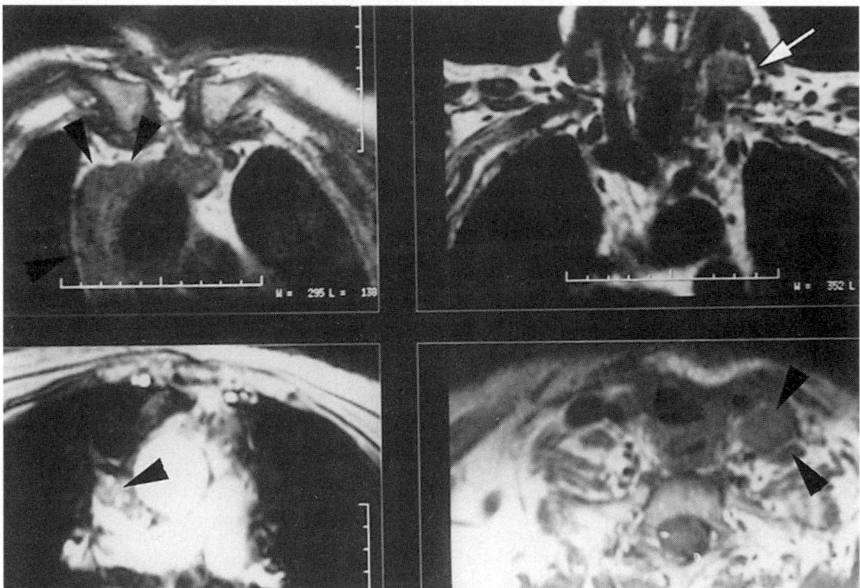

Figure 29.32 Invasive thyroid cancer. Coronal T1-weighted magnetic resonance imaging (*upper panel*), axial gradient echo (*lower left*), and axial T1-weighted views (*lower right*) show residual disease in the neck status (*arrow*) after thyroidectomy. Images on the left show large intravenous tumor thrombus (*arrowheads*) that remained *in situ* at the brachiocephalic vein and cava.

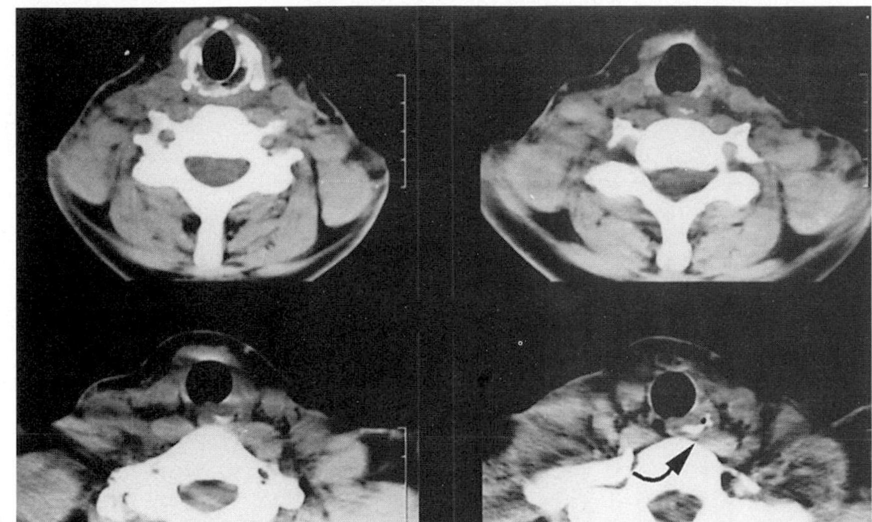

A

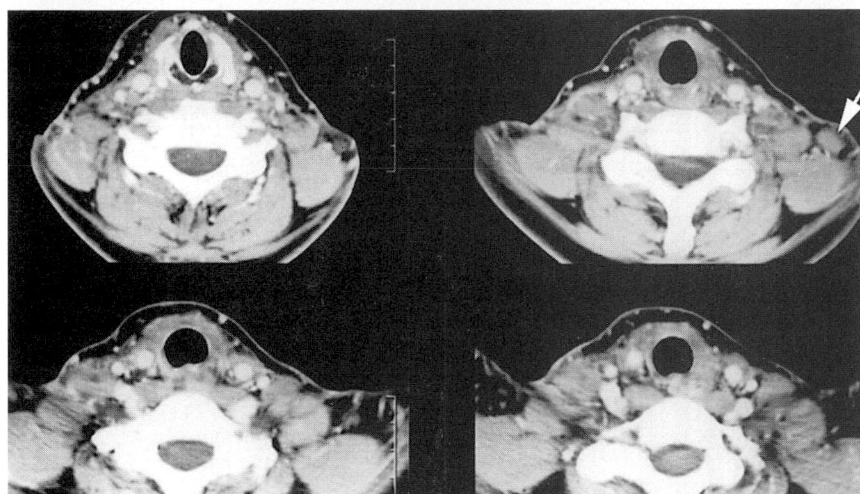

B

Figure 29.33 Postoperative follow-up. **A:** Precontrast series reveals thickening within the central compartment after thyroidectomy. Note oral contrast paste in esophagus. **B:** Postcontrast series shows no abnormality in thyroid bed. There is a suspicious lymph node at the left posterior triangle (*arrow*). [Also note common carotid artery (*curved arrow*) and internal jugular vein.]

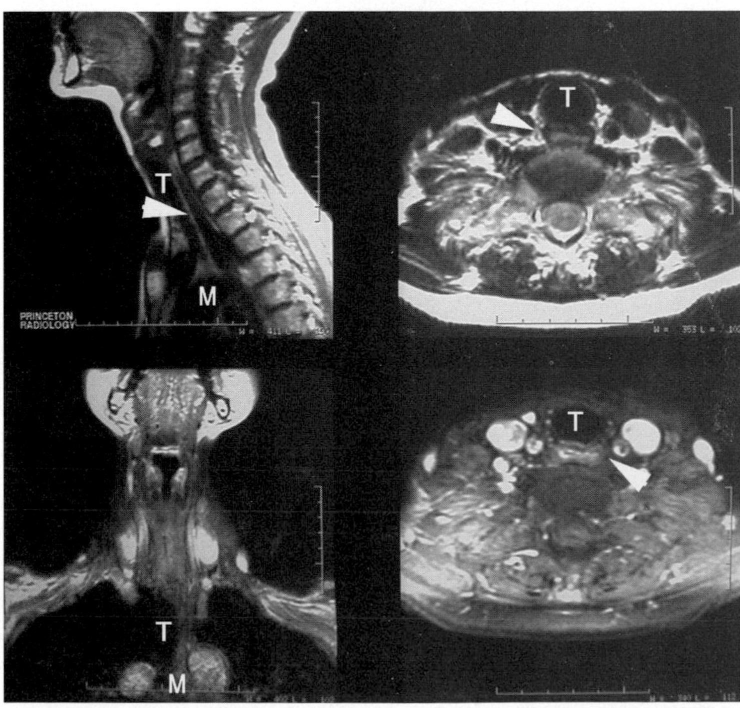

Figure 29.34 Magnetic resonance imaging surveillance. Magnetic resonance image collage from upper left includes sagittal T1, axial T2, contrast axial T1, and coronal T1. Images show excellent coverage of the tracheoesophageal groove (*arrowheads*), mediastinum (*M*), and trachea (*T*).

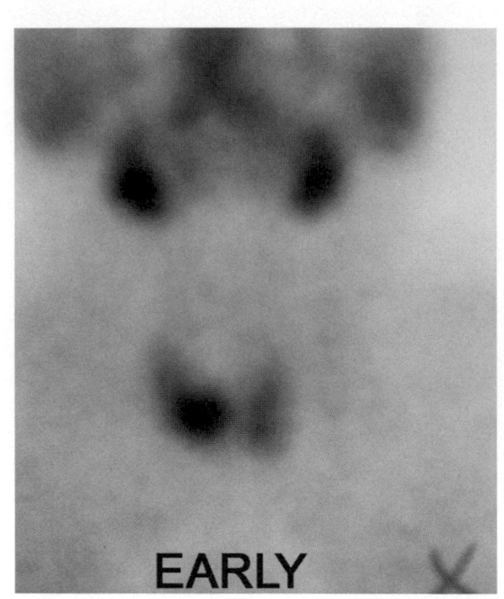

A

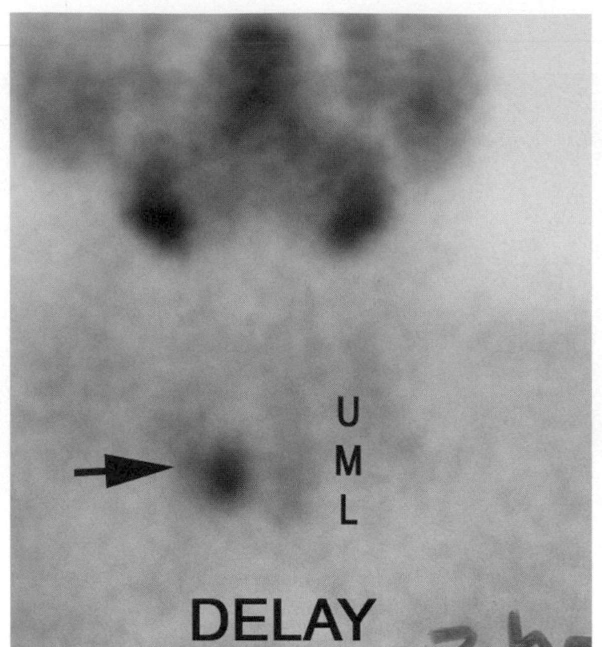

B

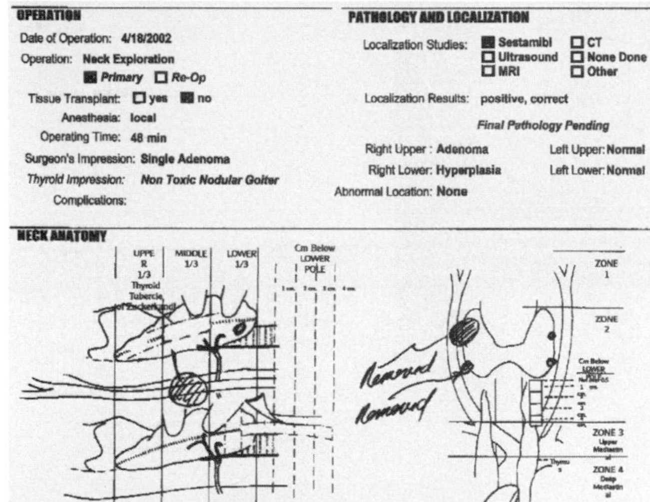

OPERATION

Date of Operation: **4/18/2002**

Operation: **Neck Exploration**

■ *Primary* □ *Re-Op*

Tissue Transplant: □ yes ■ no

Anesthesia: **local**

Operating Time: **48 min**

Surgeon's Impression: **Single Adenoma**

Thyroid Impression: ***Non Toxic Nodular Goiter***

Complications:

PATHOLOGY AND LOCALIZATION

Localization Studies: ■ Sestamibi □ CT □ Ultrasound □ None Done □ MRI □ Other

Localization Results: **positive, correct**

Final Pathology Pending

Right Upper : **Adenoma** Left Upper: **Normal**

Right Lower: **Hyperplasia** Left Lower: **Normal**

Abnormal Location: **None**

NECK ANATOMY

C

Figure 29.35 Parathyroid adenoma. Early **(A)** early and delayed **(B)** technetium sestamibi scans of the neck show persistent activity at the right thyroid bed, interpreted to be at the mid-pole. **C:** Surgical graphic sheet shows adenoma at the mid-upper pole and an unanticipated hyperplastic gland at the lower pole. (Case courtesy of Paul LoGerfo, M.D.)

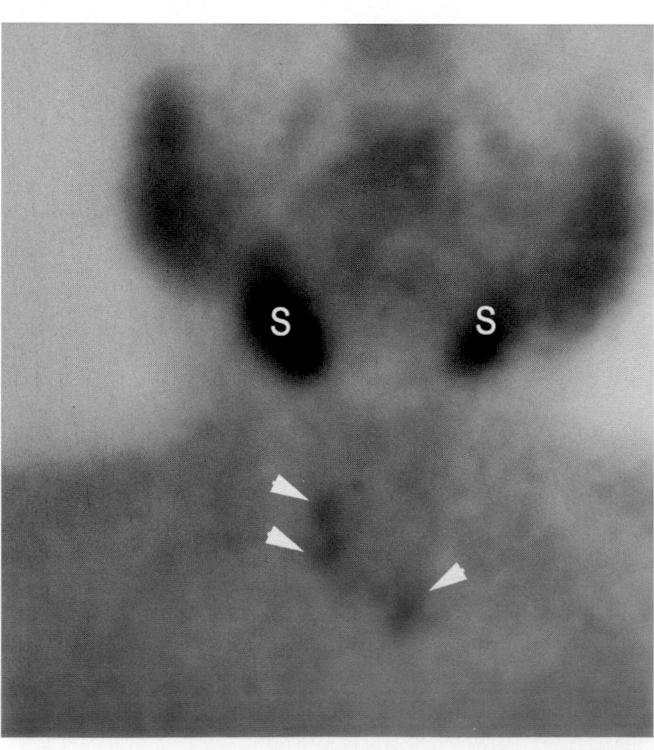

Figure 29.36 Parathyroid hyperplasia. Coronal planar view at 2-hour delay of sestamibi image shows multiple foci of activity in the thyroid bed (*arrowheads*) confirmed to be related to parathyroid hyperplasia. Background salivary tissue (*S*).

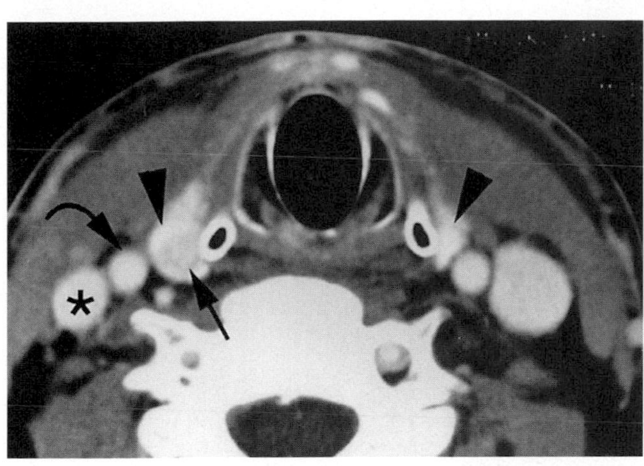

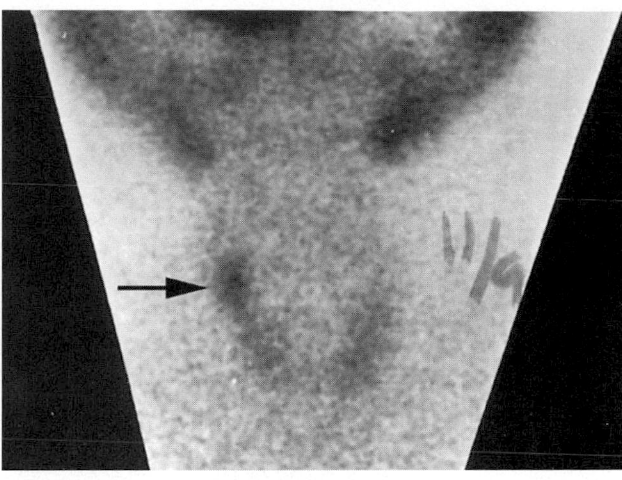

Figure 29.37 Parathyroid adenoma. **A:** Enhanced axial computed tomography of the neck after parathyroid dissection, showing a moderately enhancing, well-circumscribed lesion (*arrow*) against the intense contrast enhancement of the thyroid gland (*arrowheads*) in the upper pole. Note common carotid artery (*curved arrow*) and internal jugular vein (*asterisk*). **B:** Coronal sestamibi view confirms the solitary adenoma at the upper pole (*arrow*) seen on computed tomography.

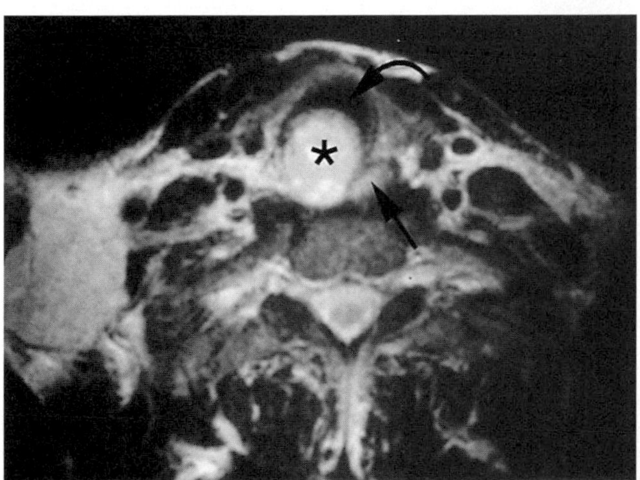

Figure 29.38 Parathyroid carcinoma. Axial T2-weighted magnetic resonance imaging shows a large submucosal lesion bulging from the tracheoesophageal groove into the tracheal lumen (*asterisk*), compromising the airway (*curved arrow*) and invading the esophagus (*arrow*).

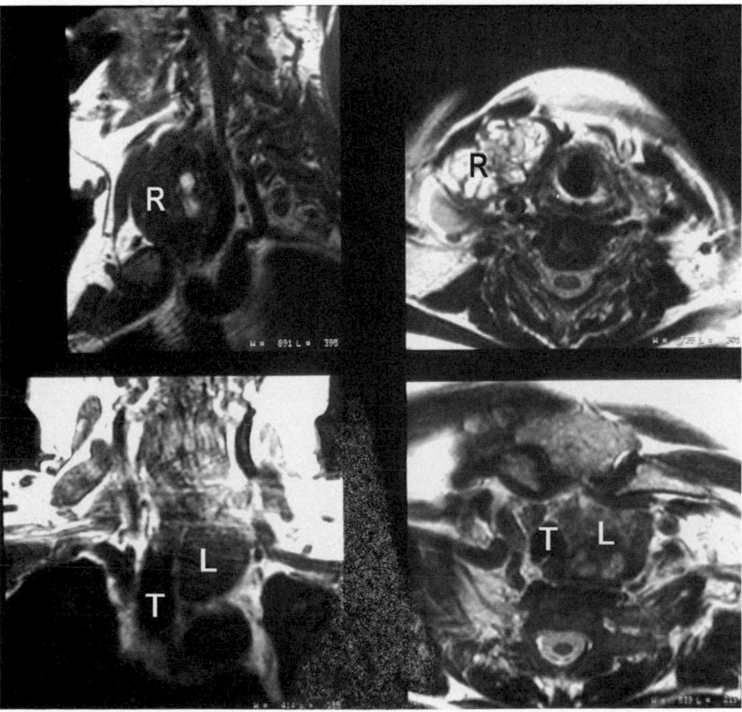

Figure 29.39 Huge chronic goiter. Magnetic resonance image collage from upper left includes sagittal T1, axial T2 lower neck, axial T2 at inlet, and coronal T1, and shows large right lobe mass (*R*) in thyroid bed and penetration of thoracic inlet by left lobe mass (*L*). Trachea (*T*) is deviated.

Figure 29.40 Acute airway compromise. (Clockwise from *upper left*) Coronal T1, midsagittal T1, axial T1, and axial T2 views obtainable only after percutaneous needle aspiration partially relieved airway distress. Surgery produced hemorrhagic adenoma. Note tracheal lumen (*asterisk*), mass (+), hemorrhage high signal (*arrow*), and esophageal mucosa (*curved arrow*).

A

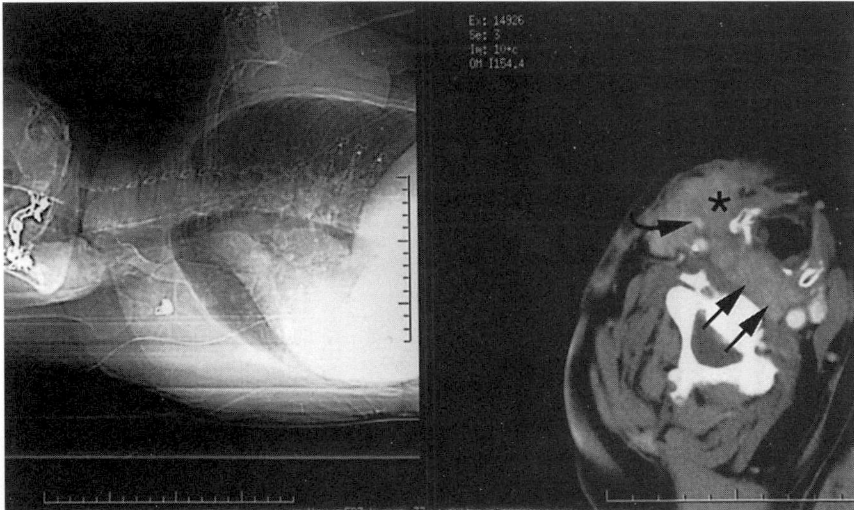

B

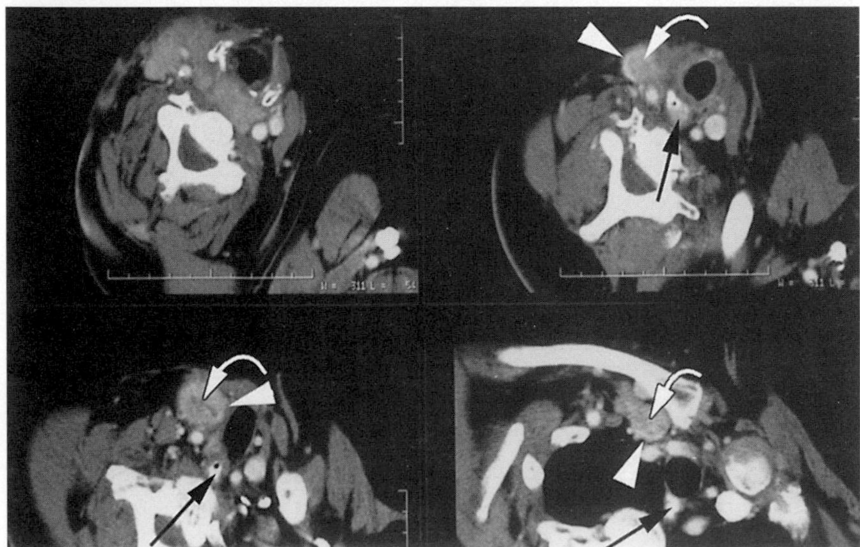

Figure 29.41 Invasive thyroid cancer. **A:** Scout lateral view (*left*) and corresponding enhanced axial view (*right*) of a patient who is in the lateral decubitus position and could not position supine. Note right thyroid mass (*asterisk*) invading the retropharyngeal space (*arrows*), and note jugular vein (*curved arrow*). **B:** Serial enhanced axial views show same findings. Note tumor thrombus within vein (*curved arrows*) outlined by contrast (*arrowheads*); also note oral contrast outlining the esophagus (*long arrows*).

REFERENCES

1. Thompson J. Historical notes. In: Smithers D, ed. *Tumors of the thyroid. Neoplastic diseases at various sites,* vol 6. Edinburgh: Churchill Livingstone, 1970.
2. Werner SC. Historical resume. In: Ingbar SH, Braverman LE, ed. *Werner's the thyroid.* Philadelphia: JB Lippincott, 1986.
3. Galen C. Definitions medical. In: Kuhn G, ed. *Bronchocele, No. 398* (cited by Thompson). 1824.
4. Reverdin J. Note sur vingtdeux operations de goitre. *Rev Med Suisse Romande* 1983;3:169.
5. Graves R. Clinical lectures. *Lond Med Surg J* (Part II) 1835;7:516.
6. Von Basedow C. Exophthalmos dutch hypertrophil ties zellgewebes in tier angankohle. *Wochenschr Heilk* 1840;6:197,220.
7. Halsted W. *Surgical papers,* vol 2. Baltimore: Johns Hopkins University Press, 1924:257.
8. Kocher T. Veberkropf sextirpation and ihre folgan. *Arch Chir* 1883;29:254.
9. Harington C, Barger G. Chemistry of thyroxine, III: constitution and synthesis of thyroxine. *Biochem J* 1927;22:169.
10. Ries L, Miller B, Hankey B, et al. *SEER cancer statistics review, 1973–1991: tables and graphs, NCI.* Publication No. 94-2789. Bethesda, MD: National Institutes of Health, 1994.
11. Boring C, Squires T, Tong T. Cancer statistics, 1993. *CA Cancer J Clin* 1993;43:7.
12. Wingo P, Tong T, Bolden S. Cancer statistics, 1995. *CA Cancer J Clin* 1995;45:8.
13. Cutler S, Young J, eds. *3rd National Cancer Survey incidence data, NCI.* Monograph No. 41. Washington, DC: Department of Health, Education and Welfare, 1975.
14. Thompson N, Nishiyama R, Harness J. Thyroid cancer. *Curr Probl Surg* 1978;25:1.
15. Parkin D, Stiller C, Draper G, et al. International incidence of childhood cancer. In: *IARC scientific publications.* Lyon: International Agency for Research on Cancer, 1988.
16. Bondeson L, Ljungberg O. Occult thyroid carcinoma at autopsy in Malmo, Sweden. *Cancer* 1981;47:319–323.
17. Lang W, Borrusch H, Bauer L. Occult carcinomas of the thyroid: evaluation of 1,020 sequential autopsies. *Am J Clin Pathol* 1988;90:72–76.
18. Sampson R. Prevalence and significance of occult thyroid cancer. In: De Groot L, Frohman L, Kaplan E, et al., eds. *Radiation associated thyroid carcinoma.* New York: Grune & Stratton, 1987:137–153.
19. Vander J, Gaston E, Dawber T. The significance of nontoxic nodules: final report of a 15 year study of the incidence of thyroid malignancy. *Ann Intern Med* 1968;69:537–540.
20. Mortensen J, Woolner L, Bennett W. Gross and microscopic findings in clinically normal thyroid glands. *J Clin Endocrinol Metab* 1955;15:1270–1280.
21. Rice C. Incidence of nodules in the thyroid: a comparative study of symptomless thyroid glands removed at autopsy and hyperfunctioning goiters operatively removed. *Arch Surg* 1932;24:505–515.
22. Fukunaga F, Lockett L. Thyroid carcinoma in the Japanese in Hawaii. *Arch Pathol* 1971;92:6.
23. Fukunaga F, Yatani R. Geographic pathology of occult thyroid carcinoma. *Cancer* 1975;36:1095.
24. Gordon D, Huvos A, Strong E. Medullary carcinoma of thyroid. *Cancer* 1973;31:915.
25. Blum M. Managing the solitary thyroid nodule: the role of needle biopsy. *Ann Intern Med* 1977;87:375.
26. Woolner LB, Beahrs O, Block B, et al. Classification and prognosis of thyroid carcinoma: a study of 885 cases observed in a 30 year period. *Am J Surg* 1961; 102:354.
27. Sampson R, Oka H, Key C, et al. Metastases from occult thyroid cancer. An autopsy study from Hiroshima and Nagasaki, Japan. *Cancer* 1970;25:803–811.
28. Nishiyami R, Ludwig G, Thompson N. The prevalence of small papillary thyroid carcinoma in 100 consecutive necropsies in an American population. In: DeGroot L, ed. *Radiation associated thyroid carcinoma.* Orlando, FL: Grune & Stratton, 1977.
29. Pottern L, Stone B, Day N, et al. Thyroid cancer in Connecticut, 1935–1975: an analysis by cell type. *Am J Epidemiol* 1980;112:764.
30. Pettersson B, Adami H, Wilander E, Coleman M. Trends in thyroid cancer incidence in Sweden, 1958–1981, by histopathologic type. *Int J Cancer* 1991;48:28.
31. Levi F, Franceschi S, Te V, et al. Descriptive epidemiology of thyroid cancer in the Swiss canton of Vaud. *J Cancer Res Clin Oncol* 1990;116:639.
32. Akslen L, Haldorsen T, Thoresen S, et al. Incidence pattern of thyroid cancer in Norway: influence of birth cohort and time period. *Int J Cancer* 1993;53: 183.
33. Glattre E, Akslen L, Thoresen S, et al. Geographic patterns and trends in the incidence of thyroid cancer in Norway, 1970–1986. *Cancer Detect Prev* 1990;14:625.
34. Hrafnkelsson J, Jonasson J, Sigurdsson G, et al. Thyroid cancer in Iceland, 1955–1984. *Acta Endocrinol* 1988;118:566.
35. LiVolsi V, Asa S. The demise of follicular carcinoma of the thyroid. *Thyroid* 1994;4:233.
36. Rallison M, Dobyns B, Keating F, et al. Thyroid nodularity in children. *JAMA* 1975;233:1069–1072.
37. Trowbridge E, Matovinovic J, McLaren G, et al. Iodine and goiter in children. *Pediatrics* 1975;56:82–90.
38. Brander A, Viikinkoski P, Nickels J, et al. Thyroid gland: US screening in a random adult population. *Radiology* 1991;181:683–687.
39. Mazzaferri E. Thyroid cancer in thyroid nodules: finding a needle in the haystack. *Am J Med* 1992;93:359–362.
40. Gupta K. Neoplasm of the thyroid. *Clin Geriatr Med* 1995;11:271–290.
41. dos Santos Silva I, Swerdlow A. Sex differences in the risks of hormone-dependent cancers. *Am J Epidemiol* 1993;138:10.
42. Cutler S, Scotto J, Devesa S, et al. 3rd National Cancer Survey. *J Marl Cancer Inst* 1974;53:1565.
43. Aldinger K, Samaan N, Ibanez M, et al. Anaplastic carcinoma of the thyroid. *Cancer* 1978;41:2267.
44. McKenzie A. The natural history of thyroid cancer. *Arch Surg* 1971;102:274.
45. Woolner L. Thyroid carcinoma: pathologic classification with data on prognosis. *Semin Nucl Med* 1971;1:481.
46. Mazzaferri E, Young R, Oertel J, et al. Papillary thyroid carcinoma: the impact of therapy in 576 patients. *Medicine* 1977;56:171.
47. Rose R, Hartfield J, Kelsey M, et al. The association of thyroid cancer and prior irradiation in infancy and childhood. *J Nucl Med* 1963;4:249.
48. Farahati J, Bucsky P, Parlowsky T, et al. Characteristics of differentiated thyroid cancer in children and adolescents with respect to age, sex, and histology. *Cancer* 1997;80:2156–2180.
49. Hayles A, Kennedy R, Beahrs O, et al. Management of the child with thyroid cancer. *JAMA* 1960;173:21.
50. Leeper R. Thyroid cancer. *Med Clin North Am* 1985;69:1079.
51. Tallroth E, Goran W. Multimodality treatment in anaplastic giant cell thyroid carcinoma. *Cancer* 1987;60:1428.
52. Duffy B, Fitzgerald P. Cancer of the thyroid in children: a report of 28 cases. *J Clin Endocrinol Metab* 1950;10:1296.
53. Shore R. Issues and epidemiological evidence regarding radiation induced thyroid cancer. *Radiat Res* 1992;131:99–111.
54. UNSCEAR (United Nations Scientific Committee on the Effects of Atomic Radiation). *Sources and effects of ionizing radiation.* Publication No. E941,IX,11. New York: United Nations, 1994.
55. Ron E, Lubin J, Shore R, et al. Thyroid cancer after exposure to external radiation: a pooled analysis of seven studies. *Radiat Res* 1995;141:259.
56. Brennan M. USSR: medical effects of Chernobyl disaster [News]. *Lancet* 1990;335:1086.
57. Baverstock K, Egloff B, Pinchera A, et al. Thyroid cancer after Chernobyl [Letter]. *Nature* 1992;359:21.
58. Malone J, Unger J, Delange F, et al. Thyroid consequences of Chernobyl accident in the countries of the European Community. *J Endocrinol Invest* 1991;14:701.
59. Schneider A, Shore-Freedman E, Ryo U, et al. Radiation-induced tumors of the head and neck following childhood irradiation. *Medicine* 1985;64:1–15.
60. Schneider A, Ron E. Carcinoma of follicular epithelium. In: Braverman LE, Utiger RD, eds. *Werner and Ingbar's the thyroid: a fundamental and clinical text,* 7th ed. Philadelphia: Lippincott-Raven, 1996:902.
61. Henderson B, Ross R, Pike M, et al. Endogenous hormones as a major factor in human cancer. *Cancer Res* 1982;42:3232.
62. Williams EL. TSH and thyroid cancer. *Horm Metab Res* 1990;23:S72.
63. Ito T, Seyama T, Iwamoto K, et al. Activated RET oncogene in thyroid cancers of children from areas contaminated by Chernobyl accident. *Lancet* 1994; 344:259.
64. Dobyns B, Sheline G, Workman J, et al. Malignant and benign neoplasms of the thyroid in patients treated for hyperthyroidism: a report of the cooperative thyrotoxicosis therapy follow-up study. *J Clin Endocrinol Metab* 1974;38:976.
65. Hall P, Berg G, Bjelkengren G, et al. Cancer mortality after iodine-131 therapy for hyperthyroidism. *Int J Cancer* 1992;50:886.
66. Hall P, Holm L, Lundell G, et al. Cancer risks in thyroid-cancer patients. *Br J Cancer* 1991;64:159.
67. Holm L, Wiklund K, Lundell G, et al. Thyroid cancer after diagnostic doses of iodine-131: a retrospective cohort study. *J Natl Cancer Inst* 1988;80:1131.
68. Franceschi S, Fassina A, Talamini R, et al. Risk factors for thyroid cancer in northern Italy. *Int J Epidemiol* 1989;18:578.
69. Preston-Martin S, Bernstein L, Pike M, et al. Thyroid cancer among young women related to prior thyroid disease and pregnancy history. *Br J Cancer* 1987;55:191.
70. Preston-Martin S, Jin F, Duda M, et al. A case-control study of thyroid cancer in women under age 55 in Shanghai (People's Republic of China). *Cancer Causes Control* 1993;4:431.
71. Ron E, Kleinerman R, Boice J, et al. A population-based case control study of thyroid cancer. *J Natl Cancer Inst* 1987;79:1.
72. Kravdal O, Glattre E, Haldorsen T. Positive correlation between parity and incidence of thyroid cancer: new evidence based on complete Norwegian birth cohorts. *Int J Cancer* 1991;49:831.
73. Belfiore A, LaRosa G, Padova G, et al. The frequency of cold thyroid nodules and thyroid malignancies in patients from an iodine-deficient area. *Cancer* 1987;60:3096.
74. Delamarre J, Capron J-P, Armand A, et al. Thyroid carcinoma in review of the literature. *J Clin Gastroenterol* 1988;10:659.
75. Gruener AC, Zhang H, Nini R, et al. The genetic basis of Cowden's syndrome: three novel mutations in PTEN/MMAC1/TEP1. *Hum Genet* 1998;102:467–473.
76. Wynford-Thomas D. Molecular basis of epithelial tumor genesis: the thyroid model. *Clin Rev Oncogenesis* 1993;4:1.
77. LiVolsi V, Merino M. Pathology of thyroid tumors. In: Thawley S, Panje W, Batsakis J, et al., eds. *Comprehensive management of head and neck tumors.* Philadelphia: WB Saunders, 1987.

78. Carcangiu M, Steeper T, Zampi G, et al. Anaplastic thyroid carcinoma: a study of 70 cases. *Am J Clin Pathol* 1985;83:135.
79. Spires J, Schwartz M, Miller R. Anaplastic thyroid carcinoma: association with differentiated thyroid cancer. *Arch Otolaryngol Head Neck Surg* 1988; 114:40.
80. Demeter J, DeJong S, Lawrence A, et al. Anaplastic thyroid carcinoma: risk factors and outcome. *Surgery* 1991;110:956.
81. Shuan L. Origin, characteristics and behavior of thyroid carcinoma. *J Clin Endocrinol Metab* 1954;14:1309.
82. Kapp D, Livolsi V, Sanders M. Anaplastic carcinoma: well differentiated thyroid cancer. *Yale J Biol Med* 1982;55:521.
83. Nishiyama R, Dunn E, Thompson N. Anaplastic spindle cell and giant cell tumors of the thyroid gland. *Cancer* 1972;30:113.
84. Baker H. Anaplastic thyroid cancer 12 years after radiation. *Cancer* 1969;23:885.
85. Hutter R, Tollefsen H, DeCosse J, et al. Spindle and giant cell metaplasia in papillary carcinoma of the thyroid. *Am J Surg* 1965;110:660.
86. Beirwaltes W. The treatment of thyroid cancer with radioactive I. *Semin Nucl Med* 1978;8:79.
87. Williams E. Pathologic and natural history. In: Duncan W, ed. *Thyroid cancer.* Berlin: Springer-Verlag, 1978:46.
88. Nel C, Van Heerden JL, Goellner J. Anaplastic carcinoma of thyroid. *Mayo Clin Proc* 1985;60:51.
89. Venkatesh Y, Ordonez N, Schultz P. Anaplastic carcinoma of thyroid. *Cancer* 1990;66:321.
90. Ito T, Seyama T, Mizano T. Unique association of p53 mutations with undifferentiated but not differentiated carcinoma of thyroid. *Cancer Res* 1992;52:1369.
91. Boyd J. Development of the human thyroid gland. In: Pitt-Rivers R, Trotter W, eds. *The thyroid,* vol 1. Washington, DC: Butterworths, 1964:9.
92. Nunez E, Gershon M. Development of follicular and parafollicular cells of the mammalian thyroid gland. In: Greenfield L, ed. *Thyroid cancer.* West Palm Beach, FL: CRC Press, 1978:1.
93. Hayes B, Anthony A, Kersham R. Anatomy and development of the thyroid gland. *Ear Nose Throat J* 1985;64:10.
94. Fisher D, Duseault J. Development of the mammalian thyroid gland. In: Greer M, Solomon D, eds. *Handbook of physiology, section 7, endocrinology, vol 3: the thyroid.* Washington, DC: American Physiological Society, 1974.
95. Shepard T. Onset of function in the human fetal thyroid: biochemical and radioautographic studies from organ culture. *J Clin Endocrinol Metab* 1967;27:945.
96. Klinck H. Structure of the thyroid. In: Veach H, Smith D, eds. *The thyroid.* Baltimore: Williams & Wilkins, 1964:1.
97. Rodgers W, Resten H. Embryological basis for thyroid tissue in the heart. *Anat Rec* 1962:142.
98. Schubert W. Uber rine akzessorische schuldrusse in der leberforte. *Zentralbl Allg Pathol* 1957;96:339.
99. Randolph J, Grunt J, Vawler G. The medical and surgical aspects of intratracheal goiter. *N Engl J Med* 1963;2698:457.
100. Kaplan M, Kauli R, Lubin E. Ectopic thyroid gland. *J Pediatr* 1978;92:205.
101. Gerard-Merchant R, Caillou B. Thyroid inclusions in cervical lymph nodes. *Clin Endocrinol Metab* 1981;10:337.
102. Meyer J, Steinberg L. Microscopically benign thyroid follicles in cervical lymph nodes: serial section study of lymph node inclusions and entire thyroid gland in 5 cases. *Cancer* 1996;24:302.
103. Roth L. Inclusions of nonneoplastic thyroid tissue within cervical lymph nodes. *Cancer* 1965;18:105.
104. Kholich R. Accessory thyroid in the lateral floor of mouth. *Oral Surg* 1965; 19:234.
105. LiVolsi V, Asa S. The demise of follicular carcinoma of the thyroid gland. *Thyroid* 1994;4:233–236.
106. Baughman R. Lingual thyroid and lingual thyroglossal tract remnants. *Oral Surg Oral Med Oral Pathol* 1972;34:781.
107. Sank J. Ectopic lingual thyroid. *J Pathol* 1971;102:239.
108. Copp D, Cockcroft D, Kuch Y. Calcitonin from ultimobranchial glands of dogfish and chickens. *Science* 1967;158:924.
109. Sessions RB, Harrison LB, Forastiere AA. Tumors of the salivary glands and paragangliomas. In: DeVita VT, Hellman S, Rosenberg SA, eds. *Cancer: principles and practice of oncology,* 5th ed. Philadelphia: Lippincott-Raven, 1996:830–847.
110. Sterling K. Thyroid hormone action at the cell level. *N Engl J Med* 1979;300: 117.
111. Schneider A, Ikekubo K, Kuma K. Iodine content of serum thyroglobulin in normal individuals and patients with thyroid tumors. *J Clin Endocrinol Metab* 1983;57:1251.
112. Schluser G, Schaffner F, Korn F. Increased serum thyroid hormone binding and decreased free hormone in chronic active liver disease. *N Engl J Med* 1978;299:510d.
113. Foster G, MacIntyre I, Pearse A. Calcitonin production and the mitochondrion: rich cells of the dog thyroid. *Nature* 1964;203:1029.
114. Pearse A. The cytochemistry of thyroid C-cells and their relationship to calcitonin. *Proc R Lond B Soc Biol Sci* 1966;164:478.
115. Williams E. A review of 17 cases of carcinoma of the thyroid and pheochromocytoma. *J Clin Pathol* 1965;18:288.
116. Melvin K, Tashjian A. The synthesis of excess thyrocalcitonin produced by medullary thyroid carcinoma. *Proc Natl Acad Sci USA* 1968;59:1210.
117. Johnson N. The blood supply of the thyroid gland. *Aust NZ J Surg* 1953;23:95.
118. Toda S, Yonemitsu N, Hikichi Y, et al. Differentiation of human thyroid follicle cells from normal subjects and Basedow's disease in three dimensional collagen gel culture. *Pathol Res Pract* 1992;188:874.
119. Nunez E, Gershon M. Cytophysiology of thyroid PFC. *Int Rev Cytol* 1978;52: 1.
120. Lietz H. C-cells: source of calcitonin. A morphological review. *Curr Top Pathol* 1971;55:109.
121. Gibson W Peng T, Croker B. C-cell nodules in adult human thyroid: a common autopsy finding. *Am J Clin Pathol* 1981;75:347.
122. Aliapoulios M, Hattner R. The hypocalcemic activity of glucagon: demonstration of independence from endogenous calcitonin secretion in the rat. *Acta Endocrinol* 1970;64:726.
123. Miller T, Abele J, Greenspan P. FNA biopsy in the management of thyroid nodules. *West J Med* 1981;134:198–205.
124. Wolfe H, Melvin K, Cervi-Skinner S, et al. C-cell hyperplasia preceding medullary thyroid carcinoma. *N Engl J Med* 1973;289:437.
125. Brunner M, LiVolsi U. Oxyphilic (Askanazy-Hurthle cell) tumors of the thyroid. *Surg Pathol* 1988;1:137.
126. Flint A, Davenport R, Lloyd RD, et al. Cytomorphologic measurements of Hurthle cell tumors of the thyroid gland. *Cancer* 1988;61:110.
127. Friedmen N. Cellular involution in the thyroid gland. *J Clin Endocrinol Metab* 1949;9:874.
128. Hollingshead W. *Anatomy for surgeons, vol 1. The head and neck.* New York: Hobes, 1954.
129. Cernea C, Ferraz A, Nishio S, et al. Surgical anatomy of the external branch of the superior laryngeal nerve. *Head Neck* 1992;14:380.
130. Klinck G, Oertel J, Winship J. Ultrastructure of normal human thyroid. *Lab Invest* 1970;22:2.
131. Feind C. Surgical anatomy. In: Ingmar S, Braverman L, eds. *Werner's the thyroid.* Philadelphia: JB Lippincott, 1986.
132. LiVolsi VA, Perzin KH, Savetsky L. Carcinoma arising in median ectopic thyroid (including thyroglossal duct tissue). *Cancer* 1974;34:1303–1315.
133. Shappey M. *Anatomie, physiologie, pathologie des vaisseaux lymphatiques.* Paris: Delahjaye & Lacrosmer, 1874.
134. Clark R, Cole V, Fuller L, et al. Thyroid. In: MacComb R, Fletcher G, eds. *Cancer of the head and neck.* Baltimore: Williams & Wilkins, 1967:293.
135. Crile G Jr. The endocrine dependency of certain thyroid cancers and danger that hypothyroidism may stimulate their growth. *Cancer* 1957;10:1119.
136. Edir A, Grant C, Egdahl R. *Manual of endocrine surgery,* 2nd ed. New York: Springer-Verlag, 1984.
137. Cady B, Sedgwick L, Meissner W, et al. Risk factor analysis in differentiated thyroid cancer. *Cancer* 1979;43:810.
138. Marchetta F, Saro K, Matskura H. Modified neck dissection for carcinoma of the thyroid gland. *Am J Surg* 1970;120:452.
139. Noguchi S, Hoguchi A, Murakani N. Papillary carcinoma of the thyroid. Developing patterns of metastasis. *Cancer* 1970;26:1053.
140. Noguchi S, Murakami N. The value of lymph node dissection in patients with differentiated thyroid cancer. *Surg Clin North Am* 1987;67:251.
141. Rosen I, Wallace C, Strawbridge H, et al. Reevaluation of needle aspiration cytology in detection of thyroid cancer. *Surgery* 1981;90:747.
142. Woolner L, McConakey W, Beahrs O, et al. Thyroid cancer. In: Young S, Inman D, eds. *Thyroid neoplasia.* New York: Academic Press, 1968:51.
143. Rouviere H. *Anatomy of the human lymphatic system.* A compendium translated from the original "Anatomie des Lymphatiques de I'Homme" and rearranged for the use of students and practitioners by M. J. Tobias. Ann Arbor, MI: Edwards Brothers, 1938.
144. Robbins K, Woodson G. Thyroid carcinoma presenting as a parapharyngeal space mass. *Head Neck Surg* 1985;7:434–436.
145. Crumley R. Repair of the recurrent laryngeal nerve. Disorders of the thyroid and parathyroid II. *Otolaryngol Clin North Am* 1990;23:529.
146. Akerstrom G, Malmaeus J, Bergstrom R. Surgical anatomy of human parathyroid glands. *Surgery* 1984;95:14–21.
147. Wang C. The anatomic basis of parathyroid surgery. *Ann Surg* 1976;183:271.
148. Meissner W, Adler A. Papillary carcinoma of thyroid. *Arch Pathol* 1958;656: 518.
149. Burman K, Ringel M, Wartofsky L. Unusual types of thyroid neoplasms. *Endocrinol Metab Clin North Am* 1996;25:49–68.
150. Rossi R, Cady B, Silverman M. Current results of conservative surgery for differentiated thyroid carcinoma. *World J Surg* 1986;10:612–662.
151. Woolner L, Lemmon M, Beahrs O. Occult papillary cancer of the thyroid gland. *J Clin Endocrinol Metab* 1960;29:89.
152. Frich L, Glattre E, Akslen LA. Familial occurrence of nonmedullary thyroid cancer: a population-based study of 5673 first-degree relatives of thyroid cancer patients from Norway. *Cancer Epidemiol Biomark Prevent* 2001;10: 113–117.
153. McConahey W, Hay I, Woolner L. Papillary thyroid cancer treated at the Mayo Clinic, 1946 through 1970: initial manifestations, pathologic findings, therapy, and outcome. *Mayo Clin Proc* 1986;61:978.
154. Frazell E, Foote F. Papillary cancer of the thyroid. *Cancer* 1958;11:895.
155. Mazzaferri E, Young R. Papillary thyroid carcinoma: a 10 year follow-up report of the impact of therapy in 576 patients. *Am J Med* 1981;70:511.
156. Meissner W, Warren S. Tumors of the thyroid gland. In: *Atlas of tumor pathology,* 2nd series, fascicle 4. Washington, DC: AFIP, 1969.
157. Lindsay S. *Carcinoma of the thyroid gland.* Springfield, IL: Charles C. Thomas, 1960.

158. Chem K, Rosai J. Follicular variant of thyroid papillary carcinoma. *Am J Surg Pathol* 1977;1:123–130.
159. Mazzaferri E. Thyroid carcinoma: papillary and follicular. In: Mazzaferri E, Samaan N, eds. *Endocrine tumors.* Cambridge, MA: Blackwell Science, 1993:278.
160. Tielens E, Sherman S, Hruban R, et al. Follicular variant of papillary thyroid carcinoma: a clinicopathologic study. *Cancer* 1994;73:424.
161. Shemen LJ. Chess Q. Fine-needle aspiration biopsy diagnosis of follicular variant of papillary thyroid cancer: therapeutic implications. *Otolaryngol Head Neck Sur* 1998;119:600–602.
162. Prendiville S, Burman KD, Ringel MD, et al. Tall cell variant: an aggressive form of papillary thyroid carcinoma. *Otolaryngol Head Neck Surg* 2000;122: 352–357.
163. Evans H. Encapsulated papillary neoplasms of the thyroid. A study of 14 cases followed for a minimum of 10 years. *Am J Surg Pathol* 1987;11:592.
164. Schroder S, Bocker W, Dralle H, et al. The encapsulated papillary carcinoma of the thyroid. A morphologic subtype of the papillary thyroid carcinoma. *Cancer* 1984;54:90.
165. Silverman ML. Path of thyroid and parathyroid glands. In: Cady B, Rossi R, eds. *Surgery of the thyroid glands,* 3rd ed. Philadelphia: WB Saunders, 1991:36.
166. Hazard J. Nomenclature of thyroid tumors. In: Young S, Inman D, eds. *Thyroid neoplasia.* London: Academic Press, 1968:3.
167. Russel W, Ibanez M, Clark R, et al. Thyroid carcinoma: classification, intraglandular dissemination and clinico-pathological study based on whole organ sections of 80 glands. *Cancer* 1963;16:1465.
168. Carcangiu M, Zampi G, Pupi A. Papillary carcinoma of the thyroid. A clinicopathologic study of 241 cases treated at the University of Florence, Italy. *Cancer* 1985;55:805.
169. LiVolsi V. Papillary lesions of the thyroid. In: *Surgical pathology of the thyroid.* Philadelphia: WB Saunders, 1990:136.
170. Mazzaferri E. Papillary thyroid carcinoma: factors influencing prognosis and current therapy. *Semin Oncol* 1987;14:315.
171. Favas M, Schneider A, Stachvra M. Thyroid cancer occurring as a consequence of head and neck irradiation. *N Engl J Med* 1976;294:1019.
172. Fralkow P. The origin and development of human tumors studied with cell markers. *N Engl J Med* 1974;291:26.
173. Emerick G, Duh Q, Siperstein A. Diagnosis, treatment, and outcome of follicular thyroid carcinoma. *Cancer* 1993;72:3287.
174. DeGroot L, Kaplan E. Second operations for completion of thyroidectomy in treatment of differentiated thyroid cancer. *Surgery* 1991;110:936.
175. Raoo R, Fakih A, Mehra A. Completion thyroidectomy for thyroid carcinoma. *Head Neck Surg* 1987;9:284.
176. Auguste L, Attie J. Completion thyroidectomy for initially misdiagnosed thyroid cancer. *Otolaryngol Clin North Am* 1990;23:429.
177. Mazzaferri E, Jhiang S. Long-term impact of initial surgical and medical therapy on papillary and follicular thyroid cancer. *Am J Med* 1994;97:418.
178. Massin J, Savoie J, Gamier H. Pulmonary metastases in differentiated thyroid carcinoma. Study of 58 cases with implications for the primary tumor treatment. *Cancer* 1984;53:982.
179. Cady B, Rossi R. An expanded view of risk-group definition in differentiated thyroid carcinoma. *Surgery* 1988;104:947.
180. Crile G Jr, Antunez A, Esselstyn C. The advantages of subtotal thyroidectomy and suppression of TSH in the primary treatment of papillary carcinoma of the thyroid. *Cancer* 1985;55:2691.
181. Gardner RE, Tuttle RM, Burman KD, et al. Prognostic importance of vascular invasion in papillary thyroid carcinoma. *Arch Otolaryngol Head Neck Surg* 2000;126:309–312.
182. Cady B, Rossi R, Silverman M, et al. Further evidence of the validity of risk group definition. *Surgery* 1985;98:1171–1178.
183. Clark O, Demling R. Management of thyroid nodules in the elderly. *Am J Surg* 1976;132:615.
184. Cady B. Changing clinical, pathologic, therapeutic and survival pattern in differentiated thyroid carcinoma. *Ann Surg* 1976;184:541.
185. Ramson R, Leeper R. Factors influencing benign versus malignant thyroid neoplasms. In: Young S, Inman D, eds. *Thyroid neoplasm.* New York: Academic Press, 1968:159.
186. Cady B, Meissner W, Sala L. Thyroid cancer for forty-one years [Letter]. *N Engl J Med* 1978;299:901.
187. DeGroot I, Kaplan E, McCormick M, et al. Natural history, treatment, and course of papillary thyroid carcinoma. *J Clin Endocrinol Metab* 1990;71:414.
188. Tscholl-Ducommun J, Hedinger C. Papillary thyroid carcinomas: morphology and prognosis. *Virchows Arch* 1982;396:19.
189. Tubiana M, Schlumberger M, Rougier P. Long-term results and prognostic factors in patients with differentiated thyroid carcinoma. *Cancer* 1985;55:794.
190. Belfiore A, Garofalo M, Giuffrida D. Increased aggressiveness of thyroid cancer in patients with Graves' disease. *J Clin Endocrinol Metab* 1990;70:830.
191. Mazzaferri E. Thyroid cancer and Graves' disease. *J Clin Endocrinol Metab* 1990;70:826.
192. Filetti S, Belfiore A, Amir S. The role of thyroid stimulating antibodies of Graves' disease in differentiated thyroid cancer. *Thyroid* 1988;318:753.
193. Belfiore A, Russo D, Vigneri R, et al. Graves' disease, thyroid nodules and thyroid cancer. *Clin Endocrinol* 2001;55:711–718.
194. Hunter R, Frazell E, Foote F. Elective radical neck dissection. *Cancer* 1970;20:87.
195. Hirabayashi R, Lindsay S. Carcinoma of the thyroid gland. *J Clin Endocrinol Metab* 1961;21:1956.
196. Hay I, Bergstralh E, Goellner J. Predicting outcome in papillary thyroid carcinoma: development of a reliable prognostic scoring system in a cohort of 1779 patients surgically treated at one institution during 1940 through 1989. *Surgery* 1993;114:1050.
197. Asanuma K, Kusama R, Maruyama M, et al. Macroscopic extranodal invasion is a risk factor for tumor recurrence in papillary thyroid cancer. *Cancer Lett* 2001;164:85–89.
198. Harwood J, Clark O, Dunphy J. Significance of lymph nodes metastasis in differentiated thyroid cancer. *Am J Surg* 1978;136:107.
199. Salvesen H, Njolstad P, Akslen L. Papillary thyroid carcinoma: a multivariate analysis of prognostic factors including an evaluation of the p-TNM staging system. *Ear J Surg* 1992;158:583.
200. Scheumann G, Gimm O, Wegener G. Prognostic significance and surgical management of locoregional lymph node metastases in papillary thyroid cancer. *World J Surg* 1994;18:559.
201. Akslen L, Haldorsen T, Thoresen S, et al. Survival and causes of death in thyroid cancer: a population based study of 2479 cases from Norway. *Cancer Res* 1991;51:1234.
202. Sellers M, Beenken S, Blankenship A. Prognostic significance of cervical lymph node metastases in differentiated thyroid cancer. *Am J Surg* 1992; 164:578.
203. Coburn M, Wanebo H. Prognostic factors and management considerations in patients with cervical metastases of thyroid cancer. *Am J Surg* 1992;164:578.
204. Clark OH. Thyroid nodules and thyroid cancer: surgical aspects. *West J Med* 1980;133:1–8.
205. Wong LL, Ewing CA, Jonklaas J. Immunochemically demonstrated micrometastases to lymph nodes in papillary thyroid cancer. Presented at the Annual Endocrine Society Meeting, Denver, CO, 2001.
206. Hung W. Well differentiated thyroid carcinomas in children and adolescents: a review. *Endocrinologist* 1994;4:117.
207. Welch Dinauer CA, Tuttle RM, Robie DK, et al. Extensive surgery improves recurrence-free survival for children and young patients with class I papillary thyroid carcinoma. *J Pediatr Surg* 1999;34:1799–1804.
208. Harness J, Thompson N, Sisson. Differentiated thyroid carcinoma: treatment of distant metastasis. *Arch Surg* 1974;108:410.
209. Buckwalter J, Thomas C, Freeman J. Is childhood thyroid cancer a lethal disease? *Ann Surg* 1975;181:632.
210. Leeper R. The effect of I-131 therapy on survival of patients with metastatic papillary or follicular thyroid carcinoma. *J Clin Endocrinol Metab* 1973;36:1143.
211. Vasilopoulos-Selin R, Schultz P. Differentiated thyroid cancer in children and adolescents: clinical outcome and mortality after very long term follow-up. *Thyroid* 1997;7(suppl 1):(abst).
211a. Welch D et al. Clinical features associated with and recurrence of differential thyroid cancer in children, adolescents, and young adults. *The clinics of endocrinology.* Oxford Press, 1998;619–628.
212. Schlumberger M, Tubiana M, De Vathaire F. Long term results of treatment of 283 patients with lung and bone metastases from differentiated thyroid carcinoma. *J Clin Endocrinol Metab* 1986;63:960–967.
213. Vassilopoulou-Selin R, Klein M, Smith T. Pulmonary metastases in children and young adults with differentiated thyroid cancer. *Cancer* 1993;71:1348.
214. Callender D, Sherman S, Gagel R, et al. Cancer of the thyroid. In: Suen J, Myers E, eds. *Cancer of the head and neck,* 3rd ed. Philadelphia: Saunders, 1996:422.
215. Hoie J, Stennig H, Kullman G, et al. Distant metastases in papillary thyroid cancer. *Cancer* 1988;61:1.
216. Prendiville S, Burman K, Ringeil M, et al. Tall cell variant: an aggressive form of papillary thyroid carcinoma. *Otolaryngol Head Neck Surg* 2000;122:352–357.
217. Donohue J, Goldfien S, Miller T. Do the prognosis of papillary and follicular thyroid cancer differ? *Am J Surg* 1984;148:168.
218. Crile G, Pontius K, Hawk W. Factors influencing the survival of patients with follicular carcinoma of the thyroid gland. *Surg Gynecol Obstet* 1985;160:409.
219. Beierwaltes W, Nishiyama R, Thompson N. Survival time and cure in papillary and follicular thyroid carcinoma with distant metastases: statistics following U. of Michigan therapy. *J Nucl Med* 1982;23:561.
220. Ruegemer J, Hay I, Bergstralh E. Distant metastases in differentiated thyroid carcinoma: a multivariate analysis of prognostic variables. *J Clin Endocrinol Metab* 1988;67:501.
221. Lang W, Choritz H, Hundeshagen H. Risk factors in follicular thyroid carcinomas: a retrospective follow-up study covering a 14 year period with emphasis on morphologic findings. *Am J Surg Pathol* 1986;10:246.
222. Brennan M, Bergstralh E, van Heerden J, et al. Follicular thyroid cancer treated at the Mayo Clinic, 1946 through 1970: initial manifestations, pathologic findings, therapy, and outcome. *Mayo Clin Proc* 1991;66:11.
223. Silverman M. Pathology of thyroid and parathyroid glands. In: Cady B, Rossi R, eds. *Surgery of the thyroid and parathyroid glands.* Philadelphia: WB Saunders, 1991:38.
224. van Heerden J, Hay I, Goellner J. Follicular thyroid carcinoma with capsular invasion alone: a nonthreatening malignancy. *Surgery* 1992;112:1130.
225. Peake R. Clinical evaluation of thyroid tumors. In: Thawley S, Panje W, Batsakis J, et al., eds. *Comprehensive management of head and neck tumors.* Philadelphia: WB Saunders, 1987.
226. Mazzaferri E. Management of a solitary thyroid nodule. *N Engl J Med* 1993;328:553.
227. Kahn N, Perzin K. Follicular carcinoma of the thyroid. *Pathol Annu* 1983;18: 221.
228. Franssila K. Prognosis in thyroid carcinoma. *Cancer* 1975;36:1138.

229. Watson R, Brennan M, van Heerden J. Invasive Hurthle cell carcinoma of the thyroid: natural history and management. *Mayo Clin Proc* 1984;59:850.
230. Belchetz G, Cheung CC, Freeman J, et al. Hurthle cell tumors: using molecular techniques to define a novel classification system. *Arch Otolaryngol Head Neck Surg* 2002;128:237–240.
231. Arganini M, Behar R, Wu T. Hurthle cell tumors: a twenty five year experience. *Surgery* 1986;100:1108.
231a. Thompson N, Dunn E, Batsacks J, et al. Cyclol cell lesions of the thyroid gland. *Surg Gynecol Obstet* 1973:139:555.
232. Samaan N, Schultz P, Haynie T, et al. Pulmonary metastasis of differentiated thyroid carcinoma: treatment results in 101 patients. *J Clin Endocrinol Metab* 1985;60:376.
233. El-Naggar A, Batsakis J, Luna M, et al. Hurthle cell tumors of the thyroid. *Arch Otolaryngol Head Neck Surg* 1988;114:520.
234. Sarker S, Pugliese P, Palestro C. Metastases from Hurthle cell thyroid cancer are far more avid for fluorodeoxyglucose than for radioiodine. American Thyroid Association Annual Meeting, Washington, DC, November 2001, abstract 53.
235. Rosai J, Carcangiu M. Pathology of thyroid tumors: some recent and old questions. *Hum Fathol* 1984;15:1008–1012.
236. Okabe T, Nomura H, Oshawa N. Establishment and characterization of a human colony stimulating factor producing cell line from a squamous cell carcinoma of the thyroid gland. *J Natl Cancer Inst* 1982;69:1235–1241.
237. Matsuzuka F, Miyauchi A, Katayama S, et al. Clinical aspects of primary thyroid lymphoma: diagnosis and treatment based on our experience of 119 cases. *Thyroid* 1993;3:93–99.
239. Tsang R, Gospodarozicz M, Sutcliffe S. Non-Hodgkin's lymphoma of the thyroid gland: prognostic factors and treatment outcome. *Inn J Radiat Oncol Biol Phys* 1993;27:559.
240. Doria R, Jekel J, Cooper D. Thyroid lymphoma: the case for combined modality therapy. *Cancer* 1994;73:200.
241. Salhany K, Pietra G. Extranodal lymphoid disorders. *Am J Clin Pathol* 1993; 99:472.
242. Shimaoka K, Badillo J, Sokal J. Clinical differentiation between thyroid cancer and benign goiter. *JAMA* 1962;181:179.
243. Souhami L, Simpson W, Carruthers J. Malignant lymphoma of the thyroid gland. *Inn J Radiat Oncol Biol Phys* 1980;6:1143.
244. Walfish P. Miscellaneous tumors of the thyroid. In: Ingbar S, Braverman L, eds. *Werner's the thyroid.* Philadelphia: JB Lippincott, 1986.
245. Harada T, Shimaoka K, Minimura T, et al. Chemotherapy for thyroid cancer. In: Andreola M, Monaco S, Robbins J, eds. *Advances in thyroid neoplasia.* Rome: Field Educational Italia, 1981.
246. Mac Pherson T, Dekker A, Kapadia S. Thyroid gland plasma cell neoplasia (plasmacytoma). *Arch Pathol Lab Med* 1981;105:570.
247. Shimaoka K, Gailani S, Tsukada Y. Plasma cell neoplasm involving the thyroid. *Cancer* 1978;41:1140–1146.
248. Chesky V, Helling C, Welch J. Fibrosarcoma of the thyroid gland. *Surg Gynecol Obstet* 1960;111:767.
249. Woolner L, McConakey W, Beahrs O, et al. Primary malignant lymphoma of the thyroid. *Am J Surg* 1966;111:502.
250. Hill C, Aldinger R. Management of anaplastic carcinoma of the thyroid. In: Greenfield L, ed. *Thyroid cancer.* West Palm Beach, FL: CRC Press, 1978:165.
251. LiVolsi V, Merino M. Histopathologic differential diagnosis of the thyroid. *Pathol Anna* 1981;16:357
252. Heimann R, Vannineuse A, De Stoover C, et al. Malignant lymphoma and undifferentiated small cell carcinoma of the thyroid. *Histopathology* 1978;2: 201.
253. Rayfeld E, Nishiyama R, Sisson J. Small cell tumors of the thyroid. *Cancer* 1971;28:1023.
254. Kostakoglu L, Leonard JP, Kuji I, et al. Comparison of fluorine-18 fluorodeoxyglucose positron emission tomography and Ga-67 scintigraphy in evaluation of lymphoma. [Clinical trial.] *Cancer* 2002;94:879–888.
255. Burke J, Butler J, Fulleri L. Malignant lymphoma of the thyroid gland. *Cancer* 1977;39:1587.
256. Hamburger J. *Nontoxic goiter.* Springfield, IL: Charles C Thomas, 1973:108.
257. Holm L, Blomgren H, Lowhagen T. Cancer risks in patients with chronic lymphocytic thyroiditis. *N Engl J Med* 1985;312:601.
258. Williams E. Malignant lymphoma thyroid. *Clin Endocrinol Metab* 1981;10:379.
259. Werner SC. Physical examination. In: Ingbar SH, Braverman LE, eds. *Werner's the thyroid.* Philadelphia: JB Lippincott, 1986.
260. Mitchell G, Huddart R, Harmer C. Phase II evaluation of high dose accelerated radiotherapy for anaplastic thyroid carcinoma. [Clinical trial, phase II.] *Radiother Oncol* 1999;50:33–38.
261. Silverberg SG, Vidone RA. Metastatic tumors in the thyroid. *Pacif Med Surg* 1966;74:175.
262. Kim J, Leeper R. Treatment of locally advanced thyroid carcinoma with combination of doxorubicin and radiation therapy. *Cancer* 1987;60:10.
263. Sokal M, Harmer C. Chemotherapy for anaplastic carcinoma of the thyroid. *Clin Oncol* 1978;4:3.
263a. Ain KB, Egorin MJ, DeSimone PA. Treatment of anaplastic thyroid carcinoma with paclitaxel: phase 2 trial using ninety-six-hour infusion. Collaborative Anaplastic Thyroid Cancer Health Intervention Trials (CATCHIT) Group. [Clinical trial, phase II.] *Thyroid* 2000;10:587–594.
264. Schlumberger M, Parmentier C, Delisle MJ, et al. Combination therapy for anaplastic giant cell thyroid carcinoma. *Cancer* 1994;74:1348.
265. Hedinger C, Williams ED, Sobin LH. *Histological typing of thyroid tumors. International histological classification of tumors,* 2nd ed. WHO. Berlin: Springer-Verlag, 1988.
266. Wychulie A, Beahrs O, Woolner L. Papillary carcinoma in associated anaplastic cancer in the thyroid gland. *Surg Gynecol Obstet* 1965;120:28.
267. Naheshawari Y, Hill C, Haynie T. I-131 therapy of differentiated carcinoma. *Cancer* 1981;47:664.
268. Tubiana M. External radiotherapy and radioiodine in the treatment of thyroid cancer. *World J Surg* 1981;5:75.
269. Winship T, Rosvoll R. Childhood thyroid cancer. *Cancer* 1961;14:734.
270. Hazard J. The C-cell of the thyroid gland and medullary thyroid carcinoma: a review. *Am J Pathol* 1977;88:214.
271. Williams E. Histogenesis of medullary thyroid cancer. *J Clin Pathol* 1966; 19:114.
272. Weichert R III. The neural ectodermal origin of the peptide-secreting endocrine glands: a unifying concept for the etiology of multiple endocrine adenomatosis and the inappropriate secretion of peptide hormone by nonendocrine tumor. *Am J Med* 1970;49:232.
273. Pearse A. The APUD cell concept and its implications in pathology. *Pathol Anna* 1974;9:27.
274. Chong F, Beahrs O, Sizemore G, et al. Medullary carcinoma of the thyroid gland. *Cancer* 1975;35:695–704.
275. Brandi ML, Gagel RF, Angeli A, et al. Guidelines for diagnosis and therapy of MEN type 1 and type 2. Consensus Development Conference. *J Clin Endocrinol Metab* 2001;86:5658–5671.
276. Schlumberger M, Caillou B. Miscellaneous tumors of the thyroid. In: Braverman LE, Utiger RD, eds. *Werner and Ingbar's the thyroid: a fundamental and clinical text,* 7th ed. Philadelphia: Lippincott-Raven, 1996:962.
277. Raue F, Frank Raue K, Grauer A. Multiple endocrine neoplasia type 2: clinical features and screening. *Endocrinol Metab Clin North Am* 1994;23:137–156.
278. Hyer SL, Vini L, A'Hern R, et al. Medullary thyroid cancer: multivariate analysis of prognostic factors influencing survival. *Eur J Surg Oncol* 2000;26: 686–690.
279. Wells S, Baylin S, Gann P. Medullary thyroid carcinoma. *Ann Surg* 1978;188: 377.
280. Melvin K, Miller H, Tashjian A. Early diagnosis of medullary carcinoma of the thyroid gland by means of calcitonin assay. *N Engl J Med* 1971;285:1115.
281. Ball D, Baylin S, Bustros AC. Medullary thyroid carcinoma. In: Braverman LE, Utiger RD, eds. *Werner and Ingbar's the thyroid: a fundamental and clinical text,* 7th ed. Philadelphia: Lippincott-Raven, 1996:946–960.
282. Ellenhorn J, Shah J, Brennan ME. Impact of therapeutic regional lymph node dissection for medullary carcinoma of thyroid gland. *Surgery* 1993;114: 1078–1082.
283. Ordonez N, Samaan N. Medullary carcinoma of the thyroid metastasis to the skin: report of two cases. *J Cutan Pathol* 1987;14:251.
284. Melvin K, Tashjian A, Miller H. Studies in familial (medullary) thyroid carcinoma. *Recent Prog Horm Res* 1972;28:399.
285. Block M, Jackson C, Tashjian A. Management of occult medullary thyroid carcinoma of thyroid: evidence only by serum calcitonin elevations after apparently adequate neck operation. *Arch Surg* 1978;113:368.
286. Block M, Jackson C, Greenwald M. Clinical characteristics distinguishing hereditary from sporadic medullary thyroid carcinoma. *Arch Surg* 1980;115: 142.
287. Jackson C, Talpos G, Block M. Clinical value of tumor doubling estimations in multiple endocrine neoplasia type II. *Surgery* 1984;96:981.
288. LiVolsi V. Surgical pathology of the thyroid. In: Bennington J, ed. *Major problems in pathology,* vol 22. Philadelphia: WB Saunders, 1990.
289. Kakudo K, Miyanchi A, Ogihara T. Medullary thyroid carcinoma. Giant cell type. *Arch Pathol Gab Med* 1978;102:445.
290. Stepanas A, Samaan N, Hill C, et al. Medullary thyroid carcinoma: importance of serial calcitonin measurements. *Cancer* 1975;43:825.
291. Ljunberg O, Lederquist E, Von Studnitz. Medullary thyroid carcinoma and pheochromocytoma: a familial chromaffinomatosis. *BMJ* 1967;1:279.
292. Franssila K. Value of histologic classification of thyroid cancer. *Acta Pathol Microbiol Scand [A]* 1971;225(suppl):1–76.
293. Melvin K. Medullary carcinoma of the thyroid. In: Ingbar S, Braverman L, eds. *Werner's the thyroid.* Philadelphia: JB Lippincott, 1986.
294. Saad ME, Ordonez NG, Rashid RK. Medullary carcinoma of the thyroid. A study of the clinical features and prognostic factors in 161 patients. *Medicine (Baltimore)* 1984;63:319–342.
295. Baylin S, Mendelsohn G. Medullary thyroid carcinoma: a model for the study of human tumor progression and cell heterogeneity. In: Owens AH, Coffey DS, Baylin SB, eds. *Tumor cell heterogeneity: origins and implications.* New York: Academic Press, 1982:12.
296. Deftos L. Simultaneous ectopic production of PTH and calcitonin. *Metabolism* 1976;25:543.
297. Baylin S, Beaver M, Buja L, et al. Histaminase and calcitonin levels in medullary thyroid carcinoma. *Lancet* 1972;1:455.
298. Roos B, Lindall A, Ells J. Increased plasma and tumor somatostatin like immunoreactivity in medullary thyroid carcinoma and small cell lung cancer. *J Clin Endocrinol Metab* 1981;52:187.
299. Melvin K, Tashjian A, Cassidy C, et al. Cushing's syndrome caused by ACTH and calcitonin secreting medullary carcinoma of the thyroid. *Metabolism* 1970;19:831.
300. Kameya T, Bessho T, Tsumuraya M. Production of gastrin releasing peptide by medullary carcinoma of the thyroid. *Virchows Arch* 1983;401:99.
301. Baylin S, Mendelsohn G. Medullary thyroid carcinoma: a model for the

study of human tumor progression and cell heterogeneity. In: Owens H, Coffey D, Baylin S, eds. *Tumor cell heterogeneity, origins, and implications.* New York: Academic Press, 1982:12.
302. Deftos I, Woloszezuk W, Krisch I. Medullary thyroid carcinomas express chromogranin A and a novel neuroendocrine protein recognized by monoclonal antibody HISL-19. *Am J Med* 1988;85:780.
303. Krisch K, Krisch I, Horvat G. The value of immunohistochemistry in medullary thyroid carcinoma: a systematic study of 30 cases. *Histopathology* 1985;9:1077.
304. Sikri K, Varndell I, Hamid Z. Medullary carcinoma of the thyroid. An immunocytochemical and histochemical study of 25 cases using eight separate markers. *Cancer* 1985;56:2481.
305. Hoff AO, Cote GJ, Gagel RF. Multiple endocrine neoplasias. *Annu Rev Physiol* 2000;62:377–411.
306. DeLellis R. Biology of disease: multiple endocrine neoplasia syndromes revisited. *Lab Invest* 1995;72:494–505.
307. Goodfellow P, Wells S. RET gene and its implication for cancer. *J Natl Cancer Inst* 1995;87:1515–1523.
308. Mallette L. Management of hyperparathyroidism in the MEN syndromes and other familial endocrinopathies. *Endocrinol Metab Clin North Am* 1994;23:19–36.
309. Halling KC, Bufill JA, Cotter M, et al. Age-related disease penetrance in a large medullary thyroid cancer family with a codon 609 RET gene mutation. *Mol Diagn* 1997;2:277–286.
310. Carlson K, Bracamotes J, Jackson C, et al. Parent of origin effects in MEN type 2B. *Am J Hum Genet* 1994;55:1076–1082.
311. Cote C, Wohllk N, Evas D, et al. RET proto-oncogene mutation in multiple endocrine neoplasia type 2 and medullary thyroid carcinoma. *Baillieres Clin Endocrinol Metab* 1995;9:609–630.
312. Easton D, Ponder M, Cummings T, et al. The clinical and screening age at onset distribution for the MEN 2 syndrome. *Am J Hum Genet* 1989;443:208–215.
313. Pacini F, Romei C, Miccoli P, et al. Early treatment of hereditary MTC after attribution of MEN 2 gene carrier status by screening for RET gene mutations. *Surgery* 1995;118:1031–1035.
314. Sipple J. The association of pheochromocytoma with carcinoma of the thyroid gland. *Am J Med* 1961;31:163–166.
315. O'Riordain D, O'Brien T, Crotty T, et al. Multiple endocrine neoplasia type 213: more than an endocrine disorder. *Surgery* 1995;118:936–942.
316. Ivy HK. Cancer metastatic to the thyroid: a diagnostic problem. *Mayo Clin Proc* 1984;59:856.
317. Green L, Ro JY, Mackay B, et al. Renal cell carcinoma metastatic to the thyroid. *Cancer* 1989;63:1810–1815.
318. Smith SA, Gharib H, Goellner JR. Fine needle aspiration. Usefulness for diagnosis and management of metastatic carcinoma to the thyroid. *Arch Intern Med* 1987;147:311.
319. Ashcraft W, VanHerle H. Management of thyroid nodules. Part I. *Head Neck Surg* 1981;3:216.
320. Hung W, August G, Randolph J. Solitary thyroid nodules in children and adolescents. *J Pediatr Surg* 1982;17:225–229.
321. Hayles A, Johnson M, Braehs B. Nodular lesions of the thyroid in children. *Am J Surg* 1963;106:735–743.
322. Kirkland RT, Kirkland JL, Rosenberg G. Solitary thyroid nodules in 30 children and a report of a child with thyroid abscess. *Pediatrics* 1973;51:85–90.
323. Belfiore A, Giuffrida D, LaRosa G. High frequency of cancer in cold thyroid nodules occurring at young age. *Acta Endocrinol (Copenh)* 1989;121:197–202.
324. Hamming J, Coslings B, Van Steenis G. The value of fine needle aspiration biopsy in patients with nodular thyroid disease divided into groups of suspicion of malignant neoplasms on clinical grounds. *Arch Intern Med* 1990;150:113–118.
325. Messaris G, Kyriakou K, Vasilopoulos P. The single thyroid nodule and carcinoma. *Br J Surg* 1974;61:943–944.
326. Belfiore A, LaRosa G, LaPorta G. Cancer risk in patients with cold thyroid nodules: relevance of iodine intake, sex, age, and multinodularity. *Am J Med* 1992;93:363–369.
327. Cole W, Majarakis J, Slaughter D. Incidence of carcinoma of the thyroid in nodular goiter. *J Clin Endocrinol* 1949;9:1007–1011.
328. Harach H, Williams E. Childhood thyroid cancer. *Br J Cancer* 1995;72:777–783.
329. Cerletti J, Guansing A, Engbring N. Radiation-related thyroid carcinoma. *Arch Surg* 1978;113:1072–1076.
330. Schneider A. Thyroid nodules following childhood irradiation: a 1989 update. *Thyroid Today* 1989;12:1–7.
331. Frankenthaler R, Sellin R, Cangir A. Lymph node metastasis from papillary-follicular thyroid carcinoma in young patients. *Am J Surg* 1990;160:341.
332. Schneider A. Radiation-induced thyroid tumors. *Endocrinol Metab Clin North Am* 1990;19:495–509.
333. DeGroot L, Reilly M, Pinnameneni K. Retrospective and prospective study of radiation-induced thyroid disease. *Am J Med* 1983;74:852–862.
334. Favus M, Schneider A, Stachura M. Thyroid cancer occurring as a late consequence of head and neck irradiation: evaluation of 1056 patients. *N Engl J Med* 1976;294:1019–1025.
335. Schneider A, Shore-Freedman E, Ryo U. Radiation-induced tumors of the head and neck following childhood irradiation. *Medicine* 1985;64:1–15.
336. Nagataki S, Shibata Y, Inoue S, et al. Thyroid diseases among atomic bomb survivors in Nagasaki. *JAMA* 1994;272:364–370.
337. Kaplan M, Garnick M, Belber R. Risk factors for thyroid abnormalities after neck irradiation for childhood cancer. *Am J Med* 1983;74:272–280.
338. Conrad R, Dibyns B, Sutow W. Thyroid neoplasia as late effect of exposure to radioactive iodine fallout. *JAMA* 1970;214:316–324.
339. Reid W, Mangano J. Thyroid cancer in the US since accident at Chernobyl. *BMJ* 1995;311:511.
340. Robbins J. Schneider AB. Thyroid cancer following exposure to radioactive iodine. *Rev Endocr Metab Disord* 2000;1:197–203.
341. Ron E, Modan B. Benign and malignant thyroid neoplasms after childhood irradiation for tinea capitus. *J Natl Cancer Inst* 1980;65:7–11.
342. Fraker D. Radiation exposure and other factors that predispose to human thyroid neoplasia. *Surg Clin North Am* 1995;75:365–375.
343. DeGroot L. Diagnostic approach and management of patients exposed to irradiation to the thyroid. *J Clin Endocrinol Metab* 1989;69:925–928.
344. Schneider A, Ron E, Lubin J. Dose-response relationships for radiation-induced thyroid cancer and thyroid nodules: evidence for the prolonged effects of radiation on the thyroid. *J Clin Endocrinol Metab* 1993;77:362–369.
345. Nauman J, Wolff J. Iodide prophylaxis in Poland after the Chernobyl reactor accident: benefits and risks. *Am J Med* 1993;94:524–532.
346. Robbins J, Adams W. Radiation effects in the Marshall Islands. In: Nagatiki S, ed. *Radiation and the thyroid.* Amsterdam: Excerpta Medica, 1989:11.
347. Conrad R. Late radiation effects in Marshall Islanders exposed to fallout 28 years ago. In: Boice JD Jr, Fraumeni J, eds. *Radiation carcinogenesis: epidemiology and biological significance.* New York: Raven Press, 1984:57.
348. Hamilton T, van Belle G, LoGerfo J. Thyroid neoplasia in Marshall Islanders exposed to nuclear fallout. *JAMA* 1987;258:629.
349. Kerber R, Till J, Simon S. A Cohort study of thyroid disease in relation to fallout from nuclear weapons testing. *JAMA* 1993;270:2076.
350. Mettler F, Williamson M, Royal H. Thyroid nodules in the population living around Chernobyl. *JAMA* 1992;268:616.
351. Stsjazhko V, Tsyb A, Tronko N, et al. Childhood thyroid cancer since accident at Chernobyl. *BMJ* 1995;310:801.
352. Williams D. Chernobyl, eight years on. *Nature* 1994;371:556.
353. Lote K, Andersen K, Nordal E. Familial occurrence of papillary thyroid carcinoma. *Cancer* 1980;46:1291.
354. Hrafnkelsson J, Tulinius H, Jonasson J. Papillary thyroid carcinoma in Iceland: a study of the occurrence in families and co-existence of other primary tumors. *Acta Oncol* 1989;28:785–788.
355. Anonymous. Patterns of cancer in five continents. *IARC Sci Publ* 1990;102:1–159.
356. Bell B, Mazzaferri E. Thyroid cancer in familial polyposis coli: case report and literature review. *Dig Dis Sci* 1993;38:185–190.
357. Ringel MD, Balducci-Silano PL, Anderson JS, et al. Quantitative reverse transcription-polymerase chain reaction of circulating thyroglobulin messenger ribonucleic acid for monitoring patients with thyroid carcinoma. *J Clin Endocrinol Metab* 1999;84:4037–4042.
358. Crile G Jr. Endocrine dependency of papillary cancer of thyroid. *JAMA* 1966;195:101.
359. Mazzaferri EL, Jhiang SM. Long-term impact of initial surgical and medical therapy on papillary and follicular thyroid cancer. [See comments.] [Erratum appears in *Am J Med* 1995;98(2):215.]. *Am J Med* 1994;97:418–428.
360. Cerise E, Randall S, Oschner A. Carcinoma of the thyroid and nontoxic nodular goiter. *Surgery* 1952;31:552–561.
361. Layfield L, Reichman A, Bottles K. Clinical determinants for the management of thyroid nodules by fine needle aspiration cytology. *Arch Otolaryngol Head Neck Surg* 1992;118:717–721.
362. McCall A, Jarosz H, Lawrence A. The incidence of thyroid carcinoma in solitary cold nodules and in multinodular goiters. *Surgery* 1986;100:1128–1132.
363. Brennan M, Bloomer W. Cancer of the endocrine system: the thyroid gland. In: DeVita V, Helman S, Rosenberg S, eds. *Cancer: principles and practice of oncology.* Philadelphia: JB Lippincott, 1982.
364. Shaba A, Alfonso AE, Jaffe BM. Operative treatment of substernal goiters. *Head Neck* 1989;11:325–330.
365. Ahuja S, Ernst H. Hyperthyroidism, and thyroid carcinoma. *Acta Endocrinol* 1991;142:146–151.
366. Intenzo C, Park C, Cohen S. Thyroid carcinoma presenting as an autonomous nodule. *Clin Nucl Med* 1990;15:313–314.
367. Van Herle A, Uller R, Matthews N. Radioimmunoassay for measurement of thyroglobulin in human serum. *J Clin Invest* 1973;52:1320–1327.
368. Anderson J. Diagnostic value of thyroid antibodies. *J Clin Endocrinol Metab* 1967;27:937.
369. Martino E. Dissociation of responsiveness to thyrotropin. Releasing hormone and thyroid suppressibility following antithyroid drug therapy of hyperthyroidism. *J Clin Endocrinol Metab* 1976;43:543.
370. Christensen S, Bondeson L, Ericsson U. Prediction of malignancy in the solitary thyroid nodule by physical examination, thyroid scan, fine needle biopsy and serum thyroglobulin: a prospective study of 100 surgically treated patients. *Acta Chir Scand* 1984;150:433.
371. Melvin K, Miller H, Tashjian A. Early diagnosis of medullary carcinoma of the thyroid gland by means of calcitonin assay. *N Engl J Med* 1971;285:1115.
372. Uwaifo GI, Remaley AT, Stene M, et al. A case of spurious hypercalcitoninemia: a cautionary tale on the use of plasma calcitonin assays in the screening of patients with thyroid nodules for neoplasia. *J Endocrinol Invest* 2001;24:361–369.
373. Ledger G, Khosla S, Lindor N. Genetic testing in the diagnosis and management of multiple endocrine neoplasia type II. *Ann Intern Med* 1995;122:118–124.
374. Eng C, Mulligan L, Smith D, et al. Low frequency of germline mutations in the RET proto-oncogene in patients with apparently sporadic medullary thyroid carcinoma. *Clin Endocrinol* 1995;43:123–127.

375. Zedenius J, Larsson C, Bergholm U, et al. Mutations of codon 918 in the RET proto-oncogene correlate to poor prognosis in sporadic medullary thyroid carcinomas. *J Clin Endocrinol Metab* 1995;80:3088–3090.
376. Mazzaferri E. Thyroid cancer in thyroid nodules: finding a needle in the haystack. *Am J Med* 1992;93:359–362.
377. Hill C, Ibanez M, Nagiub A. Medullary thyroid carcinoma. *Medicine* 1973;52: 141.
378. Schluter B, Bohuslavizki KH, Beyer W, et al. Impact of FDG PET on patients with differentiated thyroid cancer who present with elevated thyroglobulin and negative 131I scan. *J Nucl Med* 2001;42:71–76.
379. Shiga T, Tsukamoto E, Nakada K, et al. Comparison of (18)F-FDG, (131)I-Na, and (201)Tl in diagnosis of recurrent or metastatic thyroid carcinoma. *J Nucl Med* 2001;42:414–419.
380. Sollbiati L, Bolterrani L, Rizzato G. The thyroid gland with low uptake lesions: evaluation by ultrasound. *Radiology* 1985;155:187–191.
381. Simeone J, Daniels G, Mueller P. High-resolution real-time sonography of the thyroid. *Radiology* 1982;145:431–435.
382. Waiters D, Ahuja A, Evans R. Role of ultrasound in the management of thyroid nodules. *Am J Surg* 1992;164:654–657.
383. De Los Santos E, Keyhani-Rofagha S, Cunningham J. Cystic thyroid nodules: the dilemma of malignant lesions. *Arch Intern Med* 1990;150:1422–1427.
384. Wei J, Burke G. Characterization of neoplastic potential of solitary solid thyroid lesions with Tc-99m-pertechnetate and Tc-99m-sestamibi scanning. *Ann Surg Oncol* 1995;2:233–237.
385. Beahrs O, Kubista T. Diagnosis of thyroid cancer. In: American Cancer Society. *Cancer management. A special graduate course on cancer.* Philadelphia: JB Lippincott, 1968:573.
386. O'Connor M, Cullen M, Malone J. A kinetic study of 131-I and 99m TC pertechnetate in thyroid carcinoma to explain a scan discrepancy: case report. *J Nucl Med* 1977;18:796–798.
387. Shanbaugh G, Quinn J, Oyasa R. Disparate thyroid imaging: combined studies with sodium pertechnetate, 99m Tc and radioactive iodine. *JAMA* 1974; 228:866–869.
388. Hermans J, Schmitz A, Merlo P. Le thallium 201 permet-il de differencier le nodule thyroideien benin du nodule malin? *Ann Endocrinol* 1993;54:248.
389. Vickery A Jr. Needle biopsy pathology. *Clin Endocrinol Metab* 1981;10: 275–292.
390. Nishiyama R, Bigos T, Goldfarb W. The efficacy of simultaneous fine needle aspiration and large needle biopsy of the thyroid gland. *Surgery* 1986;100: 1133–1137.
391. Oertel YC, Oertel JE. Thyroid cytology and histology. *Best Pract Res Clin Endocrinol Metab* 2000;14:541–557.
392. Al-Sayer H, Krukowski Z, Williams V. Fine needle aspiration cytology in isolated thyroid swellings: a prospective two year evaluation. *BMJ* 1985;290: 1490–1492.
393. Bisi H, Camargo R, Filho A. Role of fine needle aspiration cytology in the management of thyroid nodules: review of experience with 1925 cases. *Diagn Cytopathol* 1991;8:504–510.
394. Caplan R, Kisken W, Strutt P. Fine needle aspiration biopsy of thyroid nodules: a cost effective diagnostic plan. *Postgrad Med* 1991;90:183–190.
395. Miller J, Hamburger J, Kim S. Diagnosis of thyroid nodules: use of fine needle aspiration and needle biopsy. *JAMA* 1979;242:481.
396. Asp A, Georgitis W, Waldron E. Fine néedle aspiration of the thyroid: use in an average health care facility. *Am J Med* 1987;83:489–493.
397. Hamburger J. Consistency of sequential needle biopsy findings for thyroid nodules: management implications. *Arch Intern Med* 1987;147:97–99.
398. Pepper G, Zwicker D, Rosen Y. Fine needle aspiration of the thyroid nodule: results of a start up project in a general teaching hospital setting. *Arch Intern Med* 1989;149:594–596.
399. Hamburger B, Gharib H, Melton L. Fine needle aspiration biopsy of thyroid nodules: impact on thyroid practice and cost of care. *Am J Med* 1982;73:381–384.
400. Gharib H, James E, Charboneau J. Suppressive therapy with levothyroxine for solitary thyroid nodules. A double blind controlled clinical study. *N Engl J Med* 1987;317:70–75.
401. Caruso D, Mazzaferri E. Fine needle aspiration in the management of thyroid nodules. *Endocrinologist* 1991;1:194–202.
402. Haas S, Trujilo A, Hunstle J. Fine needle aspiration of thyroid nodules in a rural setting. *Am J Med* 1993;94:357–361.
403. McIvor N, Freeman J, Salem S. Ultrasonography and ultrasound guided fine needle aspiration biopsy of head and neck lesions: a surgical perspective. *Laryngoscope* 1994;104:669–674.
404. Piromalli D, Martelli G, Del Prato I. The role of fine needle aspiration in the diagnosis of thyroid nodules: analysis of 795 consecutive cases. *J Surg Oncol* 1992;50:247–250.
405. Goellner J, Gharib H, Grant C. Fine needle aspiration cytology of the thyroid, 1980 to 1986. *Acta Cytol* 1987;31:587–590.
406. Cochand-Priollet B, Guillausseau P, Chagnon S. The diagnostic value of fine needle aspiration biopsy under ultrasonography in nonfunctional thyroid nodules: a prospective study comparing cytologic and histologic findings. *Am J Med* 1994;97:152–157.
407. Grant C. Operative and postoperative management of the patient with follicular and Hurthle cell carcinoma. *Surg Clin North Am* 1995;75:395–403.
408. Callender D, Sherman S, Gagel R, et al. Cancer of the thyroid. In: Suen J, Myers E, eds. *Cancer of the head and neck,* 3rd ed. Philadelphia: Saunders, 1996.
409. Baloch ZW, Sack MJ, Yu GH, et al. Fine-needle aspiration of thyroid: an institutional experience. *Thyroid* 1998;8:565–569.
410. Ma M, Ong G. Cystic thyroid nodules. *Br J Surg* 1975;2:205.
411. Clark OH, Okerlund MD, Cavalieri RR, et al. Diagnosis and treatment of thyroid, parathyroid and thyroglossal duct cysts. *J Clin Endocrinol Metab* 1979;48: 983–988.
412. Oertel YC. Fine-needle aspiration of the thyroid. In: Moore WT, Eastman RC, eds. *Diagnostic endocrinology.* Toronto: BC Decker 1990:149–165.
413. Rosen I, Walfish P, Bain J, et al. Secondary malignancy of the thyroid gland and its management. *Ann Surg Oncol* 1995;2:252–256.
414. Oertel Y. A pathologist's comments on diagnosis of thyroid nodules by fine needle aspiration. *J Clin Endocrinol Metab* 1995;80:1467–1468.
415. DeMicco C, Zoro P, Garcia S. Thyroid peroxidase immunodetection as a tool to assist diagnosis of thyroid nodules on fine needle aspiration biopsy. *Eur J Endocrinol* 1994;131:474–479.
416. Cheifetz R, Davis N, Robinson B. Differentiation of thyroid neoplasms by evaluating epithelial membrane antigen, Leu-7 antigen, epidermal growth factor receptor and DNA content. *Am J Surg* 1984;167:531–534.
417. Sadler B, Stapfer G, Bein B. Increased binding capacity of receptors for the epidermal growth factor in benign nodules and thyroid malignancies. *Clin Invest* 1993;71:898–902.
418. Ermak G, Gerasimov G, Troshinia K, et al. Deregulated alternative splicing of CD44 messenger RNA transcripts in neoplastic and nonneoplastic lesions of the human thyroid. *Cancer Res* 1995;55:4594–4598.
419. Roque L, Clode A, Gomes P, et al. Cytogenetic findings in 31 papillary thyroid carcinomas. *Genes Chromosomes Cancer* 1995;13:157–162.
420. Saggiorato E, Cappia S, De Giuli P, et al. Galectin-3 as a presurgical immunocytodiagnostic marker of minimally invasive follicular thyroid carcinoma. *J Clin Endocrinol Metab* 2001;86:5152–5158.
421. Viglietto G, Chiappetta G, Martinez-Tello F, et al. RET/PTC oncogene activation is an early event in thyroid carcinogenesis. *Oncogene* 1995;11: 1207–1210.
422. Greco A, Mariani C, Miranda C, et al. The DNA rearrangement that generates the TRK-T3 oncogene involves a novel gene on chromosome 3 whose product has a potential coiled-coil domain. *Mol Cell Biol* 1995;15:618–627.
423. Prevostel C, Alvaro V, de Boisvilliers F, et al. The natural protein kinase C alpha mutant is present in human thyroid neoplasms. *Oncogene* 1995;11: 669–674.
424. Van Herle A, Rich P, Ljung B. The thyroid nodule. *Ann Intern Med* 1982;96:221.
425. Tyler D, Winchester D, Caraway N. Indeterminate fine needle aspiration biopsy of the thyroid: identification of subgroups at high risk for invasive carcinoma. *Surgery* 1994;116:1054.
426. Gharib H, Mazzaferri EL. Thyroxine suppressive therapy in patients with nodular thyroid disease. *Ann Intern Med* 1998;128:386–394.
427. Pita J. Suppressive therapy with levothyroxine for solitary thyroid nodules. *N Engl J Med* 1987;317:1663.
428. Cheung P, Lee J, Boey J. Thyroxine suppressive therapy of benign solitary thyroid nodules: a randomized prospective study. *World J Surg* 1989;13: 818–822.
429. Gharib H, Goellner J, Zinsmeister A. Fine needle aspiration biopsy of the thyroid. *Ann Intern Med* 1984;101:25–28.
430. LaRosa G, Lupo L, Giuffrida D. Levothyroxine and potassium iodide are both effective in treating benign solitary solid cold nodules of the thyroid. *Ann Intern Med* 1995;122:108.
431. Papini E, Bacci V, Panunzi C. A prospective randomized trial of levothyroxine suppressive therapy for solitary thyroid nodules. *Clin Endocrinol* (Oxf) 1993;38:507–513.
432. Cooper D. Thyroxine suppression for benign nodular disease. *J Clin Endocrinol Metab* 1995;80:331–334.
433. Mandel S, Brent G, Larsen P. Levothyroxine therapy in patients with thyroid disease. *Ann Intern Med* 1993;119:492–502.
434. Faber J, Galloe A. Changes in bone mass during prolonged subclinical hyperthyroidism due to L-thyroxine treatment: a meta-analysis. *Eur J Endocrinol* 1994;130:350–356.
435. Nixon J, Anderson R, Cohen M. Alterations in left ventricular mass and performance in patients treated effectively for thyrotoxicosis: a comparative echocardiographic study. *Am J Med* 1979;67:268–276.
436. Sawin C, Geller A, Wolf P. Low serum thyrotropin concentration as a risk factor for atrial fibrillation in older persons. *N Engl J Med* 1994;331:1249–1252.
437. Rojeski M, Gharib H. Nodular thyroid disease. *N Engl J Med* 1993;313:428–436.
438. Lennquist S. Surgical strategy in thyroid carcinoma: a clinical review. *Acta Chir Scand* 1986;152:321.
439. Grant C, Hay I, Gough I. Local recurrence in papillary thyroid carcinoma: is extent of surgical resection important? *Surgery* 1988;104:954.
440. Reeve T, Delbridge K. Thyroid cancers of follicular origin: the place of radical or limited surgery. *Prog Surg* 1988;19:78.
441. Schlumberger M, Tubiana M, De Vathaire F. Long term results of treatment of 283 patients with lung and bone metastases from differentiated thyroid carcinoma. *J Clin Endocrinol Metab* 1986;63:1956.
442. Cady B. Surgery of thyroid cancer. *World J Surg* 1981;5:3.
443. Stanburg J. Familial goiter. In: Stanburg J, Wyngaarden J, Fredrickson P, eds. *The metabolic basis of inherited disease,* vol 4. New York: McGraw-Hill, 1978: 206.
444. Crile G Jr. Treatment of carcinoma of the thyroid. In: Young S, Inman D, eds. *Controversy in surgery.* Philadelphia: WB Saunders, 1976:39.
445. Mazzaferri EL, Kloos RT. Clinical review 128: current approaches to primary therapy for papillary and follicular thyroid cancer. *J Clin Endocrinol Metab* 2001;86:1447–1463.

446. Kitamura Y, Shimizu K, Nagahama M, et al. Immediate causes of death in thyroid carcinoma: clinicopathological analysis of 161 fatal cases. *J Clin Endocrinol Metab* 1999;84:4043–4049.
447. Tollefsen H, Shah J, Huvos A. Papillary cancer of the thyroid: recurrence in the gland after initial surgical treatment. *Am J Surg* 1972;124:468.
448. Siperstein AE, Clark OH. Surgical therapy. In: Braverman LE, Utiger RD, eds. *Werner and Ingbar's the thyroid: a fundamental and clinical text,* 7th ed. Philadelphia: Lippincott-Raven, 1996:920.
449. Robbins KT, Medina JE, Wolfe GT, et al. Standardizing neck dissection terminology: official report of the Academy's Committee for Head and Neck Surgery and Oncology. *Arch Otolaryngol Head Neck Surg* 1991;117:601–605.
450. Brierley JD, Tsang RW. External radiation therapy in the treatment of thyroid malignancy. *Endocrinol Metab Clin North Am* 1996;25:141–157.
451. Russel C, Van Herrden J, Sizemore G. The surgical management of medullary thyroid carcinoma. *Ann Surg* 1983:197:42.
452. Grillo A, Zannini P. Resectional management of airway invasion by thyroid carcinoma. *Ann Thorac Surg* 1986;42:287.
453. Ballantyne A. Resections of the upper aerodigestive tract for locally invasive thyroid cancer. *Am J Surg* 1994;168:636.
454. Friedman M, Shelton V, Skolnick G. Laryngotracheal invasion by thyroid carcinoma. *Ann Otol Rhinol Laryngol* 1982;91:363.
455. Lipton R, McCaffrey T, von Heerden J. Surgical treatment of invasion of the upper aerodigestive tract by well differentiated thyroid carcinoma. *Am J Surg* 1987;154:363.
456. Freidman M, Skolnick E, Baum H. Thyroid carcinoma. *Laryngoscope* 1980;90: 1991.
457. Gerwat J, Bryce D. The management of subglottic laryngeal stenosis by resection and direct anastomosis. *Laryngoscope* 1974;84:940.
458. Pearson F, Cooper J, Nelems J. Primary tracheal anastomosis after resection of cricoid cartilage with preservation of recurrent laryngeal nerves. *J Thorac Cardiovasc Surg* 1975;70:806–816.
459. Samaan N, Schultz P, Hickey R. The results of various modalities of treatment of well differentiated thyroid carcinoma: a retrospective review of 1599 patients. *J Clin Endocrinol Metab* 1992; 75:714.
460. Simpson W, Carruthers J. The role of external radiation in the management of papillary and follicular thyroid cancer. *Am J Surg* 1978;136:457.
461. Simpson W. Radioiodine and radiotherapy in the management of thyroid cancers. *Otolaryngol Clin North Am* 1990;23:509.
462. Wells S, Dilley W Famdon J. Early diagnosis and treatment of medullary thyroid carcinoma. *Arch Intern Med* 1985;145:1248.
463. Tisell L, Hansson G, Jansson S, et al. Reoperation in the treatment of asymptomatic metastasizing medullary thyroid carcinoma. *Surgery* 1986;99:60–68.
464. Moley J, Wells S, Dilley W, et al. Reoperation for recurrent or persistent medullary thyroid cancer. *Surgery* 1993;114:1090.
465. Shimaoka K, Schoenfeld D, De Wys W. A randomized trial of doxorubicin versus doxorubicin plus cisplatin in patients with advanced thyroid carcinoma. *Cancer* 1985;56:2155.
466. Tennvall J, Lundell G, Hallquist A, et al. Combined doxorubicin, hyperfractionated radiotherapy, and surgery in anaplastic thyroid carcinoma. Report on two protocols. *Cancer* 1994;74:1348.
467. Tallroth E, Wallin G, Lundell G. Multimodality treatment in anaplastic giant cell thyroid carcinoma. *Cancer* 1987;16:1428.
468. U.S. Dept. of Health and Human Services, Public Health Service. *Cancer statistics review 1973–87.* Bethesda, MD: National Institutes of Health, 1991:1,39.
469. Gordin J, Sallan S. Thyroid cancer in childhood. *Endocrinol Metab Clin North Am* 1990;19:649.
470. Goepfert H, Dichtel W, Samaan N. Thyroid cancer in children and teenagers. *Arch Otolaryngol* 1984;110:72.
471. Simpson W, Panzarella T, Carruthers J. Papillary and follicular thyroid cancer: impact of treatment in 1578 patients. *Int J Radiat Oncol Biol Phys* 1988; 14:1063.
472. Zimmerman D, Hay I, Bergstralh E. Papillary thyroid carcinoma in children. In: Robbins J, ed. *Treatment of thyroid cancer in childhood: proceedings of a workshop held September 10—11, 1992, at the NIH in Bethesda, Maryland.* DOE/EH-0406. Springfield, VA: U.S. Department of Commerce, 1992:3.
473. Ceccarelli C, Pacini F, Lippi F. Thyroid cancer in children and adolescents. *Surgery* 1988;104:1143.
474. Gupta S, Patel A, Folstad A, et al. Infiltration of differentiated thyroid carcinoma by proliferating lymphocytes is associated with improved disease-free survival for children and young adults. *J Clin Endocrinol Metab* 2001;86: 1346–1354.
475. Harness J, Thompson N, McLeod M. Differentiated thyroid carcinoma in children and adolescents. *World J Surg* 1992;16:547.
476. Burmeister L, duCret R, Mariash C. Local reactions to radioiodine in the treatment of thyroid cancer. *Am J Med* 1991;90:217.
477. Dulgeroff A, Hershman J. Medical therapy for differentiated thyroid carcinoma. *Endocr Rev* 1994;15:50.
478. Dulgeroff A, Geffner M, Koyal S. Bromocriptine and Triac therapy for hyperthyroidism due to pituitary resistance to thyroid hormone. *J Clin Endocrinol Metab* 1992;75:1071.
479. Carayon P, Guibout M, Lissitzky S. Thyrotropin receptor adenylate cyclase system in plasma membranes from normal and diseased human thyroid glands. *J Endocrinol Invest* 1987;1:321.
480. Mitsumori K, Onodera H, Takahashi M, et al. Effect of thyroid stimulating hormone on the development and progression of rat thyroid follicular cell tumors. *Cancer Lett* 1995;92:193–202.
481. Szanto J, Ringwald G, Karika Z. Follicular cancer of the thyroid gland. *Oncology* 1991;48:483.
482. Young R, Mazzaferri E, Rahe A. Pure follicular thyroid carcinoma: impact of therapy in 214 patients. *J Nucl Med* 1980;21:733.
483. McDermott MT, Perloff JJ, Kidd GS. A longitudinal assessment of bone loss in women with levothyroxine-suppressed benign thyroid disease and thyroid cancer. *Calcif Tissue Int* 1995;56:521–525.
484. Radetti G, Castellan C, Tato L. Bone mineral density in children and adolescent females treated with high doses of L-thyroxine. *Horm Res* 1993;39:127.
485. Dobyns B, Maloof F. The study and treatment of 119 cases of carcinoma of the thyroid with radioactive iodine. *J Clin Endocrinol* 1951;11:1323.
486. Edmonds C, Smith T. The long term hazards of the treatment of thyroid cancer with radioiodine. *Br J Radiol* 1986;59:45.
487. Hilts S, Hellman D, Anderson J. Serial TSH determination after T3 withdrawal or thyroidectomy in the therapy of thyroid carcinoma. *J Nucl Med* 1979;20:928.
488. Haugen BR, Pacini F, Reiners C, et al. A comparison of recombinant human thyrotropin and thyroid hormone withdrawal for the detection of thyroid remnant or cancer. Randomized controlled trial. *J Clin Endocrin Metab* 1999; 84:3877–3885.
489. Ladenson PW. Recombinant thyrotropin versus thyroid hormone withdrawal in evaluating patients with thyroid carcinoma. *Semin Nucl Med* 2000;30:98–106.
490. Meier A, Braverman L, Ebner S. Diagnostic use of recombinant human thyrotropin in patients with thyroid carcinoma (phase I/II study). *J Clin Endocrinol Metab* 1994;78:188.
491. Morris LF, Waxman AD, Braunstein GD. The nonimpact of thyroid stunning: remnant ablation rates in 131I-scanned and nonscanned individuals. *J Clin Endocrinol Metab* 2001;86:3507–3511.
492. Edmonds C, Hayes S, Kermode J, et al. Measurement of serum TSH and thyroid hormones in the management of treatment of thyroid carcinoma with radioiodine. *Br J Radiol* 1977;40:195.
493. Lakshmanan M, Schaffer A, Bobbins J. A simplified low iodine diet in I-131 scanning and therapy of thyroid cancer. *Clin Nucl Med* 1988;2:866.
494. Maxon H, Boehringer T, Drilling J. Low iodine diet in I-131 ablation of thyroid remnants. *Clin Nucl Med* 1983;8:123.
495. Maraca J, Santner S, Miller K. Prolonged iodine clearance with a depletion regimen for thyroid carcinoma: concise communication. *J Nucl Med* 1984;25:1089.
496. Wen C, Iuanow E, Oates E, et al. Post-therapy iodine-131 localization in unsuspected large renal cyst: possible mechanisms. *J Nucl Med* 1998;39: 2158–2161.
497. Bierwaltes W Rabbani R, Dmuchowski C. An analysis of ablation of thyroid remnants with I-131 in 511 patients from 1947–1984: experience at U of Michigan. *J Nucl Med* 1984;25:1287.
498. Goolden A. The indications for ablating normal thyroid tissue with 131-I in differentiated thyroid cancer. *Clin Endocrinol* 1985;23:81.
499. Van De Velde C, Hamming J, Goslings B. Report of the consensus development conference on the management of differentiated thyroid cancer in the Netherlands. *Ear J Cancer Clin Oncol* 1988;24:287.
500. Baldet L, Manderscheid J, Glinoer D. The management of differentiated thyroid cancer in Europe in 1988.Results of an international survey. *Acta Endocrinol* 1989;120:547.
501. Ronga G, Fiorentino A, Paserio E. Can iodine-131 whole body scan be replaced by thyroglobulin measurement in the postsurgical follow up of differentiated thyroid carcinoma? *Arch Surg* 1988;123:569.
502. Sisson J. Applying the radioactive eraser: I-131 to ablate normal thyroid tissue in patients from whom thyroid cancer has been resected. *J Nucl Med* 1983;24:743.
503. Schlumberger M. Can I-131 replace thyroglobulin for follow up of differentiated thyroid carcinoma? *J Nucl Med* 1992;33:172.
504. Ramanna L, Waxman A, Braunstein G. Thallium-201 scintigraphy in differentiated thyroid cancer: comparison with radioiodine scintigraphy and serum thyroglobulin determination. *J Nucl Med* 1991;32:441.
505. Mazzaferri E. Radioiodine and other treatments and outcomes. In: Braverman LE, Utiger RD, eds. *Werner and Ingbar's the thyroid: a fundamental and clinical text,* 7th ed. Philadelphia: Lippincott-Raven, 1996:922–945.
506. Eipe J, Johnson S, Kiamko R. Hypoparathyroidism following 131-I therapy for hyperthyroidism. *Arch Intern Med* 1968;121:270.
507. Nemec J, Zamrazil V, Pohunkova D, et al. Radioiodide treatment of pulmonary metastases of differentiated thyroid cancer. Results and prognostic factors. *Nuklearmedizin* 1979;18:86.
508. Varma V, Beierwaltes W, Now M. Treatment of thyroid cancer: death rates after surgery and after surgery followed by sodium iodine I-131. *JAMA* 1970; 214:437.
509. Hay I. Papillary thyroid carcinoma. *Endocrinol Metab Clin North Am* 1990;19:545.
510. Freitas J, Gross M, Ripley S. Radionuclide diagnosis and therapy of thyroid cancer: current status report. *Semin Nucl Med* 1985;15:106.
511. Dinneen S, Valimake M, Bergstralh E, et al. Distant metastases in papillary thyroid carcinoma: 100 cases observed at one institution during five decades. *J Clin Endocrinol Metab* 1995;80:2041–2045.
512. Eroglu A, Berberoglu U, Buruk F, et al. Completion thyroidectomy for differentiated thyroid carcinoma. *J Surg Oncol* 1995;59:261–266.
513. Segal K, Friedental R, Lubin E, et al. Papillary carcinoma of the thyroid. *Otolaryngol Head Neck Surg* 1995;113:356–363.
514. McHenry C, Jarosz H, Davis M. Selective postoperative radioactive iodine treatment of thyroid carcinoma. *Surgery* 1989;106:956.

515. Harbert J. Radioiodine therapy of differentiated thyroid carcinoma. In: *Nuclear medicine therapy*. New York: Thieme, 1987.
516. Rossi R, Cady B, Silverman M. Surgically incurable well-differentiated thyroid carcinoma. *Arch Surg* 1988;12:569.
517. Proye C, Dromer D, Carnaille B. Is it worthwhile to treat bone metastases from differentiated thyroid carcinoma with radioactive iodine? *World J Surg* 1992;16:640.
518. Brown A, Greening W, McCready V. Radioiodine treatment of metastatic thyroid carcinoma: the Royal Marsden Hospital experience. *Br J Radiol* 1984;57: 323.
519. Asadian A, Rosen I, Walfish P, et al. Management considerations in Hurthle cell carcinoma. *Surgery* 1995;118:711–714.
520. Pons F, Carrio 1, Estorch M. Lithium as an adjuvant of iodine-131 uptake when treating patients with well differentiated thyroid carcinoma. *Clin Nucl Med* 1987;8:644.
521. Reynolds J. Future prospects for treatment of differentiated thyroid carcinoma. *Ann Intern Med* 1991;115:133.
522. Robbins J. The role of TRH and lithium in the management of thyroid cancer. In: Andreoli M, Monaco F, Robbinsa J, eds. *Advances in thyroid neoplasia*. Rome: Field Educational Italia, 1981:233.
523. Dumas L, Wolf C, Keck F. Thyrotropin releasing hormone (TRH) metabolism and thyrotropin secretion after repeated administrations of nasal TRH. *Thyroid* 1991;1:S84.
524. Schmutzler C, Kohrle J. Retinoic acid redifferentiation therapy for thyroid cancer. *Thyroid* 2000;10:393–406.
525. Goolden A, Kam K, Fitzpatrick M. Oedema of the neck after ablation of the thyroid with radioactive iodine. *Br J Radial* 1986;59:583.
526. Allweiss P, Braunstein G, Kate A. Sialadenitis following I-131 therapy for thyroid carcinoma: concise communication. *J Nucl Med* 1984;25:755.
527. Abbatt J, Brown W, Farran H. Radiation sickness in man following the administration of therapeutic radioiodine: relationship between latent period, dose rate and body size. *Br J Radiol* 1955;28:358.
528. Glazebrook G. Effect of decicurie doses of radioactive iodine 131 on parathyroid function. *Am J Surg* 1987;154:368.
529. Casara D, Rubello D, Saladini G, et al. Thyroid cancer: potential risks and recommendations. *Eur J Nucl Med* 1993;20:192–194.
530. Dottorini M, Lomuscio G, Mazzucchelli L. Assessment of female fertility and carcinogenesis after I-131 therapy for differentiated thyroid carcinoma. *J Nucl Med* 1995;36:21.
531. Pacini F, Gasperi M, Fugazzola L, et al. Testicular function in patients with differentiated thyroid cancer treated with radioiodine. *J Nucl Med* 1994;35: 1418.
532. Haynie T, Beierwaltes W. Hematologic changes observed following therapy for thyroid carcinoma. *J Nucl Med* 1963;4:85.
533. Benua R, Cicale N, Sonenberg M. The relation of radioiodine dosimetry to results and complications in the treatment of metastatic thyroid cancer. *AJR* 1962;87:171.
534. Brincker H, Hansen H, Andersen A. Induction of leukemia by 131-I treatment of thyroid carcinoma. *Br J Cancer* 1973;28:232.
535. Hall P, Boice J, Berg G. Leukemia incidence after iodine exposure. *Lancet* 1992;340:1.
536. Rall J, Alpers J, Lewallen C. Radiation pneumonitis and fibrosis: a complication of radioiodine treatment of pulmonary metastases from cancer of the thyroid. *J Clin Endocrinol Metab* 1957;17:1263.
537. Brunt L, Wells S. Advances in the diagnosis and treatment of medullary carcinoma. *Surg Clin North Am* 1987;67:263.
538. Rougier P, Parmentier C, LaPlanche A. Medullary thyroid carcinoma: prognostic factors and treatment. *Int J Radiat Oncol Biol Phys* 1983;9:161.
539. Steinfeld A. The role of radiation therapy in medullary carcinoma of the thyroid. *Radiology* 1977;123:745.
540. Nguyen T, Chassard J, Lagarde P. Results of postoperative radiation therapy in medullary carcinoma of the thyroid: a retrospective study by the French Federation of Cancer Institutes. The Radiotherapy Cooperative Group. *Radiother Oncol* 1992;23:1.
541. Parsons J, Stringer S, Manciso A. Cancer of the thyroid. In: Million R, Cassisi N, eds. *Management of head and neck cancer,* 2nd ed. Philadelphia: JB Lippincott, 1994:785.
542. Schlumberger M, Parmentier C, deVathiere F. 131-I and external radiation in the treatment of local metastatic thyroid cancer. In: Falk S, ed. *Thyroid disease. Endocrinology, surgery, nuclear medicine and radiotherapy.* New York: Raven Press, 1990:537.
543. Samaan N, Schultz P, Hickey R. Medullary thyroid carcinoma: prognosis of familial versus sporadic disease and the role of radiotherapy. *J Clin Endocrinol Metab* 1988;67:801.
544. Benker G, Olbricht T, Reinwein D. Survival rates in patients with differentiated thyroid carcinoma: influence of postoperative external radiotherapy. *Cancer* 1990;65:1517.
545. Simpson W, Palmer J, Rosen I. Management of medullary carcinoma of the thyroid. *Am J Surg* 1982;144:420.
546. Samaan N, Yanbg K, Schultz P. Diagnosis, management, and pathogenetic studies in medullary thyroid carcinoma syndrome. *Henry Ford Hosp Med J* 1989;37:132.
547. Sarrazin D, Fontaine F, Rougier P. Role of radiotherapy in the treatment of medullary cancer of the thyroid. *Bull Cancer (Paris)* 1984;71:200.
548. Schlumberger M, Gardet F, de Vathaire. External radiotherapy and chemotherapy in MTC patients. In: Calmettes C, Guliana J, eds. *Medullary thyroid carcinoma.* Montrouge, France: Colloques INSERM/John Libbey Eurotext, 1991:213.
549. Junor E, Paul J, Reed N. Anaplastic thyroid carcinoma: 91 patients treated by surgery and radiotherapy. *Eur J Surg Oncol* 1992;18:83.
550. Tan R, Finley R, Driscoli D. Anaplastic carcinoma of the thyroid: a 24 year experience. *Head Neck* 1995;17:41.
551. Burgess M, Hill C Jr. Chemotherapy in the management of thyroid cancer. In: Greenfield L, ed. *Thyroid cancer.* Boca Raton, FL: CRC Press, 1978:233.
552. Ekman E, Lundell G, Tennvall J. Chemotherapy and multimodality treatment in thyroid carcinoma. *Otolaryngol Clin North Am* 1990;23:523.
553. Hadar T, Mor C, Shvero J. Anaplastic carcinoma of the thyroid. *Ear J Surg Oncol* 1993;19:511.
554. de Besi P, Busnardo B, Toso S. Combined chemotherapy with bleomycin, Adriamycin and platinum in advanced thyroid cancer. *J Endocrinol Invest* 1991;14:475.
555. Ozata M, Suzuki S, Miyamoto T. Serum thyroglobulin in the follow up of patients with treated differentiated thyroid cancer. *J Clin Endocrinol Metab* 1994;79:98.
556. von Sorge-van Boxtel R, van Eck-Smit B, Gosling B. Comparison of serum thyroglobulin ^{131}I and ^{201}Th scintography in the post-operative follow-up of differentiated thyroid cancer. *Nucl Med Commun* 1993;14:365–372.
557. Muller-Gartner H, Schneider C, Tenpel M. Serum thyroglobulin in der metastasendiagnostil des differenzierten schilddrusenkarzinoms. *Nucl Med Biol* 1986;25:194.
558. Szanto J, Vincze B, Sinkovics I. Postoperative thyroglobulin level determination to follow-up patients with highly differentiated thyroid cancer. *Oncology* 1989;46:99.
559. Haapala A, Soppi E, Morsky P, et al. Thyroid antibodies in association with thyroid malignancy II: qualitative properties of thyroglobulin antibodies. *Scand J Clin Lab Invest* 1995;55:317–322.
560. Erricsson U, Christensen S, Thorell J. A high prevalence of thyroglobulin autoantibodies in adults with and without thyroid disease as measured with a sensitive solid phase immunosorbent radioassay. *Clin Immunol Immunopathol* 1985;37:154.
561. Clark O, Hoefing T. Management of patients with differentiated thyroid cancer who have positive serum thyroglobulin levels and negative radioiodine scans. *Thyroid* 1994;4:501.
562. Dralle H, Schwarzrock R, Lang W. Comparison of histology and immunohistochemistry with thyroglobulin serum levels and radioiodine uptake in recurrences and metastases of differentiated thyroid carcinomas. *Acta Endocrinol (Copenh)* 1985;108:504.
563. Robbins J. Thyroid cancer: a lethal endocrine neoplasm. *Ann Intern Med* 1991; 115:133.
564. Wohlkk N, Cote G, Evans D, et al. Application of genetic screening information to the management of medullary thyroid carcinoma and multiple endocrine neoplasia type 2. *Endocrinol Metab Clin North Am* 1996;25:1–25.
565. Lore J, Kim D, Elias S. Preservation of the laryngeal nerves during total thyroid lobectomy. *Ann Otol Rhinol Laryngol* 1977;86:777.
566. Ward P, Berci G, Calcaterra T. Superior laryngeal nerve paralysis, an often overlooked entity. *Trans Am Acad Ophthalmol Otolaryngol* 1977;84:78.
567. Beahrs O. Complications of surgery of the head and neck. *Surg Clin North Am* 1977;57:823.
568. Flynn M, Lyons K, Tartar J. Local complications after surgical resection for thyroid cancer. *Am J Surg* 1994;168:404.
569. Boles R, Fritzell B. Injury and repair of the recurrent laryngeal nerves in dogs. *Laryngoscope* 1969;70:1405.
570. Crumley R, Izdensk K. Voice quality following laryngeal reinnervation by ansa hypoglossal transfer. *Laryngoscope* 1986;96:611–616.
571. Tucker H. Reinnervation of unilateral paralyzed larynx. *Ann Otol Rhinol Laryngol* 1977;86:789.
572. Dedo H. The paralyzed larynx: an electromyographic study in dogs and humans. *Laryngoscope* 1970;80:1455.
573. Isshiki N, Morita H, Okamura H. Thyroplasty as a new phonosurgical technique. *Acta Otolaryngol* 1974;78:451.
574. Isshiki N, Tanabe M, Sawada M. Arytenoid adduction for unilateral vocal cord paralysis. *Arch Otolaryngol* 1978;104:555.
575. Isshiki N. Recent advances in phonosurgery. *Folia Phoniatr* 1980;32:119.
576. Koufman J. *Laryngoplastic phonosurgery instructional courses.* St. Louis: Mosby, 1988:339.
577. Ossoff R, Sisson GA, Dunclavage JA, et al. Endoscopic laser arytenoidectomy for the treatment of bilateral vocal cord paralysis. *Laryngoscope* 1984;94:1293.
578. Kashima HK. Bilateral vocal fold motion impairment: pathophysiology and management by transverse cordotomy. *Ann Otol Rhinol Laryngol* 1991;100(9 Pt 1):717–721.
579. Parnes S, Satya-Murti S. Predictive value of laryngeal electromyography in patients with vocal cord paralysis of neurogenic origin. *Laryngoscope* 1985;95: 1323.
580. Rodriguez A, Myers B, Ford C. Laryngeal electromyography in the diagnosis of laryngeal nerve injuries. *Arch Phys Med Rehabil* 1990;71:587.
581. Troost T, Smith R, Miller S, et al. Alterations in airflow and voice after transverse cordotomy for bilateral vocal told paralysis. *Otolaryngol Head Neck Surg* 1994;111:178(abst).
582. Applebaum E, Allen G, Sisson G. Human laryngeal reinnervation. The Northwestern experience. *Laryngoscope* 1979;89:1784.
583. Moreledge D, Lauvstad W, Calcaterra T. Delayed reinnervation of paralyzed larynx. *Arch Otolaryngol* 1973;97:291.

584. May M, Lavorato A, Bleyaert A. Rehabilitation of the crippled larynx: application of the Tucker technique for muscle nerve reinnervation. *Laryngoscope* 1980;90:1.
585. Rice D. Laryngeal reinnervation. *Laryngoscope* 1982;92:1049.
586. Crumley R. Experiments in laryngeal reinnervation. *Laryngoscope* 1982;92 (suppl 30):1.
587. Crumley R, Horn K, Clendenning D. Laryngeal reinnervation using the split phrenic nerve graft procedure. *Otolaryngol Head Neck Surg* 1980;88:159–164.
588. Falk S, Birken E, Baran D. Temporary post thyroidectomy hypocalcemia. *Arch Otolaryngol Head Neck Surg* 1988;114:168.
589. Bourrel C, Uzzan B, Tisson P, et al. Transient hypocalcemia after thyroidectomy. *Ann Otol Rhinol Laryngol* 1993;102:496–501.
590. Beahrs O. Complications in thyroid and parathyroid surgery. In: Conley J, ed. *Complications in head and neck surgery.* Philadelphia: WB Saunders, 1979:239.
591. Walker R, Paloyan E, Kelley T. Parathyroid autotransplantation in patients undergoing total thyroidectomy: a review of 261 patients. *Otolaryngol Head Neck Surg* 1994;111:258.
592. Michie W Duncan T, Hamer-Hodges DW, et al. Mechanisms of hypocalcemia after thyroidectomy for thyrotoxicosis. *Lancet* 1971;1:508–514.
593. Demeester-Mirkine N, Hooghe L, Van Geertruyden J, et al. Hypocalcemia after thyroidectomy. *Arch Surg* 1992;127:854–858.
594. Watson C, Steed D, Robinson AG, et al. The role of calcitonin and parathyroid hormone in the pathogenesis of postthyroidectomy hypocalcemia. *Metabolism* 1981;30:588–589.
595. Shambaugh GE III, Khoury N, Zonschein J, et al. Hypocalcemia accompanying agranulocytosis during propylthiouracil therapy. *Ann Intern Med* 1979;91: 576–577.
596. Falk S. Metabolic complications of thyroid surgery: hypocalcemia and hypoparathyroidism; hypocalcitonemia; and hypothyroidism and hyperthyroidism. In: Falk S, ed. *Thyroid disease.* Philadelphia: Lippincott-Raven, 1997: 717.
597. McHenry C, Speroff T, Wentworth D, et al. Risk factors for hypocalcemia. *Surgery* 1994;116:641–647.
598. Wingert DJ, Friesen SR, Iliopoulos If, et al. Post-thyroidectomy hypocalcemia. Incidence and risk factors. *Am J Surg* 1986;152:606–610.
599. Szubin L, Kacker A, Kakani R, et al. The management of postthyroidectomy hypocalcemia. *Ear Nose Throat J* 1996;75:612–616.
600. Rude R. Magnesium metabolism. In: Becker K, ed. *Principles and practice of endocrinology and metabolism.* Philadelphia: JB Lippincott, 1995.
601. Reber P, Heath H. Hypocalcemic emergencies. *Med Clin North Am* 1995;79(1): 93–106.

Radiologic Imaging Concerns

602. Boland GW, Lee MJ, Mueller PR, et al. Efficacy of sonographically guided biopsy of thyroid masses and cervical lymph nodes. *AJR* 1993;161:1053–1056.
603. Dorr U, Wurstlin S, Frank-Raue K, et al. Somatostatin receptor scintigraphy and magnetic resonance imaging in recurrent medullary thyroid carcinoma: a comparative study. *Horm Metab Res Suppl* 1993;27:48–55.
604. Hopkins CR, Reading CC. Thyroid and parathyroid imaging. [Review] *Semin Ultrasound CT MR* 1995;16:279–295.
605. Scott AM, Macapinlac H, Zhang J, et al. Image registration of SPECT and CT images using an external fiduciary band and three-dimensional surface fitting in metastatic thyroid cancer. *J Nucl Med* 1995;36:100–103.
606. Mallin WH, Elgazzar AH, Maxon HR 3rd. Imaging modalities in the follow-up of non-iodine avid thyroid carcinoma. [Review] *Am J Otolaryngol* 1994;15:417–422.
607. Muros MA, Llamas-Elvira JM, Ramirez-Navarro A, et al. Utility of fluorine-18-fluorodeoxyglucose positron emission tomography in differentiated thyroid carcinoma with negative radioiodine scans and elevated serum thyroglobulin levels. *Am J Surg* 2000;179:457–461.
608. Wang W, Macapinlac H, Larson SM, et al. [18F]-2-fluoro-2-deoxy-D-glucose positron emission tomography localizes residual thyroid cancer in patients with negative diagnostic (131)I whole body scans and elevated serum thyroglobulin levels. *J Clin Endocrinol Metab* 1999;84:2291–2302.
609. Wang W, Larson SM, Fazzari M, et al. Prognostic value of [18F]fluorodeoxyglucose positron emission tomographic scanning in patients with thyroid cancer. *J Clin Endocrinol Metab* 2000;85:1107–1113.
610. Adams S, Acker P, Lorenz M, et al. Radioisotope-guided surgery in patients with pheochromocytoma and recurrent medullary thyroid carcinoma: a comparison of preoperative and intraoperative tumor localization with histopathologic findings. *Cancer* 2001;92:263–270.
611. Freitas JE, Freitas AE. Thyroid and parathyroid imaging. [Review] *Semin Nucl Med* 1994;24:234–245.
612. Shen W, Duren M, Morita E, et al. Reoperation for persistent or recurrent primary hyperparathyroidism. *Arch Surg* 1996;131:861–867; discussion 867–869.
613. Greene AK, Mowschenson P, Hodin RA. Is sestamibi-guided parathyroidectomy really cost-effective? *Surgery* 1999;126:1036–1040; discussion 1040–1031.
614. Norman J, Denham D. Minimally invasive radioguided parathyroidectomy in the reoperative neck. *Surgery* 1998;124:1088–1092; discussion 1092–1083.
615. Sanders LE, Rossi RL, Shahian DM, et al. Mediastinal goiters. The need for an aggressive approach. *Arch Surg* 1992;127:609–613.

CHAPTER 30

Soft Tissue and Bone Sarcomas of the Head and Neck

Brian O'Sullivan, Nathalie Audet, Charles N. Catton, and Patrick J. Gullane

Sarcomas are rare malignancies of mesodermal origin. The annual incidence is less than 10,000 per year in North America. Fifteen percent of cases occur in the head and neck region, comprising less than 1% of all head and neck cancers. Not only are they rare, but an excess of 40 histopathologic subtypes may affect numerous anatomic sites within the head and neck. The rarity and complex nature of these tumors warrant referral to specialized centers for multidisciplinary evaluation, including expert imaging and pathology assessment. All such consultations and evaluations should take place prior to therapy. In addition to expertise in ablative and reconstructive surgical oncology, the full sarcoma team should include radiation oncology and medical oncology, oncology nursing, radiation therapy, and medical physics. Moreover, unique challenges present themselves in the head and neck demanding special expertise in nutritional support, dental and voice rehabilitation, ophthalmology, and social support.

The management of head and neck sarcoma follows principles extrapolated from other anatomic sites where the disease is more common (1). Although primary data about the head and neck would be desirable, evidence that the biologic behavior differs by anatomic site is not apparent. What sets these lesions apart from tumors elsewhere are the unique functional and cosmetic requirements. Because of the presence of critical anatomy, both surgery and radiotherapy (RT) must be applied more precisely and with greater complexity than elsewhere in the body. Therefore, in particular, neurologic tissues (especially optic apparatus, spinal cord, and brainstem), nonexpendable vascular anatomy, organs necessary for speech and swallowing, and cosmetically sensitive tissues provide substantial challenges.

The chapter provides general information, classification, and management for both soft tissue tumors and their osseous counterparts. The discussion of adjuvant systemic treatments relies for the most part on published meta-analyses for soft tissue sarcoma (STS) and the meta-analyses (overviews) that have been undertaken in head and neck osteosarcoma. Special features include treatment and behavior of unique histologic subtypes. The general problem of salvage for recurrence and the treatment of metastases (soft tissue and bone) concludes the discussion.

PATHOLOGY AND GRADING

Soft tissue and bone sarcoma may present as any of several clinical entities that are disproportionately represented in the head and neck. Clearly, the full range of histologic subtypes seen in other body sites also exist in the head neck, but space limitations prevent a comprehensive discussion. A summary of some of the main issues to be considered in evaluating and classifying these lesions is presented. A brief description of particular clinical features of different histologic subtypes is also presented later.

Pathology of Selected Soft Tissue Sarcoma Subtypes

CLASSIFICATION

The most common classification scheme for STS is based on histogenesis, as outlined in the recent World Health Organization (WHO) classification (Table 30.1) (2). The classification is reproducible for the better-differentiated tumors. However, as the degree of histologic differentiation declines, the determination of cellular origin becomes increasingly difficult. In particular, despite advanced immunohistochemical techniques and electron microscopy, determining the cellular origin for many spindle cell and round cell soft tissue tumors is difficult, occasionally arbitrary, and sometimes impossible. In the head and neck, as elsewhere in the body, the prototypical STS is the malignant fibrous histiocytoma (MFH), but additional unique predispositions include rhabdomyosarcoma, angiosarcoma of the scalp and facial regions, hemangiopericytoma of the sinonasal region (Fig. 30.1A), and dermatofibrosarcoma protuberans of the dermal regions of the low neck and supraclavicular regions. Recently, molecular gene expression profiling of soft tissue tumors with complementary DNA (cDNA) microarrays suggests new methods for classification, which may improve on histologic means of classification (3,4). Already a number of cytogenetic findings and corresponding genetic abnormalities characterize a number of the histologic subtypes (Table 30.2).

Malignant Fibrous Histiocytoma

Traditionally, MFH has been regarded as the most common histologic type of STS. Recent evidence suggests that MFH is a more general diagnosis that can be subtyped by immunohistochemical and ultrastructural means in the majority of patients (5). The most common subclassifications are myxofibrosarcoma and leiomyosarcoma. Subclassification with attention to reclassified MFH subtypes that are of myogenic origin (leiomyosarcoma, rhabdomyosarcoma, pleomorphic myogenic sarcoma, and myogenic spindle-cell sarcoma) appears to be of prognostic significance in that patients with myogenic differentiation appear at greater risk for disease relapse than nonmyogenic reclassified subtypes of MFH.

TABLE 30.1 Principal Histologic Types of Soft Tissue Sarcoma in the WHO Classification of Bone Tumors with ICD-O Morphology Rubrics

Histologic type[a]	ICD-O morphology
Alveolar soft part sarcoma	9581/3
Angiosarcoma	9120/3
Clear cell sarcoma	9044/3
Dermatofibrosarcoma protuberans	8832/3
Epithelioid sarcoma	8804/3
Extraskeletal chondrosarcoma	9220/3
Extraskeletal osteosarcoma	9180/3
Fibrosarcoma	8810/3
Leiomyosarcoma	8890/3
Liposarcoma	8850/3
Malignant fibrous histiocytoma	8830/3
Malignant hemangiopericytoma	9150/3
Malignant mesenchymoma	8990/3
Malignant peripheral nerve sheath tumor	9540/3
Malignant schwannoma, melanotic	9560/3
Rhabdomyosarcoma	8900/3
Synovial sarcoma	9040/3
Sarcoma NOS	8800/3

ICD-O, International Classification of Disease for Oncology; NSO, not otherwise specified; WHO, World Health Organization.
[a]Types listed in alphabetical order.
Source: Weiss SW, Sobin LH. *Histologic typing of soft tissue tumors,* 2nd ed. Berlin: Springer-Verlag, 1994.

Angiosarcoma

A particular problem in the head and neck is angiosarcoma of the scalp and facial regions. This uncommon high-grade malignancy of vascular endothelial cell origin comprises less than 0.1% of all head and neck malignancies (6). Fifty percent of cutaneous angiosarcoma occur in the head and neck region (7). Typical extension is radially within the dermis of the scalp and face. Three histologic growth patterns are recognized: angiomatous (with vascular channels), spindle cell (sheets of cells), and undifferentiated (solid pattern). Immunohistochemistry is helpful in establishing the diagnosis. Factor VIII–related antigen is a marker with variable expression. *Ulex europaeus I* (UEA I) is more sensitive but not more specific. Antibodies directed against CD31 antigen have proven to be specific and sensitive for endothelial cell differentiation (8,9).

Rhabdomyosarcoma

Of great importance in the head and neck is the need to recognize classic rhabdomyosarcoma. Although one of the most common of pediatric solid tumors, it is only rarely encountered in adults. Rhabdomyosarcoma can be recognized on light microscopy by the presence of cross-striations within cytoplasmic fibrils of spindle-shaped cells that typically demonstrate immunostaining for myogenic markers (10). The disease is subdivided into embryonal (about 70% of cases), alveolar (about 20%), and pleomorphic subtypes according to histologic pattern as well as typical molecular alterations (11,12). The pleomorphic subtype is the least common, almost never seen in the pediatric population, and is not considered in those classifications; there is debate about whether it truly represents part of the disease process.

Embryonal rhabdomyosarcoma appears as a spindle or cell or mixed spindle/round cell malignancy in a myxoid or collagenous stroma (Fig. 30.2A). The hallmark is the resemblance to fetal muscle characterized by the rhabdomyoblast, a straplike cell that bears cross-striations in the most differentiated forms. Electron microscopy should show special features such as sarcomeric Z bands and thick and thin filaments.

Alveolar rhabdomyosarcoma has well-defined alveolar-like spaces separated by thick collagenous bands lined by the characteristic round tumor cells with myogenic features (Fig. 30.2B). The cytologic features are in fact sufficient to secure the diagnosis even in the absence of the classic alveolar pattern (termed the "solid alveolar" variant). In addition, the alveolar architecture does not need to predominate and even focal evidence of the pattern is sufficient for the diagnosis.

Both embryonal and alveolar rhabdomyosarcoma have been studied extensively for cytogenic and molecular genetic alterations. No consistent findings have been observed in embryonal rhabdomyosarcoma, although an abnormality at chromosome 11 may be encountered (13). In contrast, in alveolar rhabdomyosarcoma, although a characteristics t(1;13) translocation is rarely seen, the majority possess the t(2;13) aberration. Both translocations may be associated with different clinical phenotypes for the tumor (14). The translocations and the gene fusion products are characteristic for the disease, and the *PAX3* gene family involved in the disease fingerprint may also have a role in muscle development (15).

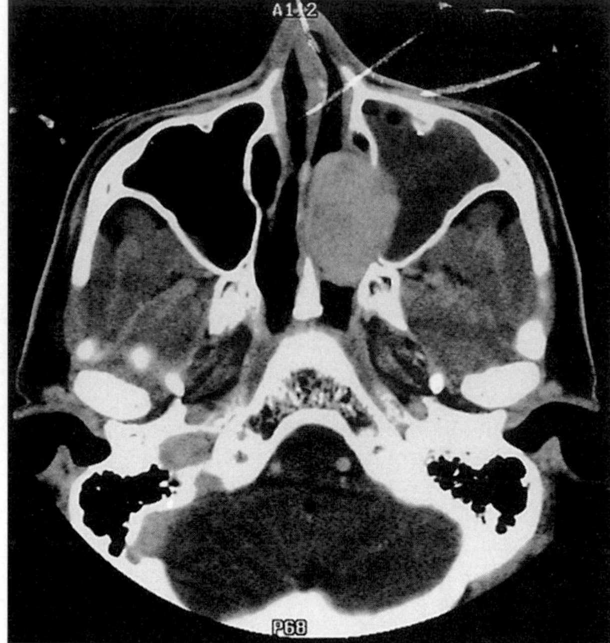

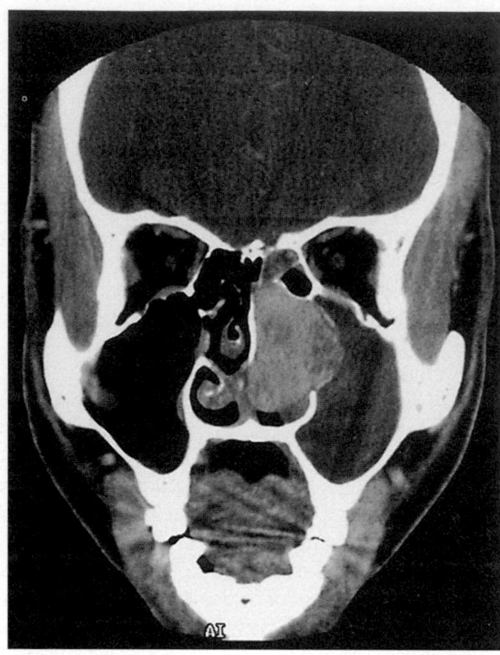

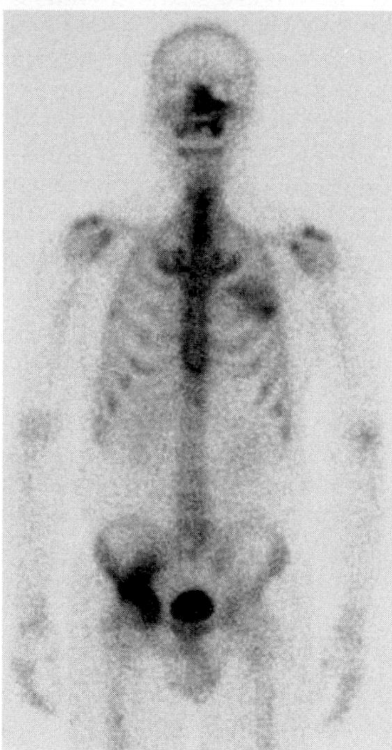

Figure 30.1 Hemangiopericytoma of the left nasal fossa in a 40-year-old man. This patient underwent resection with positive margins for well-circumscribed lesion in 1994 (**A,B**). Postoperative radiotherapy to a dose of 60 Gy achieved durable local control. Recently, after 8 years, he experienced a relapsed with two bone lesions—one in the left chest wall and one in the right pelvis without other lesions, shown on nuclide bone scan (**C**). Both lesions are being treated with combined radiotherapy and surgery. The original primary site also shows nucleotide uptake, but cross-sectional anatomic imaging and clinical examination failed to reveal recurrent tumor (see Fig. 30.8 for histology of such lesions.)

TABLE 30.2 Cytogenetic Abnormalities in Soft Tissue Sarcoma

Histologic subtype	Usual translocations	Genes involved
Alveolar sarcoma of soft parts	t(X;17)	
Chondrosarcomas extraskeletal myxoid	t(9;22),(q22;q12.2)	EWS/CHN
Clear cell sarcoma	t(12;22)(q13;q12)	EWS/ATF1
Congenital infantile fibrosarcoma	t(15;15)(p13;q25)	ETV6, NTRK3
Dermatofibrosarcoma protuberans	t(17;22)(q22;q13)	Collagen type 1 alpha-1; PDGF-B
Desmoplastic small round-cell tumor	t(11;22)(p13;q12)	EWS/WT1
Lipoma (minimal atypia)	12q abnormalities	Amplified 12q13–15
Liposarcoma (myxoid)	t(12;16)(q13;p11)	TLS/CHOP
	t(12;12)(q13;p12)	CHOP/EWS
Liposarcoma well differentiated	Rings and giant markers	Amplified 12q13–15; HMG1-C CDK4; MDM2
Rhabdomyosarcoma (alveolar)	t(2;13)(q35;q14)t(1;13)(p36,q14)	PAX3 (or 7)/FKHR
Synovial sarcoma	t(X;18)(p11.2;q11.2)	SYT/SSX1 or SSX2

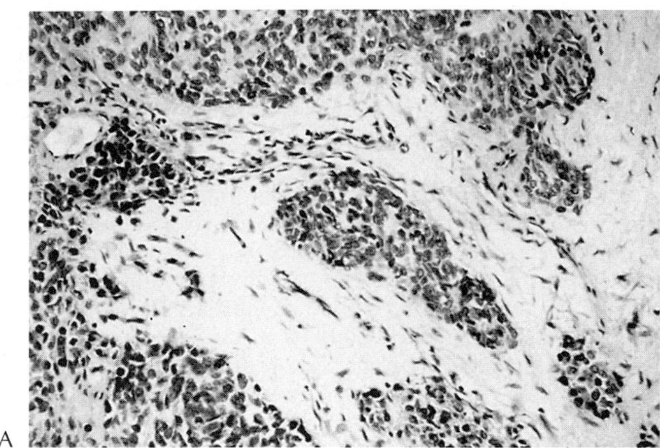
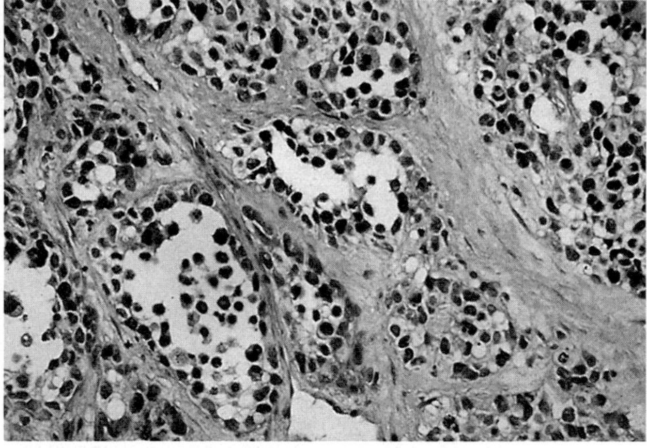

Figure 30.2 **A:** Embryonal rhabdomyosarcoma cells in a myxoid or collagenous stroma. **B:** Alveolar rhabdomyosarcoma showing alveolar-like spaces separated by thick collagenous bands lined by characteristic round tumor cells. (Courtesy of Dr. David Howarth, Staff Pathologist, Sarcoma Site Program, Princess Margaret Hospital and Mount Sinai Hospital, University of Toronto, Ontario, Canada.)

Dermatofibrosarcoma Protuberans

Although clinically this lesion is usually well circumscribed, pathologically dermatofibrosarcoma protuberans (DFSP) diffusely infiltrates the skin and subcutis. Fibrosarcomatous change with multiple recurrences may be seen over many years. Infiltration can take place along connective tissue septa, between adnexa and interdigitating with lobules of subcutaneous fat. A uniform population of slender fibroblasts is arranged in a monotonous storiform pattern with little nuclear pleomorphism and low mitotic activity. Characteristic immunohistochemical staining for CD34 suggests evidence of neural differentiation. In addition, chromosomal translocation and gene fusion products have been observed (Table 30.2). The result is that platelet-derived growth factor (PDGF) is increased locally, resulting in autocrine or paracrine tumor growth. Of importance, imatinib (STI-571, Gleevec®, Novartis, Cambridge, MA) is an inhibitor of the PDGF receptor tyrosine kinase in the same way as it has activity against the *bcr-abl* tyrosine kinase of chronic myeloid leukemia and the *c-kit* tyrosine kinase of gastrointestinal stromal tumor. Recent clinical data have shown response to imatinib in metastatic DFSP (16). This suggests the opportunity for targeted molecular therapies in the future and particularly for metastatic or locally advanced DFSP if other therapy options are limited.

Synovial Sarcoma

Unusual histologic characteristics on light microscopy and immunohistochemistry are seen in synovial sarcoma, where a biphasic cellular pattern consisting of a stroma of fibroblast spindle-like cells and epithelial-like cells in a glandular pattern is often seen. Synovial sarcoma typically has a t(x;18) translocation and demonstrates a fusion between the *SSX1* and *SYT* genes with a biphasic appearance on light microscopy in two thirds of cases, whereas the remainder show fusion between the *SSX2* and *SYT* genes with monophasic histology. The *SSX1* fusion portends a worse prognosis than the *SSX2* translocation (17).

Grading Soft Tissue Sarcoma

One of the most consistent prognostic factors in STS for the risk for distant metastasis and tumor-specific mortality is histologic grade. Despite this, there is no agreement about which grading system should be used. Two of the best known are the French Federation of Cancer Centers Sarcoma Group (18) and U.S. National Cancer Institute (NCI) systems (19). Both classify based on degrees of necrosis and mitotic rate but differ in that the American system considers histologic type or subtype, location, cellularity, and nuclear pleomorphism, whereas the French system relies more on differentiation (Table 30.3). An evaluation of both systems suggests that the French method may provide more accurate prognostic discrimination (20). In general, grading of these lesions seems to be reproducible, although peer review may contribute to better quality (21,22). The situation is further complicated by the existence of a two-grade system (e.g., high vs. low grade as used at Memorial Sloan-Kettering Cancer Center, MSKCC), and the four-grade system of the International Union Against Cancer (UICC) and the American Joint Committee on Cancer (AJCC), where grade is incorporated into the TNM classification of prognosis. The TNM stage classification (see later) uses a two-tiered grade classification (low vs. high grade). Because different grading systems are used, a translation of three- and four-tiered grading systems into a two-tiered system is required for TNM. In the most commonly employed three-tiered classification, grade 1 is considered low grade and grades 2 and 3 high grade. In the less common four-tiered systems, grade 1 and 2 are considered low grade and grades 3 and 4 high grade (23,24).

TABLE 30.3 Comparison of Histologic Variables Contributing to the FNCLCC and NCI Grading Systems for Soft Tissue Sarcoma

	FNCLCC	NCI
Histologic type	−	+
Differentiation	+	−
Mitosis	+	−
Necrosis	+	+

+, histologic variables used to elaborate the histologic grading for the system described; −, histologic variables not used to elaborate the histologic grading in comparison to the contrasting systems (FNCLCC or NCI); FNCLCC, French Federation of Cancer Centers (see ref. 18); NCI, National Cancer Institutes (see ref. 19).

Source: O'Sullivan B, Bell RS, Bramwell VHC. Sarcomas of the soft tissues. In: Souhami RL, Tannock I, Hohenberger P, et al., eds. *Oxford textbook of oncology,* 2nd ed. Oxford: Oxford University Press, 2002:2495–2523.

Pathology of Selected Bone Subtypes

CLASSIFICATION

In contrast to STS, primary malignant tumors of bone are predominantly confined to two histologic types: osteosarcoma and chondrosarcoma. Other histologies including primitive neuroectodermal tumor/Ewing sarcoma are much less frequent in the head and neck although a wide variety of histologic subtypes may be found (25) (Table 30.4).

Osteosarcoma

Osteosarcoma is a primary malignancy of osteoblastic tissue and is distinguished from all other tumors, including chondrosarcoma, by the direct formation of bone or osteoid tissue by its tumor cells. It covers a wide spectrum of lesions with distinct clinical and pathologic features. The malignant component comprises an undifferentiated stroma characterized by dense cellularity, pleomorphism, and cytologically atypical osteoblasts. Although the tumor is derived from osteoblasts and the malignant cells can be shown to contain intracytoplasmic alkaline phosphatase, it usually exhibits a mixed picture containing fibroblastic, osteoblastic, and chondroblastic areas, based on the predominant characteristic of the stroma. Tumor osteoid may be seen copiously with numerous pleomorphic tumor osteoblasts. The WHO histologic classification recognizes high- and low-grade osteosarcoma as well as distinguishing central (medullary) from lesions arising on the surface (peripheral) (25) Thus it is usual to classify according to cell type (Table 30.4) as well as origin in relation to the bone (intramedullary, surface, or extraosseous). High-grade central osteosarcoma is the commonest form of osteosarcoma and can extend through the periosteum into the soft tissues where perivascular structures including neurovascular structures can be invaded. Radiographs show corresponding sclerosis. Parosteal sarcoma (also called juxtacortical osteogenic sarcoma) is a distinct surface bone tumor with a predominantly fibroblastic surface location, without medullary involvement, and found most often in the distal femur. This lesion may be found in the skull and has a better prognosis than conventional osteosarcoma. They are typically well differentiated and characterized by relatively well-formed osteoid trabeculae within a spindle cell stroma. Occasionally they will show dedifferentiation, especially following recurrence.

TABLE 30.4 Principal Histologic Types of Bone Sarcoma Selected from the 2nd Edition (1993) of the WHO Classification of Bone Tumors

Histologic type	ICD-O morphology
Bone-forming tumors	
Conventional central osteosarcoma	9180/3
Telangiectatic osteosarcoma	9183/3
Intraosseous well-differentiated (low-grade) osteosarcoma	9180/31
Round cell osteosarcoma	9185/3
Parosteal (juxtacortical) osteosarcoma	9190/31
Periosteal osteosarcoma	9190/32
High-grade surface osteosarcoma	9190/33
Cartilage-forming tumors	9220/3
Chondrosarcoma	9220/3
Juxtacortical (periosteal) chondrosarcoma	9211/3
Mesenchymal chondrosarcoma	9240/3
Dedifferentiated chondrosarcoma	
Clear cell chondrosarcoma	
Malignant chondoblastoma	
Marrow tumors (round cell tumors)	9150/3
Ewing sarcoma	9260/3
Primitive neuroectodermal tumor of bone	9473/3
Malignant lymphoma of bone	9590/3
Myeloma	9732/3
Vascular tumors	
Angiosarcoma of bone	9120/3
Malignant hemangiopericytoma	9150/3
Other connective tumors	9040/3
Fibrosarcoma	8810/3
Leiomyosarcoma	8890/3
Liposarcoma	8850/3
Malignant fibrous histiocytoma	8830/3
Malignant mesenchymoma	8990/3
Undifferentiated sarcoma	8800/3

ICD-O, International Classification of Diseases for Oncology.
Source: Schajowicz F, Sissons HA, Sobin L. The World Health Organization's histologic classification of bone tumors. A commentary on the second edition. *Cancer* 1995;75:1208–1214.

Although the description provided is typical of common presentations of osteosarcoma, it is most frequent in the long bones. Several features distinguish craniofacial osteosarcoma. Accounting for about 5% to 10% of all osteosarcomas, they most usually affect individuals in the fourth decade of life of equal sex. The mandible and maxilla are the most frequent bones involved, although other skull bones may be affected. The majority are chondroblastic, and at least one third are of low-grade histology, a feature that may explain a lower potential for metastatic spread compared with other sites.

Chondrosarcoma

Chondrosarcoma constitutes approximately 10% of malignancies of bone and is the second most common bone sarcoma after osteosarcoma. The largest series (n < 400) of chondrosarcoma of the head and neck was reported from the National Cancer Data Base (NCDB) for the years 1985 to 1995 (26). This series comprised 0.1% of head and neck cancers during the same period and is reported to make up 1% to 12% of chondrosarcoma in various reports (26). The hallmark of chondrosarcoma is its origin from cells that form chondroid (cartilage) as opposed to osteoid. Several types exist (Table 30.4). Conventional chondrosarcoma is most common, but subtypes include the uncommon clear cell and other variants. Overall, most cases in the NCDB series were grade 1 (50%) and grade 2 (37%), whereas only a minority were grades 3 and 4. In addition, most (60%) arose from osseous tissue grouped as head and neck bones and sinonasal, the latter including 8% originating in the mandible. Almost one quarter arose from the laryngotracheal cartilages (26). Although a rare site for chondrosarcoma, the cricoid lamina of the larynx is a unique tumor. Such tumors are invariably low grade as determined by cellularity, nuclear features, and mitotic activity. Metastasis is almost never seen, and dedifferentiation to high-grade sarcoma is quite exceptional.

Central chondrosarcoma originates centrally in bone (intramedullary). Although most common in long bones, they are also seen in craniofacial bones. Two thirds of central chondrosarcoma are low grade (grade 1 and 2) at diagnosis. Dedifferentiated central chondrosarcomas in the craniofacial bones are extremely rare, as are peripheral chondrosarcomas (those originating at the surface of a bone). Mesenchymal chondrosarcoma is seen in the skull as well as the bones of the trunk. This highly malignant tumor is composed of primitive mesenchymal cells focally differentiating in cartilage. The lesion is usually osteolytic with poorly defined limits, and it permeates cortex into soft tissues. A biphasic appearance is usual with two histologic patterns comprising sheets of dense small round or oval undifferentiated cells resembling Ewing sarcoma or lymphoma, alternating with a second pattern of easily identified cartilaginous tissue. Chondroid islands may appear quite abruptly among the undifferentiated cells that mimic early chondrogenesis, although more gradual transitions are also seen. Mitoses are frequent

Although chondrosarcoma most commonly arises from either cartilaginous structures or bone derived from chondroid precursors, chondrosarcoma may also arise in areas where cartilage is not normally found. Such tumors developing in soft tissues presumably arise from cartilaginous differentiation of primitive mesenchymal cells. Some of these comprise the myxoid variant of chondrosarcoma, with conflicting reports describing these as variant of chordoma (chordoid sarcoma) as opposed to a variant of chondrosarcoma (27,28). Myxoid change in chondrosarcoma is also seen and should not be confused with the myxoid variant, making accurate classification difficult. In general, soft tissue lesions are staged (and classified) by the principles used for STSs.

Ewing Sarcoma

Ewing sarcoma also amounts to about 10% of bone tumors but is exceptionally rare in the head and neck, and experience in their management remains anecdotal. A recent cooperative Ewing sarcoma study of 301 cases recruited only six lesions affecting skull bones (2%), and three (1%) in the clavicles (29). It appears to arise from pluripotent mesenchymal tissue, although a neuroectodermal origin is suspected (30,31). The histologic features are characterized by a structureless array of small hyperchromatic cells as one of the group of small round blue cell tumors. The diagnosis is established by additional measures beyond conventional light microscopy. These include immunocytochemistry, cytogenic analysis, and molecular detection of fusion transcripts by reverse-transcriptase polymerase chain reaction. Glycogen is detectable in approximately 90% of Ewing sarcomas using periodic acid-Schiff reagent or diastase reaction. More recently refined diagnostic methods for Ewing sarcoma include immunohistochemical demonstration of the cell surface glycoprotein MIC-2 (or CD-99), which is not seen in other tumors resembling Ewing sarcoma by conventional histology. In addition, the majority of Ewing sarcomas (at least 80%) exhibit the specific translocation t(11;22)(q24;q12) between the *EWS* gene on chromosome 22 and the *FLI1* gene on chromosome 11. An *EWS-ETS* gene fusion transcript type is also characteristic. The type of gene fusion transcript appears to carry prognostic significance in patients with localized disease (32).

Grading Bone Sarcomas

As with STS, the grading of bone tumors provides an important prognostic measure and has been incorporated in the TNM staging system discussed below. As noted for STS, varying conventions exist for grading bone sarcomas including two-, three-, and four-tier systems. The same approach is adopted to create a two-tiered classification as was described above for STS when incorporating grade into the staging system (23,24) (see "Staging Classifications").

Osteosarcomas are graded according to the cell type and relative anaplasia of the stromal component of the tumor. Low-grade lesions (grade 1) may resemble parosteal osteosarcoma or fibrous dysplasia. Increasingly anaplastic tumors are given higher grades, with the least well-differentiated tumors appearing of highest grade. High-grade tumors (grade 3 or 4) generally comprise conventional (osteoblastic), telangiectatic, and dedifferentiated tumors. Chondroblastic and fibroblastic tumors are usually lower grade (grade 1 or 2).

The gross and microscopic appearance of chondrosarcoma varies according to the grade and anatomic site, which itself is often associated with grade (26). Low-grade (well-differentiated) chondrosarcomas may also be difficult to discriminate histologically from benign cartilaginous lesions because they have the consistency of hyaline cartilage. Most chondrosarcomas have a consistent grade throughout. Commonly, however, multiple foci of different grades may be present, and there is controversy about whether grading should consider only the highest grade identified within a tumor, or be the predominant grade (26). Typically grade is classified according to cellularity, nuclear features, and mitotic activity. For chondrosarcoma, well-differentiated appearance (grade 1) is associated with longevity and favorable prognosis. In the NCDB report, progression to distant metastases was three times more likely to occur among higher grade cases than the lower grade cases (26). Myxomatous changes with cystic degeneration in the tumor correlate well with a low or medium histologic grade. An absence of cartilaginous lobulation and the presence of spindle cell forms is characteristic of high-grade (grade 3) malignancy and heralds an unfavorable prognosis.

Of importance, Ewing sarcoma is always classified as high grade (and grade IV in the UICC/AJCC TNM classification).

ETIOLOGY AND SCREENING

Etiology

Apart from the diagnostic dilemma in distinguishing additional neurofibromata from metastatic lesions in patients with neurofibromatosis, the precise etiology of an individual sarcoma is of little clinical significance because it does not affect therapeutic decision making. This is not the case in those patients who have sarcomas arising in a previously irradiated field and they often cannot receive further external-beam RT. In fact, most sarcomas of the head and neck or elsewhere are without obvious cause. Of known factors, an induced STS and osteosarcoma is a long-term hazard of either iatrogenic or accidental exposure to radiation. Frequently, such tumors arise in the low-dose areas at the edge of prior radiation target volumes. Sarcomas have also been reported after chemotherapy, especially for pediatric cancers, such as acute lymphatic leukemia. The relative risk appears to increase with cumulative exposure to alkylating agents. Chemical exposure (usually occupational) is also linked to sarcoma causation being most recognized with thorotrast (x-ray technicians), vinyl chloride gas (plastics industry), phenoxyacetic acids (agricultural and forestry workers), chlorophenols (sawmill workers), and arsenic (vineyard work).

Association of rhabdomyosarcoma with genitourinary or central nervous system (CNS) anomalies has been noted, as well as links to a variety of genetic conditions (33). Multiple factors are implicated in the etiology of angiosarcoma, although the usual patient with a head and neck angiosarcoma does not manifest them; the disease typically is seen in the scalp and face of an elderly white male. In addition to prior radiation exposure, chronic infection or solar exposure have been implicated, as well as vinyl chloride, thorotrast, insecticides, and steroid exposure (8,34). Aggressive fibromatosis is associated with exposure to abnormal stimulus by estrogen, local trauma with resulting uncontrolled immature fibroblast growth, or genetic predispositions, typified by Gardner syndrome. There is up to a 10% cumulative lifetime risk for developing sarcoma (usually malignant peripheral nerve sheath tumor, MPNST) in patients with type 1 neurofibromatosis, an autosomal-dominant disease with dysfunction of the *NF1* gene on chromosome 17q11.2 (35). The *NF1* gene product (neurofibronin) appears to be a tumor suppressor gene acting through guanosine triphosphatase (GTPase) activity, with mutations leading to dysfunction and uncontrolled signaling via *ras* pathways (36–38) This may facilitate the development of MPNST.

Osteosarcoma (OS) has a number of risk factors. Exposure to radiation was noted earlier, but trauma and thorotrast exposure have also been described, as have underlying Paget disease, fibrous dysplasia, multiple osteochondromatosis, chronic osteomyelitis, and myositis ossificans. Retinoblastoma survivors provide a specific example of a dysfunctional or deleted tumor suppressor genetic element (in this case, the product of the *Rb* gene on chromosome 13q14), rendering these patients and their families at risk for STS, osteosarcoma (with or without RT), and several other malignancies including breast cancer. In patients with heritable retinoblastoma, almost half are osteosarcomas, with the head and neck providing the overwhelmingly risk (39) compared with other body sites (40). Alterations in p53 germlines are also associated with the high predisposition of families with Li-Fraumeni syndrome for the development of osteosarcoma, again with or without RT (41).

The etiology of chondrosarcoma remains obscure, although various physical and chemical agents may be implicated. Speculation concerning undetermined dietary or environmental factors was prompted by the observation of a disproportionate incidence in low-income patients, although the mesenchymal subtype was more common among higher income groups (26). Chondrosarcoma (especially in the skull base) may complicate Maffucci syndrome, a congenital nonhereditary condition associating multiple cutaneous hemangiomas, dyschondroplasia, and often enchondromas (see Fig. 30.12B) (42). Ewing sarcoma has only very rarely been reported with specific congenital anomalies or other etiologic factors.

Screening for Sarcomas

Predisposing genetic tendencies and environmental exposures associated with sarcoma development should be borne in mind when assessing patients. Genetic counseling would be appropriate to discuss issues relating to the genetic predispositions. However, no general screening is indicated beyond routine health care surveillance because of the rarity of sarcoma. A more detailed clinical evaluation in certain subjects is reasonable and with a lower threshold of intervention than one might use for general health care. For example, rapidly growing and/or symptomatic masses in patients with neurofibromatosis merit resection because of potential malignant transformation within a neurofibroma. Similarly painful and dramatic deformity in Paget disease should be viewed with concern about underlying osteosarcoma. Superficial or deep abnormalities of skin or soft tissues in patients with a history of prior RT should also be regarded with suspicion, given the known increased risk for sarcoma.

CLINICAL PRESENTATION, EVALUATION, STAGE CLASSIFICATIONS

Local Presentation

Sarcomas of the head and neck present in multiple ways depending on the numerous potential anatomic sites where disruption of function and contour may result. Local management starts with imaging and physical examination to determine whether soft tissue lesions originate superficial or deep to the investing fascia at the local site and whether bone tumors are intramedullary or have invaded into the extraosseous compartment. Evidence of bone, vascular, or neural invasion (uncommon) should be excluded.

Lesions may originate in the upper aerodigestive tract, paranasal sinus, and skull base with symptoms referable to these areas (e.g., nasal symptoms including obstruction or discharge and ocular proptosis from direct invasion in paranasal sinus tumors; cranial nerve abnormalities in lesions arising in the skull base or masticator space; alteration of voice or airway compromise for laryngeal and hypopharyngeal lesion lesions). Tumors originating in the subcutaneous tissues of the face, neck, or scalp can initially present with a superficial mass.

Approximately 5% to 10% of osteosarcomas are located in the head and neck, typically in the mandible or maxilla. Both bone and cartilage tumors often present with pain in addition to symptoms of mass and compression. Pain generally relates to infiltration and expansion of bone. In lower grade lesions pain can be of long duration, and characterized as a prolonged aching sensation, sometimes present for several years. Most often tumors present as a slow growing mass or with looseness of dentition. Because of the potential to also arise in the skull base and paranasal sinuses, a wide variety of symptoms are also possible, depending on tumor site. These include cranial neuropathy, visual disturbance (including ophthalmoplegia and proptosis), in addition to pain, the latter being evident in about half the cases.

Metastatic Manifestations

Most sarcomas present with localized disease, and metastasis is present in only 10% of cases at the time of diagnosis. Generally the patient is asymptomatic, and staging investigations are needed to demonstrate the metastatic process. The predominant risk is to the lungs. Regional lymph node involvement is unusual but is represented most frequently in certain histologic subtypes, most notably rhabdomyosarcomas, epithelioid sarcomas, alveolar soft part, and clear cell and synovial sarcomas. Rarely, remote bone marrow metastases are apparent but are seen almost exclusively in rhabdomyosarcoma with associated lymphadenopathy. In osteosarcoma, bone metastases may be present in the absence of lung involvement, but this is exceptional.

Evaluation

INITIAL ASSESSMENT

Successful outcome starts with reliance on basic principles and understanding the behavior of the disease and the necessary steps to be undertaken. The overall management of head and neck STS is summarized in the treatment algorithm (Fig. 30.3). Before embarking on treatment, histologic confirmation of the diagnosis is necessary. All soft tissue masses deep to the investing fascia should be considered to be sarcoma until proven otherwise. The same vigilance is needed for bone lesions, but here the opinion of an experienced diagnostic radiologist is required. Both bone and soft tissue lesions should be staged with cross-sectional imaging before the biopsy to avoid compromising the planning of appropriate management. Open incisional biopsy of deep tumors is preferred over excisional biopsy to minimize the difficulty of the "unplanned" excision (43,44). This results when the unsuspecting surgeon contaminates surrounding tissues following an ill-advised attempt to remove a deep-seated lesion (Fig. 30.4), and is frequently performed without full diagnostic assessments completed. It is equally important that the

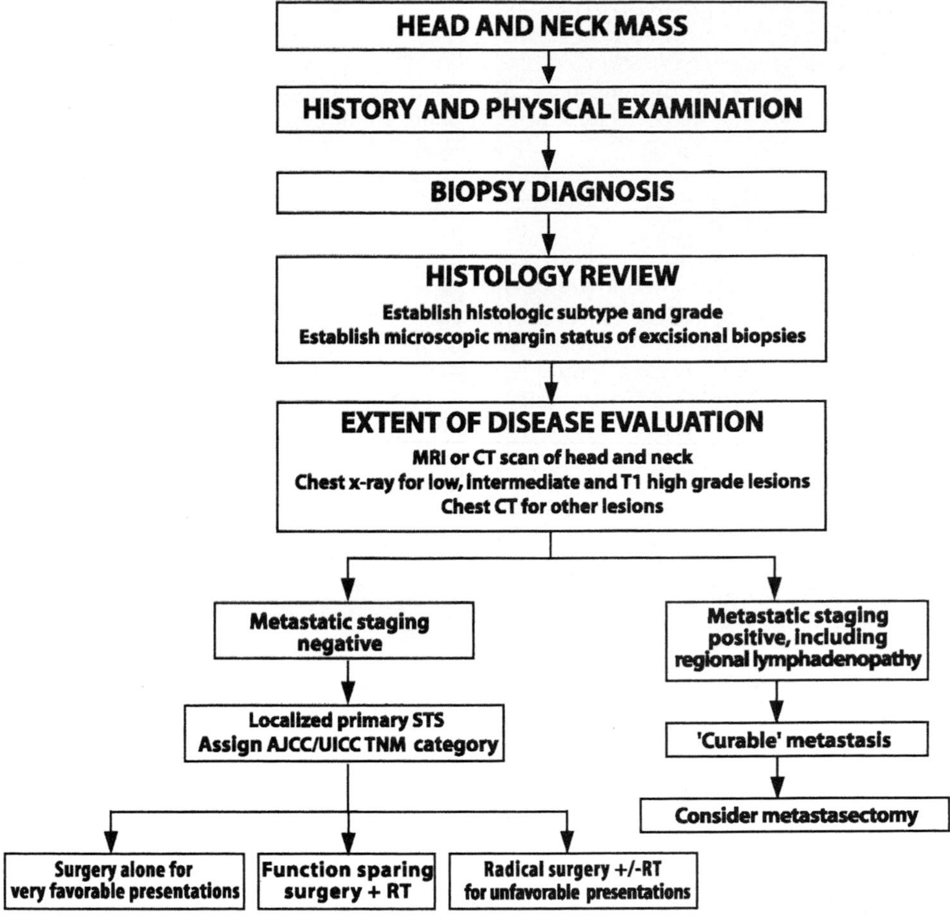

Figure 30.3 Flow schema for the assessment of soft tissue sarcoma of the head and neck. Because of the heterogeneity of tumor and anatomic sites, individualization is also needed. Thus some diseases, like rhabdomyosarcoma, may need additional investigations (e.g., bone marrow examination; see text for management details).

surgeon performing the biopsy should also perform the definitive resection (45) with full anticipation of the therapy to be undertaken.

Establishing the Diagnosis

Fine-needle aspiration biopsy (FNAB) is useful for establishing the presence of recurrence (both local and metastatic). Its use as a primary diagnostic tool, however, is controversial. Essentially, this method should be used only when a cytopathologist experienced in sarcoma is available. Core needle biopsy under local anesthesia provides a more consistent tissue specimen and cell preparation compared with FNAB. In our experience, open biopsy of STS is rarely indicated but almost always yields a diagnosis when needle biopsy is unsuccessful (about 10% of cases).

Interventional radiologists are often requested to biopsy deep-seated lesions using ultrasound or computed tomography (CT) guidance. An atraumatic biopsy close to critical structures or where the lesion is difficult to palpate can be accomplished. The radiologist should collaborate with the oncologists who will resect or irradiate the lesion. Needle tracts are potential sites of tumor contamination, and the surgeon and radiation oncologist should be involved in planning the optimal biopsy route and be aware of potential contamination.

Imaging Local Disease

Both CT scan and magnetic resonance imaging (MRI) are used widely; CT provides better bony detail than MRI, but MRI provides multiplanar images without losing specificity and is likely the best instrument for tumor definition with optimal tissue contrast. Therefore, in those situation where it is important to visualize the matrix of a lesion, CT is preferred. This usually occurs in flat bones including the calvarium. Plain radiography is also useful for bony lesions but has largely been replaced by CT. Both have the advantage of exhibiting calcification in tumor, which may be characteristic of certain histologies (e.g., chondrosarcoma and synovial sarcoma). Malignant bone lesions frequently present with marked permeative bone destruction, ill-defined transition to normal bone, aggressive periosteal reaction, and an accompanying soft tissue mass. In the end, it is our impression that MRI generally provides superior depiction of intra- and extraosseous tumor in most malignant tumors of bone. Axial imaging complemented by either coronal or sagittal imaging planes using T1- and T2-weighted spin echo sequences most often provides accurate depiction of intra- and extraosseous tumor. To improve conspicuity, these sequences could be augmented by fat-suppressed pulse sequences. The maximum dimension of the tumor must be measured prior to any treatment.

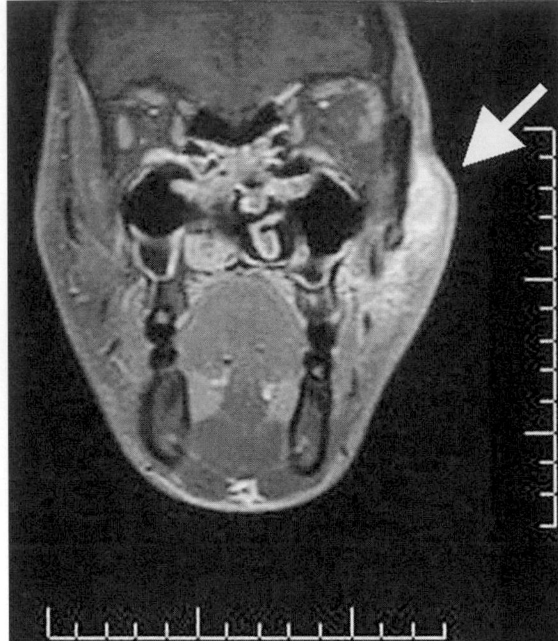
A

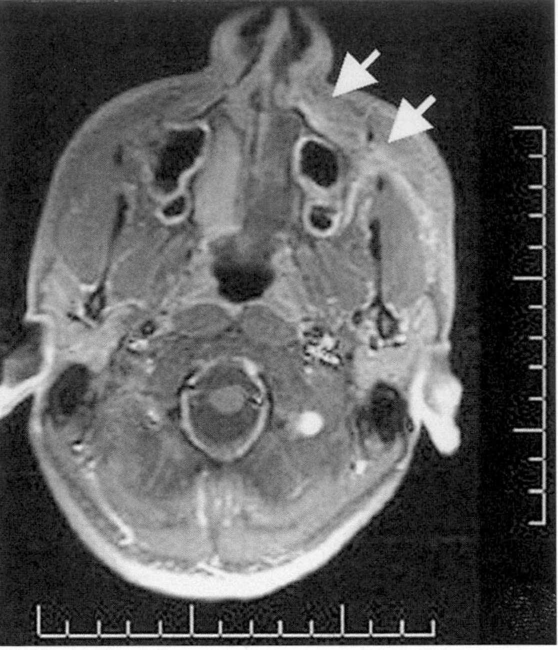
B

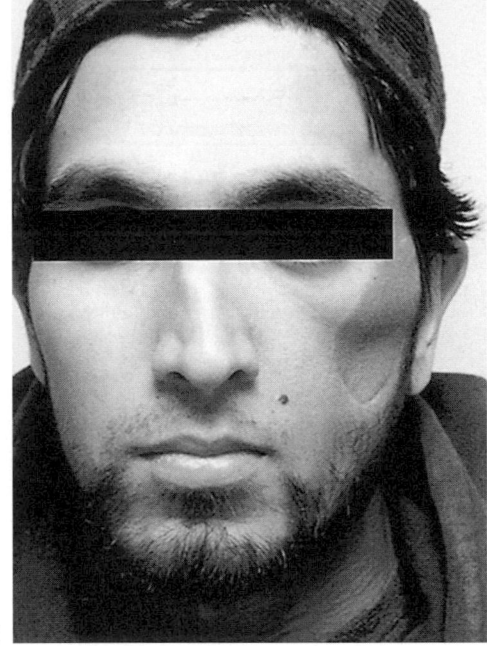
C

Figure 30.4 Example of an inappropriate excision prior to referral to a multidisciplinary center. A young man presented with a deeply located mass in the vicinity of the left zygoma. Remarkably, it was excised intraorally by an approach commencing superior to the left upper incisor to minimize cosmetic change. Regrowth of tumor (a malignant fibrous histiocytoma) had already taken place by the time of referral only a few weeks later (*arrow* on coronal magnetic resonance imaging, **A**). Grossly contaminated tissues from biopsy intrusion are evident along the anterolateral maxillary wall (two *arrows* in **B**) that extended to the upper lip and incisor region. Preoperative radiotherapy with margins surrounding the tumor regrowth and all contaminated tissues was followed by excision and reconstruction. Stigma of radiotherapy (paucity of beard hair delineating the medial field border) and the grafted site where skin was resected overlying the lesion can be seen (**C**).

In STS, low signal intensity on T1-weighted images and a high signal on T2-weighted images are the usual appearances and can be readily separated from normal soft tissue structures. Again lesion size should be recorded.

Of interest, a recent blinded study by the Radiation Diagnostic Oncology Group that compared MRI and CT in patients with malignant bone and soft tissue tumors showed no specific advantage of MRI over CT (46). Although it may true that the diagnostic evaluation may be equally served by both modalities, treatment planning (e.g., for both surgery and RT) frequently requires additional information provided by the multiplanar capability of MRI and the additional advantages of MRI/CT image fusion techniques for RT treatment planning (47,48).

Radionuclide bone scanning is a sensitive indicator of osteoblastic activity but lacks specificity. It can demonstrate multiple lesions but may also overestimate the extent of intramedullary infiltration when compared with MRI scanning.

EVALUATION OF METASTASIS

For metastatic staging, CT of the chest is required. If the underlying diagnosis is rhabdomyosarcoma, a bone marrow biopsy is also necessary as well as cerebrospinal fluid analysis in parameningeal lesions. Angiography is scarcely required in the evaluation of sarcomas. Positron emission tomography (PET) scan is also not widely used but may have applicability in identifying metastases in high-risk subsets (e.g., recurrent high-grade tumors) (49). Technetium scintigraphy is the examination of choice for evaluating the entire skeleton to determine whether there are multiple lesions, and is particularly important for diseases with high propensity for bone metastasis such as Ewing sarcoma. Occasionally, intrapulmonary osteoblastic metastases may be demonstrated.

Staging Classifications

Both soft tissue and bone sarcomas are classified according to the TNM stage classification (6th edition) (23,24). A major limitation of the staging system is that it does not take into account the anatomic and histologic heterogeneity of these lesions. The system is optimally designed to stage extremity tumors but is also applicable to the head and neck, although it lacks subtlety since the T-category size criterion dwarfs the anatomic sites of origin in the head and neck, which tend to be much smaller. An additional issue concerns rhabdomyosarcoma, where two separate descriptions of disease extent exist.

SOFT TISSUE SARCOMA

"Ordinary" Soft Tissue Sarcoma

The relative rarity of STSs, the anatomic heterogeneity of these lesions, and the presence of more than 30 recognized histologic subtypes of variable grade have made it difficult to establish a functional system that can accurately stage all forms of this disease. The UICC/AJCC TNM staging system is the most widely employed staging system for STSs. The TNM staging systems for bone and STS are exceptional insofar as they incorporate histologic grade with anatomic disease characteristics. All head and neck STS subtypes are included except dermatofibrosarcoma protuberans, because it is considered to have only borderline malignant potential. Four distinct histologic grades are recognized in the staging system, ranging from well differentiated to undifferentiated. Histologic grade and tumor size are the primary determinants of clinical stage (Table 30.5). Tumor size is further substaged as "a" (superficial tumor arising outside the investing fascia) or "b" (a deep tumor that arises beneath the fascia or invades the fascia).

TABLE 30.5 International Union Against Cancer (UICC) and American Joint Committee on Cancer (AJCC) TNM Classification (6th Edition) of Soft Tissue Sarcomas

Primary tumor (T)[a]				
TX	Primary tumor cannot be assessed			
T0	No evidence of primary tumor			
T1	Tumor 5 cm or less in greatest dimension			
	T1a superficial tumor			
	T2b deep tumor			
T2	Tumor more than 5 cm in greatest dimension			
	T2a superficial tumor			
	T2b deep tumor			
Regional lymph nodes (N)				
NX	Regional lymph nodes cannot be assessed			
N0	No regional lymph node metastasis			
N1	Regional lymph node metastasis			
Distant metastasis (M)				
MX	Distant metastasis cannot be assessed			
M0	No distant metastasis			
M1	Distant metastasis			
Stage grouping				
Stage I	G1–2	T1a, 1b, 2a, 2b	N0	M0
Stage II	G3–4	T1a, 1b, 2a	N0	M0
Stage III	G3–4	T2b	N0	M0
Stage IV	Any G	Any T	N1	M0
	Any G	Any T	N0	M1

G, grade.
[a]Superficial tumor is located exclusively above the superficial fascia without invasion of the fascia; deep tumor is located either exclusively beneath the superficial fascia, superficial to the fascia with invasion of or through the fascia, or both superficial yet beneath the fascia.
Source: Sobin L, et al. *TNM classification of malignant tumours,* 6th ed. New York: Wiley-Liss, 2002; and Greene FL, Page D, Norrow M, et al. *AJCC cancer staging manual,* 6th ed. New York: Springer, 2002.

TABLE 30.6 Intergroup Rhabdomyosarcoma Study Group (IRSG) Postsurgical Grouping Classification

Group 1: Localized disease, completely excised, and no residual microscopic disease
- A. Confined to the site of origin, completely resected
- B. Infiltrating beyond site of origin, completely resected

Group 2: Total gross resection
- A. Gross resection with evidence of microscopic local residual disease
- B. Regional disease with involved lymph nodes, completely resected with no microscopic residual disease
- C. Microscopic local and/or nodal residual disease

Group 3: Incomplete resection or biopsy with gross residual disease
Group 4: Distant metastases

Rhabdomyosarcoma

For rhabdomyosarcoma, the description of disease extent has traditionally been by a postoperative surgical classification developed by the North American Intergroup Rhabdomyosarcoma Study Group (IRSG) more than two decades ago (Table 30.6). This is not always relevant in the head and neck because such lesions are frequently treated with aggressive chemoradiotherapy protocols (Fig. 30.5). In general, the contemporary era has also seen the initiation of chemotherapy well in advance of surgery so that reliance on a surgical staging system that describes the extent of disease at diagnosis is a major problem. The International Society of Pediatric Oncology (SIOP) employs a TNM presurgical staging system more in keeping with contemporary TNM staging for STS, and both use a T-category breakpoint at 5 cm (Table 30.7) (50). This process of staging prior to treatment is also being introduced in North America (33).

BONE SARCOMA

The UICC and AJCC TNM classification of bone tumor has recently been modified substantially (Table 30.8) (23,24). It considers maximum lesion size (with a break point at 8 cm) and the presence discontinuous tumors in the same bone without other distant metastasis. Of interest, metastasis to nonpulmonary sites is distinguished from M1 disease based on lung involvement alone. One potential problem is that the existing stages may need adjustment for the impact of grade in the stage grouping algorithm. Thus discontinuous tumor in the same bone that is low grade appears to have better prognosis than if high grade. In the 6th edition TNM (23,24), both situations are considered stage III (51). A similar problem exists when considering lung vs. nonpulmonary metastases. The staging system is applicable to all primary malignant tumors of bone except multiple myeloma, malignant lymphoma (both having different natural history), and juxtacortical osteosarcoma and chondrosarcoma (both with much more favorable prognosis) (23,24).

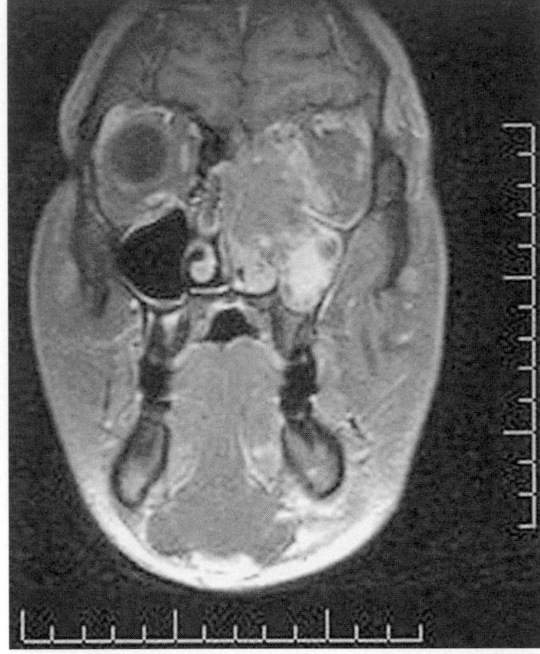
A

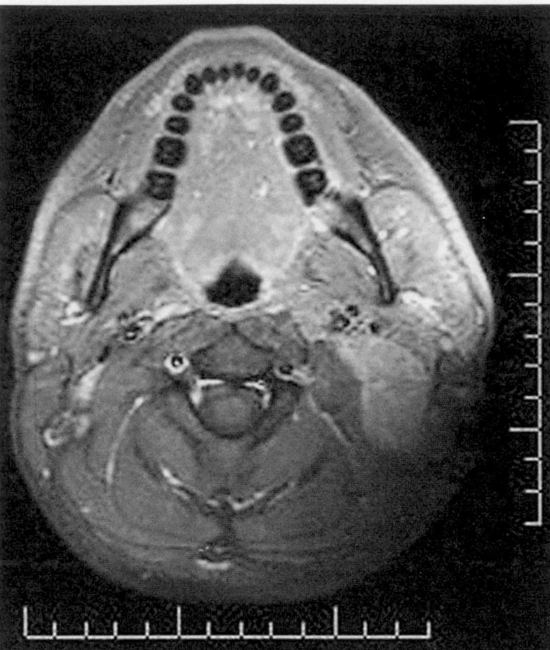
B

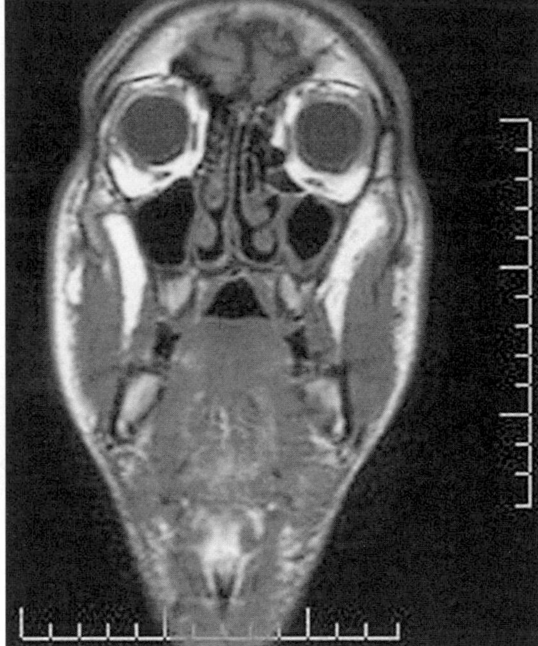
C

Figure 30.5 Magnetic resonance image of an alveolar rhabdomyosarcoma of the ethmoid sinus in a young adult. **A:** Coronal view showing extensive orbital invasion. **B:** Axial view showing concurrent extensive regional lymphadenopathy. **C:** Complete response following combination chemotherapy with cyclophosphamide, actinomycin-D, vincristine (CAV), and etoposide with ifosfamide. Although consolidation radiotherapy commonly achieves locoregional control in these responsive tumors, such patients are at extremely high risk for failure in bone marrow, lung, and leptomeningeal sites.

TABLE 30.7 International Society of Pediatric Oncology (SIOP) Presurgical Staging Classification (Clinical and Radiological Staging)

Stage	Tumor	Node	Metastases
I	T1a or T1b	N0, NX	M0
II	T2a or T2b	N0, NX	M0
III	Any T	N1	M0
IV	Any T	Any N	M1

M0, no distal metastasis; M1, metastasis present; NX, unknown nodal status; N0, no nodes present clinically; N1, regional nodes present; T1, confined to the anatomic site of origin; T2, extension and/or fixation to surrounding tissue; T2a, ≤5 cm in diameter; T2b, >5 cm in diameter.

Source: Stevens MCG. Malignant mesenchymal tumours of childhood. In: Souhami RL, Tannock I, Hohenberger P, et al., eds. *Oxford textbook of oncology,* 2nd ed. Oxford: Oxford University Press, 2002:2525–2538.

TABLE 30.8 International Union Against Cancer (IUCC) and American Joint Committee on Cancer (AJCC) TNM Classification (6th edition) of Bone Sarcomas

Primary tumor (T)				
TX	Primary tumor cannot be assessed			
T0	No evidence of primary tumor			
T1	Tumor (maximum dimension) ≤8 cm at time of diagnosis			
T2	Tumor (maximum dimension) >8 cm at time of diagnosis			
T3	Skip metastases—two discontinuous tumors in the same bone with no other distant metastases			
Regional lymph nodes (N)[a]				
NX	Regional lymph nodes cannot be assessed			
N0	No regional lymph node metastasis			
N1	Regional lymph node metastasis to be considered equivalent to distant metastatic disease (see M1b below)			
Distant metastasis (M)				
MX	Distant metastasis cannot be assessed			
M0	No distant metastasis			
M1	Distant metastasis M1a, Lung only metastases M1b, All other distant metastases including lymph nodes			
Stage grouping				
Stage IA	G1,2	T1	N0	M0
Stage IB	G1,2	T2	N0	M0
Stage IIA	G3,4	T1	N0	M0
Stage IIB	G3,4	T2	N0	M0
Stage III	Any G	T3	N0	M0
Stage IVA	Any G	Any T	N0	M1a
Stage IVB	Any G	Any T	N0/N1	M1b

G, grade.
[a]Because of the rarity of lymph node involvement in sarcomas, the designation NX may not be appropriate and could be considered N0 if no clinical involvement is evident.
Source: Sobin L, et al. *TNM classification of malignant tumours,* 6th ed. New York: Wiley-Liss, 2002; and Greene FL, Page D, Norrow M, et al. *AJCC cancer staging manual,* 6th ed. New York: Springer, 2002.

TREATMENT OF SOFT TISSUE SARCOMA

The benchmark for local control rates for extremity sarcomas is set at approximately 90% in modern series, and the overall 5-year survival of patients with STS can be expected to be in the range of 60% (52), although this will vary as a function of prognostic factors from case to case. This result is achievable with combined RT (usually administered preoperatively or postoperatively, or brachytherapy) combined with surgery, or surgery alone in selected cases (53). Unfortunately, reported series of head and neck sarcoma have usually not achieved these high local controls (Table 30.9). This has been attributed to the traditional inability to deliver aggressive treatments because of their location in the critical anatomy of the head and neck (54). It may also relate to problems in delivering care for these rare diseases, if undertaken in the absence of a full multidisciplinary team. However, properly deployed principles and approaches can achieve results in the head and neck that are comparable to similar lesions in extremity sites. Several randomized controlled trials have collectively established important milestones in the evolution of the local management of STS. With one exception, these trials have focussed on extremity lesions and around the themes of surgery and adjuvant RT. These results are also highly relevant to the head and neck because of the similarity of biologic behavior of STS across body sites, even if the different histologic subtypes are not equally distributed by site.

Surgery

MAJOR ABLATION VERSUS CONSERVATION MANAGEMENT

In the 1970s, it became apparent that RT in combination with surgery could achieve results equivalent to more ablative surgery in STS. This observation was confirmed in a trial that randomized high-grade sarcoma of the extremities to receive amputation versus a limb-sparing operation followed by adjuvant RT (55). The result of this trial combined with numerous institutional reports at a National Institutes of Health Consensus Development Conference, including one of the earliest examples of a decision analysis approach in oncology (56), heralded a new era in STS management (57).

EXTENT OF SURGERY AND CHARACTERIZATION OF MARGINS

An important component of contemporary management is the value of imaging in demonstrating the radial extent of sarcoma within the compartment or site of origin, which, together with RT, permits conservation of much of the surrounding soft tissue without increased local failure. Of more importance than the description of the type of surgery is the actual extent of viable residual disease remaining after surgery. This variable (the amount of residual viable disease remaining in the wound following resection) can never be known exactly, but is probably best represented by expert pathologic assessment of the surgi-

TABLE 30.9 Outcome in Adult Soft Tissue Sarcoma of the Head and Neck (Selected Reports)

Author and year	No.	Combined therapy	Local control (5 years)	Overall survival (5 years)
Le et al., 1997 (61)	65	61%	66%	56%
Farhood et al., 1990 (75)	176	36%	83/149 (56%)	55%
Freedman et al., 1989 (76)	352	33%	NA	68% (inc peds)
McKenna et al., 1987 (77)	16	100%	75%	75%
Farr et al., 1981 (78)	242	NA	32%	43% (inc peds)
LeVay et al., 1994 (70)	73	80%	59%	62%
Sanroman et al., 1992 (79)	14	43%	57%	56%
Kraus et al., 1994 (80)	60	26/60 (43%)	70%	71%
Eeles et al., 1993 (81)	130	41/130 (31.5%)	47%	50%
Tran et al., 1992 (82)	94	23%	52% (Sx alone) 90% (combined rx)	66% (overall)
Dudhat et al., 2000 (83)	72	38/72 (53%)	25/72 (35%)	60%

NA, not assessable (information not provided); inc peds, includes pediatric cases; rx, treatment; Sx: surgery.

cal margin. Characterization of the margin guides the need for adjuvant RT for those tumors with insufficient normal tissue at the surface to reliably prevent local recurrence. Patients with positive margins of resection have inferior local control in STS (58–60). Although generally based on extremity sarcomas, the situation is the same in the head and neck (61).

The cause of positive margins is rarely discussed. We reported a series from Princess Margaret Hospital that showed a 48% rate of involved margins in a group of extremity lesions treated by a variety of surgeons in different hospitals (62). This contrasted to a margin-positive rate of 15% in a later study at our center where all patients were operated on within the musculoskeletal oncology group (63). The policy in STS surgery should be to achieve negative surgical margins, and this is best achieved by performing surgery at an experienced referral center. More recently we have also shown, in a blinded study using a prospective database, that a small isolated positive resection margin, planned from the outset by the multidisciplinary team with the intention of sparing a critical anatomic structure (e.g., at a major nerve, vessel, or bone), has a favorable outcome [local recurrence 3.6%, 95% confidence interval (CI) 0 to 10.4] compared with an "unplanned excision" margin-positive situation (local recurrence 31.6%, 95% CI 10.7 to 52.5) (64). Radiotherapy is used in both circumstances, but substantial contamination with tumor seeding in a hypoxic environment means that subsequent RT is less successful in eliminating tumor seeding in the unplanned excision circumstance. In addition, the burden of residual disease is often underestimated (64). If undertaken, function-preserving approaches of the type described must be planned collaboratively and the involvement of diagnostic radiologists prior to local treatment, in addition to multidisciplinary consultation between the surgical and radiation oncology, is essential in the event that brachytherapy or small-volume boost RT may be needed in high-risk cases.

EVIDENCE FOR USING SURGERY ALONE

Although the evidence is compelling that major ablation is avoidable in most cases, it is also helpful to consider whether adjuvant RT is needed to achieve conservation management, in comparison with surgery alone. This issue is complicated by case heterogeneity, but a subgroup of patients undoubtedly does not need RT based on several sources of evidence, although none reported in the head and neck specifically. These sources rely on single-institution experience with practices involving degrees of selection including subcutaneous or intramuscular presentation, or extramuscular lesions with favorable resection margin status (65–68). However, most deep sarcomas in all sites are referred with lesions significantly expanding out of a single muscle unit or have undergone biopsy prior to referral and therefore need RT combined with surgery (69). The approach is less applicable in the head and neck because the proximity to critical anatomy makes it less likely to achieve sufficient clearance to have confidence that surgery alone would eradicate disease, and there remains the added concern that local failure in head and neck STS confers extremely adverse outcome. The latter includes mortality directly from progressive local disease (70), a phenomenon not relevant to extremity lesions.

Radiotherapy

ADJUVANT RADIOTHERAPY

The principle of using RT in combination with surgery is based on two facts: (a) microscopic nests of tumor can be destroyed by RT; (b) more limited surgery can be performed when RT is combined with surgery. Despite earlier views to the contrary, radiosensitivity assays performed on sarcoma cell lines grown *in vitro* have confirmed similar radiosensitivity to other malignancies such as breast cancer (71,72) and provides further support for the first premise.

Adjuvant RT with conservative surgical resection has been evaluated in two randomized clinical trials (73,74). Yang et al. (74) at the NCI randomized high-grade extremity lesions following limb-sparing surgery to receive adjuvant RT or no further treatment following the surgery. Chemotherapy was also used depending on grade. The local control for those receiving RT was 99% compared with 70% in the control group ($p < 0.0001$). The results were similar for high- and low-grade tumors. Adjuvant RT, using brachytherapy (BRT), was also evaluated in a second randomized trial at MSKCC with a similar effect in high-grade lesions (73). Of interest, no improvement in local control was evident in the low-grade tumors, potentially related to slowly cycling cells not entering the radiosensitive phases of the cycle during the short BRT dwell time (73).

For head and neck STS, relatively high rates of local relapse in different treatment settings have generally been reported by numerous institutions, as compared with extremity STS (61,70,75–83) (Table 30.9), and surgical excision is often constrained by anatomic considerations. However, if the principles used in other sites are applied in the head and neck, where tissue preservation is paramount, the results should be similar. Advantages to a combined modality approach are evident in a series where local control was 52% in those treated with surgery alone versus 90% in those treated with combined RT and surgery (82). Additional evidence from our institution indicates that head and neck STS patients with clear surgical margins or microscopic residuum had similar local control rates (26% and 30% failure, respectively), provided RT was administered (Fig. 30.6) (70). Indeed these outcomes for RT following R0/R1 resections approach those achieved in extremity sarcoma. Finally, a prospective series of high-risk cases has been treated on a consistent combined modality protocol with preoperative RT. The results are comparable to

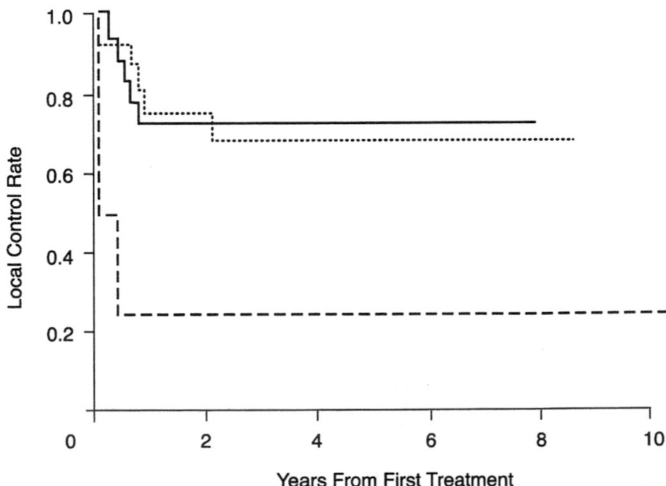

Figure 30.6 Actuarial estimate of local control rate in soft tissue sarcoma of the head and neck by surgical margins. Histopathologically clear (*solid line*), microscopically positive (*dotted line*), and gross disease (*dashed line*) are shown for patients treated with curative intent after surgical resection. (From Le Vay J, O'Sullivan B, Catton C, et al. An assessment of prognostic factors in soft-tissue sarcoma of the head and neck. *Arch Otolaryngol Head Neck Surg* 1994;120:981–986, with permission.)

extremity sarcoma of similar histology and are certainly superior to our historical series (84).

TIMING OF RADIOTHERAPY (PREOPERATIVE VS. POSTOPERATIVE RADIOTHERAPY)

Preoperative RT promotes collaboration between the surgical and radiation oncologist and facilitates a complete management plan to be fashioned prior to any surgical intervention. Preoperative RT is also delivered to an undisturbed and potentially better oxygenated tumor site (85) and permits administration of lower dosages and smaller fields of radiation without compromising local control. These observations are confirmed in our randomized trial comparing preoperative and postoperative RT in extremity STS (86). Local control was equivalent in both groups (93%), but a statistically significant overall survival advantage, mostly related to sarcoma death, in favor of preoperative RT was evident in the first report of the study (86). Others have suggested that preoperative RT has advantages in certain situations especially for gross disease at referral and large tumors (87,88). However, preoperative RT is often delivered on a partially representative biopsy and may interfere with future histopathologic analysis. Additional concerns about preoperative RT include the increased risk for wound complications in some but not all anatomic sites (86). Tissue transfer with flaps is commonly used for reconstruction and appears to minimize wound healing problems in the head and neck following preoperative radiotherapy for STS (89). In fact, in the combined modality approach to head and neck STS, preoperative RT is particularly suitable because of the smaller RT volumes and lower doses that can be delivered to critical anatomy and locations with difficult surgical access, such as base of skull (Fig. 30.7). At present, our guidelines for using preoperative RT are (a) the need to maximally restrict RT volumes in some anatomic sites (e.g., head and neck); (b) the desire to minimize RT dose in some situations (e.g., where critical neurologic tissues are in close proximity); and (c) a desire not to irradiate new tissues, especially vascular reconstructions vulnerable to the effects of high-dose postoperative RT (53).

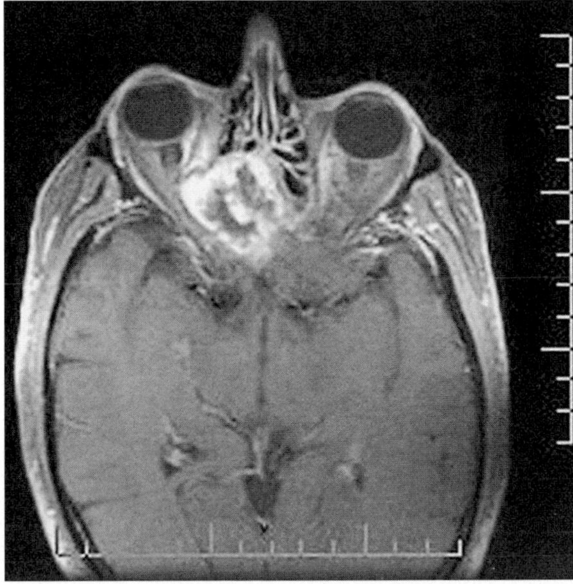

Figure 30.7 Leiomyosarcoma of the skull base with optic nerve compression. Such patients are preferentially managed at the authors' center with preoperative radiotherapy to limit both the volume of radiotherapy and the dose that is administered because of the constraints imposed by the presence of critical adjacent anatomy (i.e., the optic chiasm). In addition, chemotherapy may be added in an additional attempt to enhance local control (see Ref. 96).

RADIOTHERAPY ALONE IN SOFT TISSUE SARCOMA

Historically, patients treated with RT alone for gross disease do not achieve the same outcome. Approximately 25% are controlled (Fig. 30.6) (70). Similar observations have been made by Tran et al. (82). At the same time, in the head and neck this may be the only option of management in selected adverse presentations of head and neck lesions in which surgical management is not feasible. It is possible that the outcomes of these problematic cases may be improved by more precise delivery methods, such as intensity modulated radiotherapy (IMRT) or proton beam (see "Specialized Radiotherapy Approaches"), thereby permitting higher doses without the same danger to normal tissue. Chemotherapy may further enhance local control based on evidence from some of the randomized trials (see "Influence of Chemotherapy on Local Control").

One exception to the almost universal need for combined surgery and RT in STS is in the treatment of rhabdomyosarcoma, where control with RT alone with chemotherapy is an accepted treatment because of the unusual radioresponsive nature of these lesions. The use of a tissue-conserving approach may be preferable in such patients if surgery is very problematic, given the very high risk for distant metastasis in these patients (Fig. 30.5).

RADIOTHERAPY MODALITY

Two methods of RT delivery are commonly employed: external beam RT (EBRT) in the ambulatory setting, and brachytherapy (BRT). No randomized data compare these modalities directly, and it is unclear how similar the selection criteria are for both approaches. As noted earlier, both have been compared with surgery alone. Brachytherapy has several advantages over EBRT, including a shorter overall treatment time (4 to 6 days vs. 5 to 6.5 weeks), and treatment can be initiated sooner following surgery when clonogen numbers are at a minimum. In the head and neck, additional potential advantages include the ability to treat close to critical anatomy such as the spinal cord. The concerns about lack of effect for low-grade tumors was noted earlier, a feature not apparent with EBRT.

External beam RT may include photons or particle beam (electrons, protons, pions, or neutrons). Protons have similar radiobiologic effects to photons. Their main advantage is when tumors lie in direct proximity to critical structures due to the ability to achieve more accurate targeting (see "Specialized Radiotherapy Approaches") (90). High linear energy transfer radiation such as neutrons confers radiobiologic advantages over photons, which include reduced repair of radiation damage in tumor cells, sensitivity of cancer cells to RT throughout the cell cycle, and less protection offered to hypoxic cancer cells. However, any such advantages are tempered by late damage because the usual repair processes in action with fractionated RT do not occur and they have not become widely available. An alternative approach is the use of intraoperative RT (IORT). The major interest for IORT has been in retroperitoneal sarcoma, but experience in other sites, especially the head and neck, is minimal.

RADIOTHERAPY DOSE FRACTIONATION

External beam RT prescriptions for postoperative RT depend on the tumor grade and involvement of the surgical margin but typically use 60 and 66 Gy for low- and high-grade tumors respectively, with a "shrinking field" techniques following 50 Gy at 1.8 to 2 Gy per fraction. In the head and neck, critical structures in the target volume frequently require doses to be curtailed to 45 to 50 Gy in components of the target volume to minimize the occurrence of catastrophic sequelae (e.g., blindness or paralysis). At most institutions the preoperative dose is 50 Gy in daily fractions over approximately 5 weeks as used in a recent randomized trial (86). Sparing of late effects may be expected with smaller fraction size in altered fractionation protocols, and may be important when critical structures are irradiated. However, an improvement in therapeutic gain remains unproven from this strategy in STS.

Unresected disease being treated with the goal of long-term control should receive at least 70 Gy in 35 fractions or equivalent.

RADIATION TARGET VOLUME

Soft tissue sarcomas generally respect barriers to tumor spread in the site of origin, such as bone, interosseous membrane, major fascial planes, etc. Thus the margins of RT must be wide, especially along the direction of the involved musculature, but care must be taken to ensure that the fascial planes are appropriately recognized and encompassed in the radiation target volume. In the preoperative setting the gross tumor volume (GTV) is typically represented by the radiologically defined tumor. Some sarcomas have extensive peritumor edema, which extends along fascial planes and may lie at some distance from the primary tumor. It is not known if the edema contains viable tumor cells (91). The inclusion of edema within the GTV can influence the size of the treatment field considerably, and studies correlating the radiologic imaging to the pathologic findings are required. A zone of potential microscopic disease beyond this comprises the clinical target volume (CTV). For postoperative RT planning the high-risk target area includes the surgical field containing all the tissues handled during the surgical procedure, including scars and drain sites. Again, an additional zone beyond this comprises the CTV. Typically, in STS RT planning, the recommended CTV margins beyond high-risk areas are at least 5 cm (86), although it is recognized this is often not feasible in the complex anatomy of the head and neck. Bone, interosseus membranes, and fascial planes are considered barriers to tumor spread and permit RT margins to be narrower. Within this framework, our policy has been to use a 5-cm margin where possible, including peritumoral edema, irrespective of grade or size of the tumor, although practice in other centers is variable (53). In contrast, the BRT protocol at MSKCC uses margins of only 2 cm around the surgical bed (73), although cases may not always be selected similarly for EBT and BRT protocols. Nevertheless, it questions whether the zone of microscopic involvement may be less than previously realized, and studies examining this issue are required. Recent improvements in surgical technique may lessen the degree of intraoperative tumor dissemination, and the need to irradiate all surgically handled tissues, scars, and drain sites may be overstated today.

Other than for the individual histologic subtypes at risk for regional lymph node involvement, elective irradiation of the neck is not ordinarily recommended in STS.

Adjuvant Chemotherapy

RATIONALE

Various rationales underpin the use of adjuvant chemotherapy. First, the efficacy of cytotoxic agents can be expected to be greater in the setting of a low tumor burden (e.g., microscopic potential disease) compared with the high (visible) tumor burden associated with overt metastatic disease. Second, chemotherapy might be better tolerated in association with a low tumor burden. Third, the growth fraction is postulated to be high in tumors with a low tumor burden, and decreases with increasing tumor size. This is relevant because tumors with a high growth fraction are believed to be more sensitive to chemotherapy. Finally, although generally considered a strategy to enhance metastatic outcome, there is also the potential to improve local control in circumstances where optimal local control strategies cannot be used because of constraints resulting from sensitive anatomic locations.

META-ANALYSIS OF RANDOMIZED TRIALS

The individual data from the 1,568 patients randomized in all 14 trials that addressed the role of doxorubicin-based adjuvant chemotherapy in STS were combined in a meta-analysis (92). Problems related to the meta-analysis have been discussed (93), and there is some disagreement about whether the results should be interpreted with respect to whether or not adjuvant chemotherapy should be used routinely in STS (93,94). In the meta-analysis, the figures for distant relapse-free interval and overall recurrence-free survival were significantly in favor of the use of adjuvant chemotherapy. However, and most importantly, the difference in overall survival, the ultimate aim of adjuvant chemotherapy, was not significantly different between the chemotherapy and the control groups ($p < 0.12$) (Table 30.10). The suggested potential absolute benefit was 4% at 10 years, representing a possible survival improvement from 50% to 54% ($p < 0.12$). Thus, based on these results, routine use of chemotherapy would result in 96% of patients receiving chemotherapy with its intrinsic side effects, but with only a modest benefit accrued to the population (93).

Only three trials in the meta-analysis were of a relatively large sample size, that of the European Organization for the Research and Treatment of Cancer (EORTC), the Scandinavian Sarcoma Group (SSG), and the Gynecologic Oncology Group (GOG) (95–97). However, given the heterogeneity of STSs, even these three studies may be too small to render definitive conclusions. In part this may arise from inclusion of cases with minimal or only small risk for metastatic failure, thereby diluting the power of the studies to detect an effect that may exist only for those patients at substantial risk for metastasis. Most of the trials addressed other body sites, although head and neck STS were included to varying degrees in half of the studies, including those examining doxorubicin alone vs. controls (95,98–100) or doxorubicin combination chemotherapy vs. controls (96,101,102).

TABLE 30.10 Hazard Ratios for Individual Patient Data Meta-Analysis in 1,568 Patients for 14 Trials of Doxorubicin-based Chemotherapy in Adult Soft Tissue Sarcoma

Outcome	Hazard ratio	95% CI	*p* Value
Local RFI	0.73	0.56–0.94	0.016
Distant RFI	0.70	0.57–0.85	0.0003
Overall recurrence-free survival	0.75	0.64–0.87	0.0001
Overall survival	0.89	0.76–1.03	0.12

CI, confidence interval; RFI, recurrence-free interval.
Source: Data from sarcoma meta-analysis collaboration. Adjuvant chemotherapy for localised resectable soft-tissue sarcoma of adults: meta-analysis of individual data. *Lancet* 1997;350:1647–1654.

INFLUENCE OF CHEMOTHERAPY ON LOCAL CONTROL

Of interest, the largest trial in the meta-analysis (that of the EORTC) compared the outcome of adjuvant CYVADIC [cyclophosphamide, Oncovin (vincristine), Adriamycin (doxorubicin), and dimethyltriazeno imidazole carboxamide (DTIC) (dacarbazine)] chemotherapy compared with control in 468 patients. The relapse-free survival was significantly better after CYVADIC (56% vs. 43% for controls; $p < 0.007$) and local recurrence was significantly reduced by CYVADIC (17% vs. 31%; $p < 0.01$) (96). This favorable result in this subset analysis appeared to be confined to head, neck, and trunk tumors. In contrast, distant metastases rates were similar in both arms, as were overall survival rates (63% vs. 56%; $p < 0.64$). Thus there is the potential for adjuvant chemotherapy to improve local control in this high-risk group of STS, where local control has traditionally not been as satisfactory as with STS overall, and surgery and RT cannot be administered with the same freedom as at other anatomic sites.

ADDITIONAL DATA

Since the publication of the meta-analysis, another important study was reported from Bologna, Italy. The inclusion criteria for this trial were appropriately restricted to very adverse tumors (confined to large high-grade lesions) and a very intensive cytotoxic regimen (five cycles of 4′-epidoxorubicin 60 mg/m^2 days 1 and 2 and ifosfamide 1.8 g/m^2 days 1 through 5, with hydration, mesna, and granulocyte colony-stimulating factor) compared with no systemic treatment (103). The disease-free and overall survival rates were statistically improved at preliminary analysis, and at the time of reporting (103,104). However, by the time of publication, the metastatic rate in both arms of the randomized trial was virtually identical (44% and 45%), and it can be expected that the ultimate survival rate will eventually also be the same (103,105). Unfortunately, this raises the question of whether the potential value of aggressive chemotherapy may largely be in delaying the manifestation of distant metastasis, but not in their prevention. This study is of particular interest because a dose-intensive chemotherapy regimen was administered to a high-risk group of patients.

RECOMMENDATION FOR INDIVIDUAL PATIENTS

At this time, given the overall results of the individual patient data meta-analysis and the uncertain nature of this recent positive trial of the Bologna trial, postoperative chemotherapy cannot be considered standard therapy for patients with localized STS. We have not adopted systemic chemotherapy for routine use and have preferred to intensify local control strategies by maximizing the completeness of resection and delivering accurate and intensive adjuvant RT. On the other hand, we feel that chemotherapy should continue to be evaluated in randomized controlled trials in head and neck and other body sites wherever possible. Additional comments about individual selected histologic types are made later. Especially important among these is rhabdomyosarcoma.

Clinical Management of Selected Soft Tissue Sarcoma Subtypes

ANGIOSARCOMA

Angiosarcoma, a rare STS, is unusually well represented in the head and neck (approximately half of all angiosarcomas), and most often as a lesion in the scalp or malar skin (8,34). Patients typically present in their seventh to eighth decade, and males outnumber females by a factor 3:1. The most frequent presentation is with diffuse purple maculae on the scalp with edema and bleeding (8,34). Lesions often seem multifocal, with considerable distance between apparent separate nodules of ulceration or patchy macularity of purplish hue. Involvement of the eyelid and periorbital tissues is particularly problematic. Local control is an overwhelming problem because of the difficulty deciding the optimal extent of surgical and RT margins from gross tumor, and local recurrence beyond the treatment areas seems to be invariable. Regional node metastases (10–20% rates) is more frequent than in most other sarcoma subtypes in the head and neck. Distant metastasis is also frequent, especially to lung, but bone and liver are also affected more often than expected. As with other STSs, treatment consists of RT and surgery. It is important to perform a wide local excision, and radiation fields must also be extensive because of the poorly circumscribed, multifocal nature of the tumors (8). All too frequently these tumors fail just beyond surgical and/or RT fields. Indeed, the sinister behavior of these lesions warrants new approaches of a technical, biologic, or combined modality nature. Unfortunately, the use of chemotherapy seems unproven, although responses to newer agents such as paclitaxel may provide opportunity for the future (106). Overall, the 5-year survival ranges between 12% and 35% (8,34).

HEMANGIOPERICYTOMA

Hemangiopericytoma, with origin from the pericytes, is a rare soft tissue neoplasms, but a disproportionate number (about 20%) are located in the head and neck (107). As the name implies, pericytes are located around the capillaries and are structurally similar to smooth muscle cells and fibroblasts (108,109) (Fig. 30.8). Often unpredictable, a true diagnosis of malignant hemangiopericytoma remains a diagnosis of exclusion, and pathologists are reluctant to predict behavior, in contrast to most sarcomas where prognostic factors are relatively reliable. Sinonasal hemangiopericytoma is reputed to be a biologically less aggressive tumor than in other anatomic sites. However, we have seen adverse outcome and metastasis in such lesions and would advise against undercautious approaches to management (Fig. 30.1). Our approach generally follows that of other low-grade STS lesions, notwithstanding the difficulty in declaring them truly malignant on a histologic basis. Clear surgical margins are indicated and adjuvant RT is applied where appropriate.

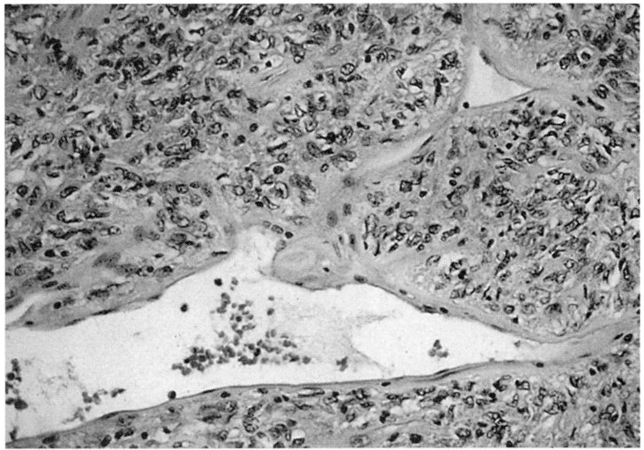

Figure 30.8 Photomicrograph of hemangiopericytoma. Dilated sinusoidal vascular channels, surrounded by tumor cells with indistinct cellular outlines ("staghorn" or "antler" configuration) is a hallmark of this tumor of "unpredictable" behavior (see Fig. 30.1). (Courtesy of Dr. David Howarth, Staff Pathologist Sarcoma Site Program, Princess Margaret Hospital and Mount Sinai Hospital, University of Toronto, Ontario, Canada.)

SYNOVIAL SARCOMA

Synovial sarcomas are of interest for several reasons. The name is a misnomer, because such lesions virtually never originate from intraarticular or synovial tissue but have origin from undifferentiated or pluripotential mesenchymal cells. Specific translocations have assisted in their classification and may have prognostic significance (see "Pathology and Grading"). Location in the prevertebral, parapharyngeal and retropharyngeal spaces is most typical but they can be seen elsewhere, including the neck and tongue. An enhanced incidence of lymph node involvement is seen. Microcalcification in the tumor is common (evident in about half of cases and often seen radiologically; therefore, care must be taken to exclude papillary thyroid carcinoma because of the epithelial appearance of biphasic tumors and the presence of calcification). Treatment approaches should follow the generic principles for the management of STS described earlier. In addition, synovial sarcoma is notably sensitive to chemotherapy, often manifesting complete responses to ifosfamide and doxorubicin, and multicenter trials of adjuvant therapy are therefore warranted (110).

KAPOSI SARCOMA

Kaposi sarcoma (KS) is often seen on the skin of the head and neck or in the oral cavity as flat, red to purple maculae that progress into nodules over time. Four different associations exist: classic, African, renal transplant associated, and epidemic (AIDS). Epidemiologic evidence reveals a marked decline in new KS since the widespread use of highly active antiretroviral therapy (111), and, correspondingly, it is our impression that the indication for intervention is significantly less that it was 10 years ago when many patients were referred for local management, especially RT. Asymptomatic disease does not require treatment. However, limited cutaneous disease may be treated for toilet or cosmetic reasons with topical alitretinoin gel, intralesional vinblastine, RT, laser therapy, or cryotherapy (111). Various low-dose radiation regimens have been evaluated with good efficacy (112). Liposomal anthracyclines (daunorubicin and doxorubicin) and paclitaxel have simplified the systemic management of patients when warranted.

DERMATOFIBROSARCOMA PROTUBERANS

Dermatofibrosarcoma protuberans, as the name suggests, is an elevated nodular (protuberant) lesion arising from the dermis with characteristic slow but persistent growth over many years. Although borderline to low grade in histologic appearance, it has a propensity for local recurrence after simple excision. Typical manifestations are of a red to purple lesion on the upper trunk, especially in proximity to the clavicular regions where it is frequent on the shoulder and supraclavicular regions of the head and neck. Not infrequently, small satellite lesions are evident at the site or bordering a skin graft following an unsuccessful previous excision. Management is best with wide surgical margins or more conservative cosmesis facilitating surgery with adjuvant EBRT, following which the recurrence rate is extremely low (113–115). Adjuvant RT should certainly be considered in cases of recurrence especially when disease is escaping control by traditional surgical approaches to prevent escalation to more adverse histology. Mohs' surgery is also advocated when feasible. The recent observation (16) that metastatic sarcoma arising in DFSP may respond to imatinib (STI 571, Gleevec®) provides fascinating possibilities for molecular target therapies in the future (see "Pathology and Grading").

AGGRESSIVE FIBROMATOSIS

Fibromatosis (also termed extraabdominal desmoid tumors or aggressive fibromatosis), although not malignant, is capable of local infiltration and destruction that is as devastating as uncontrolled true malignancy (116). About 10% of fibromatosis occur in the head and neck, often in the supraclavicular neck in proximity to the brachial plexus. It demonstrates a unique pattern of spread with infiltration widely along fascial planes and sinuous fibrotic stranding in the soft tissues at considerable distance from the main tumor mass. Wide surgical excision is the treatment of choice for this capricious disease, but recurrence was seen at the M. D. Anderson Cancer Center (MDACC) in about one third of cases treated with surgery alone at 10 years despite negative margins. The recurrence rate exceeded 50% at 10 years for surgery alone if resection margins were positive, which compared adversely with a 31% of recurrence if margin-positive cases received RT ($p < 0.007$). For patients treated with combined resection and RT, the overall 10-year actuarial relapse rate was 25%. Therefore, the addition of RT offsets the adverse impact of positive margins seen in the surgical group at MDACC (117). In fact, in patients treated with RT for gross disease, the 10-year actuarial relapse rate was 24%, making this a viable option for such patients. Because positive surgical margins are frequent, we usually advise adjuvant RT, depending on lesion location, and consideration of salvage options for any subsequent recurrence, and particularly if we anticipate its resulting in major functional deficit. As noted, these lesions are often intimately associated with the brachial plexus and intervertebral foramina, and recurrence would be very problematic (Fig. 30.9). Hormonal manipulations, EBRT, and chemotherapy can be used for symptomatic unresectable disease, although a trial of surveillance to evaluate the presence and/or pace of progression may also be considered.

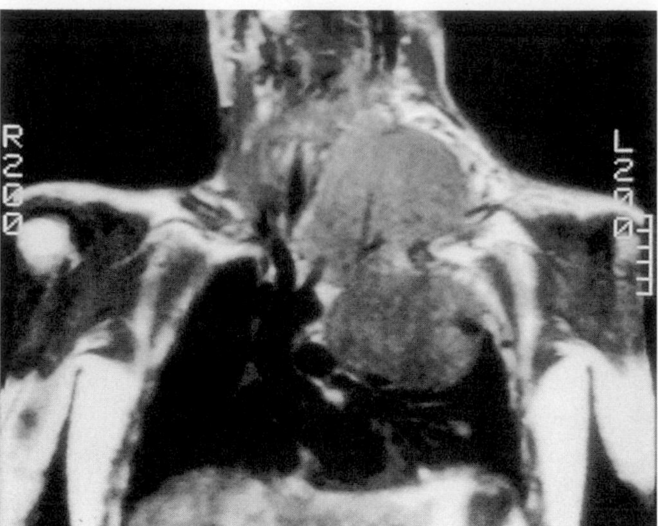

Figure 30.9 Aggressive fibromatosis with immense growth and infiltration presenting as a mass in the low neck in a 19-year-old man. This patient had progressive symptoms including pain, motor brachial plexopathy, upper extremity edema, and recent-onset Horner syndrome. He was treated with preoperative radiotherapy (50 Gy in 25 fractions) to minimize dose to heart, spinal cord, and especially lung. Resection included vascular reconstruction. He remains well and disease-free 11 years later with normal recreational and vocational activity.

LIPOSARCOMA

Although liposarcoma represents one of the most common STSs, it has no particular significance in the head and neck, and the principles of management for STS outlined later should be applied. As in other body sites, the most favorable outcome is associated with the well-differentiated subtype. The myxoid variant is present in 40% to 50% of all cases. Round cell admixture and pleomorphic histology are associated with a poor prognosis. Of interest, myxoid liposarcoma may demonstrate unusual natural history with metastasis to extrapulmonary soft tissue sites (e.g., the retroperitoneum, chest wall, pleura, and pericardium being typical) (118). Such remote metastasis to unusual sites may masquerade as isolated second sarcomas, but share identical lineage to the original primary by virtue of monoclonality confirmed by analysis of TLS-CHOP or EWS-CHOP rearrangements (119).

RHABDOMYOSARCOMA

Clinical Issues

We recommend several excellent reviews of rhabdomyosarcoma for more detailed discussion (33,50). This tumor is the fifth most common cancer in children (33). About two thirds occur in children less than 10 years old. The most common sites of origin are the head and neck (about 40%) and the genitourinary tract (about 20%) (50). Head and neck primaries typically afflict children aged 5 to 9 years, whereas genitourinary lesions appear in younger ages. Among head and neck lesions, one quarter affect the orbit, one half are parameningeal (Table 30.11), and the remainder are in other sites (50). The site of origin is important because it provides information concerning patterns of spread and relapse. Thus orbital lesions, while presenting with dramatic early orbital content displacement, rarely manifest regional node metastasis or distant disease. In contrast, parameningeal sites provide significant risk for intracranial extension and cerebrospinal fluid (CSF) metastasis as well as distant disease. The initial evaluation of rhabdomyosarcoma is similar to regular STS, but should include bone marrow examination because the risk is moderate and the prognosis unfavorable. In addition, the CSF should be sampled in parameningeal lesions.

Treatment of these children and young adults is arduous and associated with considerable cost, including the burden of therapy experienced by the individual at the time, but also the late sequelae (50). Because most of these patients are young children, the principal dilemma concerns the use of disfiguring local treatments. Surgery, an immediate and potentially major intrusion, usually results in cosmetic and function loss, but RT has a high probability for growth and tissue maldevelopment later. Philosophically, only one local treatment should be employed where feasible and with the minimum possible intensity. In many ways the role of chemotherapy has been to facilitate this, in addition to treating systemically. Current research efforts are even exploring the potential of relying on chemotherapy as the sole therapy given the devastating local sequelae that may arise in young children (50).

TABLE 30.11 Definition of Sites of Origin of Rhabdomyosarcoma of the Head and Neck

Site	Relative proportions	Definition
Orbit	25%	
Parameningeal	50%	Nasopharynx, nasal cavity, paranasal sinuses, middle ear, mastoid, pterygoid fossa, and any parameningeal site with extension into a parameningeal location
Nonparameningeal site	25%	

Source: Data from Stevens MCG. Malignant mesenchymal tumours of childhood. In: Souhami RL, Tannock I, Hohenberger P, et al., eds. *Oxford textbook of oncology,* 2nd ed. Oxford: Oxford University Press, 2002:2525–2538.

Surgery

The role of surgery is controversial given the great sensitivity of these lesions to chemotherapy and RT. It should be performed only at diagnosis in the absence of metastasis to lymph nodes or distant sites because prompt chemotherapy is the most critical intervention required to realize a favorable outcome. Secondary surgery to achieve local control following initial chemotherapy is reasonable but should be conservative. In general, RT is used most often in the head and neck sites (50). In the young adult, where growth arrest and structural abnormalities from RT are not at issue, we recommend surgery only for the smallest lesions in favorable sites in the primary nonsalvage situation. Frequently, RT would also be added to sterilize the field and treat potential lymph node regions because this risk is prodigious in our experience of treating young adults (Fig. 30.5).

Chemotherapy

Over several decades a complex and impressive series of trials addressing the role of chemotherapy predominantly have been completed through cooperative group mechanisms in North America and Europe. Unfortunately, these models of collaboration in oncology cannot be reviewed other than to comment that chemotherapy has dramatically improved the outcome of this disease. Its purpose is to both ameliorate the risk for distant metastasis manifestation and to reduce the extent of subsequent surgery or RT (or even eliminate them).

The classic drugs have been vincristine (V), actinomycin-D (A), and cyclophosphamide (C). In addition, doxorubicin (adr) has been used in some schedules, or alone, though its role in initial therapy is uncertain (50). Combinations have included VA, VAC (the most established), and VACadr. Recent approaches, especially in Europe, have involved substitution of ifosfamide for cyclophosphamide, although the superiority of one over the other remains unproven. Ifosfamide is frequently used in combination with vincristine and etoposide or with etoposide alone. These strategies are often intended to overcome drug resistance especially in advanced disease protocols. We often use the combination of ifosfamide and etoposide while RT is being administered after initial induction with VAC or VACadr because of prohibitive normal tissue sensitization with actinomycin-D or doxorubicin.

The role of autologous bone marrow transplant, or peripheral blood stem-cell support remains unestablished in either "normal" presentations or advanced disease with metastasis.

Radiotherapy

Radiotherapy alone (meaning with chemotherapy) or as an adjunct to surgery is a very effective strategy to effect local control, achieving rates on the order of 90% with doses of approximately 50 to 60 Gy at conventional daily fractionation of 2 Gy per day. However, in IRSG group 1 tumors (Table 30.6), there is no need for EBRT, which is reserved for residual or unresected disease.

In children it is highly desirable to maintain doses at a minimum. In consequence, research is exploring the lower dose limits that can be used safely. The potential to use doses less than 40 Gy is being considered, although there is also concern that this may be insufficient, especially for adverse situations such as the alveolar subtype or in the face of overt clinic disease. Other strategies have included altered fractionation employing lower dose per fraction with the potential to exploit radiobiology strategies for additional normal tissue protection. The current standard is to provide doses on the order of 50 Gy and where possible use doses in the 45-Gy range. In the full-grown patient, our usual approach is to prescribe 60 Gy to sites of gross disease, while administering 50 Gy to potential areas of involvement, including the nodal regions at risk.

Radiotherapy fields and volumes are problematic especially in parameningeal sites where local failure and leptomeningeal relapse is possible. Thus wide margins intracranially are considered but are associated with major potential sequelae, and firm guidelines to ameliorate these risks (for example, whole brain RT or intrathecal chemotherapy) do not exist in the absence of established meningeal metastasis (50). Radiotherapy volumes should also consider coverage of the lymph nodes at risk or involved in these adverse parameningeal sites. Plans developed with these goals are extremely complex and may need to consider some of the new RT technologies (see "Specialized Radiotherapy Approaches").

Results

Since the introduction of combination chemotherapy, survival outcome has improved dramatically from approximately 25% to 5-year survival rates of approximately 70%. The rates exceed 80% for embryonal lesions, and are somewhat lower for alveolar and lower again for undifferentiated lesions. Good prognostic factors include head and neck location, stage 1 or 2 lesions, and low tumor grade. Poor outcome is seen in patients younger than 1 year old, alveolar histology, and high-grade tumors. As yet unexplained is the observation that the different histologic subtypes have an intrinsically worse prognosis in adults compared with children (120). Adult tumors may manifest extremely unfavorable behavior including sanctuary site metastasis and may require bone marrow replacement not long following initial combined modality treatment including aggressive adjuvant chemotherapy.

TREATMENT OF BONE SARCOMAS OF THE HEAD AND NECK

The management of bone sarcomas in the head and neck suffers even more than that of STSs from the paucity of data because they are even more rare. Approaches are again extrapolated from the more usual body sites, predominantly the limbs. Local treatment is again compromised by the proximity to important anatomic structures, making resection and RT more challenging than they are elsewhere. The situation differs from STS in that RT is much less established as a component of treatment in bone tumors, and chemotherapy is more established in osteosarcoma and the very rarely seen Ewing tumors.

Osteosarcoma

BACKGROUND

Few centers see more than one case of head and neck osteogenic sarcoma annually, and differences in reported outcome appear to relate to the rarity of the disease, case selection, and variable practice patterns (121). Moreover, histologic grade strongly influences outcome, and comparison and prediction of outcome and behavior appear to be particularly vulnerable to treatment selection bias (122,123). Although generally considered more favorable than other osteosarcomas, possibly because of lower histologic grade, agreement is not uniform about whether the risk for metastasis is less than in long bone tumors. The pertinent data was reviewed and will not be repeated in detail (121).

TABLE 30.12 Osteosarcoma of the Head and Neck (Selected Series)

Author and year	No. of cases	Local control (5 years)	Overall survival (5 years)
Mark et al., 1991 (124)	18	10/18	50%
Ha et al., 1999 (125)	27	NA	55%
Kassir et al., 1997 (meta-analysis) (122)	173	NA	37%
Smeele et al., 1997 (meta-analysis) (123)[a]	201	NA	NA
Oda et al., 1997 (121)	13	12/13 (2/3 salvaged)	72%

NA, not assessable (data not provided).
[a]Data provided as actuarial curves for different prognostic groupings and not for the overall population (see text and ref. 123).

At the same time, local relapse in head and neck lesions remains a grave sequela. Overall reported survival rates remain disappointing, generally being in the 30% to 40% range, with occasional small series projecting survival on the order of 70% (Table 30.12) (121–125).

SURGERY

The foundation of local treatment is surgery, and as for osteosarcoma elsewhere, should be accomplished with clear resection margins. Usually surgery follows neoadjuvant chemotherapy (see later). The principles of resection and reconstruction should be observed, including anticipation of the routes of spread into difficult areas in the head and neck and skull base (Fig. 30.10). The local resection should be planned

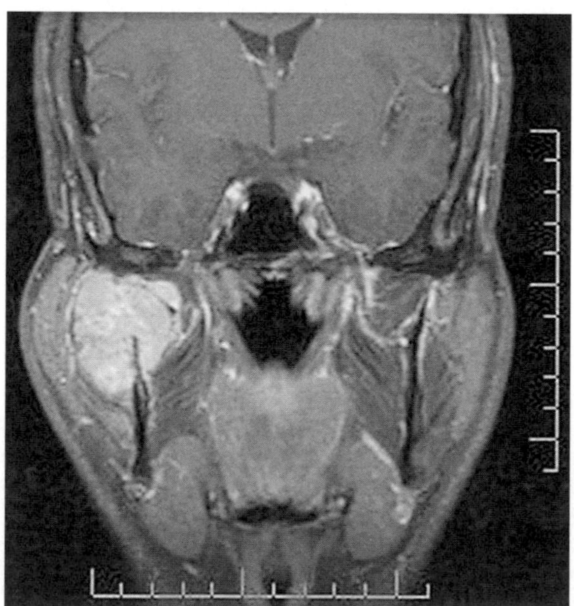

Figure 30.10 Chondroblastic osteosarcoma of the vertical mandibular ramus with temporomandibular joint destruction and invasion of masticator apparatus and infratemporal fossa in a 25-year-old man. The soft tissue component has virtually "exploded" the bone. This patient did not experience local control after postinduction chemotherapy surgery and later failed combined surgery with proton beam radiotherapy. Progressive pulmonary metastases developed that were refractory to all chemotherapy until gemcitabine achieved complete and sustained remission of local and metastatic disease.

with a very clear definition of tumor extent, particularly the intramedullary component. An MRI scan is particularly useful to delineate both intramedullary extent and any extraosseous component. Intraoperatively, tumor clearance is confirmed by pathologic examination of marrow biopsy at the resection site; similarly, verification of completeness of resection is recommended in doubtful areas such as tissues adjacent to neurovascular structures in proximity to the tumor. Any biopsy scars or other access routes for disease to track from the primary site should also be excised.

RADIOTHERAPY

Adjuvant Radiotherapy

At times only marginal resection is feasible and other options for local management must be considered. Revision surgery where feasible is advisable because the outlook for these patients is bleak. Although RT is intuitively attractive, the reality is that adjuvant RT for high-risk osteogenic sarcoma does not appear to confer the high rates of local control seen in oncology in general. Nevertheless, we feel it should be considered in these adverse situations even though it was not found to be of benefit in two systemic reviews of the literature where individual patient data were considered (122,123). As noted earlier, a significant problem affecting the literature of this disease is selection bias in the choice of adjuvant treatments, and it remains possible that RT may provide valuable delay in progression. Indeed the results of evaluation of RT indicate that it either confers no significant value (123), or is associated with worse outcome (121,122) because of selection of cases due to unresectability or residual disease after surgery.

It would seem from these retrospective results that the role of RT has not been explored adequately, even if its actual contribution is only modest. What are needed are controlled trials, but it would be most improbable that this will ever be explored in a randomized prospective fashion, even through a multicenter mechanism, because of disease rarity. At the same time the role of RT is not likely to be considered in osteogenic sarcoma of the limbs where the local control rate is at least 90% following neoadjuvant chemotherapy and limb salvage surgery, and wide application of adjuvant RT is unnecessary.

Finally, if RT is employed, it should follow identical principles described earlier for STS. In essence, routes of spread and location of tumor, including potential tissues contaminated by surgery, biopsy, and tumor invasion/incursion, should be considered in the planning volumes. Adequate doses are also necessary and should exceed 60 Gy, even when only microscopic disease is present because of the apparent deserved reputation of relative radioresistance.

Radiotherapy Alone

At the present time the literature does not provide any convincing evidence that radiation as a sole modality is useful for the local management of osteosarcoma. It therefore should be confined to the experimental approach or be reserved for palliation. Unfortunately, in our experience it has not been successful for the latter.

ADJUVANT CHEMOTHERAPY

Adjuvant Chemotherapy for Osteosarcoma

A number of trials have established the routine use of chemotherapy in extremity osteosarcoma, although initially controversy existed about whether the apparent survival benefits could relate to improvements in other aspects of the illness and not to the use of systemic treatment. Specifically, a change in natural history was posited as contributing combined with more aggressive staging and surgical intervention for metastases, as well as better local surgery. The discordant views were addressed by the completion of the Multiinstitution Osteosarcoma Study (126) in which patients were randomized to observation only (instead of systemic therapy) or multiagent chemotherapy (Rosen T10 protocol). In Rosen's protocols a variety of drugs were used (methotrexate, doxorubicin, bleomycin, actinomycin-D, and cyclophosphamide given repeatedly for up to 1 year) including cisplatin for poor responders (see later). A significant improvement in disease-free survival was observed in favor of the chemotherapy arm of the trial, although overall survival was not apparently different in the initial report of the trial. A putative influence of salvage treatment may have explained the early observation, but with later follow-up a survival advantage in favor of early chemotherapy was apparent (127).

As noted, a variety of agents have been used in the chemotherapy of osteosarcoma. Currently established protocols are high-dose methotrexate-based chemotherapy or the combination of doxorubicin/cisplatin. Because of toxicity of prolonged chemotherapy, the European Osteosarcoma Intergroup performed a multicenter randomized study comparing 12 months of multiagent methotrexate-based chemotherapy vs. six courses of doxorubicin/cisplatin. Survival appeared comparable for both groups (128). More recently, ifosfamide has emerged as an active agent, but questions remain about optimal scheduling and dosage. Ongoing trials are in progress evaluating these questions and include the use of hematopoietic growth factors such as granulocyte colony-stimulating factor (G-CSF) in intensification protocols.

There still remains uncertainty about whether neoadjuvant chemotherapy is superior to prompt postoperative chemotherapy in terms of survival benefit. Neoadjuvant chemotherapy permits the potential for early eradication of micrometastatic disease, delivery of chemotherapy to an intact blood supply, and assessment of the effectiveness of the preoperative chemotherapy regimen used. The latter has become an important principle in the management of osteogenic sarcoma through assessment of histologic response after systemic chemotherapy (129). It also appears to facilitate surgery and was pivotal in the introduction of limb preservation for osteosarcoma of limb bones. In osteosarcoma of the extremities, completeness of histologic response to neoadjuvant chemotherapy (e.g., less than 5% to 10% tumor viability at surgical resection) has been correlated with improved survival. Poor responders to neoadjuvant chemotherapy typically require more aggressive postoperative regimens and have a poorer prognosis. Because of this it is customary to adjust chemotherapy to a different regimen in an effort to shift the survival to equate with the good responders. Unfortunately, evidence that this truly takes place is more difficult to obtain.

Adjuvant Chemotherapy in Head and Neck Osteosarcoma

Although important trials have been completed in extremity osteosarcoma, prospective studies in the head and neck are lacking and treatment has been inconsistent. As a result, there is disagreement about its role in the seemingly more favorable osteosarcomas of the mandible and maxilla compared with extremity lesions. Remarkably, in this rare condition, two independent quasi–meta-analyses of the retrospective data regarding the role of adjuvant chemotherapy were reported simultaneously (122,123). In both studies the authors described their methodology in detail, which were similar in restricting cases to those where individual patient data were available in the reports chosen for analysis. In this way actuarial estimates of outcome could be calculated and proportional hazards techniques applied to estimate risk and to attempt to control for prognostic variables. Of importance, both studies report the conclusion that RT seemed to be unhelpful, bearing in mind the caveats mentioned earlier and that the inherent biases of retrospective studies cannot be completely controlled for.

In addition, however, the authors reached different conclusions regarding the efficacy of systemic chemotherapy. Kassir et al. (122) concluded that the role of chemotherapy in head and neck osteosarcoma remains unproven. In contrast, Smeele et al. (123) maintained that chemotherapy does improve survival and advocated the adoption of the same chemotherapy protocols as used for long bone primary sites. It turns out that an important distinction separates the two studies. Kassir et al. accepted all nonmetastatic patients, whereas Smeele et al. restricted entry to those studies that reported on surgical margins. Both the variables "involved margins" and "chemotherapy," when adjusted for each other, turned out to be significant (130). Although it is of interest to observe the findings by Smeele et al., we would also caution that neither the margin status nor the response to chemotherapy is known at baseline when a patient first presents at diagnosis, and the patients who performed well in their study following chemotherapy are already selected by virtue of favorable responses to surgery (i.e., clear margins). Moreover, the margin status could itself be complicated by whether there was a favorable response to preoperative chemotherapy. In other words, we still do not have strong evidence about what to recommend for a given patient presenting for the first time until after surgery has been performed, and in most cases after induction chemotherapy as well.

Recommendation for Individual Patients

Notwithstanding the discussion concerning the evidence about the role of adjuvant chemotherapy in osteogenic sarcoma and the putative more favorable behavior compared with long bone lesions, it is our view that certain of these lesions can manifest sinister behavior (Fig. 30.10), and we would routinely advise systemic chemotherapy in fit patients. This is administered using a neoadjuvant/induction approach. Of interest, despite their results suggesting a lack of benefit, Kassir et al., influenced by their observation of relatively poor prognosis for these lesions, provide similar recommendations to ours (122). Our general approach to management of head and neck osteosarcoma is summarized in an algorithm (Fig. 30.11).

Chondrosarcoma

Chondrosarcoma makes up 10% of malignant bone tumors and is the second most common sarcoma arising in bone (after osteosarcoma). Chondrosarcoma also comprises less than 10% of these primary bone malignancies in the head and neck. In this location, it presents a broad spectrum of tumors of similar histology but widely dissimilar behavior and demographic character. For example, age and sex distribution vary by histologic subtype and site. In the NCDB report, older age (>50 years) was most prevalent among laryngotracheal cases (90%) and among men (26). In contrast, women and patients younger than 50 years were more likely to be associated with lesions of the osseous head and neck skeleton including the sinonasal region. These demographic differences in a large contemporary database indicate that head and neck chondrosarcoma encompasses subgroups of dissimilar cancers, and the great heterogeneity of presentation and biology, as well as potential management strategies, makes it difficult to summarize outcome succinctly. The NCDB analysis also demonstrated that decreased survival was statistically associated with advanced stage, higher grade, and the histologic subtypes myxoid or mesenchymal.

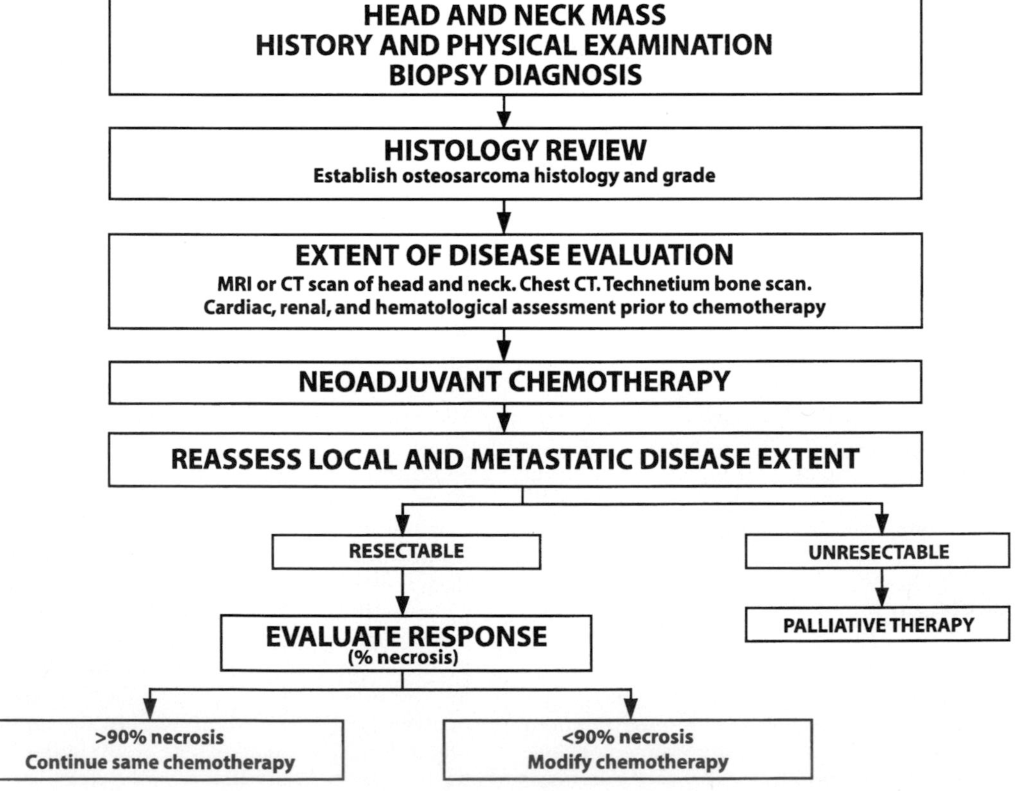

Figure 30.11 Flow diagram for the management of osteosarcoma of the head and neck using the usual approach of induction chemotherapy with pathologic response assessment.

SURGERY

All evidence about the management of chondrosarcoma of the head and neck would support the use of surgical excision as the primary treatment when possible. In addition, the surgery should concentrate on the primary tumor following the principles outlined for osteosarcoma, including adequacy and verification of complete excision and meticulous staging prior to excision. These principles are not repeated here other than to emphasize that wide excision beyond the pseudocapsule is required because chondrosarcomas tend to have microscopic fingerlike extensions and have a notorious propensity to seed the wound with later nodular recurrence if the tumor is violated. In addition, because the overall low incidence of regional metastases (approximately 5%) (26,131), neck dissection is not indicated.

ADJUVANT TREATMENT

Adjuvant Chemotherapy

The management of osteosarcoma and chondrosarcoma differs in two significant ways, both relating to the use of adjuvant treatments. First, and for reasons of efficacy, chemotherapy is not ordinarily a component of management of chondrosarcoma, in contrast with osteosarcoma. The exception is in the mesenchymal subtype where chemotherapy was used in the majority of mesenchymal chondrosarcoma cases (57.5%) in the NCDB series and has been our policy at Princess Margaret Hospital (132). By extrapolation, intense chemotherapy approaches would be used as for osteosarcoma or Ewing sarcoma.

Adjuvant Radiotherapy

Radiotherapy, usually a doubtful addition to the treatment of osteosarcoma, can be a very effective adjunct to the treatment of chondrosarcoma where there is concern about the adequacy of resection (133,134), although it is acknowledged that opinions vary as to its value. At our center we have always regarded positive resection margins as an indication for adjuvant RT (133,135), and would expect similar outcome to high-risk positive margin STS following combined surgery and RT. Both adjuvant RT and RT as a sole modality (see later) should follow similar principles regarding planning, dose-fractionation parameters, and target volumes as outlined for STS and osteosarcoma. Of interest, the use of RT is not altogether unusual, having been used as a component of management in more than 20% of cases in the large NCDB report (26), which would follow our general recommendations.

RADIOTHERAPY ALONE

Radiotherapy as sole modality is also capable of long-term control of chondrosarcomas in difficult locations, such as the clival regions, although here opinions may vary about whether this is best accomplished with proton beam RT or IMRT (see "Skull Base Chondrosarcomas" and "Specialized Radiotherapy Approaches"). In either event, 10-year control rates on the order of 70% to 80% have been reported from excellent centers using proton beam RT. Our approach is to use RT as the sole modality in cases where the lesion is not resectable without great risk to the patient. Examples would include the need to sacrifice the critical vascular supply in clival lesions and especially where the lesion is of small volume (Fig. 30.12A).

RESULTS OF MANAGEMENT OF CHONDROSARCOMA

As noted earlier, the grade of the lesion and the accessibility for treatment are important determinants of outcome. In the NCDB, survival rates appeared to be similar regardless of the site of disease and are profoundly influenced by the grade of

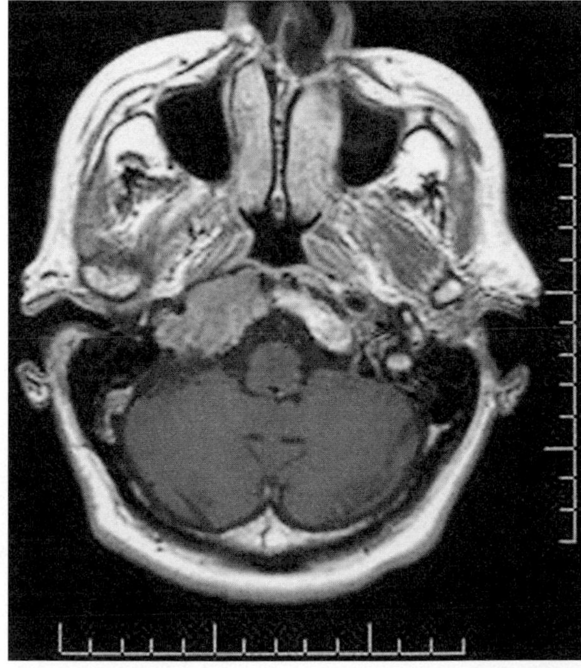
A

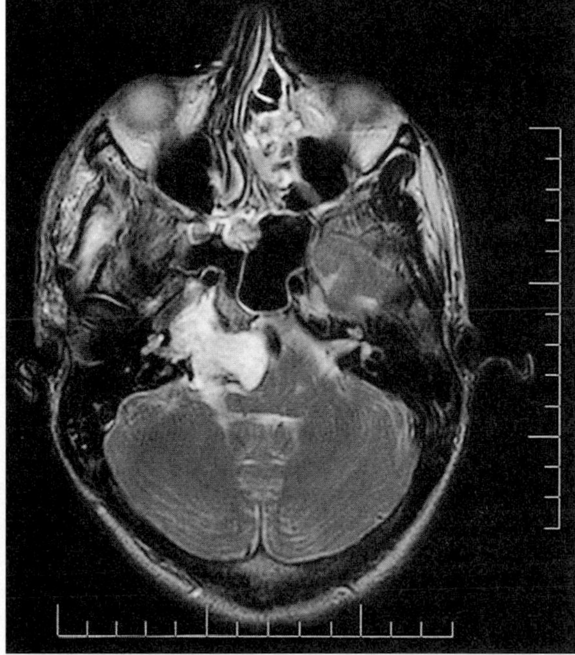
B

Figure 30.12 Magnetic resonance images of two cases of chondrosarcoma of the petroclival region. In one, an enhancing mass is seen destroying the right side of the clivus. The right internal carotid artery is incorporated within the mass at the skull base and through the petrous portion. The patient was treated with stereotactic intensity modulated radiotherapy (IMRT) to a high-fractionated dose and remains asymptomatic on follow-up examination (**A**). The second case (**B**) exhibits a chondrosarcoma of the petroclivus complicating Maffucci syndrome (see text). This 21-year-old man was managed with surgery followed by postoperative stereotactic IMRT to minimize the dose to the juxtaposed brainstem as much as possible (limit of 55 Gy fractionated to a small portion of the brainstem was achieved with this technique).

TABLE 30.13 Disease-Specific Survival Rates (%) by Grade and Anatomic Site from the National Cancer Database Report on Chondrosarcoma of the Head and Neck

	1 year	2 years	3 years	4 years	5 years	Cases (n)
Grade						
1–2	97.6	97.6	96.2	93.2	93.2	90
3–4	90.9	90.9	79.6	67.3	67.3	12
Anatomic site						
Head and neck bones	96.7	96.7	94.6	92.4	92.4	65
Laryngotracheal	95.8	95.8	93.3	88.0	88.0	51
Sinonasal	93.9	93.9	93.9	87.5	87.5	17
Head and neck soft tissue	100	93.6	93.6	80.2	80.2	21

Source: Data from Koch BB, Karnell LH, Hoffman HT, et al. National cancer database report on chondrosarcoma of the head and neck. *Head and Neck* 2000;22:408–425.

the lesion. The 5-year disease-specific rates generally exceed 80%. The beneficial outcomes are clearly related to the fact that grade 1 (50%) and grade 2 (37%) were the predominant subtypes, with grades 3 and 4 representing only 8% and 4%, respectively, since superior outcome for patients with lower-grade tumors (93.2%) compared with higher-grade tumors (67.3%) ($p < 0.0265$) (Table 30.13) (26). Individual series have not reported as favorable outcomes for the higher-grade lesions. For example, the UCLA group reported a 5-year disease-free survival of 90% for low-grade tumors and 14% for high-grade tumors (131), whereas the MDACC reported a 90% 5-year survival for grade 1 lesions versus 43% for grade 3 (136).

SPECIAL SITUATIONS IN HEAD AND NECK CHONDROSARCOMA

Chondrosarcoma of the Larynx

Chondrosarcoma is the most common sarcoma of the larynx. Usually it presents as a mass originating on the posterior cricoid lamina, eventually resulting in airway compromise and voice dysfunction (Fig. 30.13). This neoplasm is particularly indolent in behavior, carrying an extraordinarily favorable outcome in terms of survival. Generally in the older age group (>50 years), >90% of cases are low-grade lesions, and males are most frequently affected. Complete laryngectomy is virtually always curable, but a more conservative approach as suggested by the Mayo Clinic report appears more appropriate given the excellent survival rates (137,138). In that series only 14% received total laryngectomy. Despite a high recurrence rate among patients treated without total laryngectomy by either complete external removal (27% recurrence rate) or subtotal external removal (67% recurrence rate), acceptable 5-year survival (90.1%) and 10-year survival (80.9%) resulted from salvage surgery. The results when compared with expected survival for a controlled population appear to show no detriment to survival because of the chondrosarcoma (Fig. 30.14). We normally explain to patients that after surgery RT following conservation laryngeal surgery should improve the ultimate likelihood of larynx retention even though an improvement in survival cannot be realized by this approach.

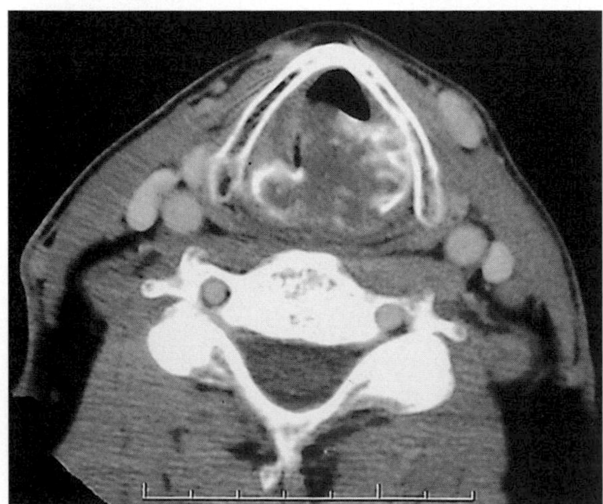

Figure 30.13 Contrast-enhanced computed tomographic axial view of a typical low-grade chondrosarcoma of the posterior cricoid lamina in a middle-aged man. Note airway reduction by the calcified and well-demarcated lesion. Although intralesional resection was recommended, with likely prospect of future and repeated reexcisions, he received postoperative radiotherapy by one of the authors (B.O'S.), at the patient's request, to minimize risk for local failure. He remains well without recurrence and with good voice 6 years later.

Skull Base Chondrosarcomas

Although rare, chondrosarcomas often arise in the skull base including clivus and petrous temporal bone. Such lesions pose particularly severe problems, including pain or gradually progressive features of brainstem compression from intracranial intrusion (e.g., cranial nerve dysfunctions, especially in the sixth nerve at the outset). The only favorable aspect is that they

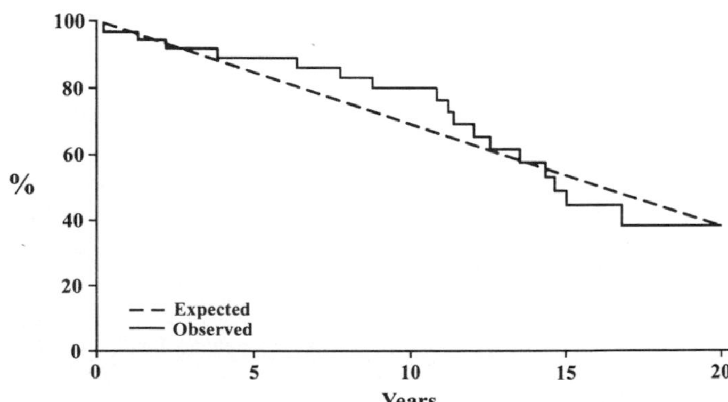

Figure 30.14 Survival curve for chondrosarcoma of the larynx treated at the Mayo clinic compared with normal population survival. (From Lewis JE, Olsen KD, Inwards CY. Cartilaginous tumors of the larynx: clinicopathologic review of 47 cases. *Ann Otol Rhinol Laryngol* 1997;106:94–100, with permission.)

TABLE 30.14 Chondrosarcoma of the Skull Base (Selected Series Treated with Precision Radiation Therapy Techniques)

Author and year	Total/ chondrosarcoma	Combined therapy	Local control (5 years)	Overall survival (5 years)
Hug et al., 1999 (139)	58/25	Sx + fractionated protons (mean 70.7 CGE)	92% (chondro)	100%
Gay et al., 1995 (152)	60/14	Sx ± EBRT	65% (chondro)	90%
Castro et al., 1994 (153)	126/27	65 CGE ± surgery	78% (chondro)	83%
Munzenrider and Liebsch, 1999 (154)	621/246	Sx + fractionated protons	94% (10 year)	88% (10 year)
Noel et al., 2001 (140)	45/11	Sx + EBRT + protons (mean 67 CGE)	90% (3 year)	90% (3 year)
Debus et al., 2000 (141)	45/8	Sx + fract stereotactic EBRT (median 64.9 Gy)	100%	100%

CGE: Cobalt Gy equivalent; chondro, chondrosarcoma; EBRT, external-beam radiotherapy; fract, fractionated; Sx, surgery.

are, like the majority of chondrosarcomas, usually of low-grade histology.

Given the grave significance of chondrosarcomas in these locations, and the inability to perform a complete excision in the majority of cases (Fig. 30.12), suitable patients with skull base primaries should be referred to specialized centers for consideration of expert skull base surgery in conjunction with specialized RT approaches, including particle beam therapy, or stereotactic photons treatments with or without IMRT (see "Specialized Radiotherapy Approaches"). A number of small series have shown that a combination of surgical debulking and high-dose precision RT results in durable local control in a large proportion of skull base chondrosarcomas (in excess of 80%) with modest late toxicity. The outcome of lesions <25 mL in volume is particularly impressive, especially if adequate doses are administered with a combination of photons and protons to approximately 70 cobalt gray equivalent (CGE) (139). Others have reported similar impressive results in smaller series with either protons or fractionated stereotactic RT (140,141). An overview of selected results is presented (Table 30.14). Such series generally also combine RT with surgery. Evaluation of this literature is problematic, because the outcome of skull base and cervical spine chordoma is frequently reported together with that of chondrosarcoma.

Mesenchymal Chondrosarcoma

This subtype tends to be more aggressive locally and has a higher rate of metastasis. Survival tends to be lower as a consequence, and it is most commonly managed with multimodality approaches. As noted earlier, this would ordinarily include a similar chemotherapy approach as used for osteosarcoma in addition to surgery and RT (132).

EWING SARCOMA

Earlier we mentioned that this tumor is exceptionally rare in the head and neck. The disease afflicts children predominantly but is rarely seen below the age of 5 and in patients older than 30 years. About 25% of patient present with distant metastasis, most often to bone.

Multimodality treatment is strongly recommended consisting of EBRT and/or surgery, and multiagent chemotherapy. We cannot emphasize too strongly the need for multidisciplinary assessments in such patients from the start, especially to make sure that the disease is adequately documented with CT and MRI before treatment is initiated. Chemotherapy is usually the first intervention and it is usually several months before RT or surgery is performed. By that time the situation will have changed and the true areas of risk may long since have been disguised in the chemotherapy response.

Although RT is highly effective, recent evidence has drawn attention to the problem of local failure is bulky disease, effects on bone growth, and second malignancies following RT (142). Therefore, surgery also should be considered in the management of different situations. We would emphasize that, with the current state of knowledge, chemotherapy alone should not be regarded as a standard to control gross tumor.

Radiotherapy

Appropriate RT portals should include the entire bone that was involved as well as any extraosseous soft tissue component of the tumor. Treatment planning should be based on the original tumor volume before chemotherapy. Classically an initial 5-cm margin beyond disease and bone has been recommended for Ewing sarcoma (143). However, as in STS and chondrosarcoma head and neck planning, this needs to be tailored to the suitability of the anatomic region. Care must be taken to protect critical organs in the head and neck, and the classic approach will rarely be used. Additional boost to the original area of visualized gross disease is also highly recommended.

Whenever a partial bone resection is undertaken, RT to the microscopic areas is indicated, and a boost applied to any gross residual disease as noted above.

Doses of RT should exceed 50 Gy in 1.8 to 2 Gy per fraction for gross disease, and need to be tailored to the critical organs at risk, the bulk of disease at the start of chemotherapy, the response to chemotherapy, and how complete any contemplated resection may be. Generally conventional daily fractionated RT is used, but studies of smaller dose per fraction altered fractionation are being tested to assess ability to minimize late-responding tissue damage.

Surgery

Surgery is indicated in expendable bones and it is hoped it would allow RT to be avoided entirely in low-volume disease. Concern about resection margins is an indication that RT is needed, which it is hoped can be administered with lower dose since the gross disease will have been resected. This may be particularly helpful in the vicinity of critical anatomy, and in that circumstance a preoperative RT approach may have advantages for the reasons described earlier for other tumors. We feel that very large volume disease is an indication for combined treatment (surgery and RT), but small volume disease is best managed with RT as the sole local modality unless disease is limited and surgery can be accomplished with wide margins obviating the need for RT. Alternatively, where RT is compromised with respect to dose and/or volume considerations, surgery should also be considered.

Chemotherapy

Chemotherapy is critical to the improvements that have been seen in the management of Ewing sarcoma in recent decades. The classic approach is a four-drug regimen consisting of vincristine, actinomycin-D, cyclophosphamide, and Adriamycin (doxorubicin) (VACA). More recent modifications have included the substitution of ifosfamide for cyclophosphamide (VAIA) especially in higher risk patients (29).

Treatment is generally administered for 12 cycles (over 36 months), and usually precedes local management as implied already. Care must be taken to avoid sensitizing agents with RT, such as actinomycin-D and doxorubicin. With these approaches, 5-year survival ranges from 50% to 75%, depending on the risk category (29). The most common site of failure remains distant disease (29). Space limitations prohibit a more detailed account of the management of this interesting but vanishingly rare head and neck tumor.

MANAGEMENT OF LOCAL RECURRENCE AND METASTASIS

This important area is discussed in the context of local recurrence following definitive local management. In some situations, this may be associated with regional lymph node (rarely) or with distant metastasis. More commonly, the first manifestation of distant metastasis is disease confined to the lungs. In general, distant metastasis at presentation should be approached using similar principles.

Local Recurrence

GENERAL APPROACH

Appropriate treatment of an isolated local sarcoma recurrence can result in cure or prolonged disease-free survival, and the approach to management should be similar to that taken with a primary tumor. However, effective management is often complex and influenced by tumor location and extent, and any prior local therapy. We have outlined an approach to the evaluation and management of locally recurrent STS (Table 30.15) (144). Assessment must include knowledge of all prior surgery, including resection margins achieved as well as previous RT and chemotherapy. A biopsy is necessary both to confirm the diagnosis and to determine change in tumor character from the original lesion.

ADJUVANT "NAIVE" RECURRENCE

In patients with STS not previously treated with RT or chemotherapy, combined modality therapy should be used, especially because these can generally be administered safely. In STS, the potential for adjuvant chemotherapy to enhance local control may mean it could have a role in local salvage because it is improbable that it was used initially. In osteogenic sarcoma this should include consideration of induction chemotherapy as described earlier for primary tumors and additional RT should be considered if resection margins remain a concern. In the case of STS and chondrosarcoma, we would generally recommend preoperative RT because of the better opportunity to spare critical structures because there is limited opportunity for tissue sparing due to prior resection of tissues in addition to contamination by previous surgery. Adequate postoperative RT following further surgery would also be appropriate but more problematic.

RECURRENCE WITH PRIOR ADJUVANT THERAPY

For previously treated lesions, individualization is needed. Prior irradiated STSs and chondrosarcomas would generally undergo tumor bed implantation with brachytherapy catheters in conjunction with a wide local excision. If resection margins are closer than 1 cm, brachytherapy is administered 5 to 7 days after surgery. Osteosarcomas should undergo chemotherapy if this is still possible, bearing in mind prior treatment. This is followed by resection, and potentially additional RT should be considered if resection margins remain a concern because RT is unlikely to have been used at the initial management.

LOCAL RECURRENCE WITH METASTASIS

Concurrent metastases are occasionally identified with local relapse. Patients who recur with multiple symptomatic metastases after a short disease-free interval are best managed with palliative approaches. Aggressive surgical palliation is rarely indicated in this situation, but local excision of a small or superficial recurrence may delay or prevent the development of local complications. The occasional patient presenting with local recurrence and limited systemic disease may benefit from aggressive treatment, especially after a long disease-free interval. This should include local salvage according to the principles outlined above, in addition to consideration of metastasectomy as described below.

Metastatic Disease

SURGERY FOR METASTASES

Sarcomas of both bone and soft tissue show an unusual predilection for metastasis to the lung, including disease isolated to the chest at presentation or recurrence. In selected cases

TABLE 30.15 Schema for the Management of Locally Recurrent Sarcoma

Context of local recurrence	Recommended approach
No prior chemotherapy and/or radiotherapy	Consider combined approach with external beam radiotherapy; in osteogenic sarcoma consider induction chemotherapy with pathologic response assessment
Prior radiotherapy	Combined approach with brachytherapy
Critical structure involvement	Consider preoperative radiotherapy Ablative approach may need to be considered
In the presence of metastases	Multiple metastases—palliative treatment possibly including aggressive local treatment Few resectable metastases—local management as for nonmetastatic context with metastasectomy

Source: Modified from Catton C, Swallow CJ, O'Sullivan B. Approaches to local salvage of soft tissue sarcoma after primary site failure. *Semin Radiat Oncol* 1999;9:378–388.

pulmonary metastasectomy has the potential to be curative, although distant disease at other sites is unlikely to be cured, excepting soft tissue metastasis in liposarcoma. Treatment of metastatic bone disease is always palliative unless representing skip metastases arising in the same bone as the primary tumor (termed T3 disease in the TNM classification).

Unfortunately, there have been no randomized trials comparing pulmonary metastasectomy with other methods of management. Frost (145), in reviewing the literature, found 697 STS patients in a number of series. Few studies provided survival data beyond 5 years, and the survival curves had a steep slope with few patients surviving at 7 years. The median 5-year survival rate for all patients undergoing resection was 25%. The 5-year survival rates ranged from 15% to 35% for first-time pulmonary metastasectomy and from 12% to 52% for subsequent pulmonary resections. The most adverse features for outcome of pulmonary metastasectomy were (a) incomplete resection, (b) tumor doubling time exceeding 40 days, (c) more than four metastatic lesions, and (d) disease-free interval shorter than 12 months. A retrospective study of 255 STS patients at the EORTC also showed 5-year disease-free and overall survival figures of 35% and 38% (146). In osteosarcoma with only a few pulmonary metastases at presentation, the median survival postmetastasectomy at MSKCC was 20 months, with 11% surviving 60 months. A better outcome was correlated with age greater than 21 years, unilateral location of lung metastases, good histologic response to preoperative chemotherapy, and completeness of resection of metastases (147). The International Registry of Lung Metastases reported 5,206 patients with pulmonary metastases resection, 2,173 of whom had bone or STS. Patients with single metastases and long disease-free intervals were recognized as having better outcome (148).

CHEMOTHERAPY FOR METASTASES

Potentially adding chemotherapy to pulmonary metastasectomy represents an additional possibility either before or after surgery, but supportive data are unavailable. In STS, a randomized trial was attempted by the EORTC, with the Eastern Cooperative Oncology Group (ECOG) and the SSG. Three cycles of doxorubicin/ifosfamide were given before surgery, and a further two cycles after surgery in patients with objective response. Unfortunately, the trial was closed early because of poor accrual.

Advanced osteosarcoma remains difficult to treat, and chemotherapy alone does not appear to be curative for inoperable metastatic disease. There have been no controlled studies designed to demonstrate the benefit of chemotherapy at recurrence in terms of adding to salvage rates. Also, unlike the case for many STS cases, many osteosarcoma patients will already have been treated with active agents.

RECOMMENDATION FOR INDIVIDUAL PATIENTS WITH METASTASES

In the absence of additional data, and in view of the potential to salvage a modest number of patients, it is our policy to advise pulmonary metastasectomy in appropriate patients. Generally we choose patients with a long disease-free interval (preferably at least 2 years from initial treatment), relatively few lesion (more than four lesions is less likely to be successful), and where clear margins are likely to be obtained. Occasionally, postoperative RT is administered for microscopic residual disease in an accessible site using similar principles to those described for RT of primary lesions. Appropriate cases should be identifiable through regular surveillance chest imaging following prior treatment of the primary tumor. We also advise resection for bilateral as well as unilateral disease, recognizing that the latter is more likely to be favorable. Chemotherapy is not routinely used, although it should be considered in advanced disease especially if symptomatic in otherwise fit and usually young patients. Resection may be considered subsequently.

In practice, it is often beneficial to allow a period of observation once metastases have been detected prior to a surgical intervention. This is because additional initial subclinical metastases may manifest subsequently, thereby permitting selection of the more favorable cases that may benefit from resection. The thoracic surgeon must also determine whether a lateral thoracotomy approach should be chosen versus a median sternotomy because the latter provides the opportunity to examine both lungs for additional palpable lesions that may not have been detected by imaging.

ADDITIONAL CONSIDERATIONS IN HEAD AND NECK SARCOMA

Radiation-Induced Sarcomas

Radiation-induced sarcoma of the head and neck (RISHN) can develop in or immediately adjacent to the fields following RT with no apparent site of predilection. Not surprisingly, MFH appears to be one of the commonest subtypes (149). Fortunately, RISHN is rare but can comprise as many as 5% of head and neck sarcomas in a given institution (150). The latency from RT to the development of RISHN is long (median of 12 years), although it can be less than a year or up to 50 years (149,150). Although the prognosis is guarded, the literature suggests that a proportion of these patients can be cured (149). Because of this, Mark et al. (150) suggest that concern about RISHN should not be a major factor influencing treatment decisions in patients with cancer. Unfortunately, the incidence of RISHN is likely to increase due to progressive aging of the population combined with improved survival in head and neck cancer patients resulting from better treatment regimes.

Diagnosis and management is extremely challenging but should follow the principles outlined for the management of local recurrence in cases who have previously received RT. Thus surgery is the mainstay of treatment, with appropriate attention to cosmesis and function preservation where possible. This requires recognition of the challenges posed by the close proximity of tumor to important regional structures and the technical difficulties of operating in an irradiated area. Judicious use of RT, potentially with brachytherapy or highly conformed external beams, may add to the outcome of the individual case. Chemotherapy may also be considered as an adjuvant, given the potential that it may enhance local control in STS when other treatments cannot be applied as aggressively as needed, and it should certainly be considered for rhabdomyosarcoma and osteosarcoma. Because there is almost no prospect for prevention, a high index of suspicion assumes great importance in the outcome of patients with RISHN (149).

Specialized Radiotherapy Approaches

Sarcomas of the head and neck are particularly suited for RT management using the superior conformal avoidance characteristics of stereotactic RT, intensity modulated RT, and particle beam therapy. In some situations these techniques represent the only means of safely delivering high doses to tumors adjacent to critical and sensitive structures, including the brain, brainstem, retina, optic nerve, optic chiasm, and spinal cord. As mentioned earlier these approaches are particularly applicable for chondrosarcoma (Table 30.14), but are equally useful for other sarcomas in difficult locations.

PARTICLE BEAM

Cyclotrons and large research accelerators produce highly energetic beams of charged particles or ions. In therapy, such ions are arrested in tissue and deposit energy rapidly over a narrow and defined range to create the Bragg peak of energy deposition. Very sharp dose gradients are possible, and intense ionization tracks of the charged particles traversing tissues are extremely effective at inducing radiation injury. Particle beam therapy requires highly specialized facilities available only at a very few centers worldwide. Until recently this approach represented the only realistic method of adequately encompassing complex tumors at the skull base with high-dose RT. This has now changed with the introduction of IMRT and stereotactic fractionated RT.

INTENSITY MODULATED RADIOTHERAPY

Intensity modulated radiotherapy is a relatively recent RT technique that delivers photons with normal linear accelerators that are especially equipped to segment the radiation beams into multiple beamlets of potentially differing intensities. Intersecting beams can create composite dose distributions of convex and concave shape ("dose sculpting") and with very steep doses gradients, or with variable dose within the target as needed ("dose painting") that are not possible with conventional RT techniques. In addition to the unique planning problems posed by these lesions where high-dose sculpted RT targets are needed adjacent to critical anatomy, head and neck STSs are also of interest because lymph node irradiation is only rarely indicated. Thus there is an added opportunity for effective preservation of salivary function with less concern compared with other head and neck sites. Specific reports about IMRT for the treatment of head and neck sarcomas are awaited.

IMRT VERSUS PROTON BEAM FOR SKULL BASE SARCOMA

The relative unavailability of particle beam therapy makes it desirable to investigate other techniques. It remains to be determined whether high precision photon irradiation such as stereotactic fractionated RT or IMRT will provide similar outcomes compared with proton therapy. Our preliminary impression is that the approaches may be equivalent on the practical side, although regular protons or intensity modulated proton beams may have theoretical superiority in providing a more precise plan, with slightly sharper dose gradient and less scatter. The latter may be of benefit in younger patients, especially children, where the theoretical risk for late malignant induction (151) needs to be factored against the enormous benefit provided by having greater access to these techniques for many more patients.

RADIOLOGIC IMAGING CONCERNS

Bernard B. O'Malley and Suresh K. Mukherji

Almost every variety of sarcoma can arise in the head and neck region. These tumors, large or small, often arise in typical locations that help identify the pathology and define the full extent of disease (Figs. 30.15 through 30.19). As a result, we suggest that imaging precede any biopsy or intervention when a sarcoma is suspected. Given that size, location, and grade of sarcomas are the most important prognostic factors (155), imaging can provide two of these three characteristics. An accurate imaging diagnosis is more often made when tumors are bulky and arise from typical locations such as the masticator space or skull base, and are less often made when sarcomas and other mesenchymal masses arise in or between soft tissue spaces (Figs. 30.20 through 30.22). Given that the completeness of resection is the primary goal for improved prognosis (156,157), imaging can help guide the surgeon through a safe comprehensive procedure and the radiation oncologist in treatment portal planning.

From an imaging standpoint, the two most important pieces of information that need to be considered to arrive at an accurate preoperative diagnosis are the site of origin and the age of the patient. Rhabdomyosarcoma is the most common solid sarcoma arising in the neck in a child. Embryonal rhabdomyosarcomas are relatively homogeneous and nearly parallel to skeletal muscle in signal and density. Parameningeal and orbital rhabdosarcomas are usually treated with chemotherapy and radiation prior to or instead of definitive surgery. Osteosarcomas and chondrosarcomas should be considered for tumors that arise in the bony regions below the skull base or for skull base tumors that have an osteoid or chondroid matrix associated with a surrounding soft tissue mass. Osteosarcomas usually have signature appearance of a bone tumor (158), even when they arise in extraosseous compartments (Fig. 30.22). Chondrosarcomas display a disorganized array of small, often-incomplete rings of calcium (Fig. 30.23) (159). Despite their malignant cell type, they are usually well circumscribed and cause more erosion than destruction of surrounding bone structures (160). In adults, sarcomas typically arise in the head and neck in areas that have a high muscle density. This region is the masticator space. The most common tumor to arise within (not invade from an adjacent region) the masticator space is a sarcoma. In our experience, the most common head and neck sarcoma is malignant fibrous histiocytomas (Fig. 30.24). Less common sarcomas in adults that occur in this region are leiomyosarcoma, synovial cell sarcoma, and neurofibrosarcomas, arising from branches of the third division of the fifth cranial nerve (161). Synovial sarcomas tend to have a homogeneous and deceivingly well-circumscribed appearance (161).

Computed tomography and MRI have complementary roles, depending on the size and location of sarcomas. The degree and extent of bone involvement with the chondro-osseous series of tumors require CT imaging for accurate estimation of resection (162). The CT must be properly planned, and the data must be correctly processed (and printed) to highlight bone information. Further processing of "raw" CT scan data is necessary if three-dimensional renderings are anticipated (Fig. 30.21). Magnetic resonance imaging is most useful to estimate the border of a lesion when edema or tumor infiltration cannot be differentiated with CT. When an oncologic margin must be determined for surgery or treatment portals, MRI is more sensitive but less specific than is CT. Often, the images predict that the tumor is "at least as deep as" a certain tissue plane, and that appropriate use of frozen-section analysis at that site should be expected. When radiation is planned for the postoperative time frame the radiologist should assist in treatment planning according to the original extent of the tumor.

The role of angiography using MRI and CT for mapping of the vascular supply is currently under evaluation in peripheral sarcomas. The exact role of this technique has not been completely agreed on. Bolus techniques with contrast CT in combination with computer postprocessing allow CT to compete with MRI for evaluation of vascular margins. Magnetic resonance imaging and magnetic resonance angiography are more accurate, however, because of better tissue discrimination and background tissue subtraction. Simpler gradient echo and "time-of-flight" magnetic resonance angiography techniques are best performed precontrast and contain more troublesome artifacts. More time-consuming "phase-contrast" magnetic resonance angiography techniques can be performed regardless of contrast parameters and can provide directional flow information. Neither technique is accurate for differentiating high-grade subtotal stenosis from complete occlusion, however.

One must be cautious in reporting a mass lesion as a malignancy, even if it is reported to be biopsy-proved. The final diagnosis is founded on a combination of imaging, pathologic, clinical, and epidemiologic parameters. Malignant-appearing lesions may be benign or perhaps nonneoplastic (Fig. 30.25). Masses developing within treatment portals may reflect recurrent disease. When the appearance of the mass is atypical for, and dissimilar to, the appearance of the original primary tumor, and the enlarging mass arises approximately 10 years after the completion of high-dose therapy, a treatment-induced lesion must be considered (Figs. 30.24 and 30.26) (163).

Follow-up imaging after surgery for sarcomas should be postponed for 6 to 12 weeks to allow swelling to resolve. These scans must be designed to highlight the site of origin and the surrounding margins with appropriate use of fat suppression on MRI (Fig. 30.27). Contrast-enhanced MRI shows early enhancement of tumor more than fibrosis from chemotherapy and/or radiation (164). The presence of diffusely low signal on T2-weighted images suggests radiation fibrosis. This allows for earlier detection of recurrence, avoiding delay of reoperation or adjuvant therapy. As treatment at the primary site becomes more intensified with combined modality therapy, the frequency of systemic progression begins to approach that of local recurrence (165). Metabolic activity of most sarcomas correlates with grade of malignancy (166). Follow-up fluorodeoxyglucose (FDG)-PET scans are useful for confirming response of sarcoma to therapy (167). This makes the use of FDG-PET attractive, although not yet proven to alter patient survival.

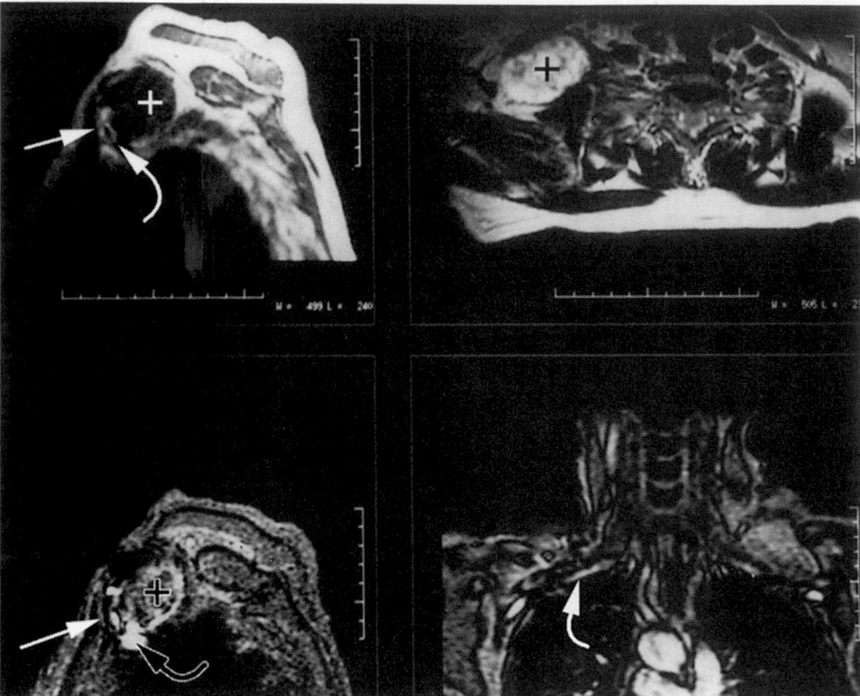

Figure 30.15 Neurofibrosarcoma. Clockwise from top left: Magnetic resonance imaging parasagittal T1, axial T2, coronal gradient echo, and parasagittal gradient echo, showing a well-circumscribed mass (+) within the right brachial plexus superior to the subclavian artery (*curved arrows*) and effaced vein (*arrows*).

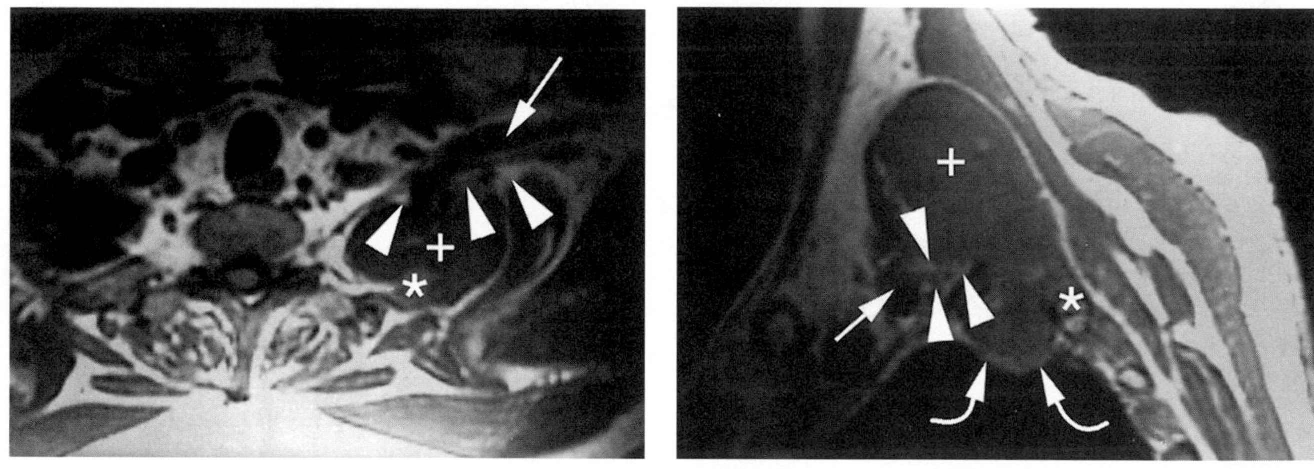

Figure 30.16 Sarcoma of scalene complex. T1 axial **(A)** and parasagittal **(B)** magnetic resonance imaging views of large mass arising within the left middle and posterior scalene muscle complex (+) as it inserts on the first and second posterior ribs (*asterisk*). Subclavian artery (*arrow*) is undisturbed, and the fibers of the brachial plexus are simply displaced (*arrowheads*). Note preserved pleural space excludes a pulmonary lesion (*curved arrows*).

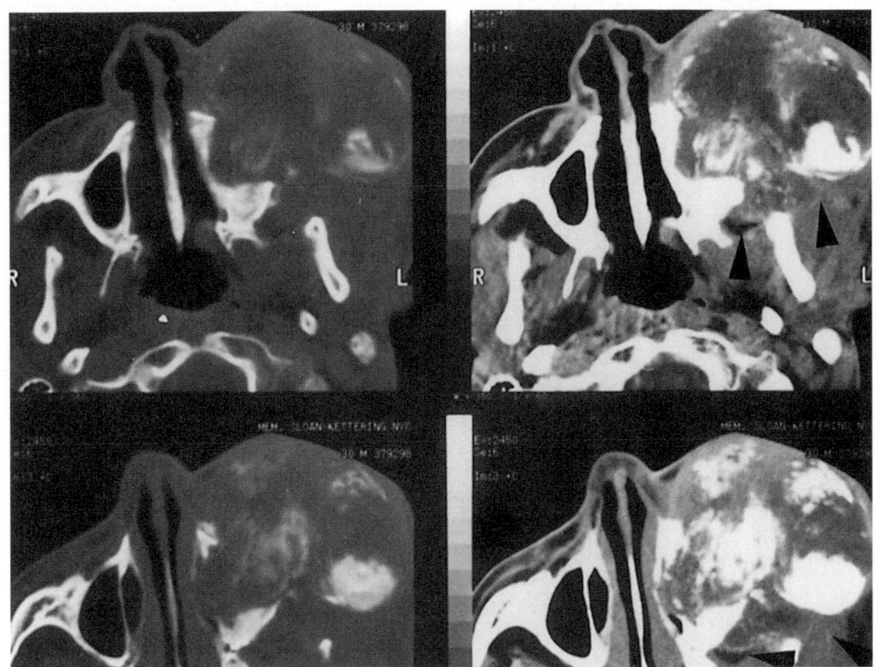

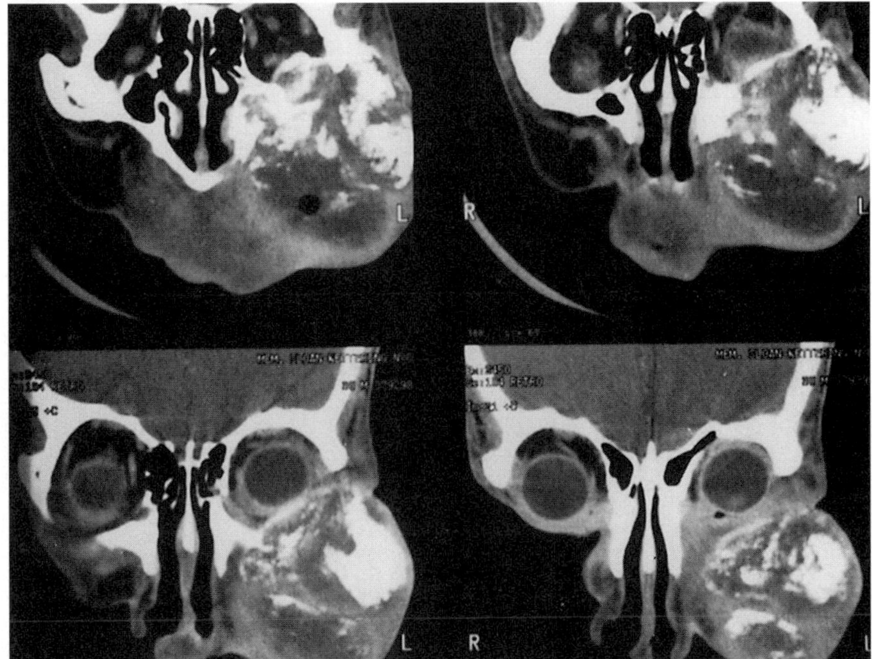

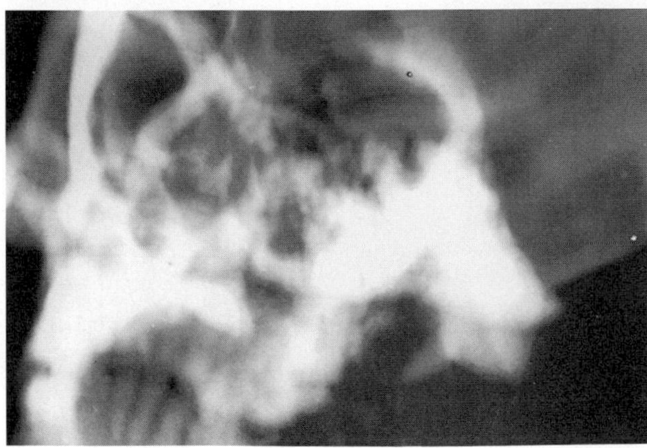

Figure 30.17 Huge osteosarcoma of maxilla. **A:** Enhanced axial view (bone and soft tissue windows). **B:** Direct coronal view. **C:** Three-dimensional rendering. Shown is a large complex lesion with "tumor bone" formation arising from lateral maxilla, with limited involvement of deep facial spaces (*arrowheads*) and lower orbit despite its size. Oblique radiographic-type three-dimensional rendering shows "blow-out" appearance of left maxilla and tumor bone at junction with zygoma.

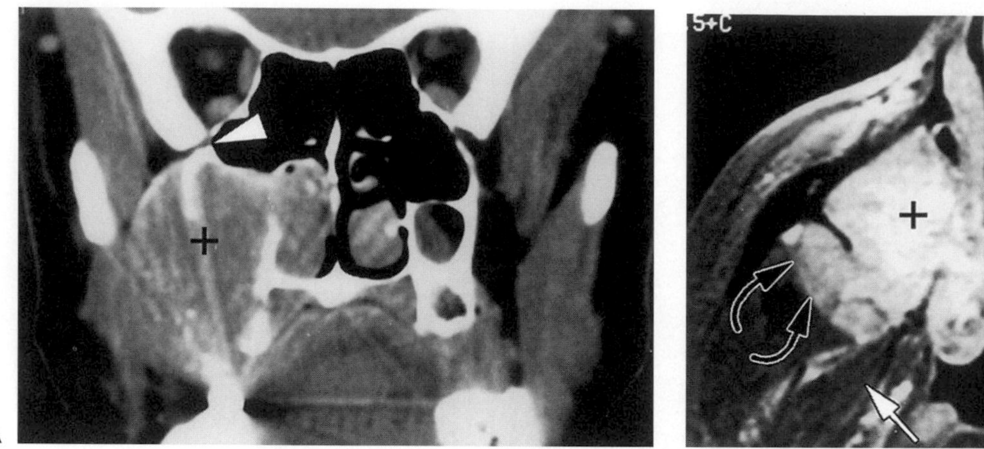

Figure 30.18 Osteosarcoma of lower maxilla. Enhanced direct coronal computed tomography **(A)** and fat-suppressed enhanced axial T1 magnetic resonance image **(B)** show well-defined upper margin of homogeneous lesion (+) approaching but not invading the inferior orbital fissure (*arrowhead*). Magnetic resonance imaging better discriminates the posterior margin, with the masticator space displacing the temporalis (*curved arrows*) but not disturbing the lateral pterygoid (*arrow*).

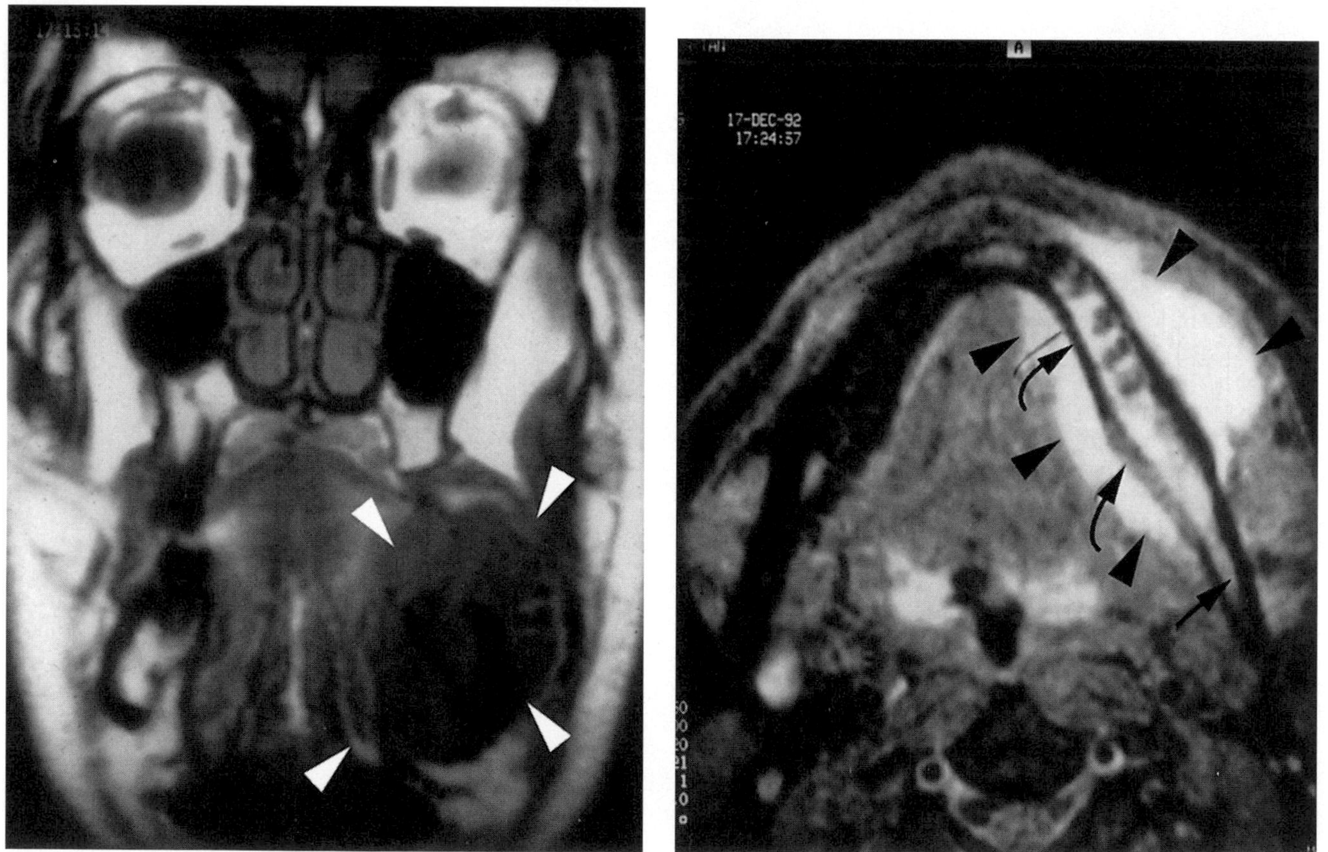

Figure 30.19 Osteosarcoma of the mandible. Direct coronal T1 **(A)** and axial fat-suppressed T2-type **(B)** magnetic resonance images show a permeative lesion expanding in all directions from body of left mandible (*arrowheads*). Note signal abnormality tracking proximally along angle of jaw (*arrow*) and apparent integrity of bone cortex (*curved arrows*).

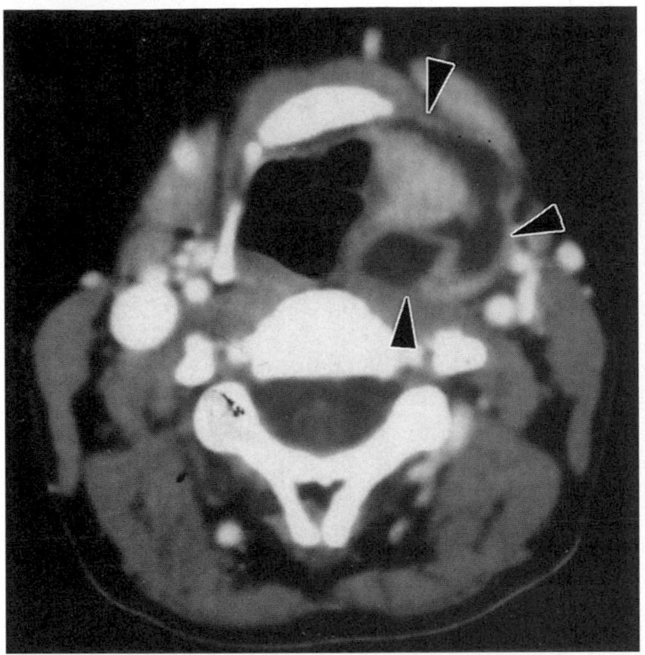

Figure 30.20 Synovial sarcoma. Enhanced axial computed tomographic scan through hyoid level shows complex heterogeneously enhancing mass of the supraglottic larynx (*arrowheads*).

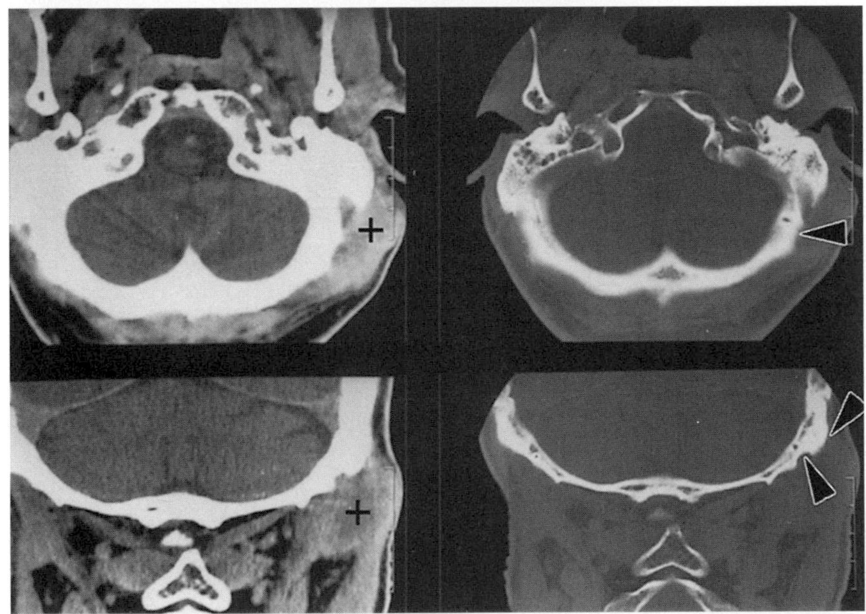

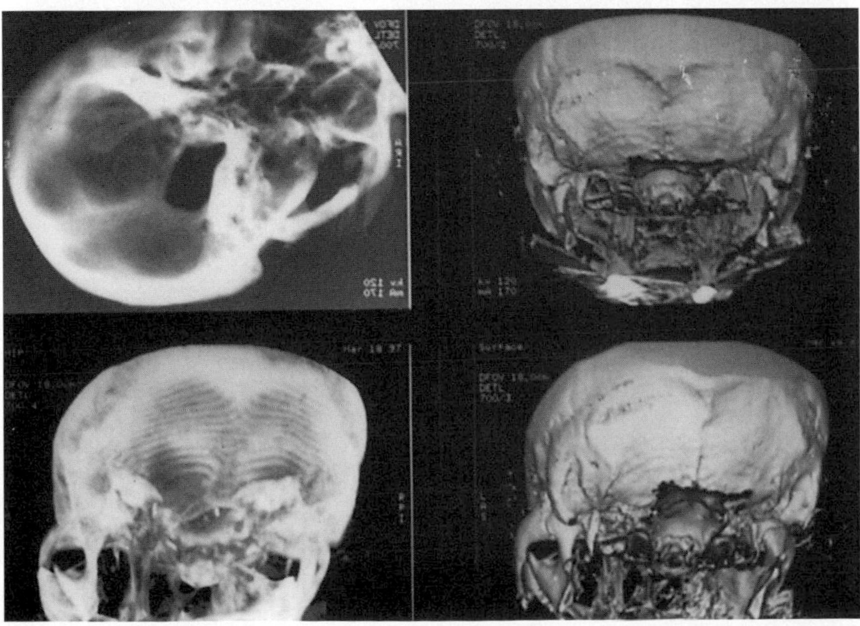

Figure 30.21 **A:** Sarcoma of submastoid region. Enhanced axial (*top panel*) and direct coronal (*bottom panel*) computed tomography soft tissue (*left*) and bone windows (*right*) show heterogeneous mass (+) with no bone destruction or intracranial extension. **B:** The apparent irregularity of the outer table (*arrowheads* in **A**) had no corresponding abnormality on the three-dimensional surface renderings (*right panels*) or radiographic style renderings (*left panels*).

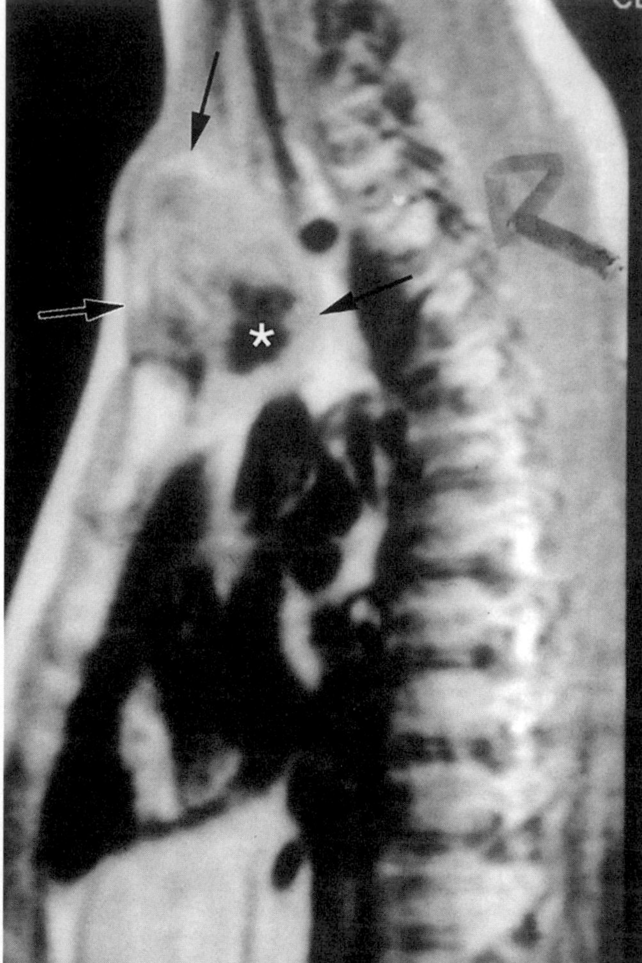

Figure 30.22 Extraosseous osteosarcoma. Axial T2 (A) and parasagittal T1 (B) magnetic resonance imaging of a complex mass within the right supraclavicular fossa (*arrows*), with extreme low signal related to tumor bone (*asterisk*).

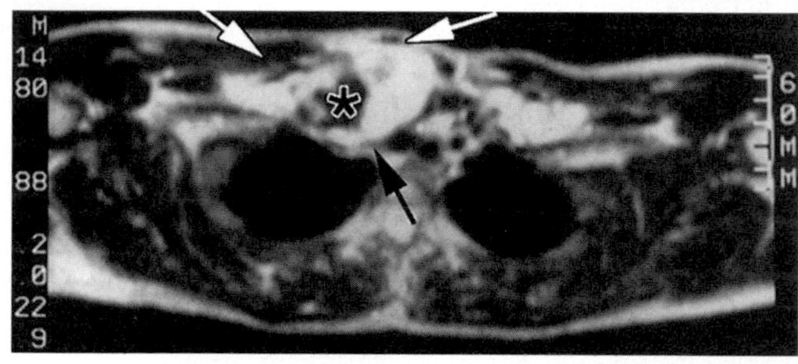
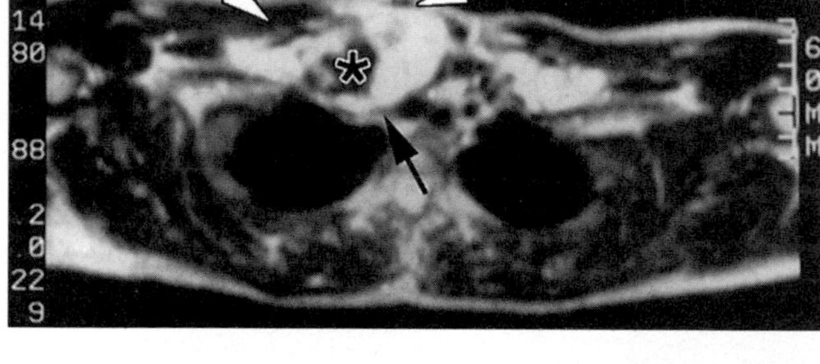

A B

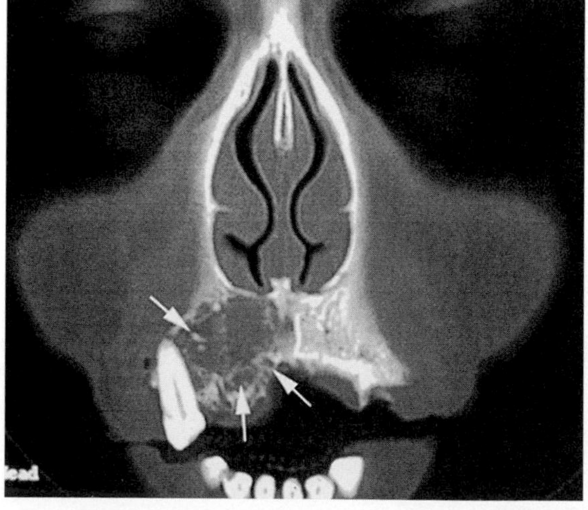

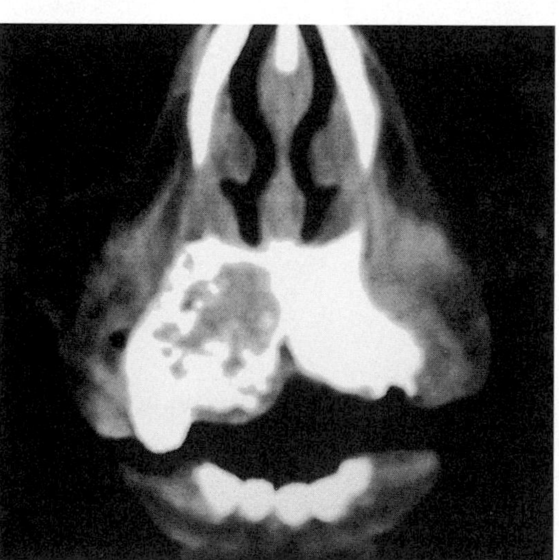

A B

Figure 30.23 Chondrosarcoma of the maxilla. **A:** Direct coronal computed tomography bone window of the maxilla shows an expansile lesion arising in bone showing a pattern of arcs and rings (*arrows*). **B:** Same image at soft tissue window shows no specific pattern of bone destruction.

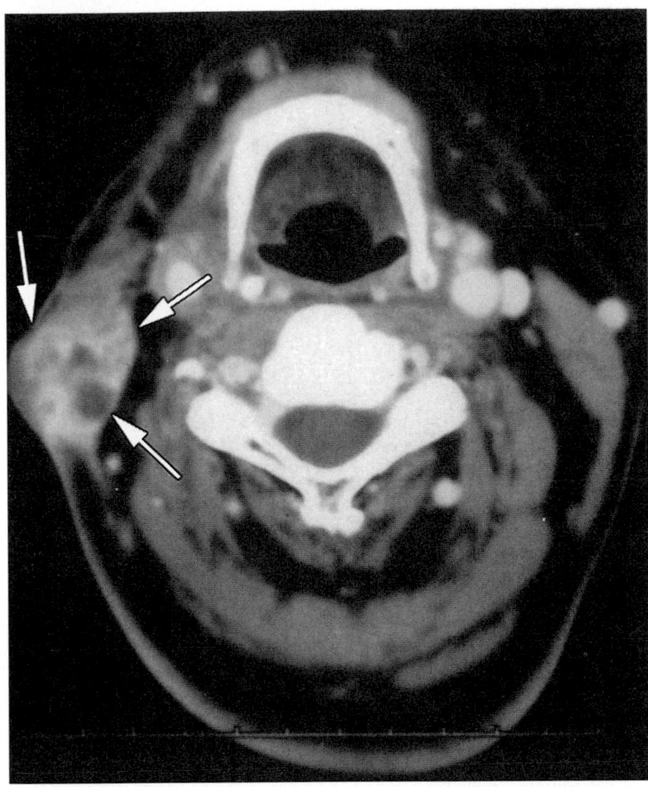

Figure 30.24 Treatment-related sarcoma. Enhanced axial computed tomography of the midneck shows a heterogeneously enhancing mass (*arrows*) that developed within the irradiated field several years after nasopharynx cancer. Neck dissection yielded malignant fibrous histiocytoma.

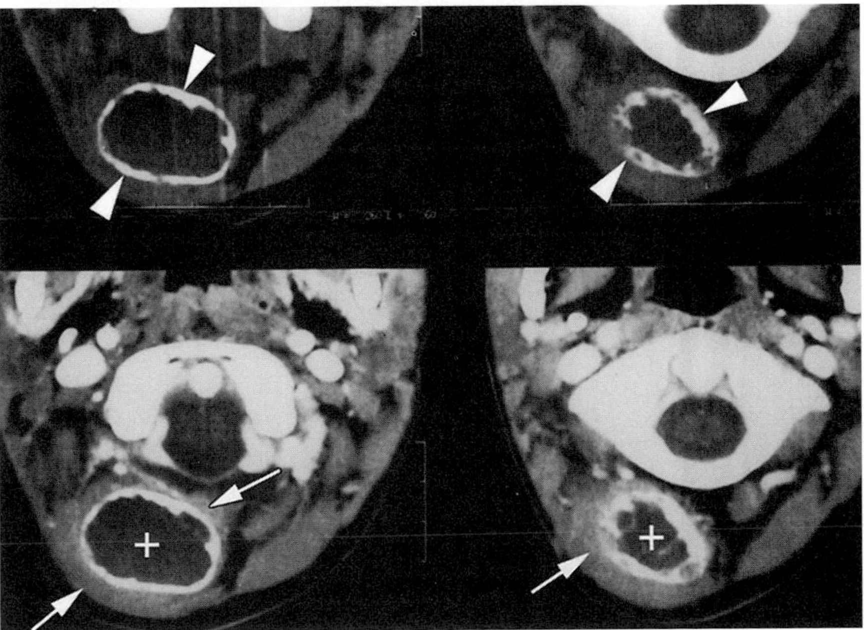

Figure 30.25 Pseudosarcoma. Axial precontrast (*top*) and enhanced views show a complex mass within the right trapezius, with a calcified margin (*arrowheads*), enhancing periphery (*arrows*), and nonenhancing center (+). *En bloc* resection yielded myositis ossificans.

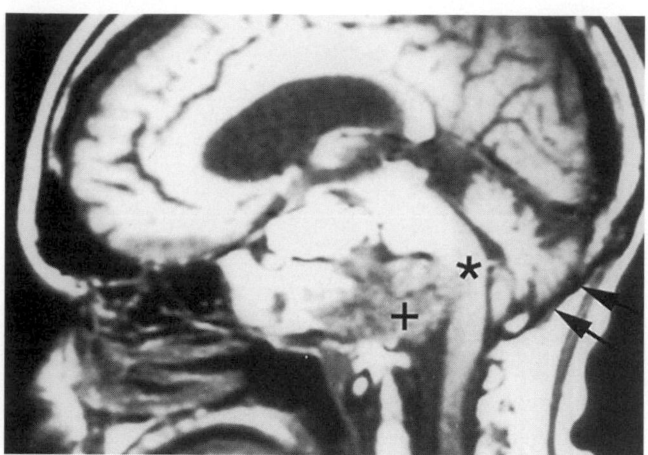

Figure 30.26 Osteogenic sarcoma. Midline sagittal magnetic resonance imaging of the head shows a complex exophytic lesion (+) expanding out of the clivus, compressing the lower brainstem (*asterisk*). The lesion developed several years after cranial irradiation for a cerebellar tumor. Note prior craniectomy behind atrophic cerebellum (*arrows*).

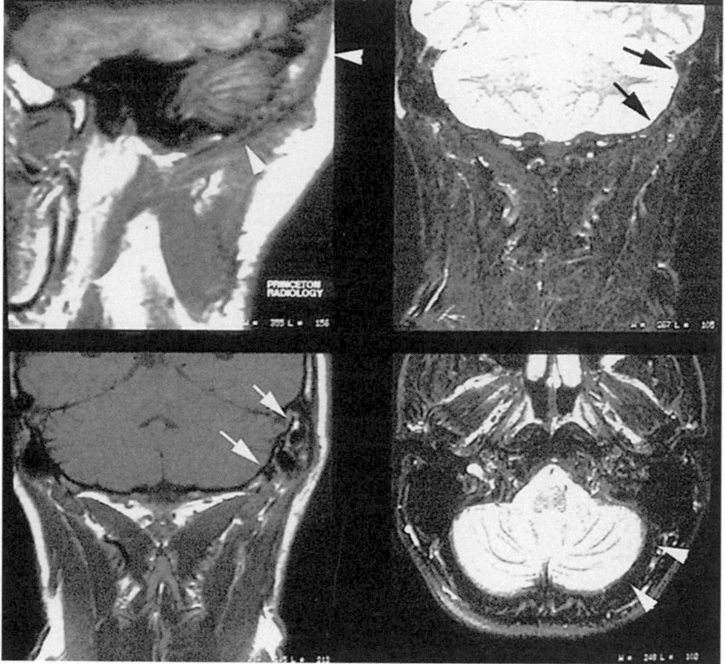

Figure 30.27 Osteogenic sarcoma follow-up. Magnetic resonance images (clockwise from top left) include sagittal T1, coronal T2, axial T2, and coronal T1 showing osteoplastic flap status post–segmental craniectomy (*arrowheads*) with no recurrence on the dural margin (*arrows*). Fat suppression on the T2 series eliminates bright signal from marrow, which could obscure tumor recurrence.

REFERENCES

1. O'Sullivan B, Bell RS, Bramwell VHC. Sarcomas of the soft tissues. In: Souhami RL, Tannock I, Hohenberger P, et al., eds. *Oxford textbook of oncology,* 2nd ed. Oxford: Oxford University Press, 2002:2495–2523.
2. Weiss SW, Sobin LH. *Histologic typing of soft tissue tumors,* 2nd ed. Berlin: Springer-Verlag, 1994.
3. Nielsen TO, West RB, Linn SC, et al. Molecular characterisation of soft tissue tumours: a gene expression study. *Lancet* 2002;359:1301–1307.
4. Dirix LY, van Oosterom AT. Gene-expression profiling to classify soft-tissue sarcomas. *Lancet* 2002;359:1263–1264.
5. Fletcher CD, Gustafson P, Rydholm A, et al. Clinicopathologic re-evaluation of 100 malignant fibrous histiocytomas: prognostic relevance of subclassification. *J Clin Oncol* 2001;19:3045–3050.
6. Maddox JC, Evans HL. Angiosarcoma of skin and soft tissue: a study of forty-four cases. *Cancer* 1981;48:1907–1921.
7. Yang JC, Rosenberg S, Glatstein E, et al. Sarcomas of soft tissue. In: DeVita VT, Hellman S, Rosenberg SA, eds. *Cancer: principles and practice of oncology.* Philadelphia: JB Lippincott, 1993:1436–1455.
8. Mark RJ, Tran LM, Sercarz J, et al. Angiosarcoma of the head and neck. The UCLA experience 1955 through 1990. *Arch Otolaryngol Head Neck Surg* 1993; 119:973–978.
9. Loudon JA, Billy ML, DeYoung BR, et al. Angiosarcoma of the mandible: a case report and review of the literature. *Oral Surg Oral Med Oral Pathol Oral Radiol Endod* 2000;89:471–476.
10. Wesche WA, Fletcher CD, Dias P, et al. Immunohistochemistry of MyoD1 in adult pleomorphic soft tissue sarcomas. *Am J Surg Pathol* 1995;19:261–269.
11. Frascella E, Toffolatti L, Rosolen A. Normal and rearranged PAX3 expression in human rhabdomyosarcoma. *Cancer Genet Cytogenet* 1998;102:104–109.
12. Barr FG, Chatten J, D'Cruz CM, et al. Molecular assays for chromosomal translocations in the diagnosis of pediatric soft tissue sarcomas. *JAMA* 1995;273:553–557.
13. Scrable H, Witte D, Shimada H, et al. Molecular differential pathology of rhabdomyosarcoma. *Genes Chromosomes Cancer* 1989;1:23–35.
14. Kelly KM, Womer RB, Sorensen PH, et al. Common and variant gene fusions predict distinct clinical phenotypes in rhabdomyosarcoma. *J Clin Oncol* 1997; 15:1831–1836.
15. Goulding M, Lumsden A, Paquette AJ. Regulation of Pax-3 expression in the dermomyotome and its role in muscle development. *Development* 1994;120: 957–971.
16. Awan RA, Dixon RH, Antonescu CR, et al. Patients with metastatic sarcoma arising from dermatofibrosarcoma protuberans (DFSP) may respond to imatinib (STI571, Gleevec). *Proc Am Soc Clin Oncol* 2002;21:1637.
17. Kawai A, Woodruff J, Healey JH, et al. SYT-SSX gene fusion as a determinant of morphology and prognosis in synovial sarcoma [see comments]. *N Engl J Med* 1998;338:153–160.
18. Trojani M, Contesso G, Coindre JM, et al. Soft-tissue sarcomas of adults; study of pathological prognostic variables and definition of a histopathological grading system. *Int J Cancer* 1984;33:37–42.
19. Costa J, Wesley RA, Glatstein E, The grading of soft tissue sarcomas. Results of a clinicohistopathologic correlation in a series of 163 cases. *Cancer* 1984;53: 530–541.
20. Guillou L, Coindre JM, Bonichon F, et al. Comparative study of the National Cancer Institute and French Federation of Cancer Centers Sarcoma Group grading systems in a population of 410 adult patients with soft tissue sarcoma. *J Clin Oncol* 1997;15:350–362.
21. Coindre JM, Trojani M, Contesso G, et al. Reproducibility of a histopathologic grading system for adult soft tissue sarcoma. *Cancer* 1986;58:306–309.
22. Alvegard TA, Berg NO. Histopathology peer review of high-grade soft tissue sarcoma: the Scandinavian Sarcoma Group experience. *J Clin Oncol* 1989;7: 1845–1851.
23. Sobin L, et al. *TNM classification of malignant tumours,* 6th ed. New York: Wiley-Liss, 2002.
24. Greene FL, Page D, Norrow M, et al. *AJCC cancer staging manual,* 6th ed. New York: Springer, 2002.
25. Schajowicz F, Sissons HA, Sobin L. The World Health Organization's histologic classification of bone tumors. A commentary on the second edition. *Cancer* 1995;75:1208–1214.
26. Koch BB, Karnell LH, Hoffman HT, et al. National cancer database report on chondrosarcoma of the head and neck. *Head Neck* 2000;22:408–425.
27. Pardo-Mindan FJ, Guillen FJ, Villas C, et al. A comparative ultrastructural study of chondrosarcoma, chordoid sarcoma, and chordoma. *Cancer* 1981;47: 2611–2619.
28. Kilpatrick SE, Inwards CY, Fletcher CD, et al. Myxoid chondrosarcoma (chordoid sarcoma) of bone: a report of two cases and review of the literature. *Cancer* 1997;79:1903–1910.
29. Paulussen M, Ahrens S, Dunst J, et al. Localized Ewing tumor of bone: final results of the cooperative Ewing's Sarcoma Study CESS 86. *J Clin Oncol* 2001; 19:1818–1829.
30. Cavazzana AO, Miser JS, Jefferson J, et al. Experimental evidence of neural origin of Ewing's sarcoma of bone. *Am J Pathol* 1987;127:508–518.
31. Womer RB. The cellular biology of bone tumours. *Clin Orthop* 1991;262:12–21.
32. Zoubek A, Dockhorn-Dworniczak B, Delattre O, et al. Does expression of different EWS chimeric transcripts define clinically distinct risk groups of Ewing tumor patients? *J Clin Oncol* 1996;14:1245–1251.
33. Ruymann FB, Grovas AC. Progress in the diagnosis and treatment of rhabdomyosarcoma and related soft tissue sarcomas. *Cancer Invest* 2000;18: 223–241.
34. Holden C, Spittle M, Jones E. Angiosarcomas of the face and scalp: prognosis and treatment. *Cancer* 1987;59:1046.
35. Pollack IF, Mulvihill JJ. Neurofibromatosis 1 and 2. *Brain Pathol* 1997;7: 823–836.
36. Barker D, Wright E, Nguyen K, et al. Gene for von Recklinghausen neurofibromatosis is in the pericentromeric region of chromosome 17. *Science* 1987; 236:1100–1102.
37. Fountain JW, Wallace MR, Bruce MA, et al. Physical mapping of a translocation breakpoint in neurofibromatosis. *Science* 1989;244:1085–1087.
38. Menon AG, Anderson KM, Riccardi VM, et al. Chromosome 17p deletions and p53 gene mutations associated with the formation of malignant neurofibrosarcomas in von Recklinghausen neurofibromatosis. *Proc Natl Acad Sci USA* 1990;87:5435–5439.
39. Sagerman RH, Cassady JR, Tretter P, et al. Radiation induced neoplasia following external beam therapy for children with retinoblastoma. *Am J Roentgenol Radium Ther Nucl Med* 1969;105:529–535.
40. Garrington GE, Scofield HH, Cornyn J, et al. Osteosarcoma of the jaws. Analysis of 56 cases. *Cancer* 1967;20:377–391.
41. Gardner GM, Steiniger JR. Family cancer syndrome: a study of the kindred of a man with osteogenic sarcoma of the mandible. *Laryngoscope* 1990;100: 1259–1263.
42. Tachibana E, Saito K, Takahashi M, et al. Surgical treatment of a massive chondrosarcoma in the skull base associated with Maffucci's syndrome: a case report. *Surg Neurol* 2000;54:165–169; discussion 169–170.
43. Noria S, Davis A, Kandel R, et al. Residual disease following unplanned excision of soft tissue sarcoma of an extremity. *J Bone Joint Surg Am* 1996;78: 650–655.
44. Davis AM, Kandel RA, Wunder JS, et al. The impact of residual disease on local recurrence in patients treated by initial unplanned resection for soft tissue sarcoma of the extremity. *J Surg Oncol* 1997;66:81–87.
45. Mankin HJ, Mankin CJ, Simon MA. The hazards of the biopsy, revisited. Members of the Musculoskeletal Tumor Society [see comments]. *J Bone Joint Surg* 1996;78A:656–663.
46. Panicek DM, Gatsonis C, Rosenthal DI, et al. CT and MR imaging in the local staging of primary malignant musculoskeletal neoplasms: report of the Radiology Diagnostic Oncology Group. *Radiology* 1997;202:237–246.
47. Austin-Seymour M, Chen GT, Rosenman J, et al. Tumor and target delineation: current research and future challenges. *Int J Radiat Oncol Biol Phys* 1995;33:1041–1052.
48. Kessler M, Pitluck S, Petti P, et al. Integration of multimodality imaging data for radiotherapy treatment planning. *Int J Radiat Oncol Biol Phys* 1991;21: 1653–1667.
49. Brennan MF, Alektiar K, Maki R. Sarcomas of soft tissue and bone. In: De Vita V, Hellman S, Rosenberg SA, eds. *Cancer: principles and practice of oncology,* 6th ed. Philadelphia: Lippincott Williams & Wilkins, 2001.
50. Stevens MCG. Malignant mesenchymal tumours of childhood. In: Souhami RL, Tannock I, Hohenberger P, et al., eds. *Oxford textbook of oncology,* 2nd ed. Oxford: Oxford University Press, 2002:2525–2538.
51. Heck RK, Stacy GS, Flaherty MJ, et al. Evaluation of the proposed new AJCC staging system for primary malignancies of bone. *Proc Muskuloskel Tumor Soc* 2002:44.
52. Pollock R, Karnell L, Menck H, et al. The National Cancer Data Base report on soft tissue sarcoma. *Cancer* 1996;78:2247–2257.
53. O'Sullivan B, Wylie J, Catton C, et al. The local management of soft tissue sarcoma. *Semin Radiat Oncol* 1999;9:328–348.
54. Patel SG, Shaha AR, Shah JP. Soft tissue sarcomas of the head and neck: an update. *Am J Otolaryngol* 2001;22:2–18.
55. Rosenberg SA, Tepper J, Glatstein E, et al. The treatment of soft-tissue sarcomas of the extremities: prospective randomized evaluations of (1) limb-sparing surgery plus radiation therapy compared with amputation and (2) the role of adjuvant chemotherapy. *Ann Surg* 1982;196:305–315.
56. Moskowitz AJ, Pauker SG. A decision analytic approach to limb-sparing treatment for adult soft tissue and osteogenic sarcoma. *Cancer Treat Symp* 1985;3:11–26.
57. Conclusion. National Institutes of Health Consensus Development Panel on limb-sparing treatment of adult soft tissue sarcomas and osteosarcomas. *Cancer Treat Symp* 1985;3:1–5.
58. Le Vay J, O'Sullivan B, Catton C, et al. Outcome and prognostic factors in soft tissue sarcoma in the adult. *Int J Radiat Oncol Biol Phys* 1993;27:1091–1099.
59. Tanabe KK, Pollock RE, Ellis LM, et al. Influence of surgical margins on outcome in patients with preoperatively irradiated extremity soft tissue sarcomas. *Cancer* 1994;73:1652–1659.
60. Sadoski C, Suit HD, Rosenberg A, et al. Preoperative radiation, surgical margins, and local control of extremity sarcomas of soft tissues. *J Surg Oncol* 1993; 52:223–230.
61. Le QT, Fu KK, Kroll S, et al. Prognostic factors in adult soft-tissue sarcomas of the head and neck. *Int J Radiat Oncol Biol Phys* 1997;37:975–984.
62. Bell RS, O'Sullivan B, Liu FF, et al. The surgical margin in soft-tissue sarcoma [see comments]. *J Bone Joint Surg* 1989;71A:370–375.
63. Wilson AN, Davis A, Bell RS, et al. Local control of soft tissue sarcoma of the extremity: the experience of a multidisciplinary sarcoma group with definitive surgery and radiotherapy. *Eur J Cancer* 1994;30A:746–751.
64. Gerrand CH, Wunder JS, Kandel RA, et al. Classification of positive margins

after resection of soft-tissue sarcoma of the limb predicts the risk of local recurrence. *J Bone Joint Surg* 2001;83B:1149–1155.
65. Rydholm A, Gustafson P, Rooser B, et al. Limb-sparing surgery without radiotherapy based on anatomic location of soft tissue sarcoma. *J Clin Oncol* 1991;9:1757–1765.
66. Karakousis C, Emrich L, Rao U, et al. Limb salvage in soft tissue sarcomas with selective combination of modalities. *Eur J Surg Oncol* 1991;17:71–80.
67. Geer RJ, Woodruff J, Casper ES, et al. Management of small soft-tissue sarcoma of the extremity in adults. *Arch Surg* 1992;127:1285–1289.
68. Baldini EH, Goldberg J, Jenner C, et al. Long-term outcomes after function-sparing surgery without radiotherapy for soft tissue sarcoma of the extremities and trunk. *J Clin Oncol* 1999;17:3252–3259.
69. Stotter A, Fallowfield M, Mott A, et al. Role of compartmental resection for soft tissue sarcoma of the limb and limb girdle. *Br J Surg* 1990;77:88–92.
70. Le Vay J, O'Sullivan B, Catton C, et al. An assessment of prognostic factors in soft-tissue sarcoma of the head and neck. *Arch Otolaryngol Head Neck Surg* 1994;120:981–986.
71. Ruka W, Taghian A, Gioioso D, et al. Comparison between the in vitro intrinsic radiation sensitivity of human soft tissue sarcoma and breast cancer cell lines. *J Surg Oncol* 1996;61:290–294.
72. Weichselbaum RR, Beckett MA, Simon MA, et al. In vitro radiobiological parameters of human sarcoma cell lines. *Int J Radiat Oncol Biol Phys* 1988;15: 937–942.
73. Pisters PW, Harrison LB, Leung DH, et al. Long-term results of a prospective randomized trial of adjuvant brachytherapy in soft tissue sarcoma. *J Clin Oncol* 1996;14:859–868.
74. Yang JC, Chang AE, Baker AR, et al. Randomized prospective study of the benefit of adjuvant radiation therapy in the treatment of soft tissue sarcomas of the extremity. *J Clin Oncol* 1998;16:197–203.
75. Farhood AI, Hajdu SI, Shiu MH, et al. Soft tissue sarcomas of the head and neck in adults. *Am J Surg* 1990;160:365–369.
76. Freedman AM, Reiman HM, Woods JE. Soft-tissue sarcomas of the head and neck. *Am J Surg* 1989;158:367–372.
77. McKenna WG, Barnes MM, Kinsella TJ, et al. Combined modality treatment of adult soft tissue sarcomas of the head and neck. *Int J Radiat Oncol Biol Phys* 1987;13:1127–1133.
78. Farr HW. Soft part sarcomas of the head and neck. *Semin Oncol* 1981;8: 185–189.
79. Sanroman JF, Alonso del Hoyo JR, Diaz FJ, et al. Sarcomas of the head and neck. *Br J Oral Maxillofac Surg* 1992;30:115–118.
80. Kraus DH, Dubner S, Harrison LB, et al. Prognostic factors for recurrence and survival in head and neck soft tissue sarcomas. *Cancer* 1994;74:697–702.
81. Eeles RA, Fisher C, A'Hern RP, et al. Head and neck sarcomas: prognostic factors and implications for treatment. *Br J Cancer* 1993;68:201–207.
82. Tran LM, Mark R, Meier R, et al. Sarcomas of the head and neck. *Cancer* 1992; 70:169–177.
83. Dudhat SB, Mistry RC, Varughese T, et al. Prognostic factors in head and neck soft tissue sarcomas. *Cancer* 2000;89:868–872.
84. O'Sullivan B, Gullane P, Irish J, et al. Preoperative radiotherapy for adult head and neck soft tissue sarcoma (sts): assessment of wound complication rates and cancer outcome in a prospective series. *Proceedings of the 5th International Conference on Head and Neck Cancer,* 2000:215.
85. Tyldesley S, Fryer K, Minchinton A, et al. Effects of debulking surgery on radiosensitivity, oxygen tension and kinetics in a mouse tumour model. *Clin Invest Med* 1997;20(4 (suppl):S83(abst).
86. O'Sullivan B, Davis A, Turcotte R, et al. Preoperative versus postoperative radiotherapy in soft-tissue sarcoma of the limbs: a randomized trial. *Lancet* 2002;359:2235–2241.
87. Pollack A, Zagars GK, Goswitz MS, et al. Preoperative vs. postoperative radiotherapy in the treatment of soft tissue sarcomas: a matter of presentation. *Int J Radiat Oncol Biol Phys* 1998;42:563–572.
88. Suit HD, Mankin HJ, Wood WC, et al. Preoperative, intraoperative, and postoperative radiation in the treatment of primary soft tissue sarcoma. *Cancer* 1985;55(11):2659–2667.
89. O'Sullivan B, Gullane P, Irish J, et al. Preoperative radiotherapy for adult head and neck soft tissue sarcoma (sts): assessment of wound complication rates and cancer outcome in a prospective series. *World J Surg (in press).*
90. Isacsson U, Hagberg H, Johansson KA, et al. Potential advantages of protons over conventional radiation beams for paraspinal tumours. *Radiother Oncol* 1997;45:63–70.
91. Manaster BJ. Musculoskeletal oncologic imaging. *Int J Radiat Oncol Biol Phys* 1991;21:1643–1651.
92. Sarcoma met-analysis collaboration. Adjuvant chemotherapy for localised resectable soft-tissue sarcoma of adults: meta-analysis of individual data. *Lancet* 1997;350:1647–1654.
93. Verweij J, Seyance C. The reason for confining the use of adjuvant chemotherapy in soft tissue sarcoma to the investigational setting. *Semin Radiat Oncol* 1999;9:352–359.
94. Benjamin RS. Evidence for using adjuvant chemotherapy as standard treatment of soft tissue sarcoma. *Semin Radiat Oncol* 1999;9:349–351.
95. Alvegard TA, Sigurdsson H, Mouridsen H, et al. Adjuvant chemotherapy with doxorubicin in high-grade soft tissue sarcoma: a randomized trial of the Scandinavian Sarcoma Group. *J Clin Oncol* 1989;7:1504–1513.
96. Bramwell V, Rouesse J, Steward W, et al. Adjuvant CYVADIC chemotherapy for adult soft tissue sarcoma—reduced local recurrence but no improvement in survival: a study of the European Organization for Research and Treatment of Cancer Soft Tissue and Bone Sarcoma Group. *J Clin Oncol* 1994;12: 1137–1149.
97. Omura GA, Blessing JA, Major F. Randomised trial of adjuvant Adriamycin in uterine sarcomas: a Gynecologic Oncology Group study. *J Clin Oncol* 1985; 3:1240–1245.
98. Wilson RE, Wood WC, Lerner HL, et al. Doxorubicin chemotherapy in the treatment of soft-tissue sarcoma. Combined results of two randomized trials. *Arch Surg* 1986;121:1354–1359.
99. Antman K, Ryan L, Borden E, et al. Pooled results from three randomized adjuvant studies of doxorubicin versus observation in soft tissue sarcoma: 10 year results and review of literature. In: *Adjuvant therapy of cancer.* Philadelphia: WB Saunders, 1990:529–543.
100. Baker LH. Adjuvant therapy for soft tissue sarcomas. In: Ryan BL Jr, ed. *Recent concepts in sarcoma treatment.* Dordecht: Kluwer Academic, 1988: 131–136.
101. Glenn J, Kinsella T, Glatstein E, et al. A randomized, prospective trial of adjuvant chemotherapy in adults with soft tissue sarcomas of the head and neck, breast, and trunk. *Cancer* 1985;55:1206–1214.
102. Ravaud A, Bui NB, Coindre JM, et al. Adjuvant chemotherapy with Cyvadic in high risk soft tissue sarcoma: a randomized prospective trial. In: *Adjuvant therapy of cancer.* Philadelphia: WB Saunders, 1990:556–566.
103. Frustaci S, Gherlinzoni F, De Paoli A, et al. Adjuvant chemotherapy for adult soft tissue sarcomas of the extremities and girdles: results of the Italian randomized cooperative trial. *J Clin Oncol* 2001;19:1238–1247.
104. Frustaci S, Gherlinzoni F, De Paoli A, et al. Preliminary results of an adjuvant randomized trial on high risk extremity soft tissue sarcomas (STS). The interim analysis. *Proc Am Soc Clin Oncol* 1997;16:496a.
105. Bramwell VH. Adjuvant chemotherapy for adult soft tissue sarcoma: Is there a standard of care? *J Clin Oncol* 2001;19:1235–1237.
106. Fata F, O'Reilly E, Ilson D, et al. Paclitaxel in the treatment of patients with angiosarcoma of the scalp or face. *Cancer* 1999;86:2034–2037.
107. Batsakis JG, Jacobs JB, Templeton AC. Hemangiopericytoma of the nasal cavity: electron-optic study and clinical correlations. *J Laryngol Otol* 1983;97: 361–368.
108. Hekkenberg RJ, Davidson J, Kapusta L, et al. hemangiopericytoma of the sinonasal tract. *J Otolaryngol* 1997;26:277–280.
109. Kowalski PJ, Paulino AFG. Proliferation index as a prognostic marker in hemangiopericytoma of the head and neck. *Head Neck* 2001;23:492–496.
110. Spillane AJ, A'Hern R, Judson IR, et al. Synovial sarcoma: a clinicopathologic, staging, and prognostic assessment. *J Clin Oncol* 2000;18:3794–3803.
111. Dezube BJ. Acquired immunodeficiency syndrome-related Kaposi's sarcoma: clinical features, staging, and treatment. *Semin Oncol* 2000;27:424–430.
112. Stelzer KJ, Griffin TW. A randomized prospective trial of radiation therapy for AIDS-associated Kaposi's sarcoma. *Int J Radiat Oncol Biol Phys* 1993;27: 1057–1061.
113. Suit H, Spiro I, Mankin HJ, et al. Radiation in management of patients with dermatofibrosarcoma protuberans. *J Clin Oncol* 1996;14:2365–2369.
114. Ballo MT, Zagars GK, Pisters P, et al. The role of radiation therapy in the management of dermatofibrosarcoma protuberans. *Int J Radiat Oncol Biol Phys* 1998;40:823–827.
115. Sun LM, Wang CJ, Huang CC, et al. Dermatofibrosarcoma protuberans: treatment results of 35 cases. *Radiother Oncol* 2000;57:175–181.
116. Catton CN, O'Sullivan B, Bell R, et al. Aggressive fibromatosis: optimisation of local management with a retrospective failure analysis. *Radiother Oncol* 1995;34:17–22.
117. Ballo MT, Zagars GK, Pollack A, et al. Desmoid tumor: prognostic factors and outcome after surgery, radiation therapy, or combined surgery and radiation therapy. *J Clin Oncol* 1999;17:158–167.
118. Pearlstone DB, Pisters PW, Bold RJ, et al. Patterns of recurrence in extremity liposarcoma: implications for staging and follow-up. *Cancer* 1999;85:85–92.
119. Antonescu CR, Elahi A, Healey JH, et al. Monoclonality of multifocal myxoid liposarcoma: confirmation by analysis of TLS-CHOP or EWS-CHOP rearrangements. *Clin Cancer Res* 2000;6:2788–2793.
120. La Quaglia MP, Heller G, Ghavimi F, et al. The effect of age at diagnosis on outcome in rhabdomyosarcoma. *Cancer* 1994;73:109–117.
121. Oda D, Bavisotto LM, Schmidt RA, et al. Head and neck osteosarcoma at the University of Washington. *Head Neck* 1997;19:513–523.
122. Kassir RR, Rassekh CH, Kinsella JB, et al. Osteosarcoma of the head and neck: meta-analysis of nonrandomized studies. *Laryngoscope* 1997;107:56–61.
123. Smeele LE, Kostense PJ, van der Waal I, et al. Effect of chemotherapy on survival of craniofacial osteosarcoma: a systematic review of 201 patients. *J Clin Oncol* 1997;15:363–367.
124. Mark RJ, Sercarz JA, Tran L, et al. Osteogenic sarcoma of the head and neck. The UCLA experience. *Arch Otolaryngol Head Neck Surg* 1991;117:761–766.
125. Ha PK, Eisele DW, Frassica FJ, et al. Osteosarcoma of the head and neck: a review of the Johns Hopkins experience. *Laryngoscope* 1999;109:964–969.
126. Link MP, Goorin AM, Miser AW, et al. The effect of adjuvant chemotherapy on relapse-free survival in patients with osteosarcoma of the extremity. *N Engl J Med* 1986;314:1600–1606.
127. Link MP, Goorin AM, Horowitz M, et al. Adjuvant chemotherapy of high-grade osteosarcoma of the extremity. Updated results of the Multi-Institutional Osteosarcoma Study. *Clin Orthop* 1991:8–14.
128. Souhami RL, Craft AW, Van der Eijken JW, et al. Randomised trial of two regimens of chemotherapy in operable osteosarcoma: a study of the European Osteosarcoma Intergroup. *Lancet* 1997;350:911–917.
129. Huvos AG, Rosen G, Marcove RC. Primary osteogenic sarcoma: pathologic

aspects in 20 patients after treatment with chemotherapy en bloc resection, and prosthetic bone replacement. *Arch Pathol Lab Med* 1977;101:14–18.
130. Smeele LE, Snow GB, van der Waal I. Osteosarcoma of the head and neck: meta-analysis of the nonrandomized studies. *Laryngoscope* 1998;108:946.
131. Mark RJ, Tran LM, Sercarz J, et al. Chondrosarcoma of the head and neck. The UCLA experience, 1955–1988. *Am J Clin Oncol* 1993;16:232–237.
132. Harwood AR, Krajbich JI, Fornasier VL. Mesenchymal chondrosarcoma: a report of 17 cases. *Clin Orthop* 1981:144–148.
133. Harwood AR, Krajbich JI, Fornasier VL. Radiotherapy of chondrosarcoma of bone. *Cancer* 1980;45:2769–2777.
134. McNaney D, Lindberg RD, Ayala AG, et al. Fifteen year radiotherapy experience with chondrosarcoma of bone. *Int J Radiat Oncol Biol Phys* 1982;8:187–190.
135. Krochak R, Harwood AR, Cummings BJ, et al. Results of radical radiation for chondrosarcoma of bone. *Radiother Oncol* 1983;1:109–115.
136. Finn DG, Goepfert H, Batsakis JG. Chondrosarcoma of the head and neck. *Laryngoscope* 1984;94(12 Pt 1):1539–1544.
137. Lewis JE, Olsen KD, Inwards CY. Cartilaginous tumors of the larynx: clinicopathologic review of 47 cases. *Ann Otol Rhinol Laryngol* 1997;106:94–100.
138. Kozelsky TF, Bonner JA, Foote RL, et al. Laryngeal chondrosarcomas: the Mayo Clinic experience. *J Surg Oncol* 1997;65:269–273.
139. Hug EB, Loredo LN, Slater JD, et al. Proton radiation therapy for chordomas and chondrosarcomas of the skull base. *J Neurosurg* 1999;91:432–439.
140. Noel G, Habrand JL, Mammar H, et al. Combination of photon and proton radiation therapy for chordomas and chondrosarcomas of the skull base: the Centre de Protontherapie D'Orsay experience. *Int J Radiat Oncol Biol Phys* 2001;51:392–398.
141. Debus J, Schulz-Ertner D, Schad L, et al. Stereotactic fractionated radiotherapy for chordomas and chondrosarcomas of the skull base. *Int J Radiat Oncol Biol Phys* 2000;47:591–596.
142. Paulussen M, Ahrens S, Lehnert M, et al. Second malignancies after Ewing tumor treatment in 690 patients from a cooperative German/Austrian/Dutch study. *Ann Oncol* 2001;12:1619–1630.
143. Razek A, Perez CA, Tefft M, et al. Intergroup Ewing's Sarcoma Study: local control related to radiation dose, volume, and site of primary lesion in Ewing's sarcoma. *Cancer* 1980;46:516–521.
144. Catton C, Swallow CJ, O'Sullivan B. Approaches to local salvage of soft tissue sarcoma after primary site failure. *Semin Radiat Oncol* 1999;9:378–388.
145. Frost DB. Pulmonary metastasectomy for soft tissue sarcomas: is it justified? *J Surg Oncol* 1995;59:110–115.
146. van Geel AN, Pastorino U, Jauch KW, et al. Surgical treatment of lung metastases: the European Organization for Research and Treatment of Cancer-Soft Tissue and Bone Sarcoma Group study of 255 patients. *Cancer* 1996;77:675–682.
147. Meyers PA, Heller G, Healey JH, et al. Osteogenic sarcoma with clinically detectable metastasis at initial presentation. *J Clin Oncol* 1993;11:449–453.
148. Friedel G, Pastorino U, Buyse M, et al. [Resection of lung metastases: long-term results and prognostic analysis based on 5206 cases—the International Registry of Lung Metastases]. *Zentralbl Chir* 1999;124:96–103.
149. Patel SG, See AC, Williamson PA, et al. Radiation induced sarcoma of the head and neck. *Head Neck* 1999;21:346–354.
150. Mark RJ, Bailet JW, Poen J, et al. Postirradiation sarcoma of the head and neck. *Cancer* 1993;72:887–893.
151. Verellen D, Vanhavere F. Risk assessment of radiation-induced malignancies based on whole-body equivalent dose estimates for IMRT treatment in the head and neck region. *Radiother Oncol* 1999;53:199–203.
152. Gay E, Sekhar LN, Rubinstein E, et al. Chordomas and chondrosarcomas of the cranial base: results and follow-up of 60 patients. *Neurosurgery* 1995;36:887–896; discussion 896–897.
153. Castro JR, Linstadt DE, Bahary JP, et al. Experience in charged particle irradiation of tumors of the skull base: 1977–1992. *Int J Radiat Oncol Biol Phys* 1994;29:647–655.
154. Munzenrider JE, Liebsch NJ. Proton therapy for tumors of the skull base. *Strahlenther Onkol* 1999;175(suppl 2):57–63.

Radiologic Imaging Concerns

155. Dudhat SB, Mistry RC, Varughese T, et al. Prognostic factors in head and neck soft tissue sarcomas. *Cancer* 2000;89:868–872.
156. Kowalski LP, San CI. Prognostic factors in head and neck soft tissue sarcomas: analysis of 128 cases. *J Surg Oncol* 1994;56:83–88.
157. Nasri S, Mark RJ, Sercarz JA, et al. Pediatric sarcomas of the head and neck other than rhabdomyosarcoma. *Am J Otolaryngol* 1995;16:165–171.
158. Varma DG, Ayala AG, Guo SQ, et al. MRI of extraskeletal osteosarcoma. *J Comput Assist Tomogr* 1993;17:414–417.
159. Wippold FJd, Smirniotopoulos JG, Moran CJ, et al. Chondrosarcoma of the larynx: CT features. *AJNR* 1993;14:453–459.
160. Lee YY, Van Tassel P. Craniofacial chondrosarcomas: imaging findings in 15 untreated cases. *AJNR* 1989;10:165–170.
161. Rangheard AS, Vanel D, Viala J, et al. Synovial sarcomas of the head and neck: CT and MR imaging findings of eight patients. *AJNR* 2001;22:851–857.
162. Mohammadi-Araghi H, Haery C. Fibro-osseous lesions of craniofacial bones. The role of imaging. *Radiol Clin North Am* 1993;31:121–134.
163. Pendlebury SC, Bilous M, Langlands AO. Sarcomas following radiation therapy for breast cancer: a report of three cases and a review of the literature. *Int J Radiat Oncol Biol Phys* 1995;31:405–410.
164. Zagdanski AM, Sigal R, Bosq J, et al. Factor analysis of medical image sequences in MR of head and neck tumors. *AJNR* 1994;15:1359–1368.
165. Kraus DH, Saenz NC, Gollamudi S, et al. Pediatric rhabdomyosarcoma of the head and neck. *Am J Surg* 1997;174:556–560.
166. Nieweg OE, Pruim J, van Ginkel RJ, et al. Fluorine-18-fluorodeoxyglucose PET imaging of soft-tissue sarcoma. *J Nucl Med* 1996;37:257–261.
167. Stokkel MP, Draisma A, Pauwels EK. Positron emission tomography with 2-[18F]-fluoro-2-deoxy-D-glucose in oncology. Part IIIb: Therapy response monitoring in colorectal and lung tumours, head and neck cancer, hepatocellular carcinoma and sarcoma. *J Cancer Res Clin Oncol* 2001;127:278–285.

CHAPTER 31

Cancer of the Orbit

Surgical Management

Gregg S. Gayre, Christopher M. DeBacker, and Jonathan J. Dutton

The eye, eyelids, ocular adnexa, and orbit are common sites for malignancies. These may arise primarily, extend secondarily from adjacent areas, or metastasize from distant sites. Malignant orbital tumors account for approximately 22% of all cases of orbital disease (1).

Early recognition and appropriate treatment are crucial to the ultimate preservation of periocular structure and visual function. Confusion with benign processes of congenital, inflammatory, or infectious origin frequently results in delayed diagnosis and increased morbidity. A high degree of clinical suspicion must be maintained, and such ancillary tests as radiography, ultrasonography, and tissue biopsy are essential.

SURGICAL ANATOMY

Eyelid

Together with the orbital rims and eyebrows, the eyelids function primarily to protect the eye. They act as a physical barrier to the outside environment and through both voluntary and involuntary movements shield the globe from foreign material and desiccation.

The eyelids form the thin outer covering of the orbital cavity. The upper eyelid merges with the eyebrow superiorly and the lower eyelid with the upper cheek inferiorly. Each eyelid is fixed to the medial and lateral orbital rims by the canthal tendons. The open interpalpebral fissure measures 7 to 11 mm vertically and 25 to 28 mm horizontally. The innermost lining of the eyelids, the palpebral conjunctiva, contacts the cornea and globe and is essential in maintaining the precorneal tear film. The caruncle is a small, fleshy mass in the medial canthus formed from specialized conjunctiva and exhibiting some features of skin.

The palpebral conjunctiva and eyelid skin merge at a mucocutaneous junction along the eyelid margin. A row of cilia emerges from the skin just anterior to this junction. Specialized sebaceous glands, known as *meibomian glands,* open along the posterior half of the eyelid margin and provide the lipid component to the tear film. Apocrine glands of Moll empty at the lid margin between the cilia, and the holocrine glands of Zeis are associated with cilia follicles.

The eyelids are best thought of as multilayered structures composed of parallel lamellae (Fig. 31.1). Anatomically, both the cutaneous and orbital structures comprise the eyelid, but physiologically the eyelid forms a single functional unit. Near the eyelid margin, the layers are (a) the eyelid skin, (b) subcutaneous areolar tissue, (c) orbicularis muscle, (d) postorbicularis areolar tissue, (e) tarsal plate, and (f) palpebral conjunctiva. At a distance of 15 mm from the upper eyelid margin, the tarsus is no longer present. Its anatomic location immediately behind the orbicularis muscles is occupied, from anterior to posterior, by

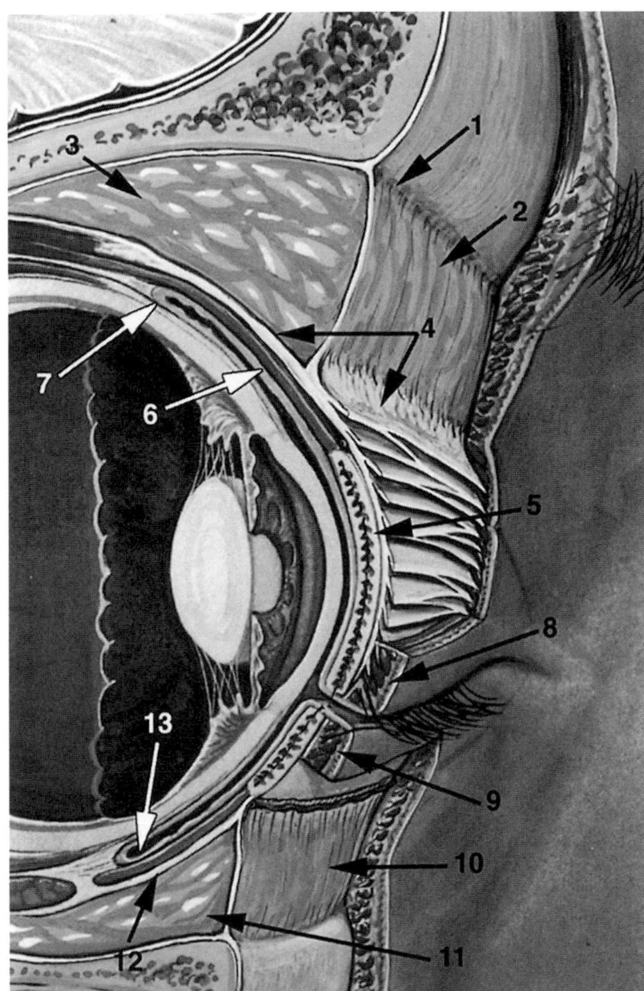

Figure 31.1 Layered sagittal cross-section through the eyelids showing the orbital septum and insertions of the levator aponeurosis. *1,* Arcus marginalis. *2,* Superior orbital septum. *3,* Preaponeurotic fat pad. *4,* Levator aponeurosis. *5,* Superior tarsal plate. *6,* Müller muscle. *7,* Superior conjunctival fornix. *8,* Superior pretarsal orbicularis muscle. *9,* Inferior pretarsal orbicularis muscle. *10,* Inferior orbital septum. *11,* Precapsulopalpebral fat pad. *12,* Capsulopalpebral fascia. *13,* Inferior conjunctival fornix. (From Dutton JJ. *Atlas of ophthalmic surgery: oculoplastic, lacrimal, and orbital surgery.* Vol 2. St. Louis: Mosby-Year Book, 1992, with permission.)

the orbital septum, preaponeurotic fat pad, the levator aponeurosis, and the sympathetic muscle of Müller.

The eyelid skin is the thinnest of the body. It is loosely attached to the underlying areolar tissue, except in its pretarsal portion and at the canthal angles. The orbicularis oculi muscle can be divided into three anatomically continuous portions (Fig. 31.2). The orbital portion originates at the medial orbital rim, fans out superiorly and inferiorly around the periphery of the orbit, and inserts near its origin at the medial orbital rim. The palpebral portion is confined to the mobile portion of the eyelids. It arises from the medial canthal tendon, arcs superiorly and inferiorly, and inserts along the lateral horizontal raphe and lateral canthal tendon. The palpebral portion is further subdivided into a pretarsal portion, overlying the anterior surface of the tarsal plates, and a preseptal portion, which overlies the orbital septum. The muscles of Riolan are delicate bands of short, striated muscle fibers along the lid margin, arising from the pretarsal orbicularis and inserting onto the tarsus. The main pretarsal orbicularis fibers pass laterally and medially into the

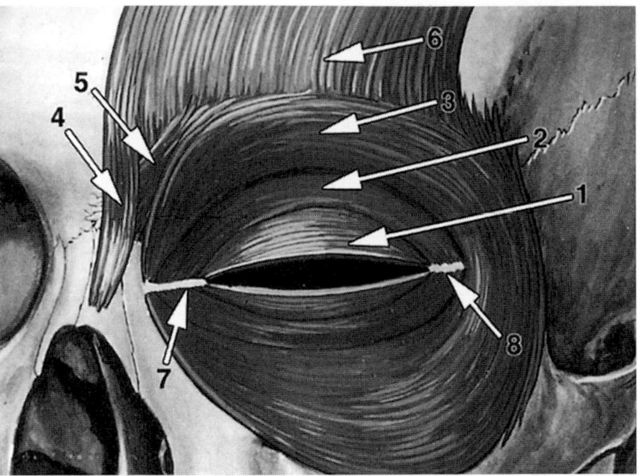

Figure 31.2 Eyelid and anterior periorbital muscular anatomy. *1,* Superior pretarsal orbicularis muscle. *2,* Superior preseptal orbicularis muscle. *3,* Superior orbital portion of orbicularis muscle. *4,* Procerus muscle. *5,* Corrugator muscle. *6,* Frontalis muscle. *7,* Anterior arm of medial canthal tendon. *8,* Lateral horizontal raphe. (From Dutton JJ. *Atlas of clinical and surgical orbital anatomy.* Philadelphia: WB Saunders, 1994, with permission.)

canthal tendons. The lateral canthal tendon inserts into the periosteum at the lateral orbital tubercle on the inner surface of the zygomatic bone. The medial canthal tendon inserts onto the periosteum of the frontal process of the maxillary bone just anterior to the anterior lacrimal crest. Small slips of orbicularis (called *Horner muscle*) pass from the deep medial portion of the pretarsal fibers and from the muscles of Riolan and insert into the periosteum of the posterior lacrimal crest. This structure contributes to the lacrimal pump system by shortening the canaliculus and compressing the lacrimal sac. The orbicularis muscle is innervated by the branches of cranial nerve VII, which run in the postorbicularis areolar plane.

The orbital septum originates along the orbital rim from the arcus marginalis, where the periosteum of the forehead and periorbita meet (Fig. 31.3). In Caucasians, the septum of the upper eyelid blends with the fibers of the levator aponeurosis 3

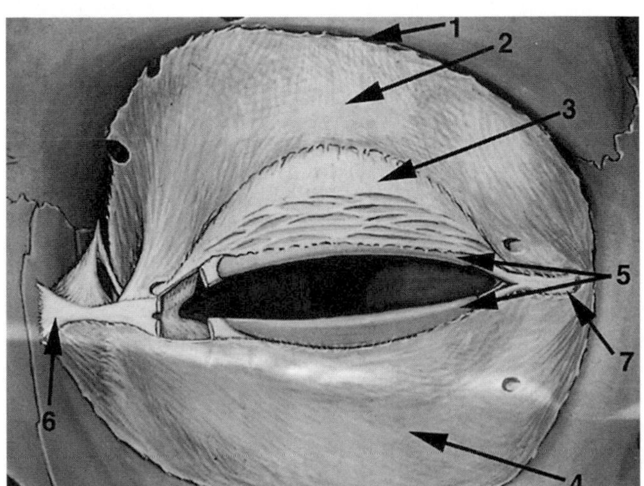

Figure 31.3 The orbital septum. *1,* Arcus marginalis. *2,* Superior orbital septum. *3,* Levator aponeurosis. *4,* Inferior orbital septum. *5,* Superior and inferior tarsal plates. *6,* Medial canthal tendon. *7,* Lateral canthal tendon. (From Dutton JJ. *Atlas of clinical and surgical orbital anatomy.* Philadelphia: WB Saunders, 1994, with permission.)

to 4 mm above the superior tarsal border; in Asians, this fusion occurs over the tarsus, closer to the eyelid margin. In the lower lid, the septum inserts onto the lower border of the tarsus in company with the lower lid retractors. Medially, the orbital septa of the upper and lower eyelids pass behind the lacrimal sac, where they blend with fibers of the medial canthal tendon before inserting onto the posterior lacrimal crest. Laterally, the septa of the upper and lower eyelids fuse and form the posterior layer of the lateral palpebral raphe. The orbital septum acts as a barrier to the spread of infection and hemorrhage and forms the anteriormost layer of the orbital space.

The preaponeurotic fat pad lies deep to the orbital septum. This represents a forward extension of the orbital extraconal fat pockets. In the upper eyelid, the fat pad immediately overlies the levator aponeurosis and is therefore a useful anatomic landmark during eyelid surgery. Weakness of the septum accounts for the herniated fat associated with baggy eyelids.

The levator palpebrae superioris muscle is the major retractor of the upper eyelid. It originates from the lesser wing of the sphenoid bone at the orbital apex, superior to the optic foramen and annulus of Zinn. As the muscle fibers approach the orbital rim, they pass into a fibrous aponeurosis that fans out horizontally into the upper eyelid. A thickened condensation of this layer (Whitnall superior suspensory ligament) extends horizontally across the upper orbit and helps to support the aponeurosis and associated fascial systems (Fig. 31.4). The aponeurosis inserts onto the anterior portion of the superior tarsus and into the sheaths of the overlying orbicularis muscle fascicles. These anterior muscular attachments unite the anterior and posterior lamellae and thus help to form the superior eyelid crease. The medial and lateral "horns" of the aponeurosis blend with the medial and lateral canthal tendons, respectively. The levator muscle receives its motor innervation from the superior division of cranial nerve III.

The capsulopalpebral fascia in the lower eyelid is the functional analog of the levator aponeurosis. It originates as a fibrous expansion from the Lockwood inferior suspensory ligament, uniting the capsules of the inferior rectus and the inferior oblique muscles, and inserts onto the inferior border of the tarsus. This mechanism allows retraction of the lower eyelid on downgaze.

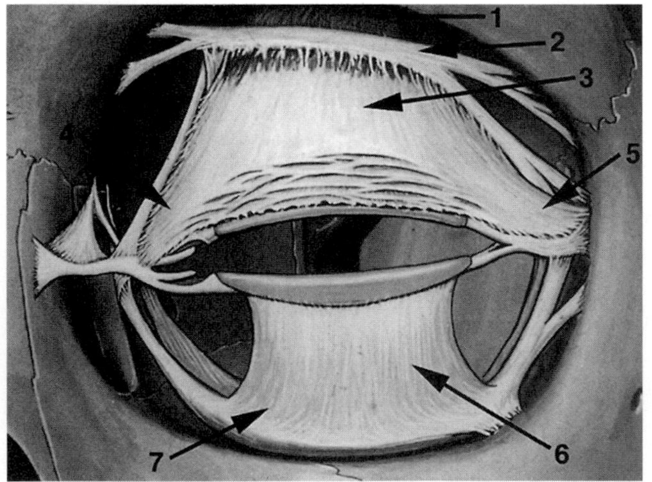

Figure 31.4 The levator aponeurosis and suspensory apparatus. *1,* Levator palpebrae superioris. *2,* Whitnall ligament. *3,* Levator aponeurosis. *4,* Medial horn of levator aponeurosis. *5,* Lateral horn of levator aponeurosis. *6,* Capsulopalpebral fascia. *7,* Lockwood ligament. (From Dutton JJ. *Atlas of clinical and surgical orbital anatomy.* Philadelphia: WB Saunders, 1994, with permission.)

The Müller muscle lies immediately posterior to the levator aponeurosis and just anterior to conjunctiva in the upper eyelid. It is a smooth muscle innervated by the sympathetic nervous system. It originates from the distal fibers of the levator palpebrae superioris muscle and from the posterior surface of the aponeurosis and inserts at the superior edge of the tarsal plate. The Müller muscle acts as an accessory retractor or perhaps as a co-tendon of the levator and contributes approximately 2 to 3 mm of lid elevation in the resting position. A similar, but less well-developed analog is present in the lower eyelid extending from the fascia of the inferior rectus muscle and inserting on the lower border of the tarsal plate. Sympathetic denervation of the Müller muscle results in Horner syndrome, characterized by mild ptosis of both upper and lower eyelids and associated with miosis and anhidrosis.

The tarsal plates are flat condensations of connective tissue that give support to the eyelids. Each plate contains 20 to 25 meibomian glands that contribute to the lipid component of the tear film.

The palpebral conjunctiva lines the posterior surface of each eyelid and is continuous across the superior and inferior fornices, with the bulbar conjunctiva lining the globe. It is a highly vascular mucous membrane containing numerous goblet cells that provide the mucous portion of the tear film. The accessory lacrimal glands of Krause and Wolfring are located in the conjunctiva as well and contribute to the aqueous portion of the tear film.

The vasculature of the eyelids is extensive. The medial superior and inferior palpebral arteries are branches of the nasofrontal artery that originates from the ophthalmic artery. They contribute to the arterial arcades that arch across the eyelids and join the lateral palpebral vessels derived from the lacrimal artery. Anastomotic branches also exist with the transverse facial and superficial temporal arteries (branches of the external carotid artery) and medially with the dorsal nasal and angular arteries.

Veins drain anterior to the tarsal plate into the angular, superficial temporal, and transverse facial veins. A deeper system from the posterior tarsus and conjunctiva drains posteriorly into tributaries of the ophthalmic vein.

Lymphatics drain from the lateral two thirds of the upper eyelid and lateral one third of the lower lid to the superficial parotid nodes. The nasal one third of the upper eyelid and nasal two thirds of the lower lid drain into the submandibular nodes.

Sensory innervation from the upper eyelid and forehead is carried in the supratrochlear and supraorbital nerves, with some contribution from the lacrimal and infratrochlear nerves. These transmit sensory information to the gasserian ganglion through the ophthalmic division of the trigeminal nerve. Sensory input from the lower eyelid is carried by the infraorbital branches of the maxillary division of the trigeminal nerve, with some contribution from the infratrochlear nerve.

Orbit

The orbits are pear-shaped cavities containing a complex array of structures subserving visual function (2). Seven bones contribute to its contour: frontal, maxillary, lacrimal, ethmoid, sphenoid, palatine, and zygomatic bones (Fig. 31.5). The inner surface of the orbit is lined by periorbita, a complex sheet composed of periosteum adjacent to the bones and several inner layers of connective tissue continuous with the orbital fascial systems. Periorbita is more firmly attached to underlying bone at the arcus marginalis along the orbital rim, at the lateral orbital tubercle, adjacent to the trochlea, around the optic fora-

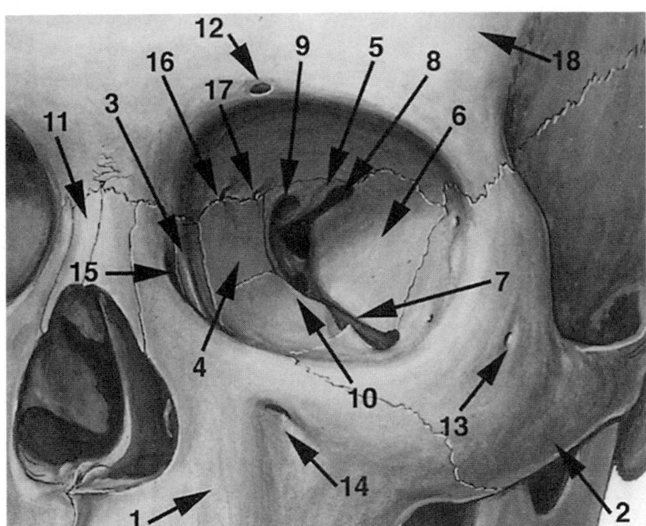

Figure 31.5 Orbital bones. *1,* Maxillary bone. *2,* Zygomatic bone. *3,* Lacrimal bone. *4,* Ethmoid bone. *5,* Lesser wing of the sphenoid. *6,* Greater wing of the sphenoid. *7,* Inferior orbital fissure. *8,* Superior orbital fissure. *9,* Optic canal. *10,* Foramen rotundum. *11,* Nasal bone. *12,* Supraorbital foramen. *13,* Zygomaticofacial foramen. *14,* Infraorbital foramen. *15,* Nasolacrimal sac fossa. *16,* Anterior ethmoidal foramen. *17,* Posterior ethmoidal foramen. *18,* Frontal bone. (From Dutton JJ. *Atlas of clinical and surgical orbital anatomy.* Philadelphia: WB Saunders, 1994, with permission.)

men, and along the superior and inferior orbital fissures. It is also fused to the dura covering the optic nerve.

The orbital roof is derived from the orbital plate of the frontal bone, with a contribution from the lesser wing of the sphenoid at the orbital apex. The roof is a thin structure separating the orbit from the frontal sinus anteriorly and from the anterior cranial fossa posteriorly. Defects may be seen in the roof with age-related dehiscence, and may be easily breached by expanding lesions of the orbit or anterior cranial compartment.

The frontal nerve and supraorbital artery run forward from the orbital apex immediately beneath the periorbita in the midline of the orbital roof. Care must be taken in opening the periorbita during superior orbital surgery to avoid injury to these structures.

Superomedially, the cartilaginous trochlea and adjacent periorbita are firmly attached to the orbital roof some 4 mm behind the orbital rim. If it is disinserted during medial orbital dissection, this layer must be reapproximated carefully to avoid superior oblique dysfunction.

The supraorbital notch lies at the junction of the medial one third and lateral two thirds of the superior orbital rim. It transmits the supraorbital vessels and nerve to the forehead. These structures are susceptible to damage during brow surgery.

The lateral wall of the orbit is derived from the orbital plate of the greater wing of the sphenoid bone posteriorly, and from the zygomatic and frontal bones anteriorly. It is bounded below by the inferior orbital fissure, and medially by the superior orbital fissure. The frontozygomatic suture line is important clinically because it is easily separated after cranial trauma. The anterior cranial fossa is situated just 1 cm above this suture line, and this is an important relationship to keep in mind when performing lateral orbital surgery. Inferiorly, the lateral rim passes into the zygomatic arch. The superior border of the arch is generally the limit of lateral wall bone removal in a lateral orbitotomy. Greater exposure may be obtained by removing the zygomatic arch; however, the structures of the inferior orbital fissure, which lies immediately medial to the arch, must be avoided.

As the orbital plate of the greater wing of the sphenoid passes back toward the apex, it is joined by the main body of the sphenoid and forms the anterior surface of the middle cranial fossa. In the removal of the more posterior portions of this wall during a lateral orbitotomy, the appearance of thick cancellous bone marks this junction and signals the imminent approach of dura. Bleeding from this bone is occasionally brisk but is easily controlled with bone wax. Low on the lateral wall, near the anterior end of the inferior orbital fissure, are the zygomaticotemporal and zygomaticofacial foramina that transmit branches of the zygomatic nerve and vessels to the temporal fossa and face, respectively. These vessels may be disrupted while elevating periorbita from the lateral wall, but this is of little consequence because of extensive anastomotic connections. More posterior in the greater wing of the sphenoid bone, at its junction with the frontal bone, is the Hyrtl canal, which transmits a branch of the middle meningeal artery into the orbit. Excessive posterior dissection of periorbita may transect this vessel, with subsequent brisk bleeding.

Lying horizontally along the middle of the lateral orbital wall immediately inside the periorbita is the lateral rectus muscle, and just above it are the lacrimal artery and nerve. Damage to these structures may result from careless opening of the periorbita during lateral orbital surgery.

The lateral orbital tubercle is a small bony prominence located just inside the lateral orbital rim, 10 mm below the frontozygomatic suture line. Attached here are the lateral canthal tendon, the lateral horn of the levator aponeurosis, the Lockwood ligament, and the tendinous check ligaments to the lateral rectus muscle sheath. These are reflected with the periorbita during lateral orbital approaches. Careful reapproximation of soft tissues to the bony rim is important to maintain normal anatomic relationships.

The orbital floor is formed primarily from the orbital plate of the maxillary bone, with small contributions from the zygomatic bone temporally and the palatine bone posteriorly. The infraorbital groove is a notch in the floor posteriorly. It runs anteriorly, becoming bridged over by a plate of bone, forming the infraorbital canal. This canal opens onto the cheek some 4 to 5 mm below the orbital rim. The infraorbital canal transmits the infraorbital artery and sensory nerve to the cheek and upper lip. Inferior orbital incisions should be made above this level to avoid transecting these structures. The maxillary sinus lies immediately below the floor and extends laterally from the maxilloethmoid suture to the inferior orbital fissure and posteriorly to the pterygopalatine fossa. The orbital floor is separated from the lateral wall by the inferior orbital fissure, which transmits the maxillary nerve and its zygomatic branch, ascending branches from the sphenopalatine ganglion, and the infraorbital branches of the internal maxillary artery.

The orbital apex lies posteriorly at the confluence of the four walls. It contains the optic canal and superior orbital fissure through which pass all the major neural and vascular elements entering the orbit from the middle cranial fossa. The relationship of these elements to one another is important in performing surgery for tumors or canal decompressions near the apex.

Just within the periorbita along the orbital floor lies the inferior rectus muscle. The inferior oblique muscle lies transversely in the anterior orbit between the periorbita and the inferior rectus, just inside the orbital rim, and is very easily injured during surgery along the orbital floor or during lower eyelid blepharoplasty.

The medial surface of the orbit is the thinnest of the orbital walls. The medial walls of the two orbits are parallel to each other and to the midsagittal plane. From front to back, the medial wall contains the frontal process of the maxillary bone, the lacrimal bone, the lamina papyracea of the ethmoid bone, and the body of the sphenoid bone. The lamina papyracea is extremely thin and separates the orbit from the ethmoid sinus air cells. It may be damaged during surgery by probing instruments and fingers and easily transmits infection and inflammation from the sinus into the orbit. In the posterior one third of the medial wall, within the frontoethmoid suture line, are the anterior and posterior ethmoidal foramina, which transmit branches of the ophthalmic artery into the nasal cavity. Rupture of these vessels after trauma results in subperiosteal hematoma. This may dissect backward to the optic canal, with subsequent optic nerve compression.

In the anterior medial orbit, between the anterior and posterior lacrimal crests, lies the lacrimal fossa containing the lacrimal drainage sac and upper duct. The medial canthal tendon attaches to the frontal process of the maxillary bone just in front of the anterior lacrimal crest. The Horner muscle is a specialized bundle of fibers originating medially from the deep head of the pretarsal orbicularis muscle. It passes posterior to the orbital septum and inserts onto the posterior lacrimal crest. This muscle compresses the lacrimal sac during eyelid closure, contributing to the tear pump mechanism.

The orbit can be divided into four conceptual surgical and physiologic spaces: the *subperiorbital* (or subperiosteal) space between orbital periosteum and orbital bones; the *peripheral* (or extraconal) space between the periorbita and the extraocular muscle cone; the *intraconal* space within the extraocular muscle cone; and the *episcleral* space lying between the Tenon capsule and the sclera of the globe. Various orbital lesions have a propensity for involving specific orbital spaces; therefore, tumor location can often be a significant factor in establishing a differential diagnosis. For example, sinus mucoceles, orbital abscesses from adjacent sinusitis, and metastatic neuroblastomas tend to involve the subperiorbital surgical space. Peripheral space lesions include lacrimal gland tumors, lymphomas, and dermoid cysts. The intraconal space is the preferred site of occurrence for cavernous hemangiomas, hemangiopericytomas, and tumors involving the optic nerve. The episcleral space is involved by contiguous spread of intraocular malignancies. Surgical spaces are not inviolate, however, and tumors frequently extend across a number of surgical planes.

The operative approach to any specific orbital lesion is determined primarily by the surgical space of primary involvement and the quadrant. Whether the tumor of interest is to be excised *en masse* or just subjected to biopsy is of importance in surgical decision making, as approaches for the two may differ. Exposure is a crucial element in orbital wall surgery and must be considered in surgical planning. Finally, consideration of the natural history of the untreated disease, the age and medical condition of the patient, and the surgical risks in management are of the utmost importance.

SURGICAL APPROACHES TO THE ORBIT

Anterior Approaches

The anterior region of the orbit can be approached through a number of different routes, depending on the surgical space of involvement and the nature of the pathologic process. Transcutaneous routes place incisions within preexisting skin creases or along natural cosmetic boundaries, such as the upper eyelid fold, the lower border of the brow, or immediately below the lower eyelid lash line.

The superior transcutaneous transseptal approach provides excellent access to the anterior superior extraconal space and yields excellent cosmetic results. The skin incision is placed along the upper eyelid fold, as for a blepharoplasty or ptosis repair (Fig. 31.6A). Beyond the entry to the suborbicularis fascial plane, the orbital septum can be identified and opened, revealing the superior extraconal fat pockets (Fig. 31.6B). Smaller lesions located within this compartment, including those of the lacrimal gland, can be biopsied or removed with little disruption of normal orbital structures. The orbital septum should not be closed, as shortening or scarring can lead to eyelid retraction and lagophthalmos. Care must be taken to avoid damage to the underlying levator aponeurosis. The grayish

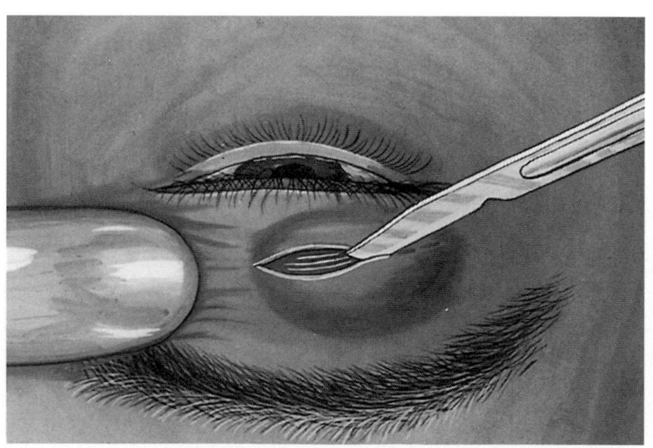
A

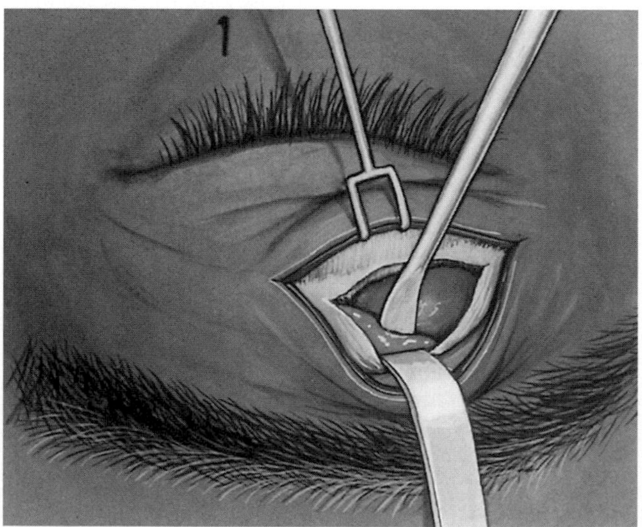

B

Figure 31.6 Transcutaneous, transseptal anterior orbitotomy. **A:** Surgical approach. Orientation as viewed by the surgeon from the patient's head. Skin incision through the upper eyelid crease overlying the lesion. Orbicularis muscle fibers are visible beneath skin. **B:** The septum has been opened, and the orbital fat is being retracted superiorly to expose the orbital tumor. (From Dutton JJ. *Atlas of ophthalmic surgery: oculoplastic, lacrimal, and orbital surgery.* Vol 2. St. Louis: Mosby-Year Book, 1992, with permission.)

orbital lobe of the lacrimal gland is located temporally and should not be confused with the more yellow preaponeurotic fat pads situated centrally and medially in the upper eyelid. Inadvertent excision of the lacrimal gland can result in a dry-eye syndrome.

The transcutaneous transperiosteal approach is similar except that dissection in the postorbicularis fascial plane is carried superiorly to the orbital rim. Here the periosteum is opened, and the dissection plane is extended over the rim into the subperiosteal orbital space for access to bony lesions involving the anterior orbital roof and rim. This eyelid crease incision avoids unsightly scars along the brow. Care must be taken to avoid damage to the supraorbital neurovascular bundle, the trochlea, and the superior oblique muscle tendon.

Transconjunctival routes to the anterior orbit are helpful in approaching tumors located in the anterior peripheral, intraconal, and episcleral surgical spaces, and they avoid any skin incisions. The conjunctiva is opened along the corneal limbus or more posteriorly, and the dissection is carried to the anterior Tenon capsule. This is opened 10 mm or more behind the limbus, to enter the anterior extraconal space. The intraconal compartment and optic nerve are accessible by disinserting one or more of the extraocular muscles. In the lower eyelid, a transconjunctival incision in the inferior fornix provides excellent access to the lower orbit and floor for blowout fracture repair or bony orbital decompression. Disinsertion of the inferior rectus muscle provides entry into the inferior intraconal compartment.

Medial Approach

Access to the medial orbit is somewhat hindered by the medial canthal tendon, nasolacrimal drainage apparatus, trochlea, and superior oblique muscle. In transcutaneous transperiosteal approaches to the medial orbit, as might be used for drainage of a subperiosteal hematoma or excision of an ethmoid mucocele, these structures can be reflected along with the periorbita. The skin incision is made 6 to 8 mm medial to the insertion of the medial canthal tendon (3). Branches of the angular vessels can generally be avoided by carrying the initial sharp dissection through skin only. Subsequent dissection is facilitated by bluntly separating underlying muscle fibers down to the periosteum.

An alternate medial orbital approach is through a transcaruncular conjunctival incision. This dissection enters the extraconal orbital space in a plane posterior to the nasolacrimal sac. Just behind the posterior lacrimal crest, the periorbita can be opened for access to the bony medial wall.

Tumors within the medial intraconal space are best approached transconjunctivally. A limbal incision is carried posteriorly in the sub-Tenon plane for access to the scleral surface and insertions of the medial rectus muscle. Disinsertion of the muscle provides limited exposure of the intraconal space adequate for biopsy or fenestration of the optic nerve sheath.

Lateral Approach

Lesions located within the lateral muscle cone, posterior to the equator of the globe, generally require a lateral orbitotomy approach. This procedure is also used for unencumbered access to the lacrimal gland. The skin incision is made in the sub-brow region and is extended temporally along the lateral orbital rim in an S-shaped fashion to follow the course of the frontozygomatic arch (Fig. 31.7A). It is carried out into a preexisting temporal laugh line. Alternatively, a horizontal incision is made, dividing the canthal angle, and is extended toward the temple for 2 to 3 cm, or an extension of the eyelid crease extension over the lateral orbital rim may be used. The periosteum is opened along the rim, and the temporalis muscle is reflected from its fossa for a distance of some 3 to 4 cm. The orbital periorbita is carefully elevated from the lateral orbital wall to expose the greater sphenoid wing. An oscillating saw is used to cut through the rim at the level of the frontozygomatic suture, parallel to the orbital roof, and again just above the zygomatic arch (Fig. 31.7B). The bony rim is then fractured outward and set aside for later replacement. The thin bone of the sphenoid wing is removed posteriorly with rongeurs to the point where cancellous bone is encountered. The periorbita then is opened carefully so as not to damage the lateral rectus muscle (Fig. 31.7C). After biopsy or removal of the lesion, the periorbita may be closed with interrupted 6-0 polyglactin sutures; however, not closing the periorbita, or intentionally leaving some gaping of the periorbita will serve to facilitate drainage of any blood from the orbit. The lateral orbital rim is then repositioned with polypropylene sutures passed through preplaced drill holes (Fig. 31.7D). Wire or metal plates are not necessary in most instances, and may interfere with future imaging studies. A low vacuum drain may be placed into the temporalis fossa and out a cutaneous puncture wound if necessary. The periosteum is then closed over the orbital rim with interrupted 4-0 polyglactin sutures, and the orbicularis muscle is reapproximated with interrupted 6-0 polyglactin suture. The skin incision is closed with interrupted vertical mattress sutures of 6-0 nylon or silk.

Operative and perioperative complications can usually be prevented by a keen understanding of the surgical anatomy of the lateral orbit. Adequate lighting with headlight illumination along with loupe magnification are mandatory in any deep orbital dissection. Traction on the lateral rectus muscle can lead to temporary paralysis and is best avoided by identifying the muscle from the outset and using broad malleable retractors rather than suture loops to displace the muscle. Any muscle weakness is usually temporary; persistence past 6 months can be repaired with strabismus surgery. Upper eyelid ptosis may also occur transiently after orbitotomy, either from edema or damage to the levator muscle. Again, this effect often resolves within the first weeks after surgery but, if persistent, may require ptosis surgery. Orbital hemorrhage can be a devastating sequel to orbital surgery, and meticulous hemostasis is critical before final closure. Compression of the optic nerve can lead to blindness if not remedied promptly. The patient should be instructed immediately to report any deep orbital pain, progressive proptosis, or decreased vision. Damage to the ciliary nerves in the deep orbit may lead to pupillary constrictor paralysis with a resultant dilated pupil. Recovery may be prolonged in these instances.

Transfrontal Craniotomy Approach

A transfrontal craniotomy approach to the orbit is necessary for all tumors occupying the superior posterior orbit and the region of the orbital apex. Once considered the procedure of choice for all orbital tumors, it is now used only in those cases not approachable by less invasive routes. After extradural exposure of the frontal bone, the orbital roof is removed, and the periorbita is opened. The frontal sinus and supraorbital nerve may be avoided by penetrating the roof more laterally. If necessary, the entire roof can be removed, providing broad access to the intraconal compartment, including nearly the entire length of the orbital optic nerve. The bony optic canal can be decompressed by unroofing it with rongeurs, leaving the dura intact. The intracranial optic nerve and chiasm are reached by opening the dura. Complications associated with the transfrontal approach to the orbit include meningitis, cere-

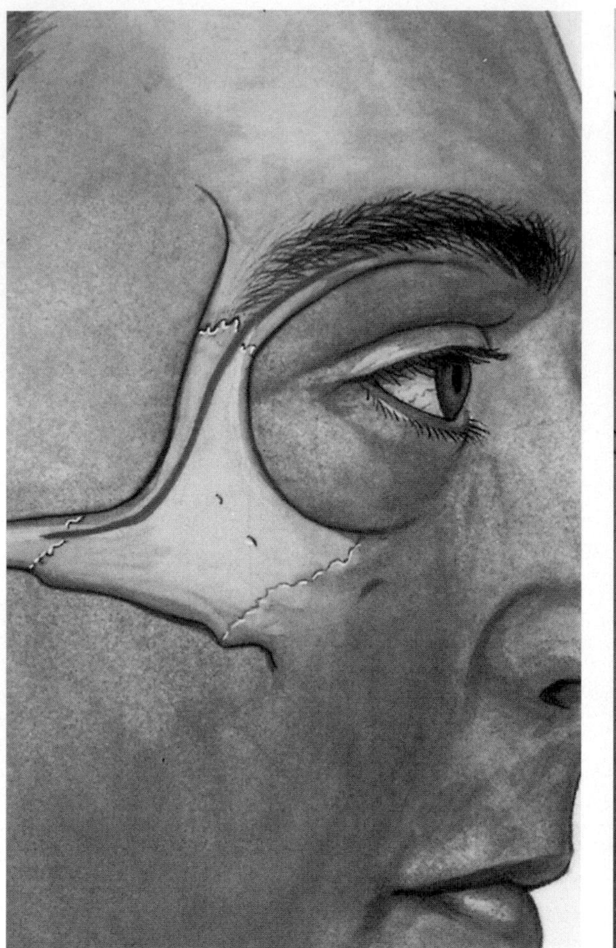

A

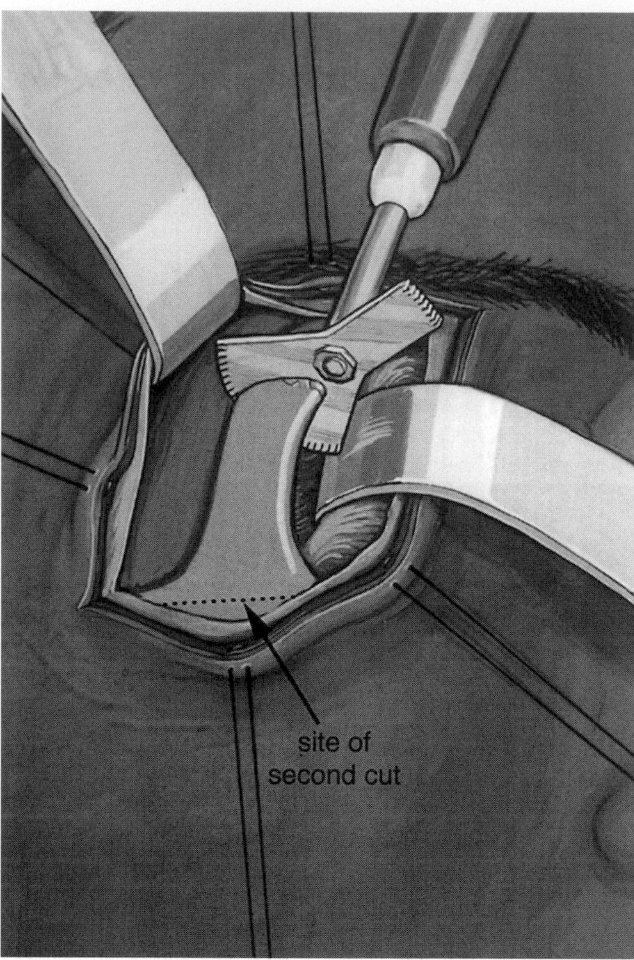

B

Figure 31.7 Lateral orbitotomy. **A:** Surgical approach. An S-shaped incision line is marked laterally from below the brow to the zygomatic arch. **B:** The skin, orbicularis muscle, and periosteum are opened, and the periosteum and temporalis muscle are reflected into the temporalis fossa. Malleable retractors protect the soft tissue as a cut is made with an oscillating saw at the level of the frontozygomatic suture line. A second cut then is made through the orbital rim just above the zygomatic arch (*dotted line*).

brospinal fluid leak, injury to orbital motor nerves, and optic nerve schemia.

Enucleation

Removal of the globe may be necessary for the management of primary intraocular malignancies and for the extirpation of malignancies involving the ocular surface. Choroidal malignant melanoma and retinoblastoma are the two most common intraocular tumors that often require enucleation. In recent years, however, more conservative methods have been advocated for the management of intraocular tumors. For instance, standard care of intraocular malignant melanoma may include observation of small dormant tumors and radiation therapy by iodine-131 episcleral plaques or external beam irradiation for larger lesions.

Under general or local anesthesia, the conjunctiva is opened for 360 degrees around the corneal limbus (Fig. 31.8A). Each rectus muscle is isolated with a muscle hook, and an absorbable 6-0 polyglactin suture is woven through the insertion (3). Each muscle is cut from the globe. Blunt dissection between the rectus muscles is performed to enter the sub-Tenon space. The globe is then rotated laterally by grasping the cut stump of the medial rectus muscle tendon, and the optic nerve is cut with scissors 3 to 4 mm from the globe (Fig. 31.8B). In cases of intraocular malignancy, some advocate a less manipulative technique in which the muscles are not hooked but simply cut from their insertions atraumatically. This approach prevents excessive pressure on the globe and the possible dissemination of malignant cells into the orbit or blood vessels. Hemostasis is obtained by packing and by direct cautery, and an orbital implant of choice is placed into the Tenon capsule (Fig. 31.8C). Meticulous closure of the Tenon capsule and conjunctiva is essential, using interrupted 5-0 polyglactin sutures and a running 6-0 plain suture, respectively (Fig. 31.8D). During the last few years, so-called integrated orbital implants, including coralline hydroxyapatite (Bio-eye®, Integrated Orbital Implants, Inc., San Diego, Calif.), bovine bone derived hydroxyapatite (M-sphere, IOP, Inc., Costa Mesa, Calif.), artificial hydroxyapatite (Bioceramic, FCI, Inc., Marshfield Hills, Mass.), and porous polyethylene (MEDPOR, Porex Surgical, Inc., Newnan, Ga.) material, either bare or wrapped in donor sclera, fascia, or polyglactin mesh have become the orbital implantation materials of choice because of their qualities of biointegration, excellent postoperative prosthetic motility, and low migration rates. The extraocular muscles are attached either directly to the implant or to its overlying wrapping material. Fibrovascular ingrowth is complete within 6 to 8 months. Commonly used

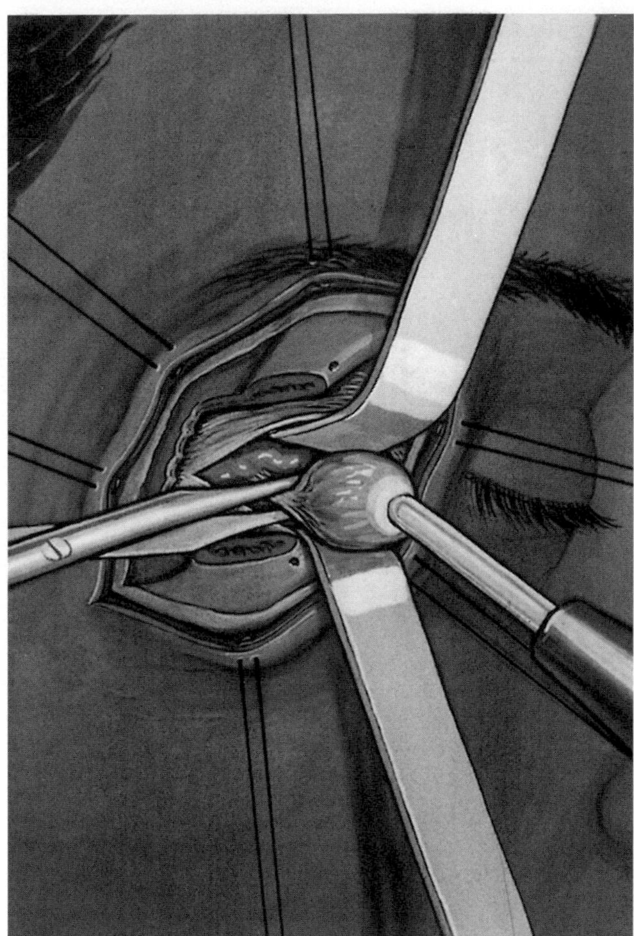

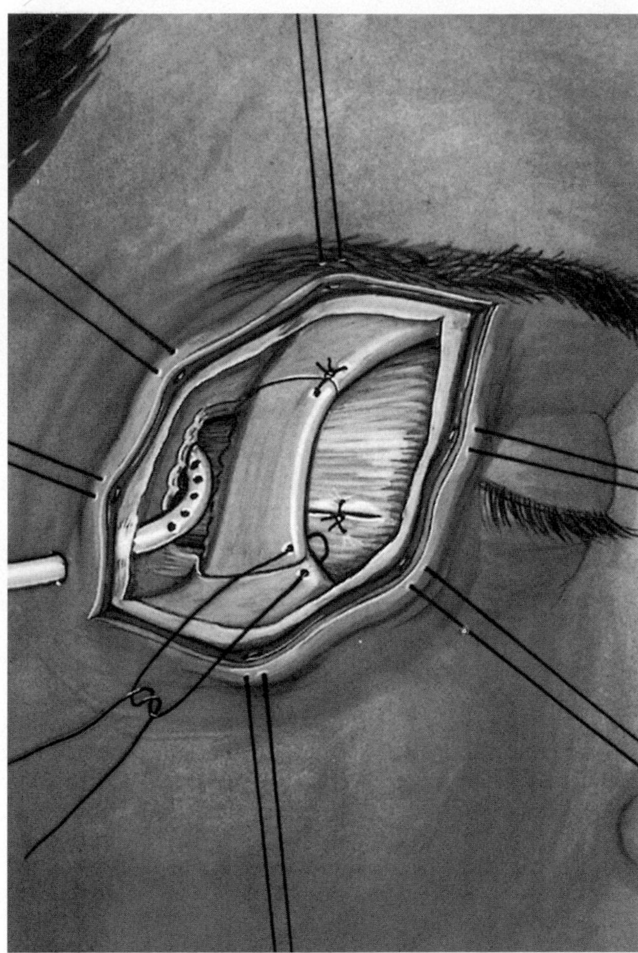

Figure 31.7 ***(continued)*** **C:** The cut portion of the orbital rim is out-fractured, and the lateral orbital wall is removed posteriorly with rongeurs. The periorbita is opened, and the tumor is engaged with the assistance of a cryoprobe. **D:** Periorbita is closed with 6–0 polyglactin sutures, and the lateral orbital rim is stabilized with 4–0 Prolene sutures passed through preplaced drill holes. A low-vacuum drain may be placed into the temporalis fossa and out through a cutaneous puncture wound. (From Dutton JJ. *Atlas of ophthalmic surgery: oculoplastic, lacrimal, and orbital surgery.* Vol 2. St. Louis: Mosby-Year Book, 1992, with permission.)

nonintegrated orbital implants include polymethylmethacrylate spheres.

Complications of enucleation include bleeding at the time of surgery or in the immediate postoperative period. Usually, this is easily controlled with pressure patching and is best avoided with a preoperative retrobulbar anesthetic injection containing epinephrine. Meticulous hemostasis during surgery will usually avoid this problem. Extrusion of orbital implants generally results from poor wound closure over the implant or from placement of an implant that is too large for the recipient tissues.

Exenteration

Orbital exenteration is a radical procedure reserved for widespread infiltrative tumors of the eyelids and orbit that are not treatable by more conservative modalities (4). In standard exenteration, the eyelids and all the soft tissues of the orbit are removed as a unit, leaving the orbital bones intact and bare. A skin graft may be placed, but healing by granulation provides an adequate cover over several months. Various forms of limited exenteration have been described with removal of the globe and varying amounts of orbital fat, muscles, and adnexa. If not involved in the pathologic process, the eyelid skin can be left intact and are closed over the shallow defect, giving a better cosmetic result. Extended exenterations include removal of orbital bone and possibly adjacent sinuses, in addition to the orbital soft tissues. Such procedures are reserved for such tumors as adenoid cystic carcinoma.

In the standard exenteration, an incision is made around the orbit just inside the orbital rim, with at least 5 mm of normal tissue surrounding the zone of pathology (Fig. 31.9A). If a more limited procedure is to be performed, the incision can be placed along the eyelash margin so that all eyelid tissues except skin are included with the orbital specimen. Dissection then is carried above the orbicularis muscle to the orbital rim (2). The periosteum is incised 2 to 4 mm outside the attachment of the orbital septum, and the medial and lateral canthal tendons are disinserted from their attachments to bone. The periorbita is separated from the orbital walls with a periosteal elevator. If the tumor involves the nasolacrimal sac and duct, the anterior wall of the canal should be removed with rongeurs, and the duct should be transected as it enters the nose; if the sac and duct are not involved, the duct may be transected as it enters the canal just inside the inferomedial orbital rim. Once the orbital contents are freed from adjacent bone to the apex, a Metzenbaum scissors is

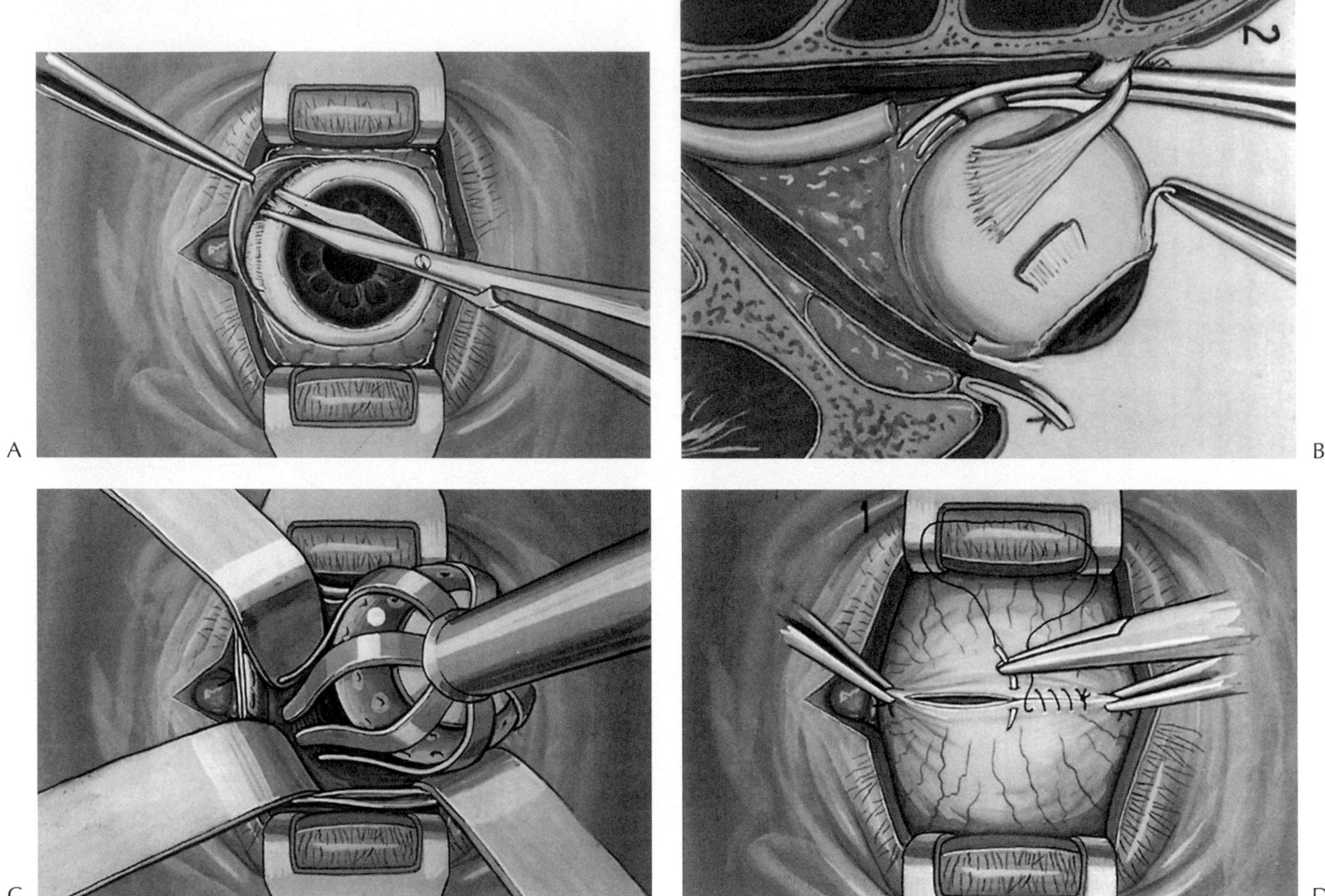

Figure 31.8 Enucleation with primary alloplastic implant placement. **A:** A 360-degree peritomy is performed to separate the conjunctiva from underlying sclera. The closed blades of a scissors are then inserted into each of the four quadrants between the rectus muscles and are spread to dissect the sclera from the overlying Tenon capsule. Each of the four rectus muscles then is cut from its insertion. **B:** The medial rectus muscle stump is grasped, and the globe is rotated temporally. An enucleation scissors is passed behind the globe, and the optic nerve is identified. The nerve is cut 3 to 4 mm behind the globe. **C:** An 18- to 20-mm methylmethacrylate or other type of sphere is placed into the orbital cavity. **D:** The anterior Tenon capsule is closed with interrupted 5–0 polyglactin sutures, and the conjunctiva is closed with a running 6–0 plain gut suture. (From Dutton JJ. *Atlas of ophthalmic surgery: oculoplastic, lacrimal, and orbital surgery.* Vol 2. St. Louis: Mosby-Year Book, 1992, with permission.)

passed posteriorly, and the orbital tissues are transected (Fig. 31.9B). Additional tissue can be excised around the superior orbital fissure if needed, and hemostasis must be ensured (Fig. 31.9C). If a skin graft is placed, the cavity is packed for 10 days. Although a temporalis muscle flap may be mobilized and transplanted into the orbit to provide soft tissue volume, this practice is discouraged, as it may conceal tumor recurrence. Potential complications of exenteration include graft failure or delayed healing, facial numbness from inevitable transection of the frontal and supratrochlear nerves, the creation of sinus–orbital fistulae, and cerebrospinal fluid leaks.

Fine-Needle Aspiration Biopsy

Diagnostic fine-needle aspiration biopsy of orbital lesions is controversial. Although fine-needle aspiration may be particularly beneficial in cases of suspected metastatic lesions, in lesions in readily accessible orbital locations, and for tumors suspected to arise from contiguous sites (i.e., sinus tumors) (5), such a procedure is ill-advised for vascular, cicatrized and, encapsulated tumors that should be removed in their entirety. A pistol-grip syringe with a 22-gauge needle is inserted into the tumor, and several core aspirations are taken without removing the needle from the orbit. Ultrasonography- or computed tomography (CT)-assisted guidance may be helpful. The material resulting from biopsy should be processed quickly for cytologic evaluation. A cytologist well acquainted with this method is necessary for accurate tissue assessment. Diagnostic yields are very surgeon-dependent. The quantity of cells obtained may be low and prohibit an accurate diagnosis. Complications include retrobulbar hemorrhage and globe perforation (6).

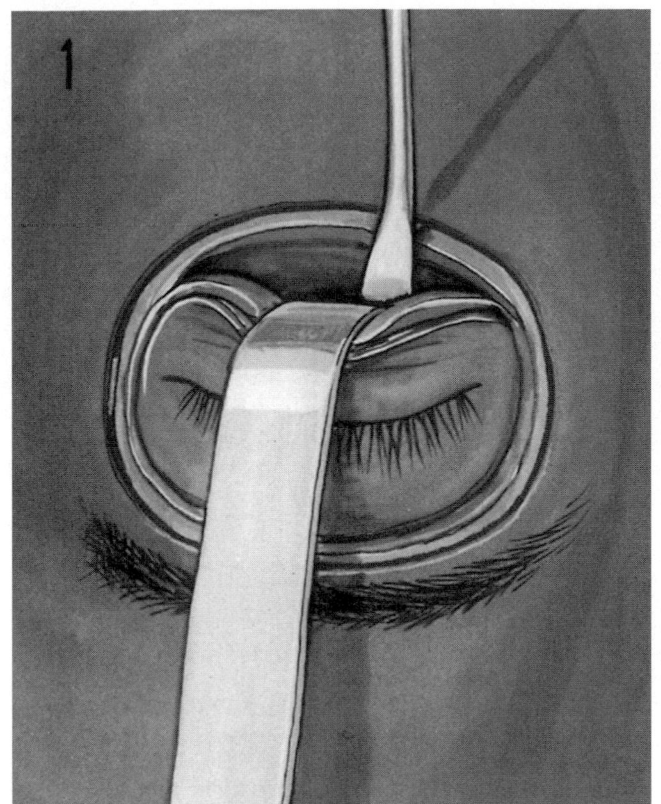

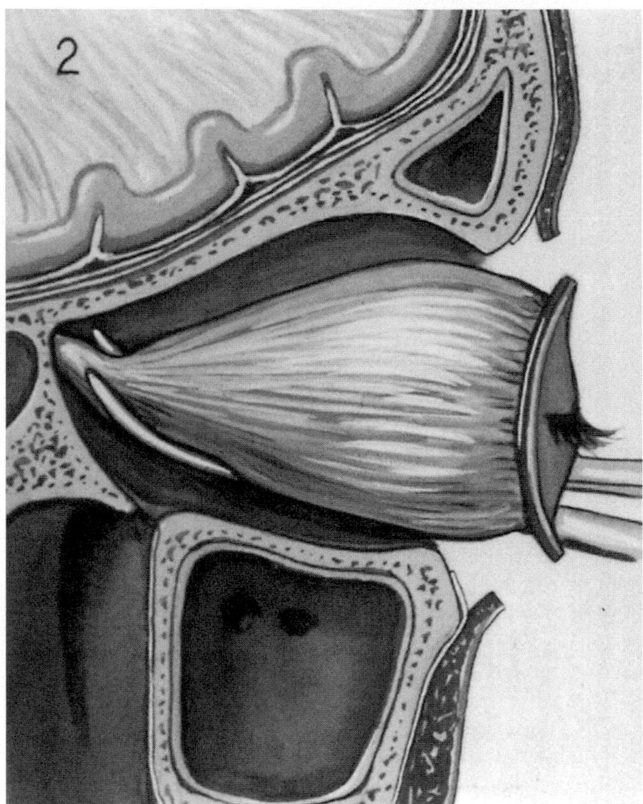

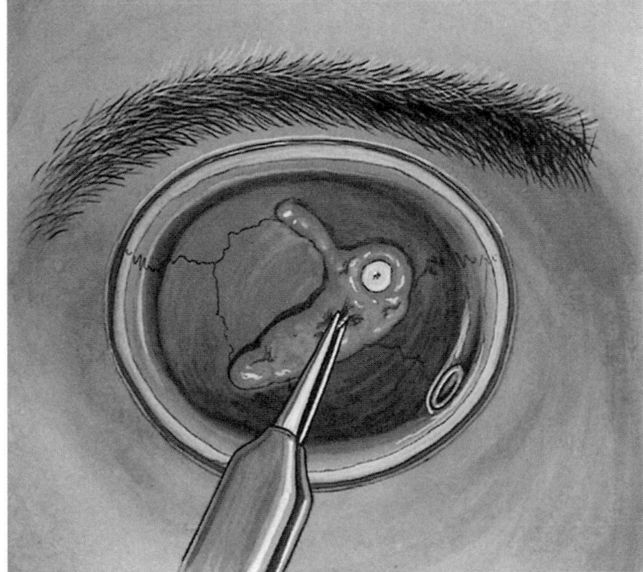

Figure 31.9 Orbital exenteration. **A:** An incision is made down to and through periosteum, just outside the orbital rim. Periosteum is carefully elevated along the orbital walls with a periosteal elevator. **B:** A Metzenbaum scissors is passed to the apex, and the tissues are transected. **C:** Hemostasis is achieved with bipolar cautery and bone wax. The orbit can be left to granulate or can be covered with a split-thickness skin graft. (From Dutton JJ. *Atlas of ophthalmic surgery: oculoplastic, lacrimal, and orbital surgery.* Vol 2. St. Louis: Mosby-Year Book, 1992, with permission.)

NATURAL HISTORY AND PATTERNS OF TUMOR SPREAD

Orbital diseases include neoplastic, vascular, inflammatory, cystic, and granulomatous processes, all of which may present clinically as mass lesions simulating malignant tumors. True neoplasms comprise 22% of all orbital disease and include both benign and malignant tumors. The majority of malignant tumors tend to be infiltrative in nature and more commonly result in functional compromise to orbital structures. Thus, compared with benign lesions, malignancies are frequently heralded by motility disturbances and diplopia, eyelid retraction or ptosis, and visual loss. They tend to grow more rapidly over months, compared with benign masses, which typically may be present for years. Though orbital pain is not a common feature of any neoplastic process, pain is more frequently associated with malignancies due to bony erosion or perineural invasion.

Some orbital malignancies, such as those of the lacrimal gland or optic nerve, may be confined to a particular anatomic orbital space, where they result in such predictable signs as medial abaxial globe displacement or papilledema. Other tumors, such as lymphomas, may invade the orbit diffusely, resulting in more widespread functional disturbances. Not uncommonly, tumors may also invade the globe or such adjacent paraorbital structures as orbital bones, nasal cavity, paranasal sinuses, and intracranial vault. Tumors may spread to the orbit or from it into distant sites through hematogenous dissemination. Lymphatic spread is not seen with deep orbital tumors because of the near absence of lymphatic channels in the orbit.

CLINICAL EVALUATION

History

The evaluation of a patient with suspected orbital tumor requires a thorough history detailing the time of onset, course of progression, presence or absence of pain, and recent or remote surgery or trauma. Very rapid progression over days to weeks is exceptional with malignant processes, except in rare cases, such as rhabdomyosarcoma. A recent history of trauma may suggest a vascular or infectious etiology, and a more distant history of trauma should alert the examiner to the possibility of mucocele, epidermal cyst, or cholesteatoma. Symptoms pointing toward systemic disorders, such as Graves disease, sarcoidosis, and tuberculosis, should be elicited. Changes in the nature of the orbital process, with alterations in body position or with straining, point toward a varix or arteriovenous malformation. Particular attention should be paid to the patient's medical history of cancers, endocrinologic disorders, infections, and immunologic diseases. Past or present medication use should be detailed.

Examination

A thorough ophthalmologic examination is mandatory and can help appreciably in diagnosis. Best corrected visual acuity, pupillary reactivity, visual field tests, intraocular pressure measurement, and measurements of ocular motility provide evidence of optic nerve compromise and extraocular muscle restriction. If diplopia is present, the ocular misalignment should be quantified with prisms. Proptosis is measured with an exophthalmometer, and eyelid positions are documented relative to the corneal limbus. Proptosis can be axial in nature (directly forward) or may show an abaxial displacement of the globe. Maxillary sinus tumors will displace the globe upward, as compared with lacrimal tumors, which displace the globe medially and downward. Resistance to retrodisplacement of the globe can provide information on the compressibility of a lesion. Measurement of cranial nerve function, both sensory and motor, can aid in pathologic localization of the orbital process. Palpation of an anterior mass can provide information on its fixation to deeper tissues, tenderness, consistency, and associated gross orbital morphologic changes. Pulsatile proptosis suggests a bony defect and communication with the cranial cavity. Auscultation of orbital processes may reveal a bruit, consistent with a high-flow carotid cavernous sinus fistula. An examination of the mouth and nose is essential to rule out involvement of these adjacent paraorbital structures.

Evaluation of the eyelids may provide information related to the orbital process. Eyelid retraction is most commonly seen with Graves orbitopathy but may be seen with infiltrative lesions affecting the levator muscle. A superior orbital mass typically results in some degree of ptosis, either through a direct mechanical effect on the muscle or a neurogenic effect on the oculomotor nerve or on sympathetic innervation to the Müller muscle. Periorbital edema, erythema, warmth, and discoloration are helpful in determining whether an inflammatory or infectious component is at work.

Slit-lamp examination of the anterior segment should be performed to assess any globe involvement. Intraocular tumors may result in anterior displacement of the iris or distortion of the lens and occasionally may be seen extending into the anterior chamber angle. A dilated fundus examination will help to assess the status of the optic nerve for evidence of atrophy (seen with lesions impinging on the optic nerve), opticociliary shunt vessels (common with some chronic optic nerve compressive lesions, particularly optic nerve sheath meningiomas), and disc hemorrhages. Choroidal folds may be seen with orbital tumors pressing on the globe and may occasionally be the earliest sign of orbital disease.

Visual field tests are helpful in detecting subtle optic nerve damage. They are especially useful for localization of contiguous intracranial involvement, frequently showing subtle abnormalities even without any other ophthalmic manifestations. Computerized visual field analyzers (such as the Humphrey Field Analyzer, Allergan Humphrey, San Leandro, Calif.) are particularly sensitive to optic nerve dysfunction. Visual field examination of the contralateral eye is necessary in evaluating tumors that may involve the optic chiasm.

Ancillary Diagnostic Imaging Tests

The most important ancillary imaging tests for orbital evaluation are CT, magnetic resonance imaging (MRI), and ultrasonography. A narrow differential diagnosis must be established prior to any imaging studies, as each examination has its own advantages and limitations. Lesions involving bone or calcification are best evaluated with CT and must include bone-window settings. Both coronal and axial orientations are essential. Magnetic resonance imaging scans are superior for evaluation of soft tissue differentiation and suspected intracranial extension. Because of its ability to distinguish fat from water-density tissues, MRI is particularly useful in differentiating optic nerve lesions. Ultrasonography is limited to the anterior one-third of the orbit because of its high 8-MHz frequency but is excellent for tissue differentiation, evaluation of tumor consistency and surface characteristics, biometry, and mobility. Ultrasonography is particularly unsurpassed for intraocular tumors such as melanomas or metastatic lesions.

SPECIFIC ORBITAL TUMORS

Orbital malignancies make up a large percentage of orbital neoplasms. In a series of more than 1,300 orbital tumors seen at the Mayo Clinic by Henderson and Farrow (7), malignant tumors outnumbered benign tumors by a ratio of 1.7:1. The most common malignancies were carcinomas and non-Hodgkin lymphoma. Carcinomas made up 22.6% of the overall tumor group, the vast majority of them being metastatic and secondary tumors. Adenocarcinoma ranks as the most common metastatic tumor, and squamous cell carcinoma is the most frequent malignant secondary tumor. Non-Hodgkin lymphoma is the most common primary malignant tumor in adults, whereas in children, the most common primary orbital malignancy is rhabdomyosarcoma.

Orbital tumors show a distinct bimodal age distribution. An initial peak occurs in the first decade, and a second larger peak occurs in the sixth to seventh decades. Certain lesions characteristically occur in childhood, whereas others most typically are found only in older adults. For example, pilocytic astrocytic gliomas of the optic nerve occur almost exclusively in the pediatric age group, whereas the malignant glioma is seen predominantly in middle-aged adults. Rhabdomyosarcomas are rarely detected in adults, but lymphomas typically occur in older adults. Malignant tumors of the orbit become more frequent in the adult population, and these are primarily metastatic and secondary tumors.

Management of orbital tumors on the basis of staging systems is much less frequently used in the orbit than in other sites of the body. This is due in large part to the relative rarity of most tumors and a consequent lack of coordinated prospective studies that could in some manner contribute to regimented treatment parameters. Nonetheless, several orbital malignancies have been granted staging criteria by the American Joint Committee on Cancer (8). Rhabdomyosarcoma is one of the few orbital malignancies that has been successfully treated on the basis of a meaningful staging system established by the Intergroup Rhabdomyosarcoma Study (9). Outcomes have improved appreciably over the last several decades.

Vascular Tumors

HEMANGIOPERICYTOMA

These relatively uncommon orbital tumors arise from pericytes of orbital blood vessels and are considered to be of mesenchymal origin. Most patients are in their third to sixth decade at presentation. Patients typically develop slowly progressive painless, unilateral, nonpulsatile proptosis (10). Because most of these tumors occur in the superior orbit, the globe is typically displaced downward. Lesions may also extend forward beneath the conjunctiva and cover the anterior globe (Fig. 31.10).

Although the vast majority of these tumors are benign, malignant hemangiopericytomas occur as well. These may arise *de novo* or by transformation of incompletely excised benign tumors. It has long been held that the cytologic appearance of these tumors does not correlate with clinical behavior, and it may be difficult to differentiate benign from malignant tumors through histologic criteria alone. Helpful indicators of malignancy include increased cellularity, nuclear atypia, and the presence of mitotic figures.

The primary goal in the management of a newly diagnosed tumor is complete excision of the lesion within its pseudocapsule. With incomplete excisions of benign tumors, there is a risk for recurrence with local invasion and malignant transformation, sometimes after a long delay. The best management of these cases is unknown, although some advocate supplemental radiation therapy. If histologic criteria suggestive of malignancy are seen, exenteration may be considered even if the tumor can apparently be completely resected. Adjunctive radiation therapy should be considered.

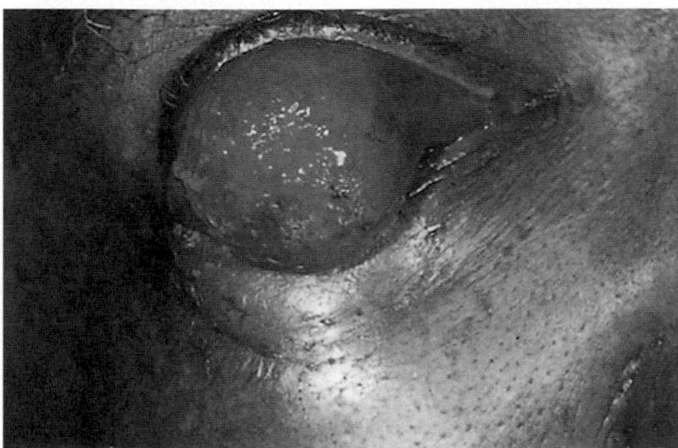

Figure 31.10 Right anterior orbital and subconjunctival hemangiopericytoma in a 76-year-old woman.

The prognosis is excellent with completely excised lesions. Mortality approaches 15% to 25% in those patients with residual tumor and subsequent recurrence (11,12). Death typically occurs from intracranial spread or distant metastases.

ANGIOSARCOMA (MALIGNANT HEMANGIOENDOTHELIOMA)

Angiosarcoma is an extremely rare malignancy (with only 14 cases reported in the literature) and is most common in the pediatric age group, although it may occur in a more lethal form in adults (13). Patients present with upper eyelid swelling of relatively short duration. The tumors tend to be fairly infiltrative, with poorly delineated margins. Management requires radical orbital exenteration and adjunctive chemotherapy. Prognosis is worse with tumors involving the posterior orbit. Death usually results from local recurrence and hematogenous spread.

Neurogenic Tumors

MALIGNANT PERIPHERAL NERVE SHEATH TUMOR

Neurofibrosarcoma, malignant schwannoma, and malignant triton tumor are very rare tumors and may originate in the orbit or from the periorbital region. The progenitor cell is not precisely known, although the majority seem to arise from Schwann cells. Perineural cells and fibroblasts have been implicated as well. These tumors may arise through malignant transformation of neurofibromas and schwannomas and may show sarcomatous characteristics. Approximately 25% of cases occur in patients with neurofibromatosis (13).

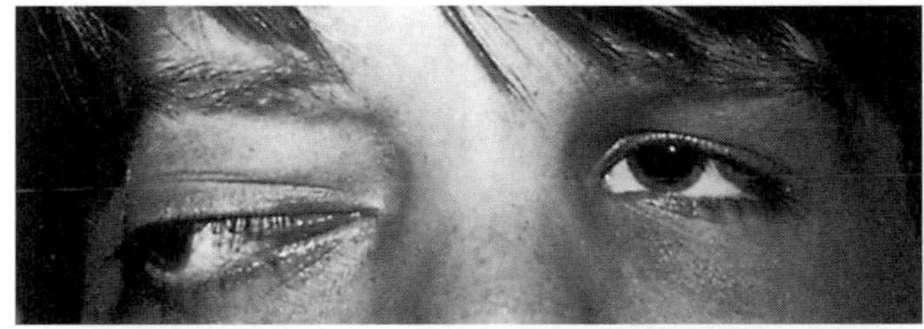

A

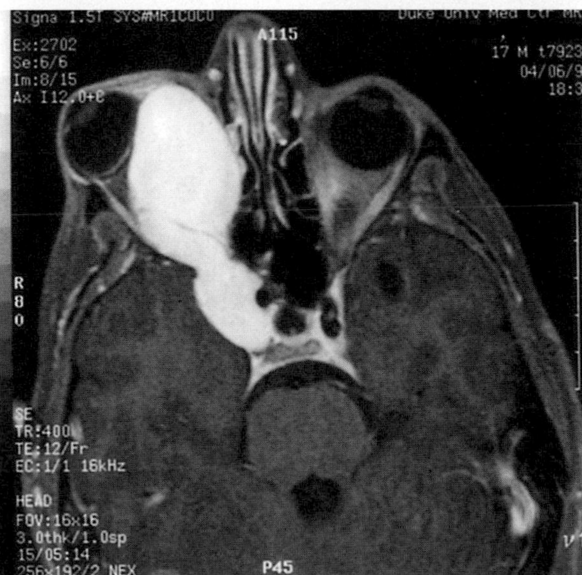

B

Figure 31.11 Malignant peripheral nerve sheath tumor. **A:** Malignant peripheral nerve sheath tumor of the right orbit in an 18-year-old man with neurofibromatosis type I. **B:** Same patient as in **A.** Gadolinium-enhanced, fat-suppressed T1-weighted image demonstrates a large tumor passing backward through the superior orbital fissure into the cavernous sinus.

These lesions usually present as an orbital or periorbital mass, with proptosis and displacement of the globe (Fig. 31.11A). On initial biopsy, these lesions frequently display benign characteristics. Multiple benign recurrences may occur before the malignant characteristics are identified. Malignant transformation is characterized by aggressive growth and a propensity for perineural extension, commonly into the middle cranial fossa. Computed tomography scan may show findings fairly similar to benign nerve sheath tumors or may demonstrate extensive bony erosion (Fig. 31.11B).

The results of treatment of malignant peripheral nerve sheath tumors are uniformly disappointing. The tumor is relatively radioresistant; therefore, surgical management has been most widely advocated. Radical resection of the soft tissue tumor and involved bone is necessary. In one study, 9 of 13 patients (69%) died within 5 years; 2 patients survived for 5 and 7 years, respectively; and 2 patients were lost to follow-up after 9 months (14).

MALIGNANT OPTIC PATHWAY GLIOMA

Malignant optic pathway glioma is an exceptionally rare tumor, with only 41 cases described in the world literature (15). It occurs primarily in middle-aged adults, with a mean age of 48 years. Two thirds of patients are male. Clinically, patients present with abrupt loss of vision progressing to complete bilateral blindness within several months. These tumors invariably arise in the optic chiasm and, in 23% of cases, extend into the orbit with subsequent proptosis and ophthalmoplegia. No treatment has proved useful, and the prognosis is uniformly fatal.

Osseous, Fibroosseous, and Cartilaginous Tumors

FIBROSARCOMA

Fibrosarcomas are very rare tumors that may occur as either primary or secondary malignancies in the orbit. A bimodal age distribution pattern exists in the primary form, with patients predominantly in the first and sixth decades. Patients generally present with proptosis of a few months' duration. The secondary form is seen in middle-aged patients with contiguous disease originating in the paranasal sinuses or nasal cavity. Fibrosarcoma may also occur in children after irradiation therapy to the orbit for retinoblastoma. In this group, fibrosarcoma is the second most common irradiation-induced secondary malignancy after osteogenic sarcoma (16).

Prognosis depends both on the extent of mitotic activity and on the duration of symptoms. In patients without evidence of metastatic disease, early aggressive surgical intervention represents the best hope for survival. Radical exenteration is generally required for total tumor removal.

OSTEOSARCOMA

Osteosarcomas are highly malignant tumors that may arise from any of the orbital bones. They are frequently associated with prior local radiation therapy or (more rarely) may arise *de novo*. Radiation-induced tumors are most commonly seen in patients previously irradiated for genomic retinoblastoma. It is now known, however, that in these children, osteosarcomas and other sarcomatous tumors may occur in distant sites not included within the field of irradiation (16). In fact, the genes for both retinoblastoma and osteosarcoma occupy chromosome 13, which may have future implications in gene therapy for both heritable and nonheritable osteosarcomas (17).

The clinical picture is one of fairly rapid onset of unilateral proptosis, displacement of the globe, orbital pain, chemosis, and eyelid edema. Computed tomography scan shows varying degrees of lysis, sclerosis, and calcification. All the histologic variants are equally aggressive. Treatment is aimed at extended resection of tumor, although it is extremely difficult to eradicate the entire tumor. Orbital exenteration and resection of all involved periorbital bone seem to offer the only hope for survival. Five-year survivals have been poor (10%), despite aggressive therapy. Adjunctive chemotherapy in combination with surgery and radiation therapy has improved survivals to as high as 50% in osteosarcoma involving the long bones. It is hoped that this will serve as a model for future treatment of orbital disease (18).

CHONDROSARCOMA

Chondrosarcomas are the second most common primary malignancy of bone after osteogenic sarcoma, primarily affecting the long bones, shoulder girdle, and pelvis. In the periocular region, they arise mainly in the nasopharynx and sinuses, with secondary involvement of the orbit. Like osteogenic sarcomas, chondrosarcomas may arise secondary to radiation therapy for retinoblastoma. They may occur in any age group, from infancy to old age. Patients usually present with symptoms related to the sites of primary tumor origin, including nasal obstruction, epistaxis, and sinusitis (7). Orbital signs and symptoms tend to occur later in the course of disease. Progressive proptosis, displacement of the globe, and motility disturbances are common (19). With more anterior lesions from the ethmoid, compression of the lacrimal sac may cause epiphora (20).

Whereas osteosarcomas tend to be rapidly growing malignancies with a definite urgency in terms of intervention, chondrosarcomas are very slowly growing lesions that rarely metastasize. Therefore, a more conservative approach can be taken in management. Treatment is aimed at complete resection of tumor without sacrificing vital ocular structures. As these tumors tend to be slow-growing over many years, radical surgery, such as exenteration, should be performed only if the tumor exhibits an aggressiveness that threatens intracranial extension. Recurrences after resection may take a number of years to manifest and are associated with local invasion, intracranial spread, and obstruction of respiratory passages. Five-year survivals vary from 43% to 90%, depending on the histologic grade of the tumor (21).

EWING SARCOMA

Ewing sarcoma is a malignant, small, round-cell neoplasm primarily affecting children in the first and second decades of life (1,22,44). The tumor classically involves the long bones of the limbs, the ribs, and the pelvis (23–25). Primary Ewing sarcoma of the head and neck region is unusual; when seen, it typically occurs in the mandible and maxillary bone (16,26). Occurrence in the orbit is exceptionally rare and, in most cases, represents metastatic disease from distant sites. Only nine unequivocal cases of primary Ewing sarcoma of bone have been described to involve the orbit. The histogenesis of this tumor remains in question.

Until recent years, the prognosis for Ewing sarcoma at all sites was uniformly dismal (27,28). With surgery and radiation therapy alone, the 5-year survival rates were only 8% and 10%, respectively (29,30). With the addition of adjuvant chemotherapy, prognosis has improved significantly (31), and 5-year survival rates have increased to 53% (32). Local recurrence has also been reduced from as high as 38% after radiation therapy alone (33) to perhaps 5% after adjunctive chemotherapy (34).

Mesenchymal Tumors

RHABDOMYOSARCOMA

Rhabdomyosarcoma is a tumor composed of cells related to striated muscle in various stages of differentiation. It was once thought that these tumors arose from mature striated muscles, but they are now believed to originate from primitive mesenchymal tissue, with the potential to differentiate into striated muscle cells (35). Rhabdomyosarcoma is the most common primary orbital malignancy of childhood, affecting boys slightly more frequently than girls in a ratio of 5:3 (36). These tumors may be primary or secondary in the orbit, the latter slightly outnumbering the former. The average age at onset is 7 to 8 years for the primary type and 14 years for the secondary type.

The classic clinical presentation is one of abrupt onset of painless proptosis, eyelid discoloration, conjunctival chemosis, and decreased ocular motility (Fig. 31.12A). This is especially true in younger patients, though older patients may present with a more insidious course. The acute presentation is often mistaken for an inflammatory process, although patients usually show no other systemic or periorbital signs suggestive of inflammation. A recent history of trauma may be elicited in some cases and may cloud the diagnostic picture. A palpable mass may sometimes be present beneath the conjunctiva or in the anterior orbit. Untreated symptoms progress rapidly to blindness and extensive orbital destruction. Hematogenous dissemination results in metastatic spread to the lungs, lymph nodes, and bones.

Once rhabdomyosarcoma is suspected, imaging studies will help to determine the extent and location of orbital involvement. Computed tomography typically reveals a well-defined to irregular soft tissue mass, sometimes with orbital bone destruction, a feature seen with very few other pediatric orbital lesions (Fig. 31.12B). Biopsy of the lesion should be performed on an urgent basis through an anterior or lateral orbitotomy approach. Histologically, rhabdomyosarcoma may be confused with other small, round-cell tumors, including lymphoma, neuroblastoma, and Ewing sarcoma, making electron microscopy and immunohistochemical analysis essential in confirming the diagnosis. A pediatric oncologist should perform a thorough physical examination and a metastatic workup, including bone

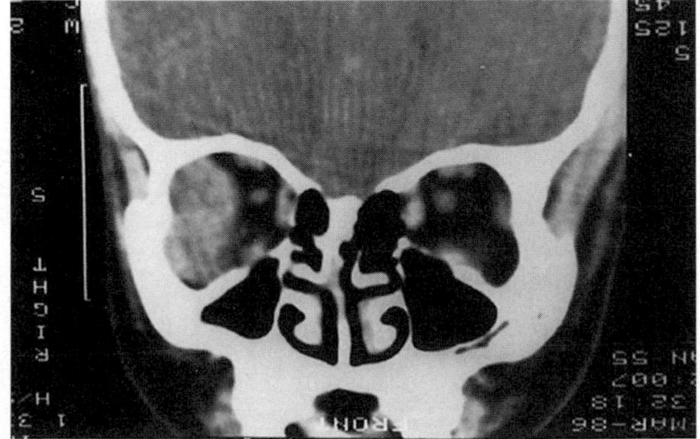

Figure 31.12 Rhabdomyosarcoma. **A:** Rapidly progressive proptosis of the right orbit in a 7-year-old girl with a rhabdomyosarcoma. **B:** Same patient as in **A.** Coronal computed tomographic scan demonstrates a well-demarcated mass in the lateral orbit.

marrow aspiration and biopsy, chest x-ray, and lumbar puncture. Metastases are most commonly to the lung.

Microscopically, these tumors have been classified into embryonal, alveolar, and pleomorphic forms. A rare botryoid form may involve the orbit secondarily from the conjunctiva or paranasal sinuses. The embryonal variant is the most common form in the orbit (37). Histologically, it is composed of spindle cells arranged in loose fascicles, with rare cross-striations. The alveolar form is the most malignant subtype and shows a greater frequency of metastasis than other variants. It is so named because of its resemblance to alveoli of the lung. This form has a predilection for the inferior orbit. The pleomorphic form typically occurs in skeletal muscles of adults and rarely involves the orbit. It is the most differentiated form and carries the most favorable prognosis.

The Intergroup Rhabdomyosarcoma Study established guidelines for staging the extent of the disease, with subsequent treatment based on this staging scheme (9). Before that study, treatment typically consisted of orbital exenteration. Despite such radical surgery, the prognosis remained poor, with survival rates of less than 20%. In recent decades, more limited surgery combined with adjunctive chemotherapy and radiation therapy (5,000–6,000 cGy) has resulted in survival rates of 90% (38). Prognosis does not appear to be affected by histologic type, as long as the tumor is confined to the orbit and does not invade adjacent bones. Lack of lymphatic drainage from the orbit and early presentation also contribute to the success in treating these orbital tumors.

The staging of orbital rhabdomyosarcoma is based on the extent of the tumor after initial resection. Stage I disease represents completely resected tumor, stage II designates resected tumor with histologic evidence of microscopic residual tumor, stage III indicates gross residual tumor, and stage IV signals documented metastatic disease. Stage II and stage III are generally treated with a chemotherapy consisting of vincristine, doxorubicin (Adriamycin), and cyclophosphamide in addition to local radiation therapy. For stage IV disease, actinomycin D is added. However, even in patients in whom the orbital tumor has apparently been completely removed (stage I), adjunctive therapy should usually be given.

No clear consensus exists regarding the extent to which tumor should be removed at the time of initial surgery. Small, well-circumscribed tumors should be removed *in toto*, and more extensive lesions should be debulked as much as possible without compromising visual function. Complications of treatment are usually related to local irradiation effects and include enophthalmos, hemifacial atrophy, cataract, retinopathy, dry-eye syndrome, and a number of other sequelae, including secondary irradiation-induced tumors. Reconstructive surgery of the face and orbit may be required later in life.

LEIOMYOSARCOMA

Leiomyosarcoma, a tumor of smooth muscle origin, may involve the orbit primarily, secondarily, or through metastasis (20). It may also arise after orbital irradiation for retinoblastoma (39). Primary orbital leiomyosarcomas are fairly rare: only eight cases have been described (40). It tends to be seen in older women, with a mean age of 57 years. Patients present with rapidly progressive proptosis, decreased vision, and diplopia (Fig. 31.13A). Computed tomography scan typically reveals a well-defined mass that may conform to other orbital structures (Fig. 31.13B). The diagnosis is usually not suspected until biopsy.

The management of these tumors remains controversial. In some cases, the tumor can easily be shelled out (Fig. 31.13C). However, the small number of reported cases illustrates the highly aggressive nature of these tumors, and most authorities

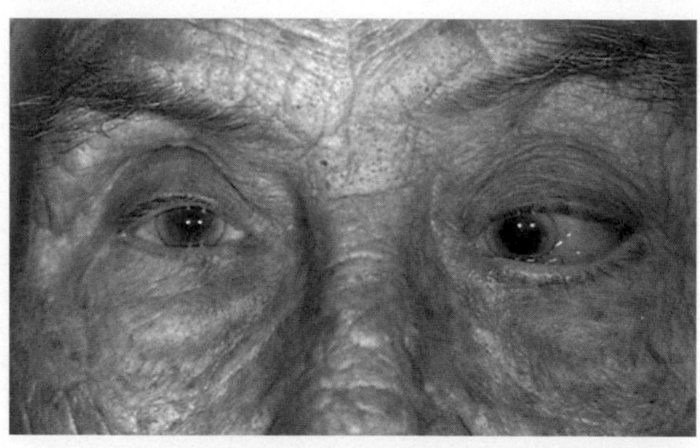
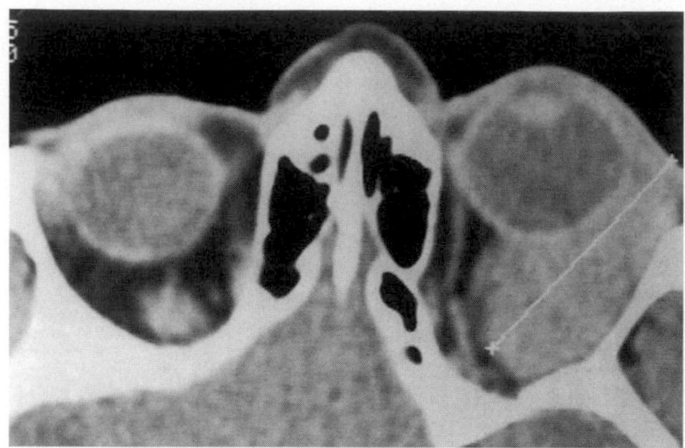
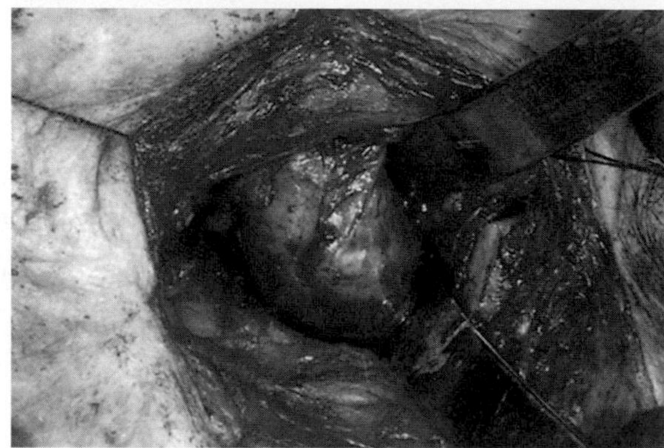

Figure 31.13 Leiomyosarcoma. **A:** Leiomyosarcoma of the left orbit in an elderly woman, resulting in long-standing proptosis with inferonasal displacement of the globe. **B:** Same patient as in **A.** Axial computed tomographic scan demonstrates an irregular mass in the lateral orbit conforming to the globe. **C:** Same patient as in **A.** Exposure of the leiomyosarcoma at lateral orbitotomy.

believe that radical orbital exenteration carries the best chances for cure. Despite intervention, recurrences are frequent, and there is a high incidence of distant metastasis.

LIPOSARCOMA

Liposarcoma is a malignant neoplasm of lipoblasts and appears to arise from primitive mesenchymal cells. Although they are one of the most common soft-tissue sarcomas, liposarcomas occur only very rarely in the orbit (20). They may be present at any age but are seen primarily in adults.

Patients present with rapidly progressive unilateral proptosis and displacement of the globe. The tumor can reach rather impressive sizes, resulting in destruction of the eye (41). Both CT and MRI are helpful in localizing the tumor and determining its extent but otherwise they offer few specific diagnostic criteria.

Clinical behavior of these tumors correlates with histologic characteristics. Histologically, liposarcomas have been grouped into pleomorphic, round-cell, myxoid, and well-differentiated types. The myxoid type is the most common variant seen in the orbit. The myxoid and well-differentiated types carry the best prognosis.

No consensus exists regarding optimal treatment. The most common approach entails removing as much of the infiltrative tumor as possible at initial surgery. The more aggressive pleomorphic and round-cell varieties may require wide excision and even exenteration. Recurrence is common after incomplete surgery, and increased risk for dedifferentiation exists with each recurrence. Radiation therapy may be used as an adjunct. Prognosis is related to the size of the tumor and the site of the initial lesion. The lung is the most common site of metastasis.

FIBROUS HISTIOCYTOMA

Fibrous histiocytoma is the most common mesenchymal tumor of the orbit. It is believed to arise from a pluripotential cell with the capacity to differentiate into both fibroblasts and histiocytes. It occurs with equal frequency in male and female populations and is more commonly seen in middle age, with a mean age of 43 years (20). Patients present with a firm orbital mass, typically in the superior or nasal quadrants. Displacement of normal structures leads to proptosis and motility disturbance and is frequently associated with decreased visual acuity from optic nerve compression.

Fibrous histiocytomas in the orbit demonstrate a spectrum of behaviors from benign to malignant. The clinical presentation generally reflects the tumor's underlying histopathology. Benign tumors (63% of cases) tend to demonstrate a cartwheel or storiform histologic pattern composed of both fibroblastic and histiocytic cells without mitoses or necrosis. Intermediate, locally aggressive tumors comprise 26% of all cases, and frankly malignant tumors account for 11%. These latter lesions show increasing cellularity, mitoses, infiltrative margins, and necrosis. Malignant fibrous histiocytomas may arise as secondary tumors after orbital irradiation for retinoblastoma or rhabdomyosarcoma (Fig. 31.14A) (42). On CT scan, these tumors show an irregular contour, with erosion of bone (Fig. 31.14B).

The management of fibrous histiocytoma is complete surgical excision. This is generally not a problem with benign tumors contained within their fibrous capsule. Intermediate and malignant tumors, however, may be more infiltrative, requiring more extensive tissue excision. Highly invasive malignant lesions should be managed by orbital exenteration. Close follow-up is important, as tumor recurrence may be delayed for many years. Recurrence is highest in instances wherein the tumor was not completely excised at initial presentation and may be seen with 31% of benign tumors (20). Benign lesions can generally be managed with repeat excisions. Recurrent lesions with borderline or malignant pathology are best managed with orbital exenteration. Neither chemotherapy nor radiation therapy has been shown to be effective (43). Survival rates are excellent in patients with benign lesions. The 10-year survival for those

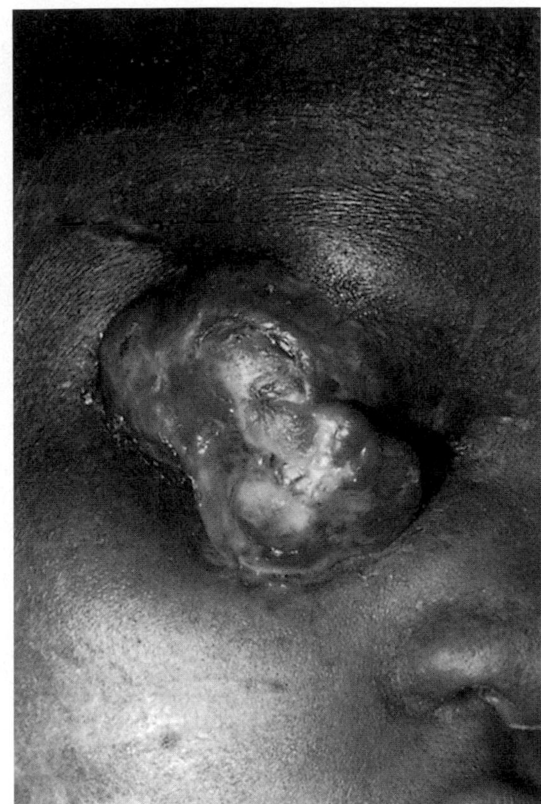

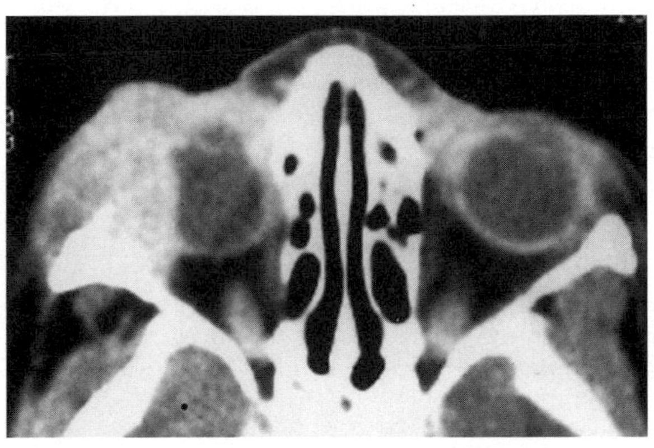

A B

Figure 31.14 Malignant fibrous histiocytoma. **A:** Malignant fibrous histiocytoma arising in the right orbit in a 13-year-old girl previously irradiated at age 2 years for retinoblastoma. **B:** Same patient as in **A.** Computed tomographic scan demonstrates a diffuse tumor in lateral orbit with erosion of the lateral orbital wall.

with locally aggressive tumors is 92% (17). Mortality in this group derives from malignant transformation of recurrent lesions with local extension. In patients with frankly malignant fibrous histiocytomas, the 10-year survival rate is only 23%. Death in these cases occurs from metastatic disease (50%) and local extension (50%).

Lymphoproliferative Tumors

MALIGNANT LYMPHOMA

Lymphoid tumors comprise approximately 11% of all orbital mass lesions (20). They are usually of the non-Hodgkin lymphoma type and predominate in older adults. Orbital lymphoma shows a predilection for the superior orbit, particularly for the lacrimal gland, but may be seen inferiorly as well (Fig. 31.15). Superiorly, they produce symptoms of painless downward displacement of the globe and often a firm, rubbery, palpable mass along the superior orbital rim. Ptosis is a common finding, but vision and ocular motility are typically normal. Although involvement is usually unilateral, bilateral occurrence may be seen.

Computed tomography scan shows a diffusely infiltrative mass molding itself around ocular structures and the orbital walls. Bony erosion is unusual. On MRI scans, lymphomas show low-signal intensity on T1-weighted images and high-signal intensity on T2-weighted sequences.

In patients with a known history of systemic lymphoma, a fine-needle aspiration biopsy of the orbital mass is adequate. However, in cases without a history, enough tissue is needed for immunohistochemical and marker studies, so an open biopsy is preferred. If the tumor is anteriorly situated, an eyelid crease incision will usually provide adequate visualization. For deeper tumors, a medial or lateral orbitotomy approach will be necessary. If positive for lymphoma, a complete systemic evaluation is necessary, including a general physical examination, chest x-ray, blood count, serum immunoglobulin electrophoresis, abdominal and bone CT, and bone marrow biopsy.

Lymphomas may be isolated to the orbit, but 60% of cases will eventually develop systemic involvement. The risk for systemic disease is greater with more undifferentiated tumors and those initially confined to the eyelid. Conjunctival lymphomas carry only a 20% risk for systemic disease.

Management depends on the extent of the disease. In the presence of systemic disease, chemotherapy is instituted with-

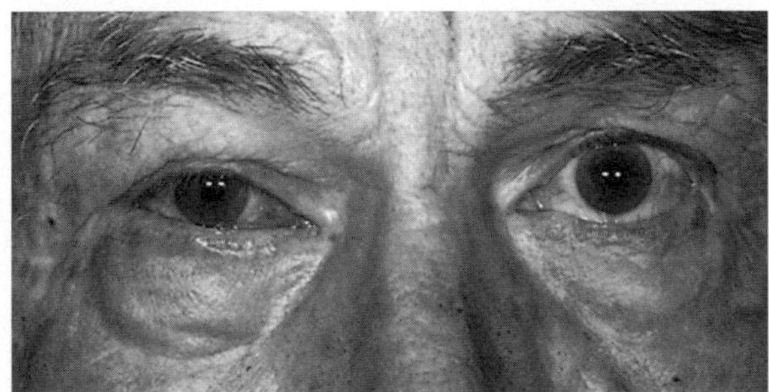

Figure 31.15 Lymphoma involving right inferior orbit and eyelid in a 67-year-old man.

out immediate local therapy to the orbit. For orbital lesions that do not respond, or for isolated lymphoma of the orbit, radiation therapy in the range of 1,500 to 3,000 cGy is indicated.

GRANULOCYTIC SARCOMA

Also referred to as chloroma or myeloid sarcoma, granulocytic sarcoma is an extramedullary solid tumor associated with acute myelogenous leukemia (AML). Although rare, it is the most common form of leukemic infiltrate involving the orbit. Granulocytic sarcoma is seen in 30% of patients with AML, and is associated with a high incidence of translocation (8,44). In up to 88% of cases of granulocytic sarcoma, the solid tumor can precede the blast phase of AML by months to years, or it may occur during periods of remission. Typical orbital lesions usually present in children with a mean age of 8 to 9 years as a rapidly enlarging mass, producing proptosis and diplopia. The lateral orbital wall is commonly involved, with medial displacement of the globe. Pain, papilledema, and retinal striae may be accompanying features. In 90% of the cases, the lesion is unilateral. Myeloperoxidase within the tumor imparts a green hue on gross examination, which accounts for the term *chloroma*.

On CT scan granulocytic sarcoma appears as an irregular, moderately defined mass of homogeneous density. Enhancement with contrast agents is minimal to moderate. Bone erosion is common. On MRI, the lesion appears isointense to cortical gray matter and muscle on T1-weighted images, and isointense to white matter and muscle on T2-weighted images. Moderate, homogenous enhancement is seen following gadolinium contrast. Radiotherapy is the treatment of choice for localized lesions although chemotherapy is warranted in individuals with documented systemic AML. The prognosis of patients with granulocytic sarcoma is generally thought to be less favorable than that in those with AML but without granulocytic sarcoma. The outcome is generally poor; only 20% of affected patients have a tumor-free survival of 5 years (44).

PLASMACYTOMA

Plamacytomas are composed of plasma cell-modified B lymphocytes and range in virulence from benign, localized, polyclonal, reactive lesions to low-grade, polyclonal, malignant lesions. In the latter form, the tumor may be solitary or may be a manifestation of systemic multiple myeloma. Males are more commonly affected than females at a ratio of 3:1 (45). The typical age at onset of symptoms is 50 to 70 years. However, primary extramedullary plasmacytoma has been described in children. Orbital involvement is very uncommon, but may be the initial manifestation of systemic disease. Lesions often present as slowly progressive painless proptosis or upper eyelid ptosis, often in association with a subconjunctival mass. Most lesions occur in the extraconal space and involvement of the adjacent paranasal sinuses with destruction of bones may occur. Rarely, the tumor may occur within the lacrimal sac. Urine protein electrophoresis typically demonstrates kappa light chains; plasma hypergammaglobulinemia may be absent.

Computed tomography scans reveal a diffuse orbital mass that is slightly denser than muscle and may not be distinguishable from the sclera or optic nerve. The mass may arise from an adjacent sinus with intervening osteolytic defects. Contrast enhancement is slight and homogeneous; in some cases, darker zones represent spontaneous intralesional hemorrhage. On MRI, plasmacytomas appear as solid, homogeneous, infiltrating masses isointense to muscle on T1-weighted images. On T2-weighted images, the lesion is isointense or slightly hypointense to fat. With intravenous administration of gadolinium, there is a slight increase in signal intensity, and the lesion appears hyperintense to muscle, but remains hypointense to fat.

Although some well-circumscribed, solitary plasmacytomas may be treated by surgical excision alone, in general, radiotherapy at 3,500 to 5,000 cGy offers good local control. Nonetheless, some tumors appear to be minimally radiosensitive. When associated with disseminated multiple myeloma, chemotherapy is warranted. Solitary lesions carry a good prognosis if treated before widespread local damage. The tumor may extend to the regional lymph nodes, and sometimes, it progresses to multiple myeloma. When associated with systemic myeloma, the prognosis is poor, and the mean survival is less than 2 years (46).

Epithelial Tumors of the Lacrimal Gland

Epithelial neoplasms of the lacrimal gland comprise a number of histopathologic types, including the benign pleomorphic adenoma and the malignant adenoid cystic carcinoma, pleomorphic adenocarcinoma, monomorphic adenocarcinoma, and mucoepidermoid carcinoma. They account for 27% to 51% of all epithelial tumors of the lacrimal gland (20,46). Malignant tumors make up only 8% of all solid lacrimal gland masses.

These tumors typically arise in young to middle-aged adults. Unilateral proptosis develops along with a downward and medial displacement of the globe. Unlike benign lacrimal gland tumors, malignant lesions more commonly are associated with orbital pain, diplopia, and upper-eyelid ptosis. The duration of symptoms is generally short, usually less than 6 months, and rarely more than 1 or 2 years. A firm mass may be palpated beneath the superotemporal orbital rim. Computed tomography scan generally demonstrates a rounded to irregular soft tissue mass in the lacrimal gland fossa that may be associated with bone erosion. Areas of calcification may be seen within the lesion.

ADENOID CYSTIC CARCINOMA

Adenoid cystic carcinomas are extremely aggressive malignancies that account for 30% of lacrimal gland cancers (20). They occur most commonly in the fifth decade of life, although patients as young as 9 years have been described.

Patients classically present with rapid onset of orbital pain and globe displacement (Fig. 31.16A), although recent reviews have found these symptoms in only a minority of patients. Radiologic studies do not demonstrate characteristic findings. Lytic destruction of bone, when present, may aid in the diagnosis.

The pathologic classification of Broders (47) provides a histologic grading scheme but has no consistent prognostic implications. The poor prognosis associated with adenoid cystic carcinoma is a result of its propensity for perineural invasion and subsequent intracranial spread. Bone invasion is probably the most common means of dissemination after the tumor cells gain access to the haversian canals.

The initial step in the management of adenoid cystic carcinoma is to obtain tissue for definitive diagnosis. A lateral orbitotomy is necessary in most cases. Further intervention should not be decided on the basis of frozen-section analysis but only after permanent sections have been reviewed. If the permanent sections demonstrate adenoid cystic carcinoma, extended exenteration is performed. A team approach with neurosurgery may be necessary to facilitate the complete removal of tumor and adjacent cranial bone (Fig. 31.16B). Postoperative radiation therapy may be beneficial as an adjunct, but it is not adequate as primary therapy. Despite heroic measures,

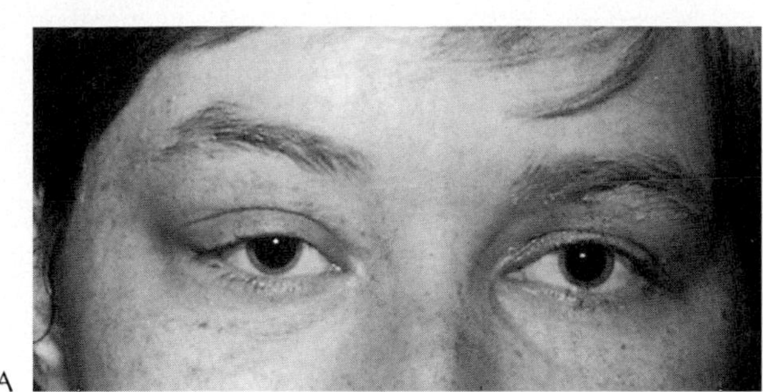

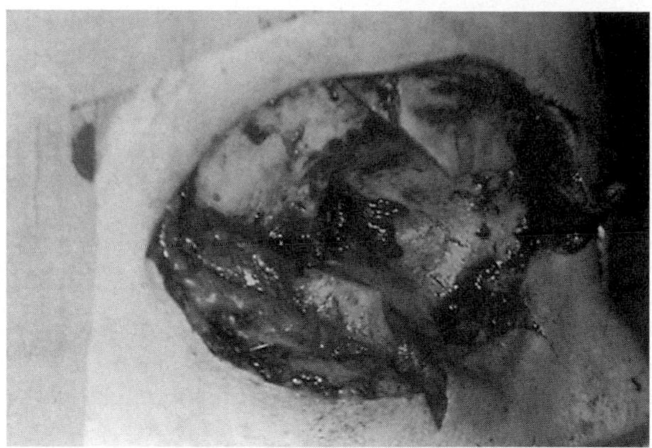

A B

Figure 31.16 Adenoid cystic carcinoma. **A:** Adenoid cystic carcinoma of the lacrimal gland presenting as a rapidly enlarging right orbital mass in a 40-year-old woman. Note ptosis of right upper eyelid and fullness in superolateral orbit. **B:** Same patient as in **A** during orbital exenteration, with removal of the lateral orbital wall and adjacent soft tissues.

the prognosis remains dismal. Average survival is in the range of 4 to 5 years, with mortality approaching 100% (48).

PLEOMORPHIC ADENOCARCINOMA (MALIGNANT MIXED TUMOR)

Approximately half of pleomorphic adenocarcinomas arise from benign lacrimal gland pleomorphic adenomas that have not been adequately removed at initial treatment. This transformation process emphasizes the necessity for complete removal of benign mixed tumors when initially encountered.

Patients are typically in their sixth decade of life and present with an acute onset of globe displacement. There may be a history of a previously excised benign pleomorphic tumor. In some patients, a long-standing orbital mass may show rapid enlargement due to malignant transformation within a previously stable benign mixed-cell tumor.

Management of pleomorphic adenocarcinoma depends on the presence or absence of bone involvement and whether the disease is localized or invasive. Bone involvement demands an extended exenteration, with bone removal. If the lesion is well circumscribed, with no evidence of bone or neuronal invasion, complete removal of the lesion is probably sufficient.

Patients with pleomorphic adenocarcinoma tend to have a much better prognosis than those with adenoid cystic carcinoma. Five-year survival approaches 70%, and 12-year survival approaches 50% (32). In Henderson and Farrow's series (49), tumor-related deaths continued to occur as long as 30 years after initial treatment.

MONOMORPHIC ADENOCARCINOMA

Monomorphic adenocarcinoma, an extremely uncommon tumor, is composed of malignant epithelial cells without mesenchymal elements. It tends to affect patients in the fifth decade of life (20). It metastasizes much earlier than does adenoid cystic carcinoma, accounting for its much poorer prognosis. Mortality approaches 100%, with a mean survival time of 1.5 years. Survival may be prolonged with extended exenteration and regional lymph node dissection.

MUCOEPIDERMOID CARCINOMA

Mucoepidermoid carcinoma is believed to arise from the duct epithelium of the lacrimal gland. It occurs commonly in the salivary glands but is rare in the lacrimal gland. Malignant grading is based on the degree of squamous differentiation and the amount of mucin production. Thus, histologic evaluation must include multiple sections for adequate diagnosis (1). Too few patients have been described to determine the best mode of therapy. It has been suggested that prognosis parallels the histologic grading and that for the more benign-appearing lesions, complete local excision may be sufficient. For the more aggressive lesions, exenteration with bone excision and adjunctive radiation therapy is more appropriate.

Secondary Tumors

Secondary orbital tumors are those that extend into the orbit by contiguous spread from adjacent anatomic regions. These tumors include intraocular tumors with extrascleral extension, such as malignant melanomas and retinoblastomas. Nasal and sinus tumors and those eroding through bone from the intracranial vault may also impinge on orbital structures. Eyelid tumors, especially after incomplete excision, may recur into the deep orbit along neurovascular pathways.

RETINOBLASTOMA

Retinoblastoma is the most common intraocular malignancy of the pediatric age group and the second most common intraocular malignancy (after choroidal malignant melanoma) in all age groups (50). Although this tumor is usually contained within the eye, extrascleral extension does occur, resulting in orbital involvement. Retinoblastoma arises from retinal sensory cells in young children, with an incidence of 1 in 14,000 to 1 in 20,000 live births. Approximately 250 new cases are reported each year in the United States. The average age at presentation is 18 months. Some 70% of cases are unilateral, and 30% are bilateral.

Orbital extension of retinoblastoma has been seen in 8% to 12% of cases (51,52). Other studies, however, reveal a much lower incidence of orbital involvement (53), most likely due to improvements in treatment. In developing countries, however, orbital involvement is still relatively common.

The genetics of retinoblastoma have been studied intensively (53). Perhaps 6% of cases have a positive family history for the disease; the other 94% are sporadic cases resulting from spontaneous mutations. The hereditary implications of retinoblastoma demand examination of asymptomatic family members and extensive genetic counseling.

The initial sign of the intraocular tumor is usually leukocoria, or a "white pupil." Children may also present with strabismus from amblyopia and with iris neovascularization. Neglected cases, as in many developing countries, may present with a reddish-black mass protruding from the orbit. Symptoms associated with orbital extension are variable and may be missed clinically if the lesion is small. With larger tumors along the optic nerve, proptosis and globe displacement are common. In orbital recurrences after enucleation, migration or extrusion of the implant may be seen.

The management of ocular retinoblastoma is well discussed in the literature (50). Extrascleral orbital involvement is a very poor prognostic indicator and carries a high incidence of intracranial spread and distant metastasis to bone. Management should include removal of as much of the orbital tumor as possible, followed by local radiation therapy if the orbit has not been irradiated previously for intraocular tumor. Chemotherapy is the mainstay of treatment for cases of metastatic or orbital disease or in cases of residual tumor at the transected optic nerve at the time of enucleation.

The presence of extrascleral extension of retinoblastoma is usually associated with distant metastasis and, therefore, carries a poor prognosis. Depending on the degree of orbital involvement, survival rates vary from 10% to 35% (52). There is an unusually high incidence of second primary malignancies in retinoblastoma patients (especially the inherited and bilateral types), which may occur years after treatment for the primary tumor (54). The incidence in bilateral retinoblastoma patients ranges from 10% to 15%. The majority are osteogenic sarcomas, which may develop in the orbit and elsewhere. These tumors were once thought to be secondary to radiation treatment but are now known to occur, like the initial retinoblastoma, because of a genetic predisposition. Once a second malignancy is diagnosed, the prognosis for survival is especially poor.

CHOROIDAL MALIGNANT MELANOMA

Malignant melanoma involving the orbit is unusual. Although primary melanomas have been described in the orbit, they are rare, and most tumors extend from the eye, nasal cavity, or paranasal sinuses. The vast majority arise from primary intraocular choroidal tumors that extend though scleral emissary canals or through the lamina cribrosa at the optic nerve head. In some cases, orbital recurrence may be seen years after enucleation of the eye (Fig. 31.17). Studies during the last century have determined the incidence of extraocular extension from primary choroidal lesions to be approximately 10%. Orbital involvement is the second most common site of malignant transformation associated with congenital oculodermal melanocytosis (55).

No universal management philosophy exists. As these tumors almost always extend from adjacent sites, patients are at high risk for metastatic disease. For orbital disease only, local excision with combined radiation therapy is appropriate, although these tumors are relatively radioresistant. Chemotherapy and immunotherapy have not proved to be of significant value.

SQUAMOUS CELL CARCINOMA

Squamous cell carcinoma is one of the most common secondary orbital malignancies (56). It typically invades the orbit from primary sites in the skin of the eyelids and forehead, nasolacrimal sac and bulbar conjunctiva, paranasal sinuses, and nasopharynx (Figs. 31.18, 31.19A). The initial presenting symptom is related to ophthalmologic problems in approximately 25% of patients. These include proptosis, diplopia, ptosis, a palpable mass, and epiphora. Patients usually will give a history of sur-

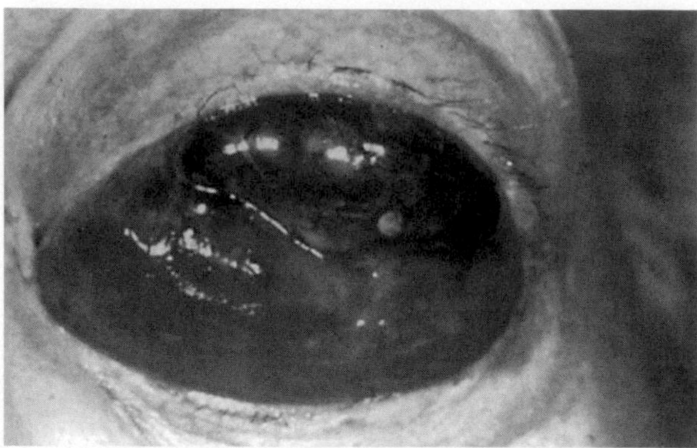

Figure 31.17 Recurrent orbital malignant melanoma in an 80-year-old woman several years after enucleation of the left eye for a choroidal melanoma.

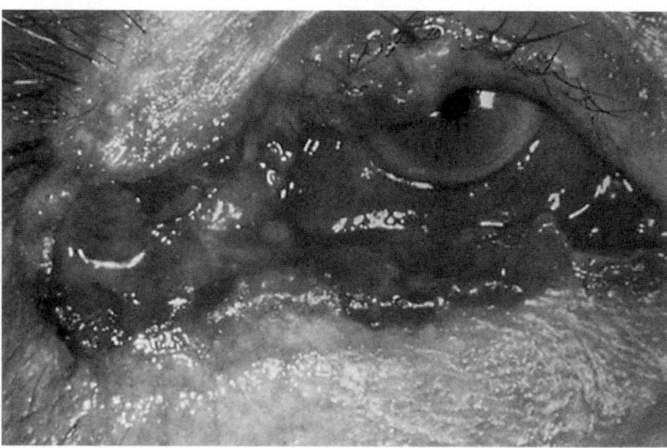

Figure 31.18 Squamous cell carcinoma of the right upper and lower eyelids with secondary orbital involvement.

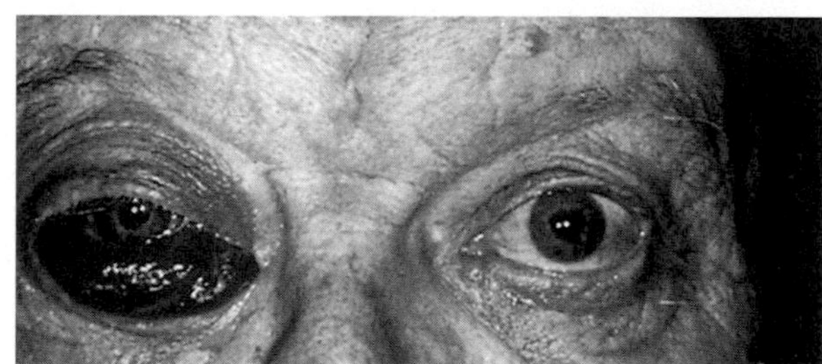

A

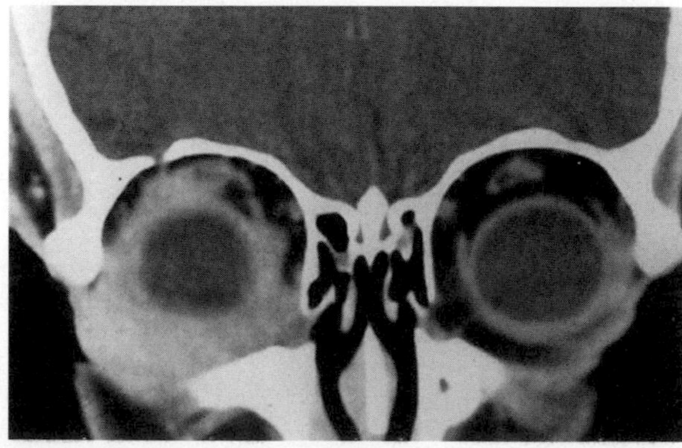

B

Figure 31.19 Squamous cell carcinoma. **A:** Squamous cell carcinoma arising in the maxillary sinus, with secondary involvement of the right orbit. **B:** Same patient as in Figure 31.10A. Coronal computed tomographic scan demonstrates extensive, diffuse orbital invasion by tumor.

gery for a cutaneous malignancy on the face. Orbital extension is more likely in cases where the original defect was covered by a thick myocutaneous flap. Computed tomography is essential for evaluating the extent of tumor invasion, sinus involvement, and possible intracranial extension (Fig. 31.19B). Occult bone involvement may be present even without evidence on CT scan.

Treatment outcome depends on a number of factors: tumor extent at the time of presentation, diffuse involvement of orbital structures, and the presence of bony or neuronal invasion. Cellular differentiation is also important, with the more anaplastic tumors having a higher propensity for aggressiveness.

Nasal and paranasal tumors are managed with extensive resection, including bone removal if necessary. Surgical intervention is also the mainstay of treatment for tumors originating from the eyelids, lacrimal sac, and epibulbar region. Orbital bone involvement is common in both of these subtypes, and orbitectomy should be anticipated in the management process. Despite aggressive therapy, tumor-related mortality is near 60%.

BASAL CELL CARCINOMA

Basal cell carcinoma is the most common eyelid neoplasm, representing 85% of all tumors of the periocular region (57). Orbital invasion is rare and usually occurs after a number of unsuccessful surgical resections to eliminate the primary lesion on the eyelids or face. Patients are typically in their seventh decade or older. Presentation is often with a painless, slowly growing mass fixed to underlying bone at the orbital rim. Depending on the degree of orbital invasion, proptosis and motility restriction may be prominent features. Computed tomography scanning may demonstrate an infiltrative mass extending along the orbital walls, extraocular muscles, and around the globe.

Treatment of orbital basal cell carcinoma is aimed at surgical extirpation of the tumor. The adjacent sinuses and intracranial vault may be involved, so orbital exenteration with concomitant removal of involved bone should be approached with a multidisciplinary team. Vascularized muscle flaps can be placed over the surgical defect to aid in later reconstruction, but such techniques may obscure further recurrences. Supplemental radiation therapy is helpful if the lesion is too extensive to be completely resected (58). Additional therapeutic modalities include 5-fluorouracil application and cisplatin, both of which may aid in tumor shrinkage before surgical removal or as a supplement to it (59). Long-term follow-up is necessary to determine adequacy of treatment.

SEBACEOUS CELL CARCINOMA

Sebaceous carcinoma is a rare tumor of the eyelids arising from the meibomian glands or accessory lacrimal glands. Orbital extension from a periorbital primary location is rare (60). More commonly, these tumors spread to regional preauricular lymph nodes. Metastatic spread occurs in a high percentage of patients. When orbital extension is seen, local resection of involved tissues is necessary if neither metastatic disease nor lymph node involvement is present. Skip lesions are common on histopathology, so wide margins of normal tissue are required.

ESTHESIONEUROBLASTOMA (OLFACTORY NEUROBLASTOMA)

Esthesioneuroblastoma is a neurogenic malignant tumor that arises from sensory epithelium in the olfactory placode. It generally presents with nasal and sinus involvement, although 13% of patients may initially present with orbital symptoms from direct orbital invasion. Overall, more than 50% of patients have some orbital involvement at initial diagnosis (61).

This tumor has a predilection for older patients, with a mean age at presentation of 40 years. Early symptoms of nasal stuffiness, discharge, epistaxis, and cerebrospinal fluid rhinorrhea bring the patient to medical attention. Ophthalmic manifestations occur later and include orbital pain, proptosis, blurred vision, and diplopia. Diagnosis can usually be made by direct nasal examination and biopsy. Magnetic resonance imaging is the single best test for demonstrating the deep extent of disease in the nose, orbit, and intracranial compartment.

Treatment options are predominantly surgical, with supplemental radiation therapy. Staging is determined according to the extent of tumor at initial presentation. Patients in stage A have tumor confined to the nasal passages, stage B patients have tumor involving the paranasal sinuses, and stage C patients have tumor extending beyond the nasal cavity and paranasal sinuses. Patients with orbital involvement fall into the stage C category and have a 5-year survival of 46.7% (62). Clinical course is often marked by extended remissions and recurrences, which can occur as late as 29 years after a remission (63).

CHORDOMA

Chordomas are rare malignancies that arise from cephalic remnants of the embryonic notochord in the region of the clivus and dorsum sella (64). Growth is slow and relentless, and they frequently result in compression of the optic chiasm and nerves to the extraocular muscles. They may extend anteriorly into the nasal cavity and orbit, producing a mass effect on structures in the orbital apex. Chordomas tend to invade and destroy the involved bone. Management is surgical, although complete removal may be difficult, owing to the tumor's poorly accessible location and diffuse growth pattern. Adjunctive radiation therapy has been used in some instances with success. These tumors tend to be slow-growing, and survival may be prolonged, especially with anteriorly situated tumors. However, the morbidity associated with orbital involvement (blindness and pain) can often diminish the patient's quality of life (65). Metastasis is quite rare.

Metastatic Tumors

Metastatic tumors to the orbit represent some 2% to 3% of all orbital mass lesions (1,20). In adults, carcinomas represent 86% of metastatic tumors, with neuroblastomas, malignant melanomas, and other sarcomas comprising the rest. In children, orbital metastases derive mainly from sarcomas and neural tumors. Metastases to the orbit arrive by hematogenous spread and usually represent a poor prognostic development. In 30% to 60% of cases, the orbital lesion may be the first indication of systemic disease (66,67). In nearly 5% of cases, orbital metastases may be bilateral.

Manifestations of orbital metastases are myriad. Most commonly, patients present with rapidly progressive proptosis, diplopia, pain, ptosis, chemosis, and loss of vision. Other symptoms may include lacrimal drainage dysfunction, eyelid edema, and eyelid retraction. Enophthalmos may be associated with scirrhous breast carcinoma, owing to fibrotic changes along the orbital fascial systems.

BREAST CARCINOMA

Breast carcinoma is by far the most common cause of metastatic disease in the orbit, representing 37% to 51% of all such lesions (20,67,68). The average age of patients on presentation is 40 to 60 years. An interval of 2 to 5 years may exist between the diagnosis and treatment of the breast cancer and the appearance of orbital metastases. Although metastases to the choroid are more

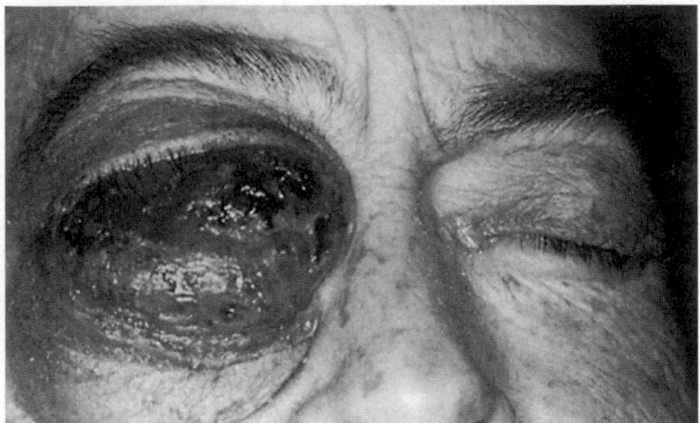

Figure 31.20 Metastatic breast carcinoma to the right orbit.

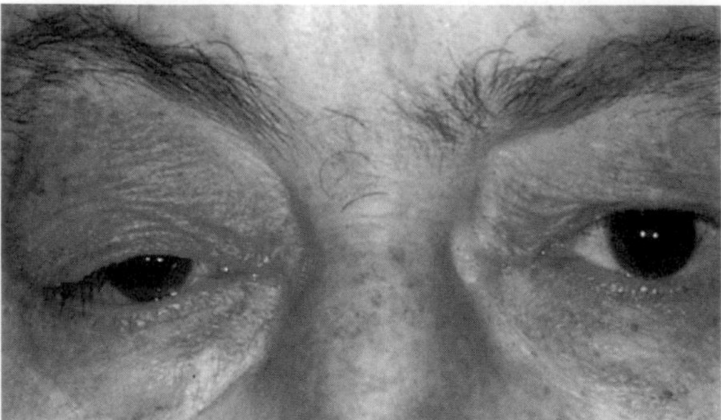

Figure 31.22 Metastatic lung adenocarcinoma involving the right orbit. Note ptosis of upper eyelid.

common, occasionally these patients present with proptosis and displacement of the globe. In neglected cases, tumor may fill the orbit (Fig. 31.20). Uncertainty in diagnosis can be aided by fine-needle aspiration biopsy of the orbital mass. Computed tomography usually shows an infiltrative lesion with molding around orbital structures (Fig. 31.21). Tumors may involve the extraocular muscles with fusiform enlargement. Bone destruction is rare.

Surgical intervention in the case of metastatic breast cancer is not warranted. Intractable pain may be treated with limited resection for palliation only. Management should include hormonal therapy or chemotherapy, combined with local radiation therapy of 3,000 to 4,000 cGy to the orbit. Orbital metastases are part of more widespread metastatic disease; thus, the prognosis is usually poor. The average survival for these patients is 21 months (69).

LUNG CARCINOMA

Carcinoma of the lung is the most common source of orbital metastases in men and lags only behind breast cancer in overall incidence. It tends to occur at a younger age than metastatic breast cancer and has a more fulminant and aggressive course, often with significant inflammatory components. This contrasts to the more gradual presentation of metastases from breast cancer. Unlike metastatic breast cancer, bronchogenic orbital metastases frequently appear before the diagnosis of the primary disease (69). Suspicion for this tumor should be high in any male patient with rapidly progressive proptosis, especially if a history of heavy smoking is elicited (Fig. 31.22). Fine-needle aspiration or open biopsy and a chest x-ray are indicated.

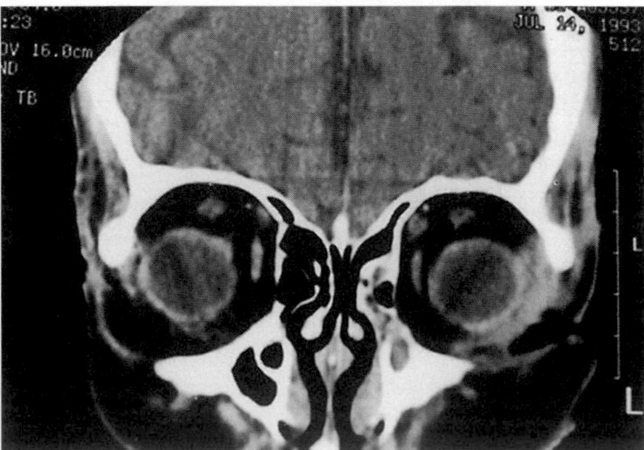

Figure 31.21 Coronal computed tomographic scan demonstrating left lateral orbital involvement by metastatic breast adenocarcinoma.

As with other metastases, surgical intervention is not warranted. In general, prognosis is poor. Bronchogenic carcinoma tends not to respond well to chemotherapy, and radiation therapy is used primarily for palliation of orbital pain. On average, life expectancy after orbital metastases is 9 months. Oat-cell carcinoma (small-cell carcinoma) may be responsive to chemotherapeutic regimens, so biopsy of the lesion is recommended for planning treatment. Both vision and life expectancy may be prolonged in these instances (70).

PROSTATE CANCER

Patients with orbital metastatic prostate cancer tend to be elderly men. The disease is the third most common carcinoma to metastasize to the orbit and occurs in patients with a known history of prostatic cancer in perhaps half of cases. Bone involvement is more common than with breast or lung metastases, which explains the more severe pain associated with this lesion (20). Computed tomography scan often reveals osteoblastic alterations in orbital bones, which can simulate a sphenoid wing meningioma. Diagnosis is aided by serum prostate-specific antigen and by immunostaining of biopsy-proved tissue with prostate-specific antigen. Hormonal therapy with diethylstilbestrol may be effective in up to 80% of patients. Orchiectomy and local radiation therapy may be helpful in those patients who fail other treatment. The 5-year survival rate for patients who develop orbital metastases is 25% (71).

RENAL CELL CARCINOMA

Renal cell carcinoma shows a predilection for adult men. Orbital metastases may present before any obvious primary disease (72) and, in 25% of patients, orbital metastases were present at the time of initial diagnosis of the renal carcinoma (27). Presentation is more insidious than for other orbital metastases (20). Renal cell carcinomas tend to be highly vascular lesions that bleed easily and can involve both soft tissues and bone. If the tumor is well defined and there is no other evidence of metastasis, local excision may be attempted (73). In other cases, radiation therapy and chemotherapy are appropriate.

METASTATIC NEUROBLASTOMA

Metastatic neuroblastoma is the most important metastatic tumor to the orbit in childhood. It is a malignant neoplasm of primitive neuroblasts arising most often in the adrenal gland or (less commonly) in the autonomic tissues of the mediastinum or sympathetic cervical ganglia. It is the second most common orbital tumor in children after rhabdomyosarcoma. In almost all cases (97%), the primary tumor is known before orbital metastases are diagnosed (74).

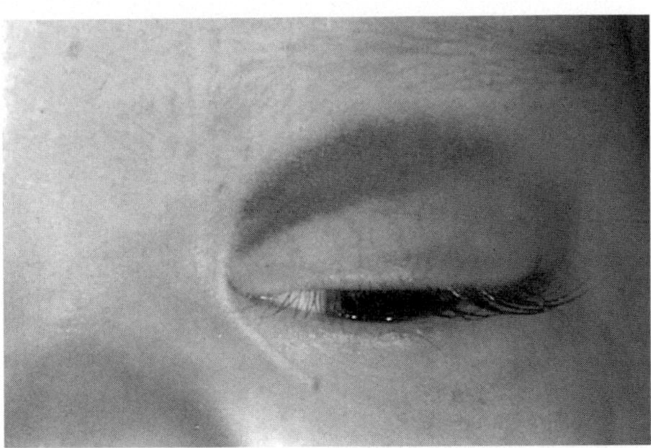

Figure 31.23 Metastatic neuroblastoma to the left orbit in a child, with ecchymosis of the left upper eyelid.

Children present with an abrupt onset of proptosis, frequently associated with eyelid ecchymoses (Fig. 31.23). In 20% to 55% of cases, the orbital lesions are bilateral (75). Most cases show signs of systemic disease. Intracranial metastases may be present with increased intracranial pressure, and bony metastases may also be present.

The management of metastatic neuroblastoma involves chemotherapy and radiation therapy. Prognosis is generally poor, with 3-year survival rates of perhaps 11% (20).

METASTATIC WILMS TUMOR

Wilms tumor is a rare neoplasm that is believed to arise from mesodermal cells in the developing kidney and retains the ability to differentiate into a variety or tissues (76). It occurs in young children in a range from birth to 5 years of age. Rapidly progressive proptosis and displacement of the globe are seen, often with ecchymosis of the eyelids and conjunctiva. Invasion of orbital bone, paranasal sinuses, and the cranial cavity is common. Treatment consists of local radiation therapy and systemic chemotherapy. Most patients also have other widespread metastases, and the prognosis is usually poor.

RADIOLOGIC IMAGING CONCERNS

Bernard B. O'Malley

Imaging of the orbits is performed for primary ocular disorders (Fig. 31.24), primary orbital disorders, and regional disorders that involve the orbits secondarily (Fig. 31.25). Primary ocular disorders are not within the scope of this chapter, and secondary involvement is discussed in Chapters 21 and 22. Imaging of the orbit and adjacent compartments is readily performed with CT or MRI. Orbital fat provides an excellent background against which disease is confidently outlined and staged. Magnetic resonance imaging allows direct acquisition of any plane through the orbit (Fig. 31.26) and is more sensitive to extension of disease to the cavernous sinus. Computed tomography shows bone changes directly and, when properly planned, can be reformatted in the same variety of planes available with MRI. Streak artifact causes minor problems in patients with permanent dental work. Field distortion from dental work can seriously compromise the fat-suppressed T2 and contrast T1 sequences.

Because of the profound cosmetic and functional impact of orbital exenteration, a prime role of imaging is to exclude the possibility of pseudotumor, lymphoma, and vascular lesions that may be managed nonsurgically or angiographically. Benign causes of proptosis, such as thyroid orbitopathy (Fig. 31.27) and carotid cavernous fistulae, can also be confirmed with imaging. Some benign tumors involving the orbit (Fig. 31.28) should not commit the patient to radical resection or ablative treatment until the pathologic diagnosis is made.

In the pediatric age group, soft tissue sarcoma is the leading type of orbital mass seen at referral centers. Accurate baseline imaging examinations are essential. Treatment portals for external beam irradiation after initial chemotherapy are planned from the original extent of disease assessment. *En bloc* surgical margins are planned from the same images.

Three-dimensional renderings contribute to complex conformal radiation therapy portals and coordination of multiple surgical teams when necessary. Despite the orbit's osseous barriers, the most important margin to image is the orbital fissure (Fig. 31.29) along which disease can spread prior to frank extraorbital extension. This is best evaluated in the direct coronal plane. Homogeneous fat suppression must be achieved if contrast or fast T2-weighted series are performed. Although the orbital fissures are well evaluated with CT (in patients who can be positioned), the next deeper compartment of spread, the cavernous sinus, is better evaluated with MRI. The cavernous sinus is challenging to image by any modality. High signal from intervening fat and alternating low and high signal within the venous channels provide a complex background against which tumor should be documented prior to overt cranial neuropathy. Furthermore, susceptibility from the air and bone interface varies with the development of the sphenoid sinus.

Both MRI and CT demonstrate perineural disease extending along the second, and less commonly, first divisions of the first nerve. Suspicious neural enhancement on MRI (Fig. 31.30) more often precedes clinically apparent symptoms than when it is shown by CT. Magnetic resonance imaging also is more sensitive for optic nerve abnormalities related to treatment injury, which is helpful when visual decline raises the specter of possible recurrent tumor (Fig. 31.31).

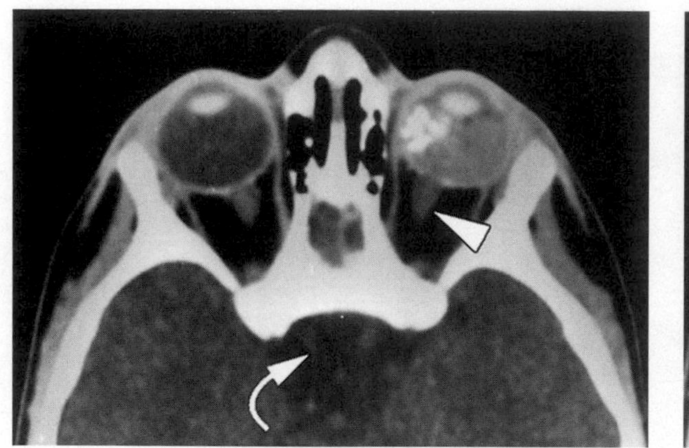

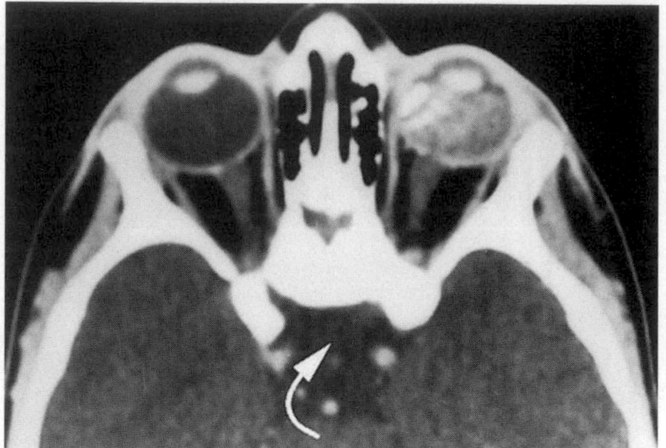

Figure 31.24 Retinoblastoma. Precontrast **(A)** axial computed tomographic view at midorbit, showing a bulky, hyperdense, partially calcified mass filling the left globe with moderate enhancement on the post-contrast **(B)** view. No evidence of optic nerve (*arrowhead) or chiasmic extension* (*curved arrow*).

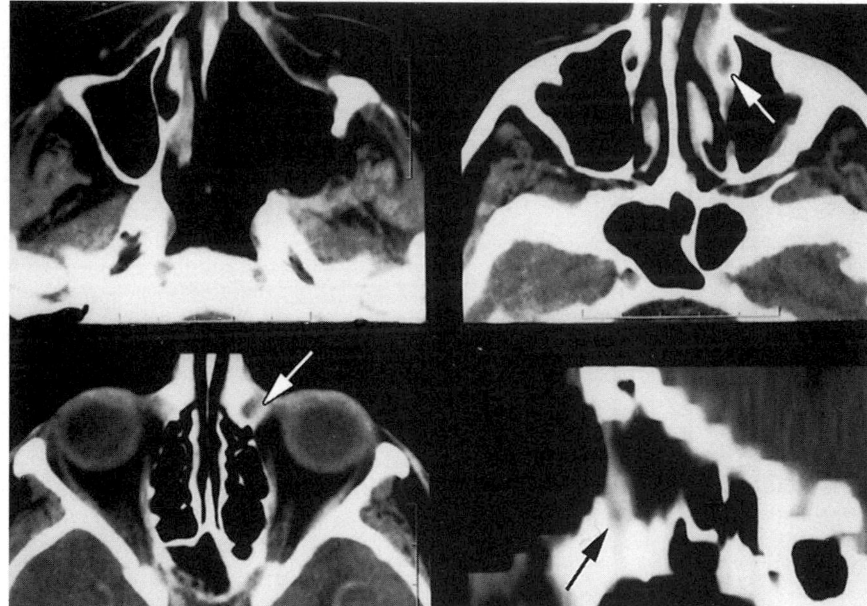

Figure 31.25 Lacrimal extension. Serial enhanced axial computed tomographic and parasagittal reformatted computed tomographic (bottom right) views of upward extension (*arrows*) of adenoid cystic carcinoma after prior maxillectomy for a primary lesion of the palate.

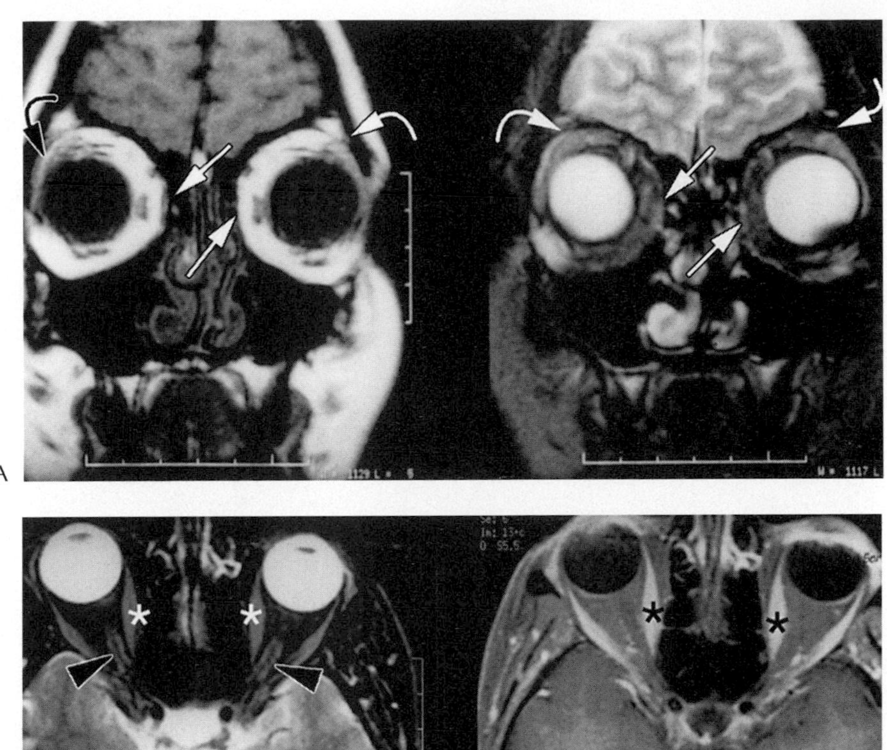

Figure 31.26 Normal magnetic resonance imaging of orbits. Coronal (**A**) T1 (left) and T2 (right) views through posterior globes and axial (**B**) fat-suppressed T2 (left) and T1 (right) views at level of lens. Orbital fat provides excellent contrast for orbital contents on T1 views and both fat-suppressed T2 and contrast T1 views. Note extraocular muscles (*asterisk*), optic nerve sheath (*arrowheads*), lamina papyracea (*arrows*), and lacrimal gland (*curved arrows*).

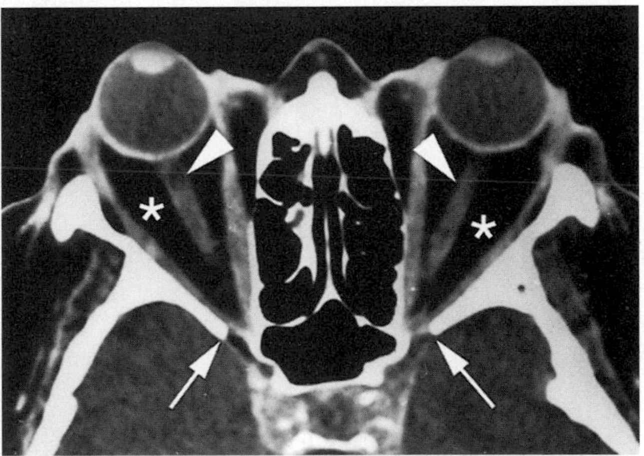

Figure 31.27 Proptosis. Fnhanced axial computed tomography at midorbit shows symmetric bilateral proptosis due to increased orbital fat content (*asterisk*), with mild stretching of optic nerves (*arrowheads*) without prolapse at the superior fissures (*arrows*).

A

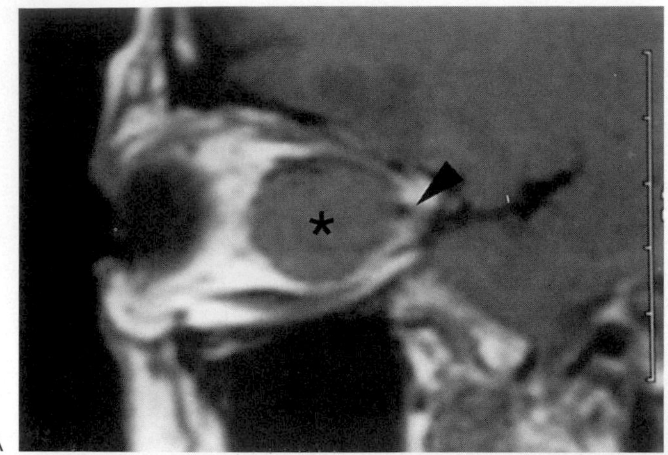

B

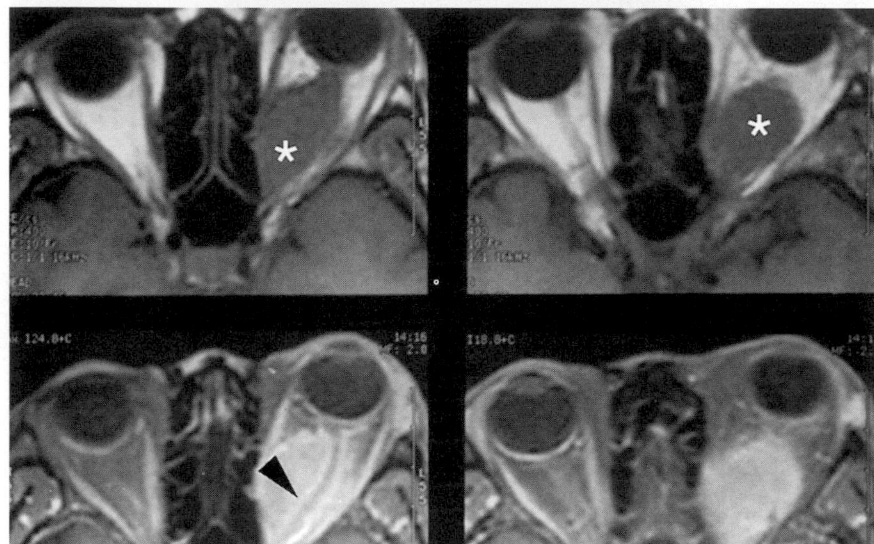

Figure 31.28 Meningioma. Sagittal T1 **(A)** and matched **(B)** axial T1 (top) and fat-suppressed contrast (bottom) axial T1 views show a large, well-circumscribed mass (*asterisk*) surrounding the optic nerve (*arrowheads*), causing mild proptosis.

A

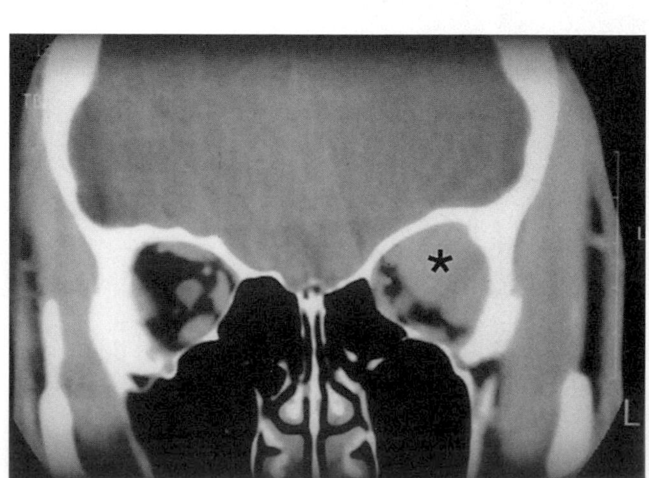

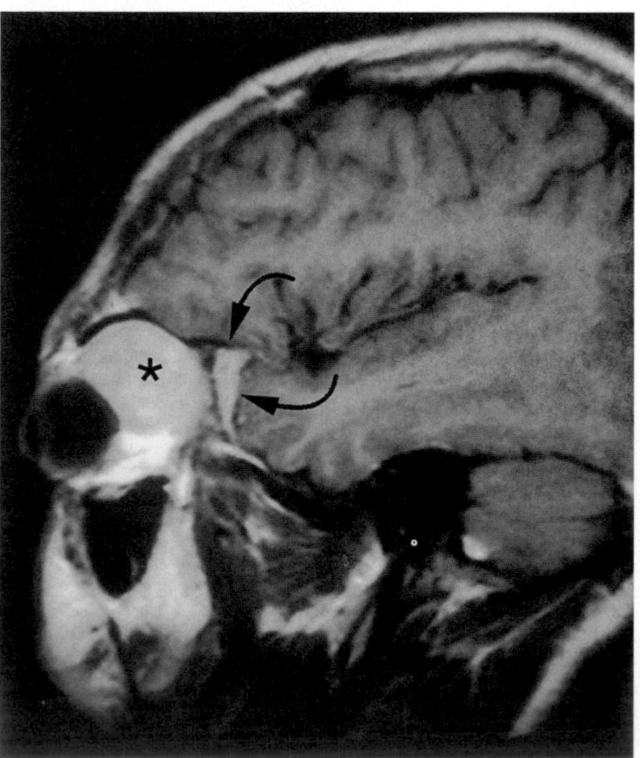

B

Figure 31.29 Lacrimal gland mass. Direct coronal computed tomography **(A)** and parasagittal contrast T1 magnetic resonance imaging **(B)** show a large adenoid cystic carcinoma of the lacrimal gland (*asterisk*) with early intracranial and extradural extension (*curved arrows*) through the superior fissure.

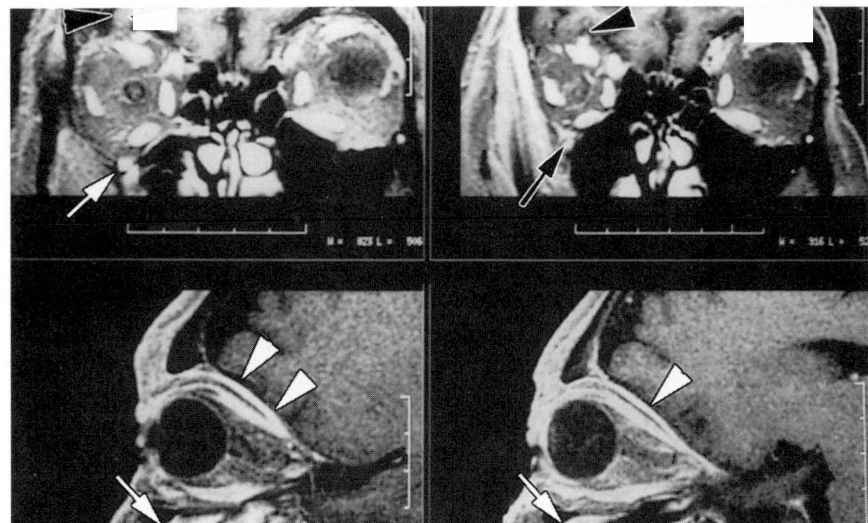

Figure 31.30 Neurotropic orbital extension. Fat-suppressed contrast coronal (top) and sagittal T1 (bottom) views of orbits show enhancing thickening of both the first (*arrowheads*) and second (*arrows*) divisions of cranial nerve V resulting from recurrent skin cancer at the medial canthus.

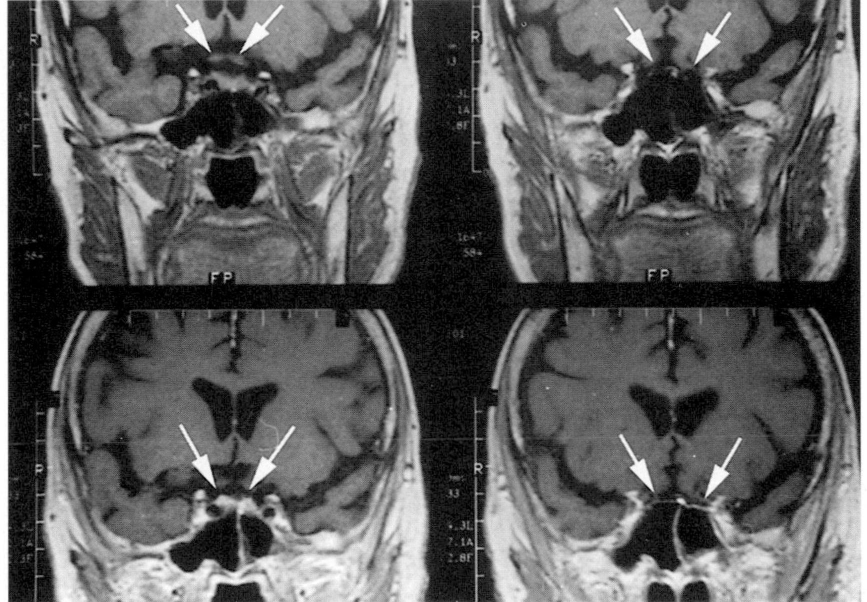

A

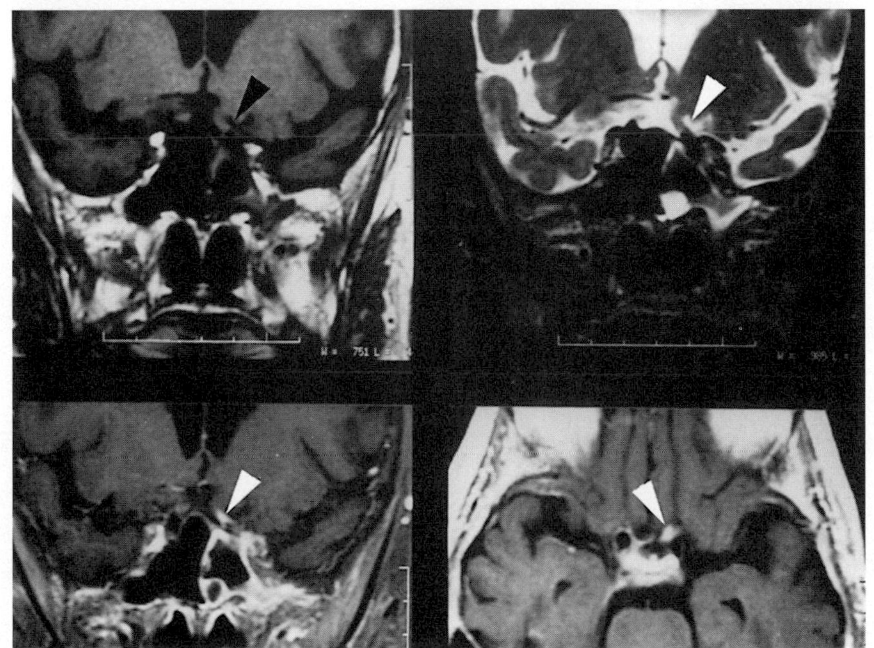

B

Figure 31.31 Optic neuritis. **A:** Pretreatment-matched coronal T1, precontrast (top) and postcontrast (right) views show normal optic nerves (*arrows*). **B:** Posttreatment collage of same patient showing pathologic enhancement of left optic nerve (*arrowheads*) within radiation portal. Clockwise from top left: Coronal T1, T2, contrast axial T1, and contrast coronal T1 views.

REFERENCES

1. Rootman J. *Diseases of the orbit: a multidisciplinary approach.* Philadelphia: JB Lippincott Co, 1988:628.
2. Dutton JJ. *Atlas of clinical and surgical orbital anatomy.* Philadelphia: WB Saunders, 1994:240.
3. Dutton JJ. *Atlas of ophthalmic surgery: oculoplastic, lacrimal and orbital surgery.* Vol 2. St. Louis: Mosby-Year Book, 1992:342.
4. Levin PS, Dutton JJ. A 20-year series of orbital exenteration. *Am J Ophthalmol* 1991;112:496.
5. Kennerdell JS, Slamovits TL, Dekker A, et al. Orbital fine-needle aspiration biopsy. *Am J Ophthalmol* 1985;99:547.
6. Liu D. Complications of fine-needle aspiration biopsy of the orbit. *Ophthalmology* 1985;92:1768.
7. Henderson JW, Farrow GM. *Orbital tumors.* New York: B. C. Decker (Thieme-Stratton), 1980.
8. American Joint Committee on Cancer. *Manual for staging of cancer,* 4th ed. Philadelphia: JB Lippincott Co, 1992.
9. Tefft M, Linberg R, Gehan E (for the Intergroup Rhabdomyosarcoma Study). Radiation of rhabdomyosarcoma in children combined with systemic chemotherapy. Local control in patients enrolled into the Intergroup Rhabdomyosarcoma Study (IRS). *Natl Cancer Inst Monogr* 1981;56:75.
10. Spaeth EB, Valders-Dapena A. Hemangiopericytoma. *Arch Ophthalmol* 1985; 60:1070.
11. Henderson JW. Vascular hamartomas, hyperplasias, and neoplasms. In: Henderson JW, ed. *Orbital tumors.* New York: Raven Press, 1994:100.
12. Croxatto JO, Font RI. Hemangiopericytoma of the orbit: a clinicopathologic study of 30 cases. *Hum Pathol* 1982;13:210.
13. Hufnagel T, Ma L, Kuo TT. Orbital angiosarcoma with subconjunctival presentation. *Ophthalmology* 1987;94:72.
14. Lyons CJ, McNab AA, Garner A, et al. Orbital malignant peripheral nerve sheath tumors. *Br J Ophthalmolv 1989;73:731.*
15. Dutton JJ. Gliomas of the anterior visual pathway. *Surv Ophthalmol* 1994;38: 427.
16. Abramson DH, Ronner HJ, Ellsworth R. Second tumors in non-irradiated bilateral retinoblastoma. *Am J Ophthalmol* 1979;87:634.
17. Dryja TP, Rapaport JM, Epstein J, et al. Chromosome 13 homozygosity in osteosarcoma without retinoblastoma. *Am J Hum Genet* 1986;38:59.
18. Rootman J, Chan KW. Osteogenic sarcoma. In: Rootman J, ed. *Diseases of the orbit: a multidisciplinary approach.* Philadelphia: JB Lippincott Co, 1988:379.
19. Holland MG, Allen JH, Ichinose H. Chondrosarcoma of the orbit. *Trans Am Acad Ophthalmol Otolaryngol* 1961;65:898.
20. Shields JA. *Diagnosis and management of orbital tumors.* Philadelphia: WB Saunders, 1989.
21. Finn DG, Goepfert H, Batsakis JG. Chondrosarcoma of the head and neck. *Laryngoscope* 1984;94:1534.
22. Coley B, Higinbotham NL, Bowden L. Endothelioma of bone (Ewing's sarcoma). *Ann Surg* 1948;128:533.
23. Ewing J. Diffuse endothelioma of bone. *Proc NY Pathol Soc* 1921;21:17.
24. Senac MOJ, Isaacs H, Gwinn JL. Primary lesions of bone in the 1st decade of life: retrospective survey of biopsy results. *Pediatr Radial* 1986;160:491.
25. Wilkins RM, Pritchard DJ, Burgett EOJ, et al. Ewing's sarcoma of bone: experience with 140 patients. *Cancer* 1986;58:2551.
26. Huvos AG. *Bone tumors: diagnosis, treatment and prognosis,* 2nd ed. Philadelphia: WB Saunders, 1991.
27. Ochsner MG. Renal cell carcinoma: 5-year follow-up study of 70 cases. *J Urol* 1965;93:361.
28. Milburn LF, O'Grady L, Hendrickson FR. Radical radiation therapy and total body irradiation in the treatment of Ewing's sarcoma. *Cancer* 1968;22:919.
29. McNab AA, Moseley I. Primary orbital liposarcoma: clinical and computed tomographic features. *Br J Ophthalmol* 1990;74:437.
30. Falk S, Alpert M. Five year survival of patients with Ewing's sarcoma. *Surg Gynecol Obstet* 1967;124:319.
31. Freeman AI, Sachatello C, Gaeta J, et al. An analysis of Ewing's tumor in children at Roswell Park Memorial Institute. *Cancer* 1972;29:1563.
32. Johnson RE, Pomeroy TC. Integrated therapy for Ewing's sarcoma. *Am J Roentgenol* 1972;114:532.
33. Suit HD. Ewing's sarcoma-treatment by radiation therapy. In: *Tumors of bone and soft tissues.* Chicago: Year Book Medical Publishers, 1965:191.
34. Fernandez CH, Linberg RD, Sutow WW, et al. Localized Ewing's sarcoma: treatment and results. *Cancer* 1974;34:143.
35. Knowles DMI, Jakobiec FA, Potter GD, et al. Ophthalmic striated muscle neoplasms. *Surv Ophthalmol* 1976;21:219.
36. Jones IS, Reese AB, Kraut J. Orbital rhabdomyosarcoma. *Am J Ophthalmol* 1966; 61:721.
37. Porterfield JF, Zimmerman LE. Rhabdomyosarcoma of the orbit. *Virchows Arch Pathol Anat* 1962;335:329.
38. Wharam M, Beltangady M, Hays D, et al. Localized orbital rhabdomyosarcoma. *Ophthalmology* 1987;94:251.
39. Font RL, Jurco SI, Brechner RJ. Postradiation leiomyosarcoma of the orbit complicating bilateral retinoblastoma. *Arch Ophthalmol* 1983;101:1557.
40. Meekins B, Dutton JJ, Praia AD. Primitive orbital leiomyosarcoma: a case report and review of the literature. *Arch Ophthalmol* 1988;106:82.
41. Quéré MA, Camin R, Baylet R. Liposarcome orbitaire. *Ann Ocul (Paris)* 1963;196:994.
42. Tewfik HH, Tewfik FA, Latourette HB. Postirradiation malignant fibrous histiocytoma. *J Surg Oncol* 1981;16:199.
43. Font RL, Hidayat AA. Fibrous histiocytoma of the orbit: a clinicopathologic study of 150 cases. *Hum Pathol* 1982;13:199.
44. Dutton JJ, Byrne SF, Proia AD. *Diagnostic atlas of orbital diseases.* Philadelphia: WB Saunders, 1994:88.
45. Dutton JJ, Byrne SF, Proia AD. *Diagnostic atlas of orbital diseases.* Philadelphia: WB Saunders, 1994:128.
46. Font RL, Gamel JW. Epithelial tumors of the lacrimal gland: an analysis of 265 cases. In: Jakobiec FA, ed. *Ocular and adnexal tumors.* Birmingham, AL: Aesculapius Publishing, 1978.
47. Broders AC. Carcinoma: grading and practical applications. *Arch Pathol* 1926; 2:376.
48. Gamel JW, Font RL. Adenoid cystic carcinoma of the lacrimal gland: the clinical significance of a basaloid histologic pattern. *Hum Pathol* 1982;13:219.
49. Henderson JW, Farrow GM. Primary malignant mixed tumors of the lacrimal gland: report of 10 cases. *Ophthalmology* 1980;87:466.
50. Shields JA, Augsburger JJ. Current approaches to the diagnosis and management of retinoblastoma. *Surv Ophthalmol* 1981;25:347.
51. Ellsworth RM. Orbital retinoblastoma. *Trans Am Ophthalmol Soc* 1974;72:79.
52. Rootman J, Hofbauer J, Ellsworth RM, et al. Invasion of the optic nerve by retinoblastoma: a clinicopathologic study. *Can J Ophthalmol* 1976;11:106.
53. Sorsby A. Bilateral retinoblastoma: a dominantly inherited affliction. *BMJ* 1972;2:580.
54. Roarty JD, McLean IW, Zimmerman LE. Incidence of second neoplasms in patients with bilateral retinoblastoma. *Ophthalmology* 1988;95:1583.
55. Dutton JJ, Anderson RL, Schelper RL, et al. Orbital malignant melanoma and oculodermal melanocytosis: report of two cases and review of the literature. *Ophthalmology* 1984;91:497.
56. Henderson JW. Secondary epithelial neoplasms. In: Henderson JW, ed. *Orbital tumors.* New York: Raven Press, 1994:343.
57. Hollander MJ, Krogh FJ. Cancer of the eyelids. *Am J Ophthalmol* 1944;27:244.
58. Anscher M, Montano G, Dutton JJ. Management of periocular basal cell carcinoma: Molts' micrographic surgery versus radiotherapy. II, III. *Surv Ophthalmol* 1993;38:193.
59. Ryan RE, Marks M, W. Topical 5-fluorouracil in the treatment of carcinoma of the nasal floor and nasal alae. *Ann Plast Surg* 1988;20:48.
60. Doxanas MT, Green WR. Sebaceous gland carcinoma: review of 40 cases. *Arch Ophthalmol* 1984;102:245.
61. Rakes SM, Yeatts RP, Campbell RJ. Ophthalmic manifestations of esthesioneuroblastoma. *Ophthalmology* 1985;92:1749.
62. Elkon D, Hightower SI, Lim ML, et al. Esthesioneuroblastoma. *Cancer* 1979;44:1087.
63. Johnson LN, Krohel GB, Yeon EB, et al. Sinus tumors invading the orbit. *Ophthalmology* 1984;91:209.
64. Unni KK. *Dahlin's tumors: general aspects of data on 11,087 cases,* 5th ed. Philadelphia: Lippincott-Raven, 1996.
65. Henderson JW. Tumors of orbital bone. In: Henderson JW, ed. *Orbital tumors.* New York: Raven Press, 1994:182.
66. Font RL, Ferry AP. Carcinoma metastatic to the eye and orbit. III. A clinicopathologic study of 28 cases metastatic to the orbit. *Cancer* 1976;38:1326.
67. Henderson JW. Metastatic carcinomas. In: Henderson JW, ed. *Orbital tumors.* New York: Raven Press, 1994:361.
68. Rootman J. Metastatic and secondary tumors of the orbit. In: Rootman J, ed. *Diseases of the orbit.* Philadelphia: JB Lippincott Co, 1988:405.
69. Shields CL, Shields JA, Peggs M. Metastatic tumors to the orbit. *Ophthal Reconstr Plast Surg* 1988;4:73.
70. Hussein AM, Fenn LG. Tumor lysis syndrome after induction chemotherapy in small cell lung carcinoma. *Am J Clin Oncol* 1989;13:10.
71. Boldt HC, Nerad JA. Orbital metastasis from prostate carcinoma. *Arch Ophthalmol* 1988;106:1403.
72. Kinderman WR, Shields JA, Eiferman RA, et al. Metastatic renal cell carcinoma to the eye and adnexa: a report of 3 cases and review of the literature. *Ophthalmology* 1982;88:1347.
73. Houghton JD. Solitary metastasis of renal cell carcinoma. *Am J Ophthalmol* 1956;41:548.
74. Albert DM, Rubenstein RA, Scheie HG. Tumor metastases to the eye. II. Clinical studies in infants and children. *Am J Ophthalmol* 1967;63:727.
75. Traboulsi EL Shammas IV, Massad M, et al. Ophthalmological aspects of metastatic neuroblastoma: report of 22 consecutive cases. *Orbit* 1984;3:247.
76. Anderson WAD, Scotti TM. *Synopsis of pathology.* St. Louis: CV Mosby, 1980.

CHAPTER 32

Cancer of the Orbit and Ocular Structures

Radiation Therapy and Management

Jorge E. Freire, Luther W. Brady, Lydia T. Komarnicky, Jerry A. Shields, and Carol L. Shields

Intraocular and orbital tumors are rarely seen in medical or ophthalmologic practice, and most patients with such tumors are referred to specialized ocular oncology centers for more accurate diagnosis and management that often includes a multimodality of treatment options such as surgery, chemotherapy, radiotherapy, cryosurgery, photocoagulation, and thermotherapy, among others.

The scope of this chapter is to outline concepts and applications of radiotherapy as one of the therapeutic modalities in the management of a variety of intraocular and orbital tumors.

ANATOMY

A brief review of the anatomy of the eye and orbit is necessary before describing the different tumors and treatment modalities.

The eye is composed of three coats, or tunicae. The outer coat consists of the cornea, located anteriorly, and the sclera, a fibrous layer that occupies four-fifths of its extension. The middle layer is the uvea, a highly vascularized coat that is formed by the choroid, ciliary body, and iris.

The innermost layer, consisting of the retina and its analogs, is the sensory layer. This coat extends from the ora serrata retinae anteriorly to the optic nerve posteriorly. The vascular supply to the posterior half of the retina derives from the central retinal artery that enters the globe through the optic nerve. The anterior half of the retina derives its blood supply from the uveal tract. The lens is suspended from the ciliary body and is posterior to the iris.

The iris divides the anterior segment of the eye in two chambers: the anterior chamber located anterior to the iris and the posterior wall of the cornea and the posterior chamber situated posterior to the iris and the anterior aspect of the lens. Both chambers are connected through the pupil which is a round, central hole in the iris. The aqueous humor circulates from the posterior to the anterior chamber and drains into the Schlemm canal. The vitreous humor fills the eye and provides support and protects the retina.

The orbit consists of two parts: the bony and the soft tissue components. The bony orbit is a cone-shaped cavity formed by seven bones: frontal, ethmoid, sphenoid, palatine, zygomatic, lacrimal, and maxillary. The cavity is pyramidal with four walls, the base that corresponds to the anterior orbital rim, and

TABLE 32.1 Current Approaches in Diagnosis of Intraocular Tumors

History
Medical evaluation
Examination of opposite eye
Indirect ophthalmoscopy
Transillumination
Fundus photography
Fluorescein angiography
Visual field examination
Ultrasonography
Computed tomography
Magnetic resonance imaging
Biopsy
p32 testing

the apex that corresponds to the optic foramen. The depth is approximately 45 mm; the height at the anterior border is 35 mm; and the horizontal width is 40 mm. The entire orbital cavity is lined by the periosteum.

Six striated muscles control the eye globe movements: superior, inferior, medial, and lateral recti and superior and inferior oblique muscles. The levator muscle of the upper eyelid controls movement of the eyelid in conjunction with the orbis ocularis.

The orbit also contains vessels: the ophthalmic artery, a branch of the internal carotid artery that is the origin of the central retinal artery, and veins such as the ophthalmic and central retinal vein. The nerves in the orbit are the optic nerve with its four portions: intraocular, intraorbital, intracanalicular, and intracranial. The ophthalmic division of the trigeminal nerve (V1) has three branches (frontal, nasociliary, and lacrimal), including the ciliary ganglion. Fat and connective tissue are present as well. The meninges—dura, arachnoid, and pia—surround the optic nerve. The lacrimal gland is located at the upper outer quadrant of the orbit in the lacrimal fossa (Tables 32.1 through 32.3).

RADIOTHERAPY CONCEPTS

There are two basic types of radiation: ionizing and non-ionizing radiation. When an atomic particle or an electromagnetic wave (photon) hits another atom or molecule, an electron or a nucleon (proton or neutron) is removed from its orbit, transforming the particle into an ion.

TABLE 32.2 Current Approaches to Management

Observation
Photocoagulation
Cryotherapy
Diathermy
Local resection
Enucleation
Exenteration
Radiation therapy
  External beam radiation therapy
  Plaque brachytherapy

TABLE 32.3 Factors Significantly Influencing Prognosis of Choroidal Melanoma

Tumor size
Cell type
Pigmentation
Degree of mitotic activity
Evidence of necrosis
Lymphocytic infiltration
Angle infiltration
Scleral infiltration
Extrascleral extension
Ciliary body infiltration
Location

Ionizing radiation is biologically important due to its ability to cause damage to DNA strands, either directly fragmenting the molecule or indirectly creating an area of ionized free radicals in the vicinity of the coiled chromatin, capable of impairing the capacity of the cells to repair or regenerate. These events form the basis of radiation therapy for cancer treatment.

Non-ionizing radiation or excitation occurs when the outermost electrons of an atom are stimulated by an electromagnetic force and remain vibrating or fluctuating within different levels of the same orbit without becoming knocked out from its orbital path. With this type of radiation the atom is not transformed into an ion which results in less biologic effect on cancer cells.

Non-ionizing radiation is being explored in conjunction with pharmaceutical sensitizers in the treatment of several cancer tumors. This modality is photodynamic therapy (PDT).

The radioactive elements emit three types of radiation, including protons and alpha particles with a positive electrical charge (helium nucleus), beta particles with a negative charge (electrons), and gamma rays as well as neutrons with no electrical charge. Gamma rays are similar to x-rays, but they originate in the atomic nucleus whereas x-rays originate from the orbiting electrons.

Radiotherapy can be generated from a remote distance (teletherapy), or at a site close to or within the target tissue (brachytherapy).

Teletherapy is produced in a linear accelerator or an isotope-loaded machine like the cobalt unit used in external beam radiotherapy. Presently, the cobalt machine is less commonly and has been replaced by the more powerful and more versatile linear accelerators due to their physical properties. Proton beam and neutrons are also used for the treatment of different tumors. Protons are particularly useful in the management of uveal melanomas.

Brachytherapy is a therapeutic modality whereby a special device loaded with an isotope is applied either inside the cavity (intracavitary) or within the target organ or tissue (interstitial).

An isotope is an unstable atom with a nucleus containing an excess of neutrons which generate an internal reaction giving off energy on the form of gamma rays, beta rays, neutrons, or other subatomic particles.

Radioactivity was discovered by Becquerel and later on identified and analyzed by Pierre and Marie Curie in 1898 while working with radium. Foster-Moore was the first to use radon-222 (^{222}Rn) seeds and later on, Stallard popularized the use of cobalt-60 (^{60}Co) plaque. After these investigators, a constant interest grew among radiation oncologists as well as ophthalmologists to investigate and try other isotopes that included palladium-103 (^{103}Pd), rhudenium-106 (^{106}Rh), iridium-192

(^{192}Ir), gold-198 (^{198}Au), and most recently, iodine-125 (^{125}I). At present, ^{125}I is the ideal isotope used extensively in the U.S., whereas ^{106}Rh is quite popular in Europe, particularly in Germany.

Other radiotherapy techniques that are occasionally employed but are not well established in the treatment of ocular tumors, include X-knife with a linear accelerator or gamma-knife radiotherapy/radiosurgery.

BENIGN OCULAR DISEASES

A variety of diseases are categorized as benign or malignant ophthalmic tumors (Table 32.4) (1). Radiation therapy of nonmalignant ocular disease is, for the most part, historically interesting, although it may still be employed to treat certain benign ocular conditions.

Pterygium

The most common benign ocular condition for which irradiation is beneficial is the pterygium. Although the primary therapy for this condition is surgical removal of the growth, the recurrence rate is high, ranging up to 67% (2). Recurrence rates are higher in women than in men and higher in patients younger than age 40. Postoperative irradiation using a strontium-90/yttrium-90 ($^{90}Sr/^{90}Y$)-emitting contact applicator significantly reduces recurrence rates to 20% or less (2–6). Post-excision–irradiation doses and application schemes reported in the literature vary widely (7–14a). Our protocol calls for weekly application of a 1,000-cGy surface dose beginning within the first 24 hours after surgery for 3 to 5 weeks, depending on the size of the surgical defect. The bare-sclera surgical excision technique appears to be associated with a higher risk for recurrence without adjuvant irradiation than the newer lamellar keratoplasty technique after excision (15,16). New surgical techniques have been developed with satisfactory results rendering the use of ^{90}Sr to very rare instances.

Capillary Hemangioma

Capillary hemangiomas of infancy are very rare benign vascular tumors that present somewhere in the body and also in the choroid. They present unique problems when they occur on the eyelids. The natural history of the lesion is a spontaneous regression over 3 to 4 years. A conservative approach of observation, therefore, is the treatment of choice (17). Occasionally, however, the lesion may be large enough to obstruct the child's vision, and amblyopia may occur. The eyelid may ulcerate because of tumor compression of the vascular supply. Historically, the best intervention was accomplished by the cautious use of steroids or low-energy x-ray or electron beam radiation therapy, delivering 500 to 750 cGy in two or three fractions (18,19). This was abandoned with the new techniques such as laser therapy.

When the choroid is affected by hemangioma like in the Sturge-Weber syndrome or the Von Hippel-Lindau syndrome, its presentation can be as a circumscribed lesion or diffuse type.

A characteristic of hemangiomas is the ability to leak fluid causing a retinal detachment or cystic changes. Some do not leak fluid and may be observed without treatment. In cases where there is subretinal fluid with associated retinal detachment, visual acuity can be impaired, particularly when the fovea and perifoveal areas are affected. Photocoagulation is effective to control leakage; however there is a high risk for recurrence that compromises vision.

A recent study at St. Bartholomew's Hospital in London, England reported a successful outcome in a group of 28 patients: 23 with circumscribed choroidal hemangioma (CCH) and 5 with diffuse choroidal hemangioma (DCH). All 5 patients with DCH had fluid reabsorbed and minimal visual impairment. All patients with CCH experienced fluid resolution, and three fourths had a visual acuity of 6/12 or better at 1 year. The study's conclusion was that plaque brachytherapy was an effective alternative in the treatment of CCH. Lens-sparing radiotherapy was equally effective in the treatment of DCH (19a).

TABLE 32.4 Incidence of Malignant Intraocular Tumors

	Incidence (%)
Primary tumor	
Pigmented tumors	75
Retinoblastoma and other neuro-ectodermal tumors of the retina	20
Epithelial–uvea	<1
Connective tissue and other mesenchymal tumors	<1
Hematopoietic	<1
Meningioma	Rare
Secondary (metastatic)	
Breast	58
Lung	15
Lymphoma or leukemia	>18

Graves Ophthalmopathy

In some patients with hyperthyroidism (thyrotoxicosis), exophthalmos may occur. The primary tissues involved are the intraocular muscles. Indications for therapy include corneal exposure secondary to proptosis and optic nerve compression, which may cause permanent visual loss. The diagnosis is made by computed tomography (CT), which may demonstrate thickened muscles. Steroid therapy is the first-line treatment, but radiation therapy can be beneficial if steroids fail. Treatment can be given by a single lateral portal excluding the ipsilateral lens. A dose of 1,500 to 2,000 cGy in 10 fractions is usually sufficient to alleviate symptoms (20–25).

Electrons, 12 to 15 MeV, were employed for the treatment of these patients. Currently, only 6 MV photons are used. In a series of 35 patients with thyroid ophthalmopathy, Sandler et al. (25) report that 71% of patients receiving 2,000 cGy in 200-cGy fractions required no further steroid therapy or surgical decompression. Of the failures, 7 (33%) of 21 patients had failed prior steroid therapy; 2 (29%) of the 7 patients had failed prior surgical decompression; and 1 (14%) of the 7 patients had no prior treatment.

The main prognostic factor for failure was an interval of less than 6 months between eye disease and radiation therapy. In a series of more than 300 patients, Peterson et al. (26) showed that 2,000 cGy in 10 fractions gave results identical to 3,000 cGy in 15 fractions and that as many as 76% of treated patients responded positively to treatment. Corneal involvement and visual loss were more likely to improve after radiation therapy than proptosis or ocular muscle impairment.

At MCP-Hahnemann University Hospital we advocate the use of 6-MV photons at lateral opposed fields, with an anterior half beam block to protect the lens and a dose of 2,000 cGy in 200 cGy fractions.

EYELID MALIGNANCIES

Malignant Melanoma

Chapter 25 contains more information on cutaneous malignant melanoma of the head and neck.

Basal and Squamous Cell Carcinomas

In the treatment of basal cell and squamous cell carcinomas of the eyelids, surgery can eradicate the disease in a high percentage of cases; however, the results sometimes are not cosmetically or functionally adequate. Radiation therapy can achieve an overall 90% to 95% cure rate. After the diagnosis is confirmed by biopsy and depending on the histology and tumor size, 4,500 to 6,000 cGy can be delivered by photon therapy from a superficial or orthovoltage machine or by low energy electron beam.

The globe may be protected by an internal eye shield. Radiation therapy may be able to provide better cosmesis than surgery while providing similar cure rates (see Chapters 24 and 25 for more information).

Meibomian Gland Carcinoma

Meibomian gland (sebaceous) carcinomas are uncommon and have a mortality rate of 30% (27). These tumors may be multicentric, which may lead to local recurrences. Radiation therapy may be used for the treatment of these tumors in selected cases, particularly if surgery would not provide acceptable cosmesis or the disease recurs after surgery. In our experience, high doses of irradiation (6,000–6,500 cGy in 6–7 weeks) are required. Pardo et al. (28) report a series of 30 patients with this tumor, 10 who received radiation therapy. Four were treated with curative intent, and the remaining six were treated after surgery for parotid metastases after initial surgery. Doses ranged from 4,500 to 6,300 cGy, but the irradiation schema varied from 4,500 cGy in four fractions over 5 days to 6,000 cGy delivered in 200-cGy fractions over 51 days. The four patients treated definitively all are free of disease at 36 to 117 months, and the patients treated after surgery for metastatic disease are all free of disease at 24 to 84 months.

CONJUNCTIVAL TUMORS

The two most important and more frequent tumors of the conjunctiva are squamous cell carcinoma and malignant melanoma. Squamous cell carcinoma is probably the most common conjunctival tumor that arises from the bulbar conjunctiva and affects the older patient. This tumor may become invasive and infiltrate other orbital tissues and, if not diagnosed or treated on time, may require orbital exenteration. Surgical resection is the standard treatment modality, with occasional need for episcleral brachytherapy for positive margins or recurrence. A fractionated plaque therapy is recommended, using ^{125}I seeds on a customized plaque applied weekly for 5 weeks with a fraction of 10 Gy per week for a total dose of 50 Gy at a calculated depth of 1 to 2 mm.

Malignant melanoma of the conjunctiva is less frequent but more aggressive than squamous cell carcinoma; when it is infiltrative to orbital tissues, it metastasizes readily through a hematogenous route to distant organs. When the tumor is confined to the conjunctiva, a complete resection followed by cryotherapy usually controls and prevents recurrence. If it recurs and a reexcision is not feasible or incomplete, similar plaque therapy (as in squamous cell carcinoma) could be applied with a higher total dose of 60 Gy in weekly applications of 10 Gy at a 1-mm depth. The control rate exceeds 80%.

UVEAL TUMORS

Metastatic Carcinoma to the Anterior and Posterior Uvea

Tumor metastases to the iris and posterior uvea were once considered rare events (29,30). However, it is now recognized that metastatic carcinoma is probably the most common malignant disease involving the eye (31). Metastatic uveal lesions arise as precocious metastases in approximately 15% of cases, as synchronous metastases in approximately 4% of cases, and as metachronous metastases in most of the remaining cases (except in 8% for which the appropriate parameters cannot be established) (32).

Uveal metastasis most commonly originates from primary neoplasms in breast or lung in women and the lung and gastrointestinal tract in men (31–33). In an autopsy series of patients with breast cancer, a third of the cases included uveal metastases (34). Uveal metastases are most often unifocal but may be multifocal within the eye or may be bilateral (35).

The aim of therapy is to return visual function to the patient, although survival time may be limited after the diagnosis of uveal metastases. Observation for small lesions may be appropriate if the patient is on an effective regimen of systemic management, which can stabilize or shrink metastatic intraocular tumors.

If the patient has visual symptoms, treatment should be started. The treatment of uveal metastasis depends largely on the systemic condition of the patient. Chemotherapy or hormonal therapy is employed to manage disseminated systemic disease, while monitoring the eye (36,37). If there is no evidence of systemic metastatic disease or if the uveal metastasis does not respond to systemic treatment, focal treatment with radiation therapy to the eye is often performed. Almost 90% of patients have positive, objective responses to their therapy (32). For patients with uveal metastases and active systemic disease, we palliate by delivering a 3,000- to 3,500-cGy tumor dose over 3 weeks to the entire ocular structure on the affected side. In the absence of active systemic disease, in the case of precocious metastases, and in patients who have breast or colon cancer and in whom the potential for long-term survival is greater, a more aggressive approach is taken.

At MCP-Hahnemann University Hospital we recommend treating the affected eye with a dose of 4,000 cGy over 4 to 5 weeks, depending on the fractionation and the use of CT scan-based three-dimensional planning to minimize irradiating healthy tissues.

Plaque radiation therapy has been employed to treat *de novo* solitary uveal metastasis as well as those who failed external beam radiation therapy (38). In a series of 36 patients with uveal metastasis treated with plaque radiation therapy, the mean time for treatment was 86 hours, and the mean therapeutic dose was 6,880 cGy to the tumor apex and 23,560 cGy to the tumor base (38). Regression of the uveal metastasis was documented in 94% of the cases. Plaque radiation therapy salvaged five of the six eyes that had failed prior external beam radiation therapy (38).

In our institution, for patients who have a diagnosis of uveal metastasis and are suitable to be treated with plaque brachytherapy, we recommend a customized plaque with a dose to the tumor apex of 3,500 to 4,000 cGy over an average of 72 to 96 hours.

Malignant Melanoma of the Posterior Uvea

Of the approximately 1,800 new cases of primary malignant tumors of the eye in 1989, almost 75% were malignant melanoma (32). The ophthalmologic community has long been familiar with the problems of uveal melanomas, but there remains considerable controversy about the optimal management of this disease. Most data have come from small series. Even the larger series have been performed in a nonprospective or nonrandomized fashion, relying on statistical matching of populations for evaluations and conclusions.

Callender developed a histologic classification of uveal tumors: spindle A, spindle B, epithelioid, and mixed. The first two have better prognosis and are less common, whereas epithelioid and mixed cellular are more common and more aggressive.

The diagnosis of malignant uveal melanoma has been rendered more precise with a variety of techniques, reducing the risk for an error that can prompt unnecessary enucleation (39). Indirect ophthalmoscopy is now combined with fluorescent angiography and ultrasonography in a standard assessment battery. The use of CT and magnetic resonance imaging (MRI) studies has also influenced assessment of uveal melanomas.

Melanomas of the anterior uvea are usually detected earlier than those located posteriorly and may be surgically removed by iridectomy or iridocyclectomy (40,41). However, lesions of the posterior uvea are not readily accessible to a biopsy, although fine-needle aspiration biopsy is possible if the diagnosis is in doubt, and the clinical diagnosis may occasionally be difficult. If there remains a degree of uncertainty about the diagnosis or if the lesion is small and relatively flat, a conservative approach of careful, sequential observation may be indicated.

Treatment of this tumor continues to be controversial. Consequently, investigators have developed an array of therapeutic modalities such as laser, thermotherapy, plaque brachytherapy, proton beam therapy, local resection, enucleation, and a periodic observation.

Posterior uveal melanoma has traditionally been treated by enucleation of the affected eyeball. The concept of enucleation has been questioned (42). In assessing the outcome of enucleation by actuarial survival tables, Zimmerman and McLean (42) suggest that the prognosis after enucleation may be worse than for an untreated patient. Some authors have postulated that tumor seeding is precipitated by the manipulation of the globe during the surgical procedure, and they advocate a "no-touch" approach to enucleation (43). Another suggestion is that radical reduction of tumor burden by enucleation alters the immune surveillance capacity, and extant micrometastases begin to grow (44). As stated by Curtin and Cavender (45), "the overall death rate of 50% does little to inspire confidence in our present management of the disease."

The melanoma treatment controversy has led to the development in the United States and Canada of the Collaborative Ocular Melanoma Study (COMS) (46). The COMS is a prospective randomized study that was designed to compare survival in patients treated either with brachytherapy or enucleation, among other aims.

The COMS report No. 18, published in July 2001, evaluates 1,317 patients accrued over 11.5 years; 660 patients were randomized to enucleation and 657 to ^{125}I plaque brachytherapy. The conclusion was that the mortality rate did not differ from those treated with enucleation followed up for 12 years. The power of this study indicates that neither treatment was likely to increase nor decrease mortality rates by as much as 25% relative to the other (46a).

For the last few years, there have been few new developments related to the management of uveal melanoma. In contrast to improved survival rates with a variety of cancers for which there is a continuing evolution toward early detection and management, the survival rate with uveal melanoma has changed little over the last few decades. The same methods of management, such as photocoagulation, radiation therapy, local resection, enucleation, orbital exenteration, chemotherapy, and immunotherapy are still being employed in selected instances (14,47–55). However, the indications for the various methods of treatment modalities as well as the technical and surgical facilities are gradually being refined and modified.

Radiation therapy has been widely employed in the treatment of choroidal melanoma. A variety of approaches have been followed (56). External beam techniques use ^{60}Co, linear accelerators, and (most recently) a gamma-knife as well as therapy with proton beam or the helium ion beam (57–69). Various isotopes have been investigated and used in brachytherapy, including ^{60}Co, ruthenium-106 (^{106}Ru)/^{106}Rh, ^{222}Rn, ^{125}I, ^{198}Au, tantalum-182 (^{182}Ta), ^{192}Ir, and ^{103}Pd (Table 32.5) (70–86).

The current relative indications for treating a posterior uveal melanoma with plaque radiation therapy are generally as follows: (a) selected small melanomas that are documented to be growing or that show clear-cut signs of activity on the first visit; (b) most medium-sized and some large choroidal and ciliary body melanomas in an eye with potential salvageable vision; and (c) almost all actively growing melanomas that occur in the patient's only useful eye. If a melanoma exceeds 15 mm in diameter and 10 mm in thickness, one should anticipate visual morbidity from radiation therapy, and enucleation should be strongly advised (87). The surgical technique of radioactive plaque application has been described in detail in the literature (87a). More recently, specially designed notched plaques have been effectively employed to surround the optic nerve and irradiate those tumors with a juxtapapillary location (87,88).

In a few articles written about the survival data of matched groups of patients treated with enucleation versus plaque radiation therapy, there does not appear to be a statistically significant difference in survival between patients treated with plaque radiation therapy (^{60}Co, ^{125}I) and those treated with enucleation (89–91). With Kaplan-Meier survival curves, the proportion of patients free of metastasis was 87% at 5 years, 84% at 10 years, and 63% at 15 years (Table 32.6) (88). Therefore, a tumor post-plaque irradiation relapse may be a manifestation of a more intrinsic malignant potential unrecognized clinically before treatment (92). The 5-year survival (87%) in relapse-free patients was significantly better than that (58%) of patients whose tumors locally recurred (92).

Moreover, there does not appear to be a major difference in local control rates among the various brachytherapy tech-

TABLE 32.5 Type of Radioactive Plaques for Treatment of Choroidal Melanoma

Isotope	No. of patients
^{60}Co	680
^{192}Ir	225
^{106}Ru	152
^{125}I	2,448
Total	3,505

Source: Wills Eye Hospital, Hahnemann University, Philadelphia, Pennsylvania, as of November 30, 1997.

TABLE 32.6 Enucleation After Conservation Radiation Therapy for Choroidal Melanoma

Treatment modality	Enucleated eyes (Total no. of treated eyes)	Percentage	Center
Plaque isotope			
^{60}Co	42 (601)	7	Wills-Hahnemann
^{106}Ru	36 (205)	17	Berlin
^{125}I	1 (42)	2	Münster
^{125}I	7 (60)	12	UNY-Downstate
^{125}I	2 (26)	8	Mayo Clinic
^{125}I	3 (21)	4.8	Wills-Hahnemann
^{192}Ir	5 (59)	1.7	Wills-Hahnemann
Charged particles			
Protons	57 (1,006)	5.7	Massachusetts General
Hospital			
Protons	22 (270)	8	Villigen
Helium ions	29 (228)	10	Berkeley

niques. Local tumor recurrence after plaque radiation therapy has been reported to occur in up to 16% of cases (88,93,94) and constitutes an important posttreatment clinical indicator of the tumor great malignant potential and the patient's increased risk for melanoma-specific mortality (92). In two series of 93 patients with juxtapapillary choroidal melanoma managed by plaque radiation therapy, local tumor recurrence was documented in 14 cases (15%) (88,93). The younger age of the patient (younger than 35 years old) and the superior and inferior location of the tumor were predictive for local tumor recurrence (88).

More than 85% of brachytherapy patients with locally controlled tumor may retain useful vision for prolonged periods (83,95). Analysis of our patients treated primarily by ^{60}Co brachytherapy shows the trend for visual and ocular survival (Figs. 32.1 through 32.5; Table 32.7). The visual outcome of an eye treatment with brachytherapy depends mainly on the tumor size and location as well as on the development of radiation retinopathy and papillopathy (94,96). Patients with tumors located near the fovea or optic disc and patients with larger tumors have a worse visual outcome (94,96). In their series of 77 patients with posterior uveal melanoma managed by ^{60}Co plaque radiation therapy, Cruess et al. (97) found that eyes receiving a radiation dose in excess of 5,000 cGy to the fovea or optic disc commonly lose a substantial amount of vision within 2 to 3 years. In a more recent Wills Eye Hospital Oncology Service series of 93 patients with choroidal melanoma touching the optic disc, the authors found an incidence of 87% retinopathy and 52% of radiation papillopathy after mean intervals of 21 and 27 months, respectively, after plaque therapy (88). Using life table analysis, the proportion of patients who experienced a decrement of at least three lines of vision was 0% by 20 months, 22% by 30 months, 45% by 40 months, and 72% by 60 months. These results were similar to those found in a series by Lommatzsch et al. (93) after ^{106}Ru/^{106}Rh plaques for juxtapapillary choroidal melanomas.

Combined plaque radiation therapy and laser photocoagulation or thermotherapy have been used to increase the likelihood of complete local tumor destruction, particularly in patients with tumor adjacent to the optic disc (98). Preliminary results have shown that hyperthermia in combination with plaque radiation therapy may decrease the adverse effects of irradiation to the retina, optic disc, and choroid (99).

The results with particle-beam radiation therapy have been reported to yield higher local control rates than with common brachytherapy techniques. The Harvard group reports an esti-

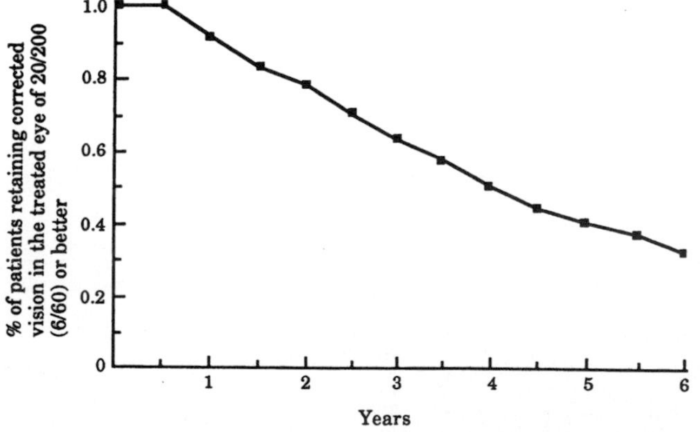

Figure 32.1 Life table assessment of visual acuity in 100 patients managed by cobalt-60 eye-plaque therapy. *x*-axis, years after therapy; *y*-axis, percentage of patients retaining corrected vision in the treated eye of 20/200 (6/60) or better.

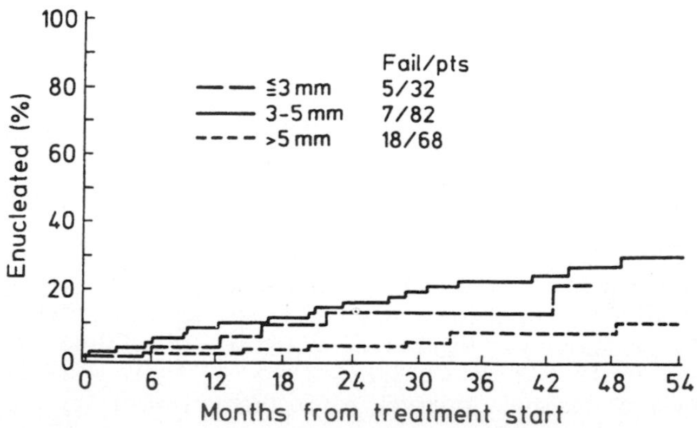

Figure 32.2 Time to enucleation (in months) according to size of tumor. pts, patients.

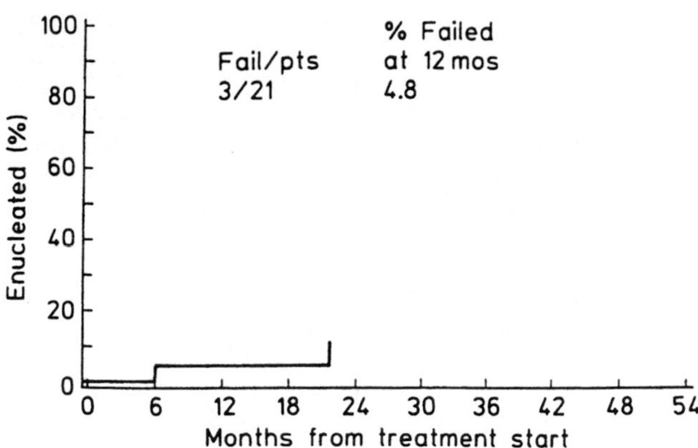

Figure 32.3 Time to enucleation (in months) for patients with small (3-mm-thick) tumors treated by iodine-125 eye-plaque therapy. pts, patients.

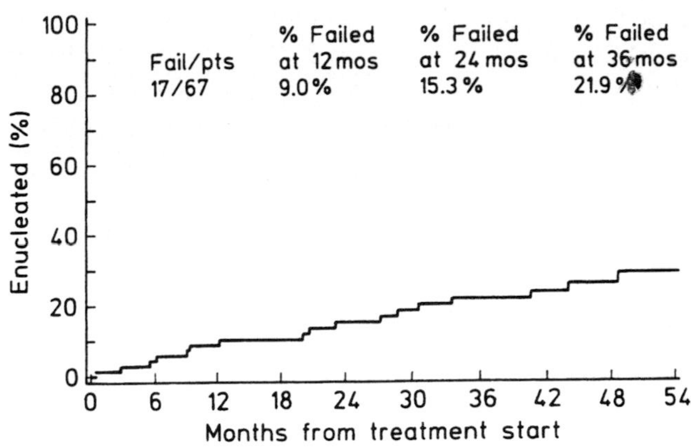

Figure 32.5 Time to enucleation (in months) for patients with large (>5-mm-thick) tumors treated by cobalt-60 eye-plaque therapy.

mated 5-year probability of local tumor control of 96.3% (70). The absolute local recurrence after helium ion therapy in patients observed for more than 5 years after treatment is given as only 2.4% (63). However, it was unclear whether all tumors were included or only those of the posterior uvea. The more anterior tumors, especially ciliary body tumors, are associated with high enucleation (60). There does not appear to be any dose–response correlation for helium ion therapy from 5,000 to 8,000 cGyE (i.e., cGy equivalent, which is equal to the physical dose in cGy multiplied by the relative biologic effectiveness factor of 1.3). A similar result with proton-beam therapy, which employed a relative biologic effectiveness factor of 1.1, has not been reported. Survival, complications, and visual acuity also did not show any dose–response association for helium ion therapy (63,100).

It is generally agreed that very large uveal melanomas and cases with massive extrascleral extension of tumor at diagnosis are not readily amenable to radiation therapy. These eyes should be managed by enucleation or exenteration, respectively. However, the arguments of Zimmerman and McLean (42) that the process of enucleation may worsen the prognosis of these patients, and the fact that the survival of patients with very large intraocular tumors has been only about 50% in classic series, have led to the investigation of preoperative radiation therapy as a means of improving survival in these patients.

The adopted schema has been 2,000 cGy delivered to the globe and proximal optic nerve (including the major draining vessels from the posterior uveal tract) in five fractions over 5 to 7 days, with enucleation within 24 to 48 hours of the last treatment fraction. Eyes thus treated have been enucleated, and cells have been harvested for tissue culture analysis. The irradiated cells did not grow and did not attach to culture vessels, demonstrating that irradiation can alter the *in vitro* growth of human ocular melanomas (101). The initial clinical report, using nonrandomized techniques, has suggested a significantly lower survival in 41 patients receiving preoperative irradiation, as compared with the survival of 31 patients treated by enucleation alone (102). However, there were significant differences between the two groups, and the results must be interpreted cautiously.

We have conducted a prospective, statistically matched study with 29 patients in each group and have shown no survival differences between preoperative radiation therapy and enucleation alone over a 5-year follow-up interval. In one study, no long-term beneficial effect on survival of patients with uveal melanoma could be found after 8-Gy preenucleation irradiation (103).

Custom-designed plaque radiation therapy appears to be an effective alternative method of controlling nonresectable diffuse iris melanoma (104). In Shields' series (104), 14 patients with nonresectable iris melanoma were treated with ^{125}I plaque radiation therapy. The mean length of treatment was 96 hours, to give a mean dose of 29,300 cGy to the base (corneal endothelium) and 10,600 cGy to the apex of the iris melanoma. Tumor control was achieved in 93% of the patients. Despite the large

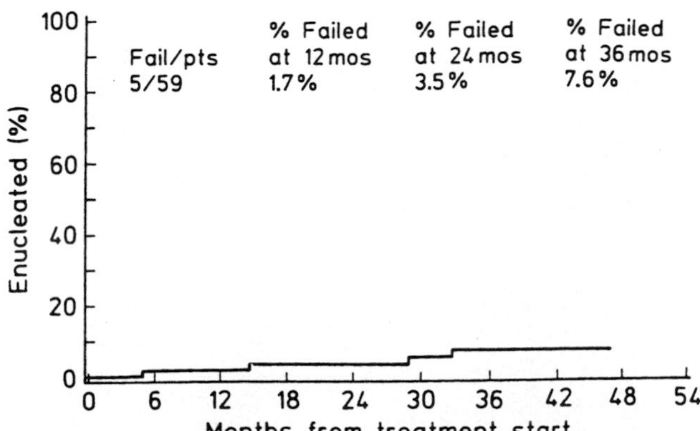

Figure 32.4 Time to enucleation (in months) for patients with medium (3- to 5-mm-thick) tumors treated by iridum-192 eye-plaque therapy.

TABLE 32.7 Adjusted Survival for Patients Treated for Melanoma[a]

Time	Enucleation	^{60}Co plaque
0	1.000	1.000
1	0.987 ± 0.007	0.936 ± 0.019
2	0.947 ± 0.015	0.883 ± 0.025
3	0.888 ± 0.021	0.829 ± 0.029
4	0.822 ± 0.026	0.780 ± 0.032
5	0.776 ± 0.029	0.733 ± 0.035
6	0.757 ± 0.030	0.694 ± 0.037
7	0.732 ± 0.034	0.683 ± 0.038
8	0.702 ± 0.039	0.642 ± 0.042

[a]Figures are fraction surviving plus or minus the standard error of the mean.
Source: Wills-Hahnemann Eye Plaque Program, Philadelphia, Pennsylvania.

dose of irradiation given transcorneally, the cornea tolerated it very well without corneal melting. Cataract developed in six patients. In all patients but one, tumor was controlled and the eye was retained (104).

An updated review of customized plaque brachytherapy in 38 patients with unresectable iris melanoma by Shields et al. (104a) found a tumor control of 92% in 5 years with an apex dose of 80 Gy. Complications included cataract formation and intraocular increased pressure.

RETINAL TUMORS

Retinoblastoma

Retinoblastoma is the most common intraocular malignancy of childhood. The incidence is approximately 1 in 15,000 to 18,000 live births, and it is seen infrequently in routine ophthalmologic practice (105–109). The disease is bilateral in 20% to 30% of patients (110). Of newly diagnosed children, 10% have a family history of retinoblastoma, and these are always heritable cases (106,110). The remaining 90% of cases are sporadic, of which 20% to 30% are bilateral, and these are heritable cases. Of the remaining 70% to 80% of apparent unilateral, sporadic cases, 10% to 12% are heritable (110). Therefore, of all cases diagnosed in the United States annually, approximately 40% to 50% are heritable.

Retinoblastoma can arise in hereditary, nonhereditary, and chromosome deletion forms, the latter occurring on the long arm of chromosome 13 (8,106,110). In general, the hereditary form is diagnosed earlier than the nonhereditary form of the disease, carries a risk for other malignancies, and can affect the offspring of the affected individual. The disease may be bilateral or unilateral. The chromosomal abnormality can result from a germinal mutation, or it may be inherited.

The nonhereditary, sporadic form is unilateral. Children of an affected individual have a 10% risk for having children with the disease, but this form of the disease is not associated with an increased risk for other malignancies (106,110). The chromosomal abnormality is from a somatic mutation (110).

As a result of newly emerging molecular genetic studies, it is now understood that the gene mutated on the long arm of chromosome 13 is a tumor-suppressor gene termed the *RB* gene. It is a large gene of perhaps 200,000 base pairs and encodes a protein whose inhibitory function is thought to be on cell growth. When the function is lost, there is increased cellular growth unopposed by any inhibitory signal. Loss of the entire RB gene, a portion of it, or a point mutation within it leading to a subtle change in the encoded protein may lead to a lack of inhibitory function. Because there are two copies of each gene—one on each of the paternally and maternally derived chromosomes—if one copy is defective or missing, the other copy is still capable of producing sufficient regulatory protein to prevent uncontrolled growth.

In the hereditary form of retinoblastoma, the mutation is thought to be in the germ cell; therefore, every cell in the body of the offspring will contain the defective gene copy. Either through spontaneous mutation or under the influence of some event (biologic, physical, chemical) that increases the probability of mutation the normal gene copy may be sufficiently damaged in the offspring during retinal development to allow for the complete inhibition of the regulatory protein, leading to the development of retinoblastoma. Whether the defective allele is, in fact, inherited from an affected parent or arises as a new mutation in a parental germ cell, the end result will be identical. In this inherited form of the disease, both bilateral and multifocal lesions are highly possible. Because the child has inherited only one defective allele in the germ cell, there is a 50% probability of transmission of this allele to any offspring.

The true sporadic disease is postulated to arise from two separate mutations, each in a separate copy of the *RB* gene within the same somatic cell. This form of the disease is not heritable, because the germ cells are not involved and not all cells in the body are affected. Therefore, the probability of multifocal and bilateral disease is low.

The conventional wisdom in the molecular genetics of cancer is that, besides inactivation of suppressor genes, such as *RB*, activation of at least one oncogene may be required. The oncogene for retinoblastoma has not been identified, but it is known that the growth promotion of the *myc* oncogene can be modulated by the protein encoded by the *RB* gene (46).

In most children, retinoblastoma is diagnosed before age 3 or 4 (although the disease may be present at birth) and rarely beyond the age of 6 years (106,111). The most common presenting signs and symptoms are leukocoria (white pupillary reflex), (Figs. 32.6 and 32.7) strabismus (squint), or a mass in the fundus noticed during ocular examination (109). Accurate diagnosis is paramount because several nonmalignant conditions can present similarly. In a series of 136 children referred for evaluation, only 44% had retinoblastoma, and the remainder had pseudoretinoblastoma (112).

Evaluation begins with an accurate history that emphasizes prenatal and parturition information, prematurity, oxygen therapy, whether leukocoria was present at birth or was noticed later, whether the child has had contact with puppies or other animals, and whether anyone in the family has had retinoblastoma. Children with retinoblastoma rarely have leukocoria or strabismus at birth, but this sign is usually noticed at 6 to 24 months of age. Leukocoria is usually detected by the child's parents or relatives or on photographs that show a white papillary reflex instead of the "red eye" which prompts the parents to seek medical attention.

A careful ophthalmologic examination of the child must be performed to rule out other diagnoses compatible with pseudoretinoblastoma. Slit-lamp biomicroscopy with the pupils dilated may reveal congenital cataract or a retrolental mem-

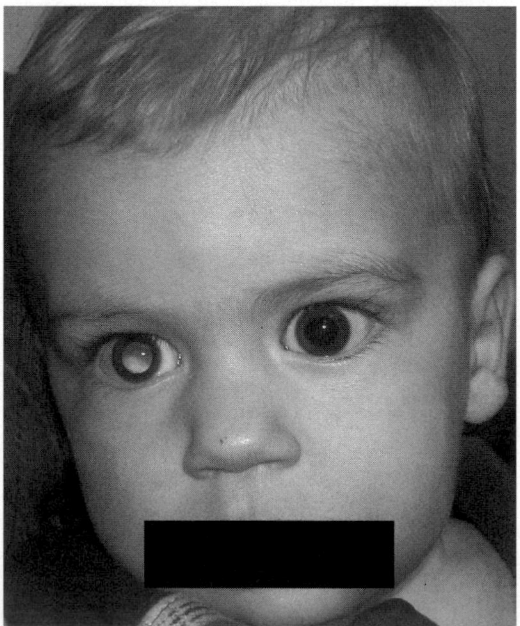

Figure 32.6 Leukocoria in a child with unilateral retinoblastoma.

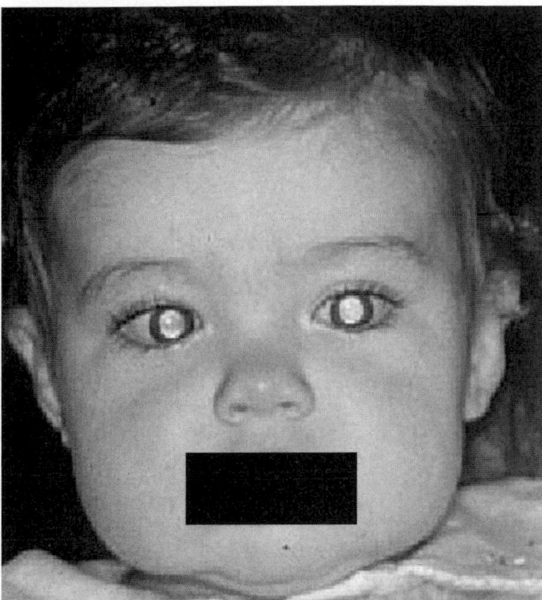

Figure 32.7 Patient with bilateral retinoblastoma.

TABLE 32.8 Reese-Ellsworth Grouping System for Retinoblastoma

Group I: Very favorable
  Solitary tumor, <4 dd[a] in size, at or beyond equator
  Multiple tumors, none >4 dd, all at or behind equator
Group II: Favorable
  Solitary tumor, 4–10 dd at or behind equator
  Multiple tumors, at or behind equator
Group III: Doubtful
  Any lesion anterior to equator
  Solitary tumors >10 dd behind equator
Group IV: Unfavorable
  Multiple tumors, some >10 dd
  Any lesion extending anteriorly to ora serrata
Group V: Very unfavorable
  Massive tumors involving more than half the retina
  Vitreous seeding

[a]1 disc diameter (dd) = 1.6 mm.
Source: Reese AB, Ellsworth RM. The evaluation and current concept of retinoblastoma therapy. *Trans Am Acad Ophthalmol Otolaryngol* 1963;67:1–4, with permission.

brane, suggesting diagnoses other than retinoblastoma, in which the lens and anterior chamber usually remain clear. Binocular indirect ophthalmoscopy seeking characteristic ophthalmic features of retinoblastoma or spontaneously regressed retinoblastoma remains the most important diagnostic tool (35).

Retinoblastoma exhibits certain ultrasonographic features that are rather typical but are not pathognomonic. On A-mode ultrasonography, the detection of very intense reflections from calcium deposits is very suggestive of retinoblastoma. B-mode ultrasonography shows a heterogeneous acoustic solidity, with highly reflective intrinsic echoes within the tumor and attenuation of orbital pattern (113).

On CT, retinoblastoma usually appears as a dense heterogeneous lesion with hyperdense foci corresponding to calcification. Computed tomography has proved to be valuable for assessing extraocular extension and invasion of the optic nerve (113). Because of its soft tissue definition and multiplanar capability, MRI appears to be helpful in differentiating retinoblastoma from simulating lesions, such as Coats disease, retinal detachment, retinopathy of prematurity, and persistent hyperplastic primary vitreous, whereas CT scan is more accurate in showing calcifications. Involvement of the optic nerve, extraocular extension, and intracranial midline neoplasm in trilateral retinoblastoma are best detected by contrast-enhanced MRI studies (113).

The final ophthalmologic procedure is accurate mapping and sizing of tumor deposits in both eyes, which is best accomplished by indirect bilateral ophthalmoscopy with the child under general anesthesia. Mapping and sizing permit visual prognostic classification using the system of Reese and Ellsworth (114) (Table 32.8). Final staging studies, usually performed by the pediatric oncologist, consist of lumbar puncture with cerebrospinal fluid analysis for malignant cells and a bone scan. The siblings of the affected child and the child's parents should also undergo bilateral indirect ophthalmoscopy to detect disease or regressed disease.

Enucleation of the involved globe has been the traditional method of therapy for unilateral disease, and early enucleation after diagnosis has been given as the major reason for the marked improvement in survival during the last half century (112). The fellow eye, although apparently normal at diagnosis, remains at risk and must be examined at frequent intervals until the child is at least school age.

Over recent decades, a substantial decrease of enucleation has occurred. In a detailed review of 324 patients managed on the oncology service at Wills Eye Hospital from 1974 to 1988, Shields et al. found that unilateral retinoblastoma was managed with enucleation in 96% patients from 1974 to 1978, in 86% cases from 1979 to 1983, and in 75% cases from 1984 to 1988. A similar decreasing trend was found with bilateral retinoblastoma. The necessity for enucleation is even less today with the advent of new modalities (114a,114b).

The therapy of bilateral disease is more complex and traditionally has consisted of enucleation of the eye with more advanced disease and radiation therapy for the lesser-involved eye. In some cases, both eyes contain advanced tumors, and there is no hope of retaining useful vision. In such cases, bilateral enucleation has been traditionally recommended. There is often asymmetric development of the disease, and one of the two eyes may be salvageable by radiation therapy. Even if the most advanced eye has more than half of the retina spared or a potential for retention of useful vision, an attempt may be made to salvage both eyes by radiation therapy, reserving enucleation for salvage of failures (112).

A multimodality approach in the management of retinoblastoma has improved the outcome and prognosis, depending on the stage and individual presentation. The current management includes: enucleation, chemotherapy, cryotherapy, laser photocoagulation, plaque brachytherapy, external beam radiotherapy, thermotherapy, chemothermotherapy (114c,114d), subconjunctival chemotherapy, and in advanced cases, orbital exenteration (114a).

If the eye contains group I or II tumors, external beam radiation therapy may be employed. An alternative to radiation therapy is ablation by cryopexy or radioactive eye plaque therapy. Group III and IV tumors can be treated by external beam radiation therapy or complex plaque techniques. Because of the severe nature of the disease in group V, there is frequent failure of radiation therapy, and enucleation may be the final outcome.

Developments with chemotherapy regimens have allowed dramatic control of intraocular retinoblastoma and play an important role in the initial management of patients. These developments are referred to as *chemoreduction.* Shields et al. (115) presently employ carboplatin, etoposide, and vincristine as initial chemotherapeutic agents for adequate tumor reduction to allow for such more focused, less damaging therapeutic measures as laser photocoagulation, cryotherapy, or thermotherapy. The goals of chemoreduction are to avoid enucleation and external beam radiation therapy (115). After 2 months of chemoreduction, there was a mean 35% decrease in tumor base and a nearly 50% decrease in tumor thickness (115a). Additional local treatments were mandatory to eradicate the residual tumor completely (115). Currently, six cycles of chemotherapy are given before evaluation and adjuvant therapy offered for residual or recurrent tumor.

EXTERNAL BEAM TECHNIQUES FOR RETINOBLASTOMA

The first successful treatment of retinoblastoma by x-rays was reported by Hilgartner in 1903 (116). External beam radiation therapy is applied if preservation of useful sight is possible and the tumor is not thought to be life-threatening. Armstrong (117) and Weiss et al. (118) described various techniques, including the classic single temporal portal and modifications, which allowed retinal irradiation and shielding of the lens and anterior chamber to minimize the development of new tumors near the ora serrata and to minimize the development of irradiation-induced cataracts. This and other lens-sparing techniques are unfortunately associated with underdosing the ora serrata with an increased incidence of recurrence and at the same time, an unacceptable incidence of cataract formation.

The modified technique uses a lateral portal, with the anterior beam edge at the equator of the globe and an anterior portal containing a 7-mm diameter central divergent block hung in a pendulum fashion along the central axis of the beam to protect the lens (118). Donaldson and Egbert (110) have recommended that the initial portal setup be done with the ophthalmologist and radiation oncologist working together to establish the posterior border of the lens, the position of the ora serrata, and other key landmarks. They advise using a Comberg contact lens at setup to delineate the cornea. For tumors located posterior to the equator, the portals were moved posteriorly to reduce the dose to the lens. Anterior portals were not necessary with this technique. Recurrences in this area, however, were frequent with seeds into the recess of the ciliary body and iris that were difficult to control.

Due to the high risk for recurrence in the past, we discourage lens-sparing techniques for external beam irradiation of retinoblastoma. McCormick et al. (119) compared a lens-sparing technique with a modified lateral technique designed to reduce the lens dose to 50% of the volume dose to the globe. The lens-sparing technique was associated with relapse in about two thirds of the treated eyes, as compared with 17% with the more recent modified techniques.

Chin et al. (120) have used three pairs of non-coplanar arcs to treat the globe and expose the lens to 30% to 35% of the target dose. No patient data were given. Foote et al. (121) report that treatment of retinoblastoma by anterior segment-sparing techniques resulted in 10 of 14 treated eyes requiring further treatment. Only 4 of 11 treated eyes required further treatment when an anterior approach was used with no attempt at lens sparing. Three of these four eyes required additional treatment for tumors in the posterior pole.

The whole-eye technique and lens-sparing technique were recently reviewed by a group at St. Bartholomew's Hospital in London (42,122). Those authors found that the eye preservation rate has improved markedly from reported older series and that the rate of ocular salvage depended on the stage of the disease (according to Reese-Ellsworth grouping) at the time of the treatment as well as on the availability of focal therapy for limited recurrences. Among the 175 eyes studied after whole-eye radiation therapy alone, the overall ocular rate was 57%, although with salvage therapy, 80% of the eyes could be preserved (122). Among the 67 eyes after lens-sparing radiation therapy with prior adjuvant treatment of anterior tumors, the overall ocular rate was 72% and, with salvage therapy, 93% of the eyes could be preserved (85). These results compare favorably with the whole-eye technique.

Schipper (123) describes various techniques for the treatment of retinoblastoma with lateral or oblique portals, depending on whether the contralateral eye was to be spared. With associates, he reports the results of several therapeutic approaches, including irradiation, with 100% (14/14 patients), 100% (9/9), 83% (10/12), 79% (11/14), and 0% (0/5) cure rates in group I through group V eyes, respectively (124). Of the eyes preserved, 95% retained useful vision.

Cassady et al. (125) report on 230 patients treated with tumor doses of 3,250 to 4,500 cGy administered in fractions ranging from 333 to 400 cGy given three times weekly. Local control was achieved in 109 (49%) of the 223 treated eyes. Doses of 4,000 to 4,500 cGy appeared as effective in achieving local control as those of 3,250 to 3,500 cGy. Combination chemotherapy was used as well, but it was not shown to improve the overall outcome. Unpublished data from Kingston et al. at St. Bartholomew's Hospital in London show that the ocular salvage rate in advanced retinoblastoma treated with external beam radiation therapy alone was 30%, whereas the ocular salvage rate in those eyes treated with chemoreduction prior to external beam radiation therapy was nearly 70%.

A group of investigators from the University of Miami recently published a paper regarding the results they obtained in the use of external beam radiation therapy in a murine transgenic retinoblastoma using hyperfractionated radiation: 1.2 Gy b.i.d. for a total of 33 Gy. This important paper opens the door for more extensive studies through clinical trials to prove the beneficial results with twice-a-day fractions and a lower total dose in retinoblastoma patients (125a).

At MCP-Hahnemann University Hospital, we use a technique that does not spare the lens for the reasons described previously, owing to underdosing the ora serrata and posterior chamber when using an anterior field edge at this level. The dose drops to 30% with this attempt, with a strong risk for recurrence at this level.

With the advent of new technology such as three-dimensional conformal radiotherapy, it is possible to minimize the dose of radiation to the surrounding tissues and maximize the dose to the target. This is the current technique used at our hospital. For unilateral cases, four-field arrangement is obtained with three-dimensional CT scan reconstructed images. In bilateral retinoblastoma patients that have failed other therapies, six fields are used with an orientation as follows: two lateral opposed fields, plus a superior–inferior and an inferior–superior for each eye.

The composite isodose distribution will show that the 98% or 95% line properly covers the eye globe and the proximal 1 cm of the optic nerve, whereas the 50% line includes the orbit and drops off posteriorly allowing decrease in dose to the optic chiasm, pituitary gland, brain, and upper posterior teeth to about 10%. We recommend a dose of 4,200 to 4,400 cGy in fractions of 180 cGy a day (Figs. 32.8 through 32.10; see Color Plates 11–13 following page 524).

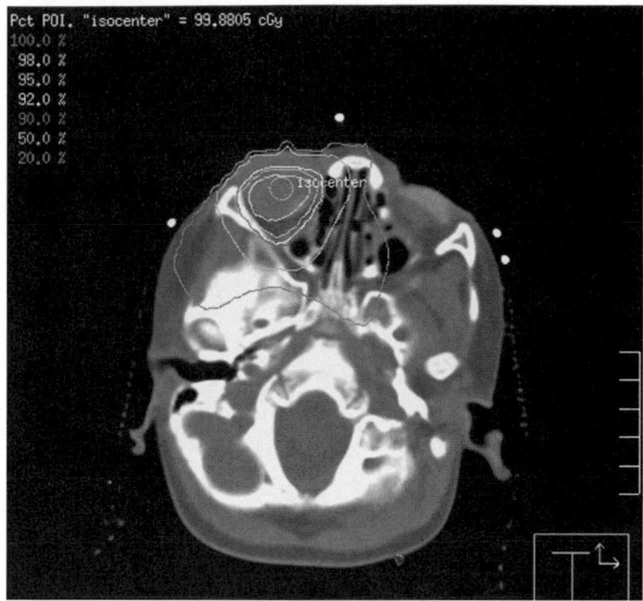

Figure 32.8 Isodose distribution obtained through computed tomographic scan three-dimensional image reconstruction showing four-field arrangement for unilateral retinoblastoma cases. Note the 50% line covers the orbit and the dose drops off fast protecting the chiasm, hypothalamus, pituitary gland, opposite eye, and so forth. (See Color Plate 11 following page 524.)

Irradiation damage to the retina, optic nerve, and lens can be challenging to manage. In a series of 10 patients (126) with macular retinoblastoma treated with external beam radiation therapy (mean dose, 4500 cGy), eight patients obtained visual acuities ranging from 20/25 to 20/100. The visual outcome has been found to depend on the size of the tumor and the involvement of the fovea (126).

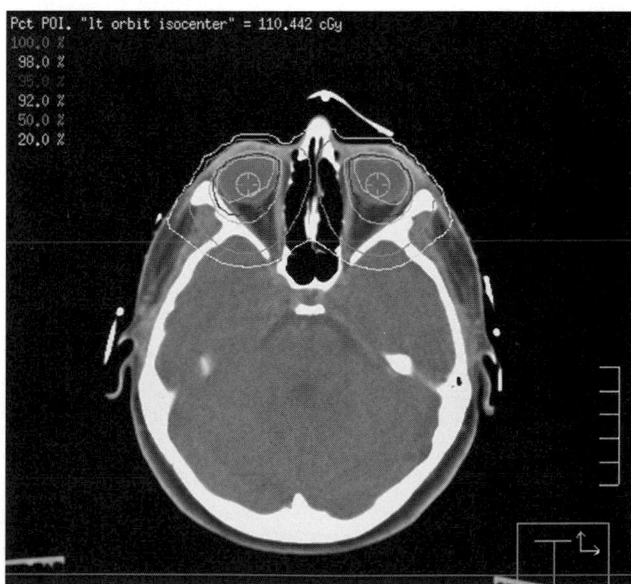

Figure 32.9 Three-dimensional reconstructed image planning for bilateral retinoblastoma using six-field arrangement. Significant sparing effect of different structures close to the eyes and orbits. (See Color Plate 12 following page 524.)

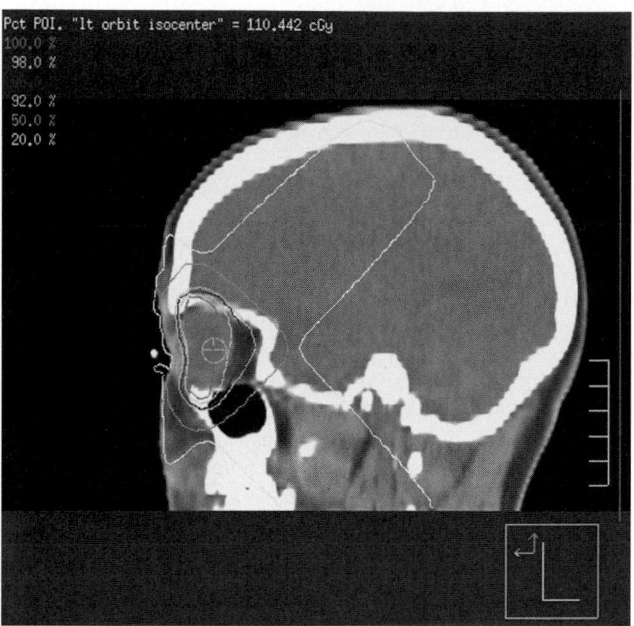

Figure 32.10 Field orientation for anterosuperior oblique and anteroinferior oblique beams used in conjunction with two additional fields: anteromedial oblique and anterolateral oblique beams in unilateral cases. (See Color Plate 13 following page 524.)

BRACHYTHERAPY FOR RETINOBLASTOMA

In 1929, Foster-Moore and Scott (10) reported their experience with radon seed implantation of retinoblastoma (85). In 1948, Stallard (127) described the development of the radium applicator that was subsequently replaced by ^{60}Co plaque. Past techniques using cobalt episcleral applicators consisted of delivering 4,000 cGy to the tumor apex, with the tumor base receiving approximately 10,000 to 20,000 cGy.

We have extended our use of episcleral applicator brachytherapy to other isotopes and employed ^{192}Ir, ^{106}Ru, and ^{125}I plaques. Plaque radiation therapy can be used either as a primary treatment or as a secondary treatment. Amendola et al. (128) report their experience with 20 patients treated with brachytherapy as a boost after external beam radiation therapy for very large tumors or for locally recurring tumors. Sixteen (80%) of the 20 patients had tumor control; the remaining four patients (20%) required enucleation for failure (128). In fact, in 70% of cases, plaque radiation therapy is used as a secondary treatment to salvage a globe after prior failed treatment, usually failed external beam radiation therapy (129,130).

In a series by Shields et al. (131), solitary plaque radiation therapy was used in 91 cases of recurrent or residual retinoblastoma in which the only other option was enucleation. Tumor control and globe salvage were achieved in 89% of these cases with plaque radiation therapy (mean dose to tumor apex, 4,100 cGy) during a mean follow-up of 52 months (131). In another series of 103 tumors treated with solitary plaque radiation therapy, there was an 87% tumor control rate with one application of plaque radiation therapy (132). Carefully selected retinoblastoma, even juxtapapillary and macular tumors, can be successfully treated with plaque radiation therapy.

The visual outcome varies with tumor size and location as well as with radiation complications of retinopathy and papillopathy (130). In a series of 103 eyes managed with plaque radiation therapy (initial or secondary treatment; mean apical dose,

4,227 cGy), the visual outcome has been reported to be good in 62% and poor in 29%, with no vision at all in 9% that required enucleation. The poor vision was a result of foveal retinoblastoma (130). Sequential, paired, opposed plaque technique has also been used as a primary treatment or a secondary treatment (128,133).

Trilateral retinoblastoma is a term describing the association of bilateral or familial retinoblastoma and neuroblastic tumor in the pineal gland or other midline structures. In the series from the Wills Eye Hospital Oncology Service, the incidence of trilateral retinoblastoma was 8% of all bilateral familial retinoblastomas and 5% of all sporadic retinoblastomas. The tumor usually occurred in children at a mean age of 23 months (134).

The disease is fatal despite aggressive treatment with chemotherapy, radiation therapy, gamma-knife therapy, and others (134,135). Trilateral retinoblastoma is a major cause of mortality in children within the first 5 years after the diagnosis of retinoblastoma (135). In asymptomatic patients, longer survival has been correlated with earlier tumor diagnosis through routine CT or MRI studies of the brain, which should be performed until 4.5 years of age (134).

Brachytherapy Physics and Technique

As described previously, over the years, different isotopes have been used for the treatment of ocular tumors such as choroidal melanoma in adults and retinoblastoma in children. Radon-222 was perhaps the first isotope used for this purpose followed by ^{60}Co, ^{192}Ir, ^{198}Au, ^{106}Ru, ^{103}Pd, and lastly, ^{125}I. The Wills Eye Hospital/Hahnemann University Plaque Program switched completely to ^{125}I since the early 1980s. The main reasons for using ^{125}I are its physical properties: a relatively long half-life of 59 days, 28 KeV–gamma-ray energy, and a half value layer (HVL) of 0.025 mm of lead which makes shielding quite simple. All of this translates into adequate treatment which is safer for the patient, surgeon, and personnel close to the patient (135a).

Cobalt-60, on the other hand, has an energy of 1.25 MeV and an HVL of 11 mm of lead, rendering it extremely difficult and cumbersome to shield and place in the orbit. A ^{60}Co plaque with less than 11 mm of lead would result in irradiation in both directions from the plaque, increasing the risk for complications in surrounding organs and tissues. Furthermore, the thickness value layer (TVL) required to reduce transmission to 10% for ^{125}I is 0.1 mm of lead. Currently, the plaque is made of a thickness of 0.3 mm of lead or more commonly, 1.0 mm of gold. The TVL of ^{60}Co would be 33.9 mm of lead.

The type of ^{125}I currently used is model 6711 (3M, New Brighton, Minn.), which has a silver rod 3 mm in length and 0.5 mm in width that is characterized by a more homogeneous isodose distribution than the old model 6702 which contained three ion exchange resin spheres impregnated with ^{125}I. The silver rod is encased in 0.05 titanium foil with welded ends. The dimensions of the seed are 4.5 mm long and 0.8 wide.

Plaques are made of gold as it is an inert metal that causes no allergic reaction, has an extended durability, resists sterilizing solutions well, and requires a thickness of 1 mm. The concave surface is a segment of a sphere with a 12-mm radius. The diameter of the plaques ranges from 10, 12, 15, 18, 20, and rarely, 22 mm. Plaques can be customized, according to tumor shape or location (Figs. 32.11 through 32.13). The ^{125}I seeds are glued to the concave surface using cyanoacrylic adhesive that, once dry, is soaked in sterilizing solution for several hours before the surgical procedure.

Planning for each plaque is done meticulously using Plaque Simulator software (Bebig, Berlin, Germany) for the proper calculation of doses to the tumor apex, base, optic disc, and fovea.

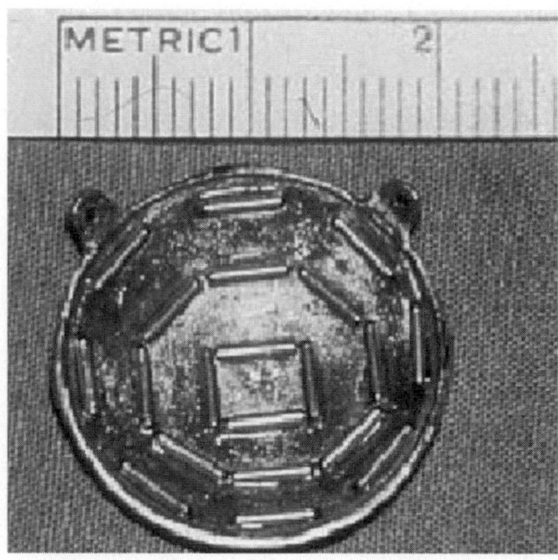

Figure 32.11 Round gold plaque with iodine-125 seeds glued on the concave surface. The seed arrangement is determined by the Plaque Simulator software (Bebig, Berlin, Germany).

The program also allows one to arrange seed orientation to optimize the final isodose distribution, number of seeds, and time of implant.

We recommend a dose of 4,000 cGy (40 Gy) prescribed at the tumor apex for retinoblastoma and 8,000 cGy (80 Gy) for choroidal melanoma. The treatment duration usually ranges from 48 to 96 hours and the plaque is removed in the operating suite under sedation and local anesthesia. The technique for plaque application in pediatric patients requires general anesthesia and in adults, local anesthesia and sedation. The entire surgical procedure is carried out by the ophthalmologist and their team, radiation oncologist, and radiation physicist. The conjunctiva is opened and dissected and the recti muscles are identified and secured with loose silk sutures to easily rotate and mobilize the globe.

Proper tumor location is identified by using a transilluminator that makes the tumor cast a shadow on the sclera which is outlined with a special marker pen. A plastic or acrylic inactive plaque, also called "dummy" plaque, identical in shape and dimension to the active plaque, is centered on the marks and loose sutures are placed through the eyelets in the exact location. The "dummy" is then replaced by the active plaque which is sutured to the sclera and the conjunctiva is closed. A lead shield is taped over the patch before the patient leaves the operating suite.

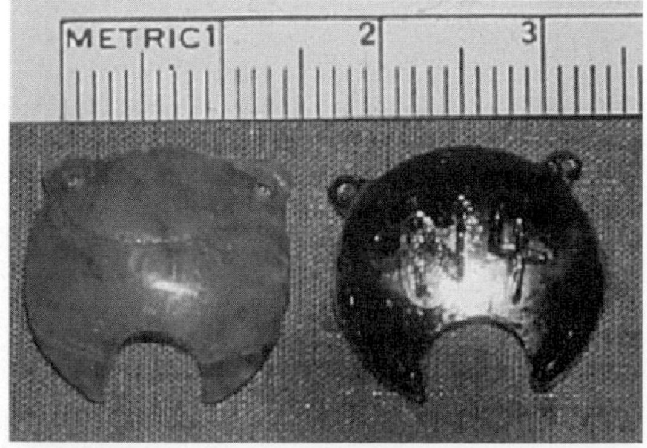

Figure 32.12 Notched plaque with identical inactive "dummy" plaque for juxtapapillary tumors. The notch slides around the optic nerve to properly cover the proximal tumor edge to the disc.

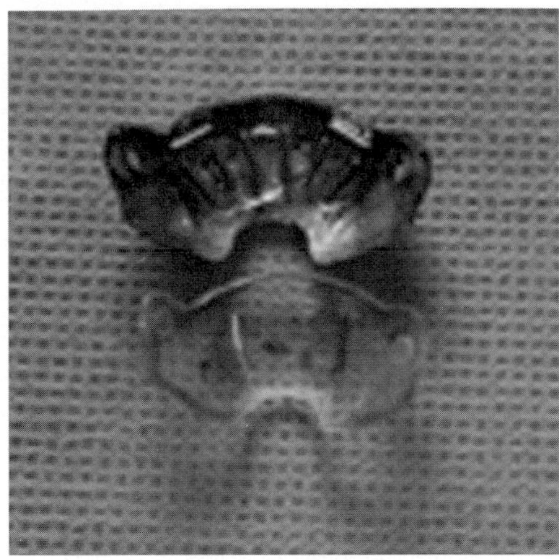

Figure 32.13 Customized "boomerang" plaque designed for the treatment of iris tumors, particularly choroidal melanoma.

The patient is kept in the hospital for the duration of the implant. This decision was made to have better control of the treatment environment and for radiation safety purposes.

After the calculated number of hours has elapsed, the plaque is removed in the operating room under general anesthesia.

In extremely rare occasions when other adjuvant therapies have failed to control the tumor and there is an isolated area which was plaqued previously when vitreous seeds conglomerated close to the retina making re-treatment with another plaque feasible, the full dose of 4,000 cGy (for retinoblastoma) and 8,000 cGy (for choroidal melanoma) should be prescribed.

Second Malignancies in Retinoblastoma

Extensive evaluation of second malignancies in retinoblastoma has been conducted. Smith et al. (136) reviewed 55 patients seen at Stanford University Medical Center between 1954 and 1986. Of 53 available patients, 8 developed 11 second primary tumors. All tumors occurred in the group of patients having the hereditary form of the disease. Three of the 11 second primary tumors were outside the area treated for the primary retinoblastoma. The actuarial incidence for development of second primary malignancies was 4.4% to 6% at 10 years after treatment for retinoblastoma, and the rate increased to 26% to 38% at 30 years (136,137). The latent period from primary therapy to development of the second primary tumor ranged from 5.2 to 36.2 years, with a median of 16 years. Aggressive multimodal treatment of the second primary disease in 5 of 8 patients was associated with 80% survival without evidence of disease at 22 to 72 months after treatment. Seven of the 11 second primary tumors were osteogenic sarcomas. Overall, the cumulative probability of death from second primary neoplasms was reported at 26% at 40 years after diagnosis of bilateral retinoblastoma (138).

Loss or mutation of both copies of the growth-control genes on chromosome 13 that cause retinoblastoma is also associated with the development of osteogenic sarcoma and other types of mesenchymal tumors (139). Schwarz et al. (139) report that second malignant tumors arising after treatment for retinoblastoma consist of osteogenic sarcoma (58%), fibrosarcoma (21%), and other sarcomas (21%). They propose a strong role for radiation induction based on the increased number of sarcomas arising in the previously irradiated field and prolonged latency periods (12.4 years), and that the predominant sites for these secondary sarcomas are not characteristic for spontaneously occurring primary sarcomas.

Hawkins et al. (140) report observing 30-fold more second primary tumors and more than 400-fold osteogenic sarcomas than would be expected in the general population after the diagnosis of retinoblastoma. In the absence of radiation therapy or chemotherapy, the inherent risk for second primary tumors after primary genetic retinoblastoma was 13-fold greater than the expected number and more than 200-fold greater than the expected number of osteogenic sarcomas.

INTRAOCULAR INVOLVEMENT WITH LEUKEMIA

Both retinal hemorrhage and infiltration of the optic nerve and retina are manifestations of childhood leukemia and may cause permanent visual damage. Treatment consists of low-dose irradiation of 1,000 to 1,500 cGy fractionated over 4 to 5 days to the eye and retrobulbar region (141).

INTRAOCULAR LYMPHOMAS

Very rarely, lymphomas may have an intraocular presentation either as an initial tumor or as a part of a systemic disease. Large-cell lymphoma is the most common type and could involve the vitreous, retina, or the uvea. The former is most frequently associated with the central nervous system and the latter with nodal and visceral involvement (87).

The initial manifestation is usually blurred vision resulting from a cellular infiltration of the vitreous cavity. In many cases, there appears to be no systemic manifestation, and the diagnosis is made either by enucleation or by vitreous biopsy (142). Michels et al. (143) treated two cases of intraocular lymphoma with 3,000-cGy external beam irradiation directed through lateral ports. We advocate treating the entire globe by a three-dimensional conformal radiotherapy technique, delivering a minimum tumor dose of 3,500 to 4,000 cGy in 180 cGy fractions over approximately 5 weeks (144).

ORBITAL TUMORS

Primary malignant tumors of the orbit are rare (145). Malignant lymphoma, rhabdomyosarcoma, and lacrimal gland tumors account for most cases (126,146). Of these, rhabdomyosarcoma has generated the most interest.

Rhabdomyosarcoma

Rhabdomyosarcoma of the orbit is most often seen in young children. It has a rapid onset, with marked proptosis and swelling of the adnexal tissue. There are three main histologic types: embryonal, alveolar, and botryoid. The former is frequently found in the head and neck area, either in the orbit or as a parameningeal tumor. Alveolar and botryoid types are most commonly seen in the genitourinary system and extremities.

Rhabdomyosarcoma of the orbit is most often seen in young children and carries a favorable prognosis. It has a rapid onset with marked proptosis and swelling of the adnexal tissue.

No entirely satisfactory staging system exists (147). The Intergroup Rhabdomyosarcoma Study (IRS) Group clinical staging system is presented in Table 32.9 (148). Previously, the recommended treatment was orbital exenteration, because many ophthalmologists thought that the tumor was radioresistant (149–151). The current recommendations are for combined radiation therapy and chemotherapy as the initial management, limiting surgical intervention to biopsy or local excision (146, 152,153).

TABLE 32.9 Intergroup Rhabdomyosarcoma Study Group Staging System for Rhabdomyosarcoma

Clinical grouping system	Stage
Group I: Localized disease, completely resected; regional nodes not involved	I
A. Confined to muscle or organ of origin	
B. Contiguous involvement or infiltration outside the muscle or organ of origin	
Group II: Regional disease	II
A. Grossly resected tumor with microscopic residual disease	
No evidence of gross residual tumor	
No clinical or microscopic evidence of regional node involvement	
B. Regional disease, completely resected (regional nodes involved completely resected with no microscopic residual)	
C. Regional disease with involved nodes, grossly resected, but with evidence of microscopic residual	
Group III: Incomplete resection or biopsy with gross residual disease	III
Group IV: Metastatic disease present at onset	IV

Source: Adapted from Maurer HM, Moon TE, Donaldson M, et al. The Intergroup Rhabdomyosarcoma Study. *Cancer* 1977;40:2015, with permission.

Lederman (154) has provided the foundations for integrated management with surgery and radiation therapy and developed guidelines for the radiation therapeutic technique and dosage. Sagerman et al. (155) suggest the necessity of higher irradiation doses. A minimum tumor dose of 4,500 to 5,000 cGy should be delivered by megavoltage equipment over 5 to 7 weeks with some protection of sensitive ocular structures. All long-term survivors exhibit late irradiation effects ranging from minimal change to phthisis bulbi, which requires enucleation.

According to the most recent recommendations of the International Rhabdomyosarcoma Group (IRSG), the IRS-IV trial for orbital rhabdomyosarcoma was reported to be superior to IRS-III. According to Wharam et al. (1997, personal communication), the former trial had 100% successful outcome compared with 83% in the latter trial. These results were thought to be explained by the use of a radiation dose of 50.4 Gy or higher and chemotherapy comprising vincristine and actinomycin-D without cyclophosphamide.

With regard to irradiation, we advocate the use of three-dimensional conformal radiotherapy whenever possible to properly treat the tumor volume with an adequate margin.

Malignant Lymphoma of the Orbit

Although clear pathologic criteria for malignant lymphomas of the orbit differentiate them from pseudolymphomas, the diagnosis is not always clear (156,157). Malignant lymphomas are characterized by diffuse or nodular lymphoid infiltrates and frequently exhibit atypical cells, mitoses, and invasion of adjacent tissues. In contrast, the pseudotumors are characterized by a polymorphic admixture of cells, including mature lymphocytes organized in reactive germinal centers with inflammatory changes. Surface markers may indicate a specific cell type.

Rao et al. (158) and Mittal et al. (159) report 23 and 22 patients, respectively, treated for malignant or indeterminate lymphomas of the orbit. Treatment was given with anterior or lateral portals covering the entire orbit and using ^{60}Co, 4- to 6-mV photons, or 15- to 16-MeV electrons. Control of the orbital tumor was achieved in 20 of 23 of the Rao group patients with doses of 3,000 to 4,000 cGy. The few patients who failed to respond received doses of less than 2,000 cGy. Fitzpatrick and Macko (160) observed tumor control in 100% of 19 patients with malignant lymphoma confined to the orbit after delivery of doses ranging from 2,500 cGy in 10 fractions to 4,500 cGy in 15 fractions. Austin-Seymour et al. (161) had comparable results in 24 patients with benign lymphomatous conditions and 8 patients with malignant lymphomas of the orbit treated with mean doses of 2,360 cGy and 3,625 cGy, respectively.

Reddy et al. (162) report 17 patients with primary orbital lymphoma. In 14 of these patients 18 eyes were treated by radiation therapy. Four of the patients were treated for local recurrence after surgery. Local control was achieved in 100%. Three of the 17 patients died of systemic progression of lymphoma, 11 died of unrelated causes, and 3 patients remain alive without evidence of disease. In a smaller series of patients with primary lymphoma of the orbit, Makepeace et al. (163) report 100% local regression after radiation therapy. However, a third of their patients developed recurrent disease. The 5-year overall survival rate was 89%.

Bessell et al. (164) treated 115 patients with orbital lymphoid tumors. Eighteen patients had high-grade malignant lymphomas, 43 had low-grade malignant lymphomas, and 54 patients were considered to have indeterminate lymphocytic lesions. The authors report that the survival of patients presenting with stage I low-grade malignant lymphoma and indeterminate lymphocytic lesions was similar to that of a normal population of the same age characteristics. However, the clinical features and dissemination pattern of the indeterminate lymphoid lesions were identical to those for low-grade malignant lesions. This suggested that most, if not all, lymphoid masses presenting in the orbit are neoplastic rather than reactive. The indication is that all cases of primary orbital lymphoma should be evaluated for a systemic component and should be staged as completely as lymphomas arising in other primary sites.

Radiation therapy is now considered the treatment of choice for localized primary orbital lymphomas (162). The suggested radiation dose is 3,500 to 4,500 cGy administered in conventional fractionation schedules.

Orbital Pseudolymphoma

Benign primary lymphoreticular tumors, if localized to the orbit, have a good prognosis, with a 5-year survival rate of 70% (165). Approximately 20% to 25% of cases of apparent pseudolymphoma may convert to malignant lymphoma (158,159). However, it is often difficult to differentiate between the pseudolymphoma and true lymphoma by biopsy specimens (156). Steroids can be effective, but radiation therapy appears to be more effective and can control cases that have been refractory to steroids (144). In our experience, surgical excision of localized pseudolymphomas has been associated with the least chance of control. Radiation therapy may consist of a single exposure of 800 cGy directed through an anterior portal (4,165,166). However, we elect to treat with 2,000 to 2,500 cGy given in 10 to 14 fractions, which can cause the condition to resolve dramatically (23,144,161). Anterior, lateral, or oblique portals similar to those employed in the therapy of malignant lymphoma of the orbit, ^{60}Co, 4- to 6-mV photons, or 15- to 16-MeV electron beams are used for treatment of these lesions. Orbital pseudolymphoma associated with a histologic picture of angiitis is refractory to this therapy, but inflammatory lymphocytic infiltration responds dramatically (161).

Lacrimal Gland Tumors

The high mortality rate of malignant lacrimal gland tumors is partially caused by the difficulty of the surgical approach and the tendency of these tumors to invade the surrounding orbital bone (167). Although relatively radioresistant, lacrimal gland tumors should routinely be irradiated after surgery to reduce postoperative recurrences (165). Tumor doses of 5,000 to 6,000 cGy are necessary, depending on the size of the lesion.

Metastatic Orbital Tumors

The most common metastatic orbital tumors are breast, lung, prostate, gastrointestinal, and other primary tumors (35,38,87). Metastatic tumors to the orbit may be treated with 3,500 to 4,500 cGy fractionated over 3 weeks (168). The treatment design depends on the location and extent of tumor within the orbit. The techniques are similar to those described for ocular metastases.

COMPLICATIONS OF THERAPY

Skin and Adnexa

Skin changes resulting from radiation therapy may include erythema, depigmentation, atrophy, telangiectasia, and ectropion or entropion of the eyelid. Although conjunctival changes are usually insignificant, a corneal abrasion may result from the formation of a keratotic plaque in a radiation-injured conjunctiva.

Loss of the cilia from the scalp, eyebrow, or eyelid may occur after radiation therapy to the ocular area (146). Hair loss from the scalp may occur at the exit area of an external beam portal if a direct anterior or oblique portal is employed. Eyebrow loss occasionally occurs when a ^{60}Co plaque has been used anteriorly and superiorly to treat choroidal malignant melanoma (70). The eyelash loss that may accompany the use of x-ray therapy in the treatment of basal cell carcinoma is usually permanent. Similar lash loss may follow radioactive plaque therapy of ciliochoroidal melanomas.

Cornea

Direct corneal injury may result from irradiation of ocular and adjacent structures (169,170). Blodi (169) classifies this damage as *pure epithelial,* with a good prognosis for recovery, or as *stromal,* with a poor prognosis. Experiments indicate that 7,200 cGy fractionated over 8 days leads to corneal perforation, but 4,800 cGy fractionated over the same time produces mostly reversible epithelial changes with minimal stromal damage.

Lens

A great concern in the treatment of ocular disease is the risk for irradiation-induced cataract (171). Merriam and Focht (172) have shown that as little as 200 cGy in a single fraction or 800 cGy fractionated and delivered at the level of the lens can significantly elevate the incidence of cataract development. At higher dosages, the percentage of lenses that develop cataracts increases to 100%. With the use of improved shielding, beam-control techniques, and more inherently sharp beams, an 80% reduction in the incidence of irradiation-induced cataracts is expected (29,116,172,173).

Retina and Choroid

Changes in the retina and choroid are observed after doses of 4,500 to 6,000 cGy (174). Vascular damage leads to infarction of tissue with the formation of exudates and hemorrhages. Decreased visual acuity may result from damage to the retinal tissue or from atrophy of the optic nerve (175). Because of the extreme radioresistance of the sclera, which may tolerate doses to 75,000 cGy or more, only a few cases of scleral necrosis have been reported (176). Enucleation is necessary in 6% of eyes treated with plaque radiation therapy for choroidal melanoma, usually for irradiation complications or tumor regrowth (41).

Lacrimal Gland and Bony Orbit

Irradiation damage to the lacrimal gland may decrease tear production and may produce irreversible corneal changes. A particularly distinctive and disfiguring orbital change that sometimes occurs in children irradiated for ocular or orbital tumors is the arrested development of the lateral orbital wall growth center, leading to a subsequent temporal osteomalacia. Another rare but disastrous complication is the development of osteogenic sarcoma of the orbit. This complication has been fatal in 100% of reported cases (177–184).

REFERENCES

1. Forrest AW. Radiotherapy of ocular lesions by x-rays and gamma rays. *Trans Am Acad Ophthalmol* 1959;63:455.
2. de Keizer RJ, Swart-van-den-Berg M, Baartse WJ. Results of pterygium excision with Sr-90 irradiation, lamellar keratoplasty and conjunctival flaps. *Doc Ophthalmol* 1987;67:33a(abst).
3. Alaniz-Camino F. The use of postoperative beta radiation in the treatment of pterygia. *Ophthalmic Surg* 1982;13:1022.
4. Grayson M. Degenerations, dystrophies and edema of the cornea. In: Duane TD, ed. *Clinical ophthalmology.* Hagerstown, MD: Harper & Row, 1976:4–5.
5. Hilgers JHC. Strontium-90 beta-irradiation, cataractongenicity and pterygium recurrence. *Arch Ophthalmol* 1966;76:329.
6. Lommatzsch P. Treatment of choroidal melanomas with 106Ru/106Rh beta-ray applicators. *Trans Ophthalmol Soc U K* 1977;97:428.
7. Assegadoo ER. Surgery, thio-tepa and corticosteroids in the treatment of pterygium. *Am J Ophthalmol* 1972;74:960.
8. Beyer DC. Single fraction postoperative beta irradiation for pterygia. Paper presented at: 31st Annual ASTRO Meeting; 1989; San Francisco.
9. Cooper JS. Postoperative irradiation of pterygia: 10 more years of experience. *Radiology* 1978;128:753.
10. Foster-Moore R, Scott RS. Clinical and pathological report of bilateral glioma retinae. *Proc R Soc Med* 1929;22:951.
11. Kiels W, Pico G. Thio-tepa therapy to prevent post-operative pterygium occurrence and neovascularization. *Am J Ophthalmol* 1973;76:371.
12. Lederman M. Radiotherapy of non-malignant diseases of the eye. In: Bushke F, ed. *Progress in radiation therapy.* New York: Grune & Stratton, 1958:256–271.
13. Lentino W, Zaret MM, Rossignol B, et al. Treatment of pterygium by surgery followed by beta irradiation. *Am J Roentgenol Radium Ther* 1949;81:93.
14. Stallard HB. Radiotherapy for malignant melanoma of the choroid. *Br J Ophthalmol* 1966;50:174.

14a. Van Den Brenk HAA. Results of prophylactic postoperative irradiation in 1300 cases of pterygium. *Am J Roentgenol Radiat Ther Nucl Med* 1968;103:723.

15. Busin M, Holliday BL, Arffa RC, et al. Precarved lyophilized tissue for lamellar keratoplasty in recurrent pterygium. *Am J Ophthalmol* 1986;102:222.

16. Laughrea PA, Arentsen JJ. Lamellar keratoplasty in the management of recurrent pterygium. *Ophthalmology* 1986;17:106.
17. Marquileth A, Museles M. Cutaneous hemangiomas in children: diagnosis and conservative management. *JAMA* 1965;1974:523.
18. de Venecia G, Lobek CC. Successful treatment of eyelid hemangioma with prednisone. *Arch Ophthalmol* 1970;84:98.
19. Jakobiec FA, Jones IS. Vascular tumors, malformations and degenerations. In: Duane TD, ed. *Clinical ophthalmology.* Vol 2. Hagerstown, MD: Harper & Row, 1976:1–40.
19a. Madreperla SA, Hungerford JL, Plowman PN et al. Choroidal hemangiomas: visual and anatomic results of treatment by photocoagulation or radiation therapy. *Ophthalmology* 1997;104:1773–1778.
20. Beierwaltes VM. X-ray treatment of malignant exophthalmos. *J Clin Endocrinol Metab* 1953;13:1090.
21. Blahut RJ, Beierwaltes VM, Lampe I. Exophthalmos response during roentgen therapy. *Am J Roentgenol Radium Ther Nucl Med* 1963;90:261.
22. Donaldson SS, McDougall IR, Egbert PR, et al. Treatment of orbital pseudotumor (idiopathic orbital inflammation) by radiation therapy. *Int J Radiat Oncol Biol Phys* 1980;6:79.
23. Knowles DM, Jacobiec FA. Orbital lymphoid neoplasms. *Cancer* 1980;46:576.
24. Ravin JG, Sisson JC, Knapp WT. Orbital radiation for the ocular changes of Graves' disease. *Am J Ophthalmol* 1975;79:285.
25. Sandler HM, Rubenstein JH, Fowble BL, et al. Results of radiotherapy for thyroid ophthalmopathy. *Int J Radiat Oncol Blot Phys* 1989;17:823.
26. Peterson IA, Donaldson SS, McDougall MB, et al. Prognostic factors in the radiotherapy of Graves' ophthalmopathy. Paper presented at: 31st Annual ASTRO Meeting; 1989; San Francisco.
27. Cavanagh HO, Gren VR, Goldberg HK. Multicentric sebaceous adenocarcinomas of the meibomian gland. *Am J Ophthalmol* 1974; 77:326.
28. Pardo FS, Wang CC, Albert D, et al. Sebaceous carcinoma of the ocular adnexa: radiotherapeutic management. *Int J Radiat Oncol Biol Phys* 1989;17: 643.
29. Gotfredsen E. On the frequency of secondary carcinoma of the choroid. *Acta Ophthalmol* (Copenh) 1944;22:394.
30. Stallard HB. Six cases of metastatic carcinoma of the choroid. *Proc R Soc Med* 1933;26:1042.
31. Ferry AP, Font RL. Carcinoma metastatic to the eye and orbit. 1. A clinicopathologic study of 227 cases. *Arch Ophthalmol* 1974;92:276.
32. Brady LW, Shields JA, Augsburger JJ, et al. Malignant intraocular tumors. *Cancer* 1982;49:578.
33. Stephens RE, Shields JA. Diagnosis and management of cancer metastatic to the uvea: a study of 70 cases. *Ophthalmology* 1979; 86:1336.
34. Bloch RS, Gartner S. The incidence of ocular metastatic carcinoma. *Arch Ophthalmol* 1971;85:673.
35. Shields JA, Stephens RA, Augsburger JJ. Metastatic tumor to the uveal tract. In: Lommatzsch PK, Blodi FC, eds. *Intraocular tumors.* Berlin: Akademie-Verlag, 1983:433–444.
36. De Potter P, Shields CL, Shields JA, Tardio DJ. Uveal metastasis from prostate carcinoma. *Cancer* 1993;71:2791–2796.
37. Letson AD, Davidorf FH, Bruce RA Jr. Chemotherapy for treatment of choroidal metastases from breast carcinoma. *Am J Ophthalmol* 1982;93:102–106.
38. Shields CL, Shields JA, De Potter P, et al. Short-term plaque radiotherapy for treatment of choroidal metastasis. *Arch Ophthalmol* 1997;115:203–209.
39. Shields JA, McDonald PR. Improvement in the diagnosis of posterior uveal melanomas. *Arch Ophthalmol* 1974;91:259.
40. Winter FC. Surgical excision of tumors of the ciliary body and iris. *Arch Ophthalmol* 1963;70:19.
41. Winter FC. Iridocyclectomy for malignant melanoma of the iris and ciliary body. In: Boniuk M, ed. *Ocular and adnexal tumors: new and controversial aspects.* St Louis: Mosby, 1964:341–352.
42. Zimmerman LE, McLean IW. Changing concepts concerning the malignancy of ocular tumors. *Arch Ophthalmol* 1975;78:487.
43. Fraunfelder FT, Boozman FW 111, Wilson DS, et al."No-touch" technique for intraocular malignant melanomas. *Arch Ophthalmol* 1977;95:616.
44. Federman JL, Lewis MG, Clark VM, et al. Tumor-associated antibodies in the serum of ocular melanoma patients. *Trans Am Acad Ophthalmol Otolaryngol* 1974;78:784.
45. Curtin VT, Cavender JC. The natural course of selected malignant melanomas of the choroid and ciliary body. *Mod Probl Ophthalmol* 1974;12: 523.
46. Straatsma BR, Fine SL, Earle JD, et al. The Collaborative Ocular Melanoma Study research group. Enucleation versus plaque irradiation for choroidal melanoma. *Ophthalmology* 1988;95:1000–1004.
46a. Collaborative Ocular Melanoma Study Group. COMS report #18. *Arch Ophthalmol* 2001;119:969–982.
47. Davidorf FH, Newman GH, Havener WH, et al. Conservative management of malignant melanoma II. Transcleral diatherapy. *Arch Ophthalmol* 1970;82: 273.
48. Foulds WS. Local excision of choroidal melanomas. *Trans Ophthalmol Soc U K* 1974;93:343.
49. Lincoff H, McLean J, Lang R. The cryosurgical treatment of intraocular tumors. *Am J Ophthalmol* 1967;63:389.
50. Long RS, Galin MA, Rotman M. Conservative treatment of intraocular melanomas. *Trans Am Acad Ophthalmol Otolaryngol* 1971;75:84.
51. Meyer-Schwickerath G. Further progress in the field of light coagulation. *Trans Ophthalmol Soc U K* 1957;77:421.
52. Peyman GA, Apple DJ. Local excision of a choroidal malignant melanoma: full thickness eye wall resection. *Arch Ophthalmol* 1974;92:216.
53. Sautter H, Naumann G. Full thickness scleral resection in iridocyclectomy and choroidectomy for anterior uveal tumors. *Ophthalmic Surg* 1973;4:25.
54. Shields JA, Shields CL, Donoso LA. Management of posterior uveal melanoma. *Surv Ophthalmol* 1991;36:161–195.
55. Vogel MH. Treatment of malignant choroidal melanoma with photocoagulation: evaluation of 10-year follow-up data. *Am J Ophthalmol* 1972;74:1.
56. Newman GH, Davidorf FH, Havener WH, et al. Conservative management of malignant melanoma. 1. Irradiation as a method of treatment for malignant melanoma of the choroid. *Arch Ophthalmol* 1970;83:21.
57. Char DH, Castro JR. Helium ion therapy for choroidal melanoma. *Arch Ophthalmol* 1982;100:935.
58. Char DH, Castro JR, Quivey JM. Helium ion charged particle therapy for choroidal melanoma. *Ophthalmology* 1982;87:565.
59. Constable IJ. Proton irradiation therapy for ocular melanoma. *Trans Ophthalmol Soc U K* 1977;97:430.
60. Decker MM, Castro JR, Linstadt DE, et al. Ciliary body melanoma treated with helium particle irradiation. Paper presented at: 31st Annual ASTRO Meeting; 1989; San Francisco.
61. Gragoudas ES, Goiten M, Verhey L, et al. Proton beam irradiation of uveal melanomas. *Arch Ophthalmol* 1982;100:928.
62. Gragoudas ES, Seddon JM, Egan K, et al. Long-term results of proton beam irradiated uveal melanomas. *Ophthalmology* 1987;94:349.
63. Kindy-Degnan NA, Char DH, Castro JR, et al. Effect of various doses of radiation for uveal melanoma on regression, visual acuity, complications, and survival. *Am J Ophthalmol* 1989;107:114.
64. Lunstadt D, Char DH, Castro JR, et al. Vision following helium ion radiotherapy of uveal melanoma: a Northern California Oncology group study. *Int J Radiat Oncol Biol Phys* 1988;15:347.
65. Munzenrider JE, Gragoudas ES, Seddon JM, et al. Conservative treatment of uveal melanoma: probability of eye retention after proton treatment. *Int J Radiat Oncol Biol Phys* 1988;15:553.
66. Munzenrider JE, Verhey LS, Gragoudas ES, et al. Conservative treatment of uveal melanoma: local recurrence after proton beam therapy. *Int J Radiat Oncol Biol Phys* 1989;17:493.
67. Rand RW, Khonsary A, Brown WJ, et al. Leksell stereotactic radiosurgery in the treatment of eye melanoma. *Neural Res* 1987; 9:142.
68. Saunders WM, Char DH, Quivey JM, et al. Precision high dose radiotherapy: helium ion treatment of uveal melanoma. *Int J Radiat Oncol Biol Phys* 1985;11: 227.
69. Seddon JM, Gragoudas ES, Egan KA, et al. Uveal melanomas near the optic disc or fovea: visual results after proton beam irradiation. *Ophthalmology* 1987;94:354.
70. Bedford MA, Bedotto C, MacFaul PA. Radiation retinopathy after application of a cobalt plaque: report of three cases. *Br J Ophthalmol* 1970;54: 505.
71. Boniuk M, Girard L. Malignant melanomas of the choroid treated with photocoagulation, transscleral diathermy and radon seed implant. *Am J Ophthalmol* 1965;59:212.
72. Bosworth JL, Packer S, Rotman M, et al. Choroidal melanoma: I-125 plaque therapy. *Radiology* 1988;169:249.
73. Chenery SG, Fitzpatrick PJ, Japp B, et al. Treatment of choroidal melanoma with radioisotopes. Paper presented at: the American Society of Therapeutic Radiology; 1978; Los Angeles.
74. Davidorf FH, Pajka JT, Makley T, et al. Radiotherapy for choroidal melanoma: an 18-year experience with radon. *Arch Ophthalmol* 1987;105:352.
75. Lommatzsch P. Treatment of choroidal melanomas with 106Rh beta ray applicators. *Surv Ophthalmol* 1974;19:85.
76. Lommatzsch P. Beta-irradiation of retinoblastoma with 106Ru/106Rh applicators. *Mod Probl Ophthalmol* 1977;18:128.
77. Lommatzsch PK. Beta irradiation with 106Ru/106Rh applicators of choroidal melanomas: sixteen years' experience. In: Lommatzsch PK, Blodi FC, eds. *Intraocular tumors.* Berlin: Academie-Verlag, 1983:290–301.
78. Lommatzsch PK, Kirsch IH. 106Ru/106Rh plaque radiotherapy for malignant melanomas of the choroid: with follow-up results more than 5 years. *Doc Ophthalmol* 1988;68:255a(abst).
79. MacFaul PA. Local radiotherapy in the treatment of malignant melanoma of the choroid. *Trans Ophthalmol Soc U K* 1977;97:421.
80. MacFaul PA, Morgan G. Histopathological changes in malignant melanomas of the choroid after cobalt plaque therapy. *Br J Ophthalmol* 1977;61:221.
81. Markoe AM, Brady LW, Shields JA, et al. Radioactive eye-plaque therapy versus enucleation for the treatment of posterior uveal malignant melanoma. *Radiology* 1985;156:801.
82. Muller RP, Busse H, Potter R, et al. Results of high dose 106 ruthenium irradiation of choroidal melanomas. *Int J Radiat Oncol Biol Phys* 1986;12:1749.
83. Packer S. Iodine 125 radiation of posterior uveal melanoma. *Ophthalmology* 1987;94:1621.
84. Stallard HB. Malignant melanoma of the choroid treated with radioactive applicators. *Trans Ophthalmol Soc U K* 1959;79:373.
85. Stallard HB. The conservative treatment of retinoblastoma. *Trans Ophthalmol Soc U K* 1962;82:473.
86. Stallard HB. Partial choroidectomy. *Br J Ophthalmol* 1966;50:660.
87. Shields JA, Shields CL. Management of posterior uveal melanoma. In: Shields JA, Shields CL, eds. *Intraocular tumors. A text and atlas.* Philadelphia: WB Saunders, 1992:171–205.

87a. Karlsson UL, Augsburger JJ, Shields JA, et al. Recurrence of posterior uveal melanoma after ^{60}Co episcleral plaque therapy. *Ophthalmology* 1989;96:382.
88. De Potter P, Shields CL, Shields JA, et al. Plaque radiotherapy for juxtapapillary choroidal melanoma: visual acuity and survival outcome. *Arch Ophthalmol* 1996;114:1357–1365.
89. Adams KS, Abramson DH, Ellsworth RM, et al. Cobalt plaque versus enucleation for uveal melanoma: comparison of survival rates. *Br J Ophthalmol* 1988;72:494–497.
90. Augsburger JJ, Gamel JW, Sardi VF, et al. Enucleation versus cobalt plaque radiotherapy for malignant melanomas of the choroid and ciliary body. *Arch Ophthalmol* 1986;104:655–661.
91. De Potter P, Shields CL, Shields JA, et al. Impact of enucleation versus plaque radiotherapy in the management of juxtapapillary choroidal melanoma on patient survival. *Br J Ophthalmol* 1994;78:109–114.
92. Vrabec TR, Augsburger JJ, Gamel JW, et al. Impact of local tumor relapse on patient's survival after cobalt 60 plaque radiotherapy. *Ophthalmology* 1991;98: 984–988.
93. Lommatzsch PK, Alberti W Lommatzsch P, et al. Radiation effects on the optic nerve observed after brachytherapy of choroidal melanomas with 106Ru/106Rh plaques. *Graefes Arch Clin Exp Ophthalmol* 1994;232:482–487.
94. Robertson DM, Earle J, Kline RW. Brachytherapy for choroidal melanoma. In: Ryan SJ, ed. *Retina,* 2nd ed. St Louis: Mosby, 1994:773–784.
95. Liggett PE. Discussion of article: recurrence of posterior uveal melanoma after ^{60}Co episcleral plaque therapy. *Ophthalmology* 1989;96:387.
96. Packer S, Stoller S, Lesser ML, et al. Long term results of iodine 125 irradiation of uveal melanoma. *Ophthalmology* 1992;99:767–774.
97. Cruess AF, Augsburger JJ, Shields JA, et al. Visual results following cobalt plaque radiotherapy for posterior uveal melanoma. *Ophthalmology* 1984;91: 131–136.
98. Augsburger JJ, Mullen D, Kleineidan M. Planned combined I-125 plaque irradiation and indirect ophthalmoscope laser therapy for choroidal melanoma. *Ophthalmol Surg* 1993;24:7681.
99. Shields CL, Shields JA, De Potter P, et al. Transpupillary thermotherapy in the management of choroidal melanoma. *Ophthalmology* 1996;103:1642–1650.
100. Brady LW, Shields JA, Augsburger JJ, et al. Posterior uveal melanomas. In: Phillips TL, Pistenmaa DA, eds. *Radiation oncology annual.* Vol 1. New York: Raven Press, 1984:233–245.
101. Kenneally CL, Farber MG, Smith ME, et al. In vitro melanoma cell growth after preenucleation radiation therapy. *Arch Ophthalmol* 1988;106:223.
102. Char DH, Phillips TL, Andeski Y, et al. Failure of pre-enucleation radiation to decrease uveal melanoma mortality. *Am J Ophthalmol* 1988;106:21.
103. Luyten GP, Mooy CM, Eijkenboom WMH, et al. No demonstrated effect of pre-enucleation irradiation on survival of patients with uveal melanoma. *Am J Ophthalmol* 1995;9:786–791.
104. Shields CL, Shields JA, De Potter P, et al. Treatment of non-resectable malignant iris tumors with custom designed plaque radiotherapy. *Br J Ophthalmol* 1995;79:306–312.
104a. Shields CL, Naseripour N, Shields JA, et al. Custom-designed plaque radiotherapy for nonresectable iris melanoma in 38 patients: tumor control and ocular complications. *Am J Ophthalmol* 2003;135:648–656.
105. Banks CN. Inheritance of retinoblastoma. *Br J Ophthalmol* 1969;53:212.
106. Donaldson SS, Smith LA. Retinoblastoma: biology, presentation and current management. *Oncology* 1989;3:45.
107. Jereb B, Koch E, Asard PE. Prognosis of retinoblastoma treated at Radiumhemmet 1926–1963. *Acta Radiol* 1967;6:369.
108. Neilson M, Goldschmidt E. Retinoblastomas among offspring of adult survivors in Denmark. *Acta Ophthalmol* (Copenh) 1968; 46:736.
109. Shields JA, Shields CL, Donoso LA, et al. Changing concepts in the management of retinoblastoma. *Ophthalmol Surg* 1990;21:72–76.
110. Donaldson SS, Egbert PR. Retinoblastoma. In: Pizzo P, ed. *Principles and practice of pediatric oncology.* Philadelphia: JB Lippincott Co, 1981.
111. Shields CL, Shields JA, Shah E. Retinoblastoma in older children. *Ophthalmology* 1991;98:395–399.
112. Shields CL, Shields JA. New treatment modalities for retinoblastoma. *Curr Opin Ophthalmol* 1997;7:20–26.
113. De Potter P, Gonzalez CF, Flanders AE, et al. Imaging studies of intraocular tumors. In: Alberti WE, Sagerman RH, eds. *Medical radiology. Radiotherapy of intraocular and orbital tumors.* Berlin: Springer-Verlag, 1993:295–309.
114. Reese AB, Ellsworth RM. The evaluation and current concept of retinoblastoma therapy. *Trans Am Acad Ophthalmol Otolaryngol* 1963;67:1–4.
114a. Shields CL and Shields JA. Recent developments in the management of retinoblastoma. *J Pediatr Ophthalmol Strabismus* 1999;36:8–18.
114b. Shields JA, Shields CL, Sivalingam V. Decreasing frequency of enucleation in patients with Retinoblastoma. *Am J Ophthalmol* 1989;108:185–188.
114c. Freire J, Miyamoto C, Brady L, et al. Retinoblastoma after chemoreduction and irradiation: preliminary results. *Front Radiat Ther Oncol* 1997;30:88–92.
114d. Gunduz K, Shields C, Shields J, et al. The outcome of chemoreduction treatment in patients with Reese-Ellsworth group V retinoblastoma. *Arch Ophthalmol* 1998;116:1613–1617.
115. Shields CL, De Potter P, Himmelstein B, et al. Chemoreduction in the initial management of intraocular retinoblastoma. *Arch Ophthalmol* 1996;114:1330–1338.
115a. Shields CL, De Potter P, Himelstein BP, et al. Chemoreduction in the initial management of intraocular retinoblastoma. *Arch Ophthalmol* 1996;114: 1330–1338.
116. Hilgartner HL. Report of a case of double glioma treated with x-ray. *Tex Med J* 1903;18:322.
117. Armstrong DI. The use of 4-6 MeV electrons for the conservative treatment of retinoblastoma. *Br J Radiol* 1974;47:326.
118. Weiss DR, Cassady JR, Petersen R. Retinoblastoma: a modification in radiation therapy technique. *Radiology* 1975;114:705.
119. McCormick B, Ellsworth R, Abramson D, et al. Radiation therapy for retinoblastoma: comparison of results with lens-sparing versus lateral beam techniques. *Int J Radiat Oncol Biol Phys* 1988;15:567.
120. Chin LM, Harter KW, Svansson GK, et al. An external-beam treatment technique for retinoblastoma. *Int J Radiat Oncol Biol Phys* 1988;15:455.
121. Foote RL, Garretson BR, Schomberg PJ, et al. External-beam irradiation for retinoblastoma: patterns of failure and dose-response analysis. *Int J Radiat Oncol Biol Phys* 1989;16:823.
122. Hungerford JL, Toma NMG, Plowman PN, et al. External beam radiotherapy for retinoblastoma: whole eye technique. *Br J Ophthalmol* 1995;79: 109–111.
123. Schipper J. An accurate and simple method for megavoltage radiation therapy of retinoblastoma. *Radiother Oncol* 1983;1:31.
124. Schipper J, Tan K-EWP, van Peperzeel HA. Treatment of retinoblastoma by precision megavoltage radiation therapy. *Radiother Oncol* 1985;3:117.
125. Cassady JR, Sagennan RH, Tretter P, et al. Radiation therapy in retinoblastoma: an analysis of 230 cases. *Radiology* 1969;93:405.
125a. Hayden B, Murray T, Cicciarelli N, et al. Hyperfractionated external beam radiation therapy in the treatment of murine transgenic Retinoblastoma. *Arch Ophthalmol* 2002;120:353–359.
126. Weiss AH, Karr DJ, Kalina RE, et al. Visual outcomes of macular retinoblastoma after external beam radiation therapy. *Ophthalmology* 1994;101: 1244–1249.
127. Stallard HB. Radiotherapy of malignant intraocular neoplasms. *Br J Ophthalmol* 1948;32:618.
128. Amendola BE, Markoe AM, Augsburger JJ, et al. Analysis of treatment results in 36 children with retinoblastoma treated by scleral plaque irradiation. *Int J Radiat Oncol Biol Phys* 1989;17:63.
129. Hernandez JC, Brady LW, Shields CL, et al. Conservative treatment of retinoblastoma. The use of plaque brachytherapy. *Am J Clin Oncol* 1993;16: 397–401.
130. Shields CL, Shields JA, De Potter P, et al. Plaque radiotherapy in the management of retinoblastoma. Use as a primary and secondary treatment. *Ophthalmology* 1993;100:216–224.
131. Shields JA, Shields CL, De Potter P, et al. Plaque radiotherapy for residual or recurrent retinoblastoma in 91 cases. *J Pediatr Ophthamol Strabismus* 1994;31: 242–245.
132. Shields CL, Shields JA, Minelli S, et al. Regression of retinoblastoma after plaque radiotherapy. *Am J Ophthalmol* 1993;115:181–187.
133. Shields JA, Giblin ME, Shields CL, et al. Episcleral plaque radiotherapy for retinoblastoma. *Ophthalmology* 1989;96:530.
134. De Potter P, Shields CL, Shields JA. Clinical variation of trilateral retinoblastoma: a report of 13 cases. *J Pediatr Ophthalmol Strabismus* 1994;31:26–31.
135. Blach LE, McCormick B, Abramson DH, et al. Trilateral retinoblastoma: incidence and outcome: a decade of experience. *Int J Radiat Oncol Biol Phys* 1994;29:729–733.
135a. Freire JE, DePotter P, Brady LW, et al. Brachytherapy in primary ocular tumors. *Semin Surg Oncol* 1997;13:167–176.
136. Smith LM, Donaldson SS, Egbert PR, et al. Aggressive management of second primary tumors in survivors of hereditary retinoblastoma. *Int J Radiat Oncol Biol Phys* 1989;17:499.
137. Roarty JD, McLean IW, Zimmerman CE. Incidence of second neoplasms in patients with bilateral retinoblastoma. *Ophthalmology* 1988;95:1583.
138. Eng C, Li FP, Abramson DH, et al. Mortality from second tumors among long-term survivors of retinoblastoma. *J Natl Cancer Inst* 1993;85:1121–1128.
139. Schwarz MB, Burgess LP, Fee WE Jr, et al. Postirradiation sarcoma in retinoblastoma: induction or predisposition. *Arch Otolaryngol Head Neck Surg* 1988;114:640.
140. Hawkins MM, Draper GJ, Kingston JE. Incidence of second primary tumors among childhood cancer survivors. *Br J Cancer* 1987;56:339.
141. Ridgeway WE, Jaffe N, Walton DS. Leukemic ophthalmopathy in children. *Cancer* 1976;38:1744.
142. Minckler DS, Font RL, Zimmerman LE. Uveitis and reticulum cell sarcoma of brain with bilateral neoplastic seeding of vitreous without retinal or uveal involvement. *Am J Ophthalmol* 1975;80:433.
143. Michels RC, Knox DL, Erozan YS, et al. Intraocular reticulum cell sarcoma: diagnosis by pars plana vitrectomy. *Arch Ophthalmol* 1975;93:1331.
144. Barthold HJ, Harvey A, Markoe AM, et al. Treatment of orbital pseudo tumor and lymphoma. *Am J Clin Oncol* 1986;9:527.
145. Shields JA, Bakewell B, Donoso L, et al. Space-occupying masses in children. A review of 250 consecutive biopsies. *Ophthalmology* 1986;93:379–384.
146. Lederman M. Radiotherapy of primary malignant tumors of the orbit. *Mod Probl Ophthalmol* 1975;14:170.
147. Pizzo PA, Miser JS, Cassady JR, et al. Solid tumors of childhood. In: Devita VT Jr, Hellman S, Rosenberg SA, eds. *Cancer: principles and practice of oncology,* 2nd ed. Philadelphia: JB Lippincott Co, 1985:1511–1589.
148. Maurer HM, Moon TE, Donaldson M, et al. The Intergroup Rhabdomyosarcoma Study. *Cancer* 1977;40:2015.
149. Calhoun FP, Reese AB. Rhabdomyosarcoma of the orbit. *Arch Ophthalmol* 1982;27:558.
150. Jones IS, Reese AB, Krout J. Orbital rhabdomyosarcoma: an analysis of 62 cases. *Trans Am Ophthalmol Soc* 1965;63:223.

151. Porterfield JF, Zimmerman LE. Rhabdomyosarcoma of the orbit: a clinicopathologic study of 55 cases. *Virchows Arch* 1962;335:329.
152. Liebner EJ. Embryonal rhabdomyosarcoma of head and neck in children: correlation of stage, radiation dose, local control and survival. *Cancer* 1976; 37:2777.
153. Sagennan RH, Cassady JR, Tretter P. Radiation therapy for rhabdomyosarcoma of the orbit. *Trans Am Acad Ophthalmol Otolaryngol* 1968;72:849.
154. Lederman M. Radiotherapy in treatment of orbital tumors. *Br J Ophthalmol* 1956;40:592.
155. Sagerman RH, Tretter P, Ellsworth RM. The treatment of orbital rhabdomyosarcoma of children with primary radiation therapy. *Am J Roentgenol Radium Ther Nucl Med* 1972;114:31.
156. Kelly AG, Rosas-Uribe A, Kraus ST. Orbital lymphomas and pseudolymphomas: a clinicopathologic study of 11 cases. *Am J Ophthalmol* 1973;76:371.
157. Rappaport H, Winter WJ, Hicks EB. Follicular lymphoma: based on a survey of 253 cases. *Cancer* 1956;9:792.
158. Rao DV, Smith M, Griffith R, et al. Orbital lymphomas and pseudolymphomas. *Int J Radiat Oncol Biol Phys* 1982;8:114.
159. Mittal B, Deutsch M, Kennerdell J, et al. Paraocular lymphoid tumors. *Radiology* 1986;159:793.
160. Fitzpatrick PJ, Macko S. Lymphoreticular tumors of the orbit. *Int J Radiat Oncol Biol Phys* 1984;10:333.
161. Austin-Seymour MM, Donaldson SS, Egbert PR, et al. Radiotherapy of lymphoid diseases of the orbit. *Int J Radiat Oncol Biol Phys* 1985;1:371.
162. Reddy BK, Bhatia P, Evans RG. Primary orbital lymphomas. *Int J Radiat Oncol Biol Phys* 1988;15:1239.
163. Makepeace AR, Fennont DC, Bennett MH. Primary non-Hodgkin's lymphoma of the orbit. *J R Soc Med* 1988;81:640.
164. Bessell EM, Henk JM, Wright JE, et al. Orbital and conjunctival lymphoma treatment and prognosis. *Radiother Oncol* 1988;13:237.
165. Franklin CIV. Primary lymphoreticular tumors in the orbit. *Clin Radiol* 1975;26:137.
166. Halnan KS. Tumors of the eye treated by radiotherapy. *Clin Radiol* 1962;13:19.
167. Shields CL, Shields JA, Eagle RL, et al. Clinicopathologic review of 142 cases of lacrimal gland lesions. *Ophthalmology* 1989;96:431–435.
168. Shields JA. *Diagnosis and management of orbital tumors.* Philadelphia: WB Saunders, 1989.
169. Blodi FC. The late effects of x-irradiation on the cornea. *Trans Am Ophthalmol Soc* 1958;56:413.
170. Blodi FC. The effects of experimental x-radiation on the cornea. *Arch Ophthalmol* 1960;63:44.
171. Cogan DG, Donaldson DD, Reese AB. Clinical and pathological characteristics of radiation cataract. *Arch Ophthalmol* 1952;47:55.
172. Merriam GR, Focht E. A clinical study of radiation cataracts and their relationship to dose. *Am J Roentgenol Radium Ther Nucl Med* 1957;77:759.
173. Ham WT. Radiation cataract. *Arch Ophthalmol* 1953;50:618.
174. MacFaul PA, Bedford MA. Ocular complications after therapeutic irradiation. *Br J Ophthalmol* 1970;54:237.
175. Ross H, Rosenberg S, Friedman AH. Delayed radiation necrosis of the optic nerve. *Am J Ophthalmol* 1973;76:683.
176. Cappin JM. Radiation scleral necrosis simulating early scleromalacia perforans. *Br J Ophthalmol* 1973;57:4525.
177. Forrest AW. Tumors following radiation about the eye. *Trans Am Acad Ophthalmol Otolaryngol* 1961;65:694.
178. Ralvio I, Tarkkanen A. Sarcoma following radiation for retinoblastoma. *Acta Ophthalmol* (Copenh) 1965;43:428.
179. Sagennan RH, Cassady JR, Tretter P, et al. Radiation-induced neoplasm following external beam therapy for children with retinoblastoma. *Am J Roentgenol Radium Ther Nucl Med* 1969;105:529.
180. Shah IC, Arlen M, Miller T. Osteogenic sarcoma developing after radiotherapy for retinoblastoma. *Am Surg* 1974;40:485.
181. Shields CL, Shields JA, Karlson U, et al. Reasons for enucleation after plaque radiotherapy for posterior uveal melanoma. *Ophthalmology* 1989;96: 919–924.
182. Soloway HB. Radiation-induced neoplasms following curative therapy for retinoblastoma. *Cancer* 1966;19:1984.
183. Tebbet RD, Vickery RD. Osteogenic sarcoma following irradiation for retinoblastoma. *Am J Ophthalmol* 1952;3:811.
184. Yoneyama T, Greenlaw RH. Osteogenic sarcoma following radiotherapy for retinoblastoma. *Radiology* 1969;93:1185.

CHAPTER 33

Unusual Tumors of the Head and Neck

Ashok R. Shaha and John F. Carew

Approximately 95% of tumors of the upper aerodigestive tract are squamous cell carcinomas. The remaining 5% of tumors seen in the head and neck region are composed of a vast array of histologic types with widely different clinical behaviors. Thus, most tumors in the head and neck, besides squamous cell carcinoma and common skin cancers, remain unusual in the day-to-day practice of a head and neck oncologist. Although seasoned head and neck oncologists of all disciplines may have a significant experience with a variety of unusual tumors, through the years they will face difficult, complex, and unusual tumors of the head and neck. The unusual nature of these lesions must also be considered with regard to the geographic and referral characteristics of the individual institution. Although tuberculosis of the parotid gland may be fairly common in India, it is extremely rare in the United States. Similarly, though Kaposi sarcoma is relatively common in Africa, it is not seen with equal frequency in other parts of the world. It is a cumbersome task to classify the plethora of unusual tumors seen in the head and neck. The general principles of evaluation and management, however, can be discussed.

Case reports of rare and unusual head and neck tumors abound in the literature. Approximately 15% to 20% of the posters presented at the annual meeting of the American Academy of Otolaryngology—Head and Neck Surgery depict unusual head and neck tumors. In a review of the literature, although many unusual tumors are reported in standard head and neck journals, only three references could be found in book reviews. In a book edited by Suen and Myers, Harrison (1) described his experience with unusual head and neck tumors and granulomatous lesions, including juvenile nasopharyngeal angiofibroma, hamartoma and hemangioma, angiosarcoma and hemangiopericytoma, chemodectoma, carotid body tumors and glomus jugulare tumors, Wegener granulomatosis, olfactory neuroblastoma, meningioma, granular cell tumor, bone tumors, osteogenic sarcoma, ameloblastoma, fibrous dysplasia, soft tissue sarcoma, chordoma, and plasmacytoma. Even though tumors as such as ameloblastoma are relatively common in a dental practice, advanced ameloblastomas of the mandible and maxilla are rare, and at times their management becomes quite complex. In a chapter written for the instruction course for the American Academy of Otolaryngology, Pratt (2) described his experience with unusual tumors of the head and neck, including such tumors as hemangioma, lymphangioma, congenital cysts and sinuses, neurofibromas, giant-cell reparative granuloma, rhabdomyosarcoma, fibrosarcoma, floor-of-mouth cysts, hemangioendothelioma, paraganglioma, pleomorphic adenoma of the upper lip, and giant lipoma of the head and neck. Hyams (3), at the Armed Forces Institute of Pathology, described a variety of conditions in the pathology of the head and neck. He described his experience with sinonasal tract polyposis, inspissated mucus, midline malignant reticulosis, papillomas of the sinonasal tract, angiofibroma, spindle-cell carcinoma, nasopharyngeal carcinoma, olfactory neuroblastomas, and primary adenomatous neoplasms of the middle ear cleft. Calcaterra (4) discussed such unusual tumors as neural tumors, vascular tumors and malformations, and fibrous and bony tumors.

Clearly, the subject of unusual tumors of the head and neck will include a variety of nonsquamous lesions of the head and neck. The decision regarding individual cases should be based on the literature review, experience of the head and neck surgeon and, often, the combined opinion of a multidisciplinary head and neck tumor board. Sarcomas of the head and neck are relatively rare and can be grouped with the unusual tumors of the head and neck. However, they form a unique group of mesenchymal tumors and can usually be treated according to a similar philosophy (described in Chapter 34). Certain basic principles related to unusual tumors of the head and neck are very important. By necessity, there may be some overlap between this chapter and other chapters in this book.

PATHOLOGY

Probably the most important issue in the management of unusual tumors in any institution is an accurate histologic diagnosis. As the individual pathologist's experience may be fairly limited in the evaluation of these unusual tumors, it is important to seek consultation from other experienced pathologists. It is also important for clinicians to discuss with the pathologist the clinical findings and clinical issues involved in the evaluation of these patients. In a majority of the small cell tumors, a variety of differential diagnoses need to be distinguished for appropriate treatment of the individual patient. For example, it is extremely important in a patient presenting with poorly differentiated or anaplastic thyroid cancer to rule out lymphoma. In a majority of cases, this distinction appears to be simple. It is not uncommon, however, for a patient to undergo a major head and neck surgical ablative procedure and, with appropriate diagnostic studies, to arrive at a diagnosis of lymphoma.

A list of differential diagnoses of poorly differentiated carcinomas is given in Table 33.1. It is apparent from this table that the management of individual tumors will differ on the basis of definite diagnosis—for example, amelanotic melanoma or neuroendocrine tumor or Kaposi sarcoma. Special immunohistochemical stains and diagnostic tests are extremely important to distinguish various head and neck tumors.

TABLE 33.1 Differential Diagnosis of Poorly Differentiated Tumors

Poorly differentiated carcinoma
Anaplastic tumor
Lymphoma
Undifferentiated tumor
Esthesioneuroblastoma
Neuroendocrine carcinoma
Merkel cell carcinoma
Malignant melanoma (amelanotic)
Eccrine carcinoma
Medullary thyroid carcinoma
Rhabdomyosarcoma
Germ-cell tumor
Kaposi sarcoma
Plasmacytoma
Ewing tumor

DIAGNOSTIC WORKUP

Obviously, complete history and physical examination are paramount in evaluation of any unusual tumor. It would be fairly appropriate to seek opinion from one of the senior colleagues in the department. Occasionally, lesions such as angiosarcoma of the scalp or adnexal tumors of the skin can be easily recognized on clinical examination, whereas tumors of the ethmoid sinus will require appropriate radiologic evaluation. Certain congenital lesions, such as lymphangiomas or hemangiomas, can be easily diagnosed on clinical examination.

Fine-Needle Aspiration

The role of fine-needle aspiration in unusual head and neck tumors is fairly limited. Even though the fine-needle aspiration can easily make a diagnosis of squamous cell carcinoma, adenocarcinoma, or thyroid carcinoma, the detailed diagnosis of individual pathology in unusual tumors by fine-needle aspiration is fairly difficult, as no cytologist has enough experience in interpretation of unusual fine-needle aspirations. Fine-needle aspiration is an easy diagnostic study that can be of great help in suspected lymphomas and neuroendocrine tumors or to rule out certain benign conditions, such as tuberculosis. It is fairly helpful for atypical lesions in the parotid region to distinguish between salivary or nonsalivary pathologies. Obviously, the final diagnosis cannot rest on the interpretation of the fine-needle aspiration alone.

Core Biopsy

Core or Tru-Cut biopsy is fairly valuable in mesenchymal and soft-tissue tumors of the head and neck. The diagnosis of fibrosarcoma, leiomyosarcoma, and osteogenic sarcoma can easily be made based on core biopsy. Due consideration should be given to injury of neurovascular structures depending on the location of the lesion.

Diagnostic Imaging

In unusual tumors of the head and neck, both computed tomography (CT) and magnetic resonance imaging (MRI) are helpful to document the extent of disease and the characteristic of the individual lesions. The soft-tissue pathology is best evaluated with MRI. Computed tomography gives better interpretation of cartilaginous and bony tumors. Angiography may be necessary for evaluation of vascular tumors or carotid body tumors. Magnetic resonance angiography has shown tremendous promise recently in the evaluation of carotid body tumors.

Open Biopsy

If previous diagnostic studies are not helpful in yielding a diagnosis, obviously open biopsy is necessary. However, before planning an open biopsy, proper consideration should be given to the future treatment plan. The incision should be placed in such a way that it can be easily included in future excision with removal of the unusual tumor. A due consideration should be given for open biopsy and appropriate surgical excision at the same time (if feasible). The majority of nonlymphomatous lesions and unusual tumors in the head and neck would require adequate surgical excision and possible adjuvant therapy.

THERAPEUTIC APPROACHES

Obviously, treatment of the unusual head and neck tumor will depend on site, pathology, and extent of disease. Certain tumors, such as parathyroid carcinoma and thyroglossal duct carcinoma, though unusual, are well described in the literature. Even though these tumors are unusual, they are not the most uncommon, and adequate literature is available to guide management. However, many other unusual tumors, such as neuroendocrine tumors of the ethmoid sinus, are fairly rare, and appropriate literature is lacking for such tumors. Decisions in such rare events are best made with multidisciplinary input from radiation oncologists, medical oncologists, and other allied head and neck specialists.

THERAPEUTIC DILEMMA

The treatment of unusual tumors of the head and neck should be individualized. A specific group of unusual tumors, however, such as angiosarcoma of the head and neck, osteogenic sarcoma of the paranasal sinuses and mandible, or unusual histology of minor salivary gland tumors, can be treated conventionally with surgery and postoperative radiation therapy when indicated. If the tumor is stage T3 or T4, meaning greater than 4 cm, it is generally fairly likely that the patient will benefit from postoperative radiation therapy. Local control in these aggressive tumors is critical. The larger the tumor is, the greater the chance of local recurrence. One of the issues that must be addressed in the management of these tumors is three-dimensional resection of the tumor. In the head and neck, even though wide margins can often be achieved on the surface, there are limitations in surgical excision of the deeper margins, such as bone, skull base, and eye. In view of this, it is likely that a substantial number of these patients will need postoperative radiation therapy. The common indications for postoperative radiation therapy are inadequate margins of resection, aggressive pathology (high-grade, perineural, or perivascular invasion) and an extirpative procedure that leaves the surgeon unhappy with its adequacy despite negative margins. Thus, preoperative consultation with the radiation oncologist is important. Occasionally, the pathologists may differ in their opinions or may be unable to provide a definitive diagnosis or the histologic variety. The critical consideration under these circumstances is to rule out lymphoma. Most of the other tumors require surgical excision.

As in other head and neck tumors, the role of chemotherapy is limited in resectable tumors. Obviously, in unresectable tumors or recurrent tumors, consultation with a medical oncologist is warranted. In unresectable tumors, consideration should be given to multimodality treatment with chemotherapy and radiation therapy in protocols designed for unresectable tumors. These protocols may include newer modalities of radiation therapy, including three-dimensional conformal therapy or hyperfractionation. Future clinical research should be directed at improving combinations of chemotherapy and radiation therapy and fractionation of radiation therapy. Brachytherapy is used for recurrent or residual tumors after gross excision of the primary lesion. Consultation with the radiation oncologist, medical oncologist, and surgical colleagues is helpful in the appropriate management of these tumors. Some examples of unusual tumors recently noted in our practice are documented in following sections.

CLASSIFICATION

The unusual tumors of the head and neck can be classified into benign and malignant tumors. Occasionally, however, tumors may be classified in the *intermediate* category. These tumors include benign tumors that are locally aggressive and malignant tumors that are slow-growing and rarely metastasize.

Benign Tumors

TERATOMAS

Teratomas of the cervical region account for approximately 2% to 4% of all teratomas (5,6). Teratomas occur in approximately 1 in 4,000 births, and there is an equal incidence among the male and female populations (7,8). Teratomas of the nasopharynx are associated with palatal and craniofacial abnormalities, whereas cervical teratomas are not associated with any other congenital anomalies (9). They are usually noted at birth or become clinically apparent soon thereafter. With routine application of fetal ultrasonography in the last several decades, prenatal diagnosis has become more common. When tumors are diagnosed prenatally, preparations can be made to secure the neonatal airway at the time of planned cesarean section (10). Although the vast majority of teratomas present before the age of 1 year, cases of adult teratomas have been reported (11). Most adult lesions, however, are malignant.

Polyhydramnios is associated with teratomas in 18% to 53% of cases (9,12). This is due to the mass effect of the teratoma on the upper aerodigestive tract preventing the fetus from swallowing amniotic fluid. Physical examination shows a firm, multilobular mass exhibiting rapid growth that does not transilluminate. The tumors usually are located in the midline but may be more prominent on one side (13). Cervical teratomas usually cause symptoms related to the structures of the aerodigestive tract, which they compress. These patients can experience dysphagia, dyspnea, stridor, and airway obstruction. The size and location of the tumor will determine its magnitude.

Mature teratomas usually demonstrate cystic regions with the density of water or fat on CT imaging. Radiographic evidence of calcification, which is virtually diagnostic of a teratoma and reflects the variety of tissue types that can be found in teratomas, has been reported in 16% of cases (5). Sometimes, a fat-fluid level can be visualized and is virtually pathognomonic of a teratoma (11). Ultrasonography will show a heterogeneous echogenicity, which can help to differentiate it from the multilocular pattern of a cystic hygroma.

The treatment of cervical teratomas includes securing the airway and prompt and complete surgical excision. Because these tumors can grow rapidly and compress the airway, early surgical removal is recommended. Often these lesions are encapsulated, enabling complete removal. An 80% mortality has been reported in patients who did not undergo expeditious surgical management during the neonatal period (14). Reports of operative mortality range from 9% to 15% in patients undergoing prompt surgical excision (12,15,16). If such tumors are treated early and are completely excised, prognosis is very good. Mortality is usually the result of delayed treatment or inability to secure the airway. The most significant factors affecting clinical course are the size and location of the teratoma. Although cervical metastasis has been reported, this occurrence is rare (17).

CYSTIC HYGROMA (LYMPHANGIOMA)

Cystic hygromas (or lymphangiomas) occur throughout the body but are most commonly found in the neck. Lymphangiomas of the cervical region comprise up to 90% of all cases (16). Incidence of lymphangiomas ranges up to 12 per 1,000 fetuses as examined on maternal ultrasonography. Approximately 50% to 60% are clinically apparent at birth, and 80% to 90% present before the age of 2 (6,17). Male and female populations are equally affected (18). Lymphangiomas have been associated with Turner syndrome and various trisomies (6). They have also been associated with other congenital anomalies, including thyroglossal duct cysts, congenital heart defects, and hand and foot deformities (7).

These tumors have been classified into three groups: (a) lymphangioma simplex (capillary-like lymphatic vessels), (b) cavernous lymphangioma (dilated lymphatic channels with one or several endothelial layers with or without an adventitial layer), and (c) cystic hygroma or cystic lymphangiomas (large multiloculated cysts) (19). The most common type is cystic hygroma, which accounts for 75% of lymphangiomas occurring in the neck (20).

Lymphangiomas present as soft, cystic, sometimes multilocular, painless masses that can be transilluminated. Within the neck, they are found most commonly in the posterior triangle but can extend anterior to the sternocleidomastoid muscle and can cross the midline. Compression of nearby structures can lead to symptoms of dysphagia, stridor, dyspnea, and sometimes pain. Cervical lesions may extend into the axilla, mediastinum, or thorax (6). When they extend into the mediastinum, they are associated with venous aneurysms that should be recognized before surgical intervention (21). The majority of lymphangiomas grow in proportion with the infant or show slowly progressive enlargement (6,9). Occasionally, infection or hemorrhage into the lymphangioma can result in rapid enlargement and potentially life-threatening airway compression (6,9).

On CT scan, lymphangiomas are low-density, non-enhancing cystic lesions that may be unilocular or multilocular. The cyst wall is thin and usually is not visualized radiographically unless previous infection or hemorrhage has caused it to thicken (17). They can displace or surround neurovascular structures and muscles but rarely are found to infiltrate on radiographic examination (17). If previous infection or hemorrhage has occurred, the cyst wall will thicken and enhance (17). On MRI, the lesions will have low intensity on T1-weighted images and high intensity on T2-weighted images. If previous hemorrhage has occurred, fluid levels may be visualized, being best seen on T2-weighted images (17).

Treatment of lymphangiomas is surgical excision. Often, these tumors can extend locally to surround neurovascular structures, making complete surgical removal challenging. Most surgeons advocate delayed removal when the infant has reached 2 to 4 years of age, unless there are symptoms of compression or the diagnosis is uncertain (7,9,18). Others, however, have advocated early surgical excision for infants born with cystic hygromas to avoid the problems of airway obstruction when hemorrhage or infection causes rapid enlargement (6). Regardless of timing, every attempt should be made to avoid rupturing the cyst during surgery to allow complete removal.

Rates of recurrence range from 5% to 10% (18). Not surprisingly, higher recurrence rates are seen with larger lymphangiomas and the cavernous type (6,9). Additionally, the location affects recurrence rates, with 81% of extraparotid suprahyoid lesions recurring, compared with only 15% of infrahyoid lesions (22). Fairly often, lymphangiomas will extend into the parotid region, and the surgeon should be prepared to excise the entire cystic hygroma with superficial parotidectomy. If not resected completely, these lesions can recur, and further surgical excision may be more difficult, endangering vital structures and nerves.

Peripheral Nerve Sheath Tumors

Approximately 45% of peripheral nerve sheath tumors occur in the head and neck region. However, these tumors are relatively rare. Schwann cells are the cells of origin of the peripheral nerve sheath tumors, including schwannomas and neurofibromas. Although schwannomas and neurofibromas share the same progenitor cell, these neoplasms display different clinical behavior and are considered separately. Interestingly, neurogenic tumors account for 17% to 25% of lesions in the parapharyngeal space (17).

Schwannoma

Schwannomas can arise anywhere in the body but have a predilection for the head and neck region. The lateral cervical region is the most common site within the head and neck, although the tumors can occur in such other areas as the internal auditory canal, where they are commonly known as acoustic neuromas or vestibular nerve schwannomas. Within the neck, they can arise from the cervical sensory nerves or cranial nerves, the cervical sympathetic chain, and the brachial plexus. Malignant degeneration is extremely rare. These tumors affect women more commonly than men and occur most commonly in the 40- to 70-year age group.

Schwannomas usually present as a solitary, slow-growing neck mass that may cause symptoms related to compression of neighboring structures. Occasionally, pain occurs and is located distal to the lesion; it can be exacerbated by pressure on the lesion. Neurologic deficits from schwannomas, however, are rare.

On CT scan, benign nerve sheath tumors are isodense to soft tissue. Both schwannomas and neurofibromas may have cystic areas. In schwannomas, this cystic appearance is due to cysts, whereas in neurofibroma it is due to fatty regions within the lesion. Although these lesions are hypovascular, they tend to enhance with intravenous contrast (17). On MRI, these lesions have intermediate intensity on T1-weighted images and high intensity on T2-weighted images (23). If they extend through foramina, nerve sheath tumors can form characteristic dumbbell-shaped tumors (24).

In the specific case in which schwannomas arise from neural structures within the parapharyngeal space or from the cervical sympathetic chain, they tend to occur in the post-styloid compartment and displace the carotid artery anteriorly (25).

Schwannomas arise from the perineural elements and histologically appear to push axons aside rather than incorporating the axons in the tumor (7,9). Surgery remains the treatment of choice. This encapsulated lesion can, on rare occasions, be dissected off the nerve of origin, with preservation of neural function. With complete excision, prognosis is good, and local recurrence is rare. The ability to excise schwannomas completely depends primarily on the size, location, and proximity of the tumor to vital structures.

Neurofibroma

Neurofibromas can be located anywhere in the head and neck region and are seen most commonly in the skin and subcutaneous tissues. Occasionally, they can be found in the upper aerodigestive tract. Malignant transformation in isolated neurofibromas is rare. Solitary neurofibromas occur equally in both sexes and most commonly in the 20- to 30-year age group.

Neurofibromas can occur as an isolated lesion, as part of the syndrome of neurofibromatosis (von Recklinghausen disease), or (rarely) as multiple neurofibromas without association with a syndrome. Additionally, mucosal neuromas can occur in association with medullary thyroid carcinoma and pheochromocytoma (multiple endocrine neoplasia type IIB).

Neurofibromatosis, or von Recklinghausen disease, is transmitted by autosomal dominant inheritance, with variable but high penetrance. It can also occur through spontaneous mutation, and positive family histories are found in only half of patients (26). Two types of neurofibromatosis—types I and II—exist, and the following discussion applies primarily to type I. A plexiform neurofibroma, which involves a major nerve trunk with the characteristic fusiform, multilobular enlargement, is characteristic of neurofibromatosis. The diagnosis of neurofibromatosis (type I) is made by the presence of two or more of the following: (a) six café-au-lait spots (light brown macules) greater than 5 mm in diameter, (b) two or more neurofibromas or one plexiform neurofibroma, (c) axillary or inguinal freckling, (d) optic gliomas, (e) two or more Lisch nodules (optic hamartomas), (f) distinctive osseous lesions (sphenoid dysplasia or thinning of long-bone cortex), and (g) first-degree relative with neurofibromatosis type I (7). Onset after 25 years of age is rare, and two thirds of patients manifest symptoms of neurofibromatosis by age 1 (7,26). The genetic abnormality resulting in neurofibromatosis has been localized to chromosome 17 (27). The other form of neurofibromatosis, type II, is associated with multiple cranial nerve neurofibromas. Sarcomatous changes have been reported in 10% of plexiform neurofibromas and in 6% to 16% of all patients with neurofibromatosis (26,28).

Neurofibromas, whether solitary or in neurofibromatosis, present as slow-growing, painless masses that are otherwise asymptomatic. Although schwannomas and neurofibromas differ histologically, their radiographic appearance on CT and MRI scans is similar.

In contrast to schwannomas that may be dissected off the nerve, neurofibromas are intimately associated with the axons of the nerve and, therefore, often require nerve sacrifice (17). Complete surgical excision is the standard treatment of solitary neurofibromas. In neurofibromatosis, surgical treatment is indicated for lesions that are large, painful, rapidly growing, or suspected of being malignant (7). These lesions are not encapsulated but are infiltrative, rendering complete excision a challenge.

Malignant Tumors

GRANULAR CELL TUMORS

The majority of granular cell tumors occur in the head and neck region. The most common sites within the head and neck region are the tongue and larynx (29). Two forms exist: an infantile form, found on the gingiva of the newborn and clinically distinct from the adult form, and a non-infantile form, the focus of this discussion. These lesions usually present as small, painless, slowly growing lesions with an intact mucosa. They can sometimes be multifocal, although this is uncommon (30). Symptoms usually are related to their location within the upper aerodigestive tract, but they can often be asymptomatic. The lesions occur most commonly in the second and third decade. Women are more commonly affected than men and African Americans are more commonly affected than other races (9).

Histologically, oval, spindle, or round cells with a pale, eosinophilic, granular cytoplasm and small nuclei are seen. Tumor cells characteristically intermingle with the adjacent stromal cells and often are intimately associated with nerves (9). Electron microscopy shows the granular nature of the cytoplasm to be the result of abundant lysosomes (31). The mucosa overlying these tumors is often hyperplastic. At times, a pseudoepitheliomatous hyperplasia covers the lesions, which may be mistaken for squamous cell carcinoma. Granular cell tumors will show positive immunohistochemical staining for S-100 protein.

The treatment of granular cell tumors is local excision. Recurrences are relatively uncommon, with rates of up to 12% reported (30). Although rare, malignant granular cell tumors do occur. The histologic distinction between benign and malignant tumors can be difficult and is sometimes more apparent from the clinical behavior as determined by their rate of growth, size, and invasiveness (31). Malignant granular cell tumors carry a very poor prognosis (9).

HEMANGIOPERICYTOMA

Hemangiopericytomas are tumors that arise from pericytes of Zimmermann and are found outside capillaries and postcapillary venules. These uncommon vascular tumors first were described by Stout and Murray in 1942 (32). Although they were well characterized, many controversies still exist regarding their malignant potential and management.

Hemangiopericytomas usually present as rapidly growing, painless masses. They are usually detected due to their rapid growth, or they may become symptomatic secondary to impingement of adjacent structures. Head and neck sites account for approximately one-fourth of all tumors, although they may be found anywhere in the body where capillaries are found (9). No sex or race predominance has been established (9). The peak incidence of hemangiopericytoma occurs in middle-aged individuals (9). Infantile hemangiopericytomas have biologically benign behavior and are regarded as a separate clinical entity (33).

These tumors usually are partially or completely encapsulated, soft to rubbery, and gray-white to translucent. Histologically, they are characterized by capillaries surrounded by an accumulation of spindle cells. Enzinger and Smith (33) described the following characteristic features of hemangiopericytomas: (a) circumscription and pseudoencapsulation; (b) a continuously ramifying vascular pattern with large channels extending from the pericapsular tissue into the tumor in a radial fashion and branching into dilated sinusoid-like spaces or vessels of precapillary or capillary size (the vessels, regardless of size, being thin-walled and thick muscular coats being unusual); (c) reticulum preparations that impart a pattern variable from tumor to tumor and within different parts of a given tumor; (d) fibrosis nearly always present and variably diffuse, localized, or primarily perivascular; (e) occasionally noted osseous and cartilaginous metaplasia; (f) necrosis, hemorrhage, and thrombosis in cellular and rapidly growing neoplasms; and (g) occasional peripheral satellitosis and vascular invasion (33).

Pericytes serve as the cell of origin of both hemangiopericytomas and glomus tumors. These cells exhibit smooth muscle origin and function in regulation of luminal size as well as mechanical support of capillaries. On electron microscopy, the glomus tumors are well differentiated and closely resemble pericytes. Hemangiopericytomas, in contrast, are poorly differentiated and have large irregular nuclei and little, poorly developed cytoplasm (9). On immunohistochemical staining, both pericytes and glomus tumors stain positively for actin, whereas hemangiopericytomas are negative (34). This difference in immunohistochemical staining supports the poor differentiation of hemangiopericytomas and may explain its malignant behavior. Hemangiopericytomas typically stain positively for vimentin and factor XIII and negatively for S-100 and desmin (34).

Hemangiopericytomas exhibit unpredictable malignant behavior, and their management remains controversial. Regional lymph node involvement is rare, and metastasis is primarily through the hematogenous route, most commonly to lung or bone. In a review of 244 cases in the literature, a total recurrence rate (local and distant recurrence) was found to be 52% (35). In 45 cases of tumors located in the head and neck region, a 40% local recurrence rate and a 10% distant recurrence rate were noted (36). Long-term follow-up is important, and 5-year cure rates do not accurately reflect the behavior of this tumor, as recurrences have been noted 26 years after treatment (35). In predicting malignant behavior, Enzinger and Smith (33) found that tumors less than 6.5 cm in diameter had improved survival (92% 10-year survival). In addition, these authors correlated mitotic activity (greater than 4 mitoses per high-power field) with a lower 10-year survival (33). Other studies have not shown an association between mitotic activity and survival (9,35).

The standard management of this neoplasm remains surgical resection. The role of radiation therapy, however, remains controversial (33,35–37). In a series of 15 patients, Staples et al. (38) report that 4 patients treated with surgery and radiation therapy (5,600–6,000 cGy) were disease-free with follow-up of 11 months to 11 years. Of the 8 patients who were treated with surgery alone, one was disease-free at 18 months. In this study, radiation therapy was also employed successfully for salvage and palliation (38). The rare occurrence and variable malignant potential of hemangiopericytomas limit attempts at determining optimal treatment and the role of adjuvant radiation therapy.

EXTRAMEDULLARY PLASMACYTOMA AND SOLITARY PLASMACYTOMA OF BONE

Extramedullary plasmacytomas and solitary plasmacytoma of bone each account for 3% of all plasma cell neoplasms (39). Eighty percent of these occur in the head and neck region, with the most common sites being the nasal cavity, paranasal sinuses, and nasopharynx (40). These lesions are usually submucosal but can also occur in the thyroid (40,41). When they occur in the bone, they are called *solitary plasmacytomas of bone* and have different clinical behaviors with regard to conversion to multiple myeloma. The main prognostic factor for both of these lesions is the rate of conversion to multiple myeloma. Fifty-eight percent of solitary plasmacytomas of bone convert to multiple myeloma, whereas 20% to 30% of extramedullary plasmacytomas convert to multiple myeloma (39). Patients should be screened for multiple myeloma by radiographic skeletal survey, serum electrophoresis (which will show a monoclonal band in multiple myeloma), urine analysis for Bence Jones proteins, and bone marrow biopsy for a plasma cell preponderance (40). It should be noted, however, that patients with extramedullary plasmacytoma can show a monoclonal band on serum electrophoresis (40).

Extramedullary plasmacytomas are more common in male than in female populations (ratio, 3:1) and occur more frequently in the older age groups. The symptoms are related to the location of the lesion.

Histologically, these lesions are made up of plasma cells with abundant, slightly basophilic cytoplasm; round eccentric nuclei; and a cartwheel pattern of chromatin within the nucleus. They can be divided into low, intermediate, or high grades (42). Immunohistochemical staining will demonstrate a monoclonal lesion, demonstrating either kappa- or lambda-light chains.

External beam radiation therapy has been advocated as the primary treatment by some authors (40,43). Most advocate treatment of the primary lesions, including the lymphatics, whereas others treat only the primary lesion. Control rates by radiation therapy have been reported to range from 67% to 94% (40,43). Control rates vary according to dose, with a 94% control rate when the radiation dose was in excess of 40 Gy and a 69% control rate for doses less than 40 Gy (43). When plasmacytomas are treated with radiation therapy, surgery is reserved for salvage of localized resectable disease. The grade of the primary lesion has been related to local recurrence but not survival (40). Additionally, the involvement of cervical lymph nodes does not affect survival or conversion to multiple myeloma (44).

MALIGNANT TERATOMA

Though benign teratomas are relatively common, malignant teratomas are rare. Of adult teratomas, reported rates of malignancy exceed 90% (45). They occur more commonly in women (46). Malignant teratomas rarely occur in the neonatal or infantile form, and the clinical significance of lymph node metastasis is unclear (46).

Malignant teratomas usually present as rapidly growing neck masses in an adult. Other symptoms may be related to nearby structures, which they invade or compress.

Computed tomography scan of malignant teratomas often shows a low attenuation, locally destructive process that can cause bone erosion. When imaged with the contrast, malignant teratomas can appear as a non-enhancing necrotic process with a zone of peripheral enhancement (47). If a dynamic CT scan is performed, it may reveal a vascular outer rim, owing to the vascularity of the capsule of this lesion (47).

With less than 20 cases of malignant teratomas reported in the literature, it is difficult to determine the optimal treatment of this rare neoplasm (46). From these reports, however, it is apparent that malignant teratomas carry a dismal prognosis, and combined surgery and radiation therapy should be considered.

Despite multimodality therapy (surgery, radiation therapy, and chemotherapy), survival remains anecdotal in patients with malignant teratomas. Locoregional recurrence and pulmonary metastases are common. Pulmonary metastases have been reported to occur through local invasion of the mediastinum and neck veins (46).

ANGIOSARCOMA

Angiosarcomas account for 2% to 3% of soft tissue sarcomas (17). Approximately half of all angiosarcomas occur in the head and neck but account for less than 0.1% of head and neck malignancies (48). Most common sites within the head and neck are the scalp and soft tissues of the neck (49). Several factors have been associated with angiosarcoma and include prior irradiation, chronic lymphedema, thorium dioxide, vinyl chloride, insecticides, anabolic steroids, and synthetic estrogens (49).

Angiosarcomas in the head and neck region commonly present as vascular, purple, macular scalp or neck lesions with poorly defined margins (49). The margins often extend laterally throughout the dermis beyond what is clinically apparent, making wide excision with negative margins difficult (50). Lesions such as angiosarcomas may be fairly vascular and associated with difficulty in obtaining hemostasis at time of biopsy. They are often mistaken for a bruise or hemangioma, resulting in a delay in diagnosis and treatment. Often, the lesion will be ulcerated (72%), and the patient will report a history of bleeding. Angiosarcomas are also often multifocal (50). Relative to other sarcomas, angiosarcomas display a high incidence of regional lymph node metastasis, with reported rates ranging from 10% to 15% (49,51).

Although this rate is relatively high, most authors agree that elective treatment of the neck is not warranted.

On CT and MRI scans, the vascularity of angiosarcomas results in significant enhancement with intravenous contrast (17). The radiographic appearance reflects their aggressive clinical behavior, and they often show bone destruction.

Angiosarcomas require multimodality treatment with wide excision followed by postoperative radiation treatment. They have a poor prognosis, with 5-year survival ranging from 12% to 33% and a propensity for local recurrence and distant dissemination (49–51). The rate of local recurrence is much higher in patients with scalp tumors larger than 10 cm (46) (see also Chapter 34).

Angiosarcoma of the head and neck is an uncommon condition, but it generally behaves in a highly aggressive manner, with an overall extremely poor prognosis. It is a rare tumor arising in the vascular structures of the skin and soft tissues. Approximately half of all angiosarcomas occur in the head and neck, but they account for less than 0.1% of all head and neck malignancies. The most common presentation is in elderly men, mainly on the scalp or face. Due to the rarity of the lesion, the clinical suspicion may be delayed and appropriate diagnostic evaluation requires immunohistochemistry to confirm the diagnosis. Most authors advocate the treatment as wide surgical excision, if the lesion is resectable, along with postoperative radiation therapy (48–51). The role of chemotherapy as an adjuvant to surgery remains investigational. However, if the lesion is surgically unresectable, a combination of chemotherapy and radiation therapy is generally advocated. The drugs of choice appear to be Adriamycin and Taxol. Despite aggressive treatment, the prognosis of angiosarcoma remains quite poor, with a median survival of 18 to 24 months and a 5-year survival of approximately 12% to 33%. The most common site of failure appears to be local area with high incidence of regional metastasis. Death is generally due to uncontrolled local disease, often with regional and distant metastasis. Even though the most common sites of head and neck primaries include the scalp and upper face, less common areas include the maxilla, the mandible, the tongue, pharynx, and laryngopharynx. The most common presentation is an ulcerated, black and blue nodule. The lesions may initially be confused with dermal conditions such as cellulitis or minor skin infections. The clinical presentation may be nodular, diffuse, or ulcerated. Bleeding and pain may be associated with larger lesions, with generally a poor prognosis. Angiosarcomas may develop in the areas of previous irradiation. Spontaneous angiosarcoma in *p53*-null mice suggests that this tumor suppressor gene may be involved in the development of angiosarcoma. The role of *p53* has not been investigated in the development of angiosarcoma, but this protein is known to play a role in repairing radiation-induced DNA damage (50). Trauma has been suggested as a causative agent, but it is more likely to bring the patient's attention to the lesion rather than any definitive etiologic factor. These lesions may be solitary or multicentric and there may be a high incidence of dermal and subdermal extension of the disease, often leading to positive margins and multicentric recurrence. Gross assessment of the lesion may be quite difficult, because high-grade lesions are more cellular and have atypical and abnormal mitosis. There appears to be a significant relationship between the tumor size and overall prognosis in angiosarcomas. The lesions above 10 cm appear to have a uniformly poor outcome, whereas better survival is reported in lesions less than 5 cm (50). Due to the multicentric nature of the disease, postoperative radiation therapy is routinely used to improve the local control. The most common indications for postoperative radiation therapy include size, extensive disease, or adverse histologic factors (such as multicentricity, close or positive margins, and deep extension of the tumor.) The incidence of regional metastasis extends from 10% to 15% and elective treatment of the neck is generally not recommended. Elective treatment of the neck (in the form of elective neck dissection) is not generally recommended except in select circumstances where the surgical procedure requires reconstructive efforts and entry into the neck. The unresectable lesions have a dismal prognosis, with the average survival being 18 months with aggressive chemotherapy and radiation therapy. Preliminary data reveal some encouraging results in selected cases, with intraarterial doxorubicin. However, the current thrust in chemotherapy appears to be on Taxol. In a series reported by Lydiatt from Memorial Sloan-Kettering Cancer Center, 16 new lesions occurred in the scalp and face (50). The overall 5-year survival was 33%, but only 20% of the patients were disease-free. The size of the tumor was an important predictor of survival. All patients with a lesion greater than 10 cm died of the disease; compared with 67% with lesions less than 10 cm. Four of the six patients treated with wide local excision for lesions less than 10 cm survived 5 years. The authors recommended surgery for resectable lesions, with postoperative radiation for unsatisfactory margin, large tumor size, deep extension, and multicentricity. Elective treatment of the neck does not appear to be warranted, according to these authors.

Other rare angiomatous lesions of the head and neck include Kaposi sarcoma and hemangiopericytoma. Kaposi sarcoma generally presents as a purplish-red or dark brown plaque-like lesion and nodule in the skin. The association between these lesions and patients with acquired immunodeficiency syndrome (AIDS) has been noted. The treatment of Kaposi sarcoma is directly related to the primary disease and there is considerable interest in managing these patients with appropriate chemotherapy related to AIDS such as azidothymidine (AZT), vincristine, and vinblastine along with radiation therapy. Again, the appropriate diagnosis of these lesions may be difficult due to the rarity of these lesions and the unawareness of human immunodeficiency virus (HIV) positivity. Hemangiopericytoma may involve the skin, subcutaneous tissue, or musculoskeletal system of the head and neck areas. As before, the most common presentation is a purplish-red lesion seen around the ear. The treatment philosophy again pertains to other aggressive skin lesions such as wide excision with radiation reserved for poor prognostic features.

Osteogenic Sarcoma

Osteogenic sarcomas located in the head and neck region account for 5% of all osteogenic sarcomas. Within the head and neck, they are found most commonly in the mandible, maxilla, and calvarium. Osteogenic sarcomas usually present with a mass or symptoms related to compression of neurovascular structures or dental complaints. In the largest study to date, the mean age was 36 years, and equal numbers in both sexes were seen (52). Reported predisposing factors include history of retinoblastoma, irradiation exposure, Paget disease, and fibrous dysplasia.

Radiographically, plain films of the mandible, maxilla, or skull will usually suggest the diagnosis of an osteogenic sarcoma. For the mandible, a Panorex and dental occlusal and periapical films often give added information. Both CT and MRI scans, however, give the most comprehensive three-dimensional representation of a bone tumor. Recent advances have allowed three-dimensional reconstructions.

Histologically, osteogenic sarcomas are characterized by abundant pleomorphic and atypical cells in a stroma that may contain cartilage and bone. They are graded on the basis of the appearance of the stromal component.

Before definitive treatment, the diagnosis of an osteogenic sarcoma must be confirmed histologically. With bone tumors, a generous specimen should be obtained to afford the pathologist ample tissue. Additionally, frozen sections are inherently difficult with bone tumors. Whenever possible, tooth extractions should be avoided, to prevent the tumor from spreading to the medullary cavity of the bone. The mainstay of treatment of osteogenic sarcomas is surgical excision with generous margins and adjuvant postoperative radiation therapy. Regional lymph node metastases are rare; therefore, elective treatment of the neck is not an issue. A meta-analysis of nonrandomized studies of osteogenic sarcoma encompassing 173 patients reported an overall 5-year survival of 37% (52). In half the patients, treatment failed locally; in 20%, it failed distantly; and in very few, it failed regionally (52). Survival was better for tumors of the mandible and maxilla, relative to other sites in the head and neck. This analysis did not show any survival benefit of adjuvant radiation therapy or chemotherapy (52). This study, however, examined retrospective studies in which a selection bias existed. Clearly, patients with high-grade histology, large lesions, and positive surgical margins were more likely to receive adjuvant treatment. Given the favorable results of adjuvant treatment in extremity osteogenic sarcoma and the several promising reports of adjuvant treatment in head and neck osteogenic sarcoma, multimodality therapy remains the mainstay of treatment (53,54) (see also Chapter 34).

RARE SKIN TUMORS

Basal cell carcinoma is the most common form of malignant skin tumor and the head and neck is the most frequently involved site. In the United States, approximately one in five individuals will develop a skin cancer in their lifetime. It is such a common cancer that the American Cancer Society has not included skin cancer in the annual statistics. It is interesting to note that the number of skin cancers developing each year in the United States is almost the same as all other types of cancers combined. Although basal cell cancer is the most common type (60%), squamous cell carcinomas form approximately 30% of skin cancers. There appears to be a steady increase in the incidence of melanoma—another aggressive form of skin cancer. The remaining 10% form the rarest types of skin cancers. Epidermal cells and many other types of cells involving the dermis and the subcutaneous tissue can give rise to various types of rare malignant skin lesions. These lesions may originate from rare neuroendocrine cells of the skin, blood vessels, and sebaceous or sweat glands. The biology and clinical behavior of these rare tumors is quite complex. Most of them behave in a very aggressive fashion. Due to the lack of understanding about some of these lesions, there may be a delay in making appropriate diagnosis and offering definite treatment to these patients. Occasionally, non-epithelial skin tumors, such as dermatofibrosarcoma protuberance, fibroxanthoma or malignant fibrous histiocytoma, are also seen. Tumors of the blood vessels include angiosarcoma, Kaposi sarcoma, and hemangiopericytoma. Other tumors in the human body may occasionally metastasize to the skin, such as breast, kidney, prostate, lung, and rare gastrointestinal tumors, whereas lymphoma may present as a subcutaneous mass—lymphoma cutis.

Merkel Cell Carcinoma

Merkel cell carcinoma is a neuroendocrine tumor arising from the trabecular cells of the skin. In 1972, Toker first described these trabecular carcinomas and approximately 1,000 cases have been described in the literature since that time (55–58). Although these were initially thought to be relatively innocuous lesions, they are generally most aggressive and potentially fatal tumors that recur locally and metastasize to the regional lymph nodes. The Merkel cell was first described in 1875 and was thought to be part of the mechanoreceptor of the skin. This lesion exhibits electron-microscopic characteristics of membrane-bound neurosecretory granules and 100- to 150-nm dense core granules scattered throughout the cytoplasm. Although these neurosecretory granules fail to demonstrate catecholamines, they are similar to the tumors (both structurally and chemically) of the APUD system. Neuron-specific enolase and isoenzyme of the glycolytic pathway are reliable markers of the neuroendocrine origin of Merkel cells. Merkel cell carcinomas occur mainly in the older adult population, in the sixth to eighth decades of life, and usually present as a painless, raised skin nodule. The malar region in the head and neck area is most commonly involved. Approximately 50% of the lesions are noted in the head and neck, but 30% may be seen in the lower extremities (59,60). These lesions present as smooth, subcutaneous nodules with skin telangiectasis with violaceous color on the surface. The size may vary from 1 to 5 cm. These lesions typically occur in older, Caucasian individuals and most commonly involve the head and neck region (approximately 50% of the cases). The most common locations in the head and neck include the cheek and malar area, upper neck, and nose. Even though the distribution of Merkel cell lesions leads to the suspicion of a relation to sun exposure, no definite association has been established. The treatment requires wide surgical margins along with regional nodal dissection. Elective node dissection is considered for larger tumors or tumors in close proximity to the draining lymphatics. It is also considered in lesions having more than 10 mitotic figures or predominantly containing small cells. The regional failure rate has been described as being as high 75%.

Local recurrence appears to be within the range of 33%, whereas regional metastasis is noted in approximately 66% of the cases and distant metastasis is noted in 33% of patients. The mortality from these lesions when they recur locoregionally is quite high. Goepfert et al. (61,62) report 29 patients with Merkel cell carcinomas of the head and neck region. Thirteen patients had clinically palpable nodes at the time of presentation, 12 of whom had positive neck disease. During the follow-up, 80% of the patients developed lymph node metastases, whereas distant metastasis occurred in 48%. Eighty-two percent of the patients died within 5 months after development of the distant metastasis. Due to the high incidence of regional metastasis, the authors recommended prophylactic removal of the regional nodes and lymphatics. Cotlar recommended postoperative radiation therapy in patients with positive regional lymph nodes and regional nodal dissection for lesions greater than 1.5 cm. There appears to be considerable controversy regarding the appropriate initial surgical management and the debate revolves around prophylactic nodal dissection. Because of the high incidence of local and regional recurrence and distant metastasis, adequate initial treatment of the primary and adjacent lymph nodes—as well as postoperative adjuvant radiation therapy—are strongly recommended (63–65). Due to the rarity of these lesions and variable clinical and biologic behavior, a randomized study has not been undertaken.

The need for chemotherapy has become more debatable as the metastatic potential of Merkel cell carcinoma has been realized. An Adriamycin-containing regimen has shown some palliative effects in patients with recurrent or progressive disease. The M. D. Anderson Hospital recently recommended adjuvant radiation therapy in patients with lesions greater than 1.5 cm, narrow margins, or in those with tumors revealing lymphatic penetration (61,62). A dose of approximately 5,000 cGy has been recommended in the adjuvant setting. The most common sites of distant metastasis include liver, bone, brain, and lung. The overall survival rate is reported to be 88% at 1 year, 72% at 2 years, 55% at 3 years, and 30% at 5 years.

In summary, Merkel cell tumors are neuroendocrine lesions presumably derived from the primordial neural crest. The biologic characteristics include (a) the presence of neurosecretory granules akin to APUD system; (b) the need of appropriate immunohistochemistry and electron microscopy to confirm the diagnosis; (c) the biosynthetic ability to produce amine and peptide hormones, even though these tumors rarely cause endocrine disturbances; and (d) deep invasion, frequent recurrence, and metastasis—leading to fatal outcome. The surgical excision of the primary and prophylactic nodal dissection is vital to the successful management of these lesions. Radiation appears to be an important component of the multidisciplinary approach and chemotherapy is used for advanced recurrent or metastatic disease for palliative efforts.

Adnexal Tumors

Although benign adnexal tumors are quite common, the malignant forms are more difficult to diagnose and treat. Adnexal tumors arise from the skin appendages and may be noted in eccrine, apocrine, or pilosebaceous differentiation. The most common benign adnexal tumors include eccrine poroma, trichoepithelioma, pilomatrixoma, syringoma, eccrine spiradenoma, cylindroma, or nevus sebaceous. Cylindroma is also known as turban tumor of the scalp. These tumors are most often multiple and may be familial with autosomal dominance. There appears to be linkage with chromosome 16-q-cyclin D1; a tumor suppressor gene is involved in both familial and sporadic types (66,67). Even though the most common lesion is a benign cylindroma, malignant transformation is well known. The presence of rapid growth or frequent recurrence raises the suspicion of malignant transformation. These tumors are locally aggressive with frequent regional and distant metastasis. All of the above benign adnexal tumors can undergo malignancy. The presence of regional metastasis confirms the malignant nature of the skin lesion. The general philosophy of treatment includes aggressive surgical excision with the use of postoperative radiation therapy. The most common malignant adnexal tumors originate from the sweat glands or the sebaceous glands. Malignant sweat gland tumors are divided into eccrine and apocrine origin. They are most common in the fifth and sixth decades of life and there appears to be a high incidence (approximately 50%) of local recurrence (68). Interestingly, apocrine gland carcinomas are frequently noted in the eyelids, where they originate in the glands of Moll. The most common presentation of eccrine carcinoma in the head and neck is a subcutaneous nodule in older individuals. The histopathologic varieties of this tumor include: syringoid, mucinous, microcystic eccrine, and adenocarcinomas. The malignant transformation may be noted due to the rapid growth in the size of the lesion. Sebaceous gland carcinomas generally arise in older adult women, near the eyelids. They may originate from the meibomian glands, the glands of Zeis, or the pilosebaceous glands. The most common site seems to be ocular areas, followed by facial regions. Prior radiation may increase the risk for developing sebaceous gland carcinomas. It is important for the clinician to initially appreciate the subcutaneous lesion as a primary skin tumor. One of the most common difficulties for the pathologist is to distinguish a primary from the metastatic lesion. The lesion may occasionally be confused as a metastatic salivary or breast carcinoma and a considerable delay may occur in making a definitive diagnosis of these lesions. A proper history, initial clinical characteristics, and other glandular pathology should lead to the suspicion of primary adnexal tumor. The treatment hinges around appropriate wide excision with postoperative radiation therapy in select circumstances, with more aggressive lesions, larger size, or close margins. Regional nodal dissection should be considered in selected cases, especially if the neck is to be entered for reconstructive techniques. Extremely close follow-up is recommended, particularly because there appears to be a high incidence of local recurrence and distant metastasis.

Other rare skin lesions include dermatofibrosarcoma protuberance. Stojadinovic et al. reviewed a large experience at Memorial Sloan-Kettering Cancer Center with these lesions in the head and neck (69). They suggest wide excision of the primary with at least a 2-cm margin. They also report a high incidence of local recurrence, due to the multicentric nature of these lesions. Even though lymphomas of the skin are rare, they may occasionally present as a long-standing or rapidly developing subcutaneous nodule. These lesions may appear as an infected skin condition, due to the direct involvement of the dermis. These lesions may be confused with other malignant skin lesions, such as squamous cell carcinoma or adnexal tumors. The systemic treatment of lymphoma is recommended after appropriate evaluation of the extent of the disease, including bone marrow evaluation.

Ameloblastoma

Ameloblastoma is a rare odontogenic tumor most commonly involving the mandible; however, occasionally it may also involve the maxilla (70,71). Generally the patient remains quite asymptomatic and this may be an incidental finding with routine dental films. There may be considerable delay in making the diagnosis and occasionally the patient may be seen in the dental office where curettage of the cystic lesion of the mandible may be performed. Rarely the tumor may break through the confines of the mandible involving the surrounding soft tissues or it may undergo malignant transformation where the incidence of local recurrence is very high. The differential diagnoses include simple dental cyst, keratocyst, metastatic tumor to the mandible, and hemangioma. The ameloblastoma is characterized by enamel epithelium, which generally clinches the diagnosis. Approximately 20% to 25% of the ameloblastomas arise in the maxilla. Even though the tumor may present in children, generally it is seen in the third and fourth decade of life. The ameloblastoma may present in various forms such as solid, unicystic, or multicystic. The unicystic lesions have excellent outcome and surgical curettage or simple excision may be satisfactory. There continues to be considerable controversy in relation to curettage or enucleation against segmental resection (72). Most of the patients seen in the dental office are generally curetted. However, if tumor recurs and it invades a considerable portion of the mandible or the entire cortex of the mandible, the patient is seen by a head and neck surgeon and segmental resection and appropriate reconstruction, preferably with fibula free flap, is recommended. The segmental resection of the mandible is generally advised for recurrent tumors. The ameloblastoma involving the maxillary alveolus will require partial maxillectomy or alveolectomy. Rarely a recurrent tumor may invade the infratemporal fossa or the orbit. The role of radiation therapy remains unclear at this time; however, it is recommended for patients in whom all of the gross tumor could not be removed or tumor involves the soft tissues of the head and neck. Metastases are very rare; however, malignant transformation is well known with multiple recurrences. If the diagnosis of malignant ameloblastoma is confirmed, postoperative radiation therapy is generally advised.

Chordoma

Chordomas are rare tumors arising from the notochord. The chordomas are most commonly noted in the clival area; however, they may occur in the coccygeal region as well (73). These tumors may present as a mass in the oropharyngeal region;

however, quite often they are noted on routine imaging studies of the head and neck. A subtype of chordoma has chondroid elements and needs to be distinguished from chordosarcoma. These tumors are generally noted in the third or fourth decade and usually are very slow-growing. Occasionally they may involve the cranial nerves near the skull base leading to a variety of symptoms related to cranial nerve involvement. They may present as a nasopharyngeal mass and differential diagnosis will include carcinoma of the nasopharynx. Due to the locale of the tumor total surgical resection is rarely possible; however, because they are slow-growing, subtotal resection does not create a major problem related to recurrent disease. The most common surgical approach includes exposure of the clival and upper cervical vertebrae either by transmaxillary or by mandibulotomy approach. One of the older approaches of median labiomandibuloglossotomy (the Trotter approach) may be used. If the disease extends into the infratemporal fossa or in a recurrent tumor, total surgical resection may be extremely difficult. Radiation therapy may be considered in these selected circumstances as a palliative effort (74). Rarely, in a recurrent tumor brachytherapy with iodine seed implantation may be considered. The overall 5-year survival is approximately 50% but it depends on the initial extent of the disease and the surgical resection. Metastases from clival chordomas are rare. The overall outcome is much better in the chondroid subtype.

RADIOLOGIC IMAGING CONCERNS

Bernard B. O'Malley

What is considered an "unusual" head and neck tumor depends on the examining institution, demographics, and referral patterns. The absolute definition of *unusual* might be a reflection of the rarity of the type of lesion or the age of the patient or the site wherein the lesion developed. Most patients arrive for imaging of a lesion that has been diagnosed by mucosal (or transmucosal) biopsy or lymph node biopsy. The majority of head and neck cancers are of the squamous type. Most of the remainder are salivary, lymphoma, and thyroid disorders. Unusual tumors are therefore usually submucosal in location or mesenchymal in etiology. Many of these tumors arise in stereotypical locations, and some have characteristic imaging features. This leaves a small minority of cases of patients with nonspecific imaging features of a process that has yet to be rendered with a biopsy-proven diagnosis. Most masses in the head and neck are neoplasms, and the first role of imaging is to stage the lesion accurately. One must be cautious, however, in labeling an imaging finding as *tumor* until tissue has been obtained.

The following cases illustrate rare lesions, rare location, and behavior of lesions.

CASE 1: Chondrosarcoma

Case History: A middle-aged man with chronic hoarseness and recent onset of respiratory difficulty presented with a bulky submucosal mass requiring a tracheostomy. Imaging features on MRI are nonspecific, but the CT scan shows coarse, irregular calcifications typical of chondrosarcoma (Fig. 33.1).

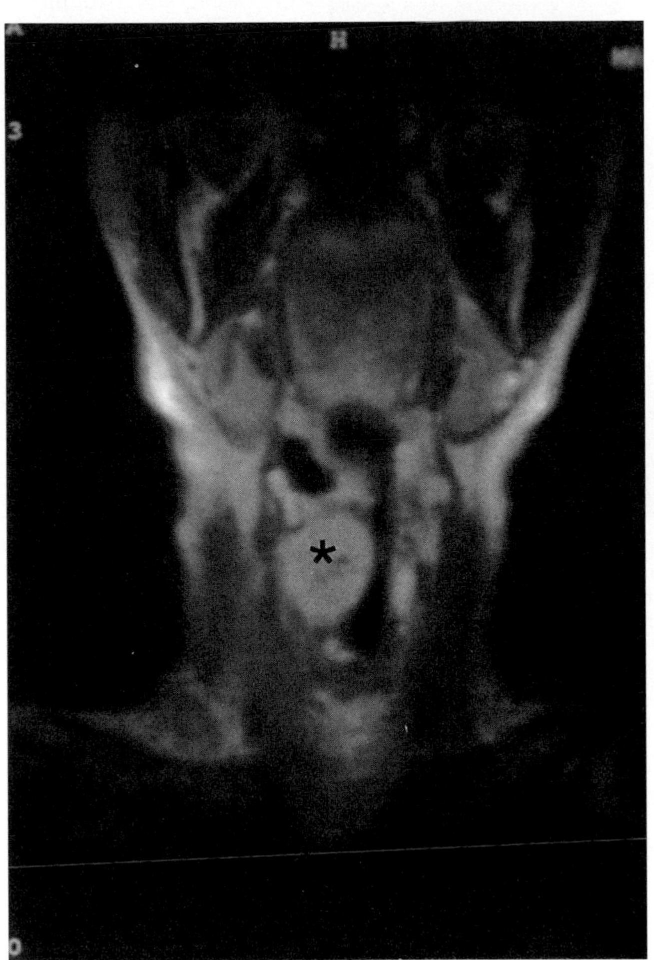

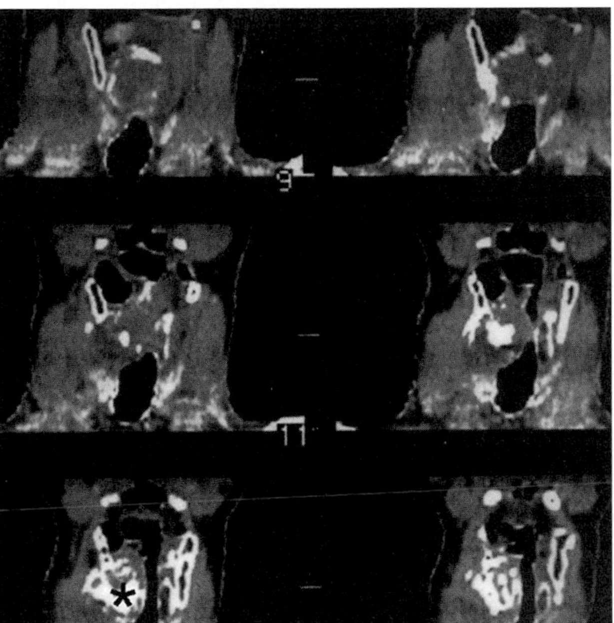

Figure 33.1 Chondrosarcoma larynx. Direct coronal T1 magnetic resonance imaging view **(A)** and reformatted coronal contrast computed tomographic view **(B)** show a heterogeneously ossified mass (*asterisk*) arising within the base of the right cricoid bulging into the larynx and deforming the glottis.

CASE 2: Neuroma of Facial Nerve

Case History: A young woman presented with progressive facial palsy and a palpable mass in the parotid bed due to a neuroma of the facial nerve (Fig. 33.2).

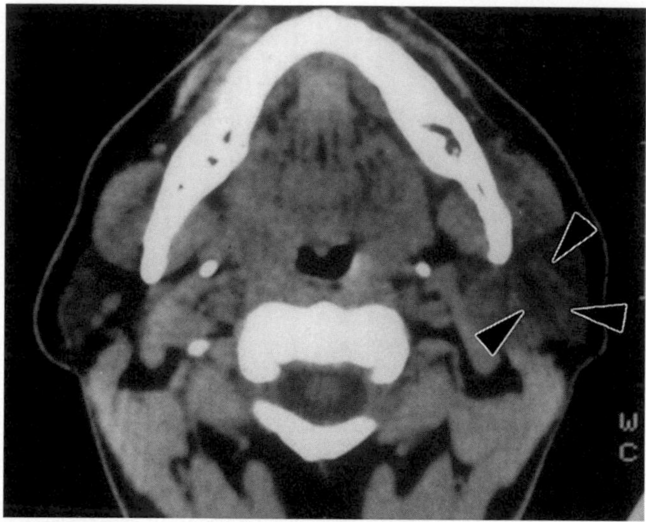

Figure 33.2 Neuroma facial nerve. Noncontrast axial computed tomographic scan shows expanded left parotid gland related to a neuroma of nerve VII (*arrowheads*). The fatty nature of parotid tissue limits conspicuity of a neural lesion, particularly without contrast.

CASE 3: Hemangioma at Base of Tongue

Case History: An older adult man with chronic dysphagia and a "hot-potato" voice quality presented with a bulky submucosal mass that was soft on palpation (Fig. 33.3).

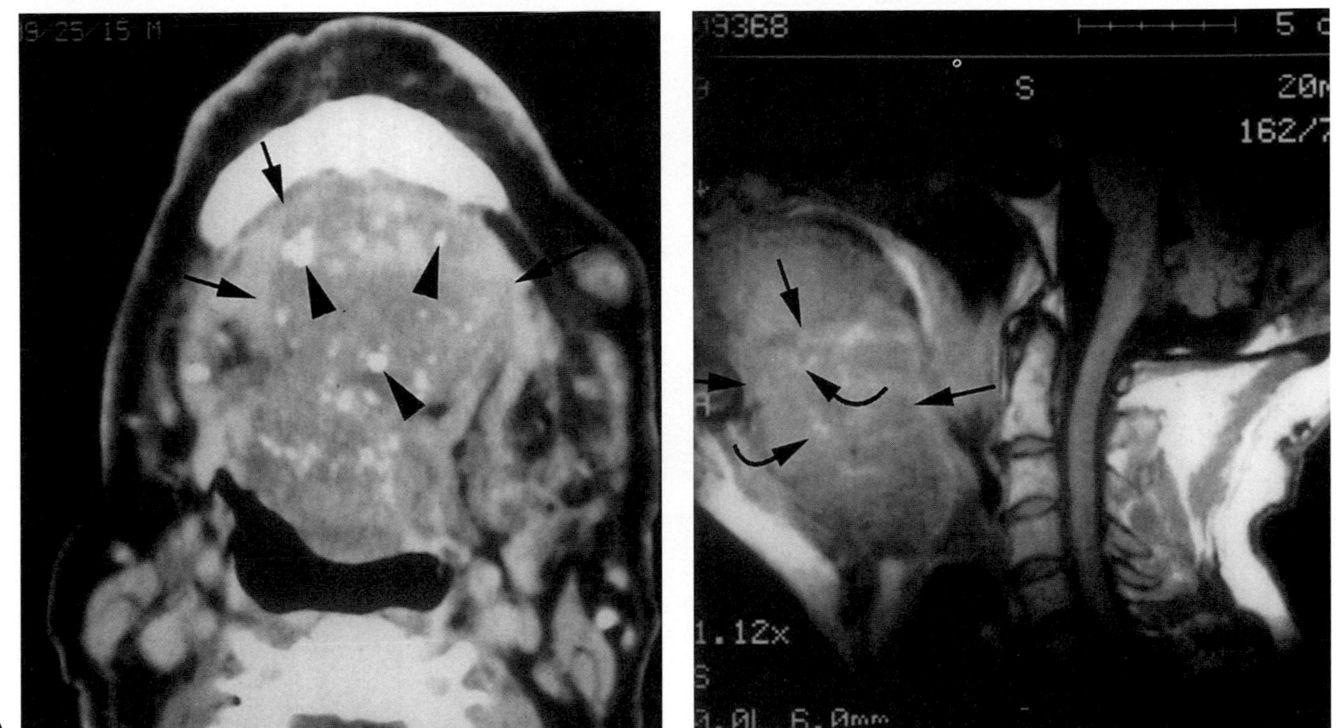

Figure 33.3 Hemangioma at base of tongue. Enhanced axial computed tomographic view **(A)** and sagittal T1 magnetic resonance imaging view **(B)** show large infiltrating mass (*arrows*) containing phleboliths (*arrowheads*) and serpiginous flow (*curved arrows*). Note preservation of preepiglottic space.

CASE 4: Angiocentric T-cell Lymphoma

Case History: A young woman presented with nasal congestion and a clinically apparent mass of the nasal septum. Endoscopic biopsy yielded angiocentric T-cell lymphoma. Systemic workup was negative (Fig. 33.4).

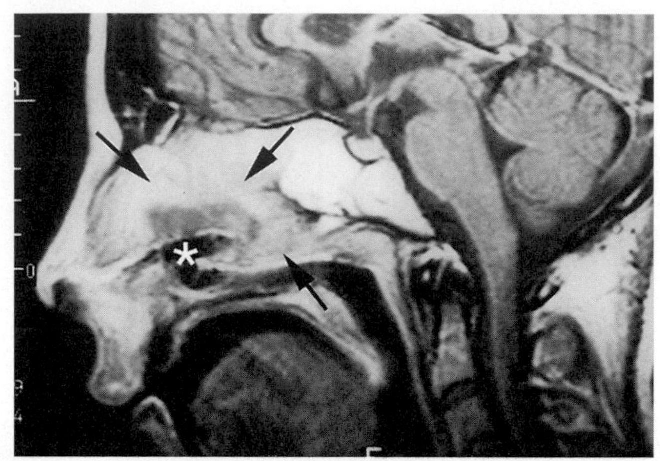

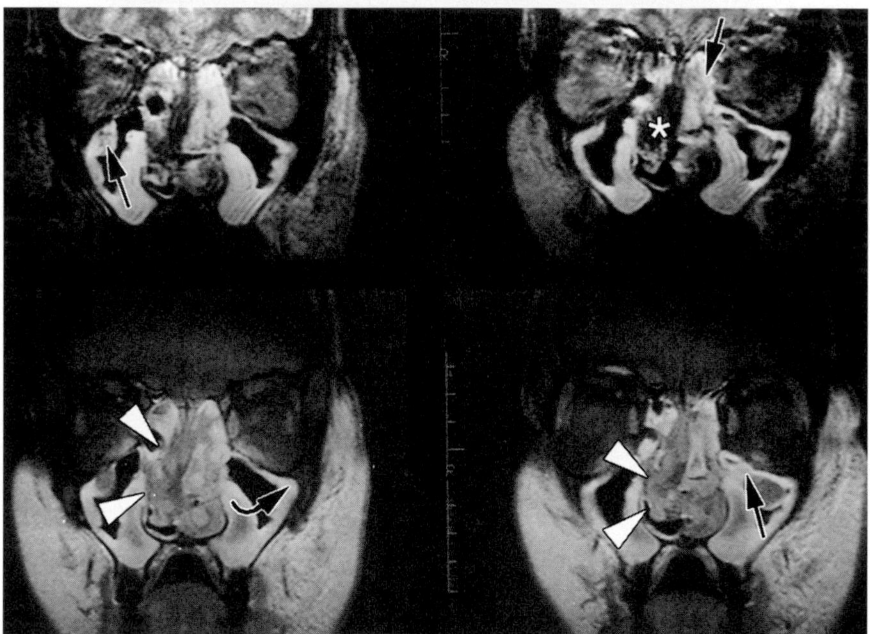

Figure 33.4 Angiocentric T-cell lymphoma (formerly known as lethal midline granuloma). Enhanced sagittal T1 view **(A)** and matched coronal T2 (top) and enhanced T1 (bottom) views **(B)** of paranasal sinuses show a defect in the anterior nasal septum (*asterisk*) secondary to a destructive lesion (*arrowheads*) of the septum. Extensive surrounding mucosal reaction (*arrows*) does not involve the orbits (*curved arrows*).

CASE 5: Castleman Disease

Case History: A middle-aged woman presented with slowly progressive lower cervical and supraclavicular adenopathy but no systemic signs or symptoms. Excisional biopsy yielded Castleman follicular lymph node hyperplasia (Fig. 33.5).

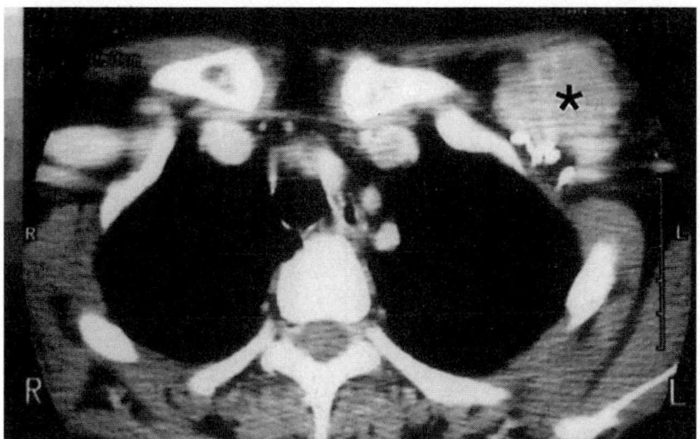

Figure 33.5 Castleman disease. Enhanced axial computed tomographic scan through the upper chest shows residual adenopathy (*asterisk*) after excisional biopsy of left supraclavicular mass revealed lymph node hyperplasia compatible with Castleman disease.

CASE 6: Neurofibroma

Case History: A teenage boy with no family history of neurocutaneous syndrome presented with progressive facial deformity due to a dominant neurofibroma of the deep face (Fig. 33.6).

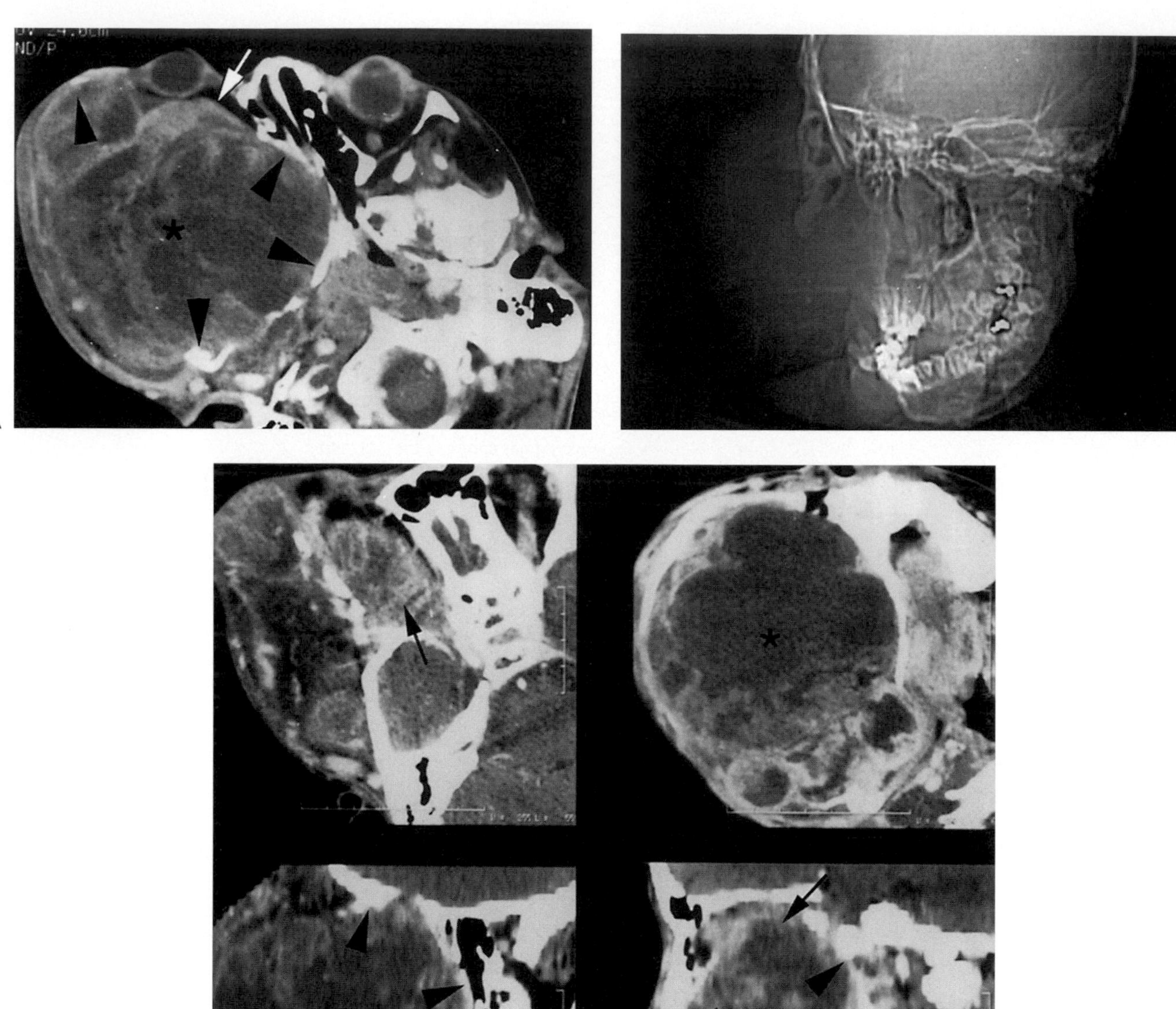

Figure 33.6 Neurofibromatosis. Enhanced axial view **(A),** frontal scout radiograph **(B),** and collage **(C)** of enhanced computed tomographic scan. Clockwise from top left: Axial, axial, parasagittal, and coronal views of a huge neuroma of the deep left face (*asterisk*) slowly deforming local bony contours (*arrowheads*) and infiltrating the right orbit (*arrows*).

CASE 7: Cystic Hygroma

Case History: A 50-year-old woman presented with a slowly enlarging soft mass at the lateral neck and no history of trauma or systemic malignancy (Fig. 33.7).

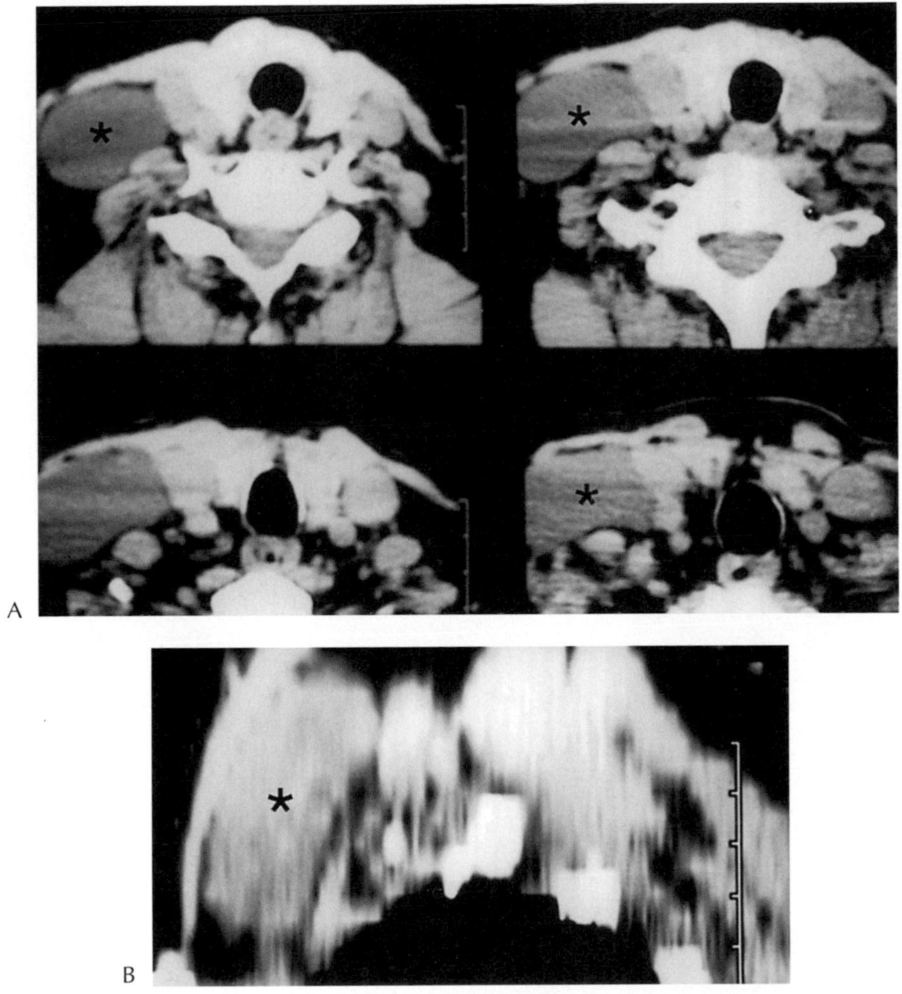

Figure 33.7 Cystic hygroma. **A:** Serial noncontrast axial computed tomographic scan of the lower neck. **B:** Parasagittal reformat views show a large, low-attenuation lateral neck mass (*asterisk*) that proved to be a cystic hygroma. Note normal homogeneous iodine concentration within the thyroid gland.

CASE 8: Neuroma of Epiglottis

Case History: A young female patient presented with a recent change in voice quality. Clinical examination revealed a submucosal lesion on the laryngeal surface of the epiglottis (Fig. 33.8).

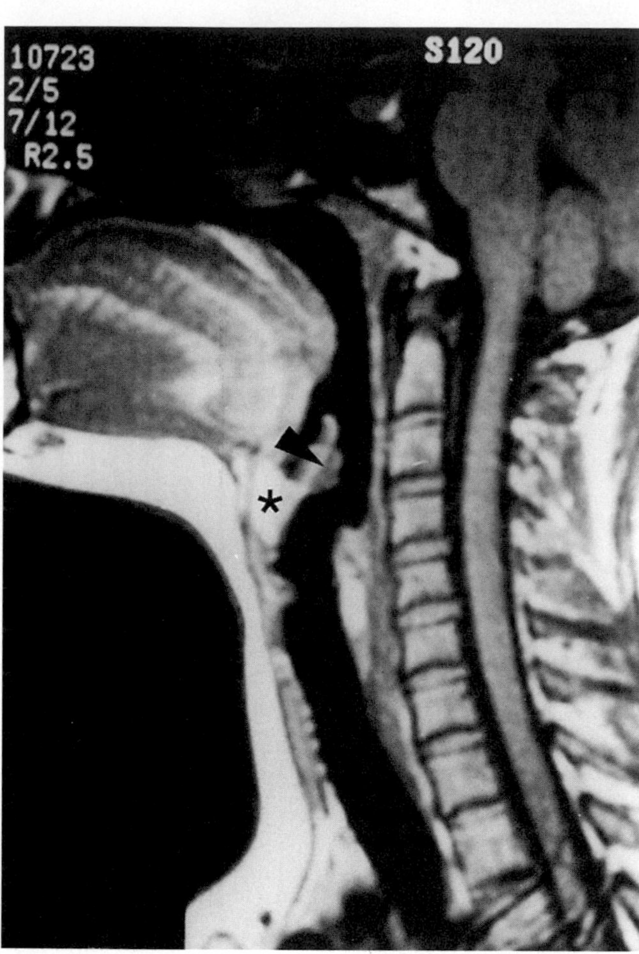

Figure 33.8 Neuroma epiglottis. Noncontrast sagittal T1 magnetic resonance imaging scan shows small, well-circumscribed lesion of the laryngeal surface of the epiglottis (*arrowhead*). Note preservation of the preepiglottic space (*asterisk*).

Case 9: Neuroendocrine Tumor-Glottis

Case History: A middle-aged man presented with hoarseness and recent hemoptysis and cervical adenopathy. Clinical examination revealed a purple-black submucosal mass of the supraglottic larynx (Fig. 33.9).

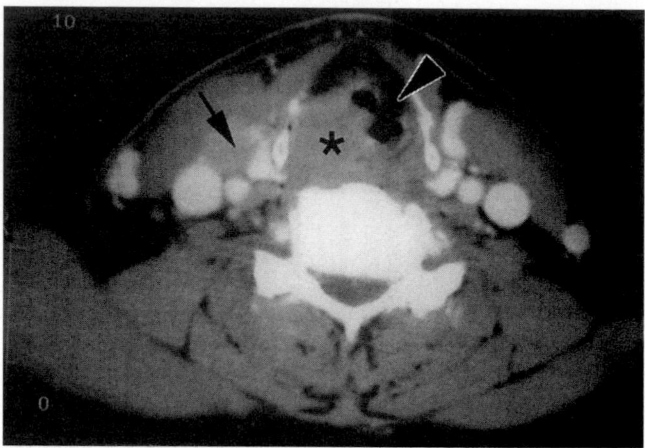

Figure 33.9 Neuroendocrine tumor of the glottis. Enhanced axial computed tomographic scan at level of false cords shows a homogeneously enhancing submucosal mass (*asterisk*) compromising the airway (*arrowhead*) with ipsilateral adenopathy (*arrow*).

CASE 10: Spindle-cell Tumor—Tongue

Case History: A young man with dysarthria and oral pain presented with a deformed tongue. Biopsy yielded spindle-cell tumor (Fig. 33.10).

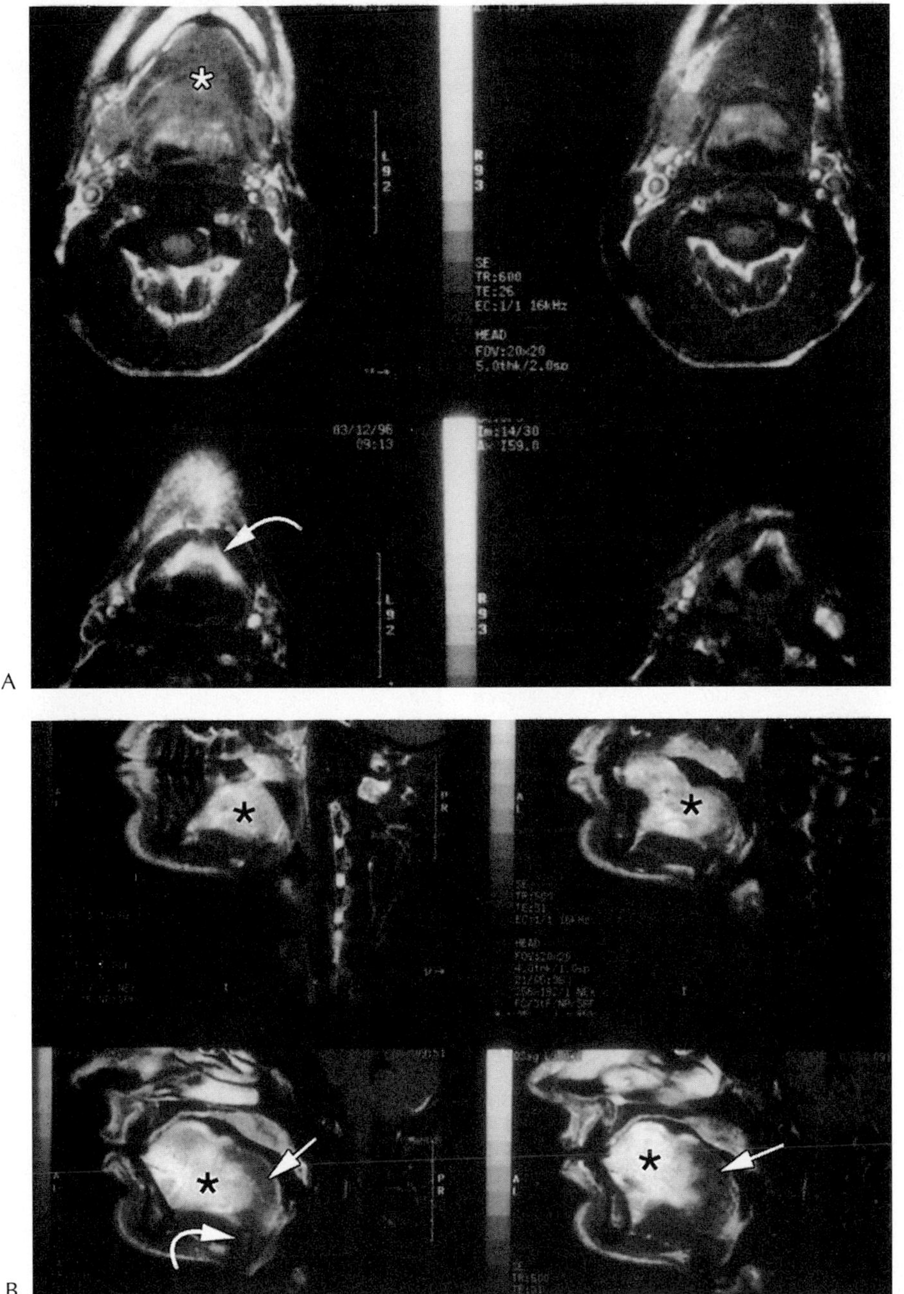

Figure 33.10 Spindle-cell tumor on tongue. Serial axial precontrast T1 views of tongue base **(A)** and serial sagittal enhanced T1 views of tongue **(B)** show large lesion involving bulk of the oral tongue (*asterisk*) sparing the tongue base (*arrows*) and preepiglottic space (*curved arrow*).

CASE 11: Neuroma—XII Nerve

Case History: An older adult presented with a right hypoglossal palsy and mild hoarseness and dysphagia. The right hemitongue was atrophic and paretic, indicating a long-standing lesion (Fig. 33.11).

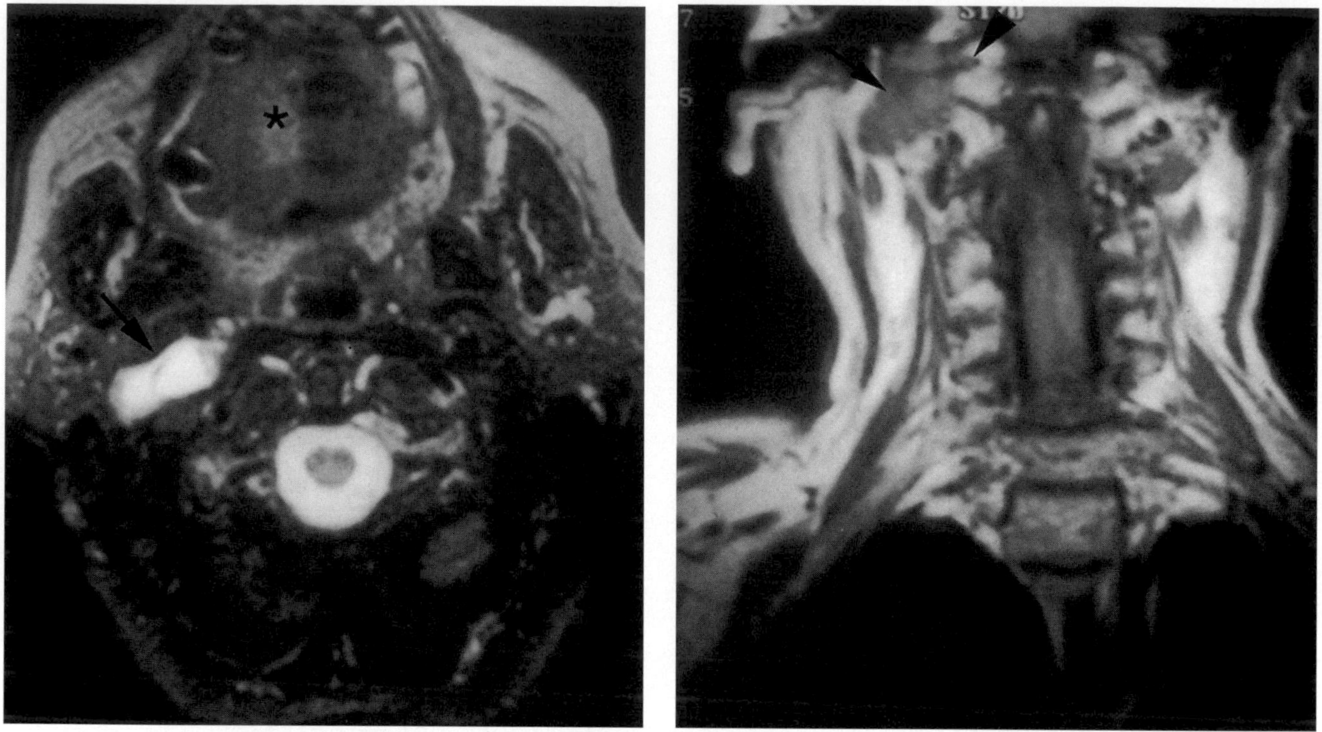

Figure 33.11 Neuroma XII. T2 axial view **(A)** and T1 coronal view **(B)** of head and neck show a well-circumscribed, hyperintense lesion of the carotid space (*arrows*) related to a hypoglossal nerve neuroma. Note expansion of hypoglossal canal (*arrowhead*) and denervation atrophy of the tongue (*asterisk*).

CASE 12: Pituitary Adenoma

Case History: A young man presented with chronic headache, progressive cranial neuropathies, and decreased libido. He had no history of systemic malignancy. Biopsy revealed pituitary adenoma (Fig. 33.12).

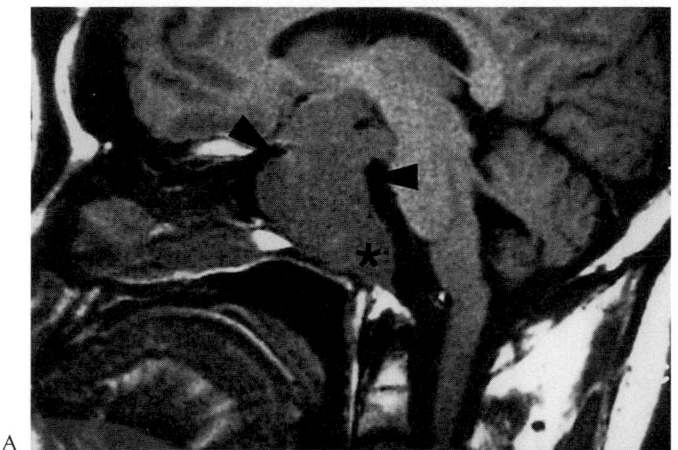

A

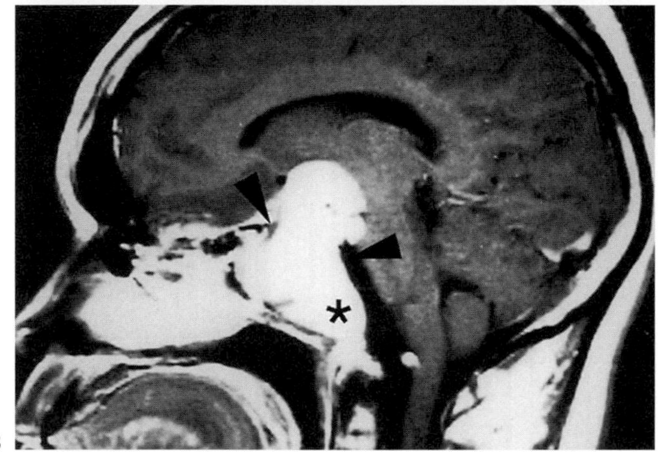

B

Figure 33.12 Pituitary adenoma. Precontrast view **(A)** and postcontrast sagittal T1 view **(B)** of a mass straddling the diaphragma sella (*arrowheads*) with infiltration of clivus (*asterisk*) greater than is typical for pituitary adenoma.

CASE 13: Adult Neuroblastoma

Case History: A 42-year-old man presented with right cranial neuropathies and no history of systemic malignancy. Biopsy revealed neuroblastoma. Bone marrow aspiration was also positive for neuroblastoma (Fig. 33.13).

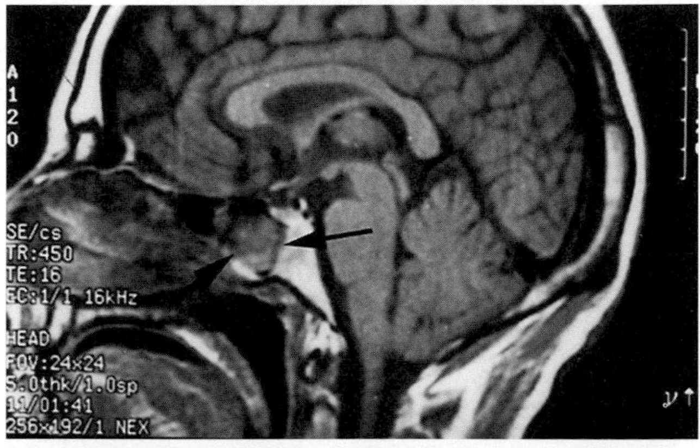

A

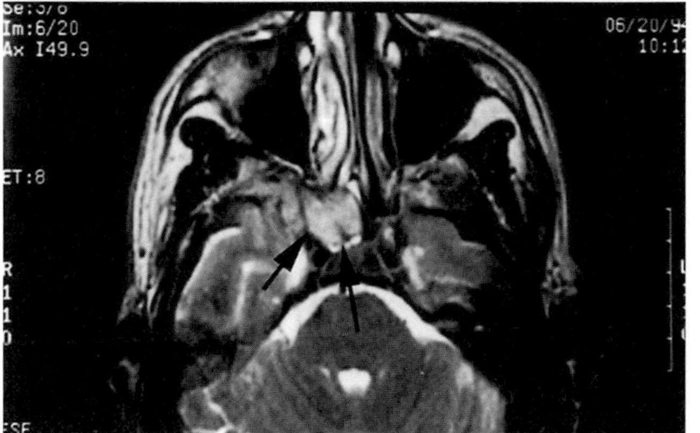

B

Figure 33.13 Adult neuroblastoma. Sagittal T1 view **(A)** and axial T2 view **(B)** show a lytic lesion of the sphenoid bone (*arrows*). Biopsy showed conventional neuroblastoma.

Case 14: Adult Neuroblastoma

Case History: A 30-year-old man presented with a mass in the right thyroid bed and ipsilateral supraclavicular adenopathy suspected to be thyroid cancer or lymphoma. Biopsy revealed neuroblastoma mixed with more mature elements (Fig. 33.14).

CASE 15: Spindle-cell Tumor at Skull Base

Case History: A young male patient presented with headache and progressive bilateral cranial neuropathies. He had no history of systemic malignancy. Biopsy revealed spindle-cell tumor (Fig. 33.15).

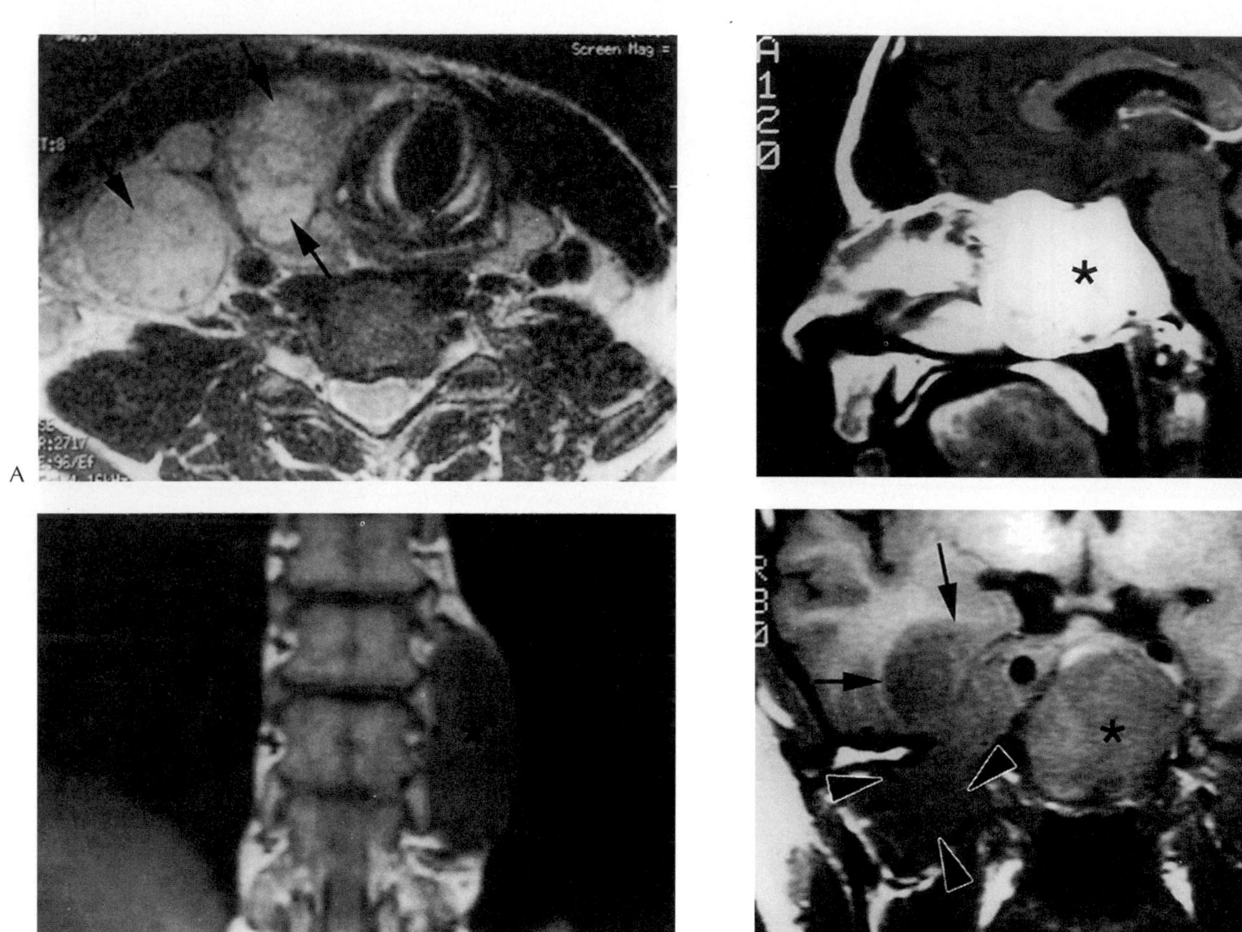

Figure 33.14 Adult neuroblastoma. Axial T2 neck view **(A)** and coronal T1 view of thoracic spine **(B)** show well-circumscribed masses (*arrows*). Neck mass thought to be of thyroid origin revealed conventional neuroblastoma. Paraspinal mass was more typical of ganglioneuroma (*asterisk*).

Figure 33.15 Spindle-cell tumor at skull base. Sagittal T1 view **(A)** and coronal T1 view **(B)** show a large expansile lesion arising within the sphenoid bone (*asterisk*) with right parasellar (*arrows*) and infratemporal extension (*arrowheads*).

CASE 16: Paget Sarcoma

Case History: A 76-year-old woman presented with a long-standing history of Paget disease and a recent decline in mental status (Fig. 33.16).

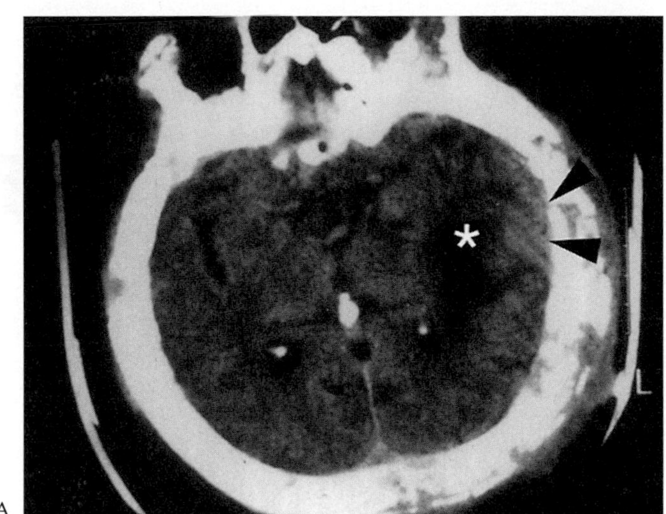

A

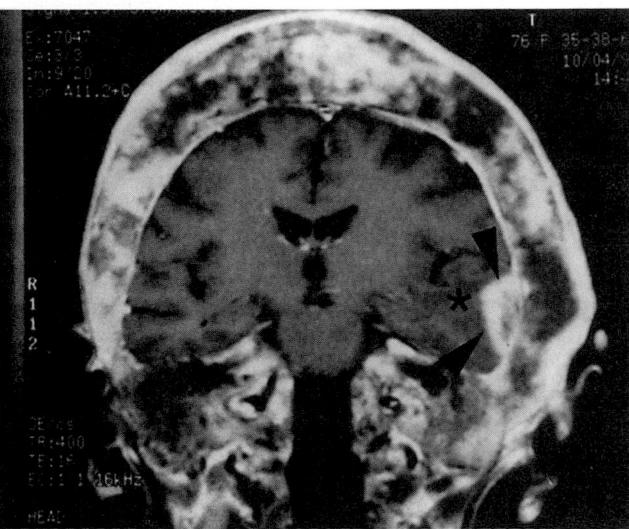

B

Figure 33.16 Paget sarcoma. Enhanced axial computed tomographic scan **(A)** and enhanced coronal T1 magnetic resonance image **(B)** show diffuse heterogeneous osseous thickening of the skull base and calvarium. There is a superimposed enhancing lesion expanding through the inner table and dura (*arrowheads*), resulting in brain edema (*asterisk*).

CASE 17: Desmoid Tumor

Case History: An older adult woman presented with neck pain and progressive swelling of the suboccipital region of the neck (Fig. 33.17).

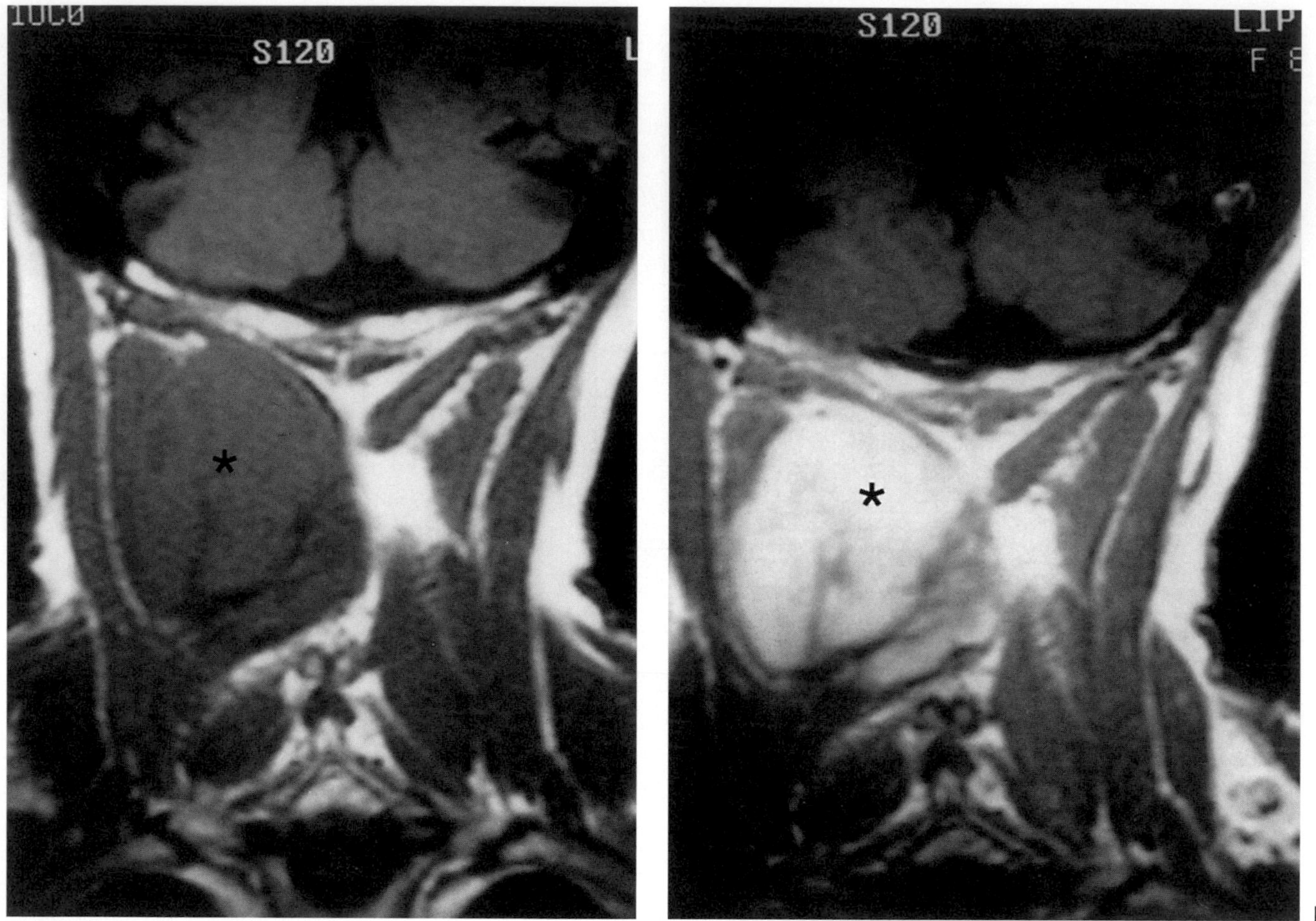

Figure 33.17 Desmoid tumor. Coronal T1 view **(A)** and enhanced coronal T1 magnetic resonance images **(B)** of large, well-circumscribed, intensely enhancing mass (*asterisk*) within the posterior paraspinous muscle complex.

CASE 18: Thymic Cyst

Case History: A young man presented with swelling in the pretracheal region of the lower neck. No systemic signs of malignancy were seen. Excisional biopsy yielded simple thymic cyst (Fig. 33.18).

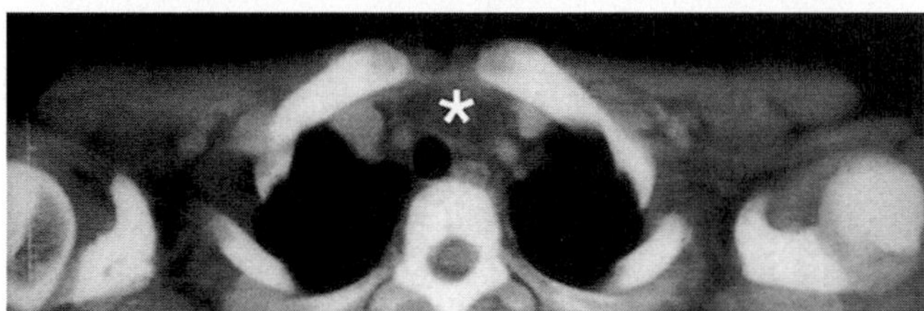

Figure 33.18 Thymic cyst. Enhanced axial computed tomographic scan through the thoracic inlet shows a complex multicystic mass (*asterisk*) bulging out of the superior mediastinum.

CASE 19: Granular Cell Tumor

Case History: A 51-year-old woman presented with neck swelling and vocal cord palsy. Resection revealed a granular cell tumor (Fig. 33.19).

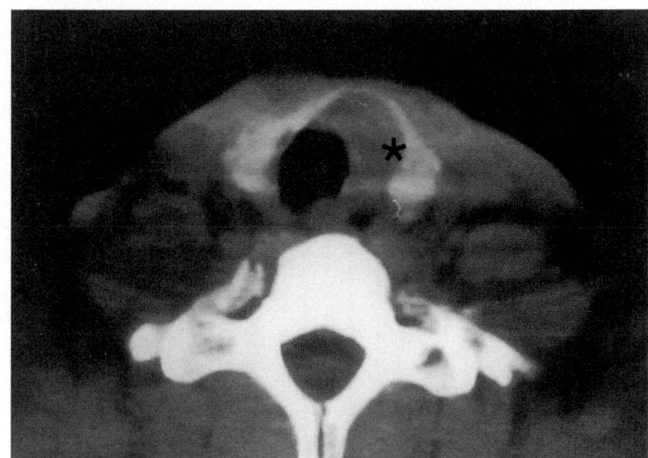

Figure 33.19 Granular cell tumor. Enhanced axial computed tomographic scan through upper trachea shows a minimally enhancing mass of the tracheal wall (*asterisk*) displacing the left lobe of the thyroid gland.

CASE 20: Ganglioneuroma

Case History: A 25-year-old woman presented with a remote history of resection of a lower cervical mass in early childhood. A screening chest roentgenogram showed scoliosis and a paraspinal mass. Incisional biopsy yielded ganglioneuroma (Fig. 33.20).

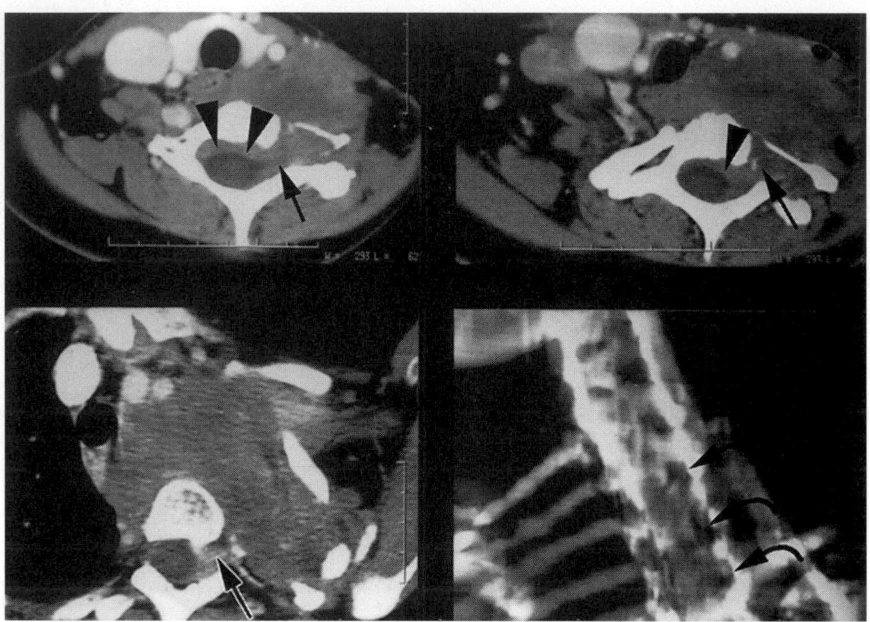

Figure 33.20 Ganglioneuroma. Serial enhanced axial computed tomography scan and three-dimensional bone rendering of a large, heterogeneous, multicompartmental, paraspinal mass presenting in the supraclavicular fossa. Note the foraminal disease (*arrows*), foraminal expansion (*curved arrows*), and epidural disease (*arrowheads*).

CASE 21: Sinus Osteoma

Case History: A middle-aged woman presented with chronic headache and unilateral proptosis (Fig. 33.21).

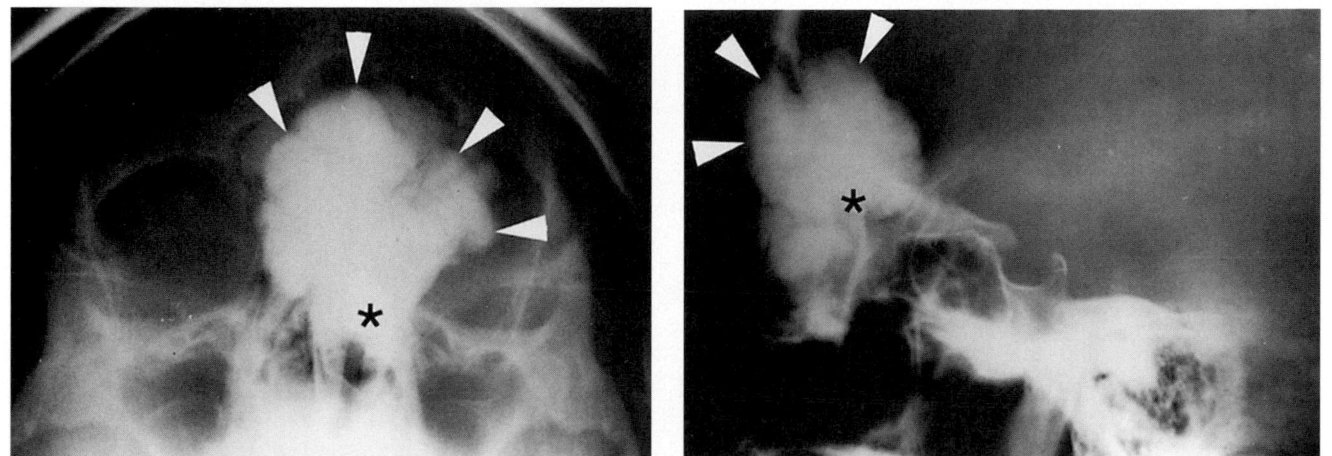

Figure 33.21 Sinus osteoma. Frontal radiograph **(A)** and lateral radiograph **(B)** of the skull show a multilobular ossified mass expanding out of the ethmoid complex (*asterisk*) into the frontal sinus (*arrowheads*).

CASE 22: Fifth Nerve Neuroma

Case History: A 57-year-old man presented with progressive facial numbness and swelling. Transfacial biopsy yielded neuroma (Fig. 33.22).

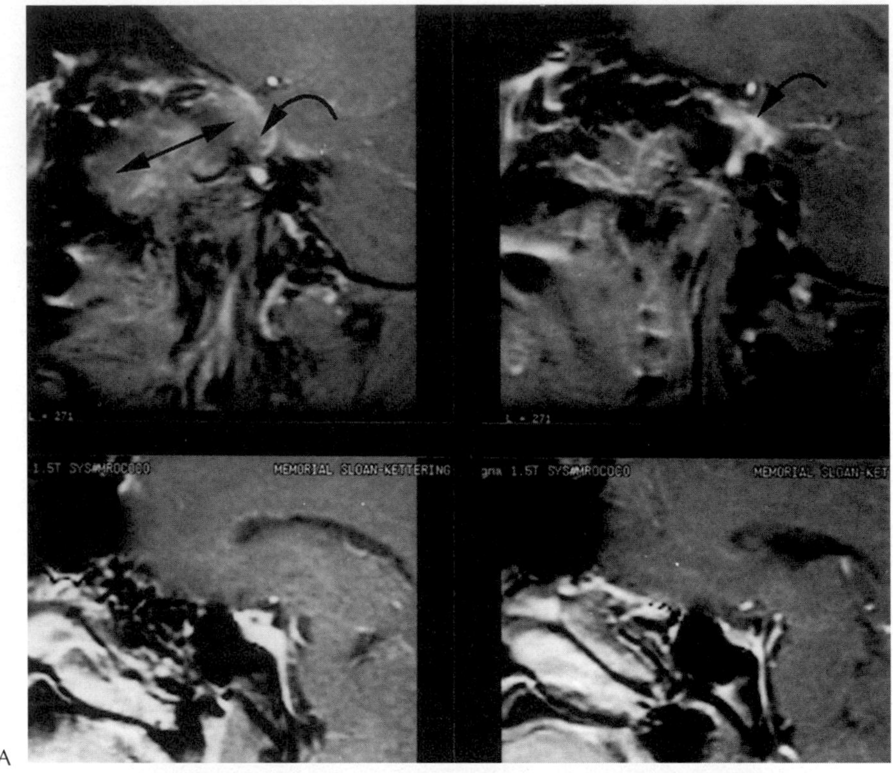

A

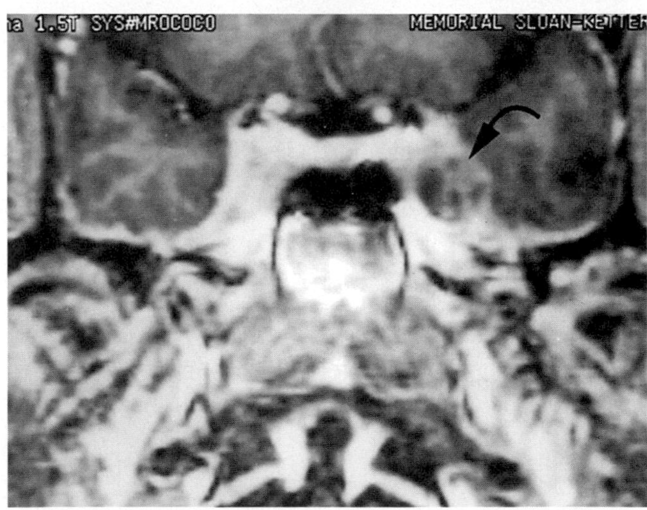

B

Figure 33.22 Fifth nerve neuroma. Serial, enhanced, parasagittal T1-weighted magnetic resonance images **(A)** through the paranasal sinuses show a mass extending along the course of the left infraorbital nerve (*double-headed arrow*) with involvement of the cavernous segment (*curved arrow*), best seen on the enhanced coronal view **(B).**

CASE 23: Fibrous Dysplasia

Case History: A 31-year-old woman presented with prior partial resection of fibrous dysplasia of the anterior and central skull base. She had experienced recent accelerated visual decline of the left eye (Fig. 33.23).

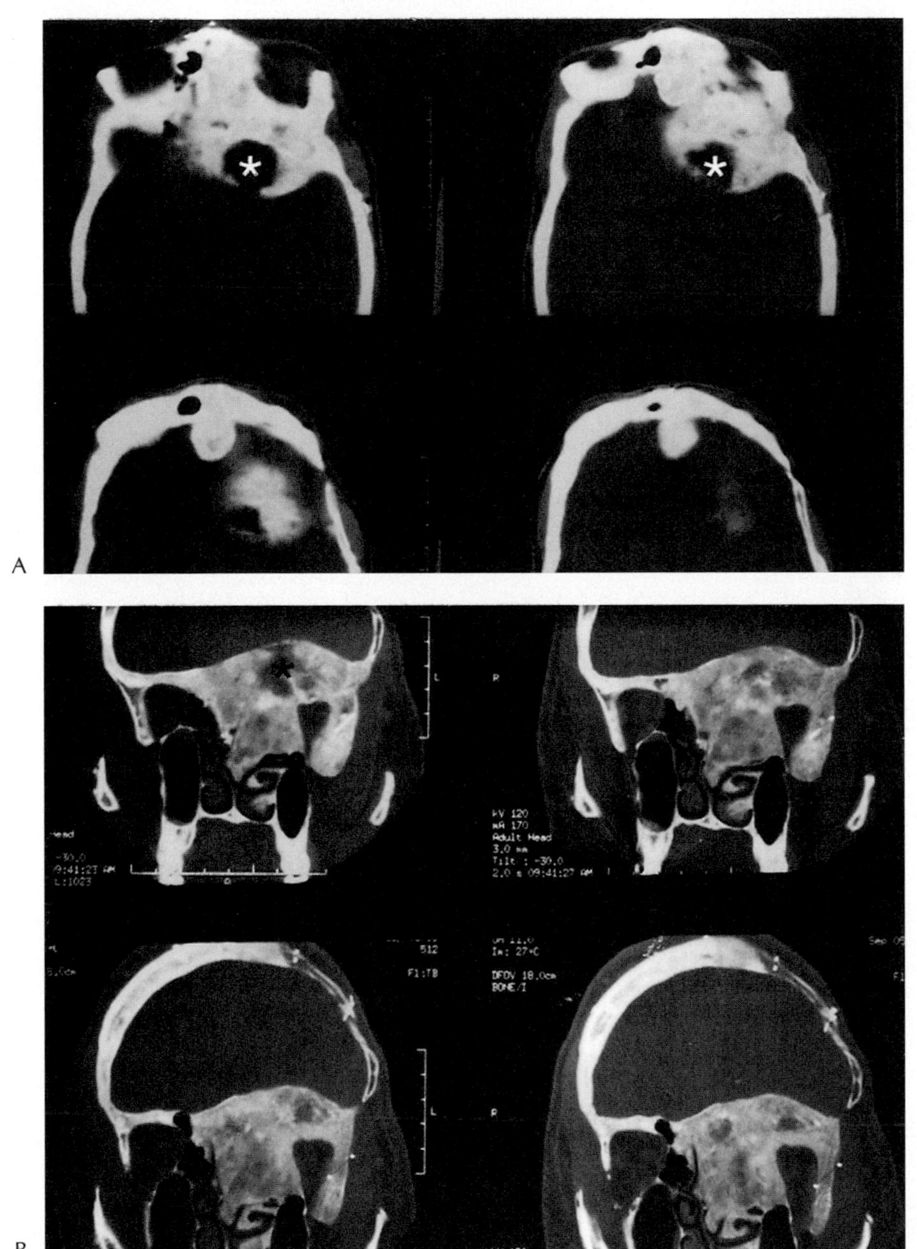

Figure 33.23 Fibrous dysplasia. Axial view **(A)** and direct coronal view **(B)** of the anterior skull base show diffuse sclerotic expansion of the skull base and calvarium. Progressive visual decline of the left eye was due to cystic degeneration of the expanded sphenoid bone (*asterisk*), not the narrowed optic foramen.

REFERENCES

1. Harrison DF. Unusual tumors. In: Suen JY, Meyers EN, eds. *Cancer of the head and neck.* New York: Churchill Livingstone, 1981:650.
2. Pratt LW. Unusual tumors of the head and neck. In: Johnson JT, Derkay CS, Mandell-Brown MK, et al., eds. *Instructional courses of the American Academy of Otolaryngology—head and neck surgery.* Vol 4. St Louis: Mosby-Year Book, 1991:118.
3. Hyams V. Unusual tumors and lesions. In: Gnepp DR, ed. *Pathology of the head and neck.* Philadelphia: WB Saunders, 1996:644.
4. Calcaterra TC. Unusual tumors. In: Meyers EN, Suen JY, eds. *Cancer of the head and neck,* 2nd ed. New York: Churchill Livingstone, 1996.
5. Jordan RB, Gauderer MWL. Cervical teratomas: an analysis, literature review and proposed classification. *J Pediatr Surg* 1988;23:583–591.
6. Filston HC. Hemangiomas, cystic hygromas and teratomas of the head and neck. *Semin Pediatr Surg* 1994;3:147–159.
7. Wenig BM. *Atlas of head and neck pathology.* Philadelphia: WB Saunders, 1993.
8. El-Sayed Y. Teratoma of the head and neck. *J Laryngol Otol* 1992;106:836–838.
9. Batsakis JG. *Tumors of the head and neck,* 2nd ed. Baltimore: Williams & Wilkins, 1979.
10. Zerella JT, Finberg FJ. Obstruction of the neonatal airway from teratomas. *Surg Gynecol Obstet* 1990; 170:126–131.
11. Kuhel WI, Yagoda M, Peterson P. Benign cervical teratomas in the adult: report of a case with dense fibrosis involving adjacent vital structures. *Otolaryngol Head Neck Surg* 1996;115:152–155.
12. Rothschild MA, Catalano P, Urken M, et al. Evaluation and management of congenital cervical teratoma. *Arch Otolaryngol Head Neck Surg* 1994;120: 444–448.
13. Ward RF, April M. Teratomas of the head and neck. *Otolaryngol Clin North Am* 1989;22:621–629.
14. Gundry SR, Wesley JR, Klein MD, et al. Cervical teratomas in the newborn. *J Pediatr Surg* 1983;18:382–386.
15. Batakis JG, Littler ER, Oberman HA. Teratomas of the neck: a clinicopathological assessment. *Arch Otolaryngol* 1964;79:619.
16. Hancok BJ, St-Vil D, Luks FL, et al. Complications of lymphangioma in children. *J Pediatr Surg* 1992;27:220–226.
17. Som PM. Head and neck imaging. In: Som PM, Curtin HD, eds. *Head and neck imaging,* 3rd ed. Vol I. New York: Mosby, 1996:533.
18. Donegan JO. Congenital neck masses. In: Cummings CW, Fredrickson JF, Harker LA, et al, eds. *Otolaryngology—head and neck surgery,* 2nd ed. Vol II. St Louis: Mosby-Year Book, 1993.
19. Stal S, Hamilton S, Spira M. Hemangiomas, lymphomangiomas and vascular malformations. *Otolaryngol Clin North Am* 1986; 19:769–796.
20. Siegel MJ, Glazer HS, St Amour TE, et al. Lymphangiomas in children: MR imaging. *Radiology* 1989;170:467.
21. Joseph AE, Donaldson JS, Reynolds M. Neck and thorax venous aneurysms: association with cystic hygromas. *Radiology* 1989;170:109–112.
22. Ricciardelli EJ, Richardson MA. Cervicofacial cystic hygromas. Patterns of recurrence and management of the difficult case. *Arch Otolaryngol Head Neck Surg* 1991;1 17:546–553.
23. Suh IS, Abenoza P, Galloway HR, et al. Peripheral nerve tumors: correlation of MR imaging and histologic findings. *Radiology* 1992;183:341.
24. Shah JP. *Head and neck surgery,* 2nd ed. London: Mosby-Wolfe, 1996.
25. Carrau RL, Myers EN, Johnson JT. Management of tumors arising in the parapharyngeal space. *Laryngoscope* 1990;100:583.
26. Myers EN, Johnson JT. Neoplasms. In: Cummings CW, Fredrickson JF, Harker LA, et al., eds. *Otolaryngology—head and neck surgery,* 2nd ed. Vol II. St Louis: Mosby-Year Book, 1993.
27. Brackman DE, Arriaga MA. Differential diagnosis of neoplasms of the posterior fossa. In: Cummings CW, Fredrickson JF, Harker LA, et al., eds. *Otolaryngology—head and neck surgery,* 2nd ed. Vol II. St Louis: Mosby-Year Book, 1993.
28. Malis LI. Neurofibromatosis (Von Recklinghausen's disease). In: Cummings CW, Fredrickson JF, Harker LA, et al., eds. *Otolaryngology—head and neck surgery.* Vol 11. St Louis: Mosby-Year Book, 1986.
29. Lack EE, Worsham GF, Callihan MD. Granular cell tumor: a clinicopathologic study of 110 patients. *J Surg Oncol* 1980;13:301–306.
30. Noonan JD, Horton CE, Old WL, et al. Granular cell myoblastoma of the head and neck. Review of the literature and 10 year experience. *Am J Surg* 1979; 138:611–614.
31. Kershisnik M, Batsalcis JG, Mackay B. Pathology consultation: granular cell tumors. *Ann Otol Rhinol Laryngol* 1994; 103:416–419.
32. Stout AP, Murray MR. Hemangiopericytomas: vascular tumor featuring Zimmermann's pericytes. *Ann Stirg* 1942; 1 16:26.
33. Enzinger FM, Smith BH. Hemangiopericytomas. An analysis of 106 cases. *Hum Pathol* 1976;7:61.
34. Zoltan N. Differentiation markers in hemangiopericytoma. *Cancer* 1992;69: 133.
35. Barkwinkel KD, Diddams JA. Hemangiopericytoma report of a case and comprehensive review of the literature. *Cancer* 1970;25:896.
36. Walike JW, Bailey BJ. Head and neck hemangiopericytomas. *Arch Otolaryngol Head Neck* 1971;93:345.
37. Mira JG, Chu FCH, Fortner JG. The role of radiotherapy in the management of malignant hemangiopericytoma. *Cancer* 1977;39:1254.
38. Staples JJ, Robinson RA, Wen BC, et al. Hemangiopericytoma—the role of radiotherapy. *Int J Radiat Oncol Biol Phys* 1990;19:445.
39. Knowling M, Harwood A, Bergasaget D. Comparison of extramedullary plasmacytoma with solitary and multiple plasma cell tumors. *J Clin Oncol* 1983;1:255–262.
40. Susnerwala SS, Shanks JH, Banerjee SS, et al. Extramedullary plasmacytoma of the head and neck region: clinicopathological correlation in 25 cases. *Br J Cancer* 1997;75:921–927.
41. Nofsinger YC, Mirza N, Rowan PT, et al. Head and neck manifestations of plasma cell neoplasms. *Laryngoscope* 1997;107:741–746.
42. Bartyl R, Frisch B, Fateh-Moghadam A, et al. Histological classification of multiple myeloma. A retrospective and prospective study of 674 cases. *Am J Clin Pathol* 1987;87:342–355.
43. Mendenhall WM, Thar TL, Million RR. Solitary plasmacytoma of the bone and soft tissue. *Int J Radiat Oncol Biol Phys* 1980;6:1497–1501.
44. Corwin J, Lindberg RD. Solitary plasmacytoma of bone versus extramedullary plasmacytoma and their relationship to multiple myeloma. *Cancer* 1979;43: 1007–1013.
45. Buckley NJ, Burch WM, Leight GS. Malignant teratoma of the thyroid gland of an adult. A case report and review of the literature. *Surgery* 1986;100: 932–937.
46. Batsakis JG, El-Naggar AK, Luna MA. Pathology consultation: teratomas of the head and neck with emphasis on malignancy. *Ann Otol Rhinol Laryngol* 1995;104:496–500.
47. Sacher M, Som PM, Lanzieri CF, et al. Malignant teratoma of the parapharyngeal space in an adult presenting as cervical cord compression. *J Comput Tomogr* 1986;10:37–40.
48. Maddox JC, Evans HL. Angiosarcoma of skin and soft tissue: a study of forty-four cases. *Cancer* 1948;48:1907–1921.
49. Mark RJ, Tran LM, Secarz J, et al. Angiosarcoma of the head and neck: the UCLA experience 1955 through 1990. *Arch Otolaryngol Head Neck Surg* 1993; 119:973–978.
50. Lydiatt WM, Shaba AR, Shah J. Angiosarcoma of the head and neck. *Am J Surg* 1994;168:451–454.
51. Hoolden CA, Spittle ME, Wilson-Jones E. Angiosarcoma for the face and scalp, prognosis and treatment. *Cancer* 19487;59:1046–1057.
52. Ramtin RK, Rassekh CH, Kinsella JB, et al. Osteosarcoma of the head and neck: meta-analysis of nonrandomized studies. *Laryngoscope* 1997;107:56–61.
53. Mark RJ, Secarz JA, Tran L, et al. Osteogenic sarcoma of the head and neck. The UCLA experience. *Arch Otolaryngol Head Neck Surg* 1991;117:761–766.
54. Geopfert H, Raymond AK, Spires JR, et al. Osteosarcoma of the head and neck. *Cancer Bull* 1990;42:347–354.
55. Smith PD, Patterson JW. Merkel cell carcinoma (neuroendocrine carcinoma of the skin). *Am J Clin Pathol* 2001;115[Suppl:S68–78].
56. Samonis G, Mantadakis E, Kononas TC, et al. Merkel cell carcinoma: a case series of twelve patients and review of the literature. *Anticancer Res* 2001;21: 4173–4177.
57. Goessling W, McKee PH, Mayer RJ. Merkel cell carcinoma. *J Clin Oncol* 2002; 20:588–598.
58. Linjawi A, Jamison WB, Meterissian S. Merkel cell carcinoma: important aspects of diagnosis and management. *Am Surg* 2001;67:943–947.
59. Coit DG. Merkel cell carcinoma. *Ann Surg Oncol* 2001;8[9 Suppl]:99S–102S.
60. Yiengpruksawan A, Coit DG, Thaler HT, et al. Merkel cell carcinoma. Prognosis and management. *Arch Surg* 1991;126:1514–1519.
61. Gillenwater AM, Hessel AC, Morrison WH, et al. Merkel cell carcinoma of the head and neck: effect of surgical excision and radiation on recurrence and survival. *Arch Otolaryngol Head Neck Surg* 2001;127:149–154.
62. Morrison WH, Peters LJ, Silva EG, et al. The essential role of radiation therapy in securing locoregional control of Merkel cell carcinoma. *Int J Radiat Oncol Biol Phys* 1990;19:583–591.
63. Medina-Franco H, Urist MM, Fiveash J, et al. Mutlimodality treatment of Merkel cell carcinoma: case series and literature review of 1024 cases. *Ann Surg Oncol* 2001;8:204–208.
64. Mann GB, Allen PJ, Coit DG. Merkel cell carcinoma. *Aust N Z J Surg* 1999;69: 87.
65. Allen, PJ, Zhang ZF, Coit DG. Surgical management of Merkel cell carcinoma. *Ann Surg* 1999;229:97–105.
66. Takata M, Hashimoto K, Mehregan P, et al. Genetic changes in sweat gland carcinomas. *J Cutaneous Pathol* 2000;27:30–35.
67. Vogelbruch M, Rutten A, Bocking A, et al. Differentiation between malignant and benign follicular adnexal tumors of the skin by DNA image cytometry. *Br J Dermatol* 2002;28:238–243.
68. Skidmore RA, Flowers FP. Non-melanoma skin cancer. *Med Clin North Am* 1998;82:1309–1323.
69. Stojadinovic A, Karpoff H, Antonescu CR, et al. Dermatofibrosarcoma protuberans of the head and neck. *Ann Surg Oncol* 2000;7:696–704.
70. Batsakis JG, Solomon AR, Rice DH. The pathology of head and neck tumors: neoplasms of cartilage, bone, and the notochord, part 7. *Head Neck Surg* 1980; 3:43–57.
71. Sehdev MK, Huvos AG, Strong EW, et al. Ameloblastoma of maxilla and mandible. *Cancer* 1974;33:324–333.
72. Crawley WA, Levin LS. Treatment of ameloblastoma: A controversy. *Cancer* 1978;42:357–363.
73. Black KL. Chordomas of the clival region. *Contemporary Neurosurgery* 1990;12: 1–8.
74. Amendola BE, Amendola MA, Oliver E, et al. Chordoma: role of radiation therapy. *Radiology* 1986;158:839–843.

CHAPTER 34

Lymphomas of the Head and Neck

M. Alma Rodriguez and Ali W. Bseiso

Lymphoma describes a heterogeneous group of lymphoproliferative disorders, classically categorized into two broad categories: Hodgkin disease (HD) and non-Hodgkin lymphoma (NHL). The most current classification system for these disorders further subcategorizes non-Hodgkin lymphoma into two types, depending on the immunophenotype of the cells: "B" cell disorders and "T" cell disorders (1). Lymphomas often present as lymphadenopathy, and it is common in the head and neck. Non-Hodgkin lymphoma, which has an incidence that is approximately five times higher than that of Hodgkin disease, constitutes approximately 5% of all head and neck cancers (2). In fact, lymphomas are the most common nonepithelial tumors in the extracranial head and neck region (3). Whereas HD rarely is accompanied by extranodal involvement in the head and neck, NHL often is. The head and neck region is the second most common site of extranodal involvement for NHL, after the gastrointestinal (GI) tract, where approximately 25% of all extranodal tumors occur (4). Lymphomas are characteristically chemosensitive and radiosensitive and are curable in a significant number of patients. Therefore, distinguishing this group of diseases from carcinomas is crucial when designing therapy and predicting outcomes.

RELEVANT ANATOMY

The lymphatic system in the head and neck drains into the deep cervical chain, which constitutes the final common drainage pathway. Lymph nodes in the head are mainly superficial, comprising the occipital, retroauricular, anterior auricular, superficial parotid, and facial nodes. The facial nodes include the infraorbital, buccal, and mandibular groups. The cervical lymph nodes can be divided into superficial and deep categories. The superficial nodes consist of the submental, submandibular, and external jugular lymph nodes. The deep cervical lymph nodes consist of the accessory chain, which follows the accessory nerve across the posterior triangle; the transverse cervical lymph nodes; and the anterior cervical chain, which extends from the superior deep cervical lymph nodes into the jugulodigastric and inferior deep cervical lymph nodes.

The Waldeyer tonsillar ring, on the other hand, forms the major extranodal group of lymphoid tissue in the head and neck and is the second most common site of extranodal lymphomas after the GI tract. The Waldeyer ring is a loosely connected lymphoid structure that is considered a primary immune barrier for ingested or inhaled antigens. The largest component of the Waldeyer ring is the palatine tonsil. It consists of a submucosal collection of lymphatic tissue between the palatoglossal and palatopharyngeal folds and is approximately 2 cm in its greatest dimension. The lingual tonsil at the base of the tongue and the pharyngeal tonsil at the upper end of the posterior wall of the nasopharynx are the other two components of the Waldeyer ring. Lymphoid tissue also exists in the salivary glands, thyroid gland, and dermis.

NATURAL HISTORY AND PATTERN OF SPREAD

The incidence of NHL has been increasing over the last four decades. Non-Hodgkin lymphoma is now the fifth leading cause of death in men and the seventh leading cause of death in women in the United States (5). The reasons for the increased incidence are unknown, but they may be explained by several factors, including the aging population; spread of viral infections such as the Epstein-Barr virus (EBV), human immunodeficiency virus (HIV), and human T-cell lymphotropic virus type 1 (HTLV-1); and exposure to chemical agents such as herbicides and pesticides. Though the incidence of NHL rises steadily with age, HD demonstrates a bimodal incidence curve, with a large peak between 15 and 30 years of age and a second, smaller peak near 50 years of age. The male–female HD ratio is 1.5:1 for patients age 10 and older, whereas the ratio is 9:1 for patients younger than 10. Non-Hodgkin lymphomas have a similar male predominance, except for follicular lymphomas, which generally occur equally among men and women. Hodgkin disease shows homogeneous predictable clinical behavior, whereas NHL has a variable clinical picture, as predicted by its histology and several clinical and laboratory parameters that constitute parts of prognostic scoring systems (6,7). The relatively young average age of HD (32 years) and NHL (42 years) patients explains why lymphomas are a leading cause of total person-years of life lost in the United States.

In general, HD generally has a better prognosis than NHL. Hodgkin disease spreads in a contiguous manner (probably indicating a unifocal origin) and, at least in the head and neck region, exhibits almost exclusive lymphatic spreading. Therefore, HD mainly involves nodes in the head and neck, and extranodal disease usually results from a break in the lymph node capsule, whereby direct extranodal extension ensues.

The non-Hodgkin lymphomas can exhibit wide variability in their clinical behavior. Although the revised European-American Lymphoma classification does not include clinical behavior in its stratification of these disorders, clinicians do refer to these as either aggressive or indolent (Table 34.1). Eighty-five percent of all NHL cases in the head and neck are aggressive, with large cell lymphoma or its variants being the most common, whereas 15% are indolent (8,9).

The designation of indolent versus aggressive depends on the survival expectation for patients with the disorder (10). Patients with indolent lymphomas have a survival expectation measured in years, even when advanced in their presentation, whereas patients with aggressive lymphomas have survival expectations of a few months if their disease is not sensitive to chemotherapy. In general, however, advanced-stage indolent lymphomas, despite their long-term natural histories, rarely are cured with conventional chemotherapy. In a large portion of the clinically more aggressive lymphomas, however, cures can be achieved with chemotherapy.

In the head and neck, 60% of all NHLs are extranodal. Although Reed-Sternberg-like cells may be seen in these lymphomas, true extranodal primary cases of HD are extremely rare. The most common nodal sites of NHL are the cervical lymph nodes, whereas the Waldeyer ring is the site of approximately two thirds of all extranodal lymphomas in the head and neck and of 5% of all NHLs (11,12). More than half of the lymphomas in the Waldeyer ring involve the palatine tonsils, 35% involve the nasopharynx, 9% involve the base of tongue, and 4% are multicentric (13). Compared with epithelial tumors, extranodal lymphomas of the head and neck are uncommon, constituting approximately 10% of cancers of the postnasal space and less than 5% of cancers of the nose, sinuses, palatine tonsils, and base of tongue (14). Among patients with "asymptomatic," localized, nodal cervical NHL, approximately one-third may demonstrate, on careful head and neck examination, unsuspected involvement of the Waldeyer ring, thus emphasizing the importance of such examinations, especially if radi-

TABLE 34.1 Revised European-American Lymphoma (REAL) Classification

B-cell neoplasms

I. Precursor B-cell neoplasms: precursor B-lymphoblastic leukemia or lymphoma[a]

II. Peripheral B-cell neoplasm

1. B-cell chronic lymphocytic leukemia or prolymphocytic leukemia or small lymphocytic leukemia
2. Lymphoplasmacytoid lymphoma or immunocytoma
3. Mantle-cell lymphoma[a]
4. Follicular-center lymphoma; follicular provisional grades: 1, small-cell; 2, mixed; 3, large-cell[a]; provisional subtype: diffuse, predominantly small-cell type
5. Marginal zone B-cell lymphoma extranodal (MALT-type ± monocytoid B cells) provisional subtype: nodal (monocytoid B-cells)
6. Provisional entity: splenic marginal zone lymphoma (± villous lymphocytes)
7. Hairy-cell leukemia
8. Plasmacytoma or plasma cell myeloma
9. Diffuse large B-cell lymphoma subtype: primary mediastinal B-cell lymphoma[a]
10. Burkitt lymphoma[a]
11. Provisional entity: high-grade B-cell lymphoma, Burkitt-like[a]

T-cell and putative NK-cell neoplasms

I. Precursor T-cell neoplasm: precursor T-lymphoblastic lymphoma or leukemia[a]

II. Peripheral T-cell and NK-cell neoplasms

1. T-cell chronic lymphocyte leukemia or prolymphocytic leukemia
2. Large granular lymphocyte leukemia: T-cell type; NK-cell type
3. Mycosis fungoides or Sézary syndrome
4. Peripheral T-cell lymphomas, unspecified[a]
5. Angioimmunoblastic T-cell lymphoma[a]
6. Angiocentric lymphoma[a]
7. Intestinal T-cell lymphoma (± enteropathy-associated)[a]
8. Adult T-cell leukemia or lymphoma[a]
9. Anaplastic large-cell lymphoma, CD30+, T- and null-cell types[a]
10. Provisional entity: anaplastic large-cell lymphoma, Hodgkin-like[a]

Hodgkin disease

I. Lymphocyte predominance

II. Nodular sclerosis

III. Mixed cellularity

IV. Lymphocyte depletion

V. Provisional entity: lymphocyte-rich classic Hodgkin disease

MALT, mucosa-associated lymphoid tissue; NK, natural killer.

[a]Clinically aggressive non-Hodgkin lymphoma.

ation therapy is being considered for inclusion in the planned treatment (15). Other frequent sites of extranodal disease include the nasal cavity, paranasal sinuses, orbit, salivary glands, thyroid gland, larynx, and even tooth extraction sites (16). In the Western hemisphere, most such extranodal lymphomas are aggressive B-cell lymphomas. Lymphomas in the orbit and salivary glands, however, mainly are of low-grade histology. This may be explained by the predominance of lymphomas arising from mucosa-associated lymphoid tissue (MALT) in these organs (17).

Unexpectedly, MALT lymphomas rarely arise in the Waldeyer ring, whereas mantle-cell lymphomas have a propensity to involve both the GI tract and the Waldeyer ring. In the Far East, T-cell lymphomas may be more common in extranodal locations in the head and neck; low-grade histology also is more common, found in more than 50% of all head and neck extranodal lymphomas in the Far East as opposed to less than 20% in the Western hemisphere (18,19).

Approximately two thirds of HD patients present with early stage disease, mainly on one side of the neck. In 70% of those patients, the disease is limited to the low-neck lymph nodes. Involvement of the supraclavicular or bilateral cervical lymph nodes predicts disease below the diaphragm in 30% to 40% of patients. In contrast, 40% to 60% of patients with head and neck NHL will have concomitant systemic disease. This is especially true for lymphomas with follicular components. Up to 70% to 80% of patients with follicular lymphomas have widespread disease at presentation, as opposed to 30% to 40% of patients who have diffuse disease. This may be related to the hematogenous and, hence, noncontiguous pattern of spread seen in NHL. Such a tendency for systemic involvement at presentation is especially common for nodal disease. Primary extranodal lymphomas tend to be more localized at diagnosis. During the course of the disease, however, lymphomas of the Waldeyer ring commonly involve the GI tract (20). In fact, up to 15% of patients who receive treatment of Waldeyer ring lymphoma with local radiation therapy alone experience relapses, usually within the GI tract (21). The GI tract relapse rate seems to decline with the incorporation of chemotherapy into the treatment program (22).

Primary NHL of the salivary glands is rare, accounting for 2.5% of all salivary gland tumors and 5% of all extranodal lymphomas (12,14). It is more common in the context of widespread disease. The parotid gland, with is rich in normal lymphoid tissue in 80% of healthy individuals (23), is probably the only salivary gland involved with true lymphoma (14). Some authors suggest that lymphomas in the salivary glands, especially the parotid, can be divided into two histologically and clinically distinct entities: those that arise from lymph nodes within the parotid gland and those that arise from lymphoid cells within the glandular parenchyma. Nodal parotid disease behaves more like nodal disease elsewhere and tends toward systemic involvement. True parotid lymphomas, on the other hand, are more likely to arise from MALT, to be more indolent and more localized, and to occur in patients with autoimmune diseases such as Sjögren syndrome (24,25). Patients with Sjögren syndrome show a 43 times greater incidence of lymphoma, almost exclusively of B-cell origin, which usually arises after myoepithelial sialadenitis (26,27). Like MALT lymphomas at other sites, the inflammatory lesions of sialadenitis and frank lymphoma form two extremes of a well-described spectrum. Progression is accompanied by the appearance of disease in cervical lymph nodes or other mucosal sites, especially in the head and neck. Such lymph nodes often have a monocytoid histologic makeup (28).

Less than 1% of all primary laryngeal cancers are of hematopoietic origin, and most occur in men older than 65 years. These cancers consist mainly of extramedullary plasmacytomas, but aggressive NHLs can also present at this site (29). Plasmacytomas are usually polypoid, nonulcerated lesions with preferential involvement of the supraglottic parts, especially the epiglottis and the aryepiglottic folds. Lymphomas, mostly NHLs, constitute approximately 2% of all thyroid malignancies and, in contrast with other head and neck lymphomas, are more common in women. This probably is related to the higher incidence of Hashimoto thyroiditis in women (30).

Nasofacial NK/T-cell lymphoma, formerly called lethal midline granuloma, is characterized by relentless ulcerative destruction of the nose or deep midfacial structures. Historically, it has been confused with other diseases including infections (e.g., syphilis, actinomycosis, tuberculosis), sarcoidosis, vasculitis (mostly Wegener granulomatosis), and nonlymphoid neoplasms (e.g., squamous cell carcinoma, adenocarcinoma, histiocytosis X, melanoma). Although the histologic diagnosis of nasofacial NK/T-cell lymphoma was difficult in the past, it has become evident that a substantial number of patients have NK- or T-cell lymphomas with an angiocentric histologic makeup. Also, EBV is detected regularly in tumor cells (31). Localized angiocentric T-cell lymphomas of the sinonasal region have been studied by Aviles et al. (32), who showed that the presence of angiocentric histology is an independent predictor of shorter disease-specific and overall survivals. Other important prognostic factors include lactate dehydrogenase (LDH) and β_2-microglobulin levels.

CLINICAL PRESENTATION

Lymphomas are the most frequent cause of unilateral neck masses in patients between 21 and 40 years of age (33). Almost always painless, these masses may become painful if the lymphoma's growth rate is rapid, causing central necrosis. Such rapid growth usually is seen in high-grade or aggressive intermediate-grade lymphomas. Hodgkin disease occurs most often as cervical nodal disease and very rarely as extranodal disease, particularly in the head and neck region. Most cervical involvement of HD occurs in the internal jugular or supraclavicular groups, usually sparing the accessory chain. The site of involvement may sometimes correlate with tumor histology; for example, lymphocyte-predominant HD tends to have upper cervical lymph node involvement. Nodes tend to be rubbery and matted but may be discrete. Approximately 40% of patients with HD have concomitant B symptoms. These consist of fever (38°C), drenching night sweats, and loss of more than 10% of the patient's original weight within 6 months. Lymph nodes affected by HD may wax and wane for a period before they acquire the progressive pattern of growth typical of malignant disease.

On physical examination, NHLs generally have nodal characteristics similar to HD, but NHLs tend to show a higher rate of growth, especially those that are aggressive. The internal jugular chain is the most common site of NHL involvement. Other lymph node groups in the head and neck tend to be more common sites of involvement with NHL than HD. These include the occipital, preauricular, submandibular, and submental lymph nodes. In contrast to patients with HD, only 10% to 15% of patients with NHL have concomitant B symptoms.

As mentioned earlier, NHL commonly occurs at extranodal sites, most notably the Waldeyer ring. The palatine tonsils and nasopharyngeal tonsils (adenoids) are the major areas of involvement with NHL. Unlike squamous cell carcinomas, NHL may cause bulky masses in those areas, commonly without causing bone destruction (30). Symptoms that may result include sore throat, a lump or sensation of fullness, dysphagia, deafness secondary to eustachian tube obstruction and, rarely, cranial nerve palsy. Such symptoms also are seen with squamous cell carcinomas. Approximately one half to two thirds of patients with Waldeyer ring involvement also have enlarged cervical lymph nodes. This is especially true for tonsillar involvement (34). The palatine tonsil often is unilaterally enlarged and has a smooth mucosal covering, a clinical picture that can be easily confused with infection. An important characteristic of extranodal lymphomas of the head and neck is multicentricity.

There is a high association of concurrent or recurrent extranodal disease within the GI tract (35). The nasal cavity and paranasal sinuses are the next most common sites of disease involvement. Symptoms from lymphomas in these areas include nasal obstruction, recurrent sinusitis, bloody discharge, and facial pain. Infraorbital hypoesthesia may occur and, in the case of invasion of the orbital floor, orbital edema and proptosis also might occur. In thyroid gland involvement, one or both lobes may be diffusely enlarged, with thyromegaly and possible airway obstruction. Patients with parotid gland involvement usually have an asymptomatic parotid mass or symptoms of parotitis. Mucosa-associated lymphoid tissue lymphoma of the orbit may present with symptoms such as eye irritation, foreign body sensation, excessive lacrimation, redness, and a mass.

DIAGNOSTIC EVALUATION AND STAGING

A patient with a neck mass must undergo a thorough examination of the head and neck to identify the site of tumor origin, whether squamous cell carcinoma or extranodal lymphoma within the Waldeyer ring. A biopsy from the primary extranodal site is preferable prior to excision of the lymph node. When tissue is required from an accessible lymph node, a fine-needle aspiration is a useful initial test to help distinguish lymphomas from carcinomas. Lymphomas almost always express the leukocyte common antigen CD45 and lack expression of keratin, melanin, protein S-100, and mucin (36,37). Material obtained through fine-needle aspiration may also be used for flow-cytometric determination of S-phase, ploidy, and RNA content and can be used for cytogenetic analysis and molecular studies (38).

For the accurate initial diagnosis of NHL and HD, however, an excisional biopsy of the lymph node is crucial. This helps to define accurately the overall architecture of the lymph node, to identify follicular lymphomas, and to differentiate lymphomas and HD from benign hyperplasia. Generally, the surgeon should obtain the specimen from the site of largest bulk, although certain lymph node groups (e.g., the parotid and submandibular groups) should preferably be avoided because of their known involvement with chronic inflammation.

In addition to pathologic and cytologic features, immunophenotypic characteristics can be determined by flow cytometry or immunohistochemistry and can be used in subclassifying lymphomas. Such studies will differentiate between T- and B-cell immunophenotypes. B-cell phenotype is characteristically positive for antigens CD19 and CD20. Light-chain restriction also indicates clonality. Antigens CD5 and CD23 are expressed in small lymphocytic lymphomas and chronic lymphocytic leukemia, whereas CD10 is a feature of indolent lymphomas of follicle-center origin. Mantle-cell lymphoma also is positive for CD5 but is negative for CD23 and positive for CD43 and FMC-7 antigens. Reed-Sternberg cells are positive for CD30. T-cell lymphomas commonly express CD45RO and CD3 (Table 34.2).

TABLE 34.2 Immunophenotypic Profile of the More Common Non-Hodgkin Lymphomas

	CD20	CD5	CD3	CD23	CD10	FMC7
B-cell/small lymphocytic	+	+	–	+	–	–
Mantle cell	+	+	–	–	–	+
Follicular	+	–	–	–	+	
Immunocytoma	+	–	–	–	–	+
Marginal zone	+	–	–	±	–	+
T-cell	–	+	+	–	–	–
"B" large cell	+	–[a]	–	–	±	–

[a]Rarely (+).

Electron microscopy rarely is needed but, in anaplastic tumors, certain features—including desmosomes, melanosomes, and neuroendocrine granules—can be of diagnostic significance. All of these help to rule out the diagnosis of lymphoma (39).

Once the diagnosis is established, staging should include careful physical examination. Special attention should be paid to the different lymph node groups, including the cervical, submandibular, submental, preauricular, retroauricular, occipital, axillary, epitrochlear, supraclavicular, infraclavicular, inguinal, and femoral lymph nodes. Splenomegaly, as well as hepatomegaly, should be noted. Careful head and neck examination by an otolaryngologist is essential, especially in situations in which the disease is believed to be localized to that region. Radiographic studies should include a computed tomographic (CT) scanning or magnetic resonance imaging (MRI) of the head and neck, a chest roentgenogram, and abdominal and pelvic CT scans. A lymphangiogram may be helpful in cases of HD, to evaluate pelvic and periaortic lymph nodes, especially when the architecture is distorted without a change in size. A lymphangiogram also provides a convenient and inexpensive way to follow up with plain films. Expertise in lymphangiography, however, has declined, and few centers in the United States perform this diagnostic procedure. Computed tomography scans of the abdomen are essential to detect mesenteric and high celiac nodes and hepatic or splenic involvement.

The goal of gathering all the aforementioned information is to allow the clinician, after initial evaluation, to predict the outcome of the illness, assess the risk for recurrence and, possibly, design therapy based on risk stratification. The Ann Arbor staging system is one strategy for reaching those goals (40) (Table 34.3). It was designed originally for HD, which spreads in a contiguous manner, making the system useful in predicting out-

TABLE 34.3 Ann Arbor Staging System

Stage	Features
I	Single node region
I(E)	Single extranodal site (E)
II	Two or more node regions on same side of the diaphragm
II(E)	Single node region and localized single extranodal site
III	Nodal involvement on both sides of the diaphragm
III(E) III(ES)	Stage III and localized single extranodal site or spleen (S) or both
IV	Diffuse involvement of extranodal sites with or without nodal disease
A	Without B symptoms
B	With B symptoms: fever, weight loss, sweats

come for that disease. However, the Ann Arbor staging system is less useful in predicting outcomes for NHLs, which disseminate hematogenously early in the course of the disease and are more heterogeneous than HD. Therefore, several other prognostic factors have been evaluated for NHL. These include tumor bulk, serum LDH, serum β_2-microglobulin level, and concomitant B symptoms. Such factors have been incorporated in different prognostic systems. The International Prognostic Index successfully predicts outcomes in intermediate-grade lymphomas and is the most widely and uniformly used today. Factors evaluated by the International Prognostic Index include age, Ann Arbor stage, serum LDH level, performance status, and number of extranodal sites (6).

Clinicians have used such scoring systems to predict outcomes and to determine therapeutic regimen intensities. Among patients with extranodal disease in the head and neck in one series, those with stage I (as opposed to stage II) or non-Waldeyer ring disease have shown significantly better disease-free and overall survival rates than have patients with stage II or Waldeyer ring diseases. This particular series (41), however, included only one patient with paranasal lymphoma, which was shown in a previous series to have a worse outcome than Waldeyer ring lymphoma. This finding probably was due to the more frequent occurrence of aggressive lymphoma in the latter group (42).

Attempts to design prognostic systems for follicular lymphoma have been less successful. However, prognostic factors similar to those used in the International Prognostic Index and tumor score systems are largely applicable. For early stage disease (stages I and II), age (<60), extranodal disease, stage II (as opposed to stage I disease), and disease of follicular mixed histology (as opposed to follicular small cleaved cell) were shown to be adverse prognostic factors, even after correction for staging diligence with laparotomy and radiation. Staging laparotomy for clinical stage I and II disease has largely been abandoned since the introduction of CT scans. However, laparotomy can identify radiographically occult disease below the diaphragm. Thus, studies using laparotomy staging demonstrate better disease-free survival rates for early stage categories. As shown in a study from Stanford University, overall survival rates also were better among stage I patients with follicular lymphoma when the stages were defined by laparotomy (43,44).

Hodgkin disease localized to the head and neck region is most often clinically stage I or II. Several clinical criteria have been identified for HD in this region to help predict outcome and thus guide treatment. The Stanford group pioneered staging laparotomy for this patient group that helped identify such criteria. Generally, 20% of patients with clinical stage I disease and 30% with clinical stage II disease had subdiaphragmatic involvement. Characteristics that do not favor subdiaphragmatic disease include women with clinical stage I disease, clinical stage I mediastinal disease only, women younger than 27 years of age with clinical stage II disease and three or fewer sites of disease involvement, and lymphocyte-predominant histology (45). Other well-established prognostic factors include tumor bulk (46,47), an elevated erythrocyte sedimentation rate (48), advanced age (49), and B-cell symptoms (50).

MANAGEMENT AND RESULTS

Nodal Indolent Lymphomas

As mentioned previously, localized, indolent NHLs are uncommon. This is demonstrated by the fact that 80% of patients with clinical stage I or II disease will have microscopic subdiaphragmatic involvement at staging laparotomy (51). In addition, the long natural history of the disease and the differences in staging workup among investigators make a comparison of data among clinical trials difficult. Another source of confusion is that many of the studies examining therapy for early stage disease are not restricted to patients with a low-grade or follicular histologic type. In general, however, radiation therapy alone can result in long-term disease-free survival in approximately half of patients with stage I or II disease and one-third of patients with stage II disease who exhibit favorable characteristics (43,52–54).

Several studies have addressed the question of whether adding chemotherapy to radiation is beneficial. Generally, patient populations in these studies are heterogeneous, and although some studies have shown improvement in disease-free survival rates (55), there is no conclusive evidence that the patients' overall survival rate is improved (55–57). Another unresolved issue is the use of total lymphoid irradiation (TLI) in limited-stage follicular lymphoma. The results of a trial conducted at Stanford University show that this modality may be superior to involved-field or extended-field radiation therapy (43). An update of the Stanford data shows that at 10 years of follow-up, only 36% of patients treated on one side of the diaphragm did not have relapses, as compared with 67% of those treated on both sides of the diaphragm. However, there was no significant difference in overall survival between the two groups (44). Thus, although TLI cannot be recommended at this time as standard therapy for patients with localized stage I or II follicular lymphomas, longer follow-up periods may eventually show a difference in survival rates. The advent of new therapeutic options with monoclonal antibodies, however, may radically change the strategy of therapy for patients with localized indolent lymphomas in the future (58).

Intermediate-Grade Lymphoma

Combined-modality therapy using chemotherapy followed by irradiation to the involved field has been clearly associated with better outcomes than radiation alone in patients with stage I and II disease (59). Chemotherapy alone, however, has gained significant support as a primary therapy because of its greater success in achieving cures. The reported 5-year disease-free survival rate in most trials is approximately 75% for combined stage I and II disease populations (60). There is a question of whether a combined-modality approach would improve outcomes over chemotherapy alone by achieving the same cure rates using fewer courses with less toxic effects (61). Another question is whether intensifying the chemotherapy portion of combined therapy would be suitable for certain subgroups of patients. The incorporation of radiation therapy clearly results in fewer local relapses within the radiation field (59), but the overall survival rate of patients receiving chemotherapy alone may not necessarily be compromised, as local relapses may be effectively treated with radiation or salvage chemotherapy (or both) (62).

To better define the role of combined-modality therapy, a recently reported Southwest Oncology Group (SWOG) study compared three cycles of CHOP (cyclophosphamide, doxorubicin, vincristine, prednisone) followed by involved-field radiation with eight cycles of CHOP without radiation in patients with stage I and nonbulky stage II intermediate- and high-grade lymphomas (63). The overall survival rate at 4 years was significantly better for the group treated with combined-modality therapy than for the group treated with CHOP alone (87% vs. 75% at 4 years; $p < 0.01$). As is the case in a previous study conducted by Jones et al. (64), disease-free survival rates were not significantly different between the two groups; the lower survival rate in the group receiving CHOP alone was attributed to mainly cardiac deaths after completion of therapy (63). A more recent update on the outcomes of this study seems to indicate, however, that the subgroup of patients with stage II disease has fared better longer term with the administration of chemotherapy only, as opposed to abbreviated chemotherapy and radiation. The addition of rituximab to the CHOP regimen (RCHOP) also appears to have a superior result to CHOP alone in patients with advanced disease (65). Thus, it is likely that RCHOP will be of greater benefit to patients with limited-stage disease as well, although the results of such studies are still not published.

From studies such as this, prognostic factors that would influence therapy can be determined. Stage II disease in the head and neck (and in general) has been associated with a significantly lower disease-free survival rate than has stage I disease (92% vs. 60%; $p < 0.03$ in one study) (62–65). Tumor bulk (64,66), age (6,62), and performance status (6,62) are also indicators of lower survival rates. As discussed earlier, such prognostic factors were included in the International Prognostic Index and tumor score. Therefore, whereas the young asymptomatic patient with stage I disease (and a low International Prognostic Index) may have excellent outcome with three cycles of CHOP followed by involved-field radiation, symptomatic patients with stage II or bulky disease may benefit from a longer or more intense chemotherapy program prior to irradiation. The issue of intensifying the chemotherapy component of combined therapy also was investigated by using a regimen of prednisone, doxorubicin (Adriamycin), methotrexate, cyclophosphamide (Cytoxan), etoposide, nitrogen mustard, vincristine, and procarbazine (Pro-MACE-MOPP) followed by radiation therapy. The patients in this study had stage I disease, however, and a very high response rate therefore was expected. At a follow-up of 42 months, no relapses were documented (67). Longer follow-up periods and the incorporation of higher-risk patients will be required to draw firm conclusions about the benefits of more intensive regimens as part of combined-modality therapy in patients with newly diagnosed early stage disease.

Extranodal Disease in the Head and Neck

Though the general principles just described should apply to extranodal intermediate-grade lymphomas in the head and neck, relatively few studies have been limited to this subgroup of patients. In Waldeyer ring lymphomas, radiation therapy has been the mainstay of treatment, but relatively poor disease-free and overall survival rates have been reported in one study (40% and 50%, respectively) (68). One single-arm trial showed an improved disease-free survival rate with combined-modality therapy as compared with irradiation alone, but the overall survival rate was unchanged (22). Indolent extranodal lymphomas in the head and neck probably are mostly MALT-related and generally show excellent disease-free and overall survival rates of 100% and 94%, respectively, when irradiation with or without chemotherapy is used (18). Patients with localized, primary paranasal sinus lymphomas may represent a special subgroup. Traditionally, these patients received involved-field radiation therapy resulting in long-term survival rates of 50% to 70% (69). More recent data suggest that patients with localized sinonasal disease may do worse than patients with other extranodal lymphomas, with one series reporting a 10-year survival rate of 50% versus more than 75% in sinonasal and Waldeyer ring lymphomas, respectively. This outcome may be related to the higher incidence of aggressive lymphomas in the sinonasal area than in the Waldeyer ring. Patients with lymphoma in the sinonasal area have benefited more from combined-modality therapy than have patients with Waldeyer ring lymphoma (42).

Nasofacial NK/T-cell Lymphoma

In the past, when the malignant nature of nasofacial NK/T-cell lymphoma was not well established, low-dose radiation therapy was a common therapeutic modality that offered limited success (70,71). Localized angiocentric lymphomas of the head and neck were compared with other localized lymphomas by Aviles et al. (32). Among 23 patients with angiocentric lymphomas treated with radiation therapy alone, the median relapse-free survival period was 16 months, as compared with a median survival period of 44 months for 42 patients having comparable lesions without angiocentric histologic makeup ($p < 0.001$). The overall survival periods were also significantly different (25 months for angiocentric lesions vs. 20 to 93 months or more; median not reached for nonangiocentric lesions, $p < 0.001$). The combination of chemotherapy plus radiation therapy results in improved overall survival rates, although results remain significantly worse than those for other extranodal head

TABLE 34.4 A Simplified Approach to Therapy for Head and Neck Non-Hodgkin Lymphomas

Histology, site	Ann Arbor stage	Therapy
Nodal low-grade lymphoma (follicular, small lymphocytic)	I/II	XRT is standard, with 5-yr DFS of 50%. Potential improvement of DFS with combined-modality treatment. TLI results in 5-year DFS of 60%.
Intermediate-grade, high-grade	Ia/II	CTP ± XRT consolidation to bulky sites with 5-year DFS of 75% in stage I or II patients. XRT alone in highly selected stage I population with 5-year DFS of 77%.
Sinus lymphoma	I/II	Radiation alone results in long-term DFS of 50%–70%. Combined-modality treatment with CTP and XRT is indicated to improve outcome in light of common occurrence of high-grade histology.
Angiocentric T-cell lymphoma	I/II	Outcome generally worse than other head and neck lymphomas. XRT alone results in median DFS of 16 months. Limited experience indicated high success in incorporating CTP.
MALT lymphoma	I	XRT alone results in excellent outcome.
	II	Combined-modality treatment with CTP and XRT helps to reduce recurrence when disease is multicentric.
Waldeyer ring	I/II	XRT alone results in modest DFS of 40%–50%. Addition of CTP seems to improve outcome and reduce incidence of gastrointestinal recurrences, especially for stage II patients.

The number and class of drugs combined in chemotherapy, as well as the combination and duration of therapy, will depend on the histology, stage, bulk, and other prognostic factors such as lactate dehydrogenase and β_2-microglobulin.
CTP, chemotherapy; DFS, disease-free survival; MALT, mucosa-associated lymphoid tissue; TLI, total lymphoid irradiation; XRT, radiation therapy.

and neck lymphomas (71). Lipford et al. (72) treated eight patients who had a high-grade histologic type of disease with aggressive chemotherapy [cyclophosphamide, mechlorethamine, vincristine, procarbazine, and prednisone (C-MOPP), ProMACE-MOPP], and seven of the eight patients achieved remission with long-term survival. It appears, therefore, that such patients should first receive chemotherapy with or without radiation therapy, though there are too few data to support a firm conclusion.

Table 34.4 summarizes the current approach to management of the various histologic subtypes of NHL and sites of involvement within the head and neck.

Hodgkin Disease

The success of radiation therapy alone in curing early stages of HD depends of the success in ruling out occult advanced disease. Thus, the results of treatment will differ depending on whether patients were clinically or pathologically staged (i.e., with laparotomy). Prognostic factors that clarify further the risk for relapse were discussed earlier. Clinically staged HD patients treated with irradiation alone have a relapse risk for 30% to 50%. If patients with adverse factors are excluded, however, extended-field radiation therapy alone can result in a 10-year relapse-free survival rate of 87% (73). One such favorable group, for example, included patients with high cervical disease of lymphocyte-predominant histology which, as compared with other histologic types, is most likely to appear as early stage disease. The cure rate is especially high in such patients receiving extended-field radiation therapy alone. All five patients treated with limited-field irradiation were disease-free in a long-term follow-up in one series (74).

In a randomized trial, extended-field irradiation has been shown to improve outcomes over involved-field radiation therapy in patients with stage I and II disease (75). In general, however, patients with clinically assessed stage IA and IIA disease are treated with mantle and paraaortic-field irradiation, without pelvic irradiation, because fewer than 5% of such patients are expected to have disease below the aortic bifurcation (47). In those patients whose disease was staged without benefit of laparotomy (i.e., clinically), the spleen also is included in the field. However, a European Organisation for Research and Treatment of Cancer (EORTC) study comparing mantle-field irradiation with mantle and paraaortic-field irradiation in patients with pathologically staged I and II disease showed no clear difference in survival rates between the two treatment modalities (76).

Patients with adverse prognostic factors such as B symptoms, stage IV disease, massive mediastinal disease, or elevated erythrocyte sedimentation rate have been shown to respond to combined-modality therapy with more durable, complete remissions. Furthermore, prospective, randomized trials have shown that chemotherapy alone offers results superior to those of radiation therapy alone in patients with poor prognostic characteristics (77). The appeal of using chemotherapy alone emerges from the reduced toxic effect encountered as compared with combined-modality therapy. Because combined-modality therapy has been associated with an increased incidence of second malignancies, particularly leukemias and NHLs, the trend is to deliver lower levels of radiation to the involved fields of bulky sites when combined-modality treatment is used.

SPECIAL ISSUES

Burkitt Lymphoma

Burkitt lymphoma (BL) is a subset of B-cell NHL originally described in tropical Africa as involving the mandible in the majority of affected African children (78). Burkitt lymphoma accounts for up to 50% to 70% of all pediatric malignancies in certain parts of Africa. It is associated with high titers of EBV in as many as 90% of patients. Similarly, viral DNA and nuclear antigens are detected in 90% of African patients. The exact role of EBV in the initiation of the disease is not clear; in many areas of the world with a high incidence of EBV, the incidence of BL is not correspondingly high. This fact suggests that other factors besides EBV infection may play a role in the pathogenesis of BL. One such factor is probably malaria, the geographic distribution of which seems to overlap that of BL in Africa.

The incidence of BL in Africa is 150 in 1 million children (79), which is markedly higher than BL in the rest of the world. African Burkitt lymphoma usually arises from the bone marrow of the jaw and carries the features of a mature B-cell, expressing surface immunoglobulin. Approximately half of all patients also have abdominal disease, and a third present with central nervous system involvement. BL has morphologic and cytogenetic characteristics identical to those of BL in Africa, but sporadic BL varies significantly in clinical presentation (80). It has no predilection for specific race (only 5% of patients are black). BL patients usually are older than those in Africa, with peak presentation at 8 to 15 years, compared with 5 to 7 years of age. Also, unlike African BL, only 20% of BL patients are seropositive for EBV antibodies at diagnosis. Their most frequent presentation is abdominal disease, whereas only 7% of patients have jaw involvement. Other head and neck extranodal sites are much less common and include the cheek, palate, maxilla, orbit, tonsil, and mastoid.

Typically, BL carries a translocation that transposes the c-myc protooncogene on chromosome 8 with the enhancer of one of the immunoglobulin heavy- or light-chain genes. Thus, the resulting translocations lead to constitutive over-expression of c-myc. With a doubting time of 24 to 48 hours, prompt diagnosis and intensive chemotherapy are imperative. The 2-year disease-free survival rate, which essentially reflects cures, is in the neighborhood of 50% with modern therapy, whereas more recent reports of intensive regimens have reported a 2-year disease-free survival rate in excess of 90% (81).

Acquired Immunodeficiency Syndrome

Although Kaposi sarcoma may be the most common tumor to occur in the head and neck region in patients with acquired immunodeficiency syndrome (AIDS) (9), NHL may develop at any point in the course of HIV infection and is the second most common neoplasm seen in the head and neck in HIV-infected patients. Human immunodeficiency virus confers a more than 25-fold increase in incidence of NHL, compared with the general population (82). Approximately 20% of long-term survivors ultimately develop lymphoma, mostly B-cell type (83) and primarily immunoblastic large-cell type (60%) or Burkitt-like (20%) (84).

Unlike other NHLs, more than 60% of HIV-associated lymphomas have an extranodal component, and up to one-third may be exclusively extranodal (84,85). The most common sites of extranodal involvement are the central nervous system and bone marrow. Therefore, the routine examination of the cerebrospinal fluid in these patients is mandatory. Initial extranodal lymphomas in the head and neck are also common (86). Reported sites of involvement include the Waldeyer ring, the gingivae, parotid gland, scalp, orbit, oral mucosa, and sinonasal area (86–88). Disease in such patients should be staged carefully, as systemic disease is common in patients infected with HIV-1.

Occasionally, benign lymphoid proliferation is noted in the head and neck region in patients with HIV. It may present as a mass in the nasopharynx or tonsils and may mimic lymphoma (89,90). Thus, careful pathologic evaluation is needed to spare the already immunocompromised patient unnecessary chemotherapy.

Prognostic factors in HIV-1–associated lymphomas depend largely on the CD4 count, extent of disease, and presence or absence of a history of opportunistic infections. Generally, aggressive chemotherapy regimens have not improved survival rates in patients with advanced HIV infection (91). Guidelines to therapy include the use of cytokine support, lower doses of chemotherapy in patients with bone marrow involvement or low CD4 counts, concomitant nonmyelosuppressive antiretroviral therapy, and the incorporation of prophylactic therapy against *Pneumocystis carinii* pneumonia, fungal infections, and *Mycobacterium avium* complex.

Plasmacytoma

Localized plasma cell tumors are classically divided into medullary and extramedullary types. Medullary plasmacytomas occur mostly in the long bones and axial spine but are rare in the head and neck. This form of disease commonly is associated with progression to multiple myeloma in more than 50% of patients within 3 to 5 years of initial therapy (92). In contrast, extramedullary plasmacytoma occurs in the submucosa of the upper aerodigestive tract in 80% of patients (93). Mostly seen in men in their sixth or seventh decades, extramedullary plasmacytoma is less likely to progress to multiple myeloma, which is seen in only 15% to 20% of patients. The nasopharynx and paranasal sinuses are involved in 75% of patients (93). Oropharyngeal involvement is seen in 12% of patients and laryngeal disease in 18% of patients. Other reported sites include the parotid gland, tongue, thyroid gland, and salivary glands. Symptoms usually result from mass effect, and airway obstruction or epistaxis may occur. Because extramedullary plasmacytoma is very radiosensitive, radiation therapy is the standard treatment; disease-free survival rates of more than 70% at 10 years have been reported with radiation therapy (94). Some cases of long-term survival have been reported after surgical excision alone (95).

RADIOLOGIC IMAGING CONCERNS

Bernard B. O'Malley and Suresh K. Mukherji

Both MRI and CT are adequate for staging HD and NHL (Fig. 34.1). Gallium scintigraphy is an adjunctive test to differentiate between active and "sterilized" disease (96). Because imaging-based differential diagnosis depends heavily on the compartment of origin, extranodal lymphoma often is not diagnosed before fine-needle aspiration. Extranodal NHL presents most commonly in the Waldeyer ring followed by the sinonasal tract (97). The differential diagnosis of an infiltrating lymphomatous process of the sinonasal tract includes the American form of Burkitt lymphoma (98). It is important to consider lymphoma as a diagnostic possibility prior to any potentially disfiguring surgical procedure.

Few neoplasms have highly characteristic imaging features on CT or even MRI. Lymphomas generally have a very homogeneous appearance in both the primary site and the lymph nodes without evidence of necrosis (Fig. 34.2) (99). The typical CT appearance of lymph node involvement with lymphoma is a homogeneously enlarged lymph node with a faint rim of capsular enhancement. Although lymph node calcification is more commonly seen in metastatic thyroid carcinomas, squamous carcinomas, and adenocarcinomas, it can be seen in treated lymphomatous adenopathy (100). It is the pattern of findings rather than any single feature that favors the diagnosis of lymphoma. That pattern is multicompartmental homogeneous lymphadenopathy in addition to the dominant mass (Fig. 34.3) (101). Atypical lymphoid infiltrate should prompt a search for MALT lymphoma (102), especially in patients with systemic connective tissue disorders such as Sjögren disease. Biopsy-confirmed malignant lymphoma should also raise the possibility of Kicuchi-Fujimoto disease (103).

Lymphoma arising at the upper aerodigestive tract primary sites is often exophytic (Figs. 34.4 and 34.5). These masses typically show moderately intense homogeneous enhancement (Figs. 34.6 and 34.7). Lymphoma of the nasal cavity and nasopharynx generally has a "soft" appearance, with minor osseous destruction (Fig. 34.8). When lymphoma does penetrate the facial bones or central or anterior skull base, it generally does so in a permeative fashion without an expansile component (104). This pattern also occurs at the calvarium (Figs. 34.9 and 34.10). Lymphomas of the oral cavity (Fig. 34.7), pharynx, and floor of mouth are readily accessible to office biopsy (105). Palpable salivary gland and thyroid gland lesions often are biopsy-confirmed as lymphoma before imaging (Fig. 34.11). Large masses of the central compartment of the neck often are inseparable from and ascribed to thyroid disease. Lymphoma arising within the thyroid bed may occur *de novo* or related to chronic thyroiditis (Fig. 34.12). Mediastinal lymphoma often bulges upward through the thoracic inlet, presenting as a low-neck mass. This is particularly true of lymphoma involving the thymus, which usually bulges into the left side of the neck.

Because supraclavicular adenopathy is such a common presenting feature of lymphoma, special attention must be paid to technical factors when imaging that compartment (Fig. 34.13). Supraclavicular disease may be a reflection of neck, chest, and even subdiaphragmatic disease. The relationship between the supraclavicular adenopathy and the brachial plexus should be carefully assessed in patients with nodal involvement in this region. This region is poorly imaged with conventional (arms up) chest CT and often not completely covered in many neck CT protocols (which use clavicular heads for the lower landmark).

Lymph node imaging requires intravenous contrast with CT, particularly on the baseline examination. Nephrotoxicity and cardiotoxicity of ongoing treatment regimens often limit the use of intravenous contrast. Survey of the neck for adenopathy is readily performed with noncontrast MRI. Magnetic resonance imaging has the additional advantage over CT of identifying marrow involvement before frank bone destruction (106). Diseased normal-sized lymph nodes cannot be differentiated from reactive nodes (Fig. 34.14), as is true of most cross-sectional imaging modalities. Some studies suggest that MRI is the most predictive imaging modality for potential relapse (107).

Bulky lymphoma adenopathy and masses usually reduce dramatically in size after, and even during treatment. Residual tissue at involved lymph node stations has long been the imaging dilemma. Patients who are clinically improved were assumed to have "sterilized disease." When necessary, nuclear gallium scintigraphy was used to support that clinical impression of cure. The negative predictive value is more useful than the more limited positive predictive value for gallium. Interval decline in activity between gallium scans that parallels a clinical improvement has been the most useful indicator. This may parallel decline in LDH and improvement in marrow histology. Gallium, however, has a relatively low spatial resolution and distracting background activity in head and neck sites. Gallium scintigraphy has been the standard method for evaluating the degree of neoplastic activity in these residual masses.

More recently, positron emission tomography (PET) scanning with fluorodeoxyglucose (FDG) has been used both in the posttreatment as well as the baseline time points (Fig. 34.15). Appropriate patient preparation including muscle relaxants is necessary to minimize background activity. All functional nuclear scans are more useful when they provide a point of comparison. Baseline scans provide supplemental baseline staging for most types of lymphoproliferative disorders (Fig. 34.16). Low-grade and small-cell malignant lymphomas and nodular sclerosing HD have a greater false-negative rate than others. These images have a very good spatial resolution, particularly when performed on dedicated whole body PET (Fig. 34.17). Currently, the follow-up scan is performed at some interval after completion of induction or consolidation (108). A potential application of early reevaluation with PET would be to scan selected patients with multiple poor risk factors after the first cycle or two of chemotherapy. Those with limited or no response or progression might be considered for alternate aggressive therapy (109).

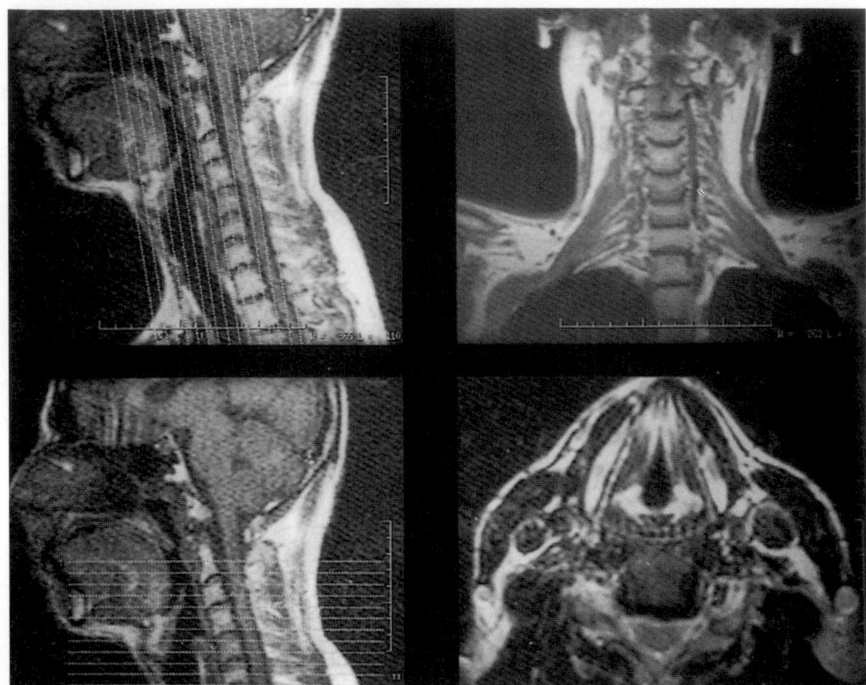

Figure 34.1 Magnetic resonance imaging examination for lymph node staging. **Top:** Sagittal T1 view and corresponding T1 coronal view show excellent tissue discrimination with noncontrast technique. **Bottom:** Sagittal T1 view and corresponding axial T2 view show normal appearance of tissue planes on routine noncontrast survey examinations.

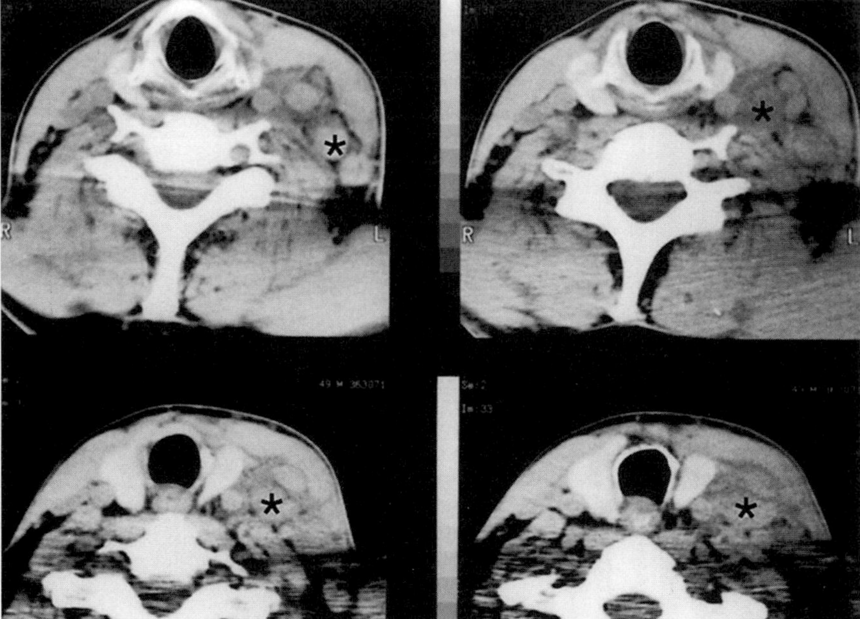

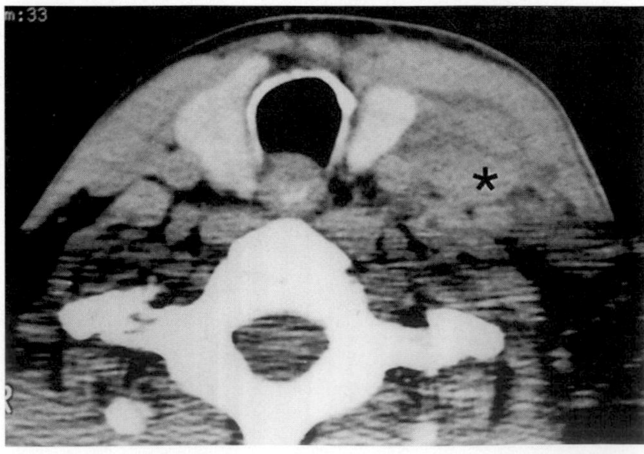

Figure 34.2 Lower cervical adenopathy. Noncontrast axial computed tomographic views show typical aggregate adenopathy limited to the left neck with homogeneous attenuation (*asterisk*).

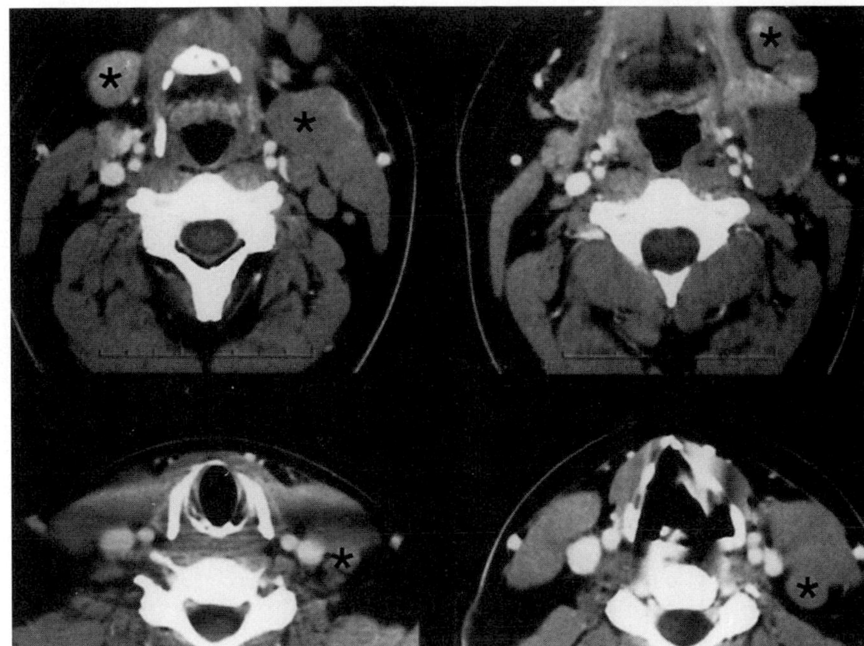

Figure 34.3 Lymphomatous adenopathy. Enhanced axial computed tomographic views show several enlarged bilateral lymph nodes (*asterisk*) that remain homogeneous and nearly isodense to muscle, typical of lymphoma.

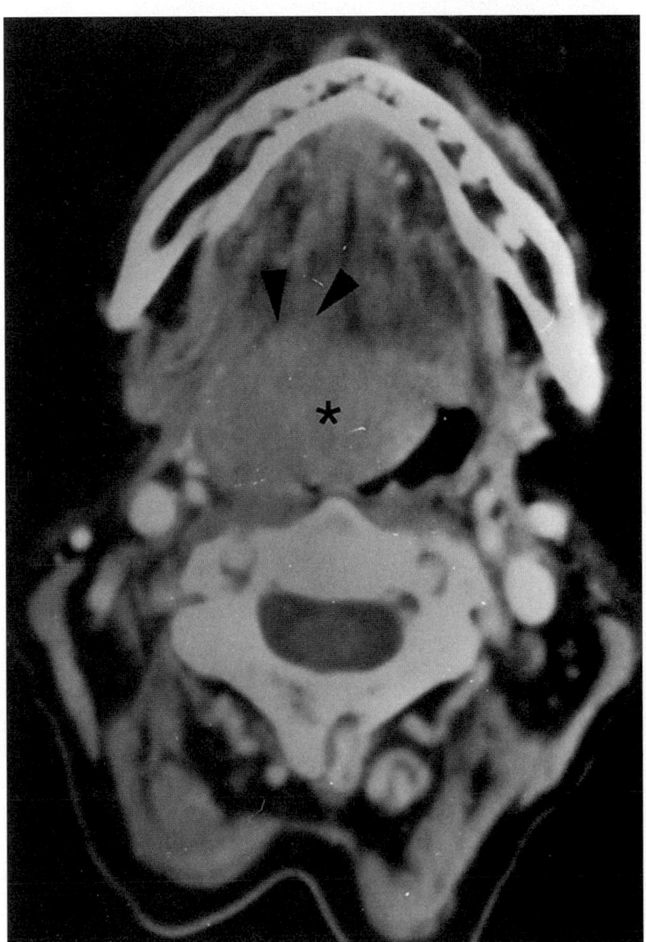

Figure 34.4 Huge tongue-base lymphoma. Enhanced axial computed tomographic view shows a large exophytic mass (*asterisk*) at the right tongue base with minimal infiltration of tongue substance (*arrowheads*).

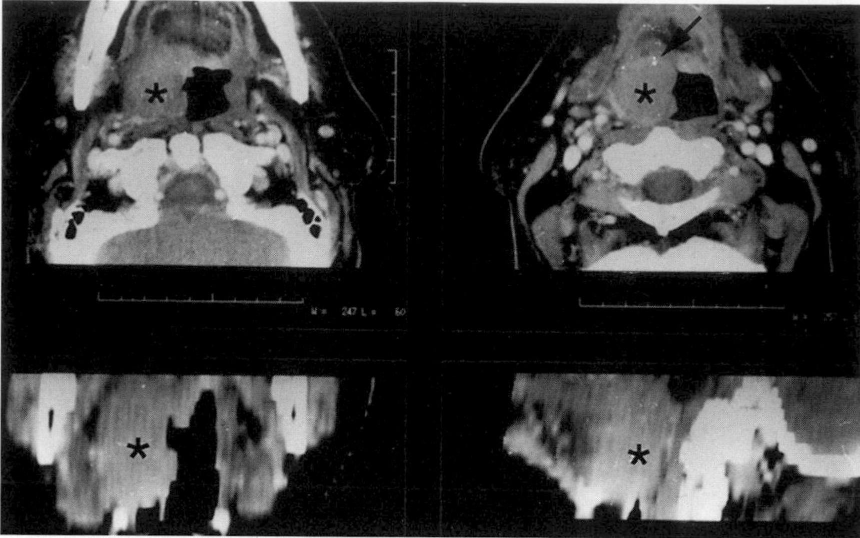

Figure 34.5 Moderate tonsillar lymphoma. Enhanced computed tomographic coronal (left) and parasagittal (right) views show a moderate-sized homogeneous mass (*asterisk*) at the base of the right tonsil involving the right tongue base (*arrow*).

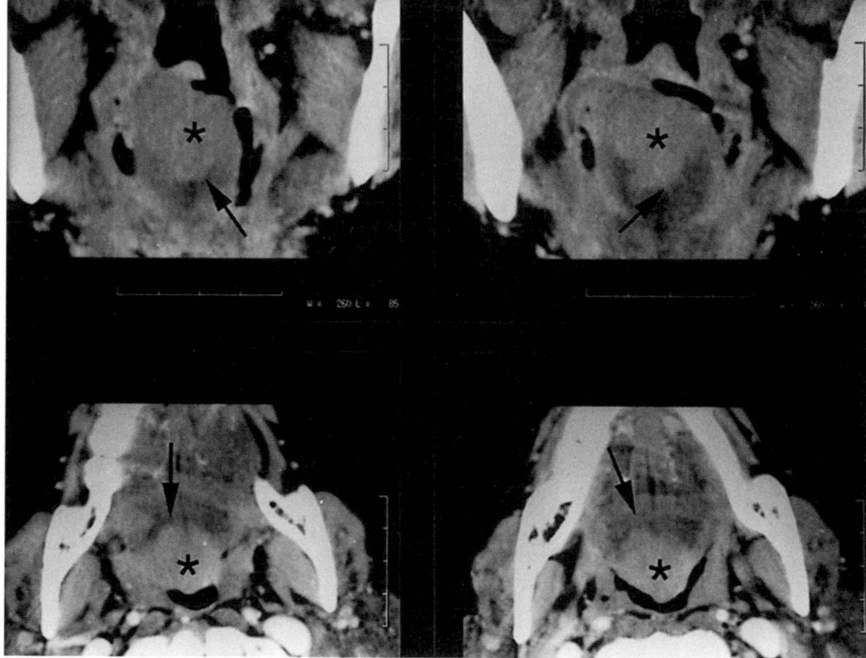

Figure 34.6 Localized tongue-base lymphoma. Enhanced direct coronal (top) and axial (bottom) computed tomographic views show homogeneous exophytic mass (*asterisk*) with minimal infiltration of tongue substance (*arrows*).

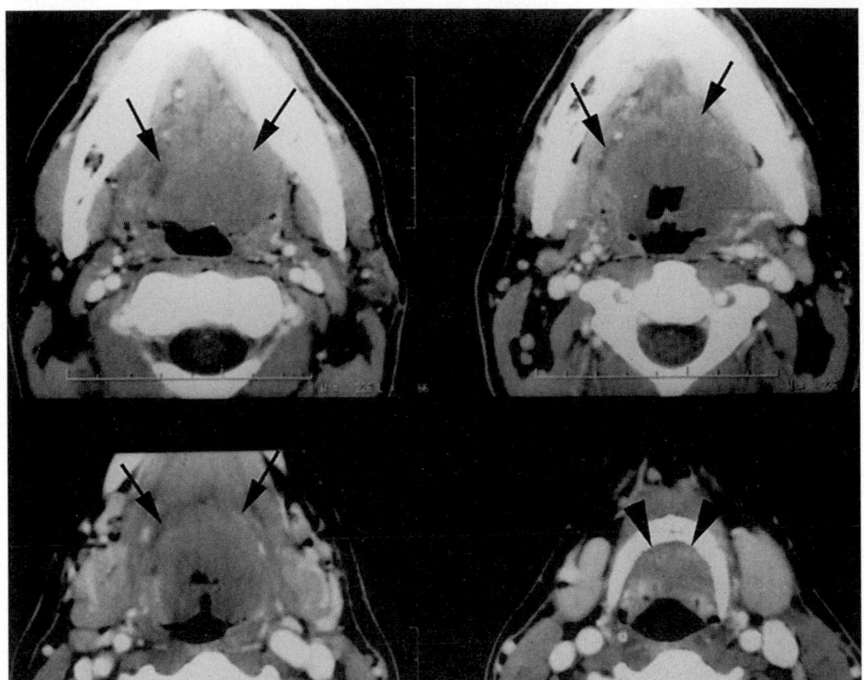

Figure 34.7 Huge tongue-base lymphoma. Enhanced axial computed tomographic views show extensive infiltrating mass involving the majority of the tongue (*arrows*) bulging into the vallecula (*arrowheads*).

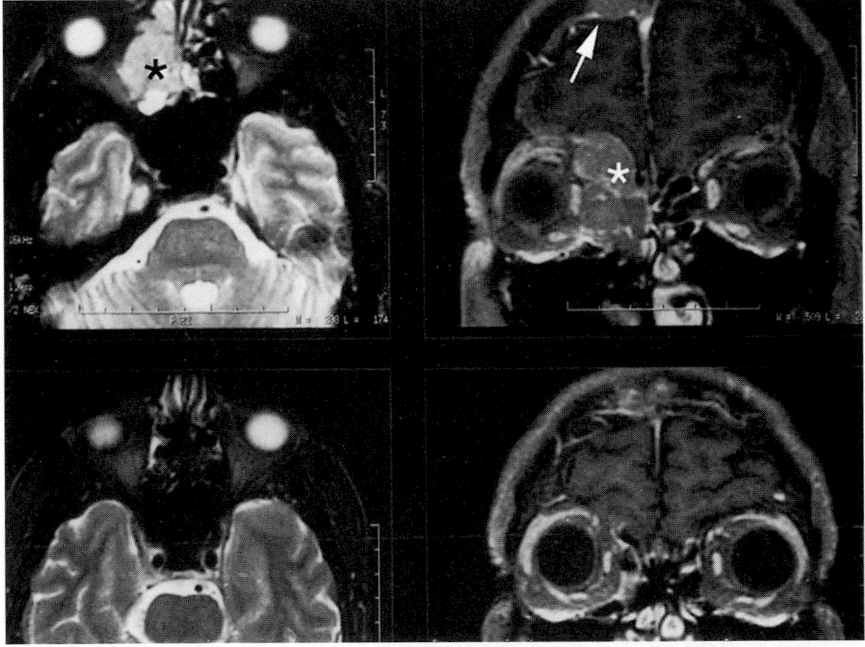

Figure 34.8 Paranasal lymphoma. Axial T2 (left) and contrast coronal T1 (right) views of the paranasal sinuses before (top) and after (bottom) treatment show typical treatment response of homogeneous, moderately enhancing masses at ethmoid sinus (*asterisk*) and frontal bone (*arrow*).

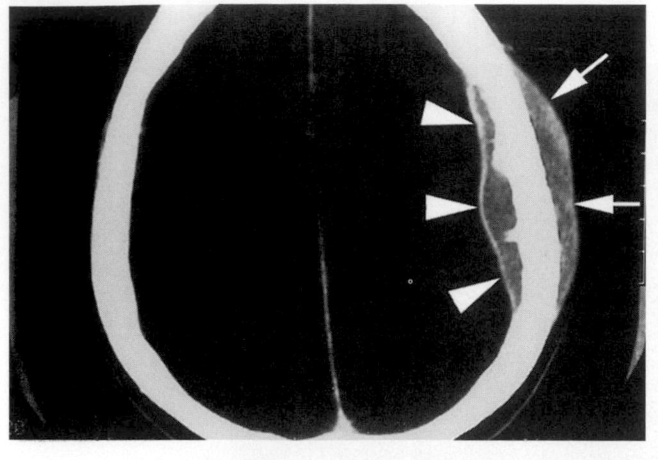

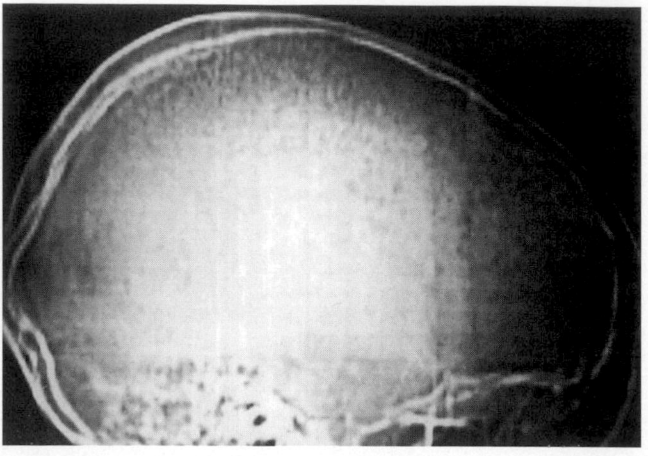

Figure 34.9 Lymphoma of calvarium. **A:** Enhanced axial head computed tomographic scan shows typical "transdiploic" mass with large intracranial (*arrowheads*) and extracranial (*arrows*) components straddling preserved-appearing calvarium. **B:** Corresponding radiographic scout image shows no lytic process.

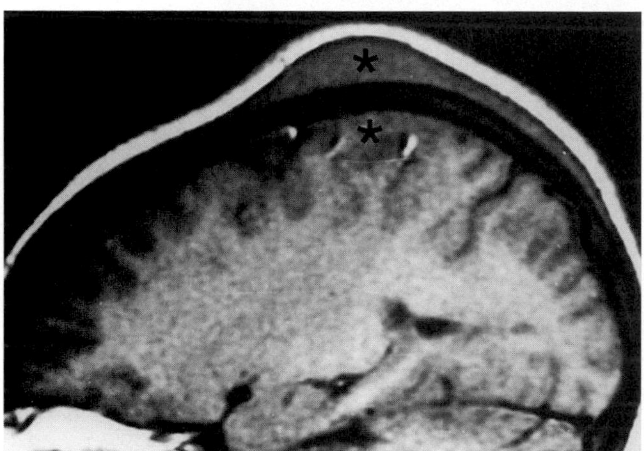

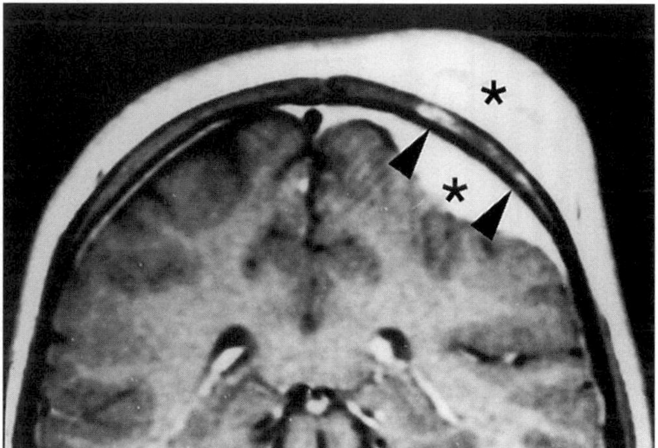

Figure 34.10 Chloroma of calvarium. Parasagittal T1 view **(A)** and coronal contrast T1 view **(B)** show homogeneous, intensely enhancing mass straddling the calvarium (*asterisk*) with intracranial and extracranial components and minimally enhancing abnormal marrow sign (*arrowheads*).

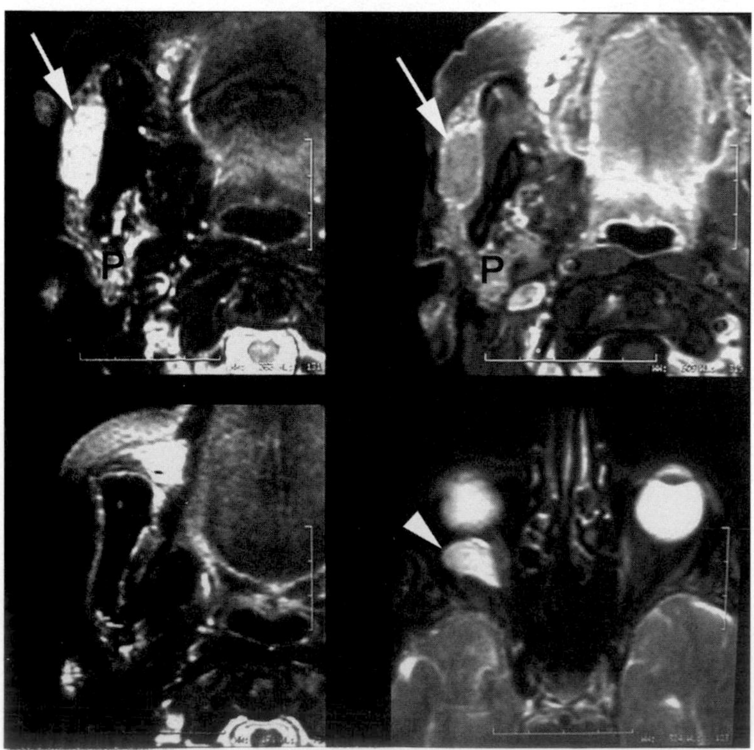

Figure 34.11 Salivary gland lymphoma. Magnetic resonance image collage from top left includes axial T2, axial contrast T1, axial T2, and contrast axial T1 showing homogeneous mass arising is the accessory parotid tissue along the Stensen duct (*arrow*). Additional component in the retrobulbar compartment of the orbit (*arrowhead*). *P,* parotid gland proper.

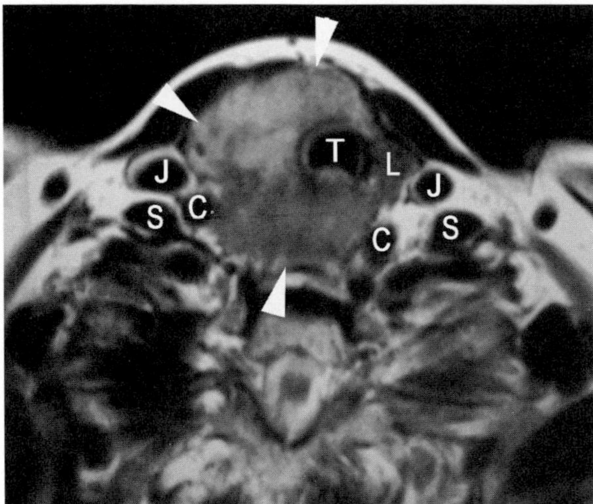

Figure 34.12 Thyroid lymphoma. Axial T2 magnetic resonance image of the thyroid bed shows displacement of the trachea (*T*) by a large mass filling the central compartment of the lower neck (*arrowheads*), spreading out the carotid arteries (*C*) and jugular veins (*J*). Note normal left thyroid lobe (*L*) and scalene muscles (*S*).

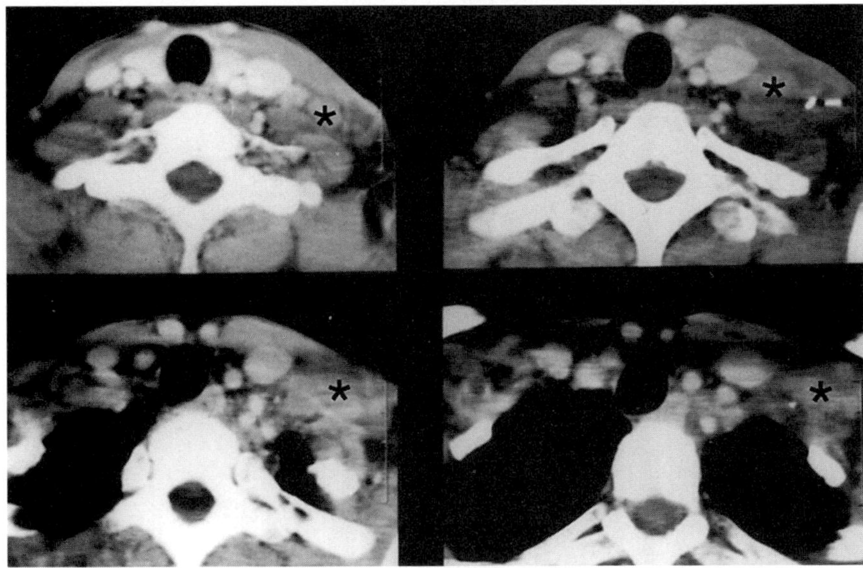

Figure 34.13 Supraclavicular adenopathy. Enhanced axial computed tomographic views show aggregate adenopathy limited to the left supraclavicular fossa (*asterisk*) and superior mediastinum status post-biopsy.

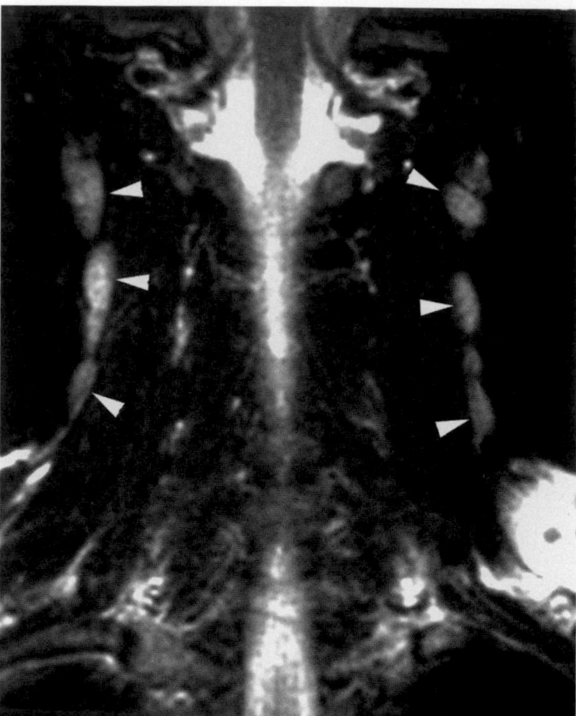

Figure 34.14 Follicular lymphoma. Coronal T2 magnetic resonance image shows several borderline-sized posterior cervical chain lymph nodes. Excisional biopsy showed follicular lymphoma.

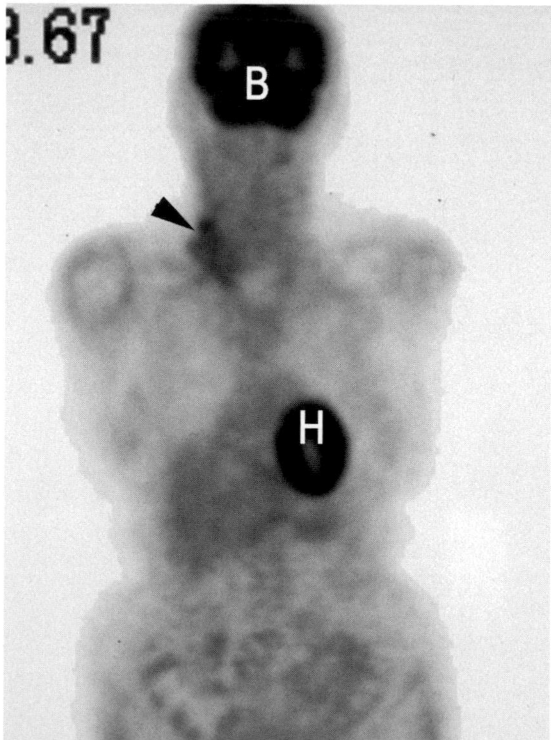

Figure 34.15 Hodgkin disease. Patient with right supraclavicular adenopathy (*arrowhead*) shows no disease outside of the right neck on fluorodeoxyglucose-positron emission tomography (FDG-PET) scan. Physiologic brain (*B*), heart (*H*), and gastrointestinal activity.

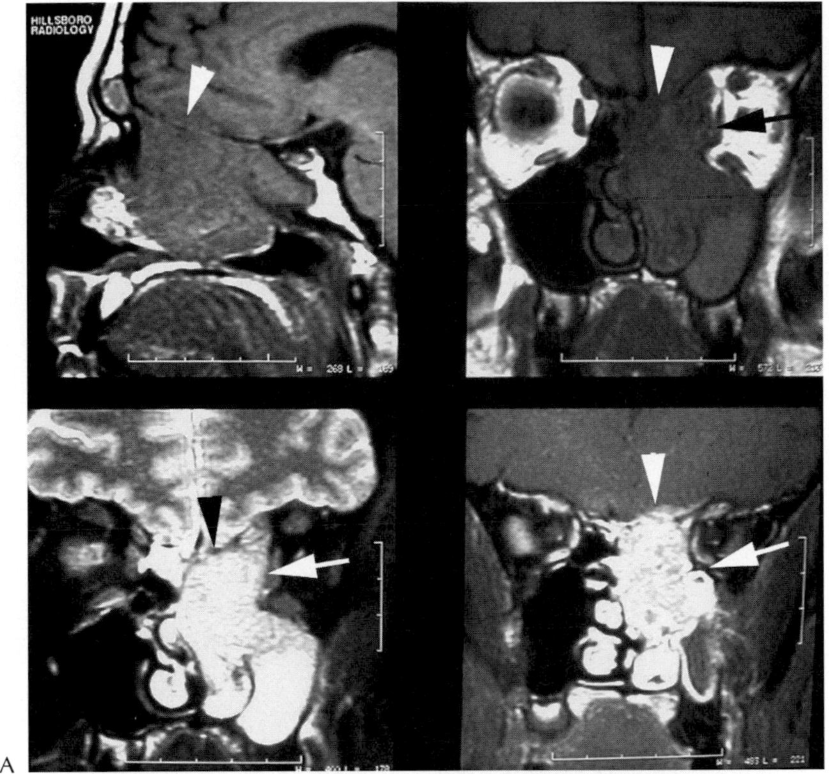

A

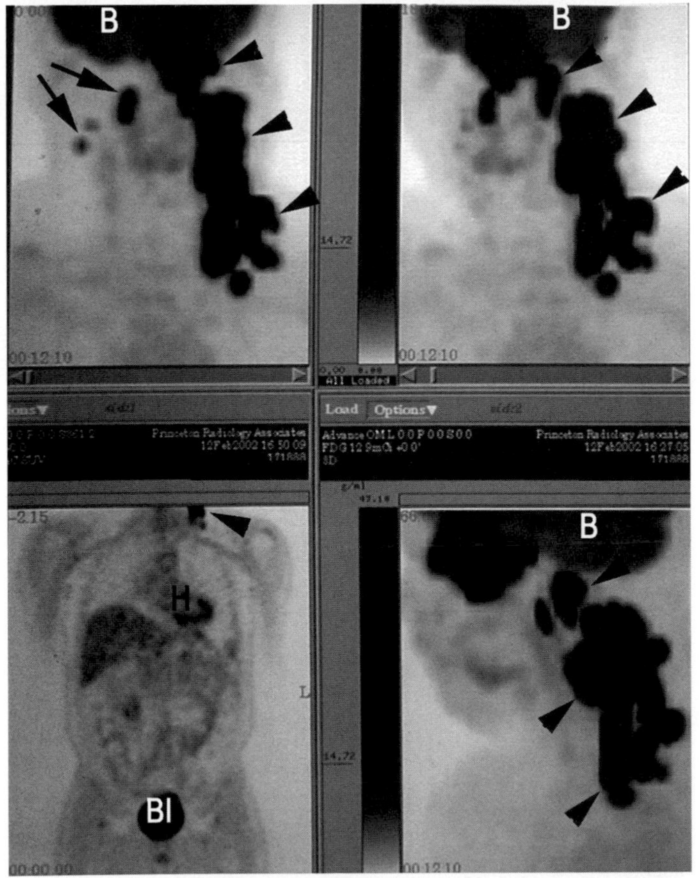

B

Figure 34.16 Sinus lymphoma. **A:** Magnetic resonance image collage from top left includes sagittal T1, coronal T1, contrast coronal T1, and coronal T2 showing a large sinonasal mass with penetration of the cribriform plate (*arrowheads*) and lamina papyracea (*arrows*). **B:** Baseline fluorodeoxyglucose-positron emission tomography (FDG-PET) scan from top left includes composite frontal, composite oblique, composite lateral, and whole body views of large central mass, right cervical (*arrows*), and left cervical (*arrowheads*) adenopathy. Physiologic activity in brain (*B*), heart (*H*), and bladder (*Bl*).

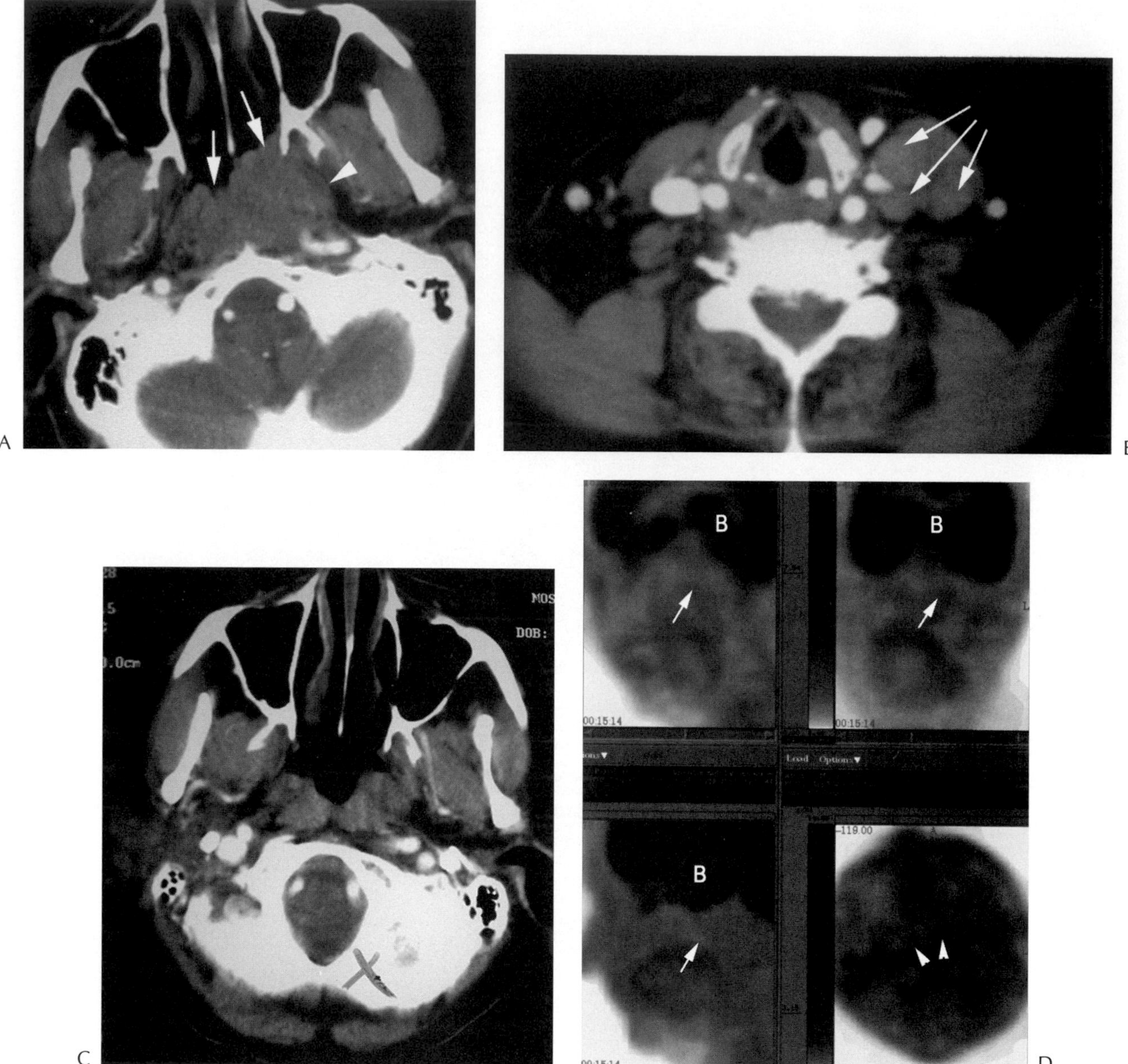

Figure 34.17 Burkitt lymphoma, positron emission tomography follow-up. **A:** Enhanced axial computed tomography (CT) scan of the nasopharynx shows a large mass (*arrows*) centered on the left. **B:** Left cervical adenopathy (*arrows*) indicative of Burkitt lymphoma. **C:** Posttreatment-enhanced axial CT scan shows resolved mass at the nasopharynx level. **D:** Fluorodeoxyglucose-positron emission tomography (FDG-PET) scan collage from top left includes sagittal, coronal, composite lateral, and axial views showing no hypermetabolic activity at primary site (*arrows*) or neck. Physiologic muscle activity (*arrowheads*).

REFERENCES

1. Harris NL, Jaffe ES, Stein H, et al. A revised European-American classification of lymphoid neoplasms: a proposal from the International Lymphoma Study Group. *Blood* 1994;84:1361.
2. Cobleigh MA, Kennedy JL. Non-Hodgkin's lymphoma of the upper aerodigestive tract and salivary glands. *Otolaryngol Clin North Am* 1986;19:685.
3. Braggi DG. Radiology of the lymphomas. *Curr Probl Diagn Radiol* 1987;16: 177.
4. Clark RM, Fitzpatrick PJ, Gospodarowicz MK. Extranodal malignant lymphomas in the head and neck. *J Otolaryngol* 1983;12:239.
5. Palackdharry CS. The epidemiology of non-Hodgkin's lymphoma: why the increased incidence? *Oncology* 1994;8:67.
6. Shipp MA, Harrington DP, Anderson JR, et al. A predictive model for aggressive NHL: the International Non-Hodgkin's Lymphoma Prognostic Factors Project. *N Engl J Med* 1993;329:987.
7. Rodriguez J, Cabanillas F, McLaughlin P, et al. A proposal for a simple staging system for intermediate grade lymphoma and immunoblastic lymphoma based on the "tumor score." *Ann Oncol* 1992;3:711.
8. Jacobs C, Weiss L, Hoppe RT. The management of extranodal head and neck lymphoma. *Arch Otolaryngol Head Neck Surg* 1986;112:654.
9. Economopoulos T, Asprou N, Stathakis N, et al. Primary extranodal non-Hodgkin's lymphoma of the head and neck. *Oncology* 1992;49:484.
10. A Clinical Evaluation of the International Lymphoma Study Group Classification of Non-Hodgkin's Lymphoma. The Non-Hodgkin's Lymphoma Classification Project. *Blood* 1997;89:3909.
11. Wong DS, Fuller LM, Butler JJ, et al. Extranodal non-Hodgkin's lymphoma of the head and neck. *AJR Am J Roentgenol* 1975;123:471–481.
12. Freeman C, Berg JW, Cutler S. Occurrence and prognosis of extranodal lymphoma. *Cancer 1972;29:252.*
13. Saul SH, Kapadia SB. Primary lymphoma of the Waldeyer's ring. Clinicopathological study of 68 cases. *Cancer* 1985;56:157.
14. Gleeson MJ, Bennett MH, Cawson LA. Lymphomas of the salivary gland. *Cancer* 1986;58:699.
15. Morton R, Sillars H, Benjamin CS. Incidence of "unsuspected" extranodal head and neck lymphoma. *Clin Otolaryngol* 1992;17:373.
16. Griffin TJ, Hurst PS, Swanson J. Non-Hodgkin's lymphoma: a case involving four third molar extraction sites. *Oral Surg Oral Med Oral Pathol* 1988;65:671.
17. Isaacson PG, Spencer J. Malignant lymphoma of mucosa-associated lymphoid tissue. *Histopathology* 1987;11:445–462.
18. Ikeda H, Inoue T, Teshima T, et al. Treatment of indolent non-Hodgkin's lymphoma localized in the head and neck. *Am J Clin Oncol* 1993;16:72.
19. Hayebuch N, Jingu K, Masaki N, et al. Analysis of non-Hodgkin's lymphomas of 210 patients with nodular and favourable histolytics: report of the Japanese lymphoma radiation therapy study group. *Jpn J Cancer Res* 1988;34: 589.
20. Morente M, Piris MA, Orradre TL, et al. Human tonsil intra-epithelial B cells: a marginal zone related subpopulation. *J Clin Pathol* 1992;45:668.
21. Makepeace AR, Fermont DL, Bennett MH. Non-Hodgkin's lymphoma of the tonsil: experience of therapy over a 27-year period. *J Laryngol Otol* 1989:101; 1151–1158.
22. Liang R, Chiu E, Todd D, et al. Combined chemotherapy and radiotherapy for lymphomas of Waldeyer's ring. *Oncology* 1991;48:36.
23. Siefert G, Gieler G. Zur pathologie der kindlichen kopfspeicheldursen. Beitrage zur pathologischen. *Anatomie Allgemeinen Pathologie* 1986;116: 1–38.
24. Schmid U, Helbran D, Lennert K. Primary malignant lymphoma localized in salivary gland. *Histopathology* 1982;6:673–687.
25. Katz J, Marmary Y, Cugarry G, et al. Primary lymphoma of the parotid gland: a report of 12 cases and a review of the literature. *Leukemia Lymphoma* 1991;5:133.
26. Kursan S, Thomas TL, Moutsopolous HM, et al. Increased risk of lymphoma in sicca syndrome. *Ann Intern Med* 1978;89:888.
27. Hvjeck E, Smith WJ, Isaacson PG. Primary B-cell lymphoma of salivary glands and its relationship to myoepithelial sialadenitis. *Hum Pathol* 1988;19: 766.
28. Sung Sik Shin, Sheibani K, Fishleder A, et al. Monocytoid B-cell lymphoma in patients with Sjögren's syndrome: a clinico-pathological study of 13 patients. *Hum Pathol* 1991;22:422.
29. Horny HP, Kaiserling E. Involvement of the larynx by hemopoietic neoplasms. An investigation of autopsy cases and review of the literature. *Pathol Res Pract* 1995;191:130.
30. De Pena CA, Van Tassel P, Lee YY. Lymphoma of the head and neck. *Radiol Clin North Am* 1990;28:723.
31. Pallesen O, Hamilton-Dutoit SJ, Zhou X. The association of Epstein-Barr virus (EBV) with T-cell lymphoproliferations and Hodgkin's disease: two new developments in the EBV field. *Adv Cancer Res* 1993;62:179.
32. Aviles A, Rodriguez L, Guzman R, et al. Angiocentric T-cell lymphoma of the nose, paranasal sinuses and hard palate. *Hematol Oncol* 1992;10:141.
33. Bergerson RT, Osborn AG, Sam PM. *Head and neck imaging excluding the brain.* St. Louis: Mosby, 1984:515.
34. Bruneton J-N, Kerboul P, Denis F. Lymphomas of the face and neck. In: Bruneton J-N, Schneider M, eds. *Radiology of lymphomas.* Berlin: Springer-Verlag, 1986:31.
35. Wultran KD, Speelman J, Pauwels SC, et al. Extranodal non-Hodgkin's lymphomas of the head and neck. *Radiother Oncol* 1987;8:199.
36. Raber M. Clinical applications of flow cytometry. *Oncology* 1994;8:67.
37. Ordonez NG. Application of immunocytochemistry in the diagnosis of poorly differentiated neoplasms and tumors of unknown origin. *Bull Cancer* 1989;41:142.
38. Sneige N, Dekmezian R, Katz R, et al. Morphologic and immunocytochemical evaluation of 220 fine needle aspirates of malignant lymphoma and lymphoid hyperplasia. *Acta Cytol* 1990;14[Suppl 3]:311.
39. MacKay B, Ordonez NG. Poorly differentiated neoplasms and tumors of unknown origin. In: Fer MF, Greco FA, Oldham RK, eds. *The role of the pathologist in the evaluation of poorly differentiated tumors and metastatic tumors of unknown origin.* Orlando, FL: Grune & Stratton, 1986:3–73.
40. Carbone P, Kaplan H, Musshoff K, et al. Report of the committee on Hodgkin's disease staging. *Cancer Res* 1971;31:1860.
41. Isaacson P. Low-grade B-cell lymphoma of MALT type in Waldeyer's ring. *Histopathology* 1994;24:1.
42. Shibuya H, Ryu-Ichi K, Wantabe I, et al. Stage I and II Waldeyer's ring, and oral-sinonasal non-Hodgkin's lymphoma. *Cancer* 1987;59:940.
43. Paryani SB, Hoppe RT, Cox RS, et al. Analysis of non-Hodgkin's lymphoma with nodular and favorable histologies, stages I and II. *Cancer* 1983;52:2300.
44. MacManus M, Hoppe R. Is radiotherapy curative for stage I and II low-grade lymphoma? Results of a long-term follow-up study of patients treated at Stanford University. *J Clin Oncol* 1996;14:1282.
45. Leibenhaut MH, Hoppe RT, Varaghese A, et al. Subdiaphragmatic Hodgkin's laparotomy and treatment results in 49 patients. *J Clin Oncol* 1987;5:1050.
46. Mauch P, Greenberg H, Lewin A, et al. Prognostic factors in patients with subdiaphragmatic Hodgkin's disease. *Hematol Oncol* 1983;1:205.
47. Mauch P, Tarbell H, Weinstein H, et al. Stage IA and IIA supradiaphragmatic Hodgkin's disease. Prognostic factors in surgically staged patients treated with mantle and paraaortic irradiation. *J Clin Oncol* 1988;6:1576.
48. Tubiana M, Henry Amar M, Burgers NV, et al. Prognostic significance of erythrocyte sedimentation rate in clinical stages I–II of Hodgkin's disease. *J Clin Oncol* 1984;3:194.
49. Walker A, Schoenfeld ER, Lowman JT, et al. Survival of the older patient compared with the younger patient with Hodgkin's disease. Influence of histologic type, staging, and treatment. *Cancer* 1990;65:1635.
50. Crnkovich MJ, Leopold K, Hoppe RT, et al. Stage I to IIB Hodgkin's disease: the combined experience at Stanford and the joint center for radiation therapy. *J Clin Oncol* 1987;5:1041.
51. Goffinett DR, Warnke R, Dunnick NR, et al. Clinical and surgical (laparotomy) evaluation of patients with non-Hodgkin's lymphoma. *Cancer Treat Res* 1977;61:981.
52. Gospodarowicz MK, Bush RS, Brown TC, et al. Prognostic factors in nodular lymphomas: a multivariate analysis based on the Princess Margaret Hospital experience. *Int J Radiat Oncol Biol Phys* 1984;10:489.
53. MacManus M, Hoppe RT. Is radiotherapy curative for stage I and II low-grade follicular lymphoma? Results of a long-term follow-up study of patients treated at Stanford University. *J Clin Oncol* 1996;14:1282.
54. Jacobs JP, Murray CJ, Wilson JF, et al. Central lymphatic irradiation for stage III nodular malignant lymphoma: long term results. *J Clin Oncol* 1993;11:233.
55. Monfardini S, Banfi A, Bonadonna G, et al. Improved 5 year survival after combined radiotherapy-chemotherapy for stage I–II non-Hodgkin's lymphoma. *Int J Radiat Oncol Biol Phys* 1980;6:125.
56. Seymour JF, McLaughlin P, Fuller LM, et al. High rate of prolonged remissions following combined modality therapy for patients with localized low-grade lymphoma. *Ann Oncol* 1996;7:157.
57. Carde P, Burgers JMV, Van Glabbeke M, et al. Combined radiotherapy-chemotherapy for early stages of non-Hodgkin's lymphoma: the 1975–1980 EORTC controlled lymphoma trial. *Radiother Oncol* 1984;2:301.
58. McLaughlin P, Grillo-Lopez A, Link B, et al. Rituximab chimeric anti-CD20 monoclonal antibody therapy for relapsed indolent lymphoma: half of patients respond to a four-dose treatment program. *J Clin Oncol* 1998;16: 2825–2833.
59. Frank C, Flentje M, Goldschmidt H, et al. Results of radiotherapy and combined modality treatment in early stage high grade non-Hodgkin's lymphoma. *Strahlenther Onkol* 1994;170:383.
60. Cabanillas F. Chemotherapy as definitive therapy of stage I–II large cell and diffuse mixed lymphomas. *Hematol Oncol* 1985;3:25.
61. Connors JM, Klimo P, Farley RN, et al. Brief chemotherapy and involved field radiation for limited stage histologically aggressive lymphoma. *Ann Intern Med* 1987;107:2530.
62. Shirato H, Tsujii H, Arimoto T, et al. Early stage head and neck non-Hodgkin's lymphoma: the effect of tumor burden on prognosis. *Cancer* 1986; 58:2312.
63. Miller TP, Dahlberg S, Cassady JR, et al. Chemotherapy alone compared with chemotherapy plus radiotherapy for localized intermediate- and high-grade non-Hodgkin's lymphoma. *N Engl J Med* 1998;339:21–26.
64. Jones SE, Miller TP, Connors JM. Long term follow-up and analysis for prognostic factors for patients with limited stage diffuse large cell lymphoma treated with initial chemotherapy with or without adjuvant radiation. *J Clin Oncol* 1989;7:1186.
65. Coiffier B, LePage E, Briere J, et al. CHOP chemotherapy plus rituximab compared with CHOP alone in elderly patients with diffuse large B-cell lymphoma. *N Engl J Med* 2002;346:235.
66. Tondini C, Zanini M, Lombardi F, et al. Combined modality treatment with primary CHOP chemotherapy followed by locoregional irradiation in stage I or II histologically aggressive non-Hodgkin's lymphomas. *J Clin Oncol* 1993;11:720–725.

67. Longo DL, Glastein E, Duffey PL, et al. Treatment of localized aggressive lymphomas with aggressive chemotherapy followed by involved field radiation therapy. *J Clin Oncol* 1989;7[Suppl 9]:1295.
68. Shimrn DS, Dosoretz DZ, Harris NL, et al. Radiation therapy of Waldeyer's ring lymphoma. *Cancer* 1984;54:426.
69. Sofferman RA, Cummings CW. Malignant lymphoma of the paranasal sinuses. *Arch Otolaryngol Head Neck Surg* 1975;101:287.
70. Jaffe ES, Chan JKC, Ho FCS, et al. Report on the workshop on nasal and related extranodal angiocentric T/natural killer cell lymphomas: definitions, differential diagnosis and epidemiology. *Am J Surg Pathol* 1996;20:103.
71. Ho FCS, Choy D, Loke SL, et al. Polymorphic reticulosis and conventional lymphomas of the nose and upper aerodigestive tract. *Hum Pathol* 1990;21: 1041.
72. Lipford E, Margolick J, Longo D, et al. Angiocentric immunoproliferative lesions: a clinicopathologic spectrum of post-thymic t-cell proliferations. *Blood* 1988;72:1674.
73. Gospodarowicz MK, Sutcliffe SB, Bergsagel DE, et al. Radiation therapy in clinical stage I and II Hodgkin's disease. *Eur J Cancer* 1992;28:1841.
74. Russel K, Hoppe R, Colby T, et al. Lymphocyte predominant Hodgkin's disease: clinical presentation and results of treatment. *Radiother Oncol* 1984;1: 197.
76. Koziner B, Myers J, Cirrincione C, et al. Treatment of stages I and II Hodgkin's disease with three different therapeutic modalities. *Am J Med* 1986;80:1067.
77. Tubiana M, Henry-Amar M, Hayat M, et al. The EORTC treatment of early stages of Hodgkin's disease: the role of radiotherapy. *Int J Radiat Oncol Biol Phys* 1984;10:197.
78. Longo D, Glastein E, Duffey P, et al. Radiation therapy versus combination chemotherapy in the treatment of early-stage Hodgkin's disease: seven-year results of a prospective randomized trial. *J Clin Oncol* 1991;6:906.
79. Burkitt DP. A sarcoma involving the jaws in African children. *Br J Surg* 1958;46:218.
80. Levine PH, Cho BR. Burkitt's lymphoma: clinical features of North American cases. *Cancer Res* 1974;34:1219–1221.
81. Burkitt DP. General features and facial tumors. In: Burkitt DP, Wright DH, eds. *Burkitt's lymphoma.* Edinburgh: Churchill Livingstone, 1970:7.
82. Magrath I, Adde M, Shad A, et al. Adults and children with small non-cleaved-cell lymphoma have a similar excellent outcome when treated with the same chemotherapy regimen. *J Clin Oncol* 1996;14:925.
83. Rabkin CS, Hilgartner MW, Hedberg KW, et al. Incidence of lymphomas and other cancers in HIV-infected and HIV-uninfected patients with hemophilia. *JAMA* 1992;267:1090.
84. Pluda J, Venzon D, Tosato G, et al. Parameters affecting the development of non-Hodgkin's lymphoma in patients with severe human immune-deficiency virus infection: review of antiretroviral therapy. *J Clin Oncol* 1993;11: 1099.
85. Kaplan LD, Abrams DI, Feigal E, et al. AIDS associated non-Hodgkin's lymphoma in San Francisco. *JAMA* 1989;216:719.
86. Knowles DM, Chamulak GA, Subar M, et al. Lymphoid neoplasia associated with the acquired immunodeficiency syndrome (AIDS): the New York University experience. *Ann Intern Med* 1988;108:744.
87. Helsper J, Formenti S, Levine A. Initial manifestation of acquired immune deficiency syndrome in the head and neck. *Am J Surg* 1986;152:403.
88. Lamb R, Gonzalez R, Myers A, et al. Aggressive non-Hodgkin's lymphoma in AIDS: the University of Colorado experience. *Am J Med Sci* 1990;300:345.
89. Shapiro A, Shechtman F, Guida R, et al. Head and neck lymphoma in patients with the acquired immune deficiency syndrome. *Otolaryngol Head Neck Surg* 1992;106:258.
90. Oksenhendler E, Lida H, D'Agag RF, et al. Tumoral nasopharyngeal hyperplasia in human immune deficiency virus infected patients. *Arch Intern Med* 1989;149:2359.
91. Shahab I, Osborne B, Butler J. Nasopharyngeal lymphoid tissue masses in patients with human immunodeficiency virus-1: histologic findings and clinical correlation. *Cancer* 1994;74:3083.
92. Karp J, Broder S. Acquired immunodeficiency syndrome and non-Hodgkin's lymphoma. *Cancer Res* 1991;51:4743.
93. Abemayor E, Canalis RF, Greenberg P, et al. Plasma cell tumors of the head and neck. *J Otolaryngol* 1988;17:376.
94. Wax M, Yun J, Omar R. Extramedullary plasmacytoma of the head and neck. *Otolaryngol Head Neck Surg* 1993;109:977.
95. Loh HS. A retrospective evaluation of 23 reported cases of solitary plasmacytoma of the mandible with an additional case report. *Br J Oral Maxillofac Surg* 1984;22:216.

Radiologic Imaging Concerns

96. Abrahamsen AF, Lien HH, Aas M, et al. Magnetic resonance imaging and 67-gallium scan in mediastinal malignant lymphoma: a prospective pilot study. *Ann Oncol* 1994;5:433–436.
97. Hanna E, Wanamaker J, Adelstein D, et al. Extranodal lymphomas of the head and neck. A 20-year experience. *Arch Otolaryngol Head Neck Surg* 1997; 123:1318–1323.
98. Wang MB, Strasnick B, Zimmerman MC. Extranodal American Burkitt's lymphoma of the head and neck. *Arch Otolaryngol Head Neck Surg* 1992;118: 193–199.
99. Chisin R, Weber AL. Imaging of lymphoma manifestations in the extracranial head and neck region [Review] [54 refs]. *Leukemia & Lymphoma* 1994;12: 177–189.
100. Eisenkraft BL, Som PM. The spectrum of benign and malignant etiologies of cervical node calcification. *AJR Am J Roentgenol* 1999;172:1433–1437.
101. Hermans R, Horvath M, De Schrijver T, et al. Extranodal non-Hodgkin lymphoma of the head and neck. *J Belge de Radiol* 1994;77:72–77.
102. Bhattacharyya N, Frankenthaler RA, Gomolin HI, et al. Clinical and pathologic characterization of mucosa-associated lymphoid tissue lymphoma of the head and neck. *Ann Otol Rhinol Laryngol* 1998;107:801–806.
103. Garcia CE, Girdhar-Gopal HV, Dorfman DM. Kikuchi-Fujimoto disease of the neck. Update. *Ann Otol Rhinol Laryngol* 1993;102:11–15.
104. Wittram C, Nixon TE, Mackenzie JM. Non-Hodgkin's lymphoma of the skull vault. *Eur J Radiol* 1994;19:7–9.
105. McGuirt WF. The neck mass. *Med Clin North Am* 1999;83:219–234.
106. Hoane BR, Shields AF, Porter BA, et al. Comparison of initial lymphoma staging using computed tomography (CT) and magnetic resonance (MR) imaging. *Am J Hematol* 1994;47:100–105.
107. Hill M, Cunningham D, MacVicar D, et al. Role of magnetic resonance imaging in predicting relapse in residual masses after treatment of lymphoma. *J Clin Oncol* 1993;11:2273–2278.
108. Jerusalem G, Beguin Y, Fassotte MF, et al. Whole-body positron emission tomography using 18F-fluorodeoxyglucose for posttreatment evaluation in Hodgkin's disease and non-Hodgkin's lymphoma has higher diagnostic and prognostic value than classical computed tomography scan imaging. *Blood* 1999;94:429–433.
109. Jerusalem G, Beguin Y, Fassotte MF, et al. Persistent tumor 18F-FDG uptake after a few cycles of polychemotherapy is predictive of treatment failure in non-Hodgkin's lymphoma. *Haematologica* 2000;85:613–618.

CHAPTER 35

Systemic Therapy for Recurrent and Metastatic Diseases

Charles Lu and Merrill S. Kies

Although approximately one third of patients with squamous cell carcinoma of the head and neck (SCCHN) present with early stage, highly curable disease, the majority manifest locally advanced disease (T3 or T4, N1–3, M0), characterized by disappointingly low long-term survival rates typically ranging from 20% to 40% (1,2). Despite aggressive surgery, radiation, or combined modality approaches, approximately 50% of patients will develop incurable locoregional or distant disease recurrence (3). In this setting, chemotherapy is an accepted treatment option. For these individuals, however, therapeutic goals remain modest. Clinical responses generally are observed in a minority, and median survival times remain approximately 6 months (4). Randomized trials have yet to demonstrate a clear survival benefit for chemotherapy in recurrent or metastatic SCCHN. Although some researchers have reported that chemotherapy appears to improve disease-related symptoms in this patient population (5), it remains clear that quality of life issues are of paramount importance and require further attention (6).

SINGLE AGENT CHEMOTHERAPY

A number of commonly used single agents have documented activity in recurrent or metastatic SCCHN. Initial clinical studies included traditional cytotoxic drugs such as methotrexate, cisplatin, carboplatin, bleomycin, and 5-fluorouracil (5-FU). Subsequent trials have focused on taxanes (paclitaxel and docetaxel) and other agents such as ifosfamide, and these studies have demonstrated that taxanes possess significant activity in SCCHN. More recent clinical studies should provide information regarding the activity of newer drugs, including topoisomerase I inhibitors, gemcitabine, and vinorelbine.

Methotrexate

Since the initial reports in the 1960s of methotrexate for the treatment of SCCHN, the use of this antimetabolite has become an accepted standard palliative therapy. Although pooled analysis of earlier trials demonstrated a single-agent response rate of 31% (7), subsequent randomized trials yielded response rates ranging from 8% to 16% (4,8–11). The standard weekly administration of 40 mg/m^2 methotrexate is generally well tolerated with relatively low rates of myelosuppression, stomatitis, and skin toxicity. Although some initial studies demonstrated increased response rates with higher doses of methotrexate with leucovorin rescue (12–14), subsequent randomized studies failed to demonstrate an improvement in overall survival compared with standard-dose weekly therapy (15–17). Browman et al. conducted a placebo-controlled randomized study comparing weekly methotrexate with or without leucovorin rescue in patients with recurrent SCCHN (18). Patients who received leucovorin demonstrated significantly lower rates of response and toxicity, suggesting that leucovorin negatively influenced the methotrexate antitumor effect.

Other Antifolates

Other antifolate analogs of methotrexate have been studied in recurrent or metastatic SCCHN, including trimetrexate, edatrexate, and piritrexim. Phase II studies have reported response rates of 26% and 27% for trimetrexate (19) and piritrexim (20), respectively. The European Organization for Research and Treatment of Cancer (EORTC) conducted a randomized trial comparing single-agent weekly edatrexate versus methotrexate in 273 patients. Similar response rates were observed for edatrexate and methotrexate (21% and 16%, respectively; $p < 0.39$), although stomatitis and skin toxicity were more pronounced with edatrexate therapy (11). The rationally designed thymidylate synthase inhibitor, nolatrexed (21), was recently compared against methotrexate in two randomized trials (22). Nolatrexed and methotrexate demonstrated similar response rates, with the former agent having more toxicity. Multitargeted antifolate (MTA) is a novel antifolate that inhibits multiple enzymes involved in purine and thymidine biosynthesis (23), and multiple phase II studies have demonstrated antitumor activity in a wide range of cancers (24). A recent phase II trial in recurrent or metastatic SCCHN reported an encouraging 33% response rate to single-agent MTA (25).

Cisplatin

Cisplatin remains one of the most widely used standard agents in recurrent or metastatic SCCHN, with an average single-agent response rate of 28% (7). Most single-agent studies have employed doses of 80 to 120 mg/m^2 administered as an intravenous bolus every 3 to 4 weeks (26). A small randomized trial compared cisplatin given as a single bolus of 120 mg/m^2 versus 20 mg/m^2/d for 5 days, with cycles repeated every 3 weeks (27). In this study activity was comparable between the two arms, and a single bolus schedule appeared more suitable for outpatient therapy. Forastiere et al. investigated the pharmacokinetic and toxicity profiles of cisplatin (total dose 150 mg/m^2) given as a 5-day continuous infusion versus an intermittent bolus (28). Exposure to drug, determined by the area under the concentration–time curve, was 1.5- to 2-fold higher with continuous infusion administration. Although myelosuppression and hypomagnesemia were increased with the continuous infusion, toxicity was judged to be clinically acceptable.

For doses that have been investigated, cisplatin does not appear to exhibit a clinically meaningful dose–response relationship in SCCHN. Several groups have examined cisplatin at total doses of 200 mg/m^2 given over 4 to 5 days. In one study 6 of 14 (46%) patients responded, with 2 responders having been previously treated with standard doses of cisplatin (29). In the other study, 11 of 16 (69%) patients with recurrent SCCHN responded, but dose-limiting neuropathy and ototoxicity led the authors not to recommend the regimen for palliation of recurrent disease (30). Veronesi et al. conducted a small, randomized trial comparing 120 mg/m^2 versus 60 mg/m^2 of cisplatin administered as a bolus (31). Response rates were similar (16.1% and 17.8% in the high- and low-dose arms, respectively) with identical median survivals (34 weeks). Several groups have compared single-agent cisplatin and methotrexate in randomized studies (9,32,33). Two of these trials demonstrated similar response rates and median survivals, suggesting comparable antitumor activity of these agents (32,33). One study, however, reported significantly longer survival in the cisplatin arm (9). Morton et al. conducted a small randomized trial of cisplatin and bleomycin using a 2×2 factorial design that included a no-chemotherapy control arm (34). In this study, cisplatin therapy significantly prolonged median survival by 10 weeks.

Cisplatin Analogs

Carboplatin is a second-generation platinum analog with an improved toxicity profile and similar spectrum of activity against a number of solid tumors compared with cisplatin (35). Single-agent phase II studies have yielded response rates of 20% to 26% in recurrent or metastatic SCCHN (36–39), suggesting antitumor activity similar to cisplatin. Although a trial directly comparing these two platinum agents has not been conducted, a Southwest Oncology Group (SWOG) study did randomize 277 patients to receive either cisplatin plus 5-FU, carboplatin plus 5-FU, or single-agent methotrexate (10). Although a formal statistical comparison of the cisplatin and carboplatin arms was not performed, subjects who received cisplatin had higher response rates compared with those who received carboplatin (32% vs. 21%). Median survival times were similar for all treatment groups. Notably, the incidence of both hematologic and nonhematologic toxicity was highest in the cisplatin plus 5-FU arm, suggesting that platinum dose-intensity may not have been equivalent. The combination of cisplatin and carboplatin has been investigated in phase II trials (40,41). Although this combination was feasible with response rates ranging from 24% to 38%, there did not appear to be a therapeutic advantage to this approach. Several other second-generation platinum compounds have been investigated, but the results of these studies have been disappointing. Phase II trials of iproplatin (38,42) and lobaplatin (43) report response rates of 0% to 12% and 7%, respectively, suggesting marginal antitumor activity.

5-Fluorouracil

As a single agent, 5-FU has limited activity in recurrent or metastatic SCCHN. Several small studies suggested that 5-FU antitumor activity may be improved with a prolonged continuous infusion schedule (44,45), although a large randomized study comparing single-agent infusional 5-FU, single-agent cisplatin, and the combination of these two agents yielded a 13% response rate in the infusional 5-FU alone arm (46). Biochemical modulation of 5-FU has been studied extensively in SCCHN. Initial preclinical data demonstrated that 5-FU, when preceded by methotrexate, resulted in synergistic antitumor activity in mice (47). Several small, randomized clinical trials subsequently examined the effects of altering the timing and sequence of administration of methotrexate and 5-FU (48–50). Although one trial demonstrated a trend toward a higher response rate with methotrexate administered prior to 5-FU (48), there were no significant differences in response rates or survival among the various regimens. A recent National Cancer Institute of Canada phase II trial examined oral therapy with the dihydropyrimidine dehydrogenase (DPD) inhibitor eniluracil and 5-FU in recurrent or metastatic SCCHN (51). Dihydropyrimidine dehydrogenase is involved in the degradation of 5-FU, and inhibition of this enzyme allows increased absorption of oral 5-FU and less interpatient variability in blood levels (52). In this study eniluracil and 5-FU produced a 15.6% response rate with a manageable toxicity, leading the investigators to recommend further development of this novel oral combination.

Bleomycin

Bleomycin is an antibiotic cytotoxic agent (53) with modest single-agent activity in SCCHN (54–56). A pooled response rate of 21% has been reported (7,57,58). Bleomycin results in mild myelosuppression with dose-limiting pulmonary toxicities manifested by pneumonitis and pulmonary fibrosis (59). Although continuous infusion administration may ameliorate the severity of pulmonary adverse effects (60,61), many investigators have opted to focus their attention on chemotherapeutic agents with more favorable toxicity profiles.

Ifosfamide

Ifosfamide, a cyclophosphamide analog, is an alkylating agent with significant antitumor activity against soft tissue sarcomas and testicular carcinomas (62). Hemorrhagic cystitis is a dose-limiting toxicity, which can be effectively prevented with uroprotectants such as mesna. A number of phase II studies in SCCHN have demonstrated activity comparable to those of other active single agents in recurrent or metastatic disease (63–68), with an average response rate of 26% (7). Several trials demonstrated minimal activity (63,65), and these results were likely attributable to the fact that these patients had received prior chemotherapy.

Paclitaxel

Paclitaxel is a diterpene plant-derived product that exerts cytotoxic effects by promoting microtubule assembly, which ultimately leads to disruption of mitosis and cell death (69). Significant single-agent activity in patients with advanced SCCHN has been demonstrated in phase II trials with encouraging response rates ranging from 20% to 40% (70–72). In the largest trial, Forastiere et al. treated 30 patients with paclitaxel 250 mg/m^2 IV over 24 hours, in addition to filgrastim support. A response rate of 40% and median survival of 9.2 months were reported, in addition to severe or life-threatening granulocytopenia in 91% of patients (72). A subsequent European randomized phase II trial compared weekly methotrexate versus paclitaxel (175 mg/m^2) administered as either a 3- or 24-hour infusion without growth factor support (73). Response rates for the methotrexate, paclitaxel 3-hour infusion, and paclitaxel 24-hour infusion arms were 9.5%, 12.5%, and 19.5%, respectively. The differences in response rates were not statistically significant, and the trial was closed due to low activity of the methotrexate and 3-hour paclitaxel infusion arms and a high rate of serious toxic events in the 24-hour paclitaxel infusion arm.

The Eastern Cooperative Oncology Group (ECOG) investigated the dose-response effects of paclitaxel combined with cisplatin in recurrent or metastatic SCCHN. Two hundred and ten patients were randomized to receive cisplatin (75 mg/m^2) with either paclitaxel 135 mg/m^2 or paclitaxel 200 mg/m^2 repeated every 3 weeks (74). Paclitaxel was administered as a 24-hour infusion, and patients received filgrastim support in the high-dose paclitaxel arm. No significant differences in outcomes were observed between the two arms. Overall response rates, median survival times, and 1-year survival rates for the high- and low-dose arms were 35% and 36%, 7.6 and 6.8 months, and 28.6% and 29.4%, respectively. Of note, hematologic toxicity was substantial in both arms, with grade 3 or 4 granulocytopenia and febrile neutropenia occurring in 70% and 78% of patients and in 27% and 39% of patients in the high- and low-dose arms, respectively. Neither of the paclitaxel regimens was recommended for further study, and ECOG decided to use paclitaxel 175 mg/m^2 (3-hour infusion) and cisplatin 75 mg/m^2 as the experimental arm for a subsequent randomized study (75).

Docetaxel

Docetaxel is a semisynthetic taxane analog that also possesses significant activity in SCCHN (76). Preclinical studies demonstrated antitumor activity in xenograft mouse models and an apparent lack of cross-resistance with cisplatin (77,78). Several single-agent phase II trials in chemotherapy-naive patients with recurrent or metastatic SCCHN revealed response rates of 21% to 42% (79–82). A European Organization for Research and Treatment of Cancer (EORTC) trial treated 43 patients with advanced or recurrent SCCHN with docetaxel 100 mg/m^2 every 3 weeks. Among 37 evaluable patients there were 12 responders, for an overall response rate of 32%. Frequent side effects included alopecia (90%), asthenia (69%), and brief grade 3 or 4 neutropenia (61% of courses). Patients did not receive premedication to prevent hypersensitivity reactions in this trial. Skin toxicity, hypersensitivity reactions, and peripheral edema occurred in 54%, 23%, and 31% of patients, respectively. Inuyama et al. employed a lower dose of docetaxel (60 mg/m^2 every 3–4 weeks) (82). A response rate of 22% was observed among 59 evaluable patients. Among 46 patients who received prior chemotherapy the response rate was 17.4%. Major hematologic toxicities included grade 3 or 4 leukopenia and neutropenia in 60% and 79% of patients, respectively. The frequency of severe nonhematologic adverse events was relatively low.

Vinorelbine

Vinorelbine is a semisynthetic vinca alkaloid whose antitumor activity is related to its ability to depolymerize microtubules and disrupt the mitotic spindle apparatus (83). Vinorelbine differs structurally from the other vinca alkaloids by substitutions on the catharinthine ring rather than on the vindoline, and its higher affinity for mitotic tubules than for axonal microtubules probably accounts for its different efficacy and toxicity profile (84). Preclinical studies have demonstrated the antitumor activity of vinorelbine against a number of human tumor cell lines, including leukemias, non-small cell lung cancer, small cell lung cancer, breast cancer, melanoma, colon cancer, and central nervous system tumors (85). Several investigators have examined vinorelbine's single-agent activity in SCCHN. Degardin et al. treated 71 patients with weekly vinorelbine at a dose of 30 mg/m^2/week (86). Two complete and seven partial responses were observed among 56 evaluable patients, for a response rate of 16%. Based on these results, further study of vinorelbine in combination with other agents was recommended. Saxman et al. conducted a phase II trial with the same weekly dose of vinorelbine (87). These investigators, however, observed a disappointingly low response rate of 7.5% in a group of 40 patients and concluded that vinorelbine had minimal activity in this setting. Another phase II study reported one response among 15 heavily pretreated patients, suggesting limited antitumor activity (88).

Gemcitabine

Gemcitabine (difluorodeoxycytidine) is a pyrimidine analog that was initially synthesized as a potential antiviral drug (89). Activation by deoxycytidine kinase eventually results in gemcitabine triphosphate, which is incorporated into DNA, resulting in chain termination (90). Gemcitabine diphosphate also inhibits ribonucleotide reductase, thereby diminishing intracellular deoxycytidine triphosphate (dCTP) and enhancing the incorporation of gemcitabine triphosphate into DNA. Gemcitabine is active against a variety of solid tumors *in vitro* and several human tumor xenografts, including SCCHN cell lines (91,92). Catimel et al. documented at least a modest degree of activity in a single-agent phase II study of weekly gemcitabine (800–1,250 mg/m^2 weekly ×3 weeks, repeated every 4 weeks) (93). Seven partial responses were observed among 54 evaluable subjects, yielding a 13% response rate.

Topoisomerase I Inhibitors

Topoisomerase I inhibitors are analogs of camptothecin, a natural alkaloid with antitumor activity extracted from the *Camptotheca acuminata* tree (94). The mechanism of action of these compounds is mediated by interactions with the topoisomerase

I enzyme, a nuclear protein necessary for normal DNA replication and transcription (95). Topoisomerase I binds to DNA to form a complex that induces single-strand DNA breaks that are essential for DNA relaxation with subsequent religation (96). Camptothecin analogs stabilize the topoisomerase I–DNA complex, resulting in single-strand breaks and inhibition of normal DNA religation. This process leads to nuclease-mediated damage of the exposed uncoiled DNA with eventual cell death (97). Topotecan, 9-aminocamptothecin, and irinotecan represent three topoisomerase I inhibitors that have been evaluated for the treatment of recurrent or metastatic SCCHN. Although the activities of topotecan and 9-aminocamptothecin appear limited, irinotecan has demonstrated more encouraging results (98).

Three phase II trials examining single-agent topotecan in recurrent or metastatic SCCHN have recently been published (99–101). Two studies administered topotecan at a dose of 1.5 mg/m^2 daily for 5 days every 3 weeks (99,100). Response rates were 13.6% and 0%. An ECOG trial employed a 1.5 mg/m^2 24-hour continuous infusion repeated weekly for 4 weeks, with cycles repeated every 5 weeks (101). In this study no responses were observed among 32 subjects. Lad et al. report no responses among 14 patients enrolled on a phase II trial of 9-aminocamptothecin delivered as a 72-hour continuous infusion every 2 weeks (102). Murphy et al. recently examined the activity of irinotecan given on a weekly basis. The initial schedule of 125 mg/m^2 repeated weekly for 4 weeks followed by a 2-week rest was too toxic, and the dose was decreased to 75 mg/m^2 weekly for 2 weeks followed by a 1-week rest (98). Modest response rates were seen for the higher and lower dose cohorts (26% and 14%, respectively), leading the investigators to design a subsequent phase II study of irinotecan combined with cisplatin.

COMBINATION CHEMOTHERAPY

Initial Studies

Numerous trials have been conducted in patients with recurrent or metastatic SCCHN examining various combinations of cytotoxic agents. One of the most active, widely used regimens is cisplatin and infusional 5-FU. Initial phase II studies of this combination reported response rates ranging from 25% to 70% (103–105), although subsequent larger phase III trials yielded response rates of approximately 30% in the cisplatin plus infusional 5-FU arms (10,46,106).

In an attempt to rigorously examine the data supporting the use of palliative chemotherapy in SCCHN, Browman et al. performed a meta-analysis of published randomized trials from 1980 to 1992 (107). A total of 15 trials were included in the meta-analysis, which concluded that combination chemotherapy resulted in significantly higher response rates compared with single agents such as methotrexate. In addition, cisplatin and infusional 5-FU resulted in higher response rates compared with other chemotherapy combinations that were examined during this time period. In these studies, however, combination chemotherapy did not significantly prolong survival. As a result, the clinical benefit of more aggressive, toxic combination therapy remained controversial, and single-agent methotrexate was considered a reasonable standard therapy (108).

Platinum and Paclitaxel Combinations

Over the past decade, combinations of platinum plus newer agents have demonstrated significant activity in recurrent or metastatic SCCHN. Several phase II trials of cisplatin plus paclitaxel yielded response rates of 32% to 48% (109,110). The ECOG and SWOG recently completed a randomized study of cisplatin (75 mg/m^2) and paclitaxel (175 mg/m^2) versus a standard control arm of cisplatin (100 mg/m^2) and 5-FU (1 mg/m^2/day continuous infusion, days 1–4) every 3 weeks in chemonaive patients (75). One hundred and ninety-four subjects were entered, and no significant differences were observed in survival times, response rates, or quality of life measures. Toxicity profiles favored cisplatin plus paclitaxel. The control and experimental arms demonstrated median survivals of 8 and 9 months and overall response rates of 22% and 28%, respectively. These findings support the use of cisplatin plus paclitaxel as another reasonable combination regimen for these patients. Two phase II studies that combined carboplatin with paclitaxel have reported response rates of 23% and 39% (111,112), suggesting that carboplatin may be substituted for cisplatin without any obvious negative impact on efficacy.

Shin et al. investigated the combination of paclitaxel, ifosfamide, and cisplatin (TIP) in a phase II trial conducted at the University of Texas M. D. Anderson Cancer Center. Based on the results of an earlier phase I study (113), 52 patients with recurrent or metastatic SCHHN were treated with paclitaxel (175 mg/m^2 over 3 hours, day 1), ifosfamide (1 mg/m^2/day, days 1–3), and cisplatin (60 mg/m^2, day 1) (114). Cycles were repeated every 3 weeks, and mesna was administered on days 1 to 3 for uroprotection. An impressive response rate of 58% was observed with a median survival time of 8.8 months. In attempt to reduce cisplatin-related toxicity, a follow-up phase II study of paclitaxel, ifosfamide, and carboplatin (TIC) was conducted (115). Similar activity to the previous TIP trial was demonstrated, with 56% of subjects responding and a median survival time of 9.1 months. Lower rates of anorexia, emesis, fatigue, and peripheral neuropathy were observed with the TIC regimen.

Platinum and Docetaxel Combinations

Similar to the development of paclitaxel-based regimens, docetaxel plus cisplatin combinations have also been investigated. Phase II studies in recurrent or metastatic SCCHN have yielded response rates of 33% to 50% (116–119). These encouraging results have prompted a three-arm, randomized, phase III trial (TAX 322) comparing docetaxel plus cisplatin versus docetaxel plus 5-FU versus a control arm of cisplatin plus 5-FU (120). The docetaxel plus 5-FU arm was discontinued due to low response rates, and the results of this trial may establish docetaxel plus cisplatin as another reasonable standard combination regimen.

Other Combinations

Platinum combined with other newer agents such as gemcitabine or vinorelbine may have modest activity in patients with recurrent or metastatic SCCHN (121–123), although definitive conclusions will require more trials. A small number of phase II studies examining various combinations of either docetaxel or paclitaxel combined with gemcitabine, vinorelbine, or 5-FU have yielded encouraging response rates ranging from 34% to 44% (124–126). Further studies of similar nonplatinum-containing regimens will help define the role of this approach in the treatment of recurrent or metastatic SCCHN.

SUMMARY

Chemotherapy options for patients with recurrent or metastatic SCCHN continue to evolve. In light of the fact that treatment goals remain palliative, surprisingly little data have been collected regarding the impact of chemotherapy on patients' symptoms and quality of life. Although combination chemotherapy yields higher response rates than those achieved with single agents, randomized studies have yet to definitively demonstrate a survival advantage for combination therapy. Recent trials have demonstrated that taxane-based combinations yield response rates comparable to the current "standard" of cisplatin and infusional 5-FU. A recent randomized trial supports cisplatin and paclitaxel as a reasonable alternative regimen, and an ongoing randomized study may provide similar data regarding cisplatin and docetaxel. While other chemotherapeutic drugs continue to be examined in SCCHN, there is clearly a need to investigate novel agents, and support of clinical trials is strongly encouraged. Recent studies of molecular targeted therapies have included promising agents such as C225, a monoclonal antibody against the epidermal growth factor receptor (EGFR) (127), OSI-774, a potent oral EGFR tyrosine kinase inhibitor (128), and SCH66336, a farnesyltransferase inhibitor (129). Developing strategies to determine the optimal way to combine these novel agents with traditional cytotoxic drugs will become one of the next challenges for clinical and translational researchers.

REFERENCES

1. Forastierre A, Koch W, Trotti A, et al. Head and neck cancer. *N Engl J Med* 2001;345:1890–1900.
2. Dimery IW, Hong WK. Overview of combined modality therapies for head and neck cancer. *J Natl Cancer Inst* 1993;85:95–111.
3. Vokes EE, Haraf DJ, Kies MS. The use of concurrent chemotherapy and radiotherapy for locoregionally advanced head and neck cancer. *Semin Oncol* 2000;27[4 Suppl 8]:34–38.
4. Pivot X, Niyikiza C, Poissonnet G, et al. Clinical prognostic factors for patients with recurrent head and neck cancer: implications for randomized trials. *Oncology* 2001;61:197–204.
5. Constenla DO, Hill ME, A'Hern RP, et al. Chemotherapy for symptom control in recurrent squamous cell carcinoma of the head and neck. *Ann Oncol* 1997;8:445–449.
6. Kies MS, Vokes EE. Does chemotherapy for head and neck cancer improve symptoms? *Ann Oncol* 1997;8:417–418.
7. Schantz SP, Harrison LB, Forastiere AA. Tumors of the nasal cavity and paranasal sinuses, nasopharynx, oral cavity, and oropharynx. In: DeVita VT, Hellman S, Rosenberg SA, eds. *Cancer principles and practice of oncology,* 5th ed. Vol 1. Philadelphia: Lippincott-Raven, 1997:741–801.
8. Vogl SE, Schoenfeld DA, Kaplan BH, et al. A randomized prospective comparison of methotrexate with a combination of methotrexate, bleomycin, and cisplatin in head and neck cancer. *Cancer* 1985;56:432–442.
9. Liverpool Head and Neck Oncology Group. A phase III randomised trial of cisplatinum, methotrexate, cisplatinum + methotrexate and cisplatinum + 5-FU in end stage squamous carcinoma of the head and neck. *Br J Cancer* 1990;61:311–315.
10. Forastiere A, Metch B, Schuller D, et al. Randomized comparison of cisplatin plus fluorouracil and carboplatin plus fluorouracil versus methotrexate in advanced squamous-cell carcinoma of the head and neck: a Southwest Oncology Group study. *J Clin Oncol* 1992;10:1245–1251.
11. Schornagel JH, Verweij J, de Mulder PH, et al. Randomized phase III trial of edatrexate versus methotrexate in patients with metastatic and/or recurrent squamous cell carcinoma of the head and neck: a European Organization for Research and Treatment of Cancer Head and Neck Cancer Cooperative Group study. *J Clin Oncol* 1995;13:1649–1655.
12. Levitt M, Mosher MB, DeConti RC, et al. Improved therapeutic index of methotrexate with "leucovorin rescue." *Cancer Res* 1973;33:1729–1734.
13. Bell R, Sullivan JR, Fleming WB, et al. Results of treatment of head and neck carcinoma with high dose methotrexate. *Clin Exp Pharmacol Physiol* 1979: 23–27.
14. Pitman SW, Miller D, Weichselbaum R. Initial adjuvant therapy in advanced squamous cell carcinoma of the head and neck employing weekly high dose methotrexate with leucovorin rescue. *Laryngoscope* 1978;88:632–638.
15. Woods RL, Fox RM, Tattersall MH. Methotrexate treatment of squamous-cell head and neck cancers: dose-response evaluation. *Br Med J (Clin Res Ed)* 1981; 282:600–602.
16. DeConti RC, Schoenfeld D. A randomized prospective comparison of intermittent methotrexate, methotrexate with leucovorin, and a methotrexate combination in head and neck cancer. *Cancer* 1981;48:1061–1072.
17. Taylor SGT, McGuire WP, Hauck WW, et al. A randomized comparison of high-dose infusion methotrexate versus standard-dose weekly therapy in head and neck squamous cancer. *J Clin Oncol* 1984;2:1006–1011.
18. Browman GP, Goodyear MD, Levine MN, et al. Modulation of the antitumor effect of methotrexate by low-dose leucovorin in squamous cell head and neck cancer: a randomized placebo-controlled clinical trial. *J Clin Oncol* 1990;8:203–208.
19. Robert F. Trimetrexate as a single agent in patients with advanced head and neck cancer. *Semin Oncol* 1988;15[2 Suppl 2]:22–26.
20. Uen WC, Huang AT, Mennel R, et al. A phase II study of piritrexim in patients with advanced squamous head and neck cancer. *Cancer* 1992;69: 1008–1011.
21. Webber S, Bartlett CA, Boritzki TJ, et al. AG337, a novel lipophilic thymidylate synthase inhibitor: in vitro and in vivo preclinical studies. *Cancer Chemother Pharmacol* 1996;37:509–517.
22. Pivot X, Wadler S, Kelly C, et al. Result of two randomized trials comparing nolatrexed (Thymitaq) versus methotrexate in patients with recurrent head and neck cancer. *Ann Oncol* 2001;12:1595–1599.
23. Shih C, Chen VJ, Gossett LS, et al. LY231514, a pyrrolo[2,3-d]pyrimidine-based antifolate that inhibits multiple folate-requiring enzymes. *Cancer Res* 1997;57:1116–1123.
24. O'Dwyer PJ, Nelson K, Thornton DE. Overview of phase II trials of MTA in solid tumors. *Semin Oncol* 1999;26[2 Suppl 6]:99–104.
25. Pivot X, Raymond E, Gedouin D, et al. Phase II trial of MTA (LY231514) in advanced or recurrent squamous cell carcinoma of the head and neck. *Proc Am Soc Clin Oncol* 1999;18:397a.
26. Clayman GL, Lippman SM, Laramore GE, et al. Neoplasms of the head and neck. In: Bast RC, Kufe DW, Pollock RE, et al, eds. *Cancer medicine,* 5th ed. Hamilton, Ontario: B.C. Decker Inc, 2000:1173–1220.
27. Sako K, Razack MS, Kalnins I. Chemotherapy for advanced and recurrent squamous cell carcinoma of the head and neck with high and low dose cis-diamminedichloroplatinum. *Am J Surg* 1978;136:529–533.
28. Forastiere AA, Belliveau JF, Goren MP, et al. Pharmacokinetic and toxicity evaluation of five-day continuous infusion versus intermittent bolus cis-diamminedichloroplatinum(II) in head and neck cancer patients. *Cancer Res* 1988;48:3869–3874.
29. Havlin KA, Kuhn JG, Myers JW, et al. High-dose cisplatin for locally advanced or metastatic head and neck cancer. A phase II pilot study. *Cancer* 1989;63:423–427.
30. Forastiere AA, Takasugi BJ, Baker SR, et al. High-dose cisplatin in advanced head and neck cancer. *Cancer Chemother Pharmacol* 1987;19:155–158.
31. Veronesi A, Zagonel V, Tirelli U, et al. High-dose versus low-dose cisplatin in advanced head and neck squamous carcinoma: a randomized study. *J Clin Oncol* 1985;3:1105–1108.
32. Hong WK, Schaefer S, Issell B, et al. A prospective randomized trial of methotrexate versus cisplatin in the treatment of recurrent squamous cell carcinoma of the head and neck. *Cancer* 1983;52:206–210.
33. Grose WE, Lehane DE, Dixon DO, et al. Comparison of methotrexate and cisplatin for patients with advanced squamous cell carcinoma of the head and neck region: a Southwest Oncology Group Study. *Cancer Treat Rep* 1985;69: 577–581.
34. Morton RP, Rugman F, Dorman EB, et al. Cisplatinum and bleomycin for advanced or recurrent squamous cell carcinoma of the head and neck: a randomised factorial phase III controlled trial. *Cancer Chemother Pharmacol* 1985; 15:283–289.
35. Alberts DS, Dorr RT. New perspectives on an old friend: optimizing carboplatin for the treatment of solid tumors. *Oncologist* 1998;3:15–34.
36. Eisenberger M, Hornedo J, Silva H, et al. Carboplatin (NSC-241-240): an active platinum analog for the treatment of squamous-cell carcinoma of the head and neck. *J Clin Oncol* 1986;4:1506–1509.
37. de Andres Basauri L, Lopez Pousa A, Alba E, et al. Carboplatin, an active drug in advanced head and neck cancer. *Cancer Treat Rep* 1986;70:1173–1176.
38. Al-Sarraf M, Metch B, Kish J, et al. Platinum analogs in recurrent and advanced head and neck cancer: a Southwest Oncology Group and Wayne State University Study. *Cancer Treat Rep* 1987;71(7–8):723–726.
39. Inuyama Y, Togawa K, Morita M, et al. [Phase II study of carboplatin in head and neck cancer]. *Gan To Kagaku Ryoho* 1988;15:2131–2138.
40. Dimery IW, Brooks BJ, Winn R, et al. Phase II trial of carboplatin plus cisplatin in recurrent and advanced squamous cell carcinoma of the head and neck. *J Clin Oncol* 1991;9:1939–1944.
41. Patton JF, Powell BL, White DR, et al. Combination cisplatin and carboplatin in advanced squamous cell carcinoma of the head and neck. *Cancer Invest* 1996;14:98–102.
42. Abele R, Clavel M, Monfardini S, et al. Phase II study of iproplatin (CHIP, JM-9) in advanced squamous cell carcinoma of the head and neck. *Eur J Cancer Clin Oncol* 1987;23:387–389.
43. Degardin M, Armand JP, Chevallier B, et al. A clinical screening cooperative group phase II evaluation of lobaplatin (ASTA D-19466) in advanced head and neck cancer. *Invest New Drugs* 1995;13:253–255.
44. Kish JA, Ensley JF, Jacobs J, et al. A randomized trial of cisplatin (CACP) + 5-fluorouracil (5-FU) infusion and CACP + 5-FU bolus for recurrent and advanced squamous cell carcinoma of the head and neck. *Cancer* 1985;56: 2740–2744.
45. Tapazoglou E, Kish J, Ensley J, et al. The activity of a single-agent 5-fluorouracil infusion in advanced and recurrent head and neck cancer. *Cancer* 1986;57:1105–1109.
46. Jacobs C, Lyman G, Velez-Garcia E, et al. A phase III randomized study comparing cisplatin and fluorouracil as single agents and in combination for advanced squamous cell carcinoma of the head and neck. *J Clin Oncol* 1992; 10:257–263.

47. Pitman SW, Kowal CD, Bertino JR. Methotrexate and 5-fluorouracil in sequence in squamous head and neck cancer. *Semin Oncol* 1983;10[2 Suppl 2]:15–19.
48. Coates AS, Tattersall MH, Swanson C, et al. Combination therapy with methotrexate and 5-fluorouracil: a prospective randomized clinical trial of order of administration. *J Clin Oncol* 1984;2:756–761.
49. Browman GP, Levine MN, Russell R, et al. Survival results from a phase III study of simultaneous versus 1-hour sequential methotrexate-5-fluorouracil chemotherapy in head and neck cancer. *Head Neck Surg* 1986;8:146–152.
50. Browman GP, Levine MN, Goodyear MD, et al. Methotrexate/fluorouracil scheduling influences normal tissue toxicity but not antitumor effects in patients with squamous cell head and neck cancer: results from a randomized trial. *J Clin Oncol* 1988;6:963–968.
51. Knowling M, Browman G, Siu L, et al. A National Cancer Institute of Canada clinical trials group phase II study of eniluracil (776C85) and oral 5-fluorouracil in patients with advanced squamous cell head and neck cancer. *Ann Oncol* 2001;12:919–922.
52. Baker SD, Khor SP, Adjei AA, et al. Pharmacokinetic, oral bioavailability, and safety study of fluorouracil in patients treated with 776C85, an inactivator of dihydropyrimidine dehydrogenase. *J Clin Oncol* 1996;14:3085–3096.
53. Crooke ST, Bradner WT. Bleomycin, a review. *J Med* 1976;7:333–428.
54. Haas CD, Coltman CA Jr, Gottlieb JA, et al. Phase II evaluation of bleomycin. A Southwest Oncology Group study. *Cancer* 1976;38:8–12.
55. Durkin WJ, Pugh RP, Jacobs E, et al. Bleomycin (NSC-125066) therapy of responsive solid tumors. *Oncology* 1976;33(5–6):260–264.
56. Bleomycin in advanced squamous cell carcinoma: a random controlled trial. Report of Medical Research Council Working Party on Bleomycin. *Br Med J* 1976;1:188–190.
57. Al-Sarraf M. Chemotherapeutic management of head and neck cancer. *Cancer Metastasis Rev* 1987;6:181–198.
58. Pinto HA, Jacobs C. Chemotherapy for recurrent and metastatic head and neck cancer. *Hematol Oncol Clin North Am* 1991;5:667–686.
59. Van Barneveld PW, Sleijfer DT, van der Mark TW, et al. Natural course of bleomycin-induced pneumonitis. A follow-up study. *Am Rev Respir Dis* 1987; 135:48–51.
60. Sikic BI, Collins JM, Mimnaugh EG, et al. Improved therapeutic index of bleomycin when administered by continuous infusion in mice. *Cancer Treat Rep* 1978;62:2011–2017.
61. Popkin JD, Hong WK, Bromer RH, et al. Induction bleomycin infusion in head and neck cancer. *Am J Clin Oncol* 1984;7:199–204.
62. Zalupski M, Baker LH. Ifosfamide. *J Natl Cancer Inst* 1988;80:556–566.
63. Verweij J, Alexieva-Figusch J, de Boer MF, et al. Ifosfamide in advanced head and neck cancer. A phase II study of the Rotterdam Cooperative Head and Neck Cancer Study Group. *Eur J Cancer Clin Oncol* 1988;24:795–796.
64. Cervellino JC, Araujo CE, Pirisi C, et al. Ifosfamide and mesna for the treatment of advanced squamous cell head and neck cancer. A GETLAC study. *Oncology* 1991;48:89–92.
65. Kish JA, Tapazoglou E, Ensley J, et al. Activity of ifosfamide in recurrent head and neck cancer patients. *Proc Am Assoc Cancer Res* 1990;31:190a.
66. Buesa JM, Fernandez R, Esteban E, et al. Phase II trial of ifosfamide in recurrent and metastatic head and neck cancer. *Ann Oncol* 1991;2:151–152.
67. Martin M, Diaz-Rubio E, Gonzalez Larriba JL, et al. Ifosfamide in advanced epidermoid head and neck cancer. *Cancer Chemother Pharmacol* 1993;31: 340–342.
68. Huber MH, Lippman SM, Benner SE, et al. A phase II study of ifosfamide in recurrent squamous cell carcinoma of the head and neck. *Am J Clin Oncol* 1996;19:379–382.
69. Rowinsky EK, Donehower RC. Paclitaxel (Taxol). *N Engl J Med* 1995;332: 1004–1014.
70. Smith RE, Thornton DE, Allen J. A phase II trial of paclitaxel in squamous cell carcinoma of the head and neck with correlative laboratory studies. *Semin Oncol* 1995;22[3 Suppl 6]:41–46.
71. Gebbia V, Testa A, Cannata G, et al. Single agent paclitaxel in advanced squamous cell head and neck carcinoma. *Eur J Cancer* 1996;32A:901–902.
72. Forastiere AA, Shank D, Neuberg D, et al. Final report of a phase II evaluation of paclitaxel in patients with advanced squamous cell carcinoma of the head and neck: an Eastern Cooperative Oncology Group trial (PA390). *Cancer* 1998;82:2270–2274.
73. Vermorken JB, Catimel G, De Mulder P, et al. Randomized phase ii trial of weekly methotrexate (mtx) versus two schedules of triweekly paclitaxel (Taxol) in patients with metastatic or recurrent squamous cell carcinoma of the head and neck (SCCHN). *Proc Am Soc Clin Oncol* 1999;18:395a.
74. Forastiere AA, Leong T, Rowinsky E, et al. Phase III comparison of high-dose paclitaxel + cisplatin + granulocyte colony-stimulating factor versus low-dose paclitaxel + cisplatin in advanced head and neck cancer: Eastern Cooperative Oncology Group Study E1393. *J Clin Oncol* 2001;19:1088–1095.
75. Murphy B, Cella D, Karnad A, et al. Phase III study comparing cisplatin (C) and 5-fluorouracil (F) versus cisplatin and paclitaxel (T) in metastatic/recurrent head and neck cancer (MHNC). *Proc Am Soc Clin Oncol* 2001;20:224a.
76. Schrijvers D, Vermorken JB. Role of taxoids in head and neck cancer. *Oncologist* 2000;5:199–208.
77. Huttmann C, Eckardt A, Fokas K, et al. [Experimental chemotherapy of xenotransplanted oral squamous epithelial carcinoma: effectiveness of docetaxel (Taxotere) in the nude mouse model]. *Mund Kiefer Gesichtschir* 1999;3:257–262.
78. Braakhuis BJ, Kegel A, Welters MJ. The growth inhibiting effect of docetaxel (Taxotere) in head and neck squamous cell carcinoma xenografts. *Cancer Lett* 1994;81:151–154.
79. Catimel G, Verweij J, Mattijssen V, et al. Docetaxel (Taxotere): an active drug for the treatment of patients with advanced squamous cell carcinoma of the head and neck. EORTC Early Clinical Trials Group. *Ann Oncol* 1994;5: 533–537.
80. Dreyfuss A, Clark J, Norris C, et al. Docetaxel: an active drug for squamous cell carcinoma of the head and neck. *J Clin Oncol* 1996;14:1672–1678.
81. Couteau C, Chouaki N, Leyvraz S, et al. A phase II study of docetaxel in patients with metastatic squamous cell carcinoma of the head and neck. *Br J Cancer* 1999;81:457–462.
82. Inuyama Y, Kataura A, Togawa K, et al. [Late phase II clinical study of RP56976 (docetaxel) in patients with advanced/recurrent head and neck cancer]. *Gan To Kagaku Ryoho* 1999;26:107–116.
83. Potier P. The synthesis of navelbine: prototype of a new series of vinblastine derivatives. *Semin Oncol* 1989;16[Suppl 4]:2.
84. Binet S, Fellous, A, Meininger, V. On site analysis of the action of navelbine on various types of microtubules using immunofluorescence. *Semin Oncol* 1989;16[Suppl]:5–8.
85. Cros S, Wright, M, Morimoto, M, et al. Experimental antitumor activity of navelbine. *Semin Oncol* 1989;16[Suppl]:15–20.
86. Degardin M, Oliveira J, Geoffrois L, et al. An EORTC-ECSG phase II study of vinorelbine in patients with recurrent and/or metastatic squamous cell carcinoma of the head and neck. *Ann Oncol* 1998;9:1103–1107.
87. Saxman S, Mann B, Canfield V, et al. A phase II trial of vinorelbine in patients with recurrent or metastatic squamous cell carcinoma of the head and neck. *Am J Clin Oncol* 1998;21:398–400.
88. Testolin A, Recher G, Cristoferi V, et al. Vinorelbine in pre-treated advanced head and neck squamous cell carcinoma. A phase II study. *Invest New Drugs* 1994;12:231–234.
89. Hertel L, Kroin, JS, Misner, JW, et al. Synthesis of 2-deoxy-2′,2′-difluoro-D-ribose and 2-deoxy-2′,2′-difluoro-D-ribofuranosyl nucleosides. *J Org Chem* 1988;53:2406–2409.
90. Huang P, Chubb, S, Hertel, LW, et al. Mechanism of action of 2′,2′difluorodeoxycytidine triphosphate on DNA synthesis. *Proc Am Assoc Cancer Res* 1990;31:426.
91. Hertel L, Boder, GB, Kroin, JS, et al. Evaluation of the antitumor activity of gemcitabine 2′,2′-difluoro-2′-deoxycytidine. *Cancer Res* 1990;50:4417–4422.
92. Braakhuis BJ, van Dongen GA, Vermorken JB, et al. Preclinical in vivo activity of 2′,2′-difluorodeoxycytidine (gemcitabine) against human head and neck cancer. *Cancer Res* 1991;51:211–214.
93. Catimel G, Vermorken JB, Clavel M, et al. A phase II study of Gemcitabine (LY 188011) in patients with advanced squamous cell carcinoma of the head and neck. EORTC Early Clinical Trials Group. *Ann Oncol* 1994;5:543–547.
94. Wall ME, Wani MC, Cook CE. Plant antitumor agents. I. The isolation and structure of camptothecin, a novel alkaloidal leukemia and tumor inhibitor from Camptotheca acuminata. *J Am Chem Soc* 1966;88:3888–3890.
95. Jaxel C, Kohn KW, Wani MC, et al. Structure-activity study of the actions of camptothecin derivatives on mammalian topoisomerase I: evidence for a specific receptor site and a relation to antitumor activity. *Cancer Res* 1989;49: 1465–1469.
96. Wang JC. DNA topoisomerases. *Annu Rev Biochem* 1985;54:665–697.
97. Schneider E, Hsiang YH, Liu LF. DNA topoisomerases as anticancer drug targets. *Adv Pharmacol* 1990;21:149–183.
98. Murphy BA, Cmelak A, Burkey B, et al. Topoisomerase I inhibitors in the treatment of head and neck cancer. *Oncology (Huntingt)* 2001;15[7 Suppl 8]:47–52.
99. Smith RE, Lew D, Rodriguez GI, et al. Evaluation of topotecan in patients with recurrent for metastatic squamous cell carcinoma of the head and neck. A phase II Southwest Oncology Group study. *Invest New Drugs* 1996;14: 403–407.
100. Robert F, Soong SJ, Wheeler RH. A phase II study of topotecan in patients with recurrent head and neck cancer. Identification of an active new agent. *Am J Clin Oncol* 1997;20:298–302.
101. Murphy BA, Leong T, Burkey B, et al. Lack of efficacy of topotecan in the treatment of metastatic or recurrent squamous carcinoma of the head and neck: an Eastern Cooperative Oncology Group Trial (E3393). *Am J Clin Oncol* 2001;24:64–66.
102. Lad T, Rosen F, Brockstein B, et al. Phase II trial of 9-aminocamptothecin (9AC/DMA) in patients with advanced squamous cell head and neck cancer. *Proc Am Soc Clin Oncol* 1998;17:392a.
103. Kish JA, Weaver A, Jacobs J, et al. Cisplatin and 5-fluorouracil infusion in patients with recurrent and disseminated epidermoid cancer of the head and neck. *Cancer* 1984;53:1819–1824.
104. Rowland KM Jr, Taylor SGT, Spiers AS, et al. Cisplatin and 5-FU infusion chemotherapy in advanced, recurrent cancer of the head and neck: an Eastern Cooperative Oncology Group Pilot Study. *Cancer Treat Rep* 1986;70: 461–464.
105. Choksi AJ, Hong WK, Dimery IW, et al. Continuous cisplatin (24-hour) and 5-fluorouracil (120-hour) infusion in recurrent head and neck squamous cell carcinoma. *Cancer* 1988;61:909–912.
106. Clavel M, Vermorken JB, Cognetti F, et al. Randomized comparison of cisplatin, methotrexate, bleomycin and vincristine (CABO) versus cisplatin and 5-fluorouracil (CF) versus cisplatin (C) in recurrent or metastatic squamous cell carcinoma of the head and neck. A phase III study of the EORTC Head and Neck Cancer Cooperative Group. *Ann Oncol* 1994;5:521–526.

107. Browman GP, Cronin L. Standard chemotherapy in squamous cell head and neck cancer: what we have learned from randomized trials. *Semin Oncol* 1994;21:311–319.
108. Clark JR, Dreyfuss AI. The role of cisplatin in treatment regimens for squamous cell carcinoma of the head and neck. *Semin Oncol* 1991;18[1 Suppl 3]:34–48.
109. Thodtmann F, Theiss F, Kemmerich M, et al. Clinical phase II evaluation of paclitaxel in combination with cisplatin in metastatic or recurrent squamous cell carcinoma of the head and neck. *Ann Oncol* 1998;9:335–357.
110. Licitra L, Capri G, Fulfaro F, et al. Biweekly paclitaxel and cisplatin in patients with advanced head and neck carcinoma. A phase II trial. *Ann Oncol* 1997;8:1157–1158.
111. Stathopoulos GP, Rigatos S, Papakostas P, et al. Effectiveness of paclitaxel and carboplatin combination in heavily pretreated patients with head and neck cancers. *Eur J Cancer* 1997;33:1780–1783.
112. Fountzilas G, Skarlos D, Athanassiades A, et al. Paclitaxel by three-hour infusion and carboplatin in advanced carcinoma of nasopharynx and other sites of the head and neck. A phase II study conducted by the Hellenic Cooperative Oncology Group. *Ann Oncol* 1997;8:451–455.
113. Benner SE, Lippman SM, Huber MH, et al. Phase I study of paclitaxel, cisplatin, and ifosfamide in patients with recurrent or metastatic squamous cell cancer of the head and neck. *Semin Oncol* 1995;22[5 Suppl 12]:22–25.
114. Shin D, Glisson B, Khuri F, et al. Phase II trial of paclitaxel, ifosfamide, and cisplatin in patients with recurrent head and neck squamous cell carcinoma. *J Clin Oncol* 1998;16:1325–1330.
115. Shin DM, Khuri FR, Glisson BS, et al. Phase II study of paclitaxel, ifosfamide, and carboplatin in patients with recurrent or metastatic head and neck squamous cell carcinoma. *Cancer* 2001;91:1316–1323.
116. Schoffski P, Catimel G, Planting AS, et al. Docetaxel and cisplatin: an active regimen in patients with locally advanced, recurrent or metastatic squamous cell carcinoma of the head and neck. Results of a phase II study of the EORTC Early Clinical Studies Group. *Ann Oncol* 1999;10:119–122.
117. Forastiere A, Glisson B, Murphy B, et al. A phase II study of docetaxel and cisplatin in patients with locally advanced, recurrent, and/or metastatic squamous cell carcinoma of the head and neck (SCCHN), not curable by standard therapy. *Proc Am Soc Clin Oncol* 1998;17:399a.
118. Specht L, Larsen SK, Hansen HS. Phase II study of docetaxel and cisplatin in patients with recurrent or disseminated squamous-cell carcinoma of the head and neck. *Ann Oncol* 2000;11:845–849.
119. Glisson BS, Murphy BA, Frenette G, et al. Phase II Trial of Docetaxel and Cisplatin Combination Chemotherapy in Patients With Squamous Cell Carcinoma of the Head and Neck. *J Clin Oncol* 2002;20:1593–1599.
120. Posner MR. Docetaxel in squamous cell cancer of the head and neck. *Anticancer Drugs* 2001;12[Suppl 1]:S21–S24.
121. Hitt R, Castellano D, Hidalgo M, et al. Phase II trial of cisplatin and gemcitabine in advanced squamous-cell carcinoma of the head and neck. *Ann Oncol* 1998;9:1347–1349.
122. Kornek V, Scheithauer W, Glaser C, et al. Vinorelbine and carboplatin in recurrent and/or metastatic squamous cell carcinoma of the head and neck. *Oncology* 1999;56:24–27.
123. Segura A, Pastor M, Santaballa A, et al. Cisplatin plus vinorelbine for patients with advanced head and neck squamous cell carcinoma. *Oncologist* 2000;5:177–178.
124. Fountzilas G, Stathopoulos G, Nicolaides C, et al. Paclitaxel and gemcitabine in advanced non-nasopharyngeal head and neck cancer: a phase II study conducted by the Hellenic Cooperative Oncology Group. *Ann Oncol* 1999;10:475–478.
125. Fillipi M, Cupissol D, Calais G, et al. A phase II study of docetaxel and 5–fluorouracil in metastatic or recurrent squamous cell carcinoma of the head and neck. *Proc Am Soc Clin Oncol* 1999;18:402a.
126. Airoldi M, Marchionatti S, Pedani F, et al. Docetaxel + vinorelbine in recurrent heavily pre-treated head and neck cancer patients. *Proc Am Soc Clin Oncol* 1999;18:402a.
127. Hong WK, Nabell A, Needle M, et al. Efficacy and safety of the anti-epidermal growth factor antibody IMC-C225 in combination with cisplatin in patients with recurrent squamous cell carcinoma of the head and neck refractory to cisplatin containing chemotherapy. *Proc Am Soc Clin Oncol* 2001; 20:224a.
128. Senzer N, Soulieres D, Siu L, et al. Phase 2 evaluation of OSI-774, a potent oral antagonist of the EGFR-TK in patients with advanced squamous cell carcinoma of the head and neck. *Proc Am Soc Clin Oncol* 2001;20:2a.
129. Kies MS, Clayman G, El-Naggar A, et al. Induction therapy with SCH 66336, a farnesyltransferase inhibitor, in squamous cell carcinoma of the head and neck. *Proc Am Soc Clin Oncol* 2001;20:225a.

PART III

Basic Science and Pathology of Head and Neck Cancer

CHAPTER 36

Molecular Biology of Head and Neck Cancer

Joseph A. Califano III and David Sidransky

Within the last decade, substantial advances in the understanding of the molecular biology of head and neck cancer have been made. Specifically, significant progress in the understanding of environmental influences, premalignant disease, tumor genetics, protein function, and molecular diagnostics has been accomplished. This chapter will outline some of these advances; however, the limited scope of this review precludes adequate discussion of some major areas of investigation, of which a few are discussed in greater detail in subsequent chapters.

It now is generally accepted that most malignant neoplasms result from a multistep process of accumulated genetic alterations that result in clonal outgrowth of transformed cells (1). These genetic alterations include a variety of changes in the structure and sequence of cellular DNA within this clonal population, resulting in activation of protooncogenes and inactivation of tumor suppressor genes (TSGs). Gene alterations may arise from spontaneous/endogenous mutations or exogenous mutations caused by potent environmental carcinogens. Often chromosomal and DNA changes are a result of the derangement of normal cellular homeostatic mechanisms caused by viral, chemical, or other exogenous influences. These genetic alterations ultimately affect the transcription of this information into mRNA intermediates, and subsequent translation into altered, increased, or absent protein products. The accumulation of these genetic changes leads to the phenotypic expression of myriad biologic characteristics of any particular neoplasm, including cell growth and death, motility, immunogenicity, and invasion. Accumulated genetic alterations also may influence normal host responses, including angiogenesis and immunologic status.

Most sporadic solid tumors are thought to require several genetic events to gain full expression of the malignant phenotype. Statistical analysis of age-specific incidence data for patients with head and neck squamous cell cancer (HNSCC) suggests that these cancers arise after six to ten independent genetic events (2). Although the precise number of events may be quite variable, these data indicate that HNSCC accumulates more genetic alterations in comparison to other solid tumors. Presumably, these genetic events are acquired over the 20- to 25-year latency period required for the development of HNSCC. During this time, exposure to carcinogens—particularly tobacco, perhaps augmented by alcohol—is believed to be the predominant cause of specific genetic alterations acquired during HNSCC progression (3).

The temporal order of specific genetic events during the initiation and progression of colorectal cancer has now become a paradigm for most human solid tumors, including brain and bladder cancer (4–7). Like colorectal cancer, HNSCC is thought to progress through a series of well-defined clinical and histopathologic stages. Association of genetic alterations with specific premalignant lesions of the head and neck has been used to construct a basic genetic progression model. (8). This model has served as a useful construct on which additional genetic and cellular alterations may be placed, to help locate additional alterations on the evolution any timeline from normal cell to invasive cancer. In this chapter, we outline the specific genetic events identified in HNSCC, the timing of these genetic events, and the current understanding of HNSCC progression. Altered cellular pathways will also be explored at the protein level as efforts increase to target these molecular pathways therapeutically. We also highlight the new understanding of field cancerization and the clinical relevance for early detection and prognostic assessment. Finally, we will touch on efforts to determine molecular prognostic factors in HNSCC.

CYTOGENETIC ALTERATIONS

Cytogenetically detectable alterations generally are gross karyotypic alterations reflecting large chromosomal deletions, amplifications, and translocations. As in most cancers, increasing aneuploidy has been associated with histopathologic progression of HNSCC (9). Technically challenging short-term cultures of primary tumors allow accurate cytogenetic analysis while minimizing the *in vitro* selection pressure that allows overgrowth of nondominant clones in culture. These studies have consistently described areas of chromosomal deletions on 3p, 5q, 8p, 9p, 18q, and 21q (10–12) and chromosomal gain or amplification on 3q,

5p, 7p, 8q, and 11q13 (10–13). Chromosomal break points have been noted at 1p36, 3q21, 5p14, 7p13, 9q32, and 11q13 (12,13), and break points at 11p22, 3p21, 8p11, and distal 14q have correlated with decreased radiosensitivity (13).

Newer cytogenetic techniques have facilitated examination of primary tumor material, eliminating the effects of *in vitro* selection pressures. Fluorescence *in situ* hybridization uses a DNA probe coupled to a fluorescent chromophore that will bind specifically to a unique chromosomal region and identify specific alterations. Gain of chromosomes 7 and 17 was noted using this technique, confirming previous studies using cytogenetic analysis (14). Comparative genomic hybridization involves the use of separately labeled tumor and normal DNA, which is then mixed and hybridized to normal metaphase chromosome spreads for evaluation of relative genomic deletion or amplification along the length of a particular chromosome. These data have largely confirmed previous conventional cytogenetic reports, observing amplification at 3q26-ter, 11q13, 12p, and copy number increases on both arms of chromosomes 3, 5, and 19 (15).

AMPLIFICATION AND PROTOONCOGENES

Protooncogenes are normal cellular genes that are activated by genetic alterations that include mutations and amplification (increased copy number of a gene encoded in DNA) and produce a phenotypic alteration characteristic of malignancy. Cytogenetic analyses point to areas of the genome that may harbor protooncogenes activated by DNA amplification (e.g., 11q13—as discussed earlier) (16,17). Direct DNA analysis has shown that cyclin D1 (also known as *PRAD1* or *CCND1*), located on 11q13, is amplified in approximately one-third of HNSCCs (18). Although other genes (*INT2* and *HST1*) located nearby may be contained within the amplified DNA segment, only cyclin D1 is amplified consistently. Further evidence for the role of cyclin D1 as a protooncogene is provided by the observations that (a) this amplification is associated with increased expression of the gene, (b) transfection of cyclin D1 in concert with other oncogenes can lead to cell transformation, and (c) cyclin D1 is required for progression through the cell cycle in some HNSCC cell lines (18,19). Amplification of cyclin D1 may correlate also with histopathologic progression in HNSCC (20). Presumably, this protooncogene functions to allow the cell to continue growth by overriding the growth-suppressive effects of the retinoblastoma (*Rb*) protein pathway.

Another putative protooncogene amplified in HNSCC is located on chromosome 3q. This gene, termed *p40/p63/AIS/CUSP,* is a homolog to *p53,* and may have diverse roles in cell cycle modulation and DNA damage response. A commonly overexpressed isotype in tumors lacking the transactivation domain was found to display opposing efforts to *p53*. *p63* has been found to be amplified in a subset of primary HNSCC, and its growth stimulatory properties may be modulated by a variety of downstream pathways that are currently under intense investigation (21,22).

Currently, evidence directly implicating other protooncogenes in the progression of HNSCC is lacking. Although increased levels of transforming growth factor-β and epidermal growth factor receptor (EGFR) mRNA and protein have been found at quite early stages of carcinogenesis and in normal mucosa from affected patients, amplification or mutation at the DNA level has rarely been seen (23,24). The genetic basis for dysregulation of these genes remains obscure. Despite the lack of characterized protooncogenes in HNSCC, continued investigation with newer and more refined techniques such as fluorescence *in situ* hybridization and comparative genomic hybridization should yield more specific genetic information, possibly leading to definitive identification of additional protooncogenes involved in the progression of HNSCC.

TUMOR SUPPRESSOR GENES AND ALLELIC LOSS

Tumor suppressor genes, under normal expression, limit the ability of a cell to express phenotypic characteristics of malignancy, including unrestrained growth, lack of cell death, and invasion. Knudson (25) hypothesizes that the differences in the age-specific incidence of inherited versus sporadic retinoblastoma are based on the necessity for inactivation of both parental copies of the *Rb* gene to initiate tumorigenesis. This hypothesis has been extended to include a two-step mechanism of inactivation for sporadic, solid tumors in adults. Inactivation of one allele of a TSG by point mutation is followed by loss of a relatively large chromosomal region that encompasses the second allele, thus completely abrogating tumor suppressor function (26). Chromosomal deletion, therefore, serves as a marker for inactivation of TSGs, and delineation of the minimal deletion area encompassed by many tumors can aid in mapping a TSG. For example, loss of 17p in colon cancer led investigators to test for mutation of p53 in the retained chromosomal arm in sporadic tumors (1). Subsequently, it was found that *p53* was the most commonly mutated gene in human cancer (27).

Polymerase chain reaction-based microsatellite marker analysis has been the basic modality to determine areas of chromosomal loss that may harbor TSGs. These markers, called *microsatellite markers,* are highly polymorphic DNA repeat units located ubiquitously throughout the genome that can be easily analyzed in fresh or archival tissues from tumor specimens. The ratio of maternal and paternal alleles in normal tissues can be compared with the ratio of these alleles in tumor cells, allowing the determination of relative gain or loss of chromosomal material within the genome of a particular tumor. Areas of chromosomal loss can be mapped to a fine degree in individual tumors, allowing precise delineation and mapping of interstitial deletions. In addition, common allelic losses may be mapped among a large number of primary tumors, allowing for precise localization of small, overlapping chromosomal regions that harbor tumor suppressor loci.

Investigators have examined all chromosomal arms using microsatellite analysis in primary HNSCC tumors, creating comprehensive allelotypes of head and neck cancer (28). The most commonly deleted region (>70%) in HNSCC is located on chromosome 9p21 (29). Other tumor types exhibit loss in this region: homozygous deletions of this region have also been observed in such tumors as melanoma, bladder cancer, lung cancer, leukemias, and brain tumors. In addition, 9p21 loss seems to be one of the earliest detectable events in HNSCC and occurs in approximately 20% of benign squamous hyperplastic (leukoplakic) lesions (8). At least one target of these losses may be a cell-cycle gene called *p16* (*CDKN2/MTS1*) (30). This gene is a critical inhibitor of cyclin CDK complexes whose inactivation is thought to permit inappropriate progression through critical G1/S cell cycle checkpoints, allowing cell division to occur unchecked (31). Although point mutations of *p16* are common in familial melanoma and sporadic pancreatic cancer, very few primary HNSCCs exhibited point mutations of the gene (32). Subsequently, two other mechanisms of inactivation of *p16* have been elucidated. Methylation of the 5′ CpG-rich promoter region of *p16* has been identified and associated with a complete block of transcription of *p16* in some primary tumors (33). In addition, homozygous deletion of *p16* has been noted in at least 50% of HNSCCs (34).

Correlation of these three mechanisms of inactivation (point mutation, chromosomal deletion, and promoter methylation) with immunohistochemical expression of p16 protein has been performed to account for all genetic events by which p16 suppressor function is lost. In approximately 80% of primary HNSCC tumors, p16 is inactivated by immunohistochemical analysis. These studies also indicate that the predominant mechanism of inactivation of p16 in HNSCC occurs by homozygous deletion, with more minor roles played by methylation and point mutation. Moreover, absence of p16 staining by immunohistochemical analysis demonstrates a near-perfect correlation with sophisticated genetic analysis (35). Further studies have been completed that assess the frequency of inactivation of p16 in early lesions and have demonstrated its functional significance during tumor progression (36).

Interestingly, a second, related mRNA transcript from the p16 locus has also been characterized (37). This gene, called *p14*^{ARF}*/p19*, forms a protein product using an alternate reading frame and an alternate first exon when compared with the p16 protein product. This protein has little amino acid homology to p16, but most likely acts as a tumor-suppressor gene by altering the subcellular location of and inactivating MDM2, a protein that binds to, and inactivates, the p53 protein. The high rate of homozygous deletion at the p16/p14 locus indicates that both these TSGs are simultaneously inactivated in HNSCC. Indeed, some studies in mice suggest that the inactivation of p14 may have effects that are more profound in terms of tumorigenesis than the inactivation of p16.

Loss of chromosome 17p was observed in more than 50% of primary HNSCCs. This observation accompanies a wealth of studies investigating the primary and common target within this region, *p53*. Mutations of *p53* increase with tumor progression in HNSCC, occurring in approximately 45% of invasive tumors (38). The p53 protein appears to be ubiquitously involved in multiple cellular functions, including cell cycling, DNA repair, and apoptosis. Studies have shown that the rate of *p53* immunohistochemical staining (indicative of abnormal or mutant protein with prolonged half-life that correlates with DNA mutation) and DNA sequence analysis of *p53* mutation both correlate with the rate of 17p loss. However, several caveats must be offered when interpreting these data—namely, that *p53* immunostaining does not always correlate with somatic mutation in individual tumors, and the proportion of positive immunostaining that is defined as significant differs widely among investigators (38). Additionally, a small minority of tumors seem to demonstrate 17p loss but lack *p53* mutation, perhaps indicating that a second gene other than *p53* is targeted by 17p loss (39).

Chromosome 3p allelic imbalance is seen in approximately 60% of HNSCCs. Rather than representing inactivation of one gene, at least two groups of investigators have mapped three separate areas of chromosomal loss, potentially representing at least three separate tumor suppressor loci (40,41). Despite intensive investigation by cancer researchers, few conclusive reports of TSG candidates from these regions exist. The *FHIT* gene was cloned from a familial breakpoint at 3p12, and altered transcripts have been observed in aerodigestive tract cancers and from HNSCC cell lines (42). However, genetic analysis has failed to demonstrate inactivation of both alleles in most primary tumors and cell lines with 3p loss. Future studies should help to elucidate the role of this gene in HNSCC progression. The target(s) of 3p loss is critical because these losses are among the earliest events in HNSCC progression.

Loss of 13q is another common genetic alteration, displayed in approximately 60% of HNSCCs. Initially, fine mapping of the minimal area of loss in this region included an excellent candidate at the *Rb* gene locus. However, very few tumors that exhibit loss of 13q also demonstrate inactivation of *Rb* by reliable, immunohistochemical analysis (43), indicating that there is most likely an alternate target of 13q loss (i.e., a second TSG located within the minimal area of loss that has not yet been identified).

Recently, the human papilloma virus (HPV) has been shown to have an etiologic role in a subset of HNSCC. Specifically, HPV subtype 16 has been shown to be present in approximately half of oropharyngeal HNSCC. In addition, a large Scandinavian population study has shown that elevated HPV-16 titers are associated with a 16-fold relative risk for oropharyngeal HNSCC, and precede the development of HNSCC on an average of 8 years (44). From a molecular perspective, the E6 and E7 protein products from the HPV genome bind to, and inactivate, the p53 and Rb protein products, respectively. In support of this, there is an inverse relationship between HPV positivity and p53 mutation in HNSCC, implying a role for HPV in the inactivation of p53 in oropharyngeal HNSCC (45). An HPV-positive tumor also exhibits a unique basaloid morphology.

Head and neck squamous cell carcinoma exhibits a substantial number of chromosomal arms that are lost with high frequency (> 30%) but for which no putative TSG or locus has been identified. These chromosomal arms include 4q, 6p, 7, 8, 14q, and 19q. Multiple other chromosomes exhibit loss slightly below this rate. This high rate of chromosomal alteration by microsatellite analysis demonstrates agreement with the hypothesis that a relatively large number of genetic events are required for HNSCC tumor progression. Many important chromosomal loci still require further mapping, identification of TSGs located within these loci, and correlation with functional biologic correlates and clinical parameters.

Other molecular alterations in HNSCC have been described that do not necessarily have a clearly defined, underlying genetic alteration on which they are based. Nevertheless, these molecular alterations appear critical to HNSCC development. In addition, many of these are well suited to therapeutic strategies, and have formed the basis for successful, molecularly based therapies in other solid tumor systems.

The epidermal growth factor pathway, known to be important as a cell division, migration, adhesion, differentiation, and apoptosis pathway, has long been known to be up-regulated in HNSCC. Described alterations include EGFR up-regulation, and alterations in subsequent downstream targets with alterations in transcriptional function. Successful clinical trials have shown activity of Herceptin, a humanized monoclonal antibody to activated *Her2neu*, in breast cancer (current trials are underway in HNSCC and have shown promise in treating cisplatin refractory diagnoses) (46). Alternative agents are currently undergoing evaluation, including small, soluble molecules that block the intracellular tyrosine kinase domain of EGFR. This area is further discussed in Chapter 38. Matrix metalloproteinases (MMPs) have recently become the objects of intense investigation in multiple tumor systems. It is likely that these molecules are active in the metastatic phenotype of tumor cells due to their proposed activity in modification of the extracellular matrix, and their role in invasion and metastasis. These targets are further discussed further in Chapter 35.

GENETIC PROGRESSION MODEL

In the last several years, tumor progression models have been constructed for a few tumor types by correlating specific genetic changes with histopathologic progression. The initial description of molecular progression proposed by Fearon and Vogel-

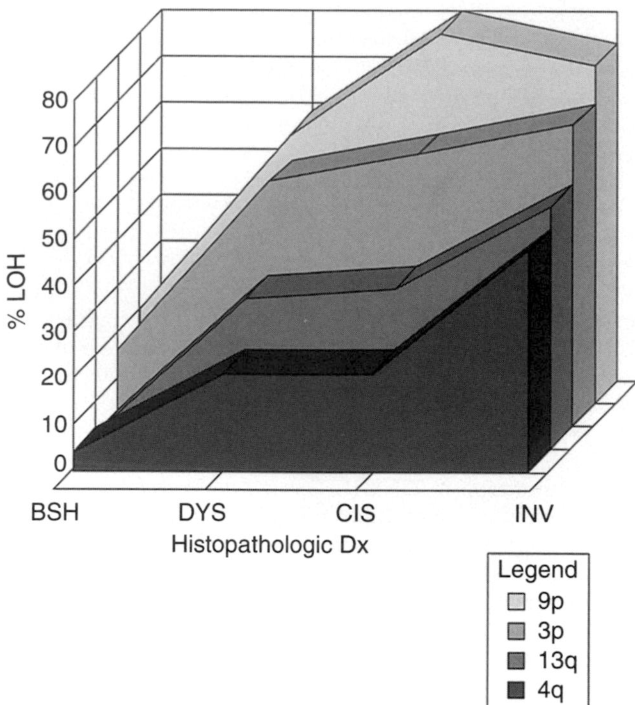

Figure 36.1 Loss of heterozygosity (*LOH*) at selected loci in head and neck squamous cell cancer (HNSCC). The LOH at 9p and 3p occurs in precursor lesions associated with progression to HNSCC, and the high frequency of loss plateaus in dysplasia. Conversely, LOH at 13q and 4q occurs at low frequency throughout progression and does not begin a significant increase in frequency until after the carcinoma *in situ* (*CIS*) stage. Thus, 9p and 3p are designated as early events in the progression of HNSCC. BSH, benign squamous hyperplasia; DYS, dysplasia; Dx, diagnosis; INV, invasive lesions.

stein (1) indicates that (a) tumors progress through the activation of oncogenes and the inactivation of TSGs, each producing a growth advantage for a clonal population of cells, (b) specific genetic events generally occur in a distinct order of progression, but (c) the order of progression is not necessarily the same for each individual tumor, and thus the accumulation of genetic events determines tumor progression.

We have described a preliminary HNSCC tumor progression model, in which allelic loss or imbalance was used as a molecular marker for inactivation of putative TSGs or to detect oncogene amplification (e.g., cyclin D1 on 11q13) (8). This model supports the initial observations of the colorectal molecular progression model, in that (a) both oncogenes and TSGs are involved in tumor progression, (b) specific events in head and neck cancer generally occur in a distinct order of progression, loss at 9p21 or 3p being among the earliest detectable events (Fig. 36.1), and (c) the accumulation and not necessarily the order of genetic events determines progression (Fig. 36.2). This model confirmed that clonal genetic changes are already present in very benign-appearing lesions, occurring "early" in the histopathologic continuum of tumor progression: 30% of histopathologically benign squamous hyperplastic lesions already consist of a clonal population of cells with shared genetic alterations characteristic of those seen in head and neck cancer. Because this malignancy requires multiple genetic alterations to develop an invasive phenotype, it might be expected that lesions involving only a few genetic events would display a rather benign morphologic phenotype.

It must be emphasized that although some benign lesions already have genetic alterations consistent with those present in a genetic progression pathway to cancer, whether their clinical behavior will differ from their behavior based on histopathologic diagnosis remains to be determined. However, identification of early events might be able to pinpoint those genetic alterations that are associated with further transformation and aggressive clinical behavior. Multiple investigators have shown that 9p21 and 3p loss are predictive of subsequent development of invasive cancer when found in noninvasive, leukoplakic lesions (47,48) or that alterations in DNA content are predictive of malignant transformation (49). Knowledge of the timing of genetic events also allows screening strategies to focus on earlier events in malignant transformation and may point out appropriate targets for early pharmacologic or genetic therapy. Early events may also be used in molecular analysis of margins or lymph nodes (discussed later in the chapter) or to identify residual clonal populations of epithelium potentially responsible for late clinical recurrence after successful primary resection.

FIELD CANCERIZATION

The term *field cancerization* originally was coined by Slaughter et al. (50) in a study of oral cancer. These authors examined resection specimens of invasive squamous cell carcinoma of the oral cavity and found histopathologic abnormalities in the epithelium surrounding the invasive cancer. These abnormalities

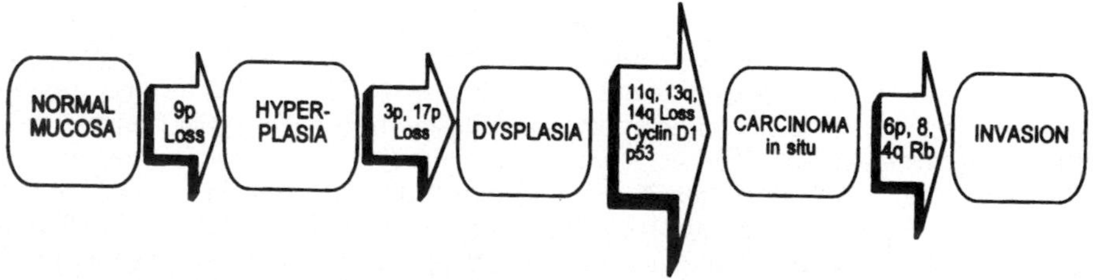

Figure 36.2 Genetic progression model of head and neck squamous cell cancer. Genetic changes associated with the histopathologic progression of head and neck squamous cell carcinoma based on loss of chromosomal material (allelic loss). Genetic alterations have been placed before the lesion at which the frequency of the particular event plateaus. The accumulation, and not necessarily the order, of genetic events determines progression. Candidate tumor suppressor genes include *p16* (9p21), *p53* (17p), and *Rb* (13q), and a candidate protooncogene includes cyclin D1 (11q13). (From Califano J, van der Riet P, Clayman G, et al. A genetic progression model for head and neck cancer: implications for field cancerization. *Cancer Res* 1996;56:2488–2492, with permission.)

included additional areas of invasive cancer, carcinoma *in situ*, dysplasia, hyperkeratosis, and epithelial hyperplasia with frequent multiple foci of more aggressive lesions (e.g., carcinoma *in situ*). Both Slaughter's group and, more recently, other investigators have reported an increased incidence of second primary head and neck, pulmonary, and esophageal cancers in patients with head and neck cancer (51–53). Based on these observations, *field cancerization* was used to describe the phenomenon by which an entire field of tissue developed malignant or premalignant change in response to prolonged exposure to a given carcinogen. Two alternative theories are posited to describe the genetic basis of this observation: First, these areas of abnormality involve separate, independent clones, each with a unique set of genetic alterations. Second, all these areas of abnormality are related genetically and are derived originally from a single cellular clone (monoclonal). In support of the latter hypothesis, previous studies in bladder cancer demonstrated that multiple tumors in a single patient actually originated from a common cellular clone.

Attempts to examine the local manifestations of field cancerization in HNSCC have also demonstrated a common (clonal) origin of these histopathologically distinct areas in premalignant lesions. Additional genetic loss was associated with progression to a more malignant phenotype. Thus, areas of histopathologic abnormality surrounding these lesions usually arise from a common progenitor clone, with variability in subsequent genetic events determining phenotypic and histopathologic diversity (8). In fact, Slaughter et al. (50) noted that "forty-three of these eighty-eight patients [with] two separate tumors occurred in the same anatomical area of the oral cavity," implying that these tumors were clonally related.

X-chromosome inactivation studies and microsatellite mapping have been used to examine synchronous and metachronous HNSCC from anatomically distinct sites (excluding any recurrent HNSCC from examination). One such study (54) also demonstrated results consistent with a common clonal origin of distant, second HNSCCs developed from spread of neoplastic cells from the original primary HNSCC, although statistical significance was not attained due to small study sample size. Conversely, there was no evidence of independent origin in any of the samples.

Although investigators have reported discordant *p53* mutations in multiple tumors, evidence indicates that several genetic events, including 3p and 9p21 loss, precede *p53* mutation (55). Thus, clonal expansion occurs through these earlier events, and subsequent events such as *p53* mutation may be merely a reflection of the genetic heterogeneity occurring late in the progression pathway of an expanding clonal population. Subsequently, cytogenetic evidence in one patient has identified the presence of a specific chromosomal marker in both of two synchronous, anatomically distinct, primary neoplasms (56). Therefore, a significant part of field cancerization in HNSCC (both its local and distant manifestations) is a reflection of the expansion and migration of clonally related cells. These events result in histopathologic abnormalities surrounding primary HNSCC and the increased incidence of distant, second primary HNSCCs.

Other epithelial premalignant states also appear to exhibit the lateral expansion of clonal, premalignant populations prior to development of invasive cancer. Specifically, altered clonal populations have been seen to spread laterally over distances of up to 17 cm in the Barrett esophagus (57,58).

MOLECULAR EPIDEMIOLOGY

The strong association of HNSCC with tobacco and alcohol exposure indicates that exposure to particular carcinogens may be responsible for DNA damage that results in subsequent malignant transformation. Specific carcinogens have shown highly specific associations with specific and sometimes unusual mutations in TSGs; for example, aflatoxin exposure is associated with a G→T transversion in codon 249 of *p53* in hepatocellular carcinoma. A report on the pattern of *p53* gene mutations in HNSCC clearly demonstrated that *p53* mutations are more frequent in patients exposed to tobacco and alcohol. Moreover, particular types of mutations were associated with exposure to these carcinogens (59). Nonsmokers and nondrinkers all were found to have mutations that occurred at CpG sites, whereas patients who rarely drank or smoked had CpG site mutations. One proposed mechanism of CpG mutation is believed to result from spontaneous deamination and methylation unrelated to exogenous mutagen exposure. These provocative results underscore the importance of tobacco and alcohol exposure as causative agents in HNSCC.

The genotypes of detoxifying enzymes in patients with HNSCC have been studied. Specifically, glutathione-S-transferase (GST) haplotypes have been examined, and observations have been made that relate an association of GST-M1with laryngeal carcinoma (60), as well as an association of poor overall survival in patients treated with neoadjuvant cisplatin-based chemotherapy with high GST-π expression (61).

MOLECULAR DIAGNOSTICS

The characterization of multiple genetic events and the timing of these events identify novel, rational targets for the development of early detection techniques. From a molecular genetics point of view, the process of transformation requires 10 to 25 years of carcinogen exposure and the accumulation of multiple genetic events. This long window of detection can be exploited in the development of diagnostic strategies that target early events of genetic progression. An intense investigation has begun to identify genetic events in premalignant lesions and new molecular biologic methods of early detection for HNSCC.

Initial diagnostic strategies centered on the identification of mutations present in primary tumor specimens. Investigators then were able to identify the same unique mutations in body fluids collected concurrently with the primary tumor (e.g., paired urine and stool samples from patients with bladder and colon cancer, respectively) (62,63). These observations were extended to include identification of *ras* and *p53* gene mutations in sputum specimens from patients with lung tumors. In one case, a mutation in one sputum sample collected 1 year before diagnosis of the primary lung tumor was identified correctly using this molecular approach (64). Similar studies identified unique *p53* gene mutations in saliva collected before surgery from patients with primary HNSCC (65).

However, the mutation detection strategies outlined previously are problematic as general screening tools. These techniques require that a unique mutation in a protooncogene or TSG be characterized by sequence analysis of the primary tumor. Subsequently, plaque hybridization approaches DNA (62,63) or mutation site-specific polymerase chain reaction (PCR) strategies must be employed on the body fluid DNA from a particular patient to determine whether a neoplastic clone is present in a clinical sample. Although these methods can be extraordinarily sensitive (able to detect 1 tumor cell in 10,000–100,000 normal cells), diagnosis and resection of a primary lesion are required before it can be performed.

To detect neoplastic clones in body fluids, investigators also have exploited the chromosomal loss present in cancer cells. Absence of one paternal polymorphic marker (microsatellite) identifies loss of a chromosomal region likely to contain a TSG. Not all genetic detection methods directly involve the identification of causative genetic events in tumor progression. In many types of cancers, small repetitive units of DNA (microsatellites) have been noted to contain more frequent expansions and deletions (alterations) of one or more repeat units. These stretches of altered microsatellite repeats in a tumor produce a novel DNA band when amplified through the PCR and indicate that a dominant clonal population of tumor cells is present (66,67). In HNSCC, chromosomal loss has been derived in paired saliva DNA without additional strategies to enrich for tumor cells. Dilution studies have shown that it is possible to detect one tumor cell in a population of several hundred normal cells. However, some complexities of this technique have yet to be resolved: only a minority of microsatellite loci analyzed in most primary tumors exhibit alterations; which factors predispose a locus to alteration in general remain unclear; and whether all HNSCC tumors exhibit these alterations is uncertain. Nevertheless, the ease of this assay and its potential adaptability to automation may surmount these obstacles. A recent study examining HNSCC patients and controls including both nonsmokers and smokers demonstrated microsatellite alterations [loss of heterozygosity (LOH) or instability] in 38 of 44 patients with HNSCC (86%) and no alterations in controls (68). Of those patients with an alteration, 35 of 38 (92%) demonstrated an alteration that was detectable in an exfoliated saliva sample, and 12 of 13 cases with Tx or T1 disease were detected.

Other methods of preselection might be useful for selecting for neoplastic cells before LOH microsatellite analysis, including the use of antibodies that target cell surface antigens specific to tumor cells, use of fluorescent-activated cell sorting (FACS) to select aneuploid cells, or use of fluorescent *in situ* hybridization to identify cells with probable LOH followed by molecular analysis (69).

More recent studies have exploited the use of TSG promoter region cytosine hypermethylation found in head and neck and other cancers. A high density of cytosines followed by guanine in promoter regions, termed *CpG islands,* occur in a characteristic pattern unique to each gene. High-density CpG island methylation is an apparent mechanism by which transcriptional repression of TSGs is accomplished. p16 methylation was detected in primary HNSCC and cell lines and can be exploited as a method of detection for rare populations of tumor DNA. Sodium metabisulfite treatment of methylated and unmethylated CpG islands results in the conversion of unmethylated cytosines to uracil. This forms the basis for a variety of PCR-based detection assays, often termed *methylation-specific PCR,* or MSP. This technique has been used to detect methylated promoter sequences present in both saliva and serum of patients with HNSCC. Using the detection of methylated promoter sequences for *p16, MGMT,* and *DAP-kinase* genes, 65% (11/17) of patients with methylation of at least one gene in a primary HNSCC showed the identical methylation patterns in a saliva sample, with only one of 30 controls positive for methylation at two target genes (70). Forty-two percent (21/50) of serum samples from patients with MSP-detectable promoter methylation in primary HNSCC also had identical methylated DNA detected in serum (71). The advent of real-time, quantitative MSP will allow for more precise quantitation of methylated DNA present in body fluids, and may be able to provide greater accuracy for these assays.

Other phenotypic characteristics of malignant cells may also be exploited for use in detection strategies. Mammalian chromosomal ends, or *telomeres,* tend to shorten as cells age and senescence approaches. Malignant cells appear to exhibit alterations in the regulation of telomeric length, and their telomeres do not shorten to a length seen in normal cells approaching senescence and cell crisis. Telomerase, an enzyme having the capability to lengthen telomeres by adding a six-base pair unit of DNA using an RNA template, can be measured using a PCR-based assay. This assay allows theoretical measurement of telomerase activity in a neoplastic cell within thousands of normal cells. Telomerase activity is seen predominantly in cells with a malignant phenotype and can be detected in a wide variety of malignant neoplasms; however, stem cells and activated lymphocytes also express telomerase activity (72). Measurement of this enzyme activity, because of its relative specificity of expression in malignant epithelial tissues, may be an excellent marker for screening sputum and for surgical margin analysis. Use of this test for analysis of occult lymph node metastasis is severely limited by the high rate of telomerase expression in benign lymph nodes by activated B and T cells. However, preliminary studies have demonstrated that 34% of oral rinses from HNSCC patients are positive for telomerase activity, whereas only 5% of normal, control patients demonstrated telomerase activity in oral rinses (73). Rapid improvements in assay and collection techniques for body fluid samples are expected to improve both sensitivity and specificity of this test. Cloning of the telomerase gene and identification of the critical protein product necessary for telomerase function may result in the development of an antibody-based test [enzyme-linked immunosorbent assay (ELISA)] that may result in greater adaptability to a clinical setting.

Analysis of surgical margins has also proven amenable to molecular biologic techniques analogous to those outlined earlier for detection of tumor cells in body fluids. Surgical margins and lymph nodes from 25 patients were analyzed by constructing unique oligonucleotide (single-stranded DNA) probes complementary to each *p53* mutation in the primary tumor (74). This molecular analysis was able to detect occult tumor cells that could not be visualized by conventional light microscopy in apparently normal tissues. After 2 years of follow-up, all patients with negative margins by molecular analysis were alive and had a statistically significant increase in disease-free survival. Real-time molecular analysis of surgical margins may be possible by using mutational probes unique to preoperative biopsy specimens and by automating the assay. Other methods (e.g., telomerase detection) may also be used to detect occult neoplastic cells in margins or lymph node specimens, as noted previously. Analysis of surgical margins using polyclonal antibodies, including those to transcription factor eIF4e, has shown promise in determining patients at risk for recurrence (75). At the time of this writing, a large, multi-institutional Eastern Cooperative Oncology Group/Intergroup trial to determine the efficacy of molecular margin analysis has just completed accrual.

CONCLUSION AND FUTURE DIRECTIONS

Molecular biologic techniques have facilitated discovery of many of the basic mechanisms underlying the genetic basis of HNSCC. Many protooncogenes and TSGs (or TSG loci) involved in HNSCC have been identified and placed in the context of a genetic progression model. The development of HNSCC is understood to be a multistep process in which a growth advantage is acquired by the accumulation of these genetic alterations. Moreover, an evolving clonal population in the upper aerodigestive tract frequently has the capacity for lateral expansion and migration. The mechanisms by which these genetic alterations result in the phenotypic characteristics of malignancy will be elucidated with increasing clarity over the next decade.

Translational approaches using molecular genetics will become increasingly applicable in the clinical setting. Molecular biologic techniques will be used to (a) profile genetic alterations in a tumor or premalignant lesion to provide prognostic information and guide treatment options; (b) indicate which patients will be more likely to develop disease based on inherent genetic makeup; (c) screen asymptomatic, high-risk patients for occult HNSCC or premalignant disease; (d) provide clues to the etiology of occult primary disease with gross nodal involvement; (e) routinely indicate when histopathologically negative surgical margins and benign-appearing lymph nodes harbor occult disease; and (f) guide gene delivery approaches in terms of appropriate genetic targets. New technology undoubtedly will expand these approaches well beyond the applications mentioned in this chapter and result in a general and important shift toward a clinical emphasis on early detection and prevention. Our understanding of the molecular genetics of HNSCC will lead to novel molecular methods that are certain to change the way we diagnose and treat affected patients.

REFERENCES

1. Fearon ER, Vogelstein B. A genetic model for colorectal tumorigenesis. *Cell* 1990;61:759–767.
2. Renan MJ. How many mutations are required for tumorigenesis? Implications from human cancer data. *Mol Carcinog* 1993;7:139.
3. Vokes EE, Weichselbaum RR, Lippman SM, et al. Head and neck cancer. *N Engl J Med* 1993;328:184–194.
4. Vogelstein B, Fearon ER, Hamilton SR, et al. Genetic alterations during colorectal tumor development. *N Engl J Med* 1988;319:525?532.
5. Sidransky D, Mikkelsen T, Schwechheimer K, et al. Clonal expansion of p53 mutant cells is associated with brain tumor progression. *Nature* 1992;355: 846–847.
6. Simoneau AR, Jones PA. Bladder cancer: the molecular progression to invasive disease. *World J Urol* 1994;12:89–95.
7. Dalbagni G, Presti J, Reuter V, et al. Genetic alterations in bladder cancer. *Lancet* 1993;342:469–471.
8. Califano J, van der Riet P, Clayman G, et al. A genetic progression model for head and neck cancer; implications for field cancerization. *Cancer Res* 1996;56: 2488–2492.
9. Zatterstrom UK, Wennerberg J, Ewers SB. Prognostic factors in head and neck cancer: histologic grading, DNA ploidy, and nodal status. *Head Neck* 1991; 13:477.
10. Carey TE, Van Dyke DL, Worsham MJ. Nonrandom chromosome aberrations and clonal populations in head and neck cancer. *Anticancer Res* 1993;13:2561.
11. Jin Y, Mertens F, Mandahl N, et al. Chromosome abnormalities in eighty-three head and neck squamous cell carcinomas: influence of culture conditions on karyotypic pattern. *Cancer Res* 1993;53:2140.
12. Van Dyke DL, Worsham MJ, Benninger MS, et al. Recurrent cytogenetic abnormalities in squamous cell carcinomas of the head and neck region. *Genes Chromosomes Cancer* 1994;9:192–206.
13. Chromosome changes characterizing *in vitro* response to radiation in human squamous cell carcinoma lines. *Cancer Res* 1993;53:5542.
14. Voravud N, Shin DM, Ro JY, et al. Increased polysomies of chromosomes 7 and 17 during head and neck multistage tumorigenesis. *Cancer Res* 1993;53: 2874.
15. Speicher MR, Howe C, Crotty P, et al. Comparative genomic hybridization detects novel deletions and amplifications in head and neck squamous cell carcinomas. *Cancer Res* 1995;55:1010–1013.
16. Berenson JR, Yan J, Micke RA. Frequent amplification of the *bcl-1* locus in head and neck squamous carcinomas. *Oncogene* 1989;4:1111–1116.
17. Somers KD, Cartwright SL, Schechter GL. Amplification of the *int-2* gene in head and neck squamous cell carcinomas. *Oncogene* 1990;5:915–920.
18. Jares P, Fernandez PL, Campo E, et al. PRAD-1/Cyclin Dl gene amplification correlates with messenger RNA overexpression and tumor progression in human laryngeal carcinomas. *Cancer Res* 1994;54:4813–4817.
19. Bartkova J, Lukas J, Muller H, et al. Abnormal patterns of D-type cyclin expression and G, regulation in human head and neck cancer. *Cancer Res* 1995; 55:949–956.
20. Callender T, El-Nagger AK, Lee MS, et al. PRAD-1 (CCND1)/cyclin Dl oncogene amplification in primary head and neck squamous cell carcinoma. *Cancer* 1994;74:152–158.
21. Yamaguchi K, Wu L, Caballero OL, et al. Frequent gain of the p40/p51/p63 gene locus in primary head and neck squamous cell carcinoma. *Int J Cancer* 2000;86:684–689.
22. Hibi K, Trink B, Patturajan M, et al. AIS is an oncogene amplified in squamous cell carcinoma. *Proc Natl Acad Sci USA* 2000;97:5462–5467.
23. Grandis JR, Tweardy DJ. Elevated levels of transforming growth factor and epidermal growth factor alpha receptor messenger RNA are early markers of carcinogenesis in head and neck cancer. *Cancer Res* 1993;53:3579–3584.
24. Garrigue-Antar L, Munoz-Antonia T, Antonia SJ, et al. Missense mutations of the transforming growth factor beta type II receptor in human head and neck squamous carcinoma cells. *Cancer Res* 1995;55:3982–3987.
25. Knudson AG. Mutation and cancer: statistical study of retinoblastoma. *Proc Natl Acad Sci USA* 1971;68:820–823.
26. Knudson AG. Hereditary cancer, oncogene, and anti-oncogenes. *Cancer Res* 1985;45:1437–1443.
27. Hollstein M, Sidransky D, Vogelstein B, et al. p53 mutations in human cancer. *Science* 1991;253:49–53.
28. Nawroz H, van der Riet P, Hruban RH, et al. Allelotype of head and neck squamous cell carcinoma. *Cancer Res* 1994;54:1152–1155.
29. van der Riet P, Nawroz H, Hruban RH, et al. Frequent loss of chromosome 9p21-22 early in head and neck cancer progression. *Cancer Res* 1994;54: 1156–1158.
30. Kamb A, Gruis NA, Weaver-Feldhaus J, et al. A cell cycle regulator potentially involved in the genesis of many tumor types. *Science* 1994;264:436–440.
31. Hartwell LH, Kastan MB. Cell cycle control and cancer. *Science* 1994;266: 1821–1828.
32. Cairns P, Mao A, Lee D, et al. Rates of p16 (MTS1) mutations in primary tumors with 9p loss. *Science* 1994;265:415–416.
33. Merlo A, Herman JG, Mao L, et al. 5′ CpG island methylation is associated with transcriptional silencing of the tumor suppressor p16/CDKN2/MTS1 in human cancers. *Nature Med* 1995;7:686–692.
34. Cairns P, Polascik TJ, Eby Y, et al. Frequency of homozygous deletion at p16/cdkn2 in primary human tumors. *Nat Genet* 1995; 11:210–212.
35. Reed AL, Califano J, Cairns P, et al. High frequency of *p16* (CDKN2/ MTS/INK4A) inactivation in head and neck squamous cell carcinoma. *Cancer Res* 1996;56:3630–3633.
36. Papadimitrakopoulou V, Izzo J, Lippman SM, et al. Frequent inactivation of p16INK4a in oral premalignant lesions. *Oncogene* 1997;14:1799–803.
37. Mao L, Merlo A, Bedi G, et al. A novel p16INK4A transcript. *Cancer Res* 1995;55:2995–2997.
38. Boyle JO, Hakim J, Koch W, et al. The incidence of *p53* mutations increases with progression of head and neck cancer. *Cancer Res* 1994:53:4477–4480.
39. Sidransky D, Hollstein M. Clinical implications of the *p53* gene. *Ann Rev Med* 1996;47:285–301.
40. Wu CL, Sloan P, Read AP, et al. Deletion mapping on the short arm of chromosome 3 in squamous cell carcinoma of the oral cavity. *Cancer Res* 1994;54: 6484–6488.
41. Maestro R, Gasparotto D, Vuksavljevic T, et al. Three discrete regions of deletion in head and neck cancers. *Cancer Res* 1993;53:5775–5779.
42. Ohta M, Inoue H, Cotticelli MG, et al. The FHIT gene, spanning the chromosome 3p14.2 fragile site and renal carcinoma-associated t(3;8) breakpoint, is abnormal in digestive tract cancers. *Cell* 1996;84: 587–597.
43. Yoo GH, Xu HJ, Brennan JA, et al. Infrequent inactivation of the retinoblastoma gene despite frequent loss of chromosome 13q in head and neck squamous cell carcinoma. *Cancer Res* 1994;54:4603–4606.
44. Mork J, Lie AK, Glattre E, et al. Human papillomavirus infection as a risk factor for squamous-cell carcinoma of the head and neck. *N Engl J Med* 2001; 344:1125–1131.
45. Gillison ML, Koch WM, Capone RB, et al. Evidence for a causal association between human papillomavirus and a subset of head and neck cancers. *J Natl Cancer Inst* 2000;92:709–720.
46. Mendelsohn J, Baselga J. The EGF receptor family as targets for cancer therapy. *Oncogene* 2000;19:6550–6565.
47. Mao L, Lee JS, Fan YH, et al. Frequent microsatellite alterations at chromosomes 9p21 and 3p14 in oral premalignant lesions and their value in cancer risk assessment. *Nat Med* 1996;2:682–685.
48. Rosin MP, Cheng X, Poh C, et al. Use of allelic loss to predict malignant risk for low-grade oral epithelial dysplasia. *Clin Cancer Res* 2000:357–362.
49. Sudbo J, Kildal W, Risberg B, et al. DNA content as a prognostic marker in patients with oral leukoplakia. *N Engl J Med* 2001;344:1270–1278.
50. Slaughter DP, Southwick HW, Smejkal W. "Field cancerization" in oral stratified squamous epithelium: clinical implications of multicentric origin. *Cancer* 1953;6:963–968.
51. Liciardello JT, Spitz MR, Hong WK. Multiple primary cancer in patients with cancer of the head and neck: second cancer of the head and neck, esophagus, and lung. *Int J Radiat Oncol Biol Phys* 1989;17:467–476.
52. Christensen P, Joergensen K, Munk J, et al. High frequency of pulmonary cancer in a population of 415 patients treated for laryngeal cancer. *Laryngoscope* 1987;97:612–614.
53. Tepperman BS, Fitzpatrick PJ. Second respiratory and upper digestive tract cancers after oral cancer. *Lancet* 1981;2:547–549.
54. Bedi G, Westra WH, Gabrielson E, et al. Multiple head and neck tumors: evidence for a common clonal origin. *Cancer Res* 1996;56:2484–2487.
55. Chung KY, Mukhopadhyay T, Kim J, et al. Discordant *p53* mutations in primary head and neck cancer and corresponding second primary cancers of the upper aerodigestive tract. *Cancer Res* 1993;53:1676–1683.
56. Worsham MJ, Wolman SR, Carey TE, et al. Common clonal origin of synchronous primary head and neck squamous cell carcinomas. *Hum Pathol* 1995;26: 251–261.

57. Raskind WH, Norwood T, Levine DS, et al. Persistent clonal areas and clonal expansion in Barrett's esophagus. *Cancer Res* 1992;52:2946–2950.
58. Prevo LJ, Sanchez CA, Galipeau PC, et al. p53-mutant clones and field effects in Barrett's esophagus. *Cancer Res* 1999;59:4784–4787.
59. Brennan JA, Boyle JO, Koch WM, et al. Association between cigarette smoking and mutation of the *p53* gene in head and neck squamous carcinoma. *N Engl J Med* 1995;332:712–717.
60. Nishimura T, Newkirk K, Sessions RB, et al. Immunohistochemical staining for glutathione S-transferase predicts response to platinum-based chemotherapy in head and neck cancer. *Clin Cancer Res* 1996;11:1859–1865.
61. Shiga H, Heath EI, Rasmussen AA, et al. Prognostic value of p53, glutathione S-transferase pi, and thymidylate synthase for neoadjuvant cisplatin-based chemotherapy in head and neck cancer. *Clin Cancer Res* 1999;12:4097–4104.
62. Sidransky D, von Eschenbach A, Tsai YC, et al. Identification of *p53* gene mutations in bladder cancers and urine samples. *Science* 1991;252:706–709.
63. Sidransky D, Tokino T, Frost P, et al. Identification of ras oncogene mutations in the stool of patients with curable colorectal tumors. *Science* 1992;256:102–105.
64. Mao L, Hruban RH, Boyle JO, et al. Detection of oncogene mutations in sputum precedes diagnosis of lung cancer. *Cancer Res* 1994;54:1634–1637.
65. Boyle JB, Mao L, Brennan JA, et al. Gene mutations in saliva as molecular markers for head and neck squamous cell carcinoma. *Am J Surg* 1994;168: 429–432.
66. Mao L, Schoenberg MP, Schicchitano M, et al. Molecular detection of primary bladder cancer by microsatellite analysis. *Science* 1996;271:659–662.
67. Mao L, Lee DJ, Tockman MS, et al. Microsatellite alterations as clonal markers in the detection of human cancer. *Proc Natl Acad Sci USA* 1994:91:9871–9875.
68. Spafford MF, Koch WM, Reed AL, et al. Detection of head and neck squamous cell carcinoma among exfoliated oral mucosal cells by microsatellite analysis. *Clin Cancer Res* 2001;3:607–612.
69. Wirtschafter A, Benninger MS, Moss TJ, et al. Micrometastatic tumor detection in patients with head and neck cancer: a preliminary report. *Otolaryngol Head Neck Surg* 2002;128:40–43.
70. Rosas SL, Koch W, da Costa Carvalho MG, et al. Promoter hypermethylation patterns of p16, O6-methylguanine-DNA-methyltransferase, and death-associated protein kinase in tumors and saliva of head and neck cancer patients. *Cancer Res* 2001;61:939–942.
71. Sanchez-Cespedes M, Esteller M, Wu L, et al. Gene promoter hypermethylation in tumors and serum of head and neck cancer patients. *Cancer Res* 2000; 60:892–895.
72. Kim NW, Piatyszek MA, Prowse KR, et al. Specific association of human telomerase activity with immortal cells and cancer. *Science* 1994;266:2011–2015.
73. Califano J, Ahrendt S, Meininger G, et al. Detection of telomerase activity in oral rinses from head and neck squamous cell cancer patients. *Cancer Res* 1996; 56:5720–5722.
74. Brennan JA, Mao L, Hruban RH, et al. Molecular assessment of histopathologic staging. *N Engl J Med* 1995;332:429–435.
75. Nathan C, Franklin S, Abreo FW, et al. Analysis of surgical margins with the molecular marker eIF4E: a prognostic factor in patients with head and neck cancer. *J Clin Oncol* 1999;17:2909–2914.

CHAPTER 37

Molecular Epidemiology and Genetic Predisposition for Head and Neck Cancer

Margaret R. Spitz, Erich M. Sturgis, and Qingyi Wei

Tobacco and alcohol exposures are the major determinants of head and neck squamous cell carcinomas (HNSCC). Blot et al. (1) estimate that tobacco use and alcohol consumption combine to account for approximately three fourths of all oral and pharyngeal cancers in the United States. However, only a fraction of exposed individuals will develop neoplastic lesions, and the role of genetic susceptibility to carcinogenic exposures must be factored into the risk assessment process. This chapter will explore some of the host factors that modulate intrinsic susceptibility to the genetic damage from these carcinogenic exposures.

DESCRIPTIVE EPIDEMIOLOGY

Worldwide, head and neck cancers account for about 6% of incident cancers or about 413,000 cases annually in men and 138,000 in women (2). In the United States in 2003, head and neck cancers will account for an estimated 2.8% of incident cancers and 2.0% of fatal cancers (3). These U.S. statistics represent 37,200 new cases and 11,000 deaths annually (3). For all stages combined, the 5-year relative survival rates for oral and pharyngeal cancers and laryngeal cancers are 56% and 64%, respectively.

SECOND PRIMARY TUMORS

A unique characteristic of HNSCCs is their high predilection for the development of second primary tumors (SPTs). These patients face an annual risk for 4% to 7% of developing a potentially fatal SPT (4–7); and the risk for developing an SPT does not decrease over time (6,8).

Cooper et al. (6) show that the highest risk for SPTs occurs in patients with the earliest stage of disease, reflecting the shorter survival time of patients with advanced stage disease. A meta-analysis of 24 studies of SPTs reports an overall rate of 14.2% (9). A population-based study suggests higher risk among patients younger than 60 years (10). In a large series of more than 3,000 patients with head and neck cancers, the median time to presentation of a second tumor was 36 months with higher risk in patients who were younger than 60 years at initial diagnosis (11).

The incidence and distribution of second cancers varies by primary tumor site, from 10% for glottic tumors to 40% in oropharyngeal primary tumors (12). About 60% of SPTs occur in the aerodigestive tract (lung, 30%; head and neck, 20%; esophagus, 8%) (13). Licciardello et al. (14) note that oral cavity cancer appears to be associated more often with subsequent head and neck SPTs and that laryngeal cancers appear so with lung SPTs.

The development of these SPTs is a consequence of field cancerization, a concept initially proposed by Slaughter et al. in 1953 (15). His concept suggested that multiple neoplastic lesions of independent origin occurred within an epithelial field in response to chronic tobacco and alcohol exposures in combination with endogenous processes (e.g., carcinogen metabolism, repair capability, inherent genetic instability). This process places whole tissue fields at increased cancer risk. Continuing carcinogen exposure leads to the accumulation of genetic damage throughout the tissue. When proliferation occurs (accentuated in association with wound healing), unrepaired DNA damage is turned into permanent genetic changes (e.g., mutations, deletions, rearrangements, loss and gain of chromosome regions, gene amplification). When specific gene regions that are functionally important for selection are altered (i.e., render cells resistant to apoptosis or differentiation, give a proliferative or survival advantage), clonal outgrowths occur throughout the field and may be clinically evident as premalignant lesions. Continued genomic change in the outgrowing clones increases their neoplastic potential.

The documentation of discordant *p53* mutations in the primary tumor and corresponding SPTs in the head and neck suggests that these cancers arise as independent events (16). Furthermore, it has been demonstrated that expression of mutated *p53* occurs in epithelia distant from the tumor, with different mutations in multiple foci, providing further molecular explanation for this concept (17). The finding of polysomies on chromosomes 7 and 17 in histologically normal epithelium adjacent to the tumor, with an increase in frequency of polysomy as tissues progress from hyperplasia to dysplasia to cancer also supports the concepts of field cancerization and multistep carcinogenesis (18).

Current local and systemic anticancer approaches are not effective against the field or multifocal cancerization processes (13). Therefore, SPTs represent a major threat to patients with early stage disease (12,14,19,20). As diagnostic and therapeutic procedures continue to improve, it is likely that the problem of second cancers will assume even greater relevance.

To detect SPTs early and successfully treat them, careful clinical surveillance is necessary. The role of chemopreventive agents, including retinoids, in prevention of SPTs is under intense investigation and with great potential (21). Thus, the ability to identify those patients at high risk for SPT development with initial HNSCC has clinical and prognostic relevance.

TOBACCO EXPOSURES

Tobacco and alcohol exposures are clearly the major determinants of these cancers, and both prospective and retrospective studies worldwide have consistently demonstrated that tobacco exposure is associated with a dose–response increase in risk for these cancers (22–26). Heavy smokers have risks 5- to 25-fold higher than those of nonsmokers (22). In our own experience at the M. D. Anderson Cancer Center, cancer risk increases linearly among men with each successive pack-year stratum from 1.8 to 4.0 to 7.5 in the heaviest smokers (23). For women, the corresponding risks were 1.5, 9.0, and 12.0.

Few prior studies have convincingly studied the impact of smoking cessation on risk for SPTs. Castigliano (27) and Schottenfeld et al. (28) report no clear benefit from such cessation after cancer diagnosis. However, the studies of Moore (29) and Silverman et al. (30) did suggest a reduced risk for SPTs among persons who stopped smoking after diagnosis of the index cancer. A population-based survey (31) of 1,090 patients with oral or pharyngeal cancer incorporated a nested case-control study design and documented significant associations between baseline tobacco and alcohol use and risk for SPTs and a dose–response relationship with intensity and duration of smoking. Current smokers at diagnosis of the index tumor experienced a fourfold increased risk for developing SPTs compared with nonsmokers and former smokers. Risk reduction was evident only after 5 years of smoking cessation following the index diagnosis. Two hospital-based studies report similar findings (32,33).

We recently reviewed data from a randomized, placebo-controlled chemoprevention trial of 1,181 patients with early stage head and neck cancer, evaluating the efficacy of low-dose 13-cis retinoic acid (13cRA) in reducing risk for SPTs. With a median follow-up time since randomization of 3.7 years (ranging between 0.1 and 7.6 years), there were 200 (16.9%) patients diagnosed with an SPT. Continued smoking and alcohol intake after the index diagnosis are factors that both emerge as simultaneous significant predictors of SPT development. There was a twofold increase in risk for SPT for patients currently smoking at randomization. There was a 16% increase in risk for SPT for every 10 years of smoking exposure and an 11% increase in risk for greater than 20 pack-years of smoking.

Molecular Genetic Changes Caused by Cigarette Smoking

Mutations in the *p53* tumor suppressor gene are the most common genetic alterations identified in human cancer. Distinct differences in the mutational frequency and type are found in different tumor types and are attributed in part to the effects of specific mutagens. The occurrence of *p53* mutations has been associated with a history of heavy smoking (34,35). Generally the frequency of *p53* mutations in head and neck cancer is similar to that for lung cancer (36), although the mutational spectrum may differ. *p53* mutations have been reported to occur less frequently in older patients and in patients with lower levels of tobacco exposure (37).

Most smoking-related mutations are transversions at GC base pairs, with about three-fourths being G to T transversions (34). Experimental studies have indicated that bulky polycyclic aromatic hydrocarbon (PAH) compounds like benzo[*a*]pyrene (B[*a*]P) induce such transversions (38). Brennan et al. (39) found mutations in 58% of 64 patients with HNSCC who smoked and used alcohol, compared with only 17% in those who were exposed to neither. The most common mutations were GCAT (31%) and GCTA (21%). In nonsmokers, mutations were at sites containing cytidine phosphate guanosine (CpG) dinucleotides (possibly representing endogenous mutations).

Cigar and Pipe Smoking

Although smokers of cigars and pipes tend to inhale smoke less than do cigarette smokers (as reflected in their lower carboxyhemoglobin levels compared with those of cigarette smokers), they are at risk for the development of oral, oropharyngeal, hypopharyngeal, and laryngeal cancers (40). The risk estimates tend to approximate those of cigarette smokers for buccal cavity but not pharyngeal malignancies (41). For laryngeal cancers, Wynder et al. (42) demonstrate a 12-fold increase in risk associated with cigar and pipe smoking compared with nonusers. Data on cigar use from the American Cancer Society's Cancer Prevention Study II cohort document significantly increased risk for mortality from both oropharyngeal cancers [relative risk (RR) < 4.0, 1.5, 10.3] and laryngeal cancers (RR < 10.3, 2.6, 41.0) (43).

Other Tobacco Products

The Advisory Committee to the Surgeon General on the Health Consequences of Smokeless Tobacco concluded that "the evidence is strong that the use of snuff can cause cancer in humans" and that "the evidence for causality is strongest for cancer of the oral cavity" (44). The committee also cited an almost 50-fold elevated risk for cheek and gum cancers in long-term snuff users. Snuff use has been implicated in the etiology of oral cavity cancer and to a lesser extent, pharyngeal cancers

(23,45). One study documented a fourfold elevated risk for oral and pharyngeal cancer in white women who used snuff; a strong dose–response relationship was also found (46). The major carcinogens identified in snuff are polonium-210 and tobacco-specific nitrosamines (47). The Advisory Committee noted that "smokeless tobacco is responsible for the development of a portion of oral leukoplakias in both teenage and adult users" (44).

Environmental Tobacco Smoke

Passive smoking exposure has also been considered to be a risk factor for these cancers (48). A recent high-profile legal case in Australia has brought significant interest in risk for HNSCC secondary to environmental tobacco smoke exposure. In May 2001 the New South Wales Supreme Court ruled that a 62-year-old nonsmoker developed HNSCC secondary to long-term exposure to environmental tobacco smoke in her job as a bar attendant (49,50). Two case-control studies supported the Court's ruling. In a study of 173 cases of HNSCC and 176 cancer-free controls, environmental tobacco smoke was associated with an increased risk for HNSCC [adjusted risk estimate or odds ratio (OR) < 2.4, (0.9–6.8)], and a dose–response relationship was also observed (OR < 2.1 and 3.6 for moderate and heavy exposures, respectively) (48). In a separate study of 44 nonsmokers with HNSCC and 132 cancer-free nonsmoker controls, environmental tobacco smoke was associated with a significantly increased risk for HNSCC (OR < 5.3), and this was particularly true for women (OR < 8.0) and for those reporting exposure at work (OR < 10.2) (51).

MARIJUANA

Marijuana use results in a greater tar burden to the respiratory tract than does a comparable cigarette; marijuana smoke and cigarette smoke are quantitatively similar. However, few reports have found direct evidence of marijuana as an etiologic factor of HNSCC because most users of marijuana are also exposed to tobacco and alcohol (52). While anecdotal evidence has long suggested marijuana as a risk factor for HNSCC (53), a case-control study including 173 patients and 176 controls noted a cigarette-adjusted risk for 2.6 (1.1, 6.6) associated with marijuana use, with evidence of a dose–response relationship (54). However, a large retrospective cohort of 64,855 health maintenance organization (HMO) members found no association with tobacco-related cancers (55). Marijuana smoking might be postulated to have a greater carcinogenic effect on the head and neck than on the lower airways, especially in light of the rapid deep inhalation used in smoking the product.

ALCOHOL

Cohort and case-control studies have consistently demonstrated increased risks for cancers of the oropharynx and larynx related to alcohol consumption (56–60). The separate effects of alcohol and tobacco have been difficult to distinguish because the two lifestyle choices are so closely correlated. An interaction between tobacco smoking and alcohol has been demonstrated consistently in head and neck cancers. This interaction appears to be multiplicative for laryngeal cancers (56). The degree of interaction for oral and pharyngeal cancers is more variable. The role of alcohol in risk for oral leukoplakia has been less extensively studied, and the results have not always been consistent (60–63).

Several studies have investigated the effect of alcohol exposure on the risk for SPT development. Alcohol has been considered to be a cofactor (63,64) or an independent risk factor for SPT development in cancers of the oral cavity or for all three sites: oral cavity, pharynx, and larynx (31,65). Baseline alcohol consumption was also associated with increased risk, and there was a suggestion of a multiplicative influence of smoking and alcohol with the effects of smoking being more pronounced (31).

DIET

Several epidemiologic studies have observed a 20% to 80% risk reduction associated with increased consumption of fruits and vegetables (24,66–71). High intake of micronutrients, including vitamin C, β-carotene, other carotenoids, and vitamin A, has been associated with reduced risk for oral and laryngeal cancers (71,72). Nomura et al. (67) used a prospective study with nested case-control design to confirm that α-carotene, β-carotene, β-cryptoxanthin, total carotenoids, and γ-tocopherol levels were significantly lower in patients with HNSCC than controls, after adjustment for smoking and alcohol intake. The role of diet–gene interactions in risk for smoking-related cancers is also an area of considerable interest (73). Considerable laboratory and epidemiologic evidence suggests that carotenoids act as dietary inhibitors of epithelial carcinogenesis. In early epidemiologic investigations of the association between vitamin A and cancer, the form of vitamin A consumed (preformed or as provitamin A carotenoids) was not distinguished.

Several case comparison investigations of dietary factor studies have been conducted in head and neck cancers. Tavani et al. (74) report that a low intake of β-carotene was associated with an increased risk for laryngeal cancer. Mackerras et al. (72) report an inverse association between carotene intake and laryngeal cancer. Marshall et al. (75) note that the risk for oral cancer was inversely associated with intake of total vitamin A and vitamin C. Men who consumed more than 3,736 IU per day of vitamin A had decreased risks of cancers of the mouth (OR < 0.65) and larynx (OR < 0.54) (76,77) after adjustment for age, smoking, and alcohol intake, compared with men who consumed less vitamin A (<2,209 IU/day). In a hospital-based case-control study in Beijing, Zheng et al. (68) found an inverse relationship between risk for oral cancer and dietary intake of total carotene, carotene intake from fruit and vegetables, and vitamin C intake. In a population-based case-control study in Shanghai, Zheng et al. (69) report a protective effect of intake of dark green and yellow vegetables, citrus fruit, and garlic against laryngeal cancer. A nested case-control study by Zheng et al. (78) confirm the inverse association between serum carotenoids (especially β-carotene) and α-tocopherol and cancer risk. A consistent protective effect was noted for each of the individual carotenoids, including β-carotene, cryptoxanthin, lutein, and lycopene. Current use of salted meat in Uruguay reported by De Stefani et al. (79) was associated with a twofold increased risk for oral and pharyngeal cancer, whereas vegetable consumption was associated with a 60% reduction in risk. In a study of 871 cases in four different areas of the United States, a protective effect of fruit consumption for oral and pharyngeal cancer was present in a dose–response manner (71).

Two large-scale intervention trials in heavy smokers however have shown possible adverse effects from β-carotene supplementation. The Alpha-Tocopherol, Beta-Carotene Lung Cancer Prevention Trial (80) showed an 18% increase in lung cancer and an 8% increase in deaths in the β-carotene arm. Investigators in the Beta-Carotene and Retinol Efficacy Trial (CARET) have noted a 28% increase in lung cancer in the β-carotene arm and a 17% higher mortality rate (81). There are no comparable data on head and neck cancer. Chemoprevention issues in HNSCC are addressed in Chapter 40.

Few studies have evaluated possible interactions between cigarette smoking and dietary factors. De Stefani et al. (82) suggest that tobacco use and low fruit intake exerted a synergistic effect in laryngeal cancer risk. A study in Texas reports that carotene exerted its protective effect among smokers who had stopped smoking 2 to 10 years previously (72). Zheng et al. (70) present data from a case-control study in China reporting that the combined effects of smoking and diet were more than additive. In the serologic investigations of Zheng et al. (78), adjustment for smoking resulted in slight attenuation of the protective associations with carotenoids. No prospective studies have comprehensively addressed how the separate and combined effects of smoking, alcohol, and diet affect the risk for SPTs.

LARYNGOPHARYNGEAL REFLUX DISEASE

Observational and anecdotal studies have long suggested that gastroesophageal reflux may be associated with laryngeal cancer (83,84). Furthermore, multiple studies have objectively documented a high prevalence of gastric reflux into the laryngopharynx by 24-hour pH probe monitoring (85–87). Recently, a retrospective case-control study of 10,140 hospitalized patients and 12,061 outpatients with laryngeal and pharyngeal cancer and 40,560 hospitalized and 48,244 outpatient controls was performed using computerized hospital and outpatient databases of the U.S. Department of Veterans Affairs (88). The diagnosis of gastroesophageal reflux disease was associated with a significantly elevated risk for laryngeal cancer after adjusting for age, sex, ethnicity, smoking, and alcohol (OR < 2.40 [2.15–2.69] and OR < 2.31 [2.10–2.53] for hospitalized and outpatient groups, respectively) and of pharyngeal cancer (OR < 2.38 [1.87–3.02] and OR < 1.92 [1.72–2.15] for hospitalized and outpatient groups, respectively).

HUMAN PAPILLOMA VIRUS INFECTION

Others have suggested that human papilloma virus (HPV) is an etiologic agent in HNSCC (89,90). Laboratory evidence supporting the role of HPV as a risk factor for HNSCC is largely circumstantial. *In vitro* experiments support the tumorigenicity of HPV types 16 and 18 in human epithelial cells, and HPV-16 and 18 viral oncoproteins E6 and E7 can inhibit *p53* function. Furthermore, HPV-16 DNA is consistently identified in HNSCC tumors using polymerase chain reaction assays. Oropharyngeal tumors and tumors in nonsmokers are the most frequently positive (91,92). Molecular epidemiologic evidence with case-control design supporting the role of HPV16 in HNSCC has been scant (93,94). However, a recent nested case-control study of 218 patients with HNSCC and 1,165 cancer-free controls demonstrated HPV-16 seropositivity to be associated with a significantly increased risk for HNSCC (adjusted OR < 2.6; [1.7–4.2]) (95).

OTHER RISK FACTORS

The evidence supporting an association between laryngeal cancer and asbestos exposure is fairly substantial, although few studies have effectively controlled for the confounding effect of tobacco exposures. These studies have been extensively reviewed (22,96), and they document RRs ranging from 1.4 to 15.0. A detailed review of this exposure and other occupation risk factors is beyond the scope of this chapter.

GENETIC SUSCEPTIBILITY

Familial Aggregation of Head and Neck Squamous Cell Carcinoma

Epidemiologic studies of familial aggregation of head and neck cancer have provided indirect evidence for the role of genetic predisposition. Foulkes et al. (97) report that the adjusted RR was 3.79 (1.11–13.0) for developing HNSCC in first-degree relatives of patients compared with the first-degree relatives of patients' spouses, and 7.89 (1.50–41.6) in first-degree relatives of patients with multiple HNSCC. A case-control study from Brazil also suggested that family history of cancer was a risk factor for HNSCC (98). A weak familial aggregation of oral and pharynx cancers was observed by Goldstein et al. (99). Other studies have also supported a familial association for HNSCC (100–102).

Metabolic Polymorphisms

The internal dose of tobacco carcinogens to which the head and neck tissue is exposed is modulated by genetic polymorphisms in enzymes responsible for activation and detoxification of these carcinogens. These polymorphisms, although generally associated with low risks for cancer, are frequent in the population (>1% allelic frequency), and therefore the attributable risks may be high. In this chapter, we will focus on select genes and pathways that are involved in the metabolism of tobacco carcinogens such as arylamines, N-nitrosamines, PAHs, and B[a]P. A comprehensive review is beyond the scope of this chapter.

Cytochrome P450 (CYP)1A1, the gene that codes for aryl hydrocarbon hydroxylase (AHH), initiates a multienzyme pathway that activates PAHs, including B[*a*]P, to highly electrophilic metabolites. Aryl hydrocarbon hydroxylase activity levels vary by up to several thousand-fold between tissues and between individuals (103). A higher prevalence of extensive metabolizers has been reported for oral, pharyngeal and larynx cancer patients (104,105) than in control subjects.

Sequencing of the *CYP1A1* gene (106,107) identified two polymorphisms that seem to have functional relevance. A restriction fragment-length polymorphism (RFLP) in the 3′ noncoding region of the gene after MspI digestion that results from a single base pair change is thought to affect *CYP1A1* mRNA stability. The polymorphism has been associated with oral cavity cancer risk in Japanese populations (108,109). Individuals with the susceptible *CYP1A1* genotype contracted smoking-induced cancers at lower levels of cigarette use than did those with other *CYP1A1* genotypes (110). Increased risk for HNSCC was also reported in two Caucasian cohorts (111,112). The prevalence of the m^2 allele ranges between 0.05 and 0.30 (113,114).

The A/G mutation on exon 7 results in a Ile/Val amino acid change (115) and is associated with elevated activity of the CYP1A1 enzyme (116). The risk genotype has a prevalence between 0.02 and 0.05 in healthy subjects in the U.S. (113). A significant association has been reported between this genotype and pharyngeal, but not oral or laryngeal cancers in Japanese populations (117,118). A study of HNSCC in a Caucasian population also reported an association (119).

A *CYP2D6 polymorphism* originally described by Ayesh et al. (120) has also been evaluated as a risk factor. CYP2D6 metabolizes a wide range of nitrogen-containing drugs, and also the tobacco-specific nitrosoamine, 4-(methylnitrosamine)-1-(3-pyridyl)-1-butanone (NNK), to mutagenic products (121). The case-control results for phenotypic status have been mixed (122,123). With genotyping (124), null alleles, slow metabolizing alleles, and a rare, ultra-rapid allele have been described. A polymorphism of the gene affects 5% to 10% of the Caucasian population (125). Agundez et al. (126) recently report a significantly increased frequency of the gene duplication in patients with laryngeal cancer. Worrall et al. (127) report an association with oral cancers only. Others found no excess risk (112,128).

CYP2E1 metabolizes benzene, N-nitrosamines, and other low-molecular-weight compounds and is readily inducible. A 50-fold variation in enzymatic activity has been observed. Two RFLPs (Rsa1 and Dra1) have been suggested as genetic risk markers, and significant ethnic differences in the distribution of allele frequencies have also been documented (129), with very low prevalences in Caucasians. Six studies have reported on risk for HNSCC with an approximately twofold increased risk associated with the c2 homozygous or heterozygous genotype in some (130–132), but not other studies (112, 116) for the *Rsa1* polymorphism. Only one study that evaluated the *Dra1* polymorphism reported an increased risk (132).

Glutathione S-transferases (GSTs) catalyze the conjugation of glutathione to several electrophilic compounds, including carcinogenic polycyclic aromatic hydrocarbons and cytotoxic drugs. Such conjugated xenobiotics are rendered harmless, and their excretion is enhanced (133). The presence or absence of the *GSTM1* gene constitutes the polymorphism and the lack of *GSTM1* (*GSTM1* < null genotype) affects approximately 50% of the Caucasian population (134). There is a 98% to 100% correlation between phenotyping and genotyping for *GSTM1* (135).

London et al. (136) performed a fairly comprehensive review of published phenotyping and genotyping studies on the *GSTM1* polymorphism and noted that stronger associations for lung cancer have been reported with phenotyping assay studies with a summary OR of 2.17 (1.61, 2.92). On the other hand, the summary OR for the genotyping studies was only 1.29 (1.09, 1.52). Much of the variation in the ORs from these studies resulted from differences in the proportion of the null genotypes among cases, and to confounding by age, race, sex, or smoking.

The *glutathione S-transferase theta (GSTT1)* gene has somewhat high activity toward epoxy and peroxide compounds (137). GSTT1 is important in the detoxification of naturally occurring monohalomethanes as well as the industrial compounds dichloromethane and aryl epoxides such as B[*a*]P found in tobacco (138). Approximately 60% to 70% of the human population are able to carry out this conjugative reaction ("conjugators"), whereas the remaining 30% to 40% are "nonconjugators." The conjugation is detoxifying with regard to monohalomethanes and ethylene oxide, but conjugation of dihalomethanes to formaldehyde yields a genotoxic intermediate (138).

In a frequency-matched case-control study of 162 patients with HNSCC and 315 cancer-free controls, *GSTM1* null and *GSTT1* null genotypes were both associated with significantly increased risk for HNSCC (adjusted OR < 1.50 [1.01–2.23] and 2.27 [1.43–3.60], respectively) (139). Having both risk genotypes was more than a threefold increased risk (OR < 3.64 (1.94–6.84). These findings confirm a previous study of 105 consecutive patients with HNSCC and 99 age- and sex-matched control subjects (140) that also reported elevated risk (above threefold) in the presence of the combined risk genotypes. Geisler and Olshan (141) recently published a review of 24 studies evaluating the risk for head and neck cancers in relation to the *GSTM1* and *GSTT1* null genotypes. They concluded that the results were inconsistent with some reporting weak or moderate associations and others reporting no association.

The *N-acetylation polymorphism* segregates individuals into rapid, intermediate, and slow acetylator phenotypes through monogenic inheritance of the *NAT2* locus. Approximately 40% to 70% of Caucasians are of the "slow acetylator" phenotype and are less efficient in the metabolism of agents containing primary aromatic amine or hydrazine groups (142). Rapid acetylation has been implicated as a risk factor for colon carcinoma.

The presence of two germline copies of any of several mutant alleles of the *NAT2* gene produces a slow acetylation phenotype (142,143). Drozdz et al. (144) report that of 120 patients with laryngeal cancer, 84% were slow acetylators, but only 60% of the control group were slow acetylators ($p < 0.001$). Gonzalez et al. (128) and Katoh et al. (145) also report that slow NAT2 activity was a risk factor. However, a recent study of 291 cases and 300 controls showed no significant differences in distribution of the fast acetylator alleles between cases and controls (146).

EPOXIDE HYDROLASE

The *mEPHX* gene is located on the long arm of chromosome 1 and is involved in detoxification reactions in which reactive compounds are converted into more water-soluble products. This cleavage is accomplished by the addition of water to a range of alkenes and arene oxides to form trans-dihydrodiols (147). Although the products of hydrolysis are less reactive than the parent epoxide, the resultant diol is sometimes a precursor to a more carcinogenic form; thus hydrolysis is not strictly a detoxification pathway (148). The *mEPHX* gene has been implicated in the metabolism of B[*a*]P. There are four *mEPHX* alleles, resulting from the presence or absence of two point mutations in the gene. On one allele, termed the "slow allele," tyrosine is replaced by histidine at residue 113 because C has been substituted for T with a 40% to 50% decrease in the enzyme activity (149). In another allele, termed the "fast allele," arginine replaces histidine at residue 139 because G has been substituted for A, with a 25% increase in enzyme activity (149,150). The third allele is the wild-type allele, which has no substitutions. The fourth allele has two mutations, one at residue 113 and the other at residue 139. The enzyme activity is normal in both cases (150). Smith and Harrison report that some individuals with particularly slow mEPHX activity (homozygotes) may be more susceptible to emphysema than those with more rapid activity (150). Thus, these polymorphic sites could also play a role in the etiology of smoking-related cancers. In fact, in a small case-control study of smoking-related cancers, Heckbert et al. (148) report a moderate protective effect of high or intermediate enzyme activity in heaviest smokers. Intermediate- and high-activity genotypes have been implicated in risk for laryngeal and oropharyngeal cancers (151). Janot et al. (152) report that epoxide hydrolase was significantly less expressed in head and neck tumors than it was in corresponding adjacent tissue.

ALCOHOL DEHYDROGENASE

Ethanol is oxidized by alcohol dehydrogenase (ADH) to acetaldehyde that has mutagenic properties. Human ADH exists as a group of enzymes placed into five classes based on structural and functional distinctions. ADH3 is polymorphic and enzymes encoded by *ADH31* allele metabolize ethanol faster that those with the *ADH32* allele (153). Harty et al. (154) found that compared with nondrinkers with ADH31-1, drinkers with the *ADH31-1*, *ADH31-2*, and *ADH32-2* genotypes had oral cancer risks of 40.1, 7.0, and 4.4, respectively. A small study in France similarly found that the *ADH31-1* was associated with increased risks for oropharyngeal and laryngeal cancers (155). A study in Japanese alcoholics found significantly higher frequencies of the mutant *ALDH-2* allele in alcoholics with HNSCC (52.9%) compared with cancer-free alcoholics (9%) (156). However in the largest study to date (229 patients and 575 controls), Sturgis et al. found no association between *ADH3* genotype and HNSCC risk (157). It is also of interest that ADH isoenzymes are capable of metabolizing retinol to retinoic acid, which controls a nuclear receptor signaling pathway and is a pleiotrophic regulator of gene expression (158).

That head and neck cancer is caused by a single explanatory gene–environmental interaction is unlikely; one marker may not have a strong effect but in conjunction with other genes may shift the risk profile in an unfavorable direction. Multiple polymorphisms must be accounted for in large, well-powered studies, to assess the true dimensions of gene–environmental interactions. McWilliams et al. found no significant relationships with *CYP1A1, GSTM1, T1* or the *p53* codon 72 polymorphism, but their study comprised only 160 cases (159). Olshan et al. (160) published data on 182 patients, but none of the markers (*GSTM1, GSTT1, GSTP1, NAT1*) achieved statistical significance.

Mutagen Sensitivity as a Marker of Risk

In vitro chromosomal analyses also have been used to study individual sensitivity to genotoxicity and cancer risk. In a cohort study of 3,182 workers occupationally exposed to mutagenic agents and evaluated for chromosomal aberrations at entry into the study, Hagmar et al. (161) report a statistically significant increase in cancer risk (RR < 2.1) in the highest stratum of baseline aberrations. Studies such as this confirm the value of using chromosomal aberrations in peripheral lymphocytes as markers of cancer risk.

Hsu et al. (162) developed a mutagen sensitivity assay based on the quantification of bleomycin-induced chromatid breaks in cultured lymphocytes to measure human susceptibility to environmental carcinogens. We demonstrated in case-control analysis that in vitro bleomycin-induced mutagen sensitivity (either as a continuous or dichotomous variable) is an independent risk factor for head and neck cancers, after adjustment for tobacco and alcohol use, with an adjusted OR of 2.5 (163,164).

A multicenter meta-analysis of three case-control studies of head and neck cancers (165) including ours cited previously confirmed this finding, demonstrating that there were no differences across institutions in the distribution of mutagen sensitivity and that age and use of tobacco and alcohol did not influence the mutagen sensitivity values. Heavy smoking in the absence of the hypersensitive phenotype posed a risk of 11.5 (5.0, 26.6). In heavy smokers who also exhibited mutagen hypersensitivity, the OR was 44.6 (17.4, 114).

This assay has been extended using B[*a*]P as the challenge mutagen. In a case-control analysis of benzo[a]pyrene diol epoxide (BPDE)-induced mutagen sensitivity and the risk for HNSCC (166), BPDE-induced chromosome breaks per cell were significantly higher in cases (n < 60) than in controls (n < 112). On multivariate analysis, BPDE-induced break per cell value was an independent risk factor for disease, with a dose–response between BPDE-induced break per cell values and risk for HNSCC. As would be expected of a phenotypic marker of genetic susceptibility, there was no significant difference among cases based on stage, site of disease, or treatment status. BDPE sensitivity and bleomycin sensitivity have a joint effect on risk for oral premalignant lesions. The underlying mechanism for mutagen sensitivity associated with cancer proneness likely reflects more than an altered repair process. However, we do not know how mutagen sensitivity as measured in lymphocytes reflects the repair capacity in the target tissue.

The host cell reactivation (HCR) assay measures the expression level of a damaged reporter gene as a marker of repair proficiency in the host cell (167). This assay uses undamaged cells, is relatively fast, and is an objective way of measuring repair. In the assay, a damaged non-replicating recombinant plasmid (pCMVcat) harboring a chloramphenicol acetyltransferase reporter gene is introduced by transfection into primary lymphocytes. Reactivated chloramphenicol acetyltransferase enzyme activity is measured as a function of nucleotide excision repair of the damaged bacterial gene. Both lymphocytes (168) and skin fibroblasts (169) from patients who have basal cell carcinoma but not xeroderma pigmentosum (XP) have lower excision repair rates of an ultraviolet-damaged reporter gene than individuals without cancer. These findings suggest that the repair capacity of lymphocytes can be considered a reflection of an individual's overall repair capacity. Using this assay, it has been demonstrated that the DNA repair capacity of HNSCC cases (n < 55) was significantly lower than that of the controls (n < 61; 8.6% vs. 12.4%, $p < 0.001$) (170). Two cell lines studies have both shown that reduced cellular DNA repair capacity was significantly correlated with increased frequency of mutagen-induced chromatid breaks (171,172).

DNA Repair Gene Polymorphisms

Genetic polymorphisms of DNA repair genes may also contribute to variation in DNA repair capacity. BPDE-induced DNA damage is effectively removed by the nucleotide excision repair (NER) pathway that involves at least 20 genes (173). The entire coding regions of several DNA repair genes on chromosome 19 [i.e., three NER genes (*ERCC1, XPD/ERCC2,* and *XPF/ERCC4*), one recombinant repair (RCR) gene (*XRCC3*), and one base excision repair (BER) gene (*XRCC1*)], have been resequenced in 12 normal individuals (174). Of these, 7 variants of *ERCC1*, 17 of *XPD/ERCC2*, 6 of *XPF/ERCC4*, 4 of *XRCC3*, and 12 of *XRCC1* were identified. Among these variants, 4 variants of *XPD/ERCC2*, 3 variants of *XRCC1*, 1 variant of *XRCC3* and one variant of *XPF/ERCC4* resulted in an amino acid change. Later, another 6 variants of *XPF/ERCC4* were identified in 38 individuals (175), 2 variants of *XPA* and 2 *XPB/ERCC3* were identified in 35 individuals, and 1 variant of *XPC* was identified (176). Although the significance of these variants is largely unknown, the implication is that variants that cause amino acid substitutions may have an impact on the function of the proteins and therefore on efficiency of DNA repair. Those variants that do not cause an amino acid change may also have an impact on the DNA repair function because they may cause mRNA instability or may be linked to genetic changes in other unknown genes (177) and therefore may affect risk for environmentally induced cancer.

ERCC1

ERCC1 is a 5′ incision subunit. It has 10 exons of 15.3 kb located in chromosome 19q 13.2-13.3. Seven polymorphisms of *ERCC1* have been identified; none of which result in an amino acid change, but one in the 3′ untranslated region (3′ UTR) is thought to affect mRNA stability (174). A recent study found that this polymorphism was not associated with head and neck cancer (178).

XPC

XPC participates in binding damaged DNA as complex. It has 15 exons located on chromosome 3p25. *XPC* has a newly identified

TABLE 37.1 DNA Repair Genotypes and Risk for Head and Neck Squamous Cell Carcinoma (SCCHN)

Genotype	Cases	Controls	p Value
XPD/ERCC2 35931			
Number	189	496	
CC genotype	16.4%	11.5%	0.086
Adjusted OR (95% CI)	1.55 (0.96–2.52)		
XRCC1 28152			
Number	203	424	
AA genotype	15.8%	10.8%	0.083
Adjusted OR (95% CI)	1.59 (0.97–2.61)		
XPC-polyAT			
Number	287	311	
XPC-polyAT +/+	17.4%	11.9%	0.056
Adjusted OR (95% CI)	1.85 (1.12–3.05)		
XRCC3 18067			
Number	238	205	
TT genotype	15.6%	9.8%	0.070
Adjusted OR (95% CI)	1.70 (0.95–3.05)		

CI, confidence interval; OR, odds ratio.

insertion/deletion variant in intron 9 that is thought to cause alternative splicing and has been shown to be in linkage disequilibrium with a single nucleotide polymorphism (SNP) in exon 15 (176). Recently, in a study of 287 cases and 311 controls, we reported that the *XPC*-PAT+ allele was associated with significantly increased risk for head and neck cancers (Table 37.1) (179).

XPD/ERCC2

XPD/ERCC2 protein is an evolutionarily conserved helicase, a subunit of transcription factor IIH (TFIIH) that is essential for transcription and NER (180). *XPD/ERCC2* has 23 exons of 54.3 kb located in chromosome 19q 13.2-13.3. Mutations in *XPD* prevent its protein from interacting with p44, another subunit of TFIIH (181), and cause decreased helicase activity, resulting in a defect in NER. Mutations at different sites result in distinct clinical phenotypes (182). For instance, mutations at different sites in *XPD* result in three distinct clinical phenotypes, XP, trichothiodystrophy, and XP combined with Cockayne syndrome. There are six variants of *XPD/ERCC2*, two of which result in an amino acid change (*Asp312Asn* and *Lys751Gln*) and one of which is a silent mutation (156Arg) (174). Six polymorphisms of the coding region of the *XPD/ERCC2* gene have been identified (174). We found the *C22541A, C23047G*, and *C23051T* polymorphisms of *XPD/ERCC2* were not of significant influence on HNSCC risk (183,184). However, the 35931CC genotype was significantly more common in 189 patients with HNSCC than 496 cancer-free control subjects (Table 37.1) (183). This genotype was associated with borderline increased risk after adjustment for age, sex, smoking, and alcohol. The *C23591A* allele was also associated with a borderline risk for HNSCC (178).

XPF/ERCC4

XPF/ERCC4 is a 5′ incision subunit, with 11 exons of 30.3 kb located on chromosome 16p 13.3-13.11. Seven polymorphisms of the *XPF/ERCC4* have been identified, but only one resulted in an amino acid change at an evolutionarily conserved region; the variant allele is relatively rare. ERCC1 forms a complex with XPF/ERCC4 in performing dual incision and cutting at the single-strand to double-strand transition 5′ of the damage (185). This complex is required for repair of interstrand crosslinks. Therefore, a null allele of *ERCC1* or *XPF/ERCC4* may be incompatible with life (186). While the *ERCC1* 3′ UTR polymorphism was reportedly associated with adult-onset glioma (187), but not HNSCC (178), a recent study of 96 lung cancer patients and 96 controls did not find an association between an *XPF4/ERCC4* (*Pro379Ser*) polymorphism and risk for lung cancer (188).

XRCC1 AND XRCC3

Five polymorphisms of the coding region of the *XRCC1* gene have been identified (174). While the *C26304T* polymorphism was not associated with risk for HNSCC, we found that the *28152AA* genotype was more common in 203 HNSCC patients than in 424 cancer-free controls and associated with borderline increased risk for HNSCC (Table 37.1) (189). One polymorphism of the coding region of the *XRCC3* gene has been identified. Individuals homozygous for the *XRCC3 18067T* variant allele were at borderline increased risk (unpublished results, Table 37.1).

Clearly, functional (phenotypic) studies of DNA repair in individuals with various genotypes of these polymorphisms are needed. However, it will be difficult to detect subtle differences in DNA repair capacity due to a single polymorphism of a single gene in a very complex pathway.

Modulation of DNA Repair Capacity by DNA Repair Genotype

We have genotyped lung cancer cases and healthy controls for two polymorphisms in the *XPD/ERCC2* gene—the *Lys751Gln* (exon 23) locus of the *XPD* gene and the *Asp312Asn* locus (190). Both variant homozygous genotypes were associated with significantly poorer DNA repair capacity as assessed by the host cell reactivation assay. Both cases and controls with the wild-type genotypes exhibited the most proficient DRC. The risk (95% confidence interval [CI]) for suboptimal DRC (defined as less than the median DRC value among the controls) was 1.57 (0.74–3.35) for those with the homozygous variant *Gln/Gln751* genotype (data not shown). For cases with the *Asn/Asn312* genotype, the risk was 3.50 (1.06–11.59). For cases who were homozygous at either locus, the risk was 2.29 (1.03–5.12) ($p < 0.048$ for trend). The pattern was less evident among the controls, although there was a nonsignificant 41% increase in risk for suboptimal DRC for controls who were homozygous at either locus. These results suggest that the two *XPD* polymorphisms have a modulating effect on DNA repair capacity (DRC), especially in the cases.

Cell Cycle Gene Polymorphisms

Because carcinogenesis of the head and neck also involves abnormalities in cell cycle control (191), polymorphisms of cell cycle genes are good candidates for investigations of genetic susceptibility. Normal cell-cycle control ensures a rest in the cell cycle allowing DNA damage to be repaired before the cell begins the process of growth, mitosis, and division.

CYCLIN D1

The transition through G1 to S phase of the cell cycle is regulated by cyclin-dependent kinases (CDKs) (192). Cyclin D1 (CCND1) is a key regulatory protein in this process, playing a critical role in the transition from the G1 phase to the S phase of the cell cycle. Activation and overexpression of CCND1 have been found in a variety of tumors, including head and neck cancers (193). There is a GA polymorphism (G870A) in exon 4 of the *CCND1* that creates an alternative splice site in its mRNA, encoding a protein with an altered C-terminal domain. Zheng et al. (194) show that this *CCND1* polymorphism modulates individual susceptibility to HNSCC in a hospital-based, case-control study of 233 HNSCC patients and 248 controls. Compared with the wild-type *CCND1 GG*, the *CCND1 AA* genotype was associated with a significantly increased risk (adjusted OR 1.77, 95% CI 1.04–3.02) for HNSCC. Among the cases, the mean age of onset was 59.0, 56.8, and 55.5 years for the *GG, GA*, and *AA* genotypes, respectively. In stratification analysis, the *CCND1 AA* variant genotype was associated with a greater than three-fold increased risk in individuals who were 50 years old (OR 3.18, 95% CI 1.19–8.46), female (3.57, 1.26–10.0), nonsmokers (3.71, 1.37–10.1) and nonusers of alcohol (4.76, 1.61–14.0). These results suggest that the *CCND1* polymorphism is associated with early onset of HNSCC and contributes to susceptibility to HNSCC. Furthermore, it has been reported that the *CCND1 GG* genotype is also an independent prognostic indicator of survival (195).

CYCLIN-DEPENDENT KINASE INHIBITOR GENE p21 (Waf1/Cip1)

The cyclin-dependent kinase inhibitor gene *p21* (*Waf1/Cip1*) induces cellular growth arrest, terminal differentiation, and apoptosis. Polymorphisms that cause amino acid change may lead to alterations in the gene function and therefore may affect regulation of cell cycle and increase susceptibility for cancer. In a recent study, Ralhan et al. (196) described a novel polymorphism in the *p21* (*Waf1/Cip1*) gene identified in an Indian population. An AG transition at codon 149 resulted in an amino acid substitution from aspartate to glycine in the proliferating cell nuclear antigen (PCNA) binding COOH-terminal domain of p21 (Waf1/Cip1) that may affect PCNA-p21 (Waf1/Cip1) interactions, thereby affecting regulation of cellular proliferation. They found that this codon 149 polymorphism variant was identified in 11 of 30 (37%) premalignant lesions (7 of 19 hyperplastic lesions and 4 of 11 dysplastic lesions) and 11 of 30 (37%) squamous cell carcinomas, whereas only 7 of 50 (14%) unrelated age- and sex-matched healthy subjects had this variant allele. This *p21* variant was more likely to be identified in those patients whose tumors did not have *p53* mutations, suggesting a *p53*-independent role for this *p21* variant in the pathogenesis of oral cancer.

Risk Prediction Model

Although smoking tobacco is clearly the dominant risk factor for HNSCC, evaluation of the interaction of tobacco with host-specific risk factors is of great importance in defining risk. Head and neck cancers occur largely in exposed individuals who are susceptible to that exposure. When important predictive variables have been identified, all variables can be evaluated together through logistic regression analysis to construct a quantitative risk assessment model.

It is most likely that multiple susceptibility factors must be accounted for to represent the true dimensions of gene–environment interactions. Thus, there is a need to capitalize on technologic advances in high throughput, automated approaches for rapid, large-scale genotyping to identify and evaluate biologic markers more selectively predictive of individual risk, disease behavior, and response to intervention. Emerging technology uses automated workstations capable of extracting DNA from blood samples and performing DNA amplification, hybridization, and detection. Though initially a high-cost endeavor, the use of such instrumentation to acquire hundreds more genotypes and protein targets 1,000-fold faster with less samples will ultimately reduce the cost of our existing assays some 100-fold while conserving precious resources. There will be a concomitant need for state-of-the-art archiving laboratories for long-term storage and tracking of human samples using individualized bar coding and tracking systems, cryogenic repositories of blood components, and room temperature-based automated storage systems for acquiring large DNA libraries. The ethical, education, social, and informatics considerations that will result are challenging.

The ability to identify smokers with the highest risks of developing cancer has substantial preventive implications. These subgroups could be targeted for the most intensive smoking cessation interventions, could be enrolled into chemoprevention trials, and might be suitable for more aggressive screening programs not appropriate for the general population. Finally, studying susceptibility to common cancers and widely prevalent exposures may provide further insights into the basic mechanisms of carcinogenesis. This knowledge is essential for the design of future epidemiologic and intervention studies.

REFERENCES

1. Blot WJ, McLaughlin JK, Winn DM, et al. Smoking and drinking in relation to oral and pharyngeal cancer. *Cancer Res* 1988;48:3282.
2. Globscan 2000: Cancer incidence, mortality, and prevalence worldwide, version 1.0 IARC Cancer Base No. 5. Lyon, IARC Press, 2001. Found at www.dep.iarc.fr/globscan/globscan.html.
3. Jemal A, Murray T, Samuels A, et al. Cancer statistics, 2003. *CA Cancer J Clin* 2003;53:5.
4. Batsakis JG. Synchronous and metachronous carcinomas in patients with head and neck cancer. *Int J Radiat Oncol Biol Phys* 1984;10:2163.
5. Boice ZD, Fraumeni ZF. Second cancer following cancer of the respiratory system in Connecticut, 1935–1982. *Natl Cancer Instit Monog* 1985;68:83.
6. Cooper JS, Pajak TF, Rubin P, et al. Second malignancies in patients who have head and neck cancers: incidence, effect on survival and implications for chemoprevention based on the RTOG experience. *Int J Radiat Oncol Biol Phys* 1989;71:449.
7. Sturgis EM, Miller RH. Second primary malignancies in the head and neck cancer patient. *Ann Otol Rhinol Laryngol* 1995;104:946.
8. Winn DM, Blot WJ. Second cancer following cancers of the buccal cavity and pharynx in Connecticut, 1935–1982. Washington, DC: National Cancer Institute, 1985:2. NIH Pub No 85-2714.
9. Haughey BH, Gates GA, Arfken CL, et al. Meta-analysis of second malignant tumors in head and neck cancer: the case for an endoscopic screening protocol. *Ann Otol Rhinol Laryngol* 1992;101:105.
10. Day GL, Blot WJ. Second primary tumors in patients with oral cancer. *Cancer* 1992;70:14.
11. Jones AS, Morar P, Phillips DE, et al. Second primary tumors in patients with head and neck squamous cell carcinoma. *Cancer* 1995;75:1343.
12. Jesse RH, Sugarbaker EV. Squamous cell carcinoma of the oropharynx: why we fail. Am J Surg 1976;132:435.
13. Lippman SM, Hong WK. Second malignant tumors in head and neck squamous cell carcinoma: the overshadowing threat for patients with early-stage disease. *Int J Radiat Oncol Biol Phys* 1989;17:691.
14. Licciardello JTW, Spitz MR, Hong WK. Multiple primary cancer in patients with cancer of the head and neck: second cancer of the head and neck, esophagus, and lung. *Int J Radiat Oncol Biol Phys* 1989;17:467.
15. Slaughter DP, Southwick HW, Smejkal W. "Field cancerization" in oral stratified squamous epithelium: clinical implications of multicentric origin. *Cancer* 1953;6:963.
16. Chung KY, Mukhopadhyay T, Kim J, et al. Discordant *p53* gene mutations in primary head and neck cancers and corresponding second primary cancers of the upper aerodigestive tract. *Cancer Res* 1993;53:1676.
17. Nees M, Homann N, Discher H, et al. Expression of mutated *p53* occurs in tumor-distant epithelia of head and neck cancer patients: a possible molecular basis for the development of multiple tumors. *Cancer Res* 1993;53:4189.
18. Voravud N, Shin DM, Ro JY, et al. Increased polysomies of chromosomes 7 and 17 during head and neck multistage tumorigenesis. *Cancer Res* 1993;53:2874.
19. Hong WK, Doos WF. Chemoprevention of head and neck cancer. *Otolaryngol Clin N Am* 1985;18:543.
20. McGuirt WF, Matthews B, Koufman JA. Multiple simultaneous tumors in patients with head and neck cancer: a prospective, sequential panendoscopic study. *Cancer* 1982;50:1195.
21. Hong WK, Lippman SM, Itri LM, et al. Prevention of second primary tumors with isotretinoin in squamous-cell carcinoma of the head and neck. *N Engl J Med* 1990;323:795.
22. Rothman KJ, Cann CI, Flanders D, et al. Epidemiology of laryngeal cancer. *Epidemiol Rev* 1980;2:195.
23. Spitz MR, Fueger JJ, Goepfert H, et al. Squamous cell carcinoma of the upper aerodigestive tract: a case comparison analysis. *Cancer* 1988;61:203.

24. Chyou PH, Nomura AM, Stemmermann GN. Diet, alcohol, smoking and cancer of the upper aerodigestive tract: a prospective study among Hawaii Japanese men. *Int J Cancer* 1995;60:616.
25. Cloos J, Steen I, Joenje H, et al. Association between bleomycin genotoxicity and non-constitutional risk factors for head and neck cancer. *Cancer Lett* 1993; 74:161.
26. Andre K, Schraub S, Mercier M, et al. Role of alcohol and tobacco in the aetiology of head and neck cancer; a case-control study in the Doubs region of France. *Eur J Cancer B Oral Oncol* 1995;31B:301.
27. Castigliano SG. Influence of continued smoking on the incidence of second primary cancers involving mouth, pharynx and larynx. *JAMA* 1968; 77:580.
28. Schottenfeld D, Gantt RD, Wynder EL. The role of alcohol and tobacco in multiple primary cancers of the upper digestive system, larynx and lung: a prospective study. *Prev Med* 1974;3:277.
29. Moore C. Cigarette smoking and cancer of the mouth, pharynx and larynx. *JAMA* 1971;218:553.
30. Silverman S Jr, Gorsky M, Greenspan D. Tobacco usage in patients with head and neck carcinomas: a follow-up study on habit change and second primary oral/oropharyngeal cancers. *J Am Dent Assoc* 1983;106:33.
31. Day GL, Blot WJ, Shore RE, et al. Second cancers following oral and pharyngeal cancers: role of tobacco and alcohol. *J Natl Cancer Inst* 1994;86:131.
32. Hsairi M, Luce D, Point D, et al. Risk factors for simultaneous carcinoma of the head and neck. *Head Neck* 1989;11:426.
33. Franco EL, Kowalski LP, Kanda JL. Risk factors for second cancers of the upper respiratory and digestive systems: a case-control study. *J Clin Epidemiol* 1991;44:615.
34. Ryberg D, Kure E, Lystad S, et al. *p53* mutations in lung tumors: relationship to putative susceptibility markers for cancer. *J Cancer Res* 1994;54:1551.
35. Field JK, Spandidos DA, Malliri A, et al. Elevated *p53* expression correlates with a history of heavy smoking in squamous cell carcinoma of the head and neck. *Br J Cancer* 1991;64:573.
36. Brachman DG, Graves D, Vokes E, et al. Occurrence of *p53* gene deletions and human papilloma virus infection in human head and neck cancer. *Cancer Res* 1992;52:4832.
37. Koch WM, Patel H, Brennan J, et al. Squamous cell carcinoma of the head and neck in the elderly. *Arch Otolaryngol* 1995;121:262.
38. Carothers AM, Grunberger D. DNA base changes in benzo[a]pyrene diol epoxide-induced dihydrofolate reductase mutants of Chinese hamster ovary cells. *Carcinogenesis* (London) 1990;11:189.
39. Brennan JA, Boyle JO, Koch WM, et al. Association between cigarette smoking and mutation of the *p53* gene in squamous-cell carcinoma of the head and heck. *N Engl J Med* 1995;332:712.
40. Tobacco Smoking: IARC Monograph on the evaluation of the carcinogenic risk for chemicals to humans. Washington, DC: IARC, 1986:380.
41. Kahn HA. The Dorn study of smoking and mortality among US veterans: report on eight and one half years of observation. *Natl Cancer Inst Monogr* 1966;19:1.
42. Wynder EL, Bross IJ, Day E. A study of environmental factors in cancer of the larynx. *Cancer* 1956;9:86.
43. Shapiro JA, Jacobs EJ, Thun MJ. Cigar smoking in men and risk for death from tobacco-related cancers. *J Natl Cancer Inst* 2000;92:333.
44. The Health Consequences of Using Smokeless Tobacco: A Report of the Advisory Committee to the Surgeon General. Washington, DC: U.S. Department of Health and Human Services, 1986, NIH Pub No 86-2874.
45. Hoffman D, Brunnemann KD, Adams JD, et al. Laboratory studies on snuff-dipping and oral cancer. *Cancer* 1986;1:10.
46. Winn DM, Blot WJ, Shy CM, et al. Snuff dipping and oral cancer among women in the southern United States. *N Engl J Med* 1981;304:745.
47. Hoffman D, Harley NH, Fisenne I, et al. Carcinogenic agents in snuff. *J Natl Cancer Inst* 1986;76:435.
48. Zhang ZF, Morgenstern H, Spitz MR, et al. Environmental tobacco smoking, mutagen sensitivity and head and neck squamous cell carcinoma. *Cancer Epidemiol Biomarkers Prev* 2000;9:1043.
49. Loff B, Cordner S. Passive smoking test case wins in Australia. *Lancet* 2001; 357:1511.
50. Chapman S. Australian bar worker wins payout in passive smoking case. *Br Med J* 2001;322:1139.
51. Tan EH, Adelstein DJ, Droughton ML, et al. Squamous cell head and neck cancer in nonsmokers. *Am J Clin Oncol* 1997;20:146.
52. Caplan GA, Brigham BA. Marijuana smoking and carcinoma of the tongue. Is there an association? *Cancer* 1990;66:1005.
53. Donald PJ. Marijuana smoking—possible cause of head and neck carcinoma in young patients. *Otolaryngol Head Neck Surg* 1986;94:517.
54. Zhang ZF, Morgenstern H, Spitz MR, et al. Marijuana use and increased risk for squamous cell carcinoma of the head and neck. *Cancer Epidemiol Biomarkers Prev* 1999;8:1071.
55. Sidney S, Quesenberry CP, Friedman GD, et al. Marijuana use and cancer incidence (California, United States). *Cancer Causes Control* 1997;8:722.
56. Saracci R. The interactions of tobacco smoking and other agents in cancer etiology. *Epidemiol Rev* 1987;9:175.
57. Jensen OM. Cancer morbidity and causes of death among Danish brewery workers. *Int J Cancer* 1979;23:454.
58. Martinez I. Factors associated with cancer of the oesophagus, mouth and pharynx in Puerto Rico. *J Natl Cancer Inst* 1969;42:1069.
59. Bundgaard T, Wildt J, Frydenberg M, et al. Case-control study of squamous cell cancer of the oral cavity in Denmark. *Cancer Causes Control* 1995;6:57.
60. Graham S, Dayal H, Rohrer T, et al. Dentition, diet, tobacco, and alcohol in the epidemiology of oral cancer. *J Natl Cancer Inst* 1977;59:1611.
61. Rothman K, Keller A. The effect of joint exposure to alcohol and tobacco on risk for cancer of the mouth and pharynx. *J Chronic Dis* 1972;25:711.
62. Mashberg A, Garfinkel L, Harris S. Alcohol as a primary risk factor in oral squamous carcinoma. *CA Cancer J Clin* 1981;31:146.
63. Wynder EL, Stellman SD. Comparative epidemiology of tobacco-related cancers. *Cancer Res* 1977;37:4608.
64. McCoy GD, Wynder EL. Etiological and preventive implications in alcohol carcinogenesis. *Cancer Res* 1979;39:2844.
65. Franceschi S, Bidoli E, Negri E, et al. Alcohol and cancers of the upper aerodigestive tract in men and women. *Cancer Epidemiol Biomarkers Prev* 1994;3:299.
66. Winn DM. Diet and nutrition in the etiology of oral cancer. *Am J Clin Nutr* 1995;61:437S.
67. Nomura AM, Ziegler RG, Stemmermann GN, et al. Serum micronutrients and upper aerodigestive tract cancer. *Cancer Epidemiol Biomarkers Prev* 1997;6: 407.
68. Zheng T, Boyle P, Willett W, et al. A case-control study of oral cancer in Beijing, People's Republic of China. Associations with nutrient intakes, foods and food groups. *Eur J Cancer Oral Oncol* 1993;29B:45.
69. Zheng W, Blot WJ, Shu X, et al. Diet and other risk factors for laryngeal cancer in Shanghai. *Am J Epidemiol* 1992;136:178.
70. Zheng W, Blot WJ, Xiao-Ou S, et al. Risk factors for oral and pharyngeal cancer in Shanghai with emphasis on diet. *Cancer Epidemiol Biomarkers Prev* 1992; 1:441.
71. McLaughlin JK, Gridley G, Block G, et al. Dietary factors in oral and pharyngeal cancer. *J Natl Cancer Inst* 1988;80:1237.
72. Mackerras D, Buffler PA, Randall DE, et al. Carotene intake and the risk for laryngeal cancer in coastal Texas. *Am J Epidemiol* 1988;128:980.
73. Spitz MR, Duphorne CM, Detry MA, et al. Dietary intake of isothiocyanates: evidence of a joint effect with glutathione S-transferase polymorphisms in lung cancer risk. *Cancer Epidemiol Biomarkers Prev* 2000;9:1017.
74. Tavani A, Negri E, Franceschi S, et al. Attributable risk for laryngeal cancer in Northern Italy. *Cancer Epidemiol Biomarkers Prev* 1994;3:121.
75. Marshall J, Graham S, Mettlin C, et al. Diet in the epidemiology of oral cancer. *Nutr Cancer* 1982;3:145.
76. Graham S. Toward a dietary prevention of cancer. *Epidemiol Rev* 1983;5:38.
77. Mettlin C, Graham S, Swanson M. Vitamin A and lung cancer. *J Natl Cancer Inst* 1979;62:1435.
78. Zheng W, Blot WJ, Diamond EL, et al. Serum micronutrients and the subsequent risk for oral and pharyngeal cancer. *Cancer Res* 1993;53:795.
79. De Stefani E, Oreggia F, Ronco A, et al. Salted meat consumption as a risk factor for cancer of the oral cavity and pharynx: a case-control study from Uruguay. *Cancer Epidemiol Biomarkers Prev* 1994;3:381.
80. ATBC (Alpha-tocopherol, Beta-carotene Prevention Study Group). The effect of vitamin E and beta-carotene on the incidence of lung cancer and other cancers in male smokers. *N Engl J Med* 1994;330:1029.
81. Omenn GS, Goodman GE, Thornquist MD, et al. Effects of a combination of beta-carotene and vitamin A on lung cancer and cardiovascular disease. *N Engl J Med* 1996;334:1150.
82. De Stefani E, Correa P, Oreggia F, et al. Risk factors for laryngeal cancer. *Cancer* 1987;60:3087.
83. Morrison MD. Is chronic gastroesophageal reflux a causative factor in glottic carcinoma? *Otolaryngol Head Neck Surg* 1988;99:370.
84. Ward PH. Hanson DG. Reflux as an etiological factor of carcinoma of the laryngopharynx. *Laryngoscope* 1988;98:1195.
85. Koufman JA. The otolaryngologic manifestations of gastroesophageal reflux disease (GERD): a clinical investigation of 225 patients using ambulatory 24-hour pH monitoring and an experimental investigation of the role of acid and pepsin in the development of laryngeal injury. *Laryngoscope* 1991;101 [Suppl 53]:1.
86. Biacabe B, Gleich LL, Laccourreye O, et al. Silent gastroesophageal reflux disease in patients with pharyngolaryngeal cancer: further results. *Head Neck* 1998;20:510.
87. Copper MP, Smit CF, Stanojcic LD, et al. High incidence of laryngopharyngeal reflux in patients with head and neck cancer. *Laryngoscope* 2000;110:1007.
88. El-Serag HB, Hepworth EJ, Lee P, et al. Gastroesophageal reflux disease is a risk factor for laryngeal and pharyngeal cancer. *Am J Gastroenterol* 2001;96: 2013.
89. McKaig RG, Baric RS, Olshan AF. Human papillomavirus and head and neck cancer: epidemiology and molecular biology. *Head Neck* 1998;20:250.
90. Gillison ML, Shah KV. Human papillomavirus-associated head and neck squamous cell carcinoma: mounting evidence for an etiologic role for human papillomavirus in a subset of head and neck cancers. *Curr Opin Oncol* 2001; 13:183.
91. Gillison ML, Koch WM, Capone RB, et al. Evidence for a causal association between human papillomavirus and a subset of head and neck cancers. *J Natl Cancer Inst* 2000;92:709.
92. Fouret P, Monceaux G, Temam S, et al. Human papillomavirus in head and neck squamous cell carcinomas in nonsmokers. *Arch Otolaryngol Head Neck Surg* 1997;123:513.
93. Smith EM, Hoffman HT, Summersgill KS, et al. Human papillomavirus and risk for oral cancer. *Laryngoscope* 1998;108:1098.

94. Maden C, Beckmann AM, Thomas DB, et al. Human papillomaviruses, herpes simplex viruses, and the risk for oral cancer in men. *Am J Epidemiol* 1992;135:1093.
95. Mork J, Lie AK, Glattre E, et al. Human papillomavirus infection as a risk factor for squamous-cell carcinoma of the head and neck. *N Engl J Med* 2001;344:1125.
96. Burch JD, Howe GR, Miller AB et al. Tobacco, alcohol, asbestos, and nickel in the etiology of cancer of the larynx: A case-control study. *J Natl Cancer Inst* 1981;67:1219
97. Foulkes WD, Brunet JS, Sieh W, et al. Familial risks of squamous cell carcinoma of the head and neck: retrospective case-control study. *Br Med J* 1996;313:716.
98. Foulkes WD, Brunet JS, Kowalski LP, et al. Family history of cancer is a risk factor for squamous cell carcinoma of the head and neck in Brazil: a case-control study. *Int J Cancer* 1995;63:769.
99. Goldstein AM, Blot WJ, Greenberg RS, et al. Familial risk in oral and pharyngeal cancer. *Eur J Cancer B Oral Oncol* 1994;30B:319.
100. Copper MP, Jovanovic A, Nauta JJ, et al. Role of genetic factors in the etiology of squamous cell carcinoma of the head and neck. *Arch Otolaryngol Head Neck Surg* 1995;121:157.
101. Yu GP, Zhang ZF, Hsu TC, et al. Family history of cancer, mutagen sensitivity and increased risk for head and neck cancer. *Cancer Lett* 1999;146:93.
102. Bondy ML, Spitz MR, Halabi S, et al. Association between family history of cancer and mutagen sensitivity in upper aerodigestive tract cancer patients. *Cancer Epidemiol Biomarkers Prev* 1993;2:103.
103. Shields PG, Caporaso NE, Falk RT, et al. Lung cancer, race and a CYP1A1 genetic polymorphism. *Cancer Epidemiol Biomarkers Prev* 1993;2:481.
104. Andreasson L, Bjorlin G, Laurell P, et al. Oral and oropharyngeal cancer aryl hydrocarbon hydroxylase inducibility and smoking. A follow-up study. *ORL J Otorhinolaryngol Relat Spec* 1985;47:131.
105. Brandenberg JH, Kellerman G. Aryl hydrocarbon hydroxylase inducibility in laryngeal carcinoma. *Arch Otolaryngol* 1978;104:151.
106. Petersen DD, McKinney CE, Ikeya K, et al. Human CYP1A1 gene: cosegregation of the enzyme inducibility phenotype and an RFLP. *Am J Hum Genet* 1991;48:720.
107. Jaiswal AK, Gonzalez FJ, Nebert DW. Human P1-450 gene sequence and correlation of mRNA with genetic differences in benzo[a]pyrene metabolism. *Nucl Acids Res* 1985;13:4503.
108. Sato M, Sato T, Izumo T, et al. Genetic polymorphism of drug-metabolizing enzymes and susceptibility to oral cancer. *Carcinogenesis* 1999;20:1927.
109. Tanimoto K, Hayashi SI, Yoshiga K, et al. Polymorphisms of the CYP1A1 and GSTM1 gene involved in oral squamous cell carcinoma in association with a cigarette dose. *Oral Oncol* 1999;35:191.
110. Nakachi K, Imai K, Hayashi S, et al. Polymorphisms of the CYP1A1 and glutathione S-transferase genes associated with susceptibility to lung cancer in relation to cigarette dose in a Japanese population. *Cancer Res* 1993;53:2994.
111. Oude-Ophuis MB, Lieshout EMM, Roelofs HMJ, et al. Glutathione S-transferase M1 and T1 and cytochrome P4501A1 polymorphisms in relation to the risk for benign and malignant head and neck lesions. *Cancer* 1998;82:936.
112. Matthias C, Bockmuhl U, Jahnke V, et al. Polymorphisms in cytochrome P450 CYP2D6, CYP1A1, CYP2E1 and glutathione S-transferase, GSTM1, GSTM3, GSTT1 and susceptibility to tobacco-related cancers: studies in upper aerodigestive tract cancers. *Pharmacogenetics* 1998;8:91.
113. Hirvonen A, Husgafvel-Pursiainen K, Karjalainen A, et al. Point-mutational MspI and Ile-Val polymorphisms closely linked in the CYP1A1 gene: lack of association with susceptibility to lung cancer in a Finnish study population. *Cancer Epidemiol Biomarkers Prev* 1992;1:485.
114. Sugimura H, Suzuki I, Hamada GS, et al. Cytochrome P4501A1 genotype in lung cancer patients and controls in Rio de Janeiro, Brazil. *Cancer Epidemiol Biomarkers Prev* 1994;3:145.
115. Hayashi S, Watanabe J, Kawajiri K. High susceptibility to lung cancer analyzed in terms of combined genotypes of P4501A1 and Mu-class glutathione S-transferase genes. *Jpn J Cancer Res* 1992;83:866.
116. Cosma G, Crofts F, Taioli E, et al. Relationship between genotype and function of the human CYP1A1 gene. *J Toxicol Environ Health* 1993;40:309.
117. Morita S, Yano M, Tsujinaka T, et al. Genetic polymorphisms of drug-metabolizing enzymes and susceptibility to head-and-neck squamous-cell carcinoma. *Int J Cancer* 1999;80:685.
118. Katoh T, Kaneko S, Kohshi K, et al. Genetic polymorphisms of tobacco and alcohol-related metabolizing enzymes and oral cavity cancer. *Int J Cancer* 1999;83:606.
119. Park JY, Muscat JE, Ren Q, et al. CYP1A1 and GSTM1 polymorphisms and oral cancer risk. *Cancer Epidemiol Biomarkers Prev* 1997;6:791.
120. Ayesh R, Idle SR, Ritchie JC, et al. Metabolic oxidation phenotypes as markers for susceptibility to lung cancer. *Nature* 1984;312:169.
121. Crespi CL, Penman BW, Gelboin HV, et al. A tobacco smoke-derived nitrosamine, 4-(methylnitrosamino)-1-(3-pyridyl)-1-butanone, is activated by multiple human cytochrome P450s including the polymorphic human cytochrome P4502D6. *Carcinogenesis* 1991;12:1197.
122. Caporaso NE, Tucker MA, Hoover RN, et al. Lung cancer and the debrisoquine metabolic phenotype. *J Natl Cancer Inst* 1990;82:1264.
123. Roots I, Drakoulis N, Ploch M, et al. Debrisoquine hydroxylation phenotype, acetylation phenotype, and ABO blood groups as genetic host factors of lung cancer risk. *Klin Wochenschr* 1988;[Suppl 66]11:87.
124. Heim M, Meyer UA. Genotyping of poor metabolizers of debrisoquine by allele-specific PCR amplification. *Lancet* 1990;336:529.
125. Spina E, Campo GM, Avenoso A, et al. CYP2D6-related oxidation polymorphism in Italy. *Pharm Res* 1994;29:281.
126. Agundez JA, Gallardo L, Ledesma MC, et al. Functionally active duplications of the CYP2D6 gene are more prevalent among larynx and lung cancer patients. *Oncology* 2001;61:59.
127. Worrall SF, Corrigan M, High A, et al. Susceptibility and outcome on oral cancer: preliminary data showing an association with polymorphism in cytochrome P450 CYP2D6. *Pharmacogenetics* 1998;8:433.
128. Gonzalez MV, Alvarez V, Pello MF, et al. Genetic polymorphism of N-acetyltransferase-2, glutathione S-transferase-M1, and cytochromes P450IIE1 and P450IID6 in the susceptibility to head and neck cancer. *Clin Pathol* 1998;51:294.
129. Stephens EA, Taylor JA, Kaplan N, et al. Ethnic variation in the CYP2E1 gene: polymorphism analysis of 695 African-Americans, European-Americans and Taiwanese. *Pharmacogenetics* 1994;4:185.
130. Hung HC, Chuang J, Chien YC, et al. Genetic polymorphisms of CYP2E1, GSTM1, and GSTT1: environmental factors and risk for oral cancer. *Cancer Epidemiol Biomarkers Prev* 1997;6:901.
131. Tan W, Song N, Wang GQ, et al. Impact of genetic polymorphisms in cytochrome P450 2E1 and glutathione S-transferases M1, T1, and P1 on susceptibility to esophageal cancer among high-risk individuals in China. *Cancer Epidemiol Biomarkers Prev* 2000; 9:551.
132. Bouchardy C, Hirvonen A, Coutelle C, et al. Role of alcohol dehydrogenase 3 and cytochrome P-4502E1 genotypes in susceptibility to cancers of the upper aerodigestive tract. *Int J Cancer* 2000;87:734.
133. Zhong S, Wyllie AH, Barnes D, et al. Relationship between the GSTM1 genetic polymorphism and susceptibility to bladder, breast and colon cancer. *Carcinogenesis* 1993;14:1821.
134. Seidegard J, Vorachek WR, Pero RW, et al. Hereditary differences in the expression of the human glutathione transferase active on trans-stilbene oxide are due to a gene deletion. *Proc Natl Acad Sci USA* 1988;85:7293.
135. Roots I, Brockmoller J, Drakoulis N, et al. Mutant genes of cytochrome P-450IID6, glutathione S-transferase class Mu, and arylamine N-acetyltransferase in lung cancer patients. *Clin Invest* 1992;70:307.
136. London SJ, Daly AK, Cooper J, et al. Polymorphism of glutathione S-transferase M1 and lung cancer risk among African Americans and Caucasians in Los Angeles County, California. *J Natl Cancer Inst* 1995;87:1246.
137. Meyer DJ, Coles B, Pemble SE, et al. Theta, a new class of glutathione transferases purified from rat and man. *Biochem J* 1991;274:409.
138. Pemble S, Schroeder KR, Spencer SR, et al. Human glutathione S-transferase theta (GSTT1): cDNA cloning and the characterization of a genetic polymorphism. *Biochem J* 1994;300:271.
139. Cheng L, Sturgis EM, Eicher SA, et al. Glutathione-S-transferase polymorphisms and risk for squamous-cell carcinoma of the head and neck. *Int J Cancer* 1999;84:220.
140. Trizna Z, Clayman GL, Spitz MR, et al. Glutathione s-transferase genotypes as risk factors for head and neck cancer. *Am J Surg* 1995;170:499.
141. Geisler SA, Olshan AF. GSTM1, GSTT1, and risk for squamous cell carcinoma of the head and neck: a mini-HuGE review. *Am J Epidemiol* 2001;154:95.
142. Blum M, Demierre A, Grant DM, et al. Molecular mechanism of slow acetylation of drugs and carcinogens in humans. *Proc Natl Acad Sci USA* 1991;88:5237.
143. Deguchi T. Sequences and expression of alleles of polymorphic arylamine N-acetyltransferase of human liver. *J Biol Chem* 1992;267:18140.
144. Drozdz M, Gierek T, Jendryczko A. N-acetyltransferase phenotype of patients with cancer of the larynx. *Neoplasia* 1987;34:481.
145. Katoh T, Kaneko S, Boissy R, et al. A pilot study testing the association between N-acetyltransferase 1 and 2 and risk for oral squamous cell carcinoma in Japanese people. *Carcinogenesis* 1998;19:1803.
146. Fronhoffs S, Bruning T, Ortiz-Pallardo E, et al. Real-time PCR analysis of the N-acetyltransferase NAT1 allele *3, *4, *10, *11, *14, and *17 polymorphism in squamous cell carcinoma of head and neck. *Carcinogenesis* 2001;22:1405.
147. Lancaster JM, Brownlee HA, Bell DA, et al. Microsomal epoxide hydrolase polymorphism as a risk factor for ovarian cancer. *Mol Carcinog* 1996;17:160.
148. Heckbert SR, Weiss NS, Hornung SK, et al. Glutathione S-transferase and epoxide hydrolase activity in human leukocytes in relation to risk for lung cancer and other smoking-related cancers. *J Natl Cancer Inst* 1992;84:414.
149. Hassett C, Aicher L, Sidhu JS, et al. Human microsomal epoxide hydrolase: genetic polymorphism and functional expression in vitro of amino acid variants. *Hum Mol Genet* 1994;3:421.
150. Smith CAD, Harrison D. Association between polymorphism in gene for microsomal epoxide hydrolase and susceptibility to emphysema. *Lancet* 1997;350:630.
151. Jourenkova-Mironova N, Mitrunen K, Bouchardy C, et al. High-activity microsomal epoxide hydrolase genotypes and the risk for oral, pharynx, and larynx cancers. *Cancer Res* 2000;60:534.
152. Janot F, Massaad L, Ribrag V, et al. Principal xenobiotic-metabolizing enzyme systems in human head and neck squamous cell carcinoma. *Carcinogenesis* 1993;14:1279.
153. Bosron WF, Li TK. Genetic polymorphism of human liver alcohol and aldehyde dehydrogenases and their relationship to alcohol metabolism and alcoholism. *Hepatology* 1998;6:502.
154. Harty LC, Caporaso NE, Hayes RB, et al. Alcohol dehydrogenase 3 genotype and risk for oral cavity and pharyngeal cancers. *J Natl Cancer Inst* 1997;89:1656.
155. Coutelle C, Ward PJ, Fleury B, et al. Laryngeal and oropharyngeal cancer,

and alcohol dehydrogenase 3 and glutathione S-transferase M1 polymorphisms. *Hum Genet* 1997;99:319.
156. Yokoyama A, Muramatsu T, Ohmori T, et al. Alcohol-related cancers and aldehyde dehydrogenase-2 in Japanese alcoholics. *Carcinogenesis* 1998;19: 1383.
157. Sturgis EM, Dahlstrom KR, Guan Y, et al. Alcohol dehydrogenase 3 genotype is not associated with risk for squamous cell carcinoma of the oral cavity and pharynx. *Cancer Epidemiol Biomarkers Prev* 2001;10:273.
158. Ang HL, Deltour L, Zgombic-Knight M, et al. Expression patterns of class I and class IV alcohol dehydrogenase genes in developing epithelia suggest a role for alcohol dehydrogenase in local retinoic acid synthesis. *Alcohol Clin Exp Res* 1996;20:1050.
159. McWilliams JE, Evans AJ, Beer TM, et al. Genetic polymorphisms in head and neck cancer risk. *Head Neck* 2000;22:609.
160. Olshan AF, Weissler MC, Watson MA, et al. GSTM1, GSTT1, GSTP1, CYP1A1, and NAT1 polymorphisms, tobacco use and the risk for head and neck cancer. *Cancer Epidemiol Biomarkers Prev* 2000;9:185.
161. Hagmar L, Brogger A, Hansteen IL, et al. Cancer risk in humans predicted by increased levels of chromosomal aberrations in lymphocytes: Nordic study group on the health risk for chromosome damage. *Cancer Res* 1994;54:2919.
162. Hsu TC, Cherry LM, Samaan NA. Differential mutagen susceptibility in cultured lymphocytes of normal individuals and cancer patients. *Cancer Genet Cytogenet* 1985;17:307.
163. Spitz MR, Fueger JJ, Beddingfield NA, et al. Chromosome sensitivity to bleomycin-induced mutagenesis, an independent risk factor for upper aerodigestive tract cancers. *Cancer Res* 1989;49:4626.
164. Hsu TC, Spitz MR, Schantz SP. Mutagen sensitivity: a biologic marker of cancer susceptibility. *Cancer Epidemiol Biomarkers Prev* 1991;1:83.
165. Cloos J, Spitz MR, Schantz SP, et al. Genetic susceptibility to head and neck squamous cell carcinoma. *J Natl Cancer Inst* 1996;88:530.
166. Wang L, Sturgis EM, Ficher SA, et al. Mutagen sensitivity to benzo[a]pyrene diol epoxide and the risk for squamous cell carcinoma of the head and neck. *Clin Cancer Res* 1998;4:1773.
167. Athas WF, Hedayati M, Matanoski GM, et al. Development and field-test validation of an assay for DNA repair in circulating lymphocytes. *Cancer Res* 1991;51:5786.
168. Wei Q, Matanoski GM, Farmer ER, et al. DNA repair and aging in basal cell carcinoma: a molecular epidemiology study. *Proc Natl Acad Sci USA* 1993;90:1614.
169. Alcalay J, Freeman SE, Goldberg LH, et al. Excision repair of pyrimidine dimers induced by simulated solar radiation in the skin of patients with basal cell carcinoma. *J Invest Dermatol* 1990;95:506.
170. Cheng L, Eicher SA, Guo Z, et al. Reduced DNA repair capacity in head and neck cancer patients. *Cancer Epidemiol Biomarkers Prev* 1998;7:465.
171. Wei Q, Spitz MR, Gu J, et al. DNA repair capacity correlates with mutagen sensitivity in lymphoblastoid cell lines. *Cancer Epidemiol Biomarkers Prev* 1996;5:199.
172. Sturgis EM, Clayman GL, Guan Y, et al. DNA repair in lymphoblastoid cell lines from patients with head and neck cancer. *Arch Otolaryngol Head Neck Surg* 1999;125:185.
173. Sancar A, Tang MS. Reduced DNA repair capacity in lung cancer patients. *Cancer Res* 1995;56:4103.
174. Shen MR, Jones IM, Mohrenweiser H. Nonconservative amino acid substitution variants exist at polymorphic frequency in DNA repair genes in healthy humans. *Cancer Res* 1998;58:604.
175. Fan F, Liu C, Tavare S, et al. Polymorphisms in the human DNA repair gene XPF. Mutat Res 1999;406:115.
176. Khan SG, Metter EJ, Tarone RE, et al. A new xeroderma pigmentosum group C poly(AT) insertion/deletion polymorphism. *Carcinogenesis* 2000;21:1821.
177. Dybdahl M, Vogel U, Frentz G, et al. Polymorphisms in the DNA repair gene XPD: Correlations with risk and age at onset of basal cell carcinoma. *Cancer Epidemiol Biomarkers Prev* 1999;8:77.
178. Sturgis EM, Dahlstrom KR, Eicher SA, et al. ERCC1 polymorphism and the risk for squamous cell carcinoma of the head and neck. *Proc Am Head Neck Society* 2001:33.
179. Shen H, Sturgis EM, Khan SG, et al. An intronic poly (AT) polymorphism of the DNA repair gene XPC and risk for squamous cell carcinoma of the head and neck: a case-control study. *Cancer Res* 2001;61:3321.
180. Coin F, Marinoni JC, Rodolfo C, et al. Mutations in the XPD helicase gene result in XP and TTD phenotypes, preventing interaction between XPD and the p44 subunit of TFIIH. *Nat Genet* 1998;20:184.
181. Taylor EM, Broughton BC, Botta E, et al. Xeroderma pigmentosum and trichothiodystrophy are associated with different mutations in the XPD (ERCC2) repair/transcription gene. *Proc Natl Acad Sci USA* 1997;94:8658.
182. Reardon JT, Ge H, Gibbs E, et al. Isolation and characterization of two human transcription factor IIH (TFIIH)-related complexes: ERCC2/CAK and TFIIH. *Proc Natl Acad Sci USA* 1996;93:6482.
183. Sturgis EM, Zheng R, Li L, et al. XPD/ERCC2 polymorphisms and risk for head and neck cancer: a case-control analysis. *Carcinogenesis* 2000;21:2219.
184. Sturgis EM, Castillo EJ, Li L, et al. *XPD/ERCC2* EXON 8 polymorphisms: rarity and lack of significance in risk for squamous cell carcinoma of the head and neck. *Eur J Cancer B Oral Oncol* 2002;38:475–477.
185. Sijbers AM, de Laat WL, Ariza RR, et al. Xeroderma pigmentosum group F caused by a defect in a structure-specific DNA repair endonuclease. *Cell* 1996;86:811.
186. de Boer J, Hoeijmakers JH. Nucleotide excision repair and human syndromes [Review]. *Carcinogenesis* 2000;2:453.
187. Chen P, Wiencke J, Aldape K, et al. Association of an ERCC1 polymorphism with adult-onset glioma. *Cancer Epidemiol Biomarkers Prev* 2000;9:843.
188. Butkiewicz D, Rusin M, Enewold L, et al. Genetic polymorphisms in DNA repair genes and risk for lung cancer. *Carcinogenesis* 2001;22:593.
189. Sturgis EM, Castillo EJ, Li L, et al. Polymorphisms of DNA repair gene *XRCC1* in squamous cell carcinoma of the head and neck. *Carcinogenesis* 1999;20:2125.
190. Spitz MR, Wu X, Wang Y, et al. Modulation of nucleotide excision repair capacity by XPD polymorphisms in lung cancer patients. *Cancer Res* 2001;61: 1354.
191. Scully C., Field JK, Tanzawa H. Genetic aberrations in oral or head and neck squamous cell carcinoma (SCCHN): 1. Carcinogen metabolism, DNA repair and cell cycle control. *Eur J Cancer B Oral Oncol* 2000;36:256.
192. Sherr CJ. Cancer cell cycles. *Science* 1996;274:1672.
193. Nakahara Y, Shintani S, Mihara M, et al. Alterations of Rb, p16(INK4A) and cyclin D1 in the tumorigenesis of oral squamous cell carcinomas. *Cancer Lett* 2000;160:3.
194. Zheng Y, Shen H, Sturgis EM, et al. Cyclin D1 polymorphism and risk for squamous cell carcinoma of the head and neck: a case-control study. *Carcinogenesis* 2001;22:1195.
195. Matthias C, Branigan K, Jahnke V, et al. Polymorphism within the cyclin D1 gene is associated with prognosis in patients with squamous cell carcinoma of the head and neck. *Clin Cancer Res* 1998;4:2411.
196. Ralhan R, Agarwal S, Mathur M, et al. Association between polymorphism in p21(Waf1/Cip1) cyclin-dependent kinase inhibitor gene and human oral cancer. *Clin Cancer Res* 2000;6:2440.

CHAPTER 38

Invasion and Metastases in Head and Neck Cancer

F. Christopher Holsinger, Janet I. Lee, Eric J. Lentsch, and Jeffrey N. Myers

Morbidity and mortality from squamous cell carcinoma (SCC) of the head and neck (HNSCC) predominantly result from local tumor invasion and regional and distant metastasis. In particular, extracapsular spread (ECS) of tumor outside of the lymph node capsule, perineural invasion, and bone invasion are associated with decreased survival. For patients with these pathologic predictors of poor outcome, postoperative radiotherapy is often recommended. Despite this and other adjuvant treatment, rates of locoregional recurrence remain high. Concomitant chemotherapy with postoperative adjuvant radiotherapy has been advocated. But often these intensification schemes result in significant morbidity and little change in survival.

Targeted molecular therapy offers an exciting, new approach to treat human cancer by basing therapy on the specific molecular abnormalities present in an individual patient's malignancy (1). Yet, despite long-standing awareness that tumor invasion and metastasis are associated with adverse outcomes in patients with HNSCC, the molecular mechanisms of invasion and metastasis are not well understood. In addition, a lack of reliable animal models for studying HNSCC has prevented significant progress in preclinical investigations of novel therapeutic strategies.

This chapter reviews the clinical significance of tumor invasion of soft tissue, nerve, and bone, and the effect of regional and distant metastases on treatment outcomes of patients with HNSCC. Current progress in determining the molecular and cellular mechanisms important in the processes of invasion and metastasis are summarized, with an emphasis on how enhanced knowledge of these mechanisms can potentially provide more rational approaches to therapy. We conclude with a discussion of preclinical animal models for oral cancer, as an ideal system to test the efficacy of novel targeted molecular therapy for HNSCC.

CLINICAL SIGNIFICANCE OF TUMOR INVASION

Soft Tissue Invasion

Studies in patients with HNSCC have shown that deeply invasive tumors are more aggressive and are associated with decreased locoregional control and survival. Although the standard American Joint Committee on Cancer (AJCC) scoring system is useful for tumor staging, it is limited in that tumor size is scored two-dimensionally with the exception of deep muscle invasion and bone invasion, which are encompassed in the T4 stage. Therefore, less drastic but clinically significant tumor invasion is not accounted for by the AJCC system, and several studies have shown that the depth of tumor invasion can be a significant predictor of local recurrence, regional metastasis, and survival. Spiro et al. (2) demonstrated the value of tumor thickness independent of T stage in predicting occult nodal metastases. In a subsequent prospective randomized trial of 70 patients with T1 or T2 N0 M0 SCC of the anterior tongue, patients with tumors greater than 4 mm in depth had an increased likelihood of nodal disease and poorer survival ($p < 0.01$). An analysis of 91 patients with SCC of the oral tongue at our institution has corroborated these earlier studies, finding that patients with a depth of invasion greater than 4 mm have a higher rate of regional metastasis and poorer survival ($p = 0.02$) (3) (Fig. 38.1).

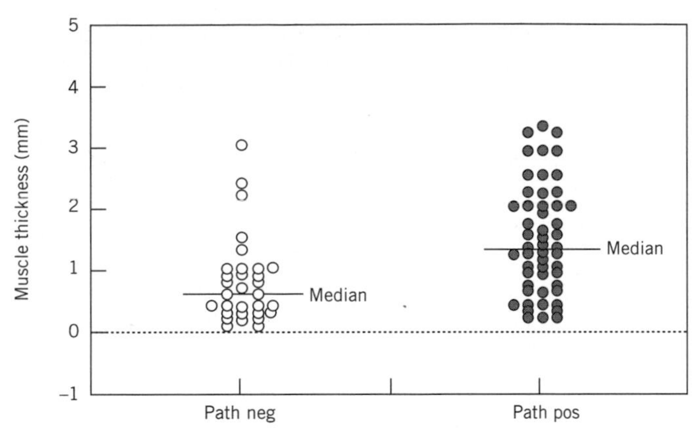

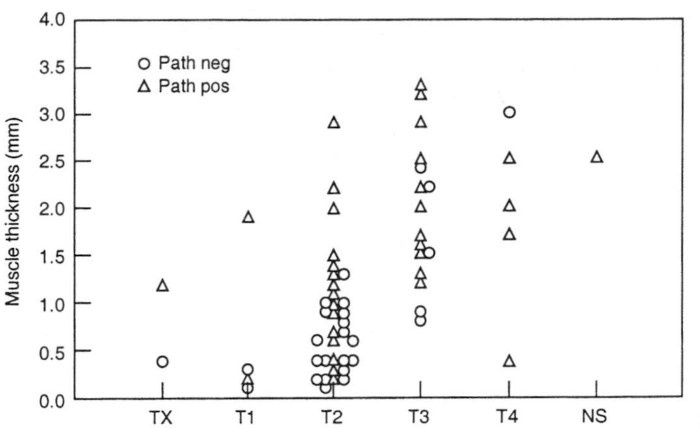

Figure 38.1 **A:** The relationship between the thickness of the primary tongue squamous cell carcinoma (SCC) and pathologic nodal disease is shown. **B:** The relationship between the thickness of the primary tongue SCC, T classification, and pathologic nodal disease is shown in this scatterplot.

Perineural Invasion

The invasion of HNSCC tumors into small and larger nerves at the primary tumor site has also been associated with higher rates of local recurrence and diminished survival. The incidence of perineural invasion has been reported to be as high as 70% in patients with head and neck cancer (4). Of the patients with pathologic evidence of invasion, only 30% to 40% present with signs or symptoms of nerve involvement. The most common initial complaint is a "crawling sensation." Late symptoms include pain, numbness, or motor deficit. The most commonly affected nerves are divisions of the trigeminal and facial nerves (5).

Invasion was initially thought to be the result of invasion of lymphatic channels in the perineurium and endoneurium (6). Ballantyne et al. (4), however, noted in their report of 70 patients that "if spread is along lymphatics, these nerves must either not have wide communication with those of the regional lymph nodes, or the cancers are incapable of growing within lymph nodes." Since then, Larson and colleagues (7) have demonstrated, using dye injections into nerves, that nerves did not communicate with lymphatics and that lymphatics draining dye did not enter the perineural space. Further studies at autopsy and surgical resections of SCC with perineural involvement have demonstrated that neoplastic cells invade the perineural space and serve as a scaffold for tumor spread in either direction (8). Immunofluorescent staining of antimyelin and antiaxonal antibodies of specimens with perineural invasion has demonstrated both axonal and myelin degeneration and segmental infarction along the nerve bundle secondary to tumor-induced hypoxia (9). The underlying mechanisms for what makes certain tumors more neurotropic have not clearly been defined. The nerve cell adhesion molecule (N-CAM), which is involved in mediating cell-to-cell and cell-to-substrate adhesions, has been implicated as a potential conduit or scaffold for perineural spread. In a study of 76 archived specimens from patients with HNSCC, N-CAM expression was significantly associated ($p < 0.002$) with tumors with perineural invasion using immunohistochemical analysis (10). Furthermore, laminin-5 expression, a basement membrane constituent involved in cell adhesion and migration, has been positively correlated with perineural invasion among HNSCCs and may play an important role in perineural invasion (11).

There have been numerous reports of perineural spread in squamous carcinomas of the head and neck, with incidences ranging from 4.9% to 52% (12–16). Yet the presence of perineural involvement has consistently been reported to be associated with more aggressive tumor behavior and local recurrence. Its prognostic implication with regional and distant spread has not been clearly defined. The incidence of perineural invasion of small peripheral nerves has been reported as high as 52% in a series of 142 patients with HNSCC from multiple sites (16). Among these patients, perineural spread was significantly associated with local recurrence and disease-specific mortality ($p < 0.02$) but not with regional or distant metastases. There was, however, an association between perineural involvement and nodal spread among oropharyngeal and oral cavity carcinomas but not among hypopharyngeal or laryngeal carcinomas (16). In a series of 239 patients with mucosal HNSCC, 64 patients (27%) had perineural involvement, again with the oral cavity being the predominant site (13). In this series, perineural involvement was a significant prognosticator for overall and disease-related survival ($p < 0.001$).

The presence of perineural invasion in cutaneous HNSCC is an indication for aggressive surgical resection of involved tissues and nerves with appropriate regional lymphadenectomy followed by postoperative adjuvant radiotherapy (17). A large series of 520 patients with cutaneous HNSCC treated between 1970 and 1979 at the M. D. Anderson Cancer Center reported an incidence rate of 14% for invasion of at least one major nerve trunk (17). In this series, perineural involvement was significantly associated with regional and distant metastases ($p < 0.0005$). In addition, patients with perineural involvement demonstrated a significantly lower overall survival rate compared with patients without perineural involvement ($p < 0.0005$).

In a historical prospective cohort of 622 patients with mucosal HNSCC treated between 1991 and 1994 at the M. D. Anderson Cancer Center, status of perineural involvement was available for 404 patients. Among these, 88 (22%) patients had perineural invasion. The presence of perineural invasion was significantly associated with both local recurrence ($p = 0.005$) and regional recurrence ($p = 0.007$). When survival analysis was performed, patients with perineural invasion had a greater disease-specific mortality than did patients without perineural invasion ($p = 0.003$), but there was no significant correlation with overall survival or development of distant metastasis. In this prospective study of 404 patients, perineural invasion was a significant predictor of local and regional recurrence and disease-specific mortality (18).

Bone Invasion

Although regional and distant metastases occur by lymphangitic and hematogenous spread, invasion of the bone occurs by direct spread and is a common problem associated with tumors of the oral cavity, oropharynx, paranasal sinuses, and nasopharynx. For tumors of the oral cavity, the incidence of pathologically confirmed bone invasion seen in resected mandible specimens ranges from 22% to 56% (19–22). These and other studies have suggested that bone invasion is more likely to occur in the edentulous patient where the cortical bone may not form a continuous layer and the alveolar canal is close to the surface (23). Most susceptible sites of invasion include areas of cortical defect, cancellous spaces, and the periodontal space.

Two distinct histologic patterns of invasion into the bone have been described: (a) an invasive and infiltrative pattern, and (b) a broad erosive tumor front with osteolysis (24–26). The infiltrative pattern is characterized by finger-like projections and tumor nests, which extend into bone in an irregular fashion, such that residual bone islands can be seen within the tumor mass. The erosive pattern is characterized by an expansive pushing front with a definable tumor-bone interface. Host osteoclasts and fibrosis are seen along the tumor front and play a role in bony erosion. Osteolytic factors, including prostaglandin E_2 and $F_{2\alpha}$, have been implicated in this process (9).

A retrospective study of 68 patients treated with mandibulectomy for mandibular invasion by oral SCC examined the correlation of histologic patterns of invasion with clinical outcome (25). In this series, the infiltrative pattern of mandibular invasion was significantly associated with higher tumor grade, history of previously failed treatment, positive bone or soft tissue margins, and postoperative recurrence. Furthermore, 90% of patients with this pattern of spread had involvement into the medullary space. In patients with tumor with the erosive pattern of spread, 69% had medullary space involvement. Patients with infiltrative lesions (30%) had a significantly worse 3-year disease-free survival rate than did patients with erosive lesions (73%) (25).

The preoperative assessment of mandibular invasion remains a clinical challenge. Surgical management of bone involvement may include segmental mandibulectomy or conservation procedures such as marginal mandibulectomy, whether horizontal or vertical. Advances in vascularized bone grafts have improved postoperative morbidity rates. For true bony invasion, segmental mandibulectomy has been advocated by most authors, with marginal mandibulectomy reserved for tumors with periosteal or limited invasion (27–29). Rapid frozen section analysis of the cancellous space has been shown to be a useful intraoperative tool in the assessment of bony margins (30). Nevertheless, an accurate preoperative assessment of bony involvement is essential in operative planning and the determination of the extent of resection. Evaluation of the mandible includes physical examination as well as radiographic modalities, including plain radiography, computed tomographic (CT) scanning, magnetic resonance imaging (MRI), bone scintigraphy, and single photon emission computed tomography (SPECT) scanning.

Plain films and CT are among the most commonly used modalities and are recognized for their specificity; however, their sensitivity remains suboptimal. In a series of 82 patients with SCC of the oral cavity and oropharynx, mandibulectomies were performed on the basis of clinical or radiographic evidence of invasion (31). Clinical invasion was defined by fixation of the tumor to the mandible. In this series, patients with oral cavity primaries were more likely to have mandible involvement. Furthermore, clinical examination showed a significant correlation with pathologically confirmed invasion, with a sensitivity of 91% and a specificity of 80%. The positive predictive value was 75% and the negative predictive value was 93%. Plain radiography, using a panoramic imaging system (Panorex, Imaging Sciences International, Hattfield, PA), was not more reliable in this study, with a sensitivity of 84% and specificity of 97%. The positive predictive value was 96% and the negative predictive value was 88% for detecting mandibular invasion (31). In a series of 40 patients with oral cavity and oropharyngeal carcinoma, preoperative utility of the Panorex system was compared with CT (32). In this series, 93% of patients with positive results from Panorex imaging for cortical invasion were found to have pathologically confirmed invasion into the periosteum and cortex, and 64% had invasion into the medulla. As expected, however, the Panorex system was less reliable in its assessment of periosteal involvement, and approximately 50% of patients with negative results for Panorex imaging had invasion into the periosteum. Positive CT scan results corresponded with 80% of patients with invasion into the periosteum. The higher false-positive rate with CT is thought to be secondary to artifacts from irregular tooth sockets, periapical dental disease, and variable bone absorption (32).

The use of bone scintigraphy, although more sensitive than conventional radiography, has not gained uniform popularity due to its high false-positive rate. The use of radionucleotide scans has been shown to have a 90% negative predictive value and an 80% positive predictive value, suggesting that it may yet be a useful tool (33). The high false positivity is due to the inability to distinguish neoplastic invasion from osteomyelitis, osteoradionecrosis, periodontal disease, and fracture. The use of MRI to evaluate bone invasion has also been investigated. Although MRI may provide improved information regarding cancellous and medullar invasion, it is still unable to accurately assess early periosteal invasion (34,35). Recently, the use of SPECT for assessing mandibular invasion has been investigated. In a prospective study of 38 patients with SCC of the oral cavity and oropharynx, the reliability of the Panorex imaging system and CT was compared with that of SPECT scanning (36); SPECT scanning demonstrated improved sensitivity at 95% over CT scan (55%) and Panorex (50%). In this series, SPECT scanning demonstrated an 87% overall accuracy in predicting bone invasion compared with 71% for clinical examination, CT, and Panorex. The use of SPECT in the routine assessment of mandibular invasion warrants further investigation.

CLINICAL SIGNIFICANCE OF REGIONAL METASTASES

The presence of nodal metastasis is the most significant clinical predictive factor for regional recurrence and death from disease. Once nodal spread has occurred, the overall survival rates are often reduced by half (37). Involvement of multiple lymph nodes and ECS of tumor outside the lymph node are associated with even poorer treatment outcomes. Given the poor outcomes associated with nodal metastases, clinicians caring for patients with HNSCC need to properly evaluate the regional lymphatics for the presence of metastases and consider whether elective or therapeutic treatment of the nodal basins at risk is indicated. The proper evaluation and management of the relevant regional nodal basins are covered in an organ-site and disease-specific manner elsewhere in this text.

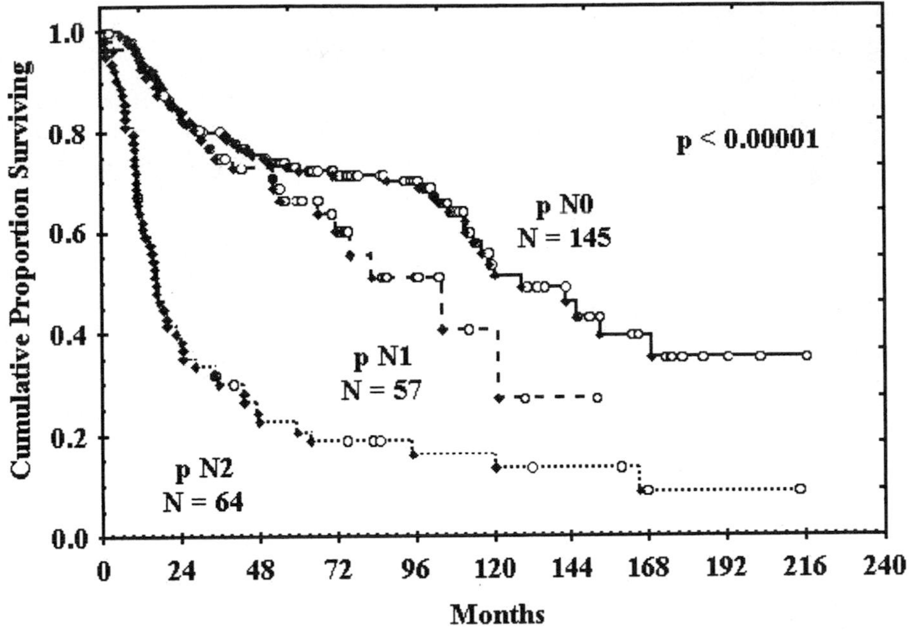

Figure 38.2 The impact of the increasing degree of nodal metastasis on survival.

Clinically Positive Lymph Nodes

The clinical finding of palpable or radiographically detectable adenopathy usually dictates aggressive treatment of the involved nodal basin and other at-risk nodal basins, yet clinical staging is not always reliable, and therefore patients with high-risk lesions in high-risk areas (such as a >4 mm depth of invasion tumor of the oral tongue) should be considered for an elective neck dissection for staging purposes. In marked contrast, significant differences were seen between patients with pN0 and pN+ disease ($p < 0.00001$), as shown in Figures 38.2 and 38.3. One possible explanation for this is a high rate of stage migration, whereas patients with cN0 or cN1 disease actually have higher nodal stage disease at the time of pathologic review, which was a frequent finding in our study. A 33.5% rate of occult nodal disease was found in the cN0 group, with 19% of occult nodes having ECS. Similarly, 40% of cN1 patients had pN2b disease, with 53% having ECS (Table 38.1). On the basis of our findings, we recommend that pathologic nodal staging based on a staging or therapeutic neck dissection be considered for patients treated for SCC of the oral tongue (SCCOT). Prospective studies are essential to validate these findings prior to inclusion of pathologic nodal staging in standard staging criteria.

EXTRACAPSULAR SPREAD AND MULTIPLE POSITIVE NODES

Extranodal extension beyond the lymph node capsule has been demonstrated to be a further predictor of poor outcome, even with adjuvant radiotherapy (39). In a retrospective review of 266 patients with SCCOT treated over a 15-year period, patients were divided into three groups: pathologically node negative, pathologically node positive but ECS negative, and pathologically node positive with ECS. Patients with pathologically positive nodes had a significantly worse 5-year overall and disease-specific survival than did patients with pathologically negative nodes, as shown in Figure 38.3. Furthermore, the presence of ECS was associated with significantly worse overall and disease-specific survival rates, with these patients having significantly higher recurrence rates, regional failure rates, and rates of distant spread (Figs. 38.4 through 38.6) (38).

To further identify high-risk patients, the extent of ECS was evaluated among these patients. There was no significant association between disease-free and overall survival rates when patients with nodes >2 mm of ECS were compared with patients with nodes ≤2 mm of ECS (Fig. 38.7). Patients with multiple positive nodes did worse than patients with one pathologically positive node, irrespective of ECS status ($p = 0.001$) (Fig. 38.8). When patients with multiple positive nodes were evaluated for extent of ECS, patients with multiple nodes with ECS had a significantly worse disease-specific and overall survival than patients with multiple nodes and only one ECS+ node (38) (Fig. 38.9).

ADJUVANT THERAPY

As discussed above, patients with tongue cancer treated at our institution with surgery and who were found to have multiple positive nodes or ECS (or both) were almost always (83–92%) treated with adjuvant radiotherapy. However, they still had unacceptably high rates of regional recurrence (16–58%) and distant metastasis. Because of outcomes such as these, a number of investigators have evaluated the role of intensification of adjuvant therapy for patients with adverse pathologic staging criteria discovered at the time of resection of the primary and regional lymphadenectomy, and several clinical trials have investigated the role of adjuvant chemoradiation therapy in high-risk patients. In a nonrandomized prospective trial (40) of 371 patients treated surgically between 1982 and 1992, all patients had negative surgical margins but positive ECS. Of these patients, 53 (14%) were treated with surgery alone, 187 (50%) were treated with surgery plus radiation therapy (50-60 Gy), and 131 (35%) were treated with surgery and radiation therapy followed by chemotherapy with 5-fluorouracil and methotrexate. With 30 months of follow-up, the disease-free survival rates were 17% for surgery only, 40% for surgery plus radiation therapy, and

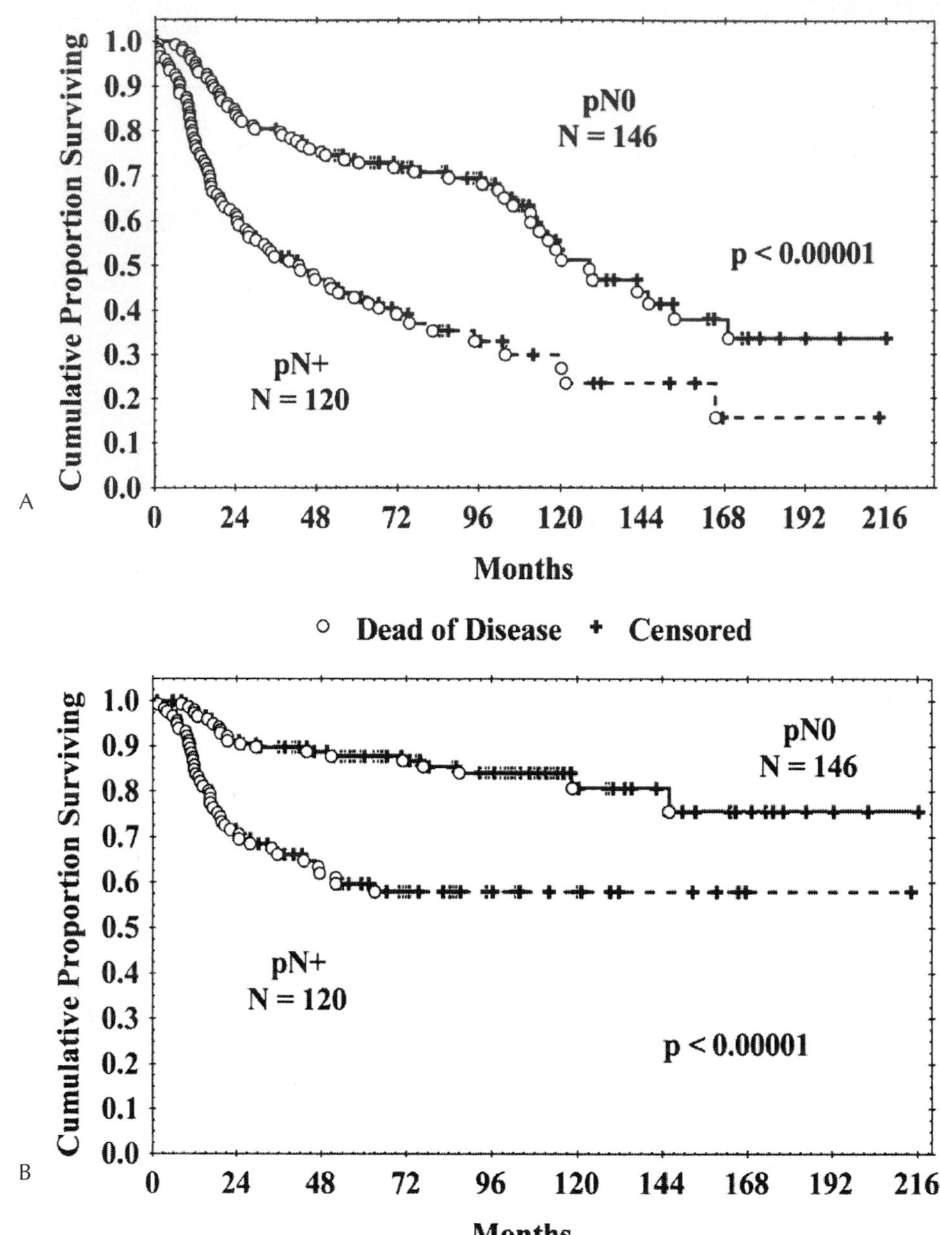

Figure 38.3 Impact of pathologically positive lymph nodes on overall **(A)** and disease-specific **(B)** survival of patients with squamous cell carcinoma of the oral tongue. pN0, node negative; pN+, node positive.

TABLE 38.1 Pathologic N Classification for Select Patients Clinically Classified as N0 and N1

	Pathologic N classification for 186 patients clinically classified as N0	
Pathologic N classification	**Prevalence of nodal metastasis**	**Presence of cN0pN+ patients with extracapsular spread**
pN0	123/186 (66.1%)	0 (0%)
pN1	39/186 (21.0%)	5/39 (12.8%)
pN2a	0/186 (0%)	0 (0%)
pN2b	21/186 (11.3%)	6/21 (28.6%)
pN2c	3/186 (1.6%)	1/3 (33%)
Total	186/266 (69.9%)	12/63 (19.0%)
	Pathologic N classification for 47 patients clinically classified as N1	
Pathologic N classification	**Prevalence of nodal metastasis**	**Presence of extracapsular spread (ECS)**
pN0	15/47 (31.9%)	0/15 (0%)
pN1	12/47 (25.5%)	5/12 (41.7%)
pN2a	0/47 (0%)	0/0 (0%)
pN2b	19/47 (40.4%)	10/19 (52.6%)
pN2c	1/47 (2.1%)	1/1 (100%)
Total	47/266 (17.7%)	16/32 (50%)

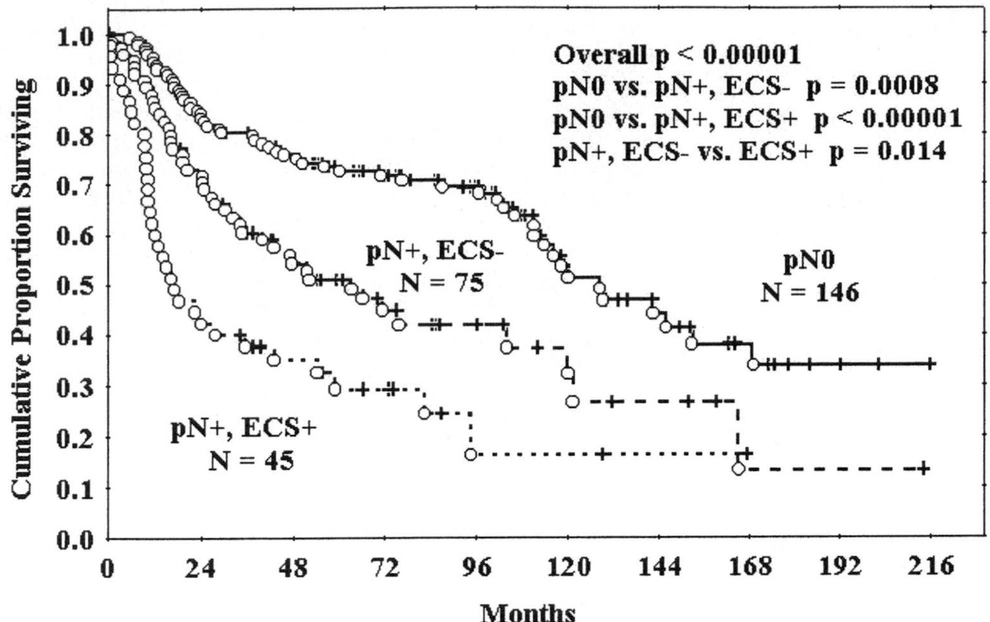

Figure 38.4 Impact of pathologically positive lymph nodes and extracapsular spread on overall survival of patients with squamous cell carcinoma of the oral tongue: composite graph.

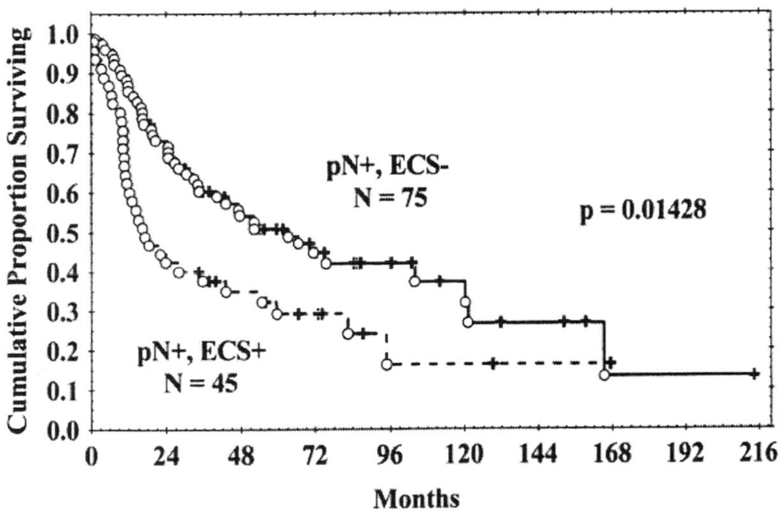

A

○ Dead of Disease + Censored

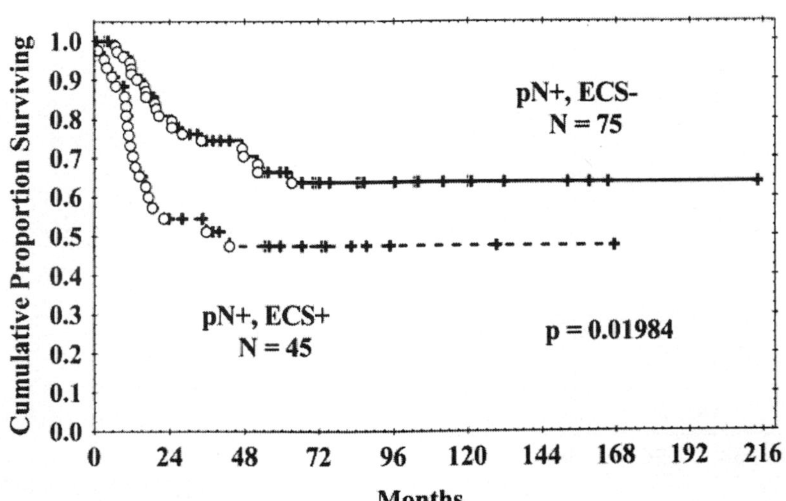

B

Figure 38.5 Impact of extracapsular spread on overall **(A)** and disease-specific survival **(B)** of patients with squamous cell carcinoma of the oral tongue.

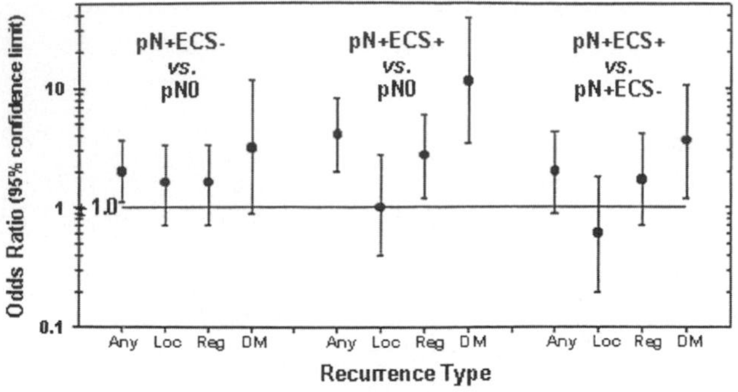

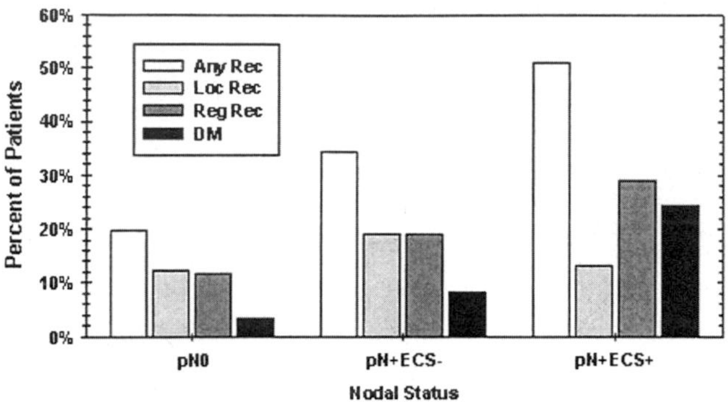

Figure 38.6 Impact on pathologic nodal status and extracapsular spread (ECS) on overall and local, regional, and distant recurrence. Crude odds ratios and confidence intervals show relative risks for recurrence between nodal and ECS groups.

58% for the surgery, radiation, and chemotherapy group ($p < 0.001$) (40).

In a prospective phase II study, Radiation Therapy Oncology Group (RTOG) 88-24, 52 surgically treated patients with stage IV HNSCC or positive margins were treated with 30 fractions over 6 weeks (total 60 Gy) and cisplatin (100 mg/m^2 per dose) on days 1, 13, and 23. Actuarial analysis at 3 years revealed a 48% overall survival rate and an 81% locoregional control rate. Severe and life-threatening toxicities, however, were found in 20% and 12% of the patients, respectively (41). On the basis of these results, the RTOG has investigated a prospective randomized trial comparing radiation therapy alone with radiation therapy with cisplatin therapy. The results of this study are still pending.

In a phase III trial conducted in France (42), 83 patients with stage III or IV HNSCC or ECS treated surgically were randomly assigned to receive radiotherapy alone (to the primary tumor and involved nodal basins) or radiation therapy plus chemotherapy, consisting of intravenous cisplatin (50 mg given weekly for seven to nine cycles). Patients who received radiation therapy with chemotherapy had significantly higher overall and disease-free survival rates compared with patients who received radiation therapy alone (42).

SIGNIFICANCE OF DISTANT METASTASIS

The term *metastasis* was first described in 1829 by French physician, Joseph Claude Récamier (43). In his treatise, *Recherches sur le traitement du cancer,* he reported the spread of cancer cells into the circulation and to distant sites in the body. Although the incidence of distant metastases in advanced head and neck cancer is relatively low compared with that for other stage-matched primary malignancies, such as breast cancer and colon cancer, once distant spread has occurred the prognosis is invariably poor. Furthermore, several studies have shown that as we obtain improved rates of locoregional control in HNSCC, higher rates of distant metastases are being observed (44,45). This highlights the need for greater understanding of the mechanisms of development of distant metastases in HNSCC and the need for identifying more effective ways to treat them.

Incidence and Outcomes

In the absence of nodal regional involvement, distant metastasis is very rare, with the exception of cases of adenoid cystic carcinoma. For SCC, the lung is the most frequent site of distant metastasis, followed by bone, liver, skin, and other sites (46–48). Clinical studies have found incidence rates for distant metastases of 4.2% (49) and 23.8% (50), whereas autopsy studies have cited higher incidences, ranging from 37 to 57% (51,52). A review of 5,019 patients treated over a 25-year period

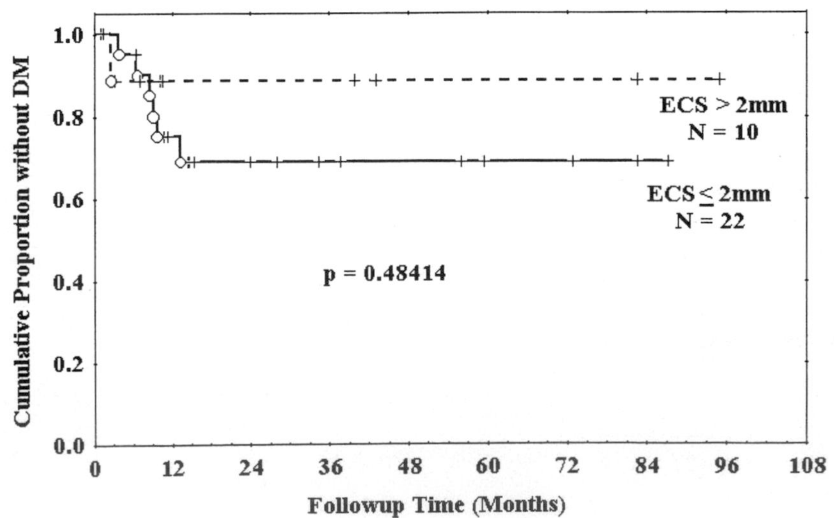

Figure 38.7 The histopathologic degree of extracapsular extension does not significantly impact on survival.

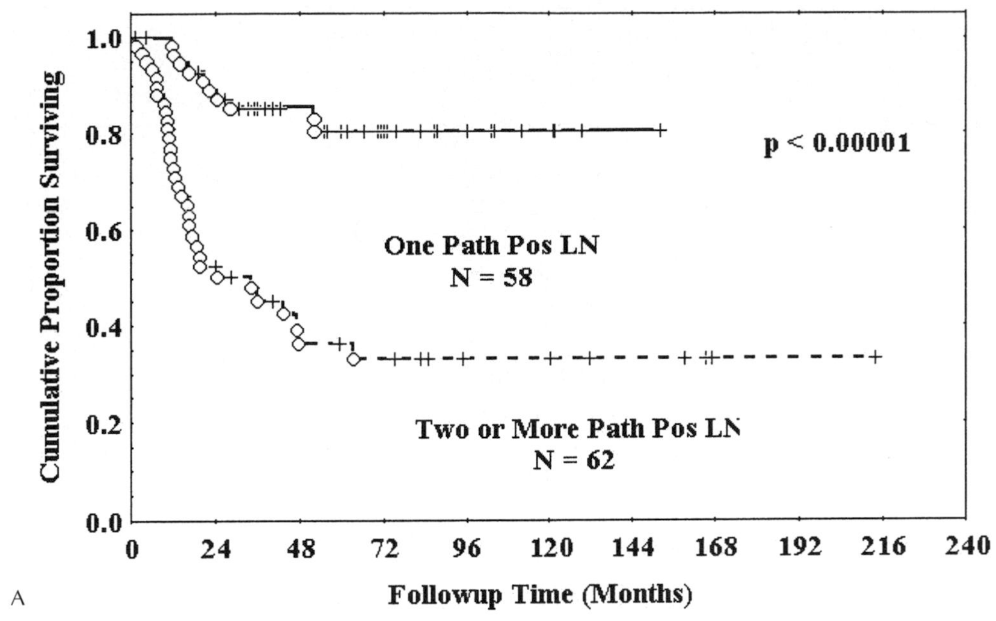

A

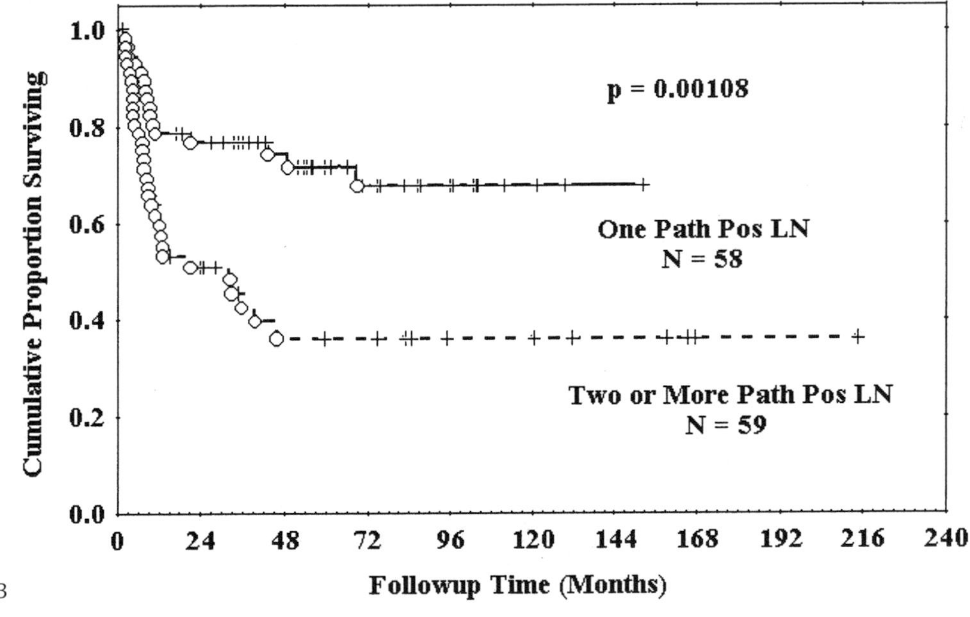

B

Figure 38.8 **A:** The impact of the multiplicity of nodal disease on overall survival in patients with squamous cell carcinoma of the oral tongue. **B:** The impact of the multiplicity of nodal disease on overall survival in patients with squamous cell carcinoma of the oral tongue.

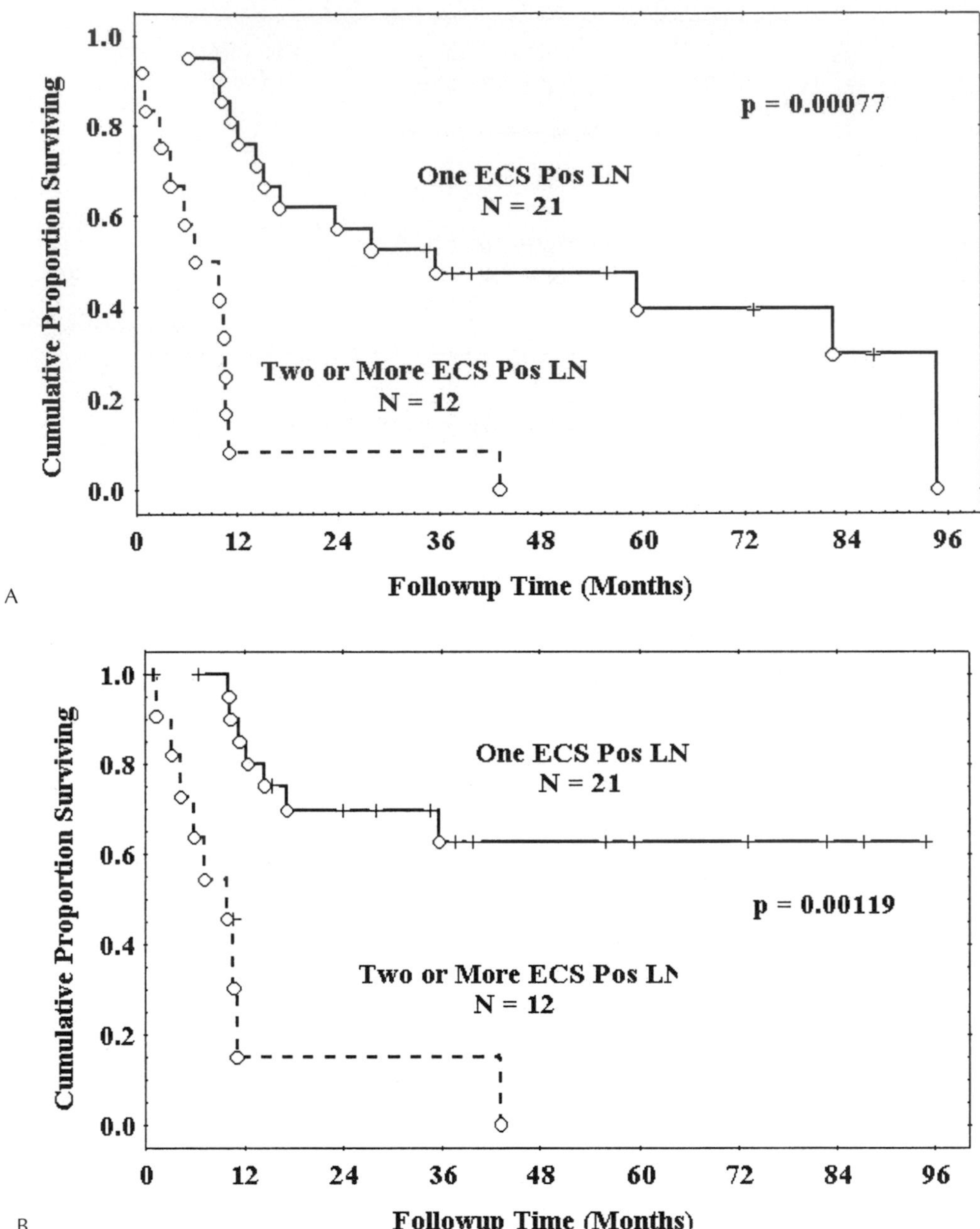

Figure 38.9 A,B: The striking impact of multiple nodes with extracapsular spread (ECS) on overall survival.

at the M. D. Anderson Cancer Center found the incidence of distant metastases to be 10.8% (46). In a retrospective review of 727 patients with HNSCC treated over a 12-year period at the University of Texas Medical Branch in Galveston, 83 (11.4%) patients developed distant metastases (47). In this series, the lung was the most common site (83.4%), followed by bone (31.1%) and liver (6.0%). The average time between initial diagnosis and presentation with distant disease was 11.7 months, with 84% of distant metastases first appearing within 24 months. Survival with distant disease averaged 4.3 months, with 86.7% patients dying within 1 year. In this series, size of the primary tumor and extent of nodal involvement were predictors of distant spread, whereas site of primary and histologic differentiation were not.

Other studies have cited variable rates of distant metastases among tumor subsites, with hypopharyngeal tumors being more likely to have distant metastases (53,54). In a retrospective review of 1,880 patients with HNSCC, 18% (115/636) of patients with local or regional relapse had distant metastases, whereas only 5% (64/1,244) of patients with locoregional control had distant metastases ($p < 0.001$) (53). In this series, neck stage and locoregional control were the most significant factors for progression to distant spread. Among patients in whom locoregional control was achieved, size of the primary (T stage) and location of the tumor at the hypopharynx and supraglottis were also significant prognostic markers for distant metastases.

CLINICOPATHOLOGIC PREDICTORS OF DISTANT METASTASES

The reason why some HNSCC behave aggressively and progress to distant metastases while others remain relatively confined is still not well understood. Recently, a panel of distinct clinical and histopathologic criteria has been proposed to identify patients at greatest risk for development of distant metastases in HNSCC

(48). In a prospective historical cohort of 622 patients with HNSCC treated between 1991 and 1994 at the M. D. Anderson Cancer Center, patients were stratified as at low, medium, and high risk for progression to distant metastases based on distinct clinical and histopathologic criteria. The overall 5-year incidence of metastases was 15.1% (94/622), with pulmonary metastases being the most common (65.9%), followed by bone (22.3%) and liver (9.5%). Although oropharyngeal and hypopharyngeal sites had higher rates of distant metastasis, the rates were not statistically significantly different from those for the larynx and oral cavity. Although the site of the primary tumor did not predict distant metastasis, when subsites were considered, particular high-risk areas could be identified. High-risk subsites include retromolar trigone and buccal mucosa within the oral cavity, base of tongue and tonsil in the oropharynx, pyriform sinus in the hypopharynx, and supraglottis in the larynx. Tumor size directly correlated with the risk for distant metastasis. As observed in other studies, the presence and extent of cervical metastasis was the most important clinical predictor for distant metastasis. Additionally, the presence of ECS and pathologically confirmed regional metastasis directly correlated with distant metastasis and extent of regional disease (Fig. 38.10).

SCREENING TESTS TO EVALUATE DISTANT METASTASES

The most common site of distant metastasis is the lung. The primary screening modality has traditionally been the chest x-ray, which has a sensitivity of 50% and a specificity of 94% (55). Computed tomography scan is more sensitive than chest x-ray. In a study of 189 patients with HNSCC, 66 patients had positive results for the CT scan, whereas only 17 of these lesions were visible on chest x-ray (56). Similar reports have supported these findings, suggesting that CT scan is a much more sensitive measure for intrathoracic metastasis and should be considered in high-risk patients (57,58).

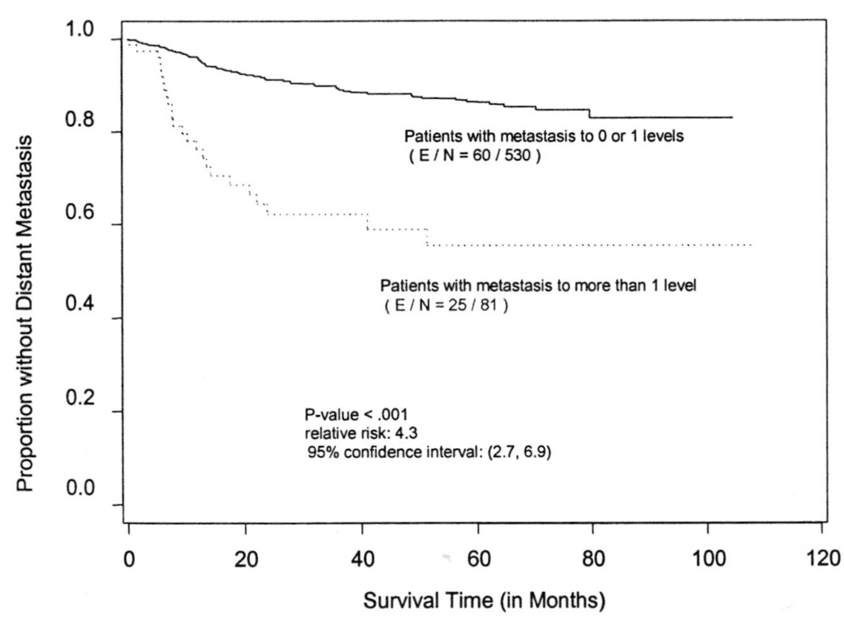

A

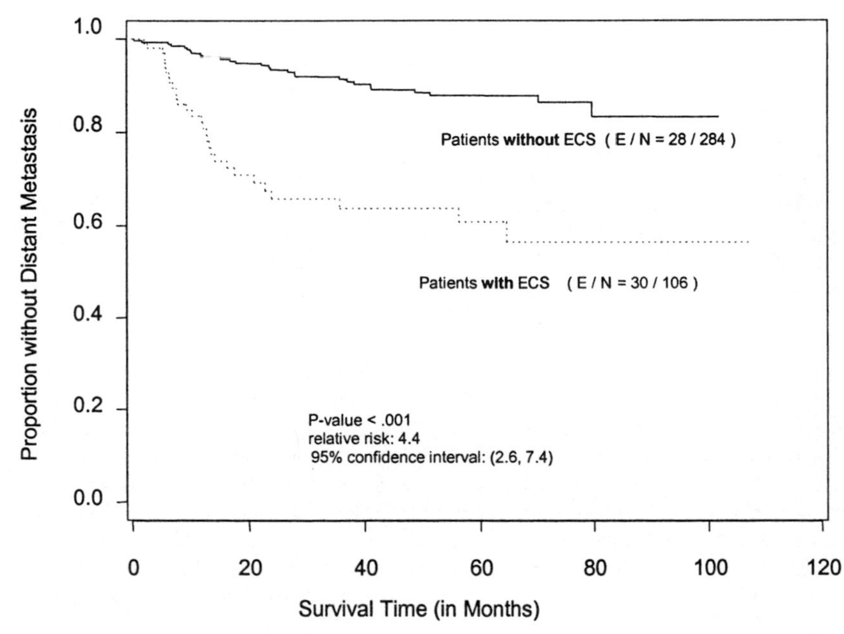

B

Figure 38.10 Kaplan–Meier actuarial curves plotting the freedom from distant metastasis (DM) for 611 patients with head and neck cancer treated at M. D. Anderson Cancer Center. **A:** Based on clinical staging, those with metastasis to more than one level of the neck (31%; 25/81) had a significantly higher rate of DM, compared with those without (11.3%; 60/530, $p < 0.001$) [relative risk (RR) 4.3; 95% confidence interval (CI) 2.7–6.9]. **B:** Of the 390 patients undergoing neck dissection, those with extracapsular spread (ECS) (28%; 30/106) had a significantly higher rate of DM, compared with those without (9.9%; 28/284, $p < 0.001$), (RR 4.4; 95% CI 2.6–7.4).

The second most common site of distant metastasis is the bone. Frequently, more than one bony site is involved, and bone metastases are almost invariably concurrent with pulmonary metastasis (59). Bone metastases from HNSCC are usually osteolytic lesions. For this reason, plasma bone-specific alkaline phosphatase, which measures osteoblastic activity, is not a sensitive screening tool for detection of distant metastasis. Overall, alkaline phosphatase has a sensitivity of only 20% and a specificity of 98% for the detection of bone metastases (60). The most sensitive diagnostic instrument for detection of bone involvement is bone scintigraphy. A positive result for a bone scan, however, is nonspecific and needs confirmation by biopsy. In a series of 172 patients with HNSCC who underwent bone scintigraphy as part of their routine workup, management was changed in only three patients. In this series, the authors concluded that routine use of bone scanning was not indicated (61).

Although liver metastases are uncommon, the liver is nevertheless the third most reported site of distant spread for HNSCC. In a series of 101 high-risk HNSCC patients, all underwent ultrasound of the abdomen and/or CT scan for metastatic evaluation. Among these patients, only one patient was discovered by routine screening to have liver metastasis (59). On the basis of these findings, the authors did not recommend routine use of imaging for screening for liver metastasis. Furthermore, serologic testing for liver metastasis is not sensitive and is very nonspecific. The HNSCC patient population has a high incidence of alcohol abuse, and underlying liver function abnormalities are therefore not uncommon.

Further screening modalities for the detection of distant metastasis are currently under investigation. These include thallium-201 SPECT, fluorine-18-fluorodeoxyglucose positron emission tomography, and radioimmunoscintigraphy.

EFFECT OF SYSTEMIC THERAPY ON DISTANT METASTASES

Once distant metastasis has occurred, the prognosis is uniformly poor, and treatment in most situations is only palliative (59). Although metastatic disease has been shown to be responsive to systemic therapy, overall survival rates have improved little. Both single-agent and multiple combination regimens have been reported (62,63). Platinum-based chemotherapy in combination with 5-fluorouracil has had higher response rates and is a commonly used regimen. Currently the addition of taxanes is being evaluated in clinical trials, with promising results (64). Taxanes behave uniquely to provide both cytotoxic and antiangiogenic effects.

EFFECT OF SURGERY ON AN ISOLATED PULMONARY METASTASES

The lung is the most common distant site of metastasis from head and neck cancer. Often spread is multifocal and not amenable to surgical resection. In evaluation of the isolated pulmonary nodule, it may be difficult to differentiate between a second primary tumor and metastatic spread from the head and neck. In the absence of surgical resection, the outcome for patients with metastatic head and neck cancer has been uniformly poor. However, for the solitary pulmonary nodule that is in a favorable location, studies have suggested that in selected patients surgical resection is beneficial, with 5-year survival rates ranging from 32% to 59% (65–68).

Only a few studies have reported the effect of surgical treatment on metastatic head and neck carcinoma. In these studies, factors predictive of survival included surgical resection of the metastasis, locoregional control of the primary, presence of an isolated pulmonary nodule, and a longer disease-free interval between treatment of the primary tumor and detection of the metastasis (65–68). Location and TNM classification of the primary tumor have not consistently been shown to be predictive of survival. However, a few studies have suggested that patients with metastatic disease from laryngeal primaries have better survival rates than do patients with tumors of the oral cavity (65,66).

In a retrospective review of 2,300 head and neck cancer patients treated between 1978 and 1994, 138 patients (6%) developed pulmonary metastases, with an overall 5-year survival rate of 13% (67). Overall, younger patients (p = 0.011), patients with a longer disease-free interval (p = 0.016), and patients with a non-SCC (p = 0.038) did significantly better. Twenty-one carefully selected patients underwent surgical resection of their pulmonary metastases; patients were considered acceptable for surgical resection if there was no locoregional recurrence, the metastasis was resectable, and baseline pulmonary function was satisfactory. In this study with an intentional selection bias, patients who underwent a surgical resection had a 5-year survival rate of 59% compared with a 4% survival rate for the nonsurgical group (p = 0.0033). Among the patients who underwent resection of their metastasis, patients who had a longer disease-free interval between treatment of their primary and detection of metastasis tended to do better. On the basis of this series, patients with locoregional control and resectable metastatic disease are potential surgical candidates with improved survival (67).

In a series of 32 patients with pulmonary metastases who underwent surgical resection (66), the 5-year survival rate was 32%. All patients underwent surgical resection of the pulmonary metastases along with mediastinal node dissection. Involvement of more than one lobe was associated with a worse 5-year survival. Although mediastinal lymph node dissection did not affect overall survival, patients with positive mediastinal lymph nodes had a significantly worse 5-year survival (p = 0.004). Pleural invasion was also a significant poor prognostic factor (p = 0.04). Results from this series reaffirm that the best surgical candidate is the patient with a single pulmonary nodule confined to one lobe without mediastinal involvement, and that surgical resection offers improved survival rates (66).

MOLECULAR AND CELLULAR MECHANISMS OF INVASION AND METASTASIS

The progression of preneoplastic lesions to invasive cancer and on to regional metastasis and finally distant metastasis represents a continuum of disease that is best explained by the interrelated concepts of multistep carcinogenesis developed by Vogelstein and Fearon et al. (69) in their studies of colon cancer and of tumor evolution as described by Nowell (70). More recently, Hanahan and Weinberg (71) have summarized six hallmark steps of cancer cells that enable tumor cells to grow, invade, and ultimately metastasize: (a) acquisition of autonomous proliferative signaling, (b) inhibition of growth inhibitory signals, (c) evasion of programmed cell death, (d) immortalization, (e) acquisition of a nutrient blood supply (angiogenesis), and (f) acquisition of the ability to invade tissue.

These biologic characteristics have been previously implicated in the metastatic process as described in the models of Fidler (72,73). On the basis of their pioneering studies with orthotopic nude mouse models of metastasis (74), Fidler and his colleagues have shown that the process of metastasis consists of a series of sequential, selective, and interdependent steps, involving transformation, angiogenesis, local invasion, detachment and embolization, attachment, and, finally, proliferation at the distant site.

Mechanisms of Tumor Invasion

Califano et al. (75) have developed an allelotype of HNSCC pathogenesis that mirrors the Fearon and Vogelstein (76) model of colon cancer progression. This construct has shown that, during HNSCC carcinogenesis, a number of specific genetic alterations occur at critical chromosomal loci that encode proteins important in the regulation of cell growth, survival, and inhibition of the cell cycle. Some of these genes are discussed further below. The precise order and number of alterations needed to develop an invasive HNSCC remains to be elucidated, but the available data suggest that the total accumulation of the alterations rather than the precise order in which they are acquired is the more critical aspect of tumorigenesis.

Unlike benign tumors, malignant tumors can break down natural host barriers and invade the surrounding host tissue. Tumor invasion and metastasis is an active process that includes loss of normal cell adhesion properties, breakdown of the basement membrane and extracellular matrix, stimulation of tumor cell migration, and angiogenesis (73,77–79). Some of the specific molecules involved in these steps have been studied in many tumor types, including HNSCC.

Attachment to the Basement Membrane

The basement membrane underlying squamous epithelium serves as a natural barrier to tumor cell invasion and has been biochemically characterized using a variety of methods. Collagen type IV, laminin, collagen type VII, and heparan sulfate proteoglycans have all been found in epithelial basement membranes (80,81). However, loss of the basement membrane has not been correlated with invasive behavior in HNSCC, as it has in other tumor types (82,83).

INTEGRINS

Both normal and neoplastic squamous cell epithelium have specific receptors for basement membrane constituents through which the cells adhere to the extracellular matrix. By raising monoclonal antibodies to human HNSCC cells, Van Waes et al. (84) isolated a tumor-expressed antigen termed A9, which was subsequently shown to be identical to the $\alpha6\beta4$ integrin. Integrins are a family of cell adhesion molecules, and the $\alpha6\beta4$ integrin is known to bind specifically to laminin. Immunohistochemical studies of normal squamous epithelium and HNSCC specimens have shown a polarized pattern of expression of the $\alpha6\beta4$ integrin on the basal pole of normal skin or mucosal keratinocytes, which are adjacent to the basement membrane, and a more diffuse staining pattern in tumors (85). When A9 antigen expression was correlated with clinical variables, increased levels of $\alpha6\beta4$ integrin expression were correlated with early recurrence and metastasis (86,87). Another integrin that has been studied in HNSCC is $\alpha V\beta5$ integrin. Unlike $\alpha6\beta4$ integrins, $\alpha V\beta5$ integrin has reduced expression in HNSCC (88). *In vitro* studies suggest that this integrin may be important in oral neoplasia since $\alpha V\beta5$-negative cell lines show a malignant phenotype that can be reversed by transfection of the missing integrin (89). Thus, it appears that integrins have important but widely varied roles in the progression of HNSCC.

E-CADHERIN

E-Cadherin is another cell-surface receptor molecule that plays a role in maintaining cell-cell contacts, an important feature of epithelial cells. By immunohistochemical methods, E-cadherin levels have been associated with differentiation in SCC (90). In other words, well-differentiated tumors express high levels of E-cadherin, whereas poorly differentiated tumors have significantly lower levels of expression (90). E-Cadherin expression has also been examined in relation to clinical outcome in patients with HNSCC (91). Although E-cadherin expression was not related to tumor size or stage, patients with increased tumor levels of E-cadherin appeared to have a more favorable survival rate. This finding was corroborated in a recent study in which patients with strong E-cadherin staining in tumors had a 5-year survival rate of 85% compared with 53% for those with weak staining (92). Lower levels of E-cadherin have also been associated with the metastatic phenotype in HNSCC cell lines (93). This relationship has been shown in tumor specimens as well (94), indicating that loss of E-cadherin may be an important step in the development of metastasis in HNSCC.

CATENINS

More recently, a group of cytoplasmic proteins called catenins, which form complexes with cadherins, has been shown to assist in the maintenance of cell–cell contacts (95). Studies in oral cavity cancers have further revealed that, as with E-cadherin, catenin levels show an inverse relationship with the degree of tumor differentiation (96). Further studies are ongoing to assess whether catenins may play a complementary role with cadherins in invasion and metastasis.

Proteolysis and Migration

Proteolysis of the extracellular matrix is thought to be a critical step for tissue invasion by tumors (97). A wide variety of proteases have been evaluated in many tumor types, and there is an expanding body of literature regarding the potential role of several specific proteolytic enzymes and their specific inhibitors in the development of tissue invasion and regional metastases of human HNSCC.

MATRIX METALLOPROTEINASES

The matrix metalloproteinases (MMPs) are a diverse group of proteinases that require metal ions for their activity, hence their name. The MMPs are important mediators of invasion and metastasis in many tumor types, including breast, colon, and prostate (98,99). In HNSCC, several individual MMPs have been studied. Using a combination of immunohistochemical, *in situ* hybridization, and zymographic methods, Sutinen and colleagues (100) found relatively increased expression of MMP-2 in oral cancer specimens compared with oral dysplastic lesions. These data have been corroborated in other studies (101,102). The expression of this enzyme, also known as 72-kDa type IV collagenase, has been correlated with the development of cervical lymph node metastases and lymphatic and vascular invasion in patients with oral cavity tumors (103).

MMP-3, also known as stromelysin-1, has also been shown to be up-regulated in approximately 50% of head and neck cancers (104). This MMP degrades laminin, fibronectin, and type IV collagen. With the use of *in situ* hybridization, MMP-3 was identified in tumor cells in 23 of 26 HNSCC samples studied, suggesting a role for MMPs in stromal invasion by HNSCC (105). These results were further substantiated in a study of 107 HNSCC samples using Northern blot analysis, in which several MMPs, including MMP-3, were found to be overexpressed (106). Further analysis by immunohistochemical staining indicated that expression of this MMP appears to be concentrated at the advancing or invasive front of the tumor (107). These studies have also demonstrated that MMP-3 is associated with higher T stage and advanced nodal status.

Another MMP implicated in the development of HNSCC is MMP-9, also known as the 92-kDa type IV collagenase. Initial investigations showed that HNSCC cell lines expressed MMP-9

(108), and subsequent analysis of fresh HNSCC biopsy specimens with antibodies to MMP-9 confirmed the presence of this protease in invasive HNSCC (109). Several studies have since verified this finding (110). The presence of increased MMP-9 activity has been associated with invasiveness in oral cavity cancer (101). In addition, suppression of MMP-9 activity has been shown to decrease tumor cell invasiveness in tongue cancer cells (111). More recent evidence points toward a new role for MMP-9 in invasion and metastasis of HNSCC. Riedel et al. (112) found that MMP-9 staining was correlated with increased microvessel density and up-regulation of vascular endothelial cell growth factor (VEGF), indicating that MMP-9 and VEGF may cooperate in the process of angiogenesis in HNSCC (112). This presents an exciting avenue for the application of MMP inhibitors that might block invasion and attenuate angiogenesis.

It has recently become evident that MMPs are regulated within the cell by various molecules, the most important of which are a group of inhibitors called tissue inhibitors of metalloproteinases (TIMPs), which participate actively in the dynamic regulation of proteolysis, and are usually produced by surrounding stromal cells in an attempt to block the proteolytic effects of MMPs (100). Only recently has this area of research been examined with respect to HNSCC. One of the few studies available suggests that both high levels of MMPs and low levels of TIMPs may be required for metastasis to occur (101). Many additional questions regarding the interaction of HNSCC with the extracellular matrix still need to be answered, and it is likely that important information about the biology of these tumors as well as clinical applications will arise from studies in this area.

UROKINASE-TYPE PLASMINOGEN ACTIVATOR

The urokinase-type plasminogen activator (uPA) system is also believed to play a role in invasion and metastasis. The uPA is known to bind to a specific receptor, urokinase-type plasminogen activator receptor (uPAR), and uPa activity can be inhibited by a specific inhibitor, plasminogen activator inhibitor (113). The uPa system has been well studied in several tumor models, including HNSCC. Early work indicated that uPA levels were significantly elevated in HNSCC cell lines, compared with levels in fibroblasts (114). In addition, uPAR has also been shown to be up-regulated in HNSCC (115). Another study of 34 primary oral cavity cancers showed that uPA and uPAR are expressed in 23.5% and 29.4% of the tumors, respectively, and that coexpression of these two molecules is associated with highly invasive tumors and lymph node metastases (116). Clayman et al. (117) were able to show that inhibition of uPA by a specific anti-uPA antibody abrogated the ability of SCC cell lines to invade. Likewise, evidence indicates that blocking the uPAR molecule also abrogates tumor metastasis (118). These data suggest that the uPa system plays an important role in the ability of HNSCC to invade and metastasize.

SERPINS

The serpin family of proteins is a group of protease inhibitors just coming to prominence for their role in carcinogenesis. Several recent studies have highlighted their importance in HNSCC (119–121). Spring et al. (119) identified and cloned a serpin member they named "headpin," which maps to chromosome 18q, a site of frequent loss of heterozygosity in HNSCC. They found headpin to be expressed in normal oral mucosa but underexpressed in oral cavity SCC. This down-regulation appeared to occur at the transcriptional level in HNSCC cell lines studied by the same group (120).

Another serpin family member, maspin, is also located on chromosome 18q and is also known to have tumor suppressor functions. Using immunohistochemical techniques, Xia et al. (121) showed that patients with oral SCC tumors that had high maspin expression had lower rates of regional metastases and better overall survival rates. Further studies are necessary to delineate the role of the serpin family of proteins in the pathogenesis of HNSCC.

Acquisition of a Blood Supply (Angiogenesis)

As tumors grow, invade, and metastasize, formation of new blood vessels is critical. Although many tumor cells have metabolic derangements, they still require essential nutrients and gas exchange for survival. Without adequate vascularization, tumors larger than 1 mm^3 may undergo necrosis. Not surprisingly, most tumors are able to overcome this impediment by stimulating endothelial cell proliferation and new blood vessel formation. This process of neovascularization, or angiogenesis, is itself a multistep process that appears to be regulated by both stimulatory and inhibitory factors (122). Steps critical to successful neovascularization include degradation of the extracellular matrix, endothelial-cell proliferation, migration, and assembly into higher-order structures. Molecules that regulate angiogenesis may affect one or more of these steps.

MICROVESSEL DENSITY

Tumor angiogenesis is quantified through the staining of blood vessels with endothelial cell markers such as factor VIII, CD31, and CD34 and the subsequent measurement of "microvessel density" (123,124). These measurements correlate with metastasis for patients with breast, ovarian, prostatic, and gastric carcinomas (73), and may serve as an independent prognostic indicator. Several studies have looked at microvessel density in relation to the clinical outcome of patients with HNSCC, but these studies have yielded conflicting results (125–128). One study of 25 patients with stage T1 lesions of the oral cavity showed a correlation between elevated microvessel density, as determined by factor VIII staining, and the development of cervical metastases (125). Another study found that patients who had HNSCC with increased microvessel density had a better prognosis, with a median survival of 69 months, than did patients with low microvessel density, with a median survival of 10 months (126). Two additional studies, of 106 patients and 19 patients, showed no correlation between microvessel density and clinical outcomes (127,128).

REGULATORS OF ANGIOGENESIS

A number of significant advances have been made in recent years to further our understanding of tumor angiogenesis, including the isolation and characterization in several tumor systems of specific angiogenic factors and their inhibitors (129). The complex interplay of both positive and negative regulators of the angiogenic process determines the degree of new blood vessel formation in and around a tumor (73,122). Studies of these molecules in the pathogenesis of HNSCC have been limited, but they indicate that angiogenesis is important for HNSCC biology, may be clinically important for prognostic information, and may be a target for biologic therapy in the future. A few of these molecules and their purported roles in the angiogenic pathway, with special reference to HNSCC, are discussed in the following subsections.

Positive Regulators of Angiogenesis

Vascular endothelial cell growth factor (VEGF). VEGF has pleiotropic angiogenic effects. Not only is VEGF a potent endothelial cell mitogen, but it also promotes cell survival, cell motility, endothelial cell organization, and permeability across endothelial cell monolayers (73). Studies have attempted to correlate VEGF overexpression with various clinical end points such as cervical nodal metastases, tumor microvessel counts, and overall survival (130,131). Thus far, the results of studies of VEGF in HNSCC are conflicting. In one study of 77 patients with oral or oropharyngeal carcinoma, VEGF was present in 41% of tumors and was identified as the most significant predictor of poor prognosis (132). Similar findings have been reported in other subsites (133). In addition, *in vitro* studies have demonstrated that down-regulation of VEGF by transfection of antisense VEGF in head and neck cancer cell lines reduced endothelial cell migration by 50% (134). However, no decrease in tumorigenicity in these cell lines was found. This supports other data that have shown no prognostic relationship between VEGF levels and tumor stage, invasiveness, or survival variables (135,136). Thus, currently no consensus exists about the role of VEGF in the pathogenesis of HNSCC.SK

Basic fibroblast growth factor (bFGF). bFGF has been found to be among the most potent of the endothelial cell mitogens (73). This molecule promotes endothelial cell motility and survival as well as the organization of endothelial cells into tubules when grown in vitro in the presence of extracellular matrix components. Basic fibroblast growth factor also up-regulates the production of the tissue proteases MMP-1 and uPA.

Basic fibroblast growth factor and its receptor FGF-2 are expressed in normal oral keratinocytes as well as in oral cancers (137). A study performed at M. D. Anderson Cancer Center on 11 head and neck cancer specimens showed high levels of bFGF in well-differentiated tumor specimens but no expression in poorly differentiated tumors (138). Furthermore, the levels of bFGF found in the tumors were similar to or less than those found in the adjacent normal mucosa. In addition, several groups have reported elevated levels of bFGF in serum and urine of patients with HNSCC and correlated this with poor prognosis (139,140).

Platelet-derived endothelial cell growth factor (PD-ECGF). PD-ECGF is an endothelial cell mitogen with in vivo angiogenic activity that also displays thymidine phosphorylase activity. PD-ECGF expression was studied in 58 patients with oral or oropharyngeal cancers and was found to be overexpressed in a high percentage of tumor cells (141). Those patients with higher percentages of tumor cells expressing PD-ECGF had higher rates of relapse and death from their disease than did those with a lesser degree of staining. However, there was no correlation between microvessel density and PD-ECGF staining.

Interleukin-8. Several lines of evidence indicate that interleukin-8 (IL-8) is a cytokine with angiogenic activity (73). Homogenates of nine fresh HNSCC tumor specimens were found to contain IL-8 by radioimmunoassay (142). Further evaluation of these tumors by immunohistochemical techniques showed that this cytokine was localized within the tumor cells. In this same study, the stimulation of cultures of HNSCC cells and established tumor cell lines with interleukin-1 or tumor necrosis factor increased IL-8 expression by the tumor cells. A follow-up study by the same research group showed that in a high percentage of HNSCC tumors, the IL-8 receptors could be detected on both cancer cells and endothelial cells within the tumor (143).

Negative Regulators of Angiogenesis

Interferons. Studies of the interferons (IFNs) have shown that the members of this family of cytokines have potent antiangiogenic activity. IFN-a and IFN-b have been particularly well studied in this regard. Both have been found to inhibit endothelial cell proliferation and migration (73). In addition, decreased IFN-b expression has been inversely correlated with microvessel density and new blood vessel formation and has been shown to down-regulate the expression of IL-8, bFGF, and MMPs (144,145). The role of IFNs in the pathogenesis of HNSCC is largely unknown at this time.SK

Thrombospondins (TSPs). TSPs are a multi-gene family of five secreted glycoproteins that are involved in the regulation of cell proliferation, adhesion, and migration. Two members of the TSP family, TSP-1 and TSP-2, are also naturally occurring inhibitors of angiogenesis (146). Evidence shows that TSP-1 inhibits angiogenesis by inducing endothelial cell apoptosis (147); therefore, programmed cell death was achieved by increased expression of Bax, decreased expression of Bcl-2, and activation of caspase-3. Little is known of the role of TSPs in the pathogenesis of HNSCC.

Others. Recent studies have also implicated nitric oxide (148) and the PTEN/MMAC1 gene (149) as angiogenesis inhibitors. MMAC1 (150) [also known as PTEN (151)] is a candidate tumor-suppressor gene located at 10q23.3 and may play an important role in the tumorigenesis of multiple tumor types (152). Based on immunohistochemical analysis in oral tongue cancer, multivariate regression analysis demonstrated that the absence of PTEN expression is an independent predictor of poor outcome when compared with tumor stage and nodal status (153).

Acquisition of Autonomous Proliferative Signaling

All normal cells require growth signals for proliferation. Growth signals can be provided in a variety of ways, including diffusible molecules (growth factors), extracellular matrix components, or cell-to-cell interactions. In general, growth signals are transmitted from the cell surface to the nucleus through various intracellular signaling pathways. A distinct characteristic of neoplastic cells is their ability to acquire autonomy from exogenous growth signaling. Several investigators have shown that aberrant expression of growth factors and growth factor receptors may play a role in the pathogenesis of HNSCC (154). In addition, other aspects of intracellular signaling may be altered in neoplastic cells, helping to provide this autonomy of growth.

EPIDERMAL GROWTH FACTOR AXIS

Cohen (155) originally purified epidermal growth factor (EGF) from mouse submandibular glands in 1962. The isolation and characterization of EGF and its receptor (EGF-R) have furthered our understanding of the regulation of normal cell proliferation and the loss of this regulation that occurs in neoplastic cell growth. Investigators have begun to study the role of EGF, EGF-R, and transforming growth factor-α (TGF-α), another ligand for the EGF-R), in the development of HNSCC.

Most studies of EGF and the EGF-R in HNSCC have involved quantification of expression at the DNA, RNA, or protein levels in cell lines or fresh tissues and the correlation of these findings to clinical variables. Although conflicting results have been obtained, some general trends have been noted. The EGF axis is up-regulated in a large proportion of HNSCC; however, the clinical significance of this up-regulation is uncertain at this time. For instance, in an immunohistochemical analysis of SCC of the tongue base, EGF-R and TGF-α were routinely seen in normal squamous mucosa adjacent to the tumors, with overexpression of the EGF-R and TGF-α seen in 60% and 35% of the tumors, respectively (15). However, overexpression appeared to have no effect on survival. Similar results were seen in an analysis of tumors of the nasal cavity and paranasal sinuses (156). Conversely, in a study of 103 laryngeal tumors, EGF-R expression was elevated, particularly in tumors that were poorly differentiated when compared with normal mucosa (157). In this study, however, the 2-year survival of patients with EGF-R–positive tumors was 58%, compared with 82% for patients with EGF-R–negative lesions. With multivariate analysis, only EGF-R status and tumor location within the larynx were identified as significant independent prognostic parameters.

To further investigate the role that TGF-α and EGF-R expression may play in the pathogenesis of HNSCC, Grandis and Tweardy (158) systematically evaluated the level of messenger RNA (mRNA) encoding these two proteins in tumors and normal mucosa from patients with HNSCC as well as in normal mucosa from patients without a history of tobacco or alcohol use. In their analysis, TGF-α mRNA was elevated in 95% of histologically normal samples in patients with HNSCC and in 87.5% of HNSCC when compared with normal mucosa from individuals without cancer. The mRNA for the EGF-R was elevated in 91% of histologically normal tissue from tumor-bearing patients and in 92% of tumors when compared with normal mucosa from tumor-free control subjects. The high levels of both the ligand and the receptor in tumors and normal mucosa from patients with head and neck cancer suggests that environmental influences, such as tobacco and alcohol usage, lead to up-regulation of growth factor production and receptor expression, which may play a role in tumor development. Correlations between growth factor and receptor levels and clinical data have begun to yield clinically meaningful results. In a detailed analysis of 91 patients, levels of EGF-R and TGF-α were quantified via immunohistochemical staining, and increased levels of both were found to be independent predictors of decreased disease-free survival (159). Other smaller studies had previously suggested these results (160,161).

Some functional data to support this hypothesis come from a study of two HNSCC cell lines that were examined for levels of EGF-R expression by immunoprecipitation of metabolically labeled cells with specific anti–EGF-R antibodies (162). In this study, the cell line that grew more efficiently in plating assays was found to have fivefold higher levels of EGF-R. The immunoprecipitated receptors were also analyzed for intrinsic tyrosine kinase activity, an enzymatic activity that is indispensable for EGF-R signal transduction, and the more rapidly proliferating cell line was found to possess greater kinase activity. Furthermore, kinase activity was increased in immunoprecipitates from both cell lines by the addition of exogenous EGF.

More recently, EGF-R and its ligands have been studied in invasion and metastasis. Increasing evidence suggests an association between an up-regulated EGF axis and activation of MMPs in HNSCC cell lines (163). In this study, up-regulation of MMP-9 was demonstrated by exposing cells to EGF-R ligands; in addition, monoclonal antibodies against EGF-R inhibited MMP-9 up-regulation and impeded tumor cell invasion. A second study confirmed these findings and also showed an up-regulation of uPA (164). These data suggest a role for the EGF axis in the regulation of invasion and metastasis of HNSCC.

SIGNAL TRANSDUCERS AND ACTIVATORS OF TRANSCRIPTION PROTEINS

Signal transducers and activators of transcription (STATs) are a family of cytoplasmic proteins that transmit signals from cell surface receptors to the nucleus where they act as transcription factors. They have been implicated as playing a role in the development of several types of tumors, including HNSCC (165). In HNSCC, STAT proteins, specifically STAT3, have been shown to play an important role in EGF/TGF-mediated cell growth (166). Activation of the EGF/TGF pathway resulted in constitutive expression of STAT3. This association was strengthened by experiments in which abrogation of STAT3 function (via mutant constructs or antisense oligonucleotides) resulted in significant growth inhibition of HNSCC cells (167). In addition, further work, also using antisense oligonucleotides, showed that STAT3 activation significantly decreases apoptosis (168). This down-regulation appears to be due to elevated levels of the antiapoptotic protein Bcl-x_L. Further studies of this downstream signaling molecule are being actively pursued.

NUCLEAR FACTOR KAPPA B

Nuclear factor kappa B (NF-κB) is a well-established transcription factor that regulates genes that drive immune and inflammatory responses. In normal cells, NF-κB remains largely in the cytoplasm, complexed to inhibitor proteins (IκBs) and therefore remains transcriptionally inactive until a cell receives an appropriate stimulus. In response to a stimulus, the IκB proteins become phosphorylated, ubiquitinated, and undergo rapid proteolysis by the 26S proteasome. This degradation of the IκB proteins results in the liberation of NF-κB, allowing this transcription factor to accumulate in the nucleus, where it activates the expression of specific genes involved in immune and inflammatory responses and in cell growth control (169).

Recently, NF-κB has been connected with the acquisition of multiple hallmarks of cancer development and progression. Through the increased transcription of genes important for mediating increased cell proliferation (cyclin D1), apoptosis evasion (c-IAP-2, XIAP), invasion (MMP-9), and angiogenesis (IL-8), NF-kB has been found to promote tumor progression in multiple ways. Evidence for the role of NF-κB in human oncogenesis was first seen in Hodgkin lymphoma (170). Other cancer types have been investigated as well (171). Duffey et al. (172) studied NF-κB function in a murine keratinocyte tumor progression model and in human HNSCC cell lines and showed that enhanced NF-κB activity is positively associated with local tumor growth and metastatic potential in animal models. More recent studies using complementary DNA (cDNA) microarrays indicated that NF-κB may activate proliferation via up-regulation of cyclin D1 and other cell cycle regulators (173,174).

HEPATOCYTE GROWTH FACTOR AXIS

Hepatocyte growth factor/scatter factor (HGF/SF) has remarkably diverse biologic functions in different tissues and has been implicated in mitogenic responses, cell motility, and angiogenesis (175). This growth factor may have a critical role in a variety of biologic processes, including normal development, wound healing, and carcinogenesis. The HGF/SF receptor (HGF-R) is coded by the c-*met* proto-oncogene. The c-*met* encoded receptor belongs to the family of transmembrane growth factor receptors with tyrosine kinase activity.

Recent evidence has implicated both HGF and c-*met* in invasion and metastasis of oral cavity cancer cell lines (176,177). It appears that this increase in invasiveness may be the result of HGF's ability to up-regulate both MMP-1 and MMP-9 (178). In addition, Dong et al. (179) have shown that HGF may play a role in angiogenesis in HNSCC via up-regulation of proangiogenic cytokines IL-8 and VEGF. Thus, HGF and c-*met* appear to play diverse and important roles in the pathogenesis of HNSCC.

Inhibition of Growth Inhibitory Signals

In the normal cell, growth and differentiation are tightly controlled. Although constitutive stimulation of cell proliferation through normal growth factors is necessary for tumor development, it is insufficient in and of itself to cause oncogenic transformation of normal cells. Another important and related step in tumorigenesis is the loss of normal antigrowth signals. A complex interplay of factors results in regulation of a cell's progression through the cell cycle. DNA replication and cell division through the cell cycle consists of several phases—G1 (growth phase 1), S (DNA synthesis), G2 (growth phase 2), and M (mitosis)—each of which is tightly controlled. Central to the control of the cell cycle is a group of molecules called cyclins and their regulators—cyclin-dependent kinases (CDKs) and cyclin-dependent kinase inhibitors (CDKIs). Any molecules that affect or regulate cyclins, CDKs, or CDKIs will have a profound effect on cell growth and are potential carcinogenic mediators. Several of these molecules are discussed below as they relate to HNSCC.

RETINOBLASTOMA GENE

The retinoblastoma (*Rb*) gene and its protein product (pRb) has been termed the gateway to the cell cycle. In its active form, pRb prevents progression through the cell cycle by binding to and inactivating the transcription factor E2F, which is vital to the expression of other genes required for DNA synthesis. Various cyclin/CDK combinations are able to respond to mitogenic stimuli and inactivate pRb via the process of phosphorylation. When it is phosphorylated, pRb releases E2F, leading to the transcription of genes critical for progression of cells from the G1 phase to the S phase of the cell cycle. This then initiates the DNA synthesis phase of the cell cycle.

Because of its critical role in cell cycle initiation, *Rb* has been intensively studied in various tumor types, including HNSCC. Examination of 60 HNSCC tumor specimens revealed loss of heterozygosity of the *Rb* region of chromosome 13 in 52% of the specimens. However, a decreased level of Rb protein expression could be detected in only 19.4% of these specimens by immunochemical analysis (180). Other studies have also demonstrated low rates of pRb alterations in HNSCC (181). These findings suggest that *Rb* inactivation is an uncommon event in the development of HNSCC and that other mechanisms of cell cycle inhibition are at work. Because several signaling molecules reside upstream of pRb, any alterations to this pathway that lead to increased phosphorylation of pRb can lead to the loss of negative growth control. Some of these molecules are discussed below.

P53 GENE

The most intensely studied gene involved in carcinogenesis is the tumor-suppressor gene *p53*. The *p53* locus is the most commonly mutated locus in human cancers. Located on the short arm of chromosome 17, p53 is a 393-amino acid protein that is evolutionarily well conserved and is expressed in all tissues of the body. Although the overall sequence of this protein in humans is nearly 82% homologous with murine p53, five regions of approximately 20 amino acids each within the protein are nearly identical across species lines (182). Mutagenesis and x-ray crystallographic studies have localized specific functions to these regions. The first 75 amino acids of p53 are involved in the activation of transcription of specific genes, whereas amino acids 120 to 290 are involved in the specific recognition of DNA sequences (183). The carboxyl terminus is believed to be important for nuclear localization and oligomerization of p53 into tetramers (184).

Although the mechanism of action of p53 is through the positive or negative regulation of gene transcription, its biologic role is to protect cells from DNA damage caused by radiation, chemical carcinogens, or other mechanisms; p53 does this either by arresting the cell cycle so that DNA repair can occur or by inducing programmed cell death (apoptosis) (185–187). Analysis of extensive data on sites of mutation of the *p53* gene in human cancers has revealed certain "hot spots" for mutations at sites that are believed to be important in performing these functions (188). The majority of these (more than 92%) are found in the five "conserved regions" of the gene. Mutations within these regions impair a cell's ability to repair its DNA, which leads to genomic instability of the cancer cell and additional alterations in oncogene and tumor-suppressor gene products. Mutations of *p53* also prevent apoptosis in response to DNA damage, which may make tumor cells resistant to treatment with irradiation or chemotherapeutic agents that act by damaging cellular DNA and triggering apoptosis. The role of this gene in the pathogenesis of HNSCC has been extensively studied; some of this work is outlined below.

Somers et al. (189) analyzed p53 in HNSCC using immunohistochemical studies and demonstrated p53 overexpression in 13 of 13 HNSCC cell lines and in 10 of 13 fresh tissue specimens. DNA sequencing of the *p53* gene revealed G to T transversions that resulted in single amino acid substitutions. Because G to T transversions can result from the interaction of DNA with benzopyrene, a component of cigarette smoke, the results of this study suggest a mechanism by which smoking may play a role in the pathogenesis of a tobacco-associated malignancy.

Numerous studies have documented overexpression and point mutations in *p53* genes from both HNSCC cell lines and fresh tumors from sites within the head and neck. As is the case with other cancer types, mutations of the *p53* gene are some of the most common abnormalities in HNSCC, with a frequency of approximately 50% (190). It seems clear that *p53* plays an important functional role in the progression of HNSCC. Early evidence for this was demonstrated by Boyle et al. (191), who found that 19% of the premalignant lesions and 43% of malignant lesions had *p53* mutations. Similar results have been seen in immunohistochemical studies performed by other groups (192,193). Work by the group at M. D. Anderson Cancer Center (194) has shown a steady increase in *p53* abnormalities during the progression of head and neck tumors, with *p53* being overexpressed in 19% of normal epithelium tissues, 29% of hyperplastic lesions, 45% of dysplastic lesions, and 58% of invasive cancers. These researchers also demonstrated a significant association between *p53* expression and genomic instability, suggesting that *p53* alterations may lead to the accumulation of genetic events during head and neck tumorigenesis.

Although *p53* can be altered through mutations, there are several other mechanisms by which *p53* function is altered that are believed to play a role in tumorigenesis. The HPV proteins E6 and E7 can bind to p53 and inactivate its function (195). The function of p53 is also altered by the cellular protein mdm-2, which binds to the transcriptional activation domain of p53, effectively blocking its ability to regulate target genes and exert its antiproliferative or apoptotic effects (196). In addition, mdm-2 appears to play a major role in *p53* degradation, thus providing a new mechanism to ensure effective termination of the *p53* signal (197). The role of mdm-2 in HNSCC remains unclear, despite preliminary studies (198,199). However, one study of *p53* inactivation found that in 95% of patients, *p53* was inactivated by mutation, HPV infection, or mdm-2 overexpression (200).

INK4 GENE FAMILY

Proteins translated from the *INK4* (*IN*hibitors of CD*K4*) family of genes, $p15^{INK4B}$, $p16^{INK4A}$, $p18^{INK4C}$, $p19^{INK4D}$, act mainly on the G1 phase of the cell cycle. By far, the most studied of this gene family is *p16*. Independent studies of the 9p21-22 region in human cancers reveal that the gene that encodes the p16 protein is important in inhibiting cells from entering the cell cycle (201). Serrano et al. (202) demonstrated that p16 binds to and inhibits the enzyme CDK4, which is important in enabling cells to pass through the cell cycle. Cell proliferation through the inactivation of a cell cycle inhibitor or the overexpression of a cell cycle activator demonstrates how quantitative and qualitative alterations in the expression of oncogenes and tumor-suppressor genes contribute to tumorigenesis.

Alterations in *p16* have been shown to be important in a variety of human cancers. Early studies on HNSCC indicated that *p16* alterations were among the most common abnormalities. Reed et al. (203) showed that *p16* activity was lost in 83% of primary tumors. Various distinct mechanisms appear to be responsible, including homozygous deletion, point mutation, and promoter methylation.

More recently, researchers have attempted to determine whether *p16* is affected early or late in the tumor progression pathway. Studies of premalignant and malignant oral cavity lesions have also shown frequent alterations of the coding region of the *p16* gene (204–206). The frequent finding of *p16* gene mutations or loss of its expression in dysplastic as well as neoplastic oral lesions indicates that this may be an early step in oral carcinogenesis (204). Because *p16* is so widely altered in head and neck cancer, it is an attractive target for newer molecular therapeutic techniques. One study showed that gene therapy directed toward the p16 protein might have potential benefit; using an adenoviral gene therapy approach, Rocco et al. (207) inhibited cell growth in human HNSCC cell lines. The same vector also stabilized or reduced tumor volumes in a nude mouse model. This work has the potential to lead to new therapies for the treatment of HNSCC.

CYCLIN D1

The cyclin family of cellular proteins, along with their partners, the CDKs, are responsible for driving cells through the cell cycle. As would be expected, proteins involved in driving the cell cycle, including cyclins, are frequently overexpressed in primary tumors (208). Of the many cell cycle regulators known to play a role in the development of cancer, cyclin D1 is most often implicated (209).

Cyclin D1 amplification has been identified in as many as 64% of HNSCC (210). Overexpression of cyclin D1 has been studied in various head and neck subsites. For instance, in oral cavity cancer, Bova et al. (211) analyzed 148 tongue cancers immunohistochemically for the expression of cyclin D1 and found it was overexpressed in 68%. This finding correlated with statistically significantly lower disease-free and overall survival rates. Another study confirmed these results and correlated high expression of cyclin D1 with lymph node metastases (212). Likewise, in a study of SCC of the larynx, amplification of cyclin D1 was identified in 37% of neoplasms, which correlated with local invasion, locoregional recurrence, and pathologic stage (213). A high correlation of cyclin D1 mRNA overexpression with gene amplification supports a role for this protein in the pathogenesis of HNSCC. Also, in studies of hypopharyngeal sites, cyclin D1 gene amplification and protein overexpression not only were correlated with prognosis but also were useful in identifying optimum treatment regimens (214); cyclin D1-negative tumors responded particularly well to multimodal treatment.

Overexpression of cyclin D1 protein in HNSCC was found to be an independent prognostic indicator of recurrence (215), a finding that was confirmed in another study (216). Further confirmation of the importance of cyclin D1 in HNSCC was provided by Nakashima and Clayman (217), who showed that transfection of antisense cyclin D1 into head and neck cancer cell lines caused lower *in vitro* growth rates and lower rates of tumorigenicity in a nude mouse model. This finding may lead to the possibility of new gene therapy approaches to HNSCC.

P21 FAMILY

The p21 family consists of p21, p27, and p57. p21 was one of the first CDK inhibitors identified (218); it was found by several different laboratories and thus has multiple names, including WAF1, CIP1, SDI1, and mda-6. p27 and p57 are also known as KIP1 and KIP2. This family is known to have a wide variety of inhibitory effects on CDKs. Currently, data concerning the role of the p21 family of proteins in the development of head and neck cancer are limited. One study evaluated p21 protein levels in tumors and found that overexpression of p21, as evaluated immunohistochemically, correlated with increasing recurrence rates and shortened disease-free and overall survival times (219). A more recent study, evaluating p27 levels in patients with oral tongue SCC, found that patients with low p27 levels, as evaluated by immunohistochemical and Western blotting techniques, had higher stage disease and lower rates of overall survival (220). A similar study by the same group in patients with hypopharyngeal SCC also showed poorer survival rates in patients with low expression levels of p27 (221). Further corroborative studies are needed to fully elucidate the role of this family of proteins in the pathogenesis of HNSCC.

Evasion of Programmed Cell Death (Apoptosis)

Programmed cell death, or apoptosis, is a critical step in cell differentiation and turnover and in tissue homeostasis (71). Intensive study in this area over the last decade has led to a greater understanding of the initiation and regulation of apoptosis (222). It is now clear that one of the requisites for cancer cells to prosper is the development of resistance to apoptosis, shifting the balance between cell division and cell death.

The biochemical process of apoptosis is one of the most studied aspects of cell biology. It has been found to be a precisely orchestrated series of steps triggered by physiologic stimuli that lead to membrane dissolution, breakdown of the nuclear and cytosolic skeletons, chromosomal degradation, and fragmentation of the nucleus (223). Currently apoptosis is thought of as a three-step process. The first step of this process is the initiation or signal step. In general, a signal, either extracellular or intracellular, triggers the apoptotic machinery. The second step is the execution or actual "program" of cell death. Within this phase, multiple effector molecules act on the signal event to cause the release of caspases, the ultimate destroyers of the cell. The third step involves the morphologic changes seen in the dying cell and the response of the surrounding cells to its death. As would be expected for such a complex process, multiple regulatory and effector molecules are needed for the successful initiation and completion of this process. Mutations of any of the genes encoding these apoptotic proteins or any changes in their levels of expression can lead to increased cell survival, a critical step in tumorigenesis.

Apoptosis can be initiated by extracellular or intracellular pathways. Extracellular initiators of the apoptotic machinery include ligands that bind cell surface receptors such as Fas, tumor necrosis factor receptor, TRAMP, TRAIL-R1, TRAIL-R2, and DR-6. These have been called "death receptors." The best studied of these is the Fas/Fas ligand complex, which may serve as a prototype for all other death receptors. The signal in this pathway is the binding of the Fas ligand to Fas, which causes clustering of Fas complexes and the subsequent intracellular binding of the Fas-associated death domain (FADD). This in turn causes the recruitment of an initiator caspase, caspase-8, which initiates apoptosis by proteolytic cleavage and activation of downstream effector caspases-3, -6, and -7. Although this pathway has been well defined and studied in other cancers (222), little is known of its role in HNSCC.

Intracellular molecules can also initiate apoptosis. By far the best-studied example is the *p53* gene. This gene and its protein product have multiple functions, as described earlier, including the induction of apoptosis in response to DNA damage. This induction appears to be mediated through Bax, a potent proapoptotic downstream effector molecule. Mutations in the *p53* gene can result in a loss of this function, which can lead to survival of cells with damaged DNA. This in turn can lead to genomic instability with the development of multiple genetic abnormalities that can foster tumor progression. Evidence for this phenomenon in HNSCC was demonstrated by Ravi et al. (224), who showed that the presence of mutant p53 protein has an inverse correlation with the extent of apoptosis in oral cavity cancer. Significant correlation was also evident between the Bax/Bcl-2 ratio and cyclin D1 levels and apoptosis. These results suggest that apoptosis decreases as histologic abnormality increases, apparently because of alterations in the levels of apoptotic regulatory proteins.

More data that support a role for p53 in the induction of apoptosis come from gene transfer studies by Clayman et al. (225) and Liu et al. (226). Using adenoviral vectors to restore wild-type *p53* to human HNSCC cell lines with *p53* alterations, these investigators were able to demonstrate a loss of tumorigenesis in nude mice and the induction of apoptosis in the wild-type *p53*-transduced tumors. Based on these preliminary data, phase I and II clinical trials of adenovirus-mediated *p53* gene therapy were begun for patients with advanced or refractory HNSCC (227,228). The initial phase I trial confirmed the safety of adenoviral mediated gene therapy and identified no significant toxicity in the 15 patients enrolled (229). Although phase II clinical trials are underway, the efficacy of this type of treatment alone or in combination with other modalities remains to be established.

Regardless of whether the apoptotic cascade is initiated by cell surface receptors or intracellular initiators, the cellular effectors of apoptosis are the caspase family of proteases. This family includes at least 13 proteins and is classically divided into three groups: *nonapoptotic caspases* (caspases 1, 4, 5, 11, 12, and 13), which appear to have no role in apoptosis; *initiator caspases* (caspases 8, 9, and 10), which function to begin and amplify the caspase cascade; and *effector caspases* (caspases 2, 3, 6, and 7), which appear to be the ultimate effectors of apoptosis. Thus, the initial step in the apoptotic cascade is the activation of a cellular receptor or intracellular initiator, which in turn activates one or more initiator caspases. This step is also the major regulatory step and is controlled by many proapoptotic and antiapoptotic proteins, which will be discussed later. Once activated, the initiator caspases process and activate one or more effector caspases, which in turn cleave cellular proteins, organelles, and chromosomes and provide the final mechanism for apoptosis.

It has become clear over the last decade that various chemotherapeutic agents exert their antitumor effect by inducing apoptosis, and several of these do so by specifically up-regulating caspases. For instance, 5-fluorouracil has been shown to specifically up-regulate caspases 1, 3, and 8 (230). Moreover, inhibitors of these caspases consistently blocked apoptosis. Likewise, in head and neck cancer cell lines, cisplatin administration selectively up-regulated caspases 3, 8, and 9 (231). Further experiments have shown that inhibitors of caspase 9 completely block apoptosis, whereas inhibitors of caspases 3 and 8 partially block apoptosis. Other chemotherapeutic agents such as 9-cis-retinoic acid (232) and arsenic trioxide (233) up-regulate various caspases.

Various regulatory molecules play a role in the apoptotic pathway. Perhaps the best studied is the Bcl-2 family of molecules, which is responsible for regulating the release of cytochrome C from the mitochondria. This family consists of proapoptotic molecules (i.e., Bax, Bak, and Bid) and antiapoptotic molecules (i.e., Bcl-2, Bcl-$_{XL}$, and Bfl-1). Complex and as yet not fully understood interactions between these regulators control the release of cytochrome C from mitochondria and the subsequent activation of the apoptotic machinery. The best-studied molecules in HNSCC are Bcl-2 and Bax, but the findings have varied. For instance, Bcl-2 overexpression has been associated with both worse (234) and better (235) overall survival rates in patients with HNSCC. Data from one study suggest that in carcinoma of the tongue, overexpression of Bcl-2 and loss of Bax expression, quantified as the Bcl-2/Bax ratio, are significantly associated with poor prognosis (236). Further studies are necessary to elucidate the role of these regulatory proteins in the pathogenesis of HNSCC.

The transcription factor NF-κB has also been shown to enhance cell survival in a variety of tumor types, including HNSCC (237). The suppression of apoptosis by NF-κB may occur through transcriptional modulation of the expression of multiple apoptosis inhibitory proteins, including c-FLIP, TRAF1, TRAF2, c-IAP1, c-IAP 2, A1/Bfl-1, Bcl-x$_L$, IEX-1, and x-IAP (238). In addition, activation of NF-κB appears to decrease p53-dependent apoptosis (239). In HNSCC, overexpression of NF-κB has been shown to decrease tumor necrosis factor-α (TNF-α)–mediated apoptosis, which is reversed by NF-κB inhibitors (239). These results indicate that inhibitors of NF-κB signaling have great therapeutic potential alone or, perhaps, in combination with apoptosis-inducing chemotherapeutic agents or radiotherapy.

Immortalization

Normal cells can replicate themselves a finite number of times before they become senescent, enter a "crisis" state, and ultimately die (240). Tumor cells, in contrast, acquire the ability to overcome this process, allowing them to replicate indefinitely. This is termed immortalization. Mechanisms by which tumors achieve immortalization are currently under investigation. Over the last decade, it has become apparent that the DNA at the ends of chromosomes, the so-called telomeric DNA or telomeres, plays an important role in cell senescence (241). These telomeres appear to act as "protective caps" at the ends of chromosomes, preventing destruction of the chromosomes. It is now known that with each replicative cycle, a small amount of telomeric DNA is lost. Over the life of the organism, therefore, the telomeres become shorter and shorter. Once enough telomeric DNA has been lost, the chromosomal ends are no longer protected, leading to the fusion of chromosomes and karyotypic abnormalities that eventually precipitate cell death. Nearly all tumor cells have acquired one or another mechanism to maintain their telomeric length (242,243). The best studied of these mechanisms is the expression of the enzyme telomerase, which extends the length of telomeres.

Several groups have investigated telomerase activity in HNSCC. In an analysis of 16 HNSCC cell lines and 29 tumor specimens, telomerase activity was found in 100% of the cell lines and 90% of the invasive cancers but was not detected in any normal tissues (206). These findings are supported by those in other published reports (244,245). At least one study has demonstrated that telomerase activity has a relationship with the degree of tumor differentiation and treatment response (246), whereas another study showed that patients with advanced cancers (those classified with T4 HNSCC) had significantly higher telomerase levels than early cancers (e.g., those classified with T1-2 HNSCC) (247). In studies of premalignant lesions, telomerase appears to be activated as well (248). These early data indicate that telomerase is important in the pathogenesis of HNSCC, that it has prognostic value, and that it may be activated early in the development of head and neck cancers.

LYMPHANGIOGENESIS

For most human cancers, metastasis to regional lymph nodes is an important index of tumor aggressiveness and is correlated with poor clinical outcomes. Although tumor cells are often found within lymphatics that are along the periphery of tumors, it is generally accepted that lymphatic vessels are not present within tumors themselves (249). However, new evidence suggests that certain tumors may induce the formation of new lymphatic capillaries in a process dubbed "lymphangiogenesis" (250).

Vascular endothelial growth factor (VEGF)-C, a novel member of the VEGF family of angiogenic growth factors, may stimulate the growth of lymphatic vascular endothelium *in vivo* (251,252). Its receptor, Flt-4, is predominantly expressed by lymphatic endothelia (253,254) in normal human tissues. VEGF-C can also activate a second receptor, VEGFR-2 (Kdr), although it is predominantly expressed by activated endothelia of blood vessels (255) and is also used by other VEGF isoforms. VEGF-D, which is structurally related to VEGF-C, also binds and activates VEGFR-2 and VEGFR-3 (256) and may play a role in lymphangiogenesis (257).

VEGF-C is expressed in a variety of human tumors, such as breast (258,259), colon (256,260), gastric (261,262), lung (263,264), and thyroid (265,266) cancers as well as melanoma (258). Recently, the expression of VEGF-C correlated with metastasis to regional lymphatics in an orthotopic murine model of breast cancer (252). In this experiment, breast cancer cells were transfected with VEGF-C and these stable transfectants had significantly higher rates of regional metastasis than did controls, providing the first evidence of a clear link between lymphangiogenesis and metastasis.

Preliminary work has been done with regard to the expression of VEGFs in HNSCC. Measured by Western blotting and enzyme-linked immunosorbent assay, VEGF-A and VEGF-C were elevated in tumor cell lines compared with normal cells (267). Although these findings are promising, they await confirmation in an animal model. Furthermore, no large-scale study for clinicopathologic correlation has been performed.

LYMPHATIC ENDOTHELIUM: NEW MARKERS

A major advance in the field of lymphangiogenesis has come with the discovery of lymphatic endothelium-specific markers (250). These include (a) podoplanin, a mucoprotein first identified in glomerular podocyte membrane (268); (b) Prox-1, a homeobox gene product that plays a role in early lymphatic development (269); and (c) LYVE-1, a lymphatic endothelial receptor for hyaluronan, the extracellular matrix/lymphatic fluid glycosaminoglycan (270). The use of these markers and the VEGF-C receptor, Flt-4, in studies to identify lymphatics within human tumors remains controversial. For instance, Flt-4 is expressed in embryonic blood vascular endothelium and reexpressed in tumor blood vessels (253,271,272). Although lymphatic metastasis is a hallmark of HNSCC, the role of lymphangiogenesis remains unknown. These initial studies, while promising, require validation and further study.

DEVELOPMENT OF AN ORTHOTOPIC NUDE MOUSE TUMOR MODEL OF ORAL CANCER

Although reductionist approaches have facilitated the investigation of the individual biologic steps important in mediating invasion and metastasis, animal models are needed to integrate these processes and to study these complex biologic processes *in vivo*.

Orthotopic nude mouse tumor models have been useful models of the metastatic process for tumors arising from a variety of sites, including melanoma and colon, breast, prostate, and bladder carcinomas (74). There have been a few prior reports of the development of orthotopic models of HNSCC using nude mice (273–278). Most of the models rely on transcutaneous injection, and thus more closely resemble heterotopic subcutaneous tumor models, which have several limitations. Subcutaneous models place tumor cells in a foreign milieu in which important growth factors and/or survival signals found in their tissue of origin may be lacking (74,279). Furthermore, these tumor models may not recapitulate the metastatic pathways seen in patients with these primary tumor types. Several reports in the literature have mentioned the use of submucosal orthotopic tumor injection in the oral cavity without describing the development of the model or specific methods used. A recent report (280) has described the use of an orthotopic model in which carcinoma cell lines induced by injecting F344 rats with 4-nitroquinoline N-oxide have been injected into the subcutaneous tissues of F344 rats and serially passaged from the lungs to generate cell lines of varying metastatic potential (282).

To study the mechanisms of invasion and metastasis in HNSCC, we have developed an orthotopic nude mouse model of oral cancer (281). In our initial studies, we showed the feasibility of submucosal lingual injection of mice by injecting the B16/BL6 melanoma into the tongues of nude mice. Direct visual inspection confirmed regional spread of the pigmented tumor cells to cervical lymph nodes within 14 days, as shown in Figure 38.11 (see also Color Plate 14 following page 524).

Having confirmed the feasibility of submucosal lingual injection, we selected three oral cavity SCC cell lines that had

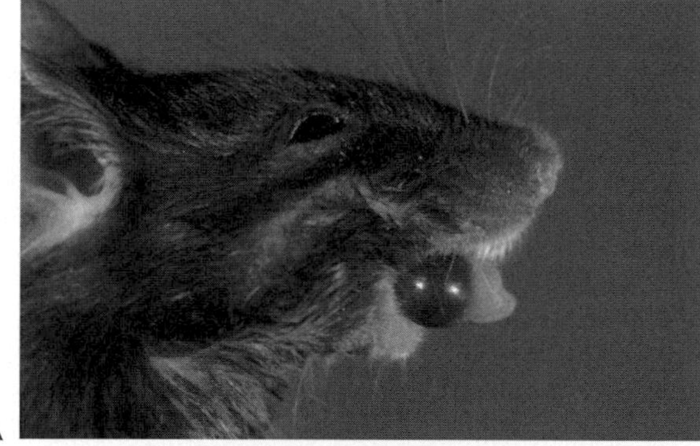
A

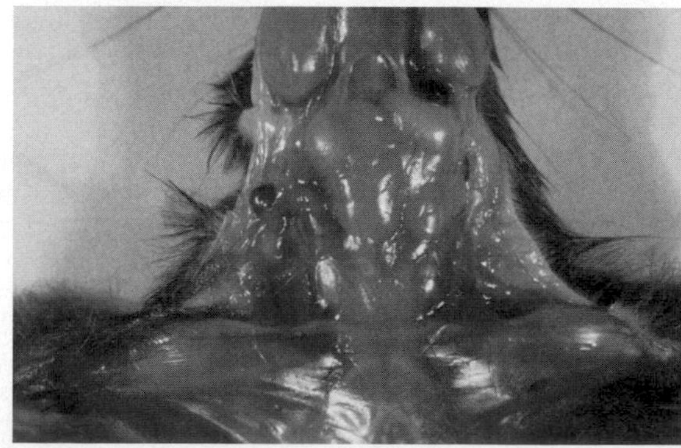
B

Figure 38.11 The tongues of C57 black mice were inoculated with syngeneic B16/BL6 melanoma cells and mice were killed after 14 days and necropsy performed. An obvious tumor is seen in the tongue. Bilateral metastases are easily identified by melanotic pigmentation within the cervical lymph nodes. (See Color Plate 14 following page 524.)

TABLE 38.2 An Orthotopic Model of Oral Cancer

Cell type: Tu167 dose (no. of cells)	Percentage of mice developing subcutaneous (flank) tumor	Percentage of mice developing submucosal (tongue) tumors
5×10^6	100%	100%
1×10^6	20%	100%
5×10^5	20%	100%
1×10^5	20%	100%

Groups of 6-week-old male nude mice were inoculated subcutaneously along the flank or submucosally in the tongue with the listed number of Tu167 cells, derived from a primary SCC of the floor of mouth; mice were then observed for tumor formation and subjected to necropsy; similar results were obtained with the MDA1986 and Tu159 cell lines.

Cell line	Mice with regional metastasis	Mice with lung metastasis
Tu167	1/45	0/45
Tu167GLN1	3/10	2/10

Groups of 6-week-old male nude mice were inoculated submucosally in the tongue with 1×10^6 cells of the squamous cell carcinoma cell line, Tu167, or the Tu167GLN1; the latter cell line was derived from *in vivo* passage of Tu167 in the orthotopic SCCOC tumor model, by placement of a cervical lymph node in culture; mice were then observed for tumor formation and subjected to necropsy and the number of mice with cervical and/or pulmonary metastases was tabulated.

previously been established in the Head and Neck Research Laboratory at M. D. Anderson. These three cell lines (MDA 1986, Tu159, and Tu167) were passaged *in vitro* and prepared for inoculation into the tongues of 6-week-old male nude mice with a dose range of 1×10^4 to 5×10^6 cells in a volume of 50 µL. Mice were also injected subcutaneously with a corresponding number of cells of each cell type, and tumorigenicity and metastatic potential were determined. In this experiment with the oral cancer line Tu167, tumors could be found in all mice injected *submucosally* with 1×10^5, 5×10^5, 1×10^6, or 5×10^6 cells, whereas only 20% of the mice developed tumors when injected *subcutaneously* with 1×10^5, 5×10^5, or 1×10^6 cells. This experiment showed that the Tu167 cell line has high tumorigenicity and revealed at least a 50-fold difference in the minimal tumorigenic dose between submucosal and subcutaneous injection with this cell line. The results of this tumorigenicity study are summarized in Table 38.2. This cell line has a low metastatic potential, as only one animal of 10 (10%) injected in the tongue with 5×10^6 cells developed a cervical metastasis of its tumor. Similar results were obtained with the MDA 1986 and Tu 159 cell lines.

To facilitate the identification and *in vivo* passage of the oral cancer cell lines using the orthotopic model, we have transfected the gene encoding the green fluorescent protein (GFP) into Tu167 cells (Fig. 38.12, see also Color Plate 15 following page 524).

To generate tumor lines of increased metastatic potential, we isolated the cervical lymph nodes from mice 3 weeks after lingual submucosal injection with 1×10^6 Tu167GFP cells, dissociated the nodes by passage through a metal sieve, and placed them in tissue culture. After 2 weeks, fibroblastic cells and tumor colonies were visualized, and the cells were treated with G418 to selectively kill all murine cells in the culture. The resultant tumor cell line Tu167GLN-1 was expanded and reinjected into the tongues of 10 mice; the mice were then killed, and the regional and distant metastases were counted. Cervical metastases were seen in 30% of the mice (Table 38.2, top), and pulmonary metastases were identified in 20% of the mice (Table 38.2, bottom). In addition, this cell line was reinjected into mice with harvesting of the lymph nodes and lungs for *in vitro* growth and further serial *in vivo* passage.

The Tu167 orthotopic nude mouse model of SCCOT has substantiated the orthotopic principle that tumor cells grow better in their tissue of origin than in a heterotopic (subcutaneous) site and has recapitulated the metastatic pathways of oral tongue cancer to cervical lymph nodes and the lungs, as seen in patients. In addition, this model has generated cell lines of

A,B

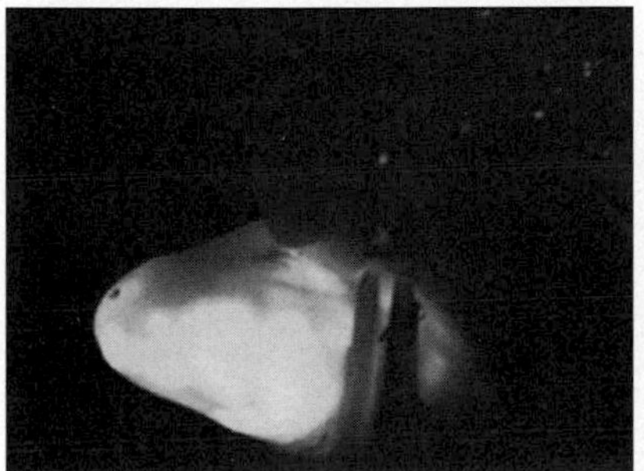

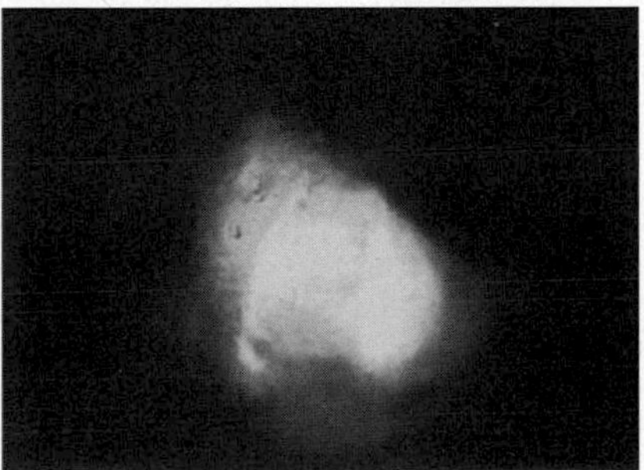

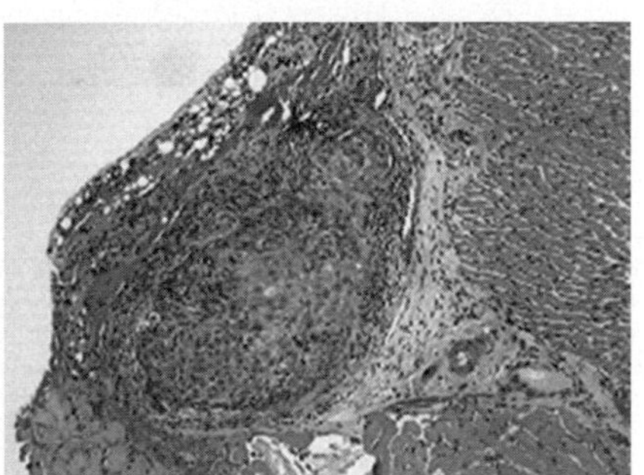

C

Figure 38.12 Photographed under a fluorescent dissecting stereomicroscope, Tu167GFP formed a tumor after injection into the anterior tongue **(A)**, which led to a submandibular metastatic deposit **(B)** that was confirmed by histologic evaluation of the resected fluorescent tissue **(C)**. (See Color Plate 15 following page 524.)

increased metastatic potential that are useful in characterizing the mechanisms of regional and distant metastases.

This animal model represents a reliable experimental system to study the mechanism of metastasis in HNSCC. More reliable prognostic indicators and ideal targets for novel molecular therapy can be identified. Finally, the model provides the opportunity to evaluate the preclinical efficacy of novel treatment schemes for head and neck cancer.

REFERENCES

1. Stephenson J. Researchers optimistic about sea change in cancer treatment. *JAMA* 2001;285:2841–2842.
2. Spiro RH, Huvos AG, Wong GY, et al. Predictive value of tumor thickness in squamous carcinoma confined to the tongue and floor of the mouth. *Am J Surg* 1986;152:345–530.
3. Byers RM, El-Naggar AK, Lee YY, et al. Can we detect or predict the presence of occult nodal metastases in patients with squamous carcinoma of the oral tongue? *Head Neck* 1998;20:138–144.
4. Ballantyne AJ, McCarten AB, Ibanez ML. The extension of cancer of the head and neck through peripheral nerves. *Am J Surg* 1963;106:651–667.
5. Mendenhall WM, Parsons JT, Mendenhall NP, et al. Carcinoma of the skin of the head and neck with perineural invasion. *Head Neck* 1989;11:301–308.
6. Ernst P. Uber das wachstum und die verbreitung bostariger geshwulste insbesondere des krebes in den lymphbahnen der nerven. *Beur Pathol Anat* 1905;7:29.
7. Larson DL, Rodin AE, Roberts DK, et al. Perineural lymphatics: myth or fact. *Am J Surg* 1966;112:488–492.
8. Carter RL, Tanner NS, Clifford P, et al. Perineural spread in squamous cell carcinomas of the head and neck: a clinicopathological study. *Clin Otolaryngol* 1979;4:271–281.
9. Carter RL, Tsao SW, Burman JF, et al. Patterns and mechanisms of bone invasion by squamous carcinomas of the head and neck. *Am J Surg* 1983;146: 451–455.
10. McLaughlin RB Jr, Montone KT, Wall SJ, et al. Nerve cell adhesion molecule expression in squamous cell carcinoma of the head and neck: a predictor of propensity toward perineural spread. *Laryngoscope* 1999;109:821–826.
11. Anderson TD, Feldman M, Weber RS, et al. Tumor deposition of laminin-5 and the relationship with perineural invasion. *Laryngoscope* 2001;111:2140–2143.
12. Byers RM. The use of postoperative irradiation—its goals and 1978 attainments. *Laryngoscope* 1979;89:567–572.
13. Soo KC, Carter RL, O'Brien CJ, et al. Prognostic implications of perineural spread in squamous carcinomas of the head and neck. *Laryngoscope* 1986;96: 1145–1148.
14. Lydiatt DD, Robbins KT, Byers RM, et al. Treatment of stage I and II oral tongue cancer. *Head Neck* 1993;15:308–312.
15. Sauter ER, Ridge JA, Gordon J, et al. p53 overexpression correlates with increased survival in patients with squamous carcinoma of the tongue base. *Am J Surg* 1992;164:651–653.
16. Fagan JJ, Collins B, Barnes L, et al. Perineural invasion in squamous cell carcinoma of the head and neck. *Arch Otolaryngol Head Neck Surg* 1998;124: 637–640.
17. Goepfert H, Dichtel WJ, Medina JE, et al. Perineural invasion in squamous cell skin carcinoma of the head and neck. *Am J Surg* 1984;148:542–547.
18. Holsinger FC, Byers RM, Bekele BN, et al. Perineural invasion predicts local recurrence and disease-specific survival in mucosal head and neck squamous cell carcinoma. *Head and Neck* 2004 *(in press)*.
19. Slaughter DP, Roeser EH, Smejkal WF. Excision of the mandible for neoplastic disease: indications and techniques. *Surgery* 1949;26:507–522.
20. O'Brien CJ, Carter RL, Soo KC, et al. Invasion of the mandible by squamous carcinomas of the oral cavity and oropharynx. *Head Neck Surg* 1986;8:247–256.
21. Gilbert S, Tzadik A, Leonard G. Mandibular involvement by oral squamous cell carcinoma. *Laryngoscope* 1986;96:96–101.
22. Tsue TT, McCulloch TM, Girod DA, et al. Predictors of carcinomatous invasion of the mandible. *Head Neck* 1994;16:116–126.
23. McGregor AD, MacDonald DG. Routes of entry of squamous cell carcinoma to the mandible. *Head Neck Surg* 1988;10:294–301.
24. Slootweg PJ, Muller H. Mandibular invasion by oral squamous cell carcinoma. *J Craniomaxillofac Surg* 1989;17:69–74.
25. Wong RJ, Keel SB, Glynn RJ, et al. Histological pattern of mandibular invasion by oral squamous cell carcinoma. *Laryngoscope* 2000;110:65–72.
26. Totsuka Y, Usui Y, Tei K, et al. Mandibular involvement by squamous cell carcinoma of the lower alveolus: analysis and comparative study of histologic and radiologic features. *Head Neck* 1991;13:40–50.
27. Wald RM Jr, Calcaterra TC. Lower alveolar carcinoma. Segmental v marginal resection. *Arch Otolaryngol* 1983;109:578–582.
28. Ord RA, Sarmadi M, Papadimitrou J. A comparison of segmental and marginal bony resection for oral squamous cell carcinoma involving the mandible. *J Oral Maxillofac Surg* 1997;55:470–477; discussion 477–478.
29. Barttelbort SW, Bahn SL, Ariyan SA. Rim mandibulectomy for cancer of the oral cavity. *Am J Surg* 1987;154:423–428.
30. Forrest LA, Schuller DE, Lucas JG, et al. Rapid analysis of mandibular margins. *Laryngoscope* 1995;105:475–477.
31. Jones AS, England J, Hamilton J, et al. Mandibular invasion in patients with oral and oropharyngeal squamous carcinoma. *Clin Otolaryngol* 1997;22: 239–245.
32. Smyth DA, O'Dwyer TP, Keane CO, et al. Predicting mandibular invasion in mouth cancer. *Clin Otolaryngol* 1996;21:265–268.
33. Kalavrezos ND, Gratz KW, Sailer HF, et al. Correlation of imaging and clinical features in the assessment of mandibular invasion of oral carcinomas. *Int J Oral Maxillofac Surg* 1996;25:439–445.
34. Ator GA, Abemayor E, Lufkin RB, et al. Evaluation of mandibular tumor invasion with magnetic resonance imaging. *Arch Otolaryngol Head Neck Surg* 1990;116:454–459.
35. Belkin BA, Papageorge MB, Fakitsas J, et al. A comparative study of magnetic resonance imaging versus computed tomography for the evaluation of maxillary and mandibular tumors. *J Oral Maxillofac Surg* 1988;46:1039–1047.
36. Imola MJ, Gapany M, Grund F, et al. Technetium 99m single positron emission computed tomography scanning for assessing mandible invasion in oral cavity cancer. *Laryngoscope* 2001;111:373–381.
37. O'Brien CJ, Smith JW, Soong SJ, et al. Neck dissection with and without radiotherapy: prognostic factors, patterns of recurrence, and survival. *Am J Surg* 1986;152:456–463.
38. Myers JN, Greenberg JS, Mo V, et al. Extracapsular spread. A significant predictor of treatment failure in patients with squamous cell carcinoma of the tongue. *Cancer* 2001;92:3030–3036.
39. Johnson JT, Barnes EL, Myers EN, et al. The extracapsular spread of tumors in cervical node metastasis. *Arch Otolaryngol* 1981;107:725–729.
40. Johnson JT, Wagner RL, Myers EN. A long-term assessment of adjuvant chemotherapy on outcome of patients with extracapsular spread of cervical metastases from squamous carcinoma of the head and neck. *Cancer* 1996;77: 181–185.
41. Al-Sarraf M, Pajak TF, Byhardt RW, et al. Postoperative radiotherapy with concurrent cisplatin appears to improve locoregional control of advanced, resectable head and neck cancers: RTOG 88-24. *Int J Radiat Oncol Biol Phys* 1997;37:777–782.
42. Bachaud JM, Cohen-Jonathan E, Alzieu C, et al. Combined postoperative radiotherapy and weekly cisplatin infusion for locally advanced head and neck carcinoma: final report of a randomized trial. *Int J Radiat Oncol Biol Phys* 1996;36:999–1004.
43. Récamier JCA. *Recherches sur le traitement du cancer,* vol 1. Paris: Gabon, 1829.
44. Vikram B, Strong EW, Shah JP, et al. Failure at distant sites following multimodality treatment for advanced head and neck cancer. *Head Neck Surg* 1984;6:730–733.
45. Goepfert H. Squamous cell carcinoma of the head and neck: past progress and future promise. *CA Cancer J Clin* 1998;48:195–198.
46. Merino OR, Lindberg RD, Fletcher GH. An analysis of distant metastases from squamous cell carcinoma of the upper respiratory and digestive tracts. *Cancer* 1977;40:145–151.
47. Calhoun KH, Fulmer P, Weiss R, et al. Distant metastases from head and neck squamous cell carcinomas. *Laryngoscope* 1994;104:1199–1205.
48. Holsinger FC, Bekele BN, Zhou X, et al. Clinical predictors of distant metastases from head and neck squamous cell carcinoma. *Arch Otolaryngol Head Neck Surg* 2004 (*in press*).
49. Bhatia R, Bahadur S. Distant metastasis in malignancies of the head and neck. *J Laryngol Otol* 1987;101:925–928.
50. Berger DS, Fletcher GH. Distant metastases following local control of squamous-cell carcinoma of the nasopharynx, tonsillar fossa, and base of the tongue. *Radiology* 1971;100:141–143.
51. Gowen GF, de Suto-Nagy G. The incidence and sites of distant metastases in head and neck carcinoma. *Surg Gynecol Obstet* 1963;47:603–607.
52. Nishijima W, Takooda S, Tokita N, et al. Analyses of distant metastases in squamous cell carcinoma of the head and neck and lesions above the clavicle at autopsy. *Arch Otolaryngol Head Neck Surg* 1993;119:65–68.
53. Leon X, Quer M, Orus C, et al. Distant metastases in head and neck cancer patients who achieved loco-regional control. *Head Neck* 2000;22:680–686.
54. Spector JG, Sessions DG, Haughey BH, et al. Delayed regional metastases, distant metastases, and second primary malignancies in squamous cell carcinomas of the larynx and hypopharynx. *Laryngoscope* 2001;111:1079–1087.
55. Troell RJ, Terris DJ. Detection of metastases from head and neck cancers. *Laryngoscope* 1995;105:247–250.
56. Reiner B, Siegel E, Sawyer R, et al. The impact of routine CT of the chest on the diagnosis and management of newly diagnosed squamous cell carcinoma of the head and neck. *AJR* 1997;169:667–671.
57. Houghton DJ, Hughes ML, Garvey C, et al. Role of chest CT scanning in the management of patients presenting with head and neck cancer. *Head Neck* 1998;20:614–618.
58. Ong TK, Kerawala CJ, Martin IC, et al. The role of thorax imaging in staging head and neck squamous cell carcinoma. *J Craniomaxillofac Surg* 1999;27: 339–344.
59. de Bree R, Deurloo EE, Snow GB, et al. Screening for distant metastases in patients with head and neck cancer. *Laryngoscope* 2000;110:397–401.
60. Leung KS, Fung KP, Sher AH, et al. Plasma bone-specific alkaline phosphatase as an indicator of osteoblastic activity. *J Bone Joint Surg* 1993;75B: 288–292.
61. Brown DH, Leakos M. The value of a routine bone scan in a metastatic survey. *J Otolaryngol* 1998;27:187–189.

62. Lam P, Yuen AP, Ho CM, et al. Prospective randomized study of post-operative chemotherapy with levamisole and UFT for head and neck carcinoma. *Eur J Surg Oncol* 2001;27:750–753.
63. Buckley JG, Ferlito A, Shaha AR, et al. The treatment of distant metastases in head and neck cancer—present and future. *ORL J Otorhinolaryngol Relat Spec* 2001;63:259–264.
64. Schoffski P, Weihkopf T, Ganser A. Advanced head and neck cancer and clinical experience of an effective new agent: docetaxel. *Anticancer Res* 1998;18: 4751–4756.
65. Mazer TM, Robbins KT, McMurtrey MJ, et al. Resection of pulmonary metastases from squamous carcinoma of the head and neck. *Am J Surg* 1988;156: 238–242.
66. Nibu K, Nakagawa K, Kamata S, et al. Surgical treatment for pulmonary metastases of squamous cell carcinoma of the head and neck. Am *J Otolaryngol* 1997;18:391–395.
67. Wedman J, Balm AJ, Hart AA, et al. Value of resection of pulmonary metastases in head and neck cancer patients. *Head Neck* 1996;18:311–316.
68. Finley RK 3rd, Verazin GT, Driscoll DL, et al. Results of surgical resection of pulmonary metastases of squamous cell carcinoma of the head and neck. *Am J Surg* 1992;164:594–598.
69. Vogelstein B, Fearon ER, Hamilton SR, et al. Genetic alterations during colorectal-tumor development. *N Engl J Med* 1988;319:525–532.
70. Nowell PC. The clonal evolution of tumor cell populations. *Science* 1976;194: 23–28.
71. Hanahan D, Weinberg RA. The hallmarks of cancer. *Cell* 2000;100:57–70.
72. Fidler IJ. Critical factors in the biology of human cancer metastasis: twenty-eighth G.H.A. Clowes memorial award lecture. *Cancer Res* 1990;50:6130–6138.
73. Fidler IJ, Kumar R, Bielenberg DR, et al. Molecular determinants of angiogenesis in cancer metastasis. *Cancer J Sci Am* 1998;4(suppl 1):S58–66.
74. Fidler IJ. Rationale and methods for the use of nude mice to study the biology and therapy of human cancer metastasis. *Cancer Metastasis Rev* 1986; 5:29–49.
75. Califano J, van der Riet P, Westra W, et al. Genetic progression model for head and neck cancer: implications for field cancerization. *Cancer Res* 1996; 56:2488–2492.
76. Fearon ER, Vogelstein B. A genetic model for colorectal tumorigenesis. *Cell* 1990;61:759–767.
77. Fidler IJ. Metastasis. In: DeVita VT, Hellman S, Rosenberg SA, et al., eds. *Cancer: principles and practice of oncology,/* vol 1. Philadelphia: Lippincott Williams & Wilkins, 2001.
78. Ridley A. Molecular switches in metastasis. *Nature* 2000;406:466–467.
79. Weiss L. Metastasis of cancer: a conceptual history from antiquity to the 1990s. *Cancer Metastasis Rev* 2000;19:I–XI, 193–383.
80. Sakr WA, Zarbo RJ, Jacobs JR, et al. Distribution of basement membrane in squamous cell carcinoma of the head and neck. *Hum Pathol* 1987;18:1043–1050.
81. Wetzels RH, van der Velden LA, Schaafsma HE, et al. Immunohistochemical localization of basement membrane type VII collagen and laminin in neoplasms of the head and neck. *Histopathology* 1992;21:459–464.
82. Carter RL, Burman JF, Barr L, et al. Immunohistochemical localization of basement membrane type IV collagen in invasive and metastatic squamous carcinomas of the head and neck. *J Pathol* 1985;147:159–164.
83. Visser R, van der Beek JM, Havenith MG, et al. Immunocytochemical detection of basement membrane antigens in the histopathological evaluation of laryngeal dysplasia and neoplasia. *Histopathology* 1986;10:171–180.
84. Van Waes C, Kozarsky KF, Warren AB, et al. The A9 antigen associated with aggressive human squamous carcinoma is structurally and functionally similar to the newly defined integrin alpha 6 beta 4. *Cancer Res* 1991;51:2395–2402.
85. Carey TE, Nair TS, Chern C, et al. Blood group antigens and integrins as biomarkers in head and neck cancer: is aberrant tyrosine phosphorylation the cause of altered alpha 6 beta 4 integrin expression? *J Cell Biochem Suppl* 1993: 223–232.
86. Wolf GT, Carey TE, Schmaltz SP, et al. Altered antigen expression predicts outcome in squamous cell carcinoma of the head and neck. *J Natl Cancer Inst* 1990;82:1566–1572.
87. Wolf GT, Carey TE. Tumor antigen phenotype, biologic staging, and prognosis in head and neck squamous carcinoma. *J Natl Cancer Inst Monogr* 1992;13: 67–74.
88. Thomas GJ, Jones J, Speight PM. Integrins and oral cancer. *Oral Oncol* 1997; 33:381–388.
89. Jones J, Sugiyama M, Speight PM, et al. Restoration of alpha v beta 5 integrin expression in neoplastic keratinocytes results in increased capacity for terminal differentiation and suppression of anchorage-independent growth. *Oncogene* 1996;12:119–126.
90. Wu H, Lotan R, Menter D, et al. Expression of E-cadherin is associated with squamous differentiation in squamous cell carcinomas. *Anticancer Res* 2000;20:1385–1390.
91. Mattijssen V, Peters HM, Schalkwijk L, et al. E-cadherin expression in head and neck squamous-cell carcinoma is associated with clinical outcome. *Int J Cancer* 1993;55:580–585.
92. Chow V, Yuen AP, Lam KY, et al. A comparative study of the clinicopathological significance of E-cadherin and catenins (alpha, beta, gamma) expression in the surgical management of oral tongue carcinoma. *J Cancer Res Clin Oncol* 2001;127:59–63.
93. Nakayama S, Sasaki A, Mese H, et al. Establishment of high and low metastasis cell lines derived from a human tongue squamous cell carcinoma. *Invasion Metastasis* 1998;18:219–228.
94. Schipper JH, Unger A, Jahnke K. E-cadherin as a functional marker of the differentiation and invasiveness of squamous cell carcinoma of the head and neck. *Clin Otolaryngol* 1994;19:381–384.
95. Gottardi CJ, Gumbiner BM. Adhesion signaling: how beta-catenin interacts with its partners. *Curr Biol* 2001;11:R792–794.
96. Lo Muzio L, Staibano S, Pannone G, et al. Beta- and gamma-catenin expression in oral squamous cell carcinomas. *Anticancer Res* 1999;19:3817–3826.
97. Liotta LA, Rao CN. Tumor invasion and metastasis. *Monogr Pathol* 1986: 183–192.
98. Yao J, Xiong S, Klos K, et al. Multiple signaling pathways involved in activation of matrix metalloproteinase-9 (MMP-9) by heregulin-beta1 in human breast cancer cells. *Oncogene* 2001;20:8066–8074.
99. Liabakk NB, Talbot I, Smith RA, et al. Matrix metalloprotease 2 (MMP-2) and matrix metalloprotease 9 (MMP-9) type IV collagenases in colorectal cancer. *Cancer Res* 1996;56:190–196.
100. Sutinen M, Kainulainen T, Hurskainen T, et al. Expression of matrix metalloproteinases (MMP-1 and -2) and their inhibitors (TIMP-1, -2 and -3) in oral lichen planus, dysplasia, squamous cell carcinoma and lymph node metastasis. *Br J Cancer* 1998;77:2239–2245.
101. Ikebe T, Shinohara M, Takeuchi H, et al. Gelatinolytic activity of matrix metalloproteinase in tumor tissues correlates with the invasiveness of oral cancer. *Clin Exp Metastasis* 1999;17:315–323.
102. Tokumaru Y, Fujii M, Otani Y, et al. Activation of matrix metalloproteinase-2 in head and neck squamous cell carcinoma: studies of clinical samples and in vitro cell lines co-cultured with fibroblasts. *Cancer Lett* 2000;150:15–21.
103. Kusukawa J, Sasaguri Y, Shima I, et al. Expression of matrix metalloproteinase-2 related to lymph node metastasis of oral squamous cell carcinoma. A clinicopathologic study. *Am J Clin Pathol* 1993;99:18–23.
104. Kusukawa J, Harada H, Shima I, et al. The significance of epidermal growth factor receptor and matrix metalloproteinase-3 in squamous cell carcinoma of the oral cavity. *Eur J Cancer B Oral Oncol* 1996;32B:217–221.
105. Polette M, Clavel C, Muller D, et al. Detection of mRNAs encoding collagenase I and stromelysin 2 in carcinomas of the head and neck by in situ hybridization. *Invasion Metastasis* 1991;11:76–83.
106. Muller D, Breathnach R, Engelmann A, et al. Expression of collagenase-related metalloproteinase genes in human lung or head and neck tumours. *Int J Cancer* 1991;48:550–556.
107. Kusukawa J, Sasaguri Y, Morimatsu M, et al. Expression of matrix metalloproteinase-3 in stage I and II squamous cell carcinoma of the oral cavity. *J Oral Maxillofac Surg* 1995;53:530–534.
108. Charous SJ, Stricklin GP, Nanney LB, et al. Expression of matrix metalloproteinases and tissue inhibitor of metalloproteinases in head and neck squamous cell carcinoma. *Ann Otol Rhinol Laryngol* 1997;106:271–278.
109. Juarez J, Clayman G, Nakajima M, et al. Role and regulation of expression of 92-kDa type-IV collagenase (MMP-9) in 2 invasive squamous-cell-carcinoma cell lines of the oral cavity. *Int J Cancer* 1993;55:10–18.
110. Pickett KL, Harber GJ, DeCarlo AA, et al. 92K-GL (MMP-9) and 72K-GL (MMP-2) are produced in vivo by human oral squamous cell carcinomas and can enhance FIB-CL (MMP-1) activity in vitro. *J Dent Res* 1999;78:1354–1361.
111. Baba Y, Tsukuda M, Mochimatsu I, et al. Inostamycin, an inhibitor of cytidine 5′-diphosphate 1,2-diacyl-sn-glycerol (CDP-DG): inositol transferase, suppresses invasion ability by reducing productions of matrix metalloproteinase-2 and -9 and cell motility in HSC-4 tongue carcinoma cell line. *Clin Exp Metastasis* 2000;18:273–279.
112. Riedel F, Gotte K, Schwalb J, et al. Expression of 92-kDa type IV collagenase correlates with angiogenic markers and poor survival in head and neck squamous cell carcinoma. *Int J Oncol* 2000;17:1099–1105.
113. Andreasen PA, Egelund R, Petersen HH. The plasminogen activation system in tumor growth, invasion, and metastasis. *Cell Mol Life Sci* 2000;57:25–40.
114. Petruzzelli GJ, Snyderman CH, Johnson JT. In vitro urokinase type plasminogen activator levels and total plasminogen activator activity in squamous cell carcinomas of the head and neck. *Arch Otolaryngol Head Neck Surg* 1994;120:989–992.
115. Schmidt M, Schler G, Gruensfelder P, et al. Urokinase receptor up-regulation in head and neck squamous cell carcinoma. *Head Neck* 2000;22:498–504.
116. Nozaki S, Endo Y, Kawashiri S, et al. Immunohistochemical localization of a urokinase-type plasminogen activator system in squamous cell carcinoma of the oral cavity: association with mode of invasion and lymph node metastasis. *Oral Oncol* 1998;34:58–62.
117. Clayman G, Wang SW, Nicolson GL, et al. Regulation of urokinase-type plasminogen activator expression in squamous-cell carcinoma of the oral cavity. *Int J Cancer* 1993;54:73–80.
118. Ignar DM, Andrews JL, Witherspoon SM, et al. Inhibition of establishment of primary and micrometastatic tumors by a urokinase plasminogen activator receptor antagonist. *Clin Exp Metastasis* 1998;16:9–20.
119. Spring P, Nakashima T, Frederick M, et al. Identification and cDNA cloning of headpin, a novel differentially expressed serpin that maps to chromosome 18q. *Biochem Biophys Res Commun* 1999;264:299–304.
120. Nakashima T, Pak SC, Silverman GA, et al. Genomic cloning, mapping, structure and promoter analysis of HEADPIN, a serpin which is down-regulated in head and neck cancer cells. *Biochim Biophys Acta* 2000;1492:441–446.
121. Xia W, Lau YK, Hu MC, et al. High tumoral maspin expression is associated with improved survival of patients with oral squamous cell carcinoma. *Oncogene* 2000;19:2398–2403.
122. Folkman J. The role of angiogenesis in tumor growth. *Semin Cancer Biol* 1992; 3:65–71.

123. Weidner N, Carroll PR, Flax J, et al. Tumor angiogenesis correlates with metastasis in invasive prostate carcinoma. *Am J Pathol* 1993;143:401–409.
124. Weidner N, Semple JP, Welch WR, et al. Tumor angiogenesis and metastasis—correlation in invasive breast carcinoma. *N Engl J Med* 1991;324:1–8.
125. Shpitzer T, Chaimoff M, Gal R, et al. Tumor angiogenesis as a prognostic factor in early oral tongue cancer. *Arch Otolaryngol Head Neck Surg* 1996;122: 865–868.
126. Zatterstrom UK, Brun E, Willen R, et al. Tumor angiogenesis and prognosis in squamous cell carcinoma of the head and neck. *Head Neck* 1995;17:312–318.
127. Dray TG, Hardin NJ, Sofferman RA. Angiogenesis as a prognostic marker in early head and neck cancer. *Ann Otol Rhinol Laryngol* 1995;104:724–729.
128. Gleich LL, Biddinger PW, Pavelic ZP, et al. Tumor angiogenesis in T1 oral cavity squamous cell carcinoma: role in predicting tumor aggressiveness. *Head Neck* 1996;18:343–346.
129. Folkman J. Seminars in medicine of the Beth Israel Hospital, Boston. Clinical applications of research on angiogenesis. *N Engl J Med* 1995;333:1757–1763.
130. Denhart BC, Guidi AJ, Tognazzi K, et al. Vascular permeability factor/vascular endothelial growth factor and its receptors in oral and laryngeal squamous cell carcinoma and dysplasia. *Lab Invest* 1997;77:659–664.
131. Salven P, Heikkila P, Anttonen A, et al. Vascular endothelial growth factor in squamous cell head and neck carcinoma: expression and prognostic significance. *Mod Pathol* 1997;10:1128–1133.
132. Smith BD, Smith GL, Carter D, et al. Prognostic significance of vascular endothelial growth factor protein levels in oral and oropharyngeal squamous cell carcinoma. *J Clin Oncol* 2000;18:2046–2052.
133. Mineta H, Miura K, Ogino T, et al. Prognostic value of vascular endothelial growth factor (VEGF) in head and neck squamous cell carcinomas. *Br J Cancer* 2000;83:775–781.
134. Nakashima T, Hudson JM, Clayman GL. Antisense inhibition of vascular endothelial growth factor in human head and neck squamous cell carcinoma. *Head Neck* 2000;22:483–488.
135. Tae K, El-Naggar AK, Yoo E, et al. Expression of vascular endothelial growth factor and microvessel density in head and neck tumorigenesis. *Clin Cancer Res* 2000;6:2821–2828.
136. Burian M, Quint C, Neuchrist C. Angiogenic factors in laryngeal carcinomas: do they have prognostic relevance? *Acta Otolaryngol* 1999;119:289–292.
137. Myoken Y, Okamoto T, Kan M, et al. Release of fibroblast growth factor-1 by human squamous cell carcinoma correlates with autocrine cell growth. *In Vitro Cell Dev Biol Anim* 1994;30A:790–795.
138. Janot F, el-Naggar AK, Morrison RS, et al. Expression of basic fibroblast growth factor in squamous cell carcinoma of the head and neck is associated with degree of histologic differentiation. *Int J Cancer* 1995;64:117–123.
139. Dietz A, Rudat V, Conradt C, et al. Prognostic relevance of serum levels of the angiogenic peptide bFGF in advanced carcinoma of the head and neck treated by primary radiochemotherapy. *Head Neck* 2000;22:666–673.
140. Leunig A, Tauber S, Spaett R, et al. Basic fibroblast growth factor in serum and urine of patients with head and neck cancer. *Oncol Rep* 1998;5:955–958.
141. Fujieda S, Sunaga H, Tsuzuki H, et al. Expression of platelet-derived endothelial cell growth factor in oral and oropharyngeal carcinoma. *Clin Cancer Res* 1998;4:1583–1590.
142. Cohen RF, Contrino J, Spiro JD, et al. Interleukin-8 expression by head and neck squamous cell carcinoma. *Arch Otolaryngol Head Neck Surg* 1995;121: 202–209.
143. Richards BL, Eisma RJ, Spiro JD, et al. Coexpression of interleukin-8 receptors in head and neck squamous cell carcinoma. *Am J Surg* 1997;174: 507–512.
144. Riedel F, Gotte K, Bergler W, et al. Expression of basic fibroblast growth factor protein and its down-regulation by interferons in head and neck cancer. *Head Neck* 2000;22:183–189.
145. Slaton JW, Perrotte P, Inoue K, et al. Interferon-alpha–mediated down-regulation of angiogenesis-related genes and therapy of bladder cancer are dependent on optimization of biological dose and schedule. *Clin Cancer Res* 1999;5:2726–2734.
146. Lawler J. The functions of thrombospondin-1 and -2. *Curr Opin Cell Biol* 2000; 12:634–640.
147. Nor JE, Mitra RS, Sutorik MM, et al. Thrombospondin-1 induces endothelial cell apoptosis and inhibits angiogenesis by activating the caspase death pathway. *J Vasc Res* 2000;37:209–218.
148. Norrby K. Constitutively synthesized nitric oxide is a physiological negative regulator of mammalian angiogenesis mediated by basic fibroblast growth factor. *Int J Exp Pathol* 2000;81:423–427.
149. Giri D, Ittmann M. Inactivation of the PTEN tumor suppressor gene is associated with increased angiogenesis in clinically localized prostate carcinoma. *Hum Pathol* 1999;30:419–424.
150. Steck PA, Pershouse MA, Jasser SA, et al. Identification of a candidate tumour suppressor gene, MMAC1, at chromosome 10q23.3 that is mutated in multiple advanced cancers. *Nat Genet* 1997;15:356–362.
151. Li J, Yen C, Liaw D, et al. PTEN, a putative protein tyrosine phosphatase gene mutated in human brain, breast, and prostate cancer. *Science* 1997;275: 1943–1947.
152. Yamada KM, Araki M. Tumor suppressor PTEN: modulator of cell signaling, growth, migration and apoptosis. *J Cell Sci* 2001;114:2375–2382.
153. Lee JI, Soria JC, Hassan KA, et al. Loss of PTEN expression as a prognostic marker for tongue cancer. *Arch Otolaryngol Head Neck Surg* 2001;127:1441–1445.
154. Grandis JR, Tweardy DJ. The role of peptide growth factors in head and neck carcinoma. *Otolaryngol Clin North Am* 1992;25:1105–1115.
155. Cohen S. Isolation of a mouse submaxillary gland protein accelerating incisor eruption and eyelid opening in the newborn animal. *J Biol Chem* 1962;237: 1555.
156. Furuta Y, Takasu T, Asai T, et al. Clinical significance of the epidermal growth factor receptor gene in squamous cell carcinomas of the nasal cavities and paranasal sinuses. *Cancer* 1992;69:358–362.
157. Maurizi M, Scambia G, Benedetti Panici P, et al. EGF receptor expression in primary laryngeal cancer: correlation with clinico-pathological features and prognostic significance. *Int J Cancer* 1992;52:862–866.
158. Grandis JR, Tweardy DJ. Elevated levels of transforming growth factor alpha and epidermal growth factor receptor messenger RNA are early markers of carcinogenesis in head and neck cancer. *Cancer Res* 1993;53:3579–3584.
159. Grandis JR, Melhem MF, Gooding WE, et al. Levels of TGF-alpha and EGFR protein in head and neck squamous cell carcinoma and patient survival. *J Natl Cancer Inst* 1998;90:824–832.
160. Dassonville O, Formento JL, Francoual M, et al. Expression of epidermal growth factor receptor and survival in upper aerodigestive tract cancer. *J Clin Oncol* 1993;11:1873–1878.
161. Formento JL, Francoual M, Ramaioli A, et al. EGF receptor, a prognostic factor in epidermoid cancers of the upper aerodigestive tracts. *Bull Cancer* 1994; 81:610–615.
162. Maxwell SA, Sacks PG, Gutterman JU et al. Epidermal growth factor receptor protein-tyrosine kinase activity in human cell lines established from squamous carcinomas of the head and neck. *Cancer Res* 1989;49:1130–1137.
163. O-charoenrat P, Modjtahedi H, Rhys-Evans P et al. Epidermal growth factor-like ligands differentially up-regulate matrix metalloproteinase 9 in head and neck squamous carcinoma cells. *Cancer Res* 2000;60:1121–1128.
164. Shibata T, Kawano T, Nagayasu H, et al. Enhancing effects of epidermal growth factor on human squamous cell carcinoma motility and matrix degradation but not growth. *Tumour Biol* 1996;17:168–175.
165. Turkson J Jr. STAT proteins: novel molecular targets for cancer drug discovery. *Oncogene* 2000;19:6613–6626.
166. Grandis JR, Drenning SD, Chakraborty A, et al. Requirement of Stat3 but not Stat1 activation for epidermal growth factor receptor-mediated cell growth In vitro. *J Clin Invest* 1998;102:1385–1392.
167. Grandis JR, Chakraborty A, Zeng Q, et al. Downmodulation of TGF-alpha protein expression with antisense oligonucleotides inhibits proliferation of head and neck squamous carcinoma but not normal mucosal epithelial cells. *J Cell Biochem* 1998;69:55–62.
168. Grandis JR, Drenning SD, Zeng Q, et al. Constitutive activation of Stat3 signaling abrogates apoptosis in squamous cell carcinogenesis in vivo. *Proc Natl Acad Sci USA* 2000;97:4227–4232.
169. Ghosh S, May MJ, Kopp EB. NF-kappa B and Rel proteins: evolutionarily conserved mediators of immune responses. *Annu Rev Immunol* 1998;16:225–260.
170. Dong G, Loukinova E, Chen Z, et al. Molecular profiling of transformed and metastatic murine squamous carcinoma cells by differential display and cDNA microarray reveals altered expression of multiple genes related to growth, apoptosis, angiogenesis, and the NF-kappaB signal pathway. *Cancer Res* 2001;61:4797–4808.
171. Sovak MA, Bellas RE, Kim DW, et al. Aberrant nuclear factor-kappaB/Rel expression and the pathogenesis of breast cancer. *J Clin Invest* 1997;100: 2952–2960.
172. Duffey DC, Chen Z, Dong G, et al. Expression of a dominant-negative mutant inhibitor-kappaBalpha of nuclear factor-kappaB in human head and neck squamous cell carcinoma inhibits survival, proinflammatory cytokine expression, and tumor growth in vivo. *Cancer Res* 1999;59:3468–3474.
173. Guttridge DC, Albanese C, Reuther JY, et al. NF-kappaB controls cell growth and differentiation through transcriptional regulation of cyclin D1. *Mol Cell Biol* 1999;19:5785–5799.
174. Dong G, Loukinova E, Chen Z, et al. Molecular profiling of transformed and metastatic murine squamous carcinoma cells by differential display and cDNA microarray reveals altered expression of multiple genes related to growth, apoptosis, angiogenesis, and the NF-kappaB signal pathway. *Cancer Res* 2001;61:4797–4808.
175. Jiang W, Hiscox S, Matsumoto K, et al. Hepatocyte growth factor/scatter factor, its molecular, cellular and clinical implications in cancer. *Crit Rev Oncol Hematol* 1999;29:209–248.
176. Bova R, Quinn D, Nankervis J, et al. Cyclin D1 and p161NK4A expression predict reduced survival in carcinoma of the anterior tongue. *Clin Cancer Res* 1999;5:2810–2819.
177. Charoenrat P, Rhys-Evans P, Eccles SA. Expression of vascular endothelial growth factor family members in head and neck squamous cell carcinoma correlates with lymph node metastasis. *Cancer* 2001: 92:556–568.
178. Hanzawa M SM, Higashino F, et al. Hepatocyte growth factor upregulates E1AF that induces oral squamous cell carcinoma cell invasion by activating matrix metalloproteinase genes. *Carcinogenesis* 2000;21:1079–1085.
179. Dong G, Chen C, Li Z, et al. Hepatocyte growth factor/scatter factor-induced activation of MEK and P13K signal pathways contributes to expression of proangiogenic cytokines interleukin-8 and vascular endothelial growth factor in head and neck squamous cell carcinoma. *Cancer Res* 2001;61:5911–5118.
180. Yoo GH, Xu HJ, Brennan JA, et al. Infrequent inactivation of the retinoblastoma gene despite frequent loss of chromosome 13q in head and neck squamous cell carcinoma. *Cancer Res* 1994;54:4603–4606.
181. Xu J, Gimenez-Conti IB, Cunningham JE, et al. Alterations of p53, cyclin D1, Rb, and H-ras in human oral carcinomas related to tobacco use. *Cancer* 1998; 83:204–212.

182. Levine AJ, Chang A, Dittmer D, et al. The p53 tumor suppressor gene. *J Lab Clin Med* 1994;123:817–822.
183. Farmer GE, Bargonetti J, Shu H, et al. Wild-type p53 activates transcription in vitro. *Nature* 1992;358:82–86.
184. Levine AJ. The p53 tumor-suppressor gene. *N Engl J Med* 1992;326:1350–1352.
185. Kastan MB, Onyekere O, Sidransky D, et al. Participation of p53 protein in the cellular response to DNA damage. *Cancer Res* 1991;6304–6311.
186. Yin Y, Tainsky MA, Bischoff FZ. Wild-type p53 restores cell cycle control and inhibits gene amplification in cells with mutant p53 alleles. *Cell* 1992;70: 937–948.
187. Yonish-Rouach E, Resnitzky D, Lotem J. Wild-type p53 induces apoptosis of myeloid leukaemic cells that are inhibited by interleukin-6. *Nature* 1991;352: 345–347.
188. Kern SE, Kinzler KW, Baker SJ, et al. Mutant p53 protein bind DNA abnormally in vitro. *Oncogene* 1991;6:131–136.
189. Somers KD, Merrick MA, Lopez ME, et al. Frequent p53 mutations in head and neck cancer. *Cancer Res* 1992;52:5997–6000.
190. Sakai I, Rikimaru K, Ueda M, et al. The p53 tumor-suppressor gene and ras oncogene mutations in oral squamous cell carcinoma. *Int J Cancer* 1992;52: 867–872.
191. Boyle JO, Hakim J, Koch W, et al. The incidence of p53 mutations increases with progression of head and neck cancer. *Cancer Res* 1993;53:4477–4480.
192. Shin DM, Kim J, Ro JY, et al. Activation of p53 gene expression in premalignant lesions during head and neck tumorigenesis. *Cancer Res* 1994;54:321–326.
193. Zhang L, Rosin M, Priddy R, et al. p53 expression during multistage human oral carcinogenesis. *Int J Oncol* 1993;3:735–739.
194. Shin DM CN, Lippman SM, et al. P53 protein accumulation and genomic instability in head and neck multistep tumorigenesis. *Cancer Epidemiol Biom Prev* 2001;10:603–609.
195. Syrjanen SM, Syrjanen K. New concepts on the role of human papillomavirus in cell cycle regulation. *Ann Med* 1999;31:175–187.
196. Oliner JD, Pietenpol PJ, Thiagalingam S, et al. Oncoprotein MDM2 conceals the activation domain of tumour suppressor p53. *Nature* 1993;362: 857–860.
197. Haupt Y Maya R, Kazaz A, et al. Mdm2 promotes the rapid degradation of p53. *Nature* 1997;387:296–299.
198. Carroll PE, Okuda M, Horn HF, et al. Centrosome hyperamplification in human cancer: chromosome instability induced by p53 mutation and/or Mdm2 overexpression. *Oncogene* 1999;18:1935–1944.
199. Millon R, Muller D, Schultz I, et al. Loss of MDM2 expression in human head and neck squamous cell carcinomas and clinical significance. *Oral Oncol* 2001;37:620–631.
200. Ganly I, Soutar D, Brown R, et al. P53 alterations in recurrent squamous cell cancer of the head and neck refractory to radiotherapy. *Br J Cancer* 2000;82: 392–398.
201. Kamb A GN, Weaver-Feldhaus J, et al. A cell cycle regulatory potentially involved in genesis of many tumor types. *Science* 1994;264:436–440.
202. Serrano M, Hannon GJ, Beach D. A new regulatory motif in cell-cycle control causing specific inhibition of cyclin D/CDK4. *Nature* 1993;366:704–707.
203. Reed A, Califano J, Cairns P, et al. High frequency of p16 (CDKN2/MTS1/INK4A) inactivation in head and neck squamous cell carcinoma. *Cancer Res* 1996;56:3630–3633.
204. Papadimitrakopoulou V, Izzo J, Lippman SM, et al. Frequent inactivation of p16^{ink4a} in oral premalignant lesions. *Oncogene* 1997;14:1799–1803.
205. El-Naggar AK, Lai S, Clayman GL. Expression of p16, Rb, and cyclin D1 gene products in oral and laryngeal squamous carcinoma: biological and clinical implications. *Hum Pathol* 1999;30:1013–1018.
206. Mao L, Fan YH, Lotan R, et al. Frequent abnormalities of FHIT, a candidate tumor suppressor gene in head and neck cancer cell lines. *Cancer Res* 1996;56:5128–5131.
207. Rocco JW, Li D, Liggett WH Jr, et al. P16INK4A adenovirus mediated gene therapy for human head and neck squamous cell cancer. *Clin Cancer Res* 1998;4:1697–1704.
208. Cordon-Cardo C. Mutations of cell cycle regulators. Biological and clinical implications for human neoplasia. *Am J Pathol* 1995;147:545–560.
209. Peters G. The D-type cyclins and their role in tumorigenesis. *J Cell Sci Suppl* 1994;18:89–96.
210. Bartkova J LJ, Muller H, et al. Abnormal patterns of D-type cyclin expression and G1 regulation in human head and neck cancer. *Cancer Res* 1995;55: 949–956.
211. Bova R, Quinn DI, Nankervis JS, et al. Cyclin D1 and p16INK4A expression predict reduced survival in carcinoma of the anterior tongue. *Clin Cancer Res* 1999;5:2810–2819.
212. Mineta H, Miura K, Takebayashi S, et al. Cyclin D1 overexpression correlates with poor prognosis in patients with tongue squamous cell carcinoma. *Oral Oncol* 2000;36:194–198.
213. Jares P, Fernandez PL, Campo E, et al. PRAD-1/Cyclin D1 gene amplification correlates with messenger RNA overexpression and tumor progression in human laryngeal carcinomas. *Cancer Res* 1994;54:4813–4817.
214. Masuda M, Hirakawa N, Nakashima T, el al. Cyclin D1 overexpression in primary hypopharyngeal carcinomas. *Cancer* 1996;78:390–395.
215. Michalides R, van Veelen N, Hart A, et al. Overexpression of cyclin D1 correlated with recurrence in a group of forty-seven operable squamous cell carcinomas of the head and neck. *Cancer Res* 1995;55:975–978.
216. Akervall JA, Michalides R, Mineta H, et al. Amplification of cyclin D1 in squamous cell carcinoma of the head and neck and the prognostic value of chromosomal abnormalities and cyclin D1 overexpression. *Cancer* 1997;79: 380–389.
217. Nakashima T, Clayman G. Antisense inhibition of cyclin D1 in human head and neck squamous cell carcinoma. *Arch Otolaryngol Head Neck Surg* 2000; 126:957–961.
218. El Deiry WS, Tokino T, Velculescu VE, et al. WAF1, a potential mediator of p53 tumor suppression. *Cell* 1993;75:817–825.
219. Erber R, Klein W, Andl T, et al. Aberrant p21 (CIP1/WAF1) protein accumulation in head and neck cancer. Int J Cancer 1997;74:383–389.
220. Mineta H Miura K, Suzuki I, et al. Low p27 expression correlates with poor prognosis for patients with oral tongue squamous cell carcinoma. *Cancer* 1999;85:1011–1017.
221. Mineta H, Miura K, Suzuki I, et al. p27 expression correlates with prognosis in patients with hypopharyngeal cancer. *Anticancer Res* 1999;19:4407–4412.
222. Green DR. Apoptotic pathways: paper wraps stone blunts scissors. *Cell* 2000;102:1–4.
223. Kumar S. *Apoptosis: biology and mechanisms.* Berlin, New York: Springer, 1999.
224. Ravi D, Ramadas K, Matthew B, et al. De novo programmed cell death in oral cancer. *Histopathology* 1999;34:241–249.
225. Clayman GL. Gene therapy for head and neck cancer. *Head Neck* 1995;17: 535–541.
226. Liu TJ, Zhang WW, Taylor DL, et al. Growth suppression of human head and neck cancer cells by the introduction of a wild-type *p53* gene via a recombinant adenovirus. *Cancer Res* 1994;54.
227. Clayman GL, el-Naggar AK, Lippman SM, et al. Adenovirus-mediated p53 gene transfer in patients with advanced recurrent head and neck squamous cell carcinoma. *J Clin Oncol* 1998;16:2221–2232.
228. Clayman GL. The current status of gene therapy. *Semin Oncol* 2000;27:39–43.
229. Clayman GL, Frank D, Bruso P, et al. Adenovirus-mediated wild-type p53 gene transfer as a surgical adjuvant in advanced head and neck cancers. *Clin Cancer Res* 1999;5:1715–1722.
230. Ohtani T, Hatori M, Ito H, et al. Involvement of caspases in 5-FU induced apoptosis in an oral cancer cell line. *Anticancer Res* 2000;20:3117–3121.
231. Kuwahara D, Tsutsumi K, Kobayashi H, et al. Caspase-9 regulates cisplatin-induced apoptosis in human head and neck squamous cell carcinoma cells. *Cancer Lett* 2000;148:65–71.
232. Hayashi K, Yokozaki H, Naka K, et al. Overexpression of retinoic acid receptor beta induces growth arrest and apoptosis in oral cancer cell liens. *Jpn J Cancer Res* 2001;92:42–50.
233. Seol JG, Park W, Kim, et al. Potential role of caspase-3 and -9 in arsenic trioxide-medicated apoptosis in PCI-1 head and neck cancer cells. *Int J Oncol* 2001;18:249–255.
234. Gallo O, Chiarelli I, Boddi V, et al. Cumulative prognostic value of p53 mutations and bcl-2 protein expression in head and neck cancer treated by radiotherapy. *Int J Cancer* 1999;84:573–579.
235. Pena JC, Thompson C, Recant W, et al. Bcl-xL and Bcl-2 expression in squamous ell carcinoma of the head and neck. *Cancer* 1999;85:164–170.
236. Xie X, Clausen O, DeAngelis P, The prognostic value of spontaneous apoptosis, Bax, Bcl-2, and p53 in oral squamous cell carcinoma of the tongue. *Cancer* 1999;86:913–920.
237. Barkett M, Gilmore T. Control of apoptosis by Rel/NF-(kappa)B transcription factors. *Oncogene* 1999;18:6910–6924.
238. Baldwin AS. Control of oncogenesis and cancer therapy resistance by the transcription factor NF-kappaB. *J Clin Invest* 2001;107:241–246.
239. Webster GA, Perkins ND. Transcriptional cross talk between NF-kappaB and p53. *Mol Cell Biol* 1999;19:3485–3495.
240. Counter C, Hahn W, Wei W, et al. Dissociation among in vitro telomerase activity, telomere maintenance, and cellular immortalization. *Proc Natl Acad Sci USA* 1998;95:14723–14728.
241. Hanahan D, Weinberg RA. The hallmarks of cancer. *Cell* 2000;100:57–70.
242. Counter CM, Hahn WC, Wei W, et al. Dissociation among in vitro telomerase activity, telomere maintenance, and cellular immortalization. *Proc Natl Acad Sci USA* 1998;95:14723–14728.
243. Counter CM. The roles of telomeres and telomerase in cell life span. *Mutat Res* 1996;366:45–63.
244. Patel M, Patel D, Parekh LJ, et al. Evaluation of telomerase activation in head and neck cancer. *Oral Oncol* 1999;35:510–515.
245. Sumida T, Hamakawa H, Sowgawa K, et al. Telomerase components as a diagnostic tool in human oral lesions. *Int J Cancer* 1999;80:1–4.
246. Mutirangura A, Supiyaphun P, Trirekapan S. Telomerase activity in oral leukoplakia and head and neck squamous cell carcinoma. *Cancer Res* 1996;56: 3530–3533.
247. Curran AJ, St Denis K, Irish J, et al. Telomerase activity in oral squamous cell carcinoma. *Arch Otolaryngol Head Neck Surg* 1998;124:784–788.
248. Kannan S, Taraha H, Yokozabi H, et al. Telomerase activity in premalignant and malignant lesions of human oral mucosa. *Cancer Epidemiol Biomarkers Prev* 1997;6:413–420.
249. Folkman J. Angiogenesis and tumor growth. [Correspondence]. *N Engl J Med* 1996;334:921.
250. Karkkainen MJ, Makinen T, Alitalo K. Lymphatic endothelium: a new frontier of metastasis research. *Nat Cell Biol* 2002;4(suppl 1):E2–5.
251. Karpanen T, Egeblad M, Karkkainen MJ, et al. Vascular endothelial growth factor C promotes tumor lymphangiogenesis and intralymphatic tumor growth. *Cancer Res* 2001;61:1786–1790.
252. Skobe M, Hawighorst T, Jackson DG, et al. Induction of tumor lymphangiogenesis by VEGF-C promotes breast cancer metastasis. *Nat Med* 2001;7:192–198.

253. Kaipainen A, Korhonen J, Mustonen T, et al. Expression of the fms-like tyrosine kinase 4 gene becomes restricted to lymphatic endothelium during development. *Proc Natl Acad Sci USA* 1995;92:3566–3570.
254. Jussila L, Valtola R, Partanen TA, et al. Lymphatic endothelium and Kaposi's sarcoma spindle cells detected by antibodies against the vascular endothelial growth factor receptor-3. *Cancer Res* 1998;58:1599–1604.
255. Joukov V, Pajusola K, Kaipainen A, et al. A novel vascular endothelial growth factor, VEGF-C, is a ligand for the Flt4 (VEGFR-3) and KDR (VEGFR-2) receptor tyrosine kinases. *EMBO J* 1996;15:1751.
256. Achen MG, Jeltsch M, Kukk E, et al. Vascular endothelial growth factor D (VEGF-D) is a ligand for the tyrosine kinases VEGF receptor 2 (Flk1) and VEGF receptor 3 (Flt4). *Proc Natl Acad Sci USA* 1998;95:548–553.
257. Stacker SA, Caesar C, Baldwin ME, et al. VEGF-D promotes the metastatic spread of tumor cells via the lymphatics. *Nat Med* 2001;7:186–191.
258. Salven P, Lymboussaki A, Heikkila P, et al. Vascular endothelial growth factors VEGF-B and VEGF-C are expressed in human tumors. *Am J Pathol* 1998; 153:103–108.
259. Kurebayashi J, Otsuki T, Kunisue H, et al. Expression of vascular endothelial growth factor (VEGF) family members in breast cancer. *Jpn J Cancer Res* 1999; 90:977–981.
260. Andre T, Kotelevets L, Vaillant JC, et al. Vegf, Vegf-B, Vegf-C and their receptors KDR, FLT-1 and FLT-4 during the neoplastic progression of human colonic mucosa. *Int J Cancer* 2000;86:174–181.
261. Yonemura Y, Endo Y, Fujita H, et al. Role of vascular endothelial growth factor C expression in the development of lymph node metastasis in gastric cancer. *Clin Cancer Res* 1999;5:1823–1829.
262. Yonemura Y, Fushida S, Bando E, et al. Lymphangiogenesis and the vascular endothelial growth factor receptor (VEGFR)-3 in gastric cancer. *Eur J Cancer* 2001;37:918–923.
263. Niki T, Iba S, Tokunou M, et al. Expression of vascular endothelial growth factors A, B, C, and D and their relationships to lymph node status in lung adenocarcinoma. *Clin Cancer Res* 2000;6:2431–2439.
264. Ohta Y, Nozawa H, Tanaka Y, et al. Increased vascular endothelial growth factor and vascular endothelial growth factor-c and decreased nm23 expression associated with microdissemination in the lymph nodes in stage I non-small cell lung cancer. *J Thorac Cardiovasc Surg* 2000;119:804–813.
265. Bunone G, Vigneri P, Mariani L, et al. Expression of angiogenesis stimulators and inhibitors in human thyroid tumors and correlation with clinical pathological features. *Am J Pathol* 1999;155:1967–1976.
266. Fellmer PT, Sato K, Tanaka R, et al. Vascular endothelial growth factor-C gene expression in papillary and follicular thyroid carcinomas. *Surgery* 1999;126:1056–1061; discussion 1061–1062.
267. O-charoenrat P, Rhys-Evans P, Eccles SA, et al. Expression of vascular endothelial growth factor family members in head and neck squamous cell carcinoma correlates with lymph node metastasis. *Cancer* 2001;92:556–568.
268. Breiteneder-Geleff S, Soleiman A, Kowalski H, et al. Angiosarcomas express mixed endothelial phenotypes of blood and lymphatic capillaries: podoplanin as a specific marker for lymphatic endothelium. *Am J Pathol* 1999;154:385–394.
269. Wigle JT, Oliver G. Prox1 function is required for the development of the murine lymphatic system. *Cell* 1999;98:769–778.
270. Banerji S, Ni J, Wang SX, et al. LYVE-1, a new homologue of the CD44 glycoprotein, is a lymph-specific receptor for hyaluronan. *J Cell Biol* 1999;144:789–801.
271. Lymboussaki A, Olofsson B, Eriksson U, et al. Vascular endothelial growth factor (VEGF) and VEGF-C show overlapping binding sites in embryonic endothelia and distinct sites in differentiated adult endothelia. *Circ Res* 1999; 85:992–999.
272. Valtola R, Salven P, Heikkila P, et al. VEGFR-3 and its ligand VEGF-C are associated with angiogenesis in breast cancer. *Am J Pathol* 1999;154:1381–1390.
273. Ezaki T, Matsuno K, Fujii H, et al. A new approach for identification of rat lymphatic capillaries using a monoclonal antibody. *Arch Histol Cytol* 1990;53:77–86.
274. Sawa Y, Mukaida A, Suzuki M, et al. Identification of lymphatic vessels by using a monoclonal antibody specific for the human thoracic duct. *Microvasc Res* 1997;53:142–149.
275. Fitch K, Somers K, Schechter G. The development of a head and neck tumor model in the nude mouse. *Otolaryngol Head Neck Surg* 1991;104:351–357.
276. Dinesman A, Haughey B, Gates GA, et al. Development of a new in vivo model for head and neck cancer. *Otolaryngol Head Neck Surg* 1990;103:766–774.
277. Simon C, Nemechek AJ, Boyd D, et al. An orthotopic floor-of-mouth cancer model allows quantification of tumor invasion. *Laryngoscope* 1998;108: 1686–1691.
278. O'Malley BW, Cope KA, Johnson CS, et al. A new immunocompetent murine model for oral cancer. *Arch Otolaryngol Head Neck Surg* 1997;123:20–24.
279. Hoffman R. Orthotopic Is Orthodox: Why are orthotopic-transplant metastatic models different from all other models? *J Cellular Biochem* 1994;56:1–3.
280. Takeuchi S, Nakanishi H, Yoshida K, et al. Isolation of differentiated squamous and undifferentiated spindle carcinoma cell lines with differing metastatic potential from a 4-nitroquinoline N-oxide-induced tongue carcinoma in a F344 rat. *Jpn J Cancer Res* 2000;91:1211–1221.
281. Myers JN, Holsinger FC, Jasser SA, et al. An orthotopic nude mouse model of oral tongue squamous cell carcinoma. *Clin Cancer Res* 2002;8:293–298.

CHAPTER 39

Human Papillomavirus and Head and Neck Cancer

Bettie M. Steinberg

Two groups of viruses play a role in the induction of at least some head and neck cancers. The first is Epstein-Barr virus (EBV). The relationship between EBV and nasopharyngeal carcinomas has been recognized since the 1970s. It is now widely accepted that EBV is present in nearly all nasopharyngeal carcinomas in Western countries as well as in China, although the molecular mechanism of EBV carcinogenesis is still not completely understood [reviewed by Pagano (1) and Niedobitek (2)]. The second group of viruses is the human papillomaviruses (HPVs). These viruses induce tumors in stratified squamous epithelium and cause between 95% and 99% of all cervical carcinomas [reviewed by Pfister (3)]. Thus, they have been suspect in causing head and neck cancers as well. However, the relationship of HPVs to head and neck cancers is not yet clear and is currently under intensive investigation. This chapter focuses on the possible role of HPVs in cancers of the head and neck.

BIOLOGY OF HUMAN PAPILLOMAVIRUSES

Papillomaviruses are small, double-stranded circular DNA viruses. The viruses are named for their natural host [e.g., cottontail rabbit papillomavirus (CRPV) and human papillomavirus (HPV)]. More than 100 types of HPV are associated with benign or malignant epithelial tumors, with HPVs 6, 11, 16, and 18 associated with nearly all genital lesions [reviewed by Pfister (3)]. The majority of HPV-induced malignancies are squamous cell carcinomas, although adenocarcinomas of the genital tract also are caused by a subset of HPVs.

Overview of the Human Papillomavirus Life Cycle

Human papillomaviruses share a common life cycle (Fig. 39.1) that can be divided into several steps. In the first step, virus particles infect squamous epithelial cells, the permissive cell type for papilloma formation. Infectious viral particles probably do not exist freely in the environment. Rather, they are packaged within squames that are shed from the surface of a wart or papilloma, are highly resistant to drying and destruction, and introduce large numbers of viral particles to a small area of epithelium. This arrangement would enhance the likelihood of infection of a single cell or small group of cells within the epithelium. Infection of stem cells must occur to establish a stable infection. If only the superficial cells of the epithelium were infected, the virus would quickly be lost as the cells are shed.

Initially, a latent infection is established, in which the tissue is clinically and histologically normal but the viral DNA is present in low copy numbers. Several alternate events can then occur. First, after a period of weeks or months a new papilloma can appear (4). Second, the latent infection can persist in the absence of disease for the life of the host (5–7). Our studies of patients with laryngeal papillomatosis have shown that HPV-6 or -11 DNA can be detected after several years in remission (5). Approximately 50% of random biopsies of uninvolved sites in the larynx of these patients are positive for HPV DNA. In any given patient, the number of sites in which papillomas occur is much more restricted, suggesting that most infected cells never form a papilloma. Finally, the infection can be cleared. Clearance probably is mediated by the immune system, but this process is still not well understood.

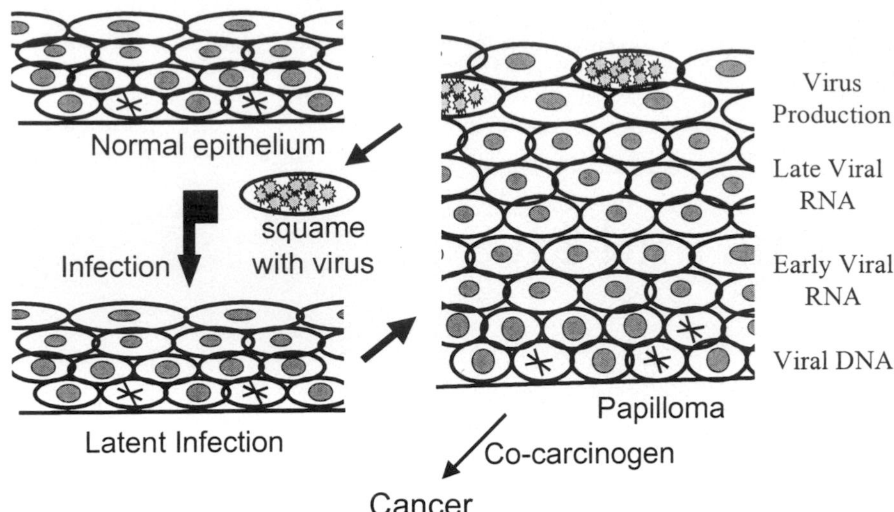

Figure 39.1 Life cycle of the human papillomaviruses (HPVs). Shown are the overall life cycle of the HPVs, the initial infection, establishment of latency, and activation to form a papilloma that initiates high-level viral RNA and DNA synthesis and virion production in a subset of cells as the epithelium matures. The possibility of malignant conversion to cancer, which requires one or more cocarcinogens to induce cellular mutations, is also indicated. Malignant conversion is a rare event, and is not directly part of the viral life cycle.

Activation of latent HPV infection in one or more cells results in formation of a papilloma. The mechanism of activation is not known, but two possibilities have been suggested by studies with animal and human papillomaviruses. First, minor irritation, wounding, exposure to ultraviolet (UV) light, or induction of cell proliferation can induce wart formation by *Mastomys* papillomavirus, CRPV, and bovine papillomavirus (8–12). Second, transient or local immunosuppression could permit viral activation and papilloma formation (11). The HPV-induced lesions are prevalent in patients with suppressed cellular immunity (13), and interferon therapy reduces or eliminates recurrence of papillomas in many patients (14). Activation of latency is accompanied by a marked increase in expression of HPV RNA in suprabasal cells, amplified synthesis of viral DNA in the upper layers, and production of new virus particles in a subset of cells in the uppermost layers. Production of viral RNAs is accompanied by increased levels of viral proteins (12), which should result in immune clearance of the infected cells. Recent evidence suggests, however, that local immune response to papillomas can be limited in patients with active disease. Respiratory papillomas show a decrease in cell surface major histocompatibility complex (MHC) class I expression (15), and the few lymphocytes that infiltrate the papilloma do not express the markers of cytotoxic T cells (16). Thus, both local proliferative induction and reduced local immune response would play a role in activation of latent infection.

Papillomas are characterized by hyperplastic epithelium surrounding cores of connective tissue. The papilloma cells are not characterized by rapid proliferation. Several years ago, we reported that the percentage of replicating basal cells was lower in papillomas than in normal tissue (17). However, the papillary structure involves a marked increase in the length of the basement membrane and increased numbers of basal cells. Therefore, expansion of tissue mass can occur even though the individual basal cells are not dividing rapidly. The squamous layer of papillomas is thickened in comparison with the normal tissue counterpart, reflecting an abnormality in differentiation (17). Most papillomas do not exhibit dysplasia, abnormal mitoses, or hyperkeratosis (18). However, a subset of cells in the upper layers of the papillomas, called *koilocytes,* contain large, clear areas surrounding abnormal nuclei. These cells produce new virus particles, which completes the life cycle. Skin warts and plantar warts produce large amounts of virus and thus are highly infectious. In contrast, laryngeal papillomas produce relatively little virus, and genital condylomas tend to be intermediate in productivity (19). The HPV types that cause mucosal and cutaneous lesions differ, and the cutaneous types may undergo more amplified replication. Alternatively, the limited viral productivity of mucosal papillomas may reflect their delayed and altered differentiation, with only a small number of cells completely differentiating, whereas cutaneous papillomas appear to differentiate more fully. A small subset of lesions can progress to dysplasias, and a rare papilloma converts to malignancy. However, this is not part of the normal life cycle. All evidence to date strongly suggests that no viral production exists in these carcinomas (3).

The altered proliferation and differentiation may reflect underlying changes in cellular signal transduction. Respiratory papillomas overexpress the epidermal growth factor receptor (EGFR) (20), have constitutively active mitogen-activated protein (MAP) kinase (21), and elevated activity of phosphoinositol-3-phosphate kinase, but reduced activation of protein kinase B due to overexpression of the tumor suppressor PTEN (22), and increased activity of nuclear factor kappa B (NF-κB) (23). Cells transformed by HPV-16 show reduced requirement for exogenous growth factors (24), suggesting that the signals normally induced by these factors binding to their cognate receptors might be constitutively "on." Interestingly, if epidermal keratinocytes from EGFR-null mice were immortalized with HPV-16 and then grafted to immunodeficient nude mice, they showed an inability to form papillomas and a marked reduction in carcinomas after treatment with tumor promoters (25). This suggests that signaling from the EGFR may be necessary for HPV-immortalized cells to form papillomas and important but not essential for formation of carcinomas.

Human Papillomavirus Organization and Gene Functions

All the papillomaviruses share a common overall genome organization and some DNA homology, especially in regions critical for viral function. Among the 100-plus HPVs, the virus types can be grouped on the basis of DNA homology, with less than 90% identity in specific regions of the virus being defined as separate types. Grouping HPV types in this way identifies closely related types and correlates with tissue site preference and risk for malignant conversion (3). For example, the group containing HPV-6 and -11 causes mucosal lesions with a low risk for malignancy (e.g., laryngeal papillomas); the groups containing HPV-16, -18, -31, and -45 cause mucosal lesions with a higher malignant potential (found in nearly all cervical cancers); and the groups containing HPV-1, -4, -60, and -65 cause strictly cutaneous lesions.

Human papillomavirus DNA is organized into three regions, with all the coding sequences for proteins located on one strand. Figure 39.2 shows the overall organization of HPV-11, an HPV type frequently found in papillomas of the upper respiratory tract. The short arcs define the individual open reading frames (ORFs), which define the individual genes. The ORFs occur in all three reading frames on the DNA and therefore are depicted on three concentric circles. The "early" region contains the ORFs for all viral functions before assembly of new viral particles. These regions are denoted by an E preceding the number defining the individual ORF. E1 and E2 are involved in viral replication (26–29), and E2 also plays a major role in regulating viral expression (30–32). E6 and E7 of the high-risk HPVs (e.g., HPV-16 and -18) can both immortalize and transform cells (33,34), and they play an essential role in the induction and persistence of carcinomas. E5 is a small, membrane-associated protein that enhances cell proliferation induced by several growth factors (35) and can alter the diacyl glycerol and phospholipase-C-gamma signaling cascade (36). Mutations in either the *E6* or *E7* gene abolish the ability of CRPV to cause warts in rabbits, and mutations in *E5* reduce efficiency of wart formation (37). The role of the E4 protein is not known entirely, but it causes alterations in the cellular cytoskeleton (38), and recent unpublished studies suggest that it may enhance viral replication and prevent entry into mitosis of cells replicating large amounts of virus.

The "late"-region genes, *L1* and *L2,* code for the viral capsid proteins. These genes are expressed only late in the viral life cycle, after the viral DNA has been amplified to high levels. The L1 and L2 proteins can assemble spontaneously into structures that appear morphologically identical to viral particles but that do not contain viral DNA (39). There is great interest in these particles, because they can be used as reagents for serologic studies of patients and might also be used to package other genes for therapeutic purposes.

The third region of the genome, the upstream regulatory region (URR), does not code for viral proteins. It contains the viral origin of replication and sequences that interact with both viral (including E1 and E2) and host proteins to regulate viral gene expression and replication [reviewed by Desaintes and Demeret (40) and McMurray et al. (41)]. This region separates the end of the late region from the beginning of the early region. Thus, because the viral RNAs are expressed from only one strand, this region is immediately "upstream" of the early region. Differences in URR sequences, interacting with cellular factors, determine tissue preference for the various HPV groups and the changes in levels of expression during epithelial differentiation.

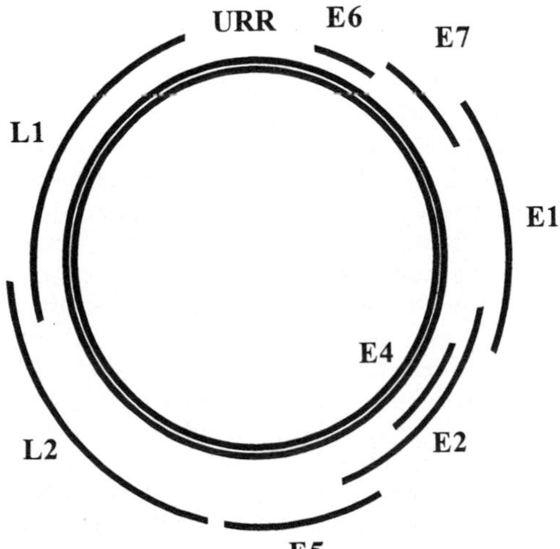

Figure 39.2 The genomic organization of human mucosal papillomavirus 11. The positions of the open reading frames (ORFs) for the "early" (*E*) and "late" (*L*) genes are marked by arcs. The ORFs are found in all three reading frames on one strand of the DNA, represented by varying distances from the closed, double-stranded circle of the DNA.

Viral Gene Transcripts

To express the various genes, viral RNAs are initiated from multiple promoters and are spliced using multiple splice donor and acceptor sites (42–45). This can be visualized on Figure 39.2, with all transcripts expressed in a clockwise fashion from the genome. In low-risk HPV-6 and -11, at least four different early promoters exist. These are located at the beginning of *E6,* generating an *E6* transcript (43); within the *E6* ORF, which generates a transcript for *E7* (44,45); within the *E7* ORF, which generates transcripts for *E1* and some of the downstream ORFs (42); and within the *E1* ORF, which also generates RNAs for the downstream ORFs (43). High-risk HPV-16 and -18 use similar promoters, except that *E6* and *E7* are expressed from the same promoter and the two proteins are produced from alternatively spliced RNAs [reviewed by Desaintes and Demeret (40)]. All early transcripts end at the junction between the end of E5 and the beginning of L2. The promoters and transcripts for the late proteins are not understood as well, although there is some evidence that the late RNAs for the mucosal HPVs are expressed from a promoter located within *E7,* with the RNAs spliced to bypass the termination signal at the end of the early region and code for the late proteins.

Changes in Human Papillomavirus Expression During the Viral Life Cycle

Very little viral RNA is expressed in latency, and it is undetectable by *in situ* or Northern blot hybridizations. Transcripts can be detected by very sensitive reverse-transcriptase polymerase chain reactions (RT-PCRs) (46). However, only a subset of transcripts is made. We have been able to detect a full-length transcript that could code for the El protein required for viral DNA replication but have been unable to detect spliced transcripts for E6 and E7 in latent infection of the respiratory tract (46). Because CRPV is unable to induce papillomas if either the *E6* or *E7* genes are mutated (47,48), absence of the homologous HPV proteins might explain why no evidence of disease is found in latent HPV infection.

Activation of the virus results in increased transcription of the early genes and induction of a papilloma. In CRPV studies (49), viral expression occurs first in stem cells and is limited to *E6* and *E7* transcripts. Only later does viral RNA appear in the epidermis, supporting the hypothesis that stem cells are the permissive cell type for initial viral expression and that *E6* and *E7* expression are required for initial papilloma induction.

In a papilloma, the full complex set of RNAs described above are present, but expression is not uniform. The levels of both viral RNA and DNA increase with cellular differentiation, reflecting a complicated interaction among cellular transcription factors that can change during differentiation, sequences within the URR that bind these factors, and viral proteins that regulate viral expression [reviewed by Desaintes and Demeret (40)]. In the basal layer, viral DNA and RNA are present at low copy numbers. In HPV-6 and -11 infections, transcripts coding for E6 proteins are located in the basal and immediate parabasal cells (50,51). The described location for initial appearance of HPV-6/11 *E7* transcripts varies, first detectable either in the lower (50) or upper (51) spinous layer. In contrast, detection of *E6* and *E7* transcripts in the lowest levels of HPV-16 induced condyloma by *in situ* hybridization is very difficult (52,53), suggesting very low abundance and possibly reflecting a more restrictive control on expression of proteins with strong transforming ability.

In the upper spinous layers, expression of *E1, E2, E4, E5,* and *E7* is markedly increased, and a subset of cells expresses the late transcripts at high levels (51–53). Because of the overlapping nature of the E2/E4/E5 RNAs (Fig. 39.2), *in situ* hybridization cannot readily distinguish between these transcripts; however, we do know that a transcript coding for E4 is the most abundant RNA in many laryngeal papillomas and genital condylomas containing HPV-6 and -11 (42). Viral DNA replication also is markedly elevated in a subset of cells in the upper spinous layer. These cells will produce new viral particles, thereby completing the viral life cycle.

HUMAN PAPILLOMAVIRUSES AND DISEASE

Biology of Tumor Induction

A biologic basis for a causal role for HPVs in some cancers is well established. Nearly all cervical cancers contain integrated HPV DNA, most commonly HPV-16 and HPV-18 [reviewed by McMurray et al. (41)], which are classified as high-risk HPVs. Presence of the high-risk HPVs alone would be only circumstantial evidence for involvement in carcinogenesis. However, cell culture studies have clearly demonstrated that the high-risk HPVs are capable of immortalizing and transforming epithelial cells from foreskin, cervix, oral cavity, and mammary gland (33,54–58). In contrast, HPV-6 and HPV-11, which are associated most often with benign lesions, do not possess this capability (59,60).

Expression of only the *E6* and *E7* ORFs of HPV-16 or -18 is sufficient for immortalization (33,61–63). These results are consistent with the findings that HPV-16 *E6* and *E7* ORFs are retained in HPV-induced cancers (64), that *E6* and *E7* are transcribed in the cancers and in cell lines derived from them (65–68), and that E6 and E7 proteins are found in these cell lines (69–71).

Interaction between high-risk HPV E6 and E7 proteins and cellular proteins is believed to be the mechanism whereby transformation occurs. Initial studies of HPV-16 E7 focused on its interaction with the tumor suppressor protein Rb, forming a complex *in vitro* (72) and *in vivo* (73). Normally, Rb acts in the early phases of the cell cycle to prevent cells from proliferating inappropriately (74). Binding to Rb overcomes the growth-suppressive activity. E7 proteins from the low-risk HPVs also bind Rb but with a fivefold (HPV-11) to 20-fold (HPV-6) lower affinity (73). HPV-16 E7 also complexes with other cell-cycle regulators [reviewed by Zwerschke and Jansen-Durr (75)], including p107 (76), p130 (77), cyclin-dependent kinase 2-cyclin A (76,78), and cyclin E (79). These interactions may be as important as, or more important than, the interaction with Rb. Most certainly they contribute to abnormal cell-cycle progression in infected cells. HPV-16 E7 also induces abnormal centrosome duplication (80), causing genomic instability. In the cytoplasm, E7 protein of both the low-risk and high-risk viruses binds the protein TAP-1 and blocks its activity (81). TAP-1 plays a critical role in presentation of peptides on the cell surface in complex with MHC class I, and inhibition by E7 may be a major mechanism of HPV escape from immune recognition.

The E6 protein of HPV-16 and HPV-18 also complexes with multiple proteins. The first identified interaction was with a second tumor suppressor protein, p53 (82). Formation of the complex results in the degradation of p53 (83). Mutations in *p53* that result in loss of function frequently are found in non–HPV-associated cancers (84). Normally, DNA damage increases the levels of p53, which then induces cell-cycle inhibition, so that damage can be repaired (85). When p53 is lost, repair before DNA replication may not occur, resulting in accumulation of mutations that could contribute to malignant conversion. Low-risk HPV E6 proteins bind p53 but do not cause its degradation, which might contribute to the distinction between high-risk and low-risk HPVs. However, E6 also has many other activities. It cooperates with E7 in abnormal centrosome duplication (80) and abrogation of the mitotic spindle checkpoint (86), binds to and inhibits coactivation by CBP and p300 (87), up-regulates transcription of *fos* and *c-jun*, down-regulates transcription of *c-HA-ras* (88), induces telomerase activity by inducing transcription of the gene *hTERT* (89), and interacts with MAGI-I (90), a cell membrane-associated protein that contributes to regulation of signal transduction. In fact, investigators are reaching the point where they speculate that it might be easier to list proteins that E6 does not bind to or alter. The important thing to remember is that the idea of E6 and E7 binding p53 and Rb is too simplistic, and many other activities may play important roles in transformation.

Clearly, HPV infection alone is not sufficient to bring about malignant transformation. Most women with HPV infections do not develop cervical cancer (91) and, in those who do, a long lag period occurs between infection and the appearance of malignancy (92). Human epithelial cells transfected with HPV-16 or -18 are immortal but not tumorigenic in nude mice (23,58,93). Prolonged passage of the cells (94,95) or treatment with carcinogens (93,96,97) can result in tumorigenic cells, presumably via cumulative genetic alterations. All the data suggest a multistep model for the development of an HPV-induced cancer, with continued expression of *E6* and *E7* being among the requisite steps (98,99).

Detection and Diagnosis of Human Papillomavirus

Human Papillomavirus infection in diseased tissues can be diagnosed in a number of ways. Clinical, cytologic, and histologic appearances can often identify active infection associated with a papillary lesion. However, cytopathology and histology do not identify latent infection. They also cannot distinguish between lesions caused by different HPV types, which requires analysis of viral DNA or RNA, and in malignant lesions of the head and neck do not distinguish between HPV-positive and HPV-negative tissues. The original gold standard for analyzing DNA was the Southern blot. Under stringent conditions, this method is very specific and informative. However, the Southern blot technique has several limitations. It is labor-intensive and not suitable for a clinical laboratory. Also, it cannot be carried out on formalin-fixed, paraffin-embedded tissue, which precludes retrospective studies. Whereas it can detect an average of less than one copy of viral DNA per cell, it requires approximately 1 million infected cells. Recently available for the clinical laboratory are new proprietary methods using hybridization in solution that reduce the amount of DNA required for assay, permitting analysis of cytologic specimens. They are, however, still limited to use of fresh or frozen material and provide HPV group identification, not specific HPV type.

In situ hybridization uses labeled probes to detect HPV RNA or DNA in sections of tissue. This can be accomplished with archival tissue specimens, and kits are available that make it feasible for use in the pathology laboratory. *In situ* hybridization has the advantage that, by adjusting conditions to detect viral RNA rather than DNA, one can determine definitively not only the HPV type but also whether the virus is being expressed at moderate to high levels. The major limitation is that 50 to 100 copies of viral DNA per cell in multiple cells are required for detection. Levels of viral RNA must be even higher. Therefore, *in situ* hybridization cannot detect latent HPV infection. It also cannot be used to detect HPVs that differ in type from the probe.

Polymerase chain reaction is now the detection method of choice for most studies. It can be used to detect and characterize small numbers of HPV molecules (100), can be used with either fresh or archival material, can be established in the clinical laboratory, can be performed with either type-specific primers or consensus primers that detect large numbers of different HPV types, and can detect a total of a few hundred molecules. This sensitivity is orders of magnitude better than that offered by the other assays. However, its very sensitivity is the major limitation of PCR. Great care must be taken in handling specimens and preparing the reactions, to eliminate contamination that results in false-positive results. Although PCR can detect a small number of infected cells, it is not clear that this is biologically meaningful. For example, a tumor in which less than 0.01% of the cells contain HPV DNA would be PCR-positive, but the likelihood that the tumor was caused by HPV infection would be extremely small. Thus, some level of positive signal must be established to suggest a relationship between HPV positivity by PCR and disease. It is now recommended that semiquantitative RT-PCR or *in situ* hybridization be used to detect E6 and/or E7 transcripts, to assure that the virus is actively expressed in tumors positive for HPV DNA by standard PCR.

ROLE OF HUMAN PAPILLOMAVIRUS IN BENIGN LESIONS OF THE HEAD AND NECK

Laryngeal Papillomas

Recurrent respiratory papillomas are benign tumors of the larynx that also can involve the trachea, bronchi, and lungs. Essentially all contain HPV DNA (5,18,101), primarily HPV-6 (102) or -11 (103). Rarely, a patient infected with HPV-16 is identified (104,105). Patients also have latent HPV infection in uninvolved sites throughout the respiratory tract (5,104,106). The incidence of laryngeal papillomas is estimated at 3.8 to 7 per million per year (107,108). In contrast, approximately 4% to 20% of biopsies from the larynx of patients with no history of HPV infection contain latent HPV DNA (109,110). Transmission of HPV from mother to child is believed to occur at the time of birth (111,112). The risk for a child's developing laryngeal papillomas from a mother with active genital HPV infection is approximately 1 in 400 (113). Because latent infection of the respiratory tract is common, perhaps most children born to mothers with clinical or subclinical condyloma become latently infected. It would then be the activation of the latent infection that is rare.

The characteristic course of laryngeal papillomatosis is multiple recurrences after surgical removal, often (but not always) interspersed with periods of remission (18). The HPV-induced lesions are limited by the immune system [reviewed by Gissmann (114) and Frazer (115)]. Our studies suggest a role for the immune system in laryngeal papillomas, although the patients clearly do not suffer general immunosuppression (15). We have seen suppression of MHC class I antigen expression in laryngeal papillomas caused by HPV-6 or -11 (15). Class I is also markedly reduced in cervical cancers caused by HPV-16 (116), apparently mediated by a decrease in the peptide transporter protein TAP-1 (117). This is consistent with our finding that HPV E7 binds to and inhibits TAP-1 (81). The effectiveness of immune surveillance of HPV infection may also be genetically restricted [reviewed by Breitburd et al. (118)]. We previously found a correlation between the class I allele human leukocyte antigen (HLA)-DQ3 and laryngeal papillomas (15) that is consistent with a report for cervical cancer (119). Together, these findings suggest a specific local suppression of response to papillomavirus infection that could contribute to the recurrent nature of laryngeal papillomatosis.

Oral and Nasal Papillomas

Benign HPV-associated lesions in the oral cavity include papillomas, focal epithelial hyperplasia, and leukoplakia (120). The papillomas contain a number of HPV types, among them HPV-6, -11, and -13, usually associated with mucosal papillomas, HPV-2, which usually is thought of as a cutaneous HPV, and HPV-16 (120–123). Focal epithelial hyperplasia often is associated with HPV-13 (124) and -32 (125), which are not usually found in lesions of other tissues.

Both exophytic and inverting nasal papillomas also contain HPVs, including types -6, -11, -16, and -57b (126–132). Most (60% to 75%) exophytic papillomas were HPV positive, whereas detection in inverting papillomas ranged from 0% to 63% (128,130–135). This wide range could reflect differences in methodology or patient populations, different and possibly novel HPV types in some populations, or different etiologies for lesions selected for study at different institutions. Interestingly, Beck et al. (131), Hwang et al. (133), and Ogura et al. (134) have all found a strong positive correlation between HPV positivity and recurrence after surgery, which suggests that there are at least two different types of lesions with similar histologic appearance but different biologic properties.

ROLE OF HUMAN PAPILLOMAVIRUS IN HEAD AND NECK CANCER

Carcinomas in Patients with Laryngeal Papilloma

The clearest evidence for malignant conversion of laryngeal papillomas is the outcome of radiation therapy, which now is strongly contraindicated. Malignant conversion occurred in 14% to 30% of radiated patients, with a lag period of 10 to 20 years (136,137). Spontaneous conversion also occurs (138–145), but at an estimated frequency of 3% (140). One study reported a rate of 19% (141). However, those patients all had a long history of heavy smoking. Perhaps the carcinogenic effects of tobacco, like radiation, increase the probability of malignant conversion.

The carcinomas usually contained the same HPV-6 or HPV-11 DNAs found in the laryngeal papillomas (142–145). Kashima et al. (144) and Lindeberg et al. (145) used *in situ* hybridization to confirm that the HPV DNA was in the carcinomas, not in possibly adjacent papillomas. Byrne et al. (142) and DiLorenzo et al. (143) analyzed the structure of the HPV DNA within two such carcinomas. Both contained HPV molecules that had undergone partial duplication, resulting in large HPV DNA molecules with two copies of the URR. Interestingly, a reconstructed HPV-11 DNA molecule containing two copies of the URR could transform cells in culture, whereas the normal HPV-11 could not (146). Although HPV-6 and -11 have been termed "low-risk" viruses, they do have the potential to cause head and neck cancers in these patients.

Verrucous Carcinoma of the Head and Neck

Verrucous carcinomas are rare, low-grade, locally invasive cancers with a papillomatous morphology and club-shaped lower margins. Cells in the upper hyperplastic layers often exhibit the koilocytotic changes seen in HPV-induced lesions. Human papillomaviruses are associated with 30% to 100% of verrucous carcinomas (147–152) and may well play a central etiologic role. Verrucous carcinomas of the larynx predominantly contain HPV-6 or -11, HPV-16, or HPV-16–related DNA (147–150). In contrast, a study of 25 oral cavity verrucous carcinomas found that 40% of the cases contained HPV-18 DNA and that only 12% of the cases contained HPV-6, -11, or -16 (151). Moreover, Adler-Storthz et al. (152) detected HPV-2 in only three of nine patients. Therefore, there might be tissue specificity in induction of verrucous carcinoma by different HPVs.

Squamous Cell Cancer of the Head and Neck

The prevalence of HPV DNA in squamous cell cancers of the head and neck has been extremely variable from one study to another, ranging from 0% to nearly 100%. In part, this might reflect differences in methodology. Some earlier studies used Southern blot or dot-blot hybridization, whereas others used *in situ* hybridization on paraffin-embedded tissue sections. Most of the more recent studies used PCR, which is a very sensitive method for determining prevalence of HPV DNA (153). However, as discussed above, false-positive results with PCR can be a major problem (154,155) and undoubtedly account for some of the very high prevalence rates in early studies. Most investigators now include appropriate negative controls to evaluate positive results properly. Another limitation of PCR that is less often appreciated is that latent infection in cells adjacent to or within the tumor specimen will elicit a positive signal. Therefore, alternative approaches must be considered. One approach is to determine prevalence data of latent HPV DNA in normal tissues from the same sites, appropriate for large epidemiologic studies but unable to determine the relationship between HPV positivity and a specific tumor. Polymerase chain reaction can be used in a simple, semiquantitative way to eliminate samples with extremely low levels of HPV DNA (e.g., less than 0.1 copy/cell) (156). Finally, positive samples can be analyzed by a second method (e.g., *in situ* hybridization) for viral RNA to distinguish between active and latent infection and confirm that the active virus is in the tumor.

Another possible explanation exists for the variation in prevalence seen in different studies. The head and neck encompass different types of epithelia that could vary in susceptibility to HPV-induced carcinomas. A representative subset of studies are presented in this chapter in which some anatomic distinction was made, samples were analyzed by PCR, no obviously strong environmental factor was present that could have altered prevalence data, and, whenever possible, normal tissue controls were included. These limitations would be expected to reduce the variability in prevalence from one study to another.

Finally, variability could reflect differences between the populations or subpopulations that were studied. There is mounting evidence, discussed above, that genetic susceptibility could play a role in HPV-induced disease. There are also differences in the use of alcohol and tobacco (and other potentially carcinogenic materials) in different populations. Thus, the variability from one study to another could have many causes. Only when we understand all of the factors that determine susceptibility to HPV-induced carcinogenesis will we be able to clearly explain the reported variation.

CANCERS OF THE ORAL CAVITY

The overall positivity of oral cancers for HPV is generally accepted to be less than 20%, but this does not take into account the variation seen with different sites. Table 39.1 summarizes studies of the prevalence of HPV DNA in three different sites within the oral cavity and oropharynx (157–167). As can be seen, there is marked difference between sites. The strongest evidence for an HPV etiology is with tonsillar cancers, and most investigators now conclude that HPV plays an etiologic role in a subset of these tumors. By far the majority of HPV-positive tonsillar cancers contained HPV-16, even when other types are also listed, consistent with the high oncogenic potential of HPV-16. Not only were a significant fraction of tonsillar cancers positive by PCR (66 of 127, 52%), but some results were also confirmed by other methods. For example, Snijders et al. (163) analyzed a subset of their PCR-positive tonsillar carcinomas by multiple methods. Four of six were positive by Southern blot analysis, whereas the Southern-blot-negative biopsies con-

TABLE 39.1 Prevalence of Human Papillomavirus (HPV) DNA in Oral Carcinomas

Location	Number positive/total (%)	HPV type	Reference
Tonsil	14/25 (56)	16, 33, 59	158
Tonsil	26/60 (43)	16	159
Tonsil	12/14 (86)	16, 33, 7, 59	161
Tonsil	3/7 (43)	ND	162
Tonsil	10/10 (100)	16, 33, ?	163
Tonsil	32/34 (94)	16, 18, 33	164
Tonsil	11/21 (52)	16	165
Tonsil, control	0/7 (0)	NA	163
Tongue	0/4 (0)	NA	157
Tongue	0/10 (0)	NA	160
Tongue	5/19 (26)	ND	162
Tongue	8/24 (33)	16, 18	167
FOM	0/1 (0)	NA	157
FOM	0/5 (0)	NA	160
FOM	1/13 (8)	ND	162

?, HPV type not known; FOM, floor of mouth; NA, not applicable; ND, not determined.

tained less than 10% carcinoma cells per sample. Three tumors with intact cellular RNA were analyzed, and all were positive for HPV RNA by both RT-PCR and *in situ* hybridization. Gillison et al. (164) also used *in situ* hybridization to confirm presence of HPV within the lesions rather than in adjacent tissues, analyzing both preinvasive and invasive tumors and associated lymph node disease, and used Southern blot to determine that patterns were consistent with integration of HPV DNA within the tumors. Interestingly, Hemminki et al. (166) reported that the risk for tonsillar cancer was elevated in men whose wives had been diagnosed with cervical cancer, suggesting a possible oral/genital route of infection in these patients.

A subset of tongue carcinomas (18 of 71, 25%) was HPV-positive. A study using Southern blot analysis (not shown in Table 39.1) also found that 18% of tongue cancers were positive (109). Balaram et al. (168) studied a group of patients who were all chewers of betel quid, which is strongly implicated in oral carcinogenesis (168,169). Tongue carcinomas were positive in nine of 11 (82%) cases. This raises questions regarding cofactors for HPV induction of oral cancers. Brandwein et al. (162) also included information on tobacco and alcohol use. Only three of 16 HPV-positive patients and six of 37 HPV-negative patients reported that they had never smoked or used alcohol, so most of the patients had been exposed to the carcinogenic effects of tobacco. However, the investigators found no correlation between HPV presence and use of tobacco and alcohol. Studies of control tissues from tonsil and tongue, included in Table 39.1, were negative for HPV. This strengthens the positive findings and suggests that HPV is not just a passenger in the oral cavity.

Floor-of-mouth cancers have a very low level of positivity, suggesting that HPVs do not play any significant role in these tumors. Thus it is important to distinguish tissue site and type in analyzing the role of HPVs in cancers the oral cavity.

CARCINOMA OF THE NOSE, SINUS, AND NASOPHARYNX

The prevalence of HPV in nasal and nasopharyngeal carcinomas has also been studied. Studies of the nasal cavity and nasal sinus have generally been limited to small numbers of samples, and used a variety of methods (109,160,170–173). One of the largest studies has recently been reported by Buchwald et al. (173), who looked at 35 cases of squamous cell carcinoma associated with sinonasal papillomas. They found four of 30 (13%) carcinomas associated with inverted papillomas were positive, and three of five (60%) associated with exophytic papillomas were positive. Although the numbers are small, there is the suggestion that a subset of sinonasal carcinomas may be caused by HPV. Overall, combining multiple studies, 22 of 121 (18%) of nasal cavity and paranasal sinus carcinomas were positive for HPV DNA. Like the oral cavity and oropharynx, HPV-16 was the most common HPV type.

Polymerase chain reaction studies of nasopharyngeal carcinomas and normal tissue are summarized in Table 39.2 (60,174–178). Overall, 83 of the 198 (42%) of carcinomas were positive for HPV DNA, and HPV-16 again predominated. One study also evaluated the prevalence of HPV in normal tissue. Tyan et al. (175) used type-specific primer sets from the E6 ORF to detect HPV-6, -11, -16, -18, or -33, confirmed positive PCR products by sequencing, and compared the prevalence of HPVs in normal nasopharynx (9%) with poorly differentiated or undifferentiated nasopharyngeal tumors (47%). Like tonsillar cancers, a high percentage of nasopharyngeal carcinomas are HPV positive.

Epstein-Barr virus has long been implicated in nasopharyngeal carcinoma. Investigators have now asked whether EBV and HPV might possibly interact in malignant induction of nasopharyngeal tumors. Tyan et al. (175) found EBV in 100% of the 30 nasopharyngeal carcinomas they assayed, and 14 of the 30 also contained HPV-16 DNA. Rassekh et al. (176) found that all of the HPV-positive tumors in their study contained EBV. Similarly, Tung et al. (178) found that 80% of their HPV-positive tumors also contained EBV DNA. Of interest, Punwaney et al. (177) analyzed 30 nasopharyngeal tumors from two different populations. Of six tumors from Caucasian Americans, two were HPV+/EBV+, one was HPV+/EBV−, and three were HPV−/EBV+. In contrast, of the 24 patients from the Orient (including one Oriental American), only four were HPV+, whereas all were EBV+. These studies suggest that, in the West, HPV and EBV may serve as cocarcinogens. It is tempting to speculate that EBV and HPV might also cooperate in tonsil cancers, because EBV is so often found in these tissues. Future studies will have to be done to address this question.

TABLE 39.2 Prevalence of Human Papillomavirus in Nasopharynx Squamous Cell Carcinomas

Tissue	Number positive/total (%)	Reference
SCC	4/16 (25)	160
SCC	4/15 (27)[a]	174
SCC	14/30 (47)[b]	175
SCC	9/17 (53)	176
SCC	7/30 (23)	177
SCC	45/88 (51)	178
Normal	1/11 (9)	175

SCC, squamous cell carcinoma.
[a]Highly differentiated, keratinizing carcinomas.
[b]Poorly differentiated carcinomas.

CARCINOMA OF THE LARYNX, BRONCHUS, AND LUNG

A final group of tumors to be considered for possible HPV etiology is carcinoma of the larynx, bronchus, and lung. Representative PCR prevalence data for laryngeal cancers and normal laryngeal tissue is shown in Table 39.3 (110,149,157,160,179–185). Human papillomavirus prevalence in studies with large numbers of samples ranged from 54% to 16% (149,160), but the study with 54% positive results also had 50% positivity in normal tissue (149). One study with a relatively high positivity rate (52%) also analyzed the HPV-positive tumors by RT-PCR, and found that only the seven that were HPV-16 positive expressed viral DNA (183). If only those were to be considered positive, the HPV

TABLE 39.3 Prevalence of Human Papillomavirus (HPV) DNA in Laryngeal Carcinomas

Tissue type	Number positive/ total (%)	HPV type	Reference
Carcinoma	26/48 (54)	16	149
Carcinoma	5/31 (16)	16, 18	160
Carcinoma	8/36 (22)	6, 11, 16	179
Carcinoma	7/34 (21)	6, 16	180
Carcinoma	22/75 (29)	16, 18, 33	182
Carcinoma	13/25 (52)	6, 16, 45	183
Carcinoma	11/44 (25)	6, 11, 16	184
Carcinoma	19/91 (21)	6, 16, 18	185
Normal	2/12 (17)	16	184
Normal	3/6 (50)	16	149
Normal	3/12 (25)	11	181
Normal	6/32 (19)	11	110

positivity rate in that study would be 25%. This would be consistent with the study by Gorgoulis et al. (185), who confirmed their PCR-positive specimens by *in situ* hybridization and found that all but one were positive. Two PCR studies evaluated HPV prevalence only in normal laryngeal tissue and found a prevalence of 19% and 25% (110,181). These results suggest that latent HPV DNA is common in the normal larynx, that much of it is either HPV-6 or -11, and that much of the HPV DNA in laryngeal carcinomas could reflect latent HPV that is unrelated to carcinogenesis. However, Smith et al. (184) found that after controlling for tobacco and alcohol, presence of oncogenic HPV types was associated with an increased risk for laryngeal cancer (odds ratio = 3.0). Thus, oncogenic HPVs could play a role in a subset of laryngeal cancers.

Studies in Europe and the United States (185–191) have generally reported that lung and bronchial carcinomas have a very low rate of HPV detection, averaging less than 3% when studies are combined. An exception to this is a study by Nuorva et al. (192) in Finland that evaluated bronchioloalveolar carcinomas, a rare type of lung cancer. They found 8/22 (36%) contained HPV DNA by both PCR and *in situ* hybridization in this unusual tumor type. However, prevalence of HPV DNA may depend on the population studied. Studies have reported a low to moderate rate of HPV presence (0–30%, but only 20% by *in situ* hybridization) in Japan (193,194), a high rate (53%, with all of 18 benign controls negative) in China (195), and a very significant rate (as high as 79%) in Okinawa (194,196). One of the Okinawa studies compared HPV prevalence on mainland Japan to Okinawa (194), confirming the difference between the two populations. A more recent study by this same group (197) reported a drop in incidence of squamous cell carcinoma between 1986 and 1998, and a parallel drop in HPV positivity from 79% to 24%, suggesting an underlying change in patterns of disease, and making Okinawa more similar to Japan. Finally, a study from Taiwan (198) addressed the etiology of lung cancer in that population, where it is the leading cause of cancer death in women although less than 10% of patients smoked. They found that 77/141 (54.6%) of the lung cancers in women were positive for HPV-16 or -18, compared with 16/60 (26.7%) of control tissues. Moreover, *in situ* hybridization of the lung cancers confirmed that the HPV DNA was in the tumor cells, not adjacent normal tissue. The odds ratio of a nonsmoking woman having HPV DNA in lung cancer in this study was 10.1, compared with nonsmoking males of only 1.98. Taken together, these studies suggest that specific populations, subpopulations, and types of lung cancer (squamous carcinoma, adenocarcinoma, or bronchioloalveolar carcinoma) may have very different prevalence of HPV.

CLINICAL IMPLICATIONS OF HUMAN PAPILLOMAVIRUS POSITIVITY

A number of recent studies have tried to address the questions of differences in outcome or molecular abnormalities in HPV-positive and HPV-negative tumors of the head and neck. HPV-positive tonsillar cancers are associated with poor differentiation (158,165), decreased expression of the cell cycle regulators cyclin D1, pRB, and p53 (157,158,165), and lower risk for relapse with increased survival (159,165). Similarly, others have reported that HPV positive head and neck squamous cell cancers had a significantly reduced disease-specific mortality (164,199–201). Lindel et al. (201) reported that HPV-positive oropharynx cancers were more sensitive to radiotherapy and had a better survival rate. Therefore, there is mounting evidence that HPV-positive tumors of the head and neck might have a different biologic behavior than comparable HPV-positive tumors. This, in turn, suggests that HPV may be the etiologic agent in many of those tumors and not just be present as a passenger.

CONCLUSION

Human papillomaviruses are clearly the etiologic agents of benign lesions of the head and neck, and some of those lesions can undergo malignant conversion. Human papillomaviruses also appear to play a significant role in the etiology of a subset of other head and neck tumors. Tonsillar cancers are strongly correlated with HPV infection, based on molecular epidemiologic data. This evidence is especially substantial, because the tumors not only contain HPV DNA in most of the cells but also express readily detectable levels of HPV RNA. Nasopharyngeal carcinomas also have relatively high levels of HPV, and both nasopharynx and tonsil are prone to EBV infection as well, which might result in cocarcinogenic activity between the two viruses. Other sites within the oral cavity, with the possible exception of base of tongue, are not associated with HPV to any significant degree. Prevalence of HPV is lower in larynx cancers than oropharynx and extremely variable in lung, depending on the population studied and pathology of the tumors. Thus it is important when discussing HPV as an etiologic factor for head and neck cancers to define the tissue site, type of carcinoma, and the population being studied.

As we learn more about the biologic basis for malignant conversion of HPV-infected cells, we better understand the complex interactions that must occur among the virus, its host cell, and environmental factors that contribute to malignancy. This knowledge may be used in the future to intervene in and prevent persistence of HPV infection and malignant conversion in those cancers where HPV plays a significant role. The potential clinical implications of HPV etiology for even a subset of cancers in the head and neck are significant. Vaccines against HPV, currently being developed, could reduce the incidence of disease. As we learn more about the pathophysiology of HPV-induced disease, we may develop specific therapies that block expression of E6 or E7 proteins. Alternatively, we could alter cellular responses to the viral transforming proteins and thus limit proliferation and progression of the cancer. The future holds the promise to more rationally treat head and neck cancers, based on this knowledge.

ACKNOWLEDGMENT

This chapter was supported in part by grant P50 DC00203 from the National Institute on Deafness and Communication Disorders.

REFERENCES

1. Pagano JS. Epstein-Barr virus: the first human tumor virus and its role in cancer. *Proc Assoc Am Physicians* 1999;111:573.
2. Niedobitek G. Epstein -Barr virus infection in the pathogenesis of nasopharyngeal carcinoma. *Mol Pathol* 2000;53:248
3. Pfister H. *Papillomaviruses and human cancer.* Boca Raton, FL: CRC Press, 1990:
4. Stoler MH, Whitbeck A, Wolinsky SM, et al. Infectious cycle of human papillomavirus type 11 in human foreskin xenografts in nude mice. *J Virol* 1990;64:3310.
5. Steinberg BM, Topp WC, Schneider PS, et al. Laryngeal papillomavirus infection during clinical remission. *N Engl J Med* 1983;308:1261.
6. Ferenczy A, Mitao M, Nagai N, et al. Latent papillomavirus and recurring genital warts. *N Engl J Med* 1985;313:784.
7. Toon PG, Arrand JR, Wilson LP, et al. Human papillomavirus infection of the

uterine cervix of women without cytological signs of neoplasia. *BMJ* 1986; 293:1261.
8. Amtmann E, Volm M, Wayss K. Tumour induction in the rodent *Mastomys natalensis* by activation of endogenous papillomavirus genomes. *Nature* 1984; 308:291.
9. Siegsmund M, Wayss K, Amtmann E. Activation of latent papillomavirus genomes by chronic mechanical irritation. *J Gen Virol* 1991;72:2787.
10. Amella CA, Lofgren LA, Ronn AM, et al. Latent infection induced with cottontail rabbit papillomavirus: a model for human papillomavirus latency. *Am J Pathol* 1994;144:1167.
11. Campo MS, Jarrett WFH, O'Neil W, et al. Latent papillomavirus infection in cattle. *Res Vet Sci* 1994;56:151.
12. Zhang P, Nouri M, Brandsma JL, et al. Induction of E6/E7 expression in cottontail rabbit papillomavirus latency following UV activation. *Virology* 1999; 263:388.
13. Benton C, Shahidullah H, Hunter JAA. Human papillomavirus in the immunosuppressed. *Papillomavirus Rep* 1992;3:23.
14. Haglund S, Lundquist PG, Cantell K, et al. Interferon therapy in juvenile laryngeal papillomatosis. *Arch Otolaryngol Head Neck Surg* 1981;107:327.
15. Bonagura VR, Siegal FP, Abramson AL, et al. Enriched HLA-DQ3 phenotype and decreased class I major histocompatibility complex antigen expression in recurrent respiratory papillomatosis. *Clin Diagn Lab Immunol* 1994;1:357.
16. Bonagura VR, Hatam L, DeVoti J, et al. Recurrent respiratory papillomatosis: altered $CD8^+$ T-cell subsets and $T_H 1/T_H 2$ cytokine imbalance. *Clin Immunol* 1999;93:302.
17. Steinberg BM, Meade R, Kalinowski S, et al. Abnormal differentiation of human papillomavirus-induced laryngeal papillomas. *Arch Otolaryngol Head Neck Surg* 1990;116:1167.
18. Abramson AL, Steinberg BM, Winkler B. Laryngeal papillomatosis: clinical, histopathologic and molecular studies. *Laryngoscope* 1987;97:678.
19. Lack EE, Jenson AB, Smith HG, et al. Immunoperoxidase localization of human papillomavirus in laryngeal papillomas. *Intervirology* 1980;14:148.
20. Vambutas A, Di Lorenzo TP, Steinberg BM. Laryngeal papilloma cells have high levels of epidermal growth factor receptor and respond to epidermal growth factor by a decrease in epithelial differentiation. *Cancer Res* 1993;53: 910.
21. Johnston D, Hall H, DiLorenzo TP, et al. Elevation of the epidermal growth factor receptor and dependent signaling in human papillomavirus-infected laryngeal papillomas. *Cancer Res* 1999;59:968.
22. Zhang P, Steinberg BM. Overexpression of PTEN/MMAC1 and decreased activation of Akt in human papillomavirus-infected laryngeal papillomas. *Cancer Res* 2000;60:1457.
23. Vancurova I, Wu W, Miskolci V, et al. Increased p50/p50 NF-κB activation in HPV 6/11-induced laryngeal papilloma tissue. *J Virol* 2002;76:1533.
24. Creek KE, Geslani G, Batova A, et al. Progressive loss of sensitivity to growth control by retinoic acid and transforming growth factor-beta at late stages of human papillomavirus type 16-initiated transformation of human keratinocytes. *Adv Exp Med Biol* 1995;375:117.
25. Woodworth CD, Gaiotti D, Michael E, et al. Targeted disruption of the epidermal growth factor receptor inhibits development of papillomas and carcinomas from human papillomavirus-immortalized keratinocytes. *Cancer Res* 2000;10:4397.
26. Chiang CM, Ustav M, Stenlund A, et al. Viral E1 and E2 proteins support replication of homologous and heterologous papillomaviral origins. *Proc Natl Acad Sci USA* 1992;89:5799.
27. Return M, Brain R, Jenkins JR. The E2 binding sites determine the efficiency of replication for the origin of human papillomavirus type 18. *Nucleic Acids Res* 1992;20:6015.
28. Del Vecchio AM, Romanczuk H, Howley PM, et al. Transient replication of human papillomavirus DNAs. *J Virol* 1992;66:5949.
29. Kuo SR, Liu JS, Broker TR, et al. Cell-free replication of the human papillomavirus DNA with homologous viral E1 and E2 proteins and human cell extracts. *J Biol Chem* 1994;269:24058.
30. McBride AA, Romanczuk H, Howley PM. The papillomavirus E2 regulatory proteins. *J Biol Chem* 1991;266:18411.
31. Chin MT, Hirochika R, Hirochika H, et al. Regulation of human papillomavirus type 11 enhancer and E6 promoter by activating and repressing proteins from the E2 open reading frame: functional and biochemical studies. *J Virol* 1988;62:2994.
32. Tan SH, Gloss B, Bernard HU. During negative regulation of the human papillomavirus-16 E6 promoter, the viral E2 protein can displace Sp1 from a proximal promoter element. *Nucleic Acids Res* 1992;20:251.
33. Woodworth CD, Bowden PE, Doniger J, et al. Characterization of normal human exocervical epithelial cells immortalized in vitro by papillomavirus types 16 and 18 DNA. *Cancer Res* 1988;48:4620.
34. Barbosa MS, Schlegel R. The *E6* and *E7* genes of HPV-18 are sufficient for inducing two-stage in vitro transformation of human keratinocytes. *Oncogeue* 1989;4:1529.
35. Straight SW, Hinkle PM, Jewers RJ, et al. The E5 oncoprotein of human papillomavirus type 16 transforms fibroblasts and effects the downregulation of the epidermal growth factor receptor in keratinocytes. *J Virol* 1993;67:4521.
36. Crusius K, Kaskin M, Kinzel V, et al. The human papillomavirus type 16 E5 protein modulates phospholipase C-gamma-1 activity and phosphatidyl inositol turnover in mouse fibroblasts. *Oncogene* 1999;19:3727.
37. Brandsma JL. Animal models of human-papillomavirus-associated oncogenesis. *Intervirology* 1994;37:189.
38. Doorbar J, Ely S, Sterling J, et al. Specific interaction between HPV-16 E1-E4 and cytokeratins results in collapse of the epithelial cell intermediate filament network. *Nature* 1991;352:824.
39. Zhou J, Sun XY, Stenzel DJ, et al. Expression of vaccinia recombinant HPV 16 L1 and L2 ORF proteins in epithelial cells is sufficient for assembly of HPV virion-like particles. *Virology* 1991;185:251.
40. Desaintes C, Demeret C. Control of papillomavirus DNA replication and transcription. *Semin Cancer Biol* 1996;7:339.
41. McMurray HR, Nguyen D, Westerbrook TF, et al. Biology of human papillomaviruses. *Int J Exp Pathol* 2001;82:15.
42. Nasseri M, Hirochika R, Broker TR, et al. A human papillomavirus type 11 transcript encoding an E1–E4 protein. *Virology* 1987;159:433.
43. Rotenberg MO, Chow LT, Broker TR. Characterization of rare human papillomavirus type 11 mRNAs coding for regulatory and structural proteins, using the polymerase chain reaction. *Virology* 1989;172:489.
44. Smotkin D, Prokoph H, Wettstein FO. Oncogenic and nononcogenic human genital papillomaviruses generate the E7 mRNA by different mechanisms. *J Virol* 1989;63:1441.
45. Ward P, Mounts P. Heterogeneity in mRNA of human papillomavirus type-6 subtypes in respiratory tract lesions. *Virology* 1989;168:1.
46. Maran A, Amella CA, DiLorenzo TP, et al. Human papillomavirus type 11 transcripts are present at low abundance in latently infected respiratory tissues. *Virology* 1995;212:285.
47. Meyers C, Harry J, Lin YL, et al. Identification of three transforming proteins encoded by cottontail rabbit papillomavirus. *J Virol* 1992;66:1655.
48. Brandsma JL, Yang ZH, Barthold SW, et al. Use of a rapid, efficient inoculation method to induce papillomas by cottontail rabbit papillomavirus DNA shows that the E7 gene is required. *Proc Natl Acad Sci USA* 1991;88:4816.
49. Schmitt A, Rochat A, Zeltner R, et al. The primary target cells of the high-risk cottontail rabbit papillomavirus colocalize with hair follicle stem cells. *J Virol* 1996;70:1912.
50. Iftner T, Oft M, Bohm S, et al. Transcription of the E6 and E7 genes of human papillomavirus type 6 in anogenital condylomata is restricted to undifferentiated cell layers of the epithelium. *J Virol* 1992;66:4639.
51. Stoler MH, Wolinsky SM, Whitbeck A, et al. Differentiation-linked human papillomavirus types 6 and 11 transcription in genital condylomata revealed by in situ hybridization with message-specific RNA probes. *Virology* 1989; 172:331.
52. Durst M, Glitz D, Schneider A, et al. Human papillomavirus type 16 (HPV16) gene expression and DNA replication in cervical neoplasia: analysis by in situ hybridization. *Virology* 1992;189:132.
53. Stoler MH, Rhodes CR, Whitbeck A, et al. Human papillomavirus type 16 and 18 gene expression in cervical neoplasias. *Hum Pathol* 1992;23:117.
54. Pirisi L, Yasumoto S, Feller M, et al. Transformation of human fibroblasts and keratinocytes with human papillomavirus type 16 DNA. *J Virol* 1987;61:1061.
55. Durst M, Dzarlieva-Petrusevska RT, Boukamp P, et al. Molecular and cytogenetic analysis of immortalized human primary keratinocytes obtained after transfection with human papillomavirus type 16 DNA. *Oncogene* 1987;1:251.
56. Park NH, Min BM, Li SL, et al. Immortalization of normal human oral keratinocytes with type 16 human papillomavirus. *Carcinogenesis* 1991;12:1627.
57. Band V, Zajchowski D, Kulesa V, et al. Human papillomavirus DNAs immortalize normal human mammary epithelial cells and reduce their growth factor requirements. *J Virol* 1990;87:463.
58. Kaur P, McDougall JK. Characterization of primary human keratinocytes transformed by human papillomavirus type 18. *J Virol* 1988;62:1917.
59. Schlegel R, Phelps WC, Zhang Y-L, et al. Quantitative keratinocyte assay detects two biological activities of human papillomavirus DNA and identifies viral types associated with cervical carcinoma. *EMBO J* 1988;7:3181.
60. Pecoraro G, Morgan D, Defendi V. Differential effects of human papillomavirus type 6, 16, and 18 DNAs on immortalization and transformation of human cervical epithelial cells. *Proc Natl Acad Sci USA* 1989;86:563.
61. Munger K, Phelps WC, Bubb V, et al. The E6 and E7 genes of the human papillomavirus type 16 together are necessary and sufficient for transformation of primary human keratinocytes. *J Virol* 1989;63:4417.
62. Hawley-Nelson P, Vousden KH, Hubbert NL, et al. HPV 16 E6 and E7 proteins cooperate to immortalize human foreskin keratinocytes. *EMBO J* 1989; 8:3905.
63. Hudson JB, Bedell MA, McCance DJ, et al. Immortalization and altered differentiation of human keratinocytes in vitro by the E6 and E7 open reading frames of human papillomavirus type 18. *J Virol* 1990;64:519.
64. Choo K-B, Pan C-C, Han S-H. Integration of human papillomavirus type 16 into cellular DNA of cervical carcinoma: preferential deletion of the E2 gene and invariable retention of the long control region and the E6/E7 open reading frames. *Virology* 1987;161:259.
65. Smotkin D, Wettstein FO. Transcription of human papillomavirus type 16 early genes in a cervical cancer and a cancer-derived cell line and identification of the E7 protein. *Proc Natl Acad Sci USA* 1986;83:4680.
66. Shirasawa H, Tomita Y, Kubota K, et al. Transcriptional differences of the human papillomavirus type 16 genome between precancerous lesions and invasive carcinomas. *J Virol* 1988;62:1022.
67. Schwarz E, Freese UK, Gissmann L, et al. Structure and transcription of human papillomavirus sequences in cervical carcinoma cells. *Nature* 1985; 314:111.
68. Baker CC, Phelps WC, Lindgren V, et al. Structural and transcriptional analysis of human papillomavirus type 16 sequences in cervical carcinoma cell lines. *J Virol* 1987;61:962.

69. Seedorf K, Oltersdorf T, Krammer G, et al. Identification of early proteins of the human papilloma viruses type 16 (HPV 16) and type 18 (HPV 18) in cervical carcinoma cells. *EMBO J* 1987; 6:139.
70. Androphy EJ, Hubbert NL, Schiller JT, et al. Identification of the HPV-16 E6 protein from transformed mouse cells and human cervical carcinoma cell lines. *EMBO J* 1987;6:989.
71. Smotkin D, Wettstein FO. The major human papillomavirus protein in cervical cancers is a cytoplasmic phosphoprotein. *J Virol* 1987;61:1686.
72. Dyson N, Howley PM, Munger K, et al. The human papilloma virus-16 E7 oncoprotein is able to bind to the retinoblastoma gene product. *Science* 1989; 243:934.
73. Munger K, Wetness BA, Dyson N, et al. Complex formation of human papillomavirus E7 proteins with the retinoblastoma tumor suppressor gene product. *EMBO J* 1989;8:4099.
74. Riley DJ, Lee EY HP, Lee W-H. The retinoblastoma protein: more than a tumor suppressor. *Annu Rev Cell Biol* 1994;10:1.
75. Zwerschke W, Jansen-Durr P. Cell transformation by the E7 oncoprotein of human papillomavirus type 16: interactions with nuclear and cytoplasmic target proteins. *Adv Cancer Res* 2000;78:1.
76. Arroyo M, Bagchi S, Raychaudhuri P. Association of the human papillomavirus type 16 E7 protein with the S-phase-specific E2F-cyclin A complex. *Mol Cell Biol* 1993;13:6537.
77. Dyson N, Guida P, Munger K, et al. Homologous sequences in adenovirus EIA and human papillomavirus E7 proteins mediate interaction with the same set of cellular proteins. *J Virol* 1992;66:6893.
78. Tommasino M, Adamczewski JP, Carlotti F, et al. HPV 16 E7 protein associates with the protein kinase $p33^{CDK2}$ and cyclin A. *Oncogene* 1993;8:195.
79. Martin LG, Demers GW, Galloway DA. Disruption of the G1/S transition in human papillomavirus type 16 E7-expressing human cells is associated with altered regulation of cyclin E. *J Virol* 1998;72:975.
80. Duensing S, Lee LY, Duensing A, et al. The human papillomavirus type 16 E6 and E7 oncoproteins cooperate to induce mitotic defects and genomic instability by uncoupling centrosome duplication from the cell division cycle. *Proc Natl Acad Sci USA* 2000;29:10002.
81. Vambutas A, DeVoti J, Pinn W, et al. Interaction of human papillomavirus type 11 E7 protein with TAP-1 results in the reduction of ATP-dependent peptide transport. *Clin Immunol* 2001;101:94.
82. Werness BA, Levine AJ, Howley PM. Association of human papillomavirus types 16 and 18 E6 proteins with p53. *Science* 1990;248:76.
83. Huibregtse JM, Scheffner M, Howley PM. Localization of the E6-AP regions that direct human papillomavirus E6 binding, association with p53, and ubiquitination of associated proteins. *Mol Cell Biol* 1993;13:4918.
84. Harris CC. p53: at the crossroads of molecular carcinogenesis and risk assessment. *Science* 1993;262:1980.
85. Pines J. Arresting developments in cell-cycle control. *Trends Biochem Sci* 1994; 19:143.
86. Thomas JT, Laimins LA. Human papillomavirus oncoproteins E6 and E7 independently abrogate the mitotic spindle checkpoint. *J Virol* 1998;72:1131.
87. Patel D, Huang SM, Baglia LA, et al. The E6 protein of human papillomavirus type 16 binds to and inhibits co-activation by CBP and p300. *EMBO J* 1999;18:5061.
88. Fogel S, Riou G. The early HPV 16 proteins can regulate mRNA levels of cell cycle genes in human cervical carcinoma cells by p53-independent mechanisms. *Virology* 1998;244:97.
89. Veldman T, Horikawa I, Barrett JC, et al. Transcriptional activation of the telomerase hTERT gene by human papillomavirus type 16 E6 oncoprotein. *J Virol* 2001;75:4467.
90. Glaunsinger BA, Lee SS, Thomas M, et al. Interactions of the PDZ-protein MAGI-I with adenovirus E4-ORF1 and high-risk papillomavirus E6 oncoproteins. *Oncogene* 2000;19:5270.
91. de Villiers E-M, Schneider A, Miklaw H, et al. Human papillomavirus infections in women with and without abnormal cervical cytology. *Lancet* 1987;2: 703.
92. zur Hansen H. Intracellular surveillance of persisting viral infections. Human genital cancer results from deficient cellular control of papillomavirus gene expression. *Lancet* 1987;2:489.
93. Kim MS, Shin K-H, Baek J-H, et al. HPV 16, tobacco-specific N-nitrosamine, and N-methyl-N′-nitro-N-nitrosoguanidine in oral carcinogenesis. *Cancer Res* 1993;53:4811.
94. Pecoraro G, Lee M, Morgan D, et al. Evolution of in vitro transformation and tumorigenesis of HPV 16 and HPV 18 immortalized primary cervical epithelial cells. *Am J Pathol* 1990;138:1.
95. Hurlin PJ, Kaur P, Smith PP, et al. Progression of human papillomavirus type 18-immortalized human keratinocytes to a malignant phenotype. *Proc Nod Acad Sci USA* 1991;88:570.
96. Garrett LR, Perez-Reyes N, Smith PP, et al. Interaction of HPV-18 and nitrosomethylurea in the induction of squamous cell carcinoma. *Carcinogenesis* 1993;14:329.
97. Kang MK, Park NH. Conversion of normal to malignant phenotype: telomere shortening, telomerase activation, and genomic instability during immortalization of human oral keratinocytes. *Crit Rev Oral Biol Med* 2001;12:38.
98. von Knebel Doeberitz M, Rittmuller F, Aengeneyndt F, et al. Reversible repression of papillomavirus oncogene expression in cervical carcinoma cells: consequences for the phenotype and E6-p53 and E7-pRB interactions. *J Virol* 1994;68:2811.
99. von Knebel Doeberitz M, Rittmuller C, zur Hansen H, et al. Inhibition of tumorigenicity of cervical cancer cells in nude mice by HPV E6-E7 anti-sense RNA. *Int J Cancer* 1992;51:831.
100. de Gravitt PE, Manos MM. Polymerase chain reaction-based methods for the detection of human papillomavirus DNA. In: Munoz N, Bosch FX, Shah, KV, et al., eds. *The epidemiology of human papillomavirus and cervical cancer*, Scientific publication No. 119. Lyon: International Agency for Research on Cancer, 1992:121.
101. Mounts P, Shaw KV, Kashima H. Viral etiology of juvenile and adult onset squamous papilloma of the larynx. *Proc Natl Acad Sci USA* 1982;79:5425.
102. De Villiers E-M, Gissmann L, zur Hansen H. Molecular cloning of viral DNA from human genital warts. *J Virol* 1981;40:932.
103. Gissmann L, Diehl V, Schultz-Coulon H-J, et al. Molecular cloning and characterization of human papillomavirus DNA derived from a laryngeal papilloma. *J Virol* 1982;44:393.
104. Rihkanen H, Aatonen L-M, Syrjanen SM. Human papillomavirus in laryngeal papillomas and in adjacent normal epithelium. *Clin Otolaryngol* 1993;18: 470.
105. Dickens P, Srivastava G, Loke SL, et al. Human papillomavirus 6, 11, and 16 in laryngeal papillomas. *J Pathol* 1991;165:243.
106. Pignatari S, Smith EM, Gray SD, et al. Detection of human papillomavirus infection in diseased and non-diseased sites of the respiratory tract in recurrent respiratory papillomatosis patients by DNA hybridization. *Ann Otol Rhinol Laryngol* 1992; 101:408.
107. Strong MS, Vaughan CW, Healy B, et al. Recurrent respiratory papillomatosis: management with the CO_2 laser. *Ann Otol Rhinol Laryngol* 1976;85:508.
108. Lindeberg H, Elbrond O. Laryngeal papillomas: the epidemiology in a Danish subpopulation, 1965–1984. *Clin Otolaryngol* 1990;15:125.
109. Brandsma JL, Abramson AL. Association of papillomavirus with cancers of the head and neck. *Arch Otolaryngol Head Neck Surg* 1989;115:621.
110. Rihkanen H, Peltomaa J, Syrjanen S. Prevalence of human papillomavirus (HPV) DNA in vocal cords without laryngeal papillomas. *Acta Otolaryngol (Stockh)* 1984;114:348.
111. Cook TA, Brunschwig JP, Butel JS, et al. Laryngeal papilloma: etiologic and therapeutic considerations. *Ann Otol Rhinol Laryngol* 1980;82:649.
112. Quick CA, Watts SL, Krzyzek RA, et al. Relationship between condylomata and laryngeal papillomata. Clinical and molecular virological evidence. *Ann Otol Rhinol Laryngol* 1980;89:467.
113. Shah K, Kashima H, Polk BF, et al. Rarity of cesarean delivery in cases of juvenile onset respiratory papillomatosis. *Obstet Gynecol* 1986;68:795.
114. Gissmann L. Immunologic responses to human papillomavirus infection. *Obstet Gynecol Clin North Am* 1996;23:625.
115. Frazer IH. Immunology of papillomavirus infection. *Curr Opin Immunol* 1996;8:484.
116. Connor ME, Stern PL. Loss of MHC class-I expression in cervical carcinomas. *Int J Cancer* 1990;46:1029.
117. Cromme FV, Airey J, Heemels MT, et al. Loss of transporter protein, encoded by the Tap-1 gene, is highly correlated with loss of HLA expression in cervical carcinomas. *J Exp Med* 1994;179:335.
118. Breitburd F, Ramoz N, Salmon J, et al. HLA control in the progression of human papillomavirus infections. *Semin Cancer Biol* 1996;7:359.
119. Wank R, Thomssen C. High risk of squamous cell carcinoma of the cervix for women with HLA-DQw3. *Nature* 1991;352:723.
120. Chang F, Syrjanen S, Kellokoski J, et al. Human papillomavirus (HPV) infections and their associations with oral disease. *J Oral Pathol Med* 1991;20:305.
121. Loning T, Reichart P, Staquet MJ, et al. Occurrence of papillomavirus structural antigens in oral papillomas and leukoplakias. *J Oral Pathol Med* 1984; 13:155.
122. Ward KA, Napier SS, Winter PC, et al. Detection of human papillomavirus DNA sequences in oral squamous cell papillomas by the polymerase chain reaction. *Oral Surg Oral Med Oral Pathol Oral Radiol Endod* 1995;80:63.
123. Jimenez C, Correnti M, Salma N, et al. Detection of human papillomavirus DNA in benign oral squamous epithelial lesions in Venezuela. *J Oral Pathol Med* 2001;30385.
124. Pfister H, Hettich I, Ronne U, et al. Characterization of human papillomavirus type 13 from focal epithelial hyperplasia Heck lesions. *J Virol* 1983; 47:363.
125. Beaudenon S, Praetorius F, Kremsdorf D, et al. A new type of human papillomavirus associated with oral focal epithelial hyperplasia. *J Invest Dermatol* 1987;88:130.
126. Sarkar FH, Visscher DW, Kintanar EB, et al. Sinonasal Schneiderian papillomas: human papillomavirus typing by polymerase chain reaction. *Mod Pathol* 1992;5:329.
127. Brandsma J, Abramson A, Sciubba J, et al. Papillomavirus infection of the nose. In: Steinberg BM, Brandsma JL, Taichman LB, eds. *Cancer cells 5: papillomaviruses.* Cold Spring Harbor, NY: Cold Spring Harbor Press, 1987:301.
128. Judd R, Zaki SR, Coffield LM, et al. Sinonasal papillomas and human papillomavirus: human papillomavirus 11 detected in fungiform Schneiderian papillomas by in situ hybridization and the polymerase chain reaction. *Hum Pathol* 1991;22:550.
129. Buchwald C, Franzmann M-B, Jacobsen GK, et al. Human papillomavirus (HPV) in sinonasal papillomas: a study of 78 cases using in situ hybridization and polymerase chain reaction. *Laryngoscope* 1995;105:66.
130. Fu YS, Hoover L, Franklin M, et al. Human papillomavirus identified by nucleic acid hybridization in concomitant nasal and genital papillomas. *Laryngoscope* 1992;102:1014.
131. Beck JC, McClatchey KD, Lesperance MM, et al. Presence of human papillo-

mavirus predicts recurrence of inverted papilloma. *Otolaryngol Head Neck Surg* 1995;113:49.
132. Kraft M, Simmen D, Casas R, et al. Significance of human papillomavirus in sinonasal papillomas. *J Laryngol Otol* 2001;115:709.
133. Hwang CS, Yang HS, Hong MK. Detection of human papillomavirus (HPV) in sinonasal inverted papillomas using polymerase chain reaction (PCR). *Am J Rhinol* 1998;12(5):363.
134. Ogura H, Fukushima K, Watanabe S. A high prevalence of human papillomavirus DNA in recurrent nasal papillomas. *J Med Microbiol* 1996;45(3):162.
135. Bernauer HS, Welkoborsky HJ, Tilling A, et al. Inverted papillomas of the paranasal sinuses and the nasal cavity: DNA indices and HPV infection. *Am J Rhinol* 1997;11:155.
136. Galloway TC, Soper GR, Elsen G. Carcinoma of the larynx after irradiation of papilloma. *Arch Otolaryngol Head Neck Surg* 1960;72:289.
137. Majoros M, Devine KD, Parkhill EM. Malignant transformation of benign laryngeal papillomas in children after radiation therapy. *Surg Clin North Am* 1963;43:1049.
138. Brach BB, Klein RC, Mathews AJ, et al. Papillomatosis of the respiratory tract: upper airway obstruction and carcinoma. *Arch Otolaryngol Head Neck Surg* 1978;104:413.
139. Zarod AP, Rutherford JD, Corbitt G. Malignant progression of laryngeal papilloma associated with human papilloma virus type 6 (HPV 6) DNA. *J Clin Pathol* 1988;41:280.
140. Yoder MG, Batsakis JG. Squamous cell carcinoma in solitary laryngeal papilloma. *Otolaryngol Head Neck Surg* 1980;88:745.
141. Singh B, Ramsaroop R. Clinical features of malignant transformation in benign laryngeal papillomata. *J Laryngol Otol* 1994;108:642.
142. Byrne JC, Tsao M-S, Fraser RS, et al. Human papillomavirus-11 DNA in a patient with chronic laryngotracheobronchial papillomatosis and metastatic squamous-cell carcinoma of the lung. *N Engl J Med* 1987;317:873.
143. DiLorenzo TP, Tamsen A, Abramson AL, et al. Human papillomavirus type 6a DNA in the lung carcinoma of a patient with recurrent laryngeal papillomatosis is characterized by a partial duplication. *J Gen Virol* 1992;73:423.
144. Kashima H, Wu T-C, Mounts P, et al. Carcinoma ex-papilloma: histologic and virologic studies in whole-organ sections of the larynx. *Laryngoscope* 1988;98: 619.
145. Lindeberg H, Syrjanen S, Karja J, et al. Human papillomavirus type 11 DNA in squamous cell carcinomas and pre-existing multiple laryngeal papillomas. *Acta Otolaryngol (Stockh)* 1989;107:141.
146. Rosen M, Auborn K. Duplication of the upstream regulatory sequences increases the transformation potential of human papillomavirus type 11. *Virology* 1991;185:484.
147. Brandsma JL, Steinberg BM, Abramson AL, et al. Presence of human papillomavirus type 16 related sequences in verrucous carcinoma of the larynx. *Cancer Res* 1986;46:2185.
148. Bryan RL, Bevan IS, Crocker J, et al. Detection of HPV 6 and 11 in tumours of the upper respiratory tract using the polymerase chain reaction. *Clin Otolaryngol* 1990;15:177.
149. Perez-Ayala M, Ruiz-Cabello F, Esteban F, et al. Presence of HPV 16 sequences in laryngeal carcinomas. *Int J Cancer* 1990;46:8.
150. Fliss DM, Noble-Topham SE, McLachlin M, et al. Laryngeal verrucous carcinoma: a clinicopathologic study and detection of human papillomavirus using polymerase chain reaction. *Laryngoscope* 1994;104:146.
151. Noble-Topham SE, Fliss DM, Hartwick WJ, et al. Detection and typing of human papillomavirus in verrucous carcinoma of the oral cavity using the polymerase chain reaction. *Arch Otolaryngol Head Neck Surg* 1993;119:1299.
152. Adler-Storthz K, Newland JR, et al. Human papillomavirus type 2 DNA in oral verrucous carcinoma. *J Oral Pathol Med* 1986;15:472.
153. Shibata DK, Arnheim N, Martin WJ. Detection of human papilloma virus in paraffin-embedded tissue using the polymerase chain reaction. *J Exp Med* 1988;167:225.
154. Kwok S, Higuchi R. Avoiding false positives with PCR. *Nature* 1989;339:237.
155. Beyer-Finkler E, Pfister H, Girardi F. Anti-contamination primers to improve specificity of polymerase chain reaction in human papillomavirus screening. *Lancet* 1990;335:1289.
156. Morrison EAB, Goldberg GL, Kadish AS, et al. Polymerase chain reaction detection of human papillomavirus: quantitation may improve clinical utility. *J Clin Microbiol* 1992;30:2539.
157. Brachman DG, Graves D, Vokes E, et al. Occurrence of p53 gene deletions and human papilloma virus infection in human head and neck cancer. *Cancer Res* 1992;52:4832.
158. Wilczynski SP, Lin BT, Xie Y, et al. Detection of human papillomavirus DNA and oncoprotein overexpression are associated with distinct morphological patterns of tonsillar squamous cell carcinoma. *Am J Pathol* 1998;152:145.
159. Mellin H, Friesland S, Lewensohn R, et al. Human papillomavirus (HPV) DNA in tonsillar cancer: clinical correlates, risk of relapse and survival. *Int J Cancer* 2000;89:300l
160. Ogura H, Watanabe S, Fukushima K, et al. Human papillomavirus DNA in squamous cell carcinomas of the respiratory and upper digestive tracts. *Jpn J Clin Oncol* 1993;23:221.
161. Snijders PJF, Steenbergen RDM, Top B, et al. Analysis of p53 status in tonsillar carcinomas associated with human papillomavirus. *J Gen Virol* 1994;75: 2769.
162. Brandwein M, Zeitlin J, Nuovo GJ, et al. HPV detection using "hot start" polymerase chain reaction in patients with oral cancer: a clinicopathological study of 64 patients. *Mod Pathol* 1994;7:720.
163. Snijders PJF, Cromme FV van den Brule AJC, et al. Prevalence and expression of human papillomavirus in tonsillar carcinomas, indicating a possible viral etiology. *Int J Cancer* 1992;51:845.
164. Gillison ML, Koch WM, Capone RB, et al. Evidence for a causal association between human papillomavirus and a subset of head and neck cancers. *J Natl Cancer Inst* 2000;92:709.
165. Andl T, Kahn T, Pfuhl A, et al. Etiological involvement of oncogenic human papillomavirus in tonsillar squamous cell carcinomas lacking retinoblastoma cell cycle control. *Cancer Res* 1998;58:5.
166. Hemminki K, Dong C, Frisch M. Tonsillar and other upper aerodigestive tract cancers among cervical cancer patients and their husbands. *Eur J Cancer Prev* 2000;9:433.
167. Shindoh M, Sawada Y, Kohgo T, et al. Detection of human papillomavirus DNA sequences in tongue squamous-cell carcinoma utilizing the polymerase chain reaction method. *Int J Cancer* 1992;50:167.
168. Balaram P, Nalinakumari KR, Abraham E, et al. Human papillomaviruses in 91 oral cancers from Indian betel quid chewers—high prevalence and multiplicity of infections. *Int J Cancer* 1995;61:450.
169. Chang KW, Chang CS, Lai KS, et al. High prevalence of human papillomavirus infection and possible association with betel quid chewing and smoking in oral epidermoid carcinomas in Taiwan. *J Med Virol* 1989;28:57.
170. Syrjanen S, Happonen R-P, Virolainen E, et al. Detection of human papillomavirus (HPV) structural antigens and DNA types in inverted papillomas and squamous cell carcinomas of the nasal cavities and paranasal sinuses. *Acta Otolaryngol (Stockh)* 1987;104:334.
171. Furuta Y, Takasu T, Asai T, et al. Detection of human papillomavirus DNA in carcinomas of the nasal cavities and paranasal sinuses by polymerase chain reaction. *Cancer* 1992;69:353.
172. Judd R, Zaki SR, Coffield LM, et al. Human papillomavirus type 6 detected by the polymerase chain reaction in invasive sinonasal papillary squamous cell carcinoma. *Arch Pathol Lab Med* 1991;115:1150.
173. Buchwald C, Lindeberg H, Pedersen BL, et al. Human papilloma virus and p53 expression in carcinomas associated with sinonasal papillomas: a Danish epidemiological study 1980–1998. *Laryngoscope* 2001;111:1104.
174. Hording U, Winther HW, Daugaard S, et al. Human papillomavirus types 11 and 16 detected in nasopharyngeal carcinomas by the polymerase chain reaction. *Laryngoscope* 1994;104:99.
175. Tyan Y-S, Liu S-T, Ong W-R, et al. Detection of Epstein-Barr virus and human papillomavirus in head and neck tumors. *J Clin Microbiol* 1993;31:53.
176. Rassekh CH, Rady PL, Arany I, et al. Combined Epstein-Barr virus and human papillomavirus infection in nasopharyngeal carcinoma. *Laryngoscope* 1998;108(3):362.
177. Punwaney R, Brandwein MS, Zhang DY, et al. Human papillomavirus may be common within nasopharyngeal carcinoma of Caucasian Americans: investigation of Epstein-Barr virus and human papillomavirus in eastern and western nasopharyngeal carcinoma using ligation-dependent polymerase chain reaction. *Head Neck* 1999;21:21.
178. Tung YC, Lin KH, Chu PY, et al. Detection of human papilloma virus and Epstein-Barr virus DNA in nasopharyngeal carcinoma by polymerase chain reaction. *Kaohsiung J Med Sci* 1999;15:256.
179. Salam MA, Rockett J, Morris A. General primer-mediated polymerase chain reaction for simultaneous detection and typing of human papillomavirus DNA in laryngeal squamous cell carcinomas. *Clin Otolaryngol* 1995;20:84.
180. Hoshikawa T, Nakajima T, Uhara H, et al. Detection of human papillomavirus DNA in laryngeal squamous cell carcinomas by polymerase chain reaction. *Laryngoscope* 1990;100:647.
181. Nunez DA, Astley SM, Lewis FA, et al. Human papilloma viruses: a study of their prevalence in the normal larynx. *J Laryngol Otol* 1994;108:319.
182. Cattani P, Hohaus S, Bellacosa A, et al. Association between cyclin D1 (CCND1) gene amplification and human papillomavirus infection in human laryngeal squamous cell carcinoma. *Clin Cancer Res* 1998;4:2585.
183. Venuti A, Manni V, Morello R, et al. Physical state and expression of human papillovirus in laryngeal carcinoma and surrounding normal mucosa. *J Med Virol* 2000;60:396.
184. Smith EM, Summersgill KF, Allen J, et al. Human papillomavirus and risk of laryngeal cancer. *Ann Otol Rhinol Laryngol* 2000;109:1069.
185. Gorgoulis VG, Zacharotos P, Kotsinas A, et al. Human papilloma virus (HPV) is possibly involved in laryngeal but not in lung carcinogenesis. *Hum Pathol* 1999;30:274.
186. Stremlau A, Gissmann L, Ikenberg H, et al. Human papillomavirus type 16 related DNA in an anaplastic carcinoma of the lung. *Cancer* 1985:55:1737.
187. Yousem SA, Ohori NP, Sonmez-Alpan E. Occurrence of human papillomavirus DNA in primary lung neoplasms. *Cancer* 1992;69:693.
188. Shamanin V, Delius H, de Villiers E-M. Development of a broad spectrum PCR assay for papillomaviruses and its application in screening lung cancer biopsies. *J Gen Virol* 1994;75:1149.
189. Thomas P, De Lamballerie X, Garbe L, et al. Detection of human papillomavirus DNA in primary lung carcinoma by nested polymerase chain reaction. *Cell Mol Biol* 1995;41:1093.
190. Welt A, Hummel M, Niedobitek G, et al. Human papillomavirus infection is not associated with bronchial carcinoma: evaluation by in situ hybridization and the polymerase chain reaction. *J Pathol* 1997;181:276.
191. Bohlmeyer T, Le TN, Shroyer AL, et al. Detection of human papillomavirus in squamous cell carcinomas of the lung by polymerase chain reaction. *Am J Respir Cell Mol Biol* 1998;18:265.
192. Nuorva K, Soini Y, Kamel D, et al. p53 protein accumulation and the presence

of human papillomavirus DNA in bronchiolo-alveolar carcinoma correlate with poor prognosis. *Int J Cancer* 1995;64:424.
193. Szabo I, Sepp R, Nakamoto K, et al. Human papillomavirus not found in squamous and large cell lung carcinomas by polymerase chain reaction. *Cancer* 1994;73:2740.
194. Hirayasu T, Iwamasa T, Kamada Y, et al. Human papillomavirus DNA in squamous cell carcinoma of the lung. *J Clin Pathol* 1996;49:810.
195. Li Q, Hu K, Pan X, et al. Detection of human papillomavirus types 16, 18 DNA related sequences in bronchogenic carcinoma by polymerase chain reaction. *Chin Med J (Engl)* 1995;108:610.
196. Tsuhako K, Nakazato I, Hirayasu T, et al. Human papillomavirus DNA in adenosquamous carcinoma of the lung. *J Clin Pathol* 1998;51:741.
197. Miyagi J, Tsuhako K, Kinjo T, et al. Recent striking changes in histological differentiation and rate of human papillomavirus infection in squamous cell carcinoma of the lung in Okinawa, a subtropical island in southern Japan. *J Clin Pathol* 2000;53:647.
198. Cheng YW, Chiou HL, Sheu GT, et al. The association of human papillomavirus 16/18 infection with lung cancer among nonsmoking Taiwanese women. *Cancer Res* 2001;61:2799.
199. Schwartz Sr, Yueh B, McDougall JK, et al. Human papillomavirus infection and survival in oral squamous cell cancer: a population-based study. *Otolaryngol Head Neck Surg* 2001;125:1.
200. Sisk EA, Bradford CR, Jacob A, et al. Human papillomavirus infection in "young" versus "old" patients with squamous cell carcinoma of the head and neck. *Head Neck* 2000;22:649.
201. Lindel K, Beer KT, Laissue J, et al. Human papillomavirus positive squamous cell carcinoma of the oropharynx: a radiosensitive subgroup of head and neck carcinoma. *Cancer* 2001;92:805.

CHAPTER 40

Chemoprevention of Head and Neck Cancer

Vassiliki A. Papadimitrakopoulou, Dong M. Shin, and Waun Ki Hong

Head and neck epithelial carcinogenesis is a process characterized by the progressive accumulation of genetic and phenotypic damage to carcinogen-exposed tissues that ultimately results in the development of invasive head and neck cancer. Head and neck squamous cell carcinomas (HNSCCs) are a substantial public health problem worldwide (1). Despite the curability of early-stage disease with surgery and/or radiation therapy, the majority of patients present with advanced disease. Survival in the setting of advanced HNSCC has improved little in the last two decades, although increasingly sophisticated combined modality approaches have been explored (2). Interfering with the carcinogenic process early before the establishment of invasive cancer could therefore represent a promising approach to reducing the incidence and mortality of this disease. In fact, head and neck tumorigenesis was one of the first settings in which seminal chemoprevention trials were performed.

Chemoprevention is the administration of agents to block or reverse carcinogenesis (3). Chemoprevention in head and neck cancer has been directed toward the reversal of premalignant lesions in a group of patients with risk factors such as tobacco exposure and toward the prevention of second primary tumors (SPTs), which represent the major threat to patients whose initial early-stage head and neck cancers are cured (4–7). The biologic concepts of chemoprevention stem from an understanding of the multistep nature of head and neck epithelial carcinogenesis and of field cancerization, whereby diffuse epithelial injury from carcinogen exposure results in the development of multiple premalignant and malignant lesions and an increased risk for SPTs within the upper aerodigestive tract. A large body of research has accumulated over the last 10 years as a result of clinical chemoprevention trials conducted in an effort to define the biology underlying the tumorigenesis process in the upper aerodigestive tract. Consequently, several of the critical specific cellular and molecular events in this multistep process have been identified.

The chemoprevention strategies used in initial and more recent clinical trials have involved retinoids chosen for their important anticarcinogenic and differentiating properties (8), and substantial progress has been made in defining their activities. Newer agents targeting specifically prevalent tumorigenic pathways have been developed over the last 3 years, and several clinical trials are in progress. The dynamic interplay between environmental and genetic factors in tumorigenesis and the mechanisms of action of chemopreventive agents are also important areas of current study. Advances in molecular biology, epidemiology, and genetics; their integration in clinical chemoprevention studies; and the new directions in research in this field are described in this chapter.

BIOLOGY

Head and Neck Tumorigenesis: Basic Concepts

Understanding the biologic processes that drive carcinogenesis is necessary for the rational development of chemoprevention approaches in head and neck cancer. The evolving concepts of field cancerization and multistep carcinogenesis have guided basic research in a translational setting associated with clinical chemoprevention studies. Field cancerization is the diffuse epithelial injury that results from exposure to mostly inhaled carcinogens, and places the entire anatomic field at risk for development of cancer (9). Abundant clinical, histologic, and molecular evidence supports this concept, including the occurrence of premalignant lesions and multiple primary tumors within the exposed field (10).

The theory of multistep carcinogenesis (11) states that the clonal evolution of neoplasia is associated with multiple types of genetic changes or events that occur early in the neoplastic process and drive it, and that these changes continue to accumulate as the progression to invasive cancer continues. Thus, continuing carcinogenic exposure, in conjunction with exogenous (e.g., viral) and endogenous factors, leads to a critical accumulation of genetic changes that are permanent and functionally important (e.g., confer resistance to apoptosis and a survival advantage) and that may lead to aberrant clonal outgrowth throughout the field. These genetic changes are thought to result in dysfunctional processes, which reflect on cell growth, function, and differentiation, and in phenotypic changes that appear in histologic studies as a progression from hyperplasia to dysplasia to invasive cancer with metastatic potential. The concept is illustrated clinically by the presence of premalignant lesions (e.g., leukoplakia and erythroplakia) that often precede, but are not necessarily the precursors of, oral squamous cell carcinomas (SCCs) (12–15). These lesions occur in up to 30% of oral SCCs, harbor histologic features of hyperplasia and dysplasia, have a malignant transformation rate of 17.5% at 8 years, with the risk increasing to 36% for dysplastic lesions (16).

Progress in molecular biology has made possible the identification of key genotypic alterations that lead to the development of malignant clones and of molecular markers of specific stages in multistep carcinogenesis. Such identification may be useful for establishing valid intermediate end points for chemoprevention trials.

Biomarkers

The concept of using biomarkers as intermediate end points for risk and efficacy assessment is closely linked to both basic science research and to the design and development of clinical chemoprevention trials. The definitive end point of these trials is the demonstration of a decrease in cancer incidence. However, this requires years of study of thousands of patients, which makes these trials very expensive and limits both the number of chemopreventive agents that can be tested and the determination of their proper doses and schedules (17). The use of phenotypic and genotypic changes that accurately reflect the tumorigenesis process could overcome these problems of current clinical trials by significantly diminishing study duration, numbers of patients needed, and cost (18–20). Efforts in chemoprevention research have consequently concentrated on development and validation of biomarkers that (a) can identify high-risk individuals who would be more likely to benefit from clinical intervention, and (b) provide an assessment of the mechanism and efficacy of the intervention. Obviously, the study of biomarkers provides the opportunity simultaneously to make valuable insights into the mechanisms and biology of head and neck tumorigenesis (21–23) and to identify of tumorigenic pathways that could become specific targets for chemopreventive intervention.

Biologic Basis of Chemoprevention

Characterization of the events underlying head and neck tumorigenesis has been tied to translational research in the setting of chemoprevention trials. As a result of intensive research and the use of several new molecular biology techniques, a panel of general and more specific genotypic and phenotypic alterations has emerged (Table 40.1), and we are now beginning to unravel the prognostic significance of these alterations *in vivo*.

TABLE 40.1 Candidate Biomarkers of Head and Neck Tumorigenesis

Genetic damage or instability
Chromosomal number changes / ∝ neuploidy
Specific genotypic markers
Proto-oncogenes
ErbB1/EGrR
Cyclin D1
Tumor suppressor genes
p53
p16
3p (unidentified)
PTEN
Proliferation markers (PCNA, Ki67)
Nuclear retinoid receptors (RARs and RXRs)
Genetic susceptibility markers
Gene promoter methylation

PCNA, proliferating cell nuclear antigen; RARs, retinoic acid receptors; RXRs, retinoid X receptors.

Genetic Susceptibility

The main genotypic alteration of interest is genetic predisposition. The interaction between genetic predisposition and lifetime carcinogen exposure (as in the case of head and neck cancer due to tobacco and alcohol use) exposure results in markedly different risks of cancer development among individuals. The rate of accumulation of genetic damage reflects the interaction between cells and carcinogens and the cells' capacity to repair DNA damage (24). One of the methods developed to assess an individual's genetic sensitivity to environmental carcinogens is the mutagen sensitivity assay (25,26), which quantifies bleomycin-induced breaks in lymphocytes. Two studies have found mutagen sensitivity (defined as >0.8 chromosomal break per cell after *in vitro* exposure to bleomycin) to be a significant independent risk factor for cancer of the head and neck and found that smoking and mutagen sensitivity together increase the risk for such cancer (27,28).

Studies of mutagen sensitivity with benzo[*a*]pyrene diol epoxide (BPDE), the most etiologically appropriate mutagen for smoking-induced cancers, have suggested that a high rate of BPDE-induced chromatid breaks per cell in lymphocytes is an independent risk factor for HNSCC (29). Moreover, subjects with sensitivity to both BPDE and bleomycin have a 19.2-fold increased risk for cancer compared with those not sensitive to either agent (30). Studies concentrating on the role of independent genes in susceptibility to tobacco-related cancers have suggested that low expression of *hMLH1* and *hGTBP/hMSH6* (31) and the *XPC-PAT+* allele (32), both implicated in DNA repair capacity, are associated with an increased risk for head and neck cancer.

In addition to the findings in primary HNSCC, two studies in patients with head and neck cancer demonstrated that mutagen hypersensitivity (>1.0 break per cell) was associated with a higher relative risk for developing a second primary tumor (33) and that a higher mean number of chromatid breaks are seen in patients who develop second primaries compared with those who do not (33,34).

Further molecular epidemiology studies of specific genes and polymorphisms may identify those that are associated with an inherent susceptibility to head and neck cancer.

Genotypic Changes

The development of technologies for analyzing genes and gene products from even minute amounts of human tissue has found a number of genetic alterations. Genetic alterations are semantically divided into general and specific. One established measure of general carcinogen-induced genetic damage by micronuclei is frequency (35). Micronuclei are chromosomal or chromatid fragments formed during cell division by chromosome nondisjunction as a result of carcinogen-induced DNA damage; they can be detected in exfoliated epithelial cells. Micronuclei frequency has been shown to correlate with target-tissue cancer risk in smokers and was effectively decreased by retinoids in prevention studies, although not consistently in association with clinical response (36–39).

Another measure of accumulated genetic damage or instability and ongoing genetic damage during the multistep head and neck carcinogenesis process is chromosome polysomy (i.e., the presence of three or more copies of a chromosome per cell). *In situ* hybridization (ISH), using DNA probes that recognize single-copy genes or specific sequences or chromosome segments, has detected chromosome polysomy in head and neck cancers and premalignant lesions. Used to explore the nature of genetic damage and genetic instability in the epithelial field exposed to carcinogen, chromosome ISH has provided evidence that genetic instability increases with histologic progression from normal epithelium to tumor and that it is a risk factor for eventual malignant transformation of oral premalignant lesions (40,41) and laryngeal premalignant lesions (42). One recent study confirmed the strong predictive role of aneuploidy as a risk factor for malignant transformation in a large patient sample (43).

Another technique used to detect structural chromosomal alterations, deletions, and amplifications is comparative genomic hybridization (CGH). The genetic abnormalities are seen as changes in the ratio of two fluorochromes along target chromosomes of differentially labeled tumor DNA and normal DNA by simultaneous hybridization with normal metaphase spreads (44). Several studies have found deletions in chromosomes 3p, 5q, and 19 and high-level amplification of chromosomes 3q26 and 11q13 (45,46). An evolution of the CGH technique is the application of array technology to CGH, either by hybridizing DNA to complementary DNA (cDNA) arrays or by creating microarrays using genomic sequences from bacterial artificial chromosome (BAC) clones. This has greatly improved the resolution and throughput of the technique greatly (47). Large-scale studies in head and neck cancer and premalignant lesions are now possible using this new technology.

Traditional cytogenetics have revealed several consistent alterations in short-term tumor cultures, including losses on chromosomes 3p, 5q, 8p, 9p, 18q, and 21q; amplification of chromosomes 3q, 5p, 7p, 8q, and 11q13; and break points at lp36, 3q21, 5p14, 7p13, 9q32, and 1q13 (48–51).

Techniques based on the polymerase chain reaction (PCR) allow specific analysis of DNA from minute specimens and the identification of allelic losses or deletions leading to the inactivation of tumor suppressor genes. The discovery of microsatellite markers (small, highly polymorphic DNA repeat units that occur throughout the human genome) has greatly facilitated the allelotyping of tumors. Allelotypes of HNSCCs have been established using a large panel of microsatellite markers analyzed after PCR amplification (52–54). Allelic losses were found mainly on chromosomes 3, 4, 5, 6, 8, 9, 11, 13, 17, and 19. The most frequently encountered regions of loss of heterozygosity (LOH) are chromosomes 3p, 5q, 9p, 11q, 13q, and 17p.

Polymerase chain reaction analysis of microdissected epithelium and ISH, which allows visualization of specific chromosomal changes directly on whole cells and tissue sections, have contributed greatly to the understanding of the genetic events associated with head and neck tumorigenesis. The concept of genetic instability as a driving force behind the multistep tumorigenesis process has evolved through a number of these studies. This concept includes generalized genomic instability as manifested in the polysomy frequency observed throughout the tissue field and the clonal outgrowth of cell populations with specific, functionally important gene alterations. Advances in cDNA microarray analysis have already revealed differences in genomic and transcriptional profiles between tumor types and have been used to identify subsets in morphologically homogeneous tumors (55,56). It is hoped that in the near future unique tumor fingerprints will be available, and this technology will be even further useful in identifying unique profiles of premalignant lesions at increased risk for cancer development. Proteomic analysis (57) will also be potentially useful in identifying the critical proteins or network of proteins necessary and sufficient for cancer development and could help guide the way to more rational and targeted approaches.

Knowledge of the specific genetic events and their timing during the tumorigenesis process will enable researchers to better characterize the carcinogenic risk for any individual lesion and the field that accompanies it, based on the number and type of genetic alterations present. A brief description of specific genetic alterations involving both oncogenes and tumor suppressor genes follows.

ONCOGENES

Epidermal Growth Factor Receptor

The epidermal growth factor receptor (EGFR), a transmembrane glycosylated phosphoprotein with tyrosine kinase activity, binds and mediates signal transduction for both epidermal growth factor (EGF) and transforming growth factor-α (TGF-α) in one of the most important pathways for cancer development identified to date (58). The epidermal growth factor receptor regulates cell growth in cell lines and in a variety of human tumors, where its overexpression in transfected cells results in transforming potential (59). Gene amplification and overexpression of EGFR through autocrine pathways (60,61) are frequently observed in HNSCCs and their cell lines (62–65).

Transforming growth factor-α, an EGFR ligand, is also up-regulated in HNSCC (66,67). Epidermal growth factor receptor messenger RNA (mRNA) and protein up-regulation cannot be accounted for by gene dosage alone (62), but rather is due to activated gene transcription, which can be modulated by retinoic acid treatment (61).

Epidermal growth factor receptor overexpression has been associated with shorter relapse-free intervals and overall survival in patients with HNSCC (68–70). Elevated EGFR has been associated with larger tumor size, advanced stage, and worse prognosis (60). Expression of TGF-α and EGFR in primary tumors also appears to be significantly associated with decreased disease-specific survival, independent of cervical lymph node metastasis, thus emphasizing the biologic importance of this autocrine growth pathway in HNSCC progression (71).

Our group (72) and others (73,74) have examined the changes in EGFR expression and their correlation with growth regulation during earlier steps in the multistep tumorigenesis process. It has been demonstrated that TGF-α and EGFR mRNA and protein levels are up-regulated in histologically normal mucosa specimens from patients with HNSCC compared with normal control mucosa from patients without HNSCC. This suggests in turn that activation of TGF-α/EGFR gene transcription is an early event in HNSCC carcinogenesis.

These findings suggest that alterations in growth factor signal transduction, as expressed through elevation of both TGF-α and EGFR mRNA levels in histologically normal but carcinogen-exposed "condemned" mucosa, contribute to proliferative dysregulation early in the carcinogenic process. This may indicate points at which early intervention may block the process. Epidermal growth factor receptor blockade as anticancer therapy has been increasingly explored over the last decade using monoclonal antibodies and small-molecule EGFR tyrosine kinase inhibitors (TKIs) (75). This has led to the recent development of chemoprevention studies with the EGFR TKIs.

Cyclin D1

Amplification of the chromosome 11q13 region is a frequent genetic alteration in several malignancies (76). Cytogenetic analysis of HNSCCs has identified frequent abnormalities in this region, including rearrangements and regions of homogeneous staining that imply amplification (51). Although a number of genes lie in this amplified region of the genome (*INT2, HST1, GST-π, bcl*-1 [locus], cyclin D1, and *EMS1*), the most important molecular target and a possible driving force behind this amplification appears to be the cyclin Dl gene (77,78). The cyclin D1 gene has been implicated in the pathogenesis of parathyroid adenomas and centrocytic lymphomas by flanking reciprocal chromosomal translocation (79) and in a variety of solid tumors, including head and neck carcinomas, by gene amplification (80).

Cyclin D1 plays a central role in the G_1-S transition by contributing to phosphorylation and inactivation of the *Rb* gene product, thereby releasing E2F, which drives transcription of downstream targets. The latter process is negatively regulated by the cdk4/6 inhibitor *p16* (81,82). Concomitant abnormalities of cyclin D1 and *p16* in human cancer cell lines suggest that these two genes may cooperate in the carcinogenic process (83). When the third member of this cell-cycle regulating pathway, *pRb*, is inactivated, affected cells no longer require cyclin D1 for progression through the cell cycle (84,85). Cells that overexpress cyclin D1 have abnormal proliferative characteristics including a shortened G_1 phase and less dependence on growth factors (86). Transfection studies have demonstrated that *PRAD1* (or cyclin D1) may function as a cooperating oncogene in the malignant transformation of cells (87,88). Approximately 30% to 50% of primary HNSCCs manifest *PRAD1* amplification (89,90), which has been correlated with high histologic grade and infiltrative growth pattern, high proliferative activity (89), advanced local invasion and tumor stage (90), and lymph node involvement (91,92). Overexpression of cyclin D1 has been associated with more rapid and more frequent recurrences of HNSCC and shortened disease-free and overall survival times (93) and has emerged as a significant independent prognostic factor in laryngeal cancer (94). Gene amplification and protein overexpression have now been described in earlier stages of the head and neck carcinogenic process (95,96). The underlying mechanism for the protein overexpression has been investigated. One possible mechanism appears to be the presence of a AA or AG genotype based on a common polymorphism A/G at codon 242 of the cyclin D1 gene that results in a spliced protein with altered (slower) turnover (97). The presence of these polymorphisms appears to hinder this process. Retinoid-dependent cyclin D1 proteolysis has been suggested as a candidate intermediate marker for effective retinoid chemoprevention (98). Cyclin D1 overexpression has been identified as an adverse prognostic factor for malignant transformation in oral and laryngeal premalignant lesions (96,99). Thus, cyclin D1 overexpression may serve not only as a biomarker of risk but also as a potential target of future chemopreventive interventions.

Other Oncogenes

***Ras*.** The *ras* protooncogene products are membrane-associated, guanine nucleotide-binding proteins that serve as molecular switches for signal transduction pathways. Genes of the ras family, which includes H-*ras*, K-*ras*, and N-*ras*, and mutated (mainly at codons 12, 13, or 61) in 10% to 15% of all human cancers (100), notably in pancreatic and lung adenocarcinomas (101), and often in smokers. However, few ras mutations have been identified in head and neck cancers in Caucasians (102–104). Saranath et al. (105) observed frequent mutations of H-*ras* in an Indian population, possibly reflecting an underlying betel-nut chewing habit in this population as confirmed in other studies (106) or a genetic predisposition. Alternatively, overexpression of even normal ras alleles might contribute to malignant transformation. In one study, overexpression of H-*ras*, K-*ras*, and N-*ras* was identified in 86%, 78%, and 57%, of SCCs of the larynx respectively (107).

bcl-2. The *bcl*-2 gene product is the prototype of a number of oncogenes that inhibit apoptosis and provide a selective growth advantage in many tumor types (108,109). *bcl*-2 is expressed in bone marrow progenitor cells, in epithelial stem cells in the intestine and skin, and in hormonally responsive epithelium but characteristically absent from terminally differentiated cells, which suggests that apoptosis is actively suppressed in proliferating cells (110). Consequently, persistence of *bcl*-2 expression in epithelial cells may be a mechanism for abnormal accumulation (an oncogenic effect) and for survival of stem cells.

Studies of *bcl*-2 expression in head and neck tumors (111,112) found that the rate of *bcl*-2–positive tumors is around 20%, and found a statistically significant association between *bcl*-2 expression and failure of primary radiation therapy treatment in patients with early-stage head and neck cancer (111). In addition, *bcl*-2 protein expression has been associated with higher risk for recurrence and shorter survival time, contrary to the findings in lung cancer (113). It has been hypothesized that early activation of *bcl*-2 during carcinogenesis may result in prolonged survival of cells, leading to tumors resistant to apoptosis-induced cytotoxicity (111). No studies to date have identified early alterations of either *ras* or *bcl*-2 in head and neck tumorigenesis. Therefore, their role in premalignancy is unclear.

Tumor Suppressor Genes

As for head and neck cancers, allelotyping of premalignant lesions in the head and neck has revealed that alterations in multiple loci occur early in the carcinogenic process (114–117). Loss of heterozygosity (LOH) at 3p and 9p in particular is not only frequent in premalignant lesions but also a predictor of progression to invasive cancer (114,118,119). Moreover, detection of LOH has genetically confirmed the concept of field cancerization through identification of clonally related transformed cells in large areas of mucosa (115) and coincided with toluidine blue staining of oral lesions (OraTest; Zila, Phoenix, Az.), suggesting the potential use of the OraTest to detect cancer or establish the malignant transformation potential of premalignant lesions (120). Loss of heterozygosity at certain of these loci usually implicates tumor suppressor genes. We will deal separately with the most commonly identified alterations of such genes.

p53. The consistent identification of 17p loss in head and neck cancers suggests a localized event at the p53 locus, consistent with previous estimates of p53 mutations in many cases of HNSCC. Of all the specific genetic abnormalities identified to date in premalignant lesions and head and neck cancers, alterations in the *p53* gene are among the most common and best studied. The gene encodes a nuclear protein with transcription factor activity that is a necessary component of the G1-S transition checkpoint, thus contributing to cell cycle control, DNA repair and synthesis, and genomic integrity (121,122). The wild-type p53 protein can induce either programmed cell death or growth arrest at the Gl phase of the cell cycle. p53 alterations impair the cell's ability to repair and undergo apoptosis in response to DNA damage and thus lead to genomic instability.

Many types of alterations (i.e., rearrangements, deletions, insertions, or point mutations) have been observed in a wide variety of cell lines and tumors, the most frequent being point mutations confined primarily to exons 5 to 8. The pattern of *p53* mutations in patients with head and neck cancer correlates strongly with cigarette smoking (33%) or smoking in combination with alcohol use (58%) and with a prevalence of particular types of mutation at nonendogenous sites (123). Several investigators have demonstrated that *p53* inactivation occurs frequently in HNSCCs (124–127). *p53* alterations of various degrees and frequencies have been identified in preinvasive tissue surrounding malignant tissue (128–131). The demonstration that *p53* alterations increase following the histologic progression of premalignant lesions to cancer (131) and the identification of distinct *p53* mutations in tumor-distant epithelia (132) suggest that *p53* is a useful molecular marker of the field wide and multifocal nature of the head and neck carcinogenic process. Use of *p53* as a molecular marker has suggested that multiple primary head and neck tumors originate independently (133) and that distinct *p53* alterations may help to differentiate between an SPT and primary tumor recurrence or metastasis (134,135). Microsatellite analysis of chromosomes 9p, 3p, 17p, 8p, 13q, and 18q and mutation analysis of *p53* have shown that genetically altered mucosa still remains after treatment in a significant proportion of HNSCC patients, a finding with potentially significant implications for the management of patients (136). These findings confirmed earlier feasibility studies of *p53* alterations as a tool for molecular staging and fingerprinting of head and neck tumors. In those studies, identical clonal tumor cells were identified in 52% (13/25) of surgical margins and 21% (6/28) of nodes that were negative by standard light microscopy, and their presence predicted recurrence (137).

Along the same lines, we have shown that *p53* overexpression in initial head and neck tumors is a marker for increased incidence of SPTs and recurrence of primary tumors (138). In chemoprevention studies with retinoids, we have shown that p53 overexpression, high levels of chromosome polysomy, and lack of RAR-β up-regulation are predictors of retinoid resistance (139).

p16. One of the most frequent findings during allelotyping of head and neck cancer is LOH on chromosome 9p2l-22 (52,53,116), which is the locus of the recently identified tumor suppressor gene *p16*/MTS1/CDKN2 (140,141). This gene encodes for a cell-cycle regulator protein, p16, which controls cell proliferation by binding to cdk4 and inhibiting the interaction of the cyclin D1–cdk4 complex with pRb (81,82). Point mutations of p16 have been linked to neoplastic progression in several human systems. Systematic study, however, has found p16 point mutations only rarely in primary cancers of the head and neck exhibiting LOH at 9p, which suggests a different mechanism for p16 inactivation or the involvement of a different suppressor gene on 9p2l-22 in these cancers (142,143). Indeed, methylation of the gene promoter (142,144) and homozygous deletions (145,146) are the most frequent mechanisms for inactivating p16 in HNSCC. Loss of p16 expression occurs early in the oral premalignancy stage (147). Cyclin D1 amplification and overexpression often occur concomitantly with p16 loss in HNSCC, suggesting the cooperation of these two events in G1-S progression and tumorigenesis (148).

The 3p chromosomal region harbors several candidate tumor suppressor genes in three distinct juxtaposed hot spots (149–152). One of these, the fragile histidine triad (*FHIT*) gene, is altered at the DNA, RNA, and protein level in a subset of HNSCCs (153). As mentioned above, LOH at 3p is a frequent event in premalignant lesions (114,115).

Loss of chromosome 5q involves the *APC/MCC* region (5q21), which is involved in colorectal carcinoma, esophageal cancer, and breast cancer (154,155), but it has not yet been associated with head and neck cancer (156). Similarly, 13q loss occurs in 50% of HNSCC, but few of these tumors exhibit *Rb* inactivation (157).

PTEN. PTEN is one of the most frequently mutated tumor suppressors in human cancer. It functions primarily as a lipid phosphatase to regulate crucial signal transduction pathways and has as a key target phosphatidylinositol 3,4,5-triphosphate (158–160). Phosphatidylinositol 3-kinase (PI3K) phosphorylates and the PTEN product dephosphorylates the same 3′ site in the inositol ring of membrane phosphatidylinositols. PTEN functions in the regulation of many normal cell processes, including growth, adhesion, migration, invasion, and apoptosis. Abnormalities of PTEN on 10q23.3 have been identified at the gene (161) or protein level (162) in 20% to 70% of tumors studied.

Epigenetic Changes

An important mechanism for gene transcriptional inactivation is hypermethylation at the cytidine phosphate guanosine (CpG) islands within the promoter regions (163). This mechanism has been investigated in HNSCC. In one study, (164) promoter hypermethylation in at least one of four genes studied [*p16*, O^6-methylguanine-DNA-methyltransferase, death-associated protein (DAP) kinase, and glutathione S-transferase P1] was hypermethylated in 55% of the head and neck tumors examined; a statistically significant correlation was made between the presence of DAP-kinase gene promoter hypermethylation and lymph node involvement and advanced disease stage. Moreover, this study provided evidence that the methylation patterns found in tumors could be used as molecular markers for cancer in paired serum DNA samples, because almost half of the HNSCC patients with methylated tumors showed these changes in their paired samples. Studies by our own group (165) have confirmed methylation in the promoter region of genes critical for head and neck tumorigenesis, such as *p16* in premalignant lesions.

Phenotypic Changes

Because abnormal proliferation is considered a hallmark of tumorigenesis, a number of proliferative markers have been studied in tumors and premalignant epithelia of the head and neck. Proliferating cell nuclear antigen (PCNA) is an essential accessory factor to the δ-polymerase that is required both for leading-strand DNA replication and for DNA repair (166,167). Shin et al. (168) elucidated the multistep process of proliferative dysregulation by PCNA immunostaining of HNSCC specimens containing adjacent premalignant lesions. Proliferating cell nuclear antigen expression increased as tissue progressed from normal epithelium adjacent to tumor through premalignant lesions to cancer. Because PCNA is also a component of a DNA repair pathway that might be active in smoking-exposed epithelia (169), other tissue markers of proliferative status such as Ki67 have been developed (170).

CHEMOPREVENTION AGENTS—RATIONALE

Retinoids

BIOLOGY OF RETINOIDS

Mechanisms of Action

Animal, biochemical, epidemiologic, and clinical studies have shown that retinoids, a group of naturally occurring and synthetic analogs of vitamin A, play a role in preventing the development of tobacco-related epithelial malignancies. The rationale for using retinoids in cancer prevention is based on the knowledge that these compounds are critical regulators of numerous physiologic developmental and morphogenic processes (171) and that they exert regulatory control over cellular differentiation and proliferation in essentially all normal epithelial tissues. The antiproliferative and differentiation-inducing activity of retinoids has been demonstrated in a broad range of transformed cell types (172,173). A major physiologic function of vitamin A is to prevent abnormal squamous differentiation of epithelial cells in nonkeratinizing tissues (174).

Retinoids have been shown to suppress carcinogenesis in various epithelial tissues, including skin, bladder, oral cavity, lung, and mammary gland, in experimental animal model systems (175–177). A retinol-deficient diet has long been associated with an increased incidence of preneoplastic lesions; exogenous supplementation of retinol has been shown to reverse preneoplastic lesions in vitamin A–deficient animals (175,178). Furthermore, retinoids exert modulatory effects on dysplastic and neoplastic cell growth differentiation and apoptosis (177,179,180). In clinical trials, their chemopreventive efficacy has been shown in patients with cervical dysplasia, bronchial metaplasia, actinic keratosis, oral leukoplakia, and SPTs of the aerodigestive tract and in xeroderma pigmentosum patients with skin cancer (181–184).

Retinoic Acid Receptors

The discovery that retinoid control of gene transcription is a receptor-mediated event laid the framework for elucidation of the retinoid signaling pathway and for identification of nuclear retinoid receptors (185–188). After ligand transactivation, retinoid receptors form homodimers or heterodimers that bind to specific DNA sequences known as *response elements* in the promoter region of genes (including growth factors, cell regulatory kinases, oncogenes, and tumor suppressor genes). Two subfamilies of retinoid receptors have been identified, the RARs and the RXRs. Each subfamily has three subtypes designated α, β, and γ.

The physiology of retinoids is thought to overlap that of many other regulatory molecules. Of particular note is the ability of RXR molecules to form heterodimers with vitamin D or thyroid hormone receptor. Each retinoid receptor subtype controls a series of overlapping and unique target genes, and differences in tissue distribution and identification of RXR-specific target genes as well as transactivating domains suggest distinct roles for retinoid receptors in transduction of retinoid responses (188). In addition, other retinoid pathways might exist. For instance, fenretinide, a synthetic active retinoid, does not bind to either receptor class (189). The discovery of molecular lesions in the *RAR-α* gene in human promyelocytic leukemia (190), in the *RAR-γ* gene in teratocarcinoma (191), and in the *RAR-β* gene in oral carcinogenesis (192) provided further linked retinoid deficiency with carcinogen susceptibility. Studies of the expression patterns of retinoid receptors in normal, premalignant, and malignant tissues provide important clues for their roles in cancer development and the tissue response to retinoids. Loss of *RAR-β* expression may play a major role in aerodigestive tract carcinogenesis (192–194). The *RAR-β* gene is located on chromosome 3p24, close to a region that often is deleted in head and neck cancer. Even though no deletions or mutations of the gene have been identified, there is now evidence that gene promoter methylation is a mechanism of its inactivation (195). *In situ* mRNA hybridization analysis of RARs and RXRs on tissue specimens from seven normal volunteers and 31 patients with HNSCC (the latter selected for the presence of sequential progression from premalignant lesions to hyperplasia to tumor) revealed loss of *RAR-β* mRNA in 30% of adjacent normal and hyperplastic lesions, in 44% of dysplastic lesions, and in 65% of carcinomas. These observations were extended in a study of *RAR-β* expression in premalignant oral lesions in patients without cancer enrolled in a chemoprevention trial of isotretinoin (196). *RAR-β* was detected in only 21 (40%) of 52 oral leukoplakia specimens, but in all normal tissue specimens. Treatment with isotretinoin restored *RAR-β* expression to 90% of the lesions. Levels of *RAR-β* mRNA increased in tissue specimens from 18 of 22 responders and in specimens from 8 of 17 nonresponders. This association of restored *RAR-β* expression with clinical response indicates that *RAR-β* may mediate the response to retinoids and that it may be a very useful intermediate biomarker for chemoprevention studies in oral carcinogenesis (192).

RETINOIDS AND RETINAMIDES

Until recently, only four retinoids had undergone substantial clinical investigations: vitamin A (retinol) and its esters all-*trans*-retinoic acid, 13-*cis*-retinoic acid (isotretinoin, 13-cRA), and etretinate (an aromatic ethyl ester derivative of retinoic acid) (Table 40.2). The best-studied retinoid agent is 13-cRA, which has clinical activity against oral leukoplakia and in the prevention of SPTs in patients with head and neck cancer (181,182). Another class of retinoids used in prevention trials is the retinamides. One example is *N*-(4-hydroxyphenyl)-retinamide (4-HPR or fenretinide). Fenretinide has received considerable interest as a potential chemopreventive agent. It has demonstrated activity against mammary gland and urinary bladder tumors chemically induced in animal models (176,197). Although studies in animal models of lung carcinogenesis have produced conflicting results (198,199), the favorable toxicity profile of fenretinide has prompted further study. The agent has also demonstrated efficacy in oral premalignancy studies. Detailed results are analyzed later in this chapter (see Clinical Studies).

Carotenoids

The most studied carotenoid agent is β-carotene. The initial use of β-carotene as a chemopreventive agent was based on epidemiologic data, mostly related to lung cancer, that suggested an independent protective effect for the unconverted carotene fraction (200–202). On the basis of these observations as well as its low toxicity, β-carotene was entered immediately into phase II and III trials. As is analyzed later in this chapter (see Clinical Studies), β-carotene has shown activity in oral premalignancy, although there is compelling evidence that 13-cRA in a randomized setting is a superior treatment of oral leukoplakia (196). This fact, along with the negative results of three large important randomized trials in lung, colon, and skin carcinogenesis (203–205), has halted the development of β-carotene as a chemopreventive agent in head and neck cancer.

TABLE 40.2 Selected Nonrandomized Chemoprevention Trials in Oral Premalignancy

Study	Agent	No. of patients	Clinical response (%)
Wolf, 1957 (238)	Vitamin A	20	90
Silverman et al., 1963 (258)	Vitamin A	16	44
Silverman et al., 1965 (239)	Vitamin A	6	83
Ryssel et al., 1971 (259)	β-All-*trans*-retinoic acid	10	70
Stuttgen, 1975 (260)	β-All-*trans*-retinoic acid	8	100
Raque et al., 1975 (261)	β-All-*trans*-retinoic acid	5	100
Koch, 1978, 1981 (240,262)	β-All-*trans*-retinoic acid	27	59
	13-*cis*-retinoic acid	24	87
	Etretinate	24	92
	Etretinate (oral and topical)	24	83
	Etretinate	21	71
Cordero et al., 1981 (263)	Etretinate	3	100
Shah et al., 1983 (264)	13-*cis*-retinoic acid	11	100
Stich et al., 1988 (37)	β-Carotene	27	15
	β-Carotene and vitamin A	51	28
	Placebo	33	3
Garewal et al., 1990 (249)	β-Carotene	24	71
Toma et al., 1992 (251)	β-Carotene	24	27
	Selenium	25	33
Malaker et al., 1991 (250)	β-Carotene	18	44
Benner et al., 1993 (253)	α-Tocopherol	43	46
Kaugars et al., 1994 (254)	β-Carotene, vitamins E and C	79	57
Armstrong et al., 2000 (257)	Bowman-Birk inhibitor concentrate	32	31

Vitamin E

Vitamin E is important in enzymatic activation of hematopoiesis, drug metabolism, and pollutant detoxification. That it has anticarcinogenic activity has been suggested by epidemiologic and laboratory studies (206). When applied topically, it effectively reduces oral cancer progression in a hamster buccal pouch model (207). Antioxidant activity has been postulated as its main mechanism of action (208).

Retinoid Toxicity and Amelioration

The major toxicities observed with high-dose 13-cRA therapy include skin dryness, cheilitis, hypertriglyceridemia, and conjunctivitis. These toxic effects often required dose reduction or temporary discontinuation of therapy in prior chemoprevention trials. The addition of agents to ameliorate retinoid-induced side effects, allowing delivery of full-dose treatment and optimizing patient compliance, might enhance the preventive effects of retinoids. Retinoid toxicity in patients with myelodysplasia was ameliorated with the addition of α-tocopherol (209), a finding confirmed in a trial of combined high-dose 13-cRA and α-tocopherol in a mixed population of patients with head and neck, skin, or lung cancer, and in patients with premalignant lesions (210). In addition, the two agents have a demonstrated synergy, providing further support for the combination of an antioxidant, which might inhibit the ongoing process of DNA damage in the early stages of epithelial carcinogenesis, with a retinoid, which can reverse phenotypic changes associated with later stages of the process.

Epidermal Growth Factor Receptor Inhibitors

As described in more detail earlier in this chapter, the EGFR is a commonly overexpressed oncogene in head and neck cancers (63–65,73). Its overexpression is associated with shorter relapse-free intervals and decreased overall survival of head and neck cancer patients (60,68–71). Up-regulation of EGFR and its ligand TGF-α is an early event in the multistep process of head and neck carcinogenesis, as occurs with increasing frequency in advancing stages of dysplasia, and is present in the majority of established head and neck cancers. In addition, EGFR expression in premalignant lesions appears to be a sensitive predictor of the neoplastic potential of premalignant lesions (73,74,211). Based on these data and the need for new agents for treating smoking-related malignancies of the upper aerodigestive tract, inhibition of EGFR is an attractive target for reversal of the carcinogenesis process. Among the EGFR inhibitors, small-molecule inhibitors of the tyrosine kinase activity of EGFR are the most attractive for use in prevention trials because of their oral bioavailability, favorable side-effect profile, and apparent clinical activity in established cancers. Among these is LD 1839, a potent specific inhibitor of EGFR tyrosine kinase activity and a potent apoptosis inducer that has shown activity against neoplastic cells in several cell systems and significant clinical activity in completed phase I and phase II trials (212). It has already been proposed for use in chemoprevention trials.

Cyclooxygenase-2 Inhibitors

Some current chemoprevention strategies are focusing on the development of agents that inhibit the activity of cyclooxygenase-2 (Cox-2). One strategy for modulating carcinogenesis is to prevent the up-regulation of prostaglandin synthesis in premalignant and malignant tissue. The rationale is that Cox catalyzes the synthesis of prostaglandins and the production of mutagenic electrophiles (213,214). Increased levels of prostaglandins have been detected in several epithelial cancers including those of head and neck origin (215), and it is well known that prostaglandins affect cell proliferation and promote angiogenesis (216).

There are two Cox enzymes: Cox-1 and Cox-2. Cox-2 is an inducible isoform encoded by an early response gene that is induced by growth factors, tumor promoters, oncogenes, and carcinogens (217–221). Overexpression of Cox-2 in epithelial cells inhibits apoptosis (216), which increases the tumorigenic potential of initiated cells. The theoretical antitumor benefits of inhibiting Cox have been confirmed in experimental models. There is strong evidence that inhibitors of Cox, including nonsteroidal antiinflammatory drugs (NSAIDs), protect against colon, mammary, and oral cancers in experimental animals (222–224) and humans (225). In addition, Cox-2 null mutations have been associated with a marked reduction in the number and size of intestinal polyps in $Apc^{\Delta716}$ knockout mice, a model of human familial adenomatous polyposis (FAP). Treatment with a novel selective inhibitor of Cox-2 also reduced the numbers of polyps in these mice, a finding particularly relevant for chemoprevention strategies (217). These facts, along with the observation that chronic inflammation is associated with an increased risk for epithelial malignancy (226), stress the potential importance of employing Cox-2 inhibition as a chemopreventive strategy for epithelial tumors. In addition, strong support for the chemopreventive use of the Cox-2 inhibitor celecoxib comes from the recent approval of the agent by the Food and Drug Administration (FDA) for use in FAP patients to prevent colonic polyps from developing (227).

Most relevant to head and neck cancer chemoprevention is the finding that Cox-2 expression is up-regulated in HNSCC (228). Mean levels of Cox-2 mRNA were increased 150-fold in HNSCC and 50-fold in normal-appearing epithelium adjacent to HNSCC when compared with normal oral mucosa from healthy volunteers. These data suggest that Cox-2 inhibition is a reasonable target for chemoprevention in upper aerodigestive tract carcinogenesis. Because selective inhibitors of Cox-2 such as celecoxib also appear to be safer than nonselective NSAIDs in terms of gastrointestinal side effects, their long-term use in chemoprevention of cancer appears feasible and attractive.

Farnesyltransferase Inhibitors

The low-molecular-weight guanine triphosphatases (GTPases) Ras, RhoA, Rac-1, and Cdc42 have been implicated in the promotion of tumorigenesis, invasion, and metastasis (229). Oncogenic mutations of *Ras* are estimated to occur in up to 30% of all human cancers (230). All the GTPases require a lipid post-translational modification catalyzed by farnesyltransferase (Ftase) or geranylgeranyltransferase I (GGTase I), and Ras requires farnesylation to exert its cancer-causing activity (231). Therefore, Ftase inhibitors (FTI) have been developed as anticancer therapeutics (232). Although FTIs have many substrates and it is not yet exactly known which of these farnesylated proteins are critical for the maintenance of the malignant phenotype, they have shown activity in cell lines and animal models. They have also advanced in clinical trials, whose preliminary data suggest activity both at the molecular and clinical level in HNSCC (233). On the basis of these data, a phase IIB trial chemoprevention of using FTIs and EGFR TKIs in former and current smokers with a history of tobacco-induced malignancies (prior stage I non–small-cell lung cancer, stage I or II head and neck or esophageal cancer, limited-stage small-cell lung cancer, or locally advanced transitional carcinoma of the urothelium). Both trials are being funded by National Cancer Institute Specialized Programs of Research Excellence (SPORE) grants and by Lung Cancer Biomarkers and Chemoprevention Consortium (LCBCC) grants (234).

CLINICAL STUDIES

As described in the introduction of this chapter, the need for an effective strategy to prevent head and neck cancer becomes obvious on review of patient survival statistics. Primary prevention through carcinogen avoidance should not be overlooked because chemoprevention trials cannot achieve their long-term goal (i.e., reduction in head and neck cancer incidence) without a successful strategy to eliminate exposure to carcinogens. Because tobacco and alcohol are the major risk factors, numerous attempts at public education and numerous programs for smoking cessation have been employed and are being actively pursued. However, active intervention with agents thought to be capable of interfering with the carcinogenic process is also becoming an increasingly important strategy. This approach remains experimental and has not yet been established as standard practice, but the design of chemoprevention trials is still evolving. Phase I and phase II trials serve primarily to determine preliminary drug activity and toxicity. The end point in these trials is to determine the impact of the intervention of cancer incidence, but the use of validated biomarkers as intermediate end points would allow them to be completed in relatively shorter periods of time. Phase IIa studies consist of one arm only, whereas phase IIb studies also include a control arm. Phase III trials use cancer incidence as the definitive end point and thus must include thousands of subjects and take several years to complete.

Selection of patients to be enrolled in such a trial often is difficult because the population at risk, if it is defined as individuals with significant tobacco and alcohol exposure, includes many healthy subjects who are not necessarily motivated to comply with preventive treatment. An excellent model for chemoprevention therefore has been the oral premalignancy model because patients with this condition have a well-defined and documented risk for cancer development. The adjuvant studies for prevention of SPTs include a population of patients who are strongly motivated to participate and who are easily identified and recruited. Nevertheless, even among these high-risk groups, the willingness to commit to the chemopreventive intervention is fairly low.

Another critical issue, especially in phase III trials, is participant noncompliance. Statistical analysis requires that even noncompliant participants be included in efficacy evaluations. The identification of noncompliant patients by the use of a run-in period of chemopreventive agent administration before randomization is an effective strategy that has been used by our group and others.

Yet another concern is the occurrence and severity of side effects associated with each agent. Toxicity in chemoprevention trials should be evaluated much more critically than, for example, chemotherapy-associated toxicity because chemoprevention is aimed at otherwise healthy individuals for whom even mild toxic effects might be unacceptable. This is particularly well illustrated by the toxicity associated with retinoids, especially at high doses. In our early trials, the toxic effects contributed to a significant dropout rate even though the agents were very effective. Finally, from an ethical viewpoint, participants must demonstrate a thorough understanding of the potential benefits and risks of participation before they are enrolled in the study.

Trials in Oral Premalignancy

The oral premalignancy model is an excellent research model for several reasons. First, oral leukoplakia and erythroplakia are clearly associated with cancer. Clinically defined as a white patch in the oral cavity that cannot be scraped off or classified clinically as any other disorder (235), oral leukoplakia is associated with the development of oral cancer. Erythroplakia (a red, velvety plaque) carries a markedly increased risk for subsequent malignant transformation and is frequently associated with *in situ* or invasive carcinoma. Leukoplakia and erythroplakia may harbor different degrees of hyperplasia and dysplasia histologically. In the United States, they are most often found among tobacco users (cigarette smokers or users of chewing tobacco or snuff). Alcohol abuse is another risk factor. Different exposures, such as betel-nut chewing, are important risk factors in other parts of the world (236). The natural history of leukoplakia is variable, with improvement occurring spontaneously in many cases. Nevertheless, the frequency of progression to invasive cancer has been well documented, up to 18% at 7 years (36% for dysplasia) in the largest reported U.S. series (16), and depends primarily on the degree of dysplasia, on the clinical characteristics of the lesion, and on marginal improvement in the resolution rate of these lesions with smoking cessation. These data, along with the fact that surgical excision cannot cure extensive, multiple lesions or address the development of new lesions, suggest that additional intervention is needed (16,43,237).

Second, oral leukoplakia lesions can be safely monitored clinically and histologically. They are easily accessible for biomarker studies and provide an exceptional model for determining the efficacy of chemoprevention agents because they directly reflect the condition of the rest of the upper aerodigestive tract. Third, and perhaps most importantly, oral premalignant lesions represent markers of fieldwide injury and increased risk for cancer development elsewhere in the aerodigestive tract. Therefore, interventions effective in this model could have wider implications. Studies of oral premalignancy have been extremely important for the development of cancer chemoprevention. Several agents have been investigated in this model, but among them the retinoid trials stand out.

RETINOID TRIALS

The first chemoprevention trials of systemic and topical vitamin A were conducted in the late 1950s (238–240) and showed some evidence of efficacy. Later trials continued to evaluate vitamin A and explored the efficacy of other natural and synthetic agents with higher preclinical therapeutic indexes. All produced promising single-arm results, but only vitamin A, 13-cRA, *N*-4-(hydroxycarbophenyl)retinamide, and 4-HPR have advanced beyond these initial trials to randomized trials that confirmed their efficacy (37,181,196,241–243).

In 1986, Hong et al. (181) reported the first double-blind, placebo-controlled trial of high-dose 13-cRA (1–2 mg/kg/d) in the oral premalignancy model. This study highlighted many important aspects of retinoid therapy in oral premalignancy. The 44 participants in the study received treatment for 3 months and were followed for 6 months. The clinical response rate was 67% in the retinoid arm and 10% in the placebo arm ($p = 0.0002$). The rate of histologic improvement was significantly better in the retinoid arm (54% vs. 10%; $p = 0.01$). Two important issues arose from this high-dose, short-term regimen. First, toxic effects were frequent and severe, with two thirds of the 13-cRA–treated patients experiencing mucocutaneous toxicity and hypertriglyceridemia. Nearly half of the patients treated at 2 mg/kg/d required dose reductions to 1 mg/kg/d. The toxicity was clearly dose-related and was reversible with treatment cessation. Second, remission was short-lived, with more than half the patients relapsing within 3 months of treatment cessation.

These issues were addressed in the design of the study that followed, which examined the effect of low-dose 13-cRA (0.5 mg/kg/d) versus β-carotene (30 mg/kg/d) for short-term maintenance after induction with high-dose 13-cRA (196). The primary end point of this randomized, phase IIb maintenance trial, conducted by Lippman et al. (196), was relapse during the maintenance phase. The trial consisted of a 3-month induction phase with high-dose 13-cRA (1.5 mg/kg/d), followed by randomization of patients whose lesions responded or remained stable to the maintenance therapy. The low-dose 13-cRA arm was intended to maintain the good responses obtained with high-dose 13-cRA while minimizing toxicity; the β-carotene arm was based on epidemiologic evidence and results of positive uncontrolled clinical studies. Consistent with the results of Hong's trial, the clinical response rate after induction therapy was 55%, with reversal of dysplasia in 43% of these responders. Fifty-three patients were fully assessable after maintenance. Further lesion response was observed in 33% and 10% of patients in the 13-cRA and the β-carotene groups, respectively. The rate of disease progression during or after low-dose 13-cRA maintenance therapy was only 8% versus 55% in the β-carotene arm ($p < 0.001$). The low-dose maintenance decreased the intensity and severity of toxic effects, although they still were significantly greater than those seen in the β-carotene group. This study established that induction with 13-cRA followed by low-dose maintenance is effective and useful in preventing the recurrence associated with treatment cessation, with acceptable toxicity. After a median follow-up of 66 months, rates of malignant transformation were similar in both arms (23% in the 13-cRA group vs. 27% in the β-carotene group) (196), although a trend toward extended latency was seen in the 13-cRA group (244). These findings further underscored the need for long-term intervention to suppress premalignant lesions (244).

The findings of Lippman et al. (196) formed the basis of a long-term randomized trial of low-dose 13-cRA (0.5 mg/kg/d for 1 year, followed by 0.25 mg/kg/d for 2 years) versus the combination of retinyl palmitate and β-carotene for 3 years. β-Carotene was deleted halfway into the accrual phase of the study and the target patient sample was modified, based on information from the α-Tocopherol/β-Carotene (ATBC) study (203) and the β-Carotene and Retinol Efficacy Trial (CARET) (245), showing the negative influence of β-carotene on the incidence of lung cancer in smokers, and data from in the Physicians' Health Study, showing that β-carotene had no impact on cancer incidence (246). The trial completed patient accrual in 2001 ($n = 184$), and results are eagerly awaited. Both the maintenance study (196) and the long-term trial in the oral premalignant model incorporated several laboratory correlates that may serve as validated biomarkers in the future (41,114,192).

Two subsequent randomized trials have confirmed the efficacy of retinoids. In a 6-month study, Stich et al. (247) confirmed that vitamin A alone is significantly more effective than placebo in producing remission (56% complete response rate) and halting of progression of oral leukoplakia lesions in Asian betel-nut chewers. In 4-month placebo-controlled study, Han et al. (241) revealed the significant activity of 4-HPR in reversing oral premalignant lesions. In a maintenance trial of the ability of 12 months of fenretinide treatment to prevent relapse compared with no treatment, Italian researchers enrolled 170 patients whose premalignant lesions had undergone complete laser resection (189,242). The relapse rate in the retinoid arm was remarkably lower than in the nontreatment arm at 12 months (8% vs. 29%). The toxic effects were minimal, prompting further study of this promising agent in 13-cRA–resistant lesions, which demonstrated modest activity (248).

NONRETINOID TRIALS

Several trials have explored the use of β-carotene in oral leukoplakia. In the 1980s, Stich et al. (36) conducted a pioneering series of trials of β-carotene in high-risk groups (snuff or betel-nut users) in which they introduced the concept of using micronucleated cell frequency as an early intermediate end point. In the first trial of β-carotene, dose was 180 mg/week. The subsequent three-arm study (placebo, β-carotene, and β-carotene plus retinol) in 130 patients indicated that the combination was twice as active as β-carotene alone in inducing the remission of established leukoplakias (37). The single-arm trials with β-carotene that followed reported an unexplained inverse relationship between escalating doses and decreasing response rates. Though all of these trials confirmed the minimal toxicity of the agent, none were randomized, and none of the histologic responses were documented with biopsies (249–251). In view of the negative results obtained with β-carotene in the CARET and ATBC trials, no further trials of β-carotene have been planned.

Several other agents were used in nonrandomized trials in oral leukoplakia. A trial of selenium produced a 33% response rate (252), and a trial of α-tocopherol produced a 46% response rate (253); of interest were responses observed in some retinoid-resistant lesions. A clinical trial of antioxidant supplements (β-carotene, ascorbic acid, and α-tocopherol) produced clinical improvement in 57% of leukoplakia lesions treated (254). Combinations of naturally occurring chemopreventive agents have also been clinically tested. In a study performed in Uzbekistan, the prevalence odds ratio of oral leukoplakia significantly decreased to 62% in subjects given a combination of retinal (100,000 IU), β-carotene, and vitamin E compared with subjects given a combination of riboflavin, retinal, β-carotene, and vitamin E (255). Another agent recently tested in oral leukoplakia is Bowman-Birk inhibitor concentrate (BBIC), a soybean-derived serine protease inhibitor with both trypsin and chymotrypsin inhibitory activities, which prevents development of malignancy in a large number of animal model systems (256). In a phase II trial in 32 subjects, BBIC taken orally for 1 month resulted in a 31% response rate and decreased protease activity in oral mucosal cells (257). Selected nonrandomized studies (37,238–240,250,252-254,258–264) in chemoprevention of oral premalignancy are presented in Table 40.3.

In the setting of oral premalignancy, retinoid studies have been encouraging, but the optimal dose, form, and schedule of chemoprevention regimens remain to be established. New agents with a potentially better toxicity profile and better-defined targets are being studied as discussed above, including selective Cox-2 inhibitors (celecoxib); the ONYX-015 virus (265), which targets cells with defects in the p53 pathway; and EGFR TKIs. Despite the encouraging results of these studies, the ultimate goal of chemoprevention—reduction of cancer risk—remains to be demonstrated.

Rationale of Combination Therapy

Several lines of evidence suggest that in the near future rationally targeted combination chemoprevention trials will be needed to address the multifaceted chemoprevention process (266–268). Initial trials with combinations of 13-cRA and α-interferon in dysplastic lesions of the upper aerodigestive tract (269) have been completed or are in progress. Combination therapy has also been tried in retinoid-resistant tumors including advanced premalignant lesions of the oral cavity and larynx (mild to severe dysplasia or carcinoma *in situ*). These lesions are very unlikely to be reversed with either antioxidant or single-agent retinoid therapy and almost inevitably develop into invasive squamous carcinomas. In our retinoid chemoprevention studies in these lesions (139), *p53* overexpression, high levels of polysomy, and lack of RAR-β up-regulation were predictors of retinoid resistance.

The combination of retinoids and interferon (IFN) has shown effectiveness *in vitro* and in clinical trials. In particular, 13-cRA and α-IFN have been shown to be effective in combination against skin and cervical cancer (270,271). In addition, they are individually active against human papillomavirus-transformed cells *in vitro* and human papillomavirus-induced diseases such as recurrent respiratory papillomatosis and cervical dysplasia (272–274), suggesting that the combination may be effective against advanced premalignant lesions of the upper aerodigestive tract. A trial of 13-cRA and α-interferon in combination with α-tocopherol, a modulator of retinoid toxicity (210) that can reverse advanced premalignancy of the upper aerodigestive tract, found the combination to be active in preventing progression of laryngeal lesions but not oral lesions to cancer. After 12 months of treatment with this combination, 50% of laryngeal sites but no oral sites showed complete histologic reversal of dysplasia. Based on these findings and the fact that 9p21 loss persisted in post-treatment specimens despite complete response (275), a new study is underway in which patients with laryngeal dysplasia are being treated for 1 year with the combination of 13-cRA, α-interferon, and α-tocopherol, and then randomized to receive 2 years of maintenance with 4-HPR or placebo. This study is also examining the contribution of gastroesophageal and laryngopharyngeal acid reflux to laryngeal premalignancy and the effects of antireflux medications on the reversal of dysplastic lesions.

Adjuvant Chemoprevention of Second Primary Tumors

Patients who have undergone successful treatment of head and neck cancer are at increased risk for the development of additional primary neoplasms, have a lifetime risk for SPT exceeding 20%, and have a constant annual SPT rate of 4% to 6% for at least 8 years after diagnosis of the primary cancer (2,7,276). Multiple primary tumors are a clinical manifestation of field cancerization and are not addressed by definitive local therapy. Second primary tumors are a major cause of death after surgical cure of head and neck cancer and are the leading cause of death in patients with early-stage disease, surpassing recur-

TABLE 40.3 Completed Randomized Chemoprevention Trials in Oral Premalignancy

Study	Design (phase)	No. of patients	Agent (dose)	Results
Hong et al., 1986 (181)	IIb	44	Isotretinoin (1–2 mg/kg/d)	Positive
Stich et al., 1988 (247)	IIb	65	Vitamin A (200,000 U/wk)	Positive
Stich et al., 1988 (37)	IIb	103	β-carotene + retinol (100,000 IU/wk) (180 mg/wk)	Positive
Han et al., 1990 (241)	IIb	61	Retinamide (40 mg/d)	Positive
Lippman et al., 1993 (196)	IIb (maintenance)	70	Isotretinoin (0.5 mg/kg/d)	Positive
Costa et al., 1994 (189); Chiesa et al., 1993 (243)	IIb (maintenance)	153	Fenretinide (200 mg/d)	Positive
Zaridze et al., 1993 (255)	IIb	675	β-carotene (40 mg/d) + retinol (100,000 IU/wk) + vitamin E (8 oz/wk)	Positive
Lippman et al. (personal communication)	IIb	189	13-cRA vs. retinol	Pending

cRA, 13-*cis*-retinoic acid.

rence (277–281). The effectiveness of smoking cessation in preventing SPTs is unknown (282). These facts, along with the known activity of retinoids in oral premalignancy, have provided the conceptual basis for the development of adjuvant chemoprevention trials in head and neck cancer.

The first phase III adjuvant chemoprevention trial was reported in 1990 by Hong et al. (182). They prospectively studied 103 patients with stages I to IV (M0) head and neck cancer who, after definitive therapy, were randomized to receive either high-dose 13-cRA (100 mg/m^2/d) or placebo. The dose of 13-cRA was reduced to 50 mg/m^2/d after 13 of the first 44 patients experienced intolerable toxic effects. The major end points were primary disease recurrence and SPT development. The retinoid treatment was not associated with any reduction in recurrence of the initial primary tumor or suppression of regional or distant metastases. However, after a median follow-up of 32 months, patients in the 13-cRA arm had significantly fewer SPTs than did patients in the placebo group (4% vs. 24%; $p = 0.005$). This difference was still after with 55 months of follow-up (283), even though a decrease in the protective effect of 13-cRA narrowed the difference between the two groups (14% vs. 31%; $p = 0.04$). More important, the chemopreventive effect of 13-cRA on tobacco-related SPTs (i.e., SPTs occurring in the aerodigestive tract) was similarly significant (7% vs. 33% placebo; $p = 0.008$). Furthermore, SPTs in the retinoid-treated patients took significantly longer to develop. Though this decrease did not translate into an increase in survival in our study, we do believe that it reflects the early detection and effective surgical salvage of patients with SPT (which occurred more often in the placebo group), the lack an impact on recurrence, and the high dropout rate in the retinoid arm secondary to toxic effects. That only two thirds of the retinoid-treated patients completed the full 12 months of intervention underscores the importance of these results.

On the basis of this adjuvant study as well as the successful experience with maintenance of remission in oral premalignancy, the National Cancer Institute sponsored the largest multicenter, phase III (double-blinded, placebo-controlled) trial in head and neck cancer to date. Patients were randomized to receive low-dose 13-cRA for 3 years versus placebo, and the primary end point was prevention of SPTs. This trial was different from the initial trial in that it used a lower dose of 13-cRA, included only early-stage (T1,2 N0) patients, and had a different period of intervention (3 years with a 4-year follow-up). The trial was closed to accrual in June 1999 after enrolling more than 1,200 participants. An interim analysis found annual SPT rates of 5.1%, 4.1%, and 3% in active, former, and never smokers, respectively ($p = 0.06$ for active versus never smokers) (234). There was no significant difference in overall survival, or SPT- or recurrence-free survival, and although decreased recurrences in the isotretinoin arm were observed during active intervention, this effect was lost after treatment stopped (285a).

Meanwhile, another randomized adjuvant chemoprevention trial using low-dose etretinate has been completed in France (284). After therapy for early-stage (T1,2 N0,1) SCCs of the oral cavity and pharynx, 316 patients were randomized to receive either etretinate (50 mg/d for 1 month, then 25 mg/d for 24 months) or placebo. The study found that etretinate had no impact on overall survival, primary disease recurrence, or SPT rate. However, drawing definitive conclusions is difficult because no data on patient compliance were kept and the diagnostic criteria for SPTs were not reported. This study did, however, confirm the high incidence of SPTs observed in our previous studies, as well as the location of the majority of SPTs within the carcinogen-exposed field of the aerodigestive tract. Second primary tumors developed in 24% of the placebo group and 38% of the etretinate group at 41 months of follow-up, and in 80% of the cases they were located in the head and neck, lungs, or esophagus.

The Euroscan study (285) was based on the favorable findings of Pastorino et al. (286), who compared retinyl palmitate treatment for 12 months with observation of patients after resection of stage I non–small-cell lung cancer and found a statistically significant difference in time to development of SPTs within the carcinogen-exposed field ($p = 0.045$) in favor of the retinoid-treated group. The Euroscan study consisted of two parallel clinical trials of two high-risk populations: patients with completely resected non–small-cell lung cancer and patients with head and neck cancer after curative treatment. The agents used were *N*-acetylcysteine and retinyl palmitate, and a 2×2 factorial design was employed. The study found no benefit in either study in terms of survival, event-free survival, or SPT rates (285).

In phase III chemoprevention trial, the Northern California Oncology Group (NCOG) in conjunction with the Eastern Cooperative Oncology Group (ECOG), involving patients with stage I or II head and neck cancer to receive either low-dose 13-cRA (0.15 mg/kg/d) or placebo for 2 years. The chemopreventive intervention was started as adjuvant primary therapy shortly after the completion of surgery or radiation therapy. One hundred eighty-nine patients were enrolled. Thirty SPTs and four third primary tumors developed, at an overall annual rate of 3.4%. There was no difference between the 13-cRA and placebo groups in terms of occurrence of second or third primary tumors (287).

Again, these retinoid trials point up the need for novel targeted interventions that can overcome retinoid toxicity. This need is being addressed with newer studies employing agents such as EGFR TKIs and farnesyltransferase inhibitors. A summary of completed and ongoing trials of randomized chemo-

TABLE 40.4 Completed Randomized Chemoprevention Trials in HNSCC to Prevent Second Primary Tumors

Study	Design (phase)	No. of patients	Agent (dose)	Results
Hong et al., 1990; Benner et al., 1994 (182,283)	III	103	Isotretinoin (50–100 mg/m^2/d)	Positive
Bolla et al., 1994 (284)	III	316	Etretinate (50–25 mg/d)	Negative
Euroscan, 2000 (285)	I	2,592	1. Retinyl palmitate (300,000 IU/daily for 1 year followed by 150,000 IU for a 2nd year) 2. *N*-acetylcysteine 600 mg/d for 2 years	No difference in SPT rate, event-free survival, or overall survival between the four arms
RTOG 91–15 (285a)	III	1,191	13-cRA 30 m^2/d for 3 years	Pending

HNSCC, head and neck squamous cell carcinoma; RTOG, Radiation Therapy Oncology Group; SPT, Second primary tumor.

TABLE 40.5 Ongoing Randomized Head and Neck Chemoprevention Trials

Agent	Design	Status	Mouthwash	No. of patients
Ketorolac	II	Completed accrual	10 mL 0.1% solvent placebo randomization to 100 mg po b.i.d., 200 mg po b.i.d.	57
Celecoxib	II	Ongoing	400 mg po b.i.d.	84
ONYX-015	II	Ongoing	1 × 10" daily × 5 then weekly × 5	20
Adenovirus *p53* gene therapy	I/II	Pending activation		33
EGFR TKI (Iressa)	IIb	Pending activation	250 mg po daily × 3 months randomization to 3 dose levels 500 mg/m^2 t.i.d., 750 mg/m^2 t.i.d., 1 g/m^2 po t.i.d.	92
GTE	II	Pending activation		36
EGFR TKI (Iressa) vs. placebo	III	Pending activation	250 mg po daily × 6 months	120
R115777	III	Pending activation	200 mg po b.i.d. 3 weeks on/1 week off	

EGFR TKI, epidermoid growth factor receptor tyrosine kinase inhibitor; GTE, green tea extract.

prevention trials in oral premalignancy and in prevention of SPTs is provided in Tables 40.4 and 40.5.

CONCLUSION

The field of head and neck cancer chemoprevention has matured over the last 20 years. A number of critical studies have been completed. Thanks to technologic advances in the field of molecular biology, important progress has been made in dissecting the molecular and phenotypic determinants of the tumorigenic process. These determinants might represent intermediate end points for future studies and might be used as screening tools for selection of suitable populations for study and intervention. As newer, better targeted, and relatively nontoxic agents emerge, novel studies will continue to be launched. It is hoped that one or several of these approaches will be incorporated into the standard clinical practice and result in true reductions in the incidence and mortality of head and neck cancer.

REFERENCES

1. Jemal A, Thomas A, Murray T, et al. Cancer statistics, 2002. *CA: Cancer J Clin* 2002;52:23–47.
2. Vokes EE, Weichselbaum RR, Lippman SM, et al. Head and neck cancer. *N Engl J Med* 1993;328:184–194.
3. Lippman SM, Benner SE, Hong WK. Cancer chemoprevention. *J Clin Oncol* 1994;12:851–873.
4. Hong WK, Lippman SM, Hittelman WN, et al. Retinoid chemoprevention of aerodigestive cancer: from basic research to the clinic. *Clin Cancer Res* 1995;1:677–686.
5. Lippman SM, Hong WK. Retinoid chemoprevention of upper aerodigestive tract carcinogenesis. *Important Adv Oncol* 1992;93–109.
6. Hong WK,Lippman SM, Wolf GT. Recent advances in head and neck cancer—larynx preservation and cancer chemoprevention: the Seventeenth Annual Richard and Hinda Rosenthal Foundation Award Lecture. *Clin Cancer Res* 1993;53:5113–5120.
7. Cooper JS, Pajak TF, Rubin P, et al. Second malignancies in patients who have head and neck cancers: incidence, effect on survival and implications for chemoprevention based on the RTOG experience. *Int J Radiat Oncol Biol Phys* 1989;17:449–456.
8. Lippman SM, Spitz MR, Huber MH, et al. Strategies for chemoprevention study of premalignancy and second primary tumors in the head and neck. *Curr Opin Oncol* 1995;7:234–241.
9. Slaughter DP, Southwick HW, Smejkal W."Field cancerization" in oral stratified squamous epithelium: clinical implications of multicentric origin. *Cancer* 1953;6:963–968.
10. Auerbach O, Stout A, Hammond E, et al. Changes in bronchial epithelium in relation to cigarette smoking and in relation to lung cancer. *N Engl J Med* 1961;265:253–267.
11. Farber E. The multistep nature of cancer development. *Clin Cancer Res* 1984; 44:4217–4223.
12. Bouquot JE, Weiland LH, Kurland LT. Leukoplakia and carcinoma in situ synchronously associated with invasive oral/oropharyngeal carcinoma in Rochester, Minn., 1935–1984. *Oral Surg Oral Med Oral Pathol Oral Radiol Endodont* 1988;65:199–207.
13. Einhorn J, Wersall J. Incidence of oral carcinoma in patients with leukoplakia of the oral mucosa. *Cancer* 1967;20:2189–2193.
14. Mashberg A. Erythroplasia vs. leukoplasia in the diagnosis of early asymptomatic oral squamous carcinoma. *N Engl J Med* 1977;297:109–110.
15. Shklar GS. Oral leukoplakia. *N Engl J Med* 1986;315:1544–1546.
16. Silverman SJ, Gorsky M, Lozada F. Oral leukoplakia and malignant transformation. A follow-up study of 257 patients. *Cancer* 1984;53:563–568.
17. Zelen M. Are primary cancer prevention trials feasible? *J Natl Cancer Inst* 1988;80:1442–1444.
18. Schatzkin A, Freedman LS, Schiffman MH, et al. Validation of intermediate end points in clinical cancer research. *J Natl Cancer Inst* 1990;82:1746–1752.
19. Tockman MS, Gupta PK, Pressman NJ, et al. Considerations in bringing a cancer biomarker to clinical application. *Clin Cancer Res* 1992;52:2711s–2718s.
20. Lippman SM, Lee JS, Lotan R, et al. Biomarkers as intermediate end points in chemoprevention trials. *J Natl Cancer Inst* 1990;82:555–560.
21. Lippman SM, Benner SE, Hong WK. The chemoprevention of cancer. In: Greenwald P, Kramer RS, Weed DL, ed. *Cancer prevention and control.* New York: Marcel Dekker, 1995:329–352.
22. Sharma S, Stutzman JD, Kelloff GJ, et al. Screening of potential chemopreventive agents using biochemical markers of carcinogenesis. *Clin Cancer Res* 1994;54:5848–5855.
23. Shin DM, Hittelman WN, Hong WK. Biomarkers in upper aerodigestive tract tumorigenesis: a review. *Cancer Epidemiol Biomark Prevent* 1994;3:697–709.
24. Harris CC. Interindividual variation among humans in carcinogen metabolism, DNA adduct formation, and DNA repair. *Carcinogenesis* 1989;10: 1563–1566.
25. Spitz MR. Epidemiology and risk factors for head and neck cancer. *Semin Oncol* 1994;21:281–288.
26. Lippman SM, Spitz M, Trizna Z, et al. Epidemiology, biology, and chemoprevention of aerodigestive cancer. *Cancer* 1994;74:2719–2725.
27. Spitz MR, Fueger JJ, Beddingfield NA, et al. Chromosome sensitivity to bleomycin-induced mutagenesis, an independent risk factor for upper aerodigestive tract cancers. *Clin Cancer Res* 1989;49:4626–4628.
28. Spitz MR, Fueger JJ, Halabi S, et al. Mutagen sensitivity in upper aerodigestive tract cancer: a case-control analysis. *Cancer Epidemiol Biomark Prevent* 1993;2:329–333.
29. Li D, Firozi PF, Chang P, et al. In vitro BPDE-induced DNA adducts in peripheral lymphocytes as a risk factor for squamous cell carcinoma of the head and neck. *Int J Cancer* 2001;93:436–440.
30. Wang LE, Sturgis EM, Eicher SA, et al. Mutagen sensitivity to benzo(a)pyrene diol epoxide and the risk of squamous cell carcinoma of the head and neck. *Clin Cancer Res* 1998;4:1773–1778.
31. Wei Q, Eicher SA, Guan Y, et al. Reduced expression of hMLH1 and hGTBP/hMSH6: a risk factor for head and neck cancer. *Cancer Epidemiol Biomark Prevent* 1998;7:309–314.
32. Shen H, Sturgis EM, Khan SG, et al. An intronic poly (AT) polymorphism of the DNA repair gene XPC and risk of squamous cell carcinoma of the head and neck: a case-control study. *Clin Cancer Res* 2001;61:3321–3325.
33. Spitz MR, Hoque A, Trizna Z, et al. Mutagen sensitivity as a risk factor for second malignant tumors following malignancies of the upper aerodigestive tract. *J Natl Cancer Inst* 1994;86:1681–1684.
34. Cloos J, Braakhuis BJ, Steen I, et al. Increased mutagen sensitivity in head-and-neck squamous-cell carcinoma patients, particularly those with multiple primary tumors. *Int J Cancer* 1994;56:816–819.
35. Stich HF. Micronucleated exfoliated cells as indicators for genotoxic damage and as markers in chemoprevention trials. *J Nat Growth Cancer* 1987;4:9–18.
36. Stich HF, Rosin MP, Vallejera MO. Reduction with vitamin A and beta-carotene administration of proportion of micronucleated buccal mucosal cells in Asian betel nut and tobacco chewers. *Lancet* 1984;1:1204–1206.
37. Stich HF, Rosin MP, Hornby AP, et al. Remission of oral leukoplakias and micronuclei in tobacco/betel quid chewers treated with beta-carotene and with beta-carotene plus vitamin A. *Int J Cancer* 1988;42:195–199.
38. Munoz N, Hayashi M, Bang U, et al. Effect of riboflavin, retinol, and zinc on

micronuclei of buccal mucosa and of esophagus: a randomized double-blind intervention study in China. *J Natl Cancer Inst* 1987;79:687–691.
39. Benner SE, Lippman SM, Wargovich MJ, et al. Micronuclei, a biomarker for chemoprevention trials: results of a randomized study in oral pre-malignancy. *Int J Cancer* 1994;59:457–459.
40. Voravud N, Shin DM, Ro JY, et al. Increased polysomies of chromosomes 7 and 17 during head and neck multistage tumorigenesis. *Clin Cancer Res* 1993;53:2874–2883.
41. Lee JS, Kim SY, Hong WK, et al. Detection of chromosomal polysomy in oral leukoplakia, a premalignant lesion. *J Natl Cancer Inst* 1993;85:1951–1954.
42. Veltman JA, Bot FJ, Huynen FC, et al. Chromosome instability as an indicator of malignant progression in laryngeal mucosa. *J Clin Oncol* 2000;18: 1644–1651.
43. Sudbo J, Kildal W, Risberg B, et al. DNA content as a prognostic marker in patients with oral leukoplakia. *N Engl J Med* 2001;344:1270–1278.
44. Kallioniemi A, Kallioniemi OP, Sudar D, et al. Comparative genomic hybridization for molecular cytogenetic analysis of solid tumors. *Science* 1992;258:818–821.
45. Speicher MR, Howe C, Crotty P, et al. Comparative genomic hybridization detects novel deletions and amplifications in head and neck squamous cell carcinomas. *Clin Cancer Res* 1995;55:1010–1013.
46. Brzoska PM, Levin NA, Fu KK, et al. Frequent novel DNA copy number increase in squamous cell head and neck tumors. *Clin Cancer Res* 1995;55: 3055–3059.
47. Pollack JR, Perou CM, Alizadeh AA, et al. Genome-wide analysis of DNA copy-number changes using cDNA microarrays. *Nat Genet* 1999;23:41–46.
48. Carey TE, Van Dyke DL, Worsham MJ. Nonrandom chromosome aberrations and clonal populations in head and neck cancer. *Anticancer Res* 1993;13: 2561–2567.
49. Van Dyke DL, Worsham MJ, Benninger MS, et al. Recurrent cytogenetic abnormalities in squamous cell carcinomas of the head and neck region. *Genes Chromosomes Cancer* 1994;9:192–206.
50. Cowan JM, Beckett MA, Ahmed-Swan S, et al. Cytogenetic evidence of the multistep origin of head and neck squamous cell carcinomas. *J Natl Cancer Inst* 1992;84:793–797.
51. Williams ME, Gaffey MJ, Weiss LM, et al. Chromosome 11q13 amplification in head and neck squamous cell carcinoma. *Arch Otolaryngol Head Neck Surg* 1993;119:1238–1243.
52. Ah-See KW, Cooke TG, Pickford IR, et al. An allelotype of squamous carcinoma of the head and neck using microsatellite markers. *Clin Cancer Res* 1994;54:1617–1621.
53. Nawroz H, van der Riet P, Hruban R, et al. Allelotype of head and neck squamous cell carcinoma. *Clin Cancer Res* 1994;54:1152–1155.
54. el-Naggar AK, Hurr K, Batsakis JG, et al. Sequential loss of heterozygosity at microsatellite motifs in preinvasive and invasive head and neck squamous carcinoma. *Clin Cancer Res* 1995;55:2656–2659.
55. Alizadeh AA, Eisen MB, Davis RE, et al. Distinct types of diffuse large B-cell lymphoma identified by gene expression profiling. *Nature* 2000;403:503–511.
56. Perou CM, Sorlie T, Eisen MB, et al. Molecular portraits of human breast tumours. *Nature* 2000;406:747–752.
57. Page MJ, Amess B, Townsend RR, et al. Proteomic definition of normal human luminal and myoepithelial breast cells purified from reduction mammoplasties. *Proc Natl Acad Sci USA* 1999;96:12589–12594.
58. Derynck R. Transforming growth factor alpha. *Cell* 1988;54:593–595.
59. Velu TJ, Beguinot L, Vass WC, et al. Epidermal-growth-factor-dependent transformation by a human EGF receptor proto-oncogene. *Science* 1987;238: 1408–1410.
60. Todd R, Donoff BR, Gertz R, et al. TGF-alpha and EGF-receptor mRNAs in human oral cancers. *Carcinogenesis* 1989;10:1553–1556.
61. Grandis JR, Zeng Q, Tweardy DJ. Retinoic acid normalizes the increased gene transcription rate of TGF-alpha and EGFR in head and neck cancer cell lines. *Nature Med* 1996;2:237–240.
62. Eisbruch A, Blick M, Lee JS, et al. Analysis of the epidermal growth factor receptor gene in fresh human head and neck tumors. *Clin Cancer Res* 1987;47:3603–3605.
63. Maxwell SA, Sacks PG, Gutterman JU, et al. Epidermal growth factor receptor protein-tyrosine kinase activity in human cell lines established from squamous carcinomas of the head and neck. *Clin Cancer Res* 1989;49: 1130–1137.
64. Ozanne B, Richards CS, Hendler F, et al. Over-expression of the EGF receptor is a hallmark of squamous cell carcinomas. *J Pathol* 1986;149:9–14.
65. Kawamoto T, Takahashi K, Nishi M, et al. Quantitative assay of epidermal growth factor receptor in human squamous cell carcinomas of the oral region by an avidin-biotin method. *Jpn J Cancer Res* 1991;82:403–410.
66. Partridge M, Green MR, Langdon JD, et al. Production of TGF-alpha and TGF-beta by cultured keratinocytes, skin and oral squamous cell carcinomas—potential autocrine regulation of normal and malignant epithelial cell proliferation. *Br J Cancer* 1989;60:542–548.
67. Yoshida K, Kyo E, Tsuda T, et al. EGF and TGF-alpha, the ligands of hyperproduced EGFR in human esophageal carcinoma cells, act as autocrine growth factors. *Int J Cancer* 1990;45:131–135.
68. Dassonville O, Formento JL, Francoual M, et al. Expression of epidermal growth factor receptor and survival in upper aerodigestive tract cancer. *J Clin Oncol* 1993;11:1873–1878.
69. Formento JL, Francoual M, Ramaioli A, et al. [EGF receptor, a prognostic factor in epidermoid cancers of the upper aerodigestive tracts]. *Bull Cancer* 1994;81:610–615.
70. Issing WJ, Liebich C, Wustrow TP, et al. Coexpression of epidermal growth factor receptor and TGF-alpha and survival in upper aerodigestive tract cancer. *Anticancer Res* 1996;16:283–288.
71. Grandis JR, Melhem MF, Gooding WE, et al. Levels of TGF-alpha and EGFR protein in head and neck squamous cell carcinoma and patient survival. *J Natl Cancer Inst* 1998;90:824–832.
72. Shin D, Ro J, Hong W, et al. Dysregulation of epidermal growth factor receptor expression in premalignant lesions during head and neck tumorigenesis. *Clin Cancer Res* 1994;54:3153–3159.
73. Grandis JR, Tweardy DJ. Elevated levels of transforming growth factor alpha and epidermal growth factor receptor messenger RNA are early markers of carcinogenesis in head and neck cancer. *Clin Cancer Res* 1993;53:3579–3584.
74. Grandis JR, Tweardy DJ, Melhem MF. Asynchronous modulation of transforming growth factor alpha and epidermal growth factor receptor protein expression in progression of premalignant lesions to head and neck squamous cell carcinoma. *Clin Cancer Res* 1998;4:13–20.
75. Herbst RS, Langer CJ. Epidermal growth factor receptors as a target for cancer treatment: the emerging role of IMC-C225 in the treatment of lung and head and neck cancers. *Semin Oncol* 2002;29:27–36.
76. Lammie GA, Peters G. Chromosome 11q13 abnormalities in human cancer. *Cancer Cells* 1991;3:413–420.
77. Berenson JR, Yang J, Mickel RA. Frequent amplification of the bcl-1 locus in head and neck squamous cell carcinomas. *Oncogene* 1989;4:1111–1116.
78. Lammie GA, Fantl V, Smith R, et al. D11S287, a putative oncogene on chromosome 11q13, is amplified and expressed in squamous cell and mammary carcinomas and linked to BCL-1. *Oncogene* 1991;6:439–444.
79. Rosenberg CL, Wong E, Petty EM, et al. PRAD1, a candidate BCL1 oncogene: mapping and expression in centrocytic lymphoma. *Proc Natl Acad Sci USA* 1991;88:9638–9642.
80. Motokura T, Bloom T, Kim HG, et al. A novel cyclin encoded by a bcl1-linked candidate oncogene. *Nature* 1991;350:512–515.
81. Sherr CJ. G1 phase progression: Cycling on cue. *Cell* 1994;79:551–555.
82. Hunter T, Pines J. Cyclins and cancer. II: Cyclin D and CDK inhibitors come of age. *Cell* 1994;79:573–582.
83. Lukas J, Aagaard L, Strauss M, et al. Oncogenic aberrations of p16INK4/CDKN2 and cyclin D1 cooperate to deregulate G1 control. *Clin Cancer Res* 1995;55:4818–4823.
84. Dowdy SF, Hinds PW, Louie K, et al. Physical interaction of the retinoblastoma protein with human D cyclins. *Cell* 1993;73:499–511.
85. Bates S, Parry D, Bonetta L, et al. Absence of cyclin D/cdk complexes in cells lacking functional retinoblastoma protein. *Oncogene* 1994;9:1633–1640.
86. Jiang W, Kahn SM, Zhou P, et al. Overexpression of cyclin Dl in rat fibroblasts causes abnormalities in growth control, cell cycle progression and gene expression. *Oncogene* 1993;8:3447–3457.
87. Quelle DE, Ashmun RA, Shurtleff SA, et al. Overexpression of mouse D-type cyclins accelerates G1 phase in rodent fibroblasts. *Genes Dev* 1993;7: 1559–1571.
88. Hinds PW, Dowdy SF, Eaton EN, et al. Function of a human cyclin gene as an oncogene. *Proc Natl Acad Sci USA* 1994;91:709–713.
89. Callender T, el-Naggar AK, Lee MS, et al. PRAD-1 (CCND1)/cyclin D1 oncogene amplification in primary head and neck squamous cell carcinoma. *Cancer* 1994;74:152–158.
90. Jares P, Fernandez PL, Campo E, et al. PRAD-1/cyclin Dl gene amplification correlates with messenger RNA overexpression and tumor progression in human laryngeal carcinomas. *Clin Cancer Res* 1994;54:4813–4817.
91. Parise O, Janot F, Guerry R, et al. Chromosome 11q13 gene amplification in head and neck squamous cell carcinomas: Relation with lymph node invasion. *Int J Oncol* 1994;5:309–313.
92. Muller D, Millon R, Lidereau R, et al. Frequent amplification of 11q13 DNA markers is associated with lymph node involvement in human head and neck squamous cell carcinomas. *Eur J Cancer B Oral Oncol* 1994;30B:113–120.
93. Michalides R, van Veelen N, Hart A, et al. Overexpression of cyclin D1 correlates with recurrence in a group of forty-seven operable squamous cell carcinomas of the head and neck. *Clin Cancer Res* 1995;55:975–978.
94. Bellacosa A, Almadori G, Cavallo S, et al. Cyclin DI gene amplification in human laryngeal squamous cell carcinomas: prognostic significance and clinical implications. *Clin Cancer Res* 1996;2:175–180.
95. Izzo JG, Papadimitrakopoulou VA, Li XQ, et al. Dysregulated cyclin D1 expression early in head and neck tumorigenesis: in vivo evidence for an association with subsequent gene amplification. *Oncogene* 1998;17:2313–2322.
96. Papadimitrakopoulou V, Izzo J, Mao L, et al. Cyclin D1 and p16 alterations in advanced premalignant lesions of the upper aerodigestive tract: role in response to chemoprevention and cancer development. *Clin Cancer Res* 2001; 7:3127–3134.
97. Izzo J, Babenko I, Hollander P, et al. Cyclin D1 genotypes: impact on expression and risk of cancer development in the upper aerodigestive tract (UADT). Proceedings of the American Association for Cancer Research Meeting, New Orleans, LA, 2001.
98. Boyle JO, Langenfeld J, Lonardo F, et al. Cyclin Dl proteolysis: a retinoid chemoprevention signal in normal, immortalized, and transformed human bronchial epithelial cells. *J Natl Cancer Inst* 1999;91:373–379.
99. Uhlman DL, Adams G, Knapp D, et al. Immunohistochemical staining for markers of future neoplastic progression in the larynx. *Clin Cancer Res* 1996;56:2199–2205.
100. Bos JL. Ras oncogenes in human cancer: review. *Clin Cancer Res* 1989;49: 4682–4689.
101. Rodenhuis S, Slebos RJ, Boot AJ, et al. Incidence and possible clinical signif-

icance of K-ras oncogene activation in adenocarcinoma of the human lung. *Clin Cancer Res* 1988;48:5738–5741.
102. Sheng ZM, Barrois M, Klijanienko J, et al. Analysis of the c-Ha-ras-1 gene for deletion, mutation, amplification and expression in lymph node metastases of human head and neck carcinomas. *Br J Cancer* 1990;62:398–404.
103. Rumsby G, Carter RL, Gusterson BA. Low incidence of ras oncogene activation in human squamous cell carcinomas. *Br J Cancer* 1990;61:365–368.
104. Hirano T, Steele PE, Gluckman JL. Low incidence of point mutation at codon 12 of K-ras proto-oncogene in squamous cell carcinoma of the upper aerodigestive tract. *Ann Otol Rhinol Laryngol* 1991;100:597–599.
105. Saranath D, Chang SE, Bhoite LT, et al. High frequency mutation in codons 12 and 61 of H-ras oncogene in chewing tobacco-related human oral carcinoma in India. *Br J Cancer* 1991;63:573–578.
106. Kuo MY, Chang HH, Hahn LJ, et al. Elevated ras p21 expression in oral premalignant lesions and squamous cell carcinoma in Taiwan. *J Oral Pathol Med* 1995;24:255–260.
107. Kiaris H, Spandidos D. Analysis of H-ras, K-ras, and N-ras genes for expression, mutation, and amplification in laryngeal tumors. *Int J Oncol* 1995;7: 75–80.
108. Vaux DL. Toward an understanding of the molecular mechanisms of physiological cell death. *Proc Natl Acad Sci USA* 1993;90:786–789.
109. Korsmeyer SJ. Bcl-2 initiates a new category of oncogenes: Regulators of cell death. *Blood* 1992;80:879–886.
110. Hockenbery DM, Zutter M, Hickey W, et al. BCL2 protein is topographically restricted in tissues characterized by apoptotic cell death. *Proc Natl Acad Sci USA* 1991;88:6961–6965.
111. Gallo O, Bianchi S, Porfirio B. Bcl-2 overexpression and smoking history in head and neck cancer. *J Natl Cancer Inst* 1995;87:1024–1025.
112. Gallo O, Boddi V, Calzolari A, et al. *bcl*-2 protein expression correlates with recurrence and survival in early stage head and neck cancer treated by radiotherapy. *Clin Cancer Res* 1996;2:261–267.
113. Pezzella F, Turley H, Kuzu I, et al. *bcl*-2 protein in non-small-cell lung carcinoma. *N Engl J Med* 1993;329:690–694.
114. Mao L, Lee JS, Fan YH, et al. Frequent microsatellite alterations at chromosomes 9p21 and 3p14 in oral premalignant lesions and their value in cancer risk assessment. *Nature Med* 1996;2:682–685.
115. Califano J, van der Riet P, Westra W, et al. Genetic progression model for head and neck cancer: implications for field cancerization. *Clin Cancer Res* 1996;56:2488–2492.
116. van der Riet P, Nawroz H, Hruban RH, et al. Frequent loss of chromosome 9p21-22 early in head and neck cancer progression. *Clin Cancer Res* 1994;54:1156–1158.
117. Partridge M, Emilion G, Pateromichelakis S, et al. Allelic imbalance at chromosomal loci implicated in the pathogenesis of oral precancer, cumulative loss and its relationship with progression to cancer. *Oral Oncol* 1998;34:77–83.
118. Partridge M, Pateromichelakis S, Phillips E, et al. A case-control study confirms that microsatellite assay can identify patients at risk of developing oral squamous cell carcinoma within a field of cancerization. *Clin Cancer Res* 2000;60:3893–3898.
119. Rosin MP, Cheng X, Poh C, et al. Use of allelic loss to predict malignant risk for low-grade oral epithelial dysplasia. *Clin Cancer Res* 2000;6:357–362.
120. Guo Z, Yamaguchi K, Sanchez-Cespedes M, et al. Allelic losses in OraTest-directed biopsies aerodigestive tract malignancy. *Clin Cancer Res* 2001;7: 1963–1968.
121. Harris CC, Hollstein M. Clinical implications of the p53 tumor-suppressor gene. *N Engl J Med* 1993;329:1318–1327.
122. Hartwell LH, Kastan MB. Cell cycle control and cancer. *Science* 1994;266: 1821–1828.
123. Brennan J, Boyle J, Koch W, et al. Association between cigarette smoking and mutation of the p53 gene in squamous-cell carcinoma of the head and neck. *N Engl J Med* 1995;332:712–717.
124. Brachman DG, Graves D, Vokes E, et al. Occurrence of p53 gene deletions and human papilloma virus infection in human head and neck cancer. *Clin Cancer Res* 1992;52:4832–4836.
125. Field JK, Spandidos DA, Malliri A, et al. Elevated P53 expression correlates with a history of heavy smoking in squamous cell carcinoma of the head and neck. *Br J Cancer* 1991;64:573–577.
126. Maestro R, Dolcetti R, Gasparotto D, et al. High frequency of p53 gene alterations associated with protein overexpression in human squamous cell carcinoma of the larynx. *Oncogene* 1992;7:1159–1166.
127. Somers KD, Merrick MA, Lopez ME, et al. Frequent p53 mutations in head and neck cancer. *Clin Cancer Res* 1992;52:5997–6000.
128. Gusterson BA, Anbazhagan R, Warren W, et al. Expression of p53 in premalignant and malignant squamous epithelium. *Oncogene* 1991;6:1785–1789.
129. Boyle JO, Hakim J, Koch W, et al. The incidence of p53 mutations increases with progression of head and neck cancer. *Clin Cancer Res* 1993;53:4477–4480.
130. el-Naggar AK, Lai S, Luna MA, et al. Sequential p53 mutation analysis of pre-invasive and invasive head and neck squamous carcinoma. *Int J Cancer* 1995;64:196–201.
131. Shin D, Kim J, Ro J, et al. Activation of p53 gene expression in premalignant lesions during head and neck tumorigenesis. *Clin Cancer Res* 1994;54:321–326.
132. Nees M, Homann N, Discher H, et al. Expression of mutated p53 occurs in tumor-distant epithelia of head and neck cancer patients: a possible molecular basis for the development of multiple tumors. *Clin Cancer Res* 1993; 53:4189–4196.
133. Chung KY, Mukhopadhyay T, Kim J, et al. Discordant p53 gene mutations in primary head and neck cancers and corresponding second primary cancers of the upper aerodigestive tract. *Clin Cancer Res* 1993;53:1676–1683.
134. Zariwala M, Schmid S, Pfaltz M, et al. p53 gene mutations in oropharyngeal carcinomas: a comparison of solitary and multiple primary tumours and lymph-node metastases. *Int J Cancer* 1994;56:807–811.
135. Gasparotto D, Maestro R, Barzan L, et al. Recurrences and second primary tumours in the head and neck region: differentiation by p53 mutation analysis. *Ann Oncol* 1995;6:933–939.
136. Tabor MP, Brakenhoff RH, van Houten VM, et al. Persistence of genetically altered fields in head and neck cancer patients: biological and clinical implications. *Clin Cancer Res* 2001;7:1523–1532.
137. Brennan J, Mao L, Hruban R, et al. Molecular assessment of histopathological staging in squamous-cell carcinoma of the head and neck. *N Engl J Med* 1995;332:429–435.
138. Shin DM, Lee JS, Lippman SM, et al. p53 expressions: Predicting recurrence and second primary tumors in head and neck squamous cell carcinoma. *J Natl Cancer Inst* 1996;88:519–529.
139. Lippman S, Shin D, Lee J, et al. p53 and retinoid chemoprevention of oral carcinogenesis. *Clin Cancer Res* 1995;55:16–19.
140. Kamb A, Gruis NA, Weaver-Feldhaus J, et al. A cell cycle regulator potentially involved in genesis of many tumor types. *Science* 1994;264:436–440.
141. Serrano M, Hannon GJ, Beach D. A new regulatory motif in cell-cycle control causing specific inhibition of cyclin D/CDK4. *Nature* 1993;366:704–707.
142. Reed AL, Califano J, Cairns P, et al. High frequency of p16 (CDKN2/MTS-1/INK4A) inactivation in head and neck squamous cell carcinoma. *Clin Cancer Res* 1996;56:3630–3633.
143. Cairns P, Mao L, Merlo A, et al. Rates of p16 (MTS1) mutations in primary tumors with 9p loss. *Science* 1994;265:415–417.
144. Merlo A, Herman JG, Mao L, et al. 5′ CpG island methylation is associated with transcriptional silencing of the tumour suppressor p16/CDKN2/MTS1 in human cancers. *Nature Med* 1995;1:686–692.
145. Cairns P, Polascik TJ, Eby Y, et al. Frequency of homozygous deletion at p16/CDKN2 in primary human tumours. *Nat Genet* 1995;11:210–212.
146. Wu CL, Roz L, McKown S, et al. DNA studies underestimate the major role of CDKN2A inactivation in oral and oropharyngeal squamous cell carcinomas. *Genes Chromosomes Cancer* 1999;25:16–25.
147. Papadimitrakopoulou V, Izzo J, Lippman SM, et al. Frequent inactivation of p161NK4a in oral premalignant lesions. *Oncogene* 1997;14:1799–1803.
148. Okami K, Reed AL, Cairns P, et al. Cyclin D1 amplification is independent of p16 inactivation in head and neck squamous cell carcinoma. *Oncogene* 1999; 18:3541–3545.
149. Hibi K, Takahashi T, Yamakawa K, et al. Three distinct regions involved in 3p deletion in human lung cancer. *Oncogene* 1992;7:445–449.
150. Killary AM, Wolf ME, Giambernardi TA, et al. Definition of a tumor suppressor locus within human chromosome 3p21-p22. *Proc Natl Acad Sci USA* 1992;89:10877–10881.
151. Maestro R, Gasparotto D, Vukosavljevic T, et al. Three discrete regions of deletion at 3p in head and neck cancers. *Clin Cancer Res* 1993;53:5775–5779.
152. Wu CL, Sloan P, Read AP, et al. Deletion mapping on the short arm of chromosome 3 in squamous cell carcinoma of the oral cavity. *Clin Cancer Res* 1994;54:6484–6488.
153. Kisielewski AE, Xiao GH, Liu SC, et al. Analysis of the FHIT gene and its product in squamous cell carcinomas of the head and neck. *Oncogene* 1998;17: 83–91.
154. Kinzler KW, Nilbert MC, Su LK, et al. Identification of FAP locus genes from chromosome 5q21. *Science* 1991;253:661–665.
155. Thompson AM, Morris RG, Wallace M, et al. Allele loss from 5q21 (APC/MCC) and 18q21 (DCC) and DCC mRNA expression in breast cancer. *Br J Cancer* 1993;68:64–68.
156. Uzawa K, Yoshida H, Suzuki H, et al. Abnormalities of the adenomatous polyposis coli gene in human oral squamous-cell carcinoma. *Int J Cancer* 1994;58:814–817.
157. Yoo G, Xu H, Brennan J, et al. Infrequent inactivation of the retinoblastoma gene despite frequent loss. *Clin Cancer Res* 1994;54:4603–4606.
158. Ali IU, Schriml LM, Dean M. Mutational spectra of PTEN/MMAC1 gene: a tumor suppressor with lipid phosphatase activity. *J Natl Cancer Inst* 1999;91: 1922–1932.
159. Steck PA, Pershouse MA, Jasser SA, et al. Identification of a candidate tumour suppressor gene, MMAC1, at chromosome 10q23.3 that is mutated in multiple advanced cancers. *Nat Genet* 1997;15:356–362.
160. Simpson L, Parsons R. PTEN: life as a tumor suppressor. *Exp Cell Res* 2001;264:29–41.
161. Poetsch M, Lorenz G, Kleist B. Detection of new PTEN/MMAC1 mutations in head and neck squamous cell carcinomas with loss of chromosome 10. *Cancer Genet Cytogenet* 2002;132:20–24.
162. Lee JI, Soria JC, Hassan KA, et al. Loss of PTEN expression as a prognostic marker for tongue cancer. *Arch Otolaryngol Head Neck Surg* 2001;127:1441–1445.
163. Baylin SB, Herman JG, Graff JR, et al. Alterations in DNA methylation: a fundamental aspect of neoplasia. *Adv Cancer Res* 1998;72:141–196.
164. Sanchez-Cespedes M, Esteller M, Wu L, et al. Gene promoter hypermethylation in tumors and serum of head and neck cancer patients. *Clin Cancer Res* 2000;60:892–895.
165. Papadimitrakopoulou V, Izzo J, Mao L, et al. Cyclin Dl and p16 alterations in advanced premalignant lesions of the upper aerodigestive tract: role in response to chemoprevention and cancer development. *Clin Cancer Res* 2001;7:3127–3134.

166. Bravo R, Frank R, Blundell PA, et al. Cyclin/PCNA is the auxiliary protein of DNA polymerase-delta. *Nature* 1987;326:515–517.
167. Celis JE, Celis A. Cell cycle-dependent variations in the distribution of the nuclear protein cyclin proliferating cell nuclear antigen in cultured cells: subdivision of S phase. *Proc Natl Acad Sci USA* 1985;82:3262–3266.
168. Shin DM, Voravud N, Ro JY, et al. Sequential increases in proliferating cell nuclear antigen expression in head and neck tumorigenesis: a potential biomarker. *J Natl Cancer Inst* 1993;85:971–978.
169. McCormick D, Hall PA. The complexities of proliferating cell nuclear antigen. *Histopathology* 1992;21:591–594.
170. Yu CC, Woods AL, Levison DA. The assessment of cellular proliferation by immunohistochemistry: a review of currently available methods and their applications. *Histochem J* 1992;24:121–131.
171. Leroy P, Krust A, Kastner P. Retinoic acid receptors. In: Morriss-Kay G, ed. *Retinoids in normal development and teratogenesis.* New York: Oxford University Press, 1992:77.
172. Lotan R, Nicolson GL. Inhibitory effects of retinoic acid or retinyl acetate on the growth of untransformed, transformed, and tumor cells in vitro. *J Natl Cancer Inst* 1977;59:1717–1722.
173. Breitman TR, Selonick SE, Collins SJ. Induction of differentiation of the human promyelocytic leukemia cell line (HL-60) by retinoic acid. *Proc Natl Acad Sci USA* 1980;77:2936–2940.
174. Thiele CJ, Deutsch LA, Israel MA. The expression of multiple proto-oncogenes is differentially regulated during retinoic acid-induced maturation of human neuroblastoma cell lines. *Oncogene* 1988;3:281–288.
175. Jetten AM. Multistep process of squamous differentiation of tracheobronchial epithelial cells: role of retinoids. *Dermatologica* 1987;175(suppl 1):37–44.
176. Moon RC, Mehta RG. Retinoid inhibition of experimental carcinogenesis. In: Dawson M, Okamura W, eds. *Chemistry and biology of synthetic retinoids.* Boca Raton, FL: CRC Press 1990:501.
177. Lippman SM, Kessler JF, Meyskens FLJ. Retinoids as preventive and therapeutic anticancer agents (Part II). *Cancer Treat Rep* 1987;71:493–515.
178. Harris CC, Kaufman DG, Sporn MB, et al. Histogenesis of squamous metaplasia and squamous cell carcinoma of the respiratory epithelium in an animal model. *Cancer Chemother Rep 3* 1973;4:43–47.
179. Gudas L, Spron M, Roberts A. Cellular biology and biochemistry of the retinoids. In: Sporn MB, Roberts AB, Goodman DS, eds. *The retinoids: biology, chemistry, and medicine.* New York: Raven Press, 1994:443.
180. Lotan R. Different susceptibilities of human melanoma and breast carcinoma cell lines to retinoic acid-induced growth inhibition. *Clin Cancer Res* 1979;39:1014–1019.
181. Hong WK, Endicott J, Itri LM, et al. 13-cis-retinoic acid in the treatment of oral leukoplakia. *N Engl J Med* 1986;315:1501–1505.
182. Hong WK, Lippman SM, Itri LM, et al. Prevention of second primary tumors with isotretinoin in squamous-cell carcinoma of the head and neck. *N Engl J Med* 1990;323:795–801.
183. Meyskens FL Jr, Surwit E, Moon TE, et al. Enhancement of regression of cervical intraepithelial neoplasia II (moderate dysplasia) with topically applied all-trans-retinoic acid: a randomized trial. *J Natl Cancer Inst* 1994;86:539–543.
184. Kraemer KH, DiGiovanna JJ, Moshell AN, et al. Prevention of skin cancer in xeroderma pigmentosum with the use of oral isotretinoin. *N Engl J Med* 1988;318:1633–1637.
185. Mangelsdorf DJ, Ong ES, Dyck JA, et al. Nuclear receptor that identifies a novel retinoic acid response pathway. *Nature* 1990;345:224–229.
186. Petkovich M, Brand NJ, Krust A, et al. A human retinoic acid receptor which belongs to the family of nuclear receptors. *Nature* 1987;330:444–450.
187. Roberts AB, Spom MB. Mechanistic interrelationships between two superfamilies: the steroid/retinoid receptors and transforming growth factor-beta. *Cancer Surv* 1992;14:205–220.
188. Leid M, Kastner P, Chambon P. Multiplicity generates diversity in the retinoic acid signaling pathways. *Trends Biochem Sci* 1992;17:427–433.
189. Costa A, Formelli F, Chiesa F, et al. Prospects of chemoprevention of human cancers with the synthetic retinoid fenretinide. *Clin Cancer Res* 1994;54: 2032s–2037s.
190. de The H, Lavau C, Marchio A, et al. The PML-RAR alpha fusion mRNA generated by the t(15;17) translocation in acute promyelocytic leukemia encodes a functionally altered RAR. *Cell* 1991;66:675–684.
191. Moasser MM, DeBlasio A, Dmitrovsky E. Response and resistance to retinoic acid are mediated through the retinoic acid nuclear receptor gamma in human teratocarcinomas. *Oncogene* 1994;9:833–840.
192. Lotan R, Xu XC, Lippman SM, et al. Suppression of retinoic acid receptor-beta in premalignant oral lesions and its up-regulation by isotretinoin. *N Engl J Med* 1995;332:1405–1410.
193. Xu XC, Ro JY, Lee JS, et al. Differential expression of nuclear retinoid receptors in normal, premalignant, and malignant head and neck tissues. *Clin Cancer Res* 1994;54:3580–3587.
194. Hu L, Crowe DL, Rheiwald JG, et al. Abnormal expression of retinoic acid receptors and keratin 19 by human oral and epidermal squamous cell carcinoma cell lines. *Clin Cancer Res* 1991;51:3972–3981.
195. Widschwendter M, Berger J, Hermann M, et al. Methylation and silencing of the retinoic acid receptor-beta2 gene in breast cancer. *J Natl Cancer Inst* 2000;92:826–832.
196. Lippman SM, Batsakis JG, Toth BB, et al. Comparison of low-dose isotretinoin with beta carotene to prevent oral carcinogenesis. *N Engl J Med* 1993;328:15–20.
197. Malone WF, Kelloff GJ, Pierson H, et al. Chemoprevention of bladder cancer. *Cancer* 1987;60:650–657.
198. Stinson SF, Reznik G, Donahoe R. Effect of three retinoids on tracheal carcinogenesis with *N*-methyl-*N*-nitrosourea in hamsters. *J Natl Cancer Inst* 1981;66:947–951.
199. Grubbs CJ, Becci PJ, Moon RC. Characterization of 1-methyl-nitrosourea (MNU)-induced tracheal carcinogenesis and the effect of feeding the retinoid *N*-(4-hydroxyphenyl) retinamide (4-HPR). *Proc Am Assoc Cancer Res* 1980;21: 102.
200. Zeigler RG. A review of epidemiologic evidence that carotenoids reduce the risk of cancer. *J Nutr* 1989;119:116–122.
201. Menkes MS, Comstock GW, Vuilleumier JP, et al. Serum beta-carotene, vitamins A and E, selenium, and the risk of lung cancer. *N Engl J Med* 1986;315: 1250–1254.
202. Peto R, Doll R, Buckley JD, et al. Can dietary beta-carotene materially reduce human cancer rates? *Nature* 1981;290:201–208.
203. The Alpha-Tocopherol BCCPSG. The effect of vitamin E and beta carotene on the incidence of lung cancer and other cancers in male smokers. *N Engl J Med* 1994;330:1029–1035.
204. Greenberg ER, Baron JA, Tosteson TD, et al. A clinical trial of antioxidant vitamins to prevent colorectal adenoma. Polyp Prevention Study Group. *N Engl J Med* 1994;331:141–147.
205. Greenberg ER, Baron JA, Stukel TA, et al. A clinical trial of beta carotene to prevent basal-cell and squamous-cell cancers of the skin. The Skin Cancer Prevention Study Group. *N Engl J Med* 1990;323:789–795.
206. Calhoun KH, Stanley D, Stiernberg CM, et al. Vitamins A and E do protect against oral carcinoma. *Arch Otolaryngol Head Neck Surg* 1989;115:484–488.
207. Shklar G. Oral mucosal carcinogenesis in hamsters: inhibition by vitamin E. *J Natl Cancer Inst* 1982;68:791–797.
208. Coombs GE, Scott ML. Antioxidant effects of selenium and vitamin E function in the chick. *J Nutr* 1974; 104:1297–1303.
209. Besa EC, Abrahm JL, Bartholomew MJ, et al. Treatment with 13-cis-retinoic acid in transfusion-dependent patients with myelodysplastic syndrome and decreased toxicity with addition of alpha-tocopherol. *Am J Med* 1990;89: 739–747.
210. Dimery I, Shirinian M, Heyne K, et al. Reduction in toxicity of high dose 13-cRA with alpha-tocopherol (AT). *Proc Am Soc Clin Oncol* 1992;11:145.
211. Shin DM, Ro JY, Hong WK, et al. Dysregulation of epidermal growth factor receptor expression in premalignant lesions during head and neck tumorigenesis. *Clin Cancer Res* 1994;54:3153–3159.
212. Baselga J, Herbst RS, LoRusso P, et al. Continuous administration of ZD1839 (Iressa), novel oral epidermal growth factor receptor tyrosine kinase inhibitor (EGFR-TKI), in patients with five selected tumor types: evidence of activity and good tolerability (abstract 686). Proceedings of American Society of Clinical Oncology 36th Annual Meeting, New Orleans, LA, 2000.
213. Eling TE, Thompson DC, Foureman GL, et al. Prostaglandin H synthase and xenobiotic oxidation. *Annu Rev Pharmacol Toxicol* 1990;30:1–45.
214. Eling TE, Curtis JF. Xenobiotic metabolism by prostaglandin H synthase. *Pharmacol Ther* 1992;53:261–273.
215. Jung TT, Berlinger NT, Juhn SK. Prostaglandins in squamous cell carcinoma of the head and neck: a preliminary study. *Laryngoscope* 1985;95:307–312.
216. Tsujii M, DuBois RN. Alterations in cellular adhesion and apoptosis in epithelial cells overexpressing prostaglandin endoperoxide synthase 2. *Cell* 1995;83:493–501.
217. Oshima M, Dinchuk JE, Kargman SL, et al. Suppression of intestinal polyposis in Apc delta716 knockout mice by inhibition of cyclooxygenase 2 (COX-2). *Cell* 1996;87:803–809.
218. Kujubu DA, Fletcher BS, Varnum BC, et al. TIS 10, a phorbol ester tumor promoter-inducible mRNA from Swiss 3T3 cells, encodes a novel prostaglandin synthase/cyclooxygenase homologue. *J Biol Chem* 1991;266:12866–12872.
219. O'Banion MK, Sadowski HB, Winn V, et al. A serum- and glucocorticoid-regulated 4-kilobase mRNA encodes a cyclooxygenase-related protein. *J Biol Chem* 1991;266:23261–23267.
220. DuBois RN, Awad J, Morrow J, et al. Regulation of eicosanoid production and mitogenesis in rat intestinal epithelial cells by transforming growth factor-alpha and phorbol ester. *J Clin Invest* 1994;93:493–498.
221. Kelley DJ, Mestre JR, Subbaramaiah K, et al. Benzo[a]pyrene up-regulates cyclooxygenase-2 gene expression in oral epithelial cells. *Carcinogenesis* 1997;18:795–799.
222. Rao CV, Rivenson A, Simi B, et al. Chemoprevention of colon carcinogenesis by sulindac, a nonsteroidal anti-inflammatory agent. *Clin Cancer Res* 1995;55: 1464–1472.
223. McCormick DL, Moon RC. Inhibition of mammary carcinogenesis by flurbiprofen, a non-steroidal antiinflammatory agent. *Br J Cancer* 1983;48:859–861.
224. Kawamori T, Rao CV, Seibert K, et al. Chemopreventive activity of celecoxib, a specific cyclooxygenase-2 inhibitor, against colon carcinogenesis. *Clin Cancer Res* 1998;58:409–412.
225. Giardiello FM, Hamilton SR, Krush AJ, et al. Treatment of colonic and rectal adenomas with sulindac in familial adenomatous polyposis. *N Engl J Med* 1993;328:1313–1316.
226. Weitzman SA, Gordon LI. Inflammation and cancer: Role of phagocyte-generated oxidants in carcinogenesis. *Blood* 1990;76:655–663.
227. Steinbach G, Lynch PM, Phillips RK, et al. The effect of celecoxib, a cyclooxygenase-2 inhibitor, in familial adenomatous polyposis. *N Engl J Med* 2000; 342:1946–1952.
228. Chan G, Boyle JO, Yang EK, et al. Cyclooxygenase-2 expression is up-regu-

lated in squamous cell carcinoma of the head and neck. *Clin Cancer Res* 1999;59:991–994.
229. Zohn IM, Campbell SL, Khosravi-Far R, et al. Rho family proteins and Ras transformation: the RHOad less traveled gets congested. *Oncogene* 1998;17: 1415–1438.
230. Barbacid M. Ras genes. *Annu Rev Biochem* 1987;56:779–827.
231. Bollag G, McCormick F. Regulators and effectors of ras proteins. *Annu Rev Cell Biol* 1991;7:601–632.
232. Sebti SM, Hamilton AD. Farnesyltransferase and geranylgeranyltransferase I inhibitors in cancer therapy: important mechanistic and bench to bedside issues. *Expert Opin Invest Drugs* 2000;9:2767–2782.
233. Kies MS, Clayman G, El-Naggar AK, et al. Induction therapy with SCH 66336, a farnesyltransferase inhibitor, in squamous cell carcinoma (SCC) of the head and neck (abstract 896). *Proceedings of the American Society of Clinical Oncology 37th Annual Meeting*, San Francisco, CA, 2001
234. Khuri FR, Kim ES, Lee JJ, et al. The impact of smoking status, disease stage, and index tumor site on second primary tumor incidence and tumor recurrence in the head and neck retinoid chemoprevention trial. *Cancer Epidemiol Biomark Prevent* 2001;10:823–829.
235. Definition of leukoplakia and related lesions: an aid to studies on precancer. *Oral Surg Oral Med Oral Pathol Oral Radiol Endodont* 1978;46:517–539.
236. Silverman SJ, Shillitoe EJ. Etiology and predisposing factors. In: Silverman S, ed. *Oral cancer.* Atlanta: American Cancer Society, 1988:7.
237. Bouquot JE, Gorlin RJ. Leukoplakia, lichen planus, and other oral keratoses in 23,616 white Americans over the age of 35 years. *Oral Surg Oral Med Oral Pathol Oral Radiol Endodont* 1986;61:373–381.
238. Wolf K. Zur vitamin A behandlung der leukoplakien [On use of vitamin A in treatment of leukoplakia]. *Arch Klin Exp Derm* 1957;206:495–498.
239. Silverman S, Eisenberg E, Renstrup G. A study of the effects of high-dose of vitamin A on oral leukoplakia (hyperkeratosis), including toxicity, liver function, and skeletal metabolism. *J Oral Ther Phamacol* 1965;2:9–23.
240. Koch HE. Effect of retinoids on precancerous lesions of oral mucosa. In: Orfanos CE, Braun-Falco O, Farber EM, eds. *Retinoids: advances in basic research and therapy.* Berlin: Springer-Verlag, 1981:307.
241. Han J, Jiao L, Lu Y, et al. Evaluation of *N*-4-(hydroxycarbophenyl) retinamide as a cancer prevention agent and as a cancer chemotherapeutic agent. *In Vivo* 1990;4:153–160.
242. Chiesa F, Tradati N, Marazza M, et al. Prevention of local relapses and new localisations of oral leukoplakias with the synthetic retinoid fenretinide (4-HPR): preliminary results. *Eur J Cancer B Oral Oncol* 1992;28B:97–102.
243. Chiesa F, Tradati N, Marazza M, et al. Fenretinide (4-HPR) in chemoprevention of oral leukoplakia. *J Cellular Biochem Suppl* 1993;17F:255–261.
244. Papadimitrakopoulou VA, Lippman SM, Lee JS, et al. Long term follow-up of low-dose isotretinoin (13-cRA) versus beta carotene to prevent oral carcinogenesis. *Proc Am Assoc Cancer Res* 1996;15:340.
245. Omenn GS, Goodman GE, Thornquist MD, et al. Effects of a combination of beta carotene and vitamin A on lung cancer and cardiovascular disease. *N Engl J Med* 1996;334:1150–1155.
246. Hennekens CH, Buring JE, Manson JE, et al. Lack of effect of long-term supplementation with beta carotene on the incidence of malignant neoplasms and cardiovascular disease. *N Engl J Med* 1996;334:1145–1149.
247. Stich BF, Hornby AP, Mathew B, et al. Response of oral leukoplakias to the administration of vitamin A. *Cancer Lett* 1988;40:93–101.
248. Lotan R, Lee J, Martin J, et al. Retinamide activity in retinoid-resistant oral premalignant lesions (OPLS): translational correlative studies. *Proceedings of the American Society of Clinical Oncology 36th Annual Meeting*, New Orleans, LA, 2000.
249. Garewal HS, Meyskens FL Jr, Killen D, et al. Response of oral leukoplakia to beta-carotene. *J Clin Oncol* 1990;8:1715–1720.
250. Malaker K, Anderson BJ, Beecroft WA, et al. Management of oral mucosal dysplasia with beta-carotene retinoic acid: a pilot cross-over study. *Cancer Detect Prevent* 1991;15:335–340.
251. Toma S, Benso S, Albanese E, et al. Treatment of oral leukoplakia with beta-carotene. *Oncology* 1992;49:77–81.
252. Toma S, Coialbu T, Collecchi P, et al. [Biological aspects and perspectives applicable to the chemoprevention of cancer of the upper respiratory-digestive tract]. *Acta Otorhinolaryngol Ital* 1990;10(suppl 27):41–54.
253. Benner SE, Winn RJ, Lippman SM, et al. Regression of oral leukoplakia with alpha-tocopherol: a community clinical oncology program chemoprevention study. *J Natl Cancer Inst* 1993;85:44–47.
254. Kaugars GE, Silverman S Jr, Lovas JG, et al. A clinical trial of antioxidant supplements in the treatment of oral leukoplakia. *Oral Surg Oral Med Oral Pathol Oral Radiol Endodont* 1994;78:462–468.
255. Zaridze D, Evstifeeva T, Boyle P. Chemoprevention of oral leukoplakia and chronic esophagitis in an area of high incidence of oral and esophageal cancer. *Ann Epidemiol* 1993;3:225–234.
256. Messadi DV, Billings P, Shklar G, et al. Inhibition of oral carcinogenesis by a protease inhibitor. *J Natl Cancer Inst* 1986;76:447–452.
257. Armstrong WB, Kennedy AR, Wan XS, et al. Clinical modulation of oral leukoplakia and protease activity by Bowman-Birk inhibitor concentrate in a phase IIa chemoprevention trial. *Clin Cancer Res* 2000;6:4684–4691.
258. Silverman S, Renstrup G, Pindborg JJ. Studies in oral leukoplakias: III. Effects of vitamin A comparing clinical, histopathologic, cytologic, and hematologic responses. *Acta Odontol Scand* 1963;21:271–292.
259. Ryssel HJ, Brunner KW, Bollag W. [The oral administration of vitamin-A-acid in leukoplakias, hyperkeratoses, and squamous cell carcinomas: results and tolerance]. *Schweiz Med Wochenschr* 1971;101:1027–1030.
260. Stuttgen G. Oral vitamin A acid therapy. *Acta Derm Venereol Suppl* 1975;74: 174–179.
261. Raque CJ, Biondo RV, Keeran MG, et al. Snuff dippers keratosis snuff-induced leukoplakia). *South Med J* 1975;68:565–568.
262. Koch HF. Biochemical treatment of precancerous oral lesions: the effectiveness of various analogues of retinoic acid. *J Craniomaxillofac Surg* 1978;6:59–63.
263. Cordero AA, Allevato MAJ, Barclay CA, et al. Treatment of lichen planus and leukoplakia with the oral retinoid RO 10-9359. In: Orfanos CE, ed. *Retinoids: advances in basic research and therapy.* Berlin: Springer-Verlag, 1981:273.
264. Shah JP, Strong EW, DeCosse JJ, et al. Effect of retinoids on oral leukoplakia. *Am J Surg* 1983;146:466–470.
265. Khuri FR, Nemunaitis J, Ganly I, et al. A controlled trial of intratumoral ONYX-015, a selectively-replicating adenovirus, in combination with cisplatin and 5-fluorouracil in patients with recurrent head and neck cancer. *Nature Med* 2000;6:879–885.
266. Hong WK, Sporn MB. Recent advances in chemoprevention of cancer. *Science* 1997;278:1073–1077.
267. Brenner DE. Multiagent chemopreventive agent combinations. *J Cell Biochem Suppl* 2000;34:121–124.
268. Torrance CJ, Jackson PE, Montgomery E, et al. Combinatorial chemoprevention of intestinal neoplasia. *Nature Med* 2000;6:1024–1028.
269. Papadimitrakopoulou VA, Clayman GL, Shin DM, et al. Biochemoprevention for dysplastic lesions of the upper aerodigestive tract. *Arch Otolaryngol Head Neck Surg* 1999;125:1083–1089.
270. Lippman SM, Kavanagh JJ, Paredes-Espinoza M, et al. 13-cis-retinoic acid plus interferon alpha-2a: highly active systemic therapy for squamous cell carcinoma of the cervix. *J Natl Cancer Inst* 1992;84:241–245.
271. Lippman SM, Parkinson DR, Itri LM, et al. 13-cis-retinoic acid and interferon alpha-2a: effective combination therapy for advanced squamous cell carcinoma of the skin. *J Natl Cancer Inst* 1992;84:235–241.
272. Healy GB, Gelber RD, Trowbridge AL, et al. Treatment of recurrent respiratory papillomatosis with human leukocyte interferon: results of a multicenter randomized clinical trial. *N Engl J Med* 1988;319:401–407.
273. Lippman SM, Donovan DT, Frankenthaler RA, et al. 13-cis-retinoic acid plus interferon-alpha 2a in recurrent respiratory papillomatosis. *J Natl Cancer Inst* 1994;86:859–861.
274. Toma S, Palumbo R, Gustavino C, et al. Efficacy of the association of 13-cis-retinoic acid (13cRA) and interferon a 2a (IFNa2a) in cervical intraepithelial neoplasia (CIN II-III): a pilot study. *Proc Am Soc Clin Oncol* 1994;13:258.
275. Mao L, El-Naggar AK, Papadimitrakopoulou V, et al. Phenotype and genotype of advanced premalignant head and neck lesions after chemopreventive therapy. *J Natl Cancer Inst* 1998;90:1545–1551.
276. Lippman SM, Hong WK. Not yet standard: retinoids versus second primary tumors. *J Clin Oncol* 1993;11:1204–1207.
277. Lippman SM, Hong WK. Second malignant tumors in head and neck squamous cell carcinoma: the overshadowing threat for patients with early-stage disease. *Int J Radiat Oncol Biol Phys* 1989;17:691–694.
278. Tepperman BS, Fitzpatrick PJ. Second respiratory and upper digestive tract cancers after oral cancer. *Lancet* 1981;2:547–549.
279. McDonald S, Haie C, Rubin P, et al. Second malignant tumors in patients with laryngeal carcinoma: diagnosis, treatment, and prevention. *Int J Radiat Oncol Biol Phys* 1989;17:457–465.
280. Licciardello JT, Spitz MR, Hong WK. Multiple primary cancer in patients with cancer of the head and neck: second cancer of the head and neck, esophagus, and lung. *Int J Radiat Oncol Biol Phys* 1989; 17:467–476.
281. Vikram B. Changing patterns of failure in advanced head and neck cancer. *Arch Otolaryngol Head Neck Surg* 1984;110:564–565.
282. Dan GL, Blot WJ, Shore RE, et al. Second cancers following oral and pharyngeal cancers: role of tobacco and alcohol. *J Natl Cancer Inst* 1994;86:131–137.
283. Benner SE, Pajak TF, Lippman SM, et al. Prevention of second primary tumors with isotretinoin in patients with squamous cell carcinoma of the head and neck: long-term follow-up. *J Natl Cancer Inst* 1994;86:140–141.
284. Bolla M, Lefur R, Ton Van J, et al. Prevention of second primary tumours with etretinate in squamous cell carcinoma of the oral cavity and oropharynx: results of a multicentric double-blind randomised study. *Eur J Cancer* 1994;30A:767–772.
285. van Zandwijk N, Dalesio O, Pastorino U, et al. EUROSCAN, a randomized trial of vitamin A and *N*-acetylcysteine in patients with head and neck cancer or lung cancer. For the European Organization for Research and Treatment of Cancer Head and Neck and Lung Cancer Cooperative Groups. *J Natl Cancer Inst* 2000;92:977–986.
285a. Khuri F, Lee JJ, Lippman SM, et al. Isotretinoin effects on head and neck cancer recurrence and second primary tumors. *Proc Ann Soc Clin Oncol* 2003; 22:90 (abstract).
286. Pastorino U, Infante M, Maioli M, et al. Adjuvant treatment of stage I lung cancer with high-dose vitamin A. *J Clin Oncol* 1993;11:1216–1222.
287. Pinto H, Li Y, Loprinzi C, et al. Phase III trial of low-dose 13-cis-retinoic acid for prevention of second primary cancers in stage I-II head and neck cancer: an Eastern Cooperative Oncology Group study (abstract 886). *Proceedings of American Society of Clinical Oncology 37th Annual Meeting*, San Francisco, CA, 2001.

CHAPTER 41

Molecular Targeting of the Epidermal Growth Factor Receptor in Head and Neck Cancer

Paul M. Harari, Shyh-Min Huang, Roy S. Herbst, and Harry Quon

Among the many diagnostic and therapeutic advances currently taking shape in head and neck (HN) oncology, perhaps no more promising arena exists than that now emerging from efforts to pharmacologically modulate specific molecular targets that control tumor growth. The epidermal growth factor receptor (EGFR) represents one such molecular target that appears particularly important for the growth and spread of squamous cell carcinomas (SCCs) of the head and neck (HNSCCs). Indeed, among human malignancies, the highest frequency of EGFR overexpression is found in HNSCCs. A series of high-precision molecular agents have been designed to target the EGFR for growth inhibition, and these agents are currently progressing to maturity in clinical trials around the world. Preliminary results suggest that these agents may have the capacity to augment the effectiveness of radiation and selected chemotherapy agents without enhancing toxicity profiles, and therefore may facilitate meaningful therapeutic gains for the HN cancer patient. This chapter provides an overview of the biology, rationale, and preclinical and early clinical results of the use of EGFR inhibitors in HN cancer therapy.

EPIDERMAL GROWTH FACTOR RECEPTOR FAMILY: STRUCTURE/FUNCTION

Structure

Human growth factors belong to a family of polypeptides that are capable of stimulating proliferation and/or differentiation following binding to specific cellular receptors. One of the earliest growth factors to be characterized was the epidermal growth factor (EGF) (1). The EGF receptor family is composed of four closely related transmembrane receptors. In mammals, the EGF receptor family includes ErbB1 (also called EGFR), ErbB2 (c-Neu), ErbB3, and ErbB4 (Fig. 41.1). The human EGF receptor family is also commonly referred to as the HER family. These receptors possess tyrosine kinase activity directed against tyrosine residues of the receptor itself or targeted downstream molecules. The epidermal growth factor receptor is the first ErbB receptor member to be described and sequenced (2). It is composed of a single polypeptide chain of 1,186 amino acids with three distinct regions, namely, an extracellular ligand binding region, a transmembrane lipophilic segment, and an intracellular protein kinase domain (3,4). The extracellular domain of the EGFR is characterized by a high content of cysteine residues. It is known that these two cysteine-rich domains compose the ligand binding domain. Six EGFR ligands have been well characterized, including EGF, transforming growth factor-α (TGF-α), amphiregulin, heparin-binding EGF-like growth factor (HB-EGF), betacellulin, and epiregulin (Fig. 41.1). The most widely expressed ligand for the EGFR in human tissues is TGF-α. The intracellular sequences encode tyrosine kinase and the carboxy-terminal regulatory functions. Binding of adenosine triphosphate (ATP) to a lysine residue at position 721 within the EGFR kinase domain represents the key event required to initiate tyrosine kinase activity of the receptor. All known functions of the EGFR appear to depend on the tyrosine kinase activity.

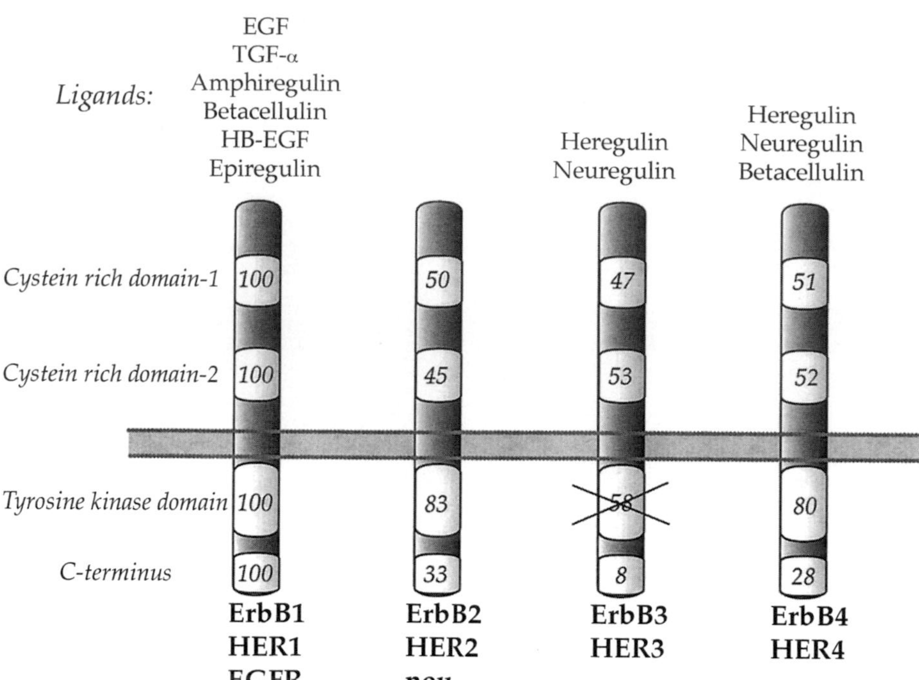

Figure 41.1 Schematic diagram of the four ErbB family members and their ligands. Numbers denote the degree (expressed as a percentage) of homology relative to ErbB1/EGFR. With the exception of the kinase-deficient ErbB3, there exists a high degree of homology in the tyrosine kinase domain. EGFR, epidermal growth factor receptor; HB-EGF, heparin-binding EGF-like growth factor; TGF-α, transforming growth factor-α. (Courtesy of AstraZeneca, Wilmington, DE.)

Signaling

Following ligand binding, the EGFR undergoes dimerization. Dimerization activates the intrinsic protein kinase via intermolecular autophosphorylation within the cytoplasmic domain. Tyrosine phosphorylation of specific residues of the EGFR creates binding sites for Src-homology 2 (SH2) and phosphotyrosine-binding (PTB)-domain–containing proteins. These proteins function as adaptors or activators that then initiate a cascade of signals from the cytoplasm to the nucleus, eventually resulting in cellular proliferation and differentiation (5,6). The best understood signaling pathway triggered by EGFR stimulation involves activation of Ras following the recruitment of SOS to the plasma membrane via adaptor proteins Grb2 and/or Shc. Once loaded with guanosine triphosphate (GTP), Ras is capable of interacting with effectors such as Raf, which ultimately lead to the activation of mitogen-activated protein kinase (MAPK) and subsequent regulation of gene transcription (Fig. 41.2). Epidermal growth factor receptor kinases are also found to trigger various signaling pathways including those involving phospholipase C-γ (PLC-γ) and its downstream protein kinase C (PKC)-mediated cascades, small guanosine triphosphatases (GTPases) such as rho, multiple STAT (signal transducer and activator of transcription) isoforms, and heterotrimeric G proteins (5,7). Therefore, signaling mediated by the EGFR cannot be considered as a simple linear pathway from cell surface to nucleus (8,9). At the terminus of these signaling cascades, activity is translated into distinct transcriptional programs. These may involve the protooncogenes *fos, jun,* and *myc,* as well as zinc-finger-containing transcription factors, such as Sp1 and Egr1 (8). Understanding the complexity of EGFR signaling networks is central to our understanding of organ development and the molecular pathogenesis of complex diseases such as cancer.

Function

Epidermal growth factor receptor signaling precipitates a wide range of effects depending on the tissue-specific origin and state of differentiation. The role of EGFR signaling in tumor cell proliferation is well recognized, but is also important in modulating tumor cell migration, angiogenesis, maturation, invasion, and apoptotic response. These factors are now recognized as critical in influencing the growth and progression of many human cancers (10). There is also evidence to suggest that EGFR signaling may be involved in the malignant transformation process (11,12), and may also drive tumor phenotypic changes that can affect cellular response to therapy (13).

Mutation

Overexpression of EGFR in human malignancy has been the subject of extensive study. Indeed, it has become increasingly apparent that structural alterations in EGFR may be as important as amplification with respect to oncogenic potential. In addition to the wild-type EGFR molecule, two alternative forms exist. One form is secreted EGFR (sEGFR), which is produced by alternative splicing just before the transmembrane domain. Evidence reveals that sEGFR levels in patient serum decline during clinical progression of ovarian cancer (14,15). However, the overall function of these soluble EGFR isoforms remains largely unknown. The other form of EGFR mutants (EGFRvI, vII, and vIII) contains distinct deletions in the extracellular domain and have been detected in several human cancers (Fig. 41.3). EGFRvIII represents the most common and best described of these mutations to date. The EGFRvIII mutation occurs in a spectrum of human cancers, most notably in patients with high-grade gliomas, but also in a cohort of patients with lung, breast, prostate, and ovarian carcinomas. This mutation is commonly overexpressed as a result of gene amplification (16–18). The gene representing the EGFRvIII mutant possesses an in-frame deletion of 801 base pairs, corresponding to exon 2 to 7 in the messenger RNA (mRNA), resulting in the deletion of amino acids 6 to 273 in the extracellular domain and the generation of a glycine at the fusion point (Fig. 41.3) (19). The resultant

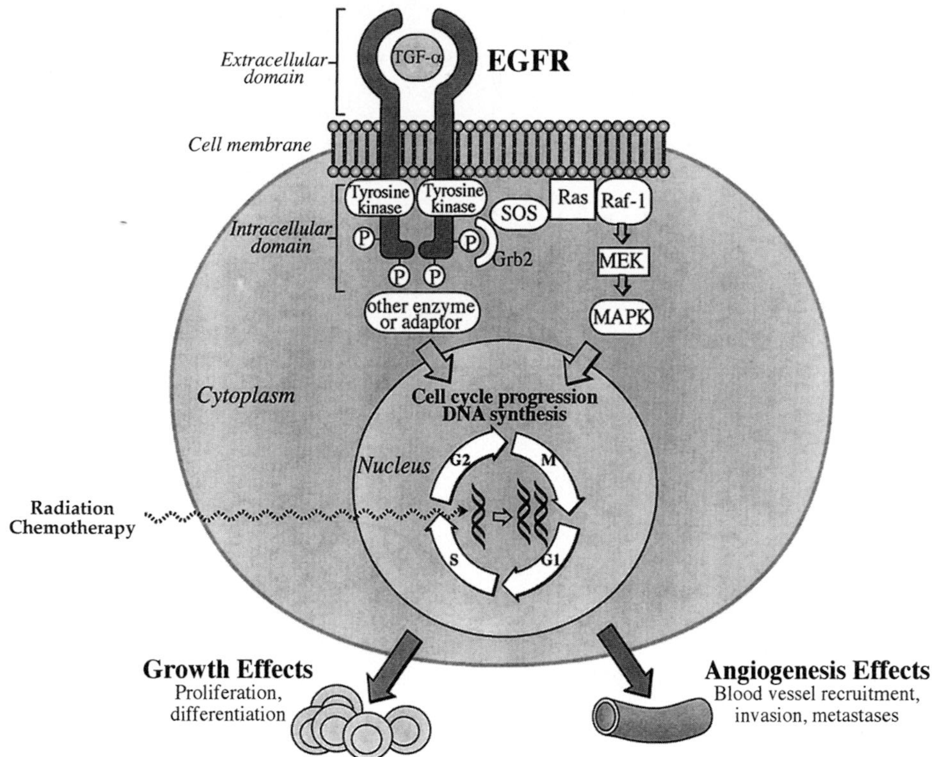

Figure 41.2 Schematic illustration of the epidermal growth factor receptor (EGFR) system depicting EGFR, mitogen-activated protein kinase (MAPK) signal transduction cascade to the nucleus, and resultant stimulation of cell cycle machinery. Potential interactions and effects of radiation and selected chemotherapy agents on the EGFR system are discussed in the text. TGF-α, transforming growth factor-α. (From Huang S-M, Harari PM. Epidermal growth factor receptor inhibition in cancer therapy: biology, rationale and preliminary clinical results. *Invest New Drugs* 1999;17:259–269, with permission.)

tumor-specific epitope is situated near the amino terminus of the receptor (extracellular domain) and can serve as a target for monoclonal antibodies. The EGFRvIII is not capable of natural ligand binding, as the deletion alters the ligand binding site. Therefore, this mutated receptor commonly shows constitutive activation, although with attenuated tyrosine kinase activity. Tumor progression may be promoted by constitutive receptor activation, impaired receptor down-regulation, activation of alternative signaling cascades, abrogation of apoptotic pathways, or other mechanisms (20–22). The EGFRvIII, which is not expressed in normal tissues, but only in cancers, has provided a highly specific internalizing target for antibody-mediated approaches in cancer therapy (19,23–26).

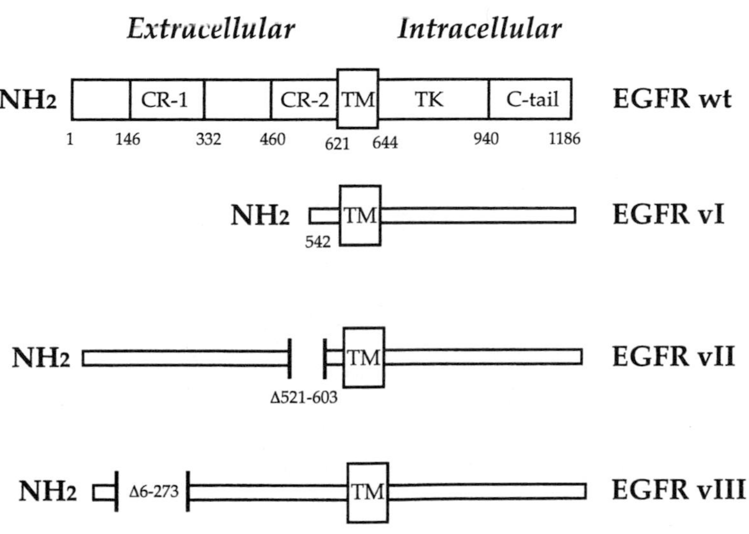

Figure 41.3 Schematic illustration of wild-type (wt) epidermal growth factor receptor (EGFR) and mutant forms. CR-1 and CR-2, cysteine-rich domains; TM, transmembrane segment; TK, tyrosine kinase domain. Amino acid residue numbers lie below the structure. (From Kuan CT, Wikstrand CJ, Bigner DD. EGF mutant receptor vIII as a molecular target in cancer therapy. *Endocr Relat Cancer* 2001;8:83–96, with permission.)

EPIDERMAL GROWTH FACTOR RECEPTOR OVEREXPRESSION AND CLINICAL IMPLICATIONS

Overexpression

Overexpression of EGFR has been identified and correlated with adverse clinical outcome across a broad spectrum of cancer patients. The precise nature of the protein overexpression remains to be fully defined. However, it is generally believed to reflect an increase in the rate of transcription (27,28), without apparent change in mRNA stability (29,30), although gene amplification is observed in some instances (31–33). Both qualitative and quantitative immunohistochemical measures of protein expression are reported with results revealing EGFR overexpression in 42% to 98% of specimens (34–38). Though the optimal assay for quantification of EGFR expression remains in evolution, current efforts focus on quantitative rather than qualitative protein expression methodologies. The former may be advantageous in reflecting not only increased EGFR cellular expression but also variations in topographic distribution throughout tissues, reflecting biologic consequences of EGFR autocrine activity.

Clinical Significance

Immunohistochemical studies characterize the topographic distribution of EGFR throughout the carcinogenic process. Based on analyses of normal and premalignant mucosa from patients with HNSCC, an early role for EGFR in the process of SCC carcinogenesis is implicated (29,39–41). Retinoids, which demonstrate therapeutic efficacy in the treatment of oral leukoplakia (42), are shown to normalize the increased transcription rate of not only EGFR but also its primary ligand, TGF-α (27,28,43).

Several studies demonstrate increased mRNA and protein expression for both EGFR and TGF-α in normal mucosa from patients with HNSCC. Grandis et al. (29,39,40) demonstrated increased expression of TGF-α throughout all layers of histologically abnormal mucosal epithelium coupled with progressively increased EGFR staining in advancing premalignant lesions (compared with normal mucosa). Similar changes in the staining pattern of advancing premalignant lesions are observed for p53 (44) and cyclin D1 (45). Grandis et al. (46) elaborated by demonstrating that wild-type p53 may function as a regulator of EGFR transcription in a temperature-sensitive p53 mutant HNSCC cell line. In addition, cells dominated by EGFR overexpression can abrogate the normal G_1 to S phase cell cycle regulatory events by increasing their expression of cyclin D1 (47).

Shin et al. (41) demonstrated that EGFR overexpression may evolve in stages, and is observed in normal epithelium adjacent to tumor in contrast to normal epithelium distant from malignancy. The level of EGFR overexpression remains elevated in hyperplastic and dysplastic premalignant lesions, consistent with a possible role in tumor initiation and promotion. There is further increase in the staining intensity of invasive lesions, suggesting a role for EGFR in the development of a malignant phenotype. These observations are consistent with preclinical studies demonstrating a relationship between EGFR overexpression and components of malignant progression. *In vitro* and *in vivo* models suggest that EGFR signaling inhibition may alter angiogenesis (48,49), adhesion (50,51), motility (51–53), and invasion (51,52,54) properties of the malignant cell.

Prognostic Significance

The clinical relevance of EGFR overexpression in HN cancer is supported by studies from Grandis et al. (55). Independent prognostic value for EGFR and TGF-α is demonstrated in a mature cohort of 91 HN cancer patients of whom 56 received postoperative radiation therapy and 16 received adjuvant chemotherapy following primary surgical resection. Protein expression is quantified by immunohistochemistry from paraffin-embedded specimens. Expression of EGFR and/or TGF-α is associated with adverse disease-free and cause-specific survival (Fig. 41.4). These observations are strengthened by the use of quantitative assays that reflect not only EGFR overexpression at the cellular level but changes in topographic distribution. The demonstration of prognostic significance independent of traditional prognostic factors, including T-stage and N-stage for both disease-free and cause-specific survival, suggests the clinical relevance and potential utility of quantitative EGFR and TGF-α assays.

Additional independent reports suggest a prognostic significance of EGFR protein overexpression (56–59). In a prospective cohort of 140 patients with laryngeal carcinomas treated primarily with surgery, Maurizi et al. (57) demonstrated a strong independent significance of EGFR protein expression for the end points of relapse-free and overall survival. These investigators identify a 5-year survival of 81% versus 25% for EGFR-negative and EGFR-positive tumors, respectively ($p < 0.0001$). Similarly, the 5-year relapse-free survival is 77% and 24%, respectively ($p < 0.01$). Dassonville et al. (58) report results for a heterogeneous group of 103 patients with advanced HNSCC treated with primary combination chemotherapy (60 patients), surgery (29 patients), or radiation therapy (six patients). A cut-

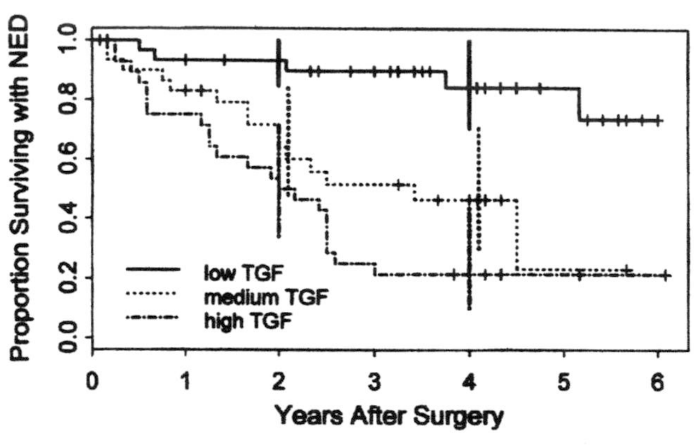

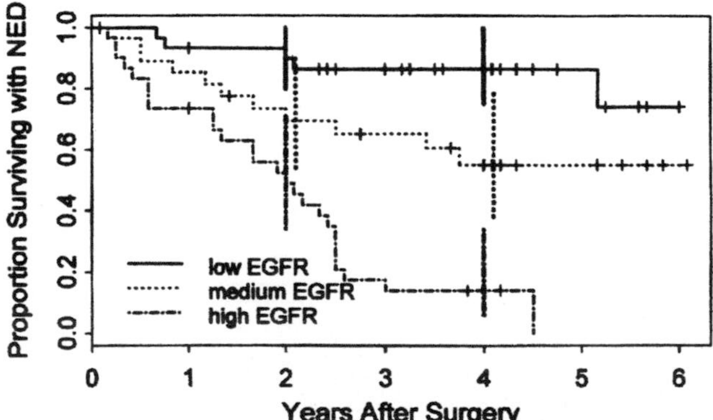

Figure 41.4 Disease-free survival plot for series of 91 head and neck cancer patients showing inverse correlation between epidermal growth factor receptor (EGFR)/transforming growth factor-α (TGF-α) protein levels and patient survival. (From Grandis JR, Melhem MF, Gooding WE, et al. Levels of TGF-alpha and EGFR protein in head and neck squamous cell carcinoma and patient survival. *J Natl Cancer Inst* 1998;90:824–832, with permission.)

off of 120 fmol/mg EGFR protein is determined to yield significant divergence in patient prognosis for both relapse-free and overall survival.

Magne et al. (56) extends the observations of Dassonville et al. by reporting significant prognostic influence for EGFR overexpression in 77 consecutively treated patients with unresectable SCC of the oropharynx and hypopharynx. This cohort of relatively homogeneously treated patients received hyperfractionated radiotherapy concurrent with three cycles of cisplatin and 5-fluorouracil (5-FU). Multivariate analysis for end points including time to progression and overall survival reveals that Karnofsky index and EGFR protein levels are significant outcome predictors, independent of traditional clinical parameters (Fig. 41.5).

Most recently, a study by K. Ang et al. (personal communication) has examined the impact of EGFR overexpression on survival and patterns of failure in patients with advanced HNSCC who received conventional radiotherapy fractionation within a phase III Radiation Therapy Oncology Group (RTOG) trial. The study cohort consisted of 155 randomized patients with sufficient pretreatment biopsy material for immunohistochemical staining of EGFR. This investigation revealed that EGFR expression was a strong independent prognostic indicator for overall and disease-free survival as well as a predictor for locoregional relapse but not for distant metastasis in advanced HN cancer patients.

Although not all reported studies capture a clear correlation between EGFR/TGF-α and clinical outcome, the preponderance of accumulating data strongly suggests that this association exists. Particularly in patients with HNSCC, a powerful linkage is emerging between EGFR/TGF-α protein levels and adverse outcome. As EGFR assay techniques are further refined and standardized across laboratories, and prospective clinical trials further define the relationship between EGFR/TGF-α expression and patient outcome, we can anticipate these parameters becoming more central to prospective design of clinical trials and individual patient treatment strategies.

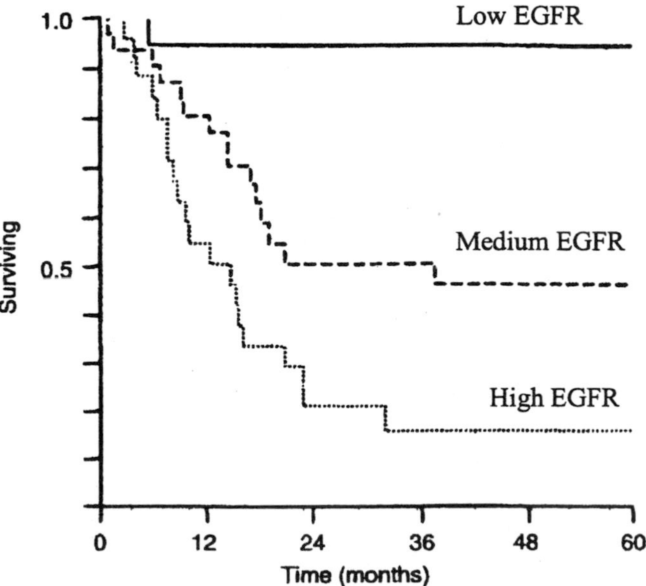

Figure 41.5 Overall survival plot for series of 77 head and neck cancer patients (advanced oropharynx and hypopharynx squamous cell carcinoma) showing inverse correlation between epidermal growth factor receptor (EGFR) protein level and survival. (From Magne N, Pivot X, Bensadoun RJ, et al. The relationship of epidermal growth factor receptor levels to the prognosis of unresectable pharyngeal cancer patients treated by chemo-radiotherapy. *Eur J Cancer* 2001;37:2169–2177, with permission.)

STRATEGIES/AGENTS FOR EPIDERMAL GROWTH FACTOR RECEPTOR INHIBITION

From the time EGFR signaling inhibition was first proposed as a promising anticancer treatment strategy (60,61) until the present, a broad array of EGFR inhibitors has been developed (62–68). For the purpose of general classification, the majority of these agents can be broadly categorized as large antibody molecules or small tyrosine kinase inhibitors (Table 41.1). Within the antibody class of EGFR inhibitors are monoclonal, bi-specific, and immunotoxin conjugate molecules (69–72). These agents have as their common molecular target the extracellular domain of the EGFR. Within the tyrosine kinase inhibitor category, there are well over a dozen agents that are commonly subcategorized as quinazolines, pyridopyrimidines/pyrrolopyrimidines, and tyrphostins based on their basic chemical structure (73–79) (Fig. 41.6). The molecular target for these small molecule EGFR inhibitors resides at the level of the intracellular tyrosine kinase domain. These agents most commonly inhibit tyrosine kinase phosphorylation through a physical interaction with either the ATP and/or the enzyme substrate binding sites (80). Although there exist a variety of promising molecular targets downstream of the EGFR, the focus of this chapter is on agents exhibiting direct interaction with the EGFR molecule itself.

The fact that EGFR inhibitors can be crudely classified as large molecules (antibodies) and small molecules (tyrosine kinase inhibitors) provides a convenient initial framework for considering routes of drug administration as well as potential toxicity profiles. The large molecule antibodies and conjugates generally require intravenous administration and possess relatively long half-lives, thereby supporting weekly administration schedules. Several potential advantages and disadvantages derive from these physical and pharmacokinetic features (Table 41.2). For example, the large size of anti-EGFR antibodies generally precludes penetration across epithelial basement membranes and thus the apparent absence of gastrointestinal (GI) toxicity in early clinical trials with these agents. On the other hand, large molecule size may present certain limitations for effective biodistribution to selected anatomic compartments (i.e., central nervous system). For the small molecule tyrosine kinase inhibitors, a potential clinical advantage is the patient convenience associated with oral bioavailability. For many agents in this class, this property enables once-daily dosing with a single tablet by mouth. A potential downside for the small molecule tyrosine kinase inhibitors is their capacity to tra-

TABLE 41.1 Epidermoid Growth Factor Receptor Inhibitory Agents (Broad Classification)

Large molecules (antibodies)
Monoclonals (e.g., C225, ABGX, mAb 806)
Bispecific
Immunotoxin conjugates
Small molecules (tyrosine kinase inhibitors)
Quinazolines (e.g., ZD1839, OSI-774, CI-1033)
Pyridopyrimidines
Pyrrolopyrimidines
Tyrphostins

Quinazolines

ZD1839 (Iressa)

OSI-774 (CP358774)

CI-1033 (PD183805)

EKB-569

Pyrrolopyrimidines

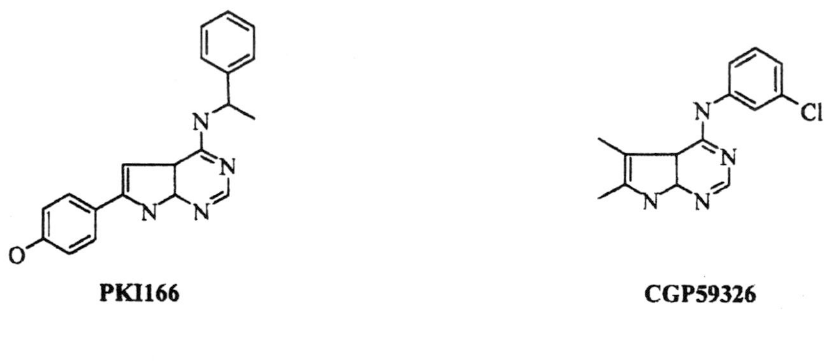

Tyrphostins

A25

RG13022

Figure 41.6 Basic chemical structure for several of the epidermal growth factor receptor selective tyrosine kinase inhibitors.

verse epithelial basement membranes and thereby precipitate GI toxicity as reflected by diarrhea as a common or dose-limiting toxicity in early clinical trials. A prototypic agent in the large molecule class is C225 (Erbitux, Cetuximab, ImClone Systems, New York, NY), which is a mouse-human chimeric anti-EGFR monoclonal antibody raised against the extracellular receptor domain. A prototypic agent in the small molecule class is ZD1839 (Iressa, Gefitinib, AstraZeneca, UK), which is a selective inhibitor of the EGFR tyrosine kinase.

At this relatively early clinical stage of EGFR inhibitor development, it remains unclear whether one particular approach (antibody) versus the other (tyrosine kinase inhibitor) is necessarily to be preferred. Having two distinct molecular targets within the EGFR molecule (extracellular domain and intracellular tyrosine kinase domain) represents a clear strength of the preclinical and early clinical research studies in this area. The maturation of clinical trials (Table 41.3) will gradually enhance our appreciation of the balance

TABLE 41.2 Theoretical Pros/Cons of Epidermoid Growth Factor Receptor (EGFR) Inhibitor Classes

	Large molecule (e.g., antibodies)	Small molecule (e.g., TK inhibitors)
Pro		
	Long half-life, less frequent administration	Oral bioavailability
	High specificity for receptor	No antibody response
	Too large to cross epithelial BM, thus absence of GI toxicity	High tissue penetration
	May recruit additional tumor toxicity	May work on truncated EGFR
Con		
	Large size may limit bioavailability/distribution to certain anatomic sites	Small size allows penetration across epithelial BM, thus GI toxicity
	Risk for allergic/anaphylactic responses	Short half-life necessitates daily dosing

ADCC, antibody dependent complement-mediated cytotoxicity; BM, basement membrane; TK, tyrosine kinase.

between efficacy and toxicity for these respective approaches. Indeed, it is certainly conceivable that effective therapeutic strategies will eventually be designed that incorporate a simultaneous attack on both the extracellular and intracellular EGFR targets.

PRECLINICAL STUDIES IN HEAD AND NECK CANCER

Proliferation/Cell Cycle Control

Inhibition of cell cycle progression is an effective mechanism for modulating the growth of tumors (81). Epidermal growth factor has been shown to induce cyclin D1 expression, a protein required for cell cycle progression from G_1 to S phase. Inhibition of EGFR signaling with either the monoclonal antibody C225 or the tyrosine kinase inhibitor ZD1839 reduces proliferation in a variety of cultured epithelial tumor cells, and blocks cell cycle progression in the G_1 phase (77,82–88). Accumulation of hypophosphorylated retinoblastoma (Rb) protein and a specific cyclin-dependent kinase (CDK2) inhibitor $p27^{KIP}$ is observed, which may contribute to this cell cycle arrest. The increased level of $p27^{KIP}$ is accompanied by an increased association with CDK2, and results in a reduction in cyclin-CDK2 kinase activity (Fig. 41.7). Cyclin-CDK2 serves to phosphorylate Rb, and therefore acts as a critical regulator for cells in their progression from G_1 to S phase. Phosphorylation of Rb in turn facilitates release of the Rb-bound transcription factor E2F, which is required for G_1 to S phase transition. When cyclin-CDK2 activity is reduced, as observed in C225 or ZD1839-treated cells, phosphorylation of Rb is similarly reduced and cells thereby arrest in the G_1 phase (82,84,89). *In vivo* xenograft studies with athymic mice further confirm that treatment with C225 results in a decline in proliferating cell nuclear antigen (PCNA) accompanied by an increase in $p27^{KIP}$ (90).

Apoptosis

Understanding the relationship between EGFR signaling and cellular apoptosis is important, since the induction of apoptosis in tumor cells can be therapeutically advantageous. It has been suggested that EGF acts as a survival factor that can inhibit apoptosis, thereby promoting tumor growth (91). Conversely, many studies now confirm that EGFR inhibition, using tyrosine kinase inhibitors or anti-EGFR antibodies, can induce apoptosis in human tumor cells. Treatment of HNSCC cells or colon DiFi cells with anti-EGFR antibody results in the induction of apoptosis (84,92,93). Additionally, the EGFR tyrosine kinase inhibitor OSI-774 is shown to promote apoptosis in

TABLE 41.3 Epidermoid Growth Factor Receptor (EGFR)-Targeted Therapeutic Agents Currently in Clinical Trials

Agent	Sponsor	Class (receptor target)	Highest development stage
IMC-C225	ImClone Systems	Human/murine chimeric anti-EGFR monoclonal antibody (EGFR/ErbB1)	Phase III
ZD1839	AstraZeneca	Small molecule tyrosine kinase inhibitor (EGFR/ErbB1)	Phase III
OSI-774	OSI Pharmaceuticals/Genentech	Small molecule tyrosine kinase inhibitor (EGFR/ErbB1)	Phase III
CI-1033	Pfizer	Small molecule tyrosine kinase inhibitor (Pan ErbB)	Phase II
ABX-EGF	Abgenix I	Humanized anti-EGFR monoclonal antibody	Phase II/III
PKI116	Novartis	Small molecule tyrosine kinase inhibitor (EGFR/ErbB1)	Phase II
h-R3	Cuban Institute of Oncology	Humanized anti-EGFR monoclonal antibody	Phase II
MDX-447	Medarex Inc.	Bispecific antibody (targets EGFR and CD64)	Phase II
EKB-569	Wyeth-Ayerst	Small molecule tyrosine kinase inhibitor (EGFR/ErbB1, some activity against other family members)	Phase I

Source: Adapted from Rowinsky EK. EGFR-targeted cancer therapies: is there a need to reconsider clinical trial design. *Signal* 2001;2:4–12, with permission.

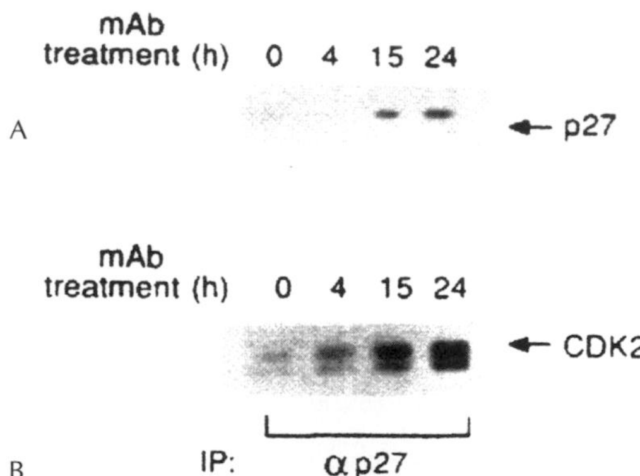

Figure 41.7 Effects of mAb C225 on the expression of p27 and its association with CDK2. **A:** p27 protein levels in C225-treated DiFi colon adenocarcinoma cells shown by Western blot analysis. **B:** C225-treated cell lysates were immunoprecipitated with anti-p27 antibody followed by Western blot analysis using anti-CDK2 antibody. (From Mendelsohn J, Baselga J. The EGF receptor family as targets for cancer therapy. *Oncogene* 2000;19:6550–6565, with permission.)

HN5 carcinoma cells (94). Similar apoptosis-inducing properties are claimed for other EGFR tyrosine kinase inhibitors, such as PD153035 in colon cancer (95) and ZD1839 in mammary epithelial cell lines (96). Taken together, these findings suggest that inhibition of EGFR signaling activates proapoptotic pathways and/or deactivates antiapoptotic pathways in tumor cells. Studies demonstrate that C225 induces an increase in the activity of caspase-3, -8, and -9 in concert with the induction of apoptosis in DiFi cells (97). A rise in Bax expression and a decrease in *bcl*-2 expression in HN cancer cells treated with C225 are observed (84). Another study reports that C225 not only enhances expression of newly synthesized Bax protein, but also triggers relocalization of Bax from the cytosol to the nucleus (98). The precise extent to which C225 induces apoptosis varies somewhat with the particular tumor cell line tested. For example, EGFR blockade with C225 does not readily induce apoptosis in prostate DU-145 cells (83). Therefore, although not universally observed, apoptosis induction appears to be a common feature triggered by EGFR inhibition in many tumor model systems.

Angiogenesis

Angiogenesis represents an important biologic process in the natural progression of human cancers, and is increasingly recognized as a promising target for anticancer therapy. Angiogenesis is controlled in part by angiogenic factors, including basic fibroblast growth factor (bFGF), cytokines such as interleukin-8 (IL-8), and vascular endothelial growth factor (VEGF) (99–102). Evidence suggests that EGFR signaling may play a role in the regulation of angiogenesis (90,103–105). Coexpression of TGF-α and EGFR shows a strong correlation with microvessel density in invasive breast cancer (106). O-charoenrat et al. (107,108) also demonstrated that TGF-α promotes the expression of VEGF family in 15 HNSCC cell lines. This up-regulation of VEGF gene expression by TGF-α is found to involve AP-1/AP-2 and EGR-1 transcription factors (109). Blockade of EGFR signaling by C225 or ZD1839 down-regulates the expression of VEGF, IL-8, and bFGF in a variety of cancers (Fig. 41.8) (48,90,110,111). The antiangiogenic influence of EGFR blocking agents facilitates potent antitumor activity in several experimental animal model systems.

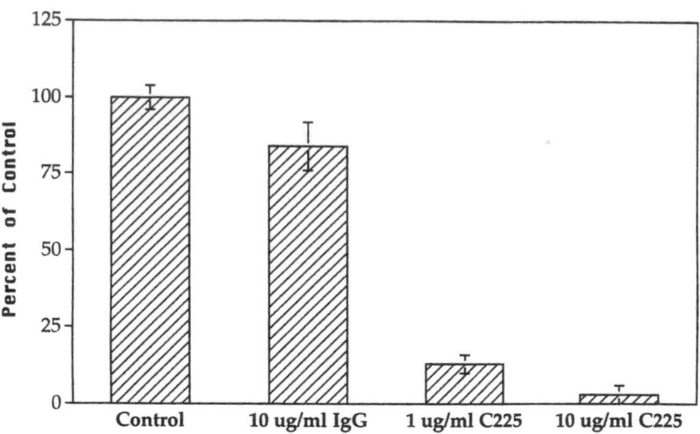

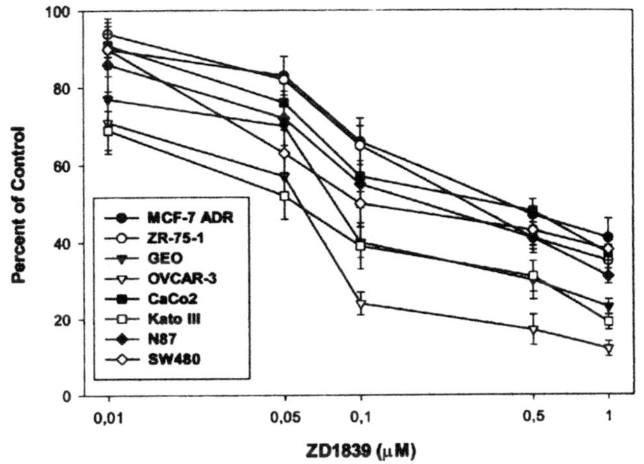

Figure 41.8 Effect of C225 or ZD1839 on the expression of vascular endothelial growth factor (VEGF) *in vitro*. VEGF level was determined by enzyme-linked immunosorbent assay and expressed in relation to untreated cells (100%). **A:** C225 inhibits VEGF production in 253J B-V cells (bladder) in a dose-dependent manner. **B:** ZD1839 inhibits VEGF production in human colon (GEO, SW480, and CaCo2), breast (ZR-75-1 and MCF-7 ADR), ovarian (OVCAR-3), and gastric (KOTO III and N87) cancer cells. (Adapted from Perrotte P, Matsumoto T, Inoue K, et al. Anti-epidermal growth factor receptor antibody C225 inhibits angiogenesis in human transitional cell carcinoma growing orthotopically in nude mice. *Clin Cancer Res* 1999;5:257–264; and Ciardiello F, Caputo R, Bianco R, et al. Inhibition of growth factor production and angiogenesis in human cancer cells by ZD1839 (Iressa), a selective epidermal growth factor receptor tyrosine kinase inhibitor. *Clin Cancer Res* 2001;7:1459–1465, with permission.)

Metastases

The HNSCCs are characterized by a marked propensity for local invasion and dissemination to cervical lymph nodes, with distant metastases developing in a minority of cases. Overexpression of EGFR and/or its ligands, as well as several matrix metalloproteinases (MMPs), is associated with the invasive or metastatic phenotype (112–115). It is shown that the EGF family ligands increase HNSCC tumor cell invasion through extracellular matrix (ECM) gel using *in vitro* Transwell invasion assay (116,117). These activities are independent of ligand effects on cell proliferation. By examining the ability of a variety of HNSCC cell lines to invade through ECM gel, a correlation is found between high levels of EGFR and tumor invasiveness (54). Furthermore, EGFR expression is found to correlate strongly with the expression and activity of MMP-9, and inversely with tissue inhibitor of metalloproteinase (TIMP-1). Matrix metalloproteinase-9 is a member of type IV collagenase/gelatinase that is involved in tumor metastases by virtue of its ability to degrade connective tissue ECM and basement membrane components. Therefore, the EGFR signaling pathway may play an important role in the invasive behavior of HNSCC via effects that specifically up-regulate MMP-9 and down-regulate TIMP-1 (117). Anti-EGFR monoclonal antibodies, C225 or others, inhibit tumor cell invasion and the expression and activity of MMP-9 (105,117).

The capacity of C225 to inhibit tumor metastases is shown in a variety of cancer models. In studies of human transitional cell carcinoma of the bladder established orthotopically in nude mice, Perrotte et al. (90) demonstrated that treatment with C225 down-regulates mRNA expression and the activity of MMP-9 in a dose-dependent manner. In addition, there is complete abrogation of lymph node and lung metastases in C225-treated mice. Similar results are observed in an orthotopic model of human pancreatic carcinoma (118). Systemic therapy with C225 alone or in combination with gemcitabine results in growth inhibition, tumor regression, and abrogation of metastases to regional lymph nodes and liver.

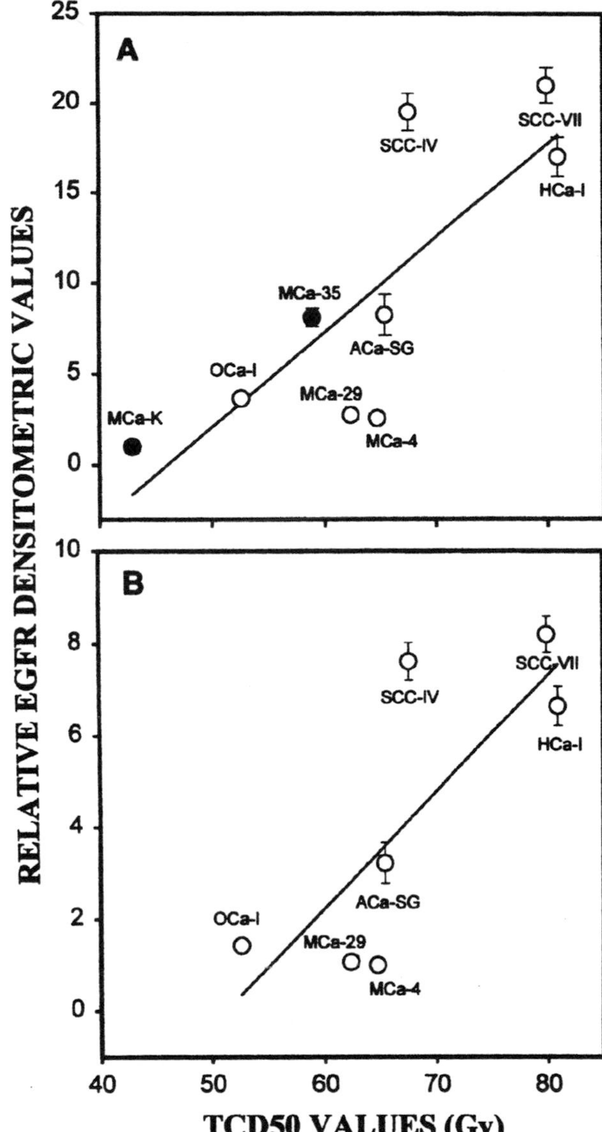

Figure 41.9 Inverse relationship between epidermal growth factor receptor expression and radiocurability of murine carcinomas. **A:** Both wild-type (V) and mutant p53 (v) tumors. **B:** Wild-type p53 tumor only. TCD_{50} constitutes the dose of radiation yielding local tumor control in 50% of irradiated animals. (From Akimoto T, Hunter NR, Buchmiller L, et al. Inverse relationship between epidermal growth factor receptor expression and radiocurability of murine carcinomas. *Clin Cancer Res* 1999;5:2884–2890, with permission.)

Radiation Interactions

Significant interest is emerging regarding the potential value of combining EGFR signal inhibitors with radiation in cancer therapy. Several studies demonstrate a positive correlation between EGFR expression level and cellular resistance to radiation (Fig. 41.9) (119–121). Squamous cells derived from HN cancer patients expressing high EGFR levels are commonly shown to be more radioresistant than those expressing low EGFR levels (120). The degree of radioresistance is found to correlate positively with the magnitude of EGFR overexpression (122). Additional studies demonstrate that cell survival and repopulation during a course of radiotherapy are influenced, in part, by activation of EGFR/TGF-α, which is induced following exposure to radiation (123,124). These results suggest that modulation of EGFR signaling activity offers promise for improving local tumor control during radiotherapy (125).

In several *in vitro* studies, EGFR blockade with C225 is shown to increase radiosensitivity across a spectrum of human cancer cells (84,126,127). Treatment of cells with C225 not only enhances cell death following radiation, but also increases the fraction of tumor cells succumbing to radiation-induced apoptosis (Fig. 41.10) (84,128). In addition, C225 is shown to augment the *in vivo* tumor response of tumor xenografts to radiation in nude mouse model systems (48,49,129,130). Treatment of well-established SCC tumor xenografts with the combination of C225 and radiation results in complete regression of tumors in nude mice over a 100-day follow-up period (Fig. 41.11) (48). Milas et al. (49) demonstrated a greater than threefold enhancement in tumor regression after single-fraction radiation exposure in mice bearing A431 xenografts that receive systemic C225 (Fig. 41.12). The potency of the antitumor effect observed, using the combination of C225 and radiation in animals, strongly suggests that mechanisms beyond simple proliferative growth inhibition are operational in the *in vivo* setting.

A very similar pattern of enhanced radiation response is now emerging from preclinical studies examining the impact of small molecular tyrosine kinase inhibitors (131–133). Treatment of human tumor cell cultures with ZD1839 is shown to increase radiation response in clonogenic survival assays, and coadministration of ZD1839 with radiation is found to significantly enhance the antitumor potency compared with ZD1839 or radiation alone in tumor xenograft models (86,89,134).

Several distinct lines of inquiry are currently under investigation in an attempt to better understand specific cellular mechanisms that may contribute to the antitumor potency of EGFR blockade in combination with radiation observed within *in vivo* model systems. Data from several laboratories suggest that EGFR blockade with C225 or ZD1839 serves to inhibit tumor angiogenesis, and this response appears to be augmented when effected in combination with radiation (48,49,105). In addition to the cell cycle effect of EGFR blockade, data are now emerging regarding the capacity of C225 and ZD1839 to modulate apoptosis, to inhibit cellular repair of radiation-induced damage, and to influence cellular migration capacity and possibly metastases (86,105,125,135). It appears that molecular down-regulation of mitogenic signal transduction pathways, including the EGFR system cascade, can disrupt cellular recovery processes following radiation injury,

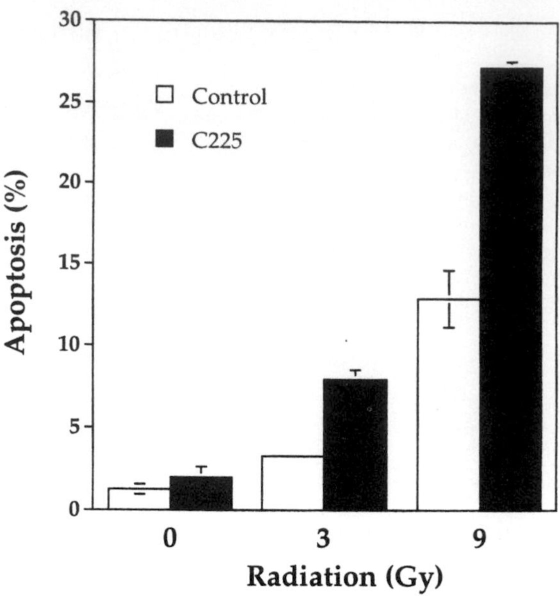

Figure 41.10 Effect of C225 on radiation-induced apoptosis. Squamous cell carcinoma was irradiated in the absence (control) or presence of C225 (30 nmol/L) at 0, 3, 9 Gy. After radiation, cells were incubated for 3 days and processed for flow cytometric analysis using propidium iodide (PI) to stain DNA. Percentage of apoptosis was determined on the basis of sub-G0 fragmented DNA content of the histogram. (From Harari PM, Huang S-M. Head and neck cancer as a clinical model for molecular targeting of therapy: combining EGFR blockade with radiation. *Int J Radiat Oncol Biol Phys* 2001;49:427–433, with permission.)

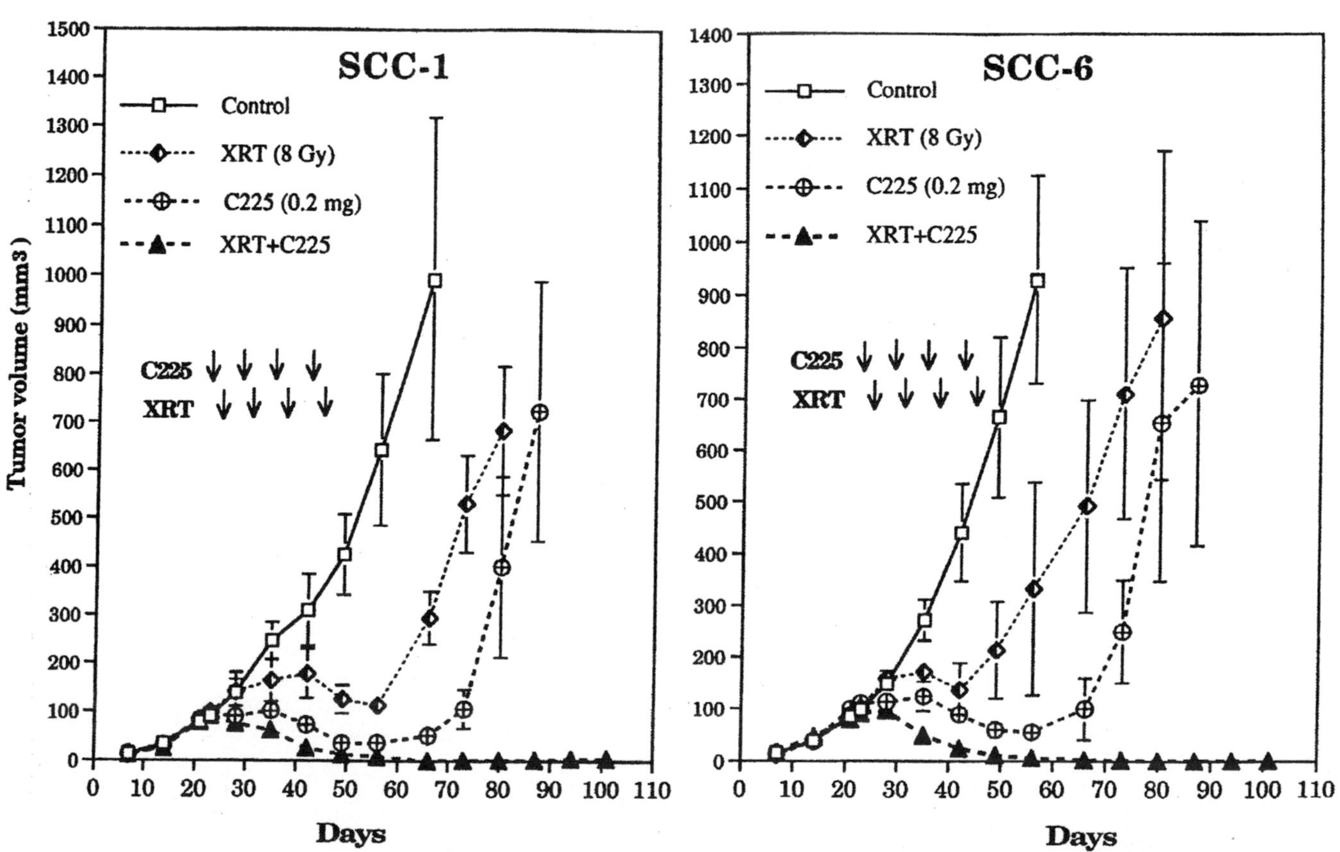

Figure 41.11 Effect of C225 on radioresponse of SCC-1 and SCC-6 tumor xenografts. Treatment was initiated by injecting 0.2 mg C225 intraperitoneally once a week for a total of four injections. The radiation (x-ray therapy, XRT)-treated group was exposed to a single 8 Gy fraction 24 hours after each injection of C225. *Arrows* depict specific days of C225 or XRT administration. (From Huang S-M, Harari PM. Modulation of radiation response following epidermal growth factor receptor blockade in squamous cell carcinomas: inhibition of damage repair, cell cycle kinetics and tumor angiogenesis. *Clin Cancer Res* 2000;6:2166–2174, with permission.)

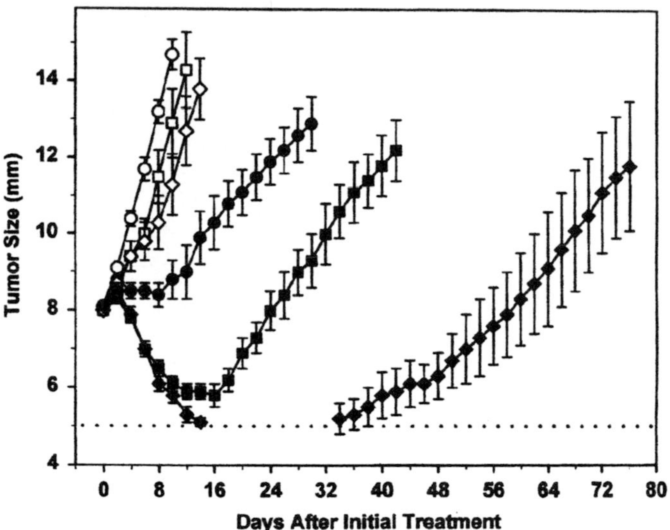

Figure 41.12 Effect of C225 on radioresponse of A431 tumor xenografts: (○), no treatment; (□), single dose of C225; (◇), three doses of C225; (●), 18 Gy radiation; (■), single dose of C225 plus 18 Gy radiation; (♦), three doses of C225 plus 18 Gy radiation. (From Milas L, Mason K, Hunter N, et al. In vivo enhancement of tumor radioresponse by C225 antiepidermal growth factor receptor antibody. *Clin Cancer Res* 2000;6:701–708, with permission.)

although the precise mechanisms for this are just beginning to be unraveled.

Chemotherapy Interactions

There is now considerable preclinical data regarding the capacity of EGFR inhibitors to enhance the effects of cytotoxic chemotherapy using *in vitro* and *in vivo* model systems. In both cell culture and in tumor xenografts, there is evidence that exposure to C225 can increase the cytotoxic response to a variety of agents including cisplatin, doxorubicin, paclitaxel, gemcitabine, irinotecan, and topotecan (118,136–142). A remarkably similar set of data emerges from preclinical studies examining EGFR signaling interruption with the tyrosine kinase inhibitor ZD1839. The same chemotherapy agents listed above, in addition to carboplatin, oxaliplatin, docetaxel, and etoposide, have been confirmed to display enhanced effects when combined with ZD1839 (110,143,144). A fairly broad spectrum of distinct tumor types has been studied with regard to EGFR inhibition plus chemotherapy, including those derived from the colon, pancreas, prostate, bladder, lung, head and neck, breast, and vulva (145–148). The expanding data set, which confirms that the effects of a diverse group of chemotherapy agents (in addition to radiation) is enhanced following EGFR inhibition, suggests that this growth factor pathway plays an important role in modulating the cellular response to cytotoxic insult.

CLINICAL STUDIES IN HEAD AND NECK CANCER

The strong EGFR biology and preclinical data established to date have stimulated design and initiation of a series of clinical trials to examine the use of EGFR-inhibitory agents in HN cancer patients (as well as in a wide variety of common human cancers including lung, prostate, breast, colon, pancreas, brain, etc.) (63,72,148–152). These studies include patients who have received monotherapy within the context of phase I trials examining the feasibility and toxicity of delivering EGFR-inhibitory agents alone, as well as a series of studies examining the use of EGFR-inhibitory agents combined with chemotherapy and/or radiotherapy. Although there are a surprising number of documented responders to monotherapy for several of the EGFR-inhibitory agents, the prevailing hypothesis is that EGFR inhibition will provide primarily growth-inhibitory as opposed to cytotoxic effects. More specifically, the currently projected future for EGFR-inhibitory strategies appears to rest in combination with conventional cytotoxic modalities such as chemotherapy and radiation. The emerging preclinical data suggest a powerful mechanistic rationale for how EGFR signaling inhibition can enhance the effectiveness of conventional cancer treatment modalities. Moreover, the frequent overexpression of EGFR (by HN cancers in particular) and the dependence of certain tumors on EGFR for their growth advantage provides a relative tumor "selectivity" to this therapeutic approach.

C225

In excess of 400 patients with advanced HNSCC have received C225 in the context of clinical trials to date. The majority of these patients have received C225 in combination with cisplatin, radiation therapy, or both (Table 41.4) (71,141,153,154). Patients have been treated in the definitive setting following newly diagnosed cancer, and in the recurrent/metastatic setting following clinical failure after conventional therapies.

In the phase I setting, C225 has been dose-escalated in combination with cisplatin for patients with recurrent/metastatic HNSCC (155). Patients received weekly C225 in combination with cisplatin (100 mg/m^2) delivered every 3 weeks. In this original 12-patient study, six of nine evaluable patients exhibited objective response (two complete and four partial) including several patients who had previously progressed during cisplatin administration. Regarding the combination with radiotherapy, a phase IB/IIA study of C225 in combination with high-dose radiation in the definitive treatment setting for advanced HN cancer patients was carried out in 16 subjects (156). Patients were treated with curative intent using either once-daily or twice-daily radiation fractionation schedules to a dose of ≥ 70 Gy. Major responses were identified in all 15 evaluable patients (13 complete and two partial). Although a majority of patients receiving high-dose radiation in the definitive setting are expected to achieve major responses, this 100% response rate was notable, and provided additional stimulus for the subsequent phase III clinical trial evaluation described further below.

In the phase II clinical trial setting, C225 has recently been examined in patients with recurrent/metastatic HNSCC (157).

TABLE 41.4 C225 Clinical Trials in Head and Neck Cancer

Trial	*n*	C225 treatment	Setting
Phase I/II	16	Plus XRT	Definitive
Phase I	12	Plus CDDP	Met/Rec
Phase II	20	Plus CDDP/XRT	Definitive
Phase II	98	Plus CDDP	Met/Rec
Phase III	416	Plus XRT	Definitive
Phase III	121	Plus CDDP	Met/Rec

CDDP, cisplatin; Met/Rec, metastatic/recurrent; XRT, radiation.

In this study, patients received two cycles of a cisplatin-containing regimen (cisplatin/paclitaxel or cisplatin/5-FU), with those patients demonstrating either progressive or stable disease going on to receive cisplatin plus C225. This study will help to identify whether recurrent/metastatic HN cancer patients who are not responding to cisplatin based therapies can respond to cisplatin delivered in combination with C225. This represents a challenging cohort of cancer patients with dismal prognosis and limited therapy options at present.

In the phase III setting there are two multiinstitutional trials to examine the impact of C225 in combination with either cisplatin or with radiation that have recently completed their enrollment phase (Fig. 41.13). In the cisplatin phase III trial, patients with recurrent/metastatic cancer of the HN were randomized to cisplatin plus placebo versus cisplatin plus C225 (158). This trial has accrued 121 patients and currently awaits follow-up maturation for analysis. In conjunction with the phase II trial described above, these studies should provide clear indication as to whether C225 will emerge as a successful therapy agent for patients with recurrent/metastatic HNSCC.

With regard to C225 plus radiation in the phase III setting, an international trial has recently completed enrollment of 416 patients treated definitively for advanced HNSCC. Patients received either high-dose radiation alone (the majority with modern hyperfractionation or concomitant boost radiation schedules) or radiation plus weekly infusions of C225 during a 7-week course of radiotherapy. This represents a very powerful clinical trial for the EGFR field in that it will provide an unencumbered assessment regarding the capacity of EGFR inhibition to modulate radiation response in a large cohort of advanced cancer patients treated with curative intent. Locoregional tumor control and overall survival will be analyzed in this randomized trial. Correlative studies will also be forthcoming from tumor materials gathered, as tissue specimens have been collected from all patients for quantitative EGFR analysis. Although EGFR status was not a prospective trial entry criterion, these data will be available to uncover potential correlations with tumor response, locoregional control, and ultimate survival outcome.

Toxicity

From the clinical data available to date, C225 appears to be quite well tolerated and accompanied by a relatively modest overall toxicity profile. The most common adverse event (AE) with C225 involves skin rash, which is observed in approximately two thirds of patients receiving the drug (71,159,160). This effect is common to many of the EGFR inhibitory agents and generally manifests clinically as an acne-like, follicular rash over the face, scalp, neck, upper torso, and arms (Fig. 41.14; see Color Plate 16 following page 524). This cutaneous manifestation is believed to reflect abundant EGFR expression in the epidermis, and appears to be self-limiting with clinical resolution several weeks to months following treatment cessation. Other reported AEs for C225 include fatigue, fever, and nausea at incidence rates of less

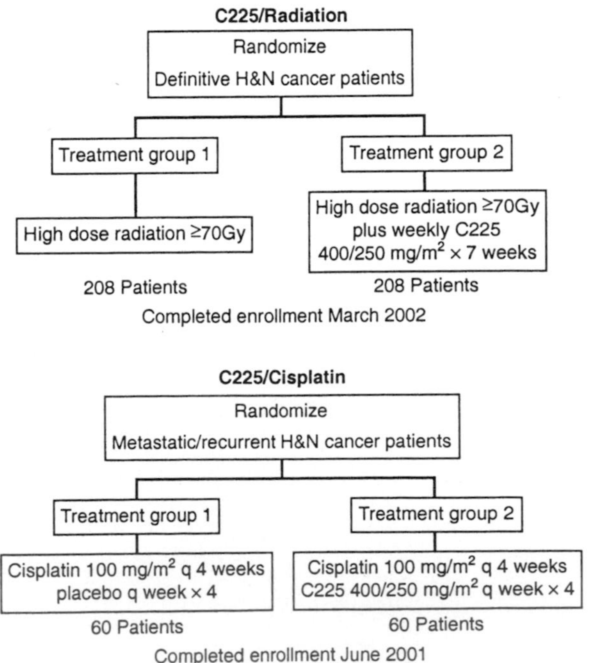

Figure 41.13 Treatment schemes for phase III C225 head and neck trials.

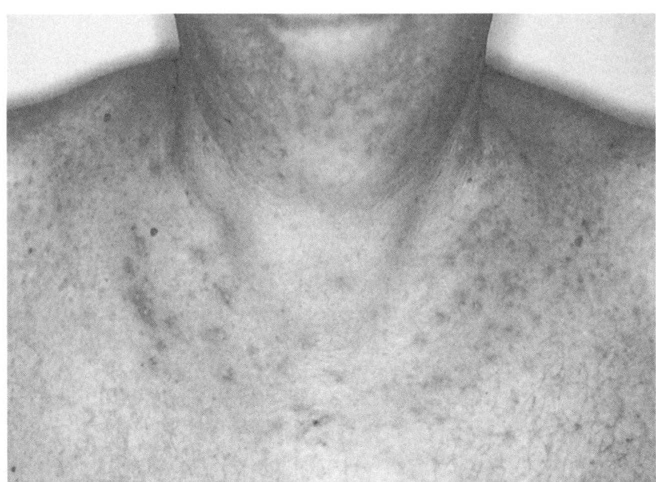

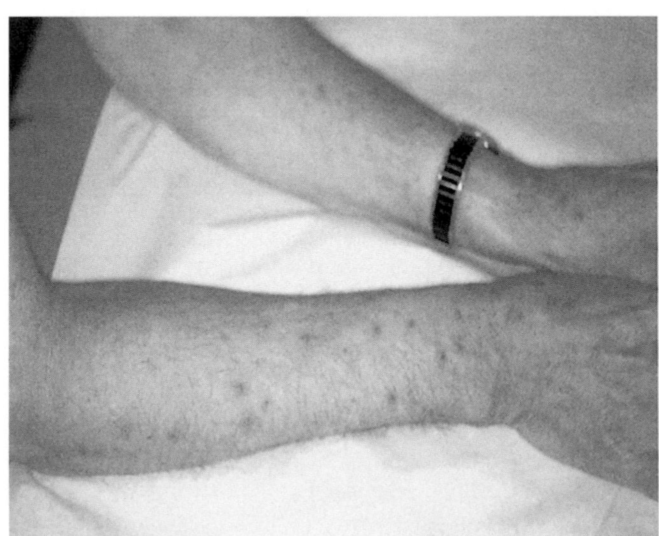

Figure 41.14 Characteristic appearance of folliculitis in a patient receiving weekly C225 during a course of head and neck radiation. This cutaneous reaction commonly manifests across the face, neck, upper torso, and arms, and resolves spontaneously over several weeks or months following completion of therapy. (From Harari PM, Huang S-M. Head and neck cancer as a clinical model for molecular targeting of therapy: combining EGFR blockade with radiation. *Int J Radiat Oncol Biol Phys* 2001; 49:427–433, with permission.) (See Color Plate 16 following page 524.)

than 20%. The majority of AEs are reported to be mild to moderate, with only 12% scored as grade 3 to 4 in severity. As with all antibody-based therapies, the potential for allergic or anaphylactic responses requires careful surveillance in early studies. In a safety analysis of 189 patients receiving C225, eight (4%) patients manifested grade 3/4 allergic reactions of which three (1.6%) were considered grade 4 anaphylactic responses (159). All patients were discontinued from further drug administration and recovered uneventfully and without sequelae. Human antichimeric antibody (HACA) response has been detected in approximately 3% (4/120) of patients receiving C225, with neutralizing antibodies identified in 2.5% (3/120) (161). However, none of these patients were observed to develop allergic or anaphylactic reactions. C225 has now been administered to several hundred patients in combination with cytotoxic chemotherapy or radiation. Preliminary observations do not suggest untoward enhancement in resultant toxicity profiles, although maturation of the clinical trials data will be required for more rigorous analysis of this issue.

ZD1839

At the time of this writing, patients with HN cancer who have received ZD1839 have done so primarily within the context of phase I studies, which include patients with a variety of disease origin sites (162–165). A recent phase II study in patients with recurrent or metastatic HN cancer shows single agent activity of ZD1839 with excellent treatment tolerance (166). There are several studies underway that will examine the use of ZD1839 combined with chemotherapy and/or radiotherapy in the treatment of HN cancer patients (149). One of these studies is described further below.

An National Cancer Institute (NCI)-sponsored multiinstitutional phase I trial examining ZD1839 plus radiation and chemotherapy for locally advanced HNSCC is underway to establish the feasibility and toxicity profile for this treatment strategy. Patients with locally advanced HNSCC will be enrolled without stratification on the basis of EGFR expression. The radiotherapy treatment schedule builds on the recently completed RTOG randomized four-arm fractionation trial demonstrating a modest improvement in disease-free survival with accelerated radiotherapy employing the concomitant boost technique (167). ZD1839 administration will commence just prior to the initiation of radiotherapy, and continue throughout the subsequent 7-week treatment course including weekends. This phase I study will limit initial accrual of patients to treatment with radiotherapy alone and escalating doses of ZD1839 from 250 to 500 mg/d before the feasibility/toxicity of adding concurrent chemotherapy is studied. Subsequent levels will incorporate weekly cisplatin dosed at 30 mg/m^2, a schedule selected for radiosensitization and for evaluation of toxicity with the addition of ZD1839. Initial study levels examining the triple therapy (radiation/ZD1839/cisplatin) will employ conventional once-daily radiotherapy before proceeding to accelerated radiation using the concomitant boost technique. Following determination of the maximum tolerated dose of ZD1839 with and without chemotherapy, patients will be further accrued to an expanded cohort to verify safety and feasibility.

Despite the lack of mature clinical trial data to date with ZD1839 combined with radiation and/or chemotherapy in HN cancer, there are certainly promising data emerging with this agent in a variety of other anatomic sites. The most mature clinical data for ZD1839 exist in lung cancer where trials as monotherapy and in combination with cytotoxic chemotherapy have been recently completed (168,169). Indeed, trials that further examine the triple therapy with radiation/ZD1839/chemotherapy are also underway. As with C225, the preliminary safety and tolerance data for ZD1839 is quite favorable (170,171). The most commonly reported adverse events with ZD1839 include skin rash (similar or identical to that observed with C225) and diarrhea (172–174). Initial reports indicate a low percentage of patients experiencing grade 3/4 adverse events, and no early indication for enhancement of toxicity profiles for the conventional treatment modalities (163). For refractory HN cancer patients, there is data to suggest that favorable response to ZD1839 correlates with the development of skin toxicity (166).

OSI-774

OSI-774 (Tarceva, Erlotinib, OSI Pharmaceuticals, New York, NY, and Genentech, San Francisco, CA) is small molecule tyrosine kinase inhibitor that has been examined in the phase I/II clinical trial setting as a single agent in patients with refractory HN cancer (151,175). In a recently reported phase II study of 114 recurrent/metastatic HN cancer patients, 150 mg/m^2 daily dosing was used showing generally good tolerance for up to 48 weeks of drug administration (176). The most common toxicities included skin rash and diarrhea, and the overall major response rate was 5.6% with 40% of patients exhibiting stable disease. This agent may progress into further clinical evaluation in combination with conventional cytotoxic therapies in HN cancer patients. Evaluation is already well underway for OSI-774 in combination with conventional cytotoxic therapies in advanced lung cancer patients (150).

Although there is an enlarging group of additional EGFR inhibitory agents in various stages of development (referred to in this chapter and in the review references), there are currently minimal data pertaining specifically to HN cancer for the remaining agents. Needless to say, several of these agents hold strong promise in HN cancer, reflecting their molecular targeting of the EGFR, which is richly overexpressed in a majority of HN tumors. As preclinical and clinical data mature, we will likely identify new EGFR inhibitors with promising activity in patients with HNSCC.

CONCLUSION

The successful integration of molecular growth inhibitors into the treatment algorithm for advanced HN cancer patients is now at hand. This approach represents an important crossroad in modern cancer therapy in that it brings molecular biology to bear on a prevalent worldwide malignancy. The coming years will afford a much clearer picture regarding the ultimate potential of EGFR signal inhibitors to modulate HN tumor growth and augment the effects of radiation and chemotherapy. If these agents are confirmed to enhance locoregional tumor control (centerpiece for successful HN cancer treatment), their potential to interrupt the metastatic process can then be aggressively pursued. The modest toxicity profile observed to date with early-generation EGFR inhibitors further suggests their potential for future development in the HN cancer chemoprevention setting. The prevalent overexpression and reliance of HN tumors on EGFR signaling for their growth advantage provides a unique opportunity for exploitation using molecular inhibitor strategies. We are fortunate as HN oncologists to have the opportunity to rigorously explore the potential of these powerful and selective growth modulators to better the long-term prospects for future HN cancer patients.

REFERENCES

1. Cohen S, Carpenter G. Human epidermal growth factor: isolation and chemical and biological properties. *Proc Natl Acad Sci USA* 1975;72:1317–1321.
2. Ullrich A, Coussens L, Hayflick JS, et al. Human epidermal growth factor receptor cDNA sequence and aberrant expression of the amplified gene in A431 epidermoid carcinoma cells. *Nature* 1984;309:418–425.
3. Carpenter G, Cohen S. Epidermal growth factor. *J Biol Chem* 1990;265: 7709–7712.
4. Wells A. EGF receptor. *Int J Biochem Cell Biol* 1999;31:637–643.
5. Moghal N, Sternberg PW. Multiple positive and negative regulators of signaling by the EGF-receptor. *Curr Opin Cell Biol* 1999;11:190–196.
6. Bogdan S, Klambt C. Epidermal growth factor receptor signaling. *Curr Biol* 2001;11:R292–295.
7. Hackel PO, Zwick E, Prenzel N, et al. Epidermal growth factor receptors: critical mediators of multiple receptor pathways. *Curr Opin Cell Biol* 1999;11: 184–189.
8. Yarden Y, Sliwkowski MX. Untangling the ErbB signalling network. *Nat Rev Mol Cell Biol* 2001;2:127–137.
9. Prenzel N, Fischer OM, Streit S, et al. The epidermal growth factor receptor family as a central element for cellular signal transduction and diversification. *Endocr Relat Cancer* 2001;8:11–31.
10. Woodburn JR. The epidermal growth factor receptor and its inhibition in cancer therapy. *Pharmacol Ther* 1999;82:241–250.
11. Dougall WC, Qian XL, Greene MI. Interaction of the neu/p185 and EGF receptor tyrosine—implications for cellular transformation and tumor therapy. *J Cell Biochem* 1993;53:61–73.
12. Maa MC, Leu TH, McCarley DJ, et al. Potentiation of epidermal growth factor receptor-mediated oncogenesis by c-src—implications for the etiology of multiple human cancers. *Proc Natl Acad Sci USA* 1995;92:6981–6985.
13. Torring N, Jorgensen PE, Sorensen BS, et al. Increased expression of heparin binding EGF (HB-EGF), amphiregulin, TGF alpha and epiregulin in androgen-independent prostate cancer cell lines. *Anticancer Res* 2000;20:91–95.
14. Maihle NJ, Flickinger TW, Raines MA, et al. Native avian c-erbB gene expresses a secreted protein product corresponding to the ligand-binding domain of the receptor. *Proc Natl Acad Sci USA* 1991;88:1825–1829.
15. Maihle NJ, Baron AT, Barrett BA, et al. *EGF/ErbB receptor family in ovarian cancer.* Boston: Kluwer Academic, 2002:247–258.
16. Wikstrand CJ, McLendon RE, Friedman AH, et al. Cell surface localization and density of the tumor-associated variant of the epidermal growth factor receptor, EGFRvIII. *Cancer Res* 1997;57:4130–4140.
17. Tang CK, Gong XQ, Moscatello DK, et al. Epidermal growth factor receptor vIII enhances tumorigenicity in human breast cancer. *Cancer Res* 2000;60: 3081–3087.
18. Nagane M, Lin H, Cavenee WK, et al. Aberrant receptor signaling in human malignant gliomas: mechanisms and therapeutic implications. *Cancer Lett* 2001;162:S17–S21.
19. Wikstrand CJ, Reist CJ, Archer GE, et al. The class III variant of the epidermal growth factor receptor (EGFRvIII): characterization and utilization as an immunotherapeutic target. *J Neurovirol* 1998;4:148–158.
20. Nagane M, Coufal F, Lin H, et al. A common mutant epidermal growth factor receptor confers enhanced tumorigenicity on human glioblastoma cells by increasing proliferation and reducing apoptosis. *Cancer Res* 1996;56:5079–5086.
21. Chu CT, Everiss KD, Wikstrand CJ, et al. Receptor dimerization is not a factor in the signalling activity of a transforming variant epidermal growth factor receptor (EGFRvIII). *Biochem J* 1997;324:855–861.
22. Huang HS, Nagane M, Klingbeil CK, et al. The enhanced tumorigenic activity of a mutant epidermal growth factor receptor common in human cancers is mediated by threshold levels of constitutive tyrosine phosphorylation and unattenuated signaling. *J Biol Chem* 1997;272:2927–2935.
23. Voldborg BR, Damstrup L, Spang-Thomsen M, et al. Epidermal growth factor receptor (EGFR) and EGFR mutations, function and possible role in clinical trials. *Ann Oncol* 1997;8:1197–1206.
24. Schmidt M, Maurer-Gebhard M, Groner B, et al. Suppression of metastasis formation by a recombinant single chain antibody-toxin targeted to full-length and oncogenic variant EGF receptors. *Oncogene* 1999;18:1711–1721.
25. Mishima K, Johns TG, Luwor RB, et al. Growth suppression of intracranial xenografted glioblastomas overexpressing mutant epidermal growth factor receptors by systemic administration of monoclonal antibody (mAb) 806, a novel monoclonal antibody directed to the receptor. *Cancer Res* 2001;61: 5349–5354.
26. Kuan CT, Wikstrand CJ, Bigner DD. EGF mutant receptor vIII as a molecular target in cancer therapy. *Endocr Relat Cancer* 2001;8:83–96.
27. Grandis JR, Zeng Q, Tweardy DJ. Retinoic acid normalizes the increased gene transcription rate of TGF-alpha and EGFR in head and neck cancer cell lines. *Nat Med* 1996;2:237–240.
28. Song JI, Lango MN, Hwang JD, et al. Abrogation of transforming growth factor-alpha/epidermal growth factor receptor autocrine signaling by an RXR-selective retinoid (LGD1069, Targretin) in head and neck cancer cell lines. *Cancer Res* 2001;61:5919–5925.
29. Grandis JR, Tweardy DJ. Elevated levels of transforming growth factor alpha and epidermal growth factor receptor messenger RNA are early markers of carcinogenesis in head and neck cancer. *Cancer Res* 1993;53:3579–3584.
30. Grandis JR, Tweardy DJ. TGF-alpha and EGFR in head and neck cancer. *J Cell Biochem* 1993;(suppl):188–191.
31. Irish JC, Bernstein A. Oncogenes in head and neck cancer. *Laryngoscope* 1993; 103:42–52.
32. O-charoenrat P, Rhys-Evans P, Eccles S. Characterization of ten newly-derived human head and neck squamous carcinoma cell lines with special reference to c-erbB proto-oncogene expression. *Anticancer Res* 2001;21:1953–1963.
33. Weichselbaum RR, Dunphy EJ, Beckett MA, et al. Epidermal growth factor receptor gene amplification and expression in head and neck cancer cell lines. *Head Neck* 1989;11:437–442.
34. Miyaguchi M, Takeuchi T, Morimoto K, et al. Correlation of epidermal growth factor receptor and radiosensitivity in human maxillary carcinoma cell lines. *Acta Otolaryngol* 1998;118:428–431.
35. Santini J, Formento JL, Francoual M, et al. Characterization, quantification, and potential clinical value of the epidermal growth factor receptor in head and neck squamous cell carcinomas. *Head Neck* 1991;13:132–139.
36. Scambia G, Panici PB, Battaglia F, et al. Receptors for epidermal growth factor and steroid hormones in primary laryngeal tumors. *Cancer* 1991;67: 1347–1351.
37. Stanton P, Richards S, Reeves J, et al. Epidermal growth factor receptor expression by human squamous cell carcinomas of the head and neck, cell lines and xenografts. *Br J Cancer* 1994;70:427–433.
38. Wen QH, Miwa T, Yoshizaki T, et al. Prognostic value of EGFR and TGF-alpha in early laryngeal cancer treated with radiotherapy. *Laryngoscope* 1996; 106:884–888.
39. Grandis JR, Melhem MF, Barnes EL, et al. Quantitative immunohistochemical analysis of transforming growth factor-alpha and epidermal growth factor receptor in patients with squamous cell carcinoma of the head and neck. *Cancer* 1996;78:1284–1292.
40. Grandis JR, Tweardy DJ, Melhem MF. Asynchronous modulation of transforming growth factor alpha and epidermal growth factor receptor protein expression in progression of premalignant lesions to head and neck squamous cell carcinoma. *Clin Cancer Res* 1998;4:13–20.
41. Shin DM, Ro JY, Hong WK, et al. Dysregulation of epidermal growth factor receptor expression in premalignant lesions during head and neck tumorigenesis. *Cancer Res* 1994;54:3153–3159.
42. Hong WK, Endicott J, Itri LM, et al. 13-cis-retinoic acid in the treatment of oral leukoplakia. *N Engl J Med* 1986;315:1501–1505.
43. Kim JS, Steck PA, Gallick GE, et al. Suppression by retinoic acid of epidermal growth factor receptor autophosphorylation and glycosylation in cultured human head and neck squamous carcinoma cells. *J Natl Cancer Inst Monogr* 1992;13:101–110.
44. Shin DM, Kim J, Ro JY, et al. Activation of p53 gene expression in premalignant lesions during head and neck tumorigenesis. *Cancer Res* 1994;54: 321–326.
45. Izzo JG, Papadimitrakopoulou VA, Li XQ, et al. Dysregulated cyclin D1 expression early in head and neck tumorigenesis: in vivo evidence for an association with subsequent gene amplification. *Oncogene* 1998;17:2313–2322.
46. Grandis JR, Zeng Q, Drenning SD, et al. Normalization of egfr mrna levels following restoration of wild-type p53 in a head and neck squamous cell carcinoma cell line. *Int J Oncol* 1998;13:375–378.
47. Aktas H, Cai H, Cooper GM. Ras links growth factor signaling to the cell cycle machinery via regulation of cyclin D1 and the Cdk inhibitor p27KIP1. *Mol Cell Biol* 1997;17:3850–3857.
48. Huang S-M, Harari PM. Modulation of radiation response following epidermal growth factor receptor blockade in squamous cell carcinomas: inhibition of damage repair, cell cycle kinetics and tumor angiogenesis. *Clin Cancer Res* 2000;6:2166–2174.
49. Milas L, Mason K, Hunter N, et al. In vivo enhancement of tumor radioresponse by C225 antiepidermal growth factor receptor antibody. *Clin Cancer Res* 2000;6:701–708.
50. Genersch E, Schneider DW, Sauer G, et al. Prevention of EGF-modulated adhesion of tumor cells to matrix proteins by specific EGF receptor inhibition. *Int J Cancer* 1998;75:205–209.
51. Lu Z, Jiang G, Blume-Jensen P, et al. Epidermal growth factor-induced tumor cell invasion and metastasis initiated by dephosphorylation and downregulation of focal adhesion kinase. *Mol Cell Biol* 2001;21:4016–4031.
52. O-charoenrat P, Rhys-Evans P, Court WJ, et al. Differential modulation of proliferation, matrix metalloproteinase expression and invasion of human head and neck squamous carcinoma cells by c-erbB ligands. *Clin Exp Metastasis* 1999;17:631–639.
53. Zolfaghari A, Djakiew D. Inhibition of chemomigration of a human prostatic carcinoma cell (TSU-pr1) line by inhibition of epidermal growth factor receptor function. *Prostate* 1996;28:232–238.
54. O-charoenrat P, Rhys-Evans P, Modjtahedi H, et al. Overexpression of epidermal growth factor receptor in human head and neck squamous carcinoma cell lines correlates with matrix metalloproteinase-9 expression and in vitro invasion. *Int J Cancer* 2000;86:307–317.
55. Grandis JR, Melhem MF, Gooding WE, et al. Levels of TGF-alpha and EGFR protein in head and neck squamous cell carcinoma and patient survival. *J Natl Cancer Inst* 1998;90:824–832.
56. Magne N, Pivot X, Bensadoun RJ, et al. The relationship of epidermal growth factor receptor levels to the prognosis of unresectable pharyngeal cancer patients treated by chemo-radiotherapy. *Eur J Cancer* 2001;37:2169–2177.
57. Maurizi M, Almadori G, Ferrandina G, et al. Prognostic significance of epidermal growth factor receptor in laryngeal squamous cell carcinoma. *Br J Cancer* 1996;74:1253–1257.
58. Dassonville O, Formento JL, Francoual M, et al. Expression of epidermal

growth factor receptor and survival in upper aerodigestive tract cancer. *J Clin Oncol* 1993;11:1873–1878.
59. Maurizi M, Scambia G, Benedetti Panici P, et al. EGF receptor expression in primary laryngeal cancer: correlation with clinico-pathological features and prognostic significance. *Int J Cancer* 1992;52:862–866.
60. Gill GN, Kawamoto T, Cochet C, et al. Monoclonal anti-epidermal growth factor receptor antibodies which are inhibitors of epidermal growth factor binding and antagonists of epidermal growth factor binding and antagonists of epidermal growth factor-stimulated tyrosine protein kinase activity. *J Biol Chem* 1984;259:7755–7760.
61. Kawamoto T, Sato JD, Le A, et al. Growth stimulation of A431 cells by epidermal growth factor: identification of high-affinity receptors for epidermal growth factor by an anti-receptor monoclonal antibody. *Proc Natl Acad Sci USA* 1983;80:1337–1341.
62. Mendelsohn J, Baselga J. The EGF receptor family as targets for cancer therapy. *Oncogene* 2000;19:6550–6565.
63. Ciardiello F, Tortora G. A novel approach in the treatment of cancer: targeting the epidermal growth factor receptor. *Clin Cancer Res* 2001;7:2958–2970.
64. Slichenmyer WJ, Fry DW. Anticancer therapy targeting the erbB family of receptor tyrosine kinases. *Semin Oncol* 2001;28:67–79.
65. Arteaga CL. The epidermal growth factor receptor: from mutant oncogene in nonhuman cancers to therapeutic target in human neoplasia. *J Clin Oncol* 2001;19:32S–40S.
66. Arteaga CL, Johnson DH. Tyrosine kinase inhibitors-ZD1839 (Iressa). *Curr Opin Oncol* 2001;13:491–498.
67. Baselga J, Albanell J. Targeting epidermal growth factor receptor in lung cancer. *Curr Oncol Rep* 2002;4:317–324.
68. de Bono JS, Rowinsky EK. The ErbB receptor family: a therapeutic target for cancer. *Trends Mol Med* 2002;8:S19–26.
69. Waksal HW. Role of an anti-epidermal growth factor receptor in treating cancer. *Cancer Metastasis Rev* 1999;18:427–436.
70. Raymond E, Faivre S, Armand JP. Epidermal growth factor receptor tyrosine kinase as a target for anticancer therapy. *Drugs* 2000;60:15–23; discussion 41–42.
71. Baselga J. The EGFR as a target for anticancer therapy—focus on cetuximab. *Eur J Cancer* 2001;37:S16–22.
72. Huang S-M, Li J, Harari PM. Monoclonal antibody blockade of the epidermal growth factor receptor in cancer therapy. In: Giaccone G, Schilsky R, Sondel P, eds. *Cancer chemotherapy and biological response modifiers annual 19*. Amsterdam: Elsevier, 2001:339–352
73. Torrance CJ, Jackson PE, Montgomery E, et al. Combinatorial chemoprevention of intestinal neoplasia. *Nat Med* 2000;6:1024–1028.
74. Traxler P, Bold G, Buchdunger E, et al. Tyrosine kinase inhibitors: from rational design to clinical trials. *Med Res Rev* 2001;21:499–512.
75. Ciardiello F. Epidermal growth factor receptor tyrosine kinase inhibitors as anticancer agents. *Drugs* 2000;60:25–32; discussion 41–42.
76. Al-Obeidi FA, Lam KS, Noonberg SB, et al. Development of inhibitors for protein tyrosine kinases. *Oncogene* 2000;19:5690–5701.
77. Lichtner RB, Menrad A, Sommer A, et al. Signaling-inactive epidermal growth factor receptor/ligand complexes in intact carcinoma cells by quinazoline tyrosine kinase inhibitors. *Cancer Res* 2001;61:5790–5795.
78. Baselga J. Targeting the epidermal growth factor receptor with tyrosine kinase inhibitors: small molecules, big hopes. *J Clin Oncol* 2002;20:2217–2219.
79. Sewell JM, Macleod KG, Ritchie A, et al. Targeting the EGF receptor in ovarian cancer with the tyrosine kinase inhibitor ZD 1839 ("Iressa"). *Br J Cancer* 2002;86:456–462.
80. Levitt ML, Koty PP. Tyrosine kinase inhibitors in preclinical development. *Invest New Drugs* 1999;17:213–226.
81. Giordano A, Rustum YM, Wenner CE. Cell cycle: molecular targets for diagnosis and therapy: tumor suppressor genes and cell cycle progression in cancer. *J Cell Biochem* 1998;70:1–7.
82. Wu X, Rubin M, Fan Z, et al. Involvement of $p27^{KIP1}$ in G1 arrest mediated by an anti-epidermal growth factor receptor monoclonal antibody. *Oncogene* 1996;12:1397–1403.
83. Peng D, Fan Z, Lu Y, et al. Anti-epidermal growth factor receptor monoclonal antibody 225 up-regulates $p27^{KIP1}$ and induces G1 arrest in prostatic cancer cell line DU145. *Cancer Res* 1996;56:3666–3669.
84. Huang S-M, Bock JM, Harari PM. Epidermal growth factor receptor blockade with C225 modulates proliferation, apoptosis, and radiosensitivity in squamous cell carcinomas of the head and neck. *Cancer Res* 1999;59:1935–1940.
85. Chan KC, Knox WF, Gandhi A, et al. Blockade of growth factor receptors in ductal carcinoma in situ inhibits epithelial proliferation. *Br J Surg* 2001;88: 412–418.
86. Huang S-M, Li J, Armstrong EA, et al. Modulation of radiation response and tumor-induced angiogenesis after epidermal growth factor receptor Inhibition by ZD1839 (Iressa). *Cancer Res* 2002;62:4300–4306.
87. Anderson NG, Ahmad T, Chan K, et al. ZD1839 (Iressa), a novel epidermal growth factor receptor (EGFR) tyrosine kinase inhibitor, potently inhibits the growth of EGFR-positive cancer cell lines with or without erbB2 overexpression. *Int J Cancer* 2001;94:774–782.
88. Kiyota A, Shintani S, Mihara M, et al. Anti-epidermal growth factor receptor monoclonal antibody 225 upregulates p27(KIP1) and p15(INK4B) and induces G1 arrest in oral squamous carcinoma cell lines. *Oncology* 2002;63:92–98.
89. Raben D, Helfrich BA, Chan D, et al. ZD1839, a selective epidermal growth factor receptor tyrosine kinase inhibitor, alone and in combination with radiation and chemotherapy as a new therapeutic strategy in non-small cell lung cancer. *Semin Oncol* 2002;29:37–46.
90. Perrotte P, Matsumoto T, Inoue K, et al. Anti-epidermal growth factor receptor antibody C225 inhibits angiogenesis in human transitional cell carcinoma growing orthotopically in nude mice. *Clin Cancer Res* 1999;5:257–264.
91. Gibson S, Tu S, Oyer R, et al. Epidermal growth factor protects epithelial cells against Fas-induced apoptosis. Requirement for Akt activation. *J Biol Chem* 1999;274:17612–17618.
92. Wu X, Fan Z, Masui H, et al. Apoptosis induced by an anti-epidermal growth factor receptor monoclonal antibody in a human colorectal carcinoma cell line and its delay by insulin. *J Clin Invest* 1995;95:1897–1905.
93. Modjtahedi H, Affleck K, Stubberfield C, et al. Egfr blockade by tyrosine kinase inhibitor or monoclonal antibody inhibits growth, directs terminal differentiation and induces apoptosis in the human squamous cell carcinoma hn5. *Int J Oncol* 1998;13:335–342.
94. Moyer JD, Barbacci EG, Iwata KK, et al. Induction of apoptosis and cell cycle arrest by CP-358,774, an inhibitor of epidermal growth factor receptor tyrosine kinase. *Cancer Res* 1997;57:4838–4848.
95. Karnes W Jr, Weller SG, Adjei PN, et al. Inhibition of epidermal growth factor receptor kinase induces protease-dependent apoptosis in human colon cancer cells. *Gastroenterology* 1998;114:930–939.
96. Gilmore AP, Valentijn AJ, Wang P, et al. Activation of BAD by therapeutic inhibition of epidermal growth factor receptor and transactivation by insulin-like growth factor receptor. *J Biol Chem* 2002;277:27643–27650.
97. Liu B, Fang M, Schmidt M, et al. Induction of apoptosis and activation of the caspase cascade by anti-EGF receptor monoclonal antibodies in DiFi human colon cancer cells do not involve the c-jun N-terminal kinase activity. *Br J Cancer* 2000;82:1991–1999.
98. Mandal M, Adam L, Mendelsohn J, et al. Nuclear targeting of Bax during apoptosis in human colorectal cancer cells. *Oncogene* 1998;17:999–1007.
99. Eisma RJ, Spiro JD, Kreutzer DL. Role of angiogenic factors: coexpression of interleukin-8 and vascular endothelial growth factor in patients with head and neck squamous carcinoma. *Laryngoscope* 1999;109:687–693.
100. Shemirani B, Crowe DL. Head and neck squamous cell carcinoma lines produce biologically active angiogenic factors. *Oral Oncol* 2000;36:61–66.
101. Smith BD, Smith GL, Carter D, et al. Prognostic significance of vascular endothelial growth factor protein levels in oral and oropharyngeal squamous cell carcinoma. *J Clin Oncol* 2000;18:2046–2052.
102. Smith BD, Haffty BG, Sasaki CT. Molecular markers in head and neck squamous cell carcinoma: their biological function and prognostic significance. *Ann Otol Rhinol Laryngol* 2001;110:221–228.
103. Petit AM, Rak J, Hung MC, Rockwell P, et al. Neutralizing antibodies against epidermal growth factor and ErbB-2/neu receptor tyrosine kinases down-regulate vascular endothelial growth factor production by tumor cells in vitro and in vivo: angiogenic implications for signal transduction therapy of solid tumors. *Am J Pathol* 1997;151:1523–1530.
104. Harris VK, Coticchia CM, Kagan BL, et al. Induction of the angiogenic modulator fibroblast growth factor-binding protein by epidermal growth factor is mediated through both MEK/ERK and p38 signal transduction pathways. *J Biol Chem* 2000;275:10802–10811.
105. Huang S-M, Li J, Harari PM. Molecular inhibition of angiogenesis and metastatic potential in human squamous cell carcinomas after epidermal growth factor receptor blockade. *Mol Cancer Ther* 2002;1:507–514.
106. Dejong JS, Vandiest PJ, Vandervalk P, et al. Expression of growth factors, growth-inhibiting factors, and their receptors in invasive breast cancer. II. Correlations with proliferation and angiogenesis. *J Pathol* 1998;184:53–57.
107. Sauter ER, Nesbit M, Watson JC, et al. Vascular endothelial growth factor is a marker of tumor invasion and metastasis in squamous cell carcinomas of the head and neck. *Clin Cancer Res* 1999;5:775–782.
108. O-charoenrat P, Rhys-Evans P, Modjtahedi H, et al. Vascular endothelial growth factor family members are differentially regulated by c-erbB signaling in head and neck squamous carcinoma cells. *Clin Exp Metastasis* 2000; 18:155–161.
109. Gille J, Swerlick RA, Caughman SW. Transforming growth factor-alpha-induced transcriptional activation of the vascular permeability factor (VPF/VEGF) gene requires AP-2-dependent DNA binding and transactivation. *EMBO J* 1997;16:750–759.
110. Ciardiello F, Caputo R, Bianco R, et al. Inhibition of growth factor production and angiogenesis in human cancer cells by ZD1839 (Iressa), a selective epidermal growth factor receptor tyrosine kinase inhibitor. *Clin Cancer Res* 2001; 7:1459–1465.
111. Hirata A, Ogawa S, Kometani T, et al. ZD1839 (Iressa) induces antiangiogenic effects through inhibition of epidermal growth factor receptor tyrosine kinase. *Cancer Res* 2002;62:2554–2560.
112. Juarez J, Clayman G, Nakajima M, et al. Role and regulation of expression of 92-kDa type-IV collagenase (MMP-9) in 2 invasive squamous-cell-carcinoma cell lines of the oral cavity. *Int J Cancer* 1993;55:10–18.
113. Kusukawa J, Harada H, Shima I, et al. The significance of epidermal growth factor receptor and matrix metalloproteinase-3 in squamous cell carcinoma of the oral cavity. *Eur J Cancer B Oral Oncol* 1996;4:217–221.
114. Quon H, Liu FF, Cummings BJ. Potential molecular prognostic markers in head and neck squamous cell carcinomas. *Head Neck* 2001;23:147–159.
115. Helliwell TR. Molecular markers of metastasis in squamous carcinomas. *J Pathol* 2001;194:289–293.
116. Price JT, Wilson HM, Haites NE. Epidermal growth factor (EGF) increases the in vitro invasion, motility and adhesion interactions of the primary renal carcinoma cell line, A704. *Eur J Cancer* 1996;32A:1977–1982.
117. O-charoenrat P, Modjtahedi H, Rhys-Evans P, et al. Epidermal growth factor-

like ligands differentially up-regulate matrix metalloproteinase 9 in head and neck squamous carcinoma cells. *Cancer Res* 2000;60:1121–1128.
118. Bruns CJ, Harbison MT, Davis DW, et al. Epidermal growth factor receptor blockade with C225 plus gemcitabine results in regression of human pancreatic carcinoma growing orthotopically in nude mice by antiangiogenic mechanisms. *Clin Cancer Res* 2000;6:1936–1948.
119. Zhu A, Shaeffer J, Leslie S, et al. Epidermal growth factor receptor: an independent predictor of survival in astrocytic tumors given definitive irradiation. *Int J Radiat Oncol Biol Phys* 1996;34:809–815.
120. Sheridan MT, O'Dwyer T, Seymour CB, et al. Potential indicators of radiosensitivity in squamous cell carcinoma of the head and neck. *Radiat Oncol Invest* 1997;5:180–186.
121. Contessa JN, Reardon DB, Todd D, et al. The inducible expression of dominant-negative epidermal growth factor receptor-CD533 results in radiosensitization of human mammary carcinoma cells. *Clin Cancer Res* 1999;5:405–411.
122. Akimoto T, Hunter NR, Buchmiller L, et al. Inverse relationship between epidermal growth factor receptor expression and radiocurability of murine carcinomas. *Clin Cancer Res* 1999;5:2884–2890.
123. Kavanagh BD, Lin PS, Chen P, et al. Radiation-induced enhanced proliferation of human squamous cancer cells in vitro: a release from inhibition by epidermal growth factor. *Clin Cancer Res* 1995;1:1557–1562.
124. Schmidt-Ullrich RK, Mikkelsen RB, Dent P, et al. Radiation-induced proliferation of the human A431 squamous carcinoma cells is dependent on EGFR tyrosine phosphorylation. *Oncogene* 1997;15:1191–1197.
125. Harari P, Huang S-M. Modulation of molecular targets to enhance radiation. *Clin Cancer Res* 2000;6:323–325.
126. Balaban N, Moni J, Shannon M, et al. The effect of ionizing radiation on signal transduction: antibodies to EGF receptor sensitize A431 cells to radiation. *Biochim Biophys Acta* 1996;1314:147–156.
127. Nasu S, Ang KK, Fan Z, et al. C225 antiepidermal growth factor receptor antibody enhances tumor radiocurability. *Int J Radiat Oncol Biol Phys* 2001;51: 474–477.
128. Bonner JA, Raisch KP, Trummell HQ, et al. Enhanced apoptosis with combination C225/radiation treatment serves as the impetus for clinical investigation in head and neck cancers. *J Clin Oncol* 2000;18:47S–53S.
129. Saleh MN, Raisch KP, Stackhouse MA, et al. Combined modality therapy of A431 human epidermoid cancer using anti-EGFr antibody C225 and radiation. *Cancer Biother Radiopharmacol* 1999;14:451–463.
130. Raben D, Buchsbaum DJ, Gillespie Y, et al. Treatment of human intracranial gliomas with chimeric monoclonal antibody against the epidermal growth factor receptor increases survival of nude mice when treated concurrently with irradiation. *Proc Am Assoc Cancer Res* 1999;40:A#1224.
131. Lawrence TS, Nyati MK. Small-molecule tyrosine kinase inhibitors as radiosensitizers. *Semin Radiat Oncol* 2002;12:33–36.
132. Harari PM, Huang S-M. Radiation response modification following molecular inhibition of epidermal growth factor receptor signaling. *Semin Radiat Oncol* 2001;11:281–289.
133. Magne N, Fischel JL, Dubreuil A, et al. Sequence-dependent effects of ZD1839 ("Iressa") in combination with cytotoxic treatment in human head and neck cancer. *Br J Cancer* 2002;86:819–827.
134. Williams KJ, Telfer BA, et al. ZD1839 ("Iressa"), a specific oral epidermal growth factor receptor-tyrosine kinase inhibitor, potentiates radiotherapy in a human colorectal cancer xenograft model. *Br J Cancer* 2002;86:1157–1161.
135. Gupta AK, McKenna WG, Weber CN, et al. Local recurrence in head and neck cancer: relationship to radiation resistance and signal transduction. *Clin Cancer Res* 2002;8:885–892.
136. Inoue K, Slaton JW, Perrotte P, et al. Paclitaxel enhances the effects of the anti-epidermal growth factor receptor monoclonal antibody ImClone C225 in mice with metastatic human bladder transitional cell carcinoma. *Clin Cancer Res* 2000;6:4874–4884.
137. Ciardiello F, Bianco R, Damiano V, et al. Antitumor activity of sequential treatment with topotecan and anti-epidermal growth factor receptor monoclonal antibody C225. *Clin Cancer Res* 1999;5:909–916.
138. Mendelsohn J, Fan Z. Epidermal growth factor receptor family and chemosensitization. *J Natl Cancer Inst* 1997;89:341–343.
139. Baselga J, Norton L, Masui H, et al. Antitumor effects of doxorubicin in combination with anti-epidermal growth factor receptor monoclonal antibodies. *J Natl Cancer Inst* 1993;85:1327–1333.
140. Fan Z, Baselga J, Masui H, et al. Antitumor effect of anti-epidermal growth factor receptor monoclonal antibodies plus cis-diaminedichloroplatinum on well established A431 cell xenografts. *Cancer Res* 1993;53:4637–4642.
141. Shin DM, Donato NJ, Perez-Soler R, et al. Epidermal growth factor receptor-targeted therapy with C225 and cisplatin in patients with head and neck cancer. *Clin Cancer Res* 2001;7:1204–1213.
142. Prewett MC, Hooper AT, Bassi R, et al. Enhanced antitumor activity of anti-epidermal growth factor receptor monoclonal antibody IMC-C225 in combination with irinotecan (CPT-11) against human colorectal tumor xenografts. *Clin Cancer Res* 2002;8:994–1003.
143. Ciardiello F, Caputo R, Bianco R, et al. Antitumor effect and potentiation of cytotoxic drugs activity in human cancer cells by ZD-1839 (Iressa), an epidermal growth factor receptor-selective tyrosine kinase inhibitor. *Clin Cancer Res* 2000;6:2053–2063.
144. Sirotnak FM, Zakowski MF, Miller VA, et al. Efficacy of cytotoxic agents against human tumor xenografts is markedly enhanced by coadministration of ZD1839 (Iressa), an inhibitor of EGFR tyrosine kinase. *Clin Cancer Res* 2000;6:4885–4892.
145. Kumar R. Targeting epidermal growth factor family members for treatment of breast cancer. *Biol Ther Breast Cancer* 2001;3:3–6.
146. Moulder SL, Yakes FM, Muthuswamy SK, et al. Epidermal growth factor receptor (HER1) tyrosine kinase inhibitor ZD1839 (Iressa) inhibits HER2/neu (erbB2)-overexpressing breast cancer cells in vitro and in vivo. *Cancer Res* 2001;61:8887–8895.
147. Ling YH, Donato NJ, Perez-Soler R. Sensitivity to topoisomerase I inhibitors and cisplatin is associated with epidermal growth factor receptor expression in human cervical squamous carcinoma ME180 sublines. *Cancer Chemother Pharmacol* 2001;47:473–480.
148. Bundred NJ, Chan K, Anderson NG. Studies of epidermal growth factor receptor inhibition in breast cancer. *Endocr Relat Cancer* 2001;8:183–189.
149. Dancey JE, Schoenfeldt M. Clinical trials referral resource. Epidermal growth factor receptor inhibitors in clinical trials. *Oncology (Huntington)* 2001;15: 748–750, 756–758.
150. Bonomi P, Perez-Soler R, Chachoua A, et al. A phase II trial of the epidermal growth factor receptor (EGFR) tyrosine-kinase inhibitor (TKI), CP-358,774, following platinum-based chemotherapy in patients (pts) with advanced non-small cell lung cancer (NSCLC). *Clin Cancer Res* 2000;6:4544s(A#386).
151. Hidalgo M, Siu LL, Nemunaitis J, et al. Phase I and pharmacologic study of OSI-774, an epidermal growth factor receptor tyrosine kinase inhibitor, in patients with advanced solid malignancies. *J Clin Oncol* 2001;19:3267–3279.
152. Barton J, Blackledge G, Wakeling A. Growth factors and their receptors: new targets for prostate cancer therapy. *Urology* 2001;58:114–122.
153. Herbst RS, Kim ES, Harari PM. IMC-C225, an anti-epidermal growth factor receptor monoclonal antibody, for treatment of head and neck cancer. *Expert Opin Biol Ther* 2001;1:719–732.
154. Baselga J, Pfister D, Cooper MR, et al. Phase I studies of anti-epidermal growth factor receptor chimeric antibody C225 alone and in combination with cisplatin. *J Clin Oncol* 2000;18:904–914.
155. Mendelsohn J, Shin DM, Donato NJ, et al. A phase I study of chimerized anti-epidermal growth factor receptor (EGFr) monoclonal antibody, C225, in combination with cisplatin (CDDP) in patients (PTS) with recurrent head and neck squamous cell carcinoma (SCC). *Proc Am Soc Clin Oncol* 1999;18:A#1502.
156. Robert F, Ezekiel MP, Spencer SA, et al. Phase I study of anti-epidermal growth factor receptor antibody cetuximab in combination with radiation therapy in patients with advanced head and neck cancer. *J Clin Oncol* 2001; 19:3234–3243.
157. Hong WK, Arquette M, Nabell L, et al. Efficacy and safety of the anti-epidermal growth factor antibody (EGFR) IMC-C225, in combination with cisplatin in patients with recurrent squamous cell carcinoma of the head and neck (SCCHN) refractory to cisplatin containing chemotherapy. *Proc Am Soc Clin Oncol* 2001;20:A#895.
158. Burtness B, Li Y, Flood W, et al. Phase III Trial comparing cisplatin (C) + placebo (P) to C + anti-epidermal growth factor antibody (EGF-R) C225 in patients (pts) with metastatic/recurrent head & neck cancer (HNC). *Proc Am Soc Clin Oncol* 2002;21:A#901.
159. Cohen RB, Falcey JW, Paulter VJ, et al. Safety profile of the monoclonal antibody (MoAb)IMC-C225, an anti-epidermal growth factor receptor (EGFr) used in the treatment of EGFr-positive tumors. *Proc Am Soc Clin Oncol* 2000;19:A#1862.
160. Busam KJ, Capodieci P, Motzer R, et al. Cutaneous side-effects in cancer patients treated with the antiepidermal growth factor receptor antibody C225. *Br J Dermatol* 2001;144:1169–1176.
161. Khazaeli AF, LoBuglio JW, Falcey JW, et al. Low immunogenicity of a chimeric monoclonal antibody (MoAb), IMC-C225, used to treat epidermal growth factor-positive tumors. *Proc Am Soc Clin Oncol* 2000;19:A#808.
162. Baselga J, LoRusso P, Herbst RS, et al. A pharmacokinetic/pharmacodynamic trial of ZD1839 (Iressa), a novel oral epidermal growth factor receptor tyrosine kinase (EGFR-TK) inhibitor, in patients with 5 selected tumor types (a phase I/II) trial of continuous once-daily treatment). *Clin Cancer Res* 1999; 5:3735s(A#29).
163. Swaisland H, Laight A, Stafford L, et al. Pharmacokinetics and tolerability of the orally active selective epidermal growth factor receptor tyrosine kinase inhibitor ZD1839 in healthy volunteers. *Clin Pharmacokinet* 2001;40:297–306.
164. Norman P. ZD-1839 (AstraZeneca). *Curr Opin Invest Drugs* 2001;2:428–434.
165. Albanell J, Rojo F, Baselga J. Pharmacodynamic studies with the epidermal growth factor receptor tyrosine kinase inhibitor ZD1839. *Semin Oncol* 2001; 28:56–66.
166. Cohen EEW, Rosen F, Stadler WM, et al. Phase II trial of ZD1839 in recurrent or metastatic squamous cell carcinoma of the head and neck. *J Clin Oncol* 2003;21:1980–1987.
167. Fu KK, Pajak TF, Trotti A, et al. A Radiation Therapy Oncology Group (RTOG) phase III randomized study to compare hyperfractionation and two variants of accelerated fractionation to standard fractionation radiotherapy for head and neck squamous cell carcinomas: First report of RTOG 9003. *Int J Radiat Oncol Biol Phys* 2000;48:7–16.
168. Baselga J, Averbuch SD. ZD1839 ("Iressa") as an anticancer agent. *Drugs* 2000;60:33–40; discussion 41–42.
169. Miller VA, Johnson D, Heelan RT, et al. A pilot trial demonstrates the safety of ZD1839 ("Iressa"), an oral epidermal growth factor receptor tyrosine kinase inhibitor (EGFR-TKI), in combination with carboplatin (C) and pacli-

taxel (P) in previously untreated advanced Non-Small Cell Lung Cancer (NSCLC). *Proc Am Soc Clin Oncol* 2001;20:A#1301.
170. Baselga J, Herbst RS, LoRusso P, et al. Continuous administration of ZD1839 (Iressa), a novel oral epidermal growth factor receptor tyrosine kinase inhibitor (EGFR-TKI), in patients with five selected tumor types: evidence of activity and good tolerability. *Proc Am Soc Clin Oncol* 2000;19:A#686.
171. Ferry D, Hammond LA, Ranson M, et al. Intermittent oral ZD1839 (Iressa), a novel epidermal growth factor receptor tyrosine kinase inhibitor (EGFR-TKI), shows evidence of good tolerability and activity: final results from a phase I study. *Proc Am Soc Clin Oncol* 2000;19:A#5E.
172. Nakagawa K, Yamamoto N, Kudoh S, et al. A phase I intermittent dose-escalation trial of ZD1839 (Iressa) in Japanese patients with solid malignant tumours. *Proc Am Soc Clin Oncol* 2000;19:A#711.
173. Albanell J, Rojo F, Averbuch S, et al. Pharmacodynamic studies of the epidermal growth factor receptor inhibitor ZD1839 in skin from cancer patients: histopathologic and molecular consequences of receptor inhibition. *J Clin Oncol* 2002;20:110–124.
174. Ranson M, Hammond LA, Ferry D, et al. ZD1839, a selective oral epidermal growth factor receptor-tyrosine kinase inhibitor, is well tolerated and active in patients with solid, malignant tumors: results of a phase I trial. *J Clin Oncol* 2002;20:2240–2250.
175. Siu LL, Soulieres D, Senzer N, et al. A Phase II, multi-center study of the epidermal growth factor receptor (EGFR) tyrosine-kinase inhibitor (TKI), CP-358,774, in patients (pts) with advanced squamous cell carcinoma of the head and neck (SCCHN). *Clin Cancer Res* 2000;6:4544s(A#387).
176. Senzer N, Soulieres D, Siu LL, et al. Phase 2 evaluation of OSI-774, a potent oral antagonist of the EGFR-TK in patients with advanced squamous cell carcinoma of the head and neck. *Proc Am Soc Clin Oncol* 2001;20:A#6.

CHAPTER 42

Gene Replacement Therapy

Randall L. Breau and Gary L. Clayman

Head and neck cancer in general and head and neck squamous cell carcinoma (HNSCC) in particular continue to present a major therapeutic challenge to physicians. Squamous cell carcinoma (SCC) accounts for 80% to 85% of tumors of the upper aerodigestive tract and affects approximately 45,000 patients annually (1). This disease process often has profound effects on multiple quality-of-life issues, including speech, swallowing, taste, and cosmetic appearance. Despite advances in radiation therapy and surgical techniques, contemporary medicine has not significantly affected the survival rate of patients with these tumors over the last 30 years. Disease recurrence among these patients is predominantly local and regional; only 10% to 15% of patients with the disease die of distant metastasis alone (2).

However, advances in biotechnology and molecular biology have allowed us to reassess these malignancies and to consider novel strategies for their management. The earliest studies in molecular therapy were gene marker protocols or studies designed to treat somewhat rare inherited diseases, such as adenosine deaminase deficiency and hemophilia (3,4). Gene therapy protocols are now being proposed to investigate not only solid malignancies, such as melanoma and SCC, but also common disorders, such as infection and arteriosclerosis (5,6). In addition, the concept of gene therapy holds promise as a prevention strategy that may reverse early premalignant events to interrupt the carcinogenic process. These trials and other pending protocols are being closely regulated for public safety by both the National Institutes of Health (NIH) Recombinant DNA Advisory Committee and the U.S. Food and Drug Administration.

This chapter discusses gene therapy and molecular intervention as a potential adjunctive treatment of head and neck solid malignancies. A historical background on the technology and efforts that have led to these treatment strategies is presented. In addition, ongoing clinical trials and major barriers to future advances in gene therapy are discussed.

HISTORICAL PERSPECTIVE

Early attempts at genetic manipulation required the introduction of a large portion of the genome (such as a chromosome). The methods used were often complex in both cellular and molecular manipulation. In addition, when a biologic response was noted, it was uncertain which part of the gene was responsible because so many genes had been introduced. Furthermore, these methods could not ensure the continued production of the introduced DNA.

Solutions to these problems have led to the current state of gene transfer technology. In the early 1970s, techniques became available for cutting and splicing DNA molecules, monitoring the cutting and joining of the fragments, and successfully altering the genetic material of host cells by introducing these spliced molecules.

The earliest studies of gene transfer (1989) at the NIH were not gene therapy protocols but rather gene marker studies. In these initial studies, a nontherapeutic gene was transferred into a patient's tumor infiltrating lymphocytes (TILs) extracorporeally and reinfused into the patient. Subsequent tumor biopsies confirmed that these TILs containing the marker gene localized to sites of metastatic tumors. These initial studies confirmed the feasibility and theoretic safety of recombinant DNA technology and paved the way for future studies (7,8). The first approved gene therapy protocol began at the NIH in 1990 and involved the extracorporeal transfer of a functioning gene for adenosine deaminase into lymphocytes of patients with an otherwise lethal defect of this enzyme (9). The resolution of the patient's immunodeficiency was temporary, however, and correlated with the expected life span of the transfused lymphocytes.

Since the initial trials, it has become apparent that gene transfer is no longer a speculative approach for treating malignancies. Now almost 100 clinical trials have been approved or are pending approval for evaluation of the safety and efficacy of these approaches in humans. As technology continues to develop, gene transfer delivery systems and approaches will progress. Because gene therapy may eventually become commonplace in the oncologic practice of the general physician, an understanding of these molecular approaches needs to be communicated to the medical community rather than remaining the province of scientists in the fields of molecular biology and genetics.

PRINCIPLES OF GENE THERAPY

Understanding gene therapy relies on a distinction first being made between somatic cells and germ cells. *Somatic cells* constitute the organs of the body, whereas *germ cells* involve those cells that produce the sperm or ovum and are passed on to an individual's offspring (10). Current guidelines for recombinant DNA prohibit genetic manipulation of the germ cells. This mandate exists to prevent manipulation of the genetic constitution of future generations, an activity that evokes safety, technical, and ethical concerns. The concept of gene therapy involves the introduction of exogenous genes into somatic cells to produce a desired therapeutic effect. Even though this sounds simple, in reality the steps required to perform this function are complex and have only recently become attainable. The selected DNA fragment must first be cleaved using restriction endonucleases. The next step in successful gene transfer is the preparation of the vector or vehicle used to transport the genetic material. The vector must first be isolated, purified, and cleaved to allow insertion of the DNA fragment. The DNA fragments must then be joined to the cleaved ends of the vector, effectively closing the molecule. This successful insertion of an exogenous DNA molecule into a vector results in a DNA chimera. These vector constructs are the basis of recombinant DNA techniques and are the first step in molecular or gene cloning. The second step involves introduction of the construct into a cell (e.g., *Escherichia coli*), allowing production of a line of genetically identical organisms all containing the DNA sequence introduced by the vector. This allows the mass production of organisms with a specifically designed genetic makeup. Finally, there must be means of assessing the effectiveness of the genetic construct and the efficiency of its expression in the desired host cell (11).

In some instances, random insertion of a normal gene may compensate for a poorly functioning or damaged gene or gene product. For example, in individuals who have hemophilia, lack a normal gene for clotting factor VIII, and have prolonged bleeding, the introduction of a normal factor VIII gene into the endothelial cells or hepatocytes could restore the ability of these cells to secrete factor VIII and normalize the person's bleeding time (12). On the other hand, a poorly functioning or abnormal gene is not necessary for gene transfer to produce a desired therapeutic effect. For example, significant overproduction of the wild-type *p53* tumor suppressor gene has been shown to induce apoptosis in SCC lines even in the presence of cancer cells possessing a normal *p53* gene (13).

Although it is often perceived that the goal of gene therapy is to introduce a therapeutic gene permanently into a patient, permanent gene therapy may not be necessary and may, at times, be undesirable. For many diseases, including cancer, insertion of a temporary gene into a patient's cells could produce the desired effect over a limited period. The theory of temporary or transient expression of a gene is desirable in recombinant DNA safety terms because the risk for permanent integration of foreign DNA is removed, thus diminishing the long-term concerns regarding the effects on germ cells (14).

GENE DELIVERY SYSTEMS

Attempts to target genes directly to somatic cells *in vivo* have made use of a variety of approaches (Table 42.1). In the past, chemical and physical techniques were the preferred methods. Examples include DNA-protein complexes for hepatocyte gene transfer, liposomes for gene transfer to airway epithelial cells, and naked DNA for gene transfer to skeletal and cardiac myocytes. At present, the therapeutic potential of most of these approaches is limited because of the lack of specificity and extremely low efficiency of gene transfer (15). Nevertheless, these methods continue to attract significant research attention as a result of the concerns regarding use of viral gene transfer.

Viral vectors were developed to enable more efficient gene transfer. Viral gene transfer involves the construction of synthetic virus particles that lack pathogenic functions, are incapable of replication, contain a therapeutic gene within the viral genome, and can deliver this gene to the cells by the process of infection.

Retroviruses

Retroviral vectors are the prototypical method of virus-mediated gene transfer. Retroviruses contain RNA genomes that are reverse-transcribed after introduction to produce a double-stranded DNA intermediate called a *provirus.* The provirus then enters the nucleus, integrating randomly into the host genome. The integration of the viral genome into the host chromosome

TABLE 42.1 Methods of Delivery of Exogenous DNA

Chemical or physical methods
Electroporation
Calcium phosphate
DEAE-dextran
Liposomes
Naked DNA
Viruses
Retroviruses
Permanently integrates DNA into host cell at random sites
Requires dividing cells
Low transduction efficiency
Adeno-associated viruses
Permanently integrates DNA into host cell on chromosome 19
High transduction efficiency
Adenovirus
Transient episomal DNA expression
High transduction efficiency
Herpesvirus
Transient expression
High transduction efficiency
Patient toxicity of virus
Systemic oligonucleotides
Short half-life
Expensive

DEAE, diethyl amino ethyl.

is an essential part of the retrovirus replication process but also poses one of the greatest theoretic concerns over recombinant DNA technology (16). Retroviruses possess properties that enhance their effectiveness in gene therapy. First, the provirus stably integrates into the host DNA of the infected cell and is retained during subsequent cell divisions (17), perpetuating the desired DNA as a permanent component of the host cell. Thus, these vectors are well suited for treating diseases that require permanent gene expression (e.g., hereditary diseases). In addition, the considerable experience obtained with animal studies and the work thus far in humans confirms that these vectors have a high margin of safety.

Several theoretic limitations in the use of retroviruses as vectors in gene therapy also exist. First, retroviruses are able to integrate only into actively dividing cells (18). This limitation presents a significant problem in the heterogeneous cell population in most solid tumors, because the cells in dormant states will be less susceptible to retrovirus infection. Another major drawback is that virus-encoded sequences are randomly integrated in the host genome. Modifications in the retrovirus have been investigated to combat this problem and thus improve their safety margin (19). One such modification is creation of a chimera with only the reverse transcriptase portion of the used virus. Other major difficulties in the use of retroviruses as vectors are their low transduction efficiency and subsequent inability to affect significant populations of cells and the difficulty in generating large numbers of virus particles.

Adenoviruses

The adenoviral vector has emerged as a leading candidate for *in vivo* gene therapy in the last several years. It enjoys an advantage over retroviral DNA transfection and transfer in its high efficiency in a wide range of host cells, its known tropism for the epithelium of the upper aerodigestive tract, and its potential to carry a large gene within its 36-kilobase (kb) DNA (20,21). Moreover, unlike the retrovirus, the adenovirus is capable of transferring genes to both nonproliferating and proliferating cells. This appears preferable because of the heterogenicity of cell cycling within the tumor microenvironment. Adenoviral DNA does not actually integrate into the chromosomal DNA and induces only transient gene expression. This allows efficient transduction of host cells, with gene expression persisting for periods ranging from 7 to 42 days (21).

Even though the adenovirus is a very useful vector, it does have its disadvantages. Unlike the retrovirus, the adenoviral vector expresses a number of viral gene products, thus potentially initiating inflammatory (reactive) responses. In addition, adenoviral vectors may become replication-competent by genetic recombination. Because many patients already have antibodies to the human adenoviruses, another concern is that preexisting immunity may reduce transduction efficiency to very low levels. Although the adenoviral vector has not been studied as extensively as the retrovirus, its long-standing use in live adenovirus vaccines in human populations suggests its safety (22–25).

Other Viral Vectors

The adeno-associated virus (AAV) and the herpes simplex virus are also being investigated for possible use as viral gene transfer vectors. The AAV is widespread in the human population, is nonpathogenic, and integrates at a specific, presumably nonessential site on chromosome 19 (26). The AAV infects the majority of its target cells, which do not have to be replicating to be infected (27). Its disadvantages center around its small reading frame, which causes it to need a helper virus to replicate in cells.

The herpes simplex virus may also have a future role as a vector in HNSCC. This virus can be propagated to high titers in the laboratory and, unlike the retroviruses, will infect nonreplicating cells. Preliminary studies are investigating whether the herpesvirus may be effective in gene transfer in head and neck carcinomas. Initial results have demonstrated high transduction efficiencies in human oral keratinocytes and skin cancer cell lines and low transduction efficiencies in SCC lines derived from oral tongue and lip sites (unpublished data). The herpes vector, however, exhibits significant growth inhibition or toxicity to infected cells, and this continues to limit its potential as a gene transfer methodology.

Non–Virus-Mediated Gene Transfer

Concerns regarding use of viral gene transfer in gene therapy have generated interest in removing viruses and viral gene products and developing nonviral methods. One of the most promising of these methods is liposome-mediated gene transfer.

Liposomes are self-assembling colloidal particles in which a lipid bilayer encapsulates a fraction of the surrounding aqueous medium. Previous attempts to use liposomes as gene carriers were limited by their rapid uptake by phagocytic cells of the immune system (28). A new generation of liposomes with reduced recognition by the immune system and improvements in their stability in a biologic environment, such as the circulation system, rejuvenated interest in liposomes (29,30). In addition, the introduction of cationic lipids increased the DNA transfection yields *in vitro* by several orders of magnitude (31). This DNA-cationic liposome complex can be added to cells *in vitro,* injected parenterally or aerosolized for pulmonary applications. Although neither the physiochemical properties of the complex nor its interaction with cells is clearly understood, the process yields reasonably efficient transfection of a variety of cells and tissues *in vitro* (28). It is hoped that future efforts will yield liposomes with improvements in both the efficiency and specificity of gene transfer.

Somatic gene delivery has also been demonstrated using intramuscular injection of a DNA plasmid. Skeletal muscle is an attractive sight for gene delivery because of its good capacity for protein synthesis, easy accessibility for injection, an ability to take up plasmid after intramuscular administration. Electroporation has also been used to increase gene expression using this approach (32).

TREATMENT STRATEGIES

Advances in molecular biology and technology have provided a number of possible therapeutic strategies for gene therapy. With the advent of the polymerase chain reaction, the discovery of oncogenes and tumor suppressor genes has become commonplace. In addition, our understanding of the immune system and its function has increased dramatically in recent years. The cancer gene therapist, therefore, may direct gene transfer efforts toward a variety of strategies, including suppressing the expression of an oncogene, restoring a defective tumor suppressor gene, inducing apoptosis, enhancing radiation or chemosensitivity, or enhancing immune surveillance. Another strategy now in favor is the introduction of drug-activating genes into tumor cells, selectively increasing their susceptibility to chemotherapeutic drugs (33–35). Most human gene therapy protocols now in use are gene transfer-labeling studies or an extension of one of these methods.

Immunomodulation

An alternative to introducing a gene directly into deficient cells is the concept of augmenting the immune system to localize and destroy cells. Activation of cellular immunity requires at least three synergistic signals including presentation of specific tumor antigens, co-stimulatory signals (B7 molecules), and propagation of the immune response via cytokine release. All of these mechanisms have been augmented by the use of gene therapy. Dendritic cell–based vaccines are gaining popularity as these cells can properly present tumor associated antigens to the immune system, thus circumventing the poor antigen-presenting qualities of tumor cells. The dendritic cells can be "loaded" with tumor-associated antigens or other molecules by a genetic modification. *Ex vivo* transduction has also been performed to allow better control of the dendritic cell quality and antigen quantity, and to allow for accurate dendritic cell reinjection (36). Inserted genes can be used to increase the expression of various cytokines: interleukins 2, 4, and 10; tumor necrosis factor (TNF); interferon-γ and -α; and granulocyte-macrophage colony-stimulating factor. Gene therapy protocols have been designed to increase the immunogenicity of the tumor (37) and increase the effectiveness of TILs (38). In one of the initial human gene transfer studies, a patient's own TILs were extracorporeally transduced with a gene coding for the cytokine TNF-α. These transfected TILs were reinfused and appeared to localize in the areas of disease and produce TNF (39).

It has also been noted that head and neck cancers have decreased expression of class I major histocompatibility complex (MHC) proteins, which are needed for presentation of tumor-associated antigens. DNA lipid complexes have been utilized to express the class I MHC human leukocyte antigen (HLA)-B7, thus initiating a tumor-specific immunologic response (40).

Tumor Suppressor Genes

A considerable amount of effort and research has been directed toward the association between tumor suppressor genes and human malignancies, including head and neck cancer. Multiple tumor suppressor genes exist, and the generated hypothesis suggests that replacement or overexpression of these genes could revert a tumor cell to a nonmalignant phenotype. Much of the current research in head and neck gene transfer therapy is directed toward the use of these genes (this topic is discussed later; see "Current Approaches in Gene Therapy").

Toxic Genes and Suicide Interventions

Multiple genes generate cytotoxic products, and this condition provides another potential method of gene intervention. Examples of such genes include those that encode diphtheria A toxin and those that encode staphylococcal enterotoxin. However, toxic gene therapy is nondiscriminatory; normal cells as well as tumor cells are destroyed. Genes that sensitize cells to drugs that are normally not toxic are referred to as *suicide genes.* One such suicide gene is the herpes simplex virus thymidine kinase gene. This gene encodes an enzyme that is not present in normal cells. The importance of herpes thymidine kinase gene transfer centers in its ability to render cells sensitive to the nucleoside analog ganciclovir. On viral transduction, the thymidine kinase gene selectively kills dividing cells by converting ganciclovir into a phosphorylated compound that terminates DNA synthesis. This property proves valuable in the treatment of rapidly growing tumors that invade normal surrounding tissues that are not dividing. The most significant concern over this approach is the potential for significant bystander effect in normal dividing cells (41,42).

Replication selective viral agents also hold promise as a novel cancer treatment platform. Onyx-015 is an E1B 55-kd gene-deleted adenovirus that efficiently replicates in and lyses tumor cells deficient in *p53* tumor suppressor activity. The 55-kd E1B protein of adenovirus binds to and inactivates the tumor suppressor protein p53, enabling the virus to infect a human host successfully and cause the common cold. Theoretically, with the *E1B* gene deleted, Onxy-015 is ineffective at replicating and killing normal cells but is fully unfectious in p53 deficient cells. Administration of Onyx-015 is predicted to result in a localized active infection leading to lysis of the infected tumor cells. Although this infection is expected to spread within the *p53* tumor cell population, its effects on *p53*-positive normal cells should be limited by the poor replication potential of the virus in these cells (43,44).

Oncogene Suppression

Multiple potential modifiers of genetic information have surfaced as possible means for correcting the molecular abnormalities in cancers. For example, gene expression can usually be inhibited by a complementary RNA sequence to the DNA strand expressing the oncogene. This "antisense" RNA can prevent the activity of several known oncogenes, including *myc, fos,* and *ras,* and can inhibit such viruses as herpes simplex virus, human papillomavirus, and the human T-lymphotropic virus (HTLV-1) (45–50). Initial results using this approach have been promising. A retroviral vector system was used to transduce a K-*ras* antisense construct into a human large-cell lung carcinoma cell line with a homozygous codon 61 K-*ras* mutation. Proliferation of this cell line was suppressed tenfold after transduction by this antisense construct (51). The limitation in this approach is that the antisense RNA strand would affect only one DNA fragment within one cell. In those tumors in which this particular gene product is significantly overexpressed, this process would not affect the overall expression of the gene product.

Another potential method of modifying genetic information is the ribozyme. Ribozymes are specialized antisense molecules that operate via an enzyme-like activity in which the target RNA is cleaved at a specific site (52,53). After RNA cleavage, the ribozyme is released and may target another specific RNA sequence. In this manner, ribozymes may cycle and affect the transcription process. A specific subtype of ribozyme that has been extensively studied is the "hammerhead" ribozyme. Ribozymes of this type have highly conserved 3-bp sequences that act as "pockets" for targeting cleavage sites. The utility of this method is in its ability to affect multiple mRNA molecules by irreversible (cleavage) events (54).

Triple-Stranded DNA

Triplex DNA consists of a hybridization between a complementary pair of nucleotides with a third strand, effectively inhibiting transcription at that site (55,56). With the progress in knowledge concerning the interaction between purine and pyrimidine nucleotides, this treatment strategy may be useful in inhibiting malignancy through an alternative gene-modifying approach.

Telomerase

Telomerase, an unusual enzyme, is a ribonucleoprotein that has been found in many tumors and is being considered as a new target for cancer therapy. It acts on the highly conserved, repeated DNA sequences (TTAGGG in humans) on the ends of chromosomes, called *telomeres* (57–60). These telomeres are thought to function in chromosome protection and stabilization (61,62).

Because DNA polymerases in somatic cells fail to replicate the 5′ end of the linear DNA molecule, chromosomes lose approximately 50 to 200 nucleotides of telomeric DNA sequence per cell division (63–66). This loss of terminal DNA sequences is thought to be the mechanism by which normal cells count their cell divisions and determine normal cellular senescence (61,64,65). Telomerase is thought to solve this end-replication problem by adding DNA sequences before each cell division (67). It has been noted that immortal cell lines possess telomerase activity, whereas mortal cell lines do not (68,69). In addition, most human tumors have been found to possess this enzyme (61). In normal human tissues, telomerase activity is observed only in germ cells, and some activity has also been detected in normal bone marrow and peripheral blood leukocytes (61,70).

The presence of telomerase in a wide range of human cancers and its absence in most normal cells point to the potential use of this enzyme as a novel treatment strategy. Telomerase-inhibiting agents have been shown to shorten telomeres effectively and to cause cell death after approximately 25 divisions (67). Further research in this area is needed to assess the future role of telomerase inhibition in cancer therapy.

Altering Radiation and Chemosensitivity

Studies have demonstrated that induction of apoptosis by chemotherapeutic drugs or ionizing irradiation may be related to the status of the *p53* gene and that DNA-damaging stimuli are able to elevate intracellular p53 protein levels in cells that are undergoing apoptosis (71–75). Preliminary experiments (76) showed that cell lines derived from human non–small-cell lung cancers with homozygous *p53* mutations were resistant to chemotherapeutic drugs, whereas those cell lines with endogenous wild-type *p53* readily showed apoptotic death after treatment with cisplatin and etoposide (VP-16). Additional *in vivo* studies in nude mice have demonstrated that a combination of adenovirus p53 (Ad-p53) with cisplatin resulted in more pronounced growth suppression than did treatment with either agent alone. These results support the potential clinical application of combining gene replacement using replication-deficient wild-type p53 adenovirus and cisplatin for treatment of human cancer.

Preclinical studies have also supported the use of Onyx-015 in chemotherapy with synergism demonstrated with Cisplatinum-based chemotherapy regimens. Onyx-015 was able to enhance the efficacy of Cisplatinum both in p53-deficient and p53-functional tumor cells in contrast to its activity as a single agent. This augmented effect may be secondary to the chemosensitivity effect of adenovirus E1A or possibly due to Onyx-015 and chemotherapy working in different tumor cell subpopulations. Another possible mechanism is an induction of higher levels of p53 protein. Other studies have noticed increased cytopathic effects of Onyx-015 in some chemoresistance cancer cell lines. This may indicate Onyx-015 may enhance the effects of chemotherapy and resensitize chemotherapy refractory patients to Cisplatinum-based chemotherapy regimens (43,77–82).

As previously mentioned, radiation sensitivity may also be related to the status of the *p53* gene. Studies have demonstrated that radiation-resistant HNSCC cell lines with a mutant *p53* gene were radiosensitized after administration of a wild-type *p53* gene via adenoviral vector. Furthermore, this radiosensitization also carried over to the *in vivo* situation where the response of xenographs to radiotherapy were markedly enhanced after treatment with adenoviral *p53* (83).

CURRENT APPROACHES IN GENE THERAPY

Various approaches for treating cancers by gene transfer have been proposed, and studies are currently underway to test these approaches. One trial employs a replication-deficient adenovirus for transmission and overexpression of a wild-type *p53* gene. Initial studies using this approach at the University of Texas M. D. Anderson Cancer Center demonstrated *in vitro* growth suppression of human head and neck cancer cells as well as *in vivo* growth suppression in xenograft animal studies (6,13). Wild-type *p53* appears to be dominant over its mutant gene and will select against proliferation when transduced into cells with the mutant gene. Further experiments at the M. D. Anderson Cancer Center have shown that transient overexpression of wild-type *p53* does not affect the growth of nonmalignant cells with endogenous wild-type *p53*. Thus, wild-type *p53* constructs might be taken up by normal cells without adverse effects.

Additional studies allowed development of a microscopic residual tumor model that mimics the postsurgical environment of head and neck cancer patients with advanced disease. In this model, tumor cells were atraumatically delivered into subcutaneous pockets in athymic nude mice. Instead of allowing the tumor cells to form nodules, molecular intervention (wild-type *p53* adenovirus) was delivered 48 hours after tumor seeding. Although no gross tumors were present, there were microscopic tumor cells within the surgical site. This situation mimics the case wherein surgical excision of all gross tumor has taken place. In this model, the establishment of tumors was prevented by transiently introducing exogenous wild-type *p53* via the adenoviral vector (Fig. 42.1) (6). This demonstrates the feasibility and the possible importance of gene therapy in patients with microscopic residual disease. When the primary tumor is removed, the tumor milieu is readily accessible for molecular therapy and is also the most likely pathway of lymphatic spread when regional lymphatic dissection is performed.

The suppression of cell growth by wild-type *p53* has been noted by other authors to be mediated by two distinct pathways, one transient and one permanent. In the case of transient suppression, *p53* serves as a cell-cycle checkpoint regulator.

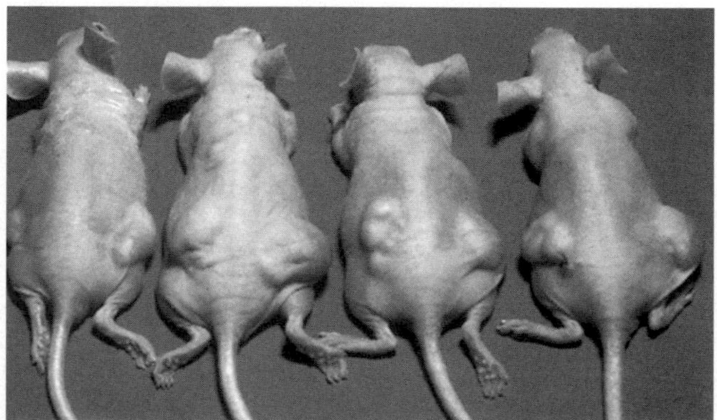

Figure 42.1 Inhibition of *in vivo* cell growth in squamous cell carcinoma of the head and neck. Representative nude mice studies for Tu-177 cell lines 20 days after therapeutic interventions. The right posterior flank received d1312, the left flank received transport medium alone, and the right anterior flap received AdCMV-p53, all 4 days after the establishment of a squamous cell tumor.

Overexpression of wild-type *p53* has been shown to induce a reversible cell-cycle arrest at the G_1-S boundary (84,85). In other instances, overexpression of wild-type *p53* resulted in growth suppression of human HNSCC *in vitro* and programmed cell death (apoptosis) *in vivo*. The mechanism of wild-type *p53*-mediated growth suppression using an adenoviral vector has been further characterized. Using *in situ* end labeling, apoptosis was clearly demonstrated *in vitro* and *in vivo* in human head and neck cancer cell lines. The results suggest that significant overexpression of the wild-type *p53* gene product plays an important role in the induction of apoptosis in human head and neck cancer cell lines and that selective induction of apoptosis in cancer cells can be exploited as a strategy for cancer gene therapy.

Other studies have demonstrated that wild-type *p53* gene therapy is capable of producing a bystander effect in HNSCC *in vitro* and that this phenomenon requires intercellular contact between wild-type *p53* transduced and nontransduced (bystander) cell populations. These data support anecdotal reports that wild-type *p53* gene therapy can produce a bystander effect, and *in vivo* experiments are currently underway to further explore these *in vitro* findings (86).

In a phase I trial with two study arms, 33 patients with incurable recurrent local or regionally metastatic HNSCC were injected intralesionally with doses of AdCMV-p53 escalating from 10^6 to 10^{11} plaque-forming units (pfu) for a maximum total dose of 3×10^{12} pfu per patient. All patients had been pretreated with surgery, radiation, or chemotherapy. Patients were entered into the surgical resection arm of the study if tumor debulking without curative potential was a treatment option; otherwise, the patients were entered into the nonresectable arm of the study. The status of the tumor p53 was not an entry criterion but was measured for each patient. A single site was selected for treatment even in patients with multiple tumor sites. Each patient received at least one course of AdCMV-p53 injections, which consisted of intralesional injection three times a week for 2 weeks. Patients in the surgical resection arm received only one course of treatment followed by two additional doses: one during surgery after resection and one 72 hours after surgery. Patients in the nonresectable arm had a 2-week rest period between each course and received up to seven courses, depending on disease progression and patient consent.

The AdCMV-p53 injections were well tolerated; injection site pain was the most common side effect, in 19 of 33 patients. Mild erythema at the injection site, transient fever, and headache were additional therapy-related adverse events. AdCMV-p53 was detected in blood, urine, and sputum samples. Because exposure of health care providers to the virus was a safety concern, the providers were monitored. No evidence of significant viral exposure was found.

Evidence of *p53* expression was detected in biopsy samples from representative patients. All patients receiving doses of greater than 10^7 pfu showed an increase in antibodies to type 5 adenovirus, but *p53* transgene expression was still detected after the antibody response in representative patients. Because one of the concerns with viral vectors is negation of the transduction and *p53* expression by the host immune response, these results suggest that the patient immune response does not block therapy.

Overall, clinical efficacy evaluated in 17 patients in the nonresectable arm showed two patients with objective tumor regression of greater than 50%, six patients with stable disease for 1 to 3.5 months, and nine patients with progressive disease. Because the indicator lesions were removed in the surgical resection arm, formal assessment of antitumor activity in the resection patients was not possible. However, one patient had a complete pathologic response and remains disease-free after 26 months, and another patient has remained disease-free for at least 24 months (87) (Table 42.2).

These results suggest the potential for Ad-p53 as a therapeutic agent in this disease and supported the initiation of a phase II international clinical trial with Ad-p53 in HNSCC. This phase II trial further established both the safety and lack of toxicity of direct injections (unpublished data). Self-limiting fevers and chills and injection site pain were the primary adverse events observed in this extensive phase II follow-up trial. Antitumor activity was observed in a small percentage of patients with stable disease (i.e., patients with a prior history of rapidly progressive recurrent disease). Separate phase III clinical trials are underway to assess the efficacy of *p53* gene therapy when combined with methotrexate or Cisplatinum/5-fluorouracil (5-FU) in patients with recurrent HNSCC.

Multiple clinical trials have been completed or are currently underway testing the use of Onyx-015 replication selective adenovirus in patients with recurrent HNSCC. In a phase II trial, patients with recurrent HNSCC received Onxy-015 at a dose of 10×10^{11} particles via intratumoral injection for either 5 consecutive days (standard) or twice daily for 2 consecutive weeks (hyperfractionated) during a 21-day cycle. Standard treatment resulted in 14% of patients showing partial to complete regression, 41% showing stable disease, and 45% showing progressive disease. Hyperfractionated treatment resulted in 10% of patients showing a complete response, 62% showing stable disease, and 29% showing progressive disease. Clinical assessments of target tumors frequently resulted in reports that the lesion became soft and fluctuant within a 7- to 14-day period following Onyx-015 injection. In some patients, these early observations were followed by mild to severe ulceration of the target tumor, central necrosis, mild to moderate swelling, or tenderness, which was reported to be closely associated with Onyx-015 treatment.

Adverse events were generally consistent with either a viral infection or flu-like illness or with cancer-related events characteristic of head and neck cancer patients. Treatment-related toxicity included mild to moderate fever (67% overall) and injection site pain.

Other trials have also noted a definite clinical response; however, durable responses and clinical benefit were seen in only a small number of patients. As predicted, p53 mutant tumors induced necrosis at a higher rate than did tumors with wild-type p53 (58% and 0%, respectively).

A phase II trial has been completed evaluating the use of Onyx-015 in conjunction with standard intravenous Cisplatinum and 5-FU in patients with recurrent HNSCC. This study design also allowed an internally controlled comparison of the efficacies of chemotherapy alone (in noninjected tumors) and the combination regimen with Onxy-015 (in injected tumors). Treatment caused tumors to shrink in 25 of 30 cases evaluated. Objective responses with a tumor reduction in injected tumors of 50% or more was noted in 63% of patients evaluated (19 of 30). There were eight (27%) complete and 11 (37%) partial responses. Median survival time for patients in this study was 10.5 months. There was no correlation between response and baseline tumor size, baseline neutralizing antibody titer, *p53* gene status, or prior treatment. Injections site pain was the most common adverse event (53%). A substantial minority of patients reported some flu-like symptoms, including fever (34%), asthenia (47%), or chills (24%).

Additional studies have been performed to assess the feasibility of IV delivery of Onyx-015. Onyx-015 was infused intravenously at escalating doses at 2×10^{10} to 2×10^{13} biweekly infusion in 21-day cycles in 10 patients with advanced cancer

TABLE 42.2 Adenovirus-Mediated *p53* Gene Transfer: Patient Profiles

Patient no.[a]	*p53* mutations[b]	*p53* immunostaining	Primary cancer	Site of injection	Treatment courses[c]	PFU per injection	Study arm
1	*arg175* to *his*	+	Floor of mouth	Neck	2	10^6	R
2	*arg267* to *pro*	+	Larynx	Neck	2	10^6	R
3	*ser127* to *tyr*	+	Pyriform sinus	Left neck mass	1	10^6	R
4	WT	+	Base of tongue	Right neck mass	2[d]	10^6	NR
5	WT	–	Unknown	Left neck mass	1	10^7	R
6	*leu257* to *gln*	+	Cervical, esophagus	Suprastoma lesion	1	10^6	NR
7	WT	–	Tonsil	Left neck mass	5[d]	10^6	NR
8	*arg248* to *trp*	+	Base of tongue	Base of tongue	1	10^6	NR
9	WT	+	Larynx	Peristomal area	1	10^7	R
10	*arg282* to *trp*	ND	Larynx	Left hypopharynx mass	1	10^8	R
11	*tyr236* to *cys*	+	Base of tongue	Base of tongue	1	10^8	R
12	*arg175* to *his*	+	Floor of mouth	Left floor on mouth, mandible	3	10^8	NR
13	WT	+	Base of tongue	Right tongue, right posterior tongue	7	10^9	NR
14	*gln167* to stop	–	Floor of mouth	Floor of mouth	2[d]	10^9	NR
15	WT	–	Mandible alveolar ridge	Left facial mass	1	10^9	NR
16	*arg282* to *trp*	+	Larynx	Left supraclavicular mass	1	10^9	R
17	WT	+	Larynx	Base of tongue, left BOT, tonsil	1	10^9	NR
18	WT	–	Left lateral pharyngeal wall	Left facial mass	4	10^9	NR
19	WT	–	Unknown	Right submental mass	1	3×10^9	R
20	WT	–	Tongue	Left neck mass	3	3×10^9	NR
21	NE	ND	Base of tongue	Right infraaurical area	5	3×10^9	NR
22	*lys132* to *asn*	+	Larynx	Anterior neck, suprastomal	3	10^{10}	NR
23	WT	+	Left mandible	Left infraauricular region	6	10^{10}	NR
24	WT	–	Left retromolar trigune	Left cheek	1	10^{10}	NR
25	*tyr126* to *cys*	+	Pharynx	Neopharynx	1	3×10^{10}	R
26	NE	–	Left oral tongue	Left lateral tongue	1	3×10^{10}	R
27	*cys275* to *trp*	+	Left tonsil	Left tonsil	1	3×10^{10}	R
28	2 bp deletion at codon 209[e]	ND	Base of tongue	Left base of tongue	1	10^{11}	R
29	NE	ND	Submental area	Submental area, base of tongue	1	10^{11}	R
30	WT	+	Left superior anterior neck dermal metastasis	Left anterior superior neck dermal mass	3	10^{11}	NR
31	*ala307* to *ser*	–	Right hypopharynx	Right hypopharynx mass	1	10^{11}	R
32	*ile232* to *ser*, *gln331* to stop	+	Left buccal mass	Left buccal mass	1	10^{11}	R
34	WT	+	Nasopharynx	Right preauricular mass	4	10^{11}	NR

Exon 6 was not sequenced. There was only sufficient tumor to sequence exon 6; it was wild-type.
+, positive; –, negative; BOT, base of tongue; chemo, chemotherapy; CR, complete histologic responses; Exp, experimental plant extract treatment in Europe; NA, not applicable; ND, not determined; NE, not evaluated; NR, nonresectable; PD, progressive disease; PFU, plaque-forming units; R, resectable; SD, stable disease; WT, wild-type; xrt, radiation therapy.
[a]Patient 33 withdrew consent before the start of treatment.
[b]Samples listed as NE (except) had insufficient tumor cells (<10%) in the biopsy for evaluation.
[c]Each course had six injections. Several patients had a partial course of one to three injections.
[d]The full set of injections was not complete in the last course.
[e]The resulting frameshift led to a stop codon at codon 214.
Source: Adapted from Clayman GL, El-Naggar AK, Lippman SM. Adenovirus-mediated p53 gene transfer in patients with advanced recurrent head and neck squamous cell carcinoma. *J Clin Oncol* 1998;16:2221, with permission.

metastatic to the lung. No dose-limiting toxicity was identified. Evidence of viral replication was detectable in three of four patients receiving Onyx-015 at doses $\geq 2 \times 10^{12}$, and intratumoral replication was confirmed in one patient, thus providing evidence as to the feasibility of this approach (88–93).

Another tumor suppressor gene, *p16,* appears to have promise for gene therapy. The *p16* gene is an attractive candidate tumor suppressor gene, because loss of its normal function as an inhibitor of cyclin-dependent kinase would be expected to lead to uncontrolled cell growth. Reports have identified a high frequency of homozygous deletions in the gene coding *p16* in cell lines derived from human tumors of diverse histologic type (94–98).

Our initial gene transfer studies of the wild-type *p16* tumor suppressor gene have shown *in vitro* growth suppression of human HNSCC lines using an adenoviral vector. Western and Northern blot analyses have confirmed the presence of *p16*-derived protein and messenger RNA (mRNA) within infected cell lines. After infection with wild-type *p16* adenovirus, flow cytometry studies identified 60% to 80% of the cellular population localized in the G_1 phase of the cell cycle. *In vivo* studies are underway to assess this approach further.

Attempts are also being made to use the retinoblastoma tumor suppressor gene (*Rb*) in gene transfer therapy. The retinoblastoma gene product is a 105-kd nuclear phosphoprotein (pRb) thought to regulate transcription and to be involved in regulating the cell's progression through its growth cycle (98–100). A distinct mechanism for these functions is unknown; however, several theories exist (101). One of the most promising is the association of pRb with several growth factors, most notably the transcription factor E2F. This E2F factor is suspected to bind to a number of host cell promoters, the activity of which it presumably regulates. Complex formation with pRb is thought to prevent E2F-promoter binding, thus altering E217 activity. Only the underphosphorylated form of pRb, which is suspected to be active in growth suppression, is able to bind E2F. These insights into the function of pRb are currently important in gene transfer studies. *In vitro* studies using pRb showed only mild growth suppression in human HNSCC cell lines. Improved results were obtained by developing an N-terminal truncated version of the *Rb* gene. This truncated fragment produced a gene product of 56 kd (pRb56), with a significant decrease in the number of potential phosphorylation sites, thus enabling pRb56 to remain in its more active underphosphorylated state. Significant growth suppression was noted in SCC cell lines using this approach with an adenoviral vector delivery system.

The use of tumor suppressor genes introduced by a recombinant adenovirus has also been investigated to potentially reduce telomerase activity. *In vitro* studies were performed in two SCC cell lines with telomerase activity examined after introduction of wild-type *p53, p21, p16,* and *E_2F-1* via a recombinant adenoviral vector. Over expression of *E_2F-1* and *p53* was noted to suppress telomerase activity in these cell lines. The mechanism of this telomerase expression and as a potential application of this suppression in gene transfers needs to be further investigated (102).

Other studies have used an adenovirus containing the murine IL-2 gene *(AdV/RSV-mIL-2)* in conjunction with the basic viral thymidine kinase therapy described above. This strategy allows a single intratumoral injection of a viral mixture that would generate a direct cytotoxic effect, through the *HSV-tk* gene product, and an enhancement of the immune response, through the *IL-2* gene product. Delivery of *IL-2* through a gene vector directly to the tumor rather than through administration of IL-2 protein eliminates the need for multiple daily injections and should reduce the severe toxicities, including chills, fever, headaches, and capillary leak syndrome, observed with systemic applications of IL-2 protein.

Using a mouse model of head and neck cancer, different combinations of the viral vectors, alone and together, followed by ganciclovir administration, were studied. Mice receiving either the *AdV/RS-tk* alone or the *AdV/RSV-tk* and *AdV/RSV-mIL-2* mixture showed significant tumor regression compared with control mice or the mice treated with *AdV/RSV-mIL-2* alone. A survival advantage for the mice treated with both *AdV/RSV-tk* and *AdV/RSV-mIL-2* compared with those treated with single agent or control therapy was also noted. Further experiments with this model suggest that the tumor cytotoxicity mediated by the *AdV/RSV-tk* and ganciclovir provides an environment for enhanced local IL-2 produced by the *AdV/RSV-mIL-2* to generate tumor-specific immune response. Further experiments are needed to clarify the potential clinical applications of this technique (103).

Direct intratumoral injection of a liposome IL-2 plasmid is under study in a phase I, single-center, single-blind, placebo-controlled dose escalation study in patients with primary untreated HNSCC. Local production of IL-2 in low levels should avoid the severe systemic side effects associated with IL-2 administration. Preliminary reports suggest that the therapy is well tolerated, but additional data are not yet available (87,103).

Allovectin 7 is a gene transfer product consisting of the *HLA-B7* gene coexpressed with the β_2-microglobulin gene. Expression of the class I MHC antigen initiates an immunologic response. This therapy is currently being developed for a variety of malignancies, with a special focus on head and neck cancer and melanoma. Phases I to II data in advanced refractory head and neck cancer patients was promising, with 10% of 60 patients achieving a partial response and 23% of patients with stable disease after one cycle of treatment. Allovectin 7 as an adjuvant treatment in earlier stages of disease evolution is planned (39,104).

Another area of interest is the application of topical gene constructs for the treatment of oral cancer (Fig. 42.2). Multiple treatment approaches have been investigated. Oral cancer cells that carry human papillomavirus may have their malignant phenotype modified by the use of antisense molecules that are directed to the transforming genes of papillomaviruses. As an alternative, the malignant phenotype of oral cancer cells may be suppressed by transduction with a wild-type *p53* gene.

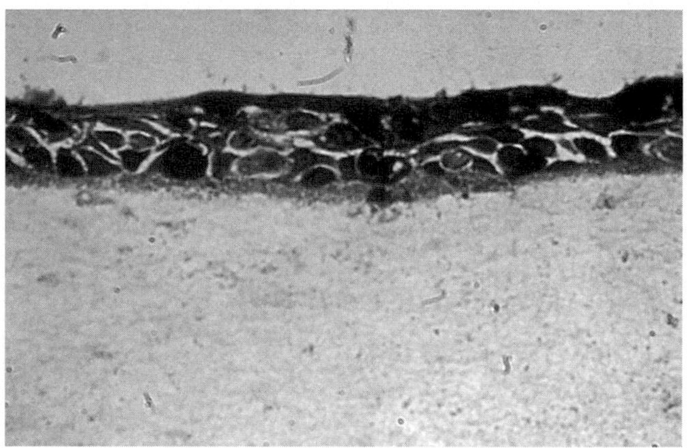

Figure 42.2 B-Gal adenovirus infection of raft culture simulating stratified epithelium. The intense staining throughout all layers of this stratified culture system indicates transduced cells.

Other approaches include the transfer of a toxic gene to oral cancer cells to induce cell death. It is clearly important that optimal delivery systems be developed for the transfer of these genetic constructs to oral mucosa and oral cancers. Thus far, results in this area have not been favorable. In studies at the M. D. Anderson Cancer Center, brief topical application of adenoviruses to the oral epithelium of mice, hamsters, or humans (*ex vivo*) did not result in direct transduction of the mucosa. Various attempts to encourage topical transduction did not result in any epithelial cells becoming transduced.

In addition, experiments were performed to assess the possibility that progression toward malignancy may induce adenoviral transduction. The Syrian hamster cheek pouch carcinogenesis model was used for this approach (105). No improvement in adenoviral transduction was seen in the different premalignant stages of SCC progression. This is unfortunate, because topical application of agents to oral mucosa is extremely simple and is an attractive mode of delivery of potential medications.

The transfer of multiple genes (combination gene therapy) is also a potentially attractive therapy and is considerably interesting. Preliminary studies in which this approach was investigated used the two tumor suppressor genes *p16* and *p21*. The simultaneous *in vitro* administration of *p16* and *p21* to HNSCC cell lines using an adenovirus vector demonstrated no improvement in growth suppression ability over that of *p16* alone (unpublished data). *In vitro* studies with combination therapy using *E$_2$F-1* and *p53* gene transfer provided similar results (106).

The potential approaches to gene therapy are too numerous to list. It is possible that the future may reveal putative oncogenes that regulate aggressive phenotypic behavior in solid malignancies such that antisense, ribozyme, or other regulators of those oncogenes may be developed as novel therapeutic approaches.

CLINICAL BARRIERS

Since the first clinical trial in 1989, it has become apparent that gene transfer is no longer a speculative approach for treating malignancies. Many methods are being evaluated for safe and efficient gene transfer. As with any new therapy, however, many clinical dilemmas face the contemporary oncologist and require further investigation.

The first challenge that exists with any gene transfer strategy is the selection of the "right" gene. As mentioned, recent advances in molecular biology and technology have presented us with a number of genes that might be used for transfer. However, for a gene to be appropriate for transfer, several criteria must be met. First, the transferred gene must have a permanent harmful effect on tumor cells. Though significant growth arrest is important in the study of cellular processes, these transient effects offer little chance for a beneficial long-term clinical response. Additionally, the appropriate gene must have minimal or no deleterious effects on normal cells. This poses a significant problem in that many genes have the potential adversely to affect normal cellular processes.

Investigators must also find ways to ensure that the therapeutic genes are consistently expressed well in the intended target. The therapeutic potential of most of the chemical and physical methods of introducing DNA into mammalian cells is limited because of the lack of specificity and low efficiency of gene transfer. Even with the improved efficiency of virus-mediated gene transfer, many pitfalls still exist. One considerable obstacle in the use of viral vectors for gene transfer is the inefficient infectivity rate seen in most vectors. Typically, only some 5% to 70% of the cellular population solid tumor will be infected. Another major theoretic limitation in the use of some viral vectors is their ability to integrate only into actively dividing cells. In the heterogeneous cellular population seen in most solid tumors, a subset of the tumor cells will remain uninfected and, consequently, untreated by the gene transfer.

Although the considerable experience with viral vectors suggests that they have an acceptable margin of safety, there are some safety concerns. The viral vectors may become replication-competent by genetic recombination. In addition, some of the vectors may express a number of gene products, thus initiating inflammatory responses. Finally, because many patients already have antibodies to these viruses, another concern is that preexisting immunity may reduce transduction efficiency to very low levels.

The presence of a gene in a cell is no guarantee that the gene will be expressed. The gene, therefore, must be delivered along with an active promoter that allows the gene to be expressed in the cell (11). There are many different kinds of promoters, differing in efficiency and activity in different cell types (107,108).

Another major limitation in current gene therapy trials is the somewhat inefficient method (i.e., needle insertion) of introducing the viral gene construct into the tumor. It is hoped that current research in other methods, such as topical transfer of genetic material, will improve on this method. The potential for systemic gene therapy trials depends on identifying safety issues regarding gene transfer and improving nonviral delivery systems.

The power to modify the genome of cells carries with it a number of risks. Exogenous DNA that integrates into the genome may interrupt essential genes, which may modify the behavior of cells in an unpredictable fashion. Conversely, genes that are close to the integration site may be unintentionally activated, which also could alter the cells in unpredictable ways (11). These clinical barriers and other obstacles must be carefully addressed as more experience with gene transfer is gained.

FUTURE CONSIDERATIONS

Over the last decade, dramatic advances have been made in our understanding of molecular biology, biochemistry, and tumor biology. Such advances in biotechnology and in our understanding of the genetic regulation of cellular differentiation, the cell cycle, and tumor progression are rapidly changing the way in which we conceptualize the management of solid malignancies.

The earliest studies in molecular therapy were directed at treating rather rare inherited diseases, such as adenosine deaminase deficiency and hemophilia. The methods used were often complex in both cellular and molecular manipulation. However, in several clinical trials, patients with cystic fibrosis are being accrued to undergo treatment with an adenoviral vector containing the cystic fibrosis transmembrane conductance regulatory gene (the defective gene in cystic fibrosis). Investigations are also underway to study the effects of several genes alone or in combination with standard chemotherapeutic agents.

As the interest in gene therapy continues to increase, it has become apparent that gene transfer is no longer a speculative approach for treating malignancies. Many methods are being evaluated for safe and efficient gene transfer. Challenges still exist, however, in identifying the best genes and delivery methods. Realistic expectations and appropriate basic, translation, and clinical research trials are necessary to advance in this arena. The application of this knowledge to the clinical dilemmas facing the contemporary oncologist is critical for continued progress in gene transfer studies.

REFERENCES

1. *Cancer facts and figures.* Publication no. 90-425, M. no. 5008-LE. Washington: American Cancer Society, 1990.
2. Whitaker DC. Clinical evaluation of tumors of the skin. In: Thawley SE, Panje WR, eds. *Comprehensive management of head and neck tumors,* vol 2. Philadelphia: WB Saunders, 1987:1158.
3. Rosenberg SA. Treatment of patients with advanced cancer using cyclophosphamide, interleukin-2, and gene-marked tumor infiltrating lymphocytes. *Hum Gene Ther* 1990;1:73.
4. Anderson WE. Human gene therapy. *Science* 1992;256:808.
5. Ohno T, Gordon D, San H, et al. Gene therapy for vascular smooth muscle cell proliferation after arterial injury. *Science* 1994;255:781.
6. Clayman GL, El-Naggar AK, Roth JA, et al. In vivo molecular therapy with p53 adenovirus for microscopic residual head and neck squamous carcinoma. *Cancer Res* 1995;55:1.
7. Mobley SR, Clayman GL. The promise of gene therapy in head and neck cancer. *Curr Opin Otolaryngol* 1996;4:82–87.
8. Rosenberg SA. Gene transfer into humans: immunotherapy of patients with advanced melanoma, using tumor infiltrating lymphocytes modified by retroviral gene transduction. *N Engl J Med* 1990;323:570.
9. Miller AD. Human gene therapy comes of age. *Nature* 1992;357:455.
10. Recombinant DNA Advisory Committee. Points to consider in the design and submission of human somatic cell gene therapy protocols. *Federal Register* 1990;54:36698.
11. Clayman GL. Gene therapy for head and neck cancer. *Head Neck* 1995;17:535.
12. O'Malley BW Jr, Ledley FD. Somatic gene therapy: methods for the present and future. *Arch Otolaryngol Head Neck Surg* 1993;119:1100.
13. Liu TJ, El-Naggar AK, McDonnell TJ, et al. Apoptosis induction mediated by wild-type p53 adenoviral gene transfer in squamous cell carcinoma of the head and neck. *Cancer Res* 1995;55:3117.
14. Breau RL, Clayman GL. Gene therapy for head and neck cancer. *Curr Opin Oncol* 1996;8:227–231.
15. Kozarsky KF, Wilson JM. Gene therapy: adenovirus vectors. *Curr Opin Genet Dev* 1993;3:499.
16. Miller AD. Retrovirus packaging cells. *Hum Gene Ther* 1990;61:5.
17. Ledley FD. Human gene therapy. In: Jacobson GK, Jolly SO, eds. *Biotechnology: a comprehensive treatise.* Weinheim, Germany: VCG Verkagsgeselischaft, 1989:399.
18. Miller DG, Adam MA, Miller AD. Gene transfer by retrovirus vectors occurs only in cells that are actively replicating at the time of infection. *Mol Cell Biol* 1990;10:4239.
19. Cometta K, Morgan RA, Anderson WE. Safety issues related to retroviral mediated gene transfer in humans. *Hum Gene Ther* 1991;2:5.
20. Liu TJ, Zhang WW, Taylor DL, et al. Growth suppression of human head and neck cancer cells by the introduction of a wild-type p53 gene via a recombinant adenovirus. *Cancer Res* 1994;54:3662.
21. Mulligan RC. The basic science of gene therapy. *Science* 1993;260:926.
22. Mittal SK, McDermott MR, Johnson DC, et al. Monitoring foreign gene expression by a human adenovirus based vector using the firefly luciferase gene as a reporter. *Virus Res* 1993;28:67.
23. Yei S, Mittereder N, Tang K. Adenovirus-mediated gene transfer for cystic fibrosis: quantitative evaluation of repeated in vivo vector administration to the lung. *Gene Ther* 1994;1:192.
24. Yang Y, Nunes FA, Berencsi K, et al. Cellular immunity to viral antigens limits E1-deleted adenoviruses for gene therapy. *Proc Natl Acad Sci USA* 1994; 91:4407.
25. Clayman GL, Trapnell BC, Mittereder N, et al. Transduction of normal and malignant oral epithelium by an adenovirus vector: the effect of dose and treatment time on transduction efficiency and tissue penetration. *Cancer Gene Ther* 1995;2:105.
26. Samulski RJ, Zhu X, Xiao X, et al. Targeted integration of adeno-associated virus (AAV) into human chromosome 19. *EMBO J* 1991;10:3941.
27. Muzyczka N. Use of adeno-associated virus as a general transduction vector for mammalian cells. *Curr Top Microbiol Immunol* 1992;158:97.
28. Lasic D, Papahadjopoulos D. Liposomes revisited. *Science* 1995; 267:1275.
29. Papahadjopoulos D, Allen TM, Gabizon A, et al. Sterically stabilized liposomes: improvements in pharmacokinetics and antitumor therapeutic efficacy. *Proc Natl Acad Sci USA* 1991;88:11460.
30. Gabizon A, Papahadjopoulos D. Liposome formulations with prolonged circulation time in blood and enhanced uptake by tumors. *Proc Natl Acad Sci USA* 1988;85:6949.
31. Felgner PL, Gadek TR, Holm M, et al. Lipofection: a highly efficient, lipid-mediated DNA-transfection procedure. *Proc Natl Acad Sci USA* 1987;84:7413.
32. Li S, Zhang X, Xia X, et al. Intramuscular electroporation delivery of IFN-α gene therapy for inhibition of tumor growth located at a distant site. *Gene Ther* 2001;8:400–407.
33. Trojan J, Blossey BK, Johnson TR, et al. Loss of tumorigenicity of rat glioblastoma directed by episome based antisense cDNA transcription of insulin-like growth factor 1. *Proc Nail Acad Sci USA* 1992; 89:4874.
34. Cheng J, Yee JK, Yeargin J, et al. Suppression of acute lymphoblastic leukaemia by the human wild-type p53 gene. *Cancer Res* 1992;52:222.
35. Pardoll D. Immunotherapy with cytokine gene transduced tumor cells: the next wave in gene therapy for cancer. *Curr Opin Oncol* 1992;4:1124.
36. Gitlitz BJ, Belldegrun AS, Figlin RA. Vaccine and gene therapy of renal cell carcinoma. *Semin Urol Oncol* 2001;19(2):141–147.
37. Townsend SE, Allison JP. Tumour rejection after costimulation of CD8+ T cells by B7-transfected melanoma cells. *Science* 1993;259:368.
38. Rosenberg SA. Immunotherapy and gene therapy of cancer. *Cancer Res* 1991; 51(suppl 18):5074.
39. Rosenberg SA. Gene therapy for cancer. *JAMA* 1992;268:2416.
40. Medline: Gleich LL, Gluckman JL, Nemunaitis J, et al. Clinical experience with HLA-B7 plasmid DNA/lipid complex in advanced squamous cell carcinoma of the head and neck. *Arch Otolaryngol Head Neck Surg* 2001;127: 775–779.
41. Moolten FL. Tumor chemosensitivity conferred by inspective cancer control strategy. *Cancer Res* 1986;46:5276.
42. Moolten FL, Wells JM, Heyman RA, et al. Lymphoma regression induced by ganciclovir in mice bearing a herpes thymidine kinase transgene. *Hum Gene Ther* 1990;1:125.
43. Bischoff JR, et al. An adenovirus mutant that replicates selectively in p53-deficient human tumor cells. *Science* 1996;274:373–376.
44. Heise C, et al. Onyx-015, an E1B gene-attenuated adenovirus, causes tumor-specific cytolysis antitumoral efficacy that can be augmented by standard chemotherapeutic agents. *Nature Med* 1997;3:639–645.
45. Wickstrom EL, Bacon TA, Gonzalez A, et al. Human promyelocytic leukemia HL-60 cell proliferation and c-myc protein expression are inhibited by an antisense pentadecadeoxynucleotide targeted against c-myc mRNA. *Proc Natl Acad Sci USA* 1988;85:1028.
46. Nishikura K, Murray JM. Anti sense RNA of protooncogene c-fos blocks renewed growth of quiescent 3T3 cells. *Mol Cell Biol* 1987;7:639.
47. Smith CC, Aurelian L, Reddy MP, et al. Antiviral effect of an oligo (nucleoside methylphosphonate) complementary to the splice junction of herpes simplex virus type I immediate early pre-mRNA's 4 and 5. *Proc Natl Acad Sci USA* 1986;83:2787.
48. von Ruden T, Gilboa E. Inhibition of human T-cell leukemia virus type I replication in primary human T cells that express antisense RNA. *J Virol* 1989; 63:677.
49. Mukhopadhyay T, Tainsky M, Cavender AC, et al. Specific inhibition of K-ras expression and tumorigenicity of lung cancer cells by antisense RNA. *Cancer Res* 1991;51:1744.
50. Steel C, Cowsert LM, Shilltoe EJ. The effects of human papillomavirus type-l8-specific antisense oligonucleotides on the transformed phenotype of human carcinoma cell lines. *Cancer Res* 1993;53:2330.
51. Zhang Y, Mukhopadhyay T, Donehower LA, et al. Retroviral vector-mediated transduction of K-ras antisense RNA into human lung cancer cells inhibits expression of the malignant phenotype. *Hum Gene Ther* 1993;4:451.
52. Forster AC, Symons RH. Self-cleavage of plus and minus RNAs of a virusoid and a structural model for the active sites. *Cell* 1987;49:211.
53. Haseloff J, Gerlach WL. Simple RNA enzymes with new and highly specific activities. *Nature* 1988;334:585.
54. Cotten M, Birnstiel ML. Ribozyme-mediated destruction of RNA in vivo. *EMBO J* 1989;8:3861.
55. Helene C. The anti-gene strategy: control of gene expression by triplex-forming-oligonucleotides. *Anticancer Drug Dev* 1991;6:569.
56. Maher LJ, Wold B, Dervan PB. Oligonucleotide-directed DNA triple-helix formation: an approach to artificial repressors? *Antisense Res Dev* 1991;1:277.
57. Bednarek A, Budunova I, Slaga TJ, et al. Increased telomerase activity in mouse skin premalignant progression. *Cancer Res* 1995;55:4566.
58. Moyzis RK, Buckingham JM, Cram S, et al. A highly conserved repetitive DNA sequence (TTAGGG), present at the telomere of human chromosomes. *Proc Natl Acad Sci USA* 1988;85:6622.
59. Meyene J, Ratliff RL, Moyzis RK. Conservation of the human telomere sequence (TTAGGG), among vertebrates. *Proc Natl Acad Sci USA* 1989;86: 7049.
60. Klobutcher LA, Swanton MT, Donini P, et al. All gene-sized DNA molecules in four species of hypotrichs have the same terminal sequence and an unusual 3′ terminus. *Proc Natl Acad Sci USA* 1981;78:3015.
61. Kim NW, Mieczyslaw A, Prowse KR, et al. Specific association of human telomerase activity with immortal cells and cancer. *Science* 1994;266:2011.
62. Blackburn EH. Structure and function of telomeres. *Nature* 1991; 350:569.
63. Blackburn EH. Telomeres: no end in sight. *Cell* 1994;77:621.
64. Allsop RC, Vaziri H, Patterson C, et al. Telomere length predicts replicative capacity of human fibroblasts. *Proc Natl Acad Sci USA* 1992;89:10114.
65. Hastie ND, Dempster M, Dunlop MG, et al. Telomerase reduction in human colorectal carcinoma and with aging. *Nature* 1990;346:866.
66. Harley CB, Futcher AB, Greider CW. Telomeres shorter during aging of human fibroblasts. *Nature* 1990;345:458.
67. Blackburn EH. Telomeres, telomerase, and cancer. *Sci Am* 1996; 274:92.
68. Morin GB. The human telomere terminal transferase enzyme is a ribonucleoprotein that synthesizes TTAGGG repeats. *Cell* 1989; 59:521.
69. Counter CM, Avilion AA, LeFeuvre CE, et al. Telomerase shortening associated with chromosome instability is arrested in immortal cells which express telomerase activity. *EMBO J* 1992;11:1921.

70. Harley CB, Andrews W, Chin CP, et al. Human telomerase inhibition and cancer. *Proc Am Assoc Cancer Res* 1995;36:671.
71. Lowe S, Schmitt EM, Smith SW, et al. p53 is required for radiation-induced apoptosis in mouse thymocytes. *Nature* 1993;362:847.
72. Clarke AR, Purdie CA, Harrison DJ, et al. Thymocyte apoptosis induced by p53-dependent and independent pathways. *Nature* 1993;362:849.
73. Fritsche M, Haessler C, Brandner G. Induction of nuclear accumulation of the tumor-suppressor protein p53 by DNA-damaging agents. *Oncogene* 1993;8:307.
74. Harper JE, Adami GR, Wei N, et al. The p21 Cdk-interacting protein Cip 1 is a potent inhibitor of GI cyclin-dependent kinases. *Cell* 1993;75:805.
75. El-Deiry WS, Tokino T, Velculescu VE, et al. WAFT, a potential mediator of p53 tumor suppression. *Cell* 1993;75:817.
76. Fujiwara T, Grimm EA, Mukhopadhyay T, et al. Induction of chemosensitivity in human lung cancer cells in vivo by adenovirus-mediated transfer of the wild-type p53 gene. *Cancer Res* 1994;54:2287–2291.
77. You L, Yang C-T, Jablons DM. Onyx-015 works synergistically with chemotherapy in lung cancer cell lines and primary cultures freshly made from lung cancer patients. *Can Res* 2000;60:2009–2013.
78. Heise C, Sampson-Johannes A, Williams A, et al. Onyx-015, an E1B-gene-attenuated adenovirus, causes tumor-specific cytolysis and antitumoral efficacy that can be augmented by standard chemotherapeutic agents. *Nature Med* 1997;6(3):639–645.
79. Sanchez-Prieto R, Quintanilla M, Cano A, et al. Carcinoma cell lines become sensitive to DNA-damaging agents by the expression of the adenovirus E1A gene. *Oncogene* 1996;13:1083–1092.
80. Heise C, Kim YT, Sampson-Johnannes A, et al. Efficacy of a replication selective adenovirus against ovarian carcinomatosis is dependent on tumor burden, viral replication, and p53 status. *Gene Ther* 2000;7:1925–1929.
81. Lowe SW, Ruley HE. Stabilization of the p53 tumor suppressor is induced by adenovirus 5 EIA and accompanies apoptosis. *Genes Dev* 1993;7:535–545.
82. Barker DD, Berk AJ. Adenovirus proteins from both E1B reading frames are required for transformation of rodent cells by viral infection and DNA transfection. *Virology* 1987;156:107–121.
83. Pirollo KF, Hao Z, Rait A, et al. p53-mediated sensitization of squamous cell carcinoma of the head and neck to radiotherapy. *Oncogene* 1997;14:1735–1746.
84. Martinez J, Georgoff I, Martinez J, et al. Cellular localization and cell cycle regulation by a temperature-sensitive p53 protein. *Genes Dev* 1991;5:151.
85. Diller L, Kassell J, Nelson CE, et al. p53 functions as a cell cycle control protein in osteosarcoma. *Mol Cell Biol* 1990;10:5772.
86. Frank DK, Frederick MJ, Liu TJ, et al. Bystander effect in the adenovirus-mediated wild-type *p53* gene therapy model of human squamous cell carcinoma of the head and neck. *Clin Cancer Res* 1998;4:2521–2527.
87. Clayman GL, DDS, Dreiling LK. Injectable modalities as local and regional strategies for head and neck cancer. *Hematol Oncol Clin North Am* 1999;13:4
88. Nemunaitis J, Khuri F, Ganly I, et al. Phase II trial of intratumoral administration of Onyx-015, a replication-selective adenovirus, in patients with refractory head and neck cancer. *J Clin Oncol* 2001;19(2):289–298.
89. Kim D, Hermiston T, McCormick F. Onyx-015: clinical data are encouraging. *Nature Med* 1998;4:1341–1342.
90. Kim D, et al. A phase II trial of intratumoral injection with an E1B-deleted adenovirus, Onyx-015, in patients with recurrent, refractory head and neck caner. *Proc Am Soc Clin Oncol* 1998;17:391a.
91. Ganly I, et al. A phase I study of Onyx-015, an E1B attenuated adenovirus, administered intratumorally to patients with recurrent head and neck cancer. *Clin Cancer Res* 2000;6:798–806.
92. Khuri FR, Nemunaitis J, Ganly I, et al. A controlled trial of intratumoral Onyx-015, a selectively-replicating adenovirus, in combination with cisplatin and 5-fluorouracil in patients with recurrent head and neck cancer. *Nature Med* 2000;6:879.
93. Nemunaitis J, Cunningham C, Buchanan A, et al. Intravenous infusion of a replication selective adenovirus (Onyx-015) in cancer patients: safety, feasibility and biological activity. *Gene Ther* 2001;8:746–759.
94. Kamb A, Gruis NA, Weaver-Feldhaus J, et al. A cell cycle regulator potentially involved in genesis of many tumor types. *Science* 1994;264:436.
95. Nobori T, Miura K, Wu DJ, et al. Deletions of the cyclin-dependent kinase-4 inhibitor gene in multiple human cancers. *Nature* 1994;370:753.
96. Spruck CH III, Gonzalez-Zulueta M, Shibata A, et al. p16 gene in uncultured tumours. *Nature* 1994;370:183.
97. Cairns P, Mao L, Merlo A, et al. Rates of p16 (MTST1) mutations in primary tumors with 9p loss. *Science* 1994;265:415.
98. Boehm T, Baer R, Lavenir I, et al. The mechanism of chromosomal translocation t(11;14) involving the T-cell receptor C delta locus on human chromosome 14g11 and a transcribed region of chromosome 11p15. *EMBO J* 1988;7:385.
99. Freyd G, Kim SK, Horvitz HR. Novel cysteine-rich motif and homeodomain in the product of the Caenorhabditis elegans cell lineage gene lin-11. *Nature* 1990;344:876.
100. Pettersson S, Cook GP, Bruggemann M, et al. A second B cell-specific enhancer 3′ of the immunoglobulin heavy-chain locus. *Nature* 1990;344:165.
101. Weinberg RA. Tumor suppressor genes. *Science* 1991;254:1138.
102. Henderson YC, Breau RL, Liu TJ, et al. Telomerase activity in head and neck tumors after introduction of wild-type P53, P21, P16, and E2F-1 genes by means of recombinant adenovirus. *Head Neck* 2000;22:347–354.
103. O'Malley BW Jr, Sewell DA, Li D, et al. The role of interleukin-2 in combination adenovirus gene therapy for head and neck cancer. *Mol Endocrinol* 1997; 11:667
104. Galanis E. Technology evaluation: Allovectin-7, Vical. *Curr Opin Mol Ther* 2002;4:80–87.
105. Gimenez-Conti IB, Slaga TJ. The hamster cheek pouch carcinogenesis model. *J Cell Biochem* 1993;17:83.
106. Frank DK, Liu TJ, Frederick MJ, et al. Combination E2F-1 and p53 gene transfer does not enhance growth inhibition in human squamous cell carcinoma of the head and neck. *Clin Cancer Res* 1998;4:2265–2272.
107. Ho DY, Mocarski ES. Beta galactosidase as a marker in the peripheral and neural tissues of the herpes simplex virus-infected mouse. *Virology* 1988;167: 279.
108. Ponder KP, Dunbar RP, Wilson DR, et al. Evaluation of relative promoter strength in primary hepatocytes using optimized lipofection. *Hum Gene Ther* 1991;2:41.

APPENDIX

Imaging Considerations for Radiation Therapy Treatment Planning

Louis B. Harrison and Bernard B. O'Malley

CERVICAL LYMPH NODES (CHAPTER 14)

It has become customary to divide the lymph nodes in the neck into various levels. As we learn more about the spread patterns, and customize surgical procedures and radiation therapy treatments, knowledge of this radiographic anatomy becomes essential to optimal treatment planning. With increasing frequency, radiation oncologists can tailor the fields of treatment, avoid contralateral nodal irradiation (also sparing salivary tissue and minimizing xerostomia), and work with surgeons to combine neck radiation and surgery. Figure A.1 shows the key lymph node levels that are important in the planning of radiation therapy. Of course, the primary site is key to this process, and the nodes of importance will vary with the primary site involved.

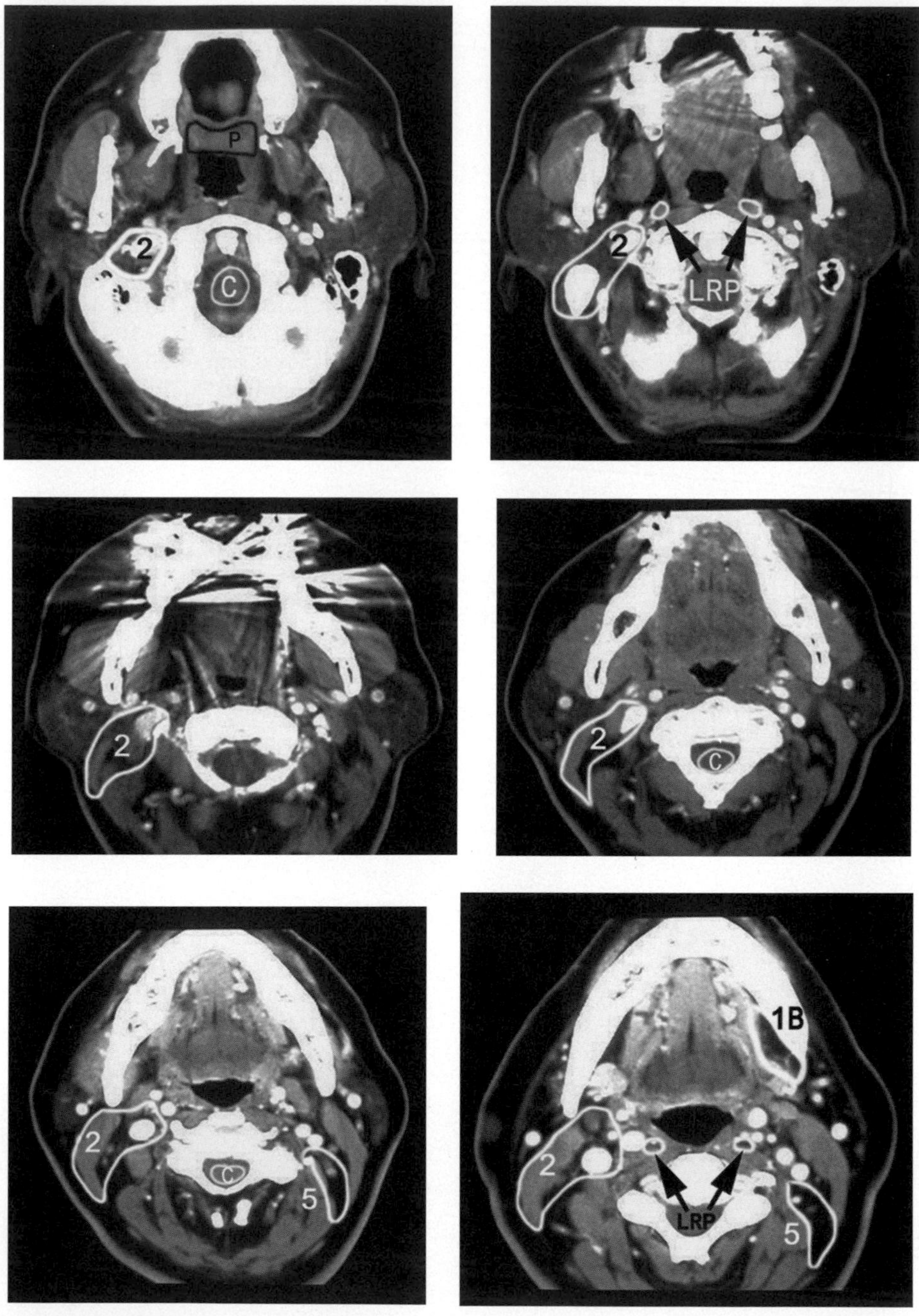

Figure A.1 Images from superior to inferior. *1A*, level I A lymph node group; *1B*, level I B lymph node group; *2*, outline of level II lymph node chain cephalad to level of hyoid bone; *2-3*, level of transition between lymph node levels II and III considered radiographically at the level of the hyoid bone (*outlined in black*); *3-4*, level of transition between lymph node levels III and IV considered radiographically at the level of the cricoid cartilage (*shaded in black*); *4*, outline of level IV lymph node group caudal to level of cricoid cartilage; *5*, outline of level V lymph node group; *C*, spinal cord; *LRP*, lateral retropharyngeal lymph nodes (see Fig. A.3 for medial retropharyngeal node); *P*, palate; *SC*, supraclavicular lymph node space.

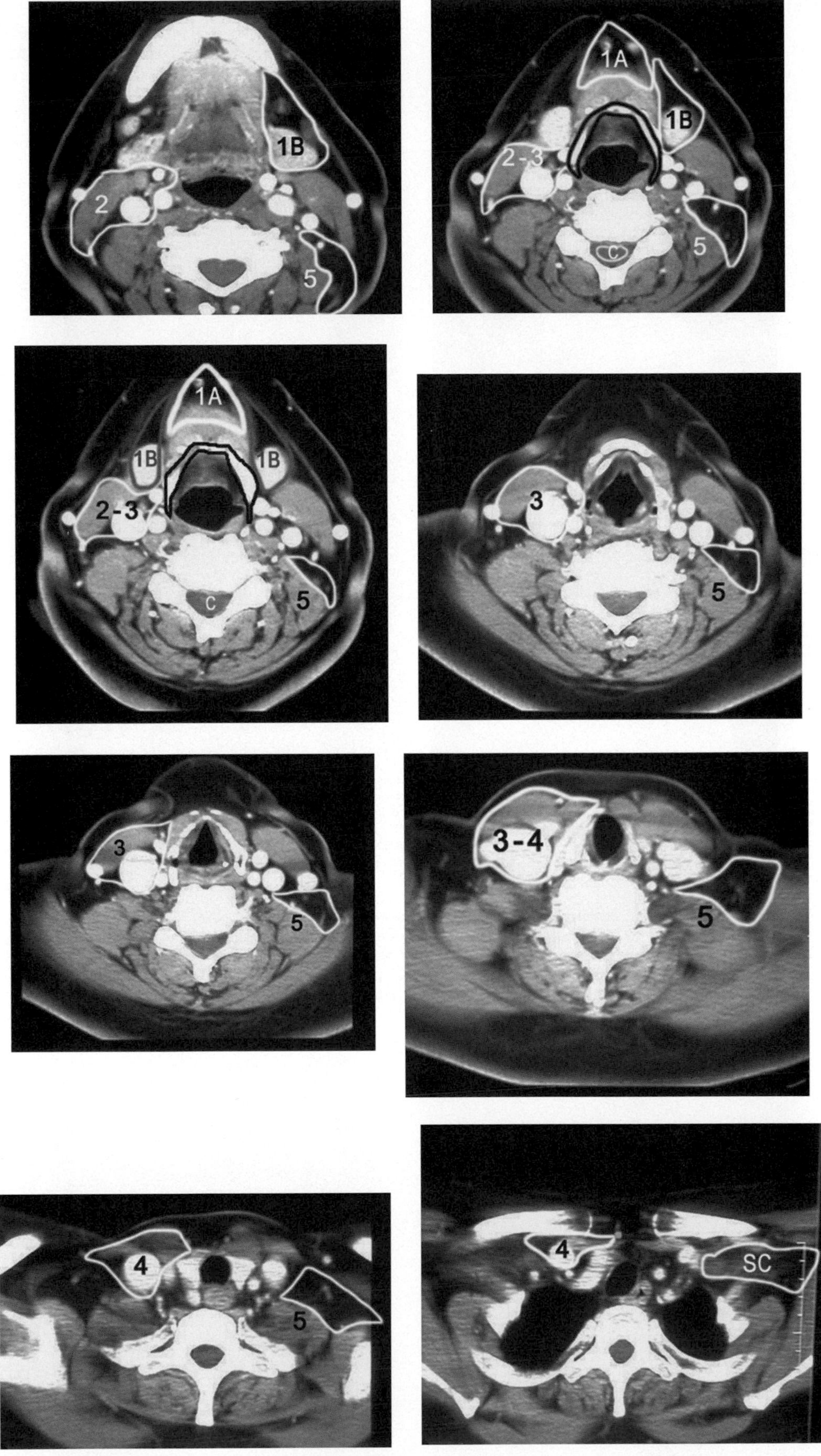

Figure A.1 *(Continued)*

ORAL CAVITY (CHAPTER 16)

The normal computed tomography (CT) anatomy of the major structures of the oral cavity are shown in Fig. A.2. Although most oral cavity tumors are currently treated with lateral opposed fields, selected buccal mucosa and retromolar trigone lesions are often treated unilaterally using CT-based planning. Figure A.1 displays the CT anatomy of the neck, showing the appropriate levels of lymphatic drainage. Levels I-III are the most important for oral cavity tumors.

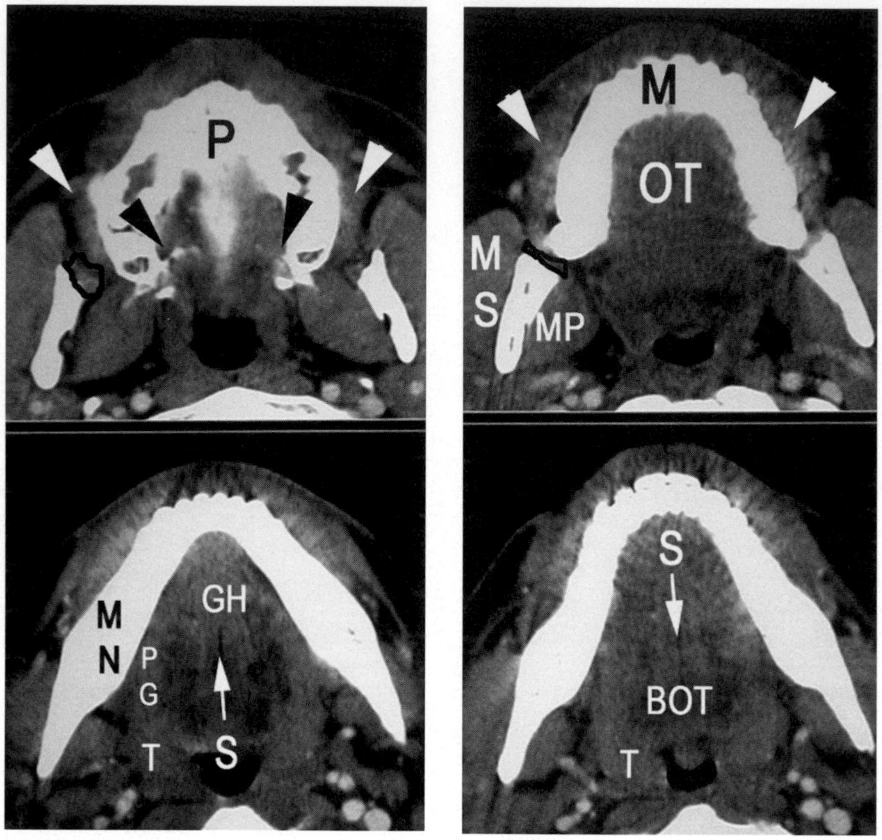

Figure A.2 Images from superior to inferior. *Black arrowheads*, palatine foraminae; *BOT*, base of tongue; *DG*, digastric muscle; *GG*, genioglossus; *GH*, geniohyoid muscles; *M*, maxillary bone; *MH*, mylohyoid; *MN*, mandible; *MP*, medial pterygoids; *MS*, masseter muscles; *OT*, oral tongue; *P*, hard palate; *PG*, palatoglossus muscles; *S*, lingual septum; *SG*, submandibular gland; *Sy*, symphysis of mandible; *T*, palatine tonsils; *white arrowheads*, buccal mucosa; *white outline*, floor of mouth.

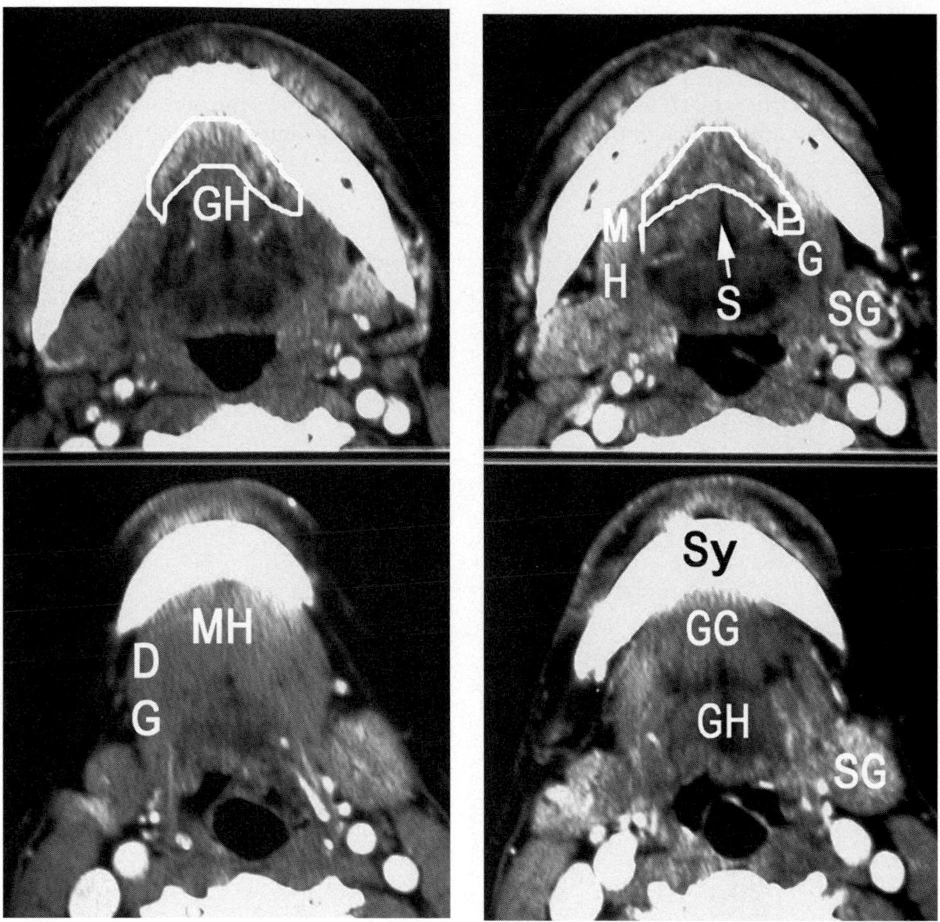

Figure A.2 *(Continued)*

OROPHARYNX (CHAPTER 17)

The oropharynx is composed of the soft palate, tonsillar pillars, tonsillar fossa, base of tongue, and pharyngeal wall. In addition, the retropharyngeal lymph nodes are a major drainage site for oropharyngeal tumors and should be included in the target volumes. Figure A.3 shows the normal anatomic areas pertinent to the oropharynx and the location of the retropharyngeal nodes. Figure A.1 shows the lymph node levels in the neck. Levels II–V are the most important, as well as the retropharyngeal nodes.

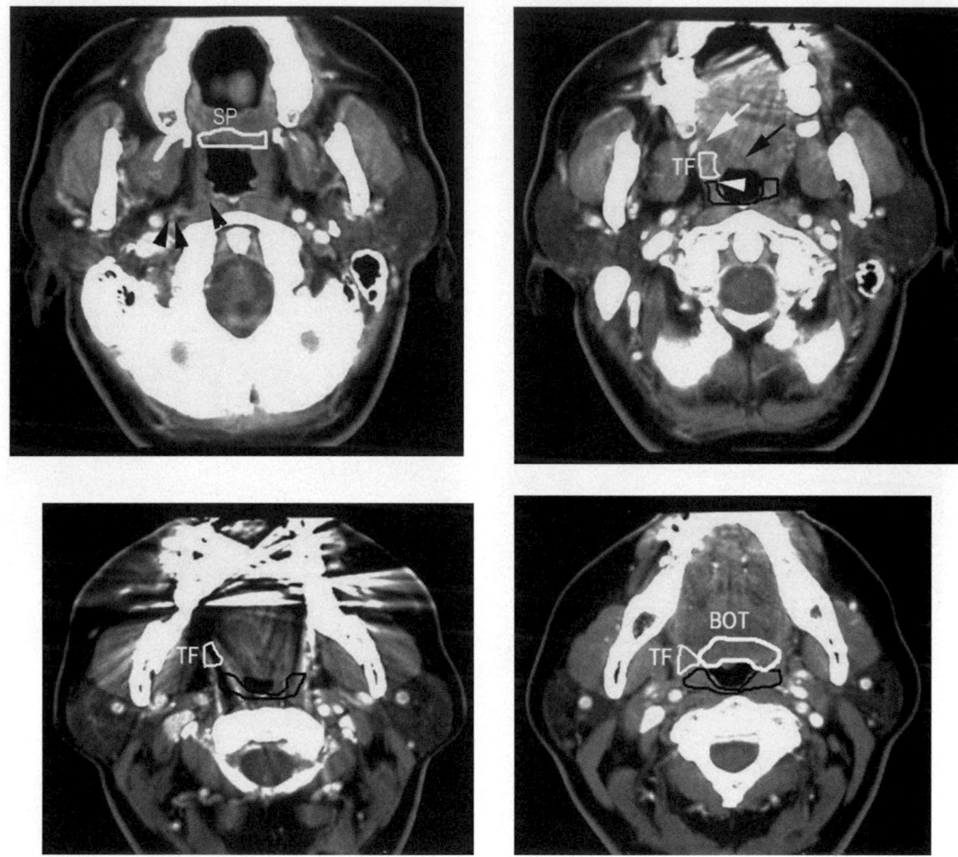

Figure A.3 Images from superior to inferior. *SP* (soft palate) *white outline*; uvula, *black arrow*; *TF* (tonsillar fossa), *white outline* (see also Fig. A.2); tonsillar pillar, *white arrow*; pharyngeal walls, *black outline*; BOT (base of tongue), *white outline*; medial retropharyngeal node, *black arrowhead*; lateral retropharyngeal node, *paired black arrowheads*.

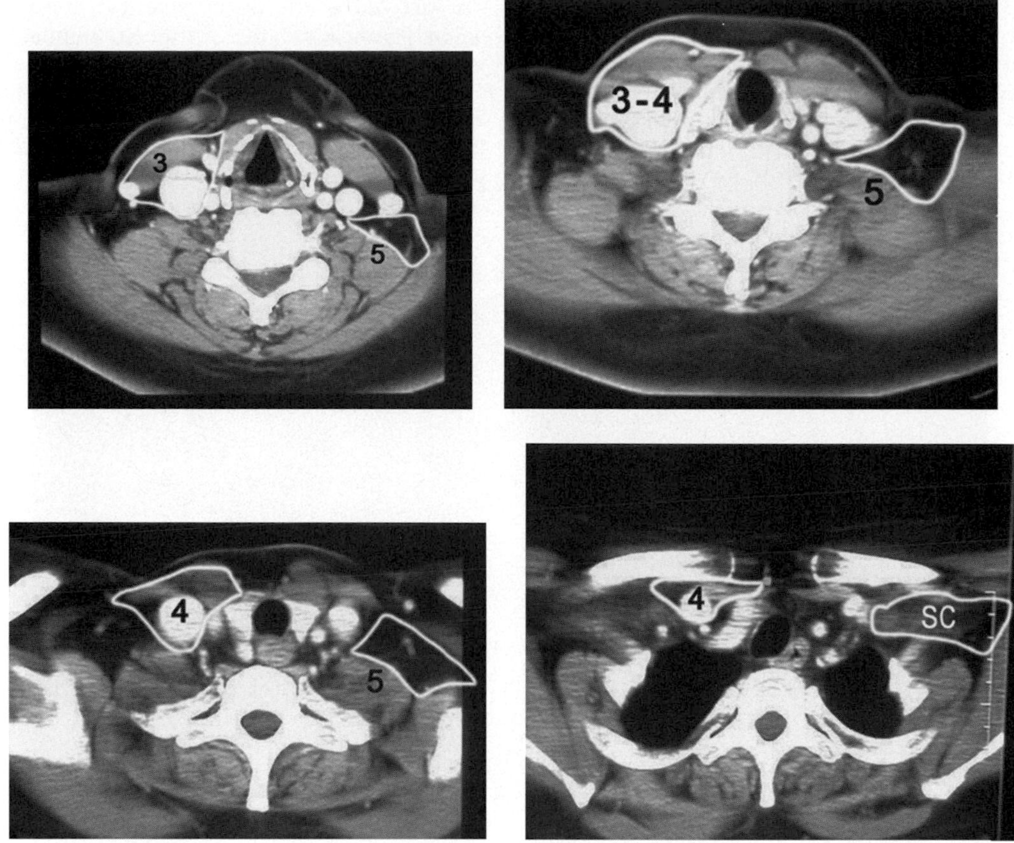

Figure A.3 *(Continued)*

LARYNX (CHAPTERS 17 AND 18)

The larynx is composed of numerous subsites. Although radiation oncologists do not regularly contour these subsites in the development of treatment plans, they may become increasingly important as our treatment planning capability continues to improve. Knowledge of the laryngeal anatomy can also aid in the development of the plans that homogeneously irradiate the entire anatomic complex that is involved with tumor. Figure A.4 shows the detailed anatomy of the larynx and its important subsites. Figure A.1 reveals the lymph node levels in the neck. Obviously, for glottic cancers that are advanced, level II, III, and IV nodes are the most important.

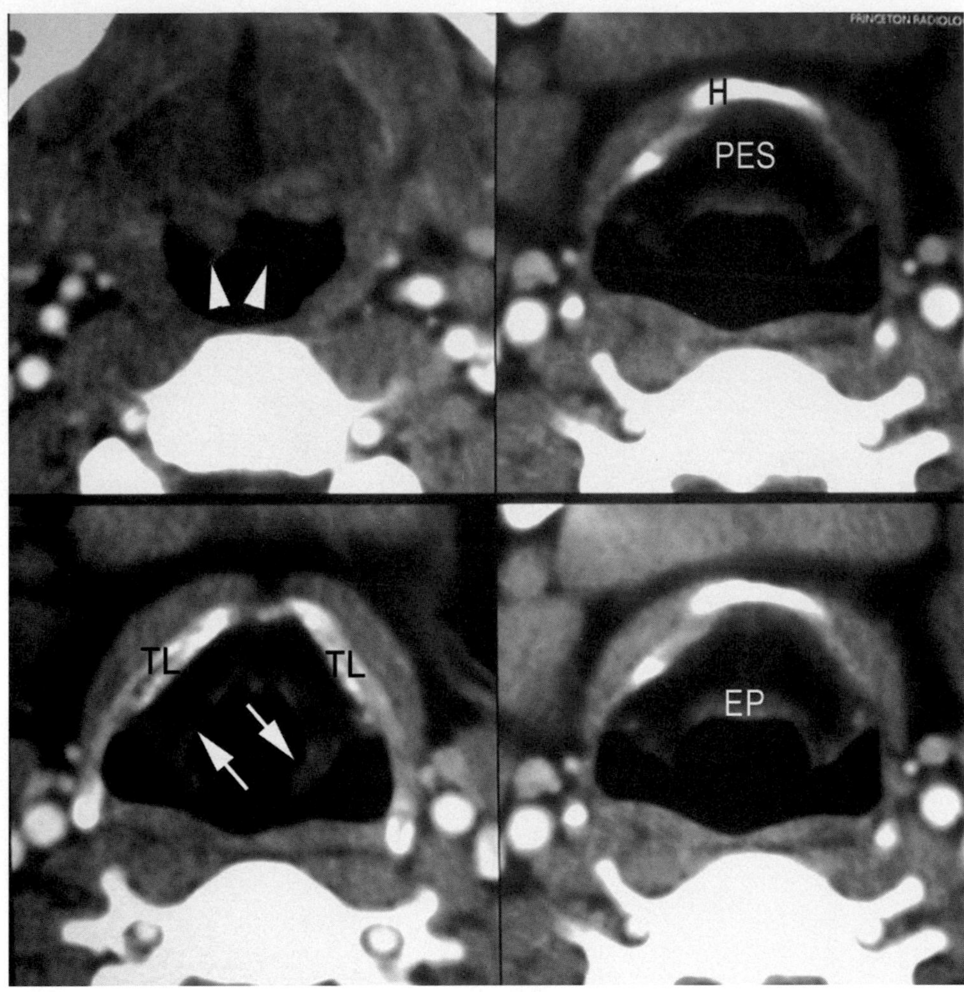

Figure A.4 Images from superior to inferior. (+), arytenoid cartilages; *A*, apex of pyriform sinus; *white arrowheads*, free edge of epiglottis; *black arrowheads*, paraglottic space; *C*, cricoid cartilage; *EP*, epiglottis proper; *FC*, level of false cords; *H*, hyoid bone; *P*, pyriform sinus; *paired black arrowheads*, anterior commisure; *paired white arrowheads*, posterior commisure; *PES*, pre-epiglottic space; *SG*, subglottic airway; *TC*, level of true vocal cords; *TL*, thyroid lamina; *white arrows*, aryepiglottic folds.

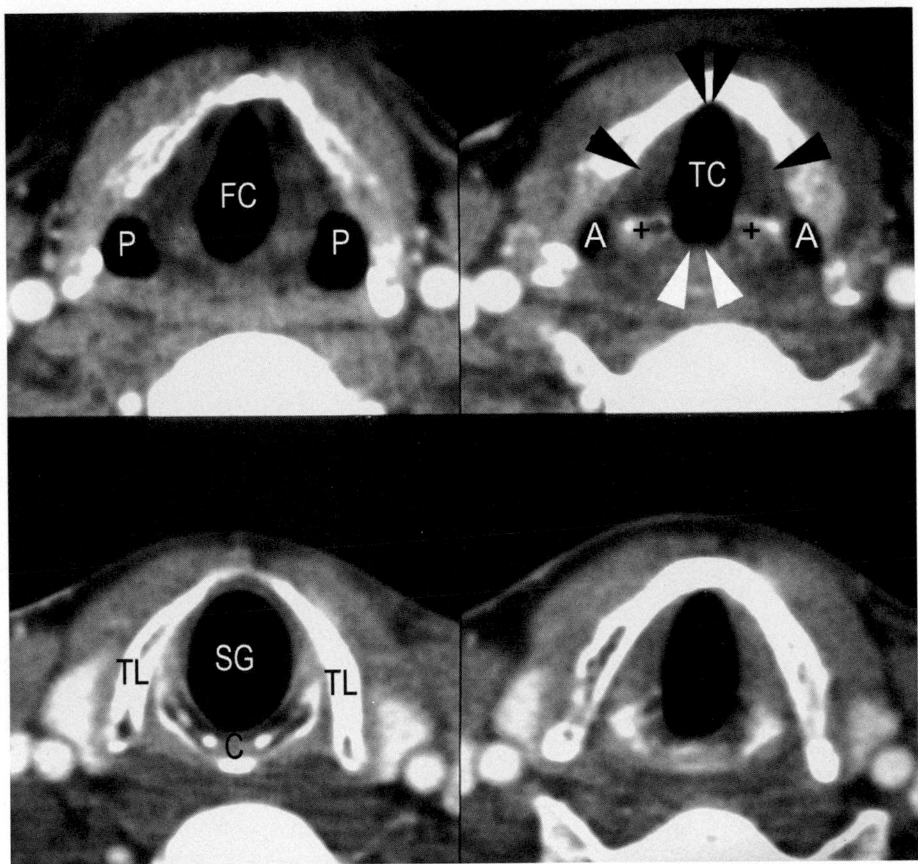

Figure A.4 *(Continued)*

HYPOPHARYNX (CHAPTER 20)

The major subsites of the hypopharynx are the pyriform sinuses, the postcricoid area, and the posterior pharyngeal wall. These structures, and the surrounding anatomy, are outlined in Fig. A.5. Most hypopharyngeal tumors are bulky, and the treatment planning encompasses the entire bilateral volume. It is important to ensure adequate and homogeneous coverage of the entire region in the treatment planning process. Also, because the neck node metastases are so important for hypopharynx cancer, Fig. A.1 reveals the radiographic anatomy of the lymph node levels in the neck.

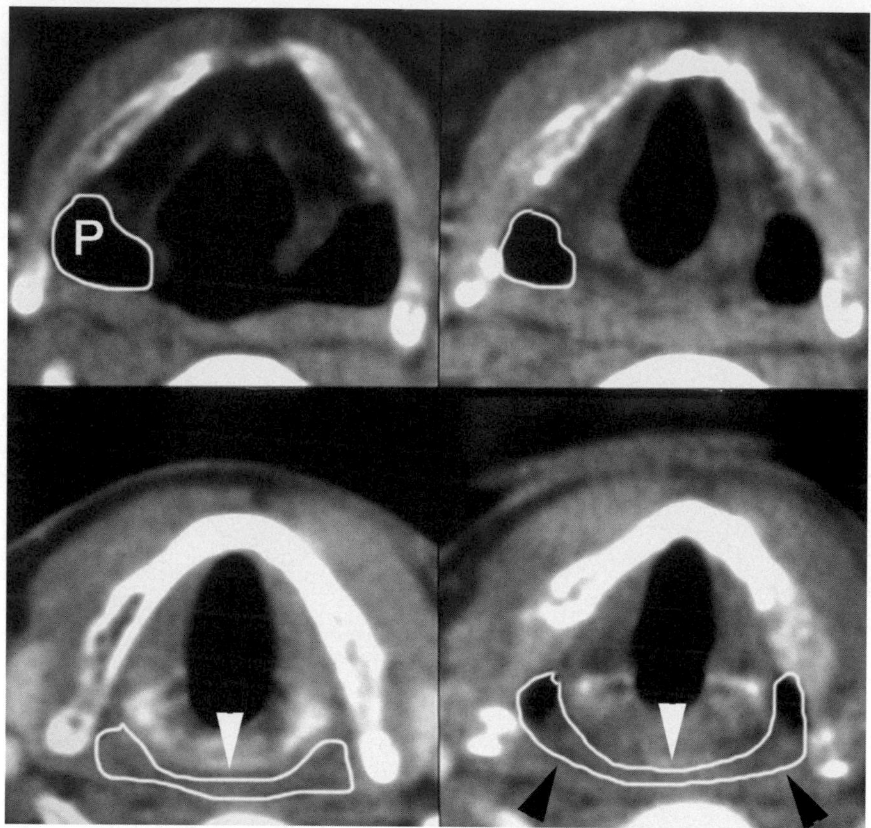

Figure A.5 Images from superior to inferior. *A*, apex of pyriform recess; *black arrowheads*, posterior pharyngeal wall; *C*, cricoid; *HE*, hypopharngo-esophageal junction; *P*, pyriform sinus; *T*, thyroid lamina; *TR*, trachea; *white arrowheads*, postcricoid hypopharynx. The hypopharynx proper is outlined with the *white line*.

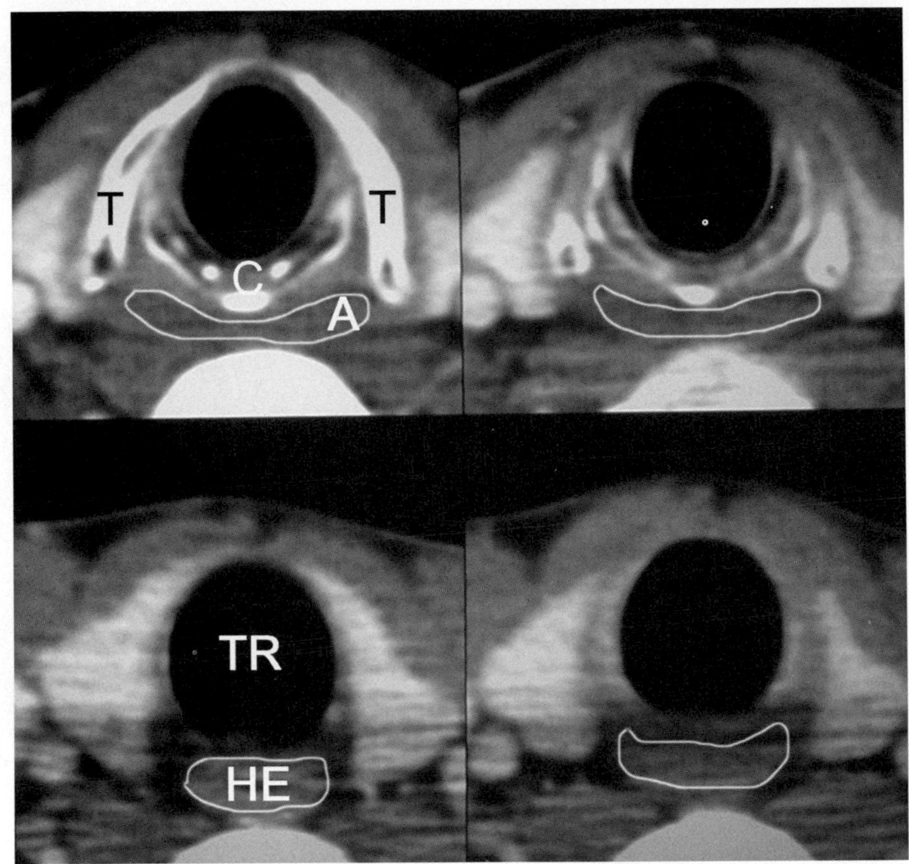

Figure A.5 *(Continued)*

NASAL CAVITY AND PARANASAL SINUSES (CHAPTER 22)

The paranasal sinuses form a complex sequence of air cavities within the facial/skull structure. The detailed anatomy of this region has been reviewed in the respective chapters on these anatomic sites.

In the treatment planning, the relationship of the sinuses to the optic nerves, optic chiasm, various cranial nerve pathways, and orbital contents, becomes a key ingredient to successful treatment planning and delivery. Figures A.6 and A.6A show the key anatomic structures that are major concerns in the planning of radiation therapy to this region, including the orbit (Fig. A.6A).

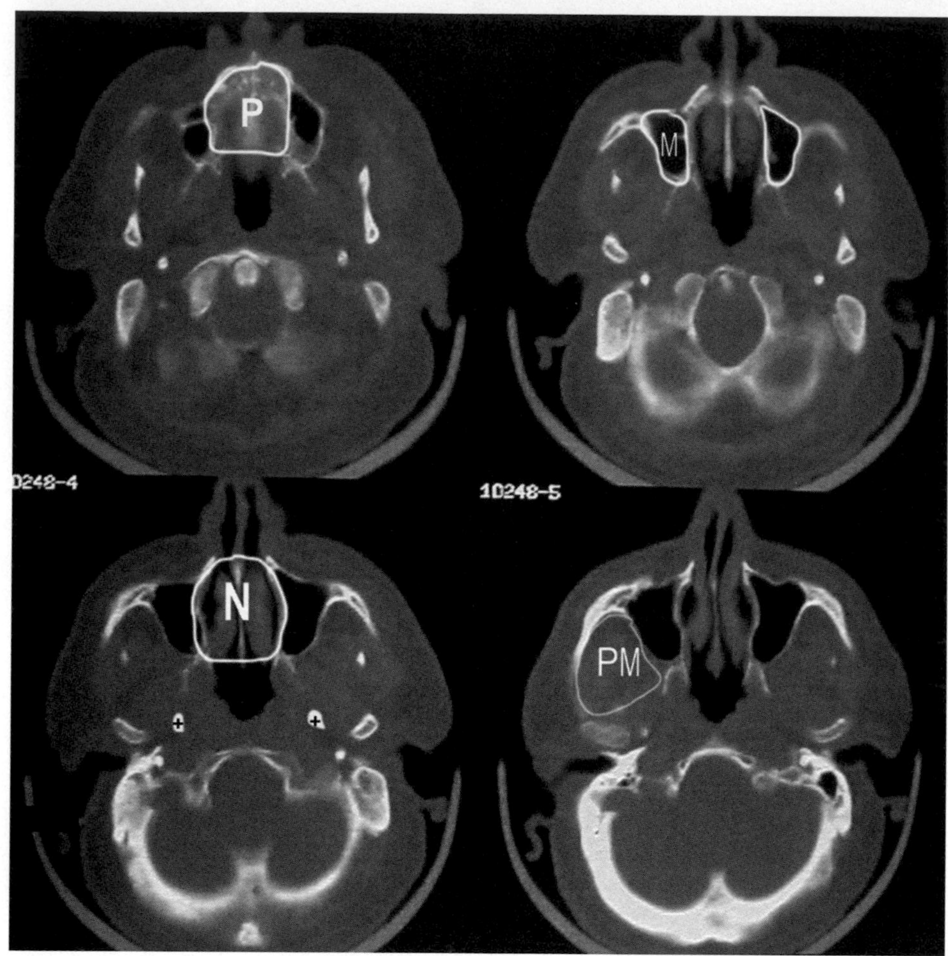

Figure A.6 Images from inferior to superior. (+), styloid processes; *arrowheads,* foraminae rotundum; *C,* clivus; *double headed arrowheads,* first divisions of trigeminal nerve; *double headed arrow,* superior orbital fissure; *DS,* dorsum sella; *E,* ethmoid sinuses; *F,* frontal sinus; *FO,* foramen ovale; *G,* globe; *I,* infraorbital groove; *IF,* inferior orbital fissure; *LF,* lacrimal fossae; *M,* maxillary sinus; *N,* nasal cavity; *OC,* optic chiasm; *OF,* optic foramen; *ON,* optic nerve; *P,* hard palate; *PC,* palatine canal; *PF,* pterygopalatine fossa; *PM,* pterygomaxillary space; *S,* sphenoid sinus; *white rectangular outline,* cribriform plate.

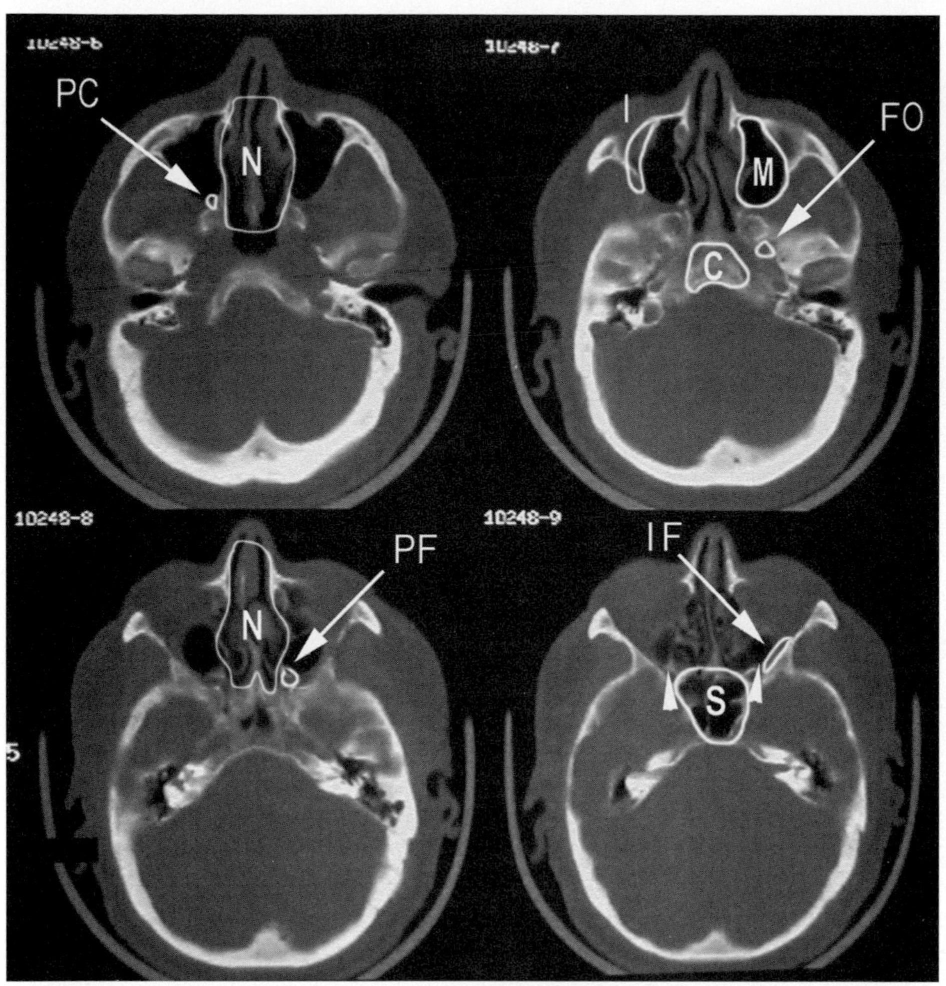

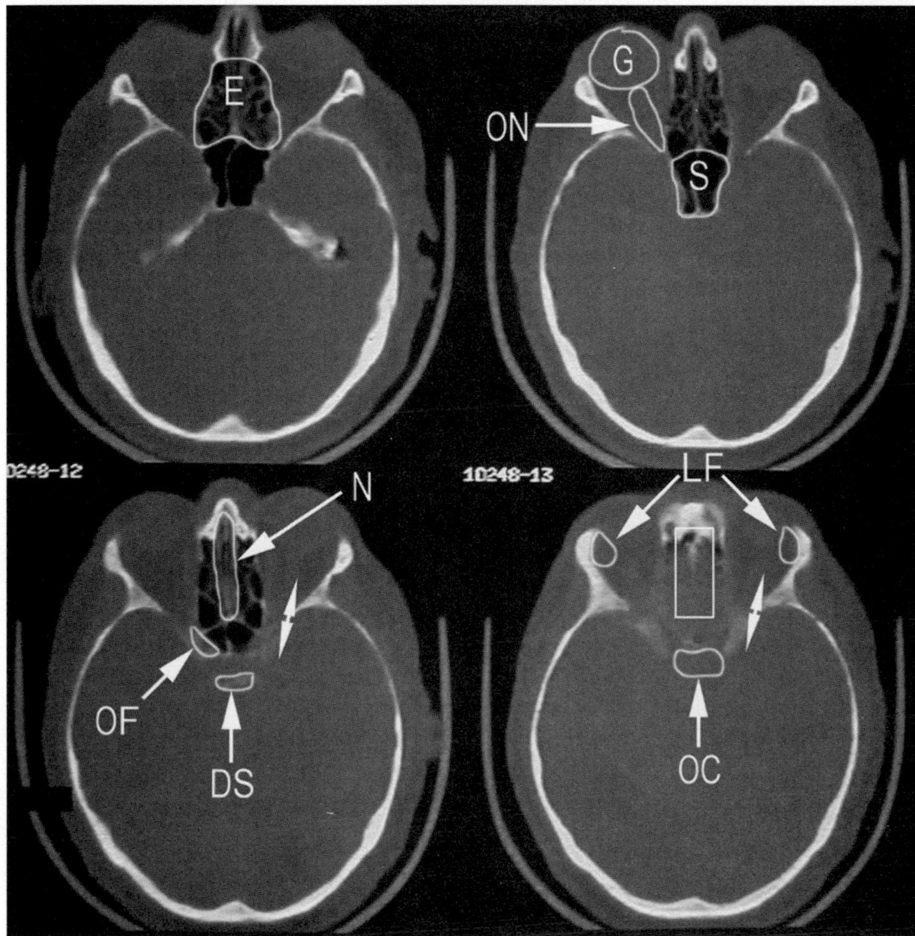

Figure A.6 *(Continued)*

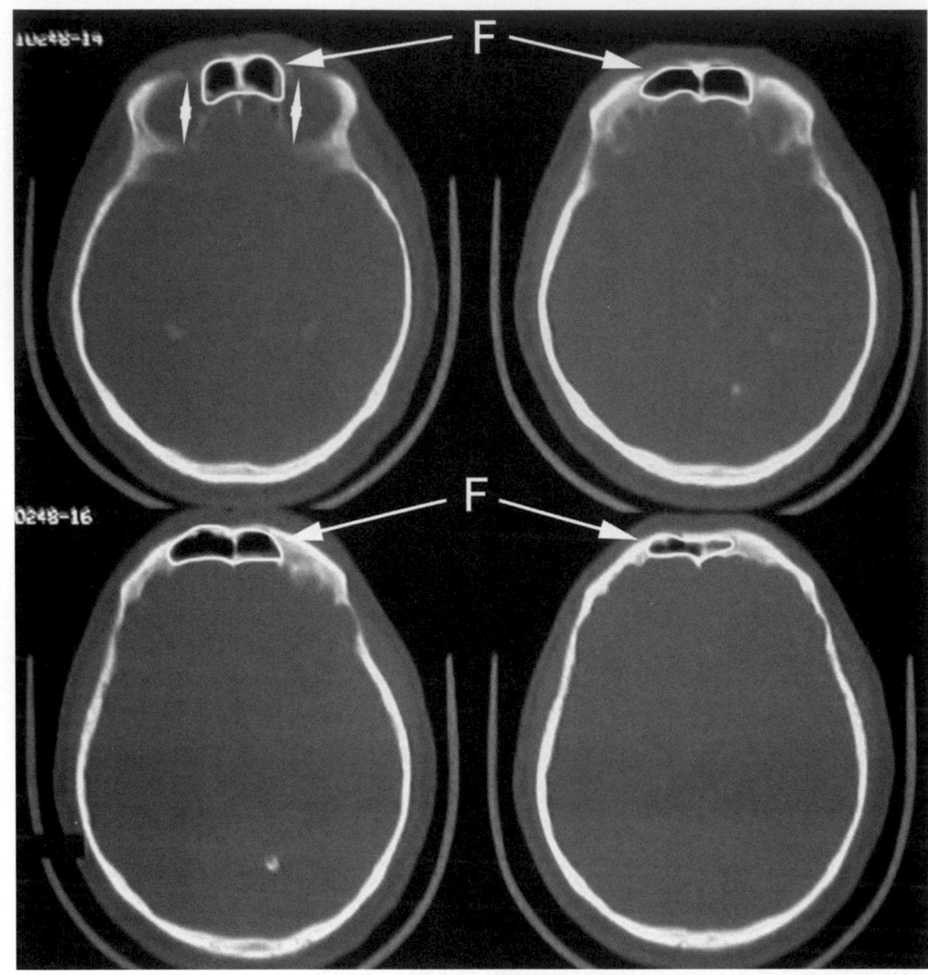

Figure A.6 *(Continued)*

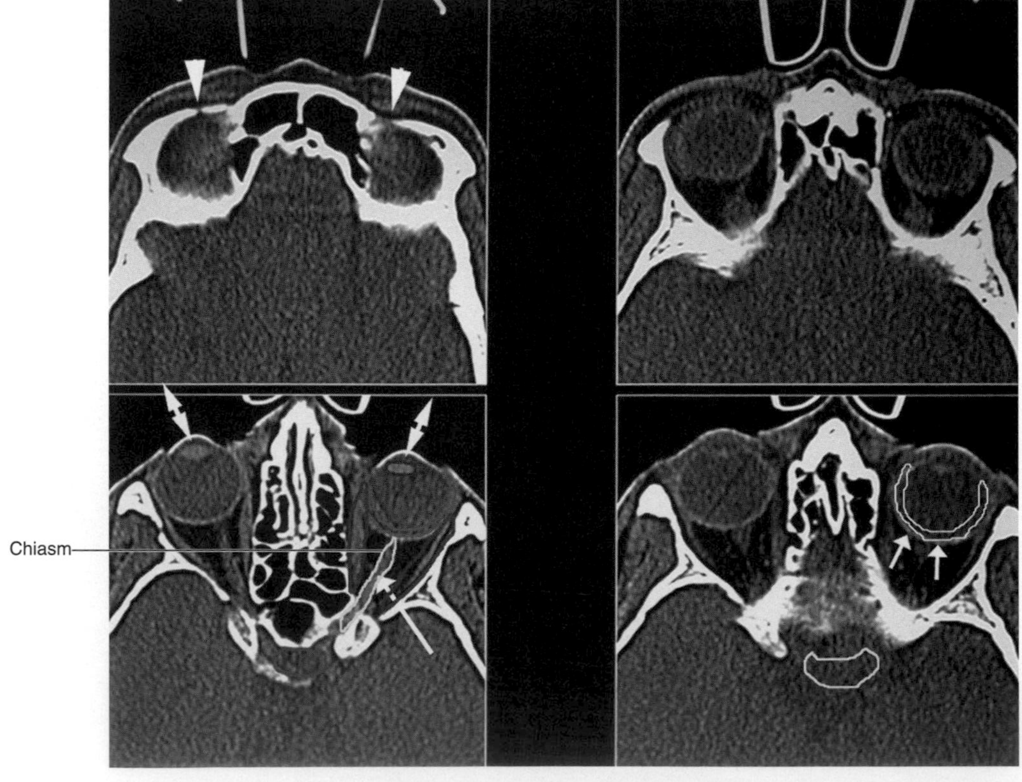

Figure A.6A Lens, *double arrowheads*; retina, *short arrows*; optic nerve, *long arrows*.

NASOPHARYNX (CHAPTER 23)

Figure A.7 shows the key anatomic structures that are integral to the treatment planning for patients with nasopharyngeal cancer. The structures that must be included in a specific case must be individualized. Obviously, the amount of parapharyngeal extension will dictate both the lateral and posterior extent of the contours for the primary site, which will be a major factor in the selected technique.

Figure A.1 shows the lymphatic drainage levels of the neck, which are clearly part of the treatment planning for all patients. Whether the primary site and the upper neck nodes are incorporated into the same fields, or junctioned fields, will depend on the selected technique.

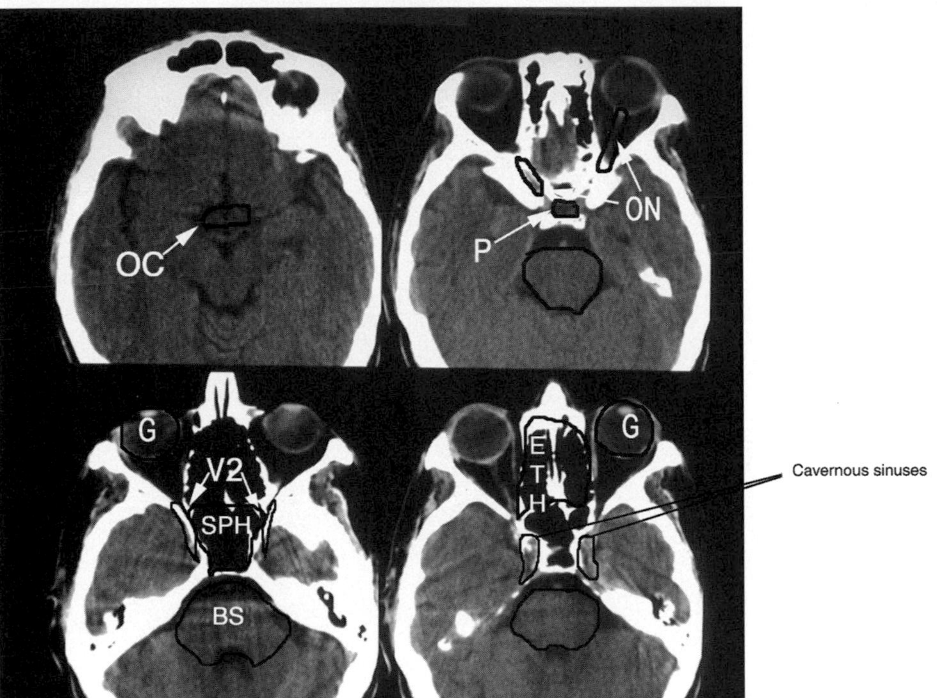

Figure A.7 Images from superior to inferior. Elements outlined include: *BS*, brainstem; *ETH*, ethmoid; *FO*, foramen ovale; *G*, globe; *LP*, lateral pterygoid; *MP*, medial pterygoid; *OC*, optic chiasm; *ON*, optic nerves; *P*, pituitary gland; *SPH*, sphenoid sinus; *V2*, maxillary nerves at foramina rotundum. *Black arrows*, petroclival fissures; *white arrowhead*, eustacian tube orifice; *white arrow*, fossa of Rosenmueller.

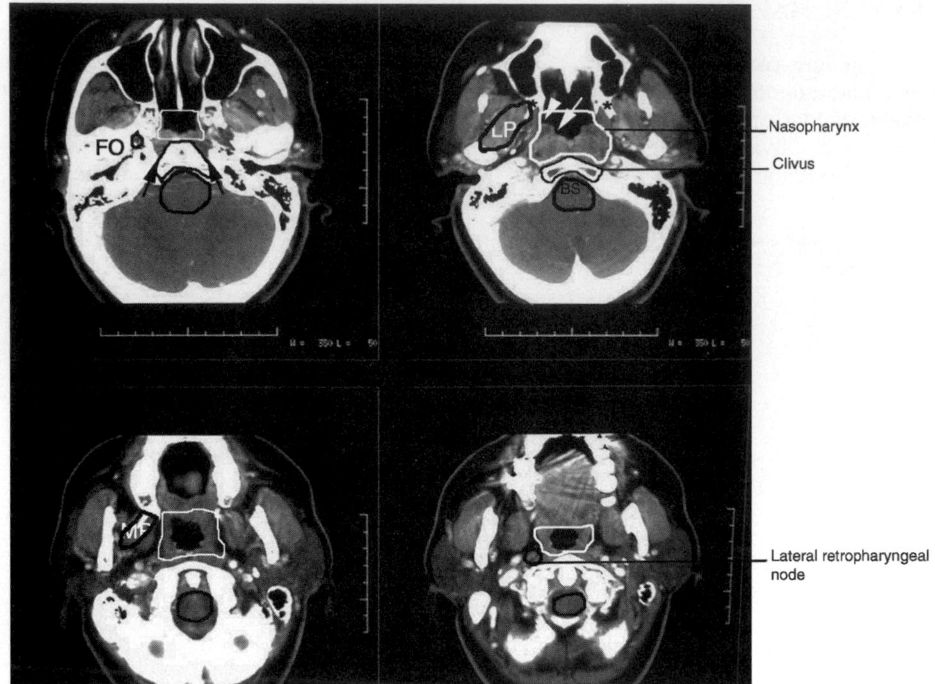

Figure A.7 *(Continued)*

SALIVARY GLANDS (CHAPTER 26)

The major salivary glands consist of the paired parotid glands, submandibular glands, and the numerous sublingual glands. The parotid gland is divided by the plane of the facial nerve into a superficial and deep lobe. For the purposes of contouring, the entire parotid gland is enclosed in the target area, and it is usually feasible to protect much of the total major salivary gland volume when treating one of these tumors. Figure A.8 outlines these structures in axial sections.

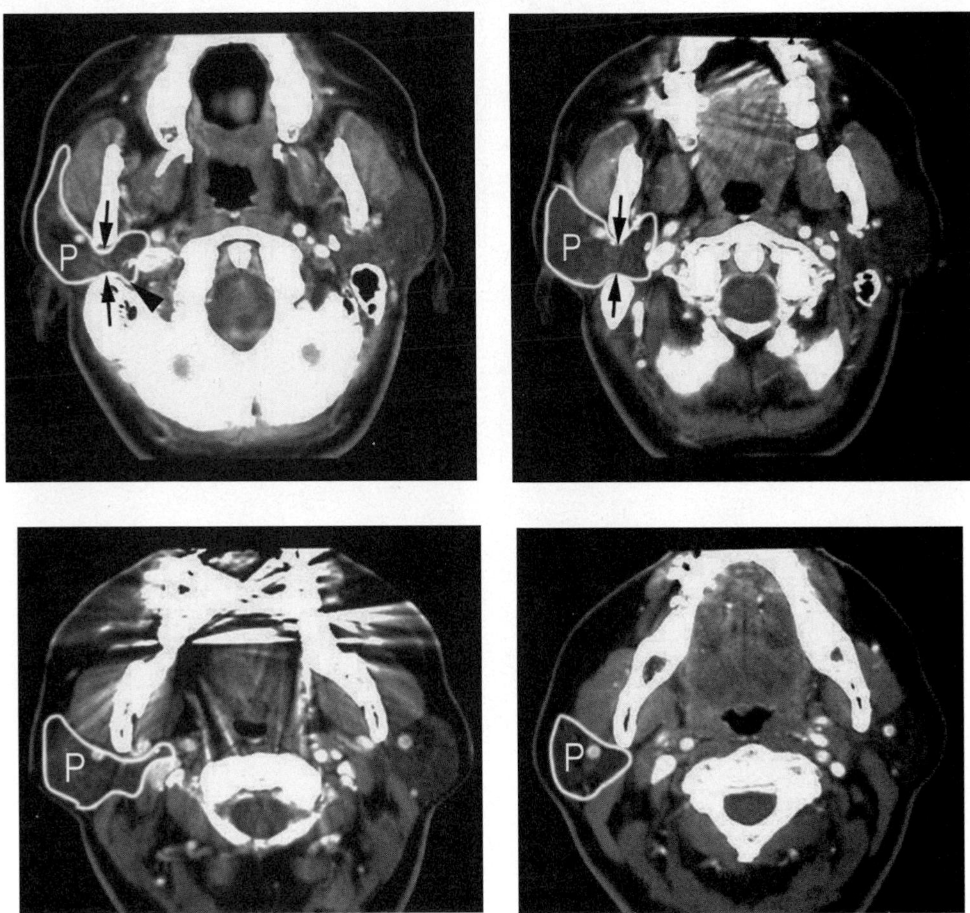

Figure A.8 Images from superior to inferior. *Black arrowhead,* stylomastoid foramen; *P,* parotid gland (*black arrows* indicate stylomandibular tunnel separating the larger superficial from the smaller deep lobe); *SL,* sublingual gland outlined in *black; SM,* submandibular gland outlined in *white.*

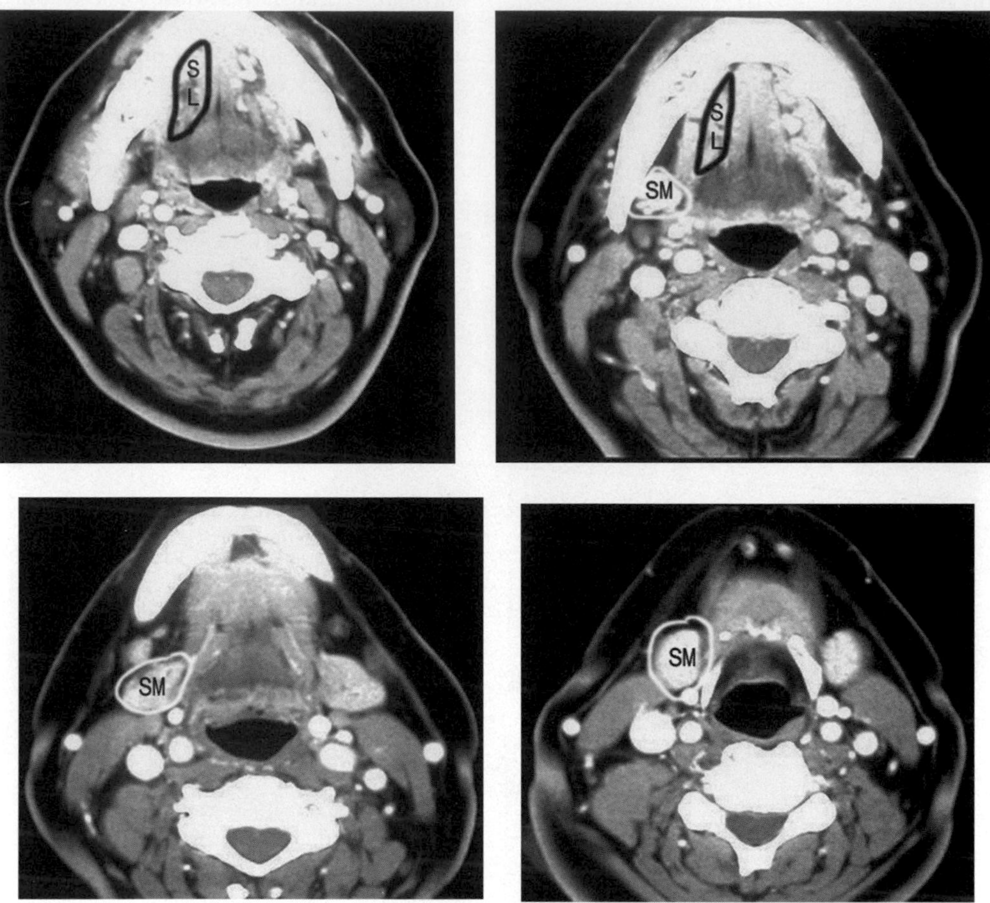

Figure A.8 *(Continued)*

SKULL BASE (CHAPTER 27)

It is important for the radiation oncologist to have a clear knowledge of important normal anatomy in the region of the skull base. Figure A.9 (see also Figs. A.6, A.6A, and A.7) outlines several important anatomic structures of interest in the planning of radiation therapy for skull base tumors.

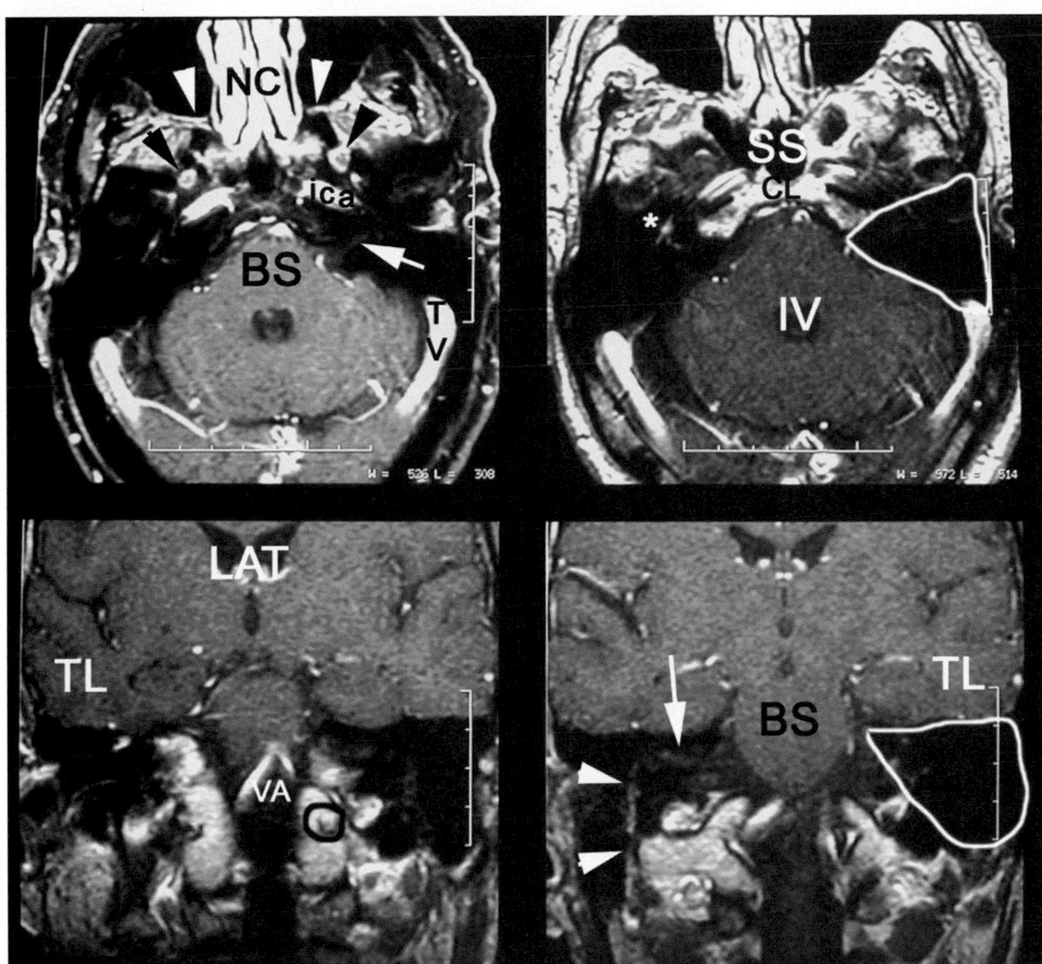

Figure A.9 MRI images (axial, *top panel*; coronal, *bottom panel*). *Black arrowheads,* foraminae ovale; *BS,* brainstem; *CL,* clivus; *double white arrowheads,* vertical segment of facial nerve; *ica,* internal carotid artery; *IV,* fourth ventricle; *LAT,* lateral ventricle; *NC,* nasal cavity; *SS,* sphenoid sinus; *TL,* temporal lobe; *TV,* transverse sinus; *VA,* vertebral arteries; *white arrowheads,* pterygopalatine fossae; *white arrow,* internal auditory canal. The right petrous pyramid is outlined by the *white triangle.* The left hypoglossal canal is outlined in *black.*

Subject Index

Page numbers followed by f indicate figures; page numbers followed by t indicate tables.

O

Q

R